Yao & Artusio's

ANESTHESIOLOGY

Problem-Oriented Patient Management

TENTH EDITION

Yao & Artusio's

ANESTHESIOLOGY

Problem-Oriented Patient Management

TENTH EDITION

Hugh C. Hemmings Jr., MD, PhD, FRCA
Senior Associate Dean for Research
Joseph F. Artusio Jr. Professor and Chair
Department of Anesthesiology
Professor of Pharmacology
Weill Cornell Medicine
Anesthesiologist-in-Chief
NewYork-Presbyterian/Weill Cornell Medical Center
New York, New York

Fun-Sun F. Yao, MD, FACA
Professor of Clinical Anesthesiology
Department of Anesthesiology
Weill Cornell Medicine
New York, New York

Peter A. Goldstein, MD
Professor of Anesthesiology
Professor of Anesthesiology in Neuroscience
Professor of Medical Ethics in Medicine
Department of Anesthesiology
Weill Cornell Medicine
New York, New York

Natalia Ivascu Girardi, MD
Stephen J. (Butch) Thomas Professor of Anesthesiology
Department of Anesthesiology
Weill Cornell Medicine
New York, New York

Vinod Malhotra, MB, BS, MD, FACA
Professor Emeritus of Clinical Anesthesiology
Department of Anesthesiology
Weill Cornell Medicine
New York, New York

Tiffany R. Tedore, MD
Chief of Regional Anesthesiology and Acute Pain Medicine
Associate Professor of Anesthesiology
Department of Anesthesiology
Weill Cornell Medicine
New York, New York

Wolters Kluwer

Philadelphia • Baltimore • New York • London
Buenos Aires • Hong Kong • Sydney • Tokyo

Acquisitions Editor: Keith Donnellan
Development Editor: Ashley Fischer
Editorial Coordinator: Chester Anthony Gonzalez
Marketing Manager: Kirsten Waturd
Senior Production Specialist: Bridgett Dougherty
Manager, Graphic Arts & Design: Stephen Druding
Manufacturing Coordinator: Lisa Bowling
Prepress Vendor: S4Carlisle Publishing Services

Tenth edition

9 8 7 6 5 4 3 2 1

Printed in Mexico

Library of Congress Cataloging-in-Publication Data

ISBN-13: 978-1-9752-1423-4

Library of Congress Control Number: 2025938876

shop.lww.com

QUADM0825

Preface

The clinical practice of anesthesiology continues to evolve in tandem with rapid advances in surgical and diagnostic procedures prompting the production of this new edition of *Yao & Artusio's Anesthesiology: Problem-Oriented Patient Management*. The remarkable popularity of the first nine editions in the anesthesiology community both in the United States and abroad encouraged us to update and expand its subject matter. The tenth edition is written to further improve anesthesia management for sophisticated modern surgery and other procedures requiring anesthesia.

As with our previous editions, *Yao & Artusio's Anesthesiology: Problem-Oriented Patient Management*, Tenth Edition was written to present important clinical entities covering the most common critical anesthetic problems encountered in daily practice. It is intended to provide logical and scientific fundamentals for individualized patient management.

In its tenth edition, *Yao & Artusio's Anesthesiology: Problem-Oriented Patient Management* is organized by organ systems into 12 sections consisting of 63 chapters. The book follows the successful format of previous editions. Each chapter begins with a brief case presentation, followed by essential problems of each disease covering four areas: (1) pathophysiology and differential diagnosis, (2) preoperative evaluation and preparation, (3) intraoperative management, and (4) postoperative anesthetic management. Using a question-and-answer format, the book is designed to stress anesthetic problems and to give anesthesia providers the opportunity to organize their own ideas for individualized patient care. A reasonable answer, with updated references, follows each question.

To maintain the fresh quality of the textbook, the tenth edition has been updated with significant new content including contributions by new authors. The text originally reflected the clinical experience of the Department of Anesthesiology at Weill Cornell Medicine and NewYork-Presbyterian Hospital/ Weill Cornell Medical Center. In this edition, experts from other prestigious institutions share their evidence-based experience and practice to make this book even more universally applicable. The book is prepared for the education of anesthesia trainees as well as anesthesia practitioners; it also serves as a review source for continuing education. The highly successful question-and-answer format and the updated content and references enhance the educational value and clinical applicability of this established and popular textbook.

Hugh C. Hemmings Jr., MD, PhD, FRCA
New York, New York

Contents

Contributors

Jaime Aaronson, MD
Associate Professor of Clinical Anesthesiology
Department of Anesthesiology
Weill Cornell Medicine
New York, New York

Sharon E. Abramovitz, MD
Associate Professor
Department of Anesthesiology
Weill Cornell Medicine
New York, New York

Diana Anca, MD
Associate Professor of Clinical Anesthesiology
Department of Anesthesiology
Weill Cornell Medicine
New York, New York

Shelby Badani, MD, MS, MSPH
Assistant Professor
Department of Anesthesiology
Weill Cornell Medicine
New York, New York

Kristin Berger, MD
Instructor in Medicine
Division of Pulmonary and Critical Care
Department of Medicine
Weill Cornell Medicine
New York, New York

Seema Brar, MD
Assistant Professor
Department of Anesthesiology
Weill Cornell Medicine
New York, New York

Joe E. L. Bryant-Huppert, MD
Assistant Professor of Clinical Anesthesiology
Department of Anesthesiology
Weill Cornell Medicine
New York, New York

Maria Bustillo, MD, FASA
Professor of Clinical Anesthesiology
Professor of Anesthesiology in Clinical Neurological Surgery
Department of Anesthesiology
Weill Cornell Medicine
New York, New York

June M. Chan, MB, BS, FANZCA
Assistant Professor
Department of Anesthesiology
Weill Cornell Medicine
New York, New York

Alan Cheng, MD
Associate Professor of Medicine and Pediatrics
Section of Cardiac Electrophysiology
Department of Medicine
Johns Hopkins University School of Medicine
Baltimore, Maryland
Chief Medical Officer
Cardiac Rhythm Management
Medtronic
Mounds View, Minnesota

Davy Cheng, MD, MSc, CCPE, FRCPC, FCAHS, DGAI (Hon), FHKCA (Hon)
Founding Dean and Presidential Chair Professor
School of Medicine
The Chinese University of Hong Kong, Shenzhen
Shenzhen, Guangdong, China
Distinguished University Professor Emeritus
Western University
London, Ontario, Canada

Justin S. Chung, MD
Department of Anesthesiology
Weill Cornell Medicine
NewYork-Presbyterian/Weill Cornell Medical Center
New York, New York

Alaeldin A. Darwich, MD
Assistant Professor of Clinical Anesthesiology
Department of Anesthesiology
Weill Cornell Medicine
New York, New York

Justin C. De Biasio, MD
Assistant Professor
Department of Anesthesiology, Perioperative Care & Pain Medicine
NYU Grossman School of Medicine
New York, New York

James A. DiNardo, MD, FAAP, FASA
Professor of Anesthesia
Harvard Medical School
Senior Associate in Cardiac Anesthesia
Boston Children's Hospital
Boston, Massachusetts

Miles Dinner, MD
Professor of Clinical Anesthesiology
Department of Anesthesiology
Weill Cornell Medicine
New York, New York

Chris R. Edmonds, MD
Clinical Assistant Professor of Anesthesiology
Department of Anesthesiology
Weill Cornell Medicine
New York, New York

James B. Eisenkraft, MD, FRCA
Professor Emeritus
Department of Anesthesiology, Perioperative and Pain Medicine
Icahn School of Medicine at Mount Sinai
New York, New York

Leif Ericksen, MD
Associate Professor
Susquehanna Anesthesia Affiliates
United Health Services
Johnson City, New York

Meghann M. Fitzgerald, MD
Assistant Professor of Clinical Anesthesiology
Department of Anesthesiology
Weill Cornell Medicine
New York, New York

Jill Fong, MD
Associate Professor of Clinical Anesthesiology
Department of Anesthesiology
Weill Cornell Medicine
Associate Attending Anesthesiologist
NewYork-Presbyterian/Weill Cornell Medical Center
New York, New York

Farida Gadalla, MB, ChB
Professor of Clinical Anesthesiology
Department of Anesthesiology
Department of Obstetrics and Gynecology
Weill Cornell Medicine
Attending Anesthesiologist
Department of Anesthesiology
NewYork-Presbyterian Hospital
New York, New York

Tong J. Gan, MD
Professor and Chair
Division Head of Anesthesiology, Critical Care, and Pain Medicine
The University of Texas MD Anderson Cancer Center
Houston, Texas

Jonathan St. George, MD
Assistant Professor of Emergency Medicine
Department of Emergency Medicine
Weill Cornell Medicine
New York, New York

Natalia Ivascu Girardi, MD
Stephen J. (Butch) Thomas Professor of Anesthesiology
Department of Anesthesiology
Weill Cornell Medicine
New York, New York

Peter A. Goldstein, MD
Professor of Anesthesiology
Professor of Anesthesiology in Neuroscience
Professor of Medical Ethics in Medicine
Department of Anesthesiology
Weill Cornell Medicine
New York, New York

Michael D. Green, MD
Assistant Professor of Anesthesiology
Division of Pediatric Anesthesiology
Department of Anesthesiology
NewYork-Presbyterian/Weill Cornell Medical Center
New York, New York

Dana L. Gurvitch, MD
Assistant Dean for Student Affairs and Student Life
Associate Professor of Clinical Anesthesiology
Department of Anesthesiology
Weill Cornell Medicine
New York, New York

Thorsten Haas, MD
Professor of Anesthesiology
Director of Patient Blood Management
Department of Anesthesiology
University of Florida College of Medicine
Gainesville, Florida

Hugh C. Hemmings Jr., MD, PhD, FRCA
Senior Associate Dean for Research
Joseph F. Artusio Jr. Professor and Chair
Department of Anesthesiology
Professor of Pharmacology
Weill Cornell Medicine
Anesthesiologist-in-Chief
NewYork-Presbyterian/Weill Cornell Medical Center
New York, New York

Charles W. Hogue, MD, FAHA
Chair
James E. Eckenhoff Professor of Anesthesiology
Professor, Anesthesiology (Cardiothoracic Anesthesiology)
Department of Anesthesiology
Feinberg School of Medicine - Northwestern University
Chicago, Illinois

Margo Hoyler, MD
Assistant Professor of Clinical Anesthesiology
Department of Anesthesiology
Weill Cornell Medicine
New York, New York

Susan A. Ironstone, MD
Department of Anesthesiology
UMass Memorial Health
Worcester, Massachusetts

Rohan Jotwani, MD, MBA
Assistant Professor of Clinical Anesthesiology
Department of Anesthesiology
Weill Cornell Medicine
New York, New York

Gunisha Kaur, MD, MA
Associate Professor
Department of Anesthesiology
Weill Cornell Medicine
New York, New York

Diana Khatib, MD
Assistant Professor of Clinical Anesthesiology
Department of Anesthesiology
Weill Cornell Medicine
New York, New York

Shreyajit R. Kumar, MD
Assistant Professor
Department of Anesthesiology
Weill Cornell Medicine
New York, New York

Philip C. Kuo, MD
Assistant Professor of Clinical Anesthesiology
Department of Anesthesiology
Weill Cornell Medicine
New York, New York

Chris C. Lee, MD, PhD, MBA
Associate Professor of Anesthesiology
Department of Anesthesiology
Washington University School of Medicine
St. Louis, Missouri

Jennifer K. Lee, MD
Assistant Professor
Department of Anesthesiology
Weill Cornell Medicine
New York, New York

Shona M. Lee, MD
Assistant Professor of Clinical Anesthesiology
Department of Anesthesiology
Weill Cornell Medicine
New York, New York

Christine M. Lennon, MD
Assistant Professor of Clinical Anesthesiology
Department of Anesthesiology
Weill Cornell Medicine
New York, New York

Adam D. Lichtman, MD, FASE
Professor of Clinical Anesthesiology
Chief, General Anesthesiology
Department of Anesthesiology
Weill Cornell Medicine
New York, New York

Janine Limoncelli, MD
Clinical Assistant Professor of Anesthesiology
Department of Anesthesiology
Weill Cornell Medicine/NewYork-Presbyterian
New York, New York
Assistant Professor of Anesthesiology
Department of Anesthesiology
Westchester County Medical Center
Valhalla, New York

Yuan-Chi Lin, MD, MPH
Associate Professor of Anesthesia and Pediatrics
Department of Anaesthesia
Harvard Medical School
Boston, Massachusetts

Jyun-you Liou, MD, PhD
Assistant Professor
Department of Anesthesiology
Weill Cornell Medicine
New York, New York

Yang Long, MD
Assistant Professor
Department of Anesthesiology and Perioperative Medicine
UMass Chan Medical School
Worcester, Massachusetts

Patricia Fogarty Mack, MD, FASA, FACHE
Professor of Clinical Anesthesiology
Department of Anesthesiology
Weill Cornell Medicine
New York, New York

Anuj Malhotra, MD
Attending Anesthesiologist
Director, Division of Pain Management
Department of Anesthesiology, Critical Care & Pain Management
Hospital for Special Surgery
New York, New York

Jaideep K. Malhotra, MD
Assistant Professor of Clinical Anesthesiology
Department of Anesthesiology
Weill Cornell Medicine
New York, New York

Vinod Malhotra, MB, BS, MD, FACA
Professor Emeritus of Clinical Anesthesiology
Department of Anesthesiology
Weill Cornell Medicine
New York, New York

Danielle McCullough, MD
Assistant Professor of Clinical Anesthesiology
Department of Anesthesiology
Weill Cornell Medicine
New York, New York

Neel D. Mehta, MD
Associate Professor of Clinical Anesthesiology
Department of Anesthesiology
Weill Cornell Medicine
New York, New York

Vivek K. Moitra, MD, MHA, FCCM
Allen I. Hyman Professor of Critical Care Anesthesiology at CUMC
Department of Anesthesiology
Columbia University Vagelos College of Physicians and Surgeons
New York City, New York

Thomas A. Moore II, MD, FASA
Professor
Department of Anesthesiology and Perioperative Medicine
Department of Neurological Surgery
University of Alabama Heersink School of Medicine
Birmingham, Alabama

Shaker J. Morcous, MD
Associate Professor
Department of Anesthesia
The University of Texas MD Anderson Cancer Center
Houston, Texas

Sagar Navare, MD
Assistant Professor
Department of Anesthesiology
University of Minnesota
Minneapolis, Minnesota

Sawyer A. Naze, MD
Assistant Professor, Anesthesiology (Cardiothoracic Anesthesiology)
Department of Anesthesiology
Feinberg School of Medicine - Northwestern University
Chicago, Illinois

Mark E. Nunnally, MD, FCCM
Professor
Department of Anesthesiology, Perioperative Care & Pain Medicine
Departments of Neurology, Surgery & Medicine
NYU School of Medicine
New York, New York

James A. Osorio, MD
Associate Professor
Department of Anesthesiology
Weill Cornell Medicine
New York, New York

Daniel Pak, MD
Associate Professor
Department of Anesthesiology, Critical Care and Pain Medicine
The University of Texas Health Science Center at Houston
Houston, Texas

Anup Pamnani, MD
Assistant Professor
Department of Anesthesiology
Weill Cornell Medicine
New York, New York

Di Pan, DO, MS
Assistant Professor of Clinical Medicine
Division of Pulmonary and Critical Care
Department of Medicine
Weill Cornell Medicine
New York, New York

Rohan K. Panchamia, MD
Assistant Professor of Clinical Anesthesiology
Department of Anesthesiology
Weill Cornell Medicine
New York, New York

Roshan Patel, MD
Assistant Professor
Department of Anesthesiology
Weill Cornell Medicine
New York, New York

Elizabeth Starker Pealy, MD
Assistant Professor of Anesthesia and Critical Care
University of Chicago Medicine
Chicago, Illinois

Alessia Pedoto, MD, FASA
Professor
Department of Anesthesiology and Critical Care Medicine
Memorial Sloan Kettering Cancer Center
New York, New York

Philip A. Petrou, MD
Assistant Professor of Clinical Anesthesiology
Department of Anesthesiology, Critical Care and Pain Medicine
Weill Cornell Medicine
New York, New York

Mohammad M. Piracha, MD, MBA, MS
Assistant Professor of Anesthesiology
Department of Anesthesiology
Weill Cornell Medicine
New York, New York

Kane O. Pryor, MB, BS
Associate Professor
Department of Anesthesiology
Weill Cornell Medicine
New York, New York

Melinda Randall, MD
Assistant Professor
Department of Anesthesiology
Weill Cornell Medicine
New York, New York

Jared Roberts, MD
Department of Anesthesiology
Feinberg School of Medicine - Northwestern University
Chicago, Illinois

Cesar A. Rodriguez-Diaz, MD
Associate Professor
Department of Anesthesiology, Perioperative and Pain Medicine
Icahn School of Medicine at Mount Sinai
New York, New York

Lisa Q. Rong, MD, MSCE
Associate Professor
Department of Anesthesiology
Weill Cornell Medicine
New York, New York

Harvey K. Rosenbaum, MD
Department of Anesthesiology
David Geffen School of Medicine
UCLA Health
Los Angeles, California

Henry Rosenberg M.D
Member Board of Directors
Malignant Hyperthermia Association of the U.S. (MHAUS)
Sherburne, NY

Olga Rozental, MD, PhD
Assistant Professor of Clinical Anesthesiology
Department of Anesthesiology
Weill Cornell Medicine
New York, New York

John E. Rubin, MD
Assistant Professor of Clinical Anesthesiology
Department of Anesthesiology
Weill Cornell Medicine
New York, New York

Seyed A. Safavynia, MD, PhD
Assistant Professor
Department of Anesthesiology
Weill Cornell Medicine
New York, New York

Jon D. Samuels, MD
Associate Professor of Clinical Anesthesiology
Department of Anesthesiology
Weill Cornell Medicine
New York, New York

Jacques H. Scharoun, MD
Assistant Professor
Department of Anesthesiology
Weill Cornell Medicine
New York, New York

Edward J. Schenck, MD, MS
Assistant Professor of Medicine
Division of Pulmonary and Critical Care
Department of Medicine
Weill Cornell Medicine
New York, New York

Aarti Sharma, MD, FASA
Associate Professor of Clinical Anesthesiology
Department of Anesthesiology
Weill Cornell Medicine
New York, New York

Liang Shen, MD, MPH
Assistant Professor of Clinical Anesthesiology
Department of Anesthesiology
Weill Cornell Medicine
New York, New York

Marc A. Sherwin, MD
Assistant Professor
Department of Anesthesiology, Perioperative and Pain Medicine
Icahn School of Medicine at Mount Sinai
New York, New York

Ralph L. Slepian, MD
Professor of Clinical Anesthesiology
Department of Anesthesiology
Weill Cornell Medicine
New York, New York

Kenneth G. Smithson, DO, PhD
Department of Anesthesiology and Critical Care
St. Louis University SSM Health
St. Louis, Illinois

Mary So, MD
Assistant Professor of Anesthesiology
Department of Anesthesiology
Will Cornell Medicine
New York, New York

Ankur Srivastava, MD
Assistant Professor
Department of Anesthesiology
Weill Cornell Medicine
New York, New York

Louise Y. Sun, MD, SM, FRCPC, FAHA
Professor and Chief
Division of Cardiothoracic Anesthesiology
Department of Anesthesiology, Perioperative and Pain Medicine
Stanford University School of Medicine
Stanford, California

Tiffany R. Tedore, MD
Chief of Regional Anesthesiology and Acute Pain Medicine
Associate Professor of Anesthesiology
Department of Anesthesiology
Weill Cornell Medicine
New York, New York

M. Angele Theard, MD
Associate Professor in Neuroanesthesiology
Department of Anesthesiology
University of Washington School of Medicine—Harborview Medical Center
Seattle, Washington

Jaroslav K. Usenko, MD
Assistant Professor
Department of Anesthesiology
Weill Cornell Medicine
New York, New York

Jennifer Landon Wagner, MD
Attending Anesthesiologist, Obstetric Anesthesia
Department of Anesthesiology
Danbury Hospital / Nuvance Health
Danbury, Connecticut

David Y. Wang, MD, MPH
Clinical Assistant Professor, Director of Chronic Pain Education
Department of Anesthesiology, Critical Care and Pain Management
Hospital for Special Surgery
New York, New York

Marissa M. Weber, MD
Assistant Professor of Anesthesiology
Department of Anesthesiology
Weill Cornell Medicine
New York, New York

Jason J. White, MD
Assistant Professor of Clinical Anesthesiology
Department of Anesthesiology
Weill Cornell Medicine
New York, New York

Robert S. White, MD, MS
Assistant Professor of Anesthesiology
Department of Anesthesiology
Weill Cornell Medicine
Assistant Attending Anesthesiologist
Department of Anesthesiology
NewYork-Presbyterian Hospital
New York, New York

David Whiting, MD
Assistant Professor of Anesthesia
Harvard Medical School
Senior Associate in Cardiac Anesthesia
Boston Children's Hospital
Boston, Massachusetts

Fun-Sun F. Yao, MD, FACA
Professor of Clinical Anesthesiology
Department of Anesthesiology
Weill Cornell Medicine
New York, New York

Albert C. Yeung, MD
Assistant Professor of Anesthesiology
Department of Anesthesiology
Weill Cornell Medicine
New York, New York

1 Asthma and Chronic Obstructive Pulmonary Disease

Jaroslav K. Usenko and Fun-Sun F. Yao

A 55-year-old male with cholelithiasis is scheduled for laparoscopic cholecystectomy. He has a long history of asthma, has smoked two packs of cigarettes a day for the past 30 years, and reports dyspnea with moderate exertion (walking uphill). He sleeps on two pillows. There is no peripheral edema. Arterial blood gas (ABG) analysis on room air shows the following: pH, 7.36; Pco_2, 60 mm Hg; Po_2, 70 mm Hg; and CO_2 content, 36 mEq/L.

A. Medical Disease and Differential Diagnosis

1. What is the differential diagnosis of dyspnea?
2. What is the prevalence of asthma and chronic obstructive pulmonary disease (COPD)?
3. What is the etiology of asthma?
4. Discuss the pathogenesis of asthma. How is asthma distinguished from COPD?
5. What are the triggers of bronchospasm?
6. What is the universal finding in ABG analysis during asthmatic attacks: hypoxemia or CO_2 retention?
7. Describe the abnormalities seen in spirometry, lung volumes, and lung capacities during an asthmatic attack.

B. Preoperative Evaluation and Preparation

1. How would you evaluate the patient preoperatively? What preoperative workup would you order?
2. How would you distinguish obstructive lung disease from restrictive lung disease by spirometry?
3. Define normal lung volumes and lung capacities. Give normal values for an average adult male.
4. What are flow-volume loops? Draw flow-volume loops for a healthy subject and for patients with COPD, restrictive lung disease, fixed obstruction of the upper airway, variable extrathoracic obstruction, and variable intrathoracic obstruction.
5. Define closing volume (CV) and closing capacity (CC). What is the normal value of CV?
6. Why is the functional residual capacity (FRC) important in oxygenation?
7. How are FRC and CC affected by age and posture? How are they affected by general anesthesia?
8. Give the equations for shunt (Q_S/Q_T) and dead space/tidal volume (V_D/V_T). What are their normal values?
9. Interpret the following ABG analysis: pH, 7.36; Pco_2, 60 mm Hg; Po_2, 70 mm Hg; and CO_2 content, 36 mEq/L.
10. What are the common physiologic causes of hypoxemia?
11. How would you prepare this patient with asthma and COPD for surgery?
12. The patient comes to your perioperative clinic 2 weeks before surgery. He wants to know if his smoking puts him at increased risk during surgery. What do you tell him? Should he quit now?
13. You discover that the patient had a recent upper respiratory infection (URI); would you postpone surgery? If so, for how long?
14. What medications would you expect the patient to have taken in the past or be taking currently?

15. The patient was on 20 mg of prednisone per day for 5 days as part of the treatment of an asthma exacerbation 3 months ago. He is currently not on corticosteroids. Should the patient receive "stress-dose" corticosteroids?
16. Should patients with reactive airway disease receive preoperative corticosteroids?
17. What is the onset of action of intravenous (IV) corticosteroid therapy in asthma?
18. You are visiting the patient in the preoperative area before coming to the operating room. How would you discuss treatment options and obtain informed consent from this patient?
19. If the patient is a 90-year-old with an order of Do-Not-Resuscitate (DNR), how would you discuss the management of a perioperative DNR order with the patient and family?

C. Intraoperative Management

1. If the patient had a severe asthmatic attack in the operating room before the induction of anesthesia, would you proceed with the anesthetic or postpone the surgery?
2. The patient did not have an asthmatic attack in the operating room, and you proceed with induction of anesthesia. How would you induce anesthesia? Would you use a supraglottic airway device instead of an endotracheal tube?
3. Would you use propofol for induction of anesthesia?
4. Would you use thiopental, methohexital, etomidate, or ketamine for induction of anesthesia?
5. Would you administer lidocaine for tracheal intubation?
6. If this were an emergency surgery and rapid sequence induction is indicated, how would you induce anesthesia in this patient?
7. Could a regional anesthetic technique be used for this surgery? Discuss the advantages and disadvantages of neuraxial anesthesia in this patient for this surgery.
8. Would you choose an inhalational or an IV technique for the maintenance of anesthesia?
9. What mechanisms produce bronchodilation by volatile anesthetics?
10. Which neuromuscular blocking agents would you use? Why?
11. How will you ventilate the patient? Will you use positive end-expiratory pressure (PEEP)? How can you detect the presence of auto-PEEP on a ventilator?
12. What is the differential diagnosis of intraoperative bronchospasm?
13. In the middle of surgery, peak inspiratory pressure (PIP) suddenly increases. How do you manage this?
14. How would you administer β_2-agonists? What is their mechanism of action in asthma?
15. If the patient does not respond to the aforementioned treatment and becomes cyanotic, what would you do?
16. If the patient does not respond to the treatments you have given, are you going to ask for help from other health care professionals? How would you do it?
17. Would you consider deep tracheal extubation for this patient?
18. If the patient cannot be extubated, what measures can you take to reduce the likelihood of bronchospasm with an endotracheal tube in place?

D. Postoperative Management

1. In patients with asthma and COPD, are there special considerations for the use of opioids and nonsteroidal anti-inflammatory drugs (NSAIDs) for postoperative pain control?
2. Would you consider using a regional anesthesia technique for analgesia?
3. The patient was breathing well and was extubated in the OR. Would you place this patient on supplemental oxygen in the recovery room? If so, how much?
4. The patient is hypoventilating in the postanesthesia care unit (PACU). Would you initiate noninvasive ventilation (NIV)?
5. The patient had a severe asthmatic attack during surgery, which was ultimately relieved by your treatment. Would you discuss the event with the patient? How would you do it?
6. Recently, many surgical cases including yours were delayed. Your department chair asked you to design a plan to improve it. What would you do?

A. Medical Disease and Differential Diagnosis

A.1. What is the differential diagnosis of dyspnea?

Dyspnea is defined as "difficult or labored breathing" and is a symptom of a broad array of underlying conditions. Although the differential diagnosis is extensive, pulmonary and cardiac conditions account for as much as 85% of the underlying causes of dyspnea. Pulmonary causes include asthma, COPD, interstitial lung disease, and chest wall deformity (kyphoscoliosis). Cardiac causes include left heart failure, sometimes called cardiac asthma, and pericardial disease (restrictive pericarditis, cardiac tamponade). Dyspnea can also be due to anemia, deconditioning, and psychological causes.

In this patient, with known asthma, the most likely causes of dyspnea are pulmonary. In patients such as this with a considerable smoking history, concomitant COPD and/or asthma is common, and airway obstruction with both reversible and irreversible components is frequently seen.

Baron RM. Dyspnea. In: Loscalzo J, Fauci AS, Kasper DL, et al, eds. *Harrison's Principles of Internal Medicine.* 21st ed. McGraw-Hill; 2022:263-266.

Israel E. Asthma. In: Loscalzo J, Fauci AS, Kasper DL, et al, eds. *Harrison's Principles of Internal Medicine.* 21st ed. McGraw-Hill; 2022:2147-2159.

Silverman EK, Crapo JD, Make BJ. Chronic obstructive pulmonary disease. In: Loscalzo J, Fauci AS, Kasper DL, et al, eds. *Harrison's Principles of Internal Medicine.* 21st ed. McGraw-Hill; 2022:2180-2189.

A.2. What is the prevalence of asthma and chronic obstructive pulmonary disease (COPD)?

Asthma is the most common chronic disease associated with significant morbidity and mortality. Globally, asthma affects up to 241 million people. The prevalence of asthma in the United States is estimated at 7.9% of the population, compared to 4.3% prevalence worldwide. Prevalence continues to increase and is associated with the transition from rural to urban living. Asthma is more prevalent among children (8.4%) than adults (7.7%). In children, the prevalence is greatest among boys (2:1 male/female ratio), with a trend toward greater prevalence in female in adulthood. COPD is estimated to affect more than 250 million people in the world. In the United States, COPD affects more than 10 million people.

Israel E. Asthma. In: Loscalzo J, Fauci AS, Kasper DL, et al, eds. *Harrison's Principles of Internal Medicine.* 21st ed. McGraw-Hill; 2022:2147-2159.

Silverman EK, Crapo JD, Make BJ. Chronic obstructive pulmonary disease. In: Loscalzo J, Fauci AS, Kasper DL, et al, eds. *Harrison's Principles of Internal Medicine.* 21st ed. McGraw-Hill; 2022:2180-2189.

A.3. What is the etiology of asthma?

Asthma is a heterogeneous disease with complex, multifactorial etiologies. The common denominator that underlies the asthmatic diathesis is a nonspecific hyperirritability of the tracheobronchial tree. Although asthma can be subdivided according to several clinical, physiologic, and pathologic variables, traditionally asthma is classified into two groups: atopic (allergic, extrinsic) and nonatopic (nonallergic, intrinsic). Atopic asthma is usually associated with a personal or family history of allergic diseases, positive skin reactions to extracts of airborne antigens, and increased levels of serum immunoglobulin E (IgE). Most patients with asthma have the atopic type. Patients with nonatopic asthma have negative skin tests for common inhalant allergens and normal serum concentrations of IgE. The patients with nonatopic asthma usually show later onset of disease and may be aspirin sensitive.

Israel E. Asthma. In: Loscalzo J, Fauci AS, Kasper DL, et al, eds. *Harrison's Principles of Internal Medicine.* 21st ed. McGraw-Hill; 2022:2147-2159.

McCracken JL, Veeranki SP, Ameredes BT, et al. Diagnosis and management of asthma in adults: a review. *JAMA.* 2017;318:279-290.

Olin JT, Wechsler ME. Asthma: pathogenesis and novel drugs for treatment. *BMJ.* 2014;349:g5517.

Silverman EK, Crapo JD, Make BJ. Chronic obstructive pulmonary disease. In: Loscalzo J, Fauci AS, Kasper DL, et al, eds. *Harrison's Principles of Internal Medicine.* 21st ed. McGraw-Hill; 2022:2180-2189.

A.4. Discuss the pathogenesis of asthma. How is asthma distinguished from COPD?

Asthma is a chronic disease characterized by reversible expiratory airflow obstruction resulting from the narrowing of the airways in response to various stimuli and a nonspecific hyperirritability of the tracheobronchial tree.

COPD is characterized by persistent respiratory symptoms and airflow limitation that is not fully reversible.

In asthma, exposure to an initiating stimulus triggers inflammatory cells (mast cells, eosinophils, T lymphocytes, macrophages, basophils, neutrophils, and platelets) and structural cells (epithelial cells, fibroblasts, and airway smooth muscle cells) to release various mediators that lead to bronchospasm, vascular congestion, increased capillary permeability (edema of bronchial mucosa), and mucus secretion.

The net result is a reduction in airway diameter, an increase in airway resistance, decreased forced expiratory volume and flow rate, hyperinflation of the lungs and thorax, increased work of breathing, alterations in respiratory tract muscle function, mismatched ventilation/perfusion, and altered ABGs.

In COPD, goblet cell hyperplasia, activation of inflammatory cells (lymphocytes, neutrophils, and macrophages), and alteration in the function of structural cells lead to increased mucus production, airway fibrosis, loss of alveolar attachments, and pulmonary vascular remodeling. Alveolar attachments are the alveolar walls radially attached to the small airways. Loss of alveolar attachments is one of the pathophysiologic features of COPD. The net result is hypersecretion of mucus, emphysema with peripheral airway collapse, impaired gas exchange, pulmonary hypertension, and right ventricular dysfunction. A minority of COPD cases are the result of a genetic deficiency in α_1 antitrypsin (α_1AT), an inhibitor of the serine protease neutrophil elastase, leading to increased lung parenchymal destruction.

Although asthma and COPD are distinct syndromes, some patients, such as this patient with an extensive smoking history, have features of COPD, such as irreversible airflow limitation. Additionally, although airway hyperresponsiveness to a variety of exogenous stimuli is one of the defining features of asthma, many patients with COPD also have airway hyperresponsiveness.

Israel E. Asthma. In: Loscalzo J, Fauci AS, Kasper DL, et al, eds. *Harrison's Principles of Internal Medicine*. 21st ed. McGraw-Hill; 2022:2147-2159.

Silverman EK, Crapo JD, Make BJ. Chronic obstructive pulmonary disease. In: Loscalzo J, Fauci AS, Kasper DL, et al, eds. *Harrison's Principles of Internal Medicine*. 21st ed. McGraw-Hill; 2022:2180-2189.

A.5. What are the triggers of bronchospasm?

- *Allergens*. Inhaled allergens activate mast cells, with bound IgE directly leading to the immediate release of bronchoconstrictor mediators. This early response is reversed by bronchodilators. Common allergens are house dust mites (*Dermatophagoides* species), pet dander, grass pollen, ragweed, and tree pollen.
- *Infections*. Respiratory tract infections are among the most common triggers of acute severe asthma exacerbations.
- *Pharmacologic agents*. Drugs that can trigger bronchospasm include β-adrenergic antagonists, aspirin and other NSAIDs, and sulfites (food preservatives). Nonspecific β-blockers should be avoided in people with asthma because their use can lead to severe bronchospasm. The ultra-short-acting β_1 selective antagonists landiolol (where available) and esmolol can be safely used perioperatively in patients with airway hyperreactivity. Aspirin-sensitive asthma is a well-defined phenotype of asthma that affects a small proportion of people with asthma. Because asthma can be triggered by cyclooxygenase (COX)-1 inhibitors, all nonselective COX inhibitors (aspirin, ibuprofen, ketorolac) should be avoided, but selective COX-2 inhibitors (celecoxib) are safe to use. Theoretically, reversal of neuromuscular blockade with anticholinesterase drugs could precipitate bronchospasm due to stimulation of postganglionic cholinergic receptors in airway smooth muscle. Adequate concomitant dosing of an anticholinergic drug is necessary to avoid this complication. Alternatively, sugammadex can be used for the reversal of rocuronium- or vecuronium-induced neuromuscular blockade.
- *Environment and air pollution*. Increased levels of sulfur dioxide, ozone, diesel particulates, and nitrogen oxides are associated with increased asthma symptoms. Dry cold air can also trigger bronchospasm in susceptible individuals.
- *Occupational factors*. Various compounds used in industry can cause asthma in susceptible individuals. Various names have been applied to this condition, such as meat wrapper's asthma, baker's asthma, and woodworker's asthma.
- *Exercise*. Asthma can be induced or exacerbated by physical exertion. The mechanism is linked to hyperventilation, which results in increased osmolality in airway lining fluid and triggers mast cell mediator release, resulting in bronchoconstriction.
- *Emotional stress*. Psychological factors can induce bronchoconstriction through the cholinergic reflex pathway.

Carron M, Zarantonello F, Tellaroli P, et al. Efficacy and safety of sugammadex compared to neostigmine for reversal of neuromuscular blockade: a meta-analysis of randomized controlled trials. *J Clin Anesth*. 2016;35:1-12.

Israel E. Asthma. In: Loscalzo J, Fauci AS, Kasper DL, et al, eds. *Harrison's Principles of Internal Medicine*. 21st ed. McGraw-Hill; 2022:2147-2159.

Tao J, Kurup V. Anesthetic considerations for obstructive lung disease. In: Hines RL, Jones SB, eds. *Stoelting's Anesthesia and Co-existing Disease*. 8th ed. Elsevier; 2022:19-36.

Yamakage M, Iwasaki S, Jeong SW, et al. Beta-1 selective adrenergic antagonist landiolol and esmolol can be safely used in patients with airway hyperreactivity. *Heart Lung*. 2009;38:48-55.

A.6. What is the universal finding in ABG analysis during asthmatic attacks: hypoxemia or CO_2 retention?

Hypoxemia is a universal finding during asthmatic attacks. Ventilatory failure with CO_2 retention is relatively uncommon because carbon dioxide has a diffusion capacity that is 20 times greater than that of oxygen. During acute asthmatic attacks, most patients try to overcome airway obstruction and hypoxemia by hyperventilation. This results in hypocarbia and respiratory alkalosis. CO_2 retention is a late finding and indicates severe and prolonged airway obstruction, as in status asthmaticus.

Israel E. Asthma. In: Loscalzo J, Fauci AS, Kasper DL, et al, eds. *Harrison's Principles of Internal Medicine*. 21st ed. McGraw-Hill; 2022:2147-2159.

Tao J, Kurup V. Anesthetic considerations for obstructive lung disease. In: Hines RL, Jones SB, eds. *Stoelting's Anesthesia and Co-existing Disease*. 8th ed. Elsevier; 2022:19-36.

A.7. Describe the abnormalities seen in spirometry, lung volumes, and lung capacities during an asthmatic attack.

There is a substantial reduction in forced expiratory volume in 1 second (FEV_1), but less reduction in forced vital capacity (FVC), resulting in a reduced FEV_1/FVC ratio. Forced expiratory flow at 25% to 75% ($FEF_{25\%-75\%}$) is sharply reduced as well. $FEF_{25\%-75\%}$ (also referred to as the maximum midexpiratory flow rate [MMEFR]) is the forced expiratory flow rate during 25% to 75% of the vital capacity (VC). Unlike FEV_1, the $FEF_{25\%-75\%}$ is independent of patient effort. Other classic spirometry findings include a decreased expiratory reserve volume (ERV), whereas the residual volume (RV), FRC, and total lung capacity (TLC) are increased.

Israel E. Asthma. In: Loscalzo J, Fauci AS, Kasper DL, et al, eds. *Harrison's Principles of Internal Medicine*. 21st ed. McGraw-Hill; 2022:2147-2159.

Tao J, Kurup V. Anesthetic considerations for obstructive lung disease. In: Hines RL, Jones SB, eds. *Stoelting's Anesthesia and Co-existing Disease*. 8th ed. Elsevier; 2022:19-36.

Woods BD, Sladen RN. Perioperative considerations for the patient with asthma and bronchospasm. *Br J Anaesth*. 2009;103:i57-i65.

B. Preoperative Evaluation and Preparation

B.1. How would you evaluate the patient preoperatively? What preoperative workup would you order?

Preoperative evaluation of patients with asthma and COPD focuses on the assessment of disease severity, the effectiveness of current medical management, and the potential need for additional therapy before surgery. The history should include an assessment of exercise tolerance, recent or current respiratory infections, sputum quantity and quality, known triggers of attacks, most recent exacerbations, current medications and time of last use, smoking history, and prior surgical and anesthetic history.

A cardiopulmonary exam should focus on detecting signs of acute bronchospasm, active lung infection, and right heart failure. Note the patient's general appearance and breathing, including the use of accessory muscles, pursed-lip exhalation, or cyanosis. Auscultation of the lungs can reveal wheezing, adventitious lung sounds, and hyperinflation. Auscultation of the heart can reveal a split-second heart sound typical of cor pulmonale or the murmur of tricuspid or pulmonary regurgitation present in some patients with long-standing pulmonary hypertension. Additionally, jugular venous distension, peripheral edema, and hepatic enlargement can be present. Cachexia might also be seen.

Laboratory testing is guided by the history and physical examination. For major surgery, it is reasonable to obtain a complete blood cell count, serum electrolytes, electrocardiogram, and chest radiograph. Additionally, these patients should have a room air Spo_2. It is not recommended to perform pulmonary function tests routinely before noncardiothoracic surgery. However, if a worsening of disease severity is suggested by the history and physical examination, additional diagnostic tests include a computed tomography scan of the chest, echocardiogram, detailed lung volume testing, and room air ABG analysis.

Lakshminarasimhachar A, Smetana GW. Preoperative evaluation: estimation of pulmonary risk. *Anesthesiol Clin.* 2016;34:71-88.

Tao J, Kurup V. Anesthetic considerations for obstructive lung disease. In: Hines RL, Jones SB, eds. *Stoelting's Anesthesia and Co-existing Disease.* 8th ed. Elsevier; 2022:19-36.

Woods BD, Sladen RN. Perioperative considerations for the patient with asthma and bronchospasm. *Br J Anaesth.* 2009;103:i57-i65.

B.2. How would you distinguish obstructive lung disease from restrictive lung disease by spirometry?

Table 1.1 summarizes the distinctions between the two types of lung disease. In restrictive lung disease (eg, pulmonary fibrosis and severe kyphoscoliosis), FVC is low because of limited expansion of the lungs or chest wall, although FEV_1 is often not reduced proportionately because airway resistance is normal. Therefore, the FEV_1/FVC ratio is normal or high.

Spirometry yields VC, FVC, and FEV_1. These values can help identify and quantify two basic types of pulmonary dysfunction: obstructive disease and restrictive disease. In obstructive lung disease, the FEV_1/FVC ratio is grossly reduced because the airway resistance is high while FVC remains normal. FEV_1/FVC of less than 70% is diagnostic of airflow obstruction. In restrictive disease, all lung volumes decrease proportionally, but FEV_1/FVC remains normal.

The TLC is increased in obstructive lung disease and decreased in restrictive lung disease. However, TLC cannot be obtained by routine screening spirometry.

Gaulton TG, Cereda M. Respiratory function in anesthesia. In: Cullen BF, Stock MC, Ortega R, et al, eds. *Barash, Cullen, and Stoelting's Clinical Anesthesia.* 9th ed. Wolters Kluwer; 2024:349-361.

Levy BD. Approach to the patient with disease of the respiratory system. In: Loscalzo J, Fauci AS, Kasper DL, et al, eds. *Harrison's Principles of Internal Medicine.* 21st ed. McGraw-Hill; 2022:2131-2132.

B.3. Define normal lung volumes and lung capacities. Give normal values for an average adult male.

There are four basic "volumes" and four derived "capacities" that are combinations of these volumes (**Figure 1.1**).

Tidal volume (V_T) is the volume of air inhaled or exhaled during normal breathing. Normal V_T is 500 mL or approximately 6 to 8 mL/kg.

Inspiratory reserve volume (IRV) is the maximum volume of gas that can be inhaled following a normal inspiration while at rest. Normal IRV is 2,500 to 3,500 mL.

ERV is the maximum volume of gas that can be exhaled after a normal expiration. Normal ERV is 1,200 mL.

RV is the volume of gas remaining in the lungs after a forced exhalation. Normal RV is 1,200 mL.

VC is the maximum amount of gas that can be exhaled after a maximum inhalation. VC is the sum of V_T, ERV, and IRV. Normal VC is 4,500 mL or approximately 60 to 70 mL/kg.

Inspiratory capacity (IC) is the maximum amount of gas that can be inhaled from the resting expiratory position after a normal exhalation. It is the sum of V_T and IRV. Normal IC is 3,500 mL.

FRC is the remaining lung volume at the end of a normal quiet expiration. It is the sum of RV and ERV. Normal FRC is 2,500 mL or 30 to 40 mL/kg.

TABLE 1.1 Differences Between Obstructive and Restrictive Lung Diseases

	Obstructive	Restrictive
FVC	N or slightly ↑	↓
FEV_1	N or slightly ↓	↓
FEV_1/FVC	↓	N
Maximum mid-expiratory flow rate	↓	N
Functional residual capacity	N or ↑ if gas trapping	↓
Total lung capacity	N or ↑ if gas trapping	↓

↓, decreased; ↑, increased; FEV_1, forced expiratory volume in 1 second; FVC, forced vital capacity; N, normal.

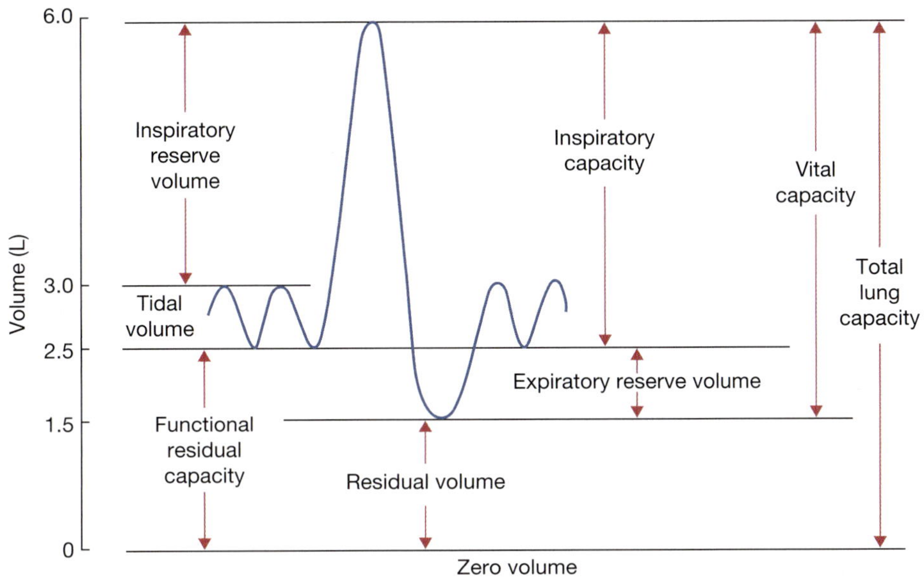

FIGURE 1.1. Lung volumes and lung capacities.

TLC is the lung volume at the end of a maximum inspiration. It is the sum of VC and RV. Normal TLC is 5,000 to 6,000 mL for an adult male and 4,000 to 5,000 mL for an adult female.

Badescu GC. Atlas of electrocardiography. In: Cullen BF, Stock MC, Ortega R, et al, eds. *Barash, Cullen, and Stoelting's Clinical Anesthesia*. 9th ed. Wolters Kluwer; 2024:1618.

Gaulton TG, Cereda M. Respiratory function in anesthesia. In: Cullen BF, Stock MC, Ortega R, et al, eds. *Barash, Cullen, and Stoelting's Clinical Anesthesia*. 9th ed. Wolters Kluwer; 2024:349-361.

Lumb AB, Thomas CR, eds. Elastic forces and lung volumes. In: *Nunn and Lumb's Applied Respiratory Physiology*. 9th ed. Elsevier; 2021:22-24.

Naureckas ET, Solway J. Disturbances of respiratory function. In: Loscalzo J, Fauci AS, Kasper DL, et al, eds. *Harrison's Principles of Internal Medicine*. 21st ed. McGraw-Hill; 2022:2133-2139.

B.4. What are flow-volume loops? Draw flow-volume loops for a healthy subject and for patients with COPD, restrictive lung disease, fixed obstruction of the upper airway, variable extrathoracic obstruction, and variable intrathoracic obstruction.

Flow-volume loops provide a graphical analysis of flow at various lung volumes. To perform the test, subjects are asked to inhale maximally (to TLC) and then to exhale as forcefully and fully as possible (to RV). This cycle is repeated. The flow (liters per second) is plotted on the y-axis and volume (liters) on the x-axis (**Figure 1.2A**). The test requires a compliant patient for accurate results—the majority of the test is effort dependent, including the entire inspiratory curve and both ends of the expiratory curve (near TLC and RV). The forced expiratory flow during 25% to 75% of VC ($FEF_{25\%-75\%}$) is reflective of the small- to medium-sized airways and is considered a relatively effort-independent value.

Normal flow-volume loop (**Figure 1.2A**). Inspiratory limb of the loop is symmetric and convex. Expiratory limb is linear. Airflow at the midpoint of IC and airflow at the midpoint of expiratory capacity are often measured and compared. Maximal inspiratory flow (MIF) at 50% FVC is greater than maximal expiratory flow (MEF) at 50% FVC because dynamic compression of the airways occurs during exhalation.

Obstructive disorder (eg, emphysema, asthma) (**Figure 1.2B**). Although all airflow is diminished, expiratory prolongation predominates, and MEF < MIF. Peak expiratory flow (PEF) is sometimes used to estimate the degree of airway obstruction but depends on patient effort.

Restrictive disorder (eg, interstitial lung disease, kyphoscoliosis) (**Figure 1.2C**). The loop is narrowed because of diminished lung volumes. Airflow is greater than normal at comparable lung volumes because the increased elastic recoil of the lungs holds the airways open.

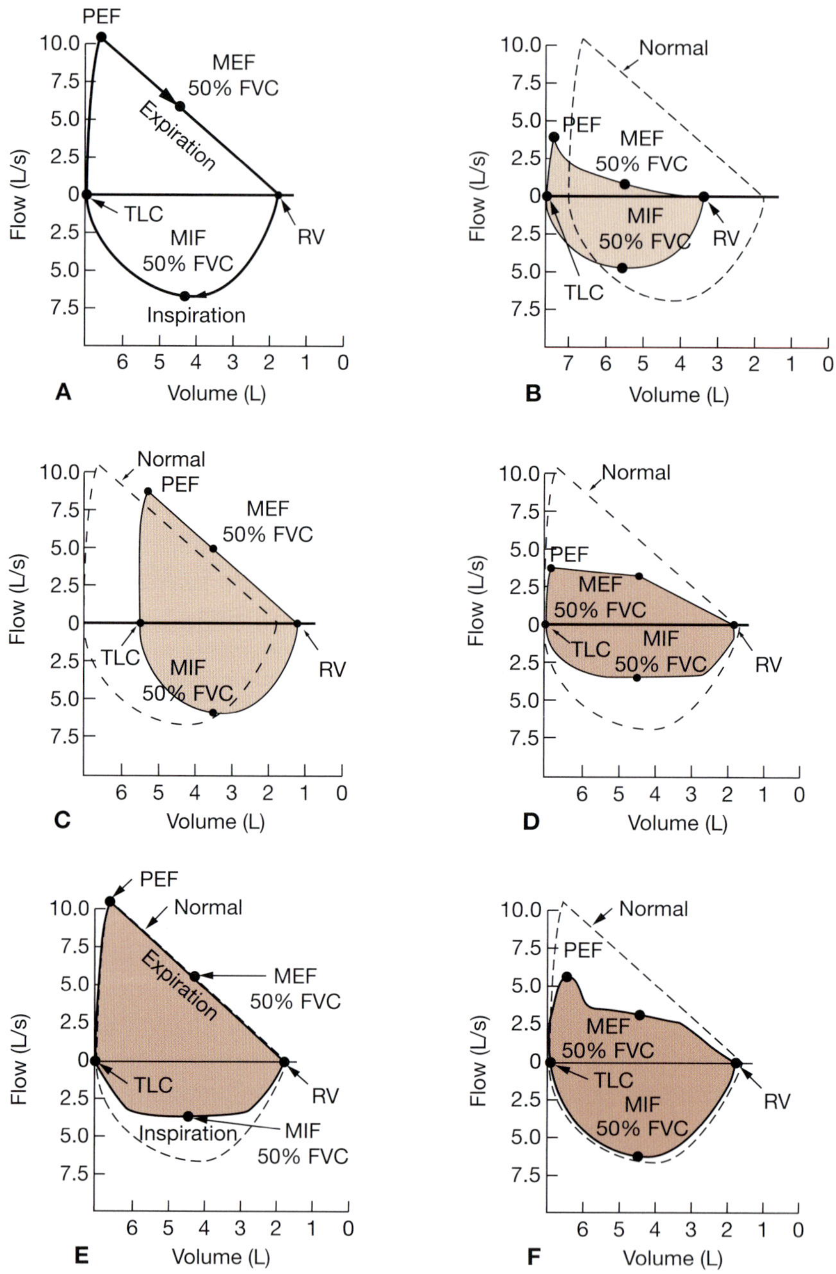

FIGURE 1.2. Flow-volume loops for a healthy person (**A**), a patient with obstructive lung disease (**B**), a patient with restrictive lung disease (**C**), a patient with a fixed obstruction (**D**), a patient with a variable extrathoracic obstruction (**E**), and a patient with a variable intrathoracic obstruction (**F**). FVC, forced vital capacity; MEF, maximal expiratory flow; MIF, maximal inspiratory flow; PEF, peak expiratory flow; RV, residual volume; TLC, total lung capacity. (Derived from Porter R. *Merck Manual Professional Version*. Merck Sharp & Dohme Corp., a subsidiary of Merck & Co, Inc. Accessed June 4, 2025. http://www.msdmanuals.com/professional)

Fixed obstruction of the upper airway (eg, tracheal stenosis, goiter) (**Figure 1.2D**). The top and bottom of the loops are flattened so that the configuration approaches that of a rectangle. Fixed obstruction limits flow equally during inspiration and expiration, and MEF = MIF.

Variable extrathoracic obstruction (eg, unilateral vocal cord paralysis, vocal cord dysfunction) (**Figure 1.2E**). When a single vocal cord is paralyzed, it moves passively with pressure gradients across the glottis. During forced inspiration, it is drawn inward, resulting in a plateau of decreased inspiratory flow. During forced expiration, it is passively blown aside, and expiratory flow is unimpaired. Therefore, MIF 50% FVC < MEF 50% FVC.

Variable intrathoracic obstruction (eg, tracheomalacia) (**Figure 1.2F**). During a forced inspiration, negative pleural pressure holds the floppy trachea open. With forced expiration, loss of structural support results in tracheal narrowing and a plateau of diminished flow. Airflow is maintained briefly before airway compression occurs.

Gaulton TG, Cereda M. Respiratory function in anesthesia. In: Cullen BF, Stock MC, Ortega R, et al, eds. *Barash, Cullen, and Stoelting's Clinical Anesthesia*. 9th ed. Wolters Kluwer; 2024:349-361.

Naureckas ET, Solway J. Disturbances of respiratory function. In: Loscalzo J, Fauci AS, Kasper DL, et al, eds. *Harrison's Principles of Internal Medicine*. 21st ed. McGraw-Hill; 2022:2133-2139.

The Merck Manual: Professional Edition. Accessed April 4, 2023. http://www.merckmanuals.com/professional/pulmonary_disorders/tests_of_pulmonary_function_pft/airflow_lung_volumes_and_flow-volume_loop.html?qt=flow%20volume%20loops&alt=sh

B.5. Define closing volume (CV) and closing capacity (CC). What is the normal value of CV?

CV is the volume above the RV at which small airways begin to close during expiration. CC is the sum of CV and RV. CC is the lung volume at which the small airways in the dependent parts of the lung begin to close. It can be measured using the single-breath nitrogen test (**Figure 1.3**) or with an inert tracer gas such as helium, xenon, or argon.

In healthy young people, CV is approximately 10% of the VC or 400 to 500 mL. CV and CC increase with age. CV is increased in patients with small airway disease and in chronic smokers.

Buist AS. New tests to assess lung function. The single-breath nitrogen test. *N Engl J Med*. 1975;293:438-440.

Gianni S, Vaporidi K, Cereda M, Berra L. Respiratory physiology and pathophysiology. In: Gropper MA, Cohen NH, Eriksson LI, et al, eds. *Miller's Anesthesia*. 10th ed. Elsevier; 2025:245-272.

Lumb AB, Thomas CR, eds. Respiratory system resistance. In: *Nunn and Lumb's Applied Respiratory Physiology*. 9th ed. Elsevier; 2021:27-41.

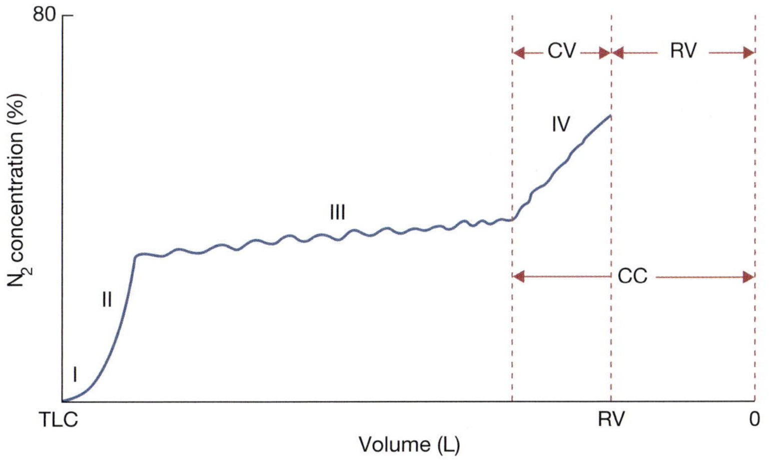

FIGURE 1.3. Closing volume (CV) measurement by single-breath nitrogen test. CC, closing capacity; RV, residual volume; TLC, total lung capacity.

B.6. Why is the functional residual capacity (FRC) important in oxygenation?

In a healthy young adult, FRC is above CC (FRC > CV + RV). Increases in CC and/or decreases in FRC can result in CC exceeding FRC and subsequent closure of the small airways during certain periods of normal tidal ventilation. Airway closure produces shunting, with perfusion of unventilated alveoli. Therefore, shunt (Q_S/Q_T) is increased and arterial oxygenation is decreased.

Perfusion to the lung occurs in both the inspiratory and expiratory phases of respiration. The FRC, or lung volume remaining at end expiration, provides surface area for gas exchange during this phase of respiration. The greater the FRC, the more oxygenation occurs. Patients in the supine position, under general anesthesia, or with acute respiratory distress syndrome all have decreased FRC to varying degrees. PEEP increases FRC, improving oxygenation in the expiratory phase and reducing small airway collapse.

FRC can be measured by helium dilution, nitrogen washout, or body plethysmography.

Gianni S, Vaporidi K, Cereda M, Berra L. Respiratory physiology and pathophysiology. In: Gropper MA, Cohen NH, Eriksson LI, et al, eds. *Miller's Anesthesia*. 10th ed. Elsevier; 2025:245-272.

Lumb AB, Thomas CR, eds. Respiratory system resistance. In: *Nunn and Lumb's Applied Respiratory Physiology*. 9th ed. Elsevier; 2021:27-41.

B.7. How are FRC and CC affected by age and posture? How are they affected by general anesthesia?

Posture has a dramatic effect on FRC. When a patient goes from an upright to a supine position, FRC decreases approximately 30%. Body position does not affect CC.

Conversely, age has a greater effect on CC than on FRC. CC increases with age, whereas FRC does not change or increases only slightly. Therefore, CC will exceed FRC in healthy adults over the age of 44 years when in the supine position and in healthy adults over the age of 75 years in the upright position.

During general anesthesia, FRC is reduced approximately 20%, whether breathing is controlled or spontaneous. The anatomic basis of the FRC reduction under anesthesia is not well understood. It is thought to be due to the cephalad shift of the diaphragm, induced by anesthesia and muscle paralysis. Although the role of the anatomic position of the diaphragm remains debatable, the current understanding is that FRC is reduced due to loss of respiratory muscle tone.

CC was previously reported to be unchanged during anesthesia, but later studies concluded that CC reduced in parallel to FRC during anesthesia.

Bergman NA, Tien YK. Contribution of the closure of pulmonary units to impaired oxygenation during anesthesia. *Anesthesiology*. 1983;59:395-401.

Gianni S, Vaporidi K, Cereda M, Berra L. Respiratory physiology and pathophysiology. In: Gropper MA, Cohen NH, Eriksson LI, et al, eds. *Miller's Anesthesia*. 10th ed. Elsevier; 2025:245-272.

Juno P, Marsh HM, Knopp TJ, et al. Closing capacity in awake and anesthetized-paralyzed man. *J Appl Physiol*. 1978;44:238.

Lumb AB, Thomas CR. Respiratory system resistance. In: *Nunn and Lumb's Applied Respiratory Physiology*. 9th ed. Elsevier; 2021a:31-32.

Lumb AB, Thomas CR. Anaesthesia. In: *Nunn and Lumb's Applied Respiratory Physiology*. 9th ed. Elsevier; 2021b:249-251.

Wahba RWM. Perioperative functional residual capacity. *Can J Anaesth*. 1991;38:384-400.

B.8. Give the equations for shunt (Q_S/Q_T) and dead space/tidal volume (V_D/V_T). What are their normal values?

$$Q_S / Q_T = \frac{C\text{c}O_2 - C\text{a}O_2}{C\text{c}O_2 - C\bar{\text{v}}O_2} \qquad V_D / V_T = \frac{P\text{a}CO_2 - P\bar{E}CO_2}{P\text{a}CO_2}$$

where CcO_2, CaO_2, and CO_2 are oxygen contents in pulmonary capillary, arterial, and mixed venous blood, respectively; Q_T is cardiac output; Q_S is shunt blood flow; and $PaCO_2$ and $P\bar{E}CO_2$ are partial pressures of CO_2 in arterial blood and mixed expired gas, respectively.

Normal Q_S/Q_T is 4% to 5%, and V_D/V_T is approximately 0.3.

Gaulton TG, Cereda M. Respiratory function in anesthesia. In: Cullen BF, Stock MC, Ortega R, et al, eds. *Barash, Cullen, and Stoelting's Clinical Anesthesia*. 9th ed. Wolters Kluwer; 2024:349-361.

Lumb AB, Thomas CR, eds. Distribution of pulmonary ventilation and perfusion. In: *Nunn and Lumb's Applied Respiratory Physiology*. 9th ed. Elsevier; 2021:99-101.

B.9. Interpret the following ABG analysis: pH, 7.36; Pco_2, 60 mm Hg; Po_2, 70 mm Hg; and CO_2 content, 36 mEq/L.

The fraction of inspired oxygen (Fio_2) is essential to evaluate Pao_2. Assume the blood sample is obtained while the patient is breathing room air. The blood gases show mild hypoxemia and respiratory acidosis, compensated by metabolic alkalosis. The blood gases are compatible with COPD.

Silverman EK, Crapo JD, Make BJ. Chronic obstructive pulmonary disease. In: Loscalzo J, Fauci AS, Kasper DL, et al, eds. *Harrison's Principles of Internal Medicine*. 21st ed. McGraw-Hill; 2022:2180-2189.

B.10. What are the common physiologic causes of hypoxemia?

From the shunt equation, arterial oxygen content is related to the change in pulmonary capillary oxygen content, venous oxygen content, and venous admixture. It is easier to classify hypoxemia into the following three categories.

Decreased Pulmonary Capillary Oxygen Tension

- Hypoventilation
- Low Fio_2
- Ventilation/perfusion mismatch from pulmonary parenchymal change
- Diffusion abnormality (rare)

Increased Shunting

- Either intrapulmonary or cardiac

Reduced Venous Oxygen Content

- Congestive heart failure—low cardiac output
- Increased metabolism—fever, hyperthyroidism, shivering
- Decreased arterial oxygen content—anemia

Chang M, Horvath R. The postanesthesia care unit. In: Gropper MA, Cohen NH, Eriksson LI, et al, eds. *Miller's Anesthesia*. 10th ed. Elsevier; 2025:2484-2511.

Gianni S, Vaporidi K, Cereda M, Berra L. Respiratory physiology and pathophysiology. In: Gropper MA, Cohen NH, Eriksson LI, et al, eds. *Miller's Anesthesia*. 10th ed. Elsevier; 2025:245-272.

Loscalzo J. Hypoxia and cyanosis. In: Loscalzo J, Fauci AS, Kasper DL, et al, eds. *Harrison's Principles of Internal Medicine*. 21st ed. McGraw-Hill; 2022:272-274.

B.11. How would you prepare this patient with asthma and COPD for surgery?

The goal of preoperative preparation is to optimize the patient for surgery and to decrease the risk of postoperative pulmonary complications (PPCs). This patient's risk factors for PPCs include preexisting pulmonary disease, cigarette smoking, abdominal surgery, and general anesthesia.

Preoperative strategies that can reduce PPC rates include smoking cessation (see Section B.12), optimizing airflow limitation in patients with obstructive lung disease (such as this patient), and treating respiratory tract infections if present.

The severity of airflow limitations is assessed during preoperative evaluation and laboratory and diagnostic studies (see Section B.1). Airflow limitation can be optimized by the continuation of anti-inflammatory and bronchodilator therapies up to the time of surgery. Additional therapy, such as systemic corticosteroids, can be initiated in patients with poorly controlled symptoms.

Elective surgery should not be performed in the presence of active respiratory infection, and symptoms should be actively treated until the patient is back to baseline status.

Additionally, preoperative lung expansion maneuvers, such as deep breathing exercises, incentive spirometry, and chest physiotherapy, are of proven benefit in reducing PPC rates.

Lakshminarasimhachar A, Smetana GW. Preoperative evaluation: estimation of pulmonary risk. *Anesthesiol Clin*. 2016;34:71-88.

Tao J, Kurup V. Anesthetic considerations for obstructive lung disease. In: Hines RL, Jones SB, eds. *Stoelting's Anesthesia and Co-existing Disease*. 8th ed. Elsevier; 2022:19-36.

Woods BD, Sladen RN. Perioperative considerations for the patient with asthma and bronchospasm. *Br J Anaesth*. 2009;103:i57-i65.

B.12. The patient comes to your perioperative clinic 2 weeks before surgery. He wants to know if his smoking puts him at increased risk during surgery. What do you tell him? Should he quit now?

Smoking results in increased levels of carboxyhemoglobin, decreased oxygen content, and decreased delivery of oxygen by hemoglobin to the tissues. These effects are dramatically improved with as little as 12 hours of smoking cessation.

Smoking also increases the risk of PPCs, which include respiratory failure, unplanned intensive care unit (ICU) admission, pneumonia, airway events during anesthesia, and increased need for postoperative respiratory support. Smokers have an increased rate of wound-related complications and decreased bone healing after surgery. Although a cessation period of at least 8 weeks prior to surgery is optimal and results in improved mucociliary clearance, decreased sputum production, and a relative risk reduction in PPCs, it is highly recommended for patients to stop smoking at any time prior to surgery.

A persistent misconception in our specialty is that short-term smoking cessation (<4 weeks) is detrimental to the patient. Some have argued that a patient smoking 2 weeks before surgery should continue smoking to avoid *increased* risks associated with cessation. There is now a preponderance of evidence that debunks this concept. Short-term smoking cessation is *not* a risk factor for long-term perioperative complications. In contrast, the long-term detrimental effects of continued smoking are well known. Anesthesiologists should be aware that admission for surgery can be a powerful motivator for patients to quit smoking, providing a "teachable moment" for smoking cessation and frequently resulting in successful long-term cessation. Therefore, this patient should be counseled to quit smoking as soon as possible.

Myers K, Hajek P, Hinds C, et al. Stopping smoking shortly before surgery and postoperative complications. *Arch Intern Med.* 2011;171:983-989.

Turan A, Mascha EJ, Roberman D, et al. Smoking and perioperative outcomes. *Anesthesiology.* 2011;114:837-846.

Warner DO. Perioperative abstinence from smoking: physiologic and clinical consequences. *Anesthesiology.* 2006;104:356-367.

Yu S, Warner DO. Surgery as a teachable moment for smoking cessation. *Anesthesiology.* 2010;112:102-107.

B.13. You discover that the patient had a recent upper respiratory infection (URI); would you postpone surgery? If so, for how long?

Respiratory tract infections are the most common trigger of acute exacerbations of asthma. Even healthy subjects have transiently increased airway responsiveness to nonspecific stimuli following a viral infection. It is unclear how long surgery should be delayed following a URI because airway hyperreactivity can last 2 to 8 weeks after the infection in both healthy subjects and patients with asthma. Cohen and Cameron reported that a child with a URI having endotracheal anesthesia has an 11-fold increased risk of respiratory complications. And Tait and Knight found that laryngospasm and bronchospasm were significantly increased in healthy children 2 weeks after a URI. However, the data are controversial. A frequently cited retrospective study by Warner et al found no increase in intraoperative bronchospasm in patients with well-controlled asthma and a recent URI.

In this patient presenting for elective surgery with multiple risk factors for PPCs, postponing surgery for 1 to 2 weeks after clinical recovery from the URI is reasonable.

Cohen MM, Cameron CB. Should you cancel the operation when a child has an upper respiratory infection? *Anesth Analg.* 1991;72:282-288.

Tait AR, Knight PR. Intraoperative respiratory complications in patients with upper respiratory tract infections. *Can J Anaesth.* 1987;34:300-303.

Vazquez AOR, Rosenbaum S. Anesthesia for adults with upper respiratory infection. *UpToDate.* Published 2021. Accessed April 8, 2023. https://www.uptodate.com/contents/anesthesia-for-adults-with-upper-respiratory-infection/print

Warner DO, Warner MA, Barnes RD, et al. Perioperative respiratory complications in patients with asthma. *Anesthesiology.* 1996;85:460-467.

Woods BD, Sladen RN. Perioperative considerations for the patient with asthma and bronchospasm. *Br J Anaesth.* 2009;103:i57-i65.

B.14. What medications would you expect the patient to have taken in the past or be taking currently?

The main drugs for asthma and COPD can be divided into rescue medications (bronchodilators) and controllers (for maintenance).

Patients with infrequent asthma symptoms are placed solely on a short-acting β_2-agonist (SABA). Alternatively, anticholinergic inhalers such as ipratropium can be given, although their slower onset of action makes them less preferred.

Patients with an increased risk for exacerbations (including smokers) and/or those with frequent symptoms should be placed on controller therapy with a low-dose inhaled corticosteroid (ICS).

In patients with severe symptoms, a long-acting β_2-agonist or a high-dose ICS is added. Acute exacerbations are treated with a short course of oral corticosteroids.

Theophylline was a widely prescribed oral controller medication for asthma but has fallen out of favor secondary to its narrow therapeutic index, multiple drug interactions, and side effect profile. It can be prescribed in patients with COPD. Patients taking theophylline require routine drug-level testing. They should continue theophylline in the perioperative period to avoid an asthma or COPD exacerbation secondary to withdrawal.

Other oral medications targeting the inflammatory component of asthma include the mast cell stabilizer cromolyn, the anti-IgE antibody omalizumab, and leukotriene receptor antagonists such as zafirlukast and montelukast. The phosphodiesterase-4 inhibitor roflumilast can be added for patients with severe COPD.

Global Initiative for Asthma. Global strategy for asthma management and prevention. Published 2022. Accessed April 8, 2022. http://www.ginasthma.org/

Global Initiative for Chronic Obstructive Lung Disease. Global strategy for the diagnosis, management, and prevention of COPD. Published 2023. Accessed April 8, 2023. http://www.goldcopd.org/

Israel E. Asthma. In: Loscalzo J, Fauci AS, Kasper DL, et al, eds. *Harrison's Principles of Internal Medicine*. 21st ed. McGraw-Hill; 2022:2147-2159.

Silverman EK, Crapo JD, Make BJ. Chronic obstructive pulmonary disease. In: Loscalzo J, Fauci AS, Kasper DL, et al, eds. *Harrison's Principles of Internal Medicine*. 21st ed. McGraw-Hill; 2022:2180-2189.

B.15. The patient was on 20 mg of prednisone per day for 5 days as part of the treatment of an asthma exacerbation 3 months ago. He is currently not on corticosteroids. Should the patient receive "stress-dose" corticosteroids?

Patients on chronic steroid therapy experience hypothalamic-pituitary-adrenal (HPA) axis suppression that can result in decreased cortisol (hydrocortisone) production, a process known as secondary adrenal insufficiency. The concern is that inadequate cortisol production in response to the stress of surgery can manifest as full-blown adrenal crisis in the perioperative period. The anesthesiologist must decide whether to administer "stress-dose" steroids to mitigate this rare but potentially life-threatening complication of chronic steroid use. However, the decision is not always clear-cut because even the recommendations found in most textbooks are inconsistent and lack class A or B evidence. There is no universally agreed dose or duration of exogenous steroids required to cause HPA axis dysfunction, although prednisone 20 mg/d for 2 weeks within the previous 6 months has been cited.

Given this patient's short duration of prednisone treatment, he should not require administration of additional corticosteroids. However, 100 mg of IV hydrocortisone (typical stress-dose for this type of surgery) should be available in the operating room in case hypotension attributable to adrenal insufficiency occurs during surgery.

Another consideration is whether the patient will receive prophylaxis for postoperative nausea/vomiting (PONV) with dexamethasone. Dexamethasone has 30 times the glucocorticoid potency of hydrocortisone, so even a modest PONV dose of 4 mg of dexamethasone is equivalent to the usual stress dose of hydrocortisone. Because there is no mineralocorticoid deficiency in secondary adrenal insufficiency, dexamethasone's absence of mineralocorticoid activity is not an issue.

Hamrahian AH, Roman S, Milan S. The management of the surgical patient taking glucocorticoids. *UpToDate*. Published 2019. Accessed April 9, 2023. https://www.uptodate.com/contents/the-management-of-the-surgical-patient-taking-glucocorticoids

Liu MM, Reidy AB, Saatee S, et al. Perioperative steroid management: approaches based on current evidence. *Anesthesiology*. 2017;127:166-172.

Wax DB. One size fits all for stress-dose steroids. *Anesthesiology*. 2018;128:680-681.

Woods BD, Sladen RN. Perioperative considerations for the patient with asthma and bronchospasm. *Br J Anaesth*. 2009;103:i57-i65.

B.16. Should patients with reactive airway disease receive preoperative corticosteroids?

The increasing understanding of the inflammatory component of reactive airway disease has led to a greater appreciation of the importance of corticosteroids in preventing and treating exacerbations. In wheezing patients, oral methylprednisolone 40 mg daily for 5 days before surgery has been shown to decrease postintubation bronchospasm. The oft-cited concern that steroids increase the rate of wound complications is not well founded. A study of patients with asthma treated with steroids preoperatively found no increase in the incidence of wound infections or wound-healing problems.

Patients with poorly controlled asthma presenting for surgery with a high risk of PPCs (open aortic aneurysm repair, thoracic, upper abdominal) that will require endotracheal intubation must be treated with utmost caution and may benefit from preoperative optimization of pulmonary function with a short course of systemic corticosteroids. On the other hand, patients with mild, well-controlled disease should not require such treatment.

Bishop MJ. Preoperative corticosteroids for reactive airway? *Anesthesiology*. 2004;100:1047-1048.

Silvanus M-T, Groeben H, Peters J. Corticosteroids and inhaled salbutamol in patients with reversible airway obstruction markedly decrease the incidence of bronchospasm after tracheal intubation. *Anesthesiology*. 2004;100:1052-1057.

Tao J, Kurup V. Anesthetic considerations for obstructive lung disease. In: Hines RL, Jones SB, eds. *Stoelting's Anesthesia and Co-existing Disease*. 8th ed. Elsevier; 2022:25-27.

Woods BD, Sladen RN. Perioperative considerations for the patient with asthma and bronchospasm. *Br J Anaesth*. 2009;103:i57-i65.

B.17. What is the onset of action of intravenous (IV) corticosteroid therapy in asthma?

Parenteral corticosteroids remain a mainstay of the treatment of acute asthma. Although the bronchial effects are not immediate and are typically seen 4 to 6 hours after initial administration, they are nonetheless indicated for severe bronchospasm that has not resolved despite intense optimal bronchodilator therapy.

Tao J, Kurup V. Anesthetic considerations for obstructive lung disease. In: Hines RL, Jones SB, eds. *Stoelting's Anesthesia and Co-existing Disease*. 8th ed. Elsevier; 2022:24.

Woods BD, Sladen RN. Perioperative considerations for the patient with asthma and bronchospasm. *Br J Anaesth*. 2009;103:i57-i65.

B.18. You are visiting the patient in the preoperative area before coming to the operating room. How would you discuss treatment options and obtain informed consent from this patient?

Discussion of treatment options with the patient should exhibit understanding and concern for the situation of the patient. Indications for proposed treatment options should be explained in lay terms. The discussion should include an explanation of the benefits and risks of the treatment options and strategies for minimizing the risks. In this patient with asthma, COPD, and extensive smoking history, the increased possibility of intraoperative bronchospasm and elevated risks of PPCs should be reviewed. Questions should be elicited from the patient and answered in lay terms. Final treatment plan should be confirmed with the patient and affirmative consent obtained.

Sweitzer BJ. Preoperative evaluation for anesthesia for noncardiac surgery. *UpToDate*. Published 2023. Accessed June 26, 2023. https://www.uptodate.com/contents/preoperative-evaluation-for-anesthesia-for-noncardiac-surgery

B.19. If the patient is a 90-year-old with an order of Do-Not-Resuscitate (DNR), how would you discuss the management of a perioperative DNR order with the patient and family?

Patients with DNR orders should not be denied anesthesia and surgery simply because of their DNR status. Policies automatically suspending DNR orders prior to procedures involving anesthetic care might not sufficiently address a patient's right to self-determination in a responsible and ethical manner. A detailed discussion of the patient's values and preferences with respect to resuscitation should take place with the patient, the family, or designated surrogate. As a result of this discussion, the status of the directives should be clarified and modified based on patient preferences. Specifically, patient acceptance of specific procedures and levels of resuscitation, such as procedures necessary for anesthesia (intubation) and treatment of hypotension related to anesthetics, should be determined and documented. Additionally, the plan for postoperative reinstatement of any existing directives should be agreed upon and documented.

American Society of Anesthesiologists. Statement on ethical guidelines for the anesthesia care of patients with do-not-resuscitate orders. Committee on Ethics. Accessed June 26, 2023. https://www.asahq.org/standards-and-practice-parameters/statement-on-ethical-guidelines-for-the-anesthesia-care-of-patients-with-do-not-resuscitate-orders

Sweitzer BJ. Preoperative evaluation for anesthesia for noncardiac surgery. *UpToDate*. Published 2023. Accessed June 26, 2023. https://www.uptodate.com/contents/preoperative-evaluation-for-anesthesia-for-noncardiac-surgery

C. Intraoperative Management

C.1. If the patient had a severe asthmatic attack in the operating room before the induction of anesthesia, would you proceed with the anesthetic or postpone the surgery?

First, medical treatment should be given to treat the asthmatic attack. Elective surgery should be postponed, the patient reevaluated carefully, and his asthma better optimized. In the case of emergency surgery, such as acute appendicitis, the surgery can be performed after the asthmatic attack is successfully treated. Regional anesthesia, if feasible, should be considered. During surgery, the medical treatment should be continued.

Dewachter P, Mouton-Faivre C, Emala CW, et al. Case scenario: bronchospasm during anesthetic induction. *Anesthesiology*. 2011;114:1200-1210.

Woods BD, Sladen RN. Perioperative considerations for the patient with asthma and bronchospasm. *Br J Anaesth*. 2009;103:i57-i65.

C.2. The patient did not have an asthmatic attack in the operating room, and you proceed with induction of anesthesia. How would you induce anesthesia? Would you use a supraglottic airway device instead of an endotracheal tube?

The principles of anesthetic management for the patient with asthma are 3-fold: to block airway reflexes before laryngoscopy and intubation, to relax airway smooth muscle, and to prevent the release of biochemical mediators.

Before induction of general anesthesia, the patient should take two or three puffs of albuterol from a metered-dose inhaler (MDI). Propofol is often used for the induction of a hemodynamically stable patient with asthma. Ketamine can be chosen for a hemodynamically unstable patient with asthma (see Sections C.3 and C.4). Then, oxygen and a potent inhalation agent, such as sevoflurane, are administered by mask to achieve an adequate depth of anesthesia that suppresses hyperreactive airway reflexes sufficiently to permit tracheal intubation without triggering bronchospasm. The lesser pungency of sevoflurane (compared with desflurane and isoflurane) might reduce the likelihood of coughing, which can induce bronchospasm. Neuromuscular blocking agents that do not release histamine, such as cisatracurium, vecuronium, and rocuronium, can be used to facilitate tracheal intubation. Prior to intubation, lidocaine can be administered (see Section C.5).

Avoidance of tracheal intubation altogether is another approach. A supraglottic airway device provides a unique opportunity for the clinician to control the airway without having to introduce a tube into the trachea. Kim and Bishop demonstrated a reversible increase in airway resistance in intubated patients under isoflurane anesthesia and showed that this increase was not present with supraglottic airway use. Therefore, it may be an ideal airway tool in the patient with asthma not at risk for reflux and aspiration.

Laparoscopic surgeries using a supraglottic airway device have been reported by multiple centers for both gynecologic surgeries and cholecystectomies. Insufflation of the abdomen and manipulation of the bowel places these patients at increased aspiration risk. However, the use of a specialized supraglottic airway such as Laryngeal mask airway (LMA) ProSeal can mitigate these effects by allowing for the placement of an orogastric tube for drainage of the stomach and a larger cuff size that reduces both the risk for gastric inflation and aspiration of refluxed gastric contents. I-Gel can be another suitable alternative to endotracheal intubation in laparoscopic surgery in appropriately selected patients.

Kim ES, Bishop MJ. Endotracheal intubation, but not laryngeal mask airway insertion, produces reversible bronchoconstriction. *Anesthesiology*. 1999;90:391-394.

Lai CJ, Liu CM, Wu CY, et al. I-Gel is a suitable alternative to endotracheal tubes in the laparoscopic pneumoperitoneum and Trendelenburg position. *BMC Anesthesiol*. 2017;17:3.

Maltby JR, Beriault MT, Watson NC, et al. The LMA-ProSeal is an effective alternative to tracheal intubation in laparoscopic cholecystectomy. *Can J Anaesth*. 2002;49:857-862.

Tanella A, Hyman JB, Rosenblatt WH. Airway management. In: Cullen BF, Stock MC, Ortega R, et al, eds. *Barash, Cullen, and Stoelting's Clinical Anesthesia*. 9th ed. Wolters Kluwer; 2024:737-777.

Tao J, Kurup V. Anesthetic considerations for obstructive lung disease. In: Hines RL, Jones SB, eds. *Stoelting's Anesthesia and Co-existing Disease*. 8th ed. Elsevier; 2022:26.

C.3. Would you use propofol for induction of anesthesia?

Propofol is the induction agent of choice for the hemodynamically stable patient with reactive airway disease. In comparison to induction with thiopental, thiamylal, or methohexital, 2.5 mg/kg propofol IV resulted in a significantly lower incidence of wheezing after tracheal intubation in patients with asthma. The incidence of wheezing was 0%, 45%, and 26% in patients who received propofol, a thiobarbiturate, or an oxybarbiturate, respectively. Another study in unselected patients found a significantly lower respiratory resistance after tracheal intubation following induction with propofol than with thiopental or etomidate. Nevertheless, propofol-induced bronchospasm has been reported in patients with allergic rhinitis, so propofol should be used with caution in patients with a high allergic tendency.

Eames WO, Rooke GA, Wu RS, et al. Comparison of the effects of etomidate, propofol, and thiopental on respiratory resistance after tracheal intubation. *Anesthesiology*. 1996;84:1307-1311.

Nishiyama T, Hanaoka K. Propofol-induced bronchoconstriction: two case reports. *Anesth Analg*. 2001;93:645-646.

Pizov R, Brown RH, Weiss YS, et al. Wheezing during induction of general anesthesia in patients with and without asthma. A randomized, blinded trial. *Anesthesiology*. 1995;82:1111-1116.

Tao J, Kurup V. Anesthetic considerations for obstructive lung disease. In: Hines RL, Jones SB, eds. *Stoelting's Anesthesia and Co-existing Disease*. 8th ed. Elsevier; 2022:26.

C.4. Would you use thiopental, methohexital, etomidate, or ketamine for induction of anesthesia?

Thiopental and thiamylal are thiobarbiturates that have been shown to release histamine. Methohexital and pentobarbital are oxybarbiturates that have not been shown to release histamine. This suggests that the sulfur atom is important in barbiturate-induced histamine release. Moreover, thiobarbiturates, but not oxybarbiturates, have been shown to lead to thromboxane-mediated tracheal constriction in guinea pigs. For these reasons, methohexital is the preferred barbiturate for induction of anesthesia in patients with extreme sensitivity to histamine (people with asthma) or increased histamine releasability (atopics).

Because it provides only suppression of airway reflexes, airway instrumentation under thiopental anesthesia alone can trigger bronchospasm. However, it can be used cautiously in people with asthma, provided that an adequate depth of anesthesia is achieved before airway stimulation.

Etomidate has not been shown to release histamine, does not depress myocardial function, and provides hemodynamic stability in critically ill patients. Both etomidate and thiopental afford no protection against wheezing after intubation and are therefore inferior to propofol in this regard.

Ketamine produces bronchodilation both through neural mechanisms and through the release of catecholamines. In an actively wheezing patient, ketamine is the induction agent of choice, particularly with unstable hemodynamics.

Eames WO, Rooke GA, Wu RS, et al. Comparison of the effects of etomidate, propofol, and thiopental on respiratory resistance after tracheal intubation. *Anesthesiology*. 1996;84:1307-1311.

Pizov R, Brown RH, Weiss YS, et al. Wheezing during induction of general anesthesia in patients with and without asthma. A randomized, blinded trial. *Anesthesiology*. 1995;82:1111-1116.

Tao J, Kurup V. Anesthetic considerations for obstructive lung disease. In: Hines RL, Jones SB, eds. *Stoelting's Anesthesia and Co-existing Disease*. 8th ed. Elsevier; 2022:26.

C.5. Would you administer lidocaine for tracheal intubation?

Administration of IV lidocaine at a dose of 1 to 1.5 mg/kg several minutes prior to tracheal intubation to prevent reflex-induced bronchospasm is a long-standing practice. However, some caution is required, as paradoxical bronchospasm can occur in patients with asthma. It appears that while IV lidocaine reduces airway responsiveness to drugs and stimuli that cause bronchospasm, lidocaine on its own does not reduce baseline airway tone and might increase it. Therefore, IV lidocaine should be administered with care in these patients.

Alternatively, topical endotracheal spray of lidocaine can be used. However, inhalation of lidocaine is itself irritating and can *provoke* bronchospasm in patients with asthma. If lidocaine spray is used to tropicalize the airway, an adequate depth of anesthesia should be achieved before lidocaine is administered.

Burches BR Jr, Warner DO. Bronchospasm after intravenous lidocaine. *Anesth Analg*. 2008;107:1260-1262.

Chang HY, Togias A, Brown RH. The effects of systemic lidocaine on airway tone and pulmonary function in asthmatic subjects. *Anesth Analg*. 2007;104:1109-1115.

McAlpine LG, Thomson NC. Lidocaine-induced bronchoconstriction in asthmatic patients. Relation to histamine airway responsiveness and effect of preservative. *Chest*. 1989;96:1012-1015.

Tao J, Kurup V. Anesthetic considerations for obstructive lung disease. In: Hines RL, Jones SB, eds. *Stoelting's Anesthesia and Co-existing Disease*. 8th ed. Elsevier; 2022:26.

Woods BD, Sladen RN. Perioperative considerations for the patient with asthma and bronchospasm. *Br J Anaesth*. 2009;103:i57-i65.

C.6. If this were an emergency surgery and rapid sequence induction is indicated, how would you induce anesthesia in this patient?

Precautions to prevent aspiration of gastric contents and asthmatic attack must be considered simultaneously. Rapid sequence induction and tracheal intubation are necessary to prevent aspiration. However, light anesthesia can precipitate severe bronchospasm.

Prior to induction, inhalation of β_2-agonists such as albuterol should be administered. The patient should then be adequately denitrogenated with 100% oxygen administered by mask. Preoxygenation is particularly important because mask ventilation is usually not performed in rapid sequence induction.

Preoxygenation is administered for 3 minutes of normal V_T breathing, or for eight deep breaths over 1 minute.

Propofol is the induction agent of choice in a hemodynamically stable patient with asthma. Ketamine and etomidate are alternatives to propofol in a patient at risk of hemodynamic instability. It is important to note that in a patient with depleted sympathetic reserve, ketamine can result in hypotension.

IV lidocaine is a useful adjunct drug to prevent reflex bronchospasm, particularly in emergency situations when deep anesthesia cannot be achieved before intubation (see Section C.5).

Traditionally, opioids were not used as part of rapid sequence induction. However, opioids reduce cardiovascular effects associated with laryngoscopy and suppress cough reflex. They also reduce the dose of induction agent required to achieve adequate depth of anesthesia. Therefore, administration of opioids that do not release histamine, such as fentanyl and remifentanil, should be considered.

A neuromuscular blocking agent is administered after the induction agent to achieve optimal intubating conditions. Unless contraindicated, succinylcholine should be used because it provides excellent intubating conditions within 30 to 60 seconds of administration. Rocuronium 1.2 mg/kg is an alternative to succinylcholine but results in a much longer neuromuscular block (although this can be reversed with an appropriate dose of sugammadex).

In a patient with asthma, efforts to achieve adequate depth of anesthesia necessary to minimize bronchospasm can result in hypotension. Therefore, medications to treat hypotension, such as phenylephrine, should be immediately available.

Tanoubi I, Drolet P, Donati F. Optimizing preoxygenation in adults. *Can J Anaesth*. 2009;56:449-466.

Tao J, Kurup V. Anesthetic considerations for obstructive lung disease. In: Hines RL, Jones SB, eds. *Stoelting's Anesthesia and Co-existing Disease*. 8th ed. Elsevier; 2022:26-27.

Thilen SR, Weigel WA, Todd MM, et al. 2023 American Society of Anesthesiologists practice guidelines for monitoring and antagonism of neuromuscular blockade: a report by the American Society of Anesthesiologists Task Force on Neuromuscular Blockade. *Anesthesiology*. 2023;138:13-41.

Tran DT, Newton EK, Mount VA, et al. Rocuronium versus succinylcholine for rapid sequence induction intubation. *Cochrane Database Syst Rev*. 2015:CD002788.

Wallace C, McGuire B. Rapid sequence induction: its place in modern anaesthesia. *Contin Educ Anaesth Crit Care Pain*. 2014;14:130-135.

Weiskopf RB, Bogetz MS, Roizen MF, et al. Cardiovascular and metabolic sequelae of inducing anesthesia with ketamine or thiopental in hypovolemic swine. *Anesthesiology*. 1984;60:214-219.

C.7. Could a regional anesthetic technique be used for this surgery? Discuss the advantages and disadvantages of neuraxial anesthesia in this patient for this surgery.

For laparoscopic surgery, regional anesthesia can be used. Typically, this is performed with epidural or combined spinal-epidural anesthesia, which allows for repeated dosing to obtain an adequate level and duration of anesthesia. Laparoscopic surgery requires a T4 to T5 dermatomal level. Even with adequate analgesia to this dermatome, patients often complain of shoulder pain, which can be treated with IV opioid administration. The advantages of regional anesthesia include avoidance of instrumenting the airway, a reduced risk of bronchospasm, and the ability to maintain the epidural postoperatively to reduce or even eliminate the need for postoperative opioids.

However, the high level required for laparoscopic surgery has multiple effects on the respiratory system. First, patients with a high blockade lose sensory input from chest wall movement and experience dyspnea, even in the presence of normal respiratory function. This feeling of dyspnea can be anxiety producing and in a patient with asthma can lead to bronchospasm.

More importantly, high segmental levels of neuraxial anesthesia should be avoided in patients with severe respiratory disease who require accessory muscle contributions in order to maintain adequate ventilation. These patients will have reduced expiratory flow and minute ventilation under high neuraxial blockade and can become hypoxemic and hypercarbic.

Newer surgical techniques, including natural orifice transluminal endoscopic surgery (NOTES), are being developed for a variety of procedures, including appendectomy, cholecystectomy, and hysterectomy. These procedures can be done with a lower dermatomal level.

Atallah S, Martin-Perez B, Keller D, Burke J, Hunter L. Natural-orifice transluminal endoscopic surgery. *Br J Surg*. 2015;102:e73-e92.

Donmez T, Erdem VM, Uzman S, et al. Laparoscopic cholecystectomy under spinal-epidural anesthesia vs. general anaesthesia: a prospective randomised study. *Ann Surg Treat Res*. 2017;92:136-142.

Tatulli F, Delcuratolo A, Caraglia A, et al. Three-trocar laparoscopic cholecystectomy under spinal anesthesia in a patient with asthma. *G Chir*. 2018;39:188-190.

Vretzakis G, Bareka M, Aretha D, et al. Regional anesthesia for laparoscopic surgery: a narrative review. *J Anesth*. 2014;28:429-446.

C.8. Would you choose an inhalational or an IV technique for the maintenance of anesthesia?

For maintenance of anesthesia, inhalation agents such as sevoflurane and isoflurane are preferred for their potent bronchodilating action. These agents are thought to be superior to desflurane, which can produce airway irritation and trigger bronchospasm. At lower doses (<1.0 minimum alveolar concentration), the currently used inhaled anesthetics inhibit chemically induced tracheal contractions in the following order: *isoflurane > sevoflurane*. More recent clinical observations in humans indicate that sevoflurane at 1.1 minimum alveolar concentration might be the most effective agent, particularly in the presence of airway instrumentation. In addition, sevoflurane can have a more rapid onset of bronchodilation than isoflurane.

Desflurane can cause increased airway resistance and tissue mechanical parameters, with markedly enhanced airway narrowing in children with asthma or a recent URI. Therefore, desflurane should be avoided in children with susceptible airways.

Nitrous oxide can be used, provided that the patient does not have pulmonary hypertension, a condition commonly present in patients with COPD.

For scenarios that require avoidance of inhaled anesthetics, such as patients with history of malignant hyperthermia or cases that require monitoring of motor and somatosensory evoked potentials, IV anesthetics can be used for maintenance. The bronchodilating properties of propofol make it a good choice as an IV anesthetic for patients with obstructive lung disease. Opioids without histamine-releasing effects and ketamine can be used as adjuncts to the IV technique.

Abola RE, Geralemou S, Szafran M, Gan TJ. Intravenous anesthetic. In: Cullen BF, Stock MC, Ortega R, et al, eds. *Barash, Cullen, and Stoelting's Clinical Anesthesia*. 9th ed. Wolters Kluwer; 2024:463-481.

Ebert TJ. Inhaled anesthetics. In: Cullen BF, Stock MC, Ortega R, et al, eds. *Barash, Cullen, and Stoelting's Clinical Anesthesia*. 9th ed. Wolters Kluwer; 2024:437-462.

Rock GA, Choi JH, Bishop MJ. The effect of isoflurane, halothane, sevoflurane, and thiopental/nitrous oxide on respiratory system resistance after tracheal intubation. *Anesthesiology*. 1997;86:1294-1299.

Tao J, Kurup V. Anesthetic considerations for obstructive lung disease. In: Hines RL, Jones SB, eds. *Stoelting's Anesthesia and Co-existing Disease*. 8th ed. Elsevier; 2022:26, 32.

Von Ungern-Sternberg BS, Saudan S, Petak F, et al. Desflurane but not sevoflurane impairs airway and respiratory tissue mechanics in children with susceptible airways. *Anesthesiology*. 2008;108:216-224.

Woods BD, Sladen RN. Perioperative considerations for the patient with asthma and bronchospasm. *Br J Anaesth*. 2009;103:i57-i65.

C.9. What mechanisms produce bronchodilation by volatile anesthetics?

Volatile anesthetics relax airway smooth muscle primarily by directly reducing smooth muscle contractility and indirectly by inhibiting reflex neural pathways. Direct effects of volatile anesthetics partially depend on the intact bronchial epithelium, suggesting that epithelial damage or inflammation secondary to asthma or a respiratory infection could lessen their bronchodilating effect.

The mechanisms responsible for the direct relaxation effects involve decreases in intracellular calcium, an important regulator of smooth muscle contraction. Several intracellular mediators responsible for the mobilization of calcium ions are potential sites of action for volatile anesthetics, but the predominant mechanism appears to be inhibition of plasma membrane voltage-gated calcium channels, an action that decreases the entry of calcium ions into the cytosol. Volatile anesthetic–induced increases in cyclic 3′,5′ adenosine monophosphate (cAMP) reduce free intracellular calcium by stimulating the efflux of calcium and increasing the uptake of calcium into the sarcoplasmic reticulum. This action contributes to airway smooth muscle relaxation. In addition, volatile anesthetics reduce calcium sensitivity by inhibition of protein kinase C activity and inhibition of G protein function.

Abola RE, Geralemou S, Szafran M, Gan TJ. Inhaled anesthetics. In: Cullen BF, Stock MC, Ortega R, et al, eds. *Barash, Cullen, and Stoelting's Clinical Anesthesia*. 9th ed. Wolters Kluwer; 2024:463-481.

Evgenov OV, Liang Y, Jiang Y. Pulmonary pharmacology and inhaled anesthetics. In: Gropper MA, Cohen NH, Eriksson LI, et al, eds. *Miller's Anesthesia*. 10th ed. Elsevier; 2025:426-456.

C.10. Which neuromuscular blocking agents would you use? Why?

Any neuromuscular blocking agents that do not release histamine, such as cisatracurium, vecuronium, rocuronium, and pancuronium, can be used. Atracurium causes histamine release, especially in high doses, and should be avoided. Succinylcholine can cause slight histamine release, but there is no evidence that succinylcholine is associated with increased airway resistance in patients with asthma.

It is advantageous to avoid long-acting pancuronium and instead to use neuromuscular blocking agents of intermediate duration of action because the earlier recovery from neuromuscular blockade might allow avoidance of reversal with an anticholinesterase, which, theoretically, could precipitate bronchospasm due to stimulation of postganglionic cholinergic receptors in airway smooth muscle. However, avoidance of anticholinesterase antagonism requires monitoring with a quantitative peripheral nerve stimulator to ensure adequate spontaneous recovery, defined as a train-of-four (TOF) ratio greater than 0.90. If an anticholinesterase is used, adequate dosing of a concomitant anticholinergic is necessary. Alternatively, sugammadex can be used for reversal of rocuronium- or vecuronium-induced neuromuscular blockade.

Basta SJ. Modulation of histamine release by neuromuscular blocking drugs. *Curr Opin Anaesthesiol.* 1992;5:572.

Brull SJ, Meistelman C, Nemes R, de Boer HD, Thilen SR, Eriksson LI. Pharmacology of neuromuscular blocking drugs and antagonists (reversal agents). In: Gropper MA, Cohen NH, Eriksson LI, et al, eds. *Miller's Anesthesia.* 10th ed. Elsevier; 2025:674-741.

Carron M, Zarantonello F, Tellaroli P, et al. Efficacy and safety of sugammadex compared to neostigmine for reversal of neuromuscular blockade: a meta-analysis of randomized controlled trials. *J Clin Anesth.* 2016;35:1-12.

Thilen SR, Weigel WA, Todd MM, et al. 2023 American Society of Anesthesiologists practice guidelines for monitoring and antagonism of neuromuscular blockade: a report by the American Society of Anesthesiologists Task Force on Neuromuscular Blockade. *Anesthesiology.* 2023;138:13-41.

C.11. How will you ventilate the patient? Will you use positive end-expiratory pressure (PEEP)? How can you detect the presence of auto-PEEP on a ventilator?

There are competing interests involved in managing the ventilation of this patient with COPD undergoing laparoscopic surgery. PIP should be kept at a minimum, end-expiratory time needs to be adequate to overcome air trapping, and hypercarbia from insufflation with CO_2 must be compensated.

A pressure control ventilation mode would be preferable to volume control because it results in lower PIP at similar V_T. However, the laparoscopic technique leads to increasing airway resistance and increasing PIP, so V_T must be watched closely since it will decrease with insufflation of the abdomen, and the PIP setting on the ventilator will need to be increased as the case proceeds.

High PIP should be avoided, especially in patients with emphysema and blebs, because pneumothorax can result from barotrauma. PIP should never be greater than 50 cm H_2O, and plateau pressures should be kept less than 30 cm H_2O to minimize barotrauma.

The inspiratory-to-expiratory time ratio (I:E ratio) can be increased in order to reduce PIP. However, in this patient, the I:E ratio will likely need to be *reduced* to allow for complete expiration in the setting of expiratory obstruction and to avoid air trapping. *Allowing an adequate expiratory time is a key component in the ventilatory management of patients with obstructive pulmonary disease.*

Adequate minute ventilation will need to be maintained and should be increased as the case proceeds and insufflated CO_2 is absorbed into the blood and exhaled through the alveoli. Minute ventilation could need to increase as much as 60% to maintain normocarbia. Absorbed CO_2 can result in hypercapnia that lingers well into the postoperative period.

Achieving adequate minute ventilation with sufficient expiratory time and reasonable PIP can be difficult. In patients with severe pulmonary disease, it might be impossible. In this scenario, alternatives to traditional laparoscopy should be discussed with the surgeon. Gasless laparoscopic techniques that do not require insufflation of the abdomen are preferable, when feasible. These techniques utilize abdominal wall lifting to avoid pneumoperitoneum.

The application of PEEP during positive pressure ventilation is a controversial issue. This type of PEEP, also referred to as extrinsic PEEP, must be differentiated from intrinsic or auto-PEEP. Intrinsic PEEP occurs in patients with COPD or asthma because outflow obstruction leads to air trapping. In ventilators equipped with an expiratory hold control, intrinsic PEEP can be measured during positive pressure ventilation. PEEP applied by the ventilator should be subtracted from the airway pressure measured during the expiratory hold in order to obtain intrinsic PEEP. When extrinsic PEEP is lower than intrinsic PEEP, it can improve ventilation, especially in spontaneously ventilating patients. Extrinsic PEEP reduces the amount of negative pressure required to generate a breath and therefore reduces the work of breathing.

However, extrinsic PEEP that exceeds intrinsic PEEP can worsen air trapping and hyperinflation. Excessive PEEP also results in reduced venous return, reduced left ventricular compliance, and increased pulmonary capillary resistance. All of these changes lead to hypotension.

Demoule A, Brochard L, Dres M, et al. How to ventilate obstructive and asthmatic patients. *Intensive Care Med.* 2020;46:2436-2449.

Gaulton TG, Cereda M. Respiratory function in anesthesia. In: Cullen BF, Stock MC, Ortega R, et al, eds. *Barash, Cullen, and Stoelting's Clinical Anesthesia*. 9th ed. Wolters Kluwer; 2024:349-361.

Slinger P. Don't make things worse with your ventilator settings: how you manage the lungs during the perioperative period affects postoperative outcomes. *Anesth Analg.* 2013;117:38-46.

C.12. What is the differential diagnosis of intraoperative bronchospasm?

The major causes of intraoperative wheezing and increased inspiratory airway pressure include the following:

- Mechanical obstruction of endotracheal tube
  - Kinking
  - Secretions or blood
- Overinflation of tracheal tube cuff
- Inadequate depth of anesthesia
- Active expiratory efforts
- Pulmonary edema
- Pneumothorax (especially in a patient with emphysema and blebs)
- Aspiration pneumonitis
- Pulmonary embolism
- Endobronchial intubation
- Acute asthmatic attack
- Anaphylaxis

Anaphylaxis is a rare event but should be considered in all patients with intraoperative bronchospasm. The most common causes of intraoperative anaphylaxis include neuromuscular blocking agents, latex, and antibiotics. Cardiovascular (hypotension) and cutaneous (flushing, urticaria) manifestations along with bronchospasm are the most common presenting signs of anaphylaxis during anesthesia. In the setting of bronchospasm with hypotension, even without cutaneous signs, anaphylaxis is high on the differential. Administration of likely inciting agents should cease; epinephrine 5 to 10 μg, diphenhydramine, and corticosteroids should be given. An infusion of epinephrine might be necessary for persistent hypotension and bronchospasm. A tryptase level should be sent to confirm the diagnosis, and the patient should be notified in writing of the potential reaction so that follow-up allergy testing can be obtained.

Hepner DL, Castells MC. Anaphylaxis during the perioperative period. *Anesth Analg.* 2003;97:1381-1395.

Tao J, Kurup V. Anesthetic considerations for obstructive lung disease. In: Hines RL, Jones SB, eds. *Stoelting's Anesthesia and Co-existing Disease*. 8th ed. Elsevier; 2022:26.

Woods BD, Sladen RN. Perioperative considerations for the patient with asthma and bronchospasm. *Br J Anaesth.* 2009;103:i57-i65.

C.13. In the middle of surgery, peak inspiratory pressure (PIP) suddenly increases. How do you manage this?

Elevation of PIP is one of the signs of intraoperative bronchospasm. One of the most common causes of bronchospasm during surgery is inadequate depth of anesthesia. The patient with asthma has an extremely sensitive tracheobronchial tree. When the level of anesthesia is too light, the patient can develop straining or coughing as a result of the endotracheal tube in the trachea, as well as bronchospasm. Therefore, during surgery, the initial treatment of bronchospasm is to increase FIO_2 and deepen anesthesia while investigating other potential causes of bronchospasm (see Section C.12).

First, increase the FIO_2 and ventilate manually in order to assess pulmonary compliance. Check the anesthesia circuit and the endotracheal tube for kinking and any other visible obstruction. Auscultate the lungs to assess for wheezing. Bilaterally diminished or absent breath sounds can be an ominous sign, suggesting critically low airflow, which can occur during severe bronchospasm or a mechanical obstruction of the tube. Unilaterally decreased breath sounds can indicate a main-stem endotracheal tube or, rarely, pneumothorax. Once bronchospasm is confirmed, prior to deepening anesthesia, measure blood pressure. If normal or high, deepen anesthesia by increasing the concentration of inhalation agents, such as sevoflurane or isoflurane which are direct bronchodilators, or administer propofol in incremental doses. This has the advantage of deepening anesthesia without relying on alveolar ventilation (which is decreased during bronchospasm) for administration. Likewise, in a patient with low to normal blood pressure, ketamine can be used as it both deepens anesthesia and bronchodilates.

Second, relieve mechanical stimulation. Pass a catheter through the endotracheal tube to suction secretions and determine whether there is an obstruction or kinking of the tube. Occasionally, the endotracheal tube migrates and stimulates the carina, causing severe bronchospasm during light anesthesia. The cuff of the endotracheal tube can be deflated, the tube pulled back 1 to 2 cm, and the cuff reinflated. Surgical stimulation, such as traction on the mesentery, intestine, or stomach, should be stopped temporarily because it stimulates a vagal reflex and can cause bronchospasm.

Third, start medical intervention if these interventions do not break the bronchospasm or anesthesia cannot be deepened secondary to hypotension. The cornerstone of treatment for intraoperative bronchospasm is the inhalation of β_2-agonists such as albuterol, which induces further bronchodilation even in the presence of adequate inhalational anesthesia. Because of "rain-out" in the endotracheal tube, a large dose (8-10 puffs) should be given to achieve adequate therapeutic levels. Epinephrine 5 to 10 μg given intravenously is highly effective, but caution should be taken as it can exacerbate tachycardia and tachyarrhythmias. If bronchospasm continues despite optimal bronchodilation therapy, high-dose IV corticosteroids are indicated (see Sections B.16 and B.17), but their onset of action is slow. Alternatively, a continuous infusion of epinephrine 0.5 to 2 μg/min in adults can provide maintenance bronchodilation with fewer adverse effects, with higher doses also effective in treating hypotension.

Fanta CH, Rossing TH, McFadden ER Jr. Glucocorticoids in acute asthma. A critical controlled trial. *Am J Med.* 1983;74:845-851.

Noseda A, De Bruyne I, De Maertelaer V, Yernault JC. Does an IV bolus of methylprednisolone relieve dyspnea in asthma exacerbations? *Chest.* 2000;118:1530-1537.

Tao J, Kurup V. Anesthetic considerations for obstructive lung disease. In: Hines RL, Jones SB, eds. *Stoelting's Anesthesia and Co-existing Disease.* 8th ed. Elsevier; 2022:25-27.

Woods BD, Sladen RN. Perioperative considerations for the patient with asthma and bronchospasm. *Br J Anaesth.* 2009;103:i57-i65.

C.14. How would you administer β_2-agonists? What is their mechanism of action in asthma?

Historically, episodes of severe asthma were treated with IV sympathomimetics such as isoproterenol. This approach is no longer used because isoproterenol infusion can induce ventricular arrhythmias and is associated with myocardial damage. Even the IV administration of β_2-selective agents such as terbutaline and albuterol offers no advantage over the inhaled route.

β_2-Agonists such as albuterol, levalbuterol, and terbutaline can be administered through MDI adapters or small-volume jet nebulizers to the anesthetic circuit. Because MDI adapters are not very efficient in the intubated patient due to "rain-out" in the endotracheal tube, 8 to 10 puffs are needed to break acute bronchospasm.

Adrenergic stimulants produce bronchodilation through action on β-adrenergic receptors. β-Agonists increase intracellular cAMP by activating adenyl cyclase, which produces cAMP from adenosine triphosphate. Increased cAMP promotes bronchial relaxation and inhibits the release of mediators from mast cells (**Figure 1.4**).

Fanta CH. Asthma. *N Engl J Med.* 2009;360:1002-1014.

Lemanske RF, Schauberger E. Beta agonists in asthma: acute administration and prophylactic use. *UpToDate.* Published 2023. Accessed April 10, 2023. https://www.uptodate.com/contents/beta-agonists-in-asthma-acute-administration-and-prophylactic-use

Tao J, Kurup V. Anesthetic considerations for obstructive lung disease. In: Hines RL, Jones SB, eds. *Stoelting's Anesthesia and Co-existing Disease.* 8th ed. Elsevier; 2022:23-25.

Woods BD, Sladen RN. Perioperative considerations for the patient with asthma and bronchospasm. *Br J Anaesth.* 2009;103:i57-i65.

C.15. If the patient does not respond to the aforementioned treatment and becomes cyanotic, what would you do?

The ABG values should be determined immediately. In a severe, prolonged asthmatic attack, there will be combined respiratory and metabolic acidosis resulting from CO_2 retention and lactic acidosis from tissue hypoxia. Hypercarbia, hypoxemia, and acidemia promote arrhythmias and impair the response to

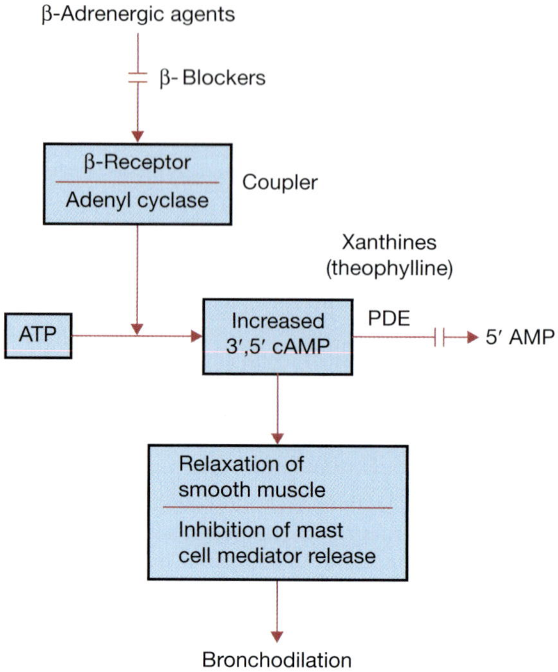

FIGURE 1.4. Cyclic adenosine monophosphate (cAMP) pathways involved in bronchodilator action. 3′,5′ cAMP, cyclic 3′,5′ adenosine monophosphate; AMP, adenosine monophosphate; ATP, adenosine triphosphate; PDE, phosphodiesterase. (Reprinted with permission from Hirshman C. Airway reactivity in humans. Anesthetic implications. *Anesthesiology.* 1983;58:170-177.)

bronchodilator therapy. Sodium bicarbonate ($NaHCO_3$) should be given to correct the acidosis because β-agonists are not effective in severe acidosis. At the same time, bronchodilator therapy should be continued or increased.

A patient with severe, refractory bronchospasm might require mechanical ventilation with a ventilator equipped to generate very high inspiratory pressures. An ICU ventilator can generate inspiratory pressures up to 120 cm H_2O. Most anesthesia machines cannot deliver adequate alveolar ventilation at these pressures because the circuit has such high compressible volume (tubing compliance) and the ventilator does not have sufficient driving power. The major disadvantage of an ICU ventilator is its inability to deliver inhalational anesthetics. Some newer anesthesia machines incorporate an ICU-type ventilator with vaporizers and oxygen mixers which could be effective for this situation.

Heliox is a helium/oxygen mixture that, secondary to its lower density than air, can permit higher flow rates at lower pressures, theoretically improving the delivery of oxygen during bronchospasm. A major limitation is that heliox mixtures only provide 21% to 30% oxygen. Although heliox facilitates ventilation, it does not reverse the underlying bronchospasm. Reports on the perioperative use of heliox remain limited.

Although not available at all centers, veno-venous extracorporeal membrane oxygenation (VV-ECMO) can adequately oxygenate the blood when other measures have failed. ECMO is expensive, requires specially trained personnel, and is an invasive treatment associated with a number of potential complications. However, it is a potentially lifesaving measure that should be considered in select cases of severe, refractory hypoxemia secondary to respiratory disease.

Katz JA, Kallet RH, Alonso JA, et al. Improved flow and pressure capabilities of the Datex-Ohmeda SmartVent anesthesia ventilator. *J Clin Anesth.* 2000;12:40-47.

Lazarus SC. Clinical practice. Emergency treatment of asthma. *N Engl J Med.* 2010;363:755-764.

Liu LL, Aldrich JM, Shimabukuro DW, et al. Special article: rescue therapies for acute hypoxemic respiratory failure. *Anesth Analg.* 2010;111:693-702.

Marks JD, Schapera A, Kraemer RW, et al. Pressure and flow limitations of anesthesia ventilators. *Anesthesiology.* 1989;71:403-408.

Woods BD, Sladen RN. Perioperative considerations for the patient with asthma and bronchospasm. *Br J Anaesth.* 2009;103:i57-i65.

C.16. If the patient does not respond to the treatments you have given, are you going to ask for help from other health care professionals? How would you do it?

It is important to know when to call for help in managing a patient. Some general criteria to request help are when the patient's condition is catastrophic, bad and getting worse, not responding to usual treatments, or known to require help to deal with. One should also request help to accomplish more in less time, when overloaded with task demands, when not sure of the diagnosis/treatment, or when in need of a second opinion.

It is useful to know in advance who is available and how to contact them. In a major hospital during regular working hours, the assistance needed may be immediately available. However, in smaller facilities, or at night or on weekends/holidays, there could be limited help available. If necessary, assistance can be requested from the emergency department, the ICU, or by calling a hospital-wide code.

Communication between team members is crucial in a crisis. The team leader must communicate the appropriate sense of urgency for a situation in a clear and professional manner, without inducing panic. Information most relevant to patient care should be prioritized. It is important to understand the concerns and perspectives of other health care professionals through active listening. Potential for conflict should be recognized and conflict resolution initiated as appropriate.

Gaba DM, Fish KJ, Howard SK, et al, eds. *Crisis Management in Anesthesiology*. 2nd ed. Elsevier; 2015:25-53.

C.17. Would you consider deep tracheal extubation for this patient?

To avoid bronchospasm triggered by coughing and straining caused by laryngeal and pharyngeal reflexes during emergence from anesthesia and tracheal extubation, patients can be extubated at surgical (deep) levels of anesthesia. However, the risks of aspiration, airway obstruction, and hypoventilation should be weighed against the benefits. With a history of severe COPD, chronic hypoxemia, and CO_2 retention, the patient is not a good candidate for extubation while deeply anesthetized. A systematic approach to emergence and extubation is illustrated in **Figure 1.5**. However, the guidelines do not include all possible patient-surgical-anesthetic conditions. Certainly, good clinical judgment is of utmost importance regarding the decision to extubate.

Lien CA, Koff H, Malhotra V, et al. Emergence and extubation: a systemic approach. *Anesth Analg*. 1997;85:1177.

Tao J, Kurup V. Anesthetic considerations for obstructive lung disease. In: Hines RL, Jones SB, eds. *Stoelting's Anesthesia and Co-existing Disease*. 8th ed. Elsevier; 2022:26.

Woods BD, Sladen RN. Perioperative considerations for the patient with asthma and bronchospasm. *Br J Anaesth*. 2009;103:i57-i65.

C.18. If the patient cannot be extubated, what measures can you take to reduce the likelihood of bronchospasm with an endotracheal tube in place?

Loading doses of lidocaine, followed by continuous infusion as described in Section C.5, can be administered intravenously to prevent bronchoconstriction induced by stimulation of the trachea by the endotracheal tube. β_2-Agonists such as albuterol can be administered through an MDI adapter to prevent bronchospasm. Dexmedetomidine, which has a favorable profile, including anxiolysis, sympatholysis, and drying of secretions without respiratory depression, can be used to sedate an agitated patient with asthma who does not meet the criteria for extubation. Alternatively, if there are no contraindications, a supraglottic airway device can be used to replace the endotracheal tube for control of ventilation and to avoid tracheal stimulation.

Bohringer C, Liu H. Is it time for an expanded role of dexmedetomidine in contemporary anesthesia practice? A clinician's perspective. *Transl Perioper Pain Med*. 2018;5:55-62.

Groeben H, Mitzner W, Brown RH. Effects of the alpha2-adrenoceptor agonist dexmedetomidine on bronchoconstriction in dogs. *Anesthesiology*. 2004;100:359-363.

Tao J, Kurup V. Anesthetic considerations for obstructive lung disease. In: Hines RL, Jones SB, eds. *Stoelting's Anesthesia and Co-existing Disease*. 8th ed. Elsevier; 2022:26.

Woods BD, Sladen RN. Perioperative considerations for the patient with asthma and bronchospasm. *Br J Anaesth*. 2009;103:i57-i65.

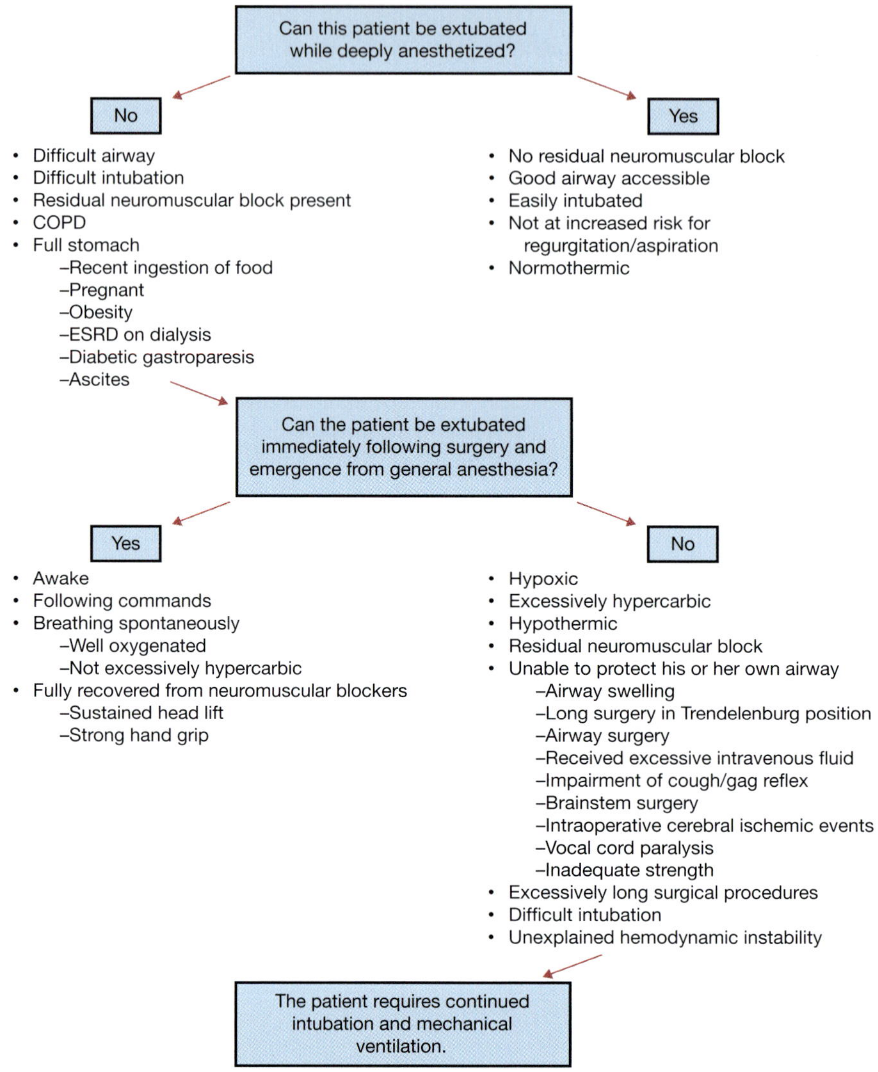

FIGURE 1.5. A systematic approach to emergence from general anesthesia and tracheal extubation. COPD, chronic obstructive pulmonary disease; ESRD, end-stage renal disease.

D. Postoperative Management

D.1. In patients with asthma and COPD, are there special considerations for the use of opioids and nonsteroidal anti-inflammatory drugs (NSAIDs) for postoperative pain control?

Morphine is avoided because of possible histamine release and increased central vagal tone, which can cause bronchospasm. Meperidine causes histamine release more frequently than most other opioids and should be avoided as well. Fentanyl is an appropriate choice for patients with asthma or other bronchospastic diseases because of its antimuscarinic, antihistaminergic, and antiserotoninergic actions. Effective analgesia is especially important in patients with respiratory disease because poor pain control can compromise respiration further due to splinting of the thoracic cage and decreased ability to cough. However, opioids should be titrated very carefully to avoid dose-dependent respiratory depression.

An estimated 5% to 10% of patients with asthma have a sensitivity toward NSAIDs, known as aspirin-exacerbated respiratory disease (AERD). NSAIDs block the COX-mediated conversion of arachidonic acid to prostaglandins, thereby shunting arachidonic acid toward the formation of bronchoconstricting leukotrienes. Patients with AERD are more likely to have an irreversible component to their obstructive airway disease, more likely to have frequent exacerbations, and more likely to have had a history of severe attacks and oral steroid use. Persistent rhinorrhea, nasal polyps, and nasal congestion are common symptoms. Most patients with AERD are unaware of the diagnosis. If a focused preoperative history reveals any of the aforementioned symptoms, NSAIDs should be avoided.

Farooque SP, Lee TH. Aspirin-sensitive respiratory disease. *Annu Rev Physiol.* 2009;71:465-487.

Hurley RW, Elkassabany NM, Wu CL. Acute postoperative pain. In: Gropper MA, Cohen NH, Eriksson LI, et al, eds. *Miller's Anesthesia.* 10th ed. Elsevier; 2025:2512-2537.

Israel E. Asthma. In: Loscalzo J, Fauci AS, Kasper DL, et al, eds. *Harrison's Principles of Internal Medicine.* 21st ed. McGraw-Hill; 2022:2147-2159.

Tao J, Kurup V. Anesthetic considerations for obstructive lung disease. In: Hines RL, Jones SB, eds. *Stoelting's Anesthesia and Co-existing Disease.* 8th ed. Elsevier; 2022:20, 26.

D.2. Would you consider using a regional anesthesia technique for analgesia?

Were this surgery to be accomplished laparoscopically, a regional technique for analgesia is typically not necessary. However, in a patient with severe respiratory disease, the complete avoidance of systemic opioids might be desired to reduce the risk of PPCs. In this case of severe COPD, epidural analgesia is preferred. An epidural catheter can be placed before surgery and used as an adjunct or alternative to general anesthesia (see Section C.7). The complete analgesia provided allows patients to avoid "splinting" secondary to abdominal pain and improves postoperative respiratory recovery.

Contraindications to epidural anesthesia include patient refusal and anticoagulation therapy. In patients unable to receive neuraxial anesthesia, an alternative is the transversus abdominis plane (TAP) block. In patients undergoing laparoscopic cholecystectomy, TAP block decreased postoperative opioid use and mean discharge time compared to conventional port site local anesthetic infiltration. A TAP block consists of two to four injections of local anesthetic (typically bupivacaine, ropivacaine, or liposomal bupivacaine) providing 12 to 36 hours of analgesia. Unlike an epidural, once the block is performed and following a period of adequate postblock monitoring, no special equipment is necessary and patients can be discharged home. However, a TAP block only covers surgical incision pain and does not affect internal surgical pain. Therefore, a multimodal pain regimen will still be required.

Macias AA, Finneran JJ. Regional anesthesia techniques for pain management for laparoscopic surgery: a review of the current literature. *Curr Pain Headache Rep. 2022*;26:33-42.

Tolchard S, Davies R, Martindale S. Efficacy of the subcostal transversus abdominis plane block in laparoscopic cholecystectomy: comparison with conventional port-site infiltration. *J Anaesthesiol Clin Pharmacol.* 2012;28:339-343.

Vretzakis G, Bareka M, Aretha D, et al. Regional anesthesia for laparoscopic surgery: a narrative review. *J Anesth.* 2014;28:429-446.

D.3. The patient was breathing well and was extubated in the OR. Would you place this patient on supplemental oxygen in the recovery room? If so, how much?

Administration of oxygen to patients with severe COPD can lead to hypercapnia. This was traditionally attributed to the impairment of hypoxic respiratory drive and subsequent hypoventilation. Although there is a transient reduction in minute ventilation when high-flow oxygen is administered to patients with COPD, this does not appear to play a major role in oxygen-induced hypercapnia.

The primary mechanism responsible for hypercapnia with oxygen administration in patients with COPD appears to be ventilation/perfusion mismatch. Under normal conditions, hypoxic pulmonary vasoconstriction helps minimize ventilation/perfusion mismatch. Oxygen therapy can reduce hypoxic pulmonary vasoconstriction in poorly ventilated areas, increasing blood flow to these areas, and decreasing blood flow to other lung regions with normal or high ventilation:perfusion ratios. These areas will then contribute further to alveolar dead space causing an increase in P_{CO_2}.

Although uncontrolled oxygen therapy in patients with COPD is potentially harmful, hypoxemic patients should receive oxygen. Carefully titrated oxygen therapy to achieve saturation of 88% to 92% is recommended.

Abdo WF, Heunks LM. Oxygen-induced hypercapnia in COPD: myths and facts. *Crit Care.* 2012;16:323.

Decalmer S, O'Driscoll BR. Oxygen: friend or for in peri-operative care? *Anaesthesia.* 2013;68:8-12.

Lumb AB, Thomas CR, eds. Airways disease. In: *Nunn and Lumb's Applied Respiratory Physiology.* 9th ed. Elsevier; 2021:333-334.

D.4. The patient is hypoventilating in the postanesthesia care unit (PACU). Would you initiate noninvasive ventilation (NIV)?

NIV refers to ventilatory support via the patient's upper airway using a mask or a similar device. NIV respiratory support ranges from continuous positive airway pressure (CPAP) to bilevel positive airway pressure (BIPAP). NIV has been shown to be safe and effective in patients with COPD and should be readily available in the PACU to treat postoperative respiratory distress. Judicious use of NIV can reduce reintubation rates after surgery.

Glossop AJ, Shephard N, Bryden DC, et al. Non-invasive ventilation for weaning, avoiding reintubation after extubation and in the postoperative period: a meta-analysis. *Br J Anaesth*. 2012;109:305-314.

Jaber S, Chanques G, Jung B. Postoperative noninvasive ventilation. *Anesthesiology*. 2010;112:453-461.

D.5. The patient had a severe asthmatic attack during surgery, which was ultimately relieved by your treatment. Would you discuss the event with the patient? How would you do it?

According to the Joint Commission, which accredits health care organizations throughout the United States, disclosure to the patient is required when the adverse event has a perceptible effect on the patient that was not discussed in advance as a known risk, necessitates a change in the patient's care, potentially poses an important risk to the patient's future health, and involves providing a treatment or procedure without the patient's consent. If the patient could not be extubated at the end of surgery, required an ICU admission, or needed additional procedures (bronchoscopy), they must be informed of the event.

Even if the event does not meet the Joint Commission requirements for disclosure, it is good practice to do a postoperative evaluation for any related residual complications and symptoms. This should be done in a manner that demonstrates understanding and concern for the patient's situation. The evaluation should elicit relevant history and include a focused physical examination. Potential causes of the event, such as asthma and current smoker status, should be reviewed with the patient. The review of the event with this patient presents another opportunity for a "teachable moment" to encourage smoking cessation. The discussion with the patient should include a plan for further evaluation and treatment if appropriate. Questions should be elicited from the patient and answered appropriately in lay terms.

Cornelissen C, Call RC, Harbell MW, et al. Enhancing a culture of safety through disclosure of adverse events. *APSF Newsl*. 2021;36:25-27.

Yu S, Warner DO. Surgery as a teachable moment for smoking cessation. *Anesthesiology*. 2010;112:102-107.

D.6. Recently, many surgical cases including yours were delayed. Your department chair asked you to design a plan to improve it. What would you do?

Timeliness is one of the six aims for quality in health care adopted by the Institute for Healthcare Improvement. The other five aims are safety, effectiveness, patient-centeredness, efficiency, and equity. Delays signal a lack of respect for a patient's time, adversely affect patient satisfaction, and reduce job satisfaction for health care personnel.

Surgical cases can be delayed by hospital-related causes (inappropriate scheduling, unavailable operating room time, etc), workup-related causes (patient not medically optimized), and patient-related causes (patient late or absent). In a recent systematic review, less than 5% of delays were anesthesia related.

Surgical delays can be tackled by the application of commonly accepted elements of quality improvement processes. These elements include:

a. measurement of current benchmarks and outcomes,
b. formulation of change in practice in collaboration with stakeholders,
c. education and training of everyone involved regarding the change in practice,
d. implementation of change in practice, and
e. measurement of outcomes after the change in practice.

Adams D. Quality improvement; part 1: introduction and overview. *BJA Educ*. 2018;18:89-94.

Buck DW, Lane-Fall MB, Varughese AM. Quality improvement in anesthesia practice and patient safety. In: Gropper MA, Cohen NH, Eriksson LI, et al, eds. *Miller's Anesthesia*. 10th ed. Elsevier; 2025:77-97.

Koushan M, Wood LC, Greatbanks R. Evaluating factors associated with the cancellation and delay of elective surgical procedures: a systematic review. *Int J Qual Health Care*. 2021;33:mzab092.

2 Bronchoscopy, Mediastinoscopy, and Thoracoscopy

Margo Hoyler and Alessia Pedoto

A 60-year-old male has suffered from cough, intermittent hemoptysis, and weight loss for 2 months. He has smoked one pack of cigarettes per day for 40 years but has recently switched to electronic cigarettes (ie, vaping). A chest radiograph 1 month ago revealed a right middle lobe infiltrate that was treated with antibiotics without clinical improvement. An obstructive lesion was suspected, which was biopsied via robotic bronchoscopy, and diagnosed as a carcinoma. He presents today for robotic-assisted thoracoscopic (RATS) lobectomy of the right middle lobe.

A. Medical Disease and Differential Diagnosis

1. How is the diagnosis of lung carcinoma made?
2. What are the major types of lung carcinoma, and how is lung cancer staged? What is the most likely type and stage of cancer for a surgical patient?
3. What are the less common manifestations of bronchogenic carcinoma?
4. The patient has a long history of cigarette smoking. What is the significance of this finding? What is the importance of the patient's current vaping habit?

B. Preoperative Evaluation and Preparation

1. How would you evaluate the patient prior to surgery?
2. What are the pulmonary function guidelines that indicate an increased risk for morbidity and mortality?
3. What are the preoperative concerns of induction immunotherapy and neoadjuvant chemotherapy?

C. Intraoperative Management

1. How would you premedicate, monitor, and anesthetize this patient presenting for endobronchial ultrasound (EBUS) for lung cancer staging?
2. What are the benefits of advanced bronchoscopy in the diagnosis of suspected lung cancer? How would you monitor and anesthetize a patient presenting for robotic bronchoscopy?
3. What other types of bronchoscopes are available, and what are the intraoperative considerations for each one?
4. What is cervical mediastinoscopy, and what are its indications and potential complications? How would you anesthetize and monitor a patient undergoing cervical mediastinoscopy?
5. The decision was made to proceed with a robotic right middle lobectomy rather than a video-assisted thoracoscopic (VATS) procedure. How would this alter your management?
6. What are the indications for one-lung ventilation (OLV), and how can it be accomplished? What complications can be associated with OLV?
7. What are the contraindications to the use of double-lumen endotracheal tubes (DLTs)?
8. Would you use a right- or left-sided DLT?
9. How do you know that the tube is in the correct position?
10. What types of bronchial blockers are available? What are the advantages and disadvantages of bronchial blockers?
11. How will systemic oxygenation be monitored during OLV?
12. The patient was placed in the lateral decubitus position. Describe the effects of lateral positioning on pulmonary blood flow and respiration.
13. What is hypoxic pulmonary vasoconstriction (HPV)?
14. What are the effects of anesthetic agents on HPV and their clinical implications?

15. Discuss pulmonary blood flow distribution, shunt flow, and Pa_{O_2} (F_{IO_2} = 1.0) during OLV in the lateral position.
16. What respiratory parameters will you target during OLV? How could you improve oxygenation during single-lung ventilation?
17. A right middle lobectomy was performed. Would you extubate the trachea at the end of the procedure?

D. Postoperative Management

1. What are the immediate life-threatening complications that follow lobectomy or pneumonectomy?
2. Why is it important to control postoperative pain? How would you achieve this?

A. Medical Disease and Differential Diagnosis

A.1. How is the diagnosis of lung carcinoma made?

Over 75% of patients with lung cancer are symptomatic at the time of diagnosis. Symptoms may suggest a pulmonary pathology (eg, cough, dyspnea, wheezing, hemoptysis) or may be nonspecific and secondary to metastatic disease. Potential lung cancer can also be identified on chest imaging. Screening imaging can lower lung cancer–related mortality and increase early-stage detection in high-risk patients. Current guidelines from the American Cancer Society recommend annual low-dose chest computed tomography (CT) scans for adults aged 50 to 80 years who have a 20 pack-year smoking history, are current smokers, or quit within the past 15 years. These recommendations, along with an overall expansion of chest imaging, have contributed to a dramatic increase in the identification of pulmonary nodules, only a minority of which proves malignant. Lung cancer diagnosis currently relies on a combination of imaging (eg, CT, magnetic resonance imaging [MRI], and positron emission imaging [PET] scanning) and tissue biopsy of the primary lesion, suspected metastatic lesions, and/or affected lymph nodes.

Diagnostic and staging procedures are performed in either the operating room (OR) or the bronchoscopy suite. Currently, most lung lesions are diagnosed via navigational image–guided flexible bronchoscopy and EBUS. Cervical mediastinoscopy for mediastinal lymph node biopsy is now done when EBUS results are inconclusive and additional tissue is needed. Pleural effusions and superficial lymph nodes in the neck or axilla can also be sampled for malignant cells. Due to its high sensitivity and specificity, minimally invasive wedge resections (either by thoracoscopy or by robotic-assisted techniques) are still the gold standard for peripheral lung biopsy, in low-resource centers or when there is a high suspicion of malignancy. Positive surgical biopsy is followed by anatomic resection in patients without contraindications to major surgery, such as metastatic disease or severe cardiopulmonary comorbidity.

Adams SJ, Stone E, Baldwin DR, et al. Lung cancer screening. *Lancet*. 2023;401:390-408.

Burks A, Rivera M. Clinical evaluation, diagnosis and staging of lung cancer. In: Grippi MI, Antin-Ozerkis DE, Dela Crus CS, Kotloff RM, Kotton C, Pack AI, eds. *Fishman's Pulmonary Diseases and Disorders*. 6th ed. McGraw Hill; 2023.

A.2. What are the major types of lung carcinoma, and how is lung cancer staged? What is the most likely type and stage of cancer for a surgical patient?

Lung cancer is the second most common cancer and leading cause of cancer death in the United States and worldwide. Bronchogenic carcinomas can be classified into four major types: small cell, large cell, squamous cell, and adenocarcinoma. For surgical purposes, lung cancers are described as non–small cell (NSCLC) or small cell (SCLC) lung cancer. Surgical resection is indicated for early-stage NSCLC. By contrast, SCLC, accounting for 15% of bronchogenic carcinomas, is characterized by aggressive growth and early metastasis and is typically inoperable. Despite advances in chemotherapy and targeted immunotherapy, the median survival for early-stage SCLC remains less than 24 months.

The TNM classification system further subclassifies lung tumors, with T = tumor site, size, and local extent; N = presence and location of regional lymph node involvement; and M = distal metastases beyond the ipsilateral hemithorax. The TNM schema is used to stage bronchogenic carcinomas, guide treatment, and determine prognosis. Five-year survival for patients with stage I NSCLC—small tumors without lymphatic or metastatic spread—is approximately 80%, and 13% to 60% for patients with stage II to stage III disease. Surgical resection is the standard of care for early-stage (eg, stage I, II, and some IIIa) NSCLC.

Adams SJ, Stone E, Baldwin DR, et al. Lung cancer screening. *Lancet*. 2023;401:390-408.

Burks A, Rivera M. Clinical evaluation, diagnosis and staging of lung cancer. In: Grippi MI, Antin-Ozerkis DE, Dela Crus CS, Kotloff RM, Kotton C, Pack AI, eds. *Fishman's Pulmonary Diseases and Disorders*. 6th ed. McGraw Hill; 2023.

Petty WJ, Paz-Ares L. Emerging strategies for the treatment of small cell lung cancer: a review. *JAMA Oncol.* 2023;9:419-429.

Thai AA, Solomon BJ, Sequist LV, et al. Lung cancer. *Lancet.* 2021;398:535-554.

A.3. What are the less common manifestations of bronchogenic carcinoma?

Less frequent manifestations of lung cancer are primarily related to mass effects or altered metabolism. In addition to bronchial obstruction and post–obstructive pneumonia (evident in this patient), mass effects include invasion into the chest wall and pleura, compression of great vessels (eg, superior vena cava syndrome) and heart, tracheobronchial displacement, and/or paresis of the recurrent laryngeal or phrenic nerves and the sympathetic chain. *Pancoast syndrome* can present with pain and upper extremity weakness secondary to invasion of the brachial plexus as well as the first and second thoracic and eighth cervical nerve roots. SCLCs are typically aggressive neuroendocrine tumors. *Metabolic manifestations* of SCLC include symptoms resembling those of Cushing syndrome as well as hypokalemia (both from ectopic adrenocorticotropic hormone production), carcinoid syndrome, hypercalcemia and hypophosphatemia (from ectopic parathyroid hormone or parathyroid hormone–related peptides), and hyponatremia (from inappropriate secretion of antidiuretic hormone and, possibly, atrial natriuretic factor). *Neurologic paraneoplastic syndromes* include Eaton-Lambert myasthenic syndrome, peripheral motor and sensory neuritis, cerebellar degeneration, retinopathy, limbic encephalopathy, and autonomic neuropathy, likely due to autoimmune pathology.

Extrathoracic spread of tumor can affect the bones, liver, adrenal glands, intra-abdominal and subcutaneous lymph nodes, brain, and spinal cord, contributing to nonspecific presentations of the cancer.

Burks A, Rivera M. Clinical evaluation, diagnosis, and staging of lung cancer. In: Grippi MA, Antin-Ozerkis DE, Dela Cruz CS, Kotloff RM, Kotton C, Pack AI, eds. *Fishman's Pulmonary Diseases and Disorders.* 6th ed. McGraw Hill; 2023.

Soomro Z, Youssef M, Yust-Katz S, et al. Paraneoplastic syndromes in small cell lung cancer. *J Thorac Dis.* 2020;12:6253-6263.

A.4. The patient has a long history of cigarette smoking. What is the significance of this finding? What is the importance of the patient's current vaping habit?

Cigarette smoking is the leading cause of lung cancer in the United States. Tobacco exposure is linked to chronic obstructive pulmonary disease (COPD) and is strongly associated with an increased incidence of stroke, myocardial infarction, and cancer (lung, oral cavity, larynx, and esophagus). Pulmonary hypertension from chronic hypoxemia and subsequent cor pulmonale can also occur.

Up to 20% of patients presenting for lung cancer resection are current smokers, and 30% to 60% of smokers will resume smoking after surgery. Active tobacco use increases the risk of postoperative respiratory failure, pneumonia, aspiration, air leak, and atelectasis, as well as 1-year mortality. Preoperative smoking cessation is strongly recommended. Carboxyhemoglobin concentration declines substantially within 12 hours of smoking cessation, and 4 weeks of abstinence decreases the incidence of surgical site infection and postoperative respiratory complications, likely because of improved mucociliary function. However, due to the risk of tumor growth and metastatic spread, deferring surgery might not be practical. Smoking cessation at any time prior to surgery is strongly recommended. A combined approach to smoking cessation therapy, including counseling and poly-pharmacology, has been shown to increase quitting success rates and decrease relapse after hospital discharge.

Vaping has increased in popularity among all ages as a smoking alternative. Nicotine and cannabis are frequently used in combination. Despite the lower dose of nicotine in vaping cartridges, the use of additives is linked to airway irritation and restrictive lung disease. On CT scan, the resulting airspace opacification in a centrilobular nodular pattern has been described as a "tree in bloom." Cannabis use, especially in high doses, has been linked with airway disease, high circulating catecholamine levels, and, in extreme cases, withdrawal syndrome when stopped abruptly.

Banks E, Yazidjoglou A, Brown S, et al. Electronic cigarettes and health outcomes: umbrella and systematic review of the global evidence. *Med J Aust.* 2023;218:267-275.

Kalininskiy A, Bach CT, Nacca NE, et al. E-cigarette, or vaping, product use associated lung injury (EVALI): case series and diagnostic approach. *Lancet Respir Med.* 2019;7:1017-1026.

Lugg ST, Tikka T, Agostini PJ, et al. Smoking and timing of cessation on postoperative pulmonary complications after curative-intent lung cancer surgery. *J Cardiothorac Surg.* 2017;12:52.

Shah S, Schwenk ES, Sondekoppam RV, et al. ASRA Pain Medicine consensus guidelines on the management of the perioperative patient on cannabis and cannabinoids. *Reg Anesth Pain Med.* 2023;48:97-117.

Stokes SM, Wakeam E, Antonoff MB, et al. Optimizing health before elective thoracic surgery: systematic review of modifiable risk factors and opportunities for health services research. *J Thorac Dis.* 2019;11:S537-S554.

Turan A, Koyuncu O, Egan C, et al. Effect of various durations of smoking cessation on postoperative outcomes: a retrospective cohort analysis. *Eur J Anaesthesiol.* 2018;35:256-265.

B. Preoperative Evaluation and Preparation

B.1. How would you evaluate the patient prior to surgery?

The main goal of preoperative evaluation is to identify patients at risk of major postoperative complications and optimize their functional status. The first step should include a complete history, physical examination, and laboratory and imaging studies (eg, complete blood count, basic metabolic profile, coagulation study, electrocardiogram, chest radiography, and CT imaging). A current or extensive smoking history, the presence of pulmonary symptoms (eg, cough, sputum, orthopnea, or dyspnea), or decreased exercise tolerance (eg, inability to climb at least three flights of stairs or walk for 6 minutes) can indicate compromised cardiopulmonary status and the inability to tolerate the stress of anesthesia and surgery. Further evaluation may be indicated to define cardiac disease or customize a prehabilitation program. Relevant tests and metrics include:

- **Respiratory mechanics**, as evaluated via forced vital capacity (FVC), forced expiratory volume in the first second (FEV_1), and the ratio between residual volume and total lung capacity (RV/TLC). Flow volume loops can help document the location of the obstruction (small vs large airway) and its severity. Postbronchodilator FEV_1 and FEV_1/FVC paired with clinical symptoms are used to determine the severity of COPD.
- **Cardiopulmonary reserve** can be evaluated by maximal oxygen uptake (Vo_2 max), stair climbing, 6-minute walk, and shuttle walk. In case of poor performance in these tests, cardiopulmonary exercise tolerance (CPET) testing can be added to identify patients who are not surgical candidates. As measured on CPET, Vo_2 max is the gold standard for aerobic capacity and cardiorespiratory fitness. Patients with Vo_2 max <10 mL/kg/min are at increased risk for postoperative morbidity and mortality.
- **Lung parenchymal function** is measured using diffusing lung capacity for carbon monoxide (DLCO), partial pressure of oxygen in the arterial blood (Pao_2), and partial pressure of arterial carbon dioxide ($Paco_2$). Predicted postoperative DLCO and FEV_1 less than 40% to 44% are significant independent predictors for increased postoperative morbidity and mortality.

Brunelli A, Gooseman MR, Pompili C. Evaluation of risk for thoracic surgery. *Surg Oncol Clin N Am.* 2020;29:497-508.

Brunelli A, Kim A, Berger KI, et al. Physiologic evaluation of the patient with lung cancer being considered for resectional surgery. Diagnosis and management of lung cancer, 3rd ed: American College of Chest Physicians evidence-based clinical practice guidelines. *Chest.* 2013;143:e166S-e190S.

B.2. What are the pulmonary function guidelines that indicate an increased risk for morbidity and mortality?

The reported mortality from lung resection is between 2% and 4%, and nearly one quarter of patients experience postoperative complications, the most common being atrial arrhythmia, pneumonia, and respiratory failure. Increased risk for postoperative complications includes advanced age and comorbid conditions, in addition to predictors calculated using the following tests:

- **Spirometry:** Spirometric parameters, such as FEV_1/FVC ratio and FEV_1 (reflective of the degree of airway obstruction), as well as static volumes (such as inspiratory and total lung capacity), are used to define the severity of COPD. A strong correlation exists between predicted postoperative FEV_1 and DLCO and a respective increase in morbidity and mortality, especially for open procedures and extensive dissection. Concerning values are summarized in **Table 2.1**.
- **Arterial blood gases:** Historically, hypercapnia ($Paco_2$ > 45 mm Hg) was considered an exclusion criterion for lung resection. However, an independent correlation between hypercapnia and increased mortality has not been demonstrated. Patients with hypercapnia often have a low predicted postoperative FEV_1 and an abnormal exercise capacity, which may preclude surgery. Preoperative hypoxemia (Pao_2 < 50 mm Hg, and percentage of available hemoglobin saturated with oxygen [Sao_2] <90%) has been associated with an increased risk of postoperative complications. However, baseline hypoxemia can result from ventilatory mismatch caused by obstructive tumors. Resection of these lesions might rarely improve gas exchange.

TABLE 2.1 Minimal Pulmonary Function Test Criteria for Various-Sized Pulmonary Resections

Test	Unit	Normal	Pneumonectomy	Lobectomy	Biopsy or Segmental
DLCO	L/min	>100	>50	>40	>25
DLCO	Percentage predicted	100%	>50%	>40%	>25%
FEV_1	Liters	>4	>2.1-1.7	>1.2-1.0	>0.6-0.9
FEV_1	Percentage	>80% FVC	>50% FVC	>40% FVC	>40% FVC
$FEV_{25\%-75\%}$	Liters	>2	>1.6	>0.6-1.6	>0.6

DLCO, diffusion capacity for carbon monoxide; FEV_1, forced expiratory volume in first second; $FEV_{25\%-75\%}$, forced expiratory volume from 25% to 75% of forced vital capacity; FVC, forced vital capacity; MBC, maximum breathing capacity.

Other factors influencing outcome include patient comorbidities and functional status, the extent and location of the proposed surgical resection, and whether the patient has undergone preoperative chemotherapy or immunotherapy.

Multiple aspects of the preoperative evaluation (eg, spirometry, ventilation-perfusion scanning, extent of planned resection, patient functional status) should be incorporated into an estimate of postoperative pulmonary function.

Fortunately, improvements in surgical and anesthesia techniques have made surgery safer for many high-risk patients. For instance, robotic and thoracoscopic lung resection techniques are associated with lower rates of postoperative morbidity and mortality compared to traditional thoracotomy, particularly in patients with reduced cardiopulmonary function. The American College of Chest Physicians recommends that high-risk patients be referred for minimally invasive approaches, when possible. In addition, "Enhanced Recovery After (Thoracic) Surgery" (ERAS/ERATS) protocols, including multimodal analgesia and early mobilization, have contributed to improved outcomes after lung resection.

Batchelor TJP, Rasburn NJ, Abdelnour-Berchtold E, et al. Guidelines for enhanced recovery after lung surgery: recommendations of the Enhanced Recovery After Surgery (ERAS®) Society and the European Society of Thoracic Surgeons (ESTS). *Eur J Cardiothorac Surg*. 2019;1:91-115.

Brunelli A, Gooseman MR, Pompili C. Evaluation of risk for thoracic surgery. *Surg Oncol Clin N Am*. 2020;29:497-508.

Fernandez FG, Kosinski AS, Furnary AP, et al. Differential effects of operative complications on survival after surgery for primary lung cancer. *J Thorac Cardiovasc Surg*. 2018;155:1254-1264.

Pennathur A, Brunelli A, Criner CJ, et al. Definition and assessment of high risk in patients considered for lobectomy for stage I non–small cell lung cancer: The American Association for Thoracic Surgery expert panel consensus document. *J Thorac Cardiovasc Surg*. 2021;162:1605-1618.e6.

Shelley B, Glass A, Keast T, et al. Perioperative cardiovascular pathophysiology in patients undergoing lung resection surgery: a narrative review. *Br J Anaesth*. 2023;130:E66-E79.

B.3. What are the preoperative concerns of induction immunotherapy and neoadjuvant chemotherapy?

Preoperative chemotherapy and stereotactic radiation can increase survival in early-stage lung cancer (IB-IIIA). The approach to chemotherapy has changed over recent decades with an increased use of immunomodulators. Lung cancer cells express abundant programmed cell death (PD-1) and programmed death ligand 1 (PD-L1) receptors, which, upon activation, decrease the function of killer T cells. Drugs that inhibit these receptors (checkpoint inhibitors, such as pembrolizumab, nivolumab, cemiplimab, atezolizumab, avelumab, and durvalumab) can increase the T-cell immune response toward cancer cells. This treatment modality has shown favorable oncologic response and outcomes but can lead to potentially life-threatening inflammation and autoimmune reactions. **Side effects** include skin reactions (diffuse rash), enteritis and diarrhea, hyperthyroidism, hypophysitis, and adrenal insufficiency as well as hepatic insufficiency. *Endocrine and hepatic* side effects can be so severe as to warrant delaying surgery. *Grade 3-4 toxicity* usually requires prednisone 1 to 2 mg/kg/d, gradually tapered to symptom improvement and discontinuation of the immunotherapy. Anti-tumor necrosis factor alpha (TNF-α) inhibitors are added in case of suboptimal response to steroids. *Interstitial pneumonitis* has been reported in patients receiving phosphoinositol-3 kinase inhibitors. When severe, it warrants intensive care unit (ICU) admission and high-dose corticosteroids (1-2 mg/kg/d) with further immunosuppression in refractory cases. *Cytokine release syndrome* (CRS) can present with encephalopathy, mental status changes, and cerebellar disease, in which case surgery should be delayed. CRS is a major concern in recipients of chimeric antigen receptor (CAR)-modified T-cell lymphocytes and checkpoint inhibitors. Altered cerebellar function, mental status, and seizures have been described after its use.

Traditional chemotherapeutics can also elevate operative risk. Neoadjuvant chemotherapy can decrease DLCO by as much as 30% and is associated with increased 30- and 90-day mortality rates following lung resection.

Brunelli A, Gooseman MR, Pompili C. Evaluation of risk for thoracic surgery. *Surg Oncol Clin N Am.* 2020;29:497-508.

Hirsch FR, Scagliotti GV, Mulshine JL, et al. Lung cancer: current therapies and new targeted treatments. *Lancet.* 2017;389:299-311.

Kroschinsky F, Stoelzl F, von Bonin S, et al. New drugs, new toxicities: severe side effects of modern targeted and immunotherapy of cancer and their management. *Crit Care.* 2017;21:89.

C. Intraoperative Management

C.1. How would you premedicate, monitor, and anesthetize this patient presenting for endobronchial ultrasound (EBUS) for lung cancer staging?

EBUS-guided lymph node biopsy is a minimally invasive and accurate tool for lung cancer diagnosis and staging, having largely replaced cervical mediastinoscopy since the mid-2010s. Mediastinal, hilar, lobar, and interlobar lymph nodes are accessible with this technique. When combined with esophageal ultrasound-guided biopsies, EBUS allows staging of the entire mediastinal lymphatic chain (from stations 1 through 11, including 8 and 9, accessible by an esophageal approach). Rapid on-site cytologic examination (ROSE) is usually performed during the procedure.

The EBUS bronchoscope is a 6.9-mm outer diameter flexible bronchoscope with a latex balloon tip, coupled with a 7.5-MHz convex ultrasound probe. When the balloon is inflated with normal saline, it allows a tight adhesion to the airway wall, facilitating ultrasound identification of lymph nodes. A 21G needle is passed through a dedicated channel in the bronchoscope for ultrasound-guided biopsy. Color Doppler is available to differentiate lymph nodes from vascular structures. In the sedated patient, or in the presence of a supraglottic airway device, it is imperative to avoid vocal cord trauma, since the positioning of the optical view is at a 30° angle.

EBUS is generally performed as an ambulatory procedure. It can be done under either sedation or general anesthesia, depending on the number and locations of lymph nodes to biopsy. Good topical anesthesia is paramount to prevent coughing and bronchospasm. Intravenous steroids can be used to reduce inflammation and edema. In nonintubated patients, local anesthetic toxicity can result from larger doses necessary to tolerate the longer procedure and abolish the cough reflex. If an endotracheal tube (ETT) is used, a size 8.5 is recommended. In the presence of precarinal lymphadenopathy, the ETT requires high placement in the trachea, leaving the balloon between the vocal cords. Trauma can occur with prolonged procedures or in the absence of paralysis.

EBUS is associated with a low risk of pneumothorax, which, in turn, depends on the location of the lymph node target or the presence of bullous disease, rather than the type of anesthesia and the ventilation modality. Bleeding is a rare complication, and in contrast to cervical mediastinoscopy, preprocedural reversal of preoperative anticoagulation is not required. Other rare complications include pneumomediastinum and hemomediastinum, pneumothorax, mediastinitis, bacteremia, and severe bronchospasm.

Abdelmalak B, Doyle DJ. Updates and controversies in anesthesia for advanced interventional pulmonology procedures. *Curr Opin Anaesthesiol.* 2021;34:455-463.

Eapen G, Shah AM, Lei X, et al. Complications, consequences and practice patterns of endobronchial ultrasound guided needle aspiration. *Chest.* 2013;143:1044.

Zhang R, Ma Y, Xu G, et al. Endobronchial ultrasound-guided transbronchial needle aspiration and cervical mediastinoscopy for mediastinal staging of non–small cell lung cancer: a retrospective comparison study. *J Thorac Dis.* 2018;10:1951-1959.

C.2. What are the benefits of advanced bronchoscopy in the diagnosis of suspected lung cancer? How would you monitor and anesthetize a patient presenting for robotic bronchoscopy?

Advanced bronchoscopy refers to a developing array of technologies designed to improve bronchial navigation to help diagnose and treat pulmonary disease. These tools can be particularly useful in the evaluation of peripheral pulmonary nodules, which are often inaccessible to traditional fiberoptic bronchoscopy (FOB) due to the anatomic complexity and small caliber of distal airways. Multiple advanced bronchoscopy technologies are currently in use. Radial probe ultrasound, a form of EBUS, enables real-time 360° grayscale imaging of distal airways and surrounding tissues. Virtual bronchoscopy utilizes preprocedural CT imaging to develop a static map of bronchial anatomy, which is then paired with live fiberoptic images. *Electromagnetic navigation bronchoscopy* utilizes a magnetic field to precisely localize the bronchoscope position in relation to the lesion on the high-resolution CT images. Advanced bronchoscopy techniques have a diagnostic yield of approximately 70%. These procedures are safe, with an overall complication rate of approximately 4%, including a 2% risk of pneumothorax. This compares favorably to a roughly 45% risk of pneumothorax reported following transthoracic needle aspiration of peripheral pulmonary lesions.

Robotic-assisted bronchoscopy (*RAB*) is the newest technology employed in sampling peripheral pulmonary lesions. Currently, three RAB platforms are US Food and Drug Administration (FDA) approved: the Monarch platform by Auris Health (2018), the Ion Endoluminal System from Intuitive Surgical (2019), and the Galaxy System by Noah Medical (March 2023). Compared to traditional FOBs, robotic bronchoscopes have greater degrees of angulation and articulation, can be locked into the desired positions, and are equipped with integrated navigation technologies, among other differences. They enable proceduralists to maneuver through smaller airways with enhanced stability and precision and to maintain visualization and/or real-time localization of suspected lesions prior to and during biopsy. Early clinical data suggest that robotic technologies can increase lesion localization rates to as high as 97%, with complication rates comparable to nonrobotic bronchoscopy techniques. However, metrics such as diagnostic yield and cost-effectiveness have yet to be evaluated.

Advanced bronchoscopy and RAB procedures are performed under general anesthesia with an ETT, ideally size 8.5 mm or greater. Total intravenous anesthesia (TIVA) is preferred. A strong emphasis is placed on the prevention of atelectasis, which is known to diminish the visibility of lung lesions on CT imaging, alter bronchial anatomy, and reduce the diagnostic yield of bronchoscopic procedures. Accordingly, relatively high tidal volumes (8-10 ml/kg of ideal body weight [IBW]), high positive end-expiratory pressure (PEEP; 8-12 cm H_2O), and low FIO_2 (eg, 40%-60% if tolerated, to reduce absorption atelectasis) are typical. Even higher tidal volumes and PEEP might be indicated in patients who are obese and those with lower lobe lesions. The risk of atelectasis during preinduction denitrogenation/preoxygenation must be balanced against individual risk factors for hypoxemia following induction. If atelectasis develops, recruitment maneuvers should be attempted but might be unsuccessful in achieving adequate and sustained patency of small, subsegmental airways. These maneuvers might also be poorly tolerated hemodynamically, due to decreased venous return and increased intrapulmonary pressures. Neuromuscular blockade is indicated to provide periods of apnea during imaging and tissue sampling and prevent coughing or spontaneous breathing. The adjustable pressure-limiting (APL) valve is used to maintain adequate PEEP or plateau pressure during breath-hold maneuvers, which are ideally timed at end inspiration during the augmented fluoroscopy.

Abdelmalak B, Doyle DJ. Updates and controversies in anesthesia for advanced interventional pulmonology procedures. *Curr Opin Anaesthesiol.* 2021;34:455-463.

De Lima A, Kheir F, Majid A, et al. Anesthesia for interventional pulmonology procedures: a review of advanced diagnostic and therapeutic bronchoscopy. *Can J Anaesth.* 2018;68:822-836.

Freyaldenhoven ST, Tsukada H. Robotics in the diagnosis and staging of lung cancer. *J Surg Oncol.* 2023;127:258-261.

Nadig T, Thomas N, Nietert P, et al. Guided bronchoscopy for the evaluation of pulmonary lesions: an updated meta-analysis. *Chest.* Jun 2023;163:1589-1598.

Pritchett MA, Lau K, Skibo S, et al. Anesthesia considerations to reduce motion and atelectasis during advanced guided bronchoscopy. *BMC Pulm Med.* 2021;21:240.

Ravikumar N, Ho E, Wagh A et al. Advanced imaging for robotic bronchoscopy: a review. *Diagnostics.* 2023;13:990.

C.3. What other types of bronchoscopes are available, and what are the intraoperative considerations for each one?

Bronchoscopes currently in use include flexible fiberoptic, robotic, EBUS, rigid ventilating, and rigid Venturi bronchoscopes. Robotic and EBUS bronchoscopes are described in the previous section.

The FOB can be used in sedated patients either under local anesthesia (allowing examination of vocal cord movements) or under general anesthesia with a supraglottic airway device or an ETT. For the awake or sedated examination, viscous lidocaine can be gargled to anesthetize the upper airway or a 2% or 4% lidocaine solution inhaled via nebulizer mask to reach the lower airway. Bilateral superior laryngeal nerve blocks or transtracheal block can be added; however, they are not as popular currently due to potential complications. Intravenous sedation can be achieved with remifentanil, propofol, or dexmedetomidine, causing amnesia without impaired ventilatory drive. If the oropharynx is adequately anesthetized, a supraglottic airway device can be inserted without discomfort in sedated patients and used to assist ventilation at higher FIO_2.

Rigid bronchoscopy usually necessitates general anesthesia. Although spontaneous ventilation has been used, the risk of tracheal trauma is high with coughing. Therefore, neuromuscular block is commonly used unless contraindicated. The rigid ventilating bronchoscope has a side-port adapter that can be attached to either the anesthesia circuit or the jet ventilator, allowing delivery of a high-flow rate. A variable air leak usually exists around the bronchoscope, so high-flow rates of inspired gases or packing of the oropharynx are needed. Significant loss of volatile anesthetic in the OR environment needs to be considered; thus, the use of TIVA is a good alternative.

The rigid Venturi-effect bronchoscope relies on an intermittent high-flow (20-60 L/min), high-pressure (50 psi) oxygen jet to entrain air and insufflate the lungs. The jet is delivered through a reducing valve (25 psi) into a 16- or 18-gauge needle inside and roughly parallel to the lumen of the bronchoscope. Major disadvantages of this technique are the lack of control of the inspired oxygen concentration and the inability to administer inhaled anesthetics. Accordingly, anesthesia should be maintained by intravenous techniques. Inadequate ventilation (with resultant hypercapnia) can occur.

Rigid bronchoscopic procedures can be relatively short and done on an outpatient basis. Patients can be fully paralyzed, with reversal of neuromuscular blockade using sugammadex, if available.

Sethi S, Cicenia J. EBUS-TBNA Bronchoscopy. In: Mehta AC, Jain P, eds. *Interventional Bronchoscopy: A Clinical Guide*. Springer Science; 2013:85-106.

José RJ, Shaefi S, Navani N. Anesthesia for bronchoscopy. *Curr Opin Anesthesiol*. 2014;27:453-457.

C.4. What is cervical mediastinoscopy, and what are its indications and potential complications? How would you anesthetize and monitor a patient undergoing cervical mediastinoscopy?

For many years, cervical mediastinoscopy was the gold standard for staging lung cancer and evaluating disease in the mediastinum. However, with the introduction of EBUS and advanced bronchoscopy, cervical mediastinoscopy has become less common. Cervical mediastinoscopy is now reserved for small lymph nodes not readily accessible through endobronchial techniques, or if additional tissue is needed after EBUS. It is generally accepted to have high sensitivity (>80%) and specificity in lung cancer staging.

In this procedure, a 3-cm incision is made in the suprasternal notch, and a plane is dissected between the left innominate vein and the sternum. A flexible or rigid mediastinoscope is then inserted anterior to the aortic arch. Accordingly, during mediastinoscopy, intermittent compression or occlusion of the right innominate artery can occur. The blood pressure cuff should be placed on the left arm and the pulse oximeter on the right hand. In the case of innominate artery compression, a dampening of the pulse oximetry trace will be evident while blood pressure measurements remain accurate. Although rare, injury to vascular structures (such as the azygos vein and innominate artery) can occur, potentially necessitating a median sternotomy and possible cardiopulmonary bypass. Patient positioning and placement of electrocardiography leads should be performed accordingly. Arterial access is not routinely used unless the patient has clinical indications for continuous hemodynamic monitoring. In this case, noninvasive continuous hemodynamic monitors, such as the FloTrac (Edwards) or ClearSight (Edwards), can also be considered. The arterial catheter or monitor should be placed in/on the left radial artery to avoid falsely low readings related to right innominate artery compression. Artifacts related to compression of the arterial line or noninvasive blood pressure monitor, especially if the arms are tucked, will affect the accuracy and precision of monitoring, making it the main limitation to its use. Despite typically being a short procedure, hypothermia can occur, especially in older patients; therefore, body temperature should be monitored, and a warming blanket applied.

Mediastinoscopy is performed under general anesthesia with full neuromuscular blockade to reduce the likelihood of accidental injury due to coughing, straining, or other patient movements. Induction, maintenance of anesthesia, and neuromuscular blockade can be achieved with relatively short-acting agents. Anesthesia can be maintained with a potent inhalational agent. Some clinicians choose to avoid the use of nitrous oxide because of the potential for the mediastinoscope to enter the pleural space and create a pneumothorax.

Because the pleural space is generally not entered intentionally, a chest tube is not indicated. Occult pneumothorax can occur as a complication, so a chest radiograph is usually obtained before discharge. Complications during mediastinoscopy occur in 1% to 2% of cases and generally result from trauma to adjacent structures (pleura, trachea, esophagus, superior vena cava, azygos vein, innominate artery, pulmonary artery, and aorta) or nerve injury (recurrent laryngeal or phrenic nerve). Should a major vascular injury occur, blood loss can be rapid and profound, necessitating emergent sternotomy. Lower extremity access would be needed due to potential packing or vascular clamping of the superior vena cava.

Ahmed-Nustrath A, Swanevelder J. Anaesthesia for mediastinoscopy. *BJA Educ*. 2007;7.

Czarnecka-Kujawa K, Yasufuku K. Mediastinoscopy: surgical versus medical. In: Turner JF Jr, Jain P, Yasufuku K, Mehta AC, eds. *From Thoracic Surgery to Interventional Pulmonology*. Humana Publishers; 2021:61-90.

Rami-Porta R, Call S. Invasive staging of mediastinal lymph nodes: mediastinoscopy and re mediastinoscopy. *Thorac Surg Clin*. 2012;22:177-189.

C.5. The decision was made to proceed with a robotic right middle lobectomy rather than a video-assisted thoracoscopic (VATS) procedure. How would this alter your management?

Robotic thoracic procedures present some unique challenges when compared to VATS, despite both being minimally invasive. In both cases, patients are positioned in the lateral decubitus position, and the bed might be flexed. Extensions for the intravenous tubing and the breathing circuit might be necessary if the bed is rotated away from the anesthesia machine, as is required for docking certain robots. Special care is required for the nondependent arm, which is suspended and sometimes abducted to facilitate motion of the robotic arms. Unnatural positioning with stretching of the brachial plexus can lead to potentially permanent damage. Direct injury can also result from the robotic arms resting on the patient's arm or head.

Optimal lung isolation and collapse are necessary to enhance lung visualization and allow full motion of the instruments in the chest cavity. Since this space remains partially closed, lung collapse is slower than for the open approach. Carbon dioxide (CO_2) insufflation can be used to expedite the process. Left DLTs are commonly used due to less chance of displacement and the ability to quickly collapse the lung. Once the patient is positioned and the robot docked, it can be difficult to gain access to the airway. Bronchial blockers are an alternative, but they often require repositioning during the case, which can be difficult due to the close proximity of the robotic arms to the patient's head.

Intravenous access should be obtained before final positioning and draping since patient access can be limited. An arterial catheter, generally in the radial artery of the dependent arm, is beneficial for hemodynamic monitoring, especially if the chest is insufflated with CO_2. The resulting "iatrogenic tension pneumothorax" can be associated with an acute increase in peak airway pressures and decreased venous return, leading to decreased lung compliance and significant hypotension. In most cases, this is transient and effectively treated with pressors and/or a temporary decrease in insufflation pressures. Suggested insufflation pressure should be less than 10 to 15 mm Hg, while peak inspiratory pressures should be less than 30 cm H_2O. Minute ventilation should be adjusted to maintain normocapnia while complying with protective lung ventilation guidelines. Low tidal volume ventilation, driving pressures (plateau pressure − PEEP), or mechanical power (mechanical power [J/min] = 0.098 × RR × Vt × (PEEP + ½[Pplat − PEEP] + [Ppeak − Pplat])) during OLV does not worsen oxygenation or pulmonary compliance and is associated with significantly reduced risk of postoperative pulmonary complications.

Hemodynamic compromise can also be caused by unexpected bleeding, arrhythmias, or, in rare cases, contralateral pneumothorax (more common during robotic esophagectomy). Bleeding can be more difficult to control in robotic cases than in VATS because the robotic arms limit access to the chest, causing delays in making an incision or performing cardiopulmonary resuscitation. Helpful maneuvers to decrease bleeding involve increasing CO_2 insufflation pressure (potentially worsening systemic hypotension), increasing PEEP, and allowing periods of apnea to decrease mediastinal movement and facilitate compression/clipping of the source of bleeding. At least one large-bore intravenous catheter is recommended.

Geraci TC, Sasankan P, Luria B, Cerfolio RJ. Intraoperative anesthetic and surgical concerns for robotic thoracic surgery. *Thorac Surg Clin*. 2020;30:293-304.

McCall P, Steven M, Shelley B. Anaesthesia for video-assisted and robotic thoracic surgery. *BJA Educ*. 2019;19:405-411.

Park M, Yoon S, Nam J-S, et al. Driving pressure-guided ventilation and postoperative pulmonary complications in thoracic surgery: a multicentre randomised clinical trial. *Br J Anaesth*. 2023;130:e106-e118.

Pedoto A, Ginsberg N. Positioning in thoracic surgery. In: Cohen E, ed. *Cohen's Comprehensive Thoracic Anesthesia*. Elsevier; 2022:133-142.

Peel JK, Funk DJ, Slinger P, et al. Tidal volume during 1-lung ventilation: a systematic review and meta-analysis. *J Thorac Cardiovasc Surg*. 2022;163:1573-1585.e1.

Santer P, Wachtendorf LJ, Suleiman A, et al. Mechanical power during general anesthesia and postoperative respiratory failure: a multicenter retrospective cohort study. *Anesthesiology*. 2022;137:41-54.

C.6. What are the indications for one-lung ventilation (OLV), and how can it be accomplished? What complications can be associated with OLV?

Absolute and relative indications for lung separation are listed in **Table 2.2**. Several techniques can be used to provide OLV, including a DLT, a bronchial blocking catheter passed inside or outside an ETT, a bronchial blocking catheter incorporated within an ETT (Univent ETT), or, rarely, a conventional ETT placed endobronchially. Other commercially available DLTs include Vivasight ET, a left DLT with a high-resolution built-in video camera at the tip of the tracheal lumen that provides a continuous view of the airway; The Silbroncho left DLT, constructed of a silicone wire–reinforced tip; and the Cliny right DLT, a device with an oblong right bronchial cuff and two ventilation slots for the right upper lobe. Currently, DLTs remain the most common method for achieving lung isolation. Several manufacturers

TABLE 2.2 Indications for One-Lung Ventilation

Absolute	
1. Isolate from spillage or contamination.	• Infection: bronchiectasis and lung abscess • Massive hemorrhage
2. Control the distribution of ventilation.	• Bronchopleural fistula • Bronchopleural cutaneous fistula • Giant unilateral lung cyst or bulla • Tracheobronchial tree disruption or trauma • Surgical procedures on major conducting airway (ie, pneumonectomy or sleeve resection) • Life-threatening hypoxemia resulting from unilateral lung disease. • Unilateral bronchopulmonary lavage (pulmonary alveolar proteinosis)
3. Facilitate surgical exposure.	• Video- and robotic-assisted thoracoscopic surgery
Relative	
1. Facilitation of surgical exposure—high priority	• Thoracic aortic aneurysm surgery • Pneumonectomy • Upper lobectomy • Mediastinal exposure • Pulmonary resection via median sternotomy
2. Facilitation of surgical exposure—low priority	• Esophageal resection • Middle and lower lobectomies and segmental resection • Procedures on the thoracic spine
3. Severe hypoxemia resulting from unilateral lung disease	

produce right and left DLTs, which are available in six sizes: 28F, 32F, 35F, 37F, 39F, and 41F (size in French = 3.14 × external diameter in millimeters or 4 × the internal diameter + 2). Average-sized males usually accommodate a 39F and average-sized females a 37F.

A variety of sizing techniques have been described based on measurements of airway size derived from radiographic, CT imaging, or ultrasound examination, but these have been questioned across sex and ethnicity. A properly sized DLT should pass atraumatically through the glottis, advance easily into the trachea and bronchus, and exhibit an air leak when the bronchial cuff is deflated.

Bronchial blockers (see Section C.10) are a good option for lung isolation in patients who have a difficult airway, when postoperative mechanical ventilation is needed, in the case of a fresh tracheostomy, or in children. Lobar blockade can also be accomplished using a blocker, especially after pneumonectomy or in case OLV is not tolerated. Disadvantages of blockers include slow lung collapse, especially in patients with severe COPD; dislodgment of the catheter tip during surgical manipulation of the hilum; and risk of being stapled in the bronchial stump. Lung deflation can be expedited by the use of 100% inhaled oxygen, which promotes diffusion atelectasis, and by ensuring that the blocker balloon is inflated at end expiration.

Independent of the technique chosen, OLV is associated with certain disadvantages and complications. The most notable is the large and variable alveolar-to-arterial oxygen tension difference ($P_{[A-a]}O_2$) that occurs because of continued perfusion to the nondependent nonventilated lung. The incidence of severe hypoxemia and hypercarbia is relatively low and often the result of DLT malposition resulting from overinflation of the endobronchial cuff, surgical manipulation of the bronchus, or head extension/flexion during positioning in the lateral decubitus position. Traumatic laryngitis and tracheobronchial rupture secondary to bronchial cuff overinflation, forceful placement, or airway pathology have also been reported as potential complication of DLT placement.

Heir SJ, Purugganan R, Jackson TA, et al. A retrospective evaluation of the use of video-capable double lumen endotracheal tubes in thoracic surgery. *J Cardiovasc Thorac Anesth*. 2014;28:870-872.

Licker M, Le Guen M, Diaper J, et al. Isolation of the lung: double lumen tubes and endobronchial blockers. *Trends Anaesth Crit Care*. 2014;4:47-54.

Pedoto A. How to choose the double lumen tube size and side: the eternal debate. *Anesthesiol Clin*. 2012;4:671-681.

Shum S, Huang A, Slinger P. Hypoxaemia during one lung ventilation. *BJA Educ*. 2023;23:328-336.

C.7. What are the contraindications to the use of double-lumen endotracheal tubes (DLTs)?

Placement of a DLT should be carefully considered in the following situations:

- Patients whose upper airway anatomy precludes safe insertion, such as recessed jaw, prominent teeth, bull neck, anterior larynx, mandibular surgery, and neck radiation
- Patients with lesions along the pathway of the tube that could be traumatized, such as airway stricture or endoluminal tumors
- Small patients for whom a 35F or 32F tube is too large to fit comfortably through the larynx and a 28F tube is considered too small
- Critically ill patients already intubated who cannot tolerate cessation of mechanical ventilation and PEEP for a short time
- Patients with known or suspected difficult airway

Under these circumstances, OLV can be achieved via an endobronchial blocker. Endobronchial placement of a single-lumen tube is an alternative but suboptimal option. The tip of the ETT can cause direct distal airway trauma and significant airway compression with potential mucosal ischemia if the cuff bulges at the carina. When placed into the right mainstem bronchus, the right upper lobe orifice will be occluded by the cuff of the tube, preventing ventilation.

Collins SR, Titus BJ, Campos JH, Blank RS. Lung isolation in the patient with a difficult airway. *Anesth Analg*. 2018;126:1968-1978.

Licker M, Le Guen M, Diaper J, et al. Isolation of the lung: double lumen tubes and endobronchial blockers. *Trends Anaesth Crit Care*. 2014;4:47-54.

C.8. Would you use a right- or left-sided DLT?

A left-sided DLT is preferred for most procedures. The left mainstem bronchus is longer than the right (5.0-5.5 cm vs 1.5-2.0 cm), allowing small movements of the tube without obstructing a bronchial division. The variable origin of the right upper lobe bronchus (1.5-2.0 cm below carina) can complicate proper positioning of a right-sided tube. A right-sided DLT is specifically indicated in the case of pathology involving the left mainstem bronchus, such as large exophytic lesions, significant bronchial stenosis, tracheobronchial disruption, endobronchial stent, or distortion by an adjacent tumor or a thoracoabdominal aneurysm. Other indications include left pneumonectomy, sleeve resection, or lung transplantation to avoid the presence of the tube in the surgical field that could be inadvertently included in the staple line or prevent suturing of the airway. At the end of a pneumonectomy, the stump can be protected from positive pressure ventilation by leaving the tracheal side clamped until the patient returns to spontaneous ventilation; for a left lung transplant or a sleeve resection, the right lung can be ventilated when the bronchus is open during the resection and reconstruction phase. The only absolute contraindications for right-sided DLT use are the presence of an anomalous take-off of the right upper bronchus above the tracheal carina, commonly referred to as a "pig bronchus," or a right mainstem lesion.

Licker M, Le Guen M, Diaper J, et al. Isolation of the lung: double lumen tubes and endobronchial blockers. *Trends Anaesth Crit Care.* 2014;4:47-54.

Pedoto A. How to choose the double lumen tube size and side: the eternal debate. *Anesthesiol Clin.* 2012;4:671-681.

C.9. How do you know that the tube is in the correct position?

Recommended insertion techniques for a DLT include direct laryngoscopy followed by fiberoptic guidance in the appropriate mainstem bronchus. Blind insertion could cause airway injury. Auscultation alone is unreliable to confirm the position of a DLT due to transmitted or diminished breath sounds, especially in patients with COPD.

During bronchoscopy, the tracheal cartilaginous rings are anterior, and the tracheal membrane is posterior. Therefore, right versus left can be discerned by the relationship of the mainstem bronchi to the anterior cartilaginous rings and the posterior membrane (**Figure 2.1A**). In addition, the right upper lobe take-off (which usually arises from the lateral aspect of the right mainstem bronchus, just below the tracheal carina) is a useful landmark when the airway anatomy has been obscured by bleeding, edema, or radiation-induced changes or has been distorted by extrinsic compression. Left DLT position and depth are confirmed by inserting the FOB in the tracheal lumen. The entire right mainstem bronchus should be visible, and the tracheal lumen orifice of the DLT should be 1 to 2 cm above the tracheal carina. When properly positioned, the upper part of the blue endobronchial cuff is visualized just below the tracheal carina in the left mainstem bronchus (**Figure 2.1B**). If a right DLT is used, correct positioning is confirmed by visualization of the bronchial cuff in the right mainstem bronchus (**Figure 2.1C**) and visualization of the right upper lobe orifice through a slot on the lateral surface of the DLT (**Figure 2.1D**). For both left- and right-sided tubes, the bronchoscope should also be inserted in the bronchial lumen to evaluate the distance between the tip of the tube and the distal bifurcation of the bronchus. DLT position should be reconfirmed after the patient is positioned laterally, before inflating the bronchial cuff and isolating the lung.

When the **Vivasight** tube is used, placement and repositioning can be facilitated by the high-resolution built-in camera. The main advantage of these left-sided tubes is the continuous visualization of the right mainstem bronchus. The main disadvantage is the fogging of the camera by secretions, especially during right-sided procedures, and the bigger outer diameter, which can cause airway injury during the placement. The lack of a camera on the bronchial side still requires the use of bronchoscopy to assess the secondary carina.

Campos JA. Lung isolation. In: Slinger P, eds. *Principle and Practice of Anesthesia for Thoracic Surgery.* Springer; 2019:283-309.

Lee GK. Airway apparatus for thoracic surgery. *Anaesth Intensive Care Med.* 2014;15:499-504.

Licker M, Le Guen M, Diaper J, et al. Isolation of the lung: double lumen tubes and endobronchial blockers. *Trends Anaesth Crit Care.* 2014;4:47-54.

C.10. What types of bronchial blockers are available? What are the advantages and disadvantages of bronchial blockers?

Several blockers are available (**Figure 2.2**), leaving ample preference of choice to the operator and the institution. Advantages and disadvantages of blockers are listed in **Table 2.3**.

- **Fogarty embolectomy catheters** can be used to isolate the lung, although not specifically made for this purpose. The 7F Fogarty catheters come with either a 12- or 20-mL high-pressure, low-volume balloon in both latex and nonlatex models and an inner metal stylet that can be bent to facilitate endobronchial placement. In case of dislodgment, the stylet can be reinserted, and the blocker repositioned. Fogarty catheters have no communicating central channel, preventing the intraoperative use of

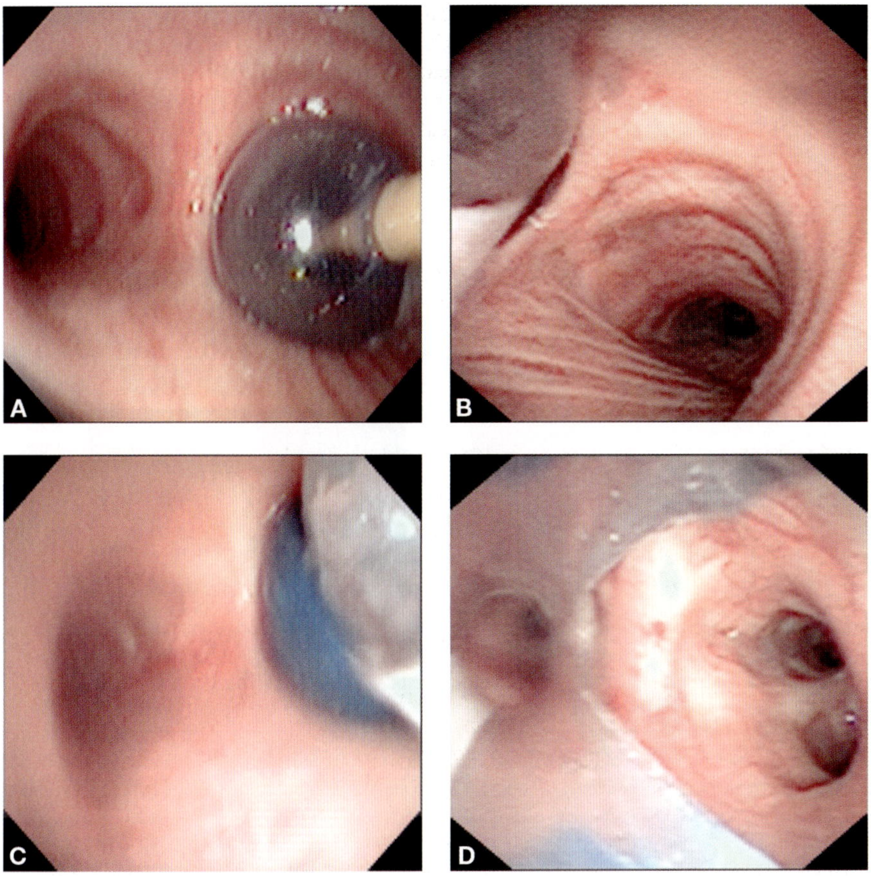

FIGURE 2.1. Representative bronchoscopic images of a bronchial blocker and double-lumen tube (DLT) placement. A. Normal tracheal anatomy with cartilaginous rings anteriorly and membranous trachea posteriorly; this helps define left versus right. A bronchial blocking catheter is seen in the right mainstem bronchus. **B.** Placement of a left-sided DLT. The upper portion of the endobronchial cuff is evident as well as the orifice of the right upper lobe just below the tracheal carina. **C.** Placement of a right-sided DLT. The upper portion of the endobronchial cuff is evident in the right mainstem bronchus. **D.** The orifice of the right upper lobe visualized through the slot on the lateral aspect of the bronchial side of a right-sided DLT.

continuous positive airway pressure (CPAP) or suction. Lung collapse occurs by absorption of oxygen. Therefore, prior to inflating the balloon, it is recommended to both discontinue ventilation and depressurize the circuit of the ventilator if the patient tolerates it. The catheters are usually placed outside a single-lumen ETT and positioned via FOB (Figure 2.1A). If placed inside the ETT, a connector such as a two-swivel adapter is needed to facilitate insertion of both the catheter and a bronchoscope.

- **Arndt blockers** (wire-guided endobronchial blocker) are available in 5F, 7F, and 9F with elliptical or spherical cuffs (low pressure, high volume), the latter particularly advantageous to isolate the right lung. They are usually inserted through the ETT via a three-way connector (catheter, bronchoscope, ventilation circuit). Positioning is facilitated by a Seldinger technique via an inner wire with a loop at the distal tip, where the flexible bronchoscope is placed. The wire is removed once the blocker is in position, leaving an inner lumen that allows for suctioning or CPAP. The wire loop can be reinserted to reposition the blocker in case of dislodgment.
- **Cohen blockers** are similar in shape to the Arndt blockers, but they use a positioning wheel to facilitate placement. By turning the wheel in a clockwise manner, the distal portion of the blocker deflects to the left. The main advantage of this blocker is for left mainstem placement, because of its steep angle. Disadvantages include cost, fragility of the wheel, and availability of only one size (9F).
- **EZ blockers** (Teleflex Life Science Ltd) are blockers with a Y-shaped bifurcation at the end fitted with two color-coded, high-pressure low-volume, inflatable cuffs and a hollow channel in the center. The blocker is placed inside an ETT, with the end on a horizontal plane to facilitate placement of the Y across carina. Final position needs be confirmed by fiberoptic visualization since both cuffs might

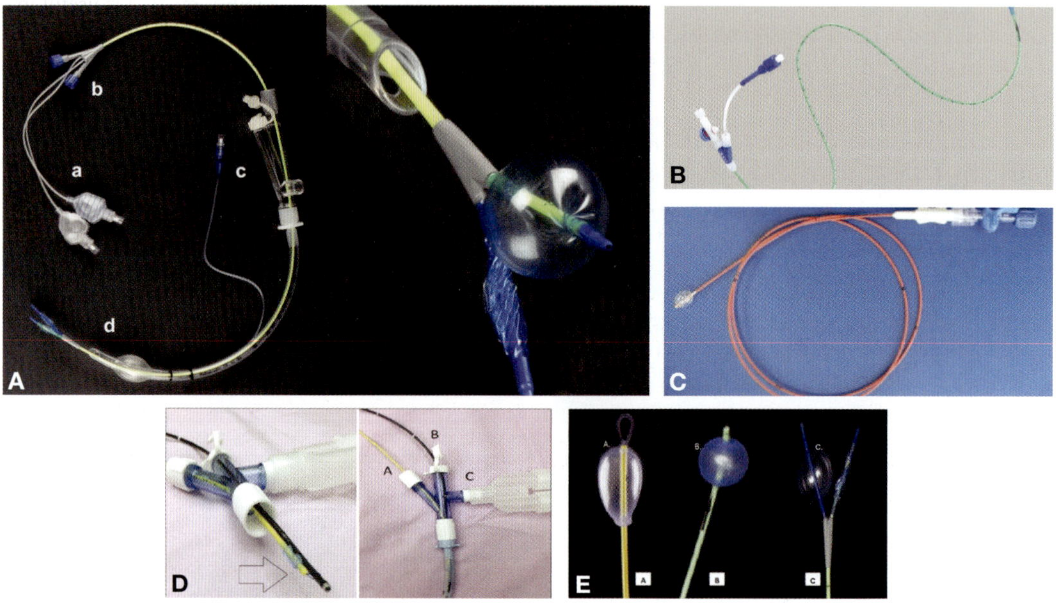

FIGURE 2.2. Commercially available bronchial blockers. A. EZ Blocker Y-shaped semirigid endobronchial blocker: (a) two separate proximal balloons; (b) central lumens; (c) connector to accommodate the blocker, the bronchoscope, and the ventilator; (d) bifurcated distal Y-shaped extension that sits at carina when the blocker is in its final position. The shaft is radio-opaque and has depth markings. **B.** Cohen FlexTip endobronchial blocker. Rotating wheel allows clockwise deflection of the distal tip of the blocker by more than 90°, facilitating placement in the desired bronchus. The distal arrow identifies the anterior part of the blocker and helps guiding the placement by differentiating right (*arrow up*) from left (*arrow down*). (Courtesy of Cook Medical.) **C.** Fogarty embolectomy catheter. Hollow catheter with a metal wire stylet that was initially designed for intravascular embolectomy. When used to isolate the lung, the catheter tip is bent to a hockey-stick shape to facilitate placement of the distal latex balloon into the desired bronchus. The product does not come with an ETT (ETT) connector; therefore, it is usually placed outside the ETT, and kept in place by the ETT inflated cuff. While rarely used in adults, this device is favored for pediatric lung isolation. (© 2024 Becton, Dickinson and Company, Irvine, CA. All rights reserved.) **D.** Arndt endobronchial blocker. Catheter with a distal loop wire that allows endobronchial placement via "Seldinger" technique via FOB. The device is placed through the proper port in the 3-way connector (image on the right) and the wire is looped around the FOB (image on the left) for the placement in the desired bronchus. For left mainstem blockade, it is important to have a tight loop around the bronchoscope, so both blocker and FOB can enter the bronchus. The blocker will preferentially go in the right mainstem due to its favorable angle. (Courtesy of Cook Medical.) **E.** Comparison of the shape and size of the distal cuffs of the Arndt (A), Cohen (B), and EZ (C) blockers.

TABLE 2.3 Advantages and Disadvantages of Bronchial Blockers

Advantages	Disadvantages
• Able to use in adults and children too small to accommodate a double-lumen tube • Difficult airway • If double-lumen tube contraindicated • Placed inside the endotracheal tube • No need to change endotracheal tube in case of postoperative mechanical ventilation • Lobar isolation	• Unable to suction efficiently • Need to be positioned via fiberoptic bronchoscopy • Lung expansion if CPAP applied • Difficult for right mainstem position and RUL isolation, when take-off is too close to the carina. • Tracheal occlusion if proximal dislodgment. • Cross ventilation if the cuff is not completely inflated. • Possible stapling in the stump if not retracted at the appropriate time

CPAP, continuous positive airway pressure; RUL, right upper lobe.

go in the right mainstem. The main advantage of this blocker is its stability, making it useful in cases where patient access is limited, or when surgery is associated with significant carinal manipulation. The presence of the two cuffs makes sequential lung isolation feasible.

Univent tubes consist of an ETT with a built-in silicon bronchial blocking catheter. The main advantage is the ability of leaving the device in place in case of postoperative mechanical ventilation. However, this device is not commonly used in the United States because of its bulkiness. The outer diameter ranges from 9.7 to 13.7 mm (for a 6.0-8.0 inner diameter tube), with the potential to cause subglottic edema and stenosis in case of long-term use. The inner diameter is quite narrow, making suctioning or FOB difficult. The silicon blocker in the Univent is available as an isolated item (**Fuji blocker**). It is a high-volume, low-pressure system with a preformed "hockey-stick" bend at the tip and a double stylet. It has a spherical cuff (ideally more suited to isolate the right mainstem bronchus) and two different sizes (5F and 9F). The **Coopdech** blocker (Daiken Medical Co, Ltd) is similar in shape to the Fuji blocker but offers the option of an autoinflate balloon via an autoinflate button, allowing the use of one hand while maneuvering the FOB.

In addition to providing lung isolation, blockers can also be used to rescue a nonfunctional DLT, by placing the device inside the lumen of the nondependent lung. This might be needed in case of rupture of the bronchial cuff in a patient already positioned, or for lobar collapse in case of DLT dislodgment and inability to appropriately reposition in the mainstem bronchus. The DLT can be left in place or withdrawn and used as a single-lumen tube.

Lee GK. Airway apparatus for thoracic surgery. *Anaesth Intensive Care Med.* 2014;15:499-504.

Licker M, Le Guen M, Diaper J, et al. Isolation of the lung: double lumen tubes and endobronchial blockers. *Trends Anaesth Crit Care.* 2014;4:47-54.

Morris BN, Fernando RJ, Garner CR et al. A randomized comparison of positional stability: the EZ-blocker versus left-sided double-lumen endobronchial tubes in adult patients undergoing thoracic surgery. *J Cardiothorac Vasc Anesth.* 2021;35:2319-2325.

C.11. How will systemic oxygenation be monitored during OLV?

Pulse oximetry is essential for monitoring arterial oxygenation during lung resection, decreasing the need for repeated measurements of arterial blood gases. (The mechanism of pulse oximetry is described in greater detail in Chapter 59: Hypoxia and Equipment Failure.) While no strict cutoffs are described, it is reasonable to target an Sao_2 greater than 88% to 90%. Strategies to manage hypoxemia are described in Section C.16.

Of note, systemic Sao_2 might not reflect cerebral oxygenation. Cerebral oximetry is a more targeted monitor of brain perfusion during thoracic and cardiac anesthesia. This technology uses near-infrared spectroscopy (NIRS) to integrate venous and arterial hemoglobin oxygen saturation signals in a ratio of 3:1. Autoregulatory mechanisms prioritize brain perfusion at the expense of other organs. Therefore, when significant cerebral desaturation occurs (<65%), it is likely that other organs have been exposed to a greater desaturation. Brain hypoperfusion seems to correlate with renal ischemia and subsequent acute renal failure (ARF) in cardiac surgery and might contribute to altered mental status after thoracic procedures. Proposed physiologic mechanisms include hypoxemia during OLV and mediastinal shift with reduced cardiac output related to the lateral decubitus position.

Campos JH, Feider A. Hypoxia during one-lung ventilation-a review and update. *J Cardiothorac Vasc Anesth.* 2018;32:2330-2338.

Hofer CK, Rex S, Ganter MT. Update on minimally invasive hemodynamic monitoring in thoracic anesthesia. *Curr Opin Anesthesiol.* 2014;27:28-35.

Mahal I, Davie S, Grocott HP. Cerebral oxymetry and thoracic surgery. *Curr Opin Anesthesiol.* 2014;27:21-27.

McCall P, Steven M, Shelley B. Anaesthesia for video-assisted and robotic thoracic surgery. *BJA Educ.* 2019;19:405-411.

C.12. The patient was placed in the lateral decubitus position. Describe the effects of lateral positioning on pulmonary blood flow and respiration.

In both upright and supine positions, the right lung receives approximately 55% of the total blood flow while the left lung receives the remaining approximately 45%. In the lateral decubitus position, gravity causes a vertical gradient in blood flow distribution of the low-pressure pulmonary system. Therefore, perfusion of the dependent lung is significantly greater than the nondependent counterpart. When the right lung is nondependent, it receives 45% of the total blood flow while 55% perfuses the dependent left

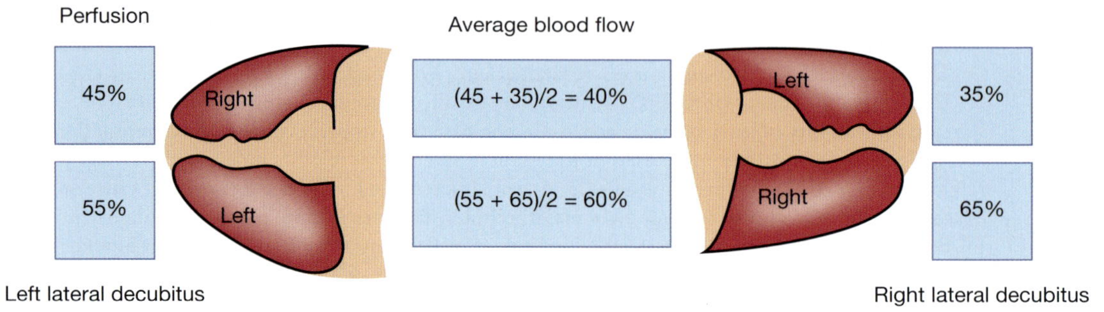

FIGURE 2.3. Changes in blood perfusion with the lateral decubitus position.

lung. When the left lung is nondependent, it receives 35% of the total blood flow, while the right lung receives 65%. Therefore, the average blood flow of the nondependent lung is approximately 40% of the total blood flow, with the dependent lung being perfused with the remaining 60% (**Figure 2.3**).

Respiratory Effects

The lateral decubitus position causes both mechanical interference with chest wall motion and a decrease in lung expansion. Specifically, the dependent chest wall is constricted by the OR table and axillary roll, the lateral movements are limited by the bolsters used to hold the patient in position, while the upper expansion is reduced by the weight of the mediastinum. The flexion at the hips causes a theoretical improvement of the diaphragmatic motion, especially in patients who are morbidly obese. However, the caudad displacement of the abdominal organs is counteracted by the negative effects of general anesthesia and muscle relaxation. The final result is a gravity-induced mismatch of ventilation and perfusion while in the lateral position, with redistribution of blood flow toward the dependent lung, which is compressed by the mediastinal contents, resulting in an increase in atelectasis and hypoventilation. In the awake, spontaneously breathing subject, the lower (dependent) diaphragm is still able to contract more efficiently, maintaining ventilation in the dependent lung and matching the increased perfusion. In contrast, when the patient is anesthetized, with or without paralysis, most of the ventilation is preferentially switched to the more compliant upper lung, while perfusion increases in the lower lung. The result is an increase in ventilation-perfusion mismatch.

Liou DZ, Berry MF. Thoracic surgery considerations in obese patients. *Thorac Surg Clin*. 2018;28:27-41.

Pedoto A, Ginsberg N. Positioning in thoracic surgery. In: Cohen E, ed. *Cohen's Comprehensive Thoracic Anesthesia*. Elsevier; 2022:133-142.

Rehder K, Hatch DJ, Sessler AD, et al. The function of each lung of anesthetized and paralyzed man during mechanical ventilation. *Anesthesiology*. 1972;37:16.

Walff KE, Aulin I. The regional lung function in the lateral decubitus position during anesthesia and operations. *Acta Anesthesiol Scand*. 1972;16:195-205.

C.13. What is hypoxic pulmonary vasoconstriction (HPV)?

HPV is an autoregulatory mechanism that reduces ventilation-perfusion mismatch and improves arterial oxygenation. Proposed mechanisms include an increase in reactive oxygen species in the pulmonary arterial smooth muscle, activation of redox-based oxygen sensors, and an increase in intracellular calcium. HPV is triggered by a decrease in PaO_2 within the lung from low FIO_2, hypoventilation, or atelectasis. The selective increase in vascular resistance in the hypoxic parenchyma diverts blood away to the better ventilated and oxygenated lung, decreasing the amount of shunt flow. This is a biphasic response that starts within 15 to 30 minutes from lung collapse, culminates at 120 minutes, and takes hours to reverse after ventilation is restored.

Increasing evidence indicates that significant systemic oxidative stress can be elicited by hyperoxic reperfusion of a lung in which HPV has been sustained. Although the subject of ongoing research, clinical data suggest an association between the magnitude of the oxidative stress and postoperative cardiopulmonary complications. Recommendations to decrease reexpansion injury include using the lowest tolerated FIO_2 during OLV, reinflating the collapsed lung with less than 100% O_2, and using protective lung strategies.

Brimioulle S, LeJeune P, Naeije R. Effects of hypoxic pulmonary vasoconstriction on pulmonary gas exchange. *Appl Physiol.* 1996;81:1535-1543.

Dunham-Snary KJ, Wu D, Sykes EA, et al. Hypoxic pulmonary vasoconstriction: from molecular mechanism to medicine. *Chest.* 2017;151:181-192.

Heerdt PM, Stowe DF. Single-lung ventilation and oxidative stress: a different perspective on a common practice. *Curr Opin Anesthesiol.* 2017;30:42-49.

Losher J, Slinger P. Lung injury after one-lung ventilation: a review of the pathophysiologic mechanisms affecting the ventilated and the collapsed lung. *Anesth Analg.* 2015;121:302-318.

Shum S, Huang A, Slinger P. Hypoxaemia during one lung ventilation. *BJA Educ.* 2023;23:328-336.

C.14. What are the effects of anesthetic agents on HPV and their clinical implications?

Any medication that causes vasodilation can inhibit HPV. Several clinical studies have failed to demonstrate a decrease in HPV during OLV and TIVA. Intravenous anesthetics, such as propofol, ketamine, morphine, and fentanyl, have no direct inhibitory effect on HPV. In contrast, volatile anesthetics inhibit HPV in a dose-related manner but usually at concentrations much higher than clinically used. Other nonanesthetic drugs such as β-agonists and antagonists, calcium channel blockers, nitro-vasodilators, and theophylline can influence the effects of inhalation anesthetics on shunting and arterial oxygenation during OLV. There is no good evidence that neuraxial blockade affects HPV, unless causing a decrease in cardiac output or systemic vasodilation.

- The result of an increased pulmonary shunt on $Pa{O_2}$ depends on the absolute level of the initial shunt and the inspired oxygen concentration used. Even when the shunt is increased, $Pa{O_2}$ usually remains well above 100 mm Hg, with minimal changes in oxygen saturation and content.
- Inhalational agents inhibit HPV, but they also decrease cardiac output and oxygen consumption and can cause a decrease in mixed venous-oxygen tension. If cardiac output decreases more than oxygen consumption, there is a decrease in $P\bar{v}{O_2}$, which is a potent stimulus for HPV. A low cardiac output results in decreased perfusion of the collapsed lung, where there is an increase in pulmonary vascular resistance as a result of HPV. Nevertheless, the presence of chronic and irreversible vascular disease in the nondependent lung can impair HPV.
- The presence of disease in the dependent lung can decrease blood flow redistribution, thereby decreasing the local HPV effect.
- Direct surgical manipulation can cause the release of vasoactive substances, such as thromboxane and prostacyclin, promoting local vasodilatation and blunting HPV, with a subsequent increase in shunt.
- Metabolic or respiratory acidosis and hypothermia are also associated with impairment of HPV.

Lumb AB, Slinger P. Hypoxic pulmonary vasoconstriction. Physiology and anesthetic implications. *Anesthesiology.* 2015;122:932-946.

Nakayama M, Murray PA. Ketamine preserves and propofol potentiates hypoxic pulmonary vasoconstriction compared with the conscious state in chronically instrumented dogs. *Anesthesiology.* 1999;91:760-771.

Shum S, Huang A, Slinger P. Hypoxaemia during one lung ventilation. *BJA Educ.* 2023;23:328-336.

C.15. Discuss pulmonary blood flow distribution, shunt flow, and $Pa{O_2}$ ($F{IO_2} = 1.0$) during OLV in the lateral position.

When the nondependent lung is collapsed, HPV will ultimately increase pulmonary vascular resistance and decrease lung blood flow to this lung. If no complicating factors exist, HPV should decrease blood flow by approximately 50%, causing a reduction from 40% to 20% of cardiac output. The resulting nondependent/dependent lung blood flow ratio during OLV should be 20%:80%.

Once atelectatic, blood flowing into the nonventilated lung is shunt flow. Therefore, OLV creates an obligatory right-to-left transpulmonary shunt that was not present during two-lung ventilation. During OLV, a total shunt flow of 20% would be expected, if no shunt existed during two-lung ventilation (ignoring the normal 1%-3% physiologic shunt from the bronchial, pleural, and thebesian circulation). $Pa{O_2}$ with a fractional inspired O_2 ratio ($F{IO_2}$) of 1 should be approximately 280 mm Hg if hemodynamic and metabolic states are normal. Clinically, $Pa{O_2}$ ($F{IO_2} = 1$) ranges from 150 to 250 mm Hg.

Lumb AB, Slinger P. Hypoxic pulmonary vasoconstriction. Physiology and anesthetic implications. *Anesthesiology*. 2015;122:932-946.

Marshall BE, Marshall C. Continuity of response to hypoxic pulmonary vasoconstriction. *J Appl Physiol*. 1980;59:189-196.

Shum S, Huang A, Slinger P. Hypoxaemia during one lung ventilation. *BJA Educ*. 2023;23:328-336.

C.16. What respiratory parameters will you target during OLV? How could you improve oxygenation during OLV?

Sao_2 greater than 90% to 92% is typically tolerated during OLV, and lung-protective strategies should be employed. Low tidal volume ventilation (eg, 4-6 mL/kg IBW during OLV) has been shown to decrease the risk of postoperative pulmonary complications without compromising intraoperative oxygenation. Optimal PEEP, including titration of PEEP to reduce driving pressure (plateau pressure—PEEP), is the subject of ongoing research. Peak inspiratory and plateau pressures should be maintained less than 30 and 20 cm H_2O, respectively. Relative hypercapnia ($Paco_2$ 40-60 mm Hg) is generally well tolerated and recommended to facilitate lung-protective ventilation.

When hypoxia occurs during OLV, the first goal is to optimize the match between ventilation and perfusion of the dependent lung first. If that is not effective, increasing the oxygen content of the shunted blood to the collapsed lung can be attempted. Methods to improve oxygenation include:

Ventilated Lung

a. Optimize ventilation:
   - Use 100% oxygen.
   - Check the position of the DLT with an FOB.
   - Ventilate manually to assess compliance and determine whether higher or lower tidal volumes or inspiratory pressures are beneficial.
   - Titrate ventilation to $Paco_2$ 40 to 60 mm Hg.
   - Apply 7 to 8 cm of PEEP, and titrate to achieve oxygenation and driving pressures (<20 cm H_2O).
   - Use intermittent two-lung ventilation.

b. Increase perfusion:
   - Selective vasodilators (inhaled nitric oxide, inhaled prostacyclin PGI_2).
   - Treat systemic hypotension (maintain mean arterial pressure [MAP] >65 mm Hg).

Collapsed Lung

a. Oxygenate shunt blood: A variety of approaches have been described but must be carefully considered for minimally invasive procedures since most involve some degree of lung reexpansion and, therefore, can affect surgical visualization.
   - Insufflate oxygen continuously: A flow of approximately 3 L/min allowed to freely circulate will often increase arterial oxygen saturation by 3% to 4% by apneic oxygenation.
   - Intermittent single breaths with oxygen.
   - Partially reexpand the nonventilated lung, then keep the DLT side closed.
   - Apply CPAP, but often leads to lung reinflation.
   - Differential CPAP to the collapsed lung and PEEP to the ventilated lung has been described but is rarely necessary and generally impractical for minimally invasive procedures.
   - Apply high-frequency ventilation to the nonventilated lung.

b. Decrease the shunt flow:
   - Use medications to augment HPV (phenylephrine, norepinephrine, almitrine).
   - Temporary clamp lobar vessels or the pulmonary artery of the nonventilated lung (rarely necessary).

Low tidal volume ventilation, in compliance with protective lung strategy and ERATS guidelines, can increase the need for the above maneuvers to maintain oxygen saturation and $Paco_2$ within acceptable ranges.

Brassard CL, Lohser J, Donati F, Bussières JS. Step-by-step clinical management of one-lung ventilation: continuing professional development. *Can J Anesth*. 2014;61:1103-1121.

Campos JH, Feider A. Hypoxia during one-lung ventilation-a review and update. *J Cardiothorac Vasc Anesth.* 2018;32:2330-2338.

Campos JH, Peacher D. Application of continuous positive airway pressure during video-assisted thoracoscopic surgery. *Curr Anesthesiol Rep. 2021*;11:446-456.

Park M, Yoon S, Nam JS et al. Driving pressure-guided ventilation and postoperative pulmonary complications in thoracic surgery: a multicentre randomised clinical trial. *Br J Anaesth.* 2023;130:e106-e118.

Peel JK, Funk DJ, Slinger P, et al. Tidal volume during 1-lung ventilation: a systematic review and meta-analysis. *J Thorac Cardiovasc Surg.* 2022;163:1573-1585.e1.

C.17. A right middle lobectomy was performed. Would you extubate the trachea at the end of the procedure?

After routine lung resection, the trachea can be extubated if the patient meets standard extubation criteria and has adequate analgesia; otherwise, postoperative mechanical support is indicated. The DLT may be exchanged to a single-lumen ETT or a supraglottic airway device prior to emergence to facilitate weaning; decrease airway edema and trauma if the DLT is left in place for prolonged periods; decrease the likelihood of dislodgment with patient movements; and improve mechanical pulmonary toilet. Spontaneous ventilation avoids the potential hazards of positive pressure on the suture lines of the new bronchial stump or parenchymal air leaks.

Hal MA, Raiten JM. Anesthetic management of post-thoracotomy complications. In: Slinger PD, ed. *Principle and Practice of Anesthesia for Thoracic Surgery*. Springer; 2019:885-923.

D. Postoperative Management

D.1. What are the immediate life-threatening complications that follow lobectomy or pneumonectomy?

Serious complications after lobectomy include lobar collapse, massive hemorrhage caused by loosening of pulmonary vessel ligatures, bronchopleural fistula from disruption of a bronchial stump, and pulmonary torsion and infarction resulting from increased mobility of the remaining lobe. Mediastinal shift, pleural effusion, hemothorax, chylothorax, empyema, and pulmonary edema can also occur. Deep venous thrombosis can lead to pulmonary embolism.

Pneumonectomy can be complicated by supraventricular arrhythmias, acute respiratory insufficiency, nerve injuries (phrenic, vagus, or recurrent laryngeal) during radical hilar dissection or excision of mediastinal tumors, cardiac herniation (in the case of intrapericardial approach), acute right heart failure, and right-to-left shunting across a patent foramen ovale due to increased pulmonary vascular resistance and increased right ventricular pressure. *Postpneumonectomy syndrome* is a rare complication characterized by mediastinal shift ipsilateral to the side of surgery with herniation of the hyperinflated lung in the same direction.

Fernandez FG, Kosinski AS, Furnary AP, et al. Differential effects of operative complications on survival after surgery for primary lung cancer. *J Thorac Cardiovasc Surg.* 2018;155:1254-1264.

Hal MA, Raiten JM. Anesthetic management of post-thoracotomy complications. In: Slinger PD, ed. *Principle and Practice of Anesthesia for Thoracic Surgery*. Springer; 2019:885-923.

Shelley B, Glass A, Keast T, et al. Perioperative cardiovascular pathophysiology in patients undergoing lung resection surgery: a narrative review. *Br J Anaesth.* 2023;130:E66-E79.

D.2. Why is it important to control postoperative pain? How would you achieve this?

Although minimally invasive lung resection can be less painful than thoracotomy, postoperative pain control remains essential. Adequate analgesia allows thoracic surgery patients to breathe deeply, cough effectively, and ambulate, helping to prevent pulmonary and nonpulmonary postoperative complications. Opioid use is independently associated with adverse outcomes after thoracic surgery, and opioid-sparing, multimodal analgesia approaches are emphasized in many enhanced recovery programs. Component strategies include thoracic epidural anesthesia (TEA), paravertebral blocks, and intercostal and chest wall blocks (eg, erector spinae and serratus plane blocks), as well as nonopioid systemic analgesics and transdermal agents (eg, lidocaine patches, capsaicin, transcutaneous electrical nerve stimulation [TENS]). Many of these analgesic techniques are also utilized for postthoracotomy pain, as described in Chapter 51: Perioperative Pain Management and Multimodal Pain Management.

Commonly used nonopioid analgesics include acetaminophen, nonsteroidal anti-inflammatory drugs (NSAIDs), and gabapentinoids. Although opioid sparing, NSAIDs can cause gastric bleeding, platelet dysfunction, and kidney injury in patients who are fluid restricted, especially the older adults. The analgesic benefits of gabapentin can be outweighed by its potential to cause sedation and respiratory depression, especially if administered with benzodiazepines.

Low-dose intravenous ketamine infusion (0.2 mg/kg/h) can be used as an adjuvant in the perioperative period, especially in patients with chronic pain. Psychotomimetic side effects are a possibility but are rare at this dose. Intravenous dexmedetomidine can be used intraoperatively to potentiate analgesia. The recommended dose is a continuous infusion of 0.2 to 0.7 μg/kg/h without loading. Its central α_2-agonism potentiates analgesia, allowing a decrease in the dose of intravenous opioids, and decreases the minimal alveolar concentration (MAC) of general anesthesia. Hypotension and bradycardia are potential side effects, as well as sedation. Lidocaine infusion (1.5-3 mg/kg/h) can also be used as an adjuvant. Despite the concern of systemic toxicity, such events appear rare. Intravenous lidocaine infusion should be considered as an alternative when neuraxial blockade is contraindicated.

Batchelor TJP, Rasburn NJ, Abdelnour-Bertchtold E, et al. Guidelines for enhanced recovery after lung surgery: recommendations of the Enhanced Recovery After Surgery (ERAS) Society and the European Society of Thoracic Surgeons (ESTS). *Eur J Cardiothorac Surg*. 2019;55:91-115.

Campos JH, Peacher D. Choosing the best method for postoperative regional analgesia after video-assisted thoracoscopic surgery. *J Cardiothorac Vasc Anesth*. 2020;34:1877-1880.

Hamilton C, Alfille P, Mountjoy J, Bao X. Regional anesthesia and acute perioperative pain management in thoracic surgery: a narrative review. *J Thorac Dis*. 2022;14:2276-2296.

3 Aspiration and Postoperative Respiratory Failure

Di Pan, Kristin Berger, and Edward J. Schenck

A 62-year-old female presents to the emergency department with small bowel obstruction. She is vomiting and hypotensive and appears to aspirate. Her trachea is emergently intubated, and she is fluid resuscitated and brought to the operating room for emergency laparotomy.

A. Aspiration

1. What are the risk factors for perioperative aspiration?
2. How does large-volume aspiration affect the respiratory system?
3. How should you manage the patient after an aspiration event?
4. How would you prevent aspiration during emergency surgery?

B. Postoperative Respiratory Failure

After successful lysis of abdominal adhesions, the patient recovers well and is extubated at the completion of surgery. Subsequently, she develops progressive hypoxemic respiratory failure while in the postanesthesia care unit.

1. How can you predict which patients will develop postoperative respiratory failure?
2. How can intraoperative anesthesia management prevent respiratory failure?
3. What is the pathogenesis of postoperative respiratory failure?
4. What is the diagnostic approach to postoperative respiratory failure?

C. Indications for Ventilator Support

The patient has worsening hypoxemia and tachypnea despite treatment with high-flow supplemental oxygen.

1. What are the indications for noninvasive positive pressure ventilation (NIPPV)?
2. What are the indications for emergency endotracheal intubation?

D. Acute Respiratory Distress Syndrome

The patient's trachea is intubated for respiratory failure. She has bilateral pulmonary infiltrates on the chest radiograph and is severely hypoxemic.

1. What is the definition and etiology of acute respiratory distress syndrome (ARDS)?
2. Explain the pathophysiology of ARDS.
3. What role does ventilator-induced lung injury (VILI) play in ARDS?

E. Management of Mechanical Ventilation

1. Which mode of mechanical ventilation will you choose? Describe the features of that mode.
2. How should you set the fraction of inspired oxygen (FIO_2)?
3. How should you set positive end-expiratory pressure (PEEP)?
4. What tidal volume and inspiratory pressure target should you set?

F. Management of Refractory Respiratory Failure

The patient remains hypoxemic on FIO_2 of 0.8.

1. What else can promote additional lung recruitment?
2. What rescue strategies can you use for refractory ARDS?

G. Adjunctive Management of Respiratory Failure

Since tracheal intubation, the patient has become hypotensive.

1. What is the cause and treatment of the hemodynamic instability associated with mechanical ventilation?
2. What is the adjunctive medical therapy for ARDS?

H. Weaning From Mechanical Ventilation

The patient slowly recovers over the next 3 days.

1. Explain the importance of the decision to extubate the patient or continue mechanical ventilation.
2. How will you prepare the patient for weaning from the ventilator?
3. How will you recognize when the patient is ready for tracheal extubation?

A. Aspiration

A.1. What are the risk factors for perioperative aspiration?

Aspiration is defined by the entry or inhalation of foreign materials, including solid foods, liquids, and gastric contents, into the airway. It can be categorized into micro-aspiration (small quantities, considered normal) or macro-aspirations (larger volume, more clinically significant). Perioperative aspiration is typically macro-aspiration.

Perioperative aspiration is a relatively rare complication of anesthesia. The reported incidence is 1 to 5 per 10,000 patients, and about half of the cases occur during induction of anesthesia. The incidence of aspiration is higher in emergency surgeries compared to elective procedures. Additionally, a difficult or failed intubation is associated with higher rates. Risk factors for perioperative aspiration are related to abnormalities of the gastrointestinal and airway anatomy and physiology, and alterations in protective airway mechanisms governed by the nervous system. Therefore, risk factors for aspiration include the full stomach, pregnancy, bowel obstruction, gastroesophageal reflux, obesity, gastrointestinal motility disorders including diabetes, neurologic conditions, and medications such as glucagon-like peptide-1 (GLP-1) agonists.

During anesthesia, the risk of aspiration can be increased by airway manipulation in an unfasted patient or an inadequate depth of anesthesia. Additionally, many anesthetics reduce lower and upper esophageal sphincter tone and diminish protective airway reflexes. However, the appropriate use of a laryngeal mask airway does not increase the risk of aspiration, although it can induce gastroesophageal reflux. Certain surgical procedures such as laparoscopic insufflation of the abdomen and bowel manipulation are associated with increased rates of aspiration.

GLP-1 agonists, such as semaglutide and liraglutide, are increasingly used for treating patients with diabetes and for weight loss. Use of GLP-1 agonists can lead to gastroparesis. In an observational study based on health claims data, which included patients prescribed semaglutide (n = 613), liraglutide (n = 4,144), or bupropion-naltrexone (n = 654) for weight loss, GLP-1 agonists were associated with an increased risk of gastroparesis compared to bupropion-naltrexone (Hazard Ratio 3.67 [95% CI, 1.15-11.90]).

Kluger MT, Short TG. Aspiration during anaesthesia: a review of 133 cases from the Australian Anaesthetic Incident Monitoring Study (AIMS). *Anaesthesia.* 1999;54:19-26.

Mandell LA, Niederman MS. Aspiration pneumonia. *N Engl J Med.* 2019;380:651-663.

Mort TC. Emergency tracheal intubation: complications associated with repeated laryngoscopic attempts. *Anesth Analg.* 2004;99:607-613.

Nason KS. Acute intraoperative pulmonary aspiration. *Thorac Surg Clin.* 2015;25:301-307.

Ng A, Smith G. Gastroesophageal reflux and aspiration of gastric contents in anesthetic practice. *Anesth Analg.* 2001;93:494-513.

Smith G, Ng A. Gastric reflux and pulmonary aspiration in anaesthesia. *Minerva Anestesiol.* 2003;69:402-406.

Sodhi M, Rezaeianzadeh R, Kezouh A, Etminan M. Risk of gastrointestinal adverse events associated with glucagon-like peptide-1 receptor agonists for weight loss. *JAMA.* 2023:e2319574.

Xiao MZ, Englesakis M, Perlas A. Gastric content and perioperative pulmonary aspiration in patients with diabetes mellitus: a scoping review. *Br J Anaesth.* 2021;127:224-235.

A.2. How does large-volume aspiration affect the respiratory system?

Aspiration of gastric and oropharyngeal contents causes three overlapping syndromes. First, aspiration of large particulate matter may obstruct the airways and lead to asphyxiation and atelectasis. Acute aspiration pneumonitis is more common and is a result of chemical damage to the tracheobronchial tree and pulmonary parenchyma by gastric and oral fluids. Finally, aspiration of bacteria from the oropharynx or superinfection of the chemical pneumonitis can result in aspiration pneumonia.

Aspiration pneumonitis was originally described by Mendelson in 1946 based on a study of 66 obstetrical patients who had aspirated gastric contents during anesthesia. Signs and symptoms range from mild (cough, fever) to severe and rapidly fatal (wheezing, hypoxic respiratory failure). While most patients improve within a short period of time, about 16.5% progress to severe pneumonitis despite initially improving. The risk of severe pneumonitis can increase in the presence of other existing systemic risk factors such as trauma, shock, or pancreatitis. The volume and pH of the aspirated fluid also play a role in the degree of lung injury. In adults, approximately 25 mL of gastric acid with a pH less than 2.5 is a clinically relevant threat for progression to severe pneumonitis.

Severe cases of aspiration pneumonitis can be characterized by radiographic findings of diffuse bilateral infiltrates typical of ARDS. Pathologically, atelectasis, peribronchial hemorrhage, pulmonary edema, and degeneration of bronchial epithelial cells occur. Subsequently, the alveoli fill with polymorphonuclear leukocytes fibrin and form hyaline membranes. The lungs become grossly edematous and hemorrhagic with alveolar consolidation.

Finally, aspiration pneumonia can result from a superimposed infection of the chemical injury or inhalation of microorganisms from the oropharynx. Poor dentition increases the risk of developing aspiration pneumonia. In community-dwelling adults, the most common organisms associated with aspiration pneumonia include *Haemophilus influenzae* and streptococcus species. In certain populations, such as those who are chronically ill or had recent hospitalizations or antibiotic exposure, the oral flora can become colonized by drug-resistant organisms. These include gram-negative bacteria such as *Pseudomonas aeruginosa*, and gram-positive bacteria such as methicillin-resistant *Staphylococcus aureus* (MRSA). These resistant organisms can further complicate the pneumonia, making treatment more difficult.

James CF, Modell JH, Gibbs CP, et al. Pulmonary aspiration—effects of volume and pH in the rat. *Anesth Analg.* 1984;63:665-668.

Mandell LA, Niederman MS. Aspiration pneumonia. *N Engl J Med.* 2019;380:651-663.

Mendelson CL. The aspiration of stomach contents into the lungs during obstetric anesthesia. *Am J Obstet Gynecol.* 1946;52:191-205.

Pan D, Niederman MS. Risk factors and algorithms for the empirical treatment of hospital-acquired pneumonia and ventilator-associated pneumonia. *Semin Respir Crit Care Med.* 2022;43:183-190.

Pan D, Nielsen E, Chung S, Niederman MS. Management of pneumonia in the critically ill. *Minerva Med.* 2023;114:667-682.

Warner MA, Warner ME, Weber JG. Clinical significance of pulmonary aspiration during the perioperative period. *Anesthesiology.* 1993;78:56-62.

A.3. How should you manage the patient after an aspiration event?

Awake patients capable of airway protection should be placed in the upright or recovery position and encouraged to cough. However, clinicians may need to suction or rescue the airway if the patient has impaired protective airway reflexes. Supplemental oxygen should be administered for hypoxemia. Clinicians should avoid noninvasive ventilation because of the risk of gastric insufflation unless there is no further risk of additional vomiting. When possible, the stomach should be emptied with a nasogastric tube. There is no evidence supporting lavage with saline or sodium bicarbonate. Gastric acid is rapidly neutralized by the physiologic response. A chest radiograph should be ordered. In select circumstances, bronchoscopy is necessary for airway clearance and evaluation especially if airway obstruction is suspected. Bronchoscopy can provide quantitative lower respiratory tract cultures from bronchoalveolar lavage or protected brushings. These techniques can distinguish aspiration pneumonitis from pneumonia.

Although some animal studies support the use of corticosteroids in aspiration pneumonitis, there is no evidence of benefit in human studies. Literature does not support the use of antibiotics immediately after aspiration. In mild-to-moderate cases, it is generally recommended to withhold antibiotics, even with radiographic abnormalities, and instead closely monitor the patient for up to 48 hours. Antibiotics are reserved for specific situations such as bowel obstruction, use of gastric acid–suppressing agents, or in severe cases with worsening or persistent respiratory failure and a higher risk of complications.

The choice of antibiotics for treating aspiration pneumonia depends on risk factors for multidrug-resistant organisms (MDROs). These risk factors include recent hospitalization or antibiotic exposure within 90 days for a minimum duration of 5 days. For individuals with minimal MDRO risk, treatment with a broad-spectrum β-lactam or cephalosporin in combination with a macrolide or fluoroquinolone monotherapy is typically sufficient.

In patients with MDRO risk factors, additional coverage for *Pseudomonas aeruginosa* and MRSA should be considered. When there is high suspicion of anaerobic infection, such as with poor dental hygiene, lower gastrointestinal tract obstruction, or in the setting of pulmonary abscess and necrotizing pneumonia, anaerobic coverage with metronidazole or clindamycin can be considered.

Allewelt M, Schüler P, Bölcskei PL, et al. Ampicillin + sulbactam vs clindamycin +/− cephalosporin for the treatment of aspiration pneumonia and primary lung abscess. *Clin Microbiol Infect.* 2004;10:163-170.

d'Escrivan T, Guery B. Prevention and treatment of aspiration pneumonia in intensive care units. *Treat Respir Med.* 2005;4:317-324.

Downs JB, Chapman RL Jr, Modell JH, et al. An evaluation of steroid therapy in aspiration pneumonitis. *Anesthesiology.* 1974;40:129-135.

Dragan V, Wei Y, Elligsen M, et al. Prophylactic antimicrobial therapy for acute aspiration pneumonitis. *Clin Infect Dis.* 2018;67:513-518.

Dudley WR, Marshall BE. Steroid treatment for acid-aspiration pneumonitis. *Anesthesiology.* 1974;40:136-141.

Ott SR, Allewelt M, Lorenz J, et al. Moxifloxacin vs ampicillin/sulbactam in aspiration pneumonia and primary lung abscess. *Infection.* 2008;36:23-30.

Pan D, Niederman MS. Risk factors and algorithms for the empirical treatment of hospital-acquired pneumonia and ventilator-associated pneumonia. *Semin Respir Crit Care Med.* 2022;43:183-190.

van Westerloo DJ, Knapp S, van't Veer C, et al. Aspiration pneumonitis primes the host for an exaggerated inflammatory response during pneumonia. *Crit Care Med.* 2005;33:1770-1778.

A.4. How would you prevent aspiration during emergency surgery?

Certain measures can help reduce the risk of perioperative aspiration. These include adequate fasting, prophylactic antiemetics, rapid sequence intubation (RSI), limited tidal volumes if bag ventilation is used, and extubation when the patient's laryngeal reflexes have returned. Antacid medications can increase gastric pH; however, their use is only supported by expert opinion.

The American Society of Anesthesiologists (ASA) released consensus guidance recognizing the increased risk of gastroparesis and perioperative aspiration associated with GLP-1 agonist medications. It is recommended that patients taking a GLP-1 agonist should withhold this medication for at least 1 week prior to the scheduled procedure.

In patients who require emergency procedures and preventive measures cannot be applied, gastric ultrasound can be utilized to visualize the presence of solid gastric contents, especially in patients taking GLP-1 agonists. This will help risk stratify patients prior to undergoing anesthesia, and additional measures such as the insertion of nasogastric tubes prior to anesthesia can be considered.

RSI involves preoxygenation followed by tracheal intubation using an induction agent and neuromuscular blockade without face-mask ventilation. RSI has been shown to decrease the time to achieve successful intubation, which can be beneficial when the risk of aspiration is high. Moreover, traditional RSI with a hypnotic followed by a neuromuscular blocking agent led to lower rates of complications, including aspiration, compared to a combination of a hypnotic plus remifentanil. The value of cricoid pressure during intubation remains controversial. A recent randomized trial did not demonstrate a reduction in aspiration with cricoid pressure but did note an increased intubation time when cricoid pressure was applied. Differing apneic oxygenation techniques such as high-flow nasal canula have not been shown to decrease the risk of aspiration.

Birenbaum A, Hajage D, Roche S, et al. Effect of cricoid pressure compared with a sham procedure in the rapid sequence induction of anesthesia: the IRIS randomized clinical trial. *JAMA Surg.* 2019;154:9-17.

Grillot N, Lebuffe G, Huet O, et al. Effect of remifentanil vs neuromuscular blockers during rapid sequence intubation on successful intubation without major complications among patients at risk of aspiration: a randomized clinical trial. *JAMA.* 2023;329:28-38.

Neilipovitz DT, Crosby ET. No evidence for decreased incidence of aspiration after rapid sequence induction. *Can J Anaesth.* 2007;54:748-764.

Ng A, Smith G. Gastroesophageal reflux and aspiration of gastric contents in anesthetic practice. *Anesth Analg.* 2001;93:494-513.

Sherwin M, Hamburger J, Katz D, DeMaria S Jr. Influence of semaglutide use on the presence of residual gastric solids on gastric ultrasound: a prospective observational study in volunteers without obesity recently started on semaglutide. *Can J Anaesth.* 2023;70:1300-1306.

Ushakumari DS, Sladen RN. ASA Consensus-based guidance on preoperative management of patients on glucagon-like peptide-1 receptor agonists. *Anesthesiology.* 2024;140:346-348.

Wallace C, McGuire B. Rapid sequence induction: its place in modern anaesthesia. *Contin Educ Anaesth Crit Care Pain.* 2013;14:130-135.

White LD, Vlok RA, Thang CY, Tian DH, Melhuish TM. Oxygenation during the apnoeic phase preceding intubation in adults in prehospital, emergency department, intensive care and operating theatre environments. *Cochrane Database Syst Rev.* 2023;8:CD013558.

B. Postoperative Respiratory Failure

After successful lysis of abdominal adhesions, the patient recovers well, and her trachea is extubated at the completion of surgery. Subsequently, she develops progressive hypoxemic respiratory failure while in the postanesthesia care unit.

B.1. How can you predict which patients will develop postoperative respiratory failure?

Respiratory failure commonly complicates the postoperative period and is strongly associated with increased mortality. A number of clinical prediction rules exist to predict the risk of postoperative pulmonary complications. Predisposing factors include a high ASA physical status classification, weight loss, extremes of body mass index, prolonged recent hospitalization, poor functional status, and hypoalbuminemia. Lung diseases such as obstructive airway dysfunction and recent respiratory infections; extrapulmonary diseases such as diabetes, liver cirrhosis, congestive heart failure, and renal failure; and current or former smoking status also predispose patients to respiratory failure. Additional risk factors include emergency indications for surgery, prolonged procedural time, and the requirement for large-volume fluid and blood product resuscitation. Intraoperative ventilatory mechanics including higher peak pressures and poor compliance are risk factors for postoperative respiratory failure. Because of their effects on respiratory mechanics, thoracoabdominal surgeries, especially aortic aneurysm repair, are particularly high-risk procedures.

Canet J, Gallart L, Gomar C, et al. Prediction of postoperative pulmonary complications in a population-based surgical cohort. *Anesthesiology*. 2010;113:1338-1350.

Fernandez-Bustamante A, Frendl G, Sprung J, et al. Postoperative pulmonary complications, early mortality, and hospital stay following noncardiothoracic surgery: a multicenter study by the Perioperative Research Network Investigators. *JAMA Surg*. 2017;152:157-166.

Schmid M, Sood A, Campbell L, et al. Impact of smoking on perioperative outcomes after major surgery. *Am J Surg*. 2015;210:221.e6-229.e6.

Serpa Neto A, Hemmes SN, Barbas CS, et al. Incidence of mortality and morbidity related to postoperative lung injury in patients who have undergone abdominal or thoracic surgery: a systematic review and meta-analysis. *Lancet Respir Med*. 2014;2:1007-1015.

Stocking JC, Drake C, Aldrich JM, et al. Outcomes and risk factors for delayed-onset postoperative respiratory failure: a multi-center case-control study by the University of California Critical Care Research Collaborative (UC3RC). *BMC Anesthesiol*. 2022;22:146.

Suleiman A, Costa E, Santer P, et al. Association between intraoperative tidal volume and postoperative respiratory complications is dependent on respiratory elastance: a retrospective, multicentre cohort study. *Br J Anaesth*. 2022;129:263-272.

B.2. How can intraoperative anesthesia management prevent respiratory failure?

An extensive literature has evaluated the role of limiting tidal volumes to prevent VILI. Observational studies have shown that ventilation with tidal volumes greater than 8 mL/kg ideal body weight (IBW) is a risk factor for postoperative pulmonary complications. These findings were supported by a randomized controlled trial that showed that restricted tidal volumes from 6 to 8 mL/kg IBW led to a decreased incidence of postoperative respiratory failure in major abdominal surgery. This trial was criticized because it included PEEP in the intervention group compared to no-PEEP and higher tidal volumes in the control group. A more recent single-center randomized controlled trial compared patients undergoing major noncardiothoracic surgery randomized to 6 mL/kg IBW to 10 mL/kg IBW with standard PEEP of 5 cm H_2O. This trial did not show reduction in postoperative respiratory failure in the lower tidal volume group, but the lower tidal volume strategy was well tolerated. Despite the conflicting evidence, the current data support targeting tidal volumes to less than 8 mL/kg IBW. However, there might be situations where lower tidal volumes are inadequate or poorly tolerated. For example, observational data suggest that the relationship between higher tidal volume and postoperative outcomes is modulated by lower lung compliance. In patients with normal or higher lung compliance and low driving pressure ($<$14 cm H_2O), higher volumes are not associated with poor outcomes. Driving pressure is calculated as the plateau pressure minus the PEEP. The driving pressure is a factor of both the tidal volume and the static compliance of the respiratory system. A high driving pressure ($>$15 cm H_2O) is associated with an increased risk of postoperative pulmonary complications. Observing the effect of ventilator settings, such as PEEP, on driving pressure can be a useful strategy. However, early prospective studies have not demonstrated a benefit in populations with normal compliance.

The optimal intraoperative PEEP is less clear. Beyond strong evidence that a no-PEEP approach should be avoided, several randomized trials during high-risk abdominal surgery did not demonstrate a benefit from high PEEP and recruitment maneuvers compared to moderate PEEP. Current evidence supports the use of moderate PEEP (~5 cm H_2O) during surgery in patients at risk of atelectasis and higher PEEP and recruitment maneuvers when the patient's physiology suggests derecruitment.

Bluth T, Serpa Neto A, Schultz M, et al. Effect of intraoperative high positive end-expiratory pressure (PEEP) with recruitment maneuvers vs low PEEP on postoperative pulmonary complications in obese patients: a randomized clinical trial. *JAMA*. 2019;321:2292-2305.

Cypel M, Fan E. Lung injury after abdominal and thoracic surgery. *Lancet Respir Med*. 2014;2:949-950.

Futier E, Constantin JM, Paugam-Burtz C, et al. A trial of intraoperative low-tidal-volume ventilation in abdominal surgery. *N Engl J Med*. 2013;369:428-437.

Hemmes SN, Gama de Abreu M, Pelosi P, et al. High versus low positive end-expiratory pressure during general anaesthesia for open abdominal surgery (PROVHILO trial): a multicentre randomised controlled trial. *Lancet*. 2014;384:495-503.

Karalapillai D, Weinberg L, Peyton P, et al. Effect of intraoperative low tidal volume vs conventional tidal volume on postoperative pulmonary complications in patients undergoing major surgery: a randomized clinical trial. *JAMA*. 2020;324:848-858.

Neto AS, Hemmes SN, Barbas CS, et al. Association between driving pressure and development of postoperative pulmonary complications in patients undergoing mechanical ventilation for general anaesthesia: a meta-analysis of individual patient data. *Lancet Respir Med*. 2016;4:272-280.

Park M, Yoon S, Nam JS, et al. Driving pressure-guided ventilation and postoperative pulmonary complications in thoracic surgery: a multicentre randomised clinical trial. *Br J Anaesth*. 2023;130:e106-e118.

Serpa Neto A, Hemmes SN, Barbas CS, et al. Incidence of mortality and morbidity related to postoperative lung injury in patients who have undergone abdominal or thoracic surgery: a systematic review and meta-analysis. *Lancet Respir Med*. 2014;2:1007-1015.

Suleiman A, Costa E, Santer P, et al. Association between intraoperative tidal volume and postoperative respiratory complications is dependent on respiratory elastance: a retrospective, multicentre cohort study. *Br J Anaesth*. 2022;129:263-272.

B.3. What is the pathogenesis of postoperative respiratory failure?

Numerous mechanisms contribute to the pathogenesis of postoperative respiratory failure (**Figure 3.1**). A combination of postoperative pain, recumbent position, anesthetics, and impaired secretion clearance leads to the collapse of dependent lung regions. Atelectasis increases shunt fraction, diminishes respiratory system compliance, and commonly contributes to postoperative respiratory insufficiency. Beyond mechanical compromise, the inflammatory effects of surgery, mechanical ventilation, and general anesthesia have also been implicated in postoperative respiratory failure.

Treating postoperative patients with high concentrations of inspired oxygen can lead to absorption atelectasis. Normally, the consumption of oxygen by peripheral tissues creates a small gradient between the gas tensions in the alveoli and pulmonary capillary blood. The gradient is normally small compared to the total gas tensions because nitrogen is the most abundant gas in both compartments. Nitrogen acts as a pneumatic splint in the lung by limiting the magnitude of the gas tension gradient between the alveoli and pulmonary capillaries. Breathing high FIO_2 denitrogenates the body and increases the partial pressure of oxygen in alveolar gas much more than in mixed venous blood. Without nitrogen, venous blood becomes hypobaric relative to alveolar gas. Therefore, high FIO_2 increases the gas tension gradient, which drives gas from the alveoli to the pulmonary capillary blood and promotes the collapse of poorly ventilated alveoli (**Figure 3.2**).

In the postoperative period, bronchospasm and impaired mucociliary clearance can decrease the rate of expiratory airflow and increase the work of breathing. Residual sedation and neuromuscular blockade can impair respiratory muscle function and diminish protective muscle tone in the upper airway. In addition to direct pulmonary causes of respiratory compromise, circulatory failure can cause acidosis and hypoperfusion of respiratory muscles, leading to respiratory failure. In particular, clinicians should consider the diagnosis of occult hemorrhage in any postoperative patient who develops respiratory failure. However, the clinician must also consider the opposite problem of hydrostatic pulmonary edema. Fluid accumulation in the lungs, chest wall, pleura, and peritoneum is a common problem and can increase shunt, decrease respiratory compliance, and worsen gas exchange. Additionally, acute pulmonary embolism can cause shock and respiratory failure and is more common in the postoperative period.

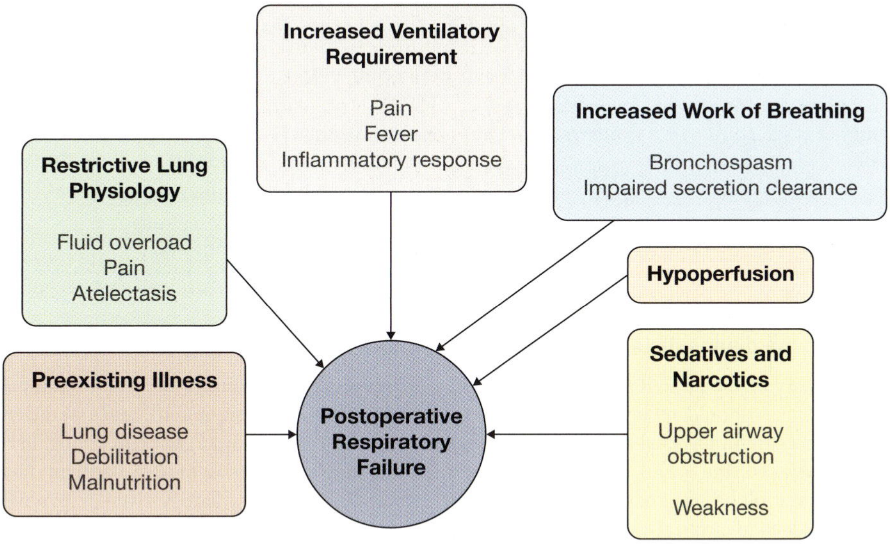

FIGURE 3.1. Pathogenesis of postoperative respiratory failure.

The systemic inflammatory response to major surgery or an acute illness increases tissue oxygen consumption and carbon dioxide (CO_2) production. The increased ventilatory requirement can impose an unsustainable burden on a respiratory system impaired by the aforementioned factors. This is especially true in the setting of frailty, malnutrition, and chronic lung disease.

Aubier M, Trippenbach T, Roussos C. Respiratory muscle fatigue during cardiogenic shock. *J Appl Physiol Respir Environ Exerc Physiol*. 1981;51:499-508.

Miskovic A, Lumb AB. Postoperative pulmonary complications. *Br J Anaesth*. 2017;118:317-334.

West JB, Luks AM. Ventilation-perfusion relationships. In: West JB, Luks AM, eds. *West's Respiratory Physiology—The Essentials*. 11th ed. Wolters Kluwer; 2021.

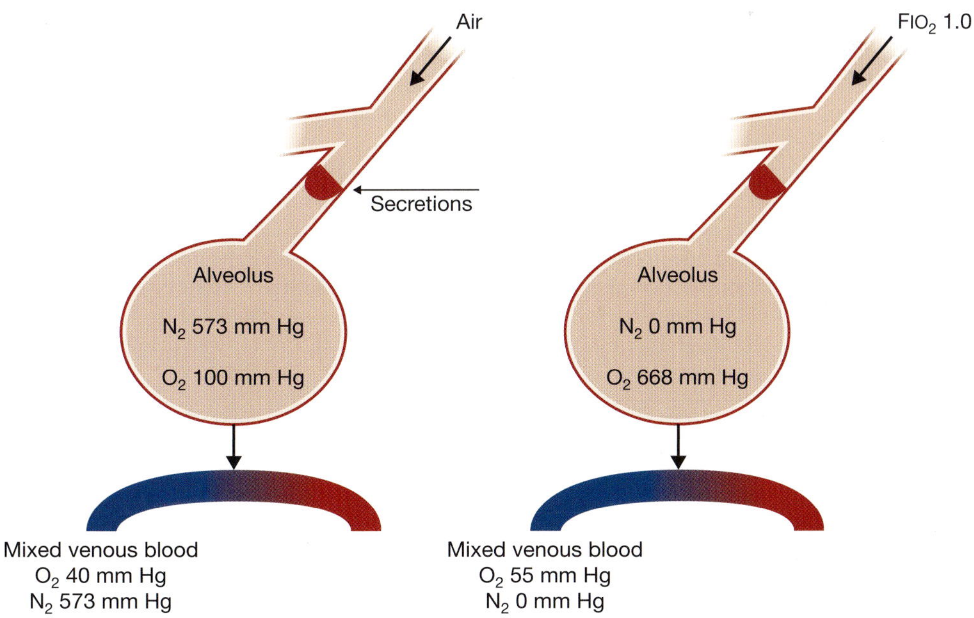

FIGURE 3.2. Nitrogen (N_2) content of inspired air prevents alveolar collapse. On the left, secretions obstruct the airway while the patient is breathing room air. There is a small oxygen (O_2) gradient between alveoli and mixed venous blood. On the right, secretions obstruct the airway after denitrogenation. As a result, mixed venous blood O_2 is hypobaric compared with the alveolus. Alveoli will tend to collapse as O_2 rapidly diffuses down its pressure gradient. CO_2 and H_2O have been omitted for simplicity. (Adapted from West JB, Luks AM. Respiratory system under stress. In: West JB, Luks AM, eds. *West's Respiratory Physiology—The Essentials*. 11th ed. Wolters Kluwer; 2021:172-194. Figure 9.4.)

TABLE 3.1 Differential Diagnosis of Postoperative Respiratory Failure

Aspiration pneumonitis	Atelectasis	Pneumonia	Bleeding and shock	Pleural effusions	Pulmonary embolism
Exacerbation of obstructive sleep apnea	Wound infections	Upper airway obstruction	Neuromuscular weakness	Exacerbation of underlying lung disorder	Pulmonary edema
	Abdominal compartment syndrome	Diaphragmatic palsy from scalene nerve block		Acute respiratory distress syndrome	

B.4. What is the diagnostic approach to postoperative respiratory failure?

The history of the patient's illness provides key evidence for determining the cause of respiratory failure. The clinician should review the past medical history, the anesthesia record, and operative reports, and perform a careful physical examination. Integration of these data should generate a short list of diagnostic possibilities (**Table 3.1**). Laboratory and radiologic testing can help exclude or confirm diagnoses.

Arterial blood gas analysis can help triage disease severity and identify alveolar hypoventilation, increased alveolar-arterial oxygen gradient, and acid-base status. Additional labs including complete blood count, metabolic profile, and coagulation parameters are an important part of the early evaluation. Chest radiography is an essential part of the diagnostic approach to respiratory failure. However, their interobserver variability is high, and their diagnostic accuracy is limited in acute respiratory failure.

Point-of-care diagnostic ultrasound can aid in the diagnosis of acute respiratory failure (**Table 3.2**). In critically ill patients, pulmonary ultrasound in the hands of a trained operator is superior to chest radiography in identifying pneumothorax, consolidation, pleural effusion, and lung edema. The use of basic bedside echocardiography to identify right or left heart dysfunction can improve diagnostic accuracy. This approach can help distinguish cardiogenic from noncardiogenic causes of pulmonary edema and raise the suspicion for pulmonary embolism. Ultrasonography, like all clinical skills, requires expert training.

Pulmonary emboli (PE) are common in the postoperative period. PE causes tachycardia, tachypnea, and mild hypoxemia. Ultrasonographic findings of smaller PE include normal aeration patterns (A-lines). The presence of right heart dilation or strain can be suggestive of a large PE that can cause shock, but a normal right heart exam does not exclude a smaller PE. An abrupt increase in arterial to end-tidal Pco_2 gradient can be a sign of increased alveolar dead space due to PE. If a clinician suspects PE, computed tomography (CT) angiography is the best test. Ventilation-perfusion scintigraphy is an alternative if CT angiography cannot be performed. Given the high case fatality rate of untreated PE, therapeutic anticoagulation is indicated when PE is strongly suspected or confirmed. Clinicians must carefully consider the risk of bleeding from surgery or neuraxial anesthesia sites.

Pneumonia is the most important postoperative infection. Surgery, hospitalization, and illness alter the host's bacterial flora and lead to pneumonia with antibiotic-resistant organisms. A chest radiograph, arterial blood gas analysis, and blood cultures should be obtained in all patients suspected of having health care–associated pneumonia. In the case of ventilator-associated pneumonia, clinical diagnosis can be inaccurate without the assistance of microbiologic data. Quantitative cultures of the lower respiratory tract obtained from bronchoalveolar lavage or protected brushings can assist in the diagnosis. The role of procalcitonin as a diagnostic tool for postoperative pneumonia is not well defined, as the physiologic stress of surgery can increase the level of procalcitonin without an infection.

American Thoracic Society, Infectious Diseases Society of America. Guidelines for the management of adults with hospital-acquired, ventilator-associated, and healthcare-associated pneumonia. *Am J Respir Crit Care Med.* 2005;171:388-416.

TABLE 3.2 Pulmonary Ultrasound Findings

Sliding lung (rules out pneumothorax)	Consolidation	A-lines (normal finding)
Lung point (rules in pneumothorax)	B-lines (interstitial edema)	Pleural effusion
Diaphragm movement (rules out diaphragmatic palsy)		

Bataille B, Riu B, Ferre F, et al. Integrated use of bedside lung ultrasound and echocardiography in acute respiratory failure: a prospective observational study in ICU. *Chest*. 2014;146:1586-1593.

Hemnes AR, Newman AL, Rosenbaum B, et al. Bedside end-tidal CO_2 tension as a screening tool to exclude pulmonary embolism. *Eur Respir J*. 2010;35:735-741.

Kearon C, Akl EA, Comerota AJ, et al. Antithrombotic therapy for VTE disease: Antithrombotic Therapy and Prevention of Thrombosis, 9th ed: American College of Chest Physicians evidence-based clinical practice guidelines. *Chest*. 2012;141:e419S-e496S.

Lichtenstein DA, Mezière GA. Relevance of lung ultrasound in the diagnosis of acute respiratory failure: the BLUE protocol. *Chest*. 2008;134:117-125.

Pepper DJ, Sun J, Rhee C, et al. Procalcitonin-guided antibiotic discontinuation and mortality in critically ill adults: a systematic review and meta-analysis. *Chest*. 2019;155:1109-1118.

van Belle A, Büller HR, Huisman MV, et al. Effectiveness of managing suspected pulmonary embolism using an algorithm combining clinical probability, D-dimer testing, and computed tomography. *JAMA*. 2006;295:172-179.

Xirouchaki N, Magkanas E, Vaporidi K, et al. Lung ultrasound in critically ill patients: comparison with bedside chest radiography. *Intensive Care Med*. 2011;37:1488-1493.

C. Indications for Ventilator Support

The patient has worsening hypoxemia and tachypnea despite treatment with high-flow supplemental oxygen.

C.1. What are the indications for noninvasive positive pressure ventilation (NIPPV)?

NIPPV may be an alternative to tracheal intubation in some situations. NIPPV can deliver high flow rates of oxygen, maintain PEEP, stent open the upper airway, and reduce the work of breathing. Careful patient selection and recognition of contraindications to its use are essential. In this patient, vomiting due to bowel obstruction is likely a contraindication to a trial of noninvasive ventilation (**Table 3.3**). Generally, the etiology of the respiratory failure and the type of mask interface are more important determinants of treatment success than the mode of NIPPV. Classical, clinical indications for NIPPV are acute cardiogenic pulmonary edema, obstructive sleep apnea, and exacerbations of chronic obstructive pulmonary disease (COPD). In cardiogenic pulmonary edema, the application of positive pressure can markedly reduce left ventricular preload and afterload. Bilevel positive airway pressure, where the inspiratory airway pressure delivered is higher than the expiratory airway pressure, and continuous positive airway pressure (CPAP) modes are both effective in cardiogenic pulmonary edema. In hypoxemic respiratory failure not due to cardiogenic pulmonary edema, use of NIPPV should be individualized as evidence for its benefit is conflicting, as shown in meta-analyses that excluded patients with pulmonary edema and COPD exacerbations. Randomized clinical trials have supported the use of NIPPV in the perioperative period. This supports the compelling physiologic rationale for the use of noninvasive ventilation for respiratory failure in the perioperative period, which is often due to neuromuscular weakness and the residual effects of anesthesia.

TABLE 3.3 Use of Noninvasive Positive Pressure Ventilation in Acute Respiratory Failure

Indications	Contraindications
Increased dyspnea	Respiratory arrest
Tachypnea	Unable to fit/wear mask
Excessive work of breathing	Progressive shock
Hypoventilation	Multiorgan dysfunction
Obstructive sleep apnea	Poor airway protection
Hypercapnia	Recent upper airway or gastrointestinal surgery
Hypoxemia	No patient cooperation
	Progressive and severe clinical instability
	Vomiting/hematemesis

Adapted from Nava S, Hill N. Non-invasive ventilation in acute respiratory failure. *Lancet*. 2009;374:250-259. Copyright © 2009 Elsevier. With permission.

The use of NIPPV in patients is more effective for the treatment of hypoxemic respiratory failure than standard oxygen therapy. The use of NIPPV also reduces atelectasis and the need for tracheal intubation with an overall mortality benefit. However, clinicians must exercise caution when using NIPPV for acute hypoxemic respiratory failure. Although it can help avoid intubation in some situations, about half of patients treated with NIPPV for ARDS or pneumonia ultimately require intubation. Patients with multiorgan dysfunction and shock are more likely to require intubation. In the subset of patients who fail NIPPV and require treatment with intubation, the rates of morbidity and mortality are high. Clinicians should be aware of the technical challenges inherent in performing tracheal intubation on patients failing NIPPV. There are higher rates of periprocedural complications including cardiac arrest in this population. This risk is likely due to the sudden derecruitment and loss of ventilation during the intubation process.

Delivery of high flow rates of warmed and humidified O_2 via nasal cannula (HFNC) is increasingly used for acute hypoxemic respiratory failure. The high flow rates limit the entrainment of room air and therefore provide more consistent FIO_2 than traditional low-flow oxygen systems. HFNC can help wash out the anatomic dead space and provide a small amount of CPAP, which can decrease the work of breathing and improve gas exchange. The role of HFNC in acute hypoxemic respiratory failure in the perioperative setting is better defined with increasing clinical experience and trial evidence. HFNC is better tolerated than NIPPV, and its use is suggested over conventional oxygen therapy in patients who cannot tolerate NIPPV. However, the concern remains that its use might delay needed tracheal intubation.

Antonelli M, Conti G, Moro ML, et al. Predictors of failure of noninvasive positive pressure ventilation in patients with acute hypoxemic respiratory failure: a multi-center study. *Intensive Care Med.* 2001;27:1718-1728.

Delclaux C, L'Her E, Alberti C, et al. Treatment of acute hypoxemic nonhypercapnic respiratory insufficiency with continuous positive airway pressure delivered by a face mask: a randomized controlled trial. *JAMA.* 2000;284:2352-2360.

Ferrer M, Esquinas A, Leon M, Gonzalez G, Alarcon A, Torres A. Noninvasive ventilation in severe hypoxemic respiratory failure: a randomized clinical trial. *Am J Respir Crit Care Med.* 2003;168:1438-1444.

Jaber S, Lescot T, Futier E, et al. Effect of noninvasive ventilation on tracheal reintubation among patients with hypoxemic respiratory failure following abdominal surgery: a randomized clinical trial. *JAMA.* 2016;315:1345-1353.

Leone M, Einav S, Chiumello D, et al; Guideline contributors. Noninvasive respiratory support in the hypoxaemic peri-operative/periprocedural patient: a joint ESA/ESICM guideline. *Intensive Care Med.* 2020;46:697-713.

Martin TJ, Hovis JD, Costantino JP, et al. A randomized, prospective evaluation of noninvasive ventilation for acute respiratory failure. *Am J Respir Crit Care Med.* 2000;161:807-13.

Monro-Somerville T, Sim M, Ruddy J, et al. The effect of high-flow nasal cannula oxygen therapy on mortality and intubation rate in acute respiratory failure: a systematic review and meta-analysis. *Crit Care Med.* 2017;45:e449-e456.

Nava S, Hill N. Non-invasive ventilation in acute respiratory failure. *Lancet.* 2009;374:250-259.

Squadrone V, Coha M, Cerutti E, et al. Continuous positive airway pressure for treatment of postoperative hypoxaemia: a randomized controlled trial. *JAMA.* 2005;293:589-595.

C.2. What are the indications for emergency endo tracheal intubation?

Tracheal intubation is performed for impending or actual respiratory failure. The possible indications for emergency tracheal intubation are shown in **Figure 3.3**. Often, a combination of problems drives the decision to intubate. In borderline situations, a need to transport the patient or a worsening trajectory of acute illness can tip the balance in favor of intubation.

Laghi F, Tobin MJ. Indications for mechanical ventilation. In: Tobin MJ, ed. *Principles and Practice of Mechanical Ventilation.* 3rd ed. McGraw-Hill; 2013:101-136.

D. Acute Respiratory Distress Syndrome

The patient's trachea is intubated for respiratory failure. She has bilateral pulmonary infiltrates on the chest radiograph and is severely hypoxemic.

D.1. What is the definition and etiology of acute respiratory distress syndrome (ARDS)?

ARDS is a clinical syndrome of rapidly progressive respiratory failure characterized by severe hypoxemia and bilateral pulmonary infiltrates. ARDS occurs after or during an insult to the lungs or other organs and is not due to hydrostatic (cardiogenic) edema. The characteristic pathologic finding is diffuse alveolar damage.

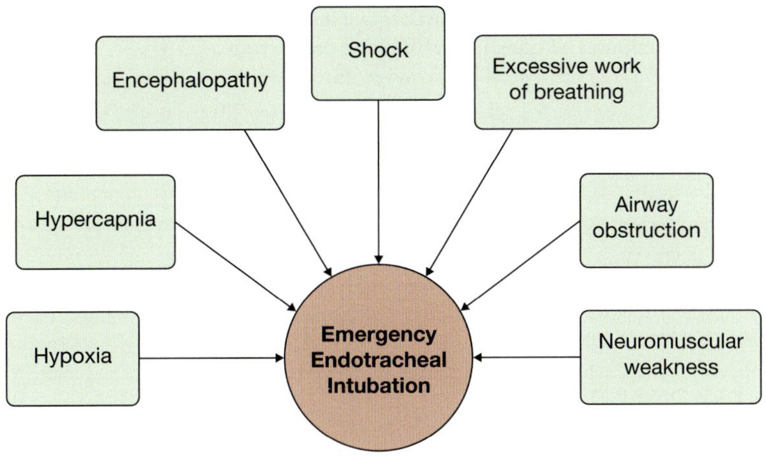

FIGURE 3.3. Indications for emergency tracheal intubation.

The research definition of ARDS has evolved over time. A previous classification did not require the use of CPAP or invasive mechanical ventilation for a patient to meet the criteria for ARDS. The current consensus called the Berlin definition of ARDS (**Figure 3.4**) requires a minimum PEEP of 5 cm H_2O through NIPPV or invasive mechanical ventilation for diagnosis. This definition removed the distinction of acute lung injury (ALI) and replaced it with mild ARDS. This case definition encompasses several distinct disease processes. A significant proportion of patients meeting the diagnostic criteria for ARDS do not have diffuse alveolar damage on biopsy or autopsy. Clinicians should be aware that there are proposed updates to the Berlin definition that incorporate high-flow nasal cannula into the minimum respiratory support returning to previous definitions that did not require minimum PEEP.

There are about 175,000 cases of ARDS each year in the United States, although the incidence has been decreasing. Worse outcomes are associated with severe hypoxemia, increased dead space, and the presence of concomitant organ failure. Prior to the COVID-19 pandemic, the case fatality rate of ARDS had decreased from approximately 40% in the late 1990s to approximately 25% in the mid-2000s; however, unadjusted mortality of those patients with severe ARDS can approach 50%. COVID-19-associated ARDS outcomes are similar to traditional ARDS. The most common etiologies of ARDS include

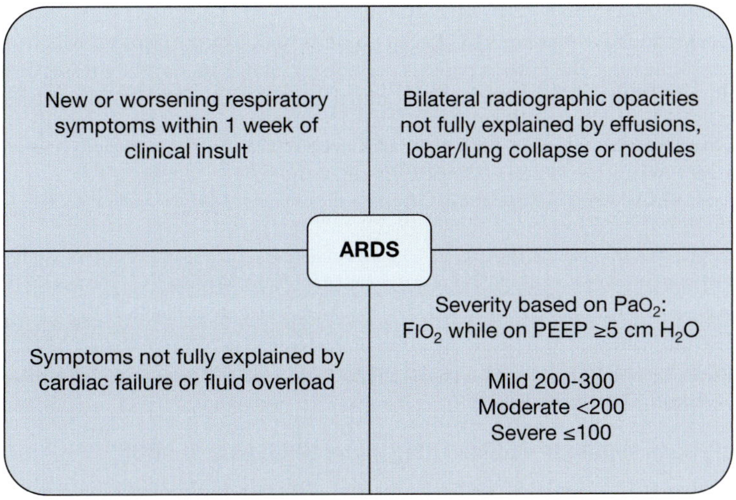

FIGURE 3.4. Definition of acute respiratory distress syndrome (ARDS). FIO_2, fraction of inspired oxygen; PaO_2, arterial partial pressure of oxygen; PEEP, positive end-expiratory pressure. (Adapted from Ranieri VM, Rubenfeld GD, Thompson BT, et al. Acute respiratory distress syndrome: the Berlin definition. *JAMA*. 2012;307:2526-2533.)

pulmonary and nonpulmonary infections, large-volume aspiration of gastric contents, trauma, acute pancreatitis, drug reactions, and transfusions of blood products.

Bellani G, Laffey JG, Pham T, et al. Epidemiology, patterns of care, and mortality for patients with acute respiratory distress syndrome in intensive care units in 50 countries. *JAMA.* 2016;315:788-800.

Ferguson ND, Fan E, Camporota L, et al. The Berlin definition of ARDS: an expanded rationale, justification, and supplementary material. *Intensive Care Med.* 2012;38:1573-1582.

Malhotra A. Low-tidal-volume ventilation in the acute respiratory distress syndrome. *N Engl J Med.* 2007;357:1113-1120.

Matthay MA, Ware LB, Zimmerman GA. The acute respiratory distress syndrome. *J Clin Invest.* 2012;122:2731-2740.

Ranieri VM, Rubenfeld GD, Thompson BT, et al. Acute respiratory distress syndrome: the Berlin definition. *JAMA.* 2012;307:2526-2533.

Rubenfeld GD, Caldwell E, Peabody E, et al. Incidence and outcomes of acute lung injury. *N Engl J Med.* 2005;353:1685-1693.

Thille AW, Esteban A, Fernández-Segoviano P, et al. Comparison of the Berlin definition for acute respiratory distress syndrome with autopsy. *Am J Respir Crit Care Med.* 2013;187:761-767.

Ware LB, Matthay MA. The acute respiratory distress syndrome. *N Engl J Med.* 2000;342:1334-1349.

D.2. Explain the pathophysiology of ARDS.

In ARDS, the alveoli have edema rich in neutrophils and proteins (**Figure 3.5**). This leads to dysfunction of both the alveolar epithelium and pulmonary capillary endothelium, causing noncardiogenic pulmonary edema. Additionally, adepletion of functioning surfactant leads to alveolar collapse.

The initial insult that triggers the development of ARDS can include pneumonia, sepsis, inhalation and aspiration, and trauma. Activation of pattern recognition receptors, such as Toll-like receptors, occurs in response to pathogen microbial products (PAMPs), or endogenous damage-associated molecular pattern molecules (DAMPs). Ultimately, the innate immune system is activated, leading to the recruitment of inflammatory cells to the lung, further propagating lung injury (**Figure 3.6**).

ARDS progresses through distinct clinical, pathologic, and radiologic phases. The acute exudative phase of ARDS is characterized by severe hypoxemia that is refractory to supplemental oxygenation and often requires invasive mechanical ventilation. Hypoxemia in this early phase is due to increased shunt fraction. Acute right-sided heart failure is common due to a marked elevation in pulmonary vascular resistance. Hypoxic and hypercapnic pulmonary vasoconstriction, regional atelectasis, and hyperinflation due to mechanical ventilation all contribute to the rise in pulmonary resistance. Radiologically, there are bilateral alveolar infiltrates. CT imaging demonstrates bilateral patchy opacities and dependent consolidation. Pleural effusions are common. ARDS caused by direct lung injury might be more responsive to higher PEEP strategies. ARDS caused by systemic inflammatory states is associated with more pronounced shock and multisystem organ dysfunction.

The acute exudative phase of ARDS can progress to fibrosing alveolitis, which appears as linear opacities on chest imaging. The fibrosis reduces pulmonary compliance and increases dead space. Patients who recover from ARDS can have normal lung function or chronic fibrotic lung disease.

Calfee CS, Delucchi K, Parsons PE, et al. Subphenotypes in acute respiratory distress syndrome: latent class analysis of data from two randomised controlled trials. *Lancet Respir Med.* 2014;2:611-620.

Matthay MA, Ware LB, Zimmerman GA. The acute respiratory distress syndrome. *J Clin Invest.* 2012;122:2731-2740.

Matthay MA, Zimmerman GA. Acute lung injury and the acute respiratory distress syndrome: four decades of inquiry into pathogenesis and rational management. *Am J Respir Cell Mol Biol.* 2005;33:319-327.

Thompson BT, Chambers RC, Liu KD. Acute respiratory distress syndrome. *N Engl J Med.* 2017;377:562-572.

Ware LB, Matthay MA. The acute respiratory distress syndrome. *N Engl J Med.* 2000;342:1334-1349.

Wiener-Kronish JP, Matthay MA. Pleural effusions associated with hydrostatic and increased permeability pulmonary edema. *Chest.* 1988;93:852-858.

D.3. What role does ventilator-induced lung injury (VILI) play in ARDS?

Mechanical ventilation injures the lungs through complex pathophysiologic processes. A variety of illnesses, particularly ARDS, increase susceptibility. Rarely, VILI leads to air leaks from the lung into the pleura or mediastinum. However, microscopic injury is a more common problem. Complications of VILI extend beyond the lungs. Excessive alveolar stretch in ARDS increases circulating inflammatory

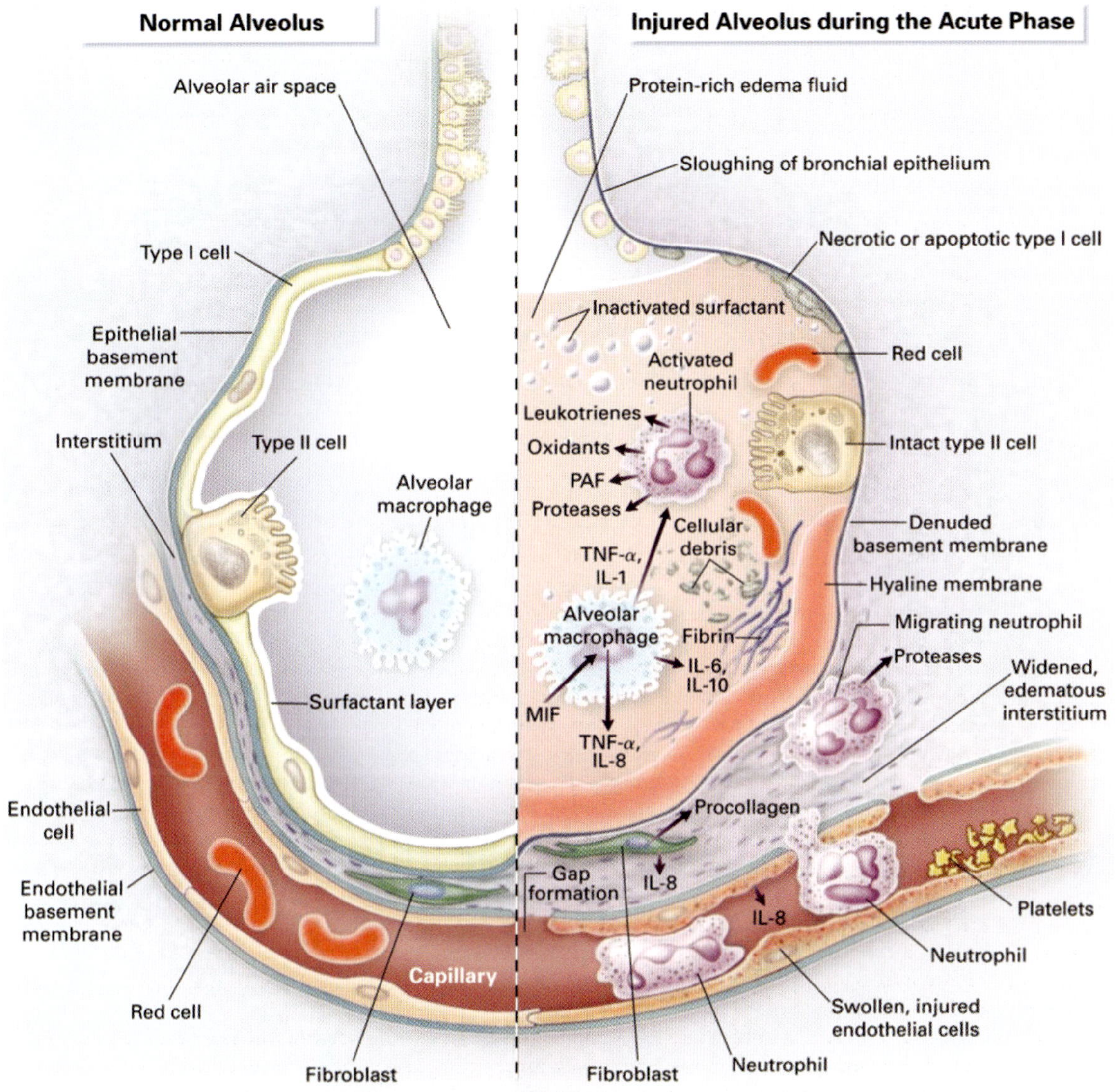

FIGURE 3.5. The pathogenesis of ARDS. ARDS, acute respiratory distress syndrome; IL, interleukin; MIF, macrophage inhibition factor; PAF, platelet-activating factor; TNF-α, tumor necrosis factor-α. (From Ware LB, Matthay MA. The acute respiratory distress syndrome. *N Engl J Med.* 2000;342:1334-1349. Figure 3. Copyright © 2000 Massachusetts Medical Society. Reprinted with permission from Massachusetts Medical Society.)

cytokines and injures small bowel and renal epithelial cells. These processes have been linked to progressive multisystem organ failure, which is the most common cause of death in ARDS.

VILI can occur through two mechanisms: (1) excessive distention of certain lung regions (volutrauma) and (2) repeated collapse and shearing of other regions (atelectotrauma).

Prevention of VILI can be challenging due to difficulties in accurately measuring the amount of air distending the lungs during mechanical ventilation. Ventilators typically display only the tidal volume, which is the amount of air delivered or exhaled, but do not measure the volume of air remaining in the lungs at end expiration, known as the functional residual capacity. The total lung volume that distends the lungs includes the tidal volume plus the functional residual capacity. Since this volume cannot be directly measured, clinicians must turn to airway pressure at the end of inspiration as a surrogate marker for maximum lung distention caused by the ventilator. To measure this pressure, clinicians must pause the

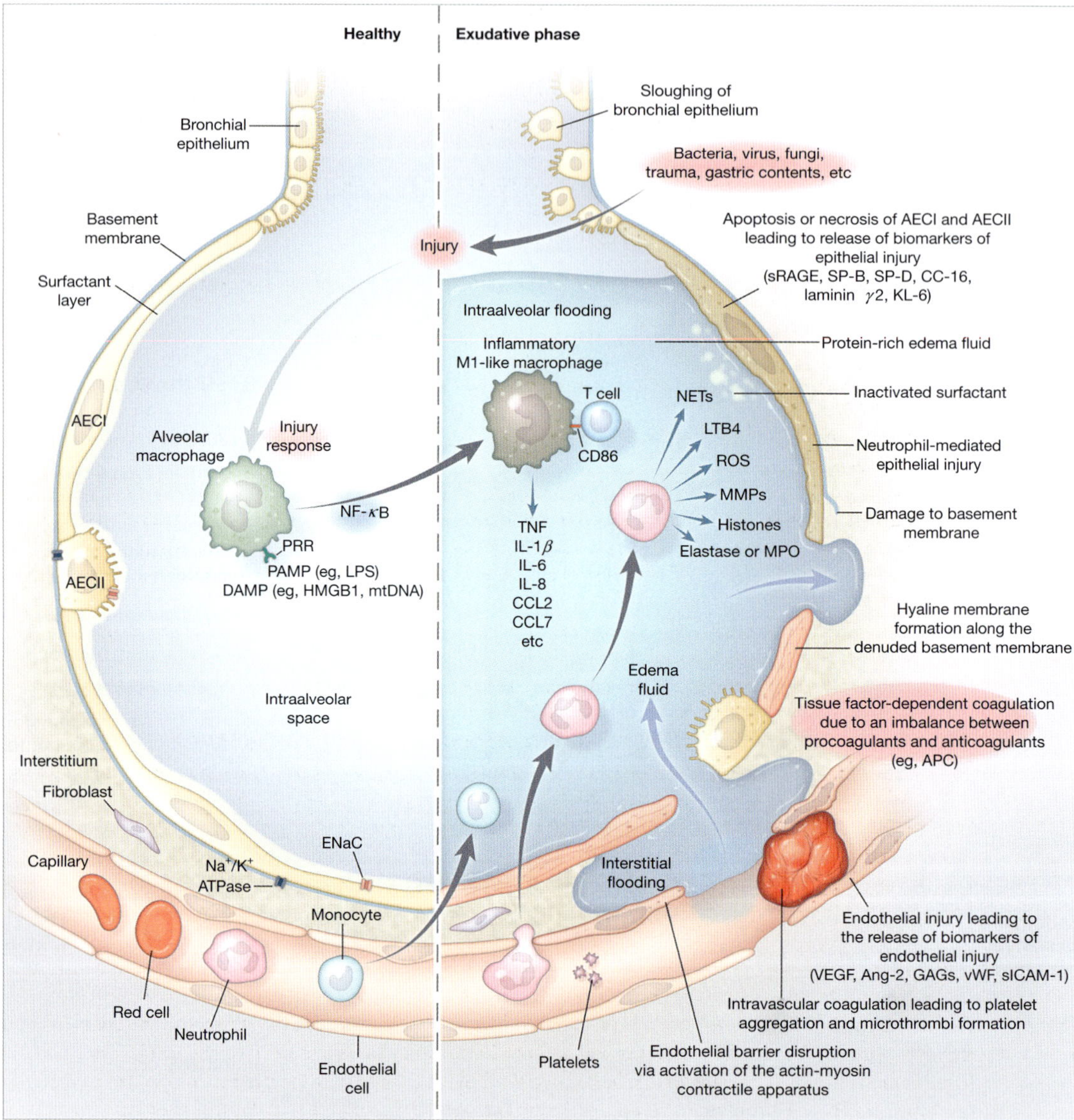

FIGURE 3.6. The exudative phase of ARDS. AECI, type I alveolar epithelial cell; AECII, type II alveolar epithelial cell; Ang-2, angiopoietin-2; APC, activated protein C; CC-16, club cell (formerly Clara cell) secretory protein 16; CCL, chemokine (CC motif) ligand; DAMP, damage-associated molecular pattern; ENaC, epithelial sodium channel; GAG, glycosaminoglycan; HMGB1, high-mobility group box 1 protein; KL-6, Krebs von den Lungen 6; LPS, lipopolysaccharide; LTB4, leukotriene B4; MMP, matrix metalloproteinase; MPO, myeloperoxidase; mtDNA, mitochondrial DNA; Na+/K+, ATPase sodium-potassium ATPase pump; NET, neutrophil extracellular trap; NF-κB, nuclear factor kappa light-chain enhancer of activated B cells; PAMP, pathogen-associated molecular pattern; PRR, pattern recognition receptor; ROS, reactive oxygen species; sICAM, soluble intercellular adhesion molecule; SP, surfactant protein; sRAGE, soluble receptor for advanced glycation end products; VEGF, vascular endothelial growth factor; vWF, von Willebrand factor. (From Thompson BT, Chambers RC, Liu KD. Acute respiratory distress syndrome. *N Engl J Med*. 2017;377:562-572. Figure 2. Copyright © 2017 Massachusetts Medical Society. Reprinted with permission from Massachusetts Medical Society.)

ventilator cycle momentarily at the end of inspiration to minimize the impact of airflow resistance. This pause also allows time for the ventilator circuit to better equilibrate with the lungs. The pressure in the ventilator circuit during this pause is known as the plateau pressure.

The plateau pressure is an imperfect surrogate for the distending pressure of the lung. It is a composite of the force in the airway that distends the lung and the forces adjacent to the lung that distend or oppose lung inflation. For example, inspiratory effort can distend the lungs while lowering plateau pressure on volume-controlled ventilation. Conversely, positive pleural pressure from intra-abdominal hypertension and gravitational effects from obesity can raise plateau pressure without increasing lung distention. Therefore, clinicians should consider both tidal volume and plateau pressure to evaluate the risk of overdistention.

Driving pressure is another way to evaluate the risk of VILI. Driving pressure reflects the relationship between the delivered tidal volume and lung compliance, and high driving pressure suggests a risk of overdistention. In an analysis of randomized trials in ARDS, higher driving pressure had a stronger correlation with mortality compared to tidal volume. Ventilator techniques that optimize lung compliance and driving pressure might offer some benefits, but early clinical trials utilizing this concept from ARDS in operative ventilator management have not shown a benefit.

Amato MB, Meade MO, Slutsky AS, et al. Driving pressure and survival in the acute respiratory distress syndrome. *N Engl J Med.* 2015;372:747.

Constantin JM, Jabaudon M, Lefrant JY, et al; AZUREA Network. Personalised mechanical ventilation tailored to lung morphology versus low positive end-expiratory pressure for patients with acute respiratory distress syndrome in France (the LIVE study): a multicentre, single-blind, randomised controlled trial. *Lancet Respir Med.* 2019;7:870-880.

Dreyfuss D, Saumon G. Ventilator-induced lung injury: lessons from experimental studies. *Am J Respir Crit Care Med.* 1998;157:294-323.

Imai Y, Parodo J, Kajikawa O, et al. Injurious mechanical ventilation and end-organ epithelial cell apoptosis and organ dysfunction in an experimental model of acute respiratory distress syndrome. *JAMA.* 2003;289:2104-2112.

Meade MO, Cook DJ, Guyatt GH, et al. Ventilation strategy using low tidal volumes, recruitment maneuvers, and high positive end-expiratory pressure for acute lung injury and acute respiratory distress syndrome: a randomized controlled trial. *JAMA.* 2008;299:637-645.

Park M, Yoon S, Nam JS, et al. Driving pressure-guided ventilation and postoperative pulmonary complications in thoracic surgery: a multicentre randomised clinical trial. *Br J Anaesth.* 2023;130:e106-e118.

Schiller HJ, Steinberg J, Halter J, et al. Alveolar inflation during generation of a quasi-static pressure/volume curve in the acutely injured lung. *Crit Care Med.* 2003;31:1126-1133.

Thompson BT, Chambers RC, Liu KD. Acute respiratory distress syndrome. *N Engl J Med.* 2017;377:562-572.

Writing Group for the Alveolar Recruitment for Acute Respiratory Distress Syndrome Trial (ART) Investigators. Effect of lung recruitment and titrated positive end-expiratory pressure (PEEP) vs low PEEP on mortality in patients with acute respiratory distress syndrome: a randomized clinical trial. *JAMA.* 2017;318:1335-1345.

E. Management of Mechanical Ventilation

E.1. Which mode of mechanical ventilation will you choose? Describe the features of that mode.

There is no proof that any one mode of mechanical ventilation is superior in any clinical situation. Aside from avoiding purely assisted modes, the choice of mode is largely dictated by physician preference. Choosing appropriate settings for a given mode is more important than the choice of the mode. Therefore, it is essential for clinicians to have a detailed understanding of the settings for the mode they are using.

With traditional controlled mechanical ventilation, the patient had no control over any aspect of the respiratory cycle. Modern controlled ventilation modes can "assist" patients' respiratory efforts. In assisted modes, the ventilator recognizes the inspiratory effort by a negative pressure deflection in the ventilator circuit. The ventilator then cycles to inspiration and forces gas into the circuit's inspiratory limb. Gas is delivered until it reaches a set target of either pressure or volume.

Assist/control with volume targeting is the most common mode in intensive care units. Inspiration begins when the ventilator recognizes the patient's inspiratory effort or at a minimum frequency set by a clinician. The ventilator compresses the gas sufficiently to deliver a set tidal volume. In general, assist/control volume targeting allows the best assessment of respiratory mechanics. The mode also guarantees delivery of a minimum minute volume. It also limits tidal volume, which can help avoid alveolar overdistention. However, assist/control with volume targeting can provide insufficient support for a patient with a strong respiratory drive. The tidal volume, duration of inspiration, and inspiratory flow rate are all set by the clinician. The ventilator cannot meet patient demand for an increased tidal volume or faster inspiratory gas flow. Patients with a strong respiratory drive can develop severe dyssynchrony and perform substantial work of breathing in this mode. Dyssynchrony is common with assist/control volume targeting and is usually due to double or ineffective triggering of inspiration.

With assist/control pressure targeting, the ventilator delivers gas until the pressure reaches a specified target. The volume and rate of gas delivered vary with patient effort and respiratory mechanics. Clinicians must set criteria for the timing of the inspiratory and expiratory cycles (either the inspiratory time or the ratio of the duration of inspiration and exhalation). The usual time of inspiration to prevent dyssynchrony is 0.8 to 1.2 seconds. A virtue of assist/control pressure targeting is that the inspiratory pressure will not exceed the upper limit. The patient with high ventilator demand can increase the volume and rate of gas delivery by making stronger inspiratory efforts. However, the ventilator does not guarantee a minimum tidal volume.

Pressure support ventilation is a form of assisted ventilation like pressure-targeted assist/control with variable delivered flow based on the set inspiratory pressure and patient effort. Unlike assist/control pressure targeting, pressure support lacks a set ventilator rate and inspiratory time. It cycles from inspiration to exhalation when inspiratory flow decreases below a set threshold. Based on this property, patients have the most control over their breathing with this mode since the rate and duration of inspiratory airflow depend on their own effort. However, this mode is inappropriate for patients with minimal respiratory effort or in situations where passive ventilator synchrony is used to optimize recruitment.

Like other pressure-targeted modes, pressure support provides increasing support to match increased inspiratory demand. In fact, oversupport is a common cause of dyssynchrony with this mode. In this situation, strong inspiratory drive causes the ventilator to deliver excessive airflow. This can lead to dynamic hyperinflation if the patient has insufficient time to exhale. Dynamic hyperinflation can lead to ineffective triggering and wasted ventilator effort. In this situation, dyssynchrony might improve by decreasing the inspiratory pressure target.

Synchronized intermittent mandatory ventilation (SIMV) is another popular mode. SIMV is a mixed mode; therefore, it shares the virtues and problems with its constituent modes. It is a combination of assist/control with spontaneous breaths. If the patient does make sufficient respiratory effort, the ventilator delivers controlled ventilation (either volume or pressure targeted). If the ventilator recognizes patient effort, it allows spontaneous ventilation. If there is PEEP, the breaths are CPAP. Many clinicians add pressure support to spontaneous breaths. Spontaneous ventilation with minimal pressure PEEP and pressure support can mitigate the hemodynamic effects of positive pressure ventilation. However, it is difficult for the patient to respond to alternating levels of support by modulating their effort on a breath-to-breath basis. Therefore, patient effort increases on controlled breaths. This will diminish the effects of spontaneous ventilation on SIMV.

A number of alternative modes are available. Many have refinements so that the ventilator adjusts flow during a breath or on subsequent breaths. Adaptive support ventilation, pressure-regulated volume control, and volume support are some of the options. Neurally adjusted ventilation assist (NAVA) uses a novel strategy; a tube is placed from the nose/mouth into the esophagus and provides electromyographic analysis of diaphragmatic effort. The ventilator synchronizes respiratory cycling and the magnitude of pressure support to diaphragmatic contraction. NAVA can improve ventilator-patient synchrony because air leaks and dynamic hyperinflation do not obscure the patient's inspiratory efforts.

High-frequency oscillating ventilation (HFOV) is an alternative mode that requires a special ventilator. The principle of HFOV is the maintenance of a high mean airway pressure with extremely brief cycling above and below the mean. The ventilator targets pressure alternating between 70 and 0 cm H_2O at a frequency of around 4 to 12 Hz (cycles per second). Because the duration of the respiratory cycle is so brief, there is insufficient time for the lungs to equilibrate with the ventilator airway pressure. This results in 1 to 2 mL/kg breaths at a rate of 4 to 12 per second. These breaths are smaller than the airway dead space; therefore, HFOV exchanges gas via alternate mechanisms. The increased hemodynamic instability found in the HFOV trial is likely due to the continuously elevated airway pressure. In particular, right ventricular failure commonly complicates HFOV for ARDS. A well-designed randomized controlled trial found that HFOV increased mortality compared with a lung protective ventilation strategy when used as a treatment for adults with ARDS. It is possible that a different HFOV protocol (such as one that targets a lower mean airway pressure) would have a benefit.

There is increasing interest in airway pressure release ventilation (APRV) as a method to improve lung recruitment. This mode provides CPAP at a high level (called "PEEP high") coupled with very brief periods of exhalation. These brief releases incompletely empty the lung and lead to dynamic hyperinflation, which raises mean airway pressures, leading to lung recruitment. Importantly, APRV allows spontaneous pressure-supported breaths during CPAP as well as during the releases (called "PEEP low"). The freedom to initiate spontaneous breaths during all phases of the respiratory cycle can improve ventilator-patient synchrony.

At present, there are no proven benefits for any of these alternative modes compared to assist/control modes. In general, pressure-targeted modes create less dyssynchrony than volume-targeted modes when the respiratory drive is strong. However, the settings on the mode affect dyssynchrony more than the choice of mode. For the patient with ARDS, unconventional modes are acceptable as long as they are employed as part of a lung protective strategy as described below.

Colombo D, Cammarota G, Bergamaschi V, et al. Physiologic response to varying levels of pressure support and neurally adjusted ventilatory assist in patients with acute respiratory failure. *Intensive Care Med.* 2008;34:2010-2018.

Esteban A, Anzueto A, Alía I, et al. How is mechanical ventilation employed in the intensive care unit? An international utilization review. *Am J Respir Crit Care Med.* 2000;161:1450-1458.

Ferguson ND, Cook DJ, Guyatt GH, et al. High-frequency oscillation in early acute respiratory distress syndrome. *N Engl J Med.* 2013;368:795-805.

Guervilly C, Forel JM, Hraiech S, et al. Right ventricular function during high-frequency oscillatory ventilation in adults with acute respiratory distress syndrome. *Crit Care Med.* 2012;40:1539-1545.

Ibarra-Estrada MÁ, García-Salas Y, Mireles-Cabodevila E, et al. Use of airway pressure release ventilation in patients with acute respiratory failure due to COVID-19: results of a single-center randomized controlled trial. *Crit Care Med.* 2022;50:586-594.

Kacmarek RM, Hess DR. Mechanical ventilation for the surgical patient. In: Longnecker DE, Newman MF, Zapol WM, et al, eds. *Anesthesiology*. 3rd ed. McGraw-Hill; 2018:1319-1335.

Piquilloud L, Vignaux L, Bialais E, et al. Neurally adjusted ventilatory assist improves patient-ventilator interaction. *Intensive Care Med.* 2011;37:263-271.

Thille AW, Cabello B, Galia F, et al. Reduction of patient-ventilator asynchrony by reducing tidal volume during pressure-support ventilation. *Intensive Care Med.* 2008;34:1477-1486.

Thille AW, Rodriguez P, Cabello B, et al. Patient-ventilator asynchrony during assisted mechanical ventilation. *Intensive Care Med.* 2006;32:1515-1522.

Zhou Y, Jin X, Lv Y, et al. Early application of airway pressure release ventilation may reduce the duration of mechanical ventilation in acute respiratory distress syndrome. *Intensive Care Med.* 2017;43:1648.

E.2. How should you set the fraction of inspired oxygen (F_{IO_2})?

The F_{IO_2} is set to maintain sufficient arterial oxygenation. Given the poor solubility of oxygen, the oxygen saturation of hemoglobin rather than the Pa_{O_2} is the more important determinant of arterial oxygen content. For example, a patient without anemia and hemoglobin that is 97% saturated with oxygen can carry 200 mL of oxygen in every liter of blood (in hemoglobin). The same patient will have a Pa_{O_2} of 90 mm Hg and just 2.7 mL of oxygen dissolved in every liter of blood (in the plasma). In ARDS, it is acceptable to target an oxygen saturation of hemoglobin greater than 88%. The F_{IO_2} should be limited as low as possible to avoid oxygen toxicity. The oxygen saturation target should be higher in situations such as intracranial hypertension, right ventricular failure, and systemic vasodilation.

Brower RG, Matthay MA, Morris A, et al. Ventilation with lower tidal volumes as compared with traditional tidal volumes for acute lung injury and the acute respiratory distress syndrome. *N Engl J Med.* 2000;342:1301-1308.

E.3. How should you set positive end-expiratory pressure (PEEP)?

PEEP can recruit atelectatic alveoli, prevent cyclical alveolar closure (atelectotrauma), and decrease shunt fraction (**Figure 3.7**). There is a potential benefit of higher levels of PEEP in severe ARDS. However, high levels of PEEP decrease venous return and cardiac output. Excessive PEEP also overdistends alveoli, leading to VILI and increased pulmonary vascular resistance. The ideal level of PEEP would maximize recruitment, respiratory system compliance, gas exchange, patient comfort, and minimize detrimental effects of overdistention on volutrauma and cardiovascular hemodynamics.

The best method to select PEEP for individual patients remains controversial. The trial that established the current standard of care for ventilation in ARDS used a table to determine PEEP based on the F_{IO_2} requirement. Multiple trials have failed to demonstrate a better method of PEEP determination than this. Some clinicians use decremental PEEP trials by serially reducing PEEP after a recruitment maneuver. However, a recent multicenter randomized clinical trial revealed significant mortality and harm with this practice. Other protocols set PEEP according to pressure-volume curves or measurement of transpulmonary gradients by esophageal probes. However, there is currently no evidence that physiologic methods effectively determine the PEEP that recruits lungs in ARDS. Some protocols emphasize hemodynamic effects such as limiting PEEP based on Doppler ultrasound analysis of pulmonary artery flow. The average PEEP used for ARDS in clinical settings is about 8 cm H_2O and 10 cm H_2O in severe cases. It is unclear whether this is ideal. An analysis of studies comparing higher versus lower PEEP settings showed no significant difference.

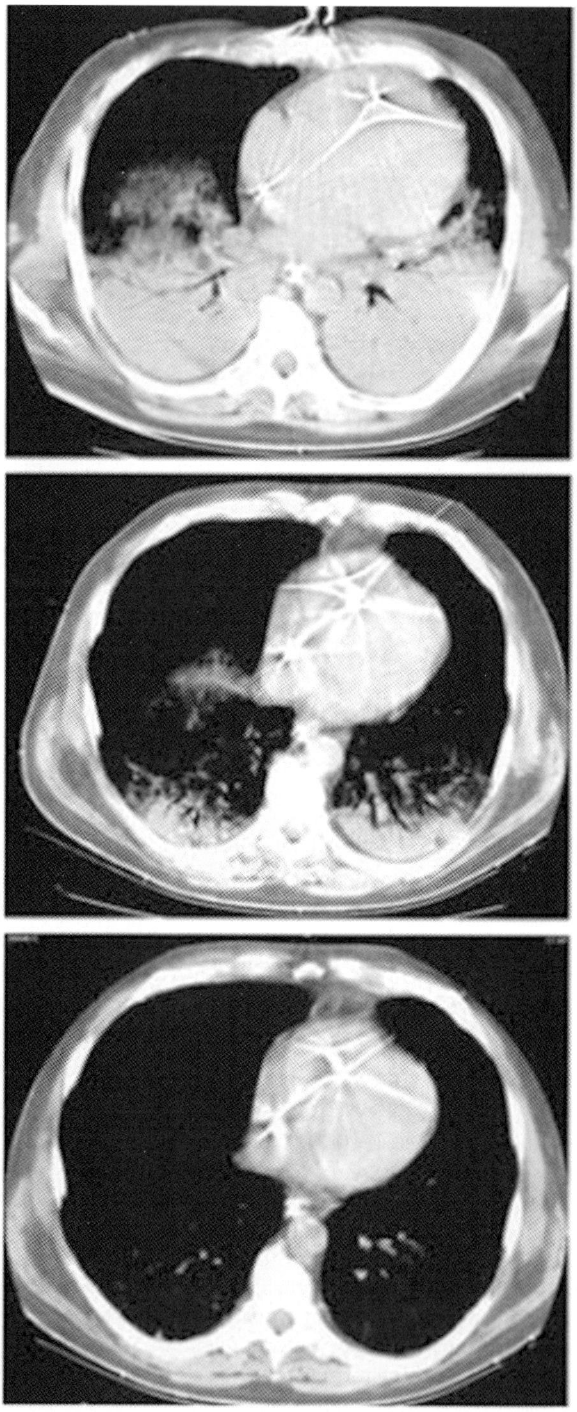

FIGURE 3.7. Lung recruitment in ARDS with progressive increase in PEEP. ARDS, acute respiratory distress syndrome; PEEP, positive end-expiratory pressure. (Reprinted with permission of the American Thoracic Society from Borges JB, Okamoto VN, Matos GF, et al. Reversibility of lung collapse and hypoxemia in early acute respiratory distress syndrome. *Am J Respir Crit Care Med.* 2006;174:268-278. Figure 7. Copyright © 2019 American Thoracic Society.)

Bellani G, Laffey JG, Pham T, et al. Epidemiology, patterns of care, and mortality for patients with acute respiratory distress syndrome in intensive care units in 50 countries. *JAMA*. 2016;315:788-800.

Brower RG, Lanken PN, MacIntyre N, et al. Higher versus lower positive end-expiratory pressures in patients with the acute respiratory distress syndrome. *N Engl J Med*. 2004;351:327-336.

Brower RG, Matthay MA, Morris A, et al. Ventilation with lower tidal volumes as compared with traditional tidal volumes for acute lung injury and the acute respiratory distress syndrome. *N Engl J Med*. 2000;342:1301-1308.

Cavalcanti AB, Suzumura ÉA, Laranjeira LN, et al. Effect of lung recruitment and titrated positive end-expiratory pressure (PEEP) vs low PEEP on mortality in patients with acute respiratory distress syndrome: a randomized clinical trial. *JAMA*. 2017;318:1335-1345.

Chiumello D, Cressoni M, Carlesso E, et al. Bedside selection of positive end-expiratory pressure in mild, moderate, and severe acute respiratory distress syndrome. *Crit Care Med*. 2014;42:252-264.

Guo R, Fan E. Beyond low tidal volumes: ventilating the patient with acute respiratory distress syndrome. *Clin Chest Med*. 2014;35:729-741.

Hager DN, Brower RG. Customizing lung-protective mechanical ventilation strategies. *Crit Care Med*. 2006;34:1554-1555.

Rubenfeld GD. How much PEEP in acute lung injury. *JAMA*. 2010;303:883-884.

Walkey AJ, Del Sorbo L, Hodgson CL, et al. Higher PEEP versus lower PEEP strategies for patients with acute respiratory distress syndrome. A systematic review and meta-analysis. *Ann Am Thorac Soc*. 2017;14:S297-S303.

E.4. What tidal volume and inspiratory pressure target should you set?

The approach of limiting tidal volume and plateau pressure has been validated in a landmark randomized controlled trial in patients with ARDS. This technique, called low tidal volume ventilation, significantly reduced organ failure and mortality. Recent data on driving pressure (plateau pressure—PEEP) have demonstrated reduced mortality with reduced driving pressure. Although low tidal volume ventilation initially worsens gas exchange, it ultimately limits lung and extrapulmonary injury. Therefore, the initial tidal volume or inspiratory pressure should be set to keep the tidal volume less than 8 mL/kg IBW and plateau pressure less than 30 cm H_2O. Tidal volume and pressure should be incrementally lowered to target 4 to 6 mL/kg IBW and plateau pressure less than 30 cm H_2O while monitoring the patient for dyssynchrony and worsening gas exchange (**Table 3.4**).

Low tidal volume ventilation can reduce alveolar ventilation and worsen hypercapnia. Increasing respiratory rate is often insufficient to maintain alveolar ventilation. In fact, the low tidal volume approach can necessitate permissive hypercapnia as a trade-off. There is conflicting evidence regarding the association between permissive hypercapnia and lower mortality, as it is difficult to distinguish whether these are the effects of low tidal volume ventilation or permissive hypercapnia. In preclinical studies, hypercapnia could reduce inflammation, decrease free alveolar protein, and even improve pulmonary compliance.

Nevertheless, it is important to acknowledge the potential adverse effects of hypercapnia. Hypercapnia can constrict pulmonary arterioles and dilate systemic and cerebral arterioles. Tidal volume restriction and hypercapnia can worsen ventilator-patient dyssynchrony and double triggering of the ventilator. In this setting, the delivered tidal volumes are much larger than the clinician sets on the ventilator. Moreover, a strong inspiratory effort can overdistend the lungs. On pressure-controlled ventilation, tidal volumes can be excessive, whereas on volume-controlled ventilation, plateau pressure can underestimate the distending pressure. Furthermore, long-term consequences for survivors of ARDS exposed to prolonged periods of permissive hypercapnia remain undetermined. Future studies to assess the benefit of incorporating extracorporeal carbon dioxide removal are needed.

Amato MB, Meade MO, Slutsky AS, et al. Driving pressure and survival in the acute respiratory distress syndrome. *N Engl J Med*. 2015;372:747-755.

Broccard AF, Hotchkiss JR, Vannay C, et al. Protective effects of hypercapnic acidosis on ventilator-induced lung injury. *Am J Respir Crit Care Med*. 2001;164:802-806.

Brower RG, Matthay MA, Morris A, et al. Ventilation with lower tidal volumes as compared with traditional tidal volumes for acute lung injury and the acute respiratory distress syndrome. *N Engl J Med*. 2000;342:1301-1308.

Fan E, Del Sorbo L, Goligher EC, et al; American Thoracic Society, European Society of Intensive Care Medicine, and Society of Critical Care Medicine. An Official American Thoracic Society/European Society of Intensive Care Medicine/Society of Critical Care Medicine Clinical Practice Guideline: Mechanical Ventilation in Adult Patients with Acute Respiratory Distress Syndrome. *Am J Respir Crit Care Med*. 2017;195:1253-1263.

Grasselli G, Calfee CS, Camporota L et al; European Society of Intensive Care Medicine Taskforce on ARDS. ESICM guidelines on acute respiratory distress syndrome: definition, phenotyping and respiratory support strategies. *Intensive Care Med*. 2023;49:727-759.

TABLE 3.4 Low-Stretch Lung Protective Ventilator Strategy for Acute Respiratory Distress Syndrome

	Allowable Combinations of PEEP and F_{IO_2}			
	F_{IO_2}	PEEP cm H_2O	F_{IO_2}	PEEP cm H_2O
Ventilator mode: assist/control volume	0.3	5	0.7	14
Initial tidal volume 6 mL/kg predicted body weight	0.4	5	0.8	14
Plateau pressure ≤30 cm H_2O	0.4	8	0.9	14
Respiratory rate 6-35 breaths per minute set to achieve pH 7.3-7.45	0.5	8	0.9	16
Ratio of inspiration to expiration 1:1-1:1.3	0.5	10	0.9	18
Oxygenation goal P_{aO_2} 55-80 mm Hg or S_{pO_2} 88%-95%	0.6	10	1.0	18
	0.7	10	1.0	20
	0.7	12	1.0	22
	0.7	14	1.0	24

F_{IO_2}, fraction of inspired oxygen; P_{aO_2}, partial pressure of oxygen; PEEP, positive end-expiratory pressure; S_{pO_2}, peripheral capillary oxygen saturation.

From Brower RG, Matthay MA, Morris A, et al. Ventilation with lower tidal volumes as compared with traditional tidal volumes for acute lung injury and the acute respiratory distress syndrome. *N Engl J Med.* 2000;342:1301-1308.

Nin N, Muriel A, Peñuelas O, et al; VENTILA Group. Severe hypercapnia and outcome of mechanically ventilated patients with moderate or severe acute respiratory distress syndrome. *Intensive Care Med.* 2017;43:200-208.

Pohlman MC, McCallister KE, Schweickert WD, et al. Excessive tidal volume from breath stacking during lung-protective ventilation for acute lung injury. *Crit Care Med.* 2008;36:3019-3023.

Vieillard-Baron A, Prin S, Augarde R, et al. Increasing respiratory rate to improve CO_2 clearance during mechanical ventilation is not a panacea in acute respiratory failure. *Crit Care Med.* 2002;30:1407-1412.

F. Management of Refractory Respiratory Failure

The patient remains hypoxemic on F_{IO_2} of 0.8.

F.1. What else can promote additional lung recruitment?

Recruitment maneuvers rely on the principle that it requires more pressure to inflate an atelectatic lung to a given volume than it does to maintain that volume after exhaling from maximum inflation. To perform a recruitment maneuver, the clinician sets a high level of CPAP for a short time interval (eg, 40 cm H_2O for 40 seconds). Alternatively, for mechanically ventilated patients, the extrinsic PEEP can be increased on the ventilator for a short duration.

Ideally, lung recruitment reduces the amount of atelectatic lung and decreases shunt fraction. The hallmark of success is an improvement in the ratio of P_{aO_2} to F_{IO_2}. Recruitment maneuvers share the deleterious effects of all treatments that raise airway pressure. The high level of airway pressure can be sufficient to obstruct venous return and reduce cardiac output as well as cause barotrauma. The potential benefit of recruitment maneuvers for patients depends on the inherent recruitability of their lungs. Recruitment maneuvers have been examined in various trials including a large multicenter clinical trial in which a high PEEP recruitment maneuver (45 cm H_2O) with decremental PEEP titration caused hemodynamic effects and increased mortality and barotrauma. Although this could be a result of poor patient selection and has not been shown with differing recruitment protocols, the current evidence suggests against routine use of recruitment maneuvers. Given the physiologic rationale and benefits of gas exchange, clinicians should consider using recruitment maneuvers on a case-by-case basis in a setting of refractory hypoxemia while considering the known potential for harm. Clinicians should await further trial evidence to define the potential role of this intervention. Some clinicians advocate for a higher PEEP strategy without a specific recruitment maneuver. A high PEEP to F_{IO_2} titration strategy has been shown to be equivalent in randomized clinical trials to the original ARDS network PEEP titration table, and higher PEEP over time can improve oxygenation in selected cases.

Pronation is a recruitment strategy that avoids the deleterious effects of increased positive airway pressure. There are a number of mechanisms by which pronation can be beneficial. Prone ventilation decreases the volume of the lung that is compressed by the heart in the supine position. Pronation also displaces the diaphragm caudally and homogenizes the distribution of the pleural pressure. In ARDS, these mechanisms can recruit lung and decrease alveolar hyperinflation. Pronation has multiple effects on hemodynamics. By reducing chest wall compliance, prone ventilation can decrease airway pressures for mechanical ventilation. Additionally, pronation can improve preload/venous return and lower pulmonary vascular resistance. A large multicenter randomized trial demonstrated a survival advantage from prone positioning in severe ARDS. The patients had Pao_2:Fio_2 ratios less than 150 mm Hg and were treated early in their illness for at least 16 hours per day for up to 3 days. Other meta-analyses have also demonstrated a survival advantage in severe ARDS.

In patients with low work of breathing, absent shock, and tolerance of mechanical ventilation with a normal sensorium, providing mechanical ventilation while they sit in a chair or walk is the ideal therapy to recruit lung. Exercise improves cardiac output, lowers pulmonary vascular resistance, and avoids sedation. Similarly, avoidance of deep sedation and neuromuscular block can improve can maintain muscle tone and preserve recruitment in selected patients.

Brower RG, Lanken PN, MacIntyre N, et al. Higher versus lower positive end-expiratory pressures in patients with the acute respiratory distress syndrome. *N Engl J Med.* 2004;351:327-336.

Cavalcanti AB, Suzumura ÉA, Laranjeira LN, et al. Effect of lung recruitment and titrated positive end-expiratory pressure (PEEP) vs low PEEP on mortality in patients with acute respiratory distress syndrome: a randomized clinical trial. *JAMA.* 2017;318:1335-1345.

Cornejo RA, Díaz JC, Tobar EA, et al. Effects of prone positioning on lung protection in patients with acute respiratory distress syndrome. *Am J Respir Crit Care Med.* 2013;188:440-448.

Fan E, Wilcox ME, Brower RG, et al. Recruitment maneuvers for acute lung injury: a systematic review. *Am J Respir Crit Care Med.* 2008;178:1156-1163.

Goligher EC, Hodgson CL, Adhikari NKJ, et al. Lung recruitment maneuvers for adult patients with acute respiratory distress syndrome. A systematic review and meta-analysis. *Ann Am Thorac Soc.* 2017;14:S304-S311.

Guérin C, Reignier J, Richard JC, et al. Prone positioning in severe acute respiratory distress syndrome. *N Engl J Med.* 2013;368:2159-2168.

Jozwiak M, Teboul JL, Anguel N, et al. Beneficial hemodynamic effects of prone positioning in patients with acute respiratory distress syndrome. *Am J Respir Crit Care Med.* 2013;188:1428-1433.

Lee JM, Bae W, Lee YJ, et al. The efficacy and safety of prone positional ventilation in acute respiratory distress syndrome: updated study-level meta-analysis of 11 randomized controlled trials. *Crit Care Med.* 2014;42:1252-1262.

Meade MO, Cook DJ, Guyatt GH, et al. Ventilation strategy using low tidal volumes, recruitment maneuvers, and high positive end-expiratory pressure for acute lung injury and acute respiratory distress syndrome: a randomized controlled trial. *JAMA.* 2008;299:637-645.

Munshi L, Del Sorbo L, Adhikari NKJ, et al. Prone position for acute respiratory distress syndrome. A systematic review and meta-analysis. *Ann Am Thorac Soc.* 2017;14:S280-S288.

F.2. What rescue strategies can you use for refractory ARDS?

Inhaled nitric oxide (NO) can improve ventilation-perfusion matching in the heterogeneous lungs of ARDS. Inhaled NO distributes to better-ventilated lung units where it relieves reflexive hypoxic and hypercapnic vasoconstriction. This effect can improve hypoxemia and reduce pulmonary vascular resistance. NO has multiple other effects that might explain the absence of a demonstrable mortality benefit in ARDS. Therefore, the role of inhaled NO, if any, in ARDS should be restricted to refractory hypoxemia. Similarly, inhaled prostacyclins have also been shown to improve oxygenation but evidence for improvement in patient outcomes is lacking.

A number of ventilator strategies have been employed to rescue patients with refractory hypoxemia. A common feature is their use of high mean airway pressure to recruit lung. HFOV, APRV, and inverse ratio ventilation all employ a brief expiratory phase. This prevents exhalation and maintains high intrathoracic pressure throughout the respiratory cycle. With HFOV and APRV, the goal is to create auto-PEEP. It is unclear if any of these ventilator strategies offer any advantage over setting a high level of extrinsic PEEP with a conventional mode of ventilation. Recruitment maneuvers can also improve oxygenation. These are brief intervals (30-40 seconds) of high PEEP or CPAP (30-40 cm H_2O). Any of the strategies using high inflation pressures for lung recruitment can cause hemodynamic instability and barotrauma and should be reserved for refractory cases.

Extracorporeal gas exchange is also being evaluated as a rescue strategy for refractory ARDS. One approach is extracorporeal CO_2 removal ($ECCO_2R$), which requires relatively low blood flow rates. CO_2 removal can theoretically increase the gas tension available for oxygen in the alveoli and allow a reduction in tidal volume. However, the routine use of $ECCO_2R$ in moderate-to-severe ARDS to facilitate lower tidal volumes demonstrated harm in a moderately sized clinical trial. There harms were related to prolonged use of neuromuscular blockade, deep sedation in the $ECCO_2R$ group, and higher rates of bleeding. A more aggressive strategy is venovenous extracorporeal membrane oxygenation (VV-ECMO). It requires high blood flow rates and can reduce the CO_2 content and raise the oxygen content of mixed venous blood. VV-ECMO can improve hemodynamics in ARDS by reducing hypoxic/hypercapnic pulmonary vasoconstriction and the magnitude of positive airway pressure required from mechanical ventilation. A randomized trial done at multiple centers in England demonstrated a survival advantage for patients with severe ARDS who were transferred to an ECMO center. There was also better than expected survival for patients with severe ARDS due to influenza when treated with ECMO. Bleeding and vascular complications are its main complications. A recent large multicenter trial was stopped for a low probability of demonstrating a benefit but showed a possible improvement in mortality in patients with severe ARDS receiving ECMO versus conventional ventilation. Patients receiving early ECMO had a higher survival as opposed to late (ie, rescue) use of ECMO. Appropriate patient selection and timing of ECMO initiation are critical factors in deriving a benefit from ECMO.

Afshari A, Brok J, Møller AM, et al. Inhaled nitric oxide for acute respiratory distress syndrome (ARDS) and acute lung injury in children and adults. *Cochrane Database Syst Rev.* 2010:CD002787.

Combes A, Hajage D, Capellier G, et al. Extracorporeal membrane oxygenation for severe acute respiratory distress syndrome. *N Engl J Med.* 2018;378:1965-1975.

Davies A, Jones D, Bailey M, et al. Extracorporeal membrane oxygenation for 2009 influenza A(H1N1) acute respiratory distress syndrome. *JAMA.* 2009;302:1888-1895.

Fuller BM, Mohr NM, Skrupky L, et al. The use of inhaled prostaglandins in patients with ARDS: a systematic review and meta-analysis. *Chest.* 2015;147:1510-1522.

Gebistorf F, Karam O, Wetterslev J, et al. Inhaled nitric oxide for acute respiratory distress syndrome (ARDS) in children and adults. *Cochrane Database Syst Rev.* 2016:CD002787.

McNamee JJ, Gillies MA, Barrett NA, et al; REST Investigators. Effect of lower tidal volume ventilation facilitated by extracorporeal carbon dioxide removal vs standard care ventilation on 90-day mortality in patients with acute hypoxemic respiratory failure: the REST randomized clinical trial. *JAMA.* 2021;326:1013-1023.

Peek GJ, Mugford M, Tiruvoipati R, et al. Efficacy and economic assessment of conventional ventilatory support versus extracorporeal membrane oxygenation for severe adult respiratory failure (CESAR): a multicentre randomised controlled trial. *Lancet.* 2009;374:1351-1363.

G. Adjunctive Management of Respiratory Failure

Since tracheal intubation, the patient has become hypotensive.

G.1. What is the cause and treatment of the hemodynamic instability associated with mechanical ventilation?

Hemodynamic instability is a common complication of emergency airway management and the institution of mechanical ventilation. Positive pressure ventilation can decrease the pressure gradient for venous return to the heart, thereby reducing cardiac filling and output. Normally, circulatory reflexes constrict the veins to restore venous return. However, sedatives and opioids used to facilitate tracheal intubation can blunt the autonomic response. Even low levels of positive pressure ventilation can reduce cardiac output in anesthetized postoperative patients, particularly if they have normal or reduced circulating blood volume. Fluid resuscitation and catecholamine vasopressors can raise venous pressure and restore the pressure gradient for venous return and cardiac output. Many patients with ARDS require a positive fluid balance during the first 48 hours of mechanical ventilation to counteract the hemodynamic effects of PEEP and sedatives/opioids.

Although diminished venous return is the most likely cause of hemodynamic instability, it is essential to consider acute cor pulmonale as an alternative explanation. The hypoxemia, hypercarbia, and regional atelectasis associated with ARDS all raise pulmonary vascular resistance. Mechanical ventilation in ARDS can lead to areas of hyperinflation in more normal lung regions. Hyperinflation raises pulmonary vascular resistance by compression of the capillaries in the alveolar septa. A severe increase in pulmonary vascular resistance can lead to right ventricular failure, particularly if the patient has had significant intravascular fluid resuscitation. The pressure increases in the right ventricle because it is unable to pump blood through the pulmonary vasculature efficiently. The incidence of acute cor pulmonale is as high as 50% in patients on mechanical ventilation for ARDS. The use of low-volume ventilation and the limitation of PEEP can lower this risk. The presence of markedly elevated central venous pressure and echocardiographic evidence of dilated right ventricular size with flattening of the interventricular septum suggest a diagnosis of acute cor pulmonale. Respirophasic variation in pulse pressure or inferior vena cava diameter does not predict an increase in cardiac output with fluid resuscitation when right-sided heart failure is present. In acute cor pulmonale, vasopressors can raise systemic blood pressure to maintain coronary perfusion to the right ventricular myocardium. Diuresis can help optimize right ventricular preload. The ventilator should be adjusted to prevent extremes of lung hyperinflation and provide sufficient PEEP to recruit poorly ventilated lung regions. Prone positioning and pulmonary vasodilators can also be beneficial.

Berlin DA, Bakker J. Understanding venous return. *Intensive Care Med.* 2014;40:1564-1566.

Jardin F, Vieillard-Baron A. Right ventricular function and positive pressure ventilation in clinical practice: from hemodynamic subsets to respirator settings. *Intensive Care Med.* 2003;29:1426-1434.

Jellinek H, Krafft P, Fitzgerald RD, et al. Right atrial pressure predicts hemodynamic response to apneic positive airway pressure. *Crit Care Med.* 2000;28:672-678.

Maas JJ, Pinsky MR, de Wilde RB, et al. Cardiac output response to norepinephrine in postoperative cardiac surgery patients: interpretation with venous return and cardiac function curves. *Crit Care Med.* 2013;41:143-150.

Mahjoub Y, Pila C, Friggeri A, et al. Assessing fluid responsiveness in critically ill patients: false-positive pulse pressure variation is detected by Doppler echocardiographic evaluation of the right ventricle. *Crit Care Med.* 2009;37:2570-2575.

Mekontso Dessap A, Charron C, Devaquet J, et al. Impact of acute hypercapnia and augmented positive end-expiratory pressure on right ventricle function in severe acute respiratory distress syndrome. *Intensive Care Med.* 2009;35:1850-1858.

Mort TC. Complications of emergency tracheal intubation: hemodynamic alterations—part I. *J Intensive Care Med.* 2007;22:157-165.

Vieillard-Baron A, Bouferrache K, Charron C. Right ventricular function evaluation in acute respiratory distress syndrome: back to the future. *Crit Care Med.* 2010;38:1909-1910.

Vieillard-Baron A, Prin S, Augarde R, et al. Increasing respiratory rate to improve CO_2 clearance during mechanical ventilation is not a panacea in acute respiratory failure. *Crit Care Med.* 2002;30:1407-1412.

Vieillard-Baron A, Prin S, Chergui K, et al. Echo-Doppler demonstration of acute cor pulmonale at the bedside in the medical intensive care unit. *Am J Respir Crit Care Med.* 2002;166:1310-1319.

G.2. What is the adjunctive medical therapy for ARDS?

After the initial resuscitation phase, many patients with ARDS require a different approach to fluid balance. The Fluids and Catheters Treatment Trial (FACTT) evaluated two fluid strategies instituted after the first 48 hours. With the restrictive fluid approach, patients received diuretics if they had oliguria and adequate perfusion. The restricted fluid approach group had better gas exchange and a shorter duration of mechanical ventilation than the liberal fluid group. There was no increase in hemodynamic instability or renal failure with a restrictive fluid approach. FACTT had a two-by-two factorial design and simultaneously demonstrated that routine use of pulmonary artery catheterization did not improve outcomes in ARDS. Therefore, clinicians should target even or slightly negative net fluid balance once patients have achieved hemodynamic stability and avoid routine use of pulmonary artery catheters.

Severe anemia can diminish oxygen delivery. However, red blood cell transfusion is linked to a wide range of complications including nosocomial pneumonia. Moreover, red blood cell transfusion has a limited capacity to improve oxygen consumption in critically ill patients. Although there is no specific randomized trial data in ARDS, it is reasonable to limit red blood cell transfusion in adequately perfused patients with isovolemic anemia unless the hemoglobin concentration is less than 7 g/dL.

Numerous trials have evaluated the ability of medications to modulate the natural history of ARDS. The support for systemic corticosteroids has waxed and waned for decades. A high-quality randomized controlled trial found that corticosteroids offered no benefit and increased mortality if started late after the first 2 weeks of ARDS. However, other analyses have shown improvement in mortality or time to resolution of ARDS. More recently, moderate-dose dexamethasone demonstrated a mortality benefit in COVID-19-associated respiratory failure treated with mechanical ventilation.

Currently, the evidence does not support the routine use of corticosteroids for ARDS in patients with mild hypoxemia or an improving trajectory. However, the Society of Critical Care Medicine (SCCM) and European Society of Intensive Care Medicine (ESICM) 2017 guidelines suggest the use of intravenous methylprednisolone 1 mg/kg/d in patients with early moderate-to-severe ARDS (Pao_2/Fio_2 <200 and within 14 days of onset). An additional indication is concomitant shock.

A number of other disease-modifying agents have been studied in ARDS. Rosuvastatin, a 3-hydroxy-3-methylglutaryl coenzyme A reductase inhibitor (statin), had no benefit in a much-anticipated trial. Recombinant activated protein C and ω-3 fatty acids also had no benefit. Theoretically, inhaled β-agonists would decrease lung edema and lung inflammation. However, no randomized trial has shown a benefit. Their use should be restricted to treating bronchospasm.

Patients with severe respiratory failure often have a strong respiratory drive due to increased metabolic rates and dead space. This high demand for minute ventilation can lead to intolerance of low-volume ventilation. In these situations, deep sedation and neuromuscular blocking agents can blunt excessive respiratory effort and enforce low-stretch ventilation. Moreover, neuromuscular blockade can reduce metabolic demand, which can be helpful when oxygen delivery and carbon dioxide clearance are inadequate. However, neuromuscular blockade and deep sedation can worsen delirium and muscular weakness, but their use in appropriate situations should not be withheld due to this concern. To help define the role of neuromuscular blockade, two high-quality randomized controlled trials of patients with early ARDS and severe hypoxemia have been performed. Both trials randomized patients to either cisatracurium besylate or placebo. Cisatracurium is useful in critical illness because it is cleared by plasma esterase. The control group of the initial study received deep sedation, whereas the control group in the second was treated with lighter sedation targets. Rescue use of neuromuscular blockade was allowed in both studies to treat double triggering and overt ventilator dyssynchrony. The first study demonstrated that cisatracurium improved gas exchange, barotrauma, and mortality compared with placebo. The second study did not confirm this benefit. As a result, the role of neuromuscular blockade in ARDS remains unclear. One approach is to avoid the routine use of cisatracurium for ARDS and reserve it for patients with severe respiratory failure as well as strong respiratory efforts and dyssynchrony with mechanical ventilation.

A growing body of evidence supports limiting sedative use in patients on mechanical ventilation. In the absence of a compelling need for sedatives (eg, status epilepticus, ventilatory dyssynchrony or increased work of breathing), clinicians should interrupt continuous sedatives and neuromuscular blocking agents at least daily. This approach is associated with a marked reduction in duration of mechanical ventilation. Reassuringly, this approach is also associated with improved long-term neuropsychiatric function among survivors of respiratory failure. Another strategy uses a detailed sedation protocol to avoid oversedation. Sedatives can contribute to delirium and disuse muscle atrophy. Sedation is not restorative sleep. Moreover, clinicians can fail to recognize that their deeply sedated patients might be able to breathe without ventilator support. Opioids are still necessary for pain and dyspnea, and neuroleptics can be used for agitated delirium. Deeper sedation can be reserved for situations when severe agitation occurs, there is a high work of breathing and ventilatory dyssynchrony, or pronation is required. Treatment plans that limit sedative use require clinicians to provide calming reassurance, repositioning, and ventilator adjustment to assure patient comfort. The study that validated the avoidance of routine sedatives for patients on mechanical ventilation used one-to-one bedside nursing and continuous presence of an intensivist in the intensive care unit.

Limiting sedation allows physical therapy. Patients can perform full physical therapy including walking while breathing through an endotracheal tube and a portable ventilator. The theoretical benefit of this approach is to decrease muscular atrophy, sedative requirements, and delirium.

The evolving treatment paradigm is to use deep sedation, opioids, and neuromuscular blockade early in the course of severe ARDS in patients with excessive ventilator demands and ventilator dyssynchrony. Patients might benefit from pronation during this phase. Clinicians should switch to the opposite approach of limited sedation as soon as there is stabilization. This includes limited or no sedation (aside from opioids for relief of pain or dyspnea) and physical therapy. This approach should also be used when the ARDS is less severe.

Alhazzani W, Alshahrani M, Jaeschke R, et al. Neuromuscular blocking agents in acute respiratory distress syndrome: a systematic review and meta-analysis of randomized controlled trials. *Crit Care.* 2013;17:R43.

Annane D, Pastores SM, Rochwerg B, et al. Guidelines for the diagnosis and management of critical illness-related corticosteroid insufficiency (CIRCI) in critically ill patients (part I): Society of Critical Care Medicine (SCCM) and European Society of Intensive Care Medicine (ESICM) 2017. *Intensive Care Med.* 2017;43:1751-1763.

Bassford CR, Thickett DR, Perkins GD. The rise and fall of β-agonists in the treatment of ARDS. *Crit Care.* 2012;16:208.

Brown EN, Lydic R, Schiff ND. General anesthesia, sleep, and coma. *N Engl J Med.* 2010;363:2638-2650.

Girard TD, Kress JP, Fuchs BD, et al. Efficacy and safety of a paired sedation and ventilator weaning protocol for mechanically ventilated patients in intensive care (Awakening and Breathing Controlled trial): a randomised controlled trial. *Lancet*. 2008;371:126-134.

Kress JP, Gehlbach B, Lacy M, et al. The long-term psychological effects of daily sedative interruption on critically ill patients. *Am J Respir Crit Care Med*. 2003;168:1457-1461.

Marik PE, Corwin HL. Efficacy of red blood cell transfusion in the critically ill: a systematic review of the literature. *Crit Care Med*. 2008;36:2667-2674.

Mehta S, Burry L, Cook D, et al. Daily sedation interruption in mechanically ventilated critically ill patients cared for with a sedation protocol: a randomized controlled trial. *JAMA*. 2012;308:1985-1992.

Meduri GU, Bridges L, Shih MC, et al. Prolonged glucocorticoid treatment is associated with improved ARDS outcomes: analysis of individual patients' data from four randomized trials and trial-level meta-analysis of the updated literature. *Intensive Care Med*. 2016;42:829-840.

Moss M, Huang D, Brower R, et al. Early neuromuscular blockade in the acute respiratory distress syndrome. *N Engl J Med*. 2019;380:1997-2008.

Needham DM. Mobilizing patients in the intensive care unit: improving neuromuscular weakness and physical function. *JAMA*. 2008;300:1685-1690.

Papazian L, Forel JM, Gacouin A, et al. Neuromuscular blockers in early acute respiratory distress syndrome. *N Engl J Med*. 2010;363:1107-1116.

Pohlman MC, Schweickert WD, Pohlman AS, et al. Feasibility of physical and occupational therapy beginning from initiation of mechanical ventilation. *Crit Care Med*. 2010;38:2089-2094.

RECOVERY Collaborative Group; Horby P, Lim WS, Emberson JR, et al. Dexamethasone in hospitalized patients with Covid-19. *N Engl J Med*. 2021;384:693-704.

Rubenfeld GD. ARDS: promising insights for a challenging syndrome. *Lancet Respir Med*. 2014;2:955-956.

Schweickert WD, Pohlman MC, Pohlman AS, et al. Early physical and occupational therapy in mechanically ventilated, critically ill patients: a randomised controlled trial. *Lancet*. 2009;373:1874-1882.

Silversides JA, Major E, Ferguson AJ, et al. Conservative fluid management or deresuscitation for patients with sepsis or acute respiratory distress syndrome following the resuscitation phase of critical illness: a systematic review and meta-analysis. *Intensive Care Med*. 2017;43:155-170.

Steinberg KP, Hudson LD, Goodman RB, et al. Efficacy and safety of corticosteroids for persistent acute respiratory distress syndrome. *N Engl J Med*. 2006;354:1671-1684.

Strøm T, Martinussen T, Toft P. A protocol of no sedation for critically ill patients receiving mechanical ventilation: a randomised trial. *Lancet*. 2010;375:475-480.

Truwit JD, Bernard GR, Steingrub J, et al. Rosuvastatin for sepsis-associated acute respiratory distress syndrome. *N Engl J Med*. 2014;370:2191-2200.

Villar J, Ferrando C, Martínez D, et al; dexamethasone in ARDS network. Dexamethasone treatment for the acute respiratory distress syndrome: a multicentre, randomised controlled trial. *Lancet Respir Med*. 2020;8:267-276.

Wheeler AP, Bernard GR, Thompson BT, et al. Pulmonary-artery versus central venous catheter to guide treatment of acute lung injury. *N Engl J Med*. 2006;354:2213-2224.

Wiedemann HP, Wheeler AP, Bernard GR, et al. Comparison of two fluid-management strategies in acute lung injury. *N Engl J Med*. 2006;354:2564-2575.

H. Weaning From Mechanical Ventilation

The patient slowly recovers over the next 3 days.

H.1. Explain the importance of the decision to extubate the patient or continue mechanical ventilation.

Unnecessarily prolonged mechanical ventilation can lead to pneumonia, delirium, and neuromuscular weakness. Unfortunately, clinicians are unable to identify which of their mechanically ventilated patients are capable of breathing without ventilator support. Conversely, the mortality rate associated with reintubation is high. Intensive care unit patients fail extubation at rates of 10% to 20%. The risk is substantially higher in patients with chronic illnesses. Patients who suffer extubation failure are much more likely to die than patients who are successfully extubated, and the survivors are much more likely to require long-term care. Reintubation is associated with nosocomial pneumonia, although it is unknown whether pneumonia is the cause or effect of reintubation. Therefore, the decision of whether or not to extubate a patient is one of the most important challenges. There is extensive literature and great controversy surrounding the topic, and the strategies employed to wean patients from mechanical ventilation vary widely.

Epstein SK, Ciubotaru RL, Wong JB. Effect of failed extubation on the outcome of mechanical ventilation. *Chest.* 1997;112:186-192.

Esteban A, Anzueto A, Alía I, et al. How is mechanical ventilation employed in the intensive care unit? An international utilization review. *Am J Respir Crit Care Med.* 2000;161:1450-1458.

Pham T, Heunks L, Bellani G, et al; WEAN SAFE Investigators. Weaning from mechanical ventilation in intensive care units across 50 countries (WEAN SAFE): a multicentre, prospective, observational cohort study. *Lancet Respir Med.* 2023;11:465-476.

Thille AW, Harrois A, Schortgen F, et al. Outcomes of extubation failure in medical intensive care unit patients. *Crit Care Med.* 2011;39:2612-2618.

H.2. How will you prepare the patient for weaning from the ventilator?

The most important aspect of weaning from mechanical ventilation is the general care of the patient and the reversal of the cause of the patient's respiratory failure. Early in the course of an acute illness, the patient must be resuscitated to preserve circulation and organ perfusion. Generally, in later stages, volume overload and hypertension should be avoided. This is especially important during the switch to negative pressure ventilation, which increases cardiac preload and left ventricular wall tension. Adequate protection against the development of coronary ischemia should be ensured by optimizing volume status and reducing sources of catecholamine surges in patients with significant coronary artery disease. Neurologic status should be optimized to maintain airway protection and patency as well as adequate respiratory drive and strength. Sedation should be limited and reversed at least daily. Delirium should be avoided, and evaluated and treated if it occurs.

Clinicians should aggressively reduce F_{IO_2} and PEEP to the minimum acceptable level. Derecruitment happens quickly after reducing PEEP, so lengthy weaning is unnecessary.

Chiumello D, Coppola S, Froio S, et al. Time to reach a new steady state after changes of positive end expiratory pressure. *Intensive Care Med.* 2013;39:1377-1385.

H.3. How will you recognize when the patient is ready for tracheal extubation?

Previously, once F_{IO_2} and PEEP were at minimal settings, clinicians would assess patients for their ability to undergo a weaning trial. Tests of weaning readiness were used to identify patients in whom it was safe to reduce ventilator support. These tests included objective measures such as the negative inspiratory force, vital capacity, and the rapid shallow breathing index (RSBI). The literature makes a clear distinction between these tests of weaning readiness and tests of extubation readiness (such as a prolonged T-tube trial as discussed below). The best validated test to predict readiness for weaning is the RSBI. This test is performed by switching from assist/control ventilation to a T-tube. A spirometer attached to the end of the endotracheal tube measures tidal volume, and respiratory rate is counted. Patients with ratios of less than 105 could safely go on to a test of extubation readiness with a T-tube trial lasting up to 2 hours. However, there is no clear advantage to performing a test of weaning readiness (such as the RSBI calculation) prior to initiating a test of extubation readiness. Instead, clinicians can perform daily clinical screening of patients on mechanical ventilation to assess them for extubation readiness (**Table 3.5**).

The purpose of clinical screening is to determine a pretest probability of extubation success. The pretest probability of success will be extremely low in the presence of clinical signs that clearly predict extubation failure. These signs include shock supported by more than minimal doses of vasopressors, severe intracranial hypertension, requirement of high F_{IO_2} or PEEP, and the absence of protective airway reflexes or spontaneous inspiratory efforts. If the pretest probability of extubation success is extremely low, there is no additional test that would be able to raise the posttest probability of success sufficiently to allow extubation. In these situations, the clinician should continue mechanical ventilation, treat the cause

TABLE 3.5 Clinical Screening Criteria for Extubation Readiness

Adequate level of alertness	Cause of respiratory failure improving
$Pa_{O_2}/F_{IO_2} \geq 150$ or $Sp_{O_2} \geq 90\%$ on $F_{IO_2} \leq 0.4$	Able to initiate an inspiratory effort
PEEP $\leq$ 5 cm H_2O	Hemodynamic stability
	Absence of refractory acidemia

F_{IO_2}, fraction of inspired oxygen; Pa_{O_2}, partial pressure of oxygen; PEEP, positive end-expiratory pressure; Sp_{O_2}, peripheral capillary oxygen saturation.

of the respiratory failure, and repeat the screening at least daily. Similarly, clinicians should not perform tests of extubation readiness in situations where the pretest probability of extubation success is very high. These situations include patients who had been intubated for a brief and uncomplicated procedure as well as those intubated for a sedative overdose that has resolved. When clinicians calculate a very high pretest probability of extubation success, they can proceed directly to extubation without testing.

When there is an intermediate pretest probability for extubation success, clinicians should consider performing tests of extubation readiness. These tests simulate the conditions of spontaneous breathing after extubation. The most common tests are T-tube, zero support or flow-by, CPAP, and pressure support ventilation. The appearance of tachypnea, hemodynamic instability, diaphoresis, anxiety, or agitation signifies failure of the test. If the patient tolerates it, the trial continues for 30 to 120 minutes. Clinicians should consider extubation if the patient passes the trial. It is unclear whether there is a single best approach to test for extubation readiness. Several recent trials support the noninferiority of pressure support ventilation compared to unassisted breathing via T-tube in moderate- and high-risk patients. Importantly, the vast majority of critically ill patients who undergo these tests are able to sustain spontaneous breathing after extubation. There is some evidence that pressure support ventilation leads to decreased time to extubation; however, this is balanced by an increased need for reintubation. There remain important physiologic differences to consider between the methods. Given the varied causes of extubation failure, the utility of the different tests can vary in different situations. For example, in patients with significant heart disease, it is important to predict the consequences of switching from positive to negative pressure ventilation that occurs with extubation. Because positive pressure ventilation decreases cardiac preload and left ventricular afterload, extubation readiness testing performed with CPAP or minimal pressure support might not predict success. Tests using T-tube or "flow-by" ventilation (with pressure support and PEEP set to 0 cm H_2O) better simulate the hemodynamic stressors of breathing after extubation (**Figure 3.8**). There are concerns about T-tubes imposing an unfair resistive load due to their narrow diameter. In one series, T-tube trials failed to identify a number of patients capable of successfully breathing after extubation. However, T-piece trials using size 7 to 8.5 endotracheal tubes accurately predict the work of breathing after extubation in critically ill patients. T-tube trials add the expense of the

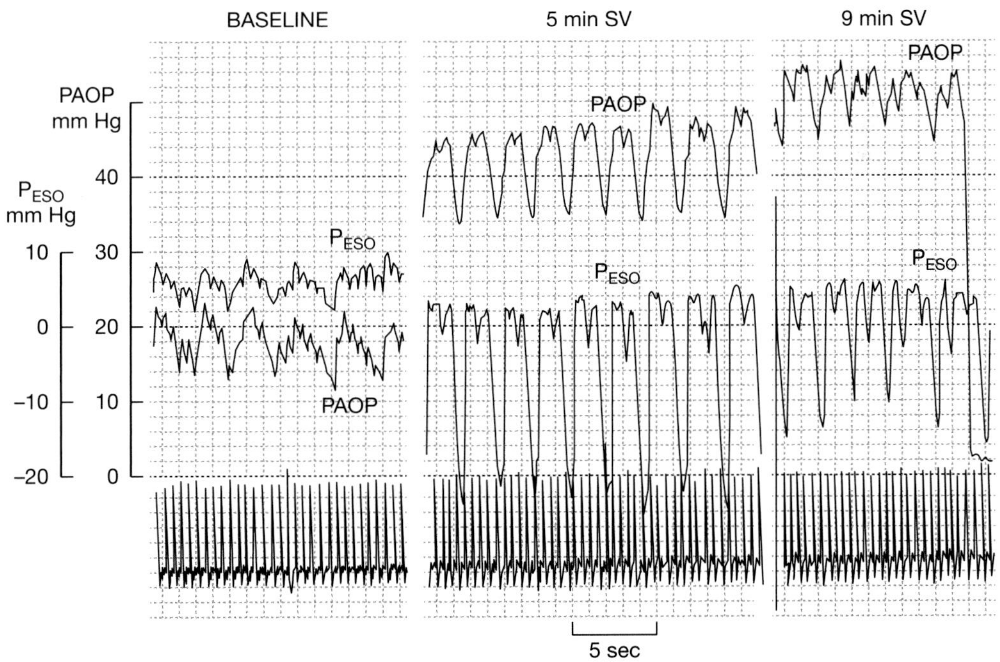

FIGURE 3.8. Ventricular failure and pulmonary edema precipitated by spontaneous ventilation. At baseline **(left)**, the patient is receiving positive pressure ventilation. During spontaneous ventilation (SV), esophageal pressure (P_{ESO}) is negative during inspiration and pulmonary artery occlusion pressure (PAOP) rises. By 9 minutes, PAOP is catastrophically elevated and respiratory muscle fatigue decreases the amplitude of P_{ESO}. (Reprinted with permission from Lemaire F, Teboul JL, Cinotti L, et al. Acute left ventricular dysfunction during unsuccessful weaning from mechanical ventilation. *Anesthesiology.* 1988;69:171-179. Figure 1.)

humidification and tubing attachments to the oxygen source. Moreover, the T-piece trials do not benefit from ventilator alarms.

Trials with pressure support overcome the resistance imposed by the ventilator circuit. However, the amount of pressure support required is unclear. These trials might underestimate the work of breathing after extubation. The opposite is also important. Pressure support can create dyssynchrony on mechanical ventilation. In particular, oversupport can induce tachypnea, which clinicians might misinterpret to mean that the patient cannot be extubated. This could lead to needlessly prolonged mechanical ventilation. Automatic tube compensation software is designed to improve the application of minimal pressure support during tests of extubation readiness. However, at present, there is no proof of the advantage of this approach in clinical trials.

In place of tests of readiness for extubation, some clinicians prefer to wean ventilator support gradually. Pressure support can be incrementally reduced or the number of controlled breaths reduced on SIMV. However, there is no proof that any ventilator strategy or weaning process trains and strengthens respiratory muscles. In clinical trials, these methods prolong the time to extubation. The importance of liberation as opposed to weaning from mechanical ventilation is illustrated by a clinical trial, which showed that pairing a once-daily awakening from sedatives with a trial of spontaneous ventilation reduced mortality.

A final step prior to extubation is to consider the risk of postextubation stridor. The cuff leak test is an imperfect predictor. Clinicians should only consider using it when there are risk factors for laryngeal edema such as prolonged intubation, a large endotracheal tube, asthma, traumatic intubation, and ventilator-patient dyssynchrony.

In situations with a higher risk of extubation failure such as morbid obesity, older age, COPD, or congestive heart failure, extubation directly to prophylactic NIPPV has been shown to reduce the need for reintubation. However, these patients must be carefully reevaluated to make sure they are not dependent on NIPPV for excessive periods of time, preventing effective nutrition and physical therapy.

Cabello B, Thille AW, Roche-Campo F, et al. Physiological comparison of three spontaneous breathing trials in difficult-to-wean patients. *Intensive Care Med.* 2010;36:1171-1179.

Cohen J, Shapiro M, Grozovski E, et al. Prediction of extubation outcome: a randomised, controlled trial with automatic tube compensation vs. pressure support ventilation. *Crit Care.* 2009;13:R21.

Conci D, Fortis S, Ramos F, et al. Factitious respiratory failure: bound to the ventilator by pressure support. *Am J Respir Crit Care Med.* 2010;182:1208-1209.

Esteban A, Frutos F, Tobin MJ, et al. A comparison of four methods of weaning patients from mechanical ventilation. Spanish Lung Failure Collaborative Group. *N Engl J Med.* 1995;332:345-350.

Girard TD, Kress JP, Fuchs BD, et al. Efficacy and safety of a paired sedation and ventilator weaning protocol for mechanically ventilated patients in intensive care (Awakening and Breathing Controlled trial): a randomised controlled trial. *Lancet.* 2008;371:126-134.

Krishna B, Sampath S, Moran JL. The role of non-invasive positive pressure ventilation in post-extubation respiratory failure: an evaluation using meta-analytic techniques. *Indian J Crit Care Med.* 2013;17:253-261.

Lemaire F, Teboul JL, Cinotti L, et al. Acute left ventricular dysfunction during unsuccessful weaning from mechanical ventilation. *Anesthesiology.* 1988;69:171-179.

Subirà C, Hernández G, Vázquez A, et al. Effect of pressure support vs T-piece ventilation strategies during spontaneous breathing trials on successful extubation among patients receiving mechanical ventilation: a randomized clinical trial. *JAMA.* 2019;321:2175-2182.

Tanios MA, Nevins ML, Hendra KP, et al. A randomized, controlled trial of the role of weaning predictors in clinical decision making. *Crit Care Med.* 2006;34:2530-2535.

Thille AW, Gacouin A, Coudroy R, et al; REVA Research Network. Spontaneous-breathing trials with pressure-support ventilation or a T-piece. *N Engl J Med.* 2022;387:1843-1854.

Thille AW, Muller G, Gacouin A, et al; HIGH-WEAN Study Group and the REVA Research Network. Effect of postextubation high-flow nasal oxygen with noninvasive ventilation vs high-flow nasal oxygen alone on reintubation among patients at high risk of extubation failure: a randomized clinical trial. *JAMA.* 2019;322:1465-1475.

Thille AW, Richard JC, Brochard L. The decision to extubate in the intensive care unit. *Am J Respir Crit Care Med.* 2013;187:1294-1302.

Tobin MJ. Extubation and the myth of "minimal ventilator settings." *Am J Respir Crit Care Med.* 2012;185:349-350.

4 Lung Transplantation

Jared Roberts, Sawyer A. Naze, and
Charles W. Hogue

A 65-year-old male with worsening dyspnea on exertion and limited functional capacity despite maximal medical treatment, pulmonary rehabilitation, and supplemental oxygen therapy is scheduled for bilateral, sequential lung transplantation. Laboratory, radiographic, and spirometry data are consistent with severe interstitial lung disease (ILD). Other significant medical findings include a 20-pack-year history of tobacco smoking (although none for 10 years), mild hypertension (145/86 mm Hg), mild pulmonary hypertension (mean pulmonary arterial pressure, 32 mm Hg), normal left and right ventricular function, and osteoarthritis.

A. Medical Disease and Differential Diagnosis

1. What are the causes and expected manifestations of ILD in this patient, and why is he a transplant candidate?
2. What other end-stage lung diseases can be treated with transplantation?
3. How many lung transplantations have been performed?
4. What are the selection criteria for recipients?
5. How is the decision made to transplant one or both lungs, and does this influence preoperative management?
6. How does a single-lung transplantation (SLT) differ technically from a bilateral-lung transplantation (BLT)?

B. Preoperative Evaluation and Preparation

1. What preoperative evaluation is desirable?
2. Would you premedicate this patient? If so, how?
3. What vascular access is appropriate?
4. Is preoperative epidural catheter placement advantageous?

C. Intraoperative Management

1. What special equipment is necessary?
2. How would you monitor this patient?
3. How would you induce anesthesia in this patient?
4. What type of endotracheal tube would you use? How would you ventilate this patient?
5. How does the physiology of one-lung ventilation (OLV) influence the procedure?
6. How does OLV affect cardiopulmonary function?
7. At what specific points in the procedure are problems anticipated?
8. How would you deal with problems related to clamping of the pulmonary artery?
9. What hemodynamic alterations would you expect during graft implantation and reperfusion? How would you correct them?
10. When is extracorporeal membrane oxygenation (ECMO) utilized for lung transplantation?
11. Should fluid administration be restricted, and are blood products commonly required?
12. Would you extubate the patient upon the conclusion of the procedure?

D. Postoperative Management

1. What are the major complications after lung transplantation?
2. How is postoperative lung ventilation managed, and for how long is it required?
3. What special precautions should be taken when a lung transplant recipient requires general anesthesia for subsequent nonpulmonary surgery?
4. What are the long-term outcomes of lung transplantation?

A. Medical Disease and Differential Diagnosis

A.1. What are the causes and expected manifestations of interstitial lung disease in this patient, and why is he a transplant candidate?

Interstitial lung disease encompasses a variety of pathologies which all result in interstitial fibrosis. The pathophysiology is complex and is dependent on the underlying cause, but generally involves some combination of abnormal cellular proliferation, interstitial inflammation, and impaired cellular repair mechanisms. The ultimate result is the destruction of alveoli leading to impaired gas exchange. ILD can arise secondary to other conditions such as hypersensitivity pneumonitis (ie, due to mold or bird exposure) or from an autoimmune or connective tissue disease such as rheumatoid arthritis, scleroderma, or pulmonary sarcoidosis. Idiopathic pulmonary fibrosis (IPF) is diagnosed when no other etiology of ILD can be identified.

Clinically, ILD is characterized by restrictive pulmonary physiology. Pulmonary function tests (PFTs) show reduced lung volumes (forced vital capacity [FVC] and total lung capacity) and impaired diffusing capacity of carbon monoxide (DL_{CO}). Ventilatory flow rates such as forced expiratory volume in 1 second (FEV_1) and FEV_1:FVC ratio are typically preserved. Comparisons of flow-volume loops representing obstructive and restrictive diseases are shown in **Figure 4.1**. The underlying disease process of ILD tends to obliterate the pulmonary microvasculature, thereby chronically increasing vascular resistance, increasing the risk of pulmonary hypertension, and predisposing to cor pulmonale.

Patients with ILD generally present with unexplained progressive exertional dyspnea with or without a chronic dry cough. This presentation is nonspecific and can initially be attributed to natural aging, cardiovascular disease, medication side effects, or a history of smoking, among other possible causes. On physical examination, patients can have "Velcro-like" crackles at the base of the lungs and frequently exhibit digital clubbing.

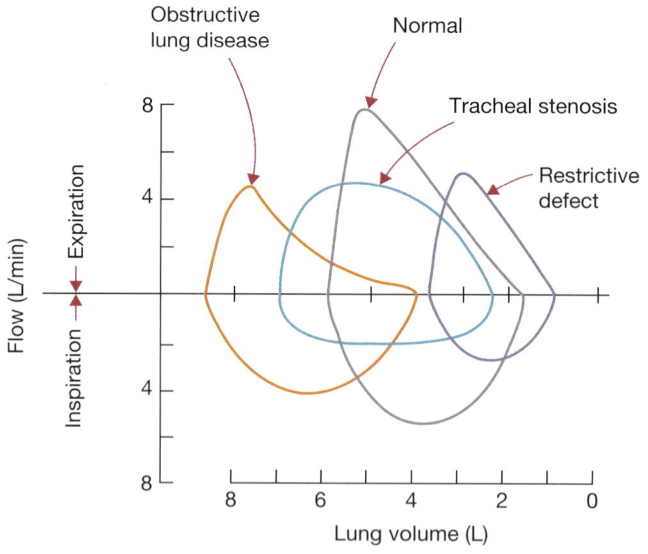

FIGURE 4.1. Representative tracings of flow-volume loops from a healthy individual, a patient with parenchymal obstructive disease, a patient with tracheal stenosis, and a patient with restrictive disease from parenchymal fibrosis. (Modified from Goudsouzian N, Karamanian A. *Physiology for the Anesthesiologist.* 2nd ed. Appleton-Century-Crofts; 1984:213.)

Disease progression of ILD varies by etiology. For the most part, IPF is an aggressive disease with a poor prognosis; the median age at diagnosis is 65 years, and the median survival from the time of diagnosis is 2 to 5 years. The antifibrotic medications nintedanib and pirfenidone slow disease progression and reduce the rate of FVC decline while reducing the frequency of acute exacerbations. Any long-term mortality benefit of these medications is yet unknown. Patients with non-IPF ILD endure a more prolonged, less predictable disease course, and medical management depends on the specific underlying disease process. Antifibrotic therapy has been shown to be effective in these patients. Nonpharmacologic treatment for ILD includes pulmonary rehabilitation and supplemental oxygen.

Lung transplantation is considered for patients with ILD when the disease is severe or continues to progress despite maximal medical management. According to The International Society of Heart and Lung Transplantation (ISHLT) guidelines, patients with ILD should be evaluated for lung transplantation if they have any of the following: FVC less than 80% predicted or DL_{CO} less than 40% predicted; if in the past 2 years they have had a relative decrease in FVC by 10%, DL_{CO} by 15%, or FVC by 5% with concomitant worsening of symptoms or radiographic progression; or if they require supplemental oxygen at rest or with exertion. A patient should be listed for transplant once they meet the following criteria: a decrease in FVC by more than 10% over 6 months, a decrease in DL_{CO} more than 10% in the past 6 months, or a decrease in FVC by more than 5% with concomitant worsening of symptoms or radiographic progression of disease; arterial desaturation (Spo_2) less than or equal to 88% on 6-minute walk test or greater than 50 m decline in 6-minute walk distance in past 6 months; pulmonary hypertension; or hospitalization due to exacerbation, decline in respiratory status, or pneumothorax. This patient's age, severity of disease, progression of disease, and lack of contraindications support consideration of lung transplantation.

Chambers DC, Perch M, Zuckermann A, et al. The International Thoracic Organ Transplant Registry of the International Society for Heart and Lung Transplantation: thirty-eighth adult lung transplantation report—2021; focus on recipient characteristics. *J Heart Lung Transplant*. 2021;40:1060-1072.

Kapnadak SG, Raghu G. Lung transplantation for interstitial lung disease. *Eur Respir Rev*. 2021;30:210017.

Leard LE, Holm AM, Valapour M, et al. Consensus document for the selection of lung transplant candidates: an update from the International Society for Heart and Lung Transplantation. *J Heart Lung Transplant*. 2021;40:1349-1379.

Richeldi L, Collard HR, Jones MG. Idiopathic pulmonary fibrosis. *Lancet*. 2017;389:1941-1952.

A.2. What other end-stage lung diseases can be treated with transplantation?

The underlying disease processes that produce chronic lung dysfunction can be broadly categorized into four categories: obstructive, restrictive, suppurative (eg, cystic fibrosis [CF] and bronchiectasis), or vascular. With the emergence of the COVID-19 pandemic in 2020 and continued advances in treatment for acute respiratory distress syndrome (ARDS), a new unofficial category of transplant recipient has emerged: a combination of suppurative and restrictive lung disease. Treatment for the latter group has been aided by the widespread implementation of extracorporeal life support (ECLS) such as veno-venous ECMO (VV-ECMO) as a bridge to transplant in patients with ARDS (**Table 4.1**).

Obstructive lung disease: Severe chronic obstructive pulmonary disease (COPD) results in increased airway resistance, reduced expiratory flow rates, and high residual lung volumes. The clinical progression of the disease is typically much slower than in restrictive or suppurative pulmonary diseases; accordingly, short- and intermediate-term survival is usually better in COPD than in other transplantable diseases. The effects on quality of life, however, can be quite profound. Significant limitations on physical activity, the need for continuous oxygen supplementation, and increased risk of infection and hospitalization contribute to diminished quality of life for those with COPD. Further, there is a point at which the expiratory airway obstruction and lung hyperinflation become so severe that the chest wall cannot physically expand to accommodate the tidal volume, resulting in restrictive physiology superimposed on obstructive disease. This condition is usually refractory to medical management and substantially limits daily activity.

The BODE index is a multivariable assessment that combines **B**ody mass index (BMI), airway **O**bstruction (FEV_1), Modified Medical Research Council **D**yspnea scale, and **E**xercise capacity (6-minute walk test) into a weighted 10-point score that is correlated to disease severity and mortality in COPD. The 2021 updated ISHLT guidelines state that to be listed for transplant, patients with COPD must meet one or more of the following criteria: (1) BODE index greater than or equal to 7, (2) FEV_1 less than 20% predicted, (3) concomitant moderate to severe pulmonary hypertension, (4) history of severe exacerbations, or (5) chronic hypercapnia.

TABLE 4.1 Lung Transplants Categorized by Indication

End-Stage Lung Disease	% of Total Lung Transplants
Idiopathic pulmonary fibrosis	29.0
Chronic obstructive pulmonary disease	26.5
Other/miscellaneous	20.3
Cystic fibrosis	14.2
Retransplant	4.1
α_1-Antitrypsin deficiency	3.1
Idiopathic pulmonary arterial hypertension	2.8

Suppurative lung disease is the most frequent indication for lung transplantation in patients 18 years or younger. Characterized by chronic infection and copious purulent secretions, patients with CF primarily exhibit obstructive functional abnormalities with increased airway reactivity. Under most circumstances, residual lung volume and functional residual capacity are increased and bronchodilators have little effect on expiratory flow rate. Cystic fibrosis transmembrane conductance regulator (CFTR) modulators are drugs that target the underlying genetic defect in CF by improving both trafficking of the CFTR protein to the plasma membrane and increasing chloride flow through the CFTR protein at the cell surface. These drugs have shown promising results with improvement in lung function, increased BMI, decreased sweat chloride values, and better subjective quality of life. Accordingly, the incidence of lung transplantation in these patients has decreased in recent years.

Pulmonary vascular disease with severe pulmonary hypertension and right ventricular dysfunction is another indication for transplantation. Pathologically, pulmonary hypertension can result from idiopathic proximal vascular processes such as primary pulmonary hypertension (PPH), secondarily from chronically increased pulmonary blood flow (eg, left-to-right intracardiac shunt, leading to Eisenmenger syndrome), or pulmonary venous hypertension from left-sided heart disease. Pulmonary hypertension can precipitate chronic hypoxemia via an intracardiac right-to-left shunt. Improved medical therapy for PPH, particularly with continuous long-term intravenous prostacyclin infusion, sildenafil, and endothelin antagonists, has reduced the number of patients undergoing lung transplantation for this disease.

ARDS develops in the setting of a variety of diseases. Common causes and risk factors include bacterial pneumonia, viral infection (eg, influenza A, COVID-19), aspiration pneumonitis, pancreatitis, amniotic fluid embolism, among others. The clinical presentation includes severe hypoxemia, bilateral radiographic chest infiltrates, and noncardiogenic pulmonary edema due to intense inflammation leading to the breakdown of the alveolocapillary membrane. Severe cases result in prolonged mechanical ventilation, the need for VV-ECMO, significant physical deconditioning, and a mortality rate greater than 30%. Less severe cases are still quite debilitating and result in chronic restrictive lung disease and the need for oxygen supplementation. ARDS has become increasingly more relevant since the onset of the COVID-19 pandemic in 2020, and lung transplantation is being utilized more and more as a last-resort treatment option for these critically ill patients.

Dickinson KM, Collaco JM. Cystic fibrosis. *Pediatr Rev*. 2021;42:55-67.

Kurihara C, Manerikar A, Querrey M, et al. Clinical characteristics and outcomes of patients with COVID-19-associated acute respiratory distress syndrome who underwent lung transplant. *JAMA*. 2022;327:652-661.

Leard LE, Holm AM, Valapour M, et al. Consensus document for the selection of lung transplant candidates: an update from the International Society for Heart and Lung Transplantation. *J Heart Lung Transplant*. 2021;40:1349-1379.

Meyer NJ, Gattinoni L, Calfee CS. Acute respiratory distress syndrome. *Lancet*. 2021;398:622-637.

Perch M, Hayes D, Cherikh WS, et al. The International Thoracic Organ Transplant Registry of the International Society for Heart and Lung Transplantation: thirty-ninth adult lung transplantation report—2022; focus on lung transplant recipients with chronic obstructive pulmonary disease. *J Heart Lung Transplant*. 2022;41:1335-1347.

A.3. How many lung transplantations have been performed?

Although the first human lung transplantation was performed in 1963, transplantation of one or both lungs did not emerge as a viable therapeutic option for patients with end-stage lung disease until the 1980s. The emergence of this procedure can be largely attributed to advances in surgical technique, anesthetic management, organ harvest and preservation, infection prevention, and immunosuppressive therapy. Since the initiation of the International Thoracic Organ Transplant Registry in the mid-1980s, the number of annual procedures has continued to rise. This is in part due to the use of extended criteria donors and ex vivo lung perfusion systems. According to the ISHLT registry, 67,493 adult lung transplants were performed globally between January 1, 1992, and June 30, 2018. In the United States, the most recent data from the Organ Procurement and Transplantation Network (OPTN) reports that there were 2,692 lung transplants and 51 heart-lung transplants performed in 2022. These numbers do not include pediatric patients or patients who received both lung and solid organ transplantation (eg, liver or kidney). Nonetheless, the number of patients awaiting lung transplantation continues to exceed the limited donor supply.

Chambers DC, Perch M, Zuckermann A, et al. The International Thoracic Organ Transplant Registry of the International Society for Heart and Lung Transplantation: thirty-eighth adult lung transplantation report—2021; focus on recipient characteristics. *J Heart Lung Transplant.* 2021;40:1060-1072.

U.S. Department of Health and Human Services. Organ procurement and transplantation network. Accessed February 11, 2023. http://optn.transplant.hrsa.gov

Valapour M, Lehr CJ, Skeans MA, et al. OPTN/SRTR 2020 annual data report: lung. *Am J Transplant.* 2022;22:438-518.

A.4. What are the selection criteria for recipients?

Historically, time spent on the lung transplant waiting list was the predominant factor contributing to donor lung allocation (in addition to ABO typing and geographic location of the donor and recipient). Mortality rates vary for different pulmonary conditions, however, so this allocation strategy was biased against sicker patients and incentivized early listing for transplantation. Long wait times then led to an unacceptable mortality rate for listed patients. In 2005, in an effort to decrease the wait-list mortality rate and improve access to organs based on patient need, the OPTN revised its allocation policies and implemented the Lung Allocation Score (LAS). Rather than emphasize time on the waiting list, this new policy prioritized illness severity and projected posttransplant survival. The result has been a decrease in both the overall size of the wait-list and the wait-list mortality rate. Another result of the revised allocation process was a change in the primary diagnosis of lung transplant recipients. By 2007, IPF, which carries the worst prognosis among the common disease indications for lung transplantation, had overtaken COPD as the leading diagnosis in lung transplant recipients in the United States.

Specific recipient criteria are dependent on primary diagnosis, but in general, lung transplantation is indicated when patients with end-stage lung disease have a more than 50% risk for mortality within 2 years. They should also have minimal disease of other organ systems and be mentally and psychologically capable of following strict regimens for rehabilitation and immunosuppressive therapy. These criteria contribute to a high (>80%) likelihood of survival for at least 90 days after transplantation. Contraindications to lung transplant are less strict now than in the past, especially at high-volume centers with greater management expertise. Multiorgan failure remains an absolute contraindication to transplantation unless the patient is being considered for multiorgan transplantation. A list of absolute contraindications can be found in **Table 4.2**.

Chambers DC, Perch M, Zuckermann A, et al. The International Thoracic Organ Transplant Registry of the International Society for Heart and Lung Transplantation: thirty-eighth adult lung transplantation report—2021; focus on recipient characteristics. *J Heart Lung Transplant.* 2021;40:1060-1072.

Leard LE, Holm AM, Valapour M, et al. Consensus document for the selection of lung transplant candidates: an update from the International Society for Heart and Lung Transplantation. *J Heart Lung Transplant.* 2021;40:1349-1379.

Weill D. Lung transplantation: indications and contraindications. *J Thorac Dis.* 2018;10:4574-4587.

A.5. How is the decision made to transplant one or both lungs, and does this influence preoperative management?

Suppurative or infective lung disease is an absolute indication for BLT rather than SLT due to the risk of cross-infection from the retained lung to the transplanted lung. BLT is typically performed for patients requiring VV-ECMO support as a bridge to transplant from severe COVID-19-related ARDS. These patients endure a prolonged duration of ICU hospitalization on mechanical ventilation and/or mechanical circulatory support prior to transplantation, compromising their physiologic reserve. As such, they need the additional functional pulmonary reserve afforded by a BLT over an SLT in order to maximize the chances of postoperative recovery.

TABLE 4.2 Absolute Contraindications to Lung Transplant

General	• Patient refusal • Limited functional status (with poor potential for posttransplant rehabilitation)
Psychosocial	• Demonstrated nonadherence to therapy • Substance abuse • Poor social support
Medical	• Malignancy (with a high risk of recurrence/death related to cancer) • GFR <40 mL/min/1.73 m^2 • Acute coronary syndrome or myocardial infarction within 30 d • Stroke within 30 d • Liver cirrhosis with portal hypertension or synthetic dysfunction • Acute liver or renal failure • Septic shock • Active extrapulmonary or disseminated infection • Active tuberculosis infection • HIV infection with detectable viral load • Other severe uncontrolled medical conditions expected to limit survival after the transplant

For all other etiologies of end-stage lung disease, either SLT or BLT can be performed. The decision for SLT or BLT remains controversial and is based on the situation, taking into account regional organ allocation policies, individual center experience, and organ availability. With a severe shortage of organs for transplant, SLT has been advocated as a way to increase the number of recipients. There are also physiologic considerations for SLT that do not pertain to BLT. Patients with restrictive disease, for example, are theoretically good candidates for SLT because the stiff, vasoconstricted native lung will receive relatively little ventilation and perfusion and can therefore usually be left without compromising the transplanted lung postoperatively. In contrast, SLT in patients with COPD creates a risk of significant postoperative ventilation/perfusion mismatch from hyperinflation of the native lung and mediastinal displacement, although experience with this group thus far limits this concern for many patients.

The data regarding outcomes for SLT versus BLT are contradictory; there are some studies showing better short-term outcomes with SLT (ie, lower rates of prolonged mechanical ventilation, less likely to need dialysis, and shorter hospital stays). The consensus is that long-term outcomes, particularly functional outcomes and survival, are better with BLT than with SLT regardless of the indication for transplant. This difference in long-term outcome can be partially attributed to selection bias, however, as BLT is often performed in younger patients with longer expected posttransplant lifespan. Rejection rates are also similar in BLT or SLT. Thus, the decision to proceed with SLT or BLT remains controversial. Patient (age, size, LAS, etc) as well as donor-specific factors (age, size, comorbidities, state of the donor organ, etc) must be considered, and the benefits must be weighed against the risk for both.

Ko RE, Oh DK, Choi SM, et al. Lung transplantation for severe COVID-19-related ARDS. *Ther Adv Respir Dis.* 2022;16:1-12.

Martin AK, Renew JR, Jayaraman AL, et al. Analysis of outcomes in lung transplantation. *J Cardiothorac Vasc Anesth.* 2019;33:1455-1466.

Ranganath NK, Malas J, Phillips KG, et al. Single and double lung transplantation have equivalent survival for idiopathic pulmonary fibrosis. *Ann Thorac Surg.* 2020;109:211-217.

Schaffer JM, Singh SK, Reitz BA, et al. Single- vs double-lung transplantation in patients with chronic obstructive pulmonary disease and idiopathic pulmonary fibrosis since the implementation of lung allocation based on medical need. *JAMA.* 2015;313:936-948.

Subramanian MP, Meyers BF. Bilateral versus single lung transplantation: are two lungs better than one? *J Thorac Dis.* 2018;10:4588-4601.

A.6. How does a single-lung transplantation (SLT) differ technically from a bilateral-lung transplantation (BLT)?

It is extremely important that anesthesiologists be broadly familiar with the surgical methods of lung transplantation because manipulation of the heart and lungs at specific points during the procedure can produce marked cardiopulmonary disturbances. The anesthesiologist should anticipate these changes and adapt anesthetic management accordingly.

BLT is usually performed with the patient in the supine position through a "clamshell" incision (bilateral anterior thoracotomies with or without transverse sternotomy). In contrast, SLT can be performed in either the lateral decubitus position through a thoracotomy incision or in the supine position through a unilateral hemi-clamshell incision. For both SLT and BLT, intermittent OLV is required during dissection and removal of the native lung. Once stable single-lung ventilation is established, dissection of the lung to be transplanted is initiated with isolation of the pulmonary artery. To assess the cardiopulmonary response to diverting the entire cardiac output through one lung, progressive temporary occlusion of the vessel is first performed manually while observing the hemodynamic response and assessment of ventricular function by transesophageal echocardiography (TEE). If well tolerated, the vessel is then clamped and stapled. After ligation of the pulmonary artery, the pneumonectomy is completed.

Implantation of the donor lung usually begins with anastomosis of the airway. In the past, the bronchial anastomosis was wrapped with an omental pedicle and mobilized through a small abdominal incision in an effort to improve blood supply to the airway and promote healing. However, the use of a "telescoping" bronchial anastomosis has now largely obviated the need for omental wrapping. The pulmonary artery branch is then attached, followed by anastomosis of a cuff of the left atrium containing the pulmonary veins. The implanted lung is then partially inflated, the left atrial cuff and pulmonary veins de-aired, and circulation to the organ restored.

In both SLT and sequential BLT, physical compression of the heart and/or great vessels (in particular, the superior vena cava) during the dissection phase can lead to profound hemodynamic instability secondary to decreases in preload and stroke volume. Clamping the pulmonary artery leads to a severe increase in right ventricular afterload, which can be poorly tolerated in patients with baseline pulmonary hypertension and right ventricular dysfunction. OLV is poorly tolerated in these patients, often resulting in refractory hypoxemia; this is typically resolved with clamping of the pulmonary artery, which eliminates the physiologic shunt by directing all pulmonary arterial blood to the ventilated lung. If any of these issues become sufficiently problematic during the dissection phase, veno-arterial (VA) ECMO or cardiopulmonary bypass (CPB) can be initiated to provide improved hemodynamic stability, oxygenation, and end-organ perfusion. This is typically performed via direct aortic and femoral venous cannulation.

Sequential implantation of the lungs is the most common method of BLT. When performing a sequential BLT without mechanical circulatory support, the most severely compromised lung (as determined by preoperative ventilation-perfusion lung scanning) is the first to be explanted while single-lung ventilation is maintained with the better contralateral lung. Implantation is achieved through a bronchial anastomosis as for SLT. The second lung is then removed and transplanted during ventilation of the new lung alone. If an en bloc technique for BLT (ie, tracheal rather than bronchial anastomosis) is used, CPB is required. This technique historically was the initial approach to lung transplantation and was performed through a median sternotomy. Although the procedure initially produced encouraging results, considerable limitations related to technical complexity, morbidity, mortality, and application to many patients with end-stage lung disease soon became apparent. Not surprisingly, the use of the procedure declined sharply and has now been largely replaced by the bilateral sequential implantation technique.

Aigner C, Klepetko W. Bilateral lung transplantation. *Oper Tech Thorac Cardiovasc Surg*. 2012;17:181-193.

Flye MW, ed. *Atlas of Organ Transplantation*. WB Saunders; 1995:296-312.

Hayanga JW, D'Cunha J. The surgical technique of bilateral sequential lung transplantation. *J Thorac Dis*. 2014;6:1063-1069.

Nagendran M, Maruthappu M, Sugand K. Should double lung transplant be performed with or without cardiopulmonary bypass? *Interact Cardiovasc Thorac Surg*. 2011;12:799-804.

B. Preoperative Evaluation and Preparation

B.1. What preoperative evaluation is desirable?

At most centers, an extensive physical examination, psychological evaluation, and numerous tests of cardiopulmonary function are performed before acceptance into the transplant program. Familiarity with PFTs, ventilation-perfusion lung scan results, heart catheterization, echocardiographic data (including evidence of intracardiac shunts), exercise tolerance, oxygen use, and dependence on continuous pulmonary vasodilator infusion (ie, prostacyclin) are beneficial for formulating an anesthetic plan. Although many of these parameters are regularly reassessed, the interval between evaluation and transplantation necessitates that a careful history and physical examination be repeated before the procedure, focusing on signs of pulmonary hypertension and cardiac dysfunction.

Bigham M, Dickstein ML, Hogue CW Jr. Cardiac and lung transplantation. In: Estafanous FG, Barash PG, Reves JG, eds. *Cardiac Anesthesia: Principles and Clinical Practice.* 2nd ed. Lippincott Williams & Wilkins; 2001:637-662.

Slinger P, Blank RS, Campos J. Lung transplantation. In: Slinger P, Blank RS, Campos J, et al, eds. *Principles and Practice of Anesthesia for Thoracic Surgery.* 2nd ed. Springer; 2019:773-790.

B.2. Would you premedicate this patient? If so, how?

As with all critically ill patients, considerations regarding preoperative sedation are governed primarily by the functional limitations imposed by the underlying disease and the potential consequences of hypercarbia and hypoxemia, which can occur as a result of the sedation. When indicated, parenteral sedation is usually chosen because of insufficient time to administer oral anxiolytics effectively. Midazolam is often sufficient, with its rapid anxiolytic onset and amnestic effects being its most useful properties, but it should be titrated to effect. Other medications that can safely be used alone or in conjunction with midazolam include dexmedetomidine, ketamine, and perhaps diphenhydramine. These medications do not negatively affect respiratory drive and are therefore generally considered safe in patients with end-stage lung disease.

Patients with pulmonary hypertension present a difficult conundrum because they often have associated right ventricular dysfunction and an increased susceptibility to the consequences of increased pulmonary vascular resistance. They also have varying degrees of reduced baseline functional status and supplemental oxygen requirements. Those who do not have hypoxemia at rest might benefit from preoperative anxiolysis to attenuate potential stress-related increases in pulmonary vascular resistance, but caution must be taken to avoid oversedation and subsequent hypercarbia/hypoxemia. Patients with more severe pulmonary vascular disease and those with significant right-to-left intracardiac shunting (ie, Eisenmenger physiology) are often cyanotic despite oxygen supplementation and might not tolerate sedation. In addition to anxiolysis, consideration should be given to immunosuppression protocols and, in appropriate patients, to supplemental bronchodilator therapy.

Hartigan PM, Pedoto A. Anesthetic considerations for lung volume reduction surgery and lung transplantation. *Thorac Surg Clin.* 2005;15:143-157.

Slinger P, Blank RS, Campos J. Lung transplantation. In: Slinger P, Blank RS, Campos J, et al, eds. *Principles and Practice of Anesthesia for Thoracic Surgery.* 2nd ed. Springer; 2019:773-790.

B.3. What vascular access is appropriate?

Typically, a large-bore intravenous catheter and central venous access for pulmonary artery catheter placement are secured before surgery. The right internal jugular vein is the most commonly chosen site of central access, given that it is the most anatomically favorable for pulmonary artery catheter placement. Consideration should be given to the type of central line used; for instance, a multiple-lumen introducer catheter can provide an access point for pulmonary artery catheter insertion, volume administration, and vasoactive infusions. For patients with chronic infectious lung disease, a history of previous lung transplant or other intrathoracic procedures, or end-stage fibrotic ARDS, placement of a second central venous line should be considered because of the potential for brisk blood loss during dissection of pleural adhesions. Direct arterial pressure monitoring is necessary, and at many institutions, a femoral arterial line is used instead of or in addition to radial arterial access because radial arterial pressures can become damped secondary to vasoactive medications or positioning of the arms. Patients on VV-ECMO will usually have venous and arterial lines in place prior to arrival in the operating room. In these cases, the anesthesiologist must thoroughly evaluate the ECMO configuration and locations of the cannulae in case additional vascular access is needed. Obtaining additional vascular access in these patients can be difficult due to their prolonged ICU stay and increased risk of venous thrombosis, among other reasons.

Flye MW, ed. *Atlas of Organ Transplantation.* WB Saunders; 1995:313-318.

Hartigan PM, Pedoto A. Anesthetic considerations for lung volume reduction surgery and lung transplantation. *Thorac Surg Clin.* 2005;15:143-157.

B.4. Is preoperative epidural catheter placement advantageous?

Pain control after lung transplantation can be critical in facilitating tracheal extubation and rehabilitation. A thoracic epidural catheter is the gold standard for postoperative pain management. Epidural catheters can be placed immediately before the procedure or postoperatively prior to extubation. If placed before the procedure, the possibility of anticoagulation and CPB during the transplantation procedure must be considered. The practice of placing preoperative epidural catheters is supported by data indicating no adverse sequelae, including in those patients who require emergent heparinization and CPB. Obvious exceptions to this approach are patients who are anticoagulated preoperatively or those in whom CPB is planned. Despite this, many centers delay the placement of the epidural catheter until the postoperative period.

Feltracco P, Barbieri S, Milevoj M, et al. Thoracic epidural analgesia in lung transplantation. *Transplant Proc.* 2010;42:1265-1269.

Hartigan PM, Pedoto A. Anesthetic considerations for lung volume reduction surgery and lung transplantation. *Thorac Surg Clin.* 2005;15:143-157.

C. Intraoperative Management

C.1. What special equipment is necessary?

For assessment and management of the airway, a flexible bronchoscope is necessary to confirm the appropriate double-lumen endobronchial tube position, to enable suctioning, and for inspection of the completed bronchial anastomoses. The anesthesia ventilator utilized should have several ventilatory mode options and be capable of delivering a wide range of inspiratory-to-expiratory (I:E) ratios. A delivery system for pulmonary arterial vasodilators such as nitric oxide or epoprostenol should be readily available. Transesophageal echocardiology should be utilized. A CPB machine and/or ECMO circuit should be immediately available. Lastly, as multiple vasopressors and inotropes are often needed, infusion pumps that allow simultaneous administration of numerous drugs should be utilized.

C.2. How would you monitor this patient?

Intraoperatively, hemodynamic and respiratory changes are often acute and profound, so extensive monitoring is imperative. In addition to standard monitors, direct arterial blood pressure monitoring, a pulmonary artery catheter, and TEE are routinely used. Right radial arterial access is often preferred, especially in the setting of peripheral veno-arterial ECMO (VA-ECMO), as differential hypoxemia may occur secondary to the ejection of hypoxemic blood from the heart mixing in the ascending aorta and aortic arch with retrograde flow from the femoral arterial cannula (ie, North-South or Harlequin syndrome). Femoral arterial access is often obtained to monitor central arterial pressure while providing rapid vascular access should the need for emergent peripheral VA-ECMO cannulation arise intraoperatively. Pulmonary artery catheters capable of providing continuous cardiac output monitoring as well as mixed venous oxygen saturation have become widely used. The surgeon should be reminded to palpate the pulmonary artery prior to cross-clamping to avoid entrapment of the pulmonary artery (PA) catheter. The role of TEE in lung transplantation is evolving. It can be used to confirm preoperative findings regarding ventricular and valvular function, evaluate for the presence of intracardiac shunts, and establish baseline pulmonary vein velocities. Increasingly, it has been used to help guide placement of ECMO cannulae and evaluate the need for extracorporeal support.

Murray AW, Boisen ML, Fritz A, et al. Anesthetic considerations in lung transplantation: past, present and future. *J Thorac Dis.* 2021;12:6550-6563.

Nicoara A, Skubas N, Ad N, et al. Guidelines for the use of transesophageal echocardiography to assist with surgical decision-making in the operating room: a surgery-based approach: from the American Society of Echocardiography in collaboration with the Society of Cardiovascular Anesthesiologists and the Society of Thoracic Surgeons. *J Am Soc Echocardiogr.* 2020;33:692-734.

Slinger P, Blank RS, Campos J. Lung transplantation. In: Slinger P, Blank RS, Campos J, et al, eds. *Principles and Practice of Anesthesia for Thoracic Surgery.* 2nd ed. Springer; 2019:773-790.

C.3. How would you induce anesthesia in this patient?

As with the induction of anesthesia in any critically ill patient, multiple techniques have been safely used for patients undergoing lung transplantation. Poor respiratory reserve can lead to rapid desaturation even after adequate preoxygenation. A slow induction is generally preferred; abrupt withdrawal of sympathetic tone in these patients with high preexisting sympathetic activity can lead to marked cardiovascular compromise, especially with the transition from spontaneous to mechanical ventilation. Rapid sequence induction should therefore be reserved for patients deemed to be at high risk of pulmonary aspiration, as large boluses of medications can cause profound hemodynamic instability. A rapid-acting induction agent to shorten the excitement stage, expedite airway management, and prevent opioid-induced truncal rigidity should be used. Propofol, etomidate, ketamine, and midazolam have all been used safely; the specific properties of each drug in the setting of patient comorbidities should be considered. For example, the sympathomimetic properties of ketamine might preclude use in the presence of pulmonary hypertension, whereas its bronchodilating effects may be beneficial in the setting of bronchospasm. Lidocaine, sufentanil or fentanyl, and succinylcholine or a nondepolarizing neuromuscular blocking agent are generally used to complete induction. The pulmonary hypertensive consequences of histamine released from some drugs (eg, atracurium, morphine) should be kept in mind in the setting of severe pulmonary hypertension.

Because of the greater potential for hemodynamic and respiratory instability in this patient population, the surgeon and perfusionist must be present during induction to initiate ECMO or CPB if needed. In patients requiring high noninvasive respiratory support or with severe pulmonary hypertension, ECMO may be instituted prior to induction. Alternatively, the groin vessels can be accessed prior to induction to facilitate initiation of ECMO or CPB after induction. Optimization of right ventricular preload, right ventricular support, and efforts to prevent increases in right ventricular afterload are keys to safe anesthesia induction. Dysrhythmias, which can lead to decreased perfusion and ischemia of the right ventricle, should be promptly treated. Especially with positive pressure ventilation, suppression of the sympathetic system, myocardial depression, and vasodilation can lead to cardiovascular collapse. Conversely, acute increases in pulmonary arterial pressures and right heart failure can result from sympathetic stimulation (eg, with intubation, acidemia, hypoxemia, hypercapnia) and should be avoided.

Kachulis B, Mitrev L, Jordan D. Intraoperative anesthetic management of lung transplantation patients. *Best Pract Res Clin Anaesthesiol.* 2017;31:261-272.

Nicoara A, Anderson-Dam J. Anesthesia for lung transplantation. *Anesthesiol Clin.* 2017;35:473-489.

Sellers D, Cassar-Demajo W, Keshavjee S, et al. The evolution of anesthesia for lung transplantation. *J Cardiothorac Vasc Anesth.* 2017;31:1071-1079.

C.4. What type of endotracheal tube would you use? How would you ventilate this patient?

After induction, the trachea is usually intubated with a left endobronchial double-lumen tube for both SLT and BLT. Use of a single-lumen endotracheal tube with either an external or an internal bronchial blocker has been described but is not clearly superior to a double-lumen tube, especially in terms of reliability of continuous lung isolation. Furthermore, an endobronchial double-lumen tube allows for differential lung ventilation if required postoperatively. One exception to this approach has been in patients with CF who exhibit thick secretions that are difficult to suction through the small-lumen suction catheters necessary for double-lumen tubes. In these patients, it is often helpful to first place a large single-lumen tube and perform extensive bronchoscopic-directed bronchial lavage and suctioning before placement of the double-lumen tube.

The transition from spontaneous to mechanical ventilation invariably produces hemodynamic alterations resulting from acute changes in intrathoracic pressure, chest wall compliance, and venous return. Individuals undergoing lung transplantation occupy a spectrum of low lung compliance in restrictive disease to high lung compliance in obstructive disease. Ventilatory strategies attempt to maximize oxygenation and removal of CO_2 while avoiding ventilator-induced lung injury. With restrictive disease, higher inspiratory pressure, positive end-expiratory pressure (PEEP), and higher than usual respiratory rates are often required. These patients can require prolonged inspiratory times with inverse I:E ratios of up to 1.5:1. Conversely, in COPD, mechanical ventilation magnifies air trapping, which can lead to auto-PEEP or "pulmonary tamponade," varying degrees of which should be expected during anesthesia induction. Treatment consists of intermittent apnea with an open ventilator circuit, adjustment of the ventilatory pattern to an I:E ratio of 1:5 or less with moderate tidal volumes, and administration of bronchodilating drugs. This complication should always be anticipated in patients with COPD. If hypotension persists, other causes of circulatory compromise must be excluded, including pneumothorax. In both obstructive and restrictive diseases, optimal balance of ventilation with hemodynamic stability often necessitates tolerating some degree of hypercapnia. In patients with pulmonary hypertension, mechanical ventilation usually produces less cardiovascular disturbance if caution is exercised to not increase pulmonary vascular resistance (eg, from hypoxia, hypercarbia, or lung hyperinflation).

Murray AW, Boisen ML, Fritz A, et al. Anesthetic considerations in lung transplantation: past, present and future. *J Thorac Dis.* 2021;12:6550-6563.

Triantafillou AN, Heerdt PM, Patterson GA. Lung transplantation. In: Youngberg JA, Lake CL, Roizen MF, et al, eds. *Cardiac, Vascular, and Thoracic Anesthesia.* Churchill Livingstone; 2000:703.

C.5. How does the physiology of one-lung ventilation (OLV) influence the procedure?

In laterally positioned patients, gravity helps redistribute blood away from the nonventilated lung during OLV and lessens the intrapulmonary shunt. In patients who are supine, this benefit is lost and OLV might not be well tolerated. If appropriately preoxygenated prior to induction and ventilated prior to OLV, patients with higher residual volumes, such as patients with severe obstructive pulmonary disease, can tolerate OLV better than patients with lower residual volumes. These patients have a higher reserve and can maintain oxygenation for the first 10 to 15 minutes of OLV. Rapid arterial desaturation can then occur once a substantial portion of the residual volume is absorbed. Conversely, patients with restrictive lung disease and a low functional residual capacity can become hypoxemic and hypercarbic rapidly if not ventilated. Multiple steps can be taken to improve oxygenation by reducing shunting through the nonventilated lung, including insufflation of oxygen or continuous positive airway pressure (CPAP) to that lung, bronchoscope-guided suctioning of the ventilated lung, careful manipulation of the ventilatory pattern, and adding PEEP to the ventilated lung. Differential PEEP/CPAP should be done cautiously, however, because increased airway pressure in the ventilated lung can divert blood toward the nonventilated lung, thereby increasing the shunt and leading to a further decrease in Pao_2. Likewise, sustained hyperinflation of the ventilated lung can lead to an increase in right ventricular afterload and preload and have severe hemodynamic consequences. In some patients, intermittent ventilation of the operative lung is necessary for adequate oxygenation. In general, oxygenation improves after clamping of the PA supplying the nonventilated lung. For oxygen desaturation not responding to the usual maneuvers, tourniquets can be placed around the PA by the surgeon as a temporizing step until dissection permits stapling of this vessel. Inhaled pulmonary arterial vasodilators can improve ventilation/perfusion matching by selective vasodilation of the alveoli being ventilated. ECMO or CPB should be initiated if the Pao_2 continues to decrease, the $Paco_2$ continues to increase, or there is progressive acidemia, despite the previously stated interventions.

Nicoara A, Anderson-Dam J. Anesthesia for lung transplantation. *Anesthesiol Clin*. 2017;35:473-489.

Slinger P, Blank RS, Campos J. Lung transplantation. In: Slinger P, Blank RS, Campos J, et al, eds. *Principles and Practice of Anesthesia for Thoracic Surgery*. 2nd ed. Springer; 2019:773-790.

C.6. How does OLV affect cardiopulmonary function?

Isolated ventilation of the dependent lung is often accompanied by a marked acute increase in peak inspiratory pressure and a subsequent gradual progressive rise in PA pressure. Because of the beneficial effect of gravity on redistributing blood away from the nondependent, nonventilated lung, single-lung ventilation is often tolerated better from a respiratory standpoint by patients undergoing SLT in the lateral position than those undergoing BLT in the supine position. Avoiding hypercarbia is desired to mitigate increases in PA pressure from elevated $Paco_2$. Close monitoring of right ventricular performance during conversion to OLV is extremely important because of the increase in afterload produced by hypoxic pulmonary vasoconstriction and redistribution of blood flow. Although unusual, if the right ventricle becomes hypokinetic and distended (by TEE imaging) or the central venous pressure (CVP) increases disproportionately to the increase in PA pressure, and if left ventricular ejection fraction decreases, ventilation might have to be altered to minimize the increase in PA pressure.

Triantafillou AN, Pasque MK, Huddleston CB, et al. Predictors, frequency, and indications for cardiopulmonary bypass during lung transplantation in adults. *Ann Thorac Surg*. 1994;57:1248-1251.

C.7. At what specific points in the procedure are problems anticipated?

Challenges encountered during lung transplantation are usually related to the underlying disease process, the complexity of the surgery, physiologic changes associated with the different stages of the procedure, patient positioning, and immediate complications such as primary graft dysfunction. COVID-19-related pulmonary fibrosis can lead to significant vascular adhesions and distortion of hilar planes, resulting in difficult surgical dissection in which massive blood loss can occur. This concern can also occur with CF. The procedure can be especially challenging at these particular points in the procedure:

- Induction of anesthesia
- Initiation of positive-pressure lung ventilation
- One-lung ventilation
- Clamping of the pulmonary artery
- Graft reperfusion

C.8. How would you deal with problems related to clamping of the pulmonary artery?

To assess the cardiopulmonary response to diverting the entire cardiac output through one lung after PA clamping, progressive occlusion of the vessel is first performed manually (**Figure 4.2**). Careful assessment of right ventricular function is performed by TEE looking for evidence of right ventricular distension or hypokinesis. If well tolerated, the vessel is then clamped and stapled. If the occlusion is poorly tolerated, the vessel is unclamped and a pulmonary vasodilator, such as prostaglandin E_1 or inhaled nitric oxide and/or a positive inotropic infusion, is begun. If severe respiratory or cardiovascular derangement persists after the reclamping of the vessel despite pharmacologic intervention, consideration is given to the use of ECMO to avoid profound hypoxia or right ventricular failure. However, for most patients undergoing SLT, hypoxemia during OLV and after PA clamping is rarely a problem, and right ventricular performance is adequately maintained.

Triantafillou AN, Heerdt PM, Patterson GA. Lung transplantation. In: Youngberg JA, Lake CL, Roizen MF, et al, eds. *Cardiac, Vascular, and Thoracic Anesthesia*. Churchill Livingstone; 2000:703.

C.9. What hemodynamic alterations would you expect during graft implantation and reperfusion? How would you correct them?

During the process of performing the vascular and bronchial anastomoses, major disturbances of cardiac filling and rhythm can be produced. Although often transient, systemic hypotension and pulmonary hypertension can ensue, and the use of vasopressors, inotropes, or an inhaled pulmonary arterial vasodilator might be necessary. Cardioversion should be used for sustained dysrhythmia causing hemodynamic instability.

The final stages of graft implantation include attaching the pulmonary veins via a left atrial cuff to the left atrium. Bleeding of the pulmonary veins, prior to doing this, facilitates de-airing and removal of graft preservatives. Transient hypotension can follow the introduction of the preservative solution from the newly perfused transplanted lung into the systemic circulation. Incomplete de-airing of the pulmonary veins can cause a coronary artery air embolism and lead to transient myocardial ischemia manifested by ST-segment elevation and regional wall motion abnormalities on TEE. These echocardiographic and electrocardiographic changes can be reversed by maintaining adequate perfusion pressure with vasopressors. Rapid intravascular volume replacement might also be necessary during this time.

After reperfusion and subsequent ventilation of the new lung, PA pressures and arterial blood gases should be closely followed. PA pressure usually falls after reperfusion of the transplanted allograft. If a substantial decrease is not observed, potential causes include anastomotic problems with the atrial cuff (pulmonary veins) or the PA, which can lead to hemodynamic instability. Echocardiography is very useful in assessing for potential obstruction of the pulmonary vessels. Turbulent high-velocity flow and/or a diameter less than 75% of the proximal PA in the left or right PA are suggestive of obstruction. When pulmonary anastomotic problems are suspected, the surgeon should palpate to assess whether the PA catheter is located proximal or distal to the anastomosis. If a proximal location is confirmed, the PA

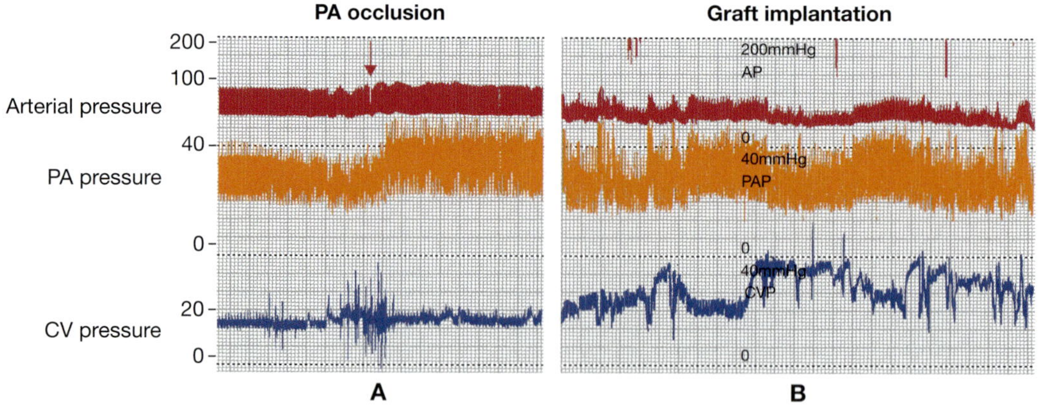

FIGURE 4.2. Tracings of femoral arterial blood pressure, along with pulmonary artery (PA) and central venous (CV) pressures, before and after occlusion of the left PA (**A**) and during implantation of a left lung graft (**B**). All pressures are in mm Hg. AP, arterial pressure; CVP, central venous pressure; PA, pulmonary artery; PAP, pulmonary artery pressure.

pressure distal to the anastomosis should be directly measured by inserting a needle and connecting it to a pressure tubing handed off the operative field. A large difference in the two measurements is suggestive of obstruction to flow. Pulmonary vein obstruction from a thrombus or suture is possible, and careful assessment must be done to assess for patency of these vessels. Pulmonary vein diameter greater than 0.5 cm and a velocity greater than 1 m/s are suggestive of obstruction. If significant obstruction of the pulmonary vasculature is detected, surgical revision/correction might be necessary because this can lead to early or late hemodynamic compromise. Anticoagulation might be necessary for obstruction secondary to thrombus. Ischemic metabolites can lead to severe vasodilation and hypotension with reperfusion, requiring treatment with vasopressors, inotropes, calcium chloride, and sodium bicarbonate. Other sources of hypotension include pneumoplegia and leaks at the vascular anastomoses. Vasopressors, inotropes, and rapid intravascular volume replacement can be helpful in these situations.

Early graft dysfunction can manifest shortly after reperfusion of the first lung as a consequence of various insults. This can result in increased alveolar-capillary permeability, transudative pulmonary edema, and severe hypoxemia with hemodynamic compromise. Supportive measures with a lung protective ventilator strategy, inhaled nitric oxide, and, if necessary, vasopressors and inotropes should be employed. ECMO should be considered for patients with refractory hypoxemia and/or hypotension despite these measures.

Batra K, Chamarthy M, Reddick M. Diagnosis and interventions of vascular complications in lung transplant. *Cardiovasc Diagn Ther*. 2018;8:378-386.

Nicoara A, Anderson-Dam J. Anesthesia for lung transplantation. *Anesthesiol Clin*. 2017;35:473-489.

C.10. When is extracorporeal membrane oxygenation (ECMO) utilized for lung transplantation?

Use of ECMO for lung transplantation can be elective or emergent, with VA-ECMO becoming the preferred intraoperative technique over CPB. ECMO can be used electively for patients who have severe PA hypertension, significant right ventricular dysfunction, are unable to tolerate OLV, or when visualization of hilar structures is poor. Some centers are now advocating the routine use of ECMO for all lung transplantation. Unplanned intraoperative use of mechanical circulatory support has been associated with increased mortality compared to planned support or elective utilization.

Intraoperatively, ECMO facilitates lung protective ventilatory strategies (low driving pressure and inspired oxygen concentration), minimizes right heart strain during clamping of the PA, and allows for controlled reperfusion of the pulmonary allograft to attenuate the effect of ischemia-reperfusion injury. However, ECMO is not without risk, as it has been associated with higher rates of intraoperative blood transfusion and activation of pro-inflammatory cytokines. This results in higher rates of nonpulmonary complications, as well as primary graft dysfunction. Evidence suggests that these disadvantages are more common with CPB compared to ECMO, though rates of primary graft dysfunction are lower in patients who do not require any mechanical circulatory support during transplantation.

Hartwig M, van Berkel V, Bharat A, et al. The American Association for Thoracic Surgery (AATS) 2022 Expert Consensus Document: the use of mechanical circulatory support in lung transplantation. *J Thorac Cardiovasc Surg*. 2023;165:301-326.

Porteous MK, Diamond JM, Christie JD. Primary graft dysfunction: lessons learned about the first 72 h after lung transplantation. *Curr Opin Organ Transplant*. 2015;20:506-514.

C.11. Should fluid administration be restricted, and are blood products commonly required?

The amount of crystalloid that can be safely administered intraoperatively without adversely affecting the newly implanted lung graft is widely variable. Although efforts should be made to minimize fluid infusion intraoperatively, many patients undergoing lung transplantation require large amounts to maintain hemodynamic stability. The transplanted lung is at risk for pulmonary edema due to lack of lymphatic drainage and inflammatory insults, direct pulmonary trauma, and inflammatory cytokine release associated with reperfusion and organ harvest.

Primary graft dysfunction occurs in 10% to 30% of patients after lung transplantation and is thought to be in part due to decreased alveolar fluid clearance. Severe (grade 3) primary graft dysfunction is a risk factor for early mortality following lung transplantation and the development of bronchiolitis obliterans syndrome. With increasing evidence that large-volume fluid administration is a modifiable risk factor for primary graft dysfunction, many providers advocate fluid restriction for lung transplantation. A retrospective cohort study of 500 patients showed that grade 3 primary graft dysfunction occurred in 25% of patients and that every liter of fluid increased the odds for grade 3 primary graft dysfunction by 22%. The patients who developed grade 3 primary graft dysfunction were transfused with more red blood cell concentrate than patients who did not develop grade 3 primary graft dysfunction. Interestingly, there was no association between the use of crystalloid or colloid (nonblood) and grade 3 primary graft dysfunction. The Lung Transplant Outcomes Group also published data showing that transfusing 1 L of red blood cell concentrate was associated with a 2-fold increase in the incidence of primary graft dysfunction. Another recent retrospective single-center study reported that transplant recipients receiving more than 1:2 fresh frozen plasma:packed red blood cells within the first 72 hours posttransplant had higher grades of primary graft dysfunction and overall transfusion requirements, including platelets and cryoprecipitate.

Before the development of the BLT procedure without CPB, patients with a history of surgery involving the lung or pleura or chronic infectious lung diseases were not deemed acceptable candidates for lung transplantation because of the anticipated excessive bleeding associated with dissecting a scarred lung after anticoagulation for CPB. Without uniform requirements for heparinization (ECMO, bilateral sequential lung transplant, etc), such patients are now generally regarded as operative candidates. Even without the need for full heparinization, these patients are at increased risk for excessive bleeding, albeit at a lower risk. Other variables reported to increase the need for blood product usage include double-lung procedures and CF. The need for CPB is a confounding factor, however. Historically, BLT patients were more likely to get planned or rescue CPB. With the advent of ECMO, new circuits, cannulas, and cannulation strategies, excessive bleeding occurs less frequently in all categories of patients.

Strategies for blood conservation should be implemented. For example, some groups have found a reduction in intraoperative bleeding in patients with a history of CF or previous intrathoracic surgery when antifibrinolytics are given continuously. ECMO, especially with heparin-bonded circuits, is a reasonable alternative to CPB because full anticoagulation is not needed. Use of ECMO for hemodynamic support also helps with reducing the amount of crystalloid and blood products being administered. Decisions regarding transfusion therapy warrant a discussion between members of the anesthesiology and surgical teams. If blood products are to be administered, the anesthesiologist must know whether the patient has antibodies to cytomegalovirus (CMV) and must closely check blood products to confirm they coincide with the patient's status.

Geube MA, Perez-Protto SE, McGrath TL, et al. Increased intraoperative fluid administration is associated with severe primary graft dysfunction after lung transplantation. *Anesth Analg*. 2016;122:1081-1088.

Martin AK, Renew JR, Jayaraman AL, et al. Analysis of outcomes in lung transplantation. *J Cardiothorac Vasc Anesth*. 2019;33:1455-1466.

Seay T, Guinn N, Maisonave Y, et al. The association of increased FFP:RBC transfusion ratio to primary graft dysfunction in bleeding lung transplantation patients. *J Cardiothorac Vasc Anesth*. 2020;34:3024-3032.

Slinger P, Blank RS, Campos J. Lung transplantation. In: Slinger P, Blank RS, Campos J, et al, eds. *Principles and Practice of Anesthesia for Thoracic Surgery*. 2nd ed. Springer; 2019:773-790.

C.12. Would you extubate the patient upon the conclusion of the procedure?

A few studies have shown that, with proper selection of patients after SLT or BLT, intraoperative or early tracheal extubation is possible and can be successful. However, most of these studies are retrospective in nature and exclude patients receiving mechanical circulatory support or the use of ex vivo lung perfusion. As such, mechanical ventilation is usually continued into the postoperative period. Unless intraoperative events suggest that postoperative differential lung ventilation will be required (eg, hyperinflation of the native lung in SLT), the double-lumen endotracheal tube is exchanged for a single-lumen tube. Excessive oropharyngeal edema or previous difficulty with intubation could also contraindicate tube exchange. Prior to exchange, thorough suctioning of the oropharynx is performed to decrease the risk of aspiration into the new graft. In many patients, the endotracheal tube change can be facilitated by the use of an exchange catheter. As the catheter is advanced, attention should be paid to the depth of placement to avoid damage to anastomoses or allograft. Bronchoscopy is then often performed to examine bronchial anastomoses and aggressively suction secretions or blood after replacement of the double-lumen tube with a single-lumen endotracheal tube.

Assenzo V, Assenzo C, Filippo R, et al. The feasibility of extubation in the operating room after bilateral lung transplantation in adult emphysema patients: an observational retrospective study. *Eur J Cardiothorac Surg*. 2018;54:1128-1133.

Felten ML, Moyer JD, Dreyfus JF, et al. Immediate postoperative extubation in bilateral lung transplantation: predictive factors and outcomes. *Br J Anaesth*. 2016;116:847-854.

D. Postoperative Management

D.1. What are the major complications after lung transplantation?

Complications from lung transplantation can occur in the immediate (<24 hours), early (24 hours to 1 week), intermediate (8 days to 2 months), or late (>2 months) postoperative period. Major immediate complications include hyperacute rejection, abnormalities due to central venous access or tracheal intubation (eg, pneumothorax, hemothorax, and hemomediastinum), and issues related to size mismatch between the donor and recipient lung. Primary graft dysfunction, wound complications such as infection or dehiscence, and pleural complications (eg, hemothorax, pneumothorax, and empyema) are the major early complications. Of these, primary graft dysfunction is by far the most significant, as it is the most common cause of early morbidity and mortality after lung transplantation. Severity can range from mild shunting and chest radiograph infiltrates to gross pulmonary edema with reduced lung compliance and intrapulmonary shunting. Management includes fluid restriction, diuretics, PEEP, inhaled nitric oxide, and ECMO for severe cases. The risk of primary graft dysfunction is increased significantly when CPB is utilized intraoperatively. Minimizing ischemic time and/or use of ex vivo perfusion systems prior to implantation can reduce the risk of primary graft dysfunction.

Intermediate complications include acute rejection, bronchial dehiscence, and *Candida* species pneumonia. Late complications include chronic rejection, infection (CMV, *Aspergillus*, mycobacteria), and bronchial stenosis. Infection and graft failure are the leading causes of death in the first posttransplant year. In later years, bronchiolitis obliterans syndrome predominates, and there are fewer cases caused by graft failure, infection, and malignancy. Bronchiolitis obliterans syndrome is perhaps the most important complication in the burden of subsequent mortality; it occurs in 10% of patients each year, and the incidence is highest at 5 years posttransplant. Retransplant patients are at the highest risk for bronchiolitis obliterans syndrome, whereas patients with CF and those with multiorgan transplants seem to be protected.

Immunosuppression is usually initiated before surgery, and the induction phase of therapy is continued for 5 to 10 days. The exact regimen varies between institutions but typically includes azathioprine, steroids, cyclosporine, and polyclonal antilymphocyte/antithymocyte globulins or interleukin-2 receptor antagonists. Acute rejection episodes are usually treated with intense steroid therapy and optimization of other immunosuppressant dosages. A challenge arises in differentiating acute rejection from infection as a source of shunting and chest radiograph infiltrates. Transbronchial biopsy is often necessary to make the distinction from histologic specimens. Bacterial pneumonia is the most frequent infection in the first 2 weeks. Although unusual in the first 2 weeks after transplantation, CMV is the second most common source of infectious pneumonitis. Broad-spectrum antibiotics are given perioperatively, and the regimen is adjusted based on the results of donor and recipient cultures. Antibiotic therapy for patients with CF is challenging, and the drug chosen is dictated by the patient's cultures and prior history of the organisms colonizing their lungs. Prophylactic acyclovir appears to be effective in reducing infections caused by herpes simplex, and trimethoprim-sulfamethoxazole is given to prevent infections from *Pneumocystis carinii*.

Bos S, Vos R, Van Raemdonck DE, et al. Survival in adult lung transplantation: where are we in 2020? *Curr Opin Organ Transplant*. 2020;25:268-273.

Chambers DC, Cherikh WS, Goldfarb SB, et al. The International Thoracic Organ Transplant Registry of the International Society for Heart and Lung Transplantation: thirty-fifth adult lung and heart-lung transplant report—2018; focus theme: multiorgan transplantation. *J Heart Lung Transplant*. 2018;37:1169-1183.

Krishnam MS, Suh RD, Tomasian A, et al. Postoperative complications of lung transplantation: radiologic findings along a time continuum. *Radiographics*. 2007;27:957-974.

D.2. How is postoperative lung ventilation managed, and for how long is it required?

After most procedures, the fraction of inspired oxygen (FIO_2) can be rapidly reduced, and weaning from the ventilator can be initiated as soon as the patient is warm and stable. An exception to this approach is the patient who has undergone SLT for pulmonary hypertension. Because of a propensity for episodes of cardiopulmonary instability during the first 24 to 48 hours postoperatively, it is advantageous to keep these patients mechanically ventilated during this period, although increasing experience is revealing the positive effects of rapid weaning protocols in those patients who tolerate it.

Lung protective ventilation strategies should be employed; patients should be ventilated with 4 to 5 mL/kg for OLV and 6 to 7 mL/kg for two-lung ventilation with PEEP to protect against lung injury. When possible, FIO_2 less than 40% should be used for the same reason. Plateau pressures greater than

30 cm H_2O should be avoided. Ventilator settings should be adjusted according to the patient's needs to achieve adequate ventilation with the lowest plateau pressure and optimal ventilation/perfusion matching.

Postoperatively, ventilation/perfusion mismatch and intrapulmonary shunt are often more pronounced after SLT than BLT. Not surprisingly, patients with restrictive disease usually display the best pulmonary function after SLT because the graft receives the majority of both ventilation and perfusion. After SLT in patients with COPD, the remaining native lung often receives a substantial portion of the tidal volume. The opposite is true in patients with pulmonary hypertension; the native lung continues to be ventilated but with limited blood flow. On rare occasions where there is a high difference in compliance between the graft and recipient lung, lung isolation and differential ventilation of the transplanted and native lung are needed after SLT for obstructive lung disease (eg, emphysematous lung disease). In these situations, the double-lumen endobronchial tube is left in place and two ventilators are employed. The native lung is ventilated with a low tidal volume (2-3 mL/kg) and rate, or even just connected to CPAP without intermittent mandatory ventilation. Nonetheless, the condition usually resolves rapidly with the return of spontaneous ventilation. Postural changes in arterial oxygen saturation are often prominent in SLT recipients. In general, patients who received a single lung for pulmonary hypertension or emphysema display better postoperative pulmonary function with the "transplant side up," whereas the opposite may be true in certain patients with restrictive lung disease. The precise etiology of this response is unclear but probably reflects positional variation in ventilation/perfusion matching.

Bigham M, Dickstein ML, Hogue CW Jr. Cardiac and lung transplantation. In: Estafanous FG, Barash PG, Reves JG, eds. *Cardiac Anesthesia: Principles and Clinical Practice*. 2nd ed. Lippincott Williams & Wilkins; 2001:637-662.

Nicoara A, Anderson-Dam J. Anesthesia for lung transplantation. *Anesthesiol Clin*. 2017;35:473-489.

D.3. What special precautions should be taken when a lung transplant recipient requires general anesthesia for subsequent nonpulmonary surgery?

After lung transplantation, patients may present to the operating room for surgeries not related to their pulmonary disease. With careful consideration and vigilance of the implications of lung transplantation, general anesthesia can be carried out with minimal issues. Aspiration precautions should be implemented, and patients should be assessed for gastritis, peptic ulcer disease, or a history of gastrointestinal bleeding especially in situations where anticoagulation is necessary. They should be evaluated for renal dysfunction, which can be caused by immunosuppressive therapy as well as hepatobiliary and/or pancreatic dysfunction. In addition to perioperative antibiotics, "stress dose" steroids and bronchodilators such as β_2-agonists should be considered; lung transplant patients usually take steroids long term and are more apt to bronchoconstriction.

Other perioperative considerations for the patient with a prior lung transplant undergoing subsequent surgery are based on whether the patient was the recipient of one or two lungs. Not surprisingly, differences in the compliance and expiratory flow rates of a native and transplanted lung after SLT for emphysema can result in alterations in intraoperative capnography. This phenomenon has been described as producing a biphasic pattern of carbon dioxide exhalation, with the first peak reflecting exhalation from the transplanted lung and the second peak exhalation from the native lung. The risk of overinflation of the native lung and resultant mediastinal shift with associated ventilation and hemodynamic consequences, although rare, must be considered when employing positive pressure ventilation.

The transplanted lung is denervated, so the cough reflex is present only in the proximal native airway and mucociliary function is impaired. In contrast, hypoxic pulmonary vasoconstriction is intact after lung transplantation and central respiratory control is unaffected. However, a blunted response to carbon dioxide can persist in patients with preoperative hypercapnia. The major factor limiting long-term survival from lung transplantation is bronchiolitis obliterans. This progressive condition characterized by progressive narrowing of small airways must be considered in patients with prior lung transplantation presenting for surgery and anesthesia after the initial recovery phase.

Bigham M, Dickstein ML, Hogue CW Jr. Cardiac and lung transplantation. In: Estafanous FG, Barash PG, Reves JG, eds. *Cardiac Anesthesia: Principles and Clinical Practice*. 2nd ed. Lippincott Williams & Wilkins; 2001:637-662.

Feltracco P, Falasco G, Barbieri S. Anesthetic considerations for nontransplant procedures in lung transplant patients. *J Clin Anesth*. 2011;23:508-516.

D.4. What are the long-term outcomes of lung transplantation?

Increased experience, improved techniques, and an increase in the number of donor organs facilitated by extended criteria donor and ex vivo perfusion systems have made lung transplantation a realistic option for more patients. The procedure, however, is not without substantial risk, and a favorable outcome is by no means ensured. Although survival has not changed over the last 5 years (84.6% 1-year, 67.8% 3-year, and 55.5% 5-year survival), the absolute number of patients living after lung transplantation has increased because more procedures are being done. From June 2009 to 2016, the median survival was 6.5 years after primary lung transplantation. For adult recipients who survive the first year after transplantation, the median postoperative survival is 8.7 years. Graft failure is the leading cause of death in the first posttransplant year and bronchiolitis obliterans predominates in later years, with lower rates of death due to graft failure, infection, and malignancies. Sex, underlying cause for lung transplantation, and type of procedure (SLT or BLT) are a few of the factors influencing outcomes. SLT recipients seem to do better in the first year after transplantation, whereas BLT recipients have a survival benefit starting the first year after transplantation. Likewise, patients with CF have better survival than patients with all other indications for lung transplantation. Female sex also confers a survival benefit.

A history of hypertension for donors is independently associated with higher 1-year survival while donor smoking, CMV mismatch, nonidentical blood type, history of diabetes mellitus, and other donor comorbidities as well as poor functional status for the donor are independently associated with lower survival at 1 year. Other factors associated with 1-year mortality include recipient age, donor age, recipient serum creatinine and bilirubin, recipient lung functional vital capacity (percentage predicted), allograft ischemic time, and transplant center volume. Risk factors that are independently associated with 5-year mortality are similar to those of 1-year mortality with a few differences. Patients with lymphangioleiomyomatosis have better survival than those with an increasing number of human leukocyte antigen mismatches who have lower 5-year survival. Likewise, extremes of recipient age, older donor age, lower transplant center volume, and higher panel reactive antibody percentage are associated with higher mortality.

Short- and long-term data are beginning to emerge for patients who received a transplant for COVID-19-associated pulmonary fibrosis or ARDS. Even though these patients typically have a greater acuity of lung disease than the general lung transplant population (ie, higher LAS scores, more preoperative days requiring mechanical ventilation and/or ECMO, worse preoperative functional status), a recent matched analysis found that patients with COVID-19 had similar rates of postoperative complications, functional status at discharge, and 6-month survival as the control population. When compared to an unmatched control population, however, patients with COVID-19 had a longer length of stay with more days requiring mechanical ventilation and/or ECMO postoperatively and were more likely to require dialysis. In-hospital mortality and mortality rates at 30 and 90 days were not significantly different.

Chambers DC, Cherikh WS, Goldfarb SB, et al. The International Thoracic Organ Transplant Registry of the International Society for Heart and Lung Transplantation: thirty-fifth adult lung and heart-lung transplant report—2018; focus theme: multiorgan transplantation. *J Heart Lung Transplant*. 2018;37:1169-1183.

Freischlag K, Lynch TJ, Ievlev V, et al. A matched survival analysis of lung transplant recipients with coronavirus disease 2019-related respiratory failure. *Ann Thorac Surg*. 2023;116:819-829.

Martin AK, Renew JR, Jayaraman AL, et al. Analysis of outcomes in lung transplantation. *J Cardiothorac Vasc Anesth*. 2019;33:1455-1466.

5 Ischemic Heart Disease and Coronary Artery Bypass Grafting

Margo Hoyler and Diana Khatib

A 57-year-old male with triple-vessel coronary artery disease (CAD), hypertension, and type 2 diabetes is scheduled for coronary artery bypass grafting (CABG). He had a myocardial infarction (MI) 7 months ago. He is currently taking metoprolol, metformin, and lisinopril. His blood pressure (BP) is 130/80 mm Hg, and his heart rate (HR) is 55 beats per minute.

A. Medical Disease and Differential Diagnosis

1. What is triple-vessel CAD? Name the branches of the coronary arteries.
2. What are the indications for CABG?
3. What is percutaneous coronary intervention (PCI)? Discuss its indications, contraindications, and results.
4. What are the expected results of CABG?

B. Preoperative Evaluation and Preparation

1. What should be included in your preoperative evaluation? Which preoperative tests would you order?
2. How would you evaluate the patient's left ventricular function?
3. Which factors determine myocardial oxygen supply?
4. What are the three major determinants of myocardial oxygen consumption? How are they measured clinically?
5. Would you continue the β-blocker (metoprolol) on the day of surgery? Why or why not? What is its half-life? What is the role of β-adrenergic blockers in treating congestive heart failure (CHF)?
6. Would you continue the angiotensin-converting enzyme (ACE) inhibitor on the day of surgery? Why or why not?
7. If the patient who is on lisinopril develops hypotension intraoperatively, how would you manage it?

C. Intraoperative Management

C.I. *Before Cardiopulmonary Bypass*

1. How will you monitor the patient?
2. Which electrocardiogram (ECG) lead has the greatest sensitivity for intraoperative myocardial ischemia?
3. How will you monitor the patient's temperature? Do you need to monitor it from multiple sites?
4. Is it necessary to monitor pulmonary artery (PA) pressure for coronary artery operations?
5. What are the possible complications of PA catheterization?
6. How do you know that the tip of the PA catheter is in the right ventricle (RV) or the PA?
7. How do you obtain pulmonary artery occlusion pressure (PAOP) and what does it represent?
8. What are the hemodynamic consequences of myocardial ischemia? How can you detect myocardial ischemia? Is PAOP a sensitive indicator of myocardial ischemia?
9. Discuss the principles and clinical applications of intraoperative two-dimensional transesophageal echocardiography (TEE).
10. How would you induce anesthesia? Is there any advantage/disadvantage to using propofol versus etomidate as the induction agent? What kind of neuromuscular blocking drug (NMBD) would you use? Why?

11. How would you maintain anesthesia? Volatile anesthesia or total intravenous anesthesia (TIVA)?
12. What are the cardiovascular effects of volatile anesthetics, morphine, and fentanyl?
13. What should you do regarding ventilation during sternotomy?
14. Would you use prophylactic nitroglycerin during CABG to prevent intraoperative myocardial ischemia or perioperative MI?
15. If ST-segment depression is seen during surgery, how would you treat it? What is the relation between perioperative myocardial ischemia and postoperative MI?
16. Discuss autologous transfusion and blood conservation for cardiac surgery.
17. What antifibrinolytic will you use to reduce blood transfusions?

C.II. *During Cardiopulmonary Bypass*

1. What anticoagulant would you give before cardiopulmonary bypass (CPB)? How much would you give? What is its mechanism?
2. What is the half-life of heparin? How is it eliminated?
3. How do you monitor heparin dosage? What is the activated coagulation time (ACT) test?
4. What is total CPB? What is partial CPB?
5. What kinds of pumps are used in CPB? Are they pulsatile or not?
6. What is the purpose of venting the left ventricle (LV)? How can it be done?
7. What are the mechanisms and features of the CPB oxygenator?
8. What kind of priming solution would you use? How much priming solution would you use? When would you prime with blood? Why?
9. What are the advantages and disadvantages of hemodilution?
10. How do you monitor the patient during CPB?
11. What should your target BP be during CPB?
12. How would you treat hypotension during CPB?
13. How would you treat hypertension (mean arterial pressure [MAP] over 80-100 mm Hg)?
14. How do you prepare an intravenous (IV) infusion of sodium nitroprusside, nicardipine, and nitroglycerin? What are the usual doses? Which do you prefer to use?
15. How much pump flow would you maintain during CPB? During hemodilution? During hypothermia?
16. How does blood viscosity change during hemodilution and hypothermia?
17. How is anesthesia provided during CPB?
18. Would you give NMBDs during CPB? How is their action affected during CPB?
19. How do you know the patient perfusion is adequate during CPB?
20. How much gas flow would you use for the oxygenator? What kind of gas would you use? Why?
21. What are the disadvantages of hypocapnia during CPB?
22. How would you preserve the myocardium during CPB?
23. What is cardioplegia? How much would you use?
24. The arterial blood gases and electrolytes during CPB are as follows: pH, 7.36; $Paco_2$, 42 mm Hg; Pao_2, 449 mm Hg; CO_2 content, 24 mEq/L; sodium (Na), 128 mEq/L; potassium (K), 5.8 mEq/L; glucose, 180 mg/dL; and hematocrit, 20%. The patient's temperature is 27 °C (80.6 °F). At what temperature are blood gases measured? How would you correct the blood gases according to the patient's body temperature? Would you treat the arterial blood gases measured at 37 °C (98.6 °F) or at the patient's body temperature?
25. How does the blood glucose level change during CPB? Why? What is optimal glucose control intraoperatively? Does hyperglycemia increase neurologic complications during CPB?
26. What are the effects of CPB on platelets and coagulation factors?
27. If the blood level of the venous reservoir is low, what would you replace it with? Blood or balanced salt solution?
28. How do you estimate the fluid balance during CPB?
29. For how long can the aorta be cross-clamped?
30. Why does the urine turn pink in some cases of CPB? What is the renal threshold for plasma hemoglobin?
31. Why does it take longer to rewarm than to cool the patient via the pump oxygenator?
32. At what temperature can the patient be weaned from CPB?
33. How would you defibrillate the heart internally during CPB?
34. If the HR is 40 beats per minute, what should you do?
35. How would you prepare for the termination of CPB?
36. How would you decide the need for inotropic support?

C.III. *After Cardiopulmonary Bypass*

1. How would you reverse heparin? How much protamine would you use? What are the other drugs used to neutralize heparin?
2. What is the mechanism of action of protamine?
3. What are the complications of too much protamine?
4. What is a protamine reaction? How can you prevent it? How do you treat it?
5. What are the indications for intra-aortic balloon pump (IABP)?
6. What are the principles of IABP?
7. What are the complications of IABP?

D. Postoperative Management

1. Would you reverse the neuromuscular blocking drug? Why?
2. When will you wean the patient from the ventilator?
3. What criteria would you use in deciding when to wean the patient from the ventilator?
4. What are the potential postoperative complications of CABG surgery?

A. Medical Disease and Differential Diagnosis

A.1. What is triple-vessel CAD? Name the branches of the coronary arteries.

Triple-vessel CAD involves progressive atherosclerosis of the major branches of the coronary arteries with eventual luminal obstruction and myocardial injury. The intimal disease is typically segmental but can be diffuse in severe cases. The major branches of the coronary arteries, shown in **Figure 5.1**, are the following:

- The right coronary artery (RCA)
- The left anterior descending (LAD) branch of the left main coronary artery (LMCA)
- The left circumflex (CX) branch of the LMCA

The coronary branches supply the cardiac conduction system with significant variability. The sinus node is supplied by the RCA in about 60% of people and the CX artery in the remaining 40%. The atrioventricular (AV) node is supplied by small branches from the posterior descending artery (PDA). Cardiac dominance is determined by which coronary artery branch supplies the PDA: 70% to 80% of people have right dominant circulation (RCA supply), while others are left dominant (CX artery supply) or codominant (RCA and CX supply).

Significant coronary stenosis is defined as greater than 70% intraluminal narrowing (50% for LMCA). The most common arteries for coronary bypass grafting are the LAD, obtuse marginal artery (branch of

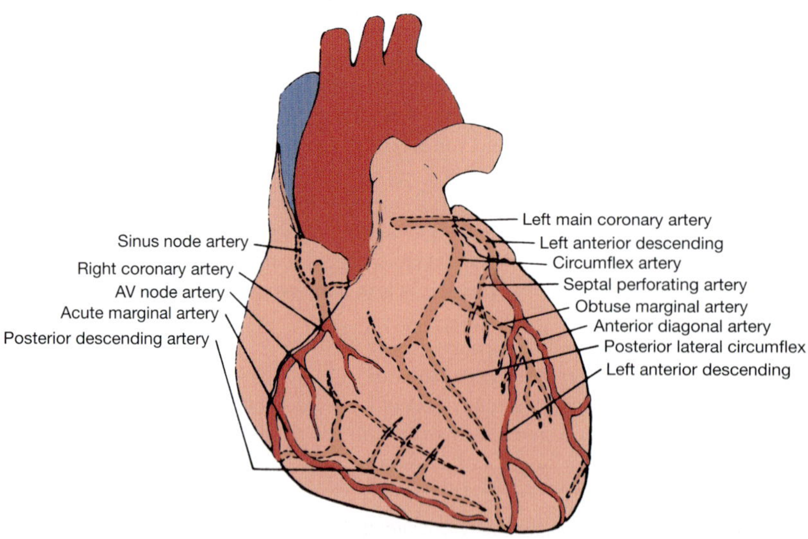

FIGURE 5.1. Branches of the coronary arteries. AV, atrioventricular.

CX), and PDA. A suitable distal target site, beyond the level of the proximal stenosis, is determined by the surgeon after a review of angiographic images, direct external inspection, and palpation.

Duncker DJ, Canty JM. Coronary blood flow and myocardial ischemia. In: Libby P, Bonow RO, Mann D, et al, eds. *Braunwald's Heart Disease: A Textbook of Cardiovascular Medicine*. 12th ed. Elsevier; 2022:609-635.

Villa ADM, Sammut E, Nair A, et al. Coronary artery anomalies overview: the normal and the abnormal. *World J Radiol*. 2016;8:537-555.

A.2. What are the indications for CABG?

Patients with significant coronary stenosis whose angina is not controlled by medical treatment or who have adverse side effects from medical management should be considered for coronary revascularization. The class I indications for CABG are:

- Left main CAD, three-vessel CAD, or two-vessel CAD with proximal LAD disease
- Multivessel CAD in patients with diabetes
- Life-threatening ventricular arrhythmia
- Concurrent with other cardiac surgical procedures

Emergent CABG should be performed after acute MI if a nonsurgical or PCI failed or the patient has persistent ischemia at rest with a large area of threatened myocardium, hemodynamic instability/cardiogenic shock, or complications such as ventricular septal defect or ruptured papillary muscle and mitral regurgitation.

Duncker DJ, Canty JM. Coronary Blood Flow and Myocardial Ischemia. In: Libby P, Bonow RO, Mann D, et al, eds. *Braunwald's Heart Disease: A Textbook of Cardiovascular Medicine*. 12th ed. Elsevier; 2022:609-635.

Lawton JS, Tamis-Holland JE, Bangalore S, et al. 2021 ACC/AHA/SCAI guideline for coronary artery revascularization: a report of the American College of Cardiology/American Heart Association Joint Committee on Clinical Practice Guidelines. *J Am Coll Cardiol*. 2022;79:197-215. Erratum in: *J Am Coll Cardiol*. 2022;79:1547.

Patel MR, Calhoon JH, Dhemer GJ, et al. ACC/AATS/AHA/ASE/ASNC/SCAI/SCCT/STS 2017 appropriate use for coronary revascularization in patients with stable ischemic heart disease: a report of the American College of Cardiology Appropriate Use Criteria Task Force, American Association for Thoracic Surgery, American Heart Association, American Society of Echocardiography, American Society of Nuclear Cardiology, Society for Cardiovascular Angiography and Interventions, Society of Cardiovascular Computed Tomography, and Society of Thoracic Surgeons. *J Am Coll Cardiol*. 2017;69:2212-2241.

A.3. What is percutaneous coronary intervention (PCI)? Discuss its indications, contraindications, and results.

PCI is performed by passing a small catheter across the stenosed coronary artery. The balloon portion of the catheter straddles the stenosis and is inflated to provide controlled coronary injury and enlarge the stenotic lumen. Following dilation, bare-metal or drug-eluting coronary stents are introduced to maintain long-term patency. PCI has redefined who is a candidate for elective surgical myocardial revascularization. The decision to perform CABG or PCI is best determined through a heart team including a cardiologist and surgeon, taking into account coronary anatomy, patient comorbidities, and patient preferences.

With the currently available technology, PCI is considered a therapeutic option in any individual with disabling ischemic symptoms despite good medical therapy and focal obstructive coronary disease regardless of cause. The indications for PCI include:

- Isolated discrete proximal single- or double-vessel disease
- Post-CABG with new stenotic lesions or stenosis at distal anastomosis
- Restenosis following PCI
- Contraindications to CABG
- Coronary stenosis following cardiac transplantation
- Occluded vessels within the last 6 months and less than 15 mm in length
- Poststreptokinase therapy for revascularization

PCI is contraindicated in the following:

- Left main CAD in which the distal coronary vessels are not protected by at least one completely patent large collateral vessel
- Multivessel severe diffuse disease
- Absence of a discrete obstructing lesion

The SYNTAX (Synergy between Percutaneous Coronary Intervention with TAXUS and Cardiac Surgery) trial compared PCI versus CABG. A SYNTAX score was developed in this trial (now SYNTAX II) and is the most widely used score to guide multivessel revascularization. A score greater than 33 is associated with favorable outcomes after CABG. The score reflects factors that increase the complexity of PCI.

The primary success rate of angioplasty alone is approximately 90%, but restenosis occurs at a rate of approximately 30%, 6 months following the procedure. Dilation can be repeated with a 90% success rate, with the artery tending to remain patent after the second angioplasty. With the introduction of coronary stents, which act as a metal scaffold, the restenosis rate after PCI has been decreasing, and fewer patients require subsequent revascularization: 10% to 15% after stenting versus 25% to 35% after angioplasty alone. The decrease in luminal diameter following stent placement is evident within the first 6 to 9 months and is the result of proliferative neointimal tissue growth in response to the associated injury and inflammation. The stent scaffold is coupled with polymers that elute or slowly release pharmacologic agents (sirolimus, an immunosuppressant, and paclitaxel, an antineoplastic) to inhibit neointimal growth. As newer-generation drug-eluting stents have become available, the need for repeat revascularization has decreased to 4% to 6%.

PCI is a different therapeutic approach than CABG. PCI targets the area of the lesion(s) only, whereas CABG bypasses the lesion areas. This is likely the reason that, at least in the intermediate term, CABG is considered superior for patients with multivessel CAD.

For isolated high-grade lesions of the LAD, Diegeler et al showed that CABG through a left anterior thoracotomy is as effective as PCI with stent placement. Although stenting provided excellent short-term results with fewer periprocedural adverse events, CABG was superior with regard to the need for repeated intervention in the target vessel and freedom from angina at 6 months of follow-up. Serruys et al compared outcomes between PCI with stent and CABG surgery; at 5 years, there was no difference in mortality between stenting and surgery for multivessel disease. Importantly, the incidence of stroke or MI was not significantly different between groups. However, the rate of major adverse cardiac and cerebrovascular events was higher in the stent group, driven by the increased need for repeat revascularization. A recent report on 10-year outcomes also showed that for treatment of unprotected LMCA disease, PCI with stenting showed similar long-term mortality and rates of death, Q-wave MI, or stroke. However, stenting, even with DES, was associated with higher rates of repeat revascularization than CABG. A recent comparison between stenting and CABG in patients with previously untreated three-vessel disease or LMCA disease concluded that CABG remains the standard of care for patients with three-vessel or LMCA disease because the use of CABG, as compared with PCI, resulted in lower rates of the combined endpoint of major adverse cardiac or cerebrovascular events at 1 year.

Diegeler A, Thiele H, Falk V, et al. Comparison of stenting with minimally invasive bypass surgery for stenosis of the left anterior descending coronary artery. *N Engl J Med.* 2002;347:561-566.

Duncker DJ, Canty JM. Coronary blood flow and myocardial ischemia. In: Libby P, Bonow RO, Mann D, et al, eds. *Braunwald's Heart Disease: A Textbook of Cardiovascular Medicine.* 12th ed. Elsevier; 2022:609-635.

Lawton JS, Tamis-Holland JE, Bangalore S, et al. 2021 ACC/AHA/SCAI guideline for coronary artery revascularization: a report of the American College of Cardiology/American Heart Association Joint Committee on Clinical Practice Guidelines. *J Am Coll Cardiol.* 2022;79:197-215. Erratum in: *J Am Coll Cardiol.* 2022;79:1547.

Moliterno DJ. Healing Achilles—sirolimus versus paclitaxel. *N Engl J Med.* 2005;353:724-727.

Park DW, Kim YH, Yun SC, et al. Long-term outcomes after stenting versus coronary artery bypass grafting for unprotected LMCA disease: 10-year results of bare-metal stents and 5-year results of drug-eluting stents from the ASAN-MAIN (ASAN Medical Center-Left MAIN Revascularization) Registry. *J Am Coll Cardiol.* 2010;56:1366-1375.

Serruys PW, Morice MC, Kappetein AP, et al. Percutaneous coronary intervention versus coronary-artery bypass grafting for severe coronary artery disease. *N Engl J Med.* 2009;360:961-972.

A.4. What are the expected results of CABG?

CABG has been shown to provide a survival benefit over medical therapy alone in the following three randomized controlled trials from the 1970s and 1980s: the Veterans Administration Cooperative Study, the European Coronary Surgery Study, and the Coronary Artery Surgery Study. A more recent systematic review comparing CABG to PCI showed that CABG resulted in lower mortality when compared to medical management at 5 years (9.2% vs 11.5%, $P < .01$). Survival was greatest for those with extensive multivessel disease (5-year mortality 11.5% in PCI group vs 8.9% in CABG group, $P < .01$), especially with coexisting diabetes (5-year mortality 15.5% vs 10%, $P < .01$).

Bypass conduits can be either arterial or venous, with arterial grafts considered superior conduits over venous grafts. The success of CABG depends on the long-term patency of the graft. The internal thoracic (mammary) artery (ITA) is the most commonly used bypass graft. The use of the ITA graft is considered a quality indicator by the Society of Thoracic Surgeons (STS). The saphenous vein is the most commonly used venous graft. Failure rates of venous grafts are related to variable size and quality.

Head SJ, Milojevic M, Daemen J, et al. Mortality after coronary artery bypass grafting versus percutaneous coronary intervention with stenting for coronary artery disease: a pooled analysis of individual patient data. *Lancet*. 2018;391:939-948. Erratum in: *Lancet*. 2018;392:476.

Lawton JS, Tamis-Holland JE, Bangalore S, et al. 2021 ACC/AHA/SCAI guideline for coronary artery revascularization: a report of the American College of Cardiology/American Heart Association Joint Committee on Clinical Practice Guidelines. *J Am Coll Cardiol*. 2022;79:197-215. Erratum in: *J Am Coll Cardiol*. 2022;79:1547.

Passamani ER, Frommer PL, Mullin S, et al. Coronary Artery Surgery Study (CASS): a randomized trial of coronary bypass surgery: survival data. *Circulation*. 1983;68:989-950.

Serruys PW, Morice MC, Kappetein AP, et al. Percutaneous coronary intervention versus coronary-artery bypass grafting for severe coronary artery disease. *N Engl J Med*. 2009;360:961-972.

Tabata M, Grab JD, Khalpey Z, et al. Prevalence and variability of internal mammary artery graft use in contemporary multivessel coronary artery bypass graft surgery: analysis of the Society of Thoracic Surgeons National Cardiac Database. *Circulation*. 2009 15;120:935-40.

Varnauskas E; European Coronary Surgery Study Group. Twelve-year follow-up of survival in the randomized European coronary surgery study. *N Engl J Med*. 1988;319:332-327.

Veterans Administration Coronary Artery Bypass Surgery Cooperative Study Group. Eleven-year survival in the Veterans Administration randomized trial of coronary bypass surgery for stable angina. *N Engl J Med*. 1984;311:1333-1339.

B. Preoperative Evaluation and Preparation

B.1. What should be included in your preoperative evaluation? Which preoperative tests would you order?

Preoperative evaluation is used for preoperative optimization and perioperative risk stratification. The STS risk model (STS score) and the European System for Cardiac Operative Risk Evaluation (EuroSCORE) are the two most widely used scores to determine the risk of major postoperative complications. In addition to the routine systemic examinations of all organ systems, special attention should be paid to the following:

- Cardiovascular function
  - Functional capacity and presence of anginal symptoms
  - Echocardiography with left ventricular and valvular assessment (from catheterization and/or echocardiography)
  - Cardiac catheterization, magnetic resonance imaging (MRI), or enhanced multidetector computed tomography (CT) to determine the location and severity of coronary disease
  - Resting and/or exercise ECG (if a stress test was performed preoperatively)
  - Presence of an implanted cardiac device with recent interrogation
  - CT for redo sternotomy to investigate the proximity of the sternum to the anterior surface of the heart
- Pulmonary function—pulmonary function tests if indicated for chronic pulmonary disease
- Hematologic function—complete blood count, prothrombin time, partial thromboplastin time, and platelet function assay (if available for patients previously receiving antiplatelet therapy)
- Gastrointestinal (GI) disease—dysphagia, recent upper GI bleed, esophageal disease precluding intraoperative TEE
- Renal function—creatinine, blood urea nitrogen, electrolytes, and blood sugar
- Hepatic function—for patients with previous history of hepatitis, jaundice, drug abuse, or right heart failure
- Neurologic disease—carotid artery duplex to evaluate concomitant cerebrovascular disease, cognitive function, and frailty assessment

Bansal M, Fuster V, Narula J, Sengupta PP. Assessment of cardiac risk and the cardiology consultation. In: Kaplan JA, Augoustides JGT, Manecke GR, et al, eds. *Kaplan's Cardiac Anesthesia for Cardiac and Noncardiac Surgery*. 7th ed. Elsevier; 2017:3-19.

B.2. How would you evaluate the patient's left ventricular function?

- Medical history: history of MI and presence or absence of angina

- Symptoms and clinical signs of left ventricular failure (dyspnea at rest or exercise, nocturnal orthopnea) and/or right heart failure (ascites, pitting edema, jugular vein distension)
- Cardiac catheterization, angiography, and/or echocardiography ejection fraction (normal 60%-65%)
- Left ventricular end-diastolic pressure (LVEDP) or PAOP (normal 6-15 mm Hg)
- Left ventricular wall motion on echocardiography—normal (wall thickening of >30%), hypokinesis (wall thickening of 10%-30%), akinesia (wall thickening of <10%), or dyskinesia (outward motion during systole) (**Figure 5.2**)
- Cardiac index (normal >2.2 L/min/m^2)
- Myocardial viability studies (contrast echocardiography, cardiac MRI, or positron emission tomography)

CAD can result in regional wall motion abnormalities (RWMA). Interruption of perfusion results in abnormal motion in the related myocardial segments. There is a gradation of wall motion abnormalities that consist of hypokinesis, akinesis, and, subsequently, dyskinesia in which a wall moves away from the center of the ventricle. Wall thickening and endocardial motion are intrinsically tied, and all RWMAs are expected initially to be associated with abnormalities of thickening as well as endocardial motion.

Bansal M, Fuster V, Narula J, Sengupta PP. Cardiovascular imaging. In: Kaplan JA, Augoustides JGT, Manecke GR, et al, eds. *Kaplan's Cardiac Anesthesia for Cardiac and Noncardiac Surgery*. 7th ed. Elsevier; 2017:20-45.

Schuleri KH, Centola M, George RT, et al. Characterization of peri-infarct zone heterogeneity by contrast-enhanced multidetector computed tomography: a comparison with magnetic resonance imaging. *J Am Coll Cardiol*. 2009;53:1699-1707.

B.3. Which factors determine myocardial oxygen supply?

$$\text{Myocardial oxygen } (O_2) \text{ supply} = \text{coronary blood flow} \times \text{arterial } O_2 \text{ content}$$

Coronary blood flow depends on the following:

- Diastolic aortic pressure (DAP)
- LVEDP
- Patency of coronary arteries
- Coronary vascular tone

Coronary blood flow can be determined by the formula:

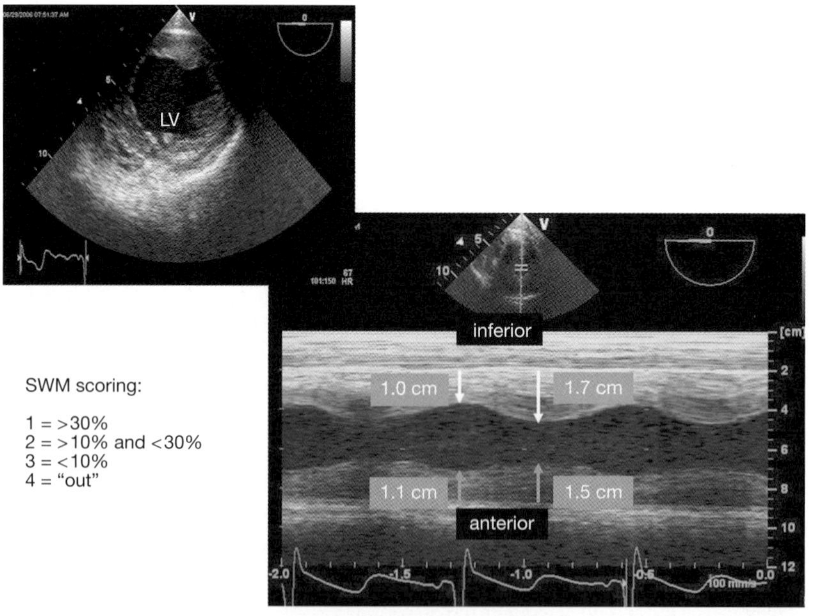

FIGURE 5.2. Echocardiographic evaluation of the left ventricle (LV). The transgastric midpapillary short-axis view of the LV is shown on the left. By placing a cursor line across the middle of the inferior **(top of the image)** and anterior **(bottom of the image)** segments of the left ventricular myocardium, the motion of the segments over time is shown in the right image. The percentage of wall thickening can be either visually estimated or measured between diastole and systole. SWM, segmental wall motion.

Coronary blood flow = coronary perfusion pressure ÷ myocardial vascular resistance, or, coronary blood flow = (DAP − LVEDP) ÷ myocardial vascular resistance.

Arterial O_2 content (Cao_2) is determined by the following equation:

$$Cao_2 = 1.34\ (\text{mL/g}) \times \text{hemoglobin concentration (g/dL)} \times O_2\ \text{saturation (\%)} + (0.0031 \times Pao_2).$$

O'Brien ERM, Nathan HJ. Coronary physiology and atherosclerosis. In: Kaplan JA, Reich DL, Savino JS, eds. *Kaplan's Cardiac Anesthesia: The Echo Era.* 6th ed. Elsevier Saunders; 2011:132-156.

B.4. What are the three major determinants of myocardial oxygen consumption? How are they measured clinically?

The three major determinants of myocardial oxygen consumption are myocardial wall tension, contractility, and HR.

Myocardial wall tension of the LV is estimated by the following:

- According to the Laplace equation, myocardial wall tension (T) is proportional to the diameter of the ventricle (R, radius) and intracavitary pressure (P) and inversely proportional to myocardial wall thickness (Th):

$$T = P \times R \div 2\text{Th}.$$

- Diastolic wall tension is related to the diastolic radius (R) of the ventricle, which is considered a surrogate of preload or left ventricular end-diastolic volume (LVEDV); the latter is estimated by the PAOP (because neither LVEDP nor left atrial pressure can be easily measured directly).
- Afterload is approximated by systolic BP, which is systolic ventricular pressure if there is no aortic stenosis.

Myocardial contractility is evaluated by:

- *Invasive*: Maximal velocity of contraction (Vmax), dP/dt (pressure time indices: how fast [dt] intraventricular pressure [dP] rises), or left ventricular end-systolic pressure/volume ratio
- *Noninvasive*: Preejection period/left ventricular ejection time and global and regional ventricular wall motion by echocardiography (**Figure 5.3**)

Pagel PS, Freed JK. Carciac physiology. In: Kaplan JA, Augoustides JGT, Manecke GR, et al, eds. *Kaplan's Cardiac Anesthesia for Cardiac and Noncardiac Surgery.* 7th ed. Elsevier; 2017:143-178.

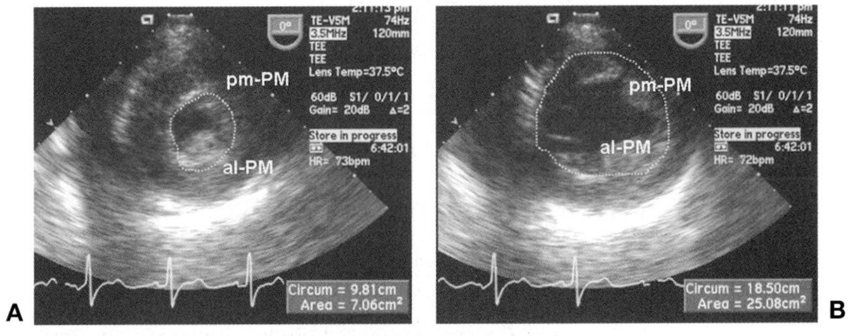

FIGURE 5.3. Echocardiographic evaluation of systolic function of the LV. The transgastric midpapillary short-axis view of the LV is shown in systole (**A**) and diastole (**B**). The endocardial border is traced (without including the endocardium of the two papillary muscles), and the end-systolic area (ESA) and end-diastolic area (EDA) are calculated. The percentage area change (fractional area change [FAC]) is calculated as FAC = (EDA − ESA)/EDA. The FAC correlates with but does not substitute the percentage ejection fraction. al-PM, anterolateral papillary muscle; pm-PM, posteromedial papillary muscle.

B.5. Would you continue the β-blocker (metoprolol) on the day of surgery? Why or why not? What is its half-life? What is the role of β-adrenergic blockers in treating congestive heart failure (CHF)?

The β-blocker (metoprolol) should be continued throughout the perioperative period. In patients with unstable angina, sudden withdrawal of a β-blocker can produce an exacerbation of symptoms and precipitate acute MI. Perioperative β-blockade in patients undergoing CABG is associated with reduced incidence of postoperative atrial fibrillation and 30-day mortality. The dose of β-blocker does not need to be reduced before surgery for fear of bradycardia, hypotension, or difficulty in weaning from CPB. The half-life of oral metoprolol is 3 hours. It is metabolized in the liver.

Reductions in HR with a β-blocker occur at lower serum levels than depression of myocardial contractility. Accordingly, as drug levels fall after discontinuation of therapy, reductions in chronotropic response last longer than reductions in inotropy. This is an important concept in treating tachycardias in patients with significant ventricular dysfunction and CHF: a small dose is appropriate and indicated, whereas a large dose can further suppress the inotropic state.

Numerous studies have confirmed improvements in cardiac function, exercise capacity, and long-term survival in patients with heart failure resulting from MI, hypertrophic cardiomyopathy, or idiopathic dilated cardiomyopathy with β-blockers. β-Blockers can also benefit patients with diastolic dysfunction secondary to hypertension.

Potential benefits of β-adrenergic blockade in heart failure include decreased HR and normalization of β-receptor function. A slower HR improves diastolic function by increasing the diastolic filling time and myocardial perfusion and by decreasing myocardial oxygen consumption. β-Adrenergic receptors are downregulated in heart failure, but their responsiveness is normalized by long-term β-blockade.

Lawton JS, Tamis-Holland JE, Bangalore S, et al. 2021 ACC/AHA/SCAI guideline for coronary artery revascularization: executive summary: a report of the American College of Cardiology/American Heart Association Joint Committee on Clinical Practice Guidelines. *Circulation.* 2022; 145:e4-e17.

Lawton JS, Tamis-Holland JE, Bangalore S, et al. 2021 ACC/AHA/SCAI guideline for coronary artery revascularization: executive summary: a report of the American College of Cardiology/American Heart Association Joint Committee on Clinical Practice Guidelines. *J Am Coll Cardiol.* 2022;79:197-215. Erratum in: *J Am Coll Cardiol.* 2022;79:1547.

Mittnacht AJC, London MJ, Puskas JD, Kaplan JA. Anesthesia for myocardial revascularization. In: Kaplan JA, Augoustides JGT, Manecke GR, et al, eds. *Kaplan's Cardiac Anesthesia for Cardiac and Noncardiac Surgery.* 7th ed. Elsevier; 2017:731-769.

B.6. Would you continue the angiotensin-converting enzyme (ACE) inhibitor on the day of surgery? Why or why not?

Major medical societies such as the American College of Cardiology and the American Heart Association recommend continuation of ACE inhibitors in the perioperative period. There is no difference in the amount of vasopressor or inotrope requirements during cardiac surgery in those patients who continue ACE inhibitors preoperatively. In fact, ACE inhibitors help control post-CPB hypertension. Patients with diabetes specifically benefit from ACE inhibitors preoperatively. Patients at risk for vasoplegia or impaired left ventricular function can experience intraoperative hypotension.

Bhatia M, Arora H, Kumar P. Pro: ACE inhibitors should be continued perioperatively and prior to cardiac surgery. *J Cardiothorac Vasc Anesth.* 2016;30:816-819.

Disque A, Neelankavil J. Con: ACE inhibitors should be stopped prior to cardiac surgery. *J Cardiothorac Vasc Anesth.* 2016;30:820-822.

Kristensen SD, Knuuti J. New ESC/ESA guidelines on noncardiac surgery: cardiovascular assessment and management. *Eur Heart J.* 2014;35:2344-2345.

Thompson A, Fleischmann KE, Smilowitz NR, et al. 2024 AHA/ACC/ACS/ASNC/HRS/SCA/SCCT/SCMR/SVM guideline for perioperative cardiovascular management for noncardiac surgery: a report of the American College of Cardiology/American Heart Association Joint Committee on Clinical Practice Guidelines. *Circulation.* 2024;150:e351-e442.

B.7. If the patient who is on lisinopril develops hypotension intraoperatively, how would you manage it?

The most common causes of intraoperative hypotension include hypovolemia, deep anesthesia, and surgical manipulation. Patients undergoing cardiac surgery are also at risk for vasoplegic syndrome, characterized by severe refractory hypotension in the absence of other identifiable causes of hypotension. Persistent hypotension increases perioperative mortality.

Three systems regulate BP: the sympathetic nervous system, the renin-angiotensin-aldosterone system (RAAS), and the vasopressinergic system. ACE inhibitors and angiotensin receptor blockers (ARBs) are RAAS antagonists. Specifically, ACE inhibitors prevent the conversion of angiotensin I to angiotensin II, resulting in lower arterial resistance and increased vascular capacitance. Many anesthetic medications affect the sympathetic system, and thus, BP relies more on the RAAS and vasopressinergic systems under anesthesia.

When conventional therapies such as volume expansion and vasopressors are ineffective, exogenous vasopressin might improve hypotension. Refractory hypotension can be treated with methylene blue, which interferes with the nitric oxide-cyclic guanosine monophosphate (cGMP) pathway. Methylene blue is contraindicated in patients with renal impairment because it is primarily eliminated by the kidneys.

Angiotensin II has been suggested as a treatment for refractory vasoplegic syndrome. In the recent Angiotensin II for the Treatment of High-Output Shock (ATHOS-3) trial, patients with vasodilatory shock requiring high doses of vasopressors had a rapid and significant decrease in vasopressor requirement upon administration of angiotensin II. As only a small subset of these patients had undergone cardiac surgery (19 out of 344 patients) and the drug can be associated with thromboembolic events, benefits should be interpreted with caution; however, it could be a useful therapeutic for patients with vasoplegic syndrome on ACE inhibitors.

Khanna A, English SW, Wang XS, et al. Angiotensin II for the treatment of vasodilatory shock. *N Engl J Med.* 2017;377:419-430.

Ortoleva J, Shapeton A, Vanneman M, Dalia AA. Vasoplegia during cardiopulmonary bypass: current literature and rescue therapy options. *J Cardiothorac Vasc Anesth.* 2020;34:2766-2775.

SECTION 2

C. Intraoperative Management

C.I. Before Cardiopulmonary Bypass

C.I-1. *How will you monitor the patient?*

- Standard American Society of Anesthesiologists (ASA) monitors
- Preinduction arterial line for continuous BP monitoring and arterial blood gas analysis. Since arteries in the upper extremity can be harvested for arterial conduits, this should be taken into account in arterial line placement.
- Central line and PA catheter (PAC) for pulmonary and central venous pressures (CVPs) and hemodynamic parameters (cardiac output, stroke volume, systemic and pulmonary vascular resistance). If the patient has good left ventricular function, a PAC might not be warranted.
- Urine output
- Temperature: esophageal (or PA) and bladder (or rectal, tympanic, or nasopharyngeal)
- Laboratory: arterial blood gases, electrolytes, hematocrit, ACT, and oxygen saturation of mixed venous blood (SVO_2)
- TEE if not contraindicated. Contraindications are esophagectomy or esophagogastrectomy, active upper gastroesophageal bleeding, oropharyngeal trauma, and the presence of esophageal pathology (tracheoesophageal fistula, stricture, trauma, tumor, scleroderma, Mallory-Weiss tear, and diverticulum). Anticipated benefits should be weighed against potential risks prior to probe placement.
- Cerebral oximetry, especially for patients with a high risk of postoperative neurologic outcomes, such as those undergoing hypothermic circulatory arrest or extensive atherosclerotic disease

Mittnacht AJC, London MJ, Puskas JD, Kaplan JA. Anesthesia for myocardial revascularization. In: Kaplan JA, Augoustides JGT, Manecke GR, et al, eds. *Kaplan's Cardiac Anesthesia for Cardiac and Noncardiac Surgery.* 7th ed. Elsevier; 2017:731-769.

C.I-2. *Which electrocardiogram (ECG) lead has the greatest sensitivity for intraoperative myocardial ischemia?*

Multiple-lead ECG monitoring provides the best clinically available method of detecting perioperative ischemia. Based primarily on results obtained from exercise treadmill testing, V_5 alone is sensitive for 75% of ischemic events. The standard combination of leads II and V_5 only increases sensitivity to 80% whereas combining leads V_4 and V_5 increases sensitivity to 90% in patients with known or suspected

CAD undergoing noncardiac surgery with general anesthesia. The sensitivity increased to 96% by combining leads II, V_4, and V_5. If only one lead can be displayed, lead V_5 should be used because it has the greatest sensitivity (see also Chapter 14: Ischemic Heart Disease and Noncardiac Surgery, Section C.3).

Salter B, Mittnacht AJC, Denault AY, Kaplan JA. Monitoring of the heart and vascular system. In: Kaplan JA, Augoustides JGT, Manecke GR, et al, eds. *Kaplan's Cardiac Anesthesia for Cardiac and Noncardiac Surgery*. 7th ed. Elsevier; 2017:283-330.

C.I-3. *How will you monitor the patient's temperature? Do you need to monitor it from multiple sites?*

In many cardiac surgery centers, temperature is measured from two or more sites in order to estimate core temperature and achieve an even distribution of body heat during cooling and rewarming by extracorporeal circulation (ECC). Esophageal, nasopharyngeal, bladder, or tympanic sites measure core temperature; the axillary and rectal sites measure peripheral temperature. Urinary bladder temperature monitoring through a urinary catheter is convenient and popular and reflects a body temperature between core and periphery; however, it is only accurate in patients who produce urine and has limited utility in patients with renal failure. During cooling and rewarming by ECC, core temperature changes rapidly, while peripheral temperature changes slowly. The opposite changes are witnessed during surface cooling or warming. Currently, single-site core temperature monitoring is the prevailing practice when ECC is conducted at near-normal body temperature.

Temperatures are measured during cooling on ECC to ensure that the organs most susceptible to potential hypoperfusion, such as the brain, receive the protective effect of the desired hypothermia. In this regard, nasopharyngeal or tympanic membrane temperatures are the best monitoring sites, although they, at times, overestimate or underestimate actual brain temperature. During rewarming, cerebral hyperthermia should be avoided (by maintaining a gradient of 5 °C between arterial blood and brain, with the brain having the lower temperature) and should be corrected immediately because hyperthermia increases cerebral oxygen consumption and can exacerbate postoperative neuropsychological dysfunction. PA or nasopharyngeal temperature can be used to wean from cardiopulmonary bypass.

Engelman R, Baker RA, Likosky DS, et al. The Society of Thoracic Surgeons, The Society of Cardiovascular Anesthesiologists, and The American Society of ExtraCorporeal Technology: clinical practice guidelines for cardiopulmonary bypass—temperature management during cardiopulmonary bypass. *J Cardiothorac Vasc Anesth*. 2015;29:1104-1113.

Mittnacht AJC, London MJ, Puskas JD, Kaplan JA. Anesthesia for myocardial revascularization. In: Kaplan JA, Augoustides JGT, Manecke GR, et al, eds. *Kaplan's Cardiac Anesthesia for Cardiac and Noncardiac Surgery*. 7th ed. Elsevier; 2017:731-769.

C.I-4. *Is it necessary to monitor pulmonary artery (PA) pressure for coronary artery operations?*

PA catheters can be used for diagnostic or therapeutic purposes including:

- Diagnosis of shock states, primary pulmonary hypertension, valvular disease, intracardiac shunts, cardiac tamponade, and pulmonary embolus
- Differentiation between high- and low-pressure pulmonary edema
- Monitoring and management of complicated acute MI
- Assessing hemodynamic response to therapies
- Management of multiorgan system failure and/or severe burns
- Management of hemodynamic instability after cardiac surgery
- Assessment of response to treatment in patients with primary pulmonary hypertension
- Therapeutic aspiration of air emboli

The indication to monitor PA pressure depends on the ventricular function. For good left ventricular function (ejection fraction >50% and normal ventricular wall motion), CVP correlates well with PAOP; therefore, PA pressure monitoring might not be necessary for this group. For patients with poor left ventricular function (ejection fractions <40% or prominent wall motion abnormalities), PA pressure monitoring is indicated. Other indications for monitoring PA pressure include pulmonary hypertension, combined coronary stenosis and valvular disease, and complex cardiac lesions.

Results of several studies involving critically ill patients consistently demonstrate that the use of a PA catheter is associated with increased mortality and morbidity or no difference in fatal and nonfatal outcomes compared to the use of CVP alone or other noninvasive monitoring. Much debate exists regarding this topic, and resolution is unlikely in the near term. Nevertheless, there has been a substantive reduction in the use of PA catheters in surgical and medical settings.

Mittnacht AJC, London MJ, Puskas JD, Kaplan JA. Anesthesia for myocardial revascularization. In: Kaplan JA, Augoustides JGT, Manecke GR, et al, eds. *Kaplan's Cardiac Anesthesia for Cardiac and Noncardiac Surgery*. 7th ed. Elsevier; 2017:731-769.

Rozental O, Thalappillil R, White RS, Tam CW. To Swan or Not to Swan: indications, alternatives, and future directions. *J Cardiothorac Vasc Anesth*. 2021;35:600-615.

C.I-5. *What are the possible complications of PA catheterization?*

Similar to central venous catheter insertion

Common Complications

- Infection/sepsis
- Hematoma
- Air embolism
- Thrombosis
- Catheter shearing and embolization

Subclavian Approach

- Pneumothorax
- Hemothorax
- Hydrothorax

Internal Jugular Approach

- Pneumothorax
- Neck hematoma/puncture of carotid artery
- Vagus nerve and brachial plexus injury
- Thoracic duct perforation from left-side approach

The basilar or cephalic vein approach has fewer complications, but the failure rate is higher.

From Pulmonary Artery Catheter Itself

- Arrhythmias/complete heart block (1.5%-11%)
- Thromboembolism
- Pulmonary infarction from continuous balloon inflation
- Massive hemorrhage from perforation of PA, right atrium, or RV
- Failure to wedge
- Hemoptysis
- Intracardiac knotting or entrapment
- Balloon rupture
- Endocardial thrombi
- Tricuspid valve injury

The incidence of PA catheter complications is related to operator experience.

Mittnacht AJC, London MJ, Puskas JD, Kaplan JA. Anesthesia for myocardial revascularization. In: Kaplan JA, Augoustides JGT, Manecke GR, et al, eds. *Kaplan's Cardiac Anesthesia for Cardiac and Noncardiac Surgery*. 7th ed. Elsevier; 2017:731-769.

Murphy GS, Vender JS. Monitoring the anesthetized patient. In: Barash PG, Cullen BF, Stoelting RK, et al, eds. *Clinical Anesthesia*. 6th ed. Lippincott Williams & Wilkins; 2009:707-708.

C.I-6. *How do you know that the tip of the PA catheter is in the right ventricle (RV) or the PA?*

There are three main differences in the pressure tracings, as shown in Figure 5.4.

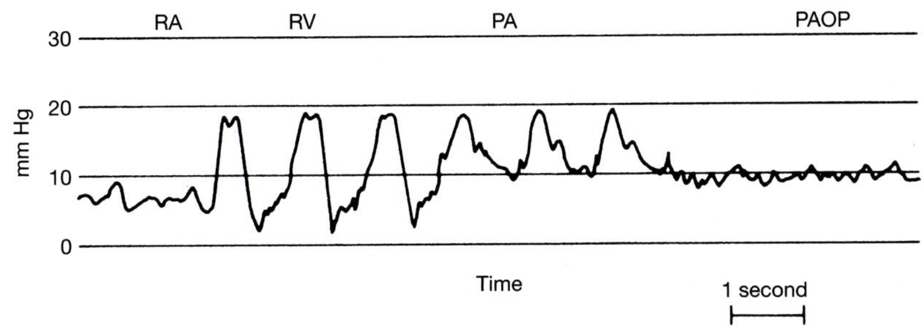

FIGURE 5.4. Pressure tracings of the right atrium (RA), right ventricle (RV), pulmonary artery (PA), and pulmonary artery occlusion pressure (PAOP).

Diastolic Step-Up

The diastolic pressure is higher in the PA than in the RV because the closed pulmonary valve maintains a diastolic gradient between the PA and the RV.

- PA pressure: 20 to 25/5 to 10 mm Hg
- Right ventricular pressure: 20 to 25/0 to 5 mm Hg

Pressure Contour

- PA pressure tracing has a dicrotic notch, created by the closure of the pulmonary valve, and is descending (decreasing) in diastole.
- Right ventricular pressure tracing has a sharp drop and a plateau in early diastole and is ascending (increasing) in diastole.

Ventricular Filling

In the late diastolic phase, PA pressure decreases because of diastolic runoff in the pulmonary circulation, whereas right ventricular pressure increases because of ventricular filling.

Salter B, Mittnacht AJC, Denault AY, Kaplan JA. Monitoring of the heart and vascular system. In: Kaplan JA, Augoustides JGT, Manecke GR, et al, eds. *Kaplan's Cardiac Anesthesia for Cardiac and Noncardiac Surgery*. 7th ed. Elsevier; 2017:283-330.

C.I-7. *How do you obtain pulmonary artery occlusion pressure (PAOP) and what does it represent?*

PAOP or pulmonary capillary wedge pressure is obtained by inflating the balloon on the PAC tip and advancing the catheter until the wave form changes, indicating position in a distal branch of the PA. The balloon should only be inflated for short periods to minimize the risk of PA injury. In the absence of pulmonary vascular disease and mitral valvular disease, PAOP is a surrogate for LVEDP and thus serves as an indicator of left ventricular preload.

- Normal—4 to 12 mm Hg
- Borderline—13 to 17 mm Hg
- Heart failure—over 18 mm Hg

Salter B, Mittnacht AJC, Denault AY, Kaplan JA. Monitoring of the heart and vascular system. In: Kaplan JA, Augoustides JGT, Manecke GR, et al, eds. *Kaplan's Cardiac Anesthesia for Cardiac and Noncardiac Surgery*. 7th ed. Elsevier; 2017:283-330.

C.I-8. *What are the hemodynamic consequences of myocardial ischemia? How can you detect myocardial ischemia? Is PAOP a sensitive indicator of myocardial ischemia?*

Acute myocardial ischemia affects systolic and diastolic cardiac function. Diastolic dysfunction usually manifests before alterations in systolic function. The immediate impact on ventricular compliance is related to the cause of the ischemic event. Decreased myocardial oxygen supply is initially accompanied by an increase in compliance. In contrast, increased myocardial oxygen demand is associated with an immediate loss of ventricular compliance (eg, the ventricle becomes stiffer). Therefore, the ventricle requires a higher filling pressure (end-diastolic pressure) to maintain a given stroke volume. A cascade of events occurs, which can include segmental wall motion abnormalities (SWMA), dysrhythmias, and conduction blocks. An 80% reduction of coronary blood flow causes akinesis (<10% of radial systolic thickening), whereas a 95% decrease causes dyskinesis (thinning, instead of thickening, during systole). If the ischemia becomes severe, the continuously elevated LVEDP leads to pulmonary edema (Figure 5.5).

The most well-recognized sign of ischemia is ECG ST-segment change. The ECG criteria for ischemia are horizontal or downsloping ST-segment depression of at least 0.1 mV at 0.06 second from the J-point, upsloping ST-segment depression of at least 0.2 mV at 0.08 second from the J-point or ST-segment elevation of at least 0.15 mV (1 mV = 10 mm). Other ECG signs of ischemia include inverted T waves and new-onset arrhythmias or conduction abnormalities.

RWMA, detected with two-dimensional echocardiography, is the earliest and most sensitive sign of myocardial ischemia. RWMAs appear with just a 25% decrease in coronary blood flow in the absence of ECG changes, whereas ECG signs of ischemia are apparent with a 50% decrease in coronary blood flow. RWMA is 4 times more sensitive than ECG ST-segment change in detecting intraoperative ischemia. Moreover, ST-segment changes cannot be analyzed if the patient has conduction disturbances, such as bundle branch block or ventricular-paced rhythms. Worsening wall motion after CABG surgery should be considered a prognostic indicator of adverse cardiovascular outcomes.

Measurement of PAOP has been suggested as an early and sensitive indicator of ischemia to be used when the ECG is not diagnostic. Although acute increases in PAOP or the development of V waves can

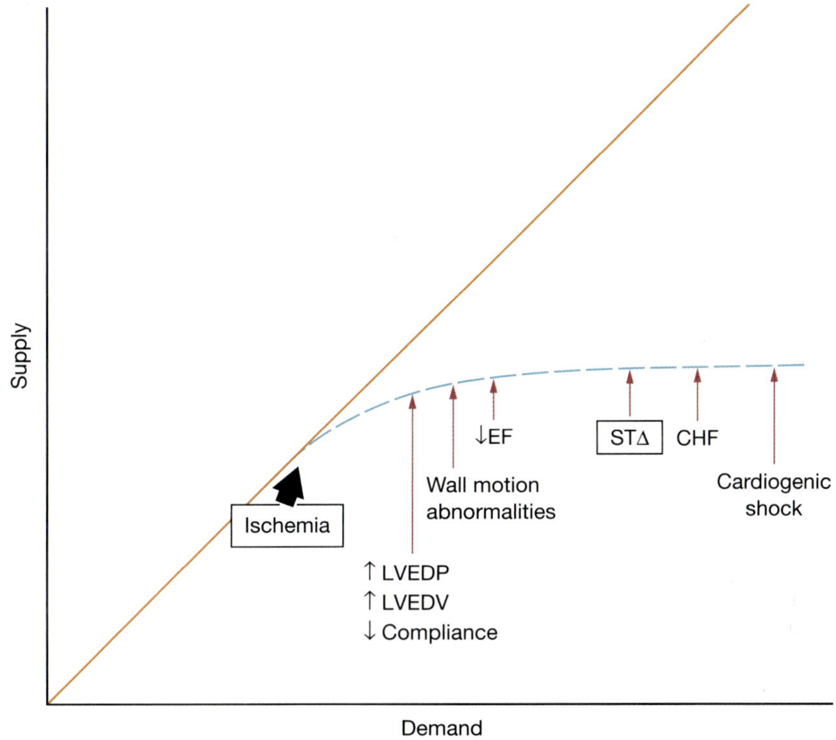

FIGURE 5.5. Hemodynamic consequences of myocardial ischemia. Ischemia occurs when demand exceeds supply. CHF, congestive heart failure; EF, ejection fraction; LVEDP, left ventricular end-diastolic pressure; LVEDV, left ventricular end-diastolic volume; STΔ, ST-segment changes. (Reprinted with permission from Barash PG. Monitoring myocardial oxygen balance: physiologic basis and clinical application. *ASA Refresher Courses Anesthesiol.* 1985;13:24.)

reflect ischemia (from decreased left ventricular compliance and/or mitral regurgitation), the absence of a change in PAOP does not ensure the absence of ischemia. Häggmark et al reported that the sensitivity, specificity, and predictive value (positive and negative) of PAOP abnormalities for ischemia were 40% to 60%. Leung et al found that 61% of TEE wall motion abnormalities in patients with CABG occurred without significant changes in HR, systolic arterial pressure, or PA pressure. Only 10% of episodes were accompanied by 5 mm Hg or greater changes in PA pressure. These studies question the value of PA catheterization and monitoring for detection of intraoperative ischemia.

Häggmark S, Hohner P, Ostman M, et al. Comparison of hemodynamic, electrocardiographic, mechanical, and metabolic indicators of intraoperative myocardial ischemia in vascular surgical patients with coronary artery disease. *Anesthesiology*. 1989;70:19-25.

Leung JM, O'Kelly B, Browner WS, et al. Prognostic importance of postbypass regional wall-motion abnormalities in patients undergoing coronary artery bypass graft surgery. SPI Research Group. *Anesthesiology*. 1989;71:16-25.

Mittnacht AJC, London MJ, Puskas JD, Kaplan JA. Anesthesia for myocardial revascularization. In: Kaplan JA, Augoustides JGT, Manecke GR, et al, eds. *Kaplan's Cardiac Anesthesia for Cardiac and Noncardiac Surgery*. 7th ed. Elsevier; 2017:731-769.

Swaminathan M, Morris RW, De Meyts DD, et al. Deterioration of regional wall motion immediately after coronary artery bypass graft surgery is associated with long-term major adverse cardiac events. *Anesthesiology*. 2007;107:739-745.

C.I-9. *Discuss the principles and clinical applications of intraoperative two-dimensional transesophageal echocardiography (TEE).*

TEE is an established technique to visualize cardiac anatomy and function. Echocardiography is based on fundamental ultrasonic principles. Ultrasound is defined as sound above the upper threshold of human hearing (>20,000 Hz). Ultrasound waves (1-7 MHz) are created by applying an alternating electric current of 500 to 1,500 pulses per second to a piezoelectric crystal. A short burst (pulse) of high-frequency, low-intensity sound is then emitted and directed through the body to detect boundaries between structures of different acoustic impedance. The ultrasound wave is partially reflected at the boundary of media with different acoustic impedance, a property that is primarily determined by slight differences in density between different tissues. The transmission of ultrasound through the heart, with detection of the returning echoes detailing the position and movement of cardiac structures, is termed *cardiac ultrasound* or *echocardiography*. Two-dimensional ultrasound reconstructs cardiac anatomy in shades of gray, from the time delay and decreased intensity of the reflected ultrasound. The ultrasound beam sweeps in an arc to give a panoramic view of the heart that results in cross-sectional images that are anatomically recognizable (see also Chapter 7: Valvular Heart Disease, Section A.6).

Doppler echocardiography blood flow is measured by applying Doppler frequency shift analysis to echoes reflected by a moving target (red blood cells or cardiac tissue). According to the Doppler principle, the frequency of the reflected ultrasound is different from the frequency of the emitted ultrasound. This change in frequency is proportional to the speed of the moving target. Color-coded Doppler flow imaging (color flow Doppler) simultaneously presents real-time images of intracardiac blood flow and moving cardiac structures in two dimensions. Color flow Doppler permits evaluation of valvular function and intracardiac shunts.

Clinical applications of intraoperative echocardiography include:

- *Monitoring ventricular volume and function.* When the left ventricular short-axis cross section is monitored at the level of the midpapillary muscles, TEE provides a direct semiquantitative method to assess left ventricular preload (left ventricular cross-sectional area at end-diastole) and ejection (difference of left ventricular cross-sectional area between end-diastole and end-systole) in real time to guide administration of fluids, inotropes, or pressors.
- *Monitoring diastolic filling patterns.* Both Doppler assessment of transmitral and transpulmonary vein flow patterns can provide important information about diastolic dysfunction that can occur in as many as 50% of patients presenting for open heart surgery, particularly those with hypertension, aortic stenosis, and hypertrophic cardiomyopathy. In patients with valvular disease, a component of left ventricular dysfunction arises from abnormal diastolic function.
- *Ischemic heart disease.* RWMAs, such as hypokinesia, akinesia, and dyskinesia, are the earliest signs of myocardial ischemia (Figures 5.2 and 5.3; Section C.I-9). Measurements of systolic wall thickening, a sensitive sign of myocardial ischemia, are not reproducible because of a difficulty in delineating the epicardial border accurately in two-dimensional echocardiography. Impairment of diastolic function can be qualitatively estimated, and filling pressures can be estimated using a combination of spectral Doppler measurements of blood flow through the transmitral and transpulmonary veins.
- *Air embolism.* In the left atrium, LV, and aorta, air embolism can be detected by TEE. Therefore, TEE can be used to help the surgeon evacuate air bubbles from the left heart before the heart ejects blood and air into the systemic circulation. This is more important when cardiac cavities are opened during surgery (aortic or valve surgery, etc).
- *Valvular regurgitation.* Valvular regurgitation can be determined intraoperatively by color Doppler echocardiography before and immediately after conservative valve repair (annuloplasty, commissurotomy) or valve replacement. The degree of valvular incompetence can be accurately measured using a combination of two-dimensional and Doppler techniques (Figures 5.6 and 5.7), and the function of the repaired or replaced valve can be quantitatively evaluated.

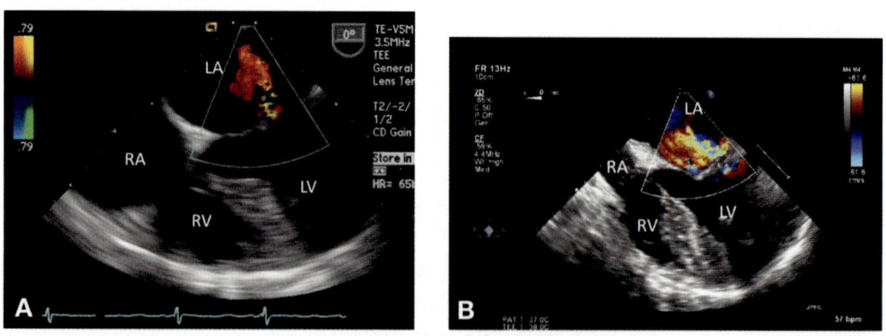

FIGURE 5.6. Color Doppler echocardiography. A. Superimposed on a two-dimensional image (here, the midesophageal view), the relative velocities of the red blood cells from a selected area (*triangle*) are visualized. Timed to the ECG (on the bottom of the sector image), normal or abnormal blood flows can be viewed as they cross orifices. In this case, a small regurgitant jet originating from the mitral valve during systole is seen. The color of the jet displays velocity and direction, according to the scale, on the left side of the figure. The mitral regurgitation jet is moving upward toward the left atrium (LA) and is colored red. **B.** In this midesophageal four-chamber view of the left ventricle (LV), a systolic mitral regurgitant jet is directed inside the LA. RA, right atrium; RV, right ventricle.

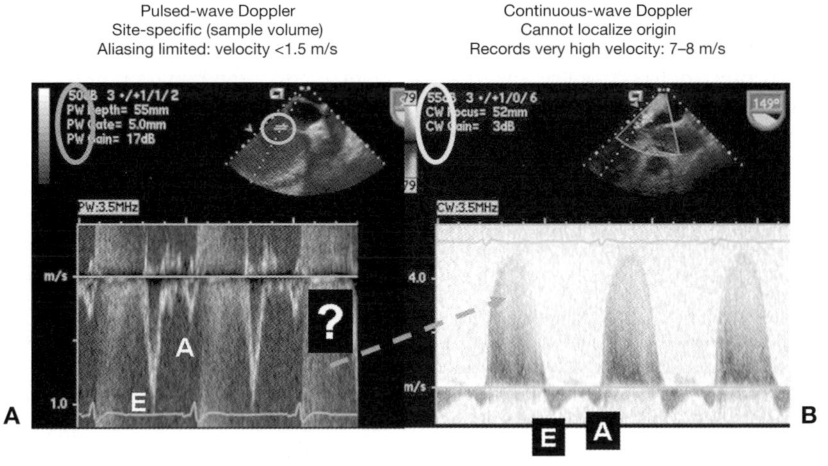

FIGURE 5.7. Doppler mode. A. A typical pulsed-wave (PW) Doppler velocity consists of a spectral recording of varying intensity, depending on the acoustic density of the reflected interface (the mass of blood cells). The most dense (or brightest) portion of the spectral tracing represents the velocity of most blood cells. The velocity is recorded from a specific site (*white circle*), and the maximum velocity recorded is limited (usually <1.5 m/s). In this PW Doppler spectrum, *E* represents the diastolic early filling, and *A* the diastolic late (due to atrial contraction) velocity. During systole, there is a broad signal (*question mark*) representing systolic flow through the mitral valve (probably mitral regurgitation). However, neither the direction nor the peak velocity can be visualized. **B.** In contrast, continuous-wave (CW) Doppler records the velocities of all the red blood cells moving along the path of the sound beam. A CW Doppler recording always consists of a full spectral envelope with the outer border corresponding to the fastest moving blood cells. The site of origin of a high-velocity jet is inferred from the particular lesion that is being examined. The maximum velocity that can be recorded can be as high as 8 m/s. Here, the direction (from bottom to top or from the LV toward the LA) as well as the maximum systolic velocity (~5 m/s) can be visualized, detailing the mitral regurgitation jet.

- *Valvular stenosis.* Spectral Doppler echocardiography can be used intraoperatively to measure the pressure gradient across a valvular stenosis and calculate the area of the diseased valve.
- *Congenital heart disease.* TEE techniques facilitate complex cardiac reconstructions, allowing visualization of the heart and adequacy of the surgical repair immediately after the procedure.
- *Thoracic aorta.* TEE can accurately diagnose thoracic aortic aneurysm, dissection, disruption, and atheroma. Epiaortic echocardiography is performed to examine the ascending aorta and arch if severe atheroma is found in the descending aorta or arch by TEE. Severe atheroma of the thoracic aorta is an independent predictor of postoperative neurologic outcome. Atheromata are graded as grade I, normal to mild intimal thickening; grade II, severe intimal thickening; grade III, atheroma protruding less than 5 mm into the lumen; grade IV, atheroma protruding greater than 5 mm; and grade V, atheroma with a mobile component (**Figure 5.8**).
- *Cardiac tumors.* Atrial myxoma can be diagnosed by TEE. Preoperative and postoperative TEE with contrast can assess the presence and severity of mitral regurgitation secondary to valve damage from a ball valve effect of the myxoma.
- *Other cardiac pathology.* Hypertrophic obstructive cardiomyopathy (HOCM) (idiopathic hypertrophic subaortic stenosis) can be identified by a combination of the systolic anterior motion of the mitral valve and left ventricular outflow obstruction. Cardiac tamponade caused by a pericardial effusion or hematoma can be detected.
- *Neurosurgery.* TEE is a sensitive monitor to detect venous air embolism during neurosurgical operations in the sitting position. Patent foramen ovale and paradoxical air embolism can be detected by TEE.
- *Monitoring for noncardiac surgery.* Recent guidelines suggest the utility of TEE in healthy patients who are acutely hemodynamically unstable during surgery, critically ill patients with significant respiratory and cardiac disease undergoing noncardiac surgery, and patients undergoing high-risk noncardiac procedures, such as orthopedic surgery and kidney and liver transplantation. TEE can be used as a hemodynamic diagnostic and monitoring tool to guide and evaluate the effectiveness of therapeutic interventions.

Agricola E, Oppizzi M, Melisurgo G, et al. Transesophageal echocardiography: a complementary view of the heart. *Expert Rev Cardiovasc Ther.* 2004;2:61-75.

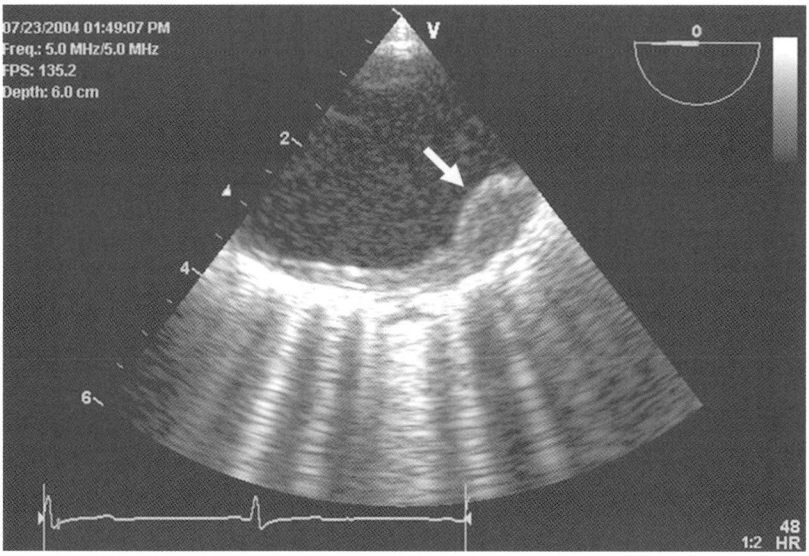

FIGURE 5.8. Atheromatous aortic disease. An echocardiographic picture of the short-axis view of the descending thoracic aorta is shown. The anterior aortic wall is irregularly thickened, and a large atheroma (8 mm) is present at 5 o'clock (*arrow*). This is a grade IV atheroma.

Kühl HP, Hanrath P. The impact of transesophageal echocardiography on daily clinical practice. *Eur J Echocardiogr*. 2004;5:455-468.

Mahmood F, Matyal R. A quantitative approach to the intraoperative echocardiographic assessment of the mitral valve for repair. *Anesth Analg*. 2015;121:34-58.

Porter TR, Shillcutt SK, Adams MS, et al. Guidelines for the use of echocardiography as a monitor for therapeutic intervention in adults: a report from the American Society of Echocardiography. *J Am Soc Echocardiogr*. 2015;28:40-56.

Shillcutt SK, Aron R, Maslow AD, et al. Transesophageal echocardiography: advanced echocardiography concepts monitoring of the heart and vascular system. In: Kaplan JA, Augoustides JGT, Manecke GR, et al, eds. *Kaplan's Cardiac Anesthesia for Cardiac and Noncardiac Surgery*. 7th ed. Elsevier; 2017:395-520.

Shapira Y, Vaturi M, Weisenberg DE, et al. Impact of intraoperative transesophageal echocardiography in patients undergoing valve replacement. *Ann Thorac Surg*. 2004;78:579-583.

C.I-10. *How would you induce anesthesia? Is there any advantage/disadvantage to using propofol versus etomidate as the induction agent? What kind of neuromuscular blocking drug (NMBD) would you use? Why?*

Perioperative hemodynamic goals for patients with coronary disease include preventing hypotension, hypertension, and tachycardia. Many techniques can achieve a smooth induction and maintain adequate coronary perfusion. Anxiety can exacerbate myocardial ischemia, so preoperative anxiolytics such as midazolam are typically given as soon as the standard ASA monitors are applied prior to arterial line insertion with local anesthetic.

For patients with good left ventricular function, anesthesia can be induced with fentanyl, 2 to 5 μγ/kg, and propofol, 1 to 2 mg/kg. Propofol can cause a reduction in MAP; however, this is less likely if it is administered at 10 mg per 40 seconds, as recommended by the manufacturer. Alternatively, etomidate 0.2 mg/kg can be administered for induction. Etomidate can cause transient adrenal insufficiency; however, this does not translate into increased vasopressor requirements or worse early outcomes. A randomized controlled trial comparing the two induction agents in the cardiac surgery population confirmed that propofol has a less favorable hemodynamic profile, although the proportion of patients receiving vasopressors was not significantly different.

After administration of a nondepolarizing neuromuscular blocking drug (vecuronium, rocuronium), the trachea is intubated. The choice of NMBD varies among practitioners. Succinylcholine is used less frequently in cardiac surgery.

For patients with poor left ventricular function, all anesthetics, including potent inhalation agents such as isoflurane, sevoflurane, and desflurane, should be used cautiously during induction of anesthesia because of their dose-dependent reduction in myocardial contractility and systemic arterial resistance.

See also Chapter 11: Hypertension, Section C.6, for other measures to prevent tachycardia and hypertension at the time of intubation.

Basciani RM, Rindlisbacher A, Begert E, et al. Anaesthetic induction with etomidate in cardiac surgery: a randomized controlled trial. *Eur J Anaesthesiol.* 2016;33:417-424.

Hannam JA, Mitchell SJ, Cumin D, et al. Haemodynamic profiles of etomidate vs propofol for induction of anaesthesia: a randomised controlled trial in patients undergoing cardiac surgery. *Br J Anaesth.* 2019;122:198-205.

Mangusan RF, Hooper V, Denslow SA, et al. Outcomes associated with postoperative delirium after cardiac surgery. *Am J Crit Care.* 2015;24:156-163.

Mittnacht AJC, London MJ, Puskas JD, Kaplan JA. Anesthesia for myocardial revascularization. In: Kaplan JA, Augoustides JGT, Manecke GR, et al, eds. *Kaplan's Cardiac Anesthesia for Cardiac and Noncardiac Surgery.* 7th ed. Elsevier; 2017:731-769.

C.I-11. *How would you maintain anesthesia? Volatile anesthesia or total intravenous anesthesia (TIVA)?*

Hemodynamic stability is essential to achieve a balance between myocardial oxygen demand and supply. Different agents and techniques can be used to accomplish this goal. A combination of fentanyl (or another synthetic opioid) and isoflurane, sevoflurane, or desflurane (or propofol) is a popular choice (balanced technique). Volatile anesthetics have cardioprotective effects through various mechanisms. A study by Landoni et al evaluating volatile anesthesia versus TIVA for CABG showed that volatile anesthetics do not improve mortality in this patient population. A recent meta-analysis comparing postoperative outcomes in patients receiving TIVA versus volatile anesthesia found no significant differences in mortality, but the volatile anesthesia group had shorter hospitalization and intensive care unit (ICU) stays. After the trachea is intubated, a mixture of 60% air and 40% oxygen is administered to lessen the possibility of oxygen toxicity subject to underlying pulmonary disease and ongoing intraoperative clinical conditions.

The depth of anesthesia must be titrated to meet the requirements of the varying intensity of surgical stimulation. Skin incision and sternal splitting are very painful. However, the strongest stimulation is usually from sternal retraction with the self-retaining retractor. Fentanyl, around 5 μγ/kg (or equivalent doses of other opioids), is given before the skin incision, before sternotomy, and intermittently throughout surgery as needed to maintain adequate analgesia. Very high doses of fentanyl or sufentanil were traditionally recommended for cardiac anesthesia due to the cardiac stability of opioids. There have been significant changes in practice over the past decade, whereby lower doses of opioids are administered to facilitate early extubation. In modern practice, maintenance of anesthesia is achieved with administration of volatile agents and smaller opioid doses. Longer-acting opioids, such as methadone, can be used to reduce the quantity of opioids administered both intraoperatively and postoperatively. Murphy et al demonstrated that methadone administration during cardiac surgery reduces postoperative opioid requirements and improves pain scores. Vasoactive agents are also used to regulate hemodynamics (HR, systemic arterial pressure, and filling pressures).

Although any volatile anesthetic can safely be used during cardiac surgery, isoflurane, desflurane, and sevoflurane have very different atmospheric half-lives, which contribute to global warming. Sevoflurane has the shortest atmospheric lifetime (1-5 years) and global warming potential compared to isoflurane (3-6 years) and desflurane (9-21 years).

Beverstock J, Park T, Alston RP, et al. A comparison of volatile anesthesia and total intravenous anesthesia (TIVA) effects on outcome from cardiac surgery: a systematic review and meta-analysis. *J Cardiothorac Vasc Anesth.* 2021;35:1096-1105.

Landoni G, Lomivorotov VV, Nigro Neto C, et al. Volatile anesthetics versus total intravenous anesthesia for cardiac surgery. *N Engl J Med.* 2019;380:1214-1225.

Mittnacht AJC, London MJ, Puskas JD, Kaplan JA. Anesthesia for myocardial revascularization. In: Kaplan JA, Augoustides JGT, Manecke GR, et al, eds. *Kaplan's Cardiac Anesthesia for Cardiac and Noncardiac Surgery.* 7th ed. Elsevier; 2017:731-769.

Murphy GS, Szokol JW, Avram MJ, et al. Intraoperative methadone for the prevention of postoperative pain: a randomized, double-blinded clinical trial in cardiac surgical patients. *Anesthesiology.* 2015;122:1112-1122.

Pagel PS. Myocardial protection by volatile anesthetics in patients undergoing cardiac surgery: a critical review of the laboratory and clinical evidence. *J Cardiothorac Vasc Anesth.* 2013;27:972-982.

Varughese S, Ahmed R. Environmental and occupational considerations of anesthesia: a narrative review and update. *Anesth Analg.* 2021;133:826-835.

C.I-12. *What are the cardiovascular effects of volatile anesthetics, morphine, and fentanyl?*

Isoflurane, desflurane, and sevoflurane all produce dose-related depression in ventricular function and vascular tone due to altered Ca^{2+} entry and sarcoplasmic reticulum function in cardiomyocytes. Out of all the volatile anesthetics, isoflurane causes the greatest reduction in vascular tone and coronary vasodilation, suggesting the possibility of a steal syndrome in patients with CAD. However, there is no conclusive evidence that isoflurane is more harmful than other anesthetics, assuming that coronary perfusion pressure is maintained. Compared to the other volatile anesthetics, desflurane causes the largest increase in HR. Isoflurane and desflurane cause tachycardia if the inspiratory concentration is increased rapidly due to increased sympathetic nervous system outflow. All volatile anesthetics decrease arterial pressure in a dose-related manner. The mechanism of BP decrease includes vasodilation, myocardial depression and decreased cardiac output, and decreased sympathetic nervous system tone.

Opioids such as morphine and fentanyl have minimal cardiovascular effects at usual doses. Both can cause bradycardia. Neither sensitizes the heart to catecholamines or depresses myocardial function. The cardiovascular effects of morphine depend on the dose. Large doses of morphine have reportedly caused myocardial lactate production and a reduction in coronary blood flow in animals. Sethna et al found that morphine sulfate, 0.25 mg/kg IV, did not produce global myocardial ischemia in patients with CAD. High doses of morphine, 1 mg/kg, produce a significant decrease in arterial BP and systemic vascular resistance (SVR) accompanied by an average 750% increase in plasma histamine. On the other hand, high doses of fentanyl, 50 μγ/kg, do not produce significant changes in BP, vascular resistance, or plasma histamine levels.

Malan TP Jr, DiNardo JA, Isner RJ, et al. Cardiovascular effects of sevoflurane compared with those of isoflurane in volunteers. *Anesthesiology*. 1995;83:918-928.

Mittnacht AJC, London MJ, Puskas JD, Kaplan JA. Anesthesia for myocardial revascularization. In: Kaplan JA, Augoustides JGT, Manecke GR, et al, eds. *Kaplan's Cardiac Anesthesia for Cardiac and Noncardiac Surgery*. 7th ed. Elsevier; 2017:731-769.

Sethna DH, Moffitt EA, Gray RJ, et al. Cardiovascular effects of morphine in patients with coronary arterial disease. *Anesth Analg*. 1982;61:109-114.

C.I-13. *What should you do regarding ventilation during sternotomy?*

It is recommended that ventilation be held to protect the lungs from injury by the electric saw for a first-time sternotomy.

C.I-14. *Would you use prophylactic nitroglycerin during CABG to prevent intraoperative myocardial ischemia or perioperative MI?*

No. It has been reported that prophylactic administration of nitroglycerin in patients undergoing CABG did not prevent myocardial ischemia or reduce the incidence of perioperative MI.

Hoshijima H, Denawa Y, Mihara T, et al. Efficacy of prophylactic doses of intravenous nitroglycerin in preventing myocardial ischemia under general anesthesia: a systematic review and meta-analysis with trial sequential analysis. *J Clin Anesth*. 2017;40:16-22.

Mittnacht AJC, London MJ, Puskas JD, Kaplan JA. Anesthesia for myocardial revascularization. In: Kaplan JA, Augoustides JGT, Manecke GR, et al, eds. *Kaplan's Cardiac Anesthesia for Cardiac and Noncardiac Surgery*. 7th ed. Elsevier; 2017:731-769.

C.I-15. *If ST-segment depression is seen during surgery, how would you treat it? What is the relation between perioperative myocardial ischemia and postoperative MI?*

ST-segment depression is indicative of myocardial oxygen supply and demand mismatch and should be treated by:

- *Increasing coronary oxygen supply*: correcting hypotension, hypoxemia, and anemia
- *Increasing coronary perfusion pressure*: most often with small boluses of a short-acting vasopressor such as phenylephrine
- *Decreasing coronary oxygen demand*: correcting hypertension, tachycardia, and increased PAOP or CVP by deepening anesthesia with a volatile agent or by using vasodilators or β-blockers. All the major determinants of decreased oxygen demand have to be considered and corrected to normal levels.

If there are no obvious changes in BP, HR, and pulmonary wedge pressure, ischemia can be due to coronary spasm in which nitroglycerin or nicardipine should be administered.

Slogoff and Keats reported that perioperative myocardial ischemia occurred in 37% of all patients undergoing CABG. Perioperative MI was almost 3 times as frequent in patients with ischemia (6.9%) compared with patients without ischemia (2.5%). Intraoperative tachycardia was associated with a higher incidence of myocardial ischemia and infarction. However, Knight et al demonstrated that 42% of patients with CABG had preoperative episodes of myocardial ischemia, 87% of which were clinically silent.

They further found that anesthesia and surgery did not worsen the preoperative ischemic pattern. Slogoff and Keats in another study postulated that approximately 90% of new myocardial ischemia observed during anesthesia was a manifestation of silent ischemia observed in the patient before the operation, and only 10% were related to anesthetic management. Therefore, the relationship between intraoperative ischemia and postoperative outcome is unsolved.

It is important to note that ST-segment changes suggestive of myocardial ischemia can be observed with alteration of patient position, particularly during retraction of the sternum for internal mammary harvesting. In addition to being attentive to the ECG, assessing for ischemia by PA catheter and echocardiography is advised. Segmental wall motion abnormalities can be detected earlier than changes in ECG.

Knight AA, Hollenberg M, London MJ, et al. Perioperative myocardial ischemia: importance of the preoperative ischemia pattern. *Anesthesiology*. 1988;68:681-688.

Mangano DT. Perioperative cardiac morbidity. *Anesthesiology*. 1990;72:153-184.

Slogoff S, Keats AS. Does perioperative myocardial ischemia lead to postoperative myocardial infarction? *Anesthesiology*. 1985;62:107-114.

Slogoff S, Keats AS. Randomized trial of primary anesthetic agents on outcome of coronary artery bypass operations. *Anesthesiology*. 1989;70:179-188.

Slogoff S, Keats AS. Myocardial ischemia revisited. *Anesthesiology*. 2006;105:214-216.

C.I-16. *Discuss autologous transfusion and blood conservation for cardiac surgery.*

Homologous blood transfusion is associated with increased morbidity and mortality including disease transmission, hepatitis, transfusion reaction, and autosensitization. There has been increased interest in blood conservation to mitigate these risks. Autologous transfusion is the collection and reinfusion of the patient's own blood or blood components.

Intraoperative normovolemic hemodilution involves the removal of blood through an arterial or venous catheter after induction of anesthesia and before CPB. Depending on patient size and hematocrit, 500 to 1,000 mL of blood is collected into blood bags containing citrate phosphate dextrose adenine (CPDA-1) anticoagulant and is kept at room temperature. This blood is spared from exposure to CPB and the resultant hemolysis, platelet destruction, and clotting factor degradation. The autologous blood is transfused after reversal of the heparin with protamine. It has been demonstrated that the effect of 1 unit of fresh whole blood on platelet aggregation after CPB is at least equal, if not superior, to the effect of 2 units of apheresis platelets. According to a recent meta-analysis by Zhou et al, maximal benefit is achieved when at least 800 mL of blood is removed. Normovolemic hemodilution is not recommended if the hematocrit is below 33% or the hemoglobin is below 11 g/dL because further decreasing the oxygen-carrying capacity can worsen myocardial ischemia. In addition, hemodilution during CPB will further decrease hematocrit to levels that require homologous blood transfusion. Normovolemic hemodilution should be performed cautiously in patients with critical left main coronary stenosis, aortic stenosis, and HOCM because sudden cardiac arrest has been observed during the procedure.

Most often, the most effective approach for blood conservation is a combination of intraoperative normovolemic hemodilution, pharmacologic treatment, and perioperative blood salvage. Preoperative autologous blood donation, preoperative use of iron and erythropoietin, and intraoperative plasmapheresis are rarely used, but should be considered in certain patient populations in whom blood transfusion is not an option.

Perioperative blood salvage involves the collection and reinfusion of blood lost during and immediately after surgery. The posttransfusion survival of perioperatively salvaged red blood cells is comparable to that of allogeneic red blood cells. At the conclusion of CPB, all blood remaining in the oxygenator and bypass circuits should be salvaged and, if needed, infused. Blood salvaged intraoperatively can be transfused directly (unwashed) or processed (washed) before infusion. Commercially available equipment exists for each option. Blood collected by intraoperative salvage represents an excellent source of red blood cells. Salvaged blood is, however, deficient in coagulation factors and platelets.

Carabini LM, Ramsey G. Hemostasis and transfusion medicine. In: Cullen BF, Stock MC, Ortega R, et al, eds. *Barash, Cullen, and Stoelting's Clinical Anesthesia*. 9th ed. Wolters Kluwer; 2024:398-436.

Henderson RA, Judd M, Strauss ER, et al. Hematologic evaluation of intraoperative autologous blood collection and allogeneic transfusion in cardiac surgery. *Transfusion*. 2021;61:788-798.

Raphael J, Mazer CD, Subramani S, Schroeder, et al. Society of Cardiovascular Anesthesiologists clinical practice improvement advisory for management of perioperative bleeding and hemostasis in cardiac surgery patients. *Anesth Analg*. 2019;129:1209-1221.

Shander A, Moskowitz D, Rijhwani TS. The safety and efficacy of "bloodless" cardiac surgery. *Semin Cardiothorac Vasc Anesth*. 2005;9:53-63.

Society of Thoracic Surgeons Blood Conservation Task Force, Ferraris VA, Brown JR, et al. 2011 update of the Society of Thoracic Surgeons and the Society of Cardiovascular Anesthesiologists blood conservation clinical practice guidelines. *Ann Thorac Surg*. 2011;91:944-982.

Spahn DR, Casutt M. Eliminating blood transfusions: new aspects and perspectives. *Anesthesiology*. 2000;93:242-255.

Van der Linden P. Perioperative blood conservation strategies: an update for clinicians. *Can J Anaesth*. 2003;50:S1-S2.

C.I-17. *What antifibrinolytic will you use to reduce blood transfusions?*

Antifibrinolytic agents include lysine analogues epsilon aminocaproic acid (EACA) and tranexamic acid (TXA). Lysine analogues block plasminogen conversion to plasmin, in turn, inhibiting fibrinolysis. These agents reduce bleeding and blood transfusions. The Society of Cardiovascular Anesthesiologists 2019 practice advisory on blood conservation strongly recommends antifibrinolytics as part of a blood conservation strategy.

Extensive dosing variability is reported for TXA. A low-dose strategy consists of a 10-mg/kg loading dose, 1 to 2 mg/kg into the CPB prime, and a 1-mg/kg/h infusion. A high-dose strategy consists of a 30-mg/kg loading dose, 2 mg/kg into the CPB prime, and a 16-mg/kg/h infusion. Up to 50% of cardiac surgical patients have renal dysfunction, and TXA is eliminated renally. High doses of TXA can also cause seizures. The mechanism of TXA-associated seizures is not fully understood, although dose is an important variable. A lower dosing strategy should be used in those patients who have renal dysfunction and/or are at risk for seizures. Jerath et al recommend a dosing strategy of a single 50 mg/kg bolus for patients with chronic renal dysfunction.

Pharmacokinetic data are also sparse for EACA. The loading dose is typically 100 mg/kg with a 5-g or 10-g bolus into the CPB prime and a 1 g/h or 30-mg/kg/h infusion. There is a risk of renal dysfunction after the administration of EACA.

The 2008 BART trial (Blood conservation using Antifibrinolytics: Randomized trial) compared three available antifibrinolytic agents available at the time: aprotinin, EACA, and TXA. The trial was terminated early due to a higher rate of death in the aprotinin group. Aprotinin was subsequently withdrawn from the market by the manufacturer and remains unavailable in the United States.

Gerstein NS, Brierley JK, Windsor J, et al. Antifibrinolytic agents in cardiac and noncardiac surgery: a comprehensive overview and update. *J Cardiothorac Vasc Anesth*. 2017;31:2183–2205.

Jerath A, Yang QJ, Pang KS, et al. Tranexamic acid dosing for cardiac surgical patients with chronic renal dysfunction: a new dosing regimen. *Anesth Analg*. 2018;127:1323-1332.

Raphael J, Mazer CD, Subramani S, et al. Society of Cardiovascular Anesthesiologists clinical practice improvement advisory for management of perioperative bleeding and hemostasis in cardiac surgery patients. *Anesth Analg*. 2019;129:1209-1221.

C.II. During Cardiopulmonary Bypass

C.II-1. *What anticoagulant would you give before cardiopulmonary bypass (CPB)? How much would you give? What is its mechanism?*

Unfractionated heparin is the most commonly used anticoagulant for CPB. Starting doses range from 300 to 500 units per kg of body weight. Therapeutic threshold is frequently defined as an activated clotting time (ACT) greater than 400 to 480 seconds. Because of marked effect heterogeneity, heparin response must be serially monitored.

Heparin acts by potentiating antithrombin III (AT III), a protease inhibitor that neutralizes several activated clotting factors, including IIa (thrombin) and Xa. Heparin binds both ATIII and clotting factors and increases the rate of thrombin-antithrombin inactivation by at least 1,000-fold. Inhibition of thrombin and factor Xa accounts for most of the anticoagulant effect of heparin.

Kunst G, Milojevic M, Boer C, et al. 2019 EACTS/EACTA/EBCP guidelines on cardiopulmonary bypass in adult cardiac surgery. *Br J Anaesth*. 2019;123:713-757.

Shore-Lesserson L, Baker RA, Ferraris VA, et al. The Society of Thoracic Surgeons, The Society of Cardiovascular Anesthesiologists, and The American Society of ExtraCorporeal Technology: clinical practice guidelines-anticoagulation during cardiopulmonary bypass. *Anesth Analg*. 2018;126:413-424.

C.II-2. *What is the half-life of heparin? How is it eliminated?*

The biologic half-life of heparin varies with dose and temperature and has remarkable individual variation. The average half-life is approximately 100 minutes in a normothermic male for the initial doses of 300 units per kg, increasing with higher doses and decreasing temperature. When 100, 400, or 800 units per kg of heparin are given intravenously, the approximate half-life is 1, 2.5, and 5 hours, respectively. Heparin concentrations decline progressively at all temperatures, but the rate of decline is delayed in hypothermia.

The primary mechanism for heparin elimination remains uncertain. Heparin appears to be cleared and degraded primarily by the reticuloendothelial system. A small amount of heparin also appears in the urine.

Spiess BD, Armour S, Horrow J, Kaplan JA. Transfusion medicine and coagulation disorders. In: Kaplan JA, Augoustides JGT, Manecke GR, et al, eds. *Kaplan's Cardiac Anesthesia for Cardiac and Noncardiac Surgery*. 7th ed. Elsevier; 2017:1248-1290.

C.II-3. *How do you monitor heparin dosage? What is the activated coagulation time (ACT) test?*

Heparin dose and effect can be assessed by partial thromboplastin time, heparin assay, heparin-protamine titration, and ACT tests. For historical and practical reasons, the gold standard for heparin monitoring on CPB is the ACT.

The ACT measures the time required for complete activation of the coagulation cascade or clot formation. In traditional ACT tests, whole blood is mixed with a particulate clot activator, and resulting clots are mechanically detected. In newer devices, electrochemical sensors detect thrombin-mediated conversion of the clotting substrate, representing the final step of the clotting cascade. The ACT is the time required to reach these endpoints. A baseline ACT value is determined before administration of heparin, and the test is repeated 3 to 5 minutes after heparin is given and at intervals of 30 to 60 minutes thereafter. Elevated ACT is confirmed prior to CPB cannula placement, and therapeutic anticoagulation is confirmed before initiation of CPB.

Measurements of plasma heparin concentration can also be used in conjunction with ACT tests. In these assays, patient plasma is incubated with factor Xa in the presence of its inhibitor, Xai. Heparin accelerates factor Xa inhibition, and residual factor Xa remaining after 2 minutes is measured and converted to a heparin concentration, expressed in units per milliliter. Measuring heparin concentration can permit more precise redosing and reversal of heparin and has been associated with laboratory markers of improved hemostatic suppression in patients on CPB. However, clinical benefits in the form of decreased blood loss or transfusion requirements have not been consistently demonstrated.

Horrow JC, Mueksch JN, Weber N, et al. Coagulation testing. In: Gravlee GP, Davis RF, Hammon J, et al, eds. *Cardiopulmonary Bypass and Mechanical Support: Principles and Practice*. 4th ed. Wolters Kluwer; 2016:452-454.

Shore-Lesserson L, Baker RA, Ferraris VA, et al. The Society of Thoracic Surgeons, The Society of Cardiovascular Anesthesiologists, and The American Society of ExtraCorporeal Technology: clinical practice guidelines-anticoagulation during cardiopulmonary bypass. *Anesth Analg*. 2018;126:413-424.

Shore-Lesserson L, Enriquez LJ, Weitzel N. Coagulation monitoring. In: Kaplan JA, Augoustides JGT, Manecke GR, et al, eds. *Kaplan's Cardiac Anesthesia for Cardiac and Noncardiac Surgery*. 7th ed. Elsevier; 2017:698-730.

C.II-4. *What is total CPB? What is partial CPB?*

Total CPB indicates that all the venous return from superior and inferior venae cavae and the coronary sinus is drained into the CPB circuit and to the oxygenator. No blood is ejected by the RV to the lungs. The PA and systemic pressure tracings become nonpulsatile. By contrast, partial CPB means that some of the blood return is still pumped by the RV across the pulmonary vasculature. The balance of venous blood is drained to the oxygenator and delivered directly to the arterial circulation. Femoral-femoral bypass, in which peripheral cannulas are typically too small to permit complete drainage of the systemic venous blood volume, is one example of partial CPB.

Matte GS, DiNardo JA. Pediatric cardiopulmonary bypass. In: Gravlee GP, Davis RF, Hammon J, et al, eds. *Cardiopulmonary Bypass and Mechanical Support: Principles and Practice*. 4th ed. Wolters Kluwer; 2016:655-682.

C.II-5. *What kinds of pumps are used in CPB? Are they pulsatile or not?*

There are three types of pumps available for modern CPB machines: the double-headed nonocclusive roller pump, the centrifugal blood pump, and the ventricular-type pneumatic or hydraulic pump. Only the first two types are in common use. Both roller pumps and centrifugal pumps generate continuous flow.

The roller pump is the most widely used. It is driven by an afterload-independent motor. Once the pump speed is set, it will continue the forward displacement of the same blood volume (or air volume) even if the resistance is increased by kinking or clamping the arterial line. This can result in the rupture of connections between sections of tubing. Pressure gauges on the arterial inflow line can help prevent this type of disaster.

The centrifugal pump is a kinetic pump that operates on the constrained vortex principle: blood is driven through the pump by centrifugal forces generated by a vortex in the pump. Centrifugal pumps are preload and afterload sensitive and consequently demonstrate variable flow (eg, decreased flow in response to an elevation in the patient's SVR). Flow meters are required to ensure adequate flow, as are valves or clamps to prevent retrograde flow. Relative to roller pumps, theoretical advantages of centrifugal pumps include decreased trauma to blood components, decreased risk of elevated line pressures (due to afterload sensitivity), flow cessation upon entrainment of large volumes of air, and decreased risk of micro air emboli (as small air bubbles are trapped in the vortex center). Although clinical benefits of centrifugal pumps have not been consistently demonstrated, centrifugal pumps may be preferable for longer CPB times.

Ventricular-type pumps, although potentially more powerful, are more cumbersome and have not been well accepted into clinical practice. This type of pump is mainly used for pulsatile bypass.

Kunst G, Milojevic M, Boer C, et al. 2019 EACTS/EACTA/EBCP guidelines on cardiopulmonary bypass in adult cardiac surgery. *Br J Anaesth*. 2019;123:713-757.

Stephenson LW, Baciewicz FA Jr. Development of cardiopulmonary bypass. In: Gravlee GP, Davis RF, Hammon J, et al, eds. *Cardiopulmonary Bypass and Mechanical Support: Principles and Practice*. 4th ed. Wolters Kluwer; 2016:3-19.

C.II-6. *What is the purpose of venting the left ventricle (LV)? How can it be done?*

The purpose of LV venting on CPB is to prevent overdistension of the LV, which can lead to myocardial injury and dysfunction, pulmonary venous hypertension, pulmonary edema, and RV strain. Venting the LV prevents myocyte injury caused by excessive myocyte stretch, minimizes myocardial oxygen demand through decreased wall stress, and facilitates subendocardial perfusion by reducing LVEDP.

LV distension can occur on full CPB because, although venous return is bypassed from the RV, 2% to 5% of cardiac output still drains to the LV. This volume represents the physiologic shunt from the bronchial, thebesian, and pleural veins. Other sources of blood flow to the left heart during CPB include aortic regurgitation from aortic insufficiency and extracardiac left-to-right shunts such as patent ductus arteriosus and Blalock-Taussig, Waterston, and Potts shunts. The left ventricular sump drain (aka "vent") prevents overdistension of the LV, which may arise due to these sources of venous blood. Venting of the LV can be accomplished by inserting a catheter or needle into the aortic root or LV apex, into the LV via the right pulmonary vein and left atrium, or into the PA or left atrium.

Matte GS, DiNardo JA. Pediatric cardiopulmonary bypass. In: Gravlee GP, Davis RF, Hammon J, et al, eds. *Cardiopulmonary Bypass and Mechanical Support: Principles and Practice*. 4th ed. Wolters Kluwer; 2016:655-682.

C.II-7. *What are the mechanisms and features of the CPB oxygenator?*

CPB oxygenators in current use are membrane oxygenators. These devices utilize countercurrent gas and blood flow across a network of hollow microtubules to achieve gas exchange. Contrary to early oxygenator models (eg, bubble oxygenators), there is no direct gas-blood interface. Advantages of membrane oxygenators include decreased risk of foaming, less trauma to blood components, reduced complement oxygenation, and independent control of oxygen and CO_2 exchange. Disadvantages include relatively large priming volumes and potential difficulty in eliminating all bubbles during priming.

Hines MH. Principles of oxygenator function: gas exchange, heat transfer, and operation. In: Gravlee GP, Davis RF, Hammon J, et al, eds. *Cardiopulmonary Bypass and Mechanical Support: Principles and Practice*. 4th ed. Wolters Kluwer; 2016:95-108.

Kunst G, Milojevic M, Boer C, et al. 2019 EACTS/EACTA/EBCP guidelines on cardiopulmonary bypass in adult cardiac surgery. *Br J Anaesth*. 2019;123:713-757.

C.II-8. *What kind of priming solution would you use? How much priming solution would you use? When would you prime with blood? Why?*

The usual priming solution includes a balanced salt solution, with or without dextrose, albumin, or mannitol. Priming volumes vary with the size of the oxygenators used and the tubing volume. Most oxygenators for adults have priming volumes of 500 to 1,000 mL, and total priming volumes are often 1,400 to 2,000 mL. In general, blood is added to the oxygenator if the patient is markedly anemic (pre-CPB hematocrit <30%) or if the priming volume is large in relation to the patient's blood volume, such as in pediatric patients. In order to maintain oxygen-carrying capacity, the hematocrit is kept above 18% to 20%. Antegrade and retrograde autologous priming, in which patient blood displaces preexisting crystalloid in venous and arterial lines following cannulation, can be used to reduce hemodilution. Autologous prime is recommended as part of a comprehensive strategy to reduce blood transfusions.

Mannitol is an osmotic diuretic that can increase renal blood flow and glomerular filtration. Historically, it was added to prime solutions to help prevent hypervolemia, tissue edema, and acute kidney injury. However, data do not support its renal protective effects, and use for renal protection is currently not advised. Heparin, 3,000 to 10,000 units, can be added to the prime depending on the size of the prime volume. This allows heparin to be distributed over the thrombogenic surfaces of the CPB circuit and provides an additional layer of protection against inadequate systemic anticoagulation.

Brown JR, Baker RA, Shore-Lesserson L, et al. The Society of Thoracic Surgeons/Society of Cardiovascular Anesthesiologists/American Society for Extracorporeal Technology clinical practice guidelines for the prevention of adult cardiac surgery-associated acute kidney injury. *Anesth Analg*. 2023;136:176-184.

Cooper JR Jr, Giesecke NM. Hemodilution and priming solutions. In: Gravlee GP, Davis RF, Hammon J, et al, eds. *Cardiopulmonary Bypass and Mechanical Support: Principles and Practice*. 4th ed. Wolters Kluwer; 2016:421-432.

Gupta S, McEwen C, Basha A, et al. Retrograde autologous priming in cardiac surgery: a systematic review and meta-analysis. *Eur J Cardiothorac Surg*. 2021;60:1245-1256.

C.II-9. *What are the advantages and disadvantages of hemodilution?*

Nonblood prime of the CPB circuit induces hemodilution. According to recent guidelines, a hematocrit of 21% to 24% can be acceptable on CPB as long as oxygen delivery is adequate. Advantages and disadvantages include the following:

Advantages of Hemodilution

- Increase in microcirculation due to a reduction of blood viscosity
- Improved oxygen delivery to tissues
- Decreased metabolic acidosis
- Reduced risk of hypertension
- Reduced blood demands
- Reduced postoperative blood loss
- Improved blood flow at lower perfusion pressure, especially during hypothermic perfusion

Disadvantages of Hemodilution

- Decreased oxygen-carrying capacity
- Postoperative extracellular fluid overload
- Possible pulmonary edema
- Increased risk of postoperative renal dysfunction
- Hypotension from decreased viscosity and peripheral resistance
- Decreased concentration of calcium, magnesium, phosphate, and zinc

Brown JR, Baker RA, Shore-Lesserson L, et al. The Society of Thoracic Surgeons/Society of Cardiovascular Anesthesiologists/American Society for Extracorporeal Technology clinical practice guidelines for the prevention of adult cardiac surgery-associated acute kidney injury. *Anesth Analg*. 2023;136:176-184.

Cooper JR Jr, Giesecke NM. Hemodilution and priming solutions. In: Gravlee GP, Davis RF, Hammon J, et al, eds. *Cardiopulmonary Bypass and Mechanical Support: Principles and Practice*. 4th ed. Wolters Kluwer; 2016:421-432.

Grocott HP, Stafford-Smith M, Mora-Mangano CT. Cardiopulmonary bypass management and organ protection. In: Kaplan JA, Augoustides JGT, Manecke GR, et al, eds. *Kaplan's Cardiac Anesthesia for Cardiac and Noncardiac Surgery*. 7th ed. Elsevier; 2017:1111-1161.

Kunst G, Milojevic M, Boer C, et al. 2019 EACTS/EACTA/EBCP guidelines on cardiopulmonary bypass in adult cardiac surgery. *Br J Anaesth*. 2019;123:713-757.

C.II-10. *How do you monitor the patient during CPB?*

Clinical Monitoring

Patients are comprehensively monitored during CPB, as follows:

- ECG
- MAP between 50 and 80 mm Hg to maintain tissue perfusion. Recent guidelines suggest no benefit from vasopressor use to increase MAP above this range.

- Bladder and esophageal temperatures are recorded (tympanic also may be used).
- CVP should be low or zero to ensure there is no obstruction to venous return from the head (when monitored from a site proximal to the RA) or there is adequate drainage of blood to the CPB circuit (when monitored from inside the RA).
- PA pressure should be low or zero to prevent overdistension of the LV.
- Urine output should be maintained above 1 mL/kg/h.
- TEE is used to evaluate ventricular function and distension, assess cannula and device placement, and identify injury (eg, dissection).
- Cerebral oximetry can be used to help monitor for adequate brain oxygen saturation (<20% change from baseline).
- Pump flow rate should be adequate for tissue perfusion and oxygenation.
- Physical exam: sweating or movement can indicate inadequate anesthetic depth or awareness; plethora of the head and neck veins may indicate inadequate venous drainage and decreased cerebral perfusion pressure.

Laboratory Monitoring at Least Once Every Hour

- Arterial blood gases are kept at normal range.
- Venous Po_2 should be 40 to 45 mm Hg.
- Hematocrit maintained between 20% and 24%
- Electrolytes Na^+, K^+, ionized Ca^{2+}
- ACT measured each hour and maintained above 400 to 480 seconds
- Glucose should be kept below 180 mg/dL.

Barry AE, Chaney MA, London MJ. Anesthetic management during cardiopulmonary bypass: a systematic review. *Anesth Analg*. 2015;120:749-769.

Grocott HP, Stafford-Smith M, Mora-Mangano CT. Cardiopulmonary bypass management and organ protection. In: Kaplan JA, Augoustides JGT, Manecke GR, et al, eds. *Kaplan's Cardiac Anesthesia for Cardiac and Noncardiac Surgery*. 7th ed. Elsevier; 2017:1111-1161.

Kunst G, Milojevic M, Boer C, et al. 2019 EACTS/EACTA/EBCP guidelines on cardiopulmonary bypass in adult cardiac surgery. *Br J Anaesth*. 2019;123:713-757.

Nelson MT, Armour SK, Butterworth JF IV. Endocrine, metabolic, and electrolyte responses to cardiac surgery and cardiopulmonary bypass. In: Gravlee GP, Davis RF, Hammon J, et al, eds. *Cardiopulmonary Bypass and Mechanical Support: Principles and Practice*. 4th ed. Wolters Kluwer; 2016:315-344.

C.II-11. *What should your target BP be during CPB?*

Controversy continues over what constitutes optimal BP for patients on CPB. BP depends on cardiac output (pump flow) and SVR. Adequate cardiac output is more important for tissue perfusion than BP. Recent guidelines suggest maintaining MAP of 50 to 80 mm Hg to ensure adequate perfusion of all end organs and minimize the risk of hypoperfusion and hyperperfusion.

Data regarding MAP and neurologic outcomes are inconsistent. Maintaining MAP within the thresholds of cerebral autoregulation could be hypothetically beneficial. Excessive MAP might be associated with an increased risk of delirium, while lower MAP can increase the risk of cerebral ischemia. However, the upper and lower limits on CPB are themselves poorly delineated. An early study by Gold et al randomized 248 patients to either low MAP (50-70 mm Hg) or high MAP (80-100 mm Hg) during CPB and found a trend toward improvement in cardiac and neurologic outcome with higher MAP. However, MAP had no significant effect on neurologic outcome in patients at low risk for cerebral embolization (normal to mild aortic atherosclerosis by TEE). Patients at high risk for adverse neurologic outcome (severe aortic atherosclerosis by TEE) had a significantly lower risk of worse neurologic outcome when randomized to higher MAP. In contrast, a recent randomized trial by Vedel et al found no difference between higher (70-80 mm Hg) and lower (40-50 mm Hg) target MAP in terms of number or volume of new cerebral infarcts.

Noninvasive monitors can help guide MAP in real time. Noninvasive cerebral oximetry utilizes near-infrared spectroscopy (NIRS) to monitor the oxygen saturation of mixed arterial and venous blood of the frontal cortex. Because this blood is predominantly venous, it reflects the balance between oxygen supply and demand in the brain. Early studies suggested that cerebral NIRS monitors were useful in recognizing cerebral ischemia and predicting adverse neurologic outcomes and other end-organ dysfunction. However, more recent studies have shown less or no significant benefit. Current guidelines suggest that NIRS can be "considered" to help improve clinical outcomes.

Gold JP, Charlson ME, Williams-Russo P, et al. Improvement of outcomes after coronary artery bypass. A randomized trial comparing intraoperative high versus low mean arterial pressure. *J Thorac Cardiovasc Surg*. 1995;110:1302-1311.

Kunst G, Milojevic M, Boer C, et al. 2019 EACTS/EACTA/EBCP guidelines on cardiopulmonary bypass in adult cardiac surgery. *Br J Anaesth*. 2019;123:713-757.

Vedel AG, Holmgaard F, Rasmussen LS, et al. High-target versus low-target blood pressure management during cardiopulmonary bypass to prevent cerebral injury in cardiac surgery patients: a randomized controlled trial. *Circulation*. 2018;137:1770-1780.

Wong ZZ, Chiong XH, Chaw SH, et al. The use of cerebral oximetry in surgery: a systematic review and meta-analysis of randomized controlled trials. *J Cardiothorac Vasc Anesth*. 2022;36:2002-2011.

SECTION 2

C.II-12. *How would you treat hypotension during CPB?*

Mean arterial pressure (MAP) = cardiac output (CO) × total peripheral resistance (TPR)

Hypotension can be caused by low cardiac output or low peripheral resistance. According to Poiseuille law, low SVR is usually due to decreased viscosity or increased vascular diameter (vasodilation). Total viscosity is reduced by hemodilution during CPB using blood-free priming solutions, although plasma viscosity is increased by hypothermia. Vasoplegia can develop in CPB due to inflammatory responses to the CPB circuit and the operation, anesthetic drugs, and residual preoperative antihypertensives. Cardiac output should first be corrected by increasing the pump flow rate. If cardiac output is adequate, then peripheral resistance can be raised by giving an α-adrenergic vasopressor, typically phenylephrine in increments of 0.1 mg to raise the MAP to 50 mm Hg. In cases of more profound vasoplegia, agents such as norepinephrine, vasopressin, angiotensin II, and methylene blue might be required. Of note, a short period of hypotension with a MAP of 30 to 40 mm Hg is often observed in the first few minutes of bypass due to the following causes:

- Autologous prime or inadequate pump flow at the beginning of bypass
- Vasodilation from vasoactive materials released because of the initial reaction of the serum proteins, blood cells, and platelets with the foreign surfaces of the heart-lung machine
- Decreased plasma levels of catecholamines by hemodilution

Grocott HP, Stafford-Smith M, Mora-Mangano CT. Cardiopulmonary bypass management and organ protection. In: Kaplan JA, Augoustides JGT, Manecke GR, et al, eds. *Kaplan's Cardiac Anesthesia for Cardiac and Noncardiac Surgery*. 7th ed. Elsevier; 2017:1111-1161.

Ortoleva J, Shapeton A, Vanneman M, Dalia AA. Vasoplegia during cardiopulmonary bypass: current literature and rescue therapy options. *J Cardiothorac Vasc Anesth*. 2020;34:2766-2775.

C.II-13. *How would you treat hypertension (mean arterial pressure [MAP] over 80-100 mm Hg)?*

Hypertension during bypass is usually the result of inadequate depth of anesthesia, which causes increased catecholamine output and increased SVR. Pump flow rate should not be reduced to lower the pressure. Low pump flow can cause tissue hypoxia even though BP is high. Treatment involves administering an inhalational agent through the vaporizer in the heart-lung machine or IV agents such as propofol, midazolam, and narcotics. Finally, vasodilator drugs might be indicated, including nitroprusside and nitroglycerin or IV calcium channel blockers (eg, nicardipine).

C.II-14. *How do you prepare an intravenous (IV) infusion of sodium nitroprusside, nicardipine, and nitroglycerin? What are the usual doses? Which do you prefer to use?*

IV solutions can be prepared by adding to 250 mL of 5% dextrose in water 50 mg of nitroglycerin or sodium nitroprusside, or 25 mg of nicardipine, to make a concentration of 200 μγ/mL (nitroglycerin or nitroprusside) or 100 μγ/mL nicardipine. The usual doses are 0.5 to 10 μγ/kg/min nitroglycerin or nitroprusside, or 0.05 μγ/kg/min nicardipine, determined by careful titration (**Table 5.1**).

Nitroglycerin or nicardipine infusion is preferred. Sodium nitroprusside dilates both arterial and venous smooth muscle. It is very effective in reducing both preload and afterload. At high doses and prolonged administration, it can cause cyanide and thiocyanate toxicity. Because nitroprusside dilates intramyocardial arterioles, intracoronary steal can occur. The solution has to be covered with aluminum foil to prevent decomposition from exposure to light. Nitroglycerin primarily causes venodilation, resulting in the reduction of preload and myocardial oxygen consumption. At higher doses, it has mild arteriolar dilation and reduces afterload. It has no known toxicity and does not produce intracoronary steal because

TABLE 5.1 Cardiac Anesthesia Intravenous Medication Preparation and Doses[a]

Drug	Amount to Add	Total Volume With D_5W	Concentration	Dosage Range
Amicar (EACA)	15 g	150 mL	1 mL = 100 mg 10 mL = 1 g	Load: 10 g over 1/2 h Maintenance: 1 g/h × 5 h
Amiodarone	450 mg	250 mL	1 mL = 1.8 mg	Initial: 150 mg over 10 min Followed by: 1 mg/min × 6 h (360 mg) Then: 0.5 mg/min × 18 h
Dexmedetomidine			1 mL = 4 μγ	Load: 0.5-1.0 μg/kg over 10 min Maintenance: 0.2-0.7 μg/kg/h
Diltiazem	25 mg	100 mL	1 mL = 0.25 mg	Load: 0.1-0.15 mg/kg Maintenance: 0.5-0.25 μg/kg/min
Dobutamine	500 mg	250 mL	1 gt = 33.3 μγ 1 mL = 2 mg	2.5-20 μg/kg/min
Dopamine	400 mg	250 mL (premixed)	1 gt = 26.6 μγ 1 mL = 1.6 mg	Renal: 1-5 μg/kg/min β: 10 μγ/kg/min α: 10-15 μg/kg/min
Epinephrine	2 mg	250 mL	8 gtt = 1 μγ	2-8 μg/min
Esmolol	5 g	250 mL	1 gt = 333 μγ 1 mL = 20 mg	50-300 μg/kg/min
Levophed	8 mg	250 mL	2 gtt = 1 μγ	2-32 μg/min
Lidocaine	2 g	500 mL (premixed)	15 gtt = 1 mg 1 mL = 4 mg	1-4 mg/min
Milrinone	20 mg	100 mL	3 gtt = 1 μγ 1 mL = 200 μγ	0.125-1 μg/kg/min
Nicardipine	25 mg	250 mL	1 gt = 1.66 μγ	Load: 5 mg/h Maintenance: Increase by 2.5 mg/h every 15 min. Maximum amount: 15 mg/h
Nitroprusside	50 mg	250 mL (premixed)	1 gt = 3.33 μγ	1-10 μg/kg/min
Nitroglycerin	50 mg	250 mL (premixed)	1 gt = 3.33 μγ	10-80 μg/min
Phenylephrine	20 mg	250 mL	19 gtt = 25 μγ	25-125 μg/min
Procainamide	2 g	500 mL (premixed)	15 gtt = 1 mg 1 mL = 4 mg	Load: 500-1,000 mg (20 mg/min) Dosage: 1-4 mg/min
Sodium bicarbonate	100 mEq	100 mL undiluted	1 mL = 1 mEq	1-3 mEq/kg/h (titrate to pH)
Tranexamic acid			1 mL = 100 mg	Load: 10 mg/kg Maintenance: 1 mg/kg/h
Vasopressin	100 units	100 mL	1 mL = 1 unit	Initial dose: 0.04 U/min, 2.4 U/h Titrate: 0.005-0.01 U/min (0.3-0.6 mL/h) every 10 min to max of 0.1 U/min or 6 U/h

D_5W, dextrose 5% in water; EACA, ε-aminocaproic acid.

[a]There are 60 gtt/mL; therefore, gtt/min = mL/h.

it dilates epicardial arteries. It can redistribute blood flow to the subendocardium and increase collateral circulation through the myocardium. Nicardipine is a systemic and coronary arterial dilator. The afterload is decreased, whereas the preload is not affected. It can cause a slight increase in HR (reflex tachycardia).

Lester L, Mitter N, Berkowitz DE, Nyhan D. Pharmacology of Anesthetic Drugs. In: Kaplan JA, Augoustides JGT, Manecke GR, et al, eds. *Kaplan's Cardiac Anesthesia for Cardiac and Noncardiac Surgery*. 7th ed. Elsevier; 2017:247-356.

C.II-15. *How much pump flow would you maintain during CPB? During hemodilution? During hypothermia?*

During CPB, pump blood flow replaces some or all of the native cardiac output and supplies oxygenated blood to tissues. Oxygen delivery (DO_2) depends on the flow volume and oxygen-carrying capacity of the blood; in turn, the adequacy of DO_2 depends on tissue oxygen demands. Increasingly, goal-directed delivery is recommended for patients on CPB. For instance, a DO_2 threshold of 272 mL/min/m^2 has been suggested as a threshold below which acute kidney injury is more likely.

The normal average cardiac output for adults is 70 mL/kg/min or 3.1 L/min/m^2. Seventy percent of normal cardiac output is usually enough to maintain tissue oxygenation. When body surface is used, both pediatric and adult patients require about the same pump flow—2.2 to 3.1 L/min/m^2. In summary, at normothermia and normal hemoglobin levels, the pump flow is as follows:

Adults 50 to 70 mL/kg/min	or	2.2 to 3.1 L/min/m^2.
Children 100 to 150 mL/kg/min	or	2.2 to 3.1 L/min/m^2.

Hemodilution reduces hemoglobin concentration and hence decreases oxygen content. In order to deliver the same amount of oxygen, pump flow has to be increased accordingly during hemodilution. For example, if hematocrit is diluted from 40% to 20% during CPB, pump flow has to be doubled (increased by a factor of 40/20 = 2). Clinically, both hypothermia and hemodilution are applied simultaneously so that the adjustment has to be done at the same time. For example, the pump flow for adults at a temperature of 30 °C (86 °F) and a hematocrit of 25% will be as follows:

$$50 \text{ to } 70 \text{ mL/kg/min} \times 50\% \times 40/25 = 40 \text{ to } 56 \text{ mL/kg/min.}$$

Hypothermia decreases oxygen consumption. Therefore, the pump flow can be decreased proportionally if the blood oxygen content does not change. The oxygen consumption at different body temperatures is as follows:

Temperature (°C)	37	32	30	28	25	20	10
O_2 consumption (%)	100	60	50	40	25–30	20	10

Because O_2 consumption at 30 °C (86 °F) is half that at 37 °C (98.6 °F), the required pump flow at 30 °C (86 °F) is 50% of the flow at 37 °C (98.6 °F) (50-70 mL/kg/min). Therefore, a pump flow of 25 to 35 mL/kg/min is adequate for adults at 30 °C (86 °F) assuming no hemodilution. From 37 °C to 30 °C (98.6 °F-86 °F), cellular metabolism decreases by approximately 7% for each 1 °C; a diminished response occurs below 30 °C (86 °F). Accordingly, every 7 °C to 8 °C (44.4 °F-46.4 °F) decrease in temperature reduces oxygen consumption by approximately 50%. During profound hypothermia (10 °C-20 °C [50 °F-68 °F]), patients can tolerate periods of total circulatory arrest without pump support. So-called deep hypothermic circulatory arrest (DHCA) can be required for surgery involving the proximal thoracic aorta. In these cases, selective cerebral perfusion is often employed to further reduce the risk of cerebral ischemia.

Brown JR, Baker RA, Shore-Lesserson L, et al. The Society of Thoracic Surgeons/Society of Cardiovascular Anesthesiologists/American Society for Extracorporeal Technology Clinical Practice Guidelines for the Prevention of Adult Cardiac Surgery-Associated Acute Kidney Injury. *Anesth Analg*. 2023;136:176-184.

Grocott HP, Stafford-Smith M, Mora-Mangano CT. Cardiopulmonary bypass management and organ protection. In: Kaplan JA, Augoustides JGT, Manecke GR, et al, eds. *Kaplan's Cardiac Anesthesia for Cardiac and Noncardiac Surgery*. 7th ed. Elsevier; 2017:1111-1161.

Isselbacher EM, Preventza O, Hamilton Black J 3rd, et al. 2022 ACC/AHA guideline for the diagnosis and management of aortic disease: a report of the American Heart Association/American College of Cardiology Joint Committee on Clinical Practice Guidelines. *Circulation*. 2022;146:e334-e482.

Magruder JT, Weiss SJ, DeAngelis KG, et al. Correlating oxygen delivery on cardiopulmonary bypass with Society of Thoracic Surgeons outcomes following cardiac surgery. *J Thorac Cardiovasc Surg*. 2022;164:997-1007.

Matte GS, DiNardo JA. Pediatric cardiopulmonary bypass. In: Gravlee GP, Davis RF, Hammon J, et al, eds. *Cardiopulmonary Bypass and Mechanical Support: Principles and Practice*. 4th ed. Wolters Kluwer; 2016:655-682.

C.II-16. *How does blood viscosity change during hemodilution and hypothermia?*

Blood viscosity varies inversely with temperature; a 2% increase occurs for each 1 °C (1.8 °F) decrease in temperature. At a hematocrit of 40%, a decrease in temperature from 37 °C to 27 °C (98.6 °F-80.6 °F) increases viscosity by approximately 25%. Hemodilution with balanced salt solution decreases blood viscosity. Decreasing hematocrit from 40% to 20% at 27 °C (80.6 °F) decreases viscosity by approximately 40%. It has been recommended that hematocrit be adjusted to the same numerical value as the core body temperature in degrees centigrade if blood viscosity is to be kept constant. For example, normal viscosity at 37 °C (98.6 °F) with a hematocrit of 40% approximates that seen at 25 °C (77 °F) with a hematocrit of 25%.

Rodrigues ES, Cook DJ. Neurologic effects of cardiopulmonary bypass. In: Gravlee GP, Davis RF, Hammon J, et al, eds. *Cardiopulmonary Bypass and Mechanical Support: Principles and Practice*. 4th ed. Wolters Kluwer; 2016:385-420.

C.II-17. *How is anesthesia provided during CPB?*

Anesthesia is maintained with intermittent administration of IV propofol, benzodiazepines, opioids, and/or volatile agents through the pump oxygenator to achieve unconsciousness and analgesia, to control BP, and to prevent shivering. IV agents are diluted by the priming solution during CPB. Hypothermia itself produces anesthesia and prolongs the duration of action of IV agents by decreasing hepatic metabolism and urinary excretion.

Patients undergoing cardiac surgery are at increased risk for intraoperative awareness. The use of processed electroencephalogram (EEG) monitors can reduce the incidence of awareness. However, these monitors have important limitations, such as unresponsiveness to certain hypnotic agents, interference artifacts, indices that are relatively unvarying, and cost-effectiveness. A large multicenter randomized trial by Avidan et al demonstrated that superiority of processed EEG monitoring such as the bispectral index is not established. Data in CPB patients are lacking.

Strategies to reduce accidental awareness include continuous monitoring of volatile anesthetic concentrations in the oxygenator exhaust line, use of multimodal anesthetic drugs, and careful monitoring of neuromuscular blockade. Processed EEG can be considered.

Avidan MS, Jacobsohn E, Glick D, et al. Prevention of intraoperative awareness in a high-risk surgical population. *N Engl J Med*. 2011;365:591-600.

Gerstein NS, Panikkath PV, Mirrakhimov AE, Lewis AE, Ram H. Cardiopulmonary Bypass Emergencies and Intraoperative Issues. *J Cardiothorac Vasc Anesth*. 2022;36:4505-4522.

C.II-18. *Would you give NMBDs during CPB? How is their action affected during CPB?*

Neuromuscular blocking drugs (NMBDs) can be utilized during CPB. NMBDs are given to prevent diaphragmatic movement that interferes with surgery and to prevent shivering during hypothermia, which increases oxygen requirements and can lead to lactic acidosis. Paralysis can help prevent displacement of lines and devices due to patient movement during defibrillation.

There remains a high risk of accidental awareness in cardiac surgery, and this risk is increased with the use of NMBDs. Involuntary movement can indicate inadequate analgesia or anesthetic depth. NMBDs should be dosed judiciously, as hypothermia is associated with decreased muscle strength and decreased metabolism and elimination of NMBDs. Continuous infusions should not be used due to the risk of residual paralysis. Neuromuscular blockade should be monitored with peripheral nerve stimulators.

Hemmerling TM, Russo G, Bracco D. Neuromuscular blockade in cardiac surgery: an update for clinicians. *Ann Card Anaesth*. 2008;11:80-90.

Kunst G, Milojevic M, Boer C, et al. 2019 EACTS/EACTA/EBCP guidelines on cardiopulmonary bypass in adult cardiac surgery. *Br J Anaesth*. 2019;123:713-757.

C.II-19. *How do you know the patient perfusion is adequate during CPB?*

Multiple endpoints are used to evaluate adequate perfusion during CPB. These include MAP, mixed venous oxygen saturation, arterial lactate levels, cerebral Sao_2 via NIRS monitors, and urine output. Pump flows are also directly measured, with typical goals greater than 2.2 L/min/m^2 of lean body weight at temperatures ranging from normothermia to moderate hypothermia. Increasingly, oxygen delivery (DO_2) is evaluated to ensure adequacy of oxygen-carrying capacity and flow. Higher pump flows can be indicated in the context of marked hemodilutional anemia.

Kunst G, Milojevic M, Boer C, et al. 2019 EACTS/EACTA/EBCP guidelines on cardiopulmonary bypass in adult cardiac surgery. *Br J Anaesth*. 2019;123:713-757.

Magruder JT, Weiss SJ, DeAngelis KG, et al. Correlating oxygen delivery on cardiopulmonary bypass with Society of Thoracic Surgeons outcomes following cardiac surgery. *J Thorac Cardiovasc Surg*. 2022;164:997-1007.

Murphy GS, Hessel EA II, Groom RC. Optimal perfusion during cardiopulmonary bypass: an evidence-based approach. *Anesth Analg*. 2009;108:1394-1417.

C.II-20. *How much gas flow would you use for the oxygenator? What kind of gas would you use? Why?*

Normal alveolar ventilation is 4 L/min, and pulmonary circulation is 5 L/min, for a ratio of 0.8. The oxygenator is not as efficient as human lungs. Usually, 2 L of gas are used for each liter of pump flow, and then gas flow rate is adjusted according to blood $Paco_2$ and Pao_2. Gas flow can be decreased if the $Paco_2$ is low and Pao_2 is too high. The ratio can be increased if $Paco_2$ is greater than 40 mm Hg or Pao_2 is less than 100 mm Hg. Air-oxygen mixtures allow for better control of oxygen tension during CPB. It is not necessary to add CO_2 to the ventilating gas during hypothermia to elevate $Paco_2$ and decrease the pH because α-stat regulation is used for acid-base management.

Hines MH. Principles of oxygenator function: gas exchange, heat transfer, and operation. In: Gravlee GP, Davis RF, Hammon J, et al, eds. *Cardiopulmonary Bypass and Mechanical Support: Principles and Practice*. 4th ed. Wolters Kluwer; 2016:95-108.

C.II-21. *What are the disadvantages of hypocapnia during CPB?*

- Cerebral blood flow decreases 2% to 4% for each mm Hg decrease in $Paco_2$ when $Paco_2$ is in the range of 20 to 60 mm Hg due to cerebral vasoconstriction. Cerebral O_2 saturation decreases approximately 1% for each mm Hg decrease in $Paco_2$.
- Respiratory alkalosis shifts the oxygen dissociation curve to the left, which increases hemoglobin O_2 affinity and decreases the release of O_2 to the tissues.
- Hypokalemia occurs because alkalosis shifts potassium intracellularly.
- Alkalosis decreases ionized calcium.

Rodrigues ES, Cook DJ. Neurologic effects of cardiopulmonary bypass. In: Gravlee GP, Davis RF, Hammon J, et al, eds. *Cardiopulmonary Bypass and Mechanical Support: Principles and Practice*. 4th ed. Wolters Kluwer; 2016:385-420.

C.II-22. *How would you preserve the myocardium during CPB?*

The most common and effective method of protecting the myocardium is to reduce myocardial oxygen demand by hypothermia and cardioplegia. Hypothermia is induced by a combination of: (1) systemic blood cooling by heat exchangers in the oxygenator; (2) local application of cold saline solution or iced slush to the external surface and chambers of the heart (if the heart is open); (3) infusion of cold cardioplegic solution through the aortic root, venous grafts, retrograde coronary sinus, and/or coronary ostium to the coronary arterial tree. Myocardial temperature can be decreased to 10 °C to 20 °C.

In addition to inducing hypothermia and using cardioplegia, one can take the following measures before aortic cross-clamping:

- Avoid tachycardia or increased contractility by discontinuing pacing at a rapid rate and discontinuing inotropes.
- Initiate rapid arrest (asystole).
- Utilize proper venting methods and ensure adequate venous drainage to the pump to avoid ventricular distension, which decreases subendocardial blood supply.
- Prevent and treat ventricular fibrillation, which increases oxygen demand in normothermic myocardium.
- Maintain adequate coronary perfusion pressure of greater than 50 mm Hg or greater than 70 mm Hg in the presence of severe coronary disease or left ventricular hypertrophy.

Barry AE, Chaney MA, London MJ. Anesthetic management during cardiopulmonary bypass: a systematic review. *Anesth Analg*. 2015;120:749-769.

Grocott HP, Stafford-Smith M, Mora-Mangano CT. Cardiopulmonary bypass management and organ protection. In: Kaplan JA, Augoustides JGT, Manecke GR, et al, eds. *Kaplan's Cardiac Anesthesia for Cardiac and Noncardiac Surgery*. 7th ed. Elsevier; 2017:1111-1161.

Kypson AP, Sanderson DA Jr, Nifong LW, et al. Cardiopulmonary bypass and myocardial protection for minimally invasive cardiac surgery. In: Gravlee GP, Davis RF, Hammon J, et al, eds. *Cardiopulmonary Bypass and Mechanical Support: Principles and Practice*. 4th ed. Wolters Kluwer; 2016:143-156.

C.II-23. *What is cardioplegia? How much would you use?*

Cardioplegic solutions are used to arrest the heart in order to achieve a still surgical field and minimize myocardial oxygen demand. These solutions typically contain high concentrations of potassium (8-20 mEq/L), which creates a depolarized arrest due to sodium channel inactivation. Cardioplegia solutions are administered antegrade (directly into the coronary arteries, into the aortic root proximal to the aortic cross-clamp, or into distal CABG grafts) or retrograde (into the coronary sinus). Retrograde delivery is indicated in the presence of significant aortic insufficiency and severe obstructive coronary lesions.

Although specific compositions vary widely, cardioplegic solutions consist of crystalloid or blood-crystalloid mixtures. When blood cardioplegia is used, four parts of bypass blood are mixed with one part of cardioplegic solution. (An exception to this is del Nido cardioplegia, which utilizes a 1:4 blood-to-crystalloid ratio, as well as lidocaine to prolong myocyte depolarization.) Although clinical outcomes appear similar between crystalloid- and blood-based solutions, blood cardioplegia might be advantageous. Blood cardioplegia helps ensure oxygen delivery to the heart peri-arrest, can reduce myocardial edema due to blood oncotic pressure, and reduces hemodilution from crystalloid solutions. Recent guidelines suggest that blood cardioplegia should be considered in patients with anemia, low body surface area (BSA) (at risk of excessive hemodilution), chronic kidney disease, or complex procedures with higher anticipated transfusion requirements.

Intermittent, continuous, or single infusions of cardioplegic solution have been used. Usually, 300 to 600 mL of cold cardioplegic solution is needed to paralyze the myocardium and cool the myocardium to 10 °C to 20 °C (50 °F-68 °F).

Chai PJ, Kussman BD. Myocardial protection for neonates and infants. In: Gravlee GP, Davis RF, Hammon J, et al, eds. *Cardiopulmonary Bypass and Mechanical Support: Principles and Practice*. 4th ed. Wolters Kluwer; 2016:683-696.

Grocott HP, Stafford-Smith M, Mora-Mangano CT. Cardiopulmonary bypass management and organ protection. In: Kaplan JA, Augoustides JGT, Manecke GR, et al, eds. *Kaplan's Cardiac Anesthesia for Cardiac and Noncardiac Surgery*. 7th ed. Elsevier; 2017:1111-1161.

Kunst G, Milojevic M, Boer C, et al. 2019 EACTS/EACTA/EBCP guidelines on cardiopulmonary bypass in adult cardiac surgery. *Br J Anaesth*. 2019;123:713-757.

C.II-24. *The arterial blood gases and electrolytes during CPB are as follows: pH, 7.36; $Paco_2$, 42 mm Hg; Pao_2, 449 mm Hg; CO_2 content, 24 mEq/L; sodium (Na), 128 mEq/L; potassium (K), 5.8 mEq/L; glucose, 180 mg/dL; and hematocrit, 20%. The patient's temperature is 27 °C (80.6 °F). At what temperature are blood gases measured? How would you correct the blood gases according to the patient's body temperature? Would you treat the arterial blood gases measured at 37 °C (98.6 °F) or at the patient's body temperature?*

Blood gases are measured at a constant temperature of 37 °C (98.6 °F). They can be corrected according to body temperature. Each 1 °C below 37 °C (98.6 °F) increases blood pH by 0.015. If pH is 7.40 at 37 °C (98.6 °F) in vitro, pH in vivo will be 7.55 at 27 °C (80.6 °F) body temperature ($7.40 + 0.015 \times [37 - 27] = 7.55$). The pH increases at lower temperatures because of increased pK_a and decreased CO_2 tension from increased CO_2 blood solubility during hypothermia. In vivo Pao_2 is decreased because of increased oxygen solubility during hypothermia. Today, blood gases are measured at 37 °C (98.6 °F) and interpreted at 37 °C (98.6 °F) without correcting to actual body temperature. Normal values of blood gases at 37 °C (98.6 °F) are as follows: pH, 7.40 ± 0.05; $Paco_2$, 40 ± 5; and Pao_2, 95 ± 5 mm Hg. During hypothermia, normal values are not the same as those at 37 °C (98.6 °F). The same blood specimen has different Po_2 values when measured at different temperatures. Yet, the oxygen content remains unchanged. It is practical to calculate oxygen content at 37 °C (98.6 °F) than at other temperatures where oxygen dissociation curves are shifted.

Optimal management of pH and $Paco_2$ for patients undergoing hypothermic CPB remains controversial. The two strategies for interpreting blood gases are the pH-stat (temperature-corrected) method and the α-stat (temperature-uncorrected) method. The pH-stat strategy aims at keeping constant arterial pH at 7.40 and $Paco_2$ at 40 mm Hg at any given temperature. A $Paco_2$ of 60 mm Hg analyzed at 37 °C

(98.6 °F) would be equivalent to a Pa_{CO_2} of 40 mm Hg if "corrected" for a body temperature of 27 °C (80.6 °F). The α-stat strategy aims at keeping a constant ratio of $[OH^-]:[H^+]$ at approximately 16:1. This is based on the premise that the pH of blood is regulated to keep the state of dissociation of the imidazole moiety (ie, the alpha of imidazole) constant. Histidine, which contains the imidazole moiety, is an integral part of the active site of many enzyme systems. The function of enzyme systems has been shown to be optimal when the ratio of $[OH^-]:[H^+]$ is approximately 16:1.

Differences between pH-stat and α-stat strategies are listed in **Table 5.2**. With the pH-stat strategy, blood gas values are corrected to the patient temperature; the patient is treated as a hibernating animal. With the α-stat strategy, blood gas values are not corrected regardless of patient temperature; the patient is treated as a poikilotherm. Studies indicate that myocardial function is better preserved when the α-stat strategy is employed. Moreover, maintenance of cerebral blood flow autoregulation appears to remain intact with α-stat management, whereas flow becomes pressure dependent with pH-stat management. The α-stat strategy preserves cerebral blood flow-metabolism coupling such that hypothermia-induced decreases in metabolic rate are accompanied by proportionate decreases in cerebral blood flow. As a result, most medical centers use α-stat management of blood gases during hypothermic CPB. However, Bashein et al found no difference in neuropsychological outcome between patients randomized to α-stat or pH-stat management.

Other studies have shown less decline in cognitive performance when α-stat management is used, especially with prolonged CPB times.

During DHCA, both animal and clinical studies have shown that pH-stat is associated with better neurologic outcome likely because of increased cerebral blood flow, leading to better brain cooling and greater cellular oxygen availability. In summary, most recent outcome studies support the utilization of α-stat for adult CPB and pH-stat for children under DHCA.

Bashein G, Townes BD, Nessly ML, et al. A randomized study of carbon dioxide management during hypothermic cardiopulmonary bypass. *Anesthesiology*. 1990;72:7-15.

Dahlbacka S, Heikkinen J, Kaakinen T, et al. pH-stat versus alpha-stat acid-base management strategy during hypothermic circulatory arrest combined with embolic brain injury. *Ann Thorac Surg*. 2005;79:1316-1325.

Grocott HP, Stafford-Smith M, Mora-Mangano CT. Cardiopulmonary bypass management and organ protection. In: Kaplan JA, Augoustides JGT, Manecke GR, et al, eds. *Kaplan's Cardiac Anesthesia for Cardiac and Noncardiac Surgery*. 7th ed. Elsevier; 2017:1111-1161.

Matte GS, DiNardo JA. Pediatric cardiopulmonary bypass. In: Gravlee GP, Davis RF, Hammon J, et al, eds. *Cardiopulmonary Bypass and Mechanical Support: Principles and Practice*. 4th ed. Wolters Kluwer; 2016:655-682.

Murkin JM. Central nervous system dysfunction after cardiopulmonary bypass. In: Kaplan JA, Reich DL, Savino JS, eds. *Kaplan's Cardiac Anesthesia: The Echo Era*. 6th ed. Elsevier Saunders; 2011:1061-1085.

C.II-25. *How does the blood glucose level change during CPB? Why? What is optimal glucose control intraoperatively? Does hyperglycemia increase neurologic complications during CPB?*

Hyperglycemia is common in cardiac surgery patients during the perioperative period. Etiologies include preexisting diabetes, increased endogenous catecholamine levels and inflammatory mediators due to the stress response to surgery, exogenous catecholamines (inotropes and vasopressors), and medications containing dextrose. On CPB, active cooling causes a marked reduction in insulin production, induces peripheral insulin resistance, and is associated with renal tubular impairment in glucose regulation. The use of dextrose-containing cardioplegia also contributes to CPB-associated hyperglycemia.

The ideal intraoperative blood glucose range remains a matter of debate, but evidence suggests euglycemia (100-180 mg/dL) is beneficial. The most recent STS guidelines from 2009 recommend maintaining glucose less than 180 mg/dL, with IV insulin as required. More recent European guidelines note that glucose less than 140 mg/dL (<7.8 mmol/L) might be appropriate for patients without diabetes and that "tight glycemic control may be considered."

It is unclear if hyperglycemia predisposes to neurologic complications during CPB. By contrast, lower blood glucose targets are associated with equivocal or inferior outcomes, including increased risk of stroke. Avoidance of hypoglycemia is therefore essential. Insulin should be dosed judiciously during periods of hypothermia. Hyperglycemia can be resistant to insulin in this setting, and excessive insulin administration can predispose to hypoglycemia on rewarming.

More recently, studies of intraoperative glucose control have focused on fluctuations in blood glucose levels. Greater glycemic variability is associated with increased mortality and morbidity (infection, stroke, kidney injury) in cardiac surgery patients.

TABLE 5.2 Hypothermic Acid-Base Regulatory Strategies

Strategy	Aim	Total CO_2 Content	pH and $Paco_2$ Maintenance	Intracellular State	α-Imidazole and Buffering	Enzyme Structure and Function	Cerebral Blood Flow and Coupling	Effect on Ischemic Tissue
pH-stat	Constant pH	Increases	Normal corrected values	Acidotic (excess H^+)	Excess (+) charge Buffering decreased	Altered and activity decreased	Flow close to normothermic ? Flow and metabolism uncoupled	? Lessens hypothermic protection
α-Stat	Constant OH^-/H^+	Constant	Normal uncorrected values	Neutral ($H^- = OH^-$)	Constant net charge Buffering constant	Normal and activity maximal	Flow decreases (appropriate) ? Flow and metabolism coupled	? Allows full hypothermic protection

?, questionable.

From Tinker JH, ed. *Cardiopulmonary Bypass: Current Concepts and Controversies*. JB Lippincott; 1989:16.

Flier S, Murkin JM. Central nervous system dysfunciton after cardiopulmonary bypass. In: Kaplan JA, Augoustides JGT, Manecke GR, et al, eds. *Kaplan's Cardiac Anesthesia for Cardiac and Noncardiac Surgery*. 7th ed. Elsevier; 2017:1374-1406.

Kunst G, Milojevic M, Boer C, et al. 2019 EACTS/EACTA/EBCP guidelines on cardiopulmonary bypass in adult cardiac surgery. *Br J Anaesth*. 2019;123:713-757.

Lazar HL, McDonnell M, Chipkin SR, et al. The Society of Thoracic Surgeons practice guideline series: blood glucose management during adult cardiac surgery. *Ann Thorac Surg*. 2009;87:663-669.

Rangasamy V, Xu X, Susheela AT, Subramaniam B. Comparison of glycemic variability indices: blood glucose, risk index, and coefficient of variation in predicting adverse outcomes for patients undergoing cardiac surgery. *J Cardiothorac Vasc Anesth*. 2020;34:1794-1802.

C.II-26. *What are the effects of CPB on platelets and coagulation factors?*

Cardiopulmonary bypass impairs coagulation by multiple mechanisms. These include hemodilution due to priming fluids and blood loss, thrombocytopenia and thrombocytopathy due to the pump and oxygenator, and absorption of clotting factors into plastic components of the CPB circuit. Activation of intrinsic and extrinsic coagulation pathways by the bypass circuit, as well as inflammation triggered by CPB, can lead to fibrinolysis and consumptive coagulopathy. Finally, preoperative antiplatelet medications and residual post-CPB heparin can exacerbate postbypass coagulopathy.

Bartoszko J, Karkouti K. Managing the coagulopathy associated with cardiopulmonary bypass. *J Thromb Haemost*. 2021;19:617-632.

C.II-27. *If the blood level of the venous reservoir is low, what would you replace it with? Blood or balanced salt solution?*

There is growing recognition of the harms and costs associated with unnecessary blood transfusions. According to recent guidelines, a hematocrit of 21% to 24% can be acceptable on CPB as long as oxygen delivery is adequate. The decision to transfuse blood should reflect the patient's overall clinical status, as opposed to a simple laboratory threshold. If hematocrit is 18% to 24%, packed red blood cells (PRBCs) can be transfused if tissue oxygenation is deemed to be inadequate. Transfusion is indicated for Hgb less than 6 g/dL (hematocrit <18%).

Cooper JR Jr, Giesecke NM. Hemodilution and priming solutions. In: Gravlee GP, Davis RF, Hammon J, et al, eds. *Cardiopulmonary Bypass and Mechanical Support: Principles and Practice*. 4th ed. Wolters Kluwer; 2016:421-432.

Kunst G, Milojevic M, Boer C, et al. 2019 EACTS/EACTA/EBCP guidelines on cardiopulmonary bypass in adult cardiac surgery. *Br J Anaesth*. Dec 2019;123:713-757.

Task Force on Patient Blood Management for Adult Cardiac Surgery of the European Association for Cardio-Thoracic Surgery, The European Association of Cardiothoracic Anaesthesiology, Boer C, et al. 2017 EACTS/EACTA Guidelines on patient blood management for adult cardiac surgery. *J Cardiothorac Vasc Anesth*. 2018;32:88-120.

C.II-28. *How do you estimate the fluid balance during CPB?*

IV fluid administration is reduced during CPB. A crystalloid carrier is infused at 50 to 100 mL/h to deliver vasopressors, antifibrinolytics, and other infusions as needed. The primary input volume consists of cardioplegia solution, volume transfused from the reservoir, and fluid or blood added to the circuit or reservoir during CPB. The output consists of blood sequestered in the reservoir, urine, insensible losses, and bleeding. Of note, shed blood is frequently recaptured, filtered, and returned to the bypass circuit or washed and readministered as RBCs.

C.II-29. *For how long can the aorta be cross-clamped?*

The myocardium receives no blood flow during periods of aortic cross-clamp. The limits of "safe" ischemic time during aortic cross-clamping are generally considered to be between 15 and 45 minutes. Despite hypothermic cardioplegia, LV venting, and other efforts to protect the myocardium, ischemic injury can occur.

Nissinen et al evaluated the impact of prolonged cardiopulmonary bypass (CBP) and aortic cross-clamp times in 3,280 patients undergoing adult cardiac surgery, with myocardial protection provided by continuous anterograde and retrograde cardioplegia. They found that cross-clamp times greater than 150 minutes and bypass times greater than 240 minutes were associated with higher 30-day mortality (1.8% vs 12.2% for increased cross-clamp times and 1.9% vs 31.5% for CPB time). Both increased cross-clamp and CBP times also correlated with increased transfusion of blood products, hospital length of stay, time to extubation, and postoperative morbidity such as stroke. More recently, Salsano and colleagues evaluated 264 patients treated surgically for infective endocarditis and found that prolonged aortic cross-clamp time (>72 minutes) was independently associated with early postoperative mortality.

Nissinen J, Biancari F, Wistbacka JO, et al. Safe time limits of aortic cross-clamping and cardiopulmonary bypass in adult cardiac surgery. *Perfusion*. 2009;24:297-305.

Salis S, Mazzanti VV, Merli G, et al. Cardiopulmonary bypass duration is an independent predictor of morbidity and mortality after cardiac surgery. *J Cardiothorac Vasc Anesth*. 2008;22:814-822.

Salsano A, Giacobbe DR, Sportelli E, et al. Aortic cross-clamp time and cardiopulmonary bypass time: prognostic implications in patients operated on for infective endocarditis. *Interact Cardiovasc Thorac Surg*. 2018;27:328-335.

C.II-30. *Why does the urine turn pink in some cases of CPB? What is the renal threshold for plasma hemoglobin?*

Pink urine is a sign of hemolysis. Hemolysis is mainly associated with the negative pressures generated by the suction apparatus and is to a lesser degree with the action of the pump. The renal threshold for hemoglobin is 100 to 150 mg per 100 mL. If significant hemolysis occurs, it is advisable to maintain a high output of alkaline urine to prevent possible tubular damage from acid hematin crystals, which are formed from hemoglobin.

Hines MH. Principles of oxygenator function: gas exchange, heat transfer, and operation. In: Gravlee GP, Davis RF, Hammon J, et al, eds. *Cardiopulmonary Bypass and Mechanical Support: Principles and Practice*. 4th ed. Wolters Kluwer; 2016:95-108.

C.II-31. *Why does it take longer to rewarm than to cool the patient via the pump oxygenator?*

It usually takes 5 to 10 minutes to cool the patient from 37 °C to 25 °C (98.6 °F-77 °F) of average body temperature, whereas it takes 20 to 40 minutes to rewarm from 28 °C to 35 °C (82.4 °F-95 °F). The speed of heat exchange by the bloodstream depends on the temperature gradient between venous blood and water in the heat exchanger, the pump blood flow rate, and the water flow rate of the heat exchanger. The initial venous blood temperature is 37 °C (98.6 °F), and the water temperature of the heat exchanger is 0 °C to 4 °C (32 °F-39.2 °F) during cooling, creating a temperature gradient of 34 °C to 37 °C (93.2 °F-98.6 °F). During rewarming, the water temperature is limited to 42 °C (107.6 °F) or less to prevent denaturation and destruction of blood proteins. In addition, the temperature gradient is limited to less than 10 °C (18 °F) to prevent gas embolism from reduced gas solubility in the blood following a sharp increase in temperature. The heat exchanger water flow does not differ much during cooling and rewarming. However, pump blood flow is usually high during initial cooling because of transient hypotension at the start of bypass. During rewarming, pump blood flow is frequently lower. Rewarming can be accelerated by administering inhalation anesthetics or employing vasodilators to decrease vascular resistance and thereby increase pump flow at the same BP. Because increased vascular resistance is often due to inadequate anesthesia during rewarming, inhalation anesthetics are preferred over vasodilators in patients with good ventricular function. In cases of poor ventricular function, inhalation agents are avoided because of potential cardiac depression after CPB.

Kurusz M, Conti VR, Davis RF. Conduct of cardiopulmonary bypass. In: Gravlee GP, Davis RF, Hammon J, et al, eds. *Cardiopulmonary Bypass and Mechanical Support: Principles and Practice*. 4th ed. Wolters Kluwer; 2016:529-556.

C.II-32. *At what temperature can the patient be weaned from CPB?*

An esophageal or nasopharyngeal temperature of 37 °C (98.6 °F) and a rectal or bladder temperature of at least 35 °C (95 °F) must be reached before the patient can be weaned from CPB. After discontinuation of the pump, surface warming should be continued in pediatric patients to prevent hypothermia due to the redistribution of heat in the body. However, in adults, the use of warming blankets and warmed humidified airway gases has not been found beneficial in preventing the expected temperature "after drop." Esophageal or nasopharyngeal temperature usually decreases and rectal or bladder temperature increases during heat redistribution. Hypothermia is associated with arrhythmia, coagulopathy, shivering and acidosis, among other adverse effects.

Royster RL, Locke AQ, Gardner JC. Termination of cardiopulmonary bypass. In: Gravlee GP, Davis RF, Hammon J, et al, eds. *Cardiopulmonary Bypass and Mechanical Support: Principles and Practice*. 4th ed. Wolters Kluwer; 2016:603-622.

C.II-33. *How would you defibrillate the heart internally during CPB?*

The heart is defibrillated via internal paddles by a direct current (DC) defibrillator, with 5 to 10 watt-seconds (joules). If the heart remains in ventricular fibrillation, blood gases, electrolytes, and temperature are rechecked, and lidocaine, 1 to 2 mg/kg, is administered before repeated DC defibrillation attempts. MAP is usually increased to 80 mm Hg. Amiodarone is occasionally added to treat intractable ventricular fibrillation.

Kaplan JA, Augoustides JGT, Manecke GR, et al, eds. *Kaplan's Cardiac Anesthesia for Cardiac and Noncardiac Surgery*. 7th ed. Elsevier; 2017:1291-1312.

C.II-34. *If the HR is 40 beats per minute, what should you do?*

A temporary AV block is often found at the end of bypass because of potassium cardioplegia and the ischemic insult that occurs during aortic cross-clamping. Although atropine can be administered to treat sinus or nodal bradycardia, a temporary epicardial pacemaker is usually employed. Atrial pacing is preferred because of improved cardiac output when the atrial kick is preserved. Ventricular pacing is necessary if there is a complete AV block or there is an atrial arrhythmia. Relative to ventricular pacing, AV sequential pacing can improve cardiac output due to AV synchrony. It is indicated when ventricular pacing does not provide adequate cardiac output.

Kaplan JA, Augoustides JGT, Manecke GR, et al, eds. *Kaplan's Cardiac Anesthesia for Cardiac and Noncardiac Surgery*. 7th ed. Elsevier; 2017:1291-1312.

C.II-35. *How would you prepare for the termination of CPB?*

Before termination of CPB, cardiac and pulmonary function must be optimized. To ensure that all important steps are not inadvertently omitted, the patient and all monitors should be carefully checked. The mnemonic LAMPS for Laboratory data, Anesthesia machine, Monitors, Patient (Pump), and Support is a useful approach. Written checklists have been shown to improve the completion of tasks before discontinuing CPB.

Laboratory Data

- Arterial pH, Pco_2, Po_2 within normal limits
- Hematocrit 20% to 25%
- K^+ 4.0 to 5.5 mEq/L
- Ionized calcium 1.1 to 1.2 mmol/L
- Pump mixed venous O_2 saturation greater than 70%

Anesthesia Machine

- Anesthesia machine functional
- Adequate depth of anesthesia

Monitors

- Alarms reactivated
- ECG stable rate and rhythm (use pacing if necessary)
- Systemic BP restored to normothermic levels
- PA catheter functional
- Transducers zeroed
- TEE out of freeze mode
- Nasopharyngeal/PA catheter temperature 36 °C to 37 °C (96.8 °F-98.6 °F)
- Bladder/rectal temperature greater than 35 °C (95 °F)

Patient/Pump

- The heart: contractility, size, rhythm, and air removed
- The lungs: atelectasis minimized, fluid in thoracic cavities drained, ventilation reinstituted

Support

- Inotropes/vasopressors/vasodilators
- Mechanical support (IABP or percutaneous ventricular assist device [VAD]) if needed

Kaplan JA, Augoustides JGT, Manecke GR, et al, eds. *Kaplan's Cardiac Anesthesia for Cardiac and Noncardiac Surgery*. 7th ed. Elsevier; 2017:1291-1312.

Kunst G, Milojevic M, Boer C, et al. 2019 EACTS/EACTA/EBCP guidelines on cardiopulmonary bypass in adult cardiac surgery. *Br J Anaesth.* 2019;123:713-757.

Royster RL, Locke AQ, Gardner JC. Termination of cardiopulmonary bypass. In: Gravlee GP, Davis RF, Hammon J, et al, eds. *Cardiopulmonary Bypass and Mechanical Support: Principles and Practice.* 4th ed. Wolters Kluwer; 2016:603-622.

C.II-36. *How would you decide the need for inotropic support?*

The need for inotropic support after CPB is usually assessed by the following (**Figure 5.9**):

- Preoperative ventricular function (ejection fraction)
- Effectiveness of intraoperative myocardial protection
- Adequacy of surgical revascularization
- Durations of aortic cross-clamping and CPB
- Appearance of ventricular function before and at the end of CPB
- Hemodynamics and evidence of low cardiac output when weaning from CPB

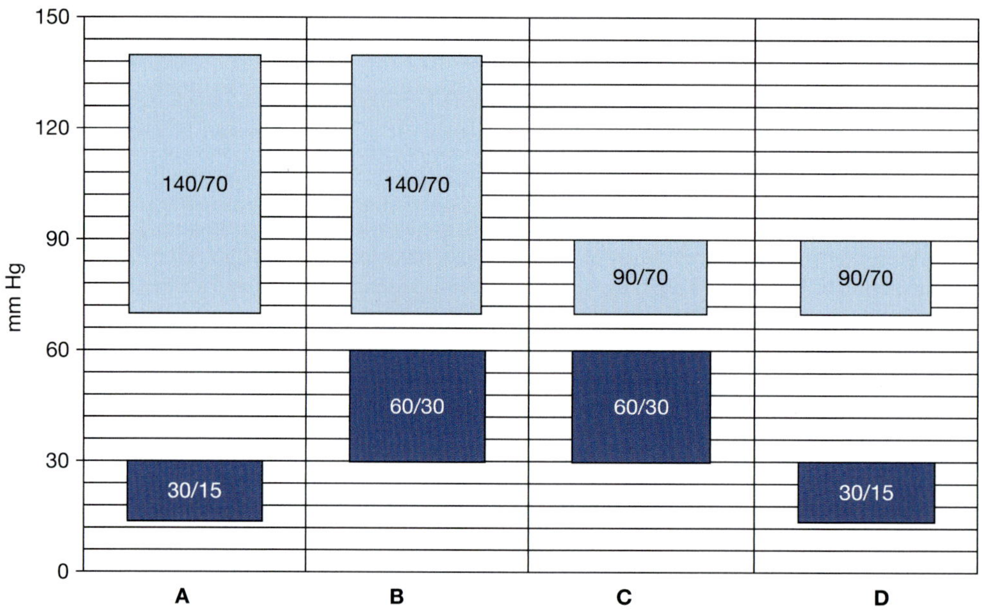

A

CO↑	CO↓
Hyperdynamic	↑↑SVR ?↓Volume
Wait ↑Depth	Dilate ± Volume

B

CO↑	CO↓
Too full	↑Vascular tone ?Contractility
Wait Dilate	Dilate ± Inotrope

C

CO↑	CO↓
↑SVR Too full	↓↓Contractility ALARM
Wait ↑Vascular tone	Adjust preload Inotrope (?IABP, LVAD) ↑Tone

D

CO↑	CO↓
↓↓SVR	↓Volume ↓Contractility ↑CVP: RV failure?
↑Tone	↑Preload Inotrope NO, PGI_2 (unload RV) (?IABP, LVAD) ↑Perfusion pressure

FIGURE 5.9. Hemodynamic management during weaning from CPB. The hemodynamic evaluation is performed by combining information from the systemic *(light shade boxes)* and pulmonary *(dark shade boxes)* arterial pressures. **A.** A combination of elevated systemic arterial and low pulmonary arterial pressure suggests either a hyperdynamic cardiac function (if cardiac output is high) or a vasoconstrictive state (if the peripheral vascular resistance is high). **B.** If systemic hypertension is accompanied by pulmonary hypertension, either the volume status is elevated (if cardiac output is high) or there is generalized vasoconstriction (if cardiac output is decreased). **C.** In the case of systemic hypotension and pulmonary hypertension, the cardiac output may be high (systemic vasodilation) or low (depressed contractility, requiring immediate intervention). **D.** When both systemic and pulmonary pressures are decreased, vasodilation (if the cardiac output is high), hypovolemia, depressed contractility, or right-sided failure is suspected (if cardiac output is decreased). The relative treatment for each hemodynamic derangement is shown in the table. CO, cardiac output; CVP, central venous pressure; IABP, intra-aortic balloon pump; LVAD, left ventricular assist device; NO, nitric oxide; PGI_2, prostacyclin; RV, right ventricle; SVR, systemic vascular resistance; ↑, increase; ↑↑, marked increase; ?, questionable.

Inotropes include epinephrine, dobutamine, and milrinone. Choice of inotrope depends on desired chronotropic, lusitropic, and inodilatory versus vasoconstrictive effects. An IABP can be placed prophylactically in patients with known low ejection fraction (eg, <25%) or in settings of difficult CPB wean. Overall, selection of vasoactive and cardioactive agents is center- and physician-specific.

Kaplan JA, Augoustides JGT, Manecke GR, et al, eds. *Kaplan's Cardiac Anesthesia for Cardiac and Noncardiac Surgery*. 7th ed. Elsevier; 2017:1291-1312.

Monaco F, Di Prima AL, Kim JH, et al. Management of challenging cardiopulmonary bypass separation. *J Cardiothorac Vasc Anesth*. 2020;34:1622-1635.

Royster RL, Locke AQ, Gardner JC. Termination of cardiopulmonary bypass. In: Gravlee GP, Davis RF, Hammon J, et al, eds. *Cardiopulmonary Bypass and Mechanical Support: Principles and Practice*. 4th ed. Wolters Kluwer; 2016:603-622.

C.III. After Cardiopulmonary Bypass

C.III-1. *How would you reverse heparin? How much protamine would you use? What are the other drugs used to neutralize heparin?*

Protamine sulfate is used to reverse heparin after discontinuation of CPB. Protamine binds unfractionated heparin and leads to disassociation of the heparin-ATIII complex. Traditionally, protamine was empirically dosed in a ratio of 0.8 to 1.0 mg per 100 units of initial heparin dose. However, calculating protamine dose according to residual heparin concentration at the end of CPB is feasible and can be associated with improved coagulation, as indicated by decreased postoperative bleeding and transfusion requirements. Excessive doses of protamine are associated with platelet inhibition, prolonged ACT, and increased risk of bleeding.

Residual heparin effect and adequate reversal can be assessed by ACT and thromboelastography testing or by protamine titration into heparinized blood samples. Although shown to correlate imperfectly with residual heparin effect, the ACT is most commonly used. The ACT is repeated 10 minutes after the administration of protamine, and if it remains significantly prolonged above baseline values, a small additional dose of protamine is often given and the ACT is remeasured. Thrombocytopenia should be considered as a cause of ACT prolongation. Additional protamine doses exert a predominantly anticoagulant effect.

Other drugs that can neutralize heparin include platelet factor 4 (PF4), heparinase, protamine variants, hexadimethrine bromide (Polybrene), and toluidine (methylene) blue. PF4 reverses heparin and does not appear to cause systemic hemodynamic effects. However, antibodies to PF4 contribute to heparin-induced thrombosis and thrombocytopenia (HITT), and exogenous PF4 could increase this risk. Heparinase neutralizes heparin by enzymatic cleavage of α-glycoside linkages at the AT III binding site. Heparinase is an effective antagonist of heparin but has been associated with an inferior safety profile compared to protamine among CPB patients. In general, protamine remains the preferred drug for heparin reversal in cardiac surgery.

Boer C, Meesters MI, Veerhoek D, Vonk ABA. Anticoagulant and side-effects of protamine in cardiac surgery: a narrative review. *Br J Anaesth*. 2018;120:914-927.

Horricks J, Comunale ME. Heparin neutralization. In: Gravlee GP, Davis RF, Hammon J, et al, eds. *Cardiopulmonary Bypass and Mechanical Support: Principles and Practice*. 4th ed. Wolters Kluwer; 2016:497-516.

Shore-Lesserson L, Baker RA, Ferraris VA, et al. The Society of Thoracic Surgeons, The Society of Cardiovascular Anesthesiologists, and The American Society of ExtraCorporeal Technology: clinical practice guidelines-anticoagulation during cardiopulmonary bypass. *Anesth Analg*. 2018;126:413-424.

Spiess BD, Armour S, Horrow J, Kaplan JA. Transfusion medicine and coagulation disorders. In: Kaplan JA, Augoustides JGT, Manecke GR, et al, eds. *Kaplan's Cardiac Anesthesia for Cardiac and Noncardiac Surgery*. 7th ed. Elsevier; 2017:1248-1290.

C.III-2. *What is the mechanism of action of protamine?*

Heparin is a strong organic acid (polyanion). Protamine is a strong organic base (polycation). They combine ionically to form a stable salt and lose their own anticoagulant activity. Protamine contains two active sites: one that neutralizes heparin and another that exerts a mild anticoagulant effect independent of heparin.

Horricks J, Comunale ME. Heparin neutralization. In: Gravlee GP, Davis RF, Hammon J, et al, eds. *Cardiopulmonary Bypass and Mechanical Support: Principles and Practice*. 4th ed. Wolters Kluwer; 2016:497-516.

Kaplan JA, Augoustides JGT, Manecke GR, et al, eds. *Kaplan's Cardiac Anesthesia for Cardiac and Noncardiac Surgery*. 7th ed. Elsevier; 2017:1248-1290.

C.III-3. *What are the complications of too much protamine?*

Protamine itself is an anticoagulant. Protamine administered in the absence of heparin interacts with platelets and with clotting proteins. It induces transient thrombocytopenia in humans. Platelet aggregation is impaired by the protamine-heparin complex, although protamine alone has no deleterious effects on platelet aggregation. Protamine can bind to thrombin and inhibit its ability to convert fibrinogen to fibrin. In summary, excessive doses of protamine are associated with platelet inhibition, prolonged ACT, and increased risk of bleeding.

Boer C, Meesters MI, Veerhoek D, Vonk ABA. Anticoagulant and side-effects of protamine in cardiac surgery: a narrative review. *Br J Anaesth.* 2018;120:914-927.

Shore-Lesserson L, Baker RA, Ferraris VA, et al. The Society of Thoracic Surgeons, The Society of Cardiovascular Anesthesiologists, and The American Society of ExtraCorporeal Technology: clinical practice guidelines-anticoagulation during cardiopulmonary bypass. *Anesth Analg.* 2018;126:413-424.

C.III-4. *What is a protamine reaction? How can you prevent it? How do you treat it?*

Protamine administration can induce immunologic and inflammatory responses with dramatic cardiopulmonary effects. Life-threatening reactions include anaphylaxis, severe anaphylactoid reactions, pulmonary edema, and severe pulmonary hypertension.

Clinical phenotypes associated with protamine reactions were initially categorized by Horrow et al as Type I—systemic hypotension from rapid injection; Type II—anaphylactic or anaphylactoid reaction (antibody or nonantibody mediated; immediate or delayed); and Type III—catastrophic pulmonary vasoconstriction with systemic hypotension. An alternative classification was proposed by Lowenstein as pharmacologic histamine release; true anaphylaxis (immunoglobulin E mediated); and anaphylactoid reactions (including pulmonary vasoconstriction and noncardiogenic pulmonary edema). Regardless of classification, appropriate management of protamine reactions depends on recognizing the primary etiology of protamine-induced hypotension, with particular attention to PA pressures and RV function.

The pharmacologic side effect of mild-to-moderate systemic hypotension is seen when protamine is given rapidly or is given to patients who are relatively hypovolemic and vasoconstricted. This response is thought to be mediated by histamine or nitric oxide and is characterized by venodilation, reduced cardiac filling pressures, and decreased vascular resistance. Mild cardiac depression by protamine is suggested but not proven. This type of hypotension can be corrected by rapid volume administration from the CPB pump while the arterial cannula is in place and by the administration of vasopressors. Slower rates of protamine infusion over 5 to 10 minutes and simultaneous maintenance of adequate blood volume have been shown to decrease the incidence of hypotension.

Anaphylactic or anaphylactoid reactions are less common. These reactions vary from mild skin flushing and urticaria to severe vascular collapse. Systemic hypotension is usually accompanied by low pulmonary arterial pressure and low right-sided and left-sided filling pressures. This type of hypotension can be treated and prevented with rapid volume infusion and administration of vasoconstrictors. Antihistamines and steroids are commonly administered; however, little published data support this practice.

Patients with diabetes taking neutral protamine Hagedorn (NPH) insulin can develop antibodies to protamine and appear to be at increased risk. However, clinical reactions do not predictably occur in these patients. Suspected cross-sensitivity in cases of fish allergy or autosensitization in males after vasectomies also does not seem to put most patients at increased risk.

Catastrophic pulmonary hypertension occurs in a subset of patients with severe protamine reactions. Acute increases in PA pressure lead to right ventricular failure, elevated CVP, low flow across the pulmonary vasculature, low left atrial pressure, and decreased cardiac output. Elevated plasma levels of anaphylatoxins and thromboxane are thought to mediate pulmonary vasoconstriction and accompany bronchoconstriction. Less severe RV dysfunction can be managed with inotropes or pulmonary vasodilators. However, in cases of severe pulmonary hypertension, acute RV failure, and impending cardiovascular collapse, protamine should be discontinued, heparin readministered, and the patient returned to CPB immediately. These maneuvers can be lifesaving.

Treatment of hypotension after protamine administration depends on pulmonary arterial pressure. Hypotension with low pulmonary arterial pressures can be corrected with rapid volume infusion and vasoconstrictors, whereas hypotension with high pulmonary arterial pressure should be treated with inotropes or immediate return to CPB. A slow infusion of diluted protamine might help prevent protamine reactions.

Boer C, Meesters MI, Veerhoek D, Vonk ABA. Anticoagulant and side-effects of protamine in cardiac surgery: a narrative review. *Br J Anaesth*. 2018;120:914-927.

Horricks J, Comunale ME. Heparin neutralization. In: Gravlee GP, Davis RF, Hammon J, et al, eds. *Cardiopulmonary Bypass and Mechanical Support: Principles and Practice*. 4th ed. Wolters Kluwer; 2016:497-516.

Horrow JC. Protamine allergy. *J Cardiothorac Anesth*. 1988;2:225-242.

Lowenstein E. Lessons from studying an infrequent event: adverse hemodynamic response associated with protamine reversal of heparin anticoagulation. *J Cardiothorac Anesth*. 1989;3:99-1071.

Shore-Lesserson L, Baker RA, Ferraris VA, et al. The Society of Thoracic Surgeons, The Society of Cardiovascular Anesthesiologists, and The American Society of ExtraCorporeal Technology: clinical practice guidelines-anticoagulation during cardiopulmonary bypass. *Anesth Analg*. 2018;126:413-424.

C.III-5. *What are the indications for intra-aortic balloon pump (IABP)?*

IABP is primarily used for pump failure and myocardial ischemia not responsive to maximal pharmacologic support. Indications include:

Ischemic Heart Disease

- Cardiogenic shock
- Acute MI
- Mechanical defects: ventricular or septal rupture, acute mitral insufficiency, or ventricular aneurysm
- Continued ischemic pain and extension of infarction
- Refractory ventricular arrhythmias
- During cardiac catheterization
- Failed PCI awaiting CABG
- Acute mitral insufficiency with CHF

Cardiac Surgery

- Before CPB and postoperatively
- After CPB: low output syndrome

Heringlake M, Berggreen AE, Paarmann H. Still a place for aortic counterpulsation in cardiac surgery and patients with cardiogenic shock? *Crit Care*. 2021;25:309.

Rocha Ferreira GS, de Almeida JP, Landoni G, et al. Effect of a perioperative intra-aortic balloon pump in high-risk cardiac surgery patients: a randomized clinical trial. *Crit Care Med*. 2018;46:e742-e750.

C.III-6. *What are the principles of IABP?*

IABP counterpulsation is designed to increase myocardial oxygen supply during diastole and to decrease myocardial oxygen demand during systole (**Figure 5.10**). The balloon is inflated during diastole to increase DAP, resulting in increased coronary blood flow. The balloon should be inflated immediately following closure of the aortic valve at the dicrotic notch of the arterial pulse. The balloon is deflated just before the next systole to decrease intra-aortic pressure and afterload, resulting in decreased myocardial oxygen consumption. Cardiac output is increased because of increased coronary perfusion (diastolic augmentation) and decreased resistance (systolic unloading). IABPs are also discussed in Chapter 7: Valvular Heart Disease.

Baldetti L, Pagnesi M, Gramegna M, et al. Intra-aortic balloon pumping in acute decompensated heart failure with hypoperfusion: from pathophysiology to clinical practice. *Circ Heart Fail*. 2021;14:e008527.

C.III-7. *What are the complications of IABP?*

IABP complications can arise from direct injury, malposition, mechanical forces, and contamination, among other causes. They include:

- Lower extremity ischemia
- Aortic dissection
- Thrombus formation and embolization
- Renal artery occlusion
- Splenic, mesenteric, and spinal cord infarction
- Internal mammary occlusion
- Thrombocytopenia
- Infection

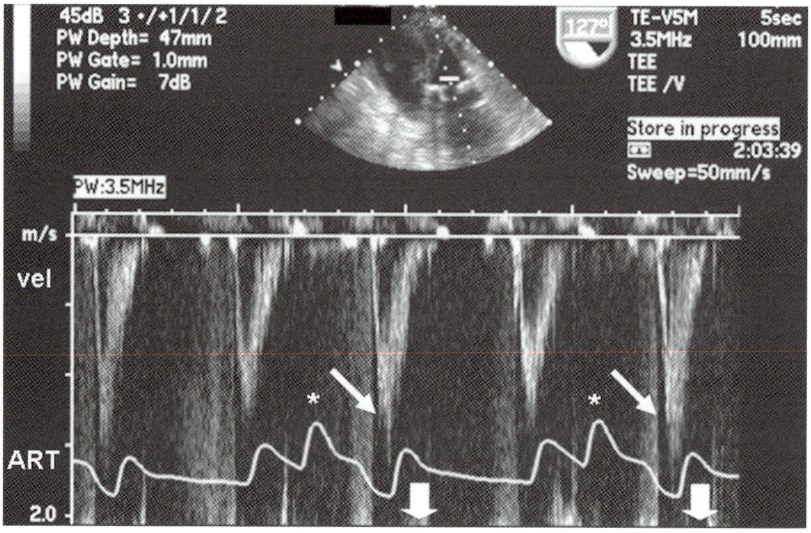

FIGURE 5.10. Function of the intra-aortic balloon pump (IABP). In this patient with an IABP in place, the velocity (vel) of the blood flow as it exits the left ventricle (LV) is recorded. The arterial waveform is shown in the following text. The IABP is set on a 1:2 ratio; that is, it inflates every other beat in diastole (*asterisks*). The velocity (and the amount) of blood exiting the LV is increased (*diagonal arrows*) after the diastolic inflation of the IABP because the LV is ejecting against lower systemic resistance. This is the reason that the systolic arterial pressure following IABP inflation is lower (*down arrows*).

- Gas embolization
- Retroperitoneal bleeding
- Arterial-venous fistula

Kaplan JA, Augoustides JGT, Manecke GR, et al, eds. *Kaplan's Cardiac Anesthesia for Cardiac and Noncardiac Surgery*. 7th ed. Elsevier; 2017:1042-1063, 1291-1312.

Webb CA, Weyker PD, Flynn BC. Management of intra-aortic balloon pumps. *Semin Cardiothorac Vasc Anesth*. 2015;19:106-121.

D. Postoperative Management

D.1. Would you reverse the neuromuscular blocking drug? Why?

It depends. Neuromuscular blocking drugs should be fully reversed in patients who are candidates for early extubation. Ongoing neuromuscular blockade can be indicated in patients who are hemodynamically unstable, profoundly hypoxemic, or who have an "open" chest. Paralyzed patients should be adequately sedated to prevent awareness.

Bainbridge D, Cheng DCH. Fast-Track Postoperative Cardiac recovery and outcomes. In: Kaplan JA, Augoustides JGT, Manecke GR, et al, eds. *Kaplan's Cardiac Anesthesia for Cardiac and Noncardiac Surgery*. 7th ed. Elsevier; 2017:1313-1326.

D.2. When will you wean the patient from the ventilator?

If the operative course is smooth and if the patient is hemodynamically stable, ventilator weaning and tracheal extubation can be performed within 6 hours after CABG surgery. In appropriate patients, early extubation helps avoid complications associated with prolonged mechanical ventilation and sedation and can also reduce health care costs. The rate of extubation within 24 hours following CABG surgery is a nationally recognized quality metric for cardiothoracic surgery centers in the United States.

Charlesworth M, Klein A. Enhanced recovery after cardiac surgery. *Anesthesiol Clin*. 2022;40:143-155.

Higgins TL, Engelman DT. Postoperative respiratory care. In: Kaplan JA, Augoustides JGT, Manecke GR, et al, eds. *Kaplan's Cardiac Anesthesia for Cardiac and Noncardiac Surgery*. 7th ed. Elsevier; 2017:1358-1373.

McCarthy C, Fletcher N. Early Extubation in enhanced recovery from cardiac surgery. *Crit Care Clin*. 2020;36:663-674.

D.3. What criteria would you use in deciding when to wean the patient from the ventilator?

- Consciousness—awake and alert
- Stable vital signs
- Acceptable arterial blood gases—pH, 7.35 to 7.45; Pao_2, over 80 mm Hg with Fio_2, 0.4; $Paco_2$, 35 to 45 mm Hg
- Acceptable respiratory mechanics
- Vital capacity greater than 10 to 15 mL/kg
- Maximal inspiratory force—greater than 20 to 25 cm H_2O
- Hemostasis—less than 100 mL/h of chest tube drainage
- Stable metabolic state—normal temperature and electrolytes

The patient should tolerate being on continuous positive airway pressure of 5 cm H_2O and pressure support of 5 cm H_2O with 40% oxygen. If the patient tolerates continuous positive airway pressure well for 30 minutes and arterial blood gases are acceptable, the patient can be extubated.

Bojar RM. Early postoperative care. In: *Manual of Perioperative Care in Adult Cardiac Surgery*. 6th ed. John Wiley & Sons; 2021:363-416.

Higgins TL, Engelman DT. Postoperative respiratory care. In: Kaplan JA, Augoustides JGT, Manecke GR, et al, eds. *Kaplan's Cardiac Anesthesia for Cardiac and Noncardiac Surgery*. 7th ed. Elsevier; 2017:1358-1373.

D.4. What are the potential postoperative complications of CABG surgery?

Neurologic

Neurologic complications include stroke (ischemic or hemorrhagic), seizure, delirium, and neurocognitive dysfunction.

Cardiovascular

Cardiovascular and hemodynamic complications include arrhythmias, low cardiac output syndrome, acute or acute-on-chronic systolic or diastolic heart failure, vasoplegia, and myocardial ischemia or infarction.

Pulmonary

Respiratory failure, acute lung injury, or adult respiratory distress syndrome due to:

- Decreased blood flow to the lung during total CPB
- Collapsed alveoli during CPB, resulting in decreased surfactant and decreased distensibility
- Fluid overload
- Hyperoxia during CPB
- Left ventricular failure
- Microemboli
- Reperfusion injury
- Inflammatory response
- Infections
- Transfusion-related lung dysfunction

Renal

Renal complications include:

- Polyuria from hemodilution and diuretics
- Oliguria from hypoperfusion
- Acute kidney injury
  - Hypoperfusion
  - Ischemia
  - Inflammatory response
  - Nephrotoxins (preoperative contrast dyes, antibiotics)
- Acute tubular necrosis
- Acute or chronic renal insufficiency

Hematologic

Bleeding and clotting complications can arise due to:

- Too much or too little protamine to reverse heparin
- Thrombocytopenia and decreased coagulation factors
- Qualitative and quantitative platelet defect
- Disseminated intravascular coagulopathy

- Fibrinolysis with low levels of fibrinogen
- Poor surgical hemostasis

Embolic events (air, destroyed or aggregated formed blood elements, fat, endogenous and exogenous debris) can also occur.

Metabolic

Metabolic derangements are common. These include hypothermia, hyperglycemia (due to dextrose-containing cardioplegia, increased catecholamine levels, and stress hyperglycemia), hypokalemia (due to hemodilution, alkalosis, and diuretics), and acidosis.

Bojar RM. Early postoperative care. In: *Manual of Perioperative Care in Adult Cardiac Surgery*. 6th ed. John Wiley & Sons; 2021:363-416.

Levy JH, Ghadimi K, Bailey JM, Ramsay JG. Postoperative cardiovascular management. In: Kaplan JA, Augoustides JGT, Manecke GR, et al, eds. *Kaplan's Cardiac Anesthesia for Cardiac and Noncardiac Surgery*. 7th ed. Elsevier; 2017:1327-1357.

6 Mechanical Circulatory Support

Lisa Q. Rong, Ankur Srivastava, and Adam D. Lichtman

A 58-year-old male presents to the hospital with acute ST-segment elevation myocardial infarction (STEMI) and is brought to the cardiac catheterization laboratory, where he undergoes angioplasty and has an intra-aortic balloon pump (IABP) placed for hemodynamic support. Overnight, the patient becomes increasingly hypotensive with reduced urine output and requires vasopressors. A pulmonary artery catheter (PAC) was placed and indicated elevated pulmonary capillary wedge pressure (25 mm Hg) and reduced cardiac output (CO; 1.8 L/min). Bedside echocardiography showed severe left ventricular dysfunction with severe central mitral regurgitation. Perfusion parameters (low CO, rising lactate, reduced urine output) remain critical despite high doses of ionotropic therapy with epinephrine and dobutamine. Cardiac surgery and interventional cardiology teams were consulted for placement of an Impella heart pump. While in the catheterization laboratory, the patient suffered cardiac arrest with ventricular tachycardia and was emergently placed on peripheral veno-arterial extracorporeal membrane oxygenation (VA-ECMO). Over the next several days, the patient's cardiac function did not recover, and he was brought back to the operating room for placement of a left ventricular assist device (LVAD).

A. Medical Disease and Differential Diagnosis

1. What is an IABP?
2. How is an IABP placed and positioned?
3. Describe IABP inflation and deflation timing.
4. How does the IABP help improve hemodynamics?
5. What are the indications and potential disadvantages of IABP placement?
6. What are the contraindications and potential complications of IABP placement?
7. What are the signs of cardiogenic shock?
8. What are the different ways to estimate CO?
9. What are the different types of temporary percutaneous ventricular assist devices (VADs)?
10. What is extracorporeal membrane oxygenation (ECMO), and what are its two main configurations?
11. What are the common indications for veno-venous (VV)-ECMO?
12. What are the common indications for VA-ECMO?
13. What are the advantages of using VA-ECMO over other temporary VADs?
14. What is the main disadvantage of VA-ECMO, and how does VA-ECMO affect myocardial recovery?
15. What is the North-South syndrome and when does it occur?
16. How do you treat North-South syndrome?
17. What are the most common complications of ECMO?
18. What are the contraindications to ECMO?
19. What are the pros and cons of peripheral versus central VA-ECMO cannula placement?
20. How can you wean off VA-ECMO?
21. How can you wean off VV-ECMO?

B. Indications for LVAD

1. What are the indications for LVAD?
2. What are the main types of LVAD, and how do they compare in terms of morbidity and mortality following implantation?

3. What are the three circumstances to consider LVAD placement?
4. What is the latest version of the most common LVAD, and why is it better than the previous version?
5. What is part of the LVAD assessment process?
6. What are the outcomes related to continuous-flow LVAD placement including survival, morbidity, and quality of life?

C. Preoperative Evaluation and Preparation

1. What is the focus of the preoperative assessment of a patient with LVAD?

D. Intraoperative Management

1. Detail the anesthetic management for a patient undergoing LVAD placement.
2. How is a patient with VAD monitored during a general anesthetic?
3. What are the most common VAD settings?
4. What are some important considerations of patients with LVAD for postoperative management?

A. Medical Disease and Differential Diagnosis

A.1. What is an IABP?

An IABP is an 8.5 to 9.5 French dual-lumen catheter with a 40 to 60 mL helium-filled balloon attached at its tip that used to assist the heart. The IABP provides diastolic counterpulsation, decreasing systolic afterload to cardiac ejection and increasing coronary perfusion pressure.

González LS, Chaney MA. Intraaortic balloon pump counterpulsation, part I: history, technical aspects, physiologic effects, contraindications, medical applications/outcomes. *Anesth Analg*. 2020;131:776-791.

Parissis H, Graham V, Lampridis S, et al. IABP: history-evolution-pathophysiology-indications: what we need to know. *J Cardiothorac Surg*. 2016;11:122.

A.2. How is an IABP placed and positioned?

An IABP is placed either percutaneously or under surgical exposure into a large peripheral artery (most commonly femoral) and directed retrograde into the thoracic aorta over a wire. The optimal position is with the tip of the balloon positioned just distal to the origin of the left subclavian artery and the proximal end of the balloon before the orifice of the renal arteries. IABPs are positioned using fluoroscopy/x-radiography, or under the guidance of transesophageal echocardiography (TEE). Incorrect placement can obstruct the cerebral or visceral arteries, which can result in cerebral or visceral organ ischemia and ineffective counterpulsation. During IABP support, patients are usually anticoagulated.

Baldetti L, Beneduce A, Boccellino A, et al. Bedside intra-aortic balloon pump insertion in cardiac intensive care unit: a single-center experience. *Catheter Cardiovasc Interv*. 2022;99:1976-1983.

Rodriguez Lima DR, Duran EJ, Rojas Díaz EL, et al. Ultrasound-guided insertion of intra-aortic balloon counterpulsation in intensive care: description of the technique. *Ultrasound J*. 2020;12:23.

A.3. Describe IABP inflation and deflation timing.

The balloon is connected to a control console that regulates inflation and deflation of the balloon at the tip of the IABP. The IABP balloon is inflated in diastole and deflated in systole. The triggers for balloon inflation are (1) the electrocardiogram (ECG) T wave; (2) the dicrotic notch on the arterial pressure waveform (as measured by a fluid-filled column), which is recorded from the tip of the IABP; and (3) in newer versions, a fiber-optic pressure manometer embedded in the tip of the IABP. Use of fiber-optic manometers and computerized waveform analysis allows better beat-to-beat cardiac support and minimizes artifacts. Balloon deflation is timed to occur prior to the ECG Q wave or the upstroke of the arterial pressure waveform (**Figure 6.1**). Improper IABP timing reduces effectiveness and can increase myocardial oxygen consumption. Early diastolic inflation of the IABP balloon (inflation is initiated during late systole) results in increased left ventricular (LV) afterload and increased myocardial oxygen consumption. Late diastolic inflation results in suboptimal coronary perfusion and diastolic augmentation. Examples of this include:

- Early inflation: inflation of the IABP before aortic valve closure (**Figure 6.2A**)
- Late inflation: inflation of the IABP after closure of the aortic valve (**Figure 6.2B**)

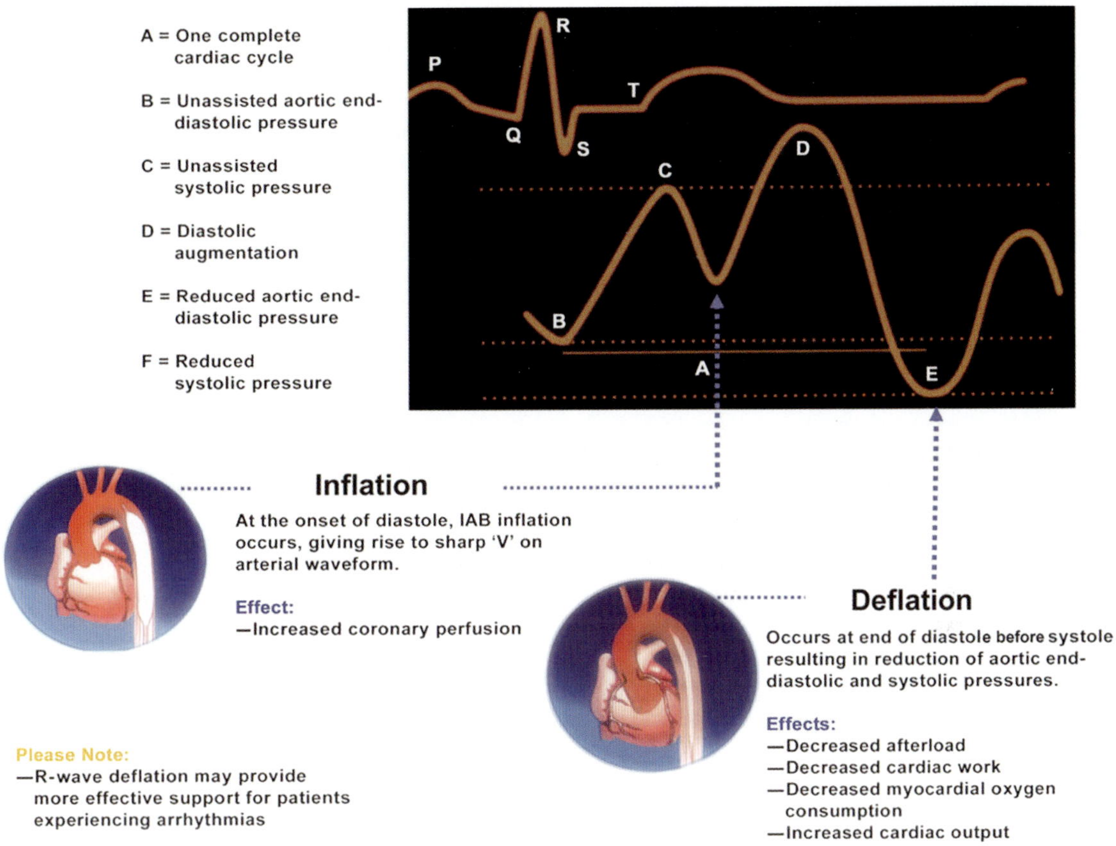

FIGURE 6.1. One complete cardiac cycle and the corresponding waveform of an intra-aortic balloon pump (IABP) during the inflation and deflation. (Reproduced with permission from Datascope®.)

- Early deflation: premature deflation of the IABP during diastole (**Figure 6.2C**)
- Late deflation: deflation of the IABP after the onset of systole (**Figure 6.2D**)

Boccellino A, Sacchi S, Pazzanese V, et al. Effects of intra-aortic balloon pump delayed deflation timing on carotid blood flow and cardiac mechanics: an ultrasound and haemodynamic study. *J Heart Lung Transplant.* 2023;42:451-455.

Yarham G, Clements A, Morris C, et al. Fiber-optic intra-aortic balloon therapy and its role within cardiac surgery. *Perfusion.* 2013;28:97-102.

A.4. How does the IABP help improve hemodynamics?

The balloon is timed to inflate in diastole, thereby augmenting diastolic pressure with a resultant increase in blood flow to the coronary arteries, great vessels, and visceral organs. The balloon deflates in systole (just prior to opening of the aortic valve), thereby causing a "void" or "potential" space in the aorta that reduces LV afterload, which in turn facilitates ventricular systolic ejection and an increase in stroke volume. The decreased systolic afterload reduces LV wall stress, decreases myocardial oxygen demand, and ameliorates the effects of coronary ischemia.

Fried JA, Nair A, Takeda K, et al. Clinical and hemodynamic effects of intra-aortic balloon pump therapy in chronic heart failure patients with cardiogenic shock. *J Heart Lung Transplant.* 2018;37:1313-1321.

González LS, Chaney MA. Balloon pump counterpulsation part II: perioperative hemodynamic support and new directions. *Anesth Analg.* 2020;131:792-807.

Nan Tie E, Dinh D, Chan W, et al. Melbourne interventional group investigators. Trends in intra-aortic balloon pump use in cardiogenic shock after the SHOCK-II trial. *Am J Cardiol.* 2023;191:125-132.

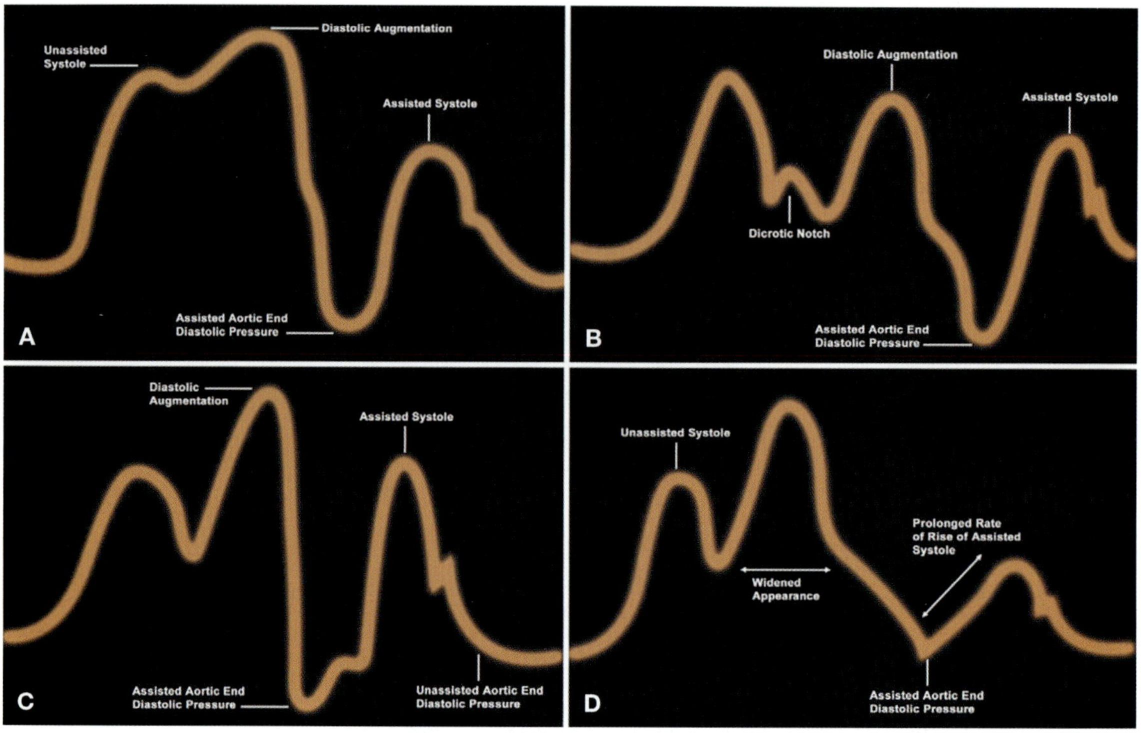

FIGURE 6.2. A. Waveform characteristics: inflation of intra-aortic balloon pump (IABP) before dicrotic notch; if diastolic augmentation encroaches onto systole, may be unable to distinguish. Physiologic effects: potential premature closure of the aortic valve; potential increase in left ventricular end-diastolic volume (LVEDV) and left ventricular end-diastolic pressure (LVEDP) or pulmonary catheter wedge pressure (PCWP); increased LV wall stress or afterload; aortic regurgitation; increased myocardial oxygen (MVO_2) demand. **B.** Waveform characteristics: inflation of IABP after the dicrotic notch; absence of sharp "V." Physiologic effects: suboptimal coronary artery perfusion. **C.** Waveform characteristics: deflation of IABP is seen as a sharp decrease after diastolic augmentation; suboptimal diastolic augmentation; assisted aortic end-diastolic pressure can be equal to or less than the unassisted aortic end-diastolic pressure; assisted systolic pressure can increase. Physiologic effects: suboptimal coronary perfusion; potential for retrograde coronary and carotid blood flow; suboptimal afterload reduction; increased MVO_2. **D.** Waveform characteristics: assisted aortic end-diastolic pressure can be equal to the unassisted aortic end-diastolic pressure; rate of increase of assisted systole is prolonged; diastolic augmentation can appear widened. Physiologic effects: afterload reduction is essentially absent; increased MVO_2 because of the LV ejecting against a greater resistance and a prolonged isovolumetric contraction phase; IABP can impede LV ejection and increase afterload. (Reproduced with permission from Datascope®.)

Zheng XY, Wang Y, Chen Y, et al. The effectiveness of intra-aortic balloon pump for myocardial infarction in patients with or without cardiogenic shock: a meta-analysis and systematic review. *BMC Cardiovasc Disord.* 2016;16:148.

A.5. What are the indications and potential disadvantages of IABP placement?

Indications include:

- Cardiogenic shock secondary to acute coronary syndrome (ACS): the most common indication for IABP placement is after ACS, such as unstable angina refractory to medical therapies and STEMI with or without acute mitral regurgitation or ventricular septal defect.
- Postcardiotomy cardiogenic shock: postcardiac surgery where a patient is unable to be separated from cardiopulmonary bypass (CPB).
- Elective high-risk percutaneous coronary interventions (PCIs) in patients with LV dysfunction and extensive coronary artery disease (CAD) to maintain coronary perfusion and CO during the intervention.
- Symptomatic severe CAD (ie, high-grade left main disease) to increase coronary perfusion before intervention.
- High-risk cardiac patients presenting for urgent noncardiac surgical procedures.

Disadvantages include:

- The main disadvantage of the IABP is it provides limited hemodynamic support of 0.5 to 1.0 L/min.

- The effects of the IABP are less effective in patients with severe cardiogenic shock, and as a result, with the introduction of new cardiac assist devices, use of the IABP may decrease in the future.

Heringlake M, Berggreen AE, Paarmann H. Still a place for aortic counterpulsation in cardiac surgery and patients with cardiogenic shock? *Crit Care*. 2021;25:309.

Pilarczyk K, Boening A, Jakob H, et al. Preoperative intra-aortic counterpulsation in high-risk patients undergoing cardiac surgery: a meta-analysis of randomized controlled trials†. *Eur J Cardiothorac Surg*. 2016;49:5-17.

Thiele H, Zeymer U, Neumann FJ, et al. Intraaortic balloon pump in cardiogenic shock II (IABP-SHOCK II) trial investigators. Intra-aortic balloon counterpulsation in acute myocardial infarction complicated by cardiogenic shock (IABP-SHOCK II): final 12-month results of a randomized, open-label trial. *Lancet*. 2013;382:1638-1645.

A.6. What are the contraindications and potential complications of IABP placement?

The contraindications to IABP placement include:

- Significant aortic insufficiency (IABP-induced increased diastolic pressure will worsen the severity of aortic valvular incompetence and increase LV diastolic pressure)
- Major aortic pathology (aneurysm, dissection, severe atherosclerotic plaque)
- Sepsis, with the risk of colonization of the IABP catheter
- Uncontrolled coagulopathy
- Cancer with metastasis

The potential complications include:

- Vascular injury at the placement site is the most common complication of IABP placement. This is especially true in patients with severe peripheral vascular disease (reported as 8%-18%, with major limb ischemia reported at 1%). Bleeding at the insertion site is another major complication.
- Thrombocytopenia has been reported in 57.9% of patients receiving IABP but has not been associated with major bleeding events or mortality.
- A rare complication is the rupture of IABP, causing a gas embolism.

Heuts S, Lorusso R, di Mauro M, et al. GIROC-investigators. Sheathless versus sheathed intra-aortic balloon pump implantation in patients undergoing cardiac surgery. *Am J Cardiol*. 2023;189:86-92.

Parissis H, Soo A, Al-Alao B. Intra aortic balloon pump: literature review of risk factors related to complications of the intraaortic balloon pump. *J Cardiothorac Surg*. 2011;6:147.

Sheng Z, Zhao H, Yan H, et al. Intra-aortic balloon pumping and thrombocytopenia in patients with acute coronary syndrome: incidence, risk factors, and prognosis. *Herz*. 2018;43:555-564.

A.7. What are the signs of cardiogenic shock?

Cardiogenic shock is a syndrome of poor organ perfusion secondary to cardiac dysfunction. Common signs include hypotension, renal dysfunction, hepatic dysfunction, lactic acidosis, cold extremities (increased systemic vascular resistance), pulmonary congestion, and altered mental status. Cardiac dysfunction is estimated by calculating CO (CO < 4 L/min) or cardiac index (CI; CO/body surface area [BSA] < 2.2 L/min) measured by transthoracic or transesophageal Doppler echocardiography, PAC thermodilution, or by diagnosing elevated cardiac filling pressures (pulmonary capillary wedge pressure > 15 mm Hg).

Vahdatpour C, Collins D, Goldberg S. Cardiogenic shock. *J Am Heart Assoc*. 2019;8:e011991.

A.8. What are the different ways to estimate CO?

CO can be measured through noninvasive and invasive methods. The gold standard CO monitor remains the PAC. Cardiogenic shock is an indication for placement of PAC to assess trends and optimization of CO medically or by mechanical support. The PAC can measure CO using thermodilution or the Fick principle. Thermodilution involves rapid injection of a crystalloid bolus at a known temperature into the superior vena cava and measuring temperature change at the tip of the PAC. The temperature change in the PA has an inverse relationship with CO. The Fick equation measures CO based on oxygen consumption. The Fick equation states that the ratio of oxygen consumption divided by the difference between arterial and venous oxygen content is equal to CO. The Fick equation requires measurement of oxygen consumption which is not possible in a critically ill patient and leads to significant error when estimates are employed. Thermodilution remains the primary method of determining CO.

The most common noninvasive methods include transthoracic echocardiography (TTE) and automated peripheral CO monitors. Doppler-derived CO by TTE usually requires calculation by a trained echocardiographer. CO can vary depending on two-dimensional or three-dimensional echocardiographic techniques, and the values obtained may not be interchangeable with PAC thermodilution. However, they can be useful to determine trends.

Peripheral CO monitors utilize bioimpedance (NCCom), bioreactance (NICOM), partial CO_2 rebreathing (INNOCOR), pulse wave transit time (EsCCO), or ultrasonic (USCOM) techniques to calculate CO. Peripheral CO monitors are not the standard of care in cardiogenic shock as they have a wide array of potential errors, including being rhythm and rate dependent, and are affected by patient body habitus and edema (NICOM). In several trials these continuous noninvasive monitors have shown poor agreement with PAC measurements. However, the trend in CO is still considered useful and often employed in patients where the risks of invasive monitors outweigh the potential benefits.

Grensemann J. Cardiac output monitoring by pulse contour analysis, the technical basics of less-invasive techniques. *Front Med (Lausanne)*. 2018;5:64.

Nguyen LS, Squara P. Non-invasive monitoring of cardiac output in critical care medicine. *Front Med (Lausanne)*. 2017;4:200.

Rali AS, Buechler T, Van Gotten B, et al. Non-invasive cardiac output monitoring in cardiogenic shock: the NICOM study. *J Card Fail*. 2020;26:160-165.

Talan JW, Mangalick K, Pradhan D, Sauthoff H. Measurement of cardiac output by point-of-care transthoracic echocardiography. *ATS Scholar*. 2022;3:631-633.

Vahdatpour C, Collins D, Goldberg S. Cardiogenic shock. *J Am Heart Assoc*. 2019;8:e011991.

A.9. What are the different types of temporary percutaneous ventricular assist devices (VADs)?

There are two systems available for percutaneous ventricular support:

- Impella system (Abiomed)
- TandemHeart (CardiacAssist)

The most common percutaneous VAD is the Impella system. It comes in several configurations for both left and right ventricular support. It consists of a catheter with an axial flow pump which provides support by propelling blood forward. There are several Impella devices available to support the LV and one device for the right ventricle (RV).

LV support: The most common LV support device is the femoral Impella CP which is usually placed percutaneously in the catheterization laboratory. It is positioned retrograde across the aortic valve to propel blood forward into the ascending aorta. The Impella CP (femoral access) can provide up to 4.3 L/min of flow.

Larger Impella devices that provide higher flows require surgical placement through femoral or axillary access. The Impella 5.5, which supports up to 6.2 L/min of flow, can be implanted surgically via a graft onto the axillary artery or ascending aorta to allow patient mobilization, as the patient does not need to be bed-bound compared to femoral artery inserted devices.

RV support: Impella RP is available for percutaneous right heart support. The Impella RP is a 22 French micro-axial pump approved by the U.S. Food and Drug Administration (FDA) for use in acute right heart failure for up to 14 days. The catheter pump is advanced antegrade under fluoroscopic guidance and positioned across the tricuspid and pulmonary valves through a sheath inserted in the femoral vein. This pump provides right heart support via propelling blood from the inferior vena cava (pump inflow) to the pulmonary artery (pump outflow) at up to 4.0 L/min of flow.

A less commonly used device is TandemHeart, which is inserted percutaneously through the femoral vein to the right atrium, across the inter-atrial septum, and into the left atrium. It can pump up to 4.0 L/min of blood through a continuous-flow centrifugal pump from the left atrium into the lower abdominal aorta or iliac arteries through a femoral arterial cannula. Hemodynamically, the TandemHeart provides a more significant increase CO and blood pressure compared to IABP and decreases RV and LV filling pressures and work. However, the complexity of placement and the high complication rate (vascular injury, bleeding leading to transfusion, sepsis/systemic inflammatory response syndrome, stroke, gastrointestinal [GI] bleeding) have limited its use and popularity.

Anderson MB, Goldstein J, Milano C, et al. Benefits of a novel percutaneous ventricular assist device for right heart failure: the prospective RECOVER RIGHT study of the Impella RP device. *J Heart Lung Transplant*. 2015;34:1549-1560.

Lampert BC. Perioperative management of the right and left ventricles. *Cardiol Clin*. 2018;36:495-506.

Ramzy D, Anderson M, Batsides G, et al. Early outcomes of the first 200 US patients treated with Impella 5.5: a novel temporary left ventricular assist device. *Innovations*. 2021;16:365-372.

Werdan K, Gielen S, Ebelt H, et al. Mechanical circulatory support in cardiogenic shock. *Eur Heart J*. 2014;35:156-167.

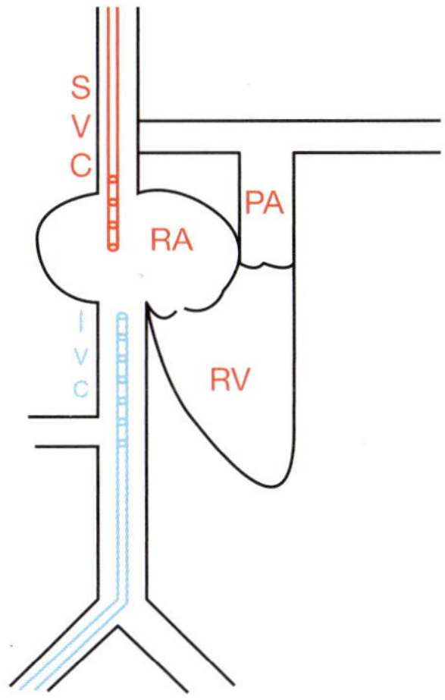

FIGURE 6.3. Cannula configuration for dual-cannula veno-venous extracorporeal membrane oxygenation (VV-ECMO). Drainage cannula is placed in the IVC and return cannula is placed in the SVC. Deoxygenated blood (blue) is drained from the femoral cannula and oxygenated blood (red) is returned to the internal jugular vein. IVC, inferior vena cava; PA, pulmonary artery; RA, right atrium; RV, right ventricle; SVC, superior vena cava; V-V, veno-venous.

A.10. What is extracorporeal membrane oxygenation (ECMO), and what are its two main configurations?

ECMO provides mechanical cardiopulmonary support. It usually consists of a centrifugal pump, heat exchanger, and membrane oxygenator. Deoxygenated blood from a drainage cannula is propelled forward with a centrifugal pump, through an oxygenator, and back into the patient through a return cannula. There are two main configurations: veno-arterial (VA) and VV-ECMO. VA-ECMO (**Figures 6.3** and **6.4**) involves draining venous blood into the pump and returning it to the arterial circulation, which helps provide both circulatory and respiratory support. VV-ECMO (**Figures 6.5** and **6.6**) drains venous blood into the pump and returns oxygenated venous blood to the right atrium, providing only pulmonary support.

ELSO Guidelines for Cardiopulmonary Extracorporeal Life Support Extracorporeal Life Support Organization, Version 1.4. Accessed May 14, 2023. www.elso.org

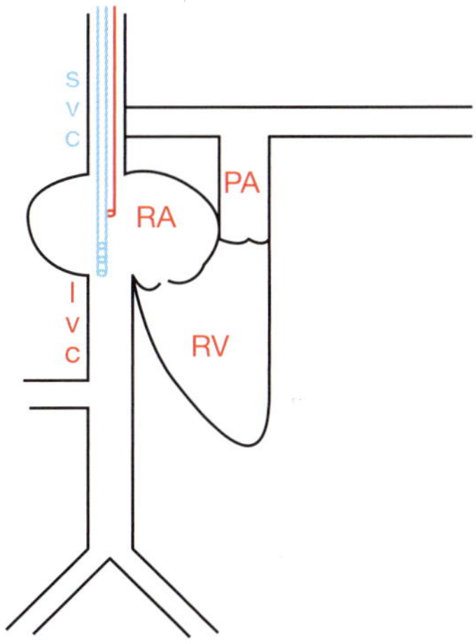

FIGURE 6.4. Cannula configuration of single-cannula (dual-lumen) veno-venous extracorporeal membrane oxygenation (VV-ECMO). Drainage lumen is positioned in the IVC while return lumen is positioned toward right atrium. Deoxygenated blood (blue) is drained from the distal lumen and oxygenated blood (red) is returned through the proximal lumen near the right atrium. IVC, inferior vena cava; PA, pulmonary artery; RA, right atrium; RV, right ventricle; SVC, superior vena cava; V-V, veno-venous.

Mazzeffi MA, Rao VK, Del Rio JM, et al. Intraoperative management of adult patients on extracorporeal membrane oxygenation: an expert consensus statement from the society of cardiovascular anesthesiologists—part I, technical aspects of extracorporeal membrane oxygenation. *J Cardiothorac Vasc Anesth.* 2021;35:3496-3512.

A.11. What are the common indications for VV-ECMO?

In VV-ECMO, an oxygenator is placed in series between a drainage cannula (usually internal jugular vein) and a venous return cannula (usually femoral vein) (**Figure 6.3**). However, using a dual-lumen cannula (**Figure 6.4**) eliminates the need for separate cannulas. Since the blood is returned to the venous circulation, CO is not augmented. After deoxygenated venous blood passes through the pump and oxygenator, it returns to the venous circulation, where it mixes with systemic venous blood and passes via the pulmonary circulation to the left side of the heart and to the systemic circulation. As such, there is no cardiac support provided by VV-ECMO. VV-ECMO is primarily used for severe acute respiratory distress syndrome (ARDS) (eg, due to COVID-19), as a bridge to lung transplantation, and as support for surgical lung or airway procedures.

ELSO Guidelines for Cardiopulmonary Extracorporeal Life Support Extracorporeal Life Support Organization, Version 1.4. Accessed May 14, 2023. www.elso.org

Combes A, Hajage D, Capellier G, et al. Extracorporeal membrane oxygenation for severe acute respiratory distress syndrome. *N Engl J Med.* 2018;378:1965-1975.

A.12. What are the common indications for VA-ECMO?

VA-ECMO is akin to conventional CPB, in which blood is drained via a cannula placed in the right atrium or inferior vena cava, routed to a pump and an oxygenator/heat exchanger, and returned to the aorta or a large artery (**Figures 6.5** and **6.6**). As a result, both cardiac and pulmonary support is achieved. The indications for VA-ECMO include post-cardiotomy shock/failure to wean from CPB, reversible cardiogenic shock, as a bridge to a durable ventricular support device, as a bridge to transplantation, and as an adjunct to advanced life support for cardiac arrest (ie, extracorporeal cardiopulmonary resuscitation [ECPR]).

ELSO Guidelines for Cardiopulmonary Extracorporeal Life Support Extracorporeal Life Support Organization, Version 1.4. Accessed May 14, 2023. www.elso.org

Mazzeffi MA, Rao VK, Del Rio JM, et al. Intraoperative management of adult patients on extracorporeal membrane oxygenation: an expert consensus statement from the society of cardiovascular anesthesiologists—Part I, technical aspects of extracorporeal membrane oxygenation. *J Cardiothorac Vasc Anesth.* 2021;35:3496-3512.

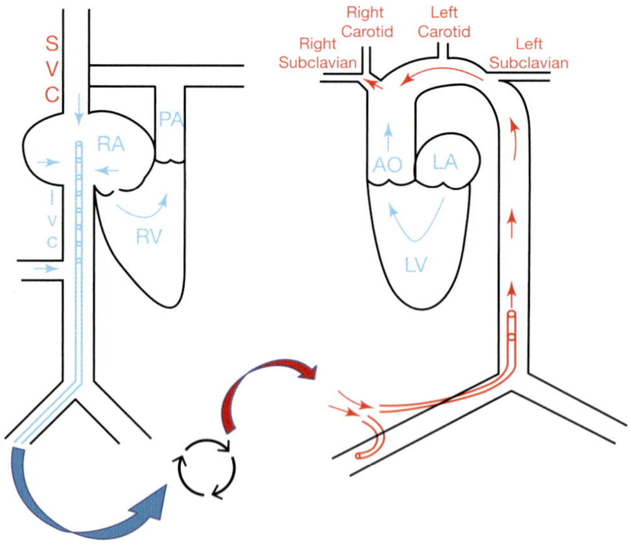

FIGURE 6.5. Peripheral femoral vein—femoral artery veno-arterial extracorporeal membrane oxygenation (VA-ECMO) cannulation. Drainage cannula is placed in the IVC and return cannula is placed in the femoral artery. Peripheral femoral vein—femoral artery V-A ECMO cannulation. Deoxygenated blood (blue) is drained from the femoral vein cannula and oxygenated blood (red) is returned to the femoral artery. AO, aorta; ECMO, extracorporeal membrane oxygenation; IVC, inferior vena cava; LA, left atrium; LV, left ventricle; PA, pulmonary artery; RA, right atrium; RV, right ventricle; SVC, superior vena cava; V-A, veno-arterial.

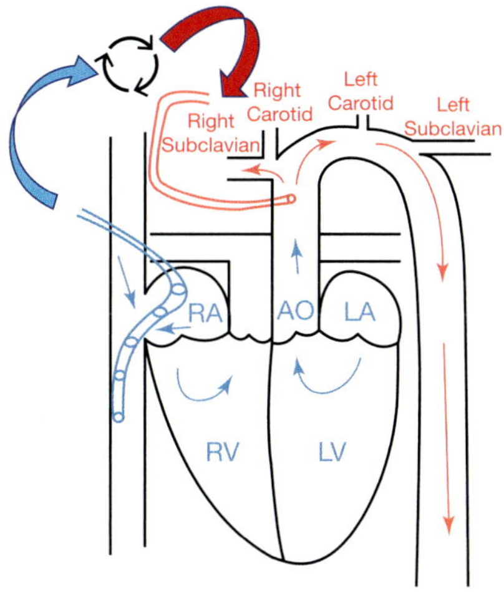

FIGURE 6.6. Cannula configuration for central veno-arterial extracorporeal membrane oxygenation (VA-ECMO). Drainage cannula is placed in right atrium and return cannula is placed in ascending aorta. Deoxygenated blood (blue) is drained from the right atrium and oxygenated blood (red) is returned to the femoral artery. AO, aorta; ECMO, extracorporeal membrane oxygenation; IVC, inferior vena cava; LA, left atrium; LV, left ventricle; PA, pulmonary artery; RA, right atrium; RV, right ventricle; SVC, superior vena cava; V-A, veno-arterial.

A.13. What are the advantages of using VA-ECMO over other temporary VADs?

The main advantages of VA-ECMO are expeditious percutaneous bedside insertion to provide full circulatory support and rapidly improve tissue perfusion in cardiogenic shock for 7 to 10 days. TEE or fluoroscopy can be used to confirm optimal positioning of the cannulae. Due to these reasons, ECMO use is increasingly popular and has the potential for wider clinical use in severe cardiogenic shock. Temporary VADs can support the LV or RV, increase perfusion in cardiogenic shock, decrease myocardial work, and provide support for up to 30 days. However, temporary VADs have a higher vascular injury rate, more hemolysis, and offer lower cardiac support.

ELSO Guidelines for Cardiopulmonary Extracorporeal Life Support Extracorporeal Life Support Organization, Version 1.4. Accessed May 14, 2023. www.elso.org

Vahdatpour C, Collins D, Goldberg S. Cardiogenic shock. *J Am Heart Assoc*. 2019;8:e011991.

A.14. What is the main disadvantage of VA-ECMO, and how does VA-ECMO affect myocardial recovery?

VA-ECMO increases myocardial perfusion but does not promote myocardial recovery. Blood is pumped retrograde into the aortic root against a poorly functioning LV, resulting in increased LV filling pressures and LV afterload. This is worsened in peripheral VA-ECMO as the oxygenated blood is delivered retrogradely from the femoral artery, which supplies the least oxygenated blood to the coronary arteries. LV filling pressures can be reduced by improving contractility, inserting an IABP, or inserting an Impella.

Mazzeffi MA, Rao VK, Del Rio JM, et al. Intraoperative management of adult patients on extracorporeal membrane oxygenation: an expert consensus statement from the society of cardiovascular anesthesiologists—part I, technical aspects of extracorporeal membrane oxygenation. *J Cardiothorac Vasc Anesth*. 2021;35:3496-3512.

A.15. What is the North-South syndrome and when does it occur?

Peripheral VA-ECMO most often uses the femoral vein and artery for cannulation. As a result, retrograde flow from the arterial cannula into the aorta can compete with the native antegrade flow through the heart. The native flow can often be deoxygenated blood, as lung function can be impaired by pulmonary edema, pneumonia, and so on. This results in differential systemic oxygenation (North/South syndrome), as the blood moving through native circulation through injured lungs has poor oxygenation while retrograde blood from the peripheral arterial cannula delivers oxygenated blood. Arterial blood gas should be checked from the right upper extremity artery to ensure proper cerebral oxygenation.

ELSO Guidelines for Cardiopulmonary Extracorporeal Life Support Extracorporeal Life Support Organization, Version 1.4. Accessed May 14, 2023. www.elso.org

Rao P, Khalpey Z, Smith R, Burkhoff D, Kociol RD. Venoarterial extracorporeal membrane oxygenation for cardiogenic shock and cardiac arrest. *Circ Heart Fail.* 2018;11:e004905.

A.16. How do you treat North-South syndrome?

Treatment usually involves a stepwise approach, considering myocardial and pulmonary recovery. This can be addressed by increasing peripheral VA-ECMO flows to divert blood away from the native flow, optimizing mechanical ventilatory support to improve native oxygenation and ventilation, or an additional venous cannula can be placed to return oxygenated blood into the native circulation.

ELSO Guidelines for Cardiopulmonary Extracorporeal Life Support Extracorporeal Life Support Organization, Version 1.4. Accessed May 14, 2023. www.elso.org

Rao P, Khalpey Z, Smith R, Burkhoff D, Kociol RD. Venoarterial extracorporeal membrane oxygenation for cardiogenic shock and cardiac arrest. *Circ Heart Fail.* 2018;11:e004905.

A.17. What are the most common complications of ECMO?

Complications of ECMO can be patient- or circuit-related. Common circuit-related complications include hemolysis, clotting, cannula-related vascular injury, bleeding due to anticoagulation, and oxygenator dysfunction. Blood clots are the most feared circuit-related complications, and can develop in any part of the ECMO circuit, including the pump, oxygenator, or tubing. Signs of clot formation include rising plasma-free hemoglobin or lactate dehydrogenase, an increasing pressure gradient across the oxygenator, and a fall in post-oxygenator oxygen saturation. Oxygenator dysfunction is often a result of clot formation that reduces gas exchange. Longer-term VV-ECMO will usually require oxygenator changes. Vascular injuries based on cannula location can result in reduced distal tissue perfusion. Most commonly, the risk of distal limb ischemia exists in peripheral femoral arterial cannulation. To prevent ischemia, a distal perfusion catheter is placed in the femoral artery distal to the arterial cannula, to provide antegrade flow to the lower leg.

Patient-related complications include bleeding (cannula site, GI, airway, intracerebral), sepsis, thrombosis, and multiorgan dysfunction.

ELSO Guidelines for Cardiopulmonary Extracorporeal Life Support Extracorporeal Life Support Organization, Version 1.4. Accessed May 14, 2023. www.elso.org

Lafç G, Budak AB, Yener AÜ, et al. Use of extracorporeal membrane oxygenation in adults. *Heart Lung Circ.* 2014;23:10-23.

Rao P, Khalpey Z, Smith R, Burkhoff D, Kociol RD. Venoarterial extracorporeal membrane oxygenation for cardiogenic shock and cardiac arrest. *Circ Heart Fail.* 2018;11:e004905.

A.18. What are the contraindications to ECMO?

The most universally agreed contraindications to ECMO support are the absence of a reversible etiology, short life expectancy due to malignancy or another terminal disease, and ongoing bleeding. Other increasingly debated contraindications include advanced age, obesity, sepsis, end-stage renal disease, end-stage hepatic disease, and coagulopathy.

ELSO Guidelines for Cardiopulmonary Extracorporeal Life Support Extracorporeal Life Support Organization, Version 1.4. Accessed May 14, 2023. www.elso.org

Mazzeffi MA, Rao VK, Del Rio JM, et al. Intraoperative management of adult patients on extracorporeal membrane oxygenation: an expert consensus statement from the society of cardiovascular anesthesiologists—part I, technical aspects of extracorporeal membrane oxygenation. *J Cardiothorac Vasc Anesth.* 2021;35:3496-3512.

A.19. What are the pros and cons of peripheral versus central VA-ECMO cannula placement?

Peripheral VA-ECMO is easier and faster to place emergently, as it can be placed bedside. However, it results in North-South syndrome and increased LV afterload and filling pressures compared to central VA-ECMO. Peripheral cannulation is also associated with an increased risk of limb ischemia and often requires a distal perfusion catheter to perfuse the leg with the arterial cannula.

Central VA-ECMO cannulation (most often placed when unable to wean from CPB) is associated with less risk of right upper extremity and right cerebral ischemia, and less risk of limb ischemia. In addition, it can unload the heart better than peripheral cannulation because of improved LV emptying and decreased afterload. However, it involves surgical removal and is associated with an increased risk of infection, increased reoperation risk for bleeding or tamponade, and higher transfusion requirements.

ELSO Guidelines for Cardiopulmonary Extracorporeal Life Support Extracorporeal Life Support Organization, Version 1.4. Accessed May 14, 2023. www.elso.org

Mariscalco G, Salsano A, Fiore A, et al. Peripheral versus central extracorporeal membrane oxygenation for postcardiotomy shock: multicenter registry, systematic review, and meta-analysis. *J Thorac Cardiovasc Surg*. 2020;160:1207-1216.e44.

Rao P, Khalpey Z, Smith R, Burkhoff D, Kociol RD. Venoarterial extracorporeal membrane oxygenation for cardiogenic shock and cardiac arrest. *Circ Heart Fail*. 2018;11:e004905.

A.20. How can you wean off VA-ECMO?

VA-ECMO requires careful weaning as cardiac and pulmonary recovery is closely evaluated. This usually involves waiting for patient recovery from severe end-organ damage (pulmonary edema, hepatic dysfunction), near resolution of vasopressor requirements and near euvolemic status. Cardiac function is evaluated with serial echocardiograms. When deemed appropriate by the multidisciplinary intensive care unit team, ECMO flow is reduced under close hemodynamic and echocardiographic monitoring. The ECMO flow rate is reduced slowly with concurrent up-titration of ionotropic support. The usual goal is to observe adequate native CO in the setting of less than ~1 to 2 L/min of ECMO flow. A small heparin bolus is usually given before flow reduction (turndown) to reduce the risk of thrombus formation at reduced ECMO flows. Lower flows are only tolerated for a short time to avoid clot formation. If the turndown is tolerated, then the patient is taken to the operating room for removal.

A.21. How can you wean off VV-ECMO?

As native lung function recovers and intrinsic gas exchange improves, the oxygen delivery and ventilation (sweep) from ECMO are weaned. Once the sweep is weaned off, lung function can be monitored briefly before decannulation to rule out deterioration. The patient can then be decannulated, which is often done at the bedside and usually requires stopping heparin infusion for a short period.

ELSO Guidelines for Cardiopulmonary Extracorporeal Life Support Extracorporeal Life Support Organization, Version 1.4. Accessed May 14, 2023. www.elso.org

Mazzeffi MA, Rao VK, Dodd-O J, et al. Intraoperative management of adult patients on extracorporeal membrane oxygenation: an expert consensus statement from the society of cardiovascular anesthesiologists—part II, intraoperative management and troubleshooting. *Anesth Analg*. 2021;133:1478-1493.

B. Indications for LVAD

B.1. What are the indications for LVAD?

Patients with advanced heart failure and New York Heart Association (NYHA) class 3 or 4 symptoms despite medical and resynchronization therapy optimization are candidates for LVAD. Current indications include severe symptomatic functional limitations, objective evidence of cardiac dysfunction, confirmation of functional impairment and worsening clinical picture with poor prognosis. The Interagency Registry for Mechanically Assisted Circulatory Support (INTERMACS) further classifies heart failure patients being considered for mechanical circulatory support (**Figure 6.7**). Implantable LVADs may be indicated for patients who have poor quality of life and medium-term prognosis. However, exclusion criteria include quickly reversible causes of heart failure, significant comorbidity, or other life-limiting illnesses.

Bhagra SK, Pettit S, Parameshwar J. Implantable left ventricular assist device: indications, eligibility and current outcomes. *Heart*. 2022;108:233-241.

B.2. What are the main types of LVAD, and how do they compare in terms of morbidity and mortality following implantation?

The two main types of implanted LVADs include (1) axial flow (HeartMate 2; HM2) and (2) centrifugal flow (Heartmate 3 [HM3] and HeartWare HVAD). **Table 6.1** lists their key differences. The axial flow device (HM 2) has largely been replaced by the centrifugal device (HM 3) based on the Momentum 3 trial which demonstrated that patients with the HeartMate 3 had improved survival and less disabling stroke or reoperation to replace or remove a malfunctioning device at 2 years, as well frequent pump removal. In 2021, Medtronic stopped the sale and distribution of the HeartWare HVAD given the risk of mortality and neurologic adverse events in patients using the device.

Mehra MR, Uriel N, Naka Y, et al. A fully magnetically levitated left ventricular assist device—final report. *N Engl J Med*. 2019;380:1618-1627.

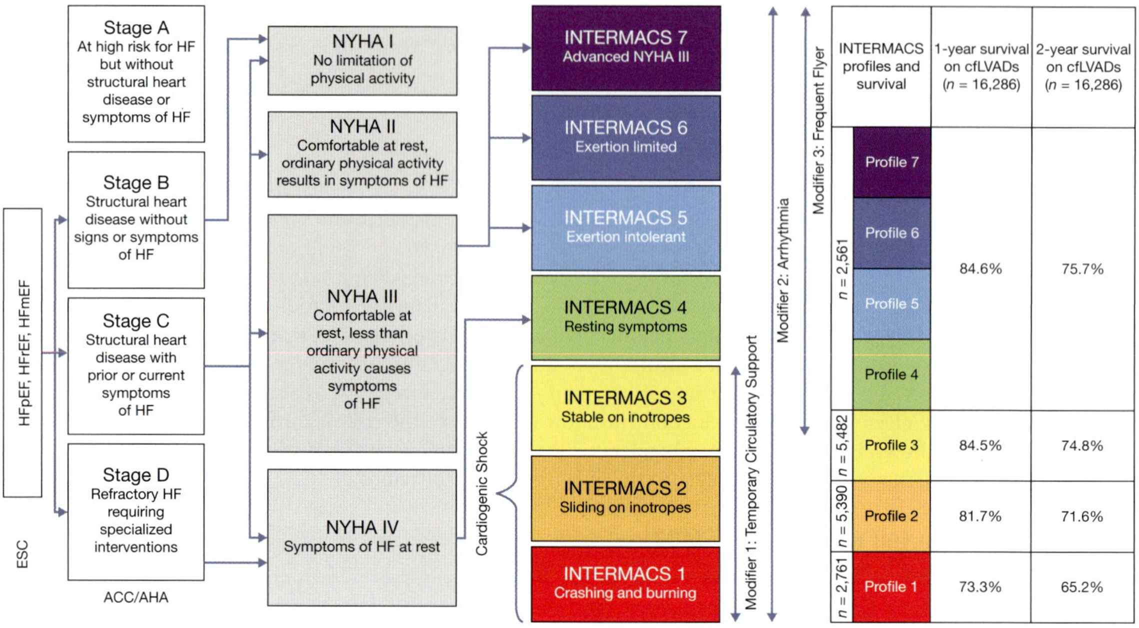

FIGURE 6.7. Categorization of patients with heart failure and 1-year and 2-year survival following LVAD implantation, stratified by INTERMACS profile. ACC/AHA, American College of Cardiology/American Heart Association; ESC, European Society of Cardiology; HF, heart failure; HFmEF, heart failure with mid-range ejection fraction; HFpEF, heart failure with preserved ejection fraction; HFrEF, heart failure with reduced ejection fraction; INTERMACS, Interagency Registry for Mechanically Assisted Circulatory Support; LVADs, continuous-flow left ventricular assist devices; NYHA, New York Heart Association. (From Goldstein DJ, Meyns B, Xie R, et al. Third annual report from the ISHLT mechanically assisted circulatory support registry: a comparison of centrifugal and axial continuous-flow left ventricular assist devices. *J Heart Lung Transplant.* 2019;38:352-363, with permission from Elsevier.)

TABLE 6.1 Key Differences Between the HeartWare, HeartMate 2, and HeartMate 3 Centrifugal Continuous-Flow LVADs

	HeartMate 2	HeartMate 3	HeartWare[a]
Pump properties	Axial flow, requires thoraco-peritoneal placement	Fully magnetically levitated rotor; wide blood flow gaps to decrease shear stress	Both passive magnetic and hydrodynamic thrust to provide contact-free rotation of wide blade impeller
Pump speed	8,800-10,000 rpm	5,000-9,000 rpm	2,400-3,200 rpm
Artificial pulse	N/A	Automatically on; rotor speed changes every 2 s produced by increase and decrease of speed of 2,000 rpm	Rotor speed decreases by 200 rpm for 2 s and increases by 200 rpm for 1 s above set speed with one cycle per minute
Regulatory approval	FDA approved for BTT (2008) and DT (2010)	FDA approved for BTT (2017) and DT (2018)	FDA approved for BTT (2012) and DT (2017), stopped sales in 2021

BTT, bridge to transplantation; DT, destination therapy; FDA, U.S. Food and Drug Administration; LVAD, left ventricular assist device; rpm, rotations per minute.

[a]Taken off the market in 2021 due to device issues.

B.3. What are the three circumstances to consider LVAD placement?

1. As a "bridge to transplantation" (BTT) for patients listed for heart transplant to maintain end-organ perfusion and improve survival to transplantation.
2. As a "bridge to transplant candidacy" (BTC) to reverse contraindications to heart transplant such as pulmonary hypertension and renal dysfunction.
3. As destination therapy (DT) for patients with advanced heart failure and contraindication to heart transplant, LVAD is used to support patients indefinitely. About 5% of these patients have LV recovery, and at 5 years have the LV explanted. For these patients, LVAD becomes a "bridge to recovery."

Teuteberg JJ, Cleveland JC, Cowger J, et al. The Society of Thoracic Surgeons Intermacs 2019 Annual Report: the changing landscape of devices and indications. *Ann Thorac Surg*. 2020;109:649-660.

B.4. What is the latest version of the most common LVAD and why is it better than the previous version?

The HeartMate 3 (HM 3), approved in 2017 by the FDA for BTT and bridge to recovery, is a fully magnetically levitated pump. The wider gap between the impeller and housing decreases shear forces on blood cells as they pass through the pump. The MOMENTUM 3 trial compared the performance of HM 3 to the HM 2 in patients with advanced heart failure, and found that 86% of patients implanted with HM 3 versus 77% of patients with HM 2 survived to 6 months (without a disabling stroke or need to replace the pump), and no HM 3 patients experienced pump thrombosis at 6-months after implantation versus 10% with HM 2.

The ENDURANCE trial demonstrated noninferiority of the intrapericardial continuous-flow HeartWare HVAD compared to the HeartMate 2 for survival in patients with advanced heart failure ineligible for heart transplantation, but stroke was more common. In 2021, Medtronic stopped the sale and distribution of the HeartWare HVAD given the risk of mortality and neurologic adverse events, and a malfunction where the device did not start, causing injuries and death.

Mehra MR, Naka Y, Uriel N, et al. A fully magnetically levitated circulatory pump for advanced heart failure. *N Engl J Med*. 2017;376:440-450.

Rogers JG, Pagani FD, Tatooles AJ, et al. Intrapericardial left ventricular assist device for advanced heart failure. *N Engl J Med*. 2017;376:451-460.

B.5. What is part of the LVAD assessment process?

Prognosis and patient selection for patients with advanced heart failure under consideration for LVAD implantation are similar to heart transplant. Briefly, this includes key assessments of cardiac function and standardized categorization of functional limitation and adverse prognostic markers. Good right heart function is essential and is assessed by echocardiography and cardiac catheterization. After LVAD implantation, the RV must be able to deliver 4 to 5 L/min of blood to the left heart while maintaining reasonable right atrial pressures to avoid renal and liver dysfunction. Poor preoperative right heart function is associated with poor postoperative outcomes after LVAD implantation. **Table 6.2** delineates important echocardiographic and hemodynamic parameters in assessing suitability of LVAD implantation.

Bhagra SK, Pettit S, Parameshwar J. Cardiac transplantation: indications, eligibility and current outcomes. *Heart*. 2019;105:252-260.

Grant ADM, Smedira NG, Starling RC, et al. Independent and incremental role of quantitative right ventricular evaluation for the prediction of right ventricular failure after left ventricular assist device implantation. *J Am Coll Cardiol*. 2012;60:521-528.

Morine KJ, Kiernan MS, Pham DT, et al. Pulmonary artery pulsatility index is associated with right ventricular failure after left ventricular assist device surgery. *J Card Fail*. 2016;22:110-116.

Vivo RP, Cordero-Reyes AM, Qamar U, et al. Increased right-to-left ventricle diameter ratio is a strong predictor of right ventricular failure after left ventricular assist device. *J Heart Lung Transplant*. 2013;32:792-799.

B.6. What are the outcomes related to continuous-flow LVAD placement including survival, morbidity, and quality of life?

Survival: Survival after LVAD continues to improve due to technological advances. In the 2019 INTERMACS report in the United States of 13,016 FDA-approved LVADs from 2014 to 2018, 1-year survival rate was significantly higher for the newer LVADs with full magnetic levitation (HM 3) versus axial flow (HM 2) (87% vs 79%, $P < .001$). Most common causes of death are neurologic (19%), multiorgan failure

TABLE 6.2 Left Ventricular Assist Device (LVAD) Considerations and Relative Contraindications and Parameters Associated With Poor Outcomes

Criteria	Relative Contraindications/Parameter Associated With Poor Outcomes
Age	>65 y
Psychosocial factors	Poor social network/noncompliance with medical advice, substance abuse
Coagulation	Bleeding disorder/unable to tolerate anticoagulation
Liver	Congested hepatopathy/elevated bilirubin
Renal	Advanced/end-stage renal dysfunction
Pulmonary function test	Advanced lung disease
Hemodynamics	CVP > 15 mm Hg
-PAPi (units)	<1.85
-RVSWi (mm Hg·L/m^2)	<0.3
-RAP/PCWP (units)	>0.63
Echocardiography parameters	
-TAPSE (units)	<7.5
-RV-to-LV end-diastolic diameter ratio	>0.75
-RV peak longitudinal strain	>−9.6%

CI, cardiac index; dPA, pulmonary artery diastolic pressure; HR, heart rate; LV, left ventricle; mPA, pulmonary artery mean pressure; PAPi, pulmonary artery pulsatility index; PCWP, pulmonary artery wedge pressure; RAP, right atrial pressure; RV, right ventricle; RVSWi, right ventricular stroke work index; sPA, pulmonary artery systolic pressure; TAPSE, tricuspid annular plane systolic excursion.

(18%), and right heart failure (10%). Short-term survival for the current generation of LVADs is now approaching that following heart transplant but patient selection is critical. Figure 6.7 shows survival stratified by the INTERMACS profile of patients supported on LVADs.

Morbidity: Despite significant improvements in survival, patients with an LVAD still have complications resulting in recurrent hospitalizations. In a US study of 2,510 LVAD recipients, 31% were hospitalized within 30 days, and 75% due to infection, bleeding, and device-related issues. The Society of Thoracic Surgeons annual report showed 2.18 readmissions per patient at 12 months. The most common complications are drive-line infection, GI bleeding, stroke, and pump thrombosis requiring pump replacement.

Quality of life: Several studies have shown improvement in patient functional capacity and quality-of-life parameters after LVAD at 3 months and continuing to at least 2 years, although some groups such as females and older patients take longer to see these improvements. Examples of improved quality of life include 6-minute walking distance increasing from 136 to 325 m at 12 months for HM 3.

Goldstein DJ, Meyns B, Xie R, et al. Third annual report from the ISHLT mechanically assisted circulatory support registry: a comparison of centrifugal and axial continuous-flow left ventricular assist devices. *J Heart Lung Transplant.* 2019;38:352-363.

Kirklin JK, Pagani FD, Kormos RL, et al. Eighth annual INTERMACS report: special focus on framing the impact of adverse events. *J Heart Lung Transplant.* 2017;36:1080-1086.

Maciver J, Ross HJ. Quality of life and left ventricular assist device support. *Circulation.* 2012;126:866-874.

Mehra MR, Uriel N, Naka Y, et al. A fully magnetically levitated left ventricular assist device—final report. *N Engl J Med.* 2019;380:1618-1627.

C. Preoperative Evaluation and Preparation

C.1. What is the focus of the preoperative assessment of a patient with LVAD?

The number of patients with LVADs is increasing mainly due to their success as a destination therapy in advanced heart failure. Therefore, these patients are increasingly encountered for noncardiac surgical procedures. Commonly encountered procedures include upper and lower GI procedures for bleeding due to arteriovenous malformation or larger and more extensive surgical procedures.

TABLE 6.3 Left Ventricular Assist Device (LVAD) Preoperative Considerations

Physical examination	Fluid status, right heart function, signs of worsening heart failure
Laboratory results	Baseline renal function, coagulation panel, hepatic function
Coagulation status	Risk of bleeding vs VAD thrombosis
Chart review	Recent Cardiology notes, echocardiogram, VAD placement, indication for device placement, VAD settings, and cardiac implantable devices settings
Perioperative care team	Cardiologist, VAD coordinator, cardiac surgeon, cardiac anesthesiologist, perfusionist

VAD, ventricular assist device.

Preoperative evaluation should include a standard evaluation assessing current state of health and changes in exercise tolerance to screen for symptoms of acute heart failure. A careful physical examination should be performed to determine fluid status, right heart function, and signs of worsening heart failure. Medications, recent cardiology notes, and laboratory results should be reviewed. The medication list should be examined for diuretics, inotropes, anticoagulants, and anti-arrhythmic therapies. Laboratory results should be reviewed for baseline renal function, coagulation panel (as all these patients should be on anticoagulation), and hepatic function (which can indicate worsening right heart function). Patients often have renal impairment, and renal precautions should be taken during surgery. Coagulation status should be carefully assessed. The risk of bleeding versus thrombosis should be assessed for each individual procedure to determine whether to stop or bridge anticoagulation perioperatively.

The most recent cardiology note should be reviewed for the type of VAD, indication for device placement, settings (including flow rate, device alarms, power elevations, and backup battery life), and any other device interrogations (ie, pacemakers and implantable cardioverter-defibrillators [ICDs]). Many of these patients have implanted defibrillators. Depending on the procedure, tachyarrhythmia therapies might need to be disabled, and the pacemaker function might need to be switched to asynchronous mode if electrocautery interference is anticipated.

The most recent echocardiogram should be reviewed for inflow cannula position, outflow graft patency, and importantly RV function and tricuspid regurgitation. The most common valvular pathologies present in patients with LVAD are aortic stenosis and insufficiency, as well as tricuspid insufficiency.

Patients with VADs should ideally be cared for at a facility that has a support team dedicated to caring for these patients perioperatively. Members of this team should include a cardiologist, a VAD coordinator, cardiac surgeons, cardiac anesthesiologists, and perfusionists. The team should be notified in advance, if possible, that the patient with a VAD will be presenting for a procedure.

Patients with LVAD require extensive support services, including coverage by a specialized nurse or physician assistant specifically assigned to the hospital VAD program. These specialists may accompany patients with VAD to the operating room in some circumstances and are knowledgeable in the intricacies of individual VADs. In addition, device manufacturers have 24-hour support services and are a source of useful clinical information. These preoperative considerations are summarized in **Table 6.3**.

Dalia AA, Cronin B, Stone ME, et al. Anesthetic management of patients with continuous-flow left ventricular assist devices undergoing noncardiac surgery: an update for anesthesiologists. *J Cardiothorac Vasc Anesth*. 2018;32:1001-1012.

Han JJ, Acker MA, Atluri P. Left ventricular assist devices. *Circulation*. 2018;138:2841-2851.

Nicolosi AC, Pagel PS. Perioperative considerations in the patient with a left ventricular assist device. *Anesthesiology*. 2003;98:565-570.

D. Intraoperative Management

D.1. Detail the anesthetic management for a patient undergoing LVAD placement

Management of patients requiring LVAD placement can be divided into the preoperative, intraoperative, and postoperative periods.

Preoperatively, a patient requiring an LVAD will, by definition, have severely reduced LV function. They may require mechanical ventilation, multiple inotropes, vasopressors, and/or an IABP. Due to chronic heart failure and its treatment, such patients can have profoundly abnormal electrolytes, liver, renal, and coagulation function tests. Preoperative echocardiography demonstrating the presence of pulmonary hypertension, impaired RV function, or tricuspid regurgitation is particularly important because these findings indicate the possible need for RV support or even placement of a right ventricular assist device. Severe irreversible pulmonary hypertension, severe tricuspid regurgitation, and severe RV dysfunction can be a contraindication for an LVAD or indicate the need for a biventricular ventricular assist device (BiVAD).

An arterial catheter is placed prior to the induction of anesthesia for monitoring. No matter the choice of anesthetic, myocardial depression or rapid changes in systemic vascular resistance must be avoided. Given patients' slow circulation, preemptive administration of vasopressors is prudent to offset unwanted side effects of induction agents. To avoid possible acute RV dysfunction due to hypoxia and hypercarbia, ventilation and tracheal intubation should be accomplished expeditiously. Early administration of neuromuscular blocking agents and controlled lung ventilation with low inspiratory airway pressure are suggested to avoid increases in intrathoracic pressure that can have a deleterious effect on the right heart. Once anesthesia is successfully induced, ICDs must be deactivated, and the pacing mode changed to allow use of intraoperative electrocautery. Large-bore peripheral and central intravenous access and a PAC should be placed. Large-bore venous access is especially important for patients who have had prior cardiac surgery because of the risk of adhesions and massive hemorrhage. Blood and blood products should be available in case of major bleeding.

Intraoperatively, the anesthetic goals are to avoid deterioration of existing cardiac function, to avoid hypovolemia and anemia, and to optimize cardiovascular status while the LVAD is implanted under CPB. Because the primary concern in a patient undergoing an LVAD implantation is RV failure, real-time monitoring of central venous pressure (and its association with pulmonary pressures) is crucial. TEE is invaluable in patients undergoing LVAD placement, and a complete echocardiographic assessment should be performed on every patient. The focus of TEE examination is assessment of (1) atrial septal defects, which can predispose to hypoxemia due to right-to-left shunting after VAD placement as left atrial pressures are decreased; (2) aortic regurgitation, which will cause a "recycling" of blood from the aorta back to the LV; (3) tricuspid regurgitation, which can cause or exacerbate RV failure; (4) mitral stenosis, which can decrease LV filling and therefore the "preload" to the LVAD; (5) an intracardiac LV thrombus; and (6) preexisting RV dysfunction.

Following LVAD implantation and following CPB, focus is placed on maintaining euvolemia, treating coagulation abnormalities, and supporting RV function. Vasoactive medications and inotropes are infused and frequently inhaled such as nitric oxide (NO) or prostacyclin, which are administered to ameliorate pulmonary hypertension. Those patients treated with pulmonary vasodilators early after LVAD placement had a decreased incidence of RV failure in observational studies. Patients with VADs require long-term anticoagulation.

Critoph C, Green G, Hayes H, et al. Clinical outcomes of patients treated with pulmonary vasodilators early and in high doses after left ventricular assist device implantation. *Artif Organs.* 2016;40:106-114.

Dalia AA, Cronin B, Stone ME, et al. Anesthetic management of patients with continuous-flow left ventricular assist devices undergoing noncardiac surgery: an update for anesthesiologists. *J Cardiothorac Vasc Anesth.* 2018;32:1001-1012.

Nicolosi AC, Pagel PS. Perioperative considerations in the patient with a left ventricular assist device. *Anesthesiology.* 2003;98:565-570.

Sparrow CT, LaRue SJ, Schilling JD. Intersection of pulmonary hypertension and right ventricular dysfunction in patients on left ventricular assist device support: is there a role for pulmonary vasodilators? *Circ Heart Fail.* 2018;11:e004255.

D.2. How is a patient with VAD monitored during a general anesthetic?

Standard American Society of Anesthesiologists monitoring is used at a minimum. Due to the continuous flow of newer VADs, noninvasive blood pressure cuffs and pulse oximeters may not function reliably in all patients. Nevertheless, mean arterial blood pressure should be monitored with noninvasive or direct measurements, and oxygenation determined by arterial blood gas measurement or continuously by cerebral oxygenation monitors. When arterial line placement is necessary, an ultrasound can help locate the vessel, as the systemic pulse is weak or nonpalpable. Monitoring central venous pressure or placement of a PAC must be individualized based on anticipated fluid shifts and risk of the procedure as well as underlying RV function. In patients with impaired RV function or for procedures involving large fluid shifts, intraoperative TEE is recommended.

No consensus guidelines currently exist to recommend whether these patients should be cared for by a cardiac or general anesthesiologist in the setting of noncardiac surgery. It is generally agreed that the anesthesiologist should be familiar with LVAD settings and specific alarms. Increasingly, these patients are cared for safely by general anesthesiologists, especially patients who are stable on their LVADs, do not require pharmacologic support, and are scheduled for noncardiac surgery where significant hemodynamic changes are not expected. Patients with LVADs on medical therapy for heart failure, have major co-morbidities, and are scheduled for high-risk surgery with likely hemodynamic instability should be cared for by a cardiac anesthesiologist.

Invasive arterial blood pressure monitoring is recommended for major surgery, given its accuracy, reliability, and ability to obtain arterial blood gases. Mean arterial pressure (MAP) should generally be kept at less than 85 mm Hg, given concerns for reduced LVAD flow, pump stasis, and risk of stroke at higher MAPs.

In the event of cardiac arrest, standard advanced cardiac life support (ACLS) should be employed including chest compressions; this policy has changed in recent years because previously chest compressions were thought to be contraindicated due to fear of disrupting or dislodging the VAD cannulas. The priority of resuscitation should be to troubleshoot the malfunctioning LVAD.

Dalia AA, Cronin B, Stone ME, et al. Anesthetic management of patients with continuous-flow left ventricular assist devices undergoing noncardiac surgery: an update for anesthesiologists. *J Cardiothorac Vasc Anesth.* 2018;32:1001-1012.

Peberdy MA, Gluck JA, Ornato JP, et al. Cardiopulmonary resuscitation in adults and children with mechanical circulatory support: a scientific statement from the American Heart Association. *Circulation.* 2017;135:e1115-e1134.

D.3. What are the most common VAD settings?

Common VAD settings: *Pulsatility index* (PI) is a dimensionless measure of LV pulsatility, ranging from 1 to 10, with an average of 5 for the HeartMate LVADs. It is increased in the setting of adequate LV preload and suggests LV systolic augmentation and a low PI represents low preload or contractility. Increasing pump speed by decompressing the LV will typically decrease PI and *vice versa.* Once a normal PI range is determined for a patient, it should not vary significantly. *Pump speed* is determined to allow adequate LV preload for intermittent LV ejection and avoid suction events. A low speed can cause pump stasis and thrombosis, and a high speed can cause hemolysis, excessive LV decompression, and suction events, as well as RV dysfunction. *Pump power,* which typically correlates directly with pump speed, can be reduced secondary to inflow cannula obstruction or reduced LV preload. An increase in pump power without increased pump flow should raise suspicion for pump thrombosis.

Dalia AA, Cronin B, Stone ME, et al. Anesthetic management of patients with continuous-flow left ventricular assist devices undergoing noncardiac surgery: an update for anesthesiologists. *J Cardiothorac Vasc Anesth.* 2018;32:1001-1012.

Nicolosi AC, Pagel PS. Perioperative considerations in the patient with a left ventricular assist device. *Anesthesiology.* 2003;98:565-570.

Stone M, Hinchey J, Sattler C, et al. Trends in the management of patients with left ventricular assist devices presenting for noncardiac surgery: a 10-year institutional experience. *Semin Cardiothorac Vasc Anesth.* 2016;20:197-204.

D.4. What are some important considerations of patients with LVAD for postoperative management?

Patients can be recovered in the standard postoperative anesthesia care unit unless intensive care is required. After arriving in the postanesthesia care unit (PACU), ensure that an ICD is reprogrammed to active therapy. Patients should be extubated when they meet criteria; however, extra care should be taken during tracheal extubation to minimize hypertension and tachycardia that can decrease LVAD output.

Adequate analgesia is important with appropriate caution to prevent hypoxia, hypercarbia, and acidosis, which can increase RV afterload and potentiate RV failure.

Reinstitution of full anticoagulation occurs when the risk of postoperative bleeding is low. Patients are usually bridged to heparin with a partial thromboplastin time (PTT) of 60 to 80 seconds until the international normalized ratio (INR) reaches a target range of 2.0 to 3.0. Postoperative bleeding is a common complication and should be monitored carefully, especially during the reinstitution of anticoagulation.

7 Valvular Heart Disease

Margo Hoyler and Natalia Ivascu Girardi

A 78-year-old male was admitted with increasing shortness of breath. He had chest pain in the past but was able to continue with normal activities. In the prior year, he experienced two episodes of syncope. On physical examination, a loud systolic murmur could be heard at the left sternal border radiating to the neck. His vital signs were blood pressure 150/90 mm Hg and heart rate 88 beats per minute and irregular. The electrocardiogram (ECG) showed sinus rhythm with atrial premature contractions and left ventricular hypertrophy (LVH) with strain. A transthoracic echocardiogram (TTE) showed a hypertrophied left ventricle (LV), and Doppler echocardiography examination demonstrated severe aortic stenosis (AS) with a mean pressure gradient of 64 mm Hg, mild aortic insufficiency (AI), and moderate mitral regurgitation (MR). He was scheduled for an aortic valve (AV) replacement and a possible mitral valve (MV) repair or replacement.

A. Medical Disease and Differential Diagnosis

1. What are the major etiologies of AS, AI, mitral stenosis (MS), and MR?
2. What are the major changes in the loading conditions of the LV that result from the four different lesions? Why do they occur? What changes result from them?
3. What are pressure-volume (*P-V*) loops? What do the different inflection points represent?
4. What are representative *P-V* loops for the four valvular lesions?
5. Draw the pressure/time curves for the LV, left atrium (LA), pulmonary artery (PA), and aorta for a normal patient and for patients with each of the four valvular lesions.
6. What are the basic principles of echocardiography? What are M-mode, B-mode, and Doppler color modalities? How are pressure gradients measured by echocardiography? How do TTE and transesophageal echocardiography (TEE) differ?
7. What are the three TEE vantage points for comprehensive imaging of the LV? How are pressure gradients measured by echocardiography? How do pressure gradients derived from Doppler echocardiography differ from those obtained in the catheterization laboratory by direct pressure measurement?
8. What is the purpose of the basic perioperative TEE examination? Describe the standard views that comprise this examination.
9. What is the role for three-dimensional (3D) echocardiography in the operating room?
10. What are the echocardiographic and cardiac catheterization criteria for the four valvular lesions?

B. Preoperative Evaluation and Preparation

1. What are the presenting signs and symptoms of the four valvular lesions listed previously?
2. What is the New York Heart Association classification of heart failure?
3. Discuss the role of premedication for patients with the four different valvular lesions.
4. How would you premedicate the patient with severe AS and MR?

C. Intraoperative Management

1. Outline the hemodynamic management goals for each of the four valvular lesions. What are the anesthetic goals with respect to heart rate and rhythm, preload, afterload, and contractility?
2. What are the hemodynamic goals for this patient with a combination of severe AS and MR?
3. How would you monitor this patient with severe AS and MR?
4. Should the patient have a PA catheter placed before induction?
5. Is a PA catheter with pacing capabilities indicated?
6. What anesthetic technique would you employ? Why?

7. What are the usual TEE findings in a patient with AS or MR? How do you grade the severity of AS by TEE? How do you quantify the severity of MR? What is the impact of AS on the severity of MR?
8. What special considerations particular to cardiopulmonary bypass (CPB) operations do you have for each of the four lesions? Focus on these concerns with respect to the induction and pre-bypass, during bypass, and post-bypass periods.
9. The patient cannot be weaned from CPB following an AV and MV replacement. What are the possible causes?
10. How would you diagnose right-sided heart failure and pulmonary hypertension? How would you treat it?
11. How does an intra-aortic balloon pump (IABP) work to benefit the failing heart?
12. What role does the IABP have in this setting?
13. What role does TEE play in the placement, timing, and demonstration of efficacy of an IABP?
14. How would you properly time the IABP cycle?
15. What are the contraindications to the use of an IABP?
16. What is the role for ventricular assist devices (VADs)?

D. Postoperative Management

1. In the intensive care unit (ICU) 4 hours later, the patient became hypotensive with a low cardiac output. How could you distinguish between cardiac tamponade and pump failure? How would the TEE images differ?
2. Would you extubate this patient early in the ICU? Why?
3. What are the advantages and disadvantages of early tracheal extubation?

E. Alternative Treatments

1. What are the transcatheter options for MV repair and replacement? How are these procedures performed? What anesthetic management is indicated?
2. What are the transcatheter options for AV replacement?
3. How is transcatheter AV replacement performed?
4. What anesthetic techniques, monitors and access are indicated? What complications can occur following transcatheter aortic valve replacement (TAVR)?
5. What is minimally invasive cardiac valve surgery?

A. Medical Disease and Differential Diagnosis

A.1. What are the major etiologies of AS, AI, mitral stenosis (MS), and MR?

AS occurs as a congenital lesion but more commonly as an acquired disease. Stenosis can develop on a previously normal AV following rheumatic fever or from progressive calcification. Congenitally bicuspid AVs are also prone to calcification with eventual stenosis. Calcification of the AV leaflets can result in incomplete closure of the valve with associated insufficiency.

AI is usually an acquired disease. The most common causes include bacterial endocarditis and rheumatic heart disease (RHD). Annular dilation with resultant AI can result from connective tissue diseases, proximal aortic aneurysms or aortic dissection.

MS is almost always caused by RHD. Although rare in high-income countries, RHD remains the leading cause of primary valvular heart disease worldwide. The inflammatory process of RHD results in thickening of the leaflets and fusion of the commissures. Other rare causes of MS include congenital stenosis and systemic diseases such as systemic lupus erythematosus and carcinoid. Pathophysiology similar to that seen with valvular MS can occur with obstructing left atrial tumors and cor triatriatum.

MR can result from defects in the leaflets, the annular ring, or the supporting chords or papillary muscles (PM) or any combination of these. Primary leaflet dysfunction occurs with RHD (ultimately leading to calcification and MS) but can also follow bacterial endocarditis, connective tissue disorders, myxomatous degeneration, and congenital malformations. Annular dilation can follow left ventricular dysfunction and dilation. MV prolapse and rupture of PM result in incomplete leaflet closure or coaptation with resultant MR. Left ventricular ischemia can affect PM contraction and lead to functional MR.

Coffey S, Roberts-Thomson R, Brown A, et al. Global epidemiology of valvular heart disease. *Nat Rev Cardiol.* 2021;18:853-864.

Otto CM, Nishimura RA, Bonow RO, et al. 2020 ACC/AHA guideline for the management of patients with valvular heart disease: executive summary: a report of the American College of Cardiology/American Heart Association Joint Committee on Clinical Practice Guidelines. *Circulation*. 2021;143:e35-e71.

Pandian NG, Kim JK, Arias-Godinez JA, et al. Recommendations for the use of echocardiography in the evaluation of rheumatic heart disease: a report from the American Society of Echocardiography. *J Am Soc Echocardiogr*. 2023;36:3-28.

A.2. What are the major changes in the loading conditions of the LV that result from the four different lesions? Why do they occur? What changes result from them?

AS represents a chronic systolic pressure load on the LV. This increases the wall tension (stress) in accordance with Laplace's law:

$$\text{Wall tension} = \frac{(\text{Pressure} \times \text{Radius})}{(2 \times \text{Wall thickness})}$$

The LV undergoes parallel duplication of muscle fibers to compensate for increased wall stress. This results in increased wall thickness (concentric hypertrophy) and some decrease in radius, thereby normalizing wall stress. If the MV remains competent, then little change occurs in the other cardiac chambers.

AI causes left ventricular diastolic volume overload due to the additional volume flowing retrograde into the LV across the incompetent AV during diastole. This results in eccentric hypertrophy and left ventricular dilation (increased muscle mass and chamber radius). However, AI decreases aortic diastolic pressure, which is the pressure that must be exceeded by the contracting LV to open the AV and result in left ventricular systolic ejection. Therefore, left ventricular work is performed against a lower outflow impedance (aortic diastolic pressure). Stroke volume and ejection fraction may be preserved until late in the disease process. As with AS, the presence of a competent MV confines the changes to the LV. However, the left ventricular dilation that follows chronic AI may result in mitral annular dilation or alteration in the PM orientations with resultant MR. Left atrial enlargement secondary to MR, or left atrial pressure overload due to increasing left ventricular end-diastolic pressure (LVEDP) in the course of AI, can occur.

MS results in a chronically underfilled LV because of progressive obstruction to left atrial emptying. This chronic underloading condition can result in diminished contractile function ("disuse atrophy"). In addition, if the cause of the MS is rheumatic, then myofibril damage can also occur. Contrary to the left ventricular pressure and volume underloading, the LA is both pressure and volume overloaded to maintain flow across the progressively narrowing mitral orifice. According to Gorlin's equation for pressure gradient,

$$\text{Pressure gradient (mm Hg)} = \left\{ \frac{\text{Valve flow rate (mL/s)}}{\left[K \times \text{valve area (cm}^2\text{)} \right]} \right\}^2$$

the pressure gradient increases by the square of any increase in flow rate or decrease in valve area. The elevated left atrial pressure leads to left atrial hypertrophy and eventually dilation that predisposes to premature atrial contractions and subsequent atrial fibrillation. The loss of atrial contraction will further diminish the flow across the stenotic MV. At the same time, elevated left atrial pressure hinders pulmonary venous flow and causes pulmonary vascular engorgement. This leads to intimal hypertrophy that induces irreversible elevations in pulmonary vascular resistance. As a consequence of pulmonary hypertension, the right ventricular (RV) systolic pressure increases and right ventricle dilates, potentially leading to RV failure and tricuspid regurgitation (TR).

MR results in volume overload of the LV. In MR, the LV ejects into both systemic circulation (across the AV; high afterload and low compliance) and retrograde to the LA (low afterload and high compliance) across the incompetent MV. This "back and forth" of the regurgitant volume results in left ventricular volume overload. However, this additional work is performed at a low pressure; therefore, left ventricular wall tension is minimally increased initially. As with AI, the volume overload results in marked left ventricular dilation and eccentric hypertrophy. At the same time, the LA is also volume overloaded and undergoes dilation. When the volume overload occurs slowly, the pulmonary pressures increase minimally despite large regurgitant volumes. In contrast, acute MR, as can occur following acute myocardial infarction with PM rupture, presents a sudden volume overload to the LA. Without time to dilate, the left atrial pressure rises rapidly, thereby limiting pulmonary drainage with resultant pulmonary engorgement and acute increase in PA pressures.

Lilly LS. Valvular heart disease. In: Lilly LS, ed. *Pathophysiology of Heart Disease: An Introduction to Cardiovascular Medicine*. 7th ed. Wolters Kluwer; 2021:202-231.

Ramakrishan H, Craner RC, Devaleria PA, Cook DJ, Housmans PR, Rehfeldt KH. Valvular heart disease: replacement and repair. In: Kaplan JA, Augustides J, Maneck GR, Maus T, eds. *Kaplan's Cardiac Anesthesia*. 7th ed. Elsevier; 2017:770-817.

A.3. What are pressure-volume (*P-V*) loops? What do the different inflection points represent?

The *P-V* loop (**Figure 7.1**) depicts the relation between ventricular volume and pressure during a single cardiac cycle. Opening and closing of the MV and AV are represented by the inflection points A, B, C, and D, respectively (**Figure 7.1**). Moving from points A to D, AB depicts left ventricular filling, BC depicts isovolumetric contraction, CD shows left ventricular ejection, and DA shows isovolumetric relaxation. Point A coincides with opening of the MV and represents left ventricular end-systolic volume and early diastolic pressure. Point B is closure of the MV and the relationship of end-diastolic pressure (LVEDP) and volume (left ventricular end-diastolic volume [LVEDV]). Point C represents the opening of the AV and coincides with systemic, aortic diastolic pressure. Finally, point D is the closure of the AV and represents left ventricular end-systolic pressure (LVESP) and volume (LVESV), coinciding with the dicrotic notch in the aortic pressure tracing (**Figure 7.1**). Left ventricular compliance is the relation between pressure and volume and is defined by the slope of the filling phase (segment AB). Preload is the *P-V* relation before the onset of contraction (LVEDP). Contractility may be illustrated by the slope of the *end-systolic pressure–volume relation* (ESPVR). The ESPVR slope is created by connecting multiple points (D) from multiple *P-V* loops generated by changing the filling volume to the LV (**Figure 7.2**). Increased contractility results in a steeper slope, whereas diminished contractility results in a shallower slope. The *P-V* loop analysis permits illustration of stroke volume and ejection fraction. Stroke volume is defined as difference in volume from the end of filling to the end of ejection (EDV–ESV), whereas the ejection fraction is the ratio of stroke volume to total volume in the heart at peak filling (SV/EDV). Therefore, the *P-V* loop analysis permits illustration of the volume-pressure relations and their changes with each of the four valvular lesions.

Bastos MB, Burkhoff D, Maly J, et al. Invasive left ventricle pressure-volume analysis: overview and practical clinical implications. *Eur Heart J*. 2020;41:1286-1297.

Hsu S, Fang JC, Borlaug BA. Hemodynamics for the heart failure clinician: a state-of-the-art review. *J Card Fail*. 2022;28:133-148.

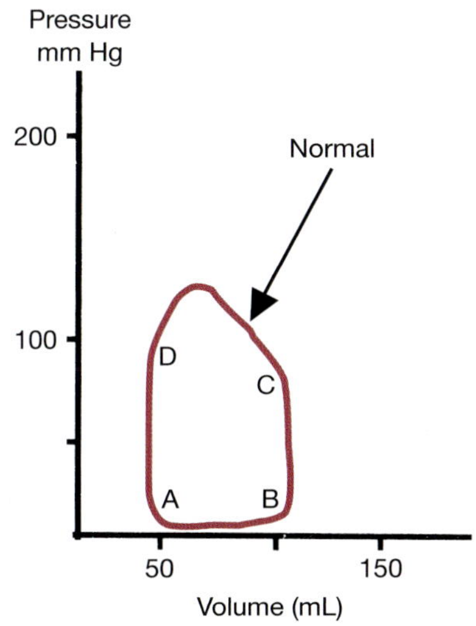

FIGURE 7.1. Normal *P-V* loop and valve positions. A, mitral valve (MV) opening; AB, left ventricular filling; B, MV closure; BC, isovolumetric contraction; C, aortic valve (AV) opening; CD, ejection; D, AV closure; DA, isovolumetric relaxation.

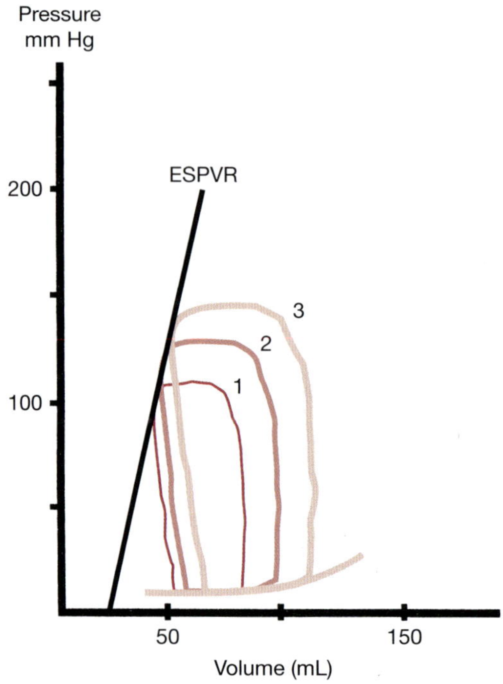

FIGURE 7.2. Contractility. ESPVR, end-systolic pressure-volume relation.

Salgado BC, Bhimaraj A. Physiological concepts of cardiogenic shock using pressure-volume loop simulations: a case-based review. *Methodist Debakey Cardiovasc J*. 2020;16:43-49.

A.4. What are representative *P-V* loops for the four valvular lesions?

The hallmarks of AS, illustrated by the *P-V* loop analysis, are an increased left ventricular systolic pressure and an upward and counterclockwise rotation in the end-diastolic *P-V* relation (AB) indicative of decreased chamber compliance (Figure 7.3). Stroke volume and ejection fraction are well preserved, but the ejection phase of the loop occurs at much higher pressures. This is accomplished by an increase in contractility (counterclockwise rotation of the ESPVR).

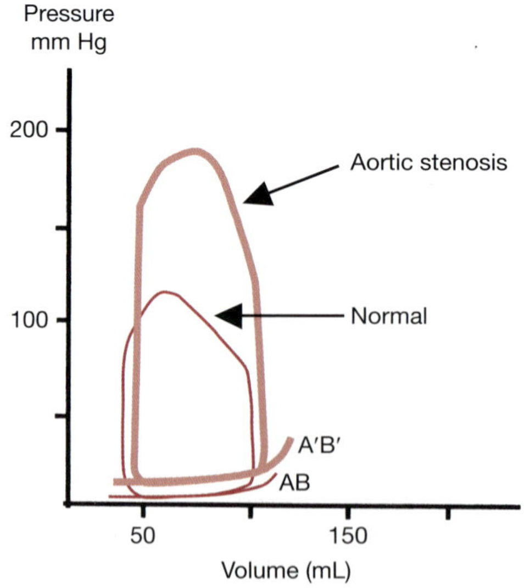

FIGURE 7.3. *P-V* loop of aortic stenosis.

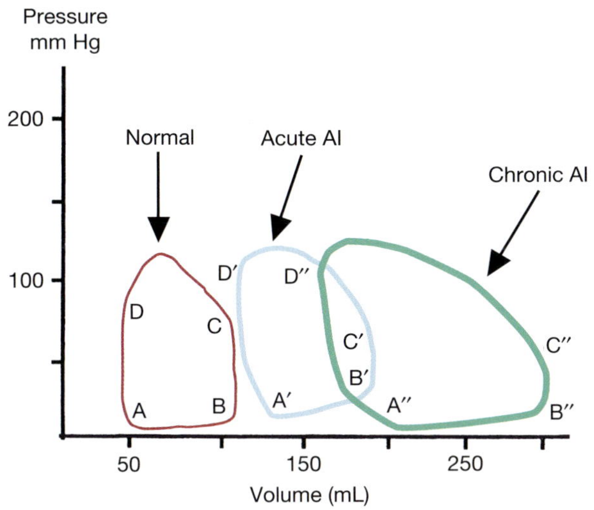

FIGURE 7.4. ***P-V*** **loops of acute and chronic aortic insufficiency (AI).**

The schematic *P-V* loop for chronic AI depicts an enlarged LV. The minimal change in LVEDP despite the large volume overload is seen by the shift in the diastolic *P-V* curve to the right (A″B″) (**Figure 7.4**). Low systemic diastolic pressures result in a brief isovolumetric phase (B″C″) and early complete ejection. The isovolumetric relaxation phase is absent because the incompetent valve permits regurgitant filling of the LV from the aorta during diastole even before opening of the MV. In contrast, when acute AI occurs, the left ventricular compliance is unchanged. Rapid increases in LVEDP from volume overload along the unshifted left ventricular diastolic *P-V* curve (A′B′) rapidly lead to increased left atrial pressure and pulmonary congestion.

The *P-V* loop of MS illustrates hypovolemia, the cause of which cannot be determined from the loop alone (**Figure 7.5**). Because the predominant impact of MS occurs proximal to the LV, the *P-V* analysis format is less useful.

In MR, the diastolic *P-V* relation (line AB) is shifted to the right, as it is in chronic AI, consistent with a marked increase in compliance (**Figure 7.6**). The isovolumetric phase (BC) is nearly absent because the LA generally serves as a low-pressure/high-compliance route for ejection through an incompetent MV. Decreases in contractility are depicted by a decrease in the slope of the ESPVR (line through D).

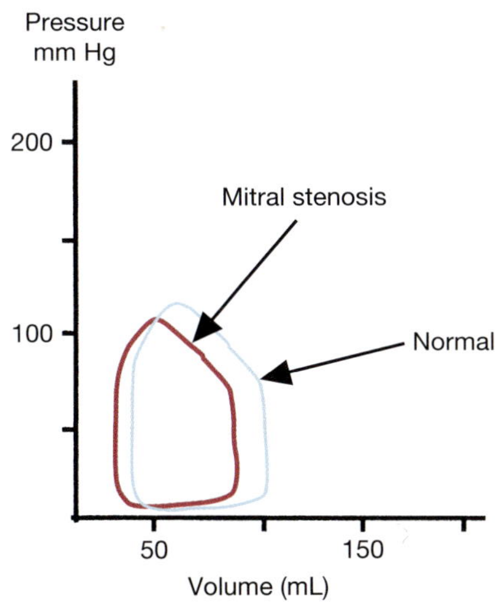

FIGURE 7.5. ***P-V*** **loops of mitral stenosis.**

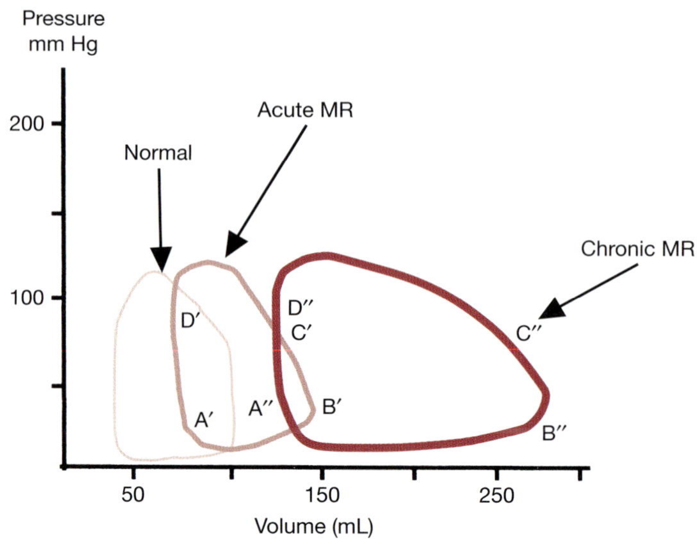

FIGURE 7.6. ***P-V* loop of acute and chronic mitral regurgitation (MR).**

Bastos MB, Burkhoff D, Maly J, et al. Invasive left ventricle pressure-volume analysis: overview and practical clinical implications. *Eur Heart J.* 2020;41:1286-1297.

Hsu S, Fang JC, Borlaug BA. Hemodynamics for the heart failure clinician: a state-of-the-art review. *J Card Fail.* 2022;28:133-148.

Nishimura RA, Carabello BA. Hemodynamics in the cardiac catheterization laboratory of the 21st century. *Circulation.* 2012;125:2138-2150.

A.5. Draw the pressure/time curves for the LV, left atrium (LA), pulmonary artery (PA), and aorta for a normal patient and for patients with each of the four valvular lesions.

Normal curves are shown in Figure 7.7. The points A, B, C, and D correspond to the same points in the *P-V* loops.

Aortic Stenosis

The additional systolic pressure work of AS can be seen in the left ventricular pressure tracing (Figure 7.8). Elevations in LVEDP (point B) can be seen to diminish the perfusion gradient for coronary flow to the LV. The augmentation in left ventricular filling late in diastole secondary to atrial contraction (left atrial "kick" from sinus rhythm) is highlighted in the inset. Rising left ventricular diastolic pressures secondary to decreased compliance necessitate elevations in left atrial pressures to permit complete left ventricular volume loading. Atrial systole provides this elevation in left atrial pressure synchronous with elevations in LVEDP while keeping left atrial pressures relatively low during the remaining cardiac cycle facilitating pulmonary venous drainage.

Aortic Insufficiency

The rapid upstroke and rapid decline of arterial pressure indicate absence of AV closure and low end-diastolic aortic pressure (Figure 7.9). Elevations in LVEDV and LVEDP are typical of AI. The early increase in LVEDP can result in left ventricular pressures exceeding those of the LA during diastole, with resultant premature closure of the MV.

Mitral Stenosis

Elevations in pressure are seen in both the left atrial and PA tracing with MS (Figure 7.10). The large gradient between left atrial and left ventricular pressures is highlighted in the inset. Chronic elevation in pulmonary volume induces changes the pulmonary arterial vascular bed and results in pulmonary hypertension.

Mitral Regurgitation

The hallmark of MR is the marked elevations of left atrial pressure during systole and the occurrence of a giant "cv" wave and elevated PA pressures (Figure 7.11).

Bowcock EM, McLean A. Bedside assessment of left atrial pressure in critical care: a multifaceted gem. *Crit Care.* 2022;26:247-263.

Pighi M, Asgar AW. Invasive hemodynamics of valvular heart disease. *Interv Cardiol Clin.* 2017;6:319-327.

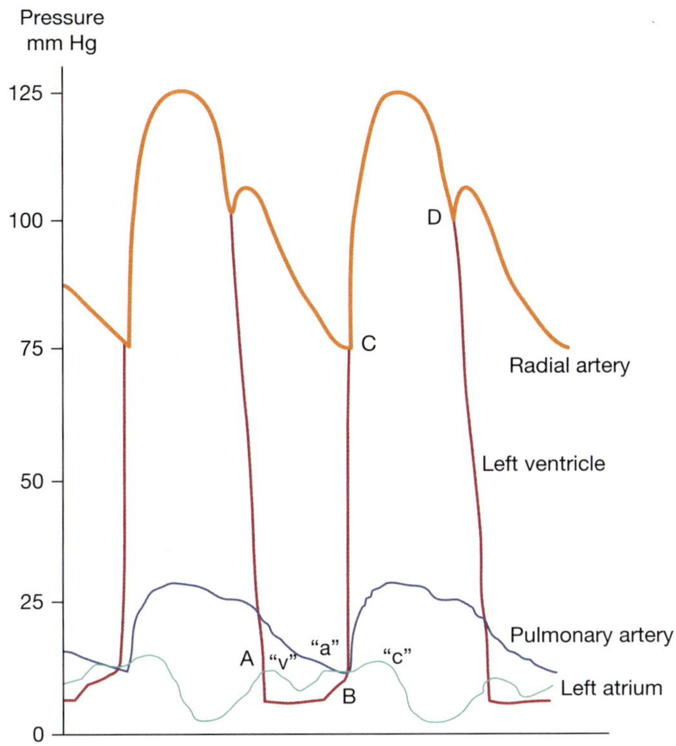

FIGURE 7.7. **Pressure curves for the LV, left atrium, pulmonary artery, and aorta in a healthy individual.**

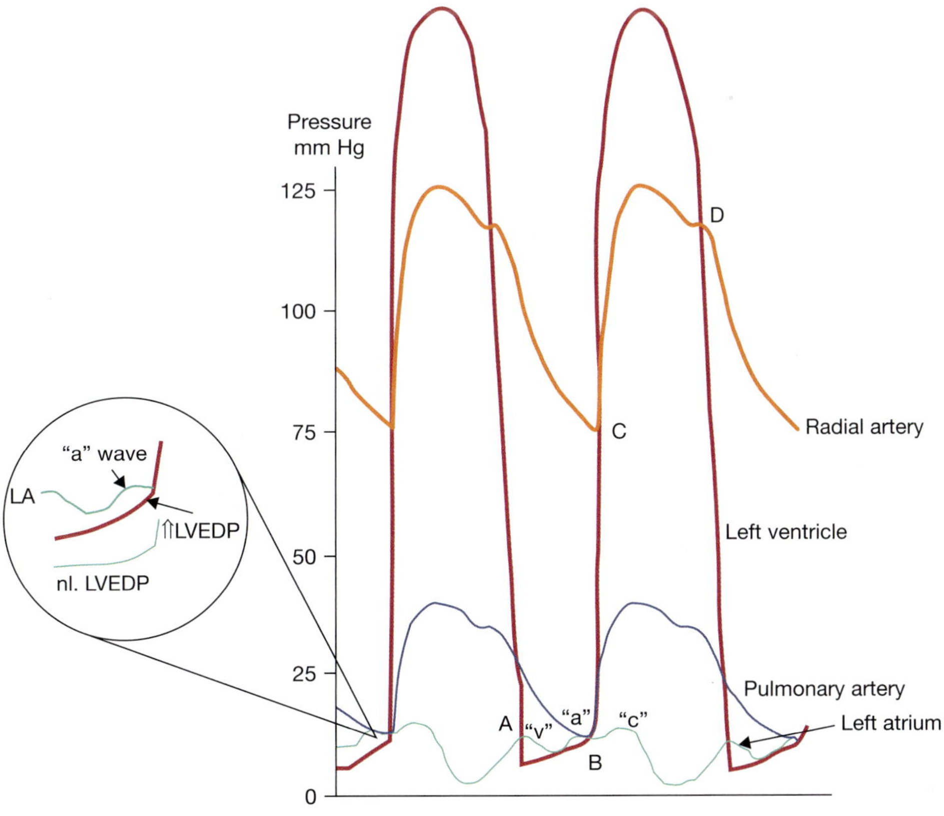

FIGURE 7.8. **Pressure curves for the LV, left atrium (LA), pulmonary artery, and aorta in patients with aortic stenosis.** LVEDP, left ventricular end-diastolic pressure.

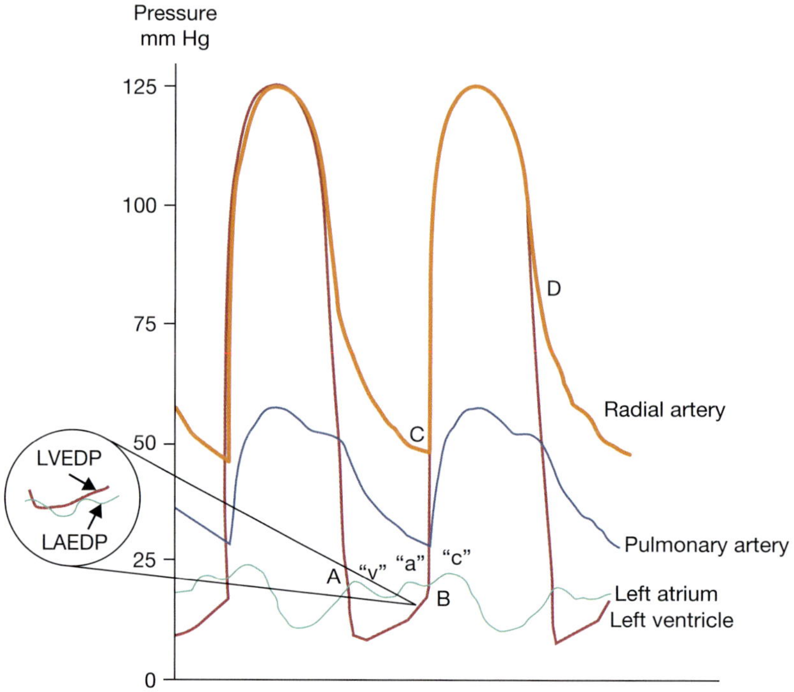

FIGURE 7.9. Pressure curves for the LV, left atrium, pulmonary artery, and aorta in patients with aortic regurgitation. LAEDP, left atrium end-diastolic pressure; LVEDP, left ventricular end-diastolic pressure.

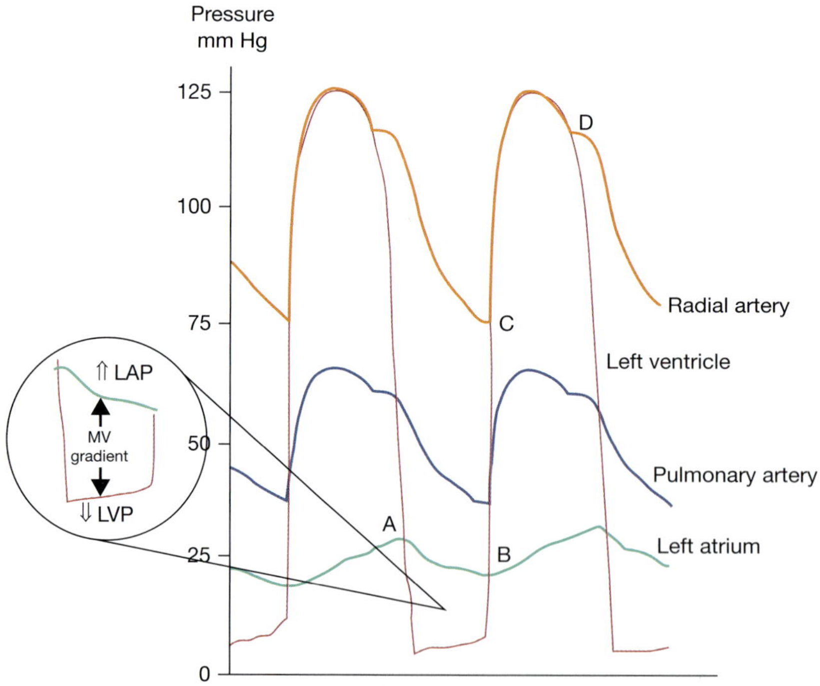

FIGURE 7.10. Pressure curves for the LV, left atrium, pulmonary artery, and aorta in patients with mitral stenosis. LAP, left atrial pressure; LVP, left ventricular pressure; MV, mitral valve.

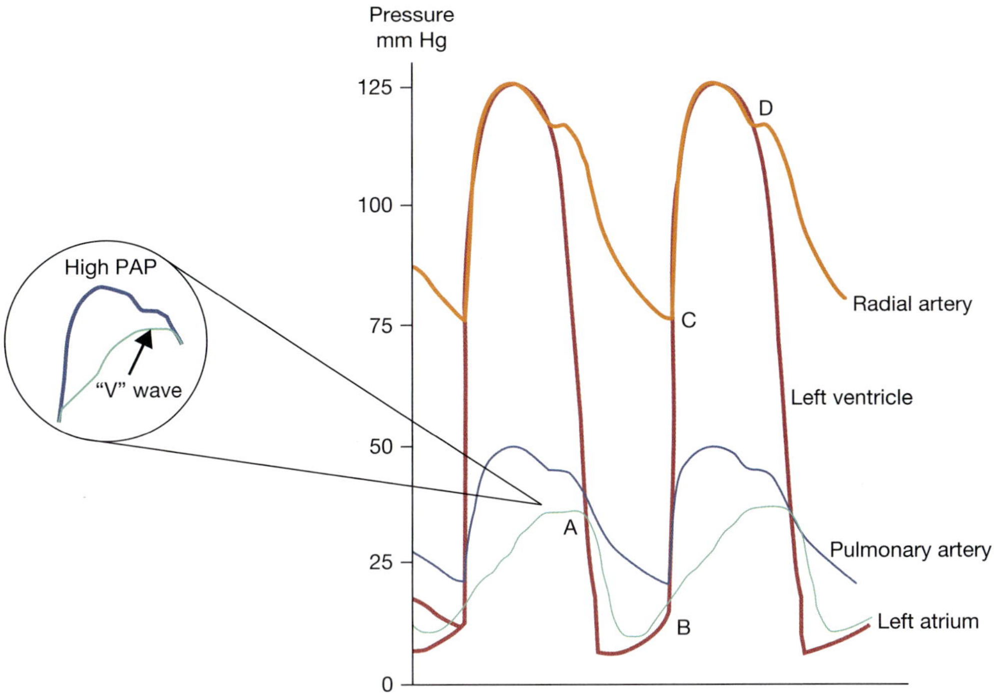

FIGURE 7.11. Pressure curves for the LV, left atrium, pulmonary artery, and aorta in patients with mitral regurgitation. PAP, pulmonary artery pressure.

A.6. What are the basic principles of echocardiography? What are M-mode, B-mode, and Doppler color modalities? How are pressure gradients measured by echocardiography? How do TTE and transesophageal echocardiography (TEE) differ?

Echocardiography is the use of ultrasound waves to image structures and blood flow within the heart and great vessels. To image tissue, sound waves are emitted from a transducer at known speeds and constant intervals. The sound packets bounce off structures in their path, and the reflected sound waves are received by the transducer during its "listening" mode. The time it takes for the reflected waves to return to the crystal is measured, and because the velocity of sound in tissues is relatively constant (1,540 m/s), solving for distance can be easily accomplished:

$$\text{Distance} = \tfrac{1}{2}\,(\text{Velocity} \times \text{Time})$$

(½ because the distance is traversed twice, once to the object and again on returning).

In this manner, the spatial orientation of cardiac structures can be determined. The strength of the returning signal can be quantified as an amplitude, thus "A" or amplitude mode (**Figure 7.12B**). The echocardiographic system codes this amplitude on a black and white scale, thereby converting the amplitude to brightness or B-mode scanning (**Figure 7.12C**). **Figure 7.12D** shows this "ice-pick" view through the LV of the heart. Each change in tissue density results in some sound waves being reflected and hence an interface. In this example, bold lines are seen at the epicardial, the endocardial-chamber, the chamber-endocardial, and the epicardial borders. If these amplitude bars are displayed in real time, then a motion or M-mode display results (**Figure 7.12E**). These images were difficult to obtain and interpret reliably because the views represent a linear slice without surrounding structural images for referencing. If the probe is moved in a sweeping mode, back and forth repetitively, then multiple M-mode images can be obtained in a given instant and a two-dimensional (2D) image formed. This rapid back-and-forth sweep of the ultrasound beam is performed electronically in a phased array transducer. The images derived in this manner appear as a cineradiographic display of myocardial movement. Echocardiography can provide information about the size, shape, location, and movement of myocardial structures.

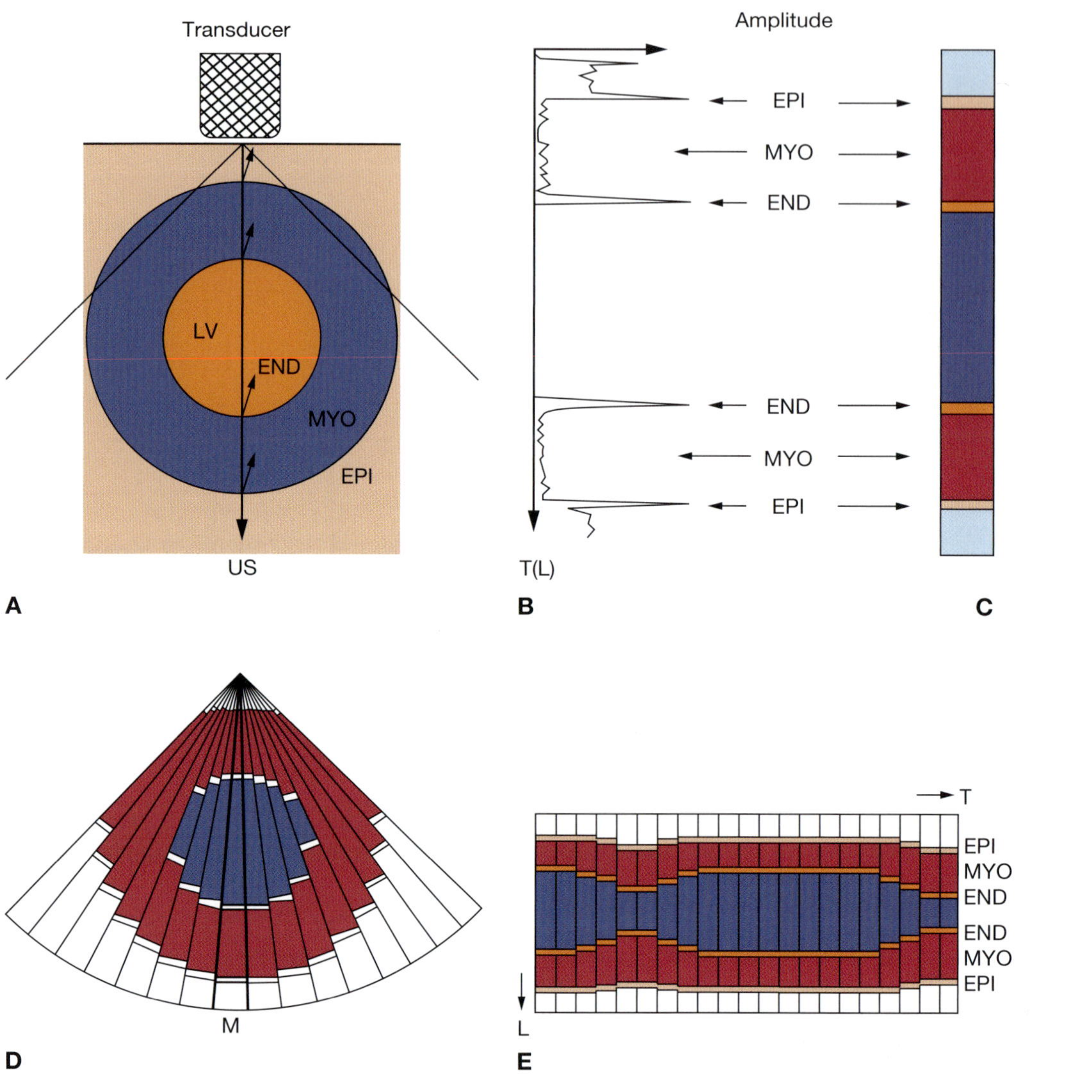

FIGURE 7.12. The process of producing the B-mode and M-mode images. A. A pulse of ultrasound is emitted into the object, and the backscattered echo is received by the same transducer. **B.** The received acoustic signal is converted to the electric signal (A-mode). **C.** The amplitude is modulated into brightness (B-mode). **D.** As subsequent pulses of ultrasound are emitted with the sequentially changing angles and the obtained one-dimensional (1D) B-mode images are compounded according to the direction of each ultrasound emission, the first frame of the sector-shaped image is formed. **E.** When the ultrasound is repeatedly transmitted in one direction, a series of 1D B-mode images is obtained. As these are arranged against time, an M-mode image is obtained. END, endocardium; EPI, epicardium; L, length; LV, left ventricle; M, motion; MYO, myocardium; T, time; US, ultrasound. (Reprinted with permission from Oka Y, Goldiner PL, eds. *Transesophageal Echocardiography*. JB Lippincott; 1992:12.)

Contact of the sound wave packet with the reflecting object (tissue, blood cells, air) also alters the wavelength of the sound packet according to the Doppler principle. When the reflecting object is moving toward the source of the ultrasound, the reflected ultrasound wavelengths are compressed (shorter). The opposite occurs when the object is moving away from the sound source. These shifts in frequency (ΔF) are proportional to the velocity of the contacted structure, and thereby, the velocity and direction of the encountered object (usually of blood flow) can be calculated. With Doppler ultrasound, only the component of blood flow parallel to the Doppler beam will be analyzed because the Doppler equation, velocity = $c\ (\Delta F)\ /\ 2\ F_T(\cos\theta)$, contains the cosine of the angle of incidence between the ultrasound beam and the moving object (F_T is the transmitted frequency). Because the cosine of 90° is zero, blood flow that is perpendicular to the ultrasound beam will not cause a Doppler shift and therefore cannot be measured.

It is important to choose an ultrasound "window" in which the expected blood flow direction is most parallel to the ultrasound. This velocity information can be displayed on a color map (Doppler color flow) or on a time/velocity scale (spectral Doppler display). Doppler-derived blood flow velocity information can identify laminar and turbulent flow patterns, regurgitant or stenotic lesions, and congenital anomalies and can permit quantification of pressure gradients.

Pressure gradients (ΔP) can be estimated from the measured blood flow velocity using the modified Bernoulli equation ($\Delta P = 4 \times \text{velocity}^2$). Simply put, the greater the velocity of blood flow, the higher is the ΔP. TTE uses imaging points or "acoustic windows" obtained with the transducer handheld on the chest wall. TTE is simple and noninvasive. Most standard echocardiograms are obtained from this position. During cardiac surgery, the chest wall is in the sterile field and therefore unavailable. The esophagus lies immediately adjacent to the heart outside of the operative field and affords an excellent imaging vantage point. The close proximity of the probe to the heart affords excellent resolution. The probe is not in the operative field, so surgery is unhindered and sterility is not at risk.

Intraoperative TEE is beneficial for quantification of cardiac contractility, for determination of the severity of regurgitant and stenotic valvular disease, for detection of intracardiac shunts and the occurrence of dissections, and as a guide for catheter and cannula placement. Accordingly, intraoperative TEE is now standard of care for open heart (eg, valve) operations, as well as a wide array of percutaneous cardiac interventions. Although invasive, the risk for esophageal injury in the anesthetized state is low. Nonetheless, prior to TEE, all patients should be screened for history of esophageal disease (eg, prior esophageal surgery, strictures or varices) or symptoms suggestive of esophageal pathology that can increase risk of injury from the probe.

American Society of Anesthesiologists and Society of Cardiovascular Anesthesiologists Task Force on Transesophageal Echocardiography. Practice guidelines for perioperative transesophageal echocardiography. An updated report by the American Society of Anesthesiologists and the Society of Cardiovascular Anesthesiologists Task Force on Transesophageal Echocardiography. *Anesthesiology*. 2010;112:1084-1096.

Otto CM. Principles of echocardiographic image acquisition and doppler analysis. In: Otto CM, ed. *Textbook of Clinical Echocardiography*. 6th ed. Elsevier; 2018:1-32.

A.7. What are the three TEE vantage points for comprehensive imaging of the LV? How are pressure gradients measured by echocardiography? How do pressure gradients derived from Doppler echocardiography differ from those obtained in the catheterization laboratory by direct pressure measurement?

The heart has two main axes: the longitudinal axis running from the base to the apex and the short axis (SAX) perpendicular to that. Multiple scan planes are required to completely image a 3D structure, such as the heart. The LV is divided into 17 segments: 6 at the basal level, 6 at the midpapillary level, 4 at the apical level, and 1 apical cap (**Figure 7.13**). By moving the TEE probe in the esophagus and rotating the crystal within the transducer tip, the LV can be comprehensively imaged. Normal ventricular motion requires that each wall segment thickens and moves toward the left ventricular cavity at systole. Segmental wall function is usually quantified as normal, hypokinesis, akinesis, or dyskinesis.

In addition to function, TEE permits the determination of wall thickness and chamber size, important parameters in understanding the pathophysiology of valvular heart disease.

Pressure gradients are derived through analysis of the Doppler profiles of blood flow. A commonly determined echocardiography gradient is that from the LV to the aorta in the setting of AS. To obtain the change in blood flow velocity across the AV with TEE, the probe is advanced far into the stomach and sharply anteflexed and left deflected to obtain the window from the apex of the heart (deep transgastric long axis [LAX]) and align the ultrasound beam most parallel to the path of blood flow. From this window, the continuous-wave Doppler cursor is directed across the left ventricular outflow tract (LVOT) and AV. An example of such a spectral Doppler display is seen in **Figure 7.14**. The large increase in blood flow velocity in this display occurs at the narrowest point along its path, which, in this case, is the stenosed orifice of the AV. Using the modified Bernoulli equation, a gradient is calculated (100 mm Hg in the example). This represents the maximum instantaneous systolic pressure difference between the LV and the aorta. AS is also quantified at the time of catheterization by measuring the pressures from within the LV and the aorta as a rapid response pressure transducer catheter is withdrawn from the LV back to the aorta across the stenotic valve. The standard pressure gradient from direct measurements is the difference between the maximum LV and aorta pressures, or "peak-to-peak" gradient. **Figure 7.15** illustrates that these peaks are not simultaneous events. Therefore, Doppler-derived AS gradients are usually higher than those derived by left heart catheterization.

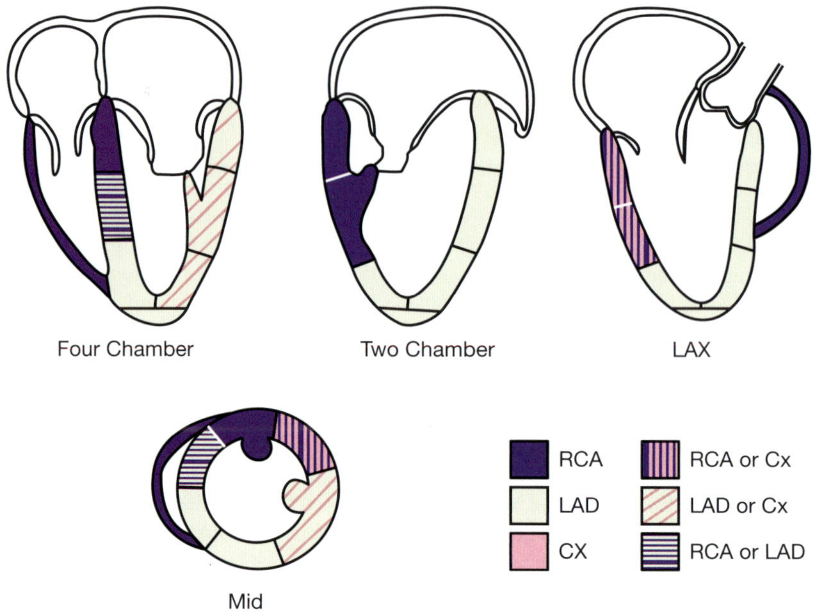

FIGURE 7.13. Wall segments of the LV. CX, circumflex; LAD, left anterior descending; LAX, long axis; LV, left ventricle; RCA, right coronary artery. (Reprinted from Lang RM, Bierig M, Devereux RB, et al. Recommendations for chamber quantification: a report from the American Society of Echocardiography's Guidelines and Standards Committee and the Chamber Quantification Writing Group, developed in conjunction with the European Association of Echocardiography, a branch of the European Society of Cardiology. *J Am Soc Echocardiogr.* 2005;18:1440-1463. Copyright © 2005 American Society of Echocardiography. With permission.)

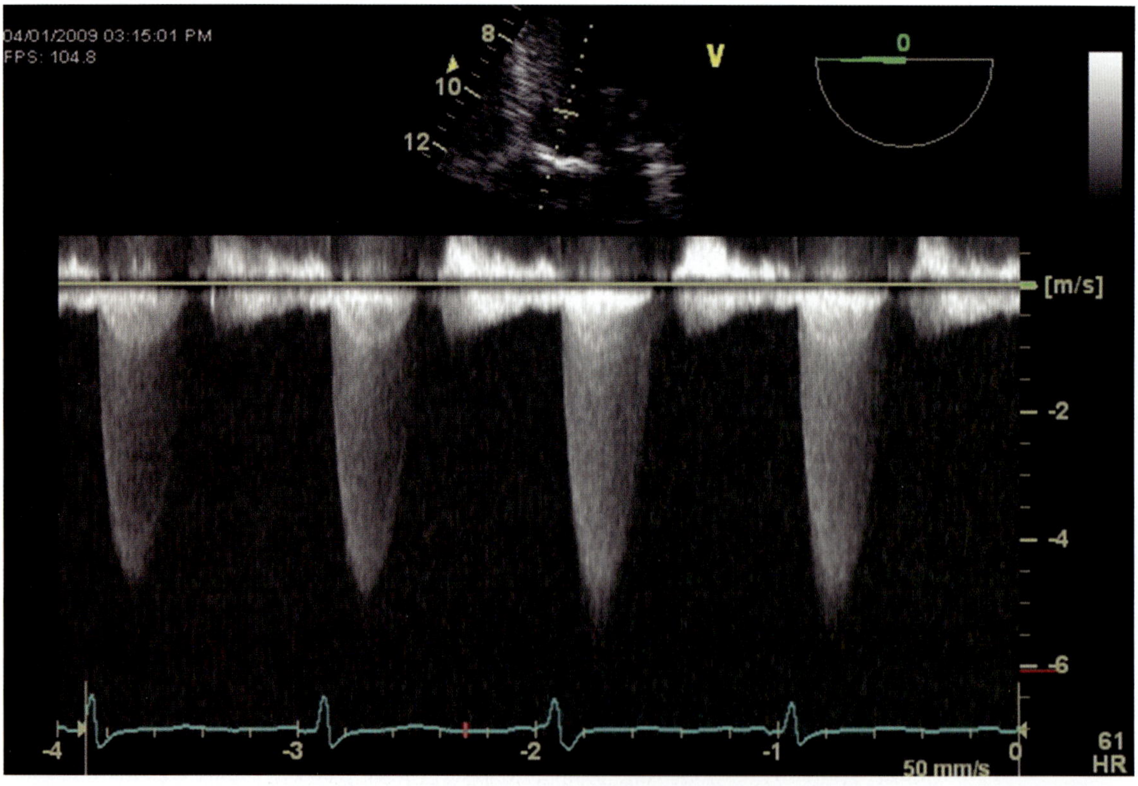

FIGURE 7.14. Continuous-wave Doppler across the aortic valve in the deep transgastric apical view from a patient with severe aortic stenosis.

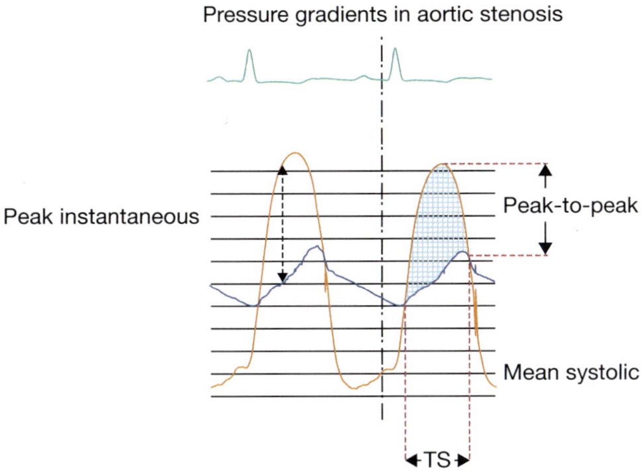

FIGURE 7.15. Pressure gradients in severe aortic stenosis are measured during systole as the difference between aortic and left ventricular pressures displayed using a scale of 0 to 20 mm Hg. The peak instantaneous gradient is the maximum gradient noted; the peak-to-peak gradient is the difference between peak left ventricular and aortic pressures. The mean systolic gradient is the average of all systolic pressure gradients noted during systolic ejection (TS). (Adapted with permission from Nanda NC, ed. *Doppler Echocardiography.* Lea & Febiger; 1993:130.)

Hahn RT, Abraham T, Adams MS, et al. Guidelines for performing a comprehensive transesophageal echocardiographic examination: recommendations from the American Society of Echocardiography and the Society of Cardiovascular Anesthesiologists. *J Am Soc Echocardiogr.* 2013;26:921-964.

Nicoara A, Skubas N, Ad N, et al. Guidelines for the use of transesophageal echocardiography to assist with surgical decision-making in the operating room: a surgery-based approach: from the American Society of Echocardiography in collaboration with the Society of Cardiovascular Anesthesiologists and the Society of Thoracic Surgeons. *J Am Soc Echocardiogr.* 2020;33:692-734.

Otto CM. Transesophogeal echocardiography. In: Otto CM, ed. *Textbook of Clinical Echocardiography.* 6th ed. Elsevier; 2018:67-95.

A.8. What is the purpose of the basic perioperative TEE examination? Describe the standard views that comprise this examination.

The basic perioperative TEE examination is comprised of 11 views. The exam is intended to enhance perioperative monitoring and enable prompt evaluation of causes of acute hemodynamic instability. To this end, the constituent views provide visualization of all cardiac chambers, LV wall segments and cardiac valves, as well as views of the great vessels.

The exam can be performed in any order. Because the majority of views are obtained at the midesophageal (ME) level (easily recognized by the presence of the LA posteriorly and adjacent to the probe), it can be practical to obtain all ME views before advancing into the stomach for transgastric views. Regardless of the chosen sequence, a systematic approach to the exam is advised.

Facility with the exam requires some practice. A variety of online simulation tools are available online, free of charge. The 11 basic views, including visualized structures and clinical applications, are as follows:

Midesophageal Four Chamber

The ME four-chamber view is obtained by advancing the probe to a depth of 30 to 35 cm until it is immediately posterior to the LA. The omniplane angle is adjusted to 0° to 20°, and the probe is rotated clockwise or counterclockwise to center the mitral valve and LV in the sector display. The LA, LV, RA, and RV should be visualized in this view. If the LVOT is visualized (an anterior structure), then the probe should be retroflexed.

The ME four chamber is extremely useful for evaluating chamber size, ventricular function, and tricuspid and mitral valvular function. Color flow Doppler over the valves is used to assess stenosis and regurgitation. Of note, the LV inferoseptal and anterolateral (AL) walls are seen in this view; new wall motion abnormalities (eg, hypokinesis, akinesis or dyskinesis) in these regions can reflect ischemia of the right coronary artery (RCA) or left anterior descending (LAD), respectively.

Midesophageal Two Chamber

From the ME four-chamber view, the omniplane angle is increased to 80° to 100° to achieve the ME two-chamber view. This view shows the LA and LA appendage, MV, LV (inferior and anterior walls), and coronary sinus (in cross-section immediately below the basal inferior segment of the LV).

Color flow Doppler over the MV may reveal stenosis or regurgitation. New regional wall motion abnormalities of the basal and mid-inferior wall can indicate ischemia of the RCA. New regional wall motion abnormalities in the apical and anterior wall segments can indicate LAD ischemia.

Midesophageal Long Axis

From the ME two-chamber view, omniplane angle is increased to 120° to 160°. The LAX view displays the LA, MV, LV (anteroseptal and inferolateral walls), LVOT, AV, and proximal ascending aorta. This view provides useful information regarding chamber volume; LV, MV, and AV function; and LVOT and proximal aortic pathology. Regional wall motion abnormalities can indicate ischemia of the RCA or left circumflex coronary artery (LCX) (basal inferolateral and mid inferolateral walls) or LAD (apical, mid- and basal anteroseptum). Color flow Doppler across the MV, LVOT, and AV can help diagnose stenosis, regurgitation, or LVOT obstruction (eg, due to ventricular hypertrophy and systolic anterior motion [SAM] of the MV).

Midesophageal Ascending Aortic Long Axis

The ME ascending aortic LAX view is obtained by withdrawing the probe from the ME LAX view. This view provides an image of the ascending aorta in LAX, as well as the right PA (in SAX). Aortic dissection and atherosclerotic plaque can be observed in this view, as can pulmonary emboli in the right PA.

Midesophageal Ascending Aortic Short Axis

From the ascending aortic LAX view, the ominplane angle is reduced to 20° to 40° to achieve the ME ascending SAX view. This view shows the ascending aorta in SAX, with the main PA on the right of the image and the right PA behind the aorta (closer to the probe). The superior vena cava (SVC) is also visualized in SAX on the left side of the image. This view can reveal a type A aortic dissection or proximal or saddle pulmonary emboli.

Midesophageal Aortic Valve Short Axis

From the ME ascending aortic SAX view, the probe is advanced to obtain the SAX AV view. Assuming a trileaflet valve, the left coronary cusp is posterior and on the right side of the screen. The right coronary cusp is anterior, adjacent to the RV and RVOT. The noncoronary cusp is adjacent to the interatrial septum. This view can identify congenital or acquired valvular abnormalities, such as a bicuspid AV or calcified and restricted valve leaflets. Color flow Doppler over the valve will identify aortic regurgitation, visible as a region of color across the cardiac cycle.

Midesophageal Right Ventricular Inflow-Outflow

From the prior view, the RV inflow-outflow view is obtained by advancing the probe, rotating slightly clockwise, and increasing the omniplane angle to 60° to 80°. The LA is closest to the probe; the RA is on the left of the screen, the RV in the middle, and the RVOT on the right of the screen. This view is useful for evaluating the tricuspid and pulmonic valves, and the systolic function of the right ventricle. Color flow Doppler can help identify tricuspid or pulmonic regurgitation or (less commonly) stenosis.

Midesophageal Bicaval

This view can be obtained by rotating the probe clockwise from the RV inflow-outflow view and increasing the omniplane angle to 90° to 110°. This view shows the SVC (on the right of the screen), the LA, RA, and RA appendage in the middle of the screen, and the inferior vena cava on the left of the screen. This view is useful for identifying correct (venous) placement of new central line wires and catheters, as well as preexisting pacemakers or other devices. Color flow Doppler at a low Nyquist setting (30 cm/s) may identify shunts across the interatrial septum, as can an injection of agitated saline ("bubble study").

Transgastric Midpapillary Short Axis

This view is obtained by advancing the probe from the ME four-chamber view, with 0° omniplane, into the stomach. The probe is then anteflexed to achieve contact with the gastric wall. The appropriate depth is determined by the visualization of the AL and posteromedial PM. The PM is typically at the 12 to 2 o'clock position on the LV, and AL PM at roughly 5 o'clock. Visualization of chords or mitral valve leaflets indicates that the probe should be advanced and/or anteflexion decreased; if no PMs are seen, then the probe is likely too deep or anteflexion inadequate.

This view is extremely useful for evaluating biventricular size and function, LV regional wall motion abnormalities, volume status, and pericardial effusion. Importantly, this is the only view in which LAD, LCX, and RCA territories can be simultaneously evaluated, albeit at a single level. The inferoseptal wall is perfused by the RCA or the LAD; the inferolateral wall by the RCA or the LCX; the anteroseptal and anterior wall segments by the LAD; and the AL wall by the LAD or the LCX. New wall motion abnormalities in any of these territories can indicate myocardial ischemia. Finally, intraventricular septal flattening during systole and diastole can indicate RV pressure or volume overload, respectively.

Descending Aortic Short Axis

The descending aorta is easily imaged by TEE, as the vessel lies adjacent and to the left of the esophagus. From the ME four-chamber view, the probe is rotated counterclockwise until the aorta appears in SAX. The probe may then be advanced and withdrawn to image the full length of the descending aorta. Type B aortic dissections, aortic aneurysms, and atherosclerotic disease can be diagnosed in this view. Left pleural effusions can also be seen.

Descending Aortic Long Axis

The descending aortic LAX view is obtained from the SAX view, described previously, by rotating the multiple to approximately 90°, such that the ultrasound beam is parallel to the vessel. The right side of the screen indicates the proximal descending aorta.

Reeves ST, Finley AC, Skubas NJ, et al. Council on Perioperative Echocardiography of the American Society of Echocardiography and the Society of Cardiovascular Anesthesiologists. Special article: basic perioperative transesophageal echocardiography examination: a consensus statement of the American Society of Echocardiography and the Society of Cardiovascular Anesthesiologists. *Anesth Analg*. 2013;117:543-558.

Vegas A. TEE views. In: Vegas A, ed. *Perioperative Two-Dimensional Transesophogeal Echocardiography: A Practical Handbook*. 2nd ed. Springer Nature; 2018:1-40.

Virtual Transesophogeal Echocardiography. Standard views: 2D TEE model. University Health Network. Peter Munk Cardiac Center. 2015. http://pie.med.utoronto.ca/tee/TEE_content/TEE_standardViews_intro.html

A.9. What is the role for three-dimensional (3D) echocardiography in the operating room?

Modern TEE technology has progressed from 2D multiplane images to real-time 3D displays of the heart. The 3D probes provide a pyramidal scanning sector (volume). There are different 3D imaging modalities used to assess cardiac anatomy (real-time, zoom, and full-volume, usually gated to ECG signal to construct an imaging dataset over multiple cardiac cycles). The 3D images can be further modified by cropping in any plane to investigate details in morphology.

3D TEE is useful for intraoperative assessment of valvular and ventricular function. Relative to 2D imaging, intraoperative assessment of the MV and AV with 3D TEE is associated with more precise assessment of leaflet pathology, more accurate measurements of valve dimensions and orifice areas, and better correlation with surgical findings. Left ventricular assessments include volume and regional wall motion. After identification of the left ventricular walls and apex from two orthogonal 2D views, a 3D model of the heart is created using endocardial border tracking. Stroke volume and ejection fraction can be automatically calculated. However, 3D echocardiography can only be combined with color, not spectral, Doppler ultrasound, and is subject to all limitations that apply to 2D echocardiography.

Otto CM. Specialized echocardiography applications. In: Otto CM, ed. *Textbook of Clinical Echocardiography*. 6th ed. Elsevier; 2018:96-119.

Rong LQ. An update on intraoperative three-dimensional transesophageal echocardiography. *J Thorac Dis*. 2017;9:S271-S282.

A.10. What are the echocardiographic and cardiac catheterization criteria for the four valvular lesions?

The TEE severity scales of the various valvular lesions are summarized in **Table 7.1**.

Aortic Stenosis

Echocardiographic criteria for AS include 2D or 3D imaging demonstrating limited AV cusp motion, a small orifice, and left ventricular concentric hypertrophy (**Figure 7.16**; **Video 7.1**). Doppler examination reveals a turbulent, high-velocity jet across the AV, and color flow Doppler demonstrates a turbulent, mosaic-appearing color map. The gradient across the AV measured at cardiac catheterization is different

TABLE 7.1 Transesophageal Echocardiography Severity Scales of Valvular Lesions

	Severity			
Measurement	**Normal**	**Mild**	**Moderate**	**Severe**
Mitral stenosis				
MVA (cm^2)	4.0-6.0	>1.5	1.0-1.5	<1.0
Mean pressure gradient (mm Hg)	<2.0	<5.0	5.0-10.0	>10.0
Aortic stenosis				
AVA (cm^2)	2.5-3.5	>1.5	1.0-1.5	<1.0
Mean pressure gradient (mm Hg)	<5	<20	20-40	>40
Mitral regurgitation				
Jet area/LA area	0	<20%	20%-40%	>40%
Jet area (cm^2)	0	<4.0	4.0-10.0	>10.0
Pulmonary vein Doppler	S wave ≫ D wave	S > D	S < D	Systolic flow reversal
Aortic insufficiency				
Jet width/LVOT width	0	<25%	25%-60%	>60%

AVA, aortic valve area; LA, left atrium; LVOT, left ventricular outflow tract; MVA, mitral valve area.

from that measured by echocardiography as discussed previously. Quantification of the Doppler-derived AS pressure gradient relies on the modified Bernoulli equation.

$$\text{Pressure gradient (mm Hg)} = 4\ (\text{transaortic valve velocity, m/s})^2$$

Because flow is an important determinant of pressure gradients, both catheterization and Doppler-derived values must be interpreted along with cardiac output. Calculations permit determination of a

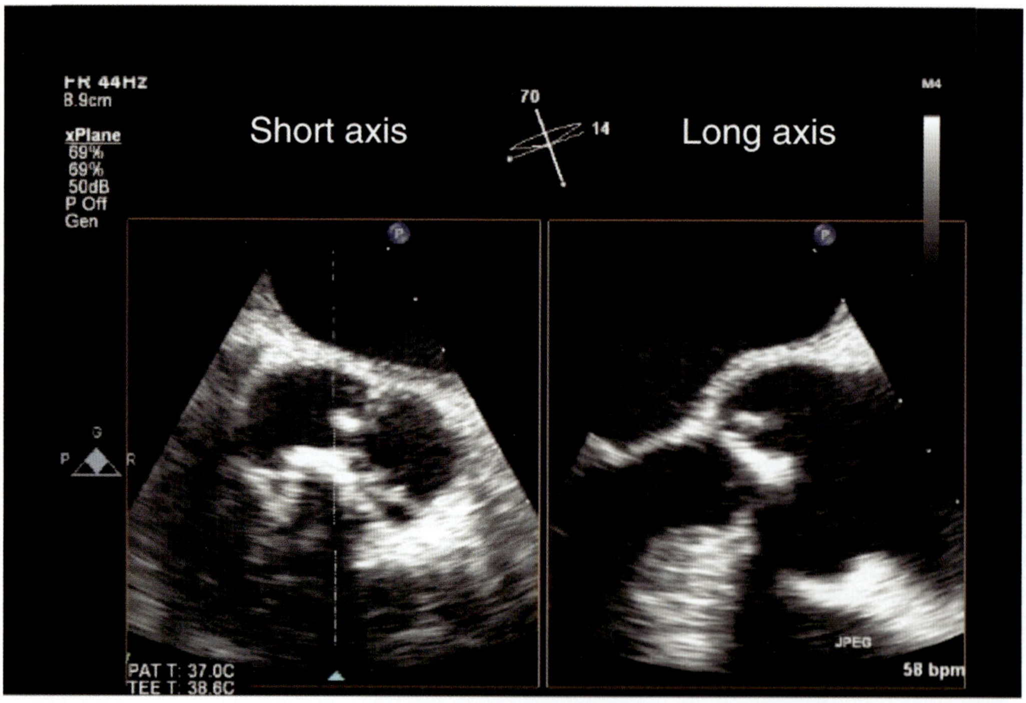

FIGURE 7.16. Transesophageal echocardiographic findings of moderate aortic stenosis (midesophageal aortic valve [AV] short-axis view [left] and long-axis view [right]). The AV cusps are calcified and demonstrate limited systolic excursion.

valve area. Severe AS is present when the mean pressure gradient exceeds 40 mm Hg or the valve area is less than 1.0 cm^2.

Aortic Insufficiency

Catheterization criteria for AI rely on the qualitative estimation of the regurgitation volume and estimation of left ventricular size and ejection fraction. Similar quantification can be made from Doppler color echocardiography–derived data. The width of the regurgitant jet at the level of the AV can be compared to the width of the LVOT. A ratio of more than 0.6 corresponds to severe AI (**Figure 7.17**; **Video 7.2**). Another sign of severe AI is diastolic flow reversal of the descending thoracic aorta, as observed on spectral Doppler.

SECTION 2

Mitral Stenosis

The severity of MS can be obtained by direct measurement of the diastolic gradient between the LA and ventricle at the time of cardiac catheterization. This requires a transatrial puncture, a procedure largely replaced by echocardiographic techniques. Echocardiographic diagnosis is based on gradient estimation by Doppler and by measuring the rate of decay in the pressure with the time spent in diastole (pressure halftime). The MV area (cm^2) can be derived from an empirical formula wherein the MV area equals 220 divided by this pressure halftime. Severe MS is present when the mean diastolic gradient exceeds 10 mm Hg, corresponding to a valve area of less than 1.0 cm^2 (**Figure 7.18**; **Video 7.3**).

Mitral Regurgitation

In the presence of MR, ventriculography demonstrates reflux of dye from the LV into the LA. Severe MR is diagnosed according to the relative volume of regurgitant flow and flow reversal in the pulmonary veins. Color Doppler echocardiography permits similar quantification, as does spectral Doppler waveforms of pulmonary venous flow (**Figure 7.19**; **Video 7.4**).

Color Doppler echocardiography is often useful in identifying the cause of the valvular lesion, its extent of involvement within and around the valve, and the associated hemodynamic changes. It is sufficient for diagnosing and grading most valvular lesions. Catheterization, however, is often performed to assess the presence of concomitant coronary artery disease, especially in patients of advanced age. Notably,

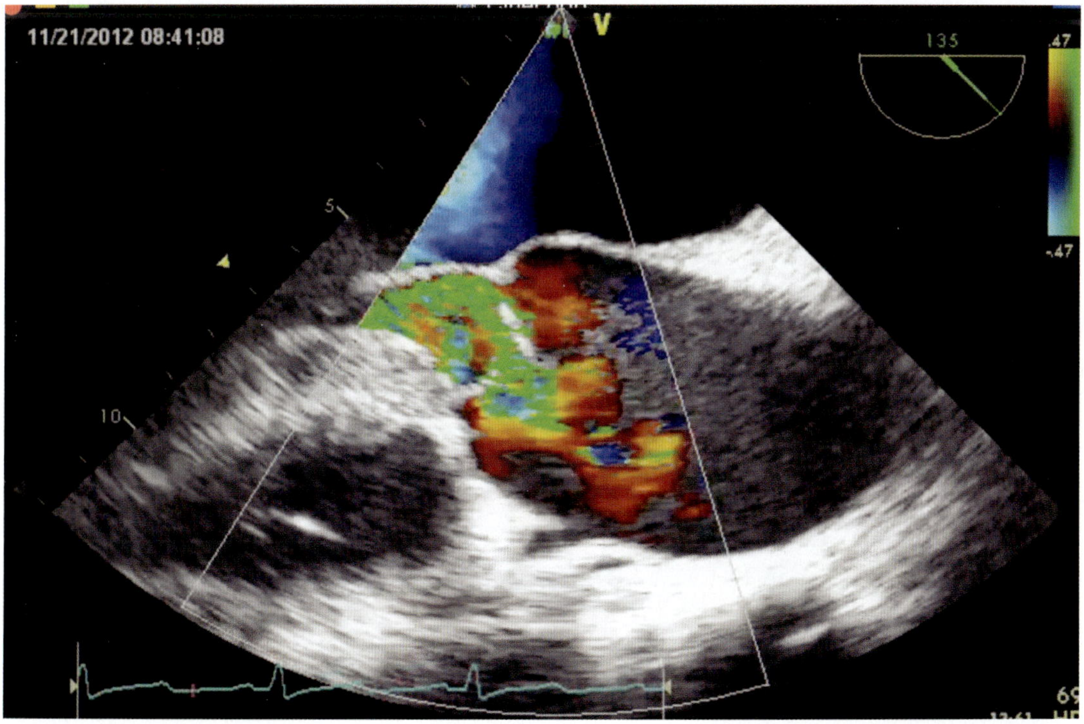

FIGURE 7.17. Transesophageal echocardiographic findings of moderate aortic regurgitation (midesophageal aortic valve long-axis view; color flow Doppler).

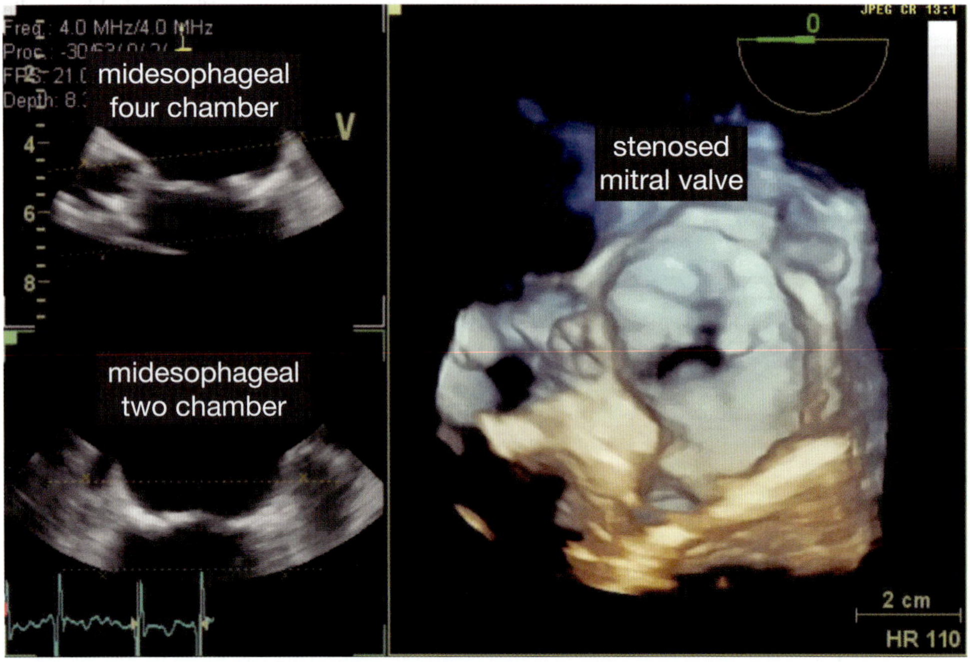

FIGURE 7.18. Transesophageal echocardiographic findings of severe mitral stenosis with 2D view (left) and 3D view (right).

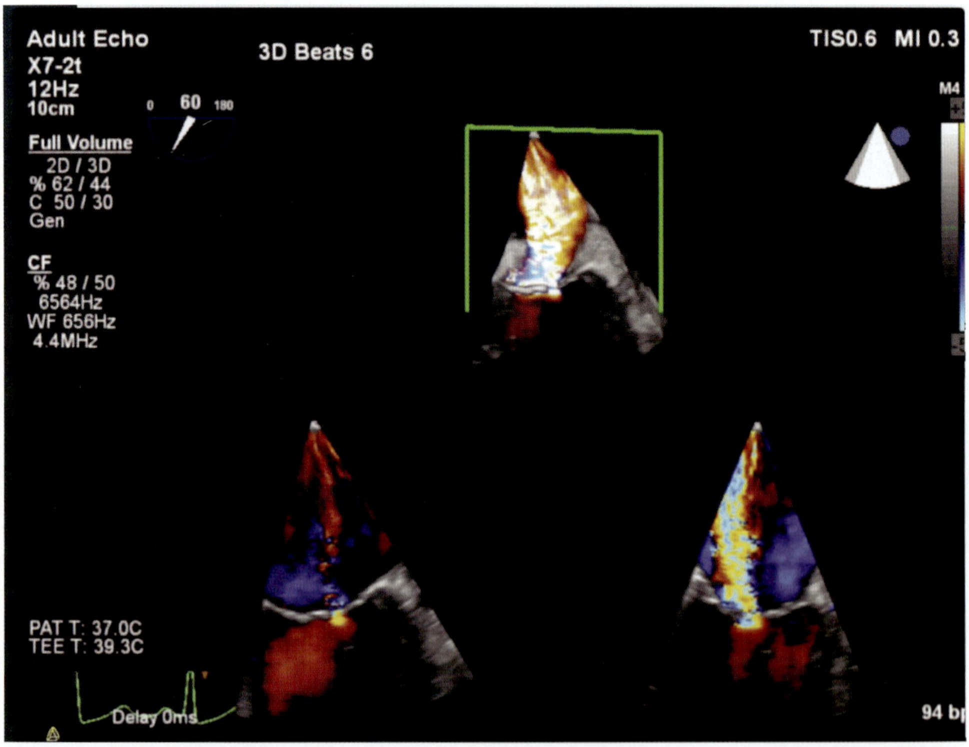

FIGURE 7.19. Transesophageal echocardiographic findings of moderate mitral stenosis (color flow Doppler) with 3D view (top) and 2D view (bottom).

diagnoses of prosthetic valve stenosis are made according to device-specific thresholds supplied by the manufacturer.

Baumgartner H, Hung J, Bermejo J, et al. Recommendations on the echocardiographic assessment of aortic valve stenosis: a focused update from the European Association of Cardiovascular Imaging and the American Society of Echocardiography. *J Am Soc Echocardiogr*. 2017;30:372-392.

Otto CM. Valvular stenosis and valvular regurgitation. In: Otto CM, ed. *Textbook of Clinical Echocardiography*. 6th ed. Elsevier; 2018:288-369.

Pandian NG, Kim JK, Arias-Godinez JA, et al. Recommendations for the use of echocardiography in the evaluation of rheumatic heart disease: a report from the American Society of Echocardiography. *J Am Soc Echocardiogr*. 2023;36:3-28.

Zoghbi WA, Adams D, Bonow RO, et al. Recommendations for noninvasive evaluation of native valvular regurgitation: a report from the American Society of Echocardiography developed in collaboration with the Society for Cardiovascular Magnetic Resonance. *J Am Soc Echocardiogr*. 2017;30:303-371.

B. Preoperative Evaluation and Preparation

B.1. What are the presenting signs and symptoms of the four valvular lesions listed previously?

See **Table 7.2.**

Aortic Stenosis

The triad of angina, syncope, and congestive heart failure represents the progression of symptoms associated with AS. These symptoms correlate directly with mortality; the 50% survival data for these symptoms are 5, 3, and 2 years from the onset of each symptom, respectively. Angina results from both increased demand and decreased supply of coronary blood flow. Increased muscle mass from LVH and the high-energy requirements to generate increased (high) systolic pressure combine to increase demand for coronary blood flow. In addition, insufficient supply secondary to decreased perfusion gradients and a decrease in coronary vasculature relative to the increased myocardial mass result in diminished relative myocardial blood supply. Therefore, up to one-third of patients with AS can have angina in the absence of significant coronary artery disease.

Aortic Insufficiency

Patients with AI have variable clinical presentations based primarily on the rapidity with which the left ventricular volume overload develops. When the volume increase occurs gradually, as in chronic AI, there is usually a long asymptomatic period. The onset of fatigue and dyspnea signals either reduced cardiac output or increased LVEDP, indicative of impairment of left ventricular contractile function. When AI occurs acutely, the ventricular compliance is unchanged; therefore, increased left ventricular diastolic volumes from regurgitant flow lead to rapid rises in LVEDP and the clinical picture of congestive failure.

Mitral Stenosis

In MS, the slow and progressive obstruction to flow across the MV leads to gradual increase in left atrial pressure and volume. Symptoms of pulmonary congestion result from elevations in left atrial pressures and *not* from poor left ventricular systolic function. Atrial fibrillation develops secondary to atrial dilation.

TABLE 7.2 Signs and Symptoms for Valvular Lesions

Lesion	Signs and Symptoms
Aortic stenosis	Angina, syncope, dyspnea/CHF
Aortic insufficiency	
Chronic	Fatigability, dyspnea
Acute	Severe pulmonary edema, CHF
Mitral stenosis	Pulmonary congestion, Afib
Mitral regurgitation	
Chronic	DOE, PND, AFib
Acute	Severe pulmonary edema, CHF

AFib, atrial fibrillation; CHF, congestive heart failure; DOE, dyspnea on exertion; PND, paroxysmal nocturnal dyspnea.

Mitral Regurgitation

The time course for the development of MR determines the severity of the symptoms. When the volume of regurgitant flow from the LV to the LA increases gradually, the LA compensates by gradual dilation. In contrast, the onset of acute MR can lead to rapid increases in left atrial pressures, severe pulmonary congestion, and congestive heart failure.

Lilly LS. Valvular heart disease. In: Lilly LS, ed. *Pathophysiology of Heart Disease: An Introduction to Cardiovascular Medicine*. 7th ed. Wolters Kluwer; 2021:202-231.

Otto CM, Nishimura RA, Bonow RO, et al. 2020 ACC/AHA guideline for the management of patients with valvular heart disease: executive summary: a report of the American College of Cardiology/American Heart Association Joint Committee on Clinical Practice Guidelines. *Circulation*. 2021;143:e35-e71.

B.2. What is the New York Heart Association classification of heart failure?

The New York Heart Association heart failure classification is based on the severity of symptoms, specifically dyspnea and fatigue:

- *Class I*—no symptoms (fatigue, palpitations, dyspnea, or angina) during ordinary physical activity; no limitations of physical activity
- *Class II*—symptoms with ordinary activity but comfortable at rest; slight limitation of physical activity
- *Class III*—symptoms with less than ordinary activity but comfortable at rest; marked limitation of physical activity
- *Class IV*—symptoms at rest; inability to carry on any physical activity without discomfort

Raphael C, Briscoe C, Davies J, et al. Limitations of the New York Heart Association functional classification system and self-reported walking distances in chronic heart failure. *Heart*. 2007;93:476-482.

B.3. Discuss the role of premedication for patients with the four different valvular lesions.

The role of premedication is to allay the anxiety of the impending surgical procedure, thereby controlling the sympathetic outflow that may accompany the stress response. Acute changes in heart rate, venous return, and systemic resistance can have profound effects on patients with valvular heart disease. Premedication is most safely administered in the operating room after placement of standard American Society of Anesthesiologists (ASA) monitors and supplemental nasal oxygen.

Patients with AS might benefit from premedication to minimize tachycardia. Concern must be taken to ensure adequate venous return and preservation of sinus rhythm (see next).

Patients with AI can similarly benefit from premedication because any increases in afterload, which accompany sympathetic stimulation, can increase regurgitant volume. Drug doses should be adjusted based on the severity of debilitation and degree of systemic hypoperfusion.

Patients with MS should be premedicated with caution. Elevations in carbon dioxide resulting from opioid-induced hypoventilation can dramatically elevate pulmonary pressures, further compromising right ventricle output. Also important, venodilation can excessively diminish filling pressures.

Patients with MR can respond similarly to those with MS, particularly when pulmonary hypertension is present. However, elevations in systemic pressure from acute preoperative stress can also compromise left ventricular output and even lead to acute pulmonary edema. Proper premedication can be delivered by careful dose selection and the provision of supplemental oxygen.

Frogel J, Galusca D. Anesthetic considerations for patients with advanced valvular heart disease undergoing noncardiac surgery. *Anesthesiol Clin*. 2010;28:67-85.

Ramakrishan H, Craner RC, Devaleria PA, Cook DJ, Housmans PR, Rehfeldt KH. Valvular heart disease: replacement and repair. In: Kaplan JA, Augustides J, Maneck GR, Maus T, eds. *Kaplan's Cardiac Anesthesia*. 7th ed. Elsevier; 2017:770-817.

B.4. How would you premedicate the patient with severe AS and MR?

Premedication of a patient with severe AS and MR must be approached with caution. The patient should receive supplemental oxygen. Small intravenous (IV) doses of sedation (eg, midazolam 0.5 mg) can be administered while the patient is closely monitored in the operating room with oxygen supplementation. It is important to remember that there can be delay in the onset of sedation secondary to pooling in the pulmonary circulation, and slow titration is essential to avoid inadvertent overdose, which can cause respiratory depression, pulmonary hypertension, and systemic hypotension. In older patients, use of benzodiazepines has been linked to postoperative delirium, which can be quite severe and difficult to treat increasing hospital length of stay and resource utilization.

Spence J, Belley-Cote E, Jacobsohn E, et al. Restricted versus liberal intraoperative benzodiazepine use in cardiac anaesthesia for reducing delirium (B-Free Pilot): a pilot, multicentre, randomised, cluster crossover trial. *Br J Anaesth.* 2020;125:38-46.

C. Intraoperative Management

C.1. Outline the hemodynamic management goals for each of the four valvular lesions. What are the anesthetic goals with respect to heart rate and rhythm, preload, afterload, and contractility?

Table 7.3 summarizes the hemodynamic goals with respect to heart rate and rhythm, preload, afterload, and contractility.

Aortic Stenosis

Patients with AS depend on left ventricular filling through adequate preload and well-timed atrial contraction. The stenotic AV is a fixed lesion that will not respond to pharmacologic intervention or decreased afterload. Reducing vascular tone will only lower diastolic coronary perfusion gradients and should be avoided. Patients with AS experiencing angina may require the administration of an α-agonist such as phenylephrine rather than nitroglycerin to increase coronary perfusion pressure.

Aortic Insufficiency

The severity of AI is determined by the size of the regurgitant orifice, the diastolic pressure gradient between the aorta and LV, and the duration of diastole. Elevated heart rates reduce the time spent in diastole and can lead to a decrease in heart size and regurgitation. Afterload reduction can lessen the regurgitant driving pressure but is limited by resulting systemic hypotension.

Mitral Stenosis

Slower heart rates permit adequate time for flow of blood from the LA to the LV across the stenotic MV. Left atrial emptying reduces left atrial pressure, thereby decreasing the pressure gradient across the MV and diminishing pulmonary congestion. Patients with MS can rapidly deteriorate in the setting of rapid heart rates. The reduced filling time exacerbates the marked elevation of left atrial pressures, and pulmonary edema can ensue. Whereas left ventricular contractility is generally preserved in MS, use of β-blockade can result in decreased RV contractility, which in the setting of pulmonary hypertension can further compromise cardiac output and systemic blood pressure. However, the loss in RV contractility is typically offset by the beneficial effects of heart rate reduction. Because an adverse response could be catastrophic, short-acting β-blockers, such as esmolol, should be used if necessary.

Mitral Regurgitation

Patients with MR can rapidly deteriorate with marked increases in systemic blood pressure, so afterload reduction is recommended. As with AI, slightly increased heart rates (80-90 beats per minute) should result in smaller left ventricular volumes. However, tachycardia should be avoided in patients with ischemic (functional) MR.

Frogel J, Galusca D. Anesthetic considerations for patients with advanced valvular heart disease undergoing noncardiac surgery. *Anesthesiol Clin.* 2010;28:67-85.

Ramakrishan H, Craner RC, Devaleria PA, Cook DJ, Housmans PR, Rehfeldt KH. Valvular heart disease: replacement and repair. In: Kaplan JA, Augustides J, Maneck GR, Maus T, eds. *Kaplan's Cardiac Anesthesia.* 7th ed. Elsevier; 2017:770-817.

TABLE 7.3 Hemodynamic Goals for Various Valvular Lesions

	Hemodynamic Goals			
Lesion	**HR and Rhythm**	**Preload**	**Afterload**	**Contractility**
Aortic stenosis	60-70, sinus	Full	Maintain	–
Aortic insufficiency	80-90	Maintain	Lower	May need support
Mitral stenosis	60-70	Full	–	–
Mitral regurgitation	80-90, sinus if possible	Maintain	Lower	May need support

HR, heart rate (beats per minute).

C.2. What are the hemodynamic goals for this patient with a combination of severe AS and MR?

In this patient with combined AS and MR, therapy benefiting AS can exacerbate the severity of MR. It is best to prioritize management based on the character of the paramount symptoms. Patients with AS and MR who present with syncope or angina are best managed for their AS, whereas patients with dyspnea and pulmonary edema are best managed for their congestive heart failure symptoms. Preoperative echocardiography and ECG findings can also be used to determine the predominant lesion. It is best to maintain the patient's usual hemodynamics. Early aggressive intervention is the key to managing these combined lesions. A lower margin for error usually exists because minor hemodynamic aberrations can rapidly lead to cardiac collapse. TEE evaluation of left ventricular performance can be helpful in distinguishing pulmonary congestion secondary to left heart failure from that due to decreased diastolic left ventricular compliance from AS.

Ajmone Marsan N, Delgado V, Shah DJ, et al. Valvular heart disease: shifting the focus to the myocardium. *Eur Heart J*. 2023;44:28-40.

Frogel J, Galusca D. Anesthetic considerations for patients with advanced valvular heart disease undergoing noncardiac surgery. *Anesthesiol Clin*. 2010;28:67-85.

Silbiger JJ. Pathophysiology and echocardiographic diagnosis of left ventricular diastolic dysfunction. *J Am Soc Echocardiogr*. 2019;32:216-232.

C.3. How would you monitor this patient with severe AS and MR?

In addition to the standard ASA monitors, the patient should have a radial artery (pre-induction) and a PA catheter (typically post-induction). Following induction of anesthesia and endotracheal intubation, a TEE probe is usually inserted to confirm the valvular pathology and to assess ventricular function. Following valve replacement, the TEE probe can be used to check for adequacy of valvular function and absence of paravalvular leaks, and to assess post-bypass ventricular function.

American Society of Anesthesiologists and Society of Cardiovascular Anesthesiologists Task Force on Transesophageal Echocardiography. Practice guidelines for perioperative transesophageal echocardiography. An updated report by the American Society of Anesthesiologists and the Society of Cardiovascular Anesthesiologists Task Force on Transesophageal Echocardiography. *Anesthesiology*. 2010;112:1084-1096.

Nicoara A, Skubas N, Ad N, et al. Guidelines for the use of transesophageal echocardiography to assist with surgical decision-making in the operating room: a surgery-based approach: from the American Society of Echocardiography in collaboration with the Society of Cardiovascular Anesthesiologists and the Society of Thoracic Surgeons. *J Am Soc Echocardiogr*. 2020;33:692-734.

C.4. Should the patient have a PA catheter placed before induction?

Intravascular volume status can be particularly difficult to assess in patients with valvular heart disease, yet is of critical importance in patient management. Patients with stenotic lesions depend on adequate filling pressures for diastolic filling of the ventricle. Patients with the volume overload lesions of AI and MR can benefit from careful reductions in pulmonary pressure guided by real-time assessment of cardiac performance, for which a PA catheter is useful. Patients with current hemodynamic stability, and without severe respiratory distress, can be safely anesthetized before placement of the PA catheter. Overall, there is no evidence that use of the PA catheter improves cardiac surgical outcomes.

American Society of Anesthesiologists and Society of Cardiovascular Anesthesiologists Task Force on Pulmonary Artery Catheterization. Practice guidelines for pulmonary artery catheterization: an updated report by the American Society of Anesthesiologists Task Force on Pulmonary Artery Catheterization. *Anesthesiology*. 2003;99:988-1014.

Joseph C, Garrubba M, Smith JA, Melder A. Does the use of a pulmonary artery catheter make a difference during or after cardiac surgery? *Heart Lung Circ*. 2018;27:952-960.

C.5. Is a PA catheter with pacing capabilities indicated?

Patients with AS can become severely compromised by loss of the atrial kick due to atrial arrhythmias or slow junctional rhythms. Patients with AI or MR can experience LV dilation in the setting of slow heart rates. A PA catheter with atrial and ventricular pacing capacity can be useful. In patients with intact conduction systems, rate manipulation can often be achieved pharmacologically. Transthoracic pacing elicits a ventricular response only and is indicated when the ability to rapidly open the pericardium and obtain epicardial pacing is limited, as occurs in reoperations or in patients with inflammatory pericardial disease. The loss of atrial contraction can lead to underfilling and hemodynamic compromise in patients dependent on the added preload from atrial systole. One of the other pacing modalities is preferable in this setting.

Before chest closure, and often prior to separation from CPB, epicardial pacing wires are placed. Atrial and ventricular wires are advisable in patients with diastolic dysfunction or who are otherwise disproportionately dependent on atrial contraction for adequate ventricular preload.

Cronin B, Dalia A, Goh R, Essandoh M, Orestes O'Brien E. Temporary epicardial pacing after cardiac surgery. *J Cardiothorac Vasc Anesth*. 2022;36:4427-4439.

Gaudino M, Di Franco A, Rong LQ, Piccini J, Mack M. Postoperative atrial fibrillation: from mechanisms to treatment. *Eur Heart J*. 2023;44:1020-1039.

C.6. What anesthetic technique would you employ? Why?

For the patient undergoing CPB and AV replacement, general anesthesia with endotracheal intubation is necessary. Opioids and IV and inhalation anesthetics can be safely administered, with careful attention to hemodynamics. Increasingly, anesthetic techniques for cardiac surgery are structured to optimize perioperative outcomes, and avoid the adverse effects of opioids and prolonged intubation. Enhanced Recovery after Cardiac Surgery (ERACS) programs emphasize the use of regional anesthesia, opioid-sparing analgesics, and readily reversible neuromuscular blockade to help reduce postoperative morbidity. These synergistic strategies can be particularly beneficial for high-risk surgical patients.

Barry AE, Chaney MA, London MJ. Anesthetic management during cardiopulmonary bypass: a systematic review. *Anesth Analg*. 2015;120:749-769.

Baxter R, Squiers J, Conner W, et al. Enhanced recovery after surgery: a narrative review of its application in cardiac surgery. *Ann Thorac Surg*. 2020;109:1937-1944.

Grant MC, Isada T, Ruzankin P, et al. Opioid-sparing cardiac anesthesia: secondary analysis of an enhanced recovery program for cardiac surgery. *Anesth Analg*. 2020;131:1852-1861.

Kelava M, Alfirevic A, Bustamante S, Hargrave J, Marciniak D. Regional anesthesia in cardiac surgery: an overview of fascial plane chest wall blocks. *Anesth Analg*. 2020;131:127-135.

C.7. What are the usual TEE findings in a patient with AS or MR? How do you grade the severity of AS by TEE? How do you quantify the severity of MR? What is the impact of AS on the severity of MR?

The *echocardiographic* severity of native valvular AS is usually determined by AV area and transaortic valve pressure gradient (**Table 7.1**). Severe AS is present when the mean pressure gradient exceeds 40 mm Hg or the valve area is less than 1.0 cm^2. Of note, in the setting of low cardiac outputs and low gradients, additional investigation might be necessary. The *clinical* severity of AS is determined by a combination of echocardiographic and clinical factors. A patient with less than severe AS by echocardiography or catheterization criteria is considered to have severe AS if their daily activities of life are reduced, they experience symptoms, or left ventricular systolic dysfunction is present.

MR is graded by the amount of blood regurgitated into the LA during systole on color Doppler. Common methods for MR quantification include analysis of the area of the regurgitant orifice (effective orifice area), the width of the MR jet (vena contracta), and pulmonary vein flow profiles. It is important to remember that the amount of regurgitant blood flow in the setting of MR is determined by the amount of time spent in systole, the size of the MV defect, and the pressure gradient across the defect. Therefore, MR severity by Doppler color flow is load dependent. Lower systemic pressure or decreased preload (relative hypovolemia) due to the anesthetic state can often mask more severe degrees of MR that are present in the awake state.

Left ventricular pressures increase in the setting of AS. Therefore, the gradient across the MV is increased often leading to more severe MR. Following replacement of the stenotic AV and elimination of the obstruction to systolic flow, left ventricular pressures are markedly reduced. In cases of functional MR without major structural defects in the MV apparatus, MR becomes less severe following replacement of AV.

Baumgartner H, Hung J, Bermejo J, et al. Recommendations on the echocardiographic assessment of aortic valve stenosis: a focused update from the European Association of Cardiovascular Imaging and the American Society of Echocardiography. *J Am Soc Echocardiogr*. 2017;30:372-392.

Mahmood F, Matyal R. A quantitative approach to the intraoperative echocardiographic assessment of the mitral valve for repair. *Anesth Analg*. 2015;121:34-58.

Zoghbi WA, Adams D, Bonow RO, et al. Recommendations for noninvasive evaluation of native valvular regurgitation: a report from the American Society of Echocardiography developed in collaboration with the Society for Cardiovascular Magnetic Resonance. *J Am Soc Echocardiogr*. 2017;30:303-371.

C.8. What special considerations particular to cardiopulmonary bypass (CPB) operations do you have for each of the four lesions? Focus on these concerns with respect to the induction and pre-bypass, during bypass, and post-bypass periods.

Aortic Stenosis

Critical to the management of a patient with AS is avoidance of hypotension, which can initiate a cascade of events leading to cardiac arrest. Hypotension decreases the gradient for coronary perfusion with resultant ischemia. Ischemia leads to diminished cardiac output and decreased blood pressure further compromising coronary perfusion. The occurrence of cardiac arrest in a patient with AS can be catastrophic because closed-chest cardiac massage will provide little gradient for blood flow across a stenotic AV.

Patients with AS are particularly dependent on their atrial "kick" for adequate ventricular filling volume and can rapidly become hypotensive and ischemic following onset of supraventricular tachycardia or atrial fibrillation. These rhythms are not uncommon during atrial cannulation. Therefore, all preparations for the initiation of CPB should be made before atrial manipulation.

The increased muscle mass of the hypertrophied LV can be more difficult to adequately protect with cardioplegia. Careful attention to surface cooling, myocardial temperature measurement, and the use of retrograde cardioplegia can be helpful. Following AV replacement, hypertension from LV output now unopposed by the stenotic valvular lesion can result in stress on suture lines and excessive bleeding. The compliance of the LV is unchanged by surgery and still critically dependent on adequate preload and sinus rhythm. Hypertension is best managed with an afterload-reducing agent, such as nicardipine, rather than a preload-reducing agent, such as nitroglycerin.

Aortic Insufficiency

Patients undergoing AV replacement for AI often present difficult management decisions. The usual treatment measures for hypotension (α-agonist) can have deleterious effects by increasing regurgitant volume. Use of combined α- and β-agonists (ephedrine, epinephrine, or infusions of dopamine or dobutamine) might be required. Although it can lessen regurgitant volume, afterload reduction is beneficial in only a subset of patients with AI. Those patients with elevated LVEDP, reduced ejection fraction, diminished cardiac output, and systemic hypertension usually benefit from afterload reduction. In contrast, those patients without this constellation can experience a decrease in cardiac output secondary to diminished preload from reduced atrial filling. Systemic hypotension usually limits the utility of targeted afterload reduction in the acute setting. The presence of AI makes initiation of CPB a critical period. Periods of bradycardia or ventricular fibrillation can lead to rapid volume overload of the LV through the incompetent AV. Pacing, electrical defibrillation, and/or cross-clamping should be performed to prevent ventricular distention. Similarly, myocardial protection is compromised by AI. Adequate root pressures are usually not obtainable; hence, delivery of cardioplegia requires aortotomy and cannulation of the coronary ostia. Use of retrograde cardioplegia is advantageous. Following AV replacement, the ventricle no longer has the lower pressure/impedance outflow afforded by the low aortic diastolic pressure, and inotropic support is often required. As with AS, the presence of an aortic suture line necessitates rapid response to hypertension to avoid bleeding and dissection.

Mitral Stenosis

Patients undergoing MV replacement for MS are particularly challenging to manage. Marked elevations in pulmonary vascular resistance can be present with associated right-sided heart failure. Stasis in the LA necessitates careful echocardiographic examination for the presence of atrial and atrial appendage thrombi. Manipulation of the heart before cross-clamping should be avoided due to risk of acute decreases in preload. Following replacement, the chronically underfilled, underworked LV might be unable to accommodate the new volume load. Inotropic support is often required for RV failure and occasionally to improve LV function. Afterload reduction and improved systemic perfusion using an IABP can be beneficial.

Mitral Regurgitation

Similarly, patients with MR can have pulmonary hypertension and right-sided heart failure. In contrast to AI, almost all patients with MR greatly benefit from afterload reduction, both pharmacologically and through an IABP. Diminution of LV systolic pressure through afterload reduction decreases the pressure gradient from the LV to the LA during systole, with a resultant decrease in regurgitant volume.

Pre-bypass assessment of LV function can be misleading. Preserved ejection fraction and elevated stroke volume can mask marked LV systolic dysfunction. In MR much of the LV volume is ejected into the low-pressure/impedance outflow path of the LA. This route is no longer available after valve replacement.

Following MV replacement, a dysfunctional LV might be unable to provide adequate cardiac output into the systemic circulation with its higher vascular resistance, which usually necessitates inotropic support.

Patients previously in atrial fibrillation without marked atrial enlargement often revert to or can be converted to sinus rhythm following valve replacement. When the diameter of the atrium is significantly enlarged; however, the likelihood of maintaining sinus rhythm dramatically decreases.

Gaudino M, Di Franco A, Rong LQ, Piccini J, Mack M. Postoperative atrial fibrillation: from mechanisms to treatment. *Eur Heart J.* 2023;44:1020-1039.

Ramakrishan H, Craner RC, Devaleria PA, Cook DJ, Housmans PR, Rehfeldt KH. Valvular heart disease: replacement and repair. In: Kaplan JA, Augustides J, Maneck GR, Maus T, eds. *Kaplan's Cardiac Anesthesia.* 7th ed. Elsevier; 2017:770-817.

C.9. The patient cannot be weaned from CPB following an AV and MV replacement. What are the possible causes?

Multiple factors can contribute to difficulty separating a patient from CPB. The adequacy of myocardial preservation should be considered. LVH without or with accompanying coronary artery disease increases myocardial oxygen demand and predisposes to demand/supply imbalance. The prolonged cross-clamp time necessitated by dual-valve replacement can lead to inadequate and/or inhomogeneous myocardial protection. In addition, there may be residual effects from the cardioplegia solution. Therefore, some degree of post-bypass LV dysfunction can be anticipated, and inotropic support required.

Although obstruction to LV ejection is acutely relieved by replacement of the stenotic valve, LV compliance is largely unchanged. Adequate preload still depends on sinus rhythm and sufficient LV filling pressures (PA occlusion pressure [PAOP] or LVEDP). Elevations in pulmonary vascular resistance can render estimation of left atrial pressure through the PA catheter inaccurate. In this setting, placement of a left atrial catheter can be useful.

TEE can be invaluable in identifying surgically correctable causes for inability to wean from CPB. Evaluation of LV filling and contractility can help resolve the situation of low cardiac output and high filling pressures. A small underfilled LV with hyperdynamic contractility and a dilated, overfilled, hypokinetic LV can both give the same hemodynamic parameters but require different pharmacologic interventions. Abnormal valve seating can compromise flow into the coronary ostia, and return to CPB might be indicated for valve inspection, repositioning or coronary artery bypass grafting. Similarly, paravalvular leaks or aortic dissection can be readily identified.

Iatrogenic injury to the circumflex artery, although rare, can occur during MV annuloplasty or replacement. The course of the circumflex artery along the posterior path of the MV annulus makes it a potential target for errant valve stitches. New regional wall motion abnormalities in the inferior-lateral territory help make this unusual diagnosis or influence the decision to pursue diagnostic testing, such as emergent cardiac catheterization. The coronary sinus can also be damaged during MV repair and replacement because the suture line is placed in the lateral mitral annulus. TEE can demonstrate abnormal echodensities in the area of the atrioventricular groove, and color flow Doppler can demonstrate high-velocity flow jets from the chambers to the sinus.

Ender J, Selbach M, Borger MA, et al. Echocardiographic identification of iatrogenic injury of the circumflex artery during minimally invasive mitral valve repair. *Ann Thorac Surg.* 2010;89:1866-1872.

Monaco F, Di Prima AL, Kim JH, et al. Management of challenging cardiopulmonary bypass separation. *J Cardiothorac Vasc Anesth.* 2020;34:1622-1635.

Nguyen L, Roth DM, Shanewise JS. Discontinuing cardiopulmonary bypass. In: Kaplan JA, Augustides J, Maneck GR, Maus T, eds. *Kaplan's Cardiac Anesthesia.* 7th ed. Elsevier; 2017:1291-1310.

C.10. How would you diagnose right-sided heart failure and pulmonary hypertension? How would you treat it?

Right-sided heart failure is diagnosed by elevations in right-sided filling pressures, specifically central venous pressure. Careful examination is required to rule out TR as the primary cause of the central venous pressure elevation, with the caveat that acute TR can also indicate a failing right ventricle. A high central venous pressure indicates the inability of the right heart to adequately pump the venous return volume into the pulmonary circulation. Elevation in PA pressures is indicative of pulmonary hypertension.

The combination of high central venous pressure and high PA pressures indicates RV dysfunction. This scenario can be difficult to manage. Attempts to elevate systemic perfusion pressure with α-agonists can worsen pulmonary hypertension. Administration of vasodilators to lower pulmonary pressures results in systemic hypotension. In this setting, it is often prudent to return to CPB, relieve ventricular distention, and improve myocardial perfusion. During this "rest period," adjustments in inotropic therapy, ventilation, and cardiac rhythm can be instituted. Optimization of acid-base status, temperature, and hemoglobin concentration should also be performed. Separation from bypass can then be attempted again.

Inotropic agents effective in this setting are those with high degrees of β-adrenergic potency and potent vasodilation in the pulmonary vasculature. Commonly employed agents include dobutamine, epinephrine, and the phosphodiesterase-III (PDE-III) inhibitors amrinone and milrinone. α-Agonists can be required to counteract systemic vasodilation. Vasopressin can also be used for systemic vasoconstriction and has little effect on the pulmonary vasculature due to absence of local vasopressin receptors.

Inhaled vasodilators are also useful for afterload reduction in the management of acute RV dysfunction. Inhaled agents selectively affect the pulmonary vasculature, thus avoiding the systemic hypotension induced by IV agents, and can improve perfusion-ventilation matching in patients with hypoxemia. Case series and small trials indicate that aerosolized vasodilators, compared to IV agents, are associated with improved RV performance in cardiac surgery. Although aerosolized milrinone, iloprost, epoprostenol, and inhaled nitric oxide (iNO) have each been evaluated in the context of cardiac surgery, iNO is common in clinical practice. Advantages of nitric oxide include its potency, extremely short half-life, and minimal systemic effects. However, methods of iNO delivery, scavenging of waste gases, and high cost remain as obstacles to its clinical utility.

Elmi-Sarabi M, Jarry S, Couture EJ, et al. Pulmonary vasodilator response of combined inhaled epoprostenol and inhaled milrinone in cardiac surgical patients. *Anesth Analg.* 2023;136:282-294.

Haddad F, Elmi-Sarabi M, Fader E, et al. Pearls and pitfalls in managing right heart failure in cardiac surgery. *Curr Opin Anaesthesiol.* 2016;2968-79.

Humbert M, Kovacs G, Hoeper MM, et al; ESC/ERS Scientific Document Group. 2022 ESC/ERS guidelines for the diagnosis and treatment of pulmonary hypertension. *Eur Respir J.* 2023;61:2200879.

Vandenheuvel M, Bouchez S, Wouters P, Mauermann E. Assessing right ventricular function in the perioperative setting, part I: echo-based measurements. *Anesthesiol Clin.* 2019;37:675-695.

C.11. How does an intra-aortic balloon pump (IABP) work to benefit the failing heart?

An IABP is a catheter with a large balloon (40-60 mL) at its tip. It is positioned in the thoracic aorta, via the femoral or axillary artery, distal to the left subclavian artery origin and proximal to the takeoff of the renal vessels. It is timed to inflate during diastole to increase diastolic perfusion pressure to the coronary arteries, great vessels, and major abdominal organs and to deflate just before systole, creating a void in volume within the aorta and thus a low end-diastolic pressure with a resultant decrease in afterload. The decreased afterload increases stroke volume, leading to decreased LVEDP and further increasing coronary perfusion pressure. In summary, an IABP improves coronary perfusion pressures while reducing myocardial oxygen demand.

Baldetti L, Pagnesi M, Gramegna M, et al. Intra-aortic balloon pumping in acute decompensated heart failure with hypoperfusion: from pathophysiology to clinical practice. *Circ Heart Fail.* 2021;14:e008527.

C.12. What role does the IABP have in this setting?

An IABP is useful because, unlike any pharmacologic intervention, it is capable of increasing mean arterial pressure during diastole, which is critical for coronary perfusion, while lowering afterload to systolic LV ejection. IABP counterpulsation can mitigate post-bypass myocardial dysfunction by reducing afterload and augmenting diastolic (eg, coronary perfusion) pressures. Although IABPs have not demonstrated a survival benefit in patients with cardiogenic shock due to acute myocardial infarction, data suggest that some subsets of cardiac surgical patients benefit from prophylactic device placement. By contrast, in observational studies, intraoperative and postoperative IABP placement has been associated with worse postoperative outcomes, likely due to underlying shock pathology. The IABP only directly improves cardiac output by about 0.5 L/min, although if cardiac function is improved by enhanced perfusion and reduced afterload, then the cardiac output can be substantially increased. The IABP can only aid patients in whom ventricular function can recover in a relatively short time. Percutaneous VADs or extracorporeal membrane oxygenation (ECMO) might be more appropriate for patients who will require longer-term support.

Heringlake M, Berggreen AE, Paarmann H. Still a place for aortic counterpulsation in cardiac surgery and patients with cardiogenic shock? *Crit Care.* 2021;25:309.

Monaco F, Di Prima AL, Kim JH, et al. Management of challenging cardiopulmonary bypass separation. *J Cardiothorac Vasc Anesth*. 2020;34:1622-1635.

Rocha Ferreira GS, de Almeida JP, Landoni G, et al. Effect of a perioperative intra-aortic balloon pump in high-risk cardiac surgery patients: a randomized clinical trial. *Crit Care Med*. 2018;46:e742-e750.

C.13. What role does TEE play in the placement, timing, and demonstration of efficacy of an IABP?

The thoracic aorta and aortic arch can be clearly imaged by TEE. Imaging of the takeoff of the left subclavian artery facilitates optimal positioning of the IABP. In addition, before insertion, the aorta can be evaluated for dissection or severe atheromatous disease; both are contraindications to IABP insertion. TEE can demonstrate the efficacy of an IABP by showing enhanced ventricular function.

Klopman MA, Chen EP, Sniecinski RM. Positioning an intraaortic balloon pump using intraoperative transesophageal echocardiogram guidance. *Anesth Analg*. 2011;113:40-43.

C.14. How would you properly time the IABP cycle?

IABP inflation can be cycled according to ECG or aortic pressure. Inflation should occur just following the dicrotic notch and deflation before the upstroke in the aortic pressure curve. Correct timing is confirmed by inspection of the arterial waveform. Early and mean diastolic pressures should increase. End-diastolic pressure (the lowest pressure in the cardiac cycle) should fall. Peak systolic pressure should also fall due to decreased LVESV and LVESP.

Webb CA, Weyker PD, Flynn BC. Management of intra-aortic balloon pumps. *Semin Cardiothorac Vasc Anesth*. 2015;19:106-121.

C.15. What are the contraindications to the use of an IABP?

The most common contraindications are moderate to severe AI and severe peripheral arterial or aortic disease (atheromatous, aneurysmal, dissection). TEE can be helpful in evaluating the effect of an IABP on overall ventricular function. End-systolic areas should decrease, and end-diastolic areas should remain unchanged or decrease. Regional wall motion abnormalities can improve in the setting of increased coronary perfusion and decreased wall stress.

Webb CA, Weyker PD, Flynn BC. Management of intra-aortic balloon pumps. *Semin Cardiothorac Vasc Anesth*. 2015;19:106-121.

C.16. What is the role for ventricular assist devices (VADs)?

VADs are used in the management of chronic heart failure after exhausting medical therapy. Both durable and temporary devices can be used as a bridge to recovery or transplantation. Durable devices can also serve as destination therapy in patients who do not qualify for transplantation.

Temporary VADs, IABPs, and veno-arterial (VA) ECMO can be used to manage refractory postcardiotomy cardiogenic shock. VA ECMO provides biventricular and respiratory support, while VADs can be used for right, left, or biventricular support. These devices are discussed in detail in Chapter 6: Mechanical Circulatory Support.

Balthazar T, Vandenbriele C, Verbrugge FH, et al. Managing patients with short-term mechanical circulatory support: JACC review topic of the week. *J Am Coll Cardiol*. 2021;77:1243-1256.

Dangl M, Albosta M, Butros H, Loebe M. Temporary mechanical circulatory support: left, right, and biventricular devices. *Curr Cardiol Rev*. 2023;19:27-42.

D. Postoperative Management

D.1. In the intensive care unit (ICU) 4 hours later, the patient became hypotensive with a low cardiac output. How could you distinguish between cardiac tamponade and pump failure? How would the TEE images differ?

Differentiation between cardiac tamponade and primary pump failure in the immediate post-bypass ICU setting can be difficult. Elevations in filling pressures, systemic hypotension, and low cardiac output are consistent with both diagnoses. The classic finding of equalization of intracardiac diastolic pressures might not be present because areas of focal compression from clot or focal effusion can markedly reduce filling of only one chamber in the absence of an intact pericardium. Echocardiography enables visualization of pericardial effusions and chamber volume and function. Diffuse or focal compression of the cardiac chambers from pericardial clot or effusion can readily be distinguished from a volume-overloaded, failing heart with poor myocardial contractility. Atrial collapse during ventricular systole with subsequent ventricular diastolic collapse is diagnostic of tamponade. TEE can be indicated, as TTE windows are frequently obscured by dressings, pacing pads, and drainage tubes. When the diagnosis is not clear, surgical reexploration can be necessary. (See Chapter 12: Cardiac Tamponade.)

Bojar RM. Mediastinal bleeding. In: Bojar RM, ed. *Manual of Perioperative Care in Adult Cardiac Surgery*. 6th ed. John Wiley & Sons; 2021:417-456.

Leiva EH, Carreño M, Bucheli FR, et al. Factors associated with delayed cardiac tamponade after cardiac surgery. *Ann Card Anaesth*. 2018;21:158-166.

Society of Thoracic Surgeons Task Force on Resuscitation After Cardiac Surgery. The Society of Thoracic Surgeons expert consensus for the resuscitation of patients who arrest after cardiac surgery. *Ann Thorac Surg*. 2017;103:1005-1020.

D.2. Would you extubate this patient early in the ICU? Why?

Likely no. Early tracheal extubation, commonly understood as extubation within 6 hours postoperatively, can be safely achieved following uncomplicated valve surgery in patients with good ventricular function. By contrast, this patient has undergone a double valve replacement, which is associated with increased duration of CPB and aortic cross-clamping, and attendant risks of systemic inflammation, myocardial dysfunction, and metabolic dysfunction. Coagulopathy and postoperative bleeding, pulmonary hypertension, and hypothermia from incomplete and nonuniform rewarming are also common in the immediate postoperative period. Sedation and mechanical ventilation can reduce systemic oxygen requirements during this early phase of recovery, minimize pulmonary hypertension secondary to hypercarbia, hypoxemia and pain, facilitate controlled assessment of patient hemodynamics, and facilitate rewarming.

Bojar RM. Early postoperative care. In: Bojar RM, ed. *Manual of Perioperative Care in Adult Cardiac Surgery*. 6th ed. John Wiley & Sons; 2021:363-416.

Charlesworth M, Klein A. Enhanced recovery after cardiac surgery. *Anesthesiol Clin*. 2022;40:143-155.

Shaw AD, Guinn NR, Brown JK, et al. Controversies in enhanced recovery after cardiac surgery. *Perioper Med (Lond)*. 2022;11:19.

D.3. What are the advantages and disadvantages of early tracheal extubation?

Early extubation can be associated with medical and financial benefits. Early extubation helps avoid complications associated with prolonged intubation such as atelectasis, diaphragmatic atrophy, retained pulmonary secretions, and pneumonia. In addition, positive pressure ventilation can have adverse hemodynamic effects due to decreased venous return, and sedatives required to maintain patient comfort while intubated can exacerbate perioperative hypotension and increase risk of delirium. Early extubation reduces these risks and can also decrease cost by lowering staffing requirements and duration of ICU stay, and helping ensure bed availability for future cardiac surgery patients.

However, early extubation is not appropriate for all patients. Post-extubation respiratory failure leads to hypoxemia, hypercarbia, and myocardial or neurologic ischemia and injury. Monetary savings realized from early extubation can be rapidly lost by one adverse event. Intraoperative and postoperative care must be coordinated to optimize patients for early cessation of invasive mechanical ventilation. Goal-directed fluid management, lung-protective ventilation, and multimodal analgesic strategies can contribute to this. Careful patient selection, with attention to underlying cardiopulmonary comorbidity and surgical complexity, is essential.

Baxter R, Squiers J, Conner W, et al. Enhanced recovery after surgery: a narrative review of its application in cardiac surgery. *Ann Thorac Surg*. 2020;109:1937-1944.

McCarthy C, Fletcher N. Early extubation in enhanced recovery from cardiac surgery. *Crit Care Clin*. 2020;36:663-674.

E. Alternative Treatments

E.1. What are the transcatheter options for MV repair and replacement? How are these procedures performed? What anesthetic management is indicated?

A growing number of transcatheter options are available for the treatment of MR. To date, these strategies are reserved for patients with moderate to severe MR who, due to comorbid disease, are deemed to have prohibitive surgical risk.

The edge-to-edge repair technique (MitraClip and PASCAL devices) directly approximates mitral valve leaflets by placing a metal clip across the middle portions of the anterior and posterior leaflets, thereby leading to double orifice valve with improved competence. This approach mimics a surgical correction known as the "Alfieri stitch," in which a suture is placed in the same position. These devices require femoral venous access and atrial septal puncture.

Percutaneous annuloplasty techniques improve MV coaptation by reducing the size of the mitral valve annulus. Adjustable bands or rings are secured adjacent to the MV in the coronary sinus, LA, or LV (Carillon, Cardioband, and Mitralign devices, respectively). These are then tightened to decrease annular dimensions and improve valvular competence. These devices are delivered via femoral venous or arterial access and might require transseptal puncture.

Nonpercutaneous, transcatheter MV replacement and repair options also exist. The Tendyne device (Abbott Medical) delivers a trileaflet, self-expanding bioprosthetic valve transapically via mini-thoracotomy. The SAPIEN 3 Ultra (Edwards Lifesciences) is a balloon-expandable trileaflet bioprosthetic valve placed femorally and via trans-septal puncture or, if vascular access is precluded, transapically. The latter device is approved for valve-in-valve replacement and treatment of bioprosthetic MR in patients at prohibitive risk of reoperation. Finally, the NeoChord device (NeoChord Inc) utilizes a mini-thoracotomy and transapical approach to place sutures (synthetic "chords") between a prolapsing posterior mitral valve leaflet and the LV apex.

With the exception of the PASCAL device, which can be placed with only fluoroscopy guidance, all of the procedures mentioned previously are performed using general anesthesia with real-time TEE imaging. Invasive blood pressure monitoring and large-bore IV or central venous access are indicated. Defibrillator pads should be placed in anticipation of arrhythmias from intracardiac device manipulation. Adjunctive regional anesthesia techniques can be considered if thoracotomy is required. Patients who are hemodynamically stable show no evidence of procedural complications and who otherwise meet standard criteria can be extubated at the end of the procedure.

Avvedimento M, Tang GHL. Transcatheter aortic valve replacement (TAVR): recent updates. *Prog Cardiovasc Dis*. 2021;69:73-83.

Khatib D, Neuburger PJ, Pan S, Rong LQ. Transcatheter mitral valve interventions for mitral regurgitation: a review of mitral annuloplasty, valve replacement, and chordal repair devices. *J Cardiothorac Vasc Anesth*. 2022;36:3887-3903.

E.2. What are the transcatheter options for AV replacement?

From the 1980s through the early 2000s, aortic balloon valvuloplasty was the sole nonsurgical intervention for severe AS. However, this procedure is associated with high restenosis rates (often within weeks or months), and no survival benefit. Its current indications include bridge to TAVR in acutely symptomatic or unstable patients, and symptom palliation in patients who are not TAVR candidates.

By contrast, TAVR has rapidly become the most common treatment for AV stenosis in the United States. It is recommended over surgical AV replacement for patients with severe AS over the age of 80 years, and is increasingly utilized in younger and lower-risk patient groups. Two types of valves are currently U.S. Food and Drug Administration (FDA)-approved and available on the US market: balloon-expandable SAPIEN valves (Edwards Lifesciences Corporation) and self-expandable CoreValves (Medtronic). Additional valve models and manufacturers are approved for use in Europe and elsewhere.

Boskovski MT, Gleason TG. Current therapeutic options in aortic stenosis. *Circ Res*. 2021;128:1398-1417.

E.3. How is transcatheter AV replacement performed?

Percutaneous TAVR devices are bioprosthetic valves mounted in nitinol stents. The valves are delivered by retrograde (eg, femoral or axillary artery) or antegrade (transapical) approaches. The latter requires mini-thoracotomy. TTE or TEE is used to confirm valve pathology prior to device placement, and echocardiographic and fluoroscopic guidance is used to ensure proper positioning during the procedure.

After venous and arterial access is obtained, a curve-tipped pigtail catheter for aortography is placed into the proximal aorta. This is followed by a straight wire across the AV, which is then exchanged for a soft-tipped rigid wire stabilized against the LV wall. The valve and deployment apparatus are advanced over this rigid wire. Balloon valvuloplasty might be required prior to valve deployment. During deployment, rapid ventricular pacing is used to decrease cardiac motion and minimize ejection pressure. Acute hypotension during valve deployment is typically followed by marked hypertension due to relief of AV stenotic obstruction.

Boskovski MT, Gleason TG. Current therapeutic options in aortic stenosis. *Circ Res*. 2021;128:1398-1417.

E.4. What anesthetic techniques, monitors and access are indicated? What complications can occur following transcatheter aortic valve replacement (TAVR)?

TAVRs are frequently performed under conscious sedation, and recent trials indicate no difference in outcomes between patients randomized to general anesthesia or sedation. However, certain cases warrant general anesthesia, such as those requiring nonstandard arterial approaches (eg, transcarotid, transaxillary, or transapical access) or complex anatomy requiring TEE guidance. Large-bore central venous access is necessary, although it is often possible to utilize the femoral venous catheter placed by the proceduralists. Similarly, radial artery catheters are placed before induction of general anesthesia, but arterial pressure can also be transduced from the arterial sheaths in patients receiving conscious sedation.

TAVR has demonstrated a favorable safety profile compared to surgical AV replacement in multiple patient groups. Nonetheless, notable complications include cerebral embolism, coronary obstruction, paravalvular leaks, and conduction abnormalities (particularly following placement of self-expanding valves). In the latter circumstance, placement of a temporary transvenous pacemaker can be required.

Feistritzer HJ, Kurz T, Stachel G, et al. Impact of anesthesia strategy and valve type on clinical outcomes after transcatheter aortic valve replacement. *J Am Coll Cardiol.* 2021;77:2204-2215.

Neuberger PJ, Patel PA. Anesthetic techniques in transcatheter aortic valve replacement and the evolving role of the anesthesiologist. *J Cardiothorac Vasc Anesth.* 2017;31:2175-2182.

E.5. What is minimally invasive cardiac valve surgery?

The Society of Thoracic Surgeons database considers "any procedure not performed with a full sternotomy and CPB support" a minimally invasive procedure. The practical applications of "mini-valve surgery" include partial sternotomy, thoracotomy, and video- and robot-assisted procedures. The downsides to minimally invasive approaches include difficulty converting to a sternotomy in the case of cannula displacement or aortic dissection, and complications of femoral artery cannulation (arterial dissection, infection, hematoma, and distal ischemia). The anesthetic management varies from standard sternotomy cases, including single-lung ventilation for thoracotomy approaches and transjugular coronary sinus catheters to provide retrograde cardioplegia. Intraoperative TEE is especially critical in these cases to monitor for cardiac distention, removal of air, and cannula placement. There is a significant learning curve to provide an equivalent surgical outcome with a "mini" versus traditional strategy. In successful procedures, patients enjoy improved cosmesis and decreased bleeding, wound infection, pain, and hospital length of stay. Unfortunately, in high-risk patients, the increased time of aortic cross-clamping and CPB can be deleterious. Complications can be severe, including aortic dissection and death. Mini-valve surgery is limited to patients with isolated valve disease.

Bouhout I, Morgant MC, Bouchard D. Minimally invasive heart valve surgery. *Can J Cardiol.* 2017;33:1129-1137.

Fitzgerald MM, Bhatt HV, Schuessler ME, et al. Robotic cardiac surgery part I: anesthetic considerations in Totally Endoscopic Robotic Cardiac Surgery (TERCS). *J Cardiothorac Vasc Anesth.* 2020;34:267-277.

Langer NB, Argenziano M. Minimally invasive cardiovascular surgery: incisions and approaches. *Methodist Debakey Cardiovasc J.* 2016;12:4-9.

8 Cardiac Implantable Electronic Devices

Diana Anca, Alan Cheng, and Fun-Sun F. Yao

A 63-year-old female with a cardiac resynchronization therapy defibrillator was diagnosed with chronic cholecystitis and is scheduled for open cholecystectomy. Her blood pressure was 110/68 mm Hg, and her heart rate was regular at 60 beats per minute. An electrocardiogram (ECG) obtained on admission indicated atrioventricular (AV) sequential pacing.

A. Medical Disease and Differential Diagnosis

1. What are the indications for permanent pacemakers (PPMs)?
2. What is sick sinus syndrome? What is chronotropic incompetence?
3. How would you diagnose first-, second-, and third-degree AV block; bifascicular block (right bundle branch block [RBBB] with left anterior fascicular hemiblock or left posterior fascicular hemiblock); and trifascicular block?
4. Is it necessary to insert a temporary pacemaker before general anesthesia for an asymptomatic patient with bifascicular or trifascicular block?
5. What are the three-letter and five-letter identification codes of the North American Society of Pacing and Electrophysiology (NASPE) and British Pacing and Electrophysiology Group (BPEG) generic (NBG) code for pacemaker classification?
6. How many modes of pacing are available in modern PPMs? How do they work? What is the difference between DDD pacing and DDI pacing?
7. The patient was mechanically hyperventilated during surgery, and her pacemaker gradually increased her heart rate. Is the pacemaker malfunctioning?
8. What are the advantages and disadvantages of atrial pacing only? What are the disadvantages of right ventricular pacing only?
9. What are the indications for, and complications associated with, AV sequential PPMs?
10. How would you know if the patient's PPM was pacing atrially, ventricularly, or atrioventricularly? What is conduction system pacing?
11. What is a biventricular PPM/ICD or cardiac resynchronization therapy (CRT) device? What are the indications for such a device?
12. What are the usual lifespans of PPMs and implantable cardioverter-defibrillators (ICDs)?
13. What is a leadless PPM? How does it work?
14. What is an ICD? How does it work? What is a subcutaneous ICD?
15. What are the indications for an ICD?
16. What is the NASPE and BPEG generic defibrillator (NBD) code?

B. Preoperative Evaluation and Preparation

1. How would you preoperatively evaluate this patient?
2. How do you determine whether the patient has a cardiac implantable electronic device (CIED) and define the type of CIED?
3. How do you determine whether the patient is dependent on pacing from the CIED?
4. How do you know if the implanted PPM or ICD is working?
5. What information would you like to obtain from interrogating this device?
6. How do you preoperatively prepare the patient for surgery and anesthesia?
7. Would you recommend reprogramming this device to asynchronously pace before surgery? What would you recommend regarding the ICD functions of the device?
8. The patient requires an abdominal magnetic resonance imaging (MRI) prior to the surgery. What considerations should you make regarding her CIED?

C. Intraoperative Management

1. How would you monitor this patient?
2. What drugs and equipment would you like to have available?
3. How would you set up the transcutaneous external pacer and defibrillator?
4. Had this patient's CRT-D been implanted the day before surgery, would you consider avoiding certain inhalational gases for anesthesia?
5. Electromagnetic interference (EMI) from electrocautery results in significant noise on your cardiac monitor. You recall that EMI also can inhibit pacing function from the PPM. In this pacemaker-dependent patient, how can you determine whether inappropriate inhibition of the PPM is occurring?
6. What are the potential responses of pacemakers and ICDs to electrocautery?
7. How would you prevent the effects of EMI from electrocautery on the pacemaker or ICD?
8. What are the effects of a magnet on pacemakers and ICDs?
9. During surgery, the patient developed hemodynamically unstable ventricular tachycardia. What would you do?
10. What precautions should be taken when a patient with a CIED is undergoing extracorporeal shock wave lithotripsy (ESWL)?
11. Is electroconvulsive therapy (ECT) contraindicated in patients with pacemakers or ICDs?
12. What precautions should be taken during radiofrequency ablation for a patient with a CIED?
13. During surgery, the patient developed frequent premature ventricular complexes, and some of these resulted in rapid ventricular pacing (see **Figure 8.10**). What is accounting for the pacemaker's behavior?

D. Postoperative Management

1. How would you monitor this patient in the postanesthesia care unit?
2. How would you confirm that the CIED is functioning properly after surgery?

A. Medical Disease and Differential Diagnosis

A.1. What are the indications for permanent pacemakers (PPMs)?

The current terminology is cardiac implantable electronic devices (CIEDs) and includes all the classic, transvenous devices as well as newer, nontransvenous pacemakers and ICD.

Artificial cardiac pacing is generally indicated for the treatment of symptomatic bradycardia or asymptomatic abnormalities in atrioventricular conduction that have a high risk for progression to complete heart block. The two main indications for permanent pacing are failure of impulse formation and failure of conduction. Sick sinus syndrome and complete heart block are the most common indications for pacemakers. The following conditions are class I and IIa indications for a PPM:

- Sinus node dysfunction with documented symptomatic bradycardia, symptomatic chronotropic incompetence, or symptomatic sinus bradycardia secondary to required drug therapy for medical conditions
- Sinus node dysfunction for heart rate less than 40 beats per minute when a clear association between symptoms consistent with bradycardia and the presence of bradycardia has not been documented
- Recurrent syncope caused by spontaneous carotid sinus hypersensitivity or more than 3-second episode of ventricular asystole induced with carotid sinus pressure
- Third-degree or advanced second-degree AV block associated with bradycardia with symptoms or ventricular arrhythmias presumed secondary to AV block
- Asymptomatic third-degree or advanced second-degree AV block in patients with sinus rhythm and documented periods of asystole more than 3 seconds, escape rate less than 40 beats per minute, or an escape rhythm that is below the AV node (suggested by a wide QRS complex)
- Ventricular pauses of more than 5 seconds in patients with persistent atrial fibrillation
- Third-degree or advanced second-degree AV block resulting from catheter ablation or cardiac surgery
- First- or second-degree AV block associated with symptoms similar to those of pacemaker syndrome or hemodynamic compromise
- Chronic bifascicular block with advanced second-degree AV block or intermittent third-degree AV block
- Chronic bifascicular block with alternating left bundle branch block (LBBB) and RBBB conduction
- High-risk patients with congenital long QT syndrome or those with documented sustained pause-dependent ventricular tachycardia
- New York Heart Association (NYHA) class III or class IV heart failure symptoms despite optimal medical therapy in patients with dilated cardiomyopathy (ejection fraction [EF] <35%), QRS duration greater than 120 ms, and sinus rhythm (eg, biventricular pacing)

Chung MK, Daubert JP. Pacemakers and cardioverter-defibrillators. In: Libby P, Bonow RO, et al, eds. *Braunwald's Heart Disease: A Textbook of Cardiovascular Medicine*. 12th ed. Elsevier; 2021:1321-1348.

A.2. What is sick sinus syndrome? What is chronotropic incompetence?

Sick sinus syndrome describes an array of clinical disorders resulting from irreversible sinus node dysfunction. This can be manifested by episodes of sinus arrest, sinus pause, or bradycardia secondary to inadequate sinus node automaticity. When the sinus node fails to generate an electrical impulse, ectopic atrial foci may fire and can result in episodes of atrial tachyarrhythmias. The diagnosis is made when a correlation is made between a patient's symptoms and electrocardiographic evidence of bradycardia. Hence, extended ambulatory cardiac telemetry such as 24- or 48-hour Holter ECG monitoring, cardiac event monitoring, or implantable loop monitors may be helpful to make a diagnosis. When episodes of tachycardia and bradycardia coexist, it is often referred to as *tachy-brady* syndrome. This is one of the most common indications for PPMs and is characterized by the following:

- Unexpected persistent symptomatic sinus bradycardia
- Episodes of sinus arrest or sinoatrial exit block
- Episodes of atrial fibrillation, atrial tachycardia, or atrial flutter
- Slow return to sinus rhythm following cardioversion (prolonged sinus node recovery time)

Chronotropic incompetence is loosely defined as the inability to achieve at least 80% to 85% of the maximum predicted heart rate (MPHR) at peak exercise. Use of medications including β-blockers, calcium channel blockers, and antiarrhythmic medications can confound this diagnosis. In the presence of these medications, a modified definition of failure to achieve at least 62% of the MPHR is sometimes used. Chronotropic incompetence increases mortality and morbidity, especially in those with heart failure. Rate-adaptive pacing is often used in these instances and increases peak oxygen consumption during exercise. Not all patients with sick sinus syndrome have chronotropic incompetence, and not all patients with chronotropic incompetence have sick sinus syndrome.

Chung MK, Daubert JP. Pacemakers and cardioverter-defibrillators. In: Libby P, Bonow RO, et al, eds. *Braunwald's Heart Disease: A Textbook of Cardiovascular Medicine*. 12th ed. Elsevier; 2021:1321-1348.

Dobrzynski H, Boyett MR, Anderson RH. New insights into pacemaker activity: promoting understanding of sick sinus syndrome. *Circulation*. 2007;115:1921-1932.

John RM, Kumar S. Sinus node and atrial arrhythmias. *Circulation*. 2016;133:1892-1900.

A.3. How would you diagnose first-, second-, and third-degree AV block; bifascicular block (right bundle branch block [RBBB] with left anterior fascicular hemiblock or left posterior fascicular hemiblock); and trifascicular block?

First-degree AV block (sometimes referred to as "delay" rather than "block" because the impulse is still conducted) is characterized by a PR interval of more than 0.20 seconds during normal sinus rhythm (**Figure 8.1**). Second-degree AV block is subdivided into Mobitz type I and II block. Mobitz type I, or Wenckebach, block is characterized by progressively lengthening PR interval until a P wave is not conducted across the AV node and a ventricular depolarization and its QRS complex is absent. The PR interval of the first beat after the blocked P wave is almost always shorter than the PR interval of the last conducted beat prior to the blocked P wave. The site of the block is usually in the AV node, and the natural history of Mobitz type I might or might not involve progression to complete heart block. Mobitz type II block is characterized by a loss of AV conduction with no progressive lengthening of the PR interval until one or more QRS complexes are absent. The PR interval of the first beat after the blocked P wave is usually the same (<25 ms) as the PR interval of the beat prior to the blocked P wave. The site of the block is typically below the AV node and within the bundle of His or in the Purkinje system. The natural history of Mobitz type II block is often progression to complete heart block. Third-degree AV block, or *complete heart block*, occurs when all electrical activity from the atrium fails to conduct to the ventricle. The site of the block can lie in either the AV node or the His-Purkinje system. Atrial and ventricular contractions are independent, with the atrial rate almost always faster than the ventricular rate. As a result, the QRS complexes seen result from an ectopic focus either in the ventricular myocardium (wide QRS complex) or in an area of the AV node/His-Purkinje system below the site of the block (narrow QRS complex). The typical rate of ventricular escape beats is between 40 and 60 beats per minute.

The term *bifascicular block* refers to a block in the right bundle and one of the two major fascicles of the left bundle. RBBB with left anterior hemiblock is present when the ECG shows an RBBB with a left axis deviation (usually >−60°) in the absence of an inferior myocardial infarction. Complete RBBB

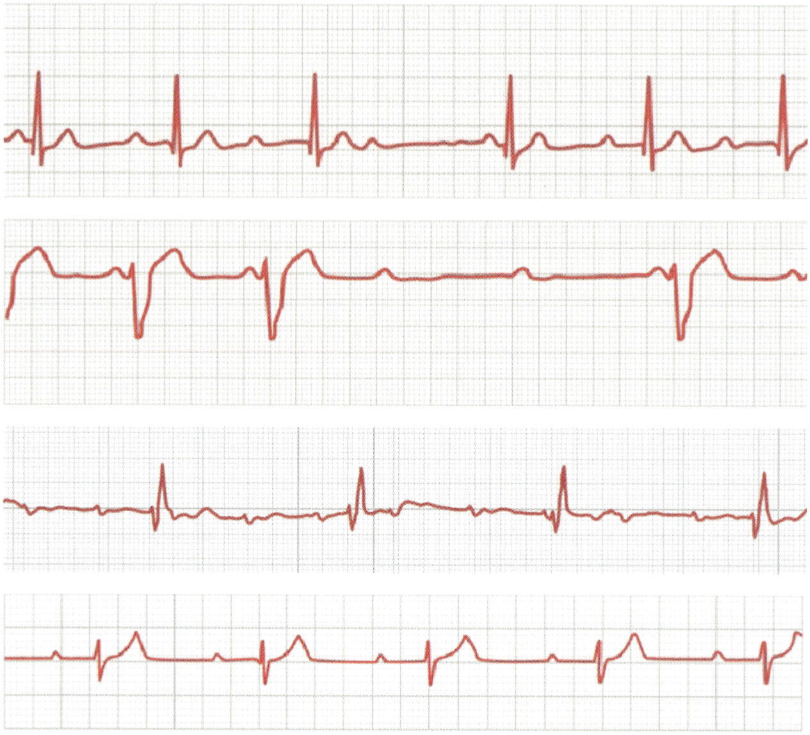

FIGURE 8.1. Atrioventricular heart block. First row: Mobitz I (Wenkebach) block. Note the PR interval of the first beat after the block is shorter than the PR interval of the conducted beat prior to the blocked P wave. Second row: Advanced second degree block. No change in the conducted PR intervals suggesting block below the AV node. Third row: Complete heart block. No communication between the atrium and ventricles. Fourth row: first degree AV block (or delay).

with right axis deviation (>90°) is indicative of RBBB and left posterior hemiblock in the absence of a lateral myocardial infarction or evidence of right-sided heart failure. The term *trifascicular block* is used to describe first-degree AV block in the presence of bifascicular block.

Chung MK, Daubert JP. Pacemakers and cardioverter-defibrillators. In: Libby P, Bonow RO, et al, eds. *Braunwald's Heart Disease: A Textbook of Cardiovascular Medicine*. 12th ed. Elsevier; 2021:1321-1348.

A.4. Is it necessary to insert a temporary pacemaker before general anesthesia for an asymptomatic patient with bifascicular or trifascicular block?

The risk of progression to complete heart block in asymptomatic patients with bifascicular block is low. No clinical characteristics have been identified that accurately predict the risk of development of complete heart block. Therefore, routine PPM implantation in patients with asymptomatic bifascicular block is not recommended. Observations made in the perioperative period suggest that the development of a complete heart block during general anesthesia is also rare; therefore, it is generally not recommended that patients undergo temporary pacemaker insertion before general anesthesia. However, it is advisable to have an external pacemaker available. The term *trifascicular block* is somewhat of a misnomer because, in truth, if all three fascicles (ie, right bundle, left anterior fascicle, and left posterior fascicle) were blocked, the patient would be in complete heart block. Although it is generally agreed that individuals with trifascicular block have a higher risk for sudden death, there is no single clinical variable that predicts a higher risk for complete heart block during surgery. Small case series have shown that the development of complete heart block in asymptomatic patients with trifascicular block is uncommon intraoperatively. Therefore, routine temporary pacemaker insertion before general anesthesia in these patients is not recommended.

Chung MK, Daubert JP. Pacemakers and cardioverter-defibrillators. In: Libby P, Bonow RO, et al, eds. *Braunwald's Heart Disease: A Textbook of Cardiovascular Medicine*. 12th ed. Elsevier; 2021:1321-1348.

Gauss A, Hübner C, Radermacher P, et al. Perioperative risk of bradyarrhythmias in patients with asymptomatic chronic bifascicular block or left bundle branch block: does an additional first-degree atrioventricular block make any difference? *Anesthesiology*. 1998;88:679-687.

A.5. What are the three-letter and five-letter identification codes of the North American Society of Pacing and Electrophysiology (NASPE) and British Pacing and Electrophysiology Group (BPEG) generic (NBG) code for pacemaker classification?

Given the complexity of current pacemaker systems, the Intersociety Commission for Heart Disease Resources established a classification code in the 1970s that is still used widely. The original nomenclature involved a three-letter identification code, as shown in the first three columns of **Table 8.1**. In 1980, this code was extended to five letters; the last two letters are omitted when not applicable. In 1987, this five-letter coding system became known as the NBG pacemaker code after being adopted by both the NASPE (now known as the *Heart Rhythm Society*) and BPEG (now referred to as the *British Heart Rhythm Society*). The first letter describes the chamber(s) that the pacemaker can pace, the second letter describes the chamber(s) that it senses, and the third letter describes the response of the pacemaker to sensed intrinsic activity. The last two letters describe additional features such as rate responsiveness that are commonly omitted when not used. For example, a VVI pacing mode paces in the ventricle, can sense intrinsic activity in the ventricle, and inhibits pacing when it senses intrinsic activity. A VOO pacing mode paces in the ventricle but does not sense intrinsic activity nor does it inhibit pacing; this is also known as asynchronous pacing.

American Society of Anesthesiologists. Practice advisory for the perioperative management of patients with cardiac implantable electronic devices: pacemakers and implantable cardioverter-defibrillators: an updated report by the American Society of Anesthesiologists Task Force on Perioperative Management of Patients with Cardiac Implantable Electronic Devices. *Anesthesiology*. 2020;132:225-252.

Chung MK, Daubert JP. Pacemakers and cardioverter-defibrillators. In: Libby P, Bonow RO, et al, eds. *Braunwald's Heart Disease: A Textbook of Cardiovascular Medicine*. 12th ed. Elsevier; 2021:1321-1348.

A.6. How many modes of pacing are available in modern PPMs? How do they work? What is the difference between DDD pacing and DDI pacing?

Modern pacemakers are programmable into one of three modes: asynchronous pacing, single-chamber demand pacing, and dual-chamber AV sequential demand pacing. Asynchronous or fixed-rate (eg, AOO, VOO, DOO [see Section A.5 for details]) modes pace at a programmable preset rate that is independent of intrinsic activity. They can be atrial, ventricular, or dual chamber. Pacing occurs without coordinating with intrinsic cardiac electrical activity and can result in pacing competition, pacemaker syndrome, and rarely induction of ventricular arrhythmias. In patients with structural heart disease, ventricular tachyarrhythmias can theoretically occur if a pacing spike is delivered during a time when the myocardium is vulnerable to arrhythmogenesis, but this is very rare.

Single-chamber demand pacing (eg, AAI, VVI) initiates at a preset rate when the spontaneous heart rate drops below the programmed preset rate. For example, if the device is programmed to VVI 70, the device would pace the ventricle only when the native beat-to-beat ventricular rate is below 70 beats per minute. If the native R-R interval exceeds a rate of 70 beats per minute, the device senses this activity

TABLE 8.1 NASPE/BPEG Generic Pacemaker Identification Code[a]

Letter I	Letter II	Letter III	Letter IV	Letter V
Chamber(s) Paced	Chamber(s) Sensed	Mode of Response	Programmability Rate Modulation	Antitachyarrhythmia Function(s)
O = None	O = None	O = None	O = None	O = None
A = Atrium	A = Atrium	T = Triggered	P = Single programmable	P = Pacing
V = Ventricle	V = Ventricle	I = Inhibited	M = Multiprogrammable	S = Shock
D = Dual (A + V)	D = Dual (A + V)	D = Dual (T + I)	C = Communicating	D = Dual (P + S)
			R = Rate modulation	

BPEG, British Pacing and Electrophysiology Group; NASPE, North American Society of Pacing and Electrophysiology.

[a]Although the pacemaker identification coding includes five letters, few modern pacemakers have antitachyarrhythmia functions. Therefore, most pacemakers are described by the first four letters of the coding system.

and inhibits pacing. Single-chamber demand pacing in the atrium functions in a similar way but is rarely used alone in the United States.

Dual-chamber AV sequential pacing requires two pacemaker leads: one in the right atrium and one in the right ventricle. The atrium is stimulated first; then, after an adjustable PR interval (also referred to as the *AV interval*), the ventricle is stimulated if no intrinsic ventricular activity is sensed by the ventricular pacing lead. For example, if the device is programmed to DDD 70 with an AV interval of 200 ms, the device would pace the atrium if the intrinsic atrial rate fell below 70 beats per minute. After the atrium has been paced, the device will wait for 200 ms to sense intrinsic ventricular activity that presumably would have been conducted down the AV node. If it does not sense intrinsic activity within 200 ms, it will then deliver an electrical impulse to the ventricle as well. DDD pacemakers can also pace the ventricle in response to intrinsic atrial activity. For example, if the intrinsic atrial rate was 80 beats per minute, the device would inhibit pacing in the atrium because the base rate was set to 70 beats per minute. But because it is a dual-chamber device programmed to inhibit and trigger pacing in both chambers (ie, the third "D" in the coding sequence), it will wait 200 ms from the time of the intrinsic atrial activity and monitor for intrinsic ventricular activity. If it detects intrinsic ventricular activity (ie, the atrial signal conducted down the AV node and to the ventricle), it will inhibit ventricular pacing. If it does not sense intrinsic ventricular activity occurring within 200 ms of the intrinsic atrial activity, the pacemaker will "trigger" the ventricular pacing lead to pace the ventricle.

Dual-chamber pacemakers programmed to DDI differ slightly from devices programmed to DDD, in that AV sequential pacing occurs only when atrial pacing is present. This is in contrast to DDD pacing in which AV sequential pacing is preserved regardless of whether atrial pacing or atrial sensing is occurring. Suppose a dual-chamber pacemaker is programmed to DDI 70 with an AV interval of 200 ms. If the sinus rate falls below 70 beats per minute, the atrial pacing lead would pace the atrium. After a 200-ms interval, if intrinsic ventricular activity was seen by the ventricular lead, the ventricular lead would be inhibited from pacing the ventricle. If ventricular activity was not seen after 200 ms, the ventricular lead would pace the ventricle. Suppose now that the sinus rate is 80 beats per minute. Because the DDI pacemaker is programmed to 70 beats per minute, atrial pacing is inhibited. Because DDI pacemakers do not track atrial sensed events, ventricular pacing would not be "triggered" after 200 ms by these atrial sensed events and ventricular pacing would only occur if the *ventricular* rate fell below the preset rate of 70 beats per minute.

Chung MK, Daubert JP. Pacemakers and cardioverter-defibrillators. In: Libby P, Bonow RO, et al, eds. *Braunwald's Heart Disease: A Textbook of Cardiovascular Medicine*. 12th ed. Elsevier; 2021:1321-1348.

A.7. The patient was mechanically hyperventilated during surgery, and her pacemaker gradually increased her heart rate. Is the pacemaker malfunctioning?

All modern pacemakers are able to adjust the pacing rate according to the patient's level of activity in an effort to obtain a more physiologic response to exercise. This is known as *rate-response* (adaptive) pacing and is denoted by an "R" in the fourth position of the NBG coding schema. This is often applied in patients with chronotropic incompetence or those with permanent atrial fibrillation who have undergone AV node ablation. Various activity-detecting systems have been developed to create a reliable rate-responsive pacemaker (eg, muscle movement, respiratory rate, minute ventilation, central venous temperature, QT interval, myocardial contractility [d*P*/d*t*], oxygen saturation and pH in mixed venous blood, and ventricular depolarization gradient), but PPMs currently used in the United States rely on sensors of motion or changes in minute ventilation through measurements of intrathoracic impedance. Because of the latter phenomenon, patients undergoing general anesthesia who are subjected to mechanical hyperventilation (eg, neurosurgery) can experience an increase in the pacing rate. Although it is generally not required to disable rate-responsive features before surgery, pacemaker-induced changes in heart rate resulting from intraoperative hyperventilation or significant motion might be mistaken for inadequate anesthesia. Hence, it is important that the anesthesia team be aware of the programmed settings of the pacemaker. If reprogramming the device to disable rate-responsive features is not readily available, a magnet can be placed over the pacemaker site to temporarily convert it to asynchronous pacing. Although the response to a magnet can be programmed off in some pacemakers, properly functioning pacemakers used in the United States have magnet-responsive features activated as a default.

Chung MK, Daubert JP. Pacemakers and cardioverter-defibrillators. In: Libby P, Bonow RO, et al, eds. *Braunwald's Heart Disease: A Textbook of Cardiovascular Medicine*. 12th ed. Elsevier; 2021:1321-1348.

Kaszala K. Evaluation, troubleshooting, and management of pacing system malfunctions. In: Ellenbogen KA, Kaszala K, eds. *Cardiac Pacing and ICDs*. 6th ed. Wiley Blackwell; 2020:265-313.

A.8. What are the advantages and disadvantages of atrial pacing only? What are the disadvantages of right ventricular pacing only?

Atrial pacing increases cardiac output by as much as 26% over ventricular-only pacing because atrial contraction normally contributes 15% to 25% to diastolic filling of the ventricle. Coronary blood flow increases and coronary resistance decreases during atrial pacing only. Atrial pacing is also associated with a reduction in the incidence of atrial fibrillation. Atrial pacing only is seldom used in the United States and often is combined with a ventricular pacing lead in the event AV block develops over time.

Ventricular pacing, occurring individually or sequentially with atrial pacing, can result in dyssynchronous left ventricular electrical activation and mechanical contraction. Under normal circumstances, electrical activation along the His-Purkinje system results in a near-simultaneous activation of the entire left ventricle. This allows for efficient contraction and is said to be synchronous. When right ventricular pacing is introduced (the lead is typically placed at the right ventricular septum or apex), the right ventricular septum is activated first, followed by passive depolarization of the left ventricle toward the free wall. This form of contraction is said to be dyssynchronous and can worsen congestive heart failure and left ventricular EF. Individuals at greatest risk for developing reductions in EF from right ventricular pacing are those who exhibit ventricular pacing over 40% of the time. Individuals requiring ventricular pacing for AV block with an EF less than 50% have a 56% risk for developing a composite endpoint of death, urgent visit for heart failure, or left ventricular dilatation over an average of 37 months. This observation has led to increased interest in finding alternative, more physiologic ways of pacing the heart; these include directly pacing the His-Purkinje system (eg, conduction system pacing (see Section A.10)) or application of cardiac resynchronization therapy. In fact, the patient in this case likely developed heart failure as a result of right ventricular pacing and underwent an upgrade to a resynchronization system to help restore left ventricular synchrony.

Curtis AB, Worley SJ, Adamson PB, et al. Biventricular pacing for atrioventricular block and systolic dysfunction. *N Engl J Med*. 2013;368:1585-1593.

Healey JS, Toff WD, Lamas GA, et al. Cardiovascular outcomes with atrial-based pacing compared with ventricular pacing: meta-analysis of randomized trials, using individual patient data. *Circulation*. 2006;114:11-17.

Vijayaraman P, Bordachar P, Ellenbogen KA. The continued search for physiological pacing: where are we now? *J Am Coll Cardiol*. 2017;69:3099-3114.

A.9. What are the indications for, and complications associated with, AV sequential PPMs?

When ventricular pacing alone cannot maintain adequate cardiac output and atrial pacing alone is not appropriate, as in a complete AV block, AV sequential pacing is indicated. Bioengineering advances such as enhanced insulation material and improved device programmability have broadened the indications for dual-chamber pacing, including sick sinus syndrome and all degrees of heart block. PPMs programmed to DDD pacing are the ultimate form of atrioventricular synchronized pacing. Programmable features include the mode of pacing, AV delay time, maximum atrial rate to which a ventricular response will occur (atrial tracking), and minimum atrial rate at which atrial pacing commences. The major advantage of such pacing is the ability to increase cardiac output. Historically, the major disadvantage of DDD pacing has been the possibility of pacemaker-mediated tachycardia (see Section C.13). Another disadvantage has been the development of ventricular dyssynchrony (see Section A.8) as a result of right ventricular-only pacing. Long-term follow-up of patients with dual-chamber pacemakers shows reductions in left ventricular EF compared to atrial pacing alone, especially in the setting of preexisting left ventricular dysfunction. A newer approach to pacing has recently gained broader adopting called conduction system pacing which early evidence suggests a lower likelihood of pacing-induced reductions in systolic function (see Section A.10).

Chung MK, Daubert JP. Pacemakers and cardioverter-defibrillators. In: Libby P, Bonow RO, et al, eds. *Braunwald's Heart Disease: A Textbook of Cardiovascular Medicine*. 12th ed. Elsevier; 2021:1321-1348.

A.10. How would you know if the patient's PPM was pacing atrially, ventricularly, or atrioventricularly? What is conduction system pacing?

Modern cardiac monitors are equipped with filters that can highlight artificial pacing potentials. In atrial pacing, an electrical spike often appears before the P wave, and the QRS complex is usually normal, provided there is normal intrinsic AV conduction. One might need to adjust the monitor so that pacing spikes are accentuated and can readily be seen. In ventricular pacing, the electrical spike is followed immediately by a widened QRS complex. Most right ventricular pacing leads are positioned at the right ventricular apex. Because of this location, pacing results in a wide QRS complex that has a QS pattern in lead V_1 and a QS pattern in the inferior limb leads (II, III, and aVF). Over the past few years, conduction system pacing has emerged as an alternative to standard ventricular pacing approaches. This technique involves placing the pacing lead near the His bundle or left bundle branch area with the goal of stimulating the conduction system and thereby allowing for more physiologic electrical activation of the heart. As a result, the QRS complex is not always wide and in fact closely resembles what is observed with intrinsic conduction through the AV node and His-Purkinje system (**Figure 8.2A-C**). Current studies are now focused on whether conduction system pacing is as good if not better than CRT.

Chung MK, Daubert JP. Pacemakers and cardioverter-defibrillators. In: Libby P, Bonow RO, et al, eds. *Braunwald's Heart Disease: A Textbook of Cardiovascular Medicine*. 12th ed. Elsevier; 2021:1321-1348.

A.11. What is a biventricular PPM/ICD or cardiac resynchronization therapy (CRT) device? What are the indications for such a device?

Individuals with interventricular conduction abnormalities have a predilection toward impaired left ventricular systolic function. One of the more common interventricular conduction delays seen in patients with congestive heart failure is LBBB. On a mechanistic level, individuals with LBBB demonstrate ventricular dyssynchrony, a phenomenon whereby the left ventricle contracts in a stepwise process rather than synchronously. Normally, the left ventricular septum and left ventricular lateral free wall are electrically activated nearly simultaneously, but patients with LBBB have a delay in the activation of the

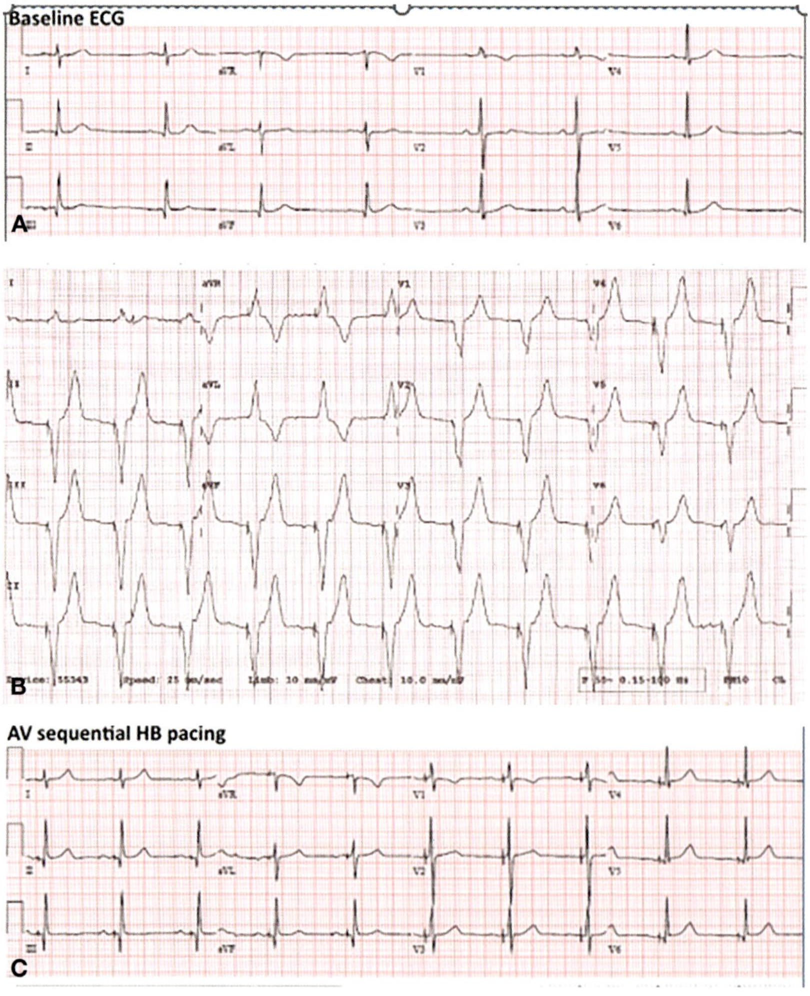

FIGURE 8.2. Normal ECG (**A**), standard right ventricular pacing (**B**), and conduction system pacing (His bundle pacing) (**C**). ECG, electrocardiogram. Note the narrowness of the QRS complex with conduction system pacing as compared to standard right ventricular pacing. This is due to the fact that electrical impulses are delivered directly into the His-Purkinje fibers allowing for a more rapid depolarization of the ventricle.

left lateral free wall. As a result, there is a marked impairment in left ventricular systolic function and increased myocardial work and oxygen consumption. One approach to correct this dyssynchrony is to "resynchronize" the heart using a biventricular pacemaker/ICD. These devices are capable of pacing both the left ventricular septum (through a pacemaker lead in the right ventricle) and the left ventricular lateral free wall simultaneously (through a pacemaker lead in the coronary sinus), thereby activating the entire left ventricle at the same time. Candidates for implantation of a biventricular device include individuals on optimal heart failure medications with

- Sinus rhythm, EF less than or equal to 35%, LBBB with QRS greater than 120 ms, NYHA II to IV symptoms
- Sinus rhythm, EF less than or equal to 35%, non-LBBB with QRS greater than 150 ms, NYHA III to IV symptoms
- Patients requiring more than 40% of ventricular pacing with EF less than or equal to 35%

Al-Khatib SM, Stevenson WG, Ackerman MJ, et al. 2017 AHA/ACC/HRS guideline for the management of patients with ventricular arrhythmias and the prevention of sudden cardiac death: executive summary [published correction appears in *Circulation*. 2018;138:e415-e418]. *Circulation*. 2018;138:e210-e271.

Jarcho JA. Biventricular pacing. *N Engl J Med*. 2006;355:288-294.

A.12. What are the usual lifespans of PPMs and implantable cardioverter-defibrillators (ICDs)?

Modern-day pacemakers are lithium battery powered and can last 10 to 15 years. The lifespan of current ICDs relies not only on the battery but also on the high-voltage capacitor. Hence, typical lifespans are 8 to 12 years. Recently, leadless pacemakers and subcutaneous ICDs have been introduced with comparable battery lives but vary across manufacturers.

Cha YM, Killu AM. Cardiac resynchronization therapy. In: Ellenbogen KA, Kaszala K, eds. *Cardiac Pacing and ICDs*. 6th ed. Wiley Blackwell; 2020:357-394.

A.13. What is a leadless PPM? How does it work?

A leadless PPM is a permanent implant anchored in the right ventricular endocardium that provides pacing support without the need for transvenous pacing leads. The first leadless pacemaker (Micra VR, Medtronic) was introduced in 2016 as a VVI-only pacemaker, which utilizes flexible nitinol tines for fixation. Since then, the Micra AV (Medtronic) and Aveir VR (Abbott) devices have been approved for use. The Micra AV device is also implanted in the right ventricle and provides ventricular-only pacing, but has the ability to synchronize AV activity through its accelerometer sensor. When the device detects that atrial filling of the ventricle has occurred, it can trigger ventricular pacing allowing for synchronized AV activity. The Aveir VR device is narrower and slightly longer than the Micra devices with a helical screw for fixation and currently provides similar functionality as the Micra VR device (**Figure 8.3A,B**). Recently, a shorter Aveir atrial leadless pacemaker was also introduced capable of synchronizing the atrium and ventricular electrical activity.

Implantation of these devices is typically done as an outpatient through a percutaneous steerable sheath introduced in the femoral vein. This obviates the need for a pacemaker pocket in the chest that is often a nidus for device infection. Given the size of these devices, the likelihood of a CIED infection is low; in the case of the Micra systems, data have shown a lower rate of complications and need for reintervention compared to standard transvenous PPMs.

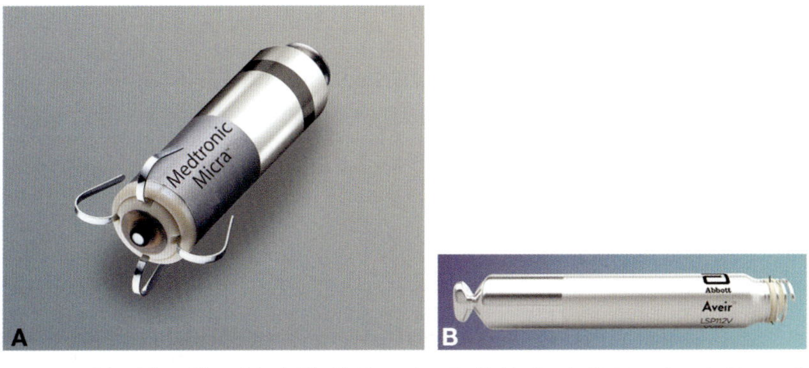

FIGURE 8.3. Leadless pacemakers, Micra (**A**) and Aveir (**B**). (**A.** Reproduced with Medtronic. **B**. Reproduced with permission from Abbott.)

Micra VR pacing modes are VVIR, VOO, and OVO. Micra AV provides AV synchronous pacing, with pacing modes: VVI, VVIR, VOO, OVO, VDD, VDI, and ODO. Aveir VR pacing modes are VVI, VOO, and OVO. Rate-responsiveness modes can be enabled. Unlike the Micra, the Aveir has a magnet response mode that can be programmed "On" or "Off."

Crossley GH, Piccini JP, Longacre C, Higuera L, Stromberg K, El-Chami MF. Leadless versus transvenous single-chamber ventricular pacemakers: 3 year follow-up of the Micra CED study. *J Cardiovasc Electrophysiol.* 2023;34:1015-1023.

Reddy VY, Exner DV, Doshi R, et al. Primary results on safety and efficacy from the LEADLESS II-Phase 2 world-wide clinical trial. *JACC Clin Electrophysiol.* 2022;8:115-117.

Reynolds D, Duray GZ, Omar R, et al. A leadless intracardiac transcatheter pacing system. *N Engl J Med.* 2016;374:533-541.

A.14. What is an ICD? How does it work? What is a subcutaneous ICD?

An ICD system consists of a pulse generator and leads for tachyarrhythmia detection and therapy. ICDs provide bradycardia pacing support, antitachycardia pacing, synchronized (cardioversion) or nonsynchronized (defibrillation) shocks, telemetry, and diagnostics including stored event ECGs and history logs. The pulse generator is a self-powered computer within a hermetically sealed titanium casing (can). A battery with high power density is used to power the pulse generator, circuitry, and storage capacitors. Most ICD designs use two capacitors in series to achieve a maximum voltage for defibrillation. A major challenge in ICD design is the large range of voltages that must be controlled in a very small package. Modern devices can charge up to 40 J of energy.

ICDs commonly use transvenous lead systems for sensing, pacing, and shocking. Epicardial leads are occasionally used in smaller-sized patients. Ventricular demand pacing for bradycardia is a standard feature of all ICDs. Modern ICDs have all the capabilities of modern PPMs, including rate-adaptive pacing and automatic mode switching. However, the response of ICDs to magnets differs from that of a PPM (see Section C.8). Almost all ICDs have telemetry-based functionality that allows for wireless communication to a bay station transponder for remote-based device monitoring.

Current ICDs have many programmable features that measure each cardiac R-R interval and categorize the rate as normal, fast (short R-R interval), or slow. When the device detects a sufficient number of short R-R intervals within a period of time (all programmable), it will declare a tachycardia episode. The internal computer decides between antitachycardia pacing (less energy use, painless therapy if programmed on) and shock based on its programmed algorithm. If shock is chosen, an internal capacitor is charged, which takes 5 to 13 seconds depending on the amount of energy to be delivered and age of the device. Most devices are programmed to reconfirm ventricular tachycardia or ventricular fibrillation immediately after charging to confirm that the arrhythmia persists. Once therapy is delivered, the ICD would redetect to determine if the therapy successfully terminated the arrhythmia. A tachycardia episode is considered terminated when sinus rhythm has been restored for a certain period (varies by manufacturer). Typically, ICDs deliver no more than six shocks for a given episode.

The subcutaneous ICD (SICD; Boston Scientific) was approved for use in the United States in 2012 and provides only defibrillation shock therapy and post-shock transcutaneous pacing (no antitachycardia pacing). Unlike traditional ICD systems, this device does not require implantation of transvenous leads within the heart. The ICD can is implanted along the left midaxillary line, and the defibrillator lead is tunneled subcutaneously across the left costal margin to the xiphoid process. From there, the lead is tunneled superiorly along the left sternal border toward the sternal notch so that the defibrillator coil is positioned alongside the sternum (**Figures 8.4** and **8.5**). The vector for defibrillation is defined between the can and the defibrillator coil. These systems provide a solution to patients who have vascular issues or may not want indwelling transvenous leads. Because sensing and defibrillation occur from the chest wall, the device has special technological requirements that limit its use in some patients. First, the size of the surface T waves can complicate device sensing, so some patients (eg, hypertrophic cardiomyopathy) are not eligible. Second, the amount of energy required for defibrillation is typically higher compared to traditional ICD systems because more energy is dissipated before reaching the heart. As a result, the battery and capacitors are larger and result in a larger device, making it a challenge in smaller-sized patients. Finally, these systems differ from traditional ICDs in that they do not provide sustained bradycardia pacing support or deliver antitachycardia pacing because of the pain that is associated with transcutaneous pacing delivery. The SICD responds to a magnet in a similar fashion as transvenous ICDs. Recently, the extravascular implantable cardioverter-defibrillator (EVICD; Medtronic) was approved for use, and similar to the SICD, it does not require implantation of the leads within the vasculature (**Figure 8.6**).

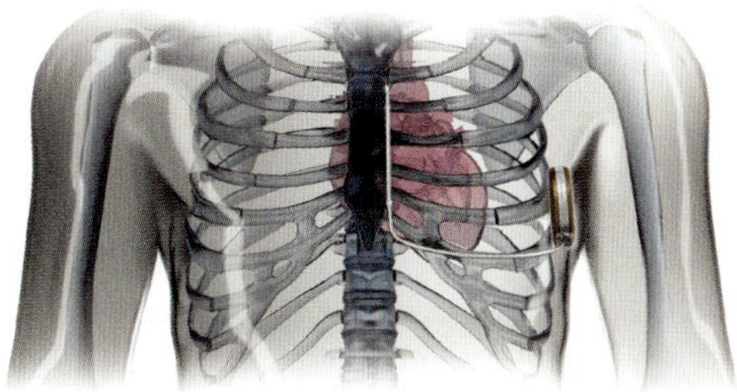

FIGURE 8.4. Subcutaneous ICD. An ICD can is implanted along the left midaxillary line, and the lead tunneled across the left lower chest to the xiphoid process. The lead is then directed superiorly along the left sternal border so that the lead's defibrillator coil is alongside the sternum. Defibrillation vector involves the can to the coil. ICD, implantable cardioverter-defibrillator. (Image provided courtesy of Boston Scientific. ©2025 Boston Scientific Corporation or its affiliates. All rights reserved.)

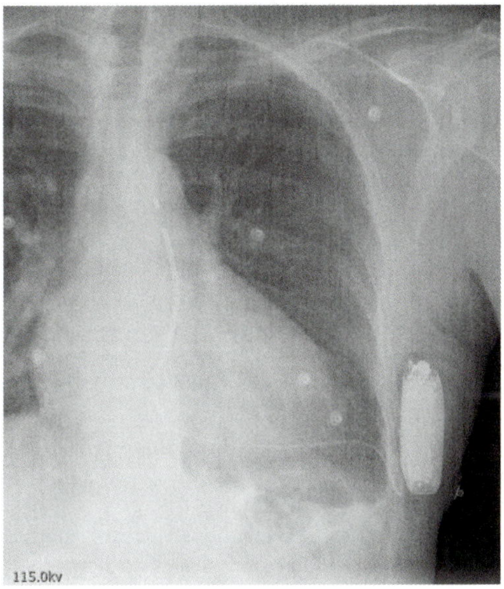

FIGURE 8.5. Chest radiograph of implanted subcutaneous ICD. ICD, implantable cardioverter-defibrillator.

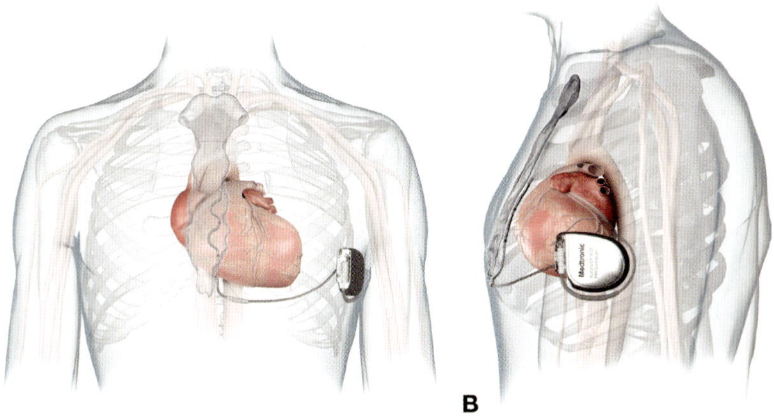

FIGURE 8.6. Front and lateral image of EVICD (with permission from Medtronic). EVICD, extravascular implantable cardioverter-defibrillator. The ICD can is smaller than the SICD and is almost identical in size to the traditional transvenous ICD cans. They are also implanted along the left midaxillary line with an epsilon shaped lead tunneled under the subcutaneous tissue to the xyphoid process. At this point, the lead is tunneled underneath the xyphoid and introduced into the mediastinal space. By placing the lead closer to the heart, less energy is required to defibrillate but pacing is possible.

The device is implanted along the left midaxillary line, but unlike the SICD, the lead is tunneled underneath the sternum within the anterior mediastinum. As a result, the device is capable of delivering antitachycardia pacing, short periods of bradycardia pacing, and requires less shock energy to defibrillate ventricular arrhythmias. The device is identical in size to a traditional transvenous defibrillator and has a battery longevity of more than 11 years. Sensing within the mediastinum has also introduced unique challenges including the possibility of inappropriate P wave sensing, especially in patients with a large atrium.

Al-Khatib SM, Stevenson WG, Ackerman MJ, et al. 2017 AHA/ACC/HRS guideline for management of patients with ventricular arrhythmias and the prevention of sudden cardiac death: executive summary [published correction appears in *Circulation*. 2018;138:e415-e418]. *Circulation*. 2018;138:e210-e271.

Bardy GH, Smith WM, Hood MA, et al. An entirely subcutaneous implantable cardioverter-defibrillator. *N Engl J Med*. 2010;363:36-44.

Burke MC, Gold MR, Knight BP, et al. Safety and efficacy of the totally subcutaneous implantable defibrillator: 2-year results from a pooled analysis of the IDE study and EFFORTLESS registry. *J Am Coll Cardiol*. 2015;65:1605-1615.

Friedman P, Murgatroyd F, Boersma LVA, et al. Efficacy and safety of an extravascular implantable cardioverter-defibrillator. *N Engl J Med*. 2022;387:1292-1302.

A.15. What are the indications for an ICD?

Initially, an ICD was indicated for hemodynamically significant ventricular tachycardia or ventricular fibrillation. Newer indications include the following and continue to evolve:

- Survivors of cardiac arrest because of ventricular tachycardia or ventricular fibrillation not resulting from a transient or reversible cause
- Spontaneous or induced at an electrophysiology study sustained ventricular tachycardia in the presence of structural heart disease
- Syncope of undetermined origin with clinically relevant, hemodynamically significant sustained ventricular tachycardia or ventricular fibrillation induced at an electrophysiology study
- Ischemic cardiomyopathy (EF ≤30%) without a myocardial infarction within the last 40 days or revascularization in the past 3 months
- Ischemic or nonischemic dilated cardiomyopathy (EF ≤35%) with NYHA class II or III heart failure symptoms
- Inherited channelopathies including Brugada syndrome (RBBB and ST-segment elevation leads V_1 to V_3), catecholaminergic polymorphic ventricular tachycardia, long QT syndrome, short QT syndrome, and idiopathic ventricular fibrillation
- Inherited or acquired high-risk states including arrhythmogenic right ventricular dysplasia, hypertrophic cardiomyopathy, cardiac sarcoidosis, or Chagas cardiomyopathy.

Al-Khatib SM, Stevenson WG, Ackerman MJ, et al. 2017 AHA/ACC/HRS guideline for management of patients with ventricular arrhythmias and the prevention of sudden cardiac death: executive summary [published correction appears in *Circulation*. 2018;138:e415-e418]. *Circulation*. 2018;138:e210-e271.

Chung MK, Daubert JP. Pacemakers and cardioverter-defibrillators. In: Libby P, Bonow RO, et al, eds. *Braunwald's Heart Disease: A Textbook of Cardiovascular Medicine*. 12th ed. Elsevier; 2021:1321-1348.

Epstein AE, DiMarco JP, Ellenbogen KA, et al. ACC/AHA/HRS 2008 guidelines for device-based therapy of cardiac rhythm abnormalities: a report of the American College of Cardiology/American Heart Association Task Force on Practice Guidelines (Writing Committee to revise the ACC/AHA/NASPE 2002 guideline update for implantation of cardiac pacemakers and antiarrhythmic devices): developed in collaboration with the American Association for Thoracic Surgery and Society of Thoracic Surgeons. *Circulation*. 2008;117:e350-e408.

Tracy CM, Epstein AE, Darbar D, et al. 2012 ACCF/AHA/HRS focused update of the 2008 guidelines for device-based therapy of cardiac rhythm abnormalities: a report of the American College of Cardiology Foundation/American Heart Association Task Force on Practice Guidelines and the Heart Rhythm Society. *J Am Coll Cardiol*. 2012;60:1297-1313.

A.16. What is the NASPE and BPEG generic defibrillator (NBD) code?

Like pacemakers, ICDs have a generic code to indicate lead placement and function. The NBD code is shown in **Table 8.2**. The most robust form of identification, referred to as the "label form," replaces the fourth letter of the NBD with the appropriate generic pacemaker code.

American Society of Anesthesiologists. Practice advisory for the perioperative management of patients with cardiac implantable electronic devices: pacemakers and implantable cardioverter-defibrillators: an updated report by the American Society of Anesthesiologists Task Force on Perioperative Management of Patients with Cardiac Implantable Electronic Devices. *Anesthesiology*. 2020;132:225-252.

TABLE 8.2 NASPE/BPEG Generic Defibrillator Code

Letter I	Letter II	Letter III	Letter IV
Shock Chamber(s)	Antitachycardia Pacing Chamber(s)	Tachycardia Detection	Antibradycardia Pacing Chamber(s)
O = None	O = None	E = Electrogram	O = None
A = Atrium	A = Atrium	H = Hemodynamic	A = Atrium
V = Ventricle	V = Ventricle	(Not yet available)	V = Ventricle
D = Dual (A + V)	D = Dual (A + V)		D = Dual (A + V)

BPEG, British Pacing and Electrophysiology Group; NASPE, North American Society of Pacing and Electrophysiology.

B. Preoperative Evaluation and Preparation

B.1. How would you preoperatively evaluate this patient?

Preoperative evaluation should include routine systemic workup, paying particular attention to cardiovascular factors. The comprehensive evaluation includes complete blood count, urinalysis, coagulation screening with prothrombin time and partial thromboplastin time, serum electrolytes, blood urea nitrogen, blood glucose, chest radiograph, and ECG. Special attention should be paid to the history, symptoms and signs of myocardial infarction, congestive heart failure, and arrhythmias. Serum electrolytes, especially potassium, must be in the normal range. For the patient with a CIED, recent guidelines recommend that all CIEDs be properly interrogated within 3 to 6 months before surgery. This evaluation should include the following:

- Establish whether a patient has a CIED—this is best accomplished by a detailed history and verified by reviewing a recent chest x-ray.
- Define the type of CIED—patients typically have a CIED information card.
- Determine dependency on the pacing function of the CIED—review recent device interrogation report.
- Determine CIED function and programming details—review recent device interrogation report.
- Determine magnet response and whether CIED requires reprogramming on the day of surgery to avoid inappropriate device behavior from EMI.

American Society of Anesthesiologists. Practice advisory for the perioperative management of patients with cardiac implantable electronic devices: pacemakers and implantable cardioverter-defibrillators: an updated report by the American Society of Anesthesiologists Task Force on Perioperative Management of Patients with Cardiac Implantable Electronic Devices. *Anesthesiology*. 2020;132:225-252.

Crossley GH, Poole JE, Rozner MA, et al. The Heart Rhythm Society (HRS)/American Society of Anesthesiologists (ASA) expert consensus statement on the perioperative management of patients with implantable defibrillators, pacemakers and arrhythmia monitors: facilities and patient management this document was developed as a joint project with the American Society of Anesthesiologists (ASA), and in collaboration with the American Heart Association (AHA), and the Society of Thoracic Surgeons (STS). *Heart Rhythm*. 2011;8:1114-1154.

B.2. How do you determine whether the patient has a cardiac implantable electronic device (CIED) and define the type of CIED?

Determining whether a patient has a CIED should be based on (1) a focused history including but not limited to a patient interview, medical records review, review of available chest radiograph, ECG, or any available monitor or rhythm strip information; and (2) a focused physical examination (eg, checking for scars, palpating for device). Of note is the availability of leadless pacemakers, which are small capsule-sized devices delivered through a catheter inserted through a jugular or femoral vein and fully implanted into the heart (see Section A.13). Therefore, there are no obvious signs of a device by physical examination, and one must review a recent chest radiograph to confirm (**Figure 8.7**).

Defining the type of device is accomplished by (1) obtaining the manufacturer's identification card from the patient, (2) ordering chest radiography if no other data are available, or (3) referring to supplemental resources (eg, manufacturer's databases, pacemaker clinic records, consultation with a cardiologist).

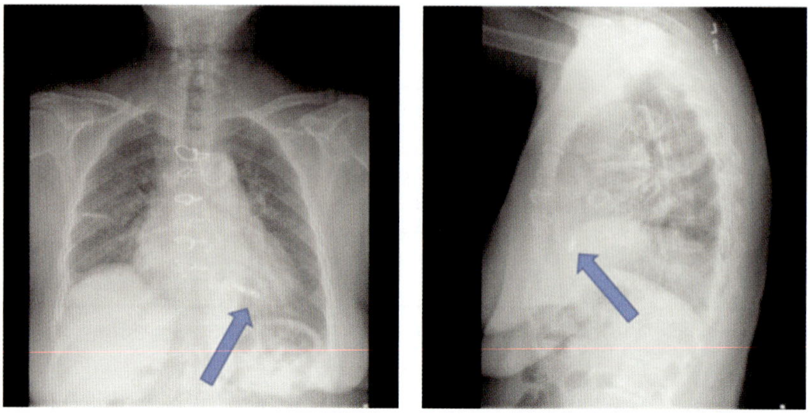

FIGURE 8.7. Chest radiograph of a Micra leadless pacemaker implanted in the right ventricle (*blue arrows*) in anterior-posterior and lateral views. (With courtesy of Hiroshi Ashikaga, MD, PhD.)

American Society of Anesthesiologists. Practice advisory for the perioperative management of patients with cardiac implantable electronic devices: pacemakers and implantable cardioverter-defibrillators: an updated report by the American Society of Anesthesiologists Task Force on Perioperative Management of Patients with Cardiac Implantable Electronic Devices. *Anesthesiology*. 2020;132:225-252.

Sideris S, Archontakis S, Dilaveris P, et al. Leadless cardiac pacemakers: current status of a modern approach in pacing. *Hellenic J Cardiol*. 2017;58:403-410.

B.3. How do you determine whether the patient is dependent on pacing from the CIED?

Pacemaker dependency is not defined by an absolute amount of pacing seen over time. Rather, it is defined by how functionally dependent a patient is on pacing support. For instance, a patient with a dual-chamber pacemaker might not pace 100% of the time. But during periods of pacing, if pacing were to be temporarily discontinued and the patient developed light-headedness or presyncope, they would be considered functionally dependent. Functional dependency on pacing support can be determined by one or more of the following: (1) verbal history or an indication in the medical record that the patient has experienced a bradyarrhythmia that has caused syncope or other symptoms requiring CIED implantation, (2) history of successful AV nodal ablation that resulted in CIED placement, or (3) CIED evaluation that shows clinically evidenced hemodynamic compromise when the pacing function of the CIED is temporarily disabled or programmed to the lowest programmable rate.

For emergency surgery, an ECG or rhythm strip should be examined for pacing spikes. If pacing spikes are noted before most or all of either the P waves or QRS complexes, then the patient should be treated as if pacemaker dependent. All pacemaker-dependent patients and patients with ICDs should have transcutaneous pacing and defibrillator pads available during anesthesia. A magnet should always be available, and its use is recommended in the pacemaker-dependent patient as well as the patient with an ICD. Regardless of the type of device, interrogation of the CIED by a provider knowledgeable in the function of devices should occur as soon as possible.

American Society of Anesthesiologists. Practice advisory for the perioperative management of patients with cardiac implantable electronic devices: pacemakers and implantable cardioverter-defibrillators: an updated report by the American Society of Anesthesiologists Task Force on Perioperative Management of Patients with Cardiac Implantable Electronic Devices. *Anesthesiology*. 2020;132:225-252.

B.4. How do you know if the implanted PPM or ICD is working?

The CIED function is best assessed by interrogating the device, which is the recommended approach. But if interrogating the device is not an option and this information is urgently needed, one can attempt to slow the intrinsic heart rate to a rate below that of the pacemaker by carotid massage or Valsalva maneuver. Carotid massage to slow the heart rate should be used cautiously because it could result in an arteriosclerotic plaque embolizing the cerebral circulation. If the rate does not slow enough for the pacemaker to take over the ventricle, the device can be tested by placing a magnet over it that will temporarily program it to a fixed-rate pacing mode. In this mode, pacing spikes march through the rhythm strip with no regard for the intrinsic electrical activity of the heart. The rate at which the pacemaker will pace in the presence of a magnet varies among device manufacturers and is dependent on the battery life.

Once the magnet is removed, the device returns to its normal programming. Of note, placing a magnet over an ICD does not temporarily program the device to pace asynchronously. The magnet on an ICD will only temporarily disable the ICD therapies and will have no effect on the pacing function. Leadless pacemakers also do not respond to the magnet by pacing asynchronously.

American Society of Anesthesiologists. Practice advisory for the perioperative management of patients with cardiac implantable electronic devices: pacemakers and implantable cardioverter-defibrillators: an updated report by the American Society of Anesthesiologists Task Force on Perioperative Management of Patients with Cardiac Implantable Electronic Devices. *Anesthesiology*. 2011;114:247-261.

Sideris S, Archontakis S, Dilaveris P, et al. Leadless cardiac pacemakers: current status of a modern approach in pacing. *Hellenic J Cardiol*. 2017;58:403-410.

B.5. What information would you like to obtain from interrogating this device?

Device interrogations provide information on the status and current programmed settings of a PPM or ICD. The important information relevant to anesthesia includes (1) battery life, (2) programmed pacing mode such as VVIR and DDDR, (3) pacemaker dependency, (4) intrinsic rhythm, (5) behavior to a magnet, (6) prior recorded arrhythmic events, and (7) pacemaker lead parameters (including pacing threshold, ability to sense intrinsic activity, and lead impedance).

American Society of Anesthesiologists. Practice advisory for the perioperative management of patients with cardiac implantable electronic devices: pacemakers and implantable cardioverter-defibrillators: an updated report by the American Society of Anesthesiologists Task Force on Perioperative Management of Patients with Cardiac Implantable Electronic Devices. *Anesthesiology*. 2020;132:225-252.

B.6. How do you preoperatively prepare the patient for surgery and anesthesia?

Preparation for patient safety and proper maintenance of the device during a procedure includes:

- Determining whether EMI is likely to occur during the planned procedure, and if so the location of the EMI
- Properly positioning the electrocautery grounding pad, so that device exposure to the path of conduction from the electrocautery instrument to the grounding pad is minimized
- Determining whether reprogramming the CIED pacing function to an asynchronous pacing mode or disabling any special algorithms, including rate-adaptive features, is needed.
- Suspending antitachyarrhythmia functions if present
- Advising the surgeon performing the procedure to minimize prolonged bursts of monopolar cautery or consider using other less EMI-generating sources of energy including bipolar electrocautery or ultrasonic (harmonic) scalpel
- Ensuring the availability of temporary pacing and defibrillation equipment
- Evaluating the possible effects of anesthetic techniques and of the procedure on CIED function and patient-CIED interactions

American Society of Anesthesiologists. Practice advisory for the perioperative management of patients with cardiac implantable electronic devices: pacemakers and implantable cardioverter-defibrillators: an updated report by the American Society of Anesthesiologists Task Force on Perioperative Management of Patients with Cardiac Implantable Electronic Devices. *Anesthesiology*. 2020;132:225-252.

B.7. Would you recommend reprogramming this device to asynchronously pace before surgery? What would you recommend regarding the ICD functions of the device?

Given the number of patients with CIEDs, recommending that all patients undergo reprogramming immediately before surgery is untenable and would significantly compromise perioperative workflow. Moreover, reports have described individuals with ICDs or PPMs who later expired because the device was not reactivated before discharge after surgery. These issues raise the need for proper triaging of patients who truly need their devices reprogrammed before surgery. The patient in this example has a CRT-D, and it is likely that the patient is functionally dependent on the CIED. Furthermore, the location of the EMI delivered in this case is close to the device system and therefore would result in inappropriate inhibition of pacing and/or sensing of EMI that the device would inappropriately mark as ventricular fibrillation. Therefore, in this patient, reprogramming the device before surgery would be recommended to deactivate the ICD and pace asynchronously for the following reasons:

- Electrocautery during surgery can inhibit pacing function.
- A magnet cannot convert the pacemaker in an ICD system to asynchronous mode pacing. A magnet placed over an ICD only disables tachycardia detection and therapy of the ICD. This is true of all

devices used in the United States. One notable exception are ICDs manufactured by LivaNova Medical, for which a magnet not only disables tachycardia detection but also converts pacing to a fixed rate at 96 beats per minute.

American Society of Anesthesiologists. Practice advisory for the perioperative management of patients with cardiac implantable electronic devices: pacemakers and implantable cardioverter-defibrillators: an updated report by the American Society of Anesthesiologists Task Force on Perioperative Management of Patients with Cardiac Implantable Electronic Devices. *Anesthesiology*. 2020;132:225-252.

B.8. The patient requires an abdominal magnetic resonance imaging (MRI) prior to the surgery. What considerations should you make regarding her CIED?

MRI has been considered contraindicated for patients with a CIED. MRI can cause rapid pacing, inhibition, resetting of DDD pacemakers, and transient switch malfunction with asynchronous pacing. Serious malfunction with no output or rapid pacing can occur because pulsed energy from MRI scanner can enter the lead by capacitive coupling and cause rapid ventricular pacing.

Current generation generators and leads have been engineered as "MRI conditional." These modern devices are equipped for the energy introduced to the CIED during the scan, which minimizes the risks of myocardial ablation and induction of arrhythmias. Hence, patients with these newer device systems can undergo MRI scanning if clinically indicated and the CIED appears to be functioning normally. Although a patient might have a CIED system that is conditionally approved to undergo MRI scanning, there are other aspects of the system that need to be evaluated to confirm that it is safe.

Precautions such as reprogramming the device to asynchronously pace and/or disabling tachyarrhythmia therapies are occasionally required. To simplify these steps, device manufacturers have developed dedicated programming settings to facilitate these changes. Rather than reprogramming each setting individually, the clinician can activate "MRI mode."

Several precautions must be observed when performing MRIs on patients with such devices:

1. The clinician needs to verify that the patient has an MRI-conditional device system.
2. An individual capable of programming the device must remain available for the duration of imaging.
3. Once MRI mode is activated, the patient must be constantly monitored throughout their time in the scanner. In most cases, ICD therapies will be disabled and pacing placed in an asynchronous pacing mode.

Once the scan has been completed, the clinician should verify that MRI mode has been deactivated.

A review of over 200 MRI examinations performed in 139 patients with one or more abandoned leads and, on average, two active leads reported minor side effects. There were no instances of change in battery voltage, power-on reset events, or pacing rate. This and similar studies question the dogma that MRIs cannot be performed in patients with CIEDs. When an MRI is needed, it is advisable to consult with a cardiologist or electrophysiologist, the diagnostic radiologist, and the CIED manufacturer.

Chung MK, Daubert JP. Pacemakers and cardioverter-defibrillators. In: Libby P, Bonow RO, et al, eds. *Braunwald's Heart Disease: A Textbook of Cardiovascular Medicine*. 12th ed. Elsevier; 2021:1321-1348.

Jung W, Jäckle S, Zvereva V. MRI and implantable cardiac electronic devices. *Curr Opin Cardiol*. 2015;30:65-73.

Roguin A, Schwitter J, Vahlhaus C, et al. Magnetic resonance imaging in individuals with cardiovascular implantable electronic devices. *Europace*. 2008;10:336-346.

Santini L, Forleo GB, Santini M, et al. Evaluating MRI-compatible pacemakers: patient data now paves the way to widespread clinical application? *Pacing Clin Electrophysiol*. 2013;36:270-278.

Schaller RD, Brunker T, Riley MP, Marchlinski FE, Nazarian S, Litt H. Magnetic resonance imaging in patients with cardiac implantable electronic devices with abandoned leads. *JAMA Cardiol*. 2021;6:549-556.

C. Intraoperative Management

C.1. How would you monitor this patient?

Intraoperative monitoring should include both continuous ECG and continuous peripheral pulse monitoring. Peripheral pulse can be monitored by palpation of the pulse, auscultation of heart sounds, pulse plethysmography or oximetry, arterial waveform, or ultrasound peripheral pulse monitoring.

Arterial and central venous or pulmonary artery pressure monitoring might need to be used in patients with poor ventricular function. Pacing detection should be enabled to detect pacing spikes on the ECG monitor. The ECG monitor should be set in diagnostic mode instead of monitoring mode.

American Society of Anesthesiologists. Practice advisory for the perioperative management of patients with cardiac implantable electronic devices: pacemakers and implantable cardioverter-defibrillators: an updated report by the American Society of Anesthesiologists Task Force on Perioperative Management of Patients with Cardiac Implantable Electronic Devices. *Anesthesiology*. 2020;132:225-252.

Crossley GH, Poole JE, Rozner MA, et al. The Heart Rhythm Society (HRS)/American Society of Anesthesiologists (ASA) expert consensus statement on the perioperative management of patients with implantable defibrillators, pacemakers and arrhythmia monitors: facilities and patient management this document was developed as a joint project with the American Society of Anesthesiologists (ASA), and in collaboration with the American Heart Association (AHA), and the Society of Thoracic Surgeons (STS). *Heart Rhythm*. 2011;8:1114-1154.

C.2. What drugs and equipment would you like to have available?

A complete array of drugs and equipment for cardiopulmonary resuscitation must be immediately available. The minimal requirements include an ECG monitor, transcutaneous external pacing and direct current (DC) defibrillator, and the usual drugs for resuscitation.

Atlee JL, Bernstein AD. Cardiac rhythm management devices (part I): indication, device selection, and function. *Anesthesiology*. 2001;95:1265-1280.

C.3. How would you set up the transcutaneous external pacer and defibrillator?

It is preferable to apply adhesive defibrillating electrode pads at the desired positions and connect to a defibrillator/pacemaker for pacing and defibrillation before surgery if possible. The electrodes should be placed as far (>15 cm) from a CIED as possible. The three recommended electrode placements are:

- *Anteroposterior placement*. The right arm (RA) electrode is placed under the left scapula and the left leg (LL) electrode at the apex of the heart (**Figure 8.8**).
- *Apex-anterior placement*. The RA electrode is placed under the right clavicle and the LL electrode at the apex of the heart (**Figure 8.9A**).
- *Apex-posterior placement*. The RA electrode is placed over the right scapula and the LL electrode at the apex of the heart (**Figure 8.9B,C**).

It is important to note that the presence of a CIED should not deter standard resuscitation efforts.

Stone KR, McPherson CA. Assessment and management of patients with pacemakers and implantable cardioverter defibrillator. *Crit Care Med*. 2004;32:S155-S165.

C.4. Had this patient's ICD been implanted the day before surgery, would you consider avoiding certain inhalational gases for anesthesia?

Nitrous oxide has been reported to cause pacemaker malfunction by increasing gas in the prepectoral pacemaker pocket. Despite air evacuation with an antibiotic solution before closure of the prepectoral pocket, a small amount of air remains entrapped in the pocket. Nitrous oxide is 35 times more soluble in blood than nitrogen. When nitrous oxide is inhaled, the volume of nitrous oxide diffusing from blood to the air pocket is greater than the amount of nitrogen diffusing from the air pocket into blood. This causes expansion of the gas in the pocket that leads to loss of anodal contact and pacing system malfunction; thus, it is advisable to avoid nitrous oxide in a patient with a newly implanted pacemaker.

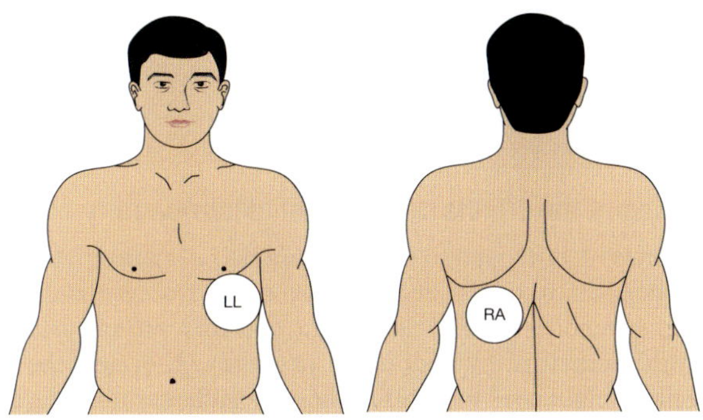

FIGURE 8.8. Anteroposterior placement of defibrillating electrodes. The right arm (RA) electrode is placed under the left scapula, and the left leg (LL) electrode is placed at the apex of the heart.

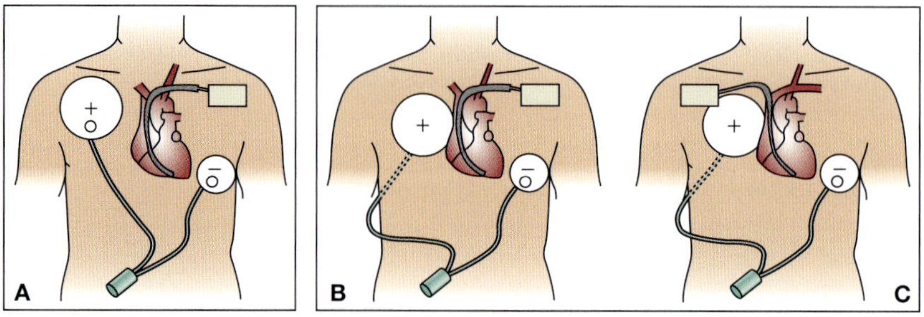

FIGURE 8.9. Placement of defibrillating electrodes. A. Apex-anterior placement with both pads placed anteriorly. **B** and **C.** Apex-posterior placement shown with the device in the left prepectoral region **(B)** and the right pectoral region **(C)**. (Adapted from Ellenbogen KA, Kay GN, Wilkoff BL, eds. *Clinical Cardiac Pacing and Defibrillation.* 2nd ed. Saunders; 2000:944. Copyright © 2000 Elsevier. With permission.)

Lamas GA, Rebecca GS, Braunwald NS, et al. Pacemaker malfunction after nitrous oxide anesthesia. *Am J Cardiol.* 1985;56:995.

C.5. Electromagnetic interference (EMI) from electrocautery results in significant noise on your cardiac monitor. You recall that EMI also can inhibit pacing function from the PPM. In this pacemaker-dependent patient, how can you determine whether inappropriate inhibition of the PPM is occurring?

During electrocautery, the ECG is frequently uninterpretable because of interference. The best monitor available to determine if inhibition is taking place is direct observation of the pulse by palpation, precordial or esophageal stethoscope, pulse oximeter, or continuous arterial pressure monitor.

American Society of Anesthesiologists. Practice advisory for the perioperative management of patients with cardiac implantable electronic devices: pacemakers and implantable cardioverter-defibrillators: an updated report by the American Society of Anesthesiologists Task Force on Perioperative Management of Patients with Cardiac Implantable Electronic Devices. *Anesthesiology.* 2020;132:225-252.

C.6. What are the potential responses of pacemakers and ICDs to electrocautery?

The potential responses of pacemakers to electrocautery or other EMI include:

- Inhibition of pacing
- Asynchronous pacing
- Reset to backup mode
- Myocardial burns, rare
- Ventricular fibrillation, rare

The responses of ICDs include:

- Inhibition of pacing
- Asynchronous pacing
- Inappropriate tachycardia therapy
- Inhibition of tachycardia therapy

Salukhe TV, Dob D, Sutton R. Pacemakers and defibrillators: anesthetic implications. *Br J Anaesth.* 2004;93:95-104.

Stone KR, McPherson CA. Assessment and management of patients with pacemakers and implantable cardioverter defibrillator. *Crit Care Med.* 2004;32:S155-S165.

C.7. How would you prevent the effects of EMI from electrocautery on the pacemaker or ICD?

The safest way to prevent intraoperative EMI response is appropriate reprogramming. The following precautions should be taken to minimize the effects of electrocautery:

- Place the cautery grounding plate as close to the operative site and as far from the CIED as possible to make sure that the current pathway does not pass through or near the CIED system. For some cases, the grounding plate might need to be placed on a site different from the thigh (eg, the superior posterior aspect of the shoulder contralateral to the CIED generator position for a head and neck case).
- Do not use cautery within 15 cm of the pacemaker because it can interfere with the battery circuitry. If in contact with a break in the insulation of the electrode, it can cauterize the myocardium at the electrode tip, rendering it insensitive to pacing impulses.

- Limit cautery to 1-second bursts every 10 seconds to prevent repetitive asystolic periods (if possible).
- If the pacemaker is inhibited by cautery, place a high-powered magnet over the demand nonprogrammable pacemaker to convert it to fixed-rate mode.
- Use bipolar electrocautery forceps or ultrasonic (harmonic) scalpel to reduce EMI.

American Society of Anesthesiologists. Practice advisory for the perioperative management of patients with cardiac implantable electronic devices: pacemakers and implantable cardioverter-defibrillators: an updated report by the American Society of Anesthesiologists Task Force on Perioperative Management of Patients with Cardiac Implantable Electronic Devices. *Anesthesiology*. 2011;114:247-261.

Salukhe TV, Dob D, Sutton R. Pacemakers and defibrillators: anaesthetic implications. *Br J Anaesth*. 2004;93:95-104.

Stone KR, McPherson CA. Assessment and management of patients with pacemakers and implantable cardioverter defibrillator. *Crit Care Med*. 2004;32:S155-S165.

C.8. What are the effects of a magnet on pacemakers and ICDs?

The effect of placing a magnet over a pacemaker or ICD varies depending on the device manufacturer, model, and individual programmed modes. This information can be obtained by consulting the device manufacturer. Most pacemakers will switch to a fixed-rate pacing mode when a magnet is placed; an exception is the Micra leadless pacemaker that does not respond to a magnet by pacing asynchronously.

The response of an ICD to magnet placement is different from the response of a pacemaker. Magnets disable tachyarrhythmia detection and therapy until the magnet is removed, except in some Boston Scientific devices. Magnets, with a few exceptions, do not affect the pacing mode or rate of ICDs. Therefore, the pacemaker in an ICD can be inappropriately inhibited by electrocautery even when a magnet is used.

Some early-generation Boston Scientific ICDs are permanently disabled when a magnet is placed for more than 30 seconds and will not be reactivated when the magnet is removed. To reactivate Boston Scientific ICDs, the magnet has to be reapplied over the ICD for more than 30 seconds and then removed. If a magnet is to be used during surgery, the magnet effects should be tested in the operating room before surgery to ensure that the desired effects will occur during surgery.

With the growing number of consumer electronic devices housing strong magnets, new sources of EMI have been reported. The Apple iPhone, for example, has a strong circular magnet array and when placed in close proximity to an ICD can result in temporary suspension of ICD therapies.

Crossley GH, Poole JE, Rozner MA, et al. The Heart Rhythm Society (HRS)/American Society of Anesthesiologists (ASA) expert consensus statement on the perioperative management of patients with implantable defibrillators, pacemakers and arrhythmia monitors: facilities and patient management this document was developed as a joint project with the American Society of Anesthesiologists (ASA), and in collaboration with the American Heart Association (AHA), and the Society of Thoracic Surgeons (STS). *Heart Rhythm*. 2011;8:1114-1154.

Nadeem F, Tran CT, Torbey E, Philbin D, Morales C, Wu M. Interference by modern smartphones and accessories with cardiac pacemakers and defibrillators. *Curr Cardiol Rep. 2022*;24:347-353.

C.9. During surgery, the patient developed unstable, ventricular tachycardia. What would you do?

For a patient with an ICD and magnet-disabled therapies:

- Advise the surgeon performing the procedure to terminate all sources of EMI.
- Remove the magnet to reenable antitachycardia therapies.
- Observe the patient and monitors for appropriate CIED therapy. This can be delayed for as long as 10 to 12 seconds as the ICD is charging.
- If these activities do not restore ICD function, proceed with emergency external defibrillation.

For a patient with an ICD and programming-disabled therapies:

- Advise the individual performing the procedure to terminate all sources of EMI while the magnet is removed.
- Reenable therapies through programming if the programmer is immediately available and ready to be used.
- Observe the patient and monitors for appropriate CIED therapy.
- If these activities do not restore ICD function, proceed with emergency external defibrillation.

For external defibrillation (see Section C.3):

- Position defibrillation/cardioversion pads or paddles as far as possible from the CIED generator.
- If it is impossible to place the pads or paddles in locations that help to protect the CIED, defibrillate/cardiovert the patient as quickly as possible and be prepared to provide pacing through other routes.
- Use a clinically appropriate energy output.

American Society of Anesthesiologists. Practice advisory for the perioperative management of patients with cardiac implantable electronic devices: pacemakers and implantable cardioverter-defibrillators: an updated report by the American Society of Anesthesiologists Task Force on Perioperative Management of Patients with Cardiac Implantable Electronic Devices. *Anesthesiology*. 2020;132:225-252.

C.10. What precautions should be taken when a patient with a CIED is undergoing extracorporeal shock wave lithotripsy (ESWL)?

ESWL is no longer contraindicated for patients with pacemakers. The only exception is for abdominally placed pacemaker generators. Because these generators are in the blast path of the shock wave, such patients should not be treated with ESWL. Nevertheless, most transvenous pacemaker generators are placed in a pectoral location that is a safe distance from the blast path. Consider preoperative disabling of atrial pacing if the lithotripsy system triggers on the R wave. Avoid focusing the lithotripsy beam near the pulse generator.

Although most pacemakers are not affected by ESWL, it can cause pacemaker malfunctions that include:

- Switching to magnet mode
- Reaching the upper rate limit
- Pacing irregularity
- Oversensing of asynchronous shocks
- Damage to the rate-sensing piezoelectric crystal
- Intermittent inhibition of ventricular output in a dual-chamber pacemaker
- EMI

There can be a rate increase in a rate-response (adaptive) pacemaker after ESWL shocks, so special precautions should be taken preoperatively. The type of pacemaker, indications for placement, degree of patient dependence, and pacemaker programmability must be determined before lithotripsy. A dedicated pacemaker programmer should be available in the lithotripsy suite should a pacemaker malfunction be caused by the shock waves. An alternative means of pacing, such as transcutaneous pacing, should also be available in case the pacemaker becomes permanently damaged. Low-energy shock waves (<16 kV) should be used initially; then the energy level is gradually increased while pacemaker function is monitored carefully. It is best to disable tachycardia detection of an ICD during ESWL and to interrogate the ICD following the procedure.

American Society of Anesthesiologists. Practice advisory for the perioperative management of patients with cardiac implantable electronic devices: pacemakers and implantable cardioverter-defibrillators: an updated report by the American Society of Anesthesiologists Task Force on Perioperative Management of Patients with Cardiac Implantable Electronic Devices. *Anesthesiology*. 2020;132:225-252.

C.11. Is electroconvulsive therapy (ECT) contraindicated in patients with pacemakers or ICDs?

It is advisable to consult with the ordering physician, the patient's cardiologist, a cardiac rhythm management device service, or the device manufacturer regarding ECT. ECT appears safe for patients with pacemakers or ICDs because little current flows within the heart due to the high impedance of body tissues. Nevertheless, the seizure and succinylcholine fasciculations can generate sufficient myopotentials for pacemaker inhibition (unipolar devices) or ventricular tracking (adaptive-rate devices). Therefore, it is advisable to program the pacemaker to a non-sensing (asynchronous) mode for pacemaker-dependent patients either by reprogramming prior to the procedure or using a magnet during the case. A magnet placed over an ICD will only disable tachytherapies and will not cause the ICD to pace asynchronously. An external pacemaker should also be available. Current guidelines suggest that all ICDs should be programmed so that tachycardia detection is disabled before ECT and reprogrammed to its original programmed parameters prior to discharge.

American Society of Anesthesiologists. Practice advisory for the perioperative management of patients with cardiac implantable electronic devices: pacemakers and implantable cardioverter-defibrillators: an updated report by the American Society of Anesthesiologists Task Force on Perioperative Management of Patients with Cardiac Implantable Electronic Devices. *Anesthesiology*. 2020;132:225-252.

C.12. What precautions should be taken during radiofrequency ablation for a patient with a CIED?

- Avoid contact of radiofrequency catheter with the CIED generator and leads.
- Radiofrequency current path as far away from the CIED generator and leads as possible.
- Discuss these concerns with the operator.

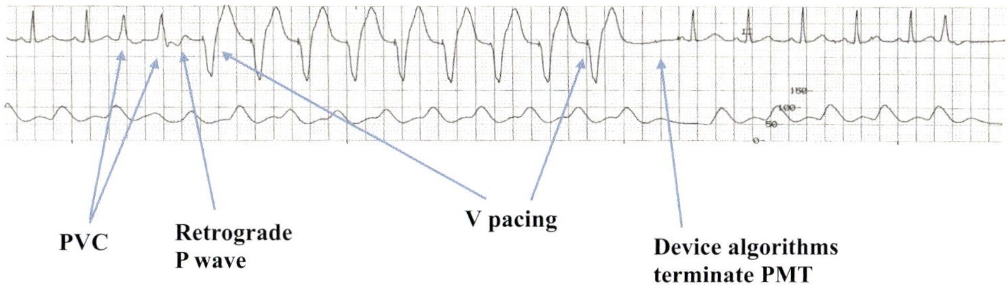

FIGURE 8.10. Rhythm strip of pacemaker-mediated tachycardia. Premature ventricular complexes (PVCs) are seen initially followed by wide complex tachycardia, with each complex preceded by a pacing spike suggesting ventricular (V) pacing. This phenomenon occurs because the PVCs are conducted through the atrioventricular node in a retrograde fashion, resulting in an atrial sensed event that the DDD device detects. Because of the DDD programming, ventricular pacing is triggered, and the paced ventricular beat perpetuates the cycle by conducting through the atrioventricular node in a retrograde fashion, resulting in another atrial sensed event. The tachycardia eventually terminates because the device has an anti-pacemaker-mediated tachycardia algorithm.

American Society of Anesthesiologists. Practice advisory for the perioperative management of patients with cardiac implantable electronic devices: pacemakers and implantable cardioverter-defibrillators: an updated report by the American Society of Anesthesiologists Task Force on Perioperative Management of Patients with Cardiac Implantable Electronic Devices. *Anesthesiology*. 2020;132:225-252.

C.13. During surgery, the patient developed frequent premature ventricular complexes, and some of these resulted in rapid ventricular pacing (see Figure 8.10). What is accounting for the pacemaker's behavior?

Ventricular ectopy can interfere with the function of a dual-chamber pacemaker or defibrillator. Premature ventricular complexes can conduct retrograde up the AV node and result in atrial sensed events that are detected by the atrial lead. Depending on when this occurs, a dual-chamber pacemaker programmed to DDD can detect this and trigger ventricular pacing, thus resulting in what is termed *pacemaker-mediated tachycardia* (**Figure 8.10**).

Current devices are equipped with algorithms that can limit the duration of these episodes. During surgery, it is important to be aware of this phenomenon and not mistake these runs of pacing-induced wide complex tachycardia as ventricular tachycardia. Look for pacing spikes in front of the wide complex beats as a quick way to determine whether they are being caused by pacing.

Sridhar ARM, Patton KK. In: Ellenbogen KA, Kaszala K, eds. *Cardiac Pacing and ICDs*. 6th ed. Wiley Blackwell; 2020:417-439.

D. Postoperative Management

D.1. How would you monitor this patient in the postanesthesia care unit?

Cardiac rate and rhythm should be continuously monitored throughout the immediate postoperative period. Backup pacing capability and cardioversion-defibrillation equipment should be immediately available.

American Society of Anesthesiologists. Practice advisory for the perioperative management of patients with cardiac implantable electronic devices: pacemakers and implantable cardioverter-defibrillators: an updated report by the American Society of Anesthesiologists Task Force on Perioperative Management of Patients with Cardiac Implantable Electronic Devices. *Anesthesiology*. 2011;114:247-261.

Crossley GH, Poole JE, Rozner MA, et al. The Heart Rhythm Society (HRS)/American Society of Anesthesiologists (ASA) expert consensus statement on the perioperative management of patients with implantable defibrillators, pacemakers and arrhythmia monitors: facilities and patient management this document was developed as a joint project with the American Society of Anesthesiologists (ASA), and in collaboration with the American Heart Association (AHA), and the Society of Thoracic Surgeons (STS). *Heart Rhythm*. 2011;8:1114-1154.

D.2. How would you confirm that the CIED is functioning properly after surgery?

Postoperative interrogation and restoration of CIED function are basic elements of postoperative management. Given the robustness of modern devices, not all CIEDs require postoperative interrogation before discharge, especially in cases in which the EMI is remote from the device system. CIEDs should be interrogated postoperatively before discharge when:

- CIEDs were reprogrammed or deactivated before surgery so that baseline settings can be restored.
- Patients underwent hemodynamically unstable procedures such as cardiac surgery or significant vascular surgery.
- Patients experienced significant intraoperative events, including cardiac arrest, requiring temporary pacing or cardiopulmonary resuscitation, and/or tachyarrhythmias requiring external electrical cardioversion during surgery.

All other individuals should have their devices evaluated as outpatients within the next 3 months.

American Society of Anesthesiologists. Practice advisory for the perioperative management of patients with cardiac implantable electronic devices: pacemakers and implantable cardioverter-defibrillators: an updated report by the American Society of Anesthesiologists Task Force on Perioperative Management of Patients with Cardiac Implantable Electronic Devices. *Anesthesiology*. 2020;132:225-252.

9 Thoracic and Thoracoabdominal Aortic Aneurysms

Olga Rozental and Meghann M. Fitzgerald

A 68-year-old male presents for surgical repair of a thoracoabdominal aortic aneurysm (TAAA). He has a significant past medical history that includes a type A aortic dissection (TAAD) 12 years ago, for which he underwent a Bentall repair; poorly controlled hypertension; chronic obstructive pulmonary disease (COPD); tobacco use (45 pack-years); and stage III chronic kidney disease (CKD). His postoperative course was complicated by end-organ ischemia, including ischemic colitis and renal failure. Since then, he has been undergoing routine surveillance of his aorta, and computed tomography (CT) now reveals his aortic aneurysm has enlarged to 5.5 cm starting at the innominate artery and extending into the abdominal aorta, proximal to the renal arteries. Chest radiography demonstrates thoracic aortic aneurysmal dilation, without compression of surrounding structures. Transthoracic echocardiogram demonstrates normal left and right ventricular function, trivial aortic insufficiency (AI), and trivial mitral insufficiency. Laboratory studies indicate a hemoglobin of 14.5 g/dL, hematocrit 44%, blood urea nitrogen (BUN) 22 mg/dL, and creatinine 1.8 mg/dL.

A. Pathophysiology and Differential Diagnosis

1. What is thoracic aortic aneurysm (TAA)? How does it typically present? How is it diagnosed?
2. How are TAAs and thoracoabdominal aneurysms (TAAAs) classified?
3. What is the pathogenesis of aortic aneurysms and what genetic conditions predispose to their formation?
4. What is the natural history and medical management of thoracic aneurysms?
5. What are the risk factors for TAA-associated mortality?
6. What is a thoracic aortic dissection? How does it typically present? How is it diagnosed?
7. How are thoracic aortic dissections classified?

B. Preoperative Evaluation and Preparation

1. What are the indications and timing of surgical intervention for TAAs?
2. Which patients are candidates for endovascular aortic repair, and what are the major advantages and disadvantages of this approach?
3. What are the preoperative considerations for the anesthesiologist before TAA repair?
4. What is the preoperative management of a patient presenting with an acute aortic dissection (AAD)?
5. What is the spinal cord blood supply?

C. Intraoperative Management

1. What are the surgical approaches to thoracic aneurysm repair?
2. How is open repair of thoracic aneurysms performed?
3. What are the specific considerations for anesthetic management and monitoring of the patient presenting for open TAAA repair?
4. What is the pathophysiology of aortic clamping and unclamping?
5. How are endovascular repairs of TAAAs performed?
6. What are the specific considerations for anesthetic management and monitoring of the patient presenting for endovascular TAAA repair?
7. What are the surgical approaches to aortic dissections?
8. Why does a coagulopathy ensue and how is it prevented/treated?

D. Postoperative Anesthetic Management

1. What are the goals of immediate postoperative care following TAAA repair?
2. Two hours following arrival in the ICU, the patient is unable to move his lower extremities. How are symptoms of spinal cord compromise or ischemia managed?
3. For how long is postoperative mechanical ventilation required?
4. On postoperative day 2, the patient's creatinine approaches 2.5 mg/dL. What is the incidence of postoperative acute kidney injury and renal failure requiring chronic hemodialysis?
5. What are the unique postoperative complications after endovascular TAAA repair?

A. Pathophysiology and Differential Diagnosis

A.1. What is thoracic aortic aneurysm (TAA)? How does it typically present? How is it diagnosed?

Thoracic Aortic Aneurysm

An arterial aneurysm is an abnormal dilation of all three layers of an artery, that is, the intima, media, and adventitia, to at least 1.5 times its expected normal diameter by convention. This definition is typically applicable to the descending thoracic and thoracoabdominal aorta, while the thresholds for aortic root and ascending thoracic aorta aneurysms vary according to the presence of associated conditions. While 60% of TAAs involve the aortic root and/or ascending aorta, 40% involve the descending aorta, 10% involve the arch, and 10% involve the thoracoabdominal aorta. The dimensions that define normal aortic size are determined by the patient's age, sex, and body surface area.

A challenge in the care of patients with thoracic aortic disease is identifying them prior to the onset of a catastrophic aortic event. Despite their propensity for life-threatening complications, TAAs are often clinically silent and diagnosed during imaging for an unrelated disorder or as part of dedicated screening for those at risk. When symptoms do occur, they are often nonspecific, and diagnosis requires a high index of clinical suspicion. Symptoms of TAAs frequently result from compression of adjacent structures. Patients may exhibit hoarseness from recurrent laryngeal nerve compression, stridor from bronchial or tracheal compression, dyspnea from lung compression, dysphagia from esophageal compression, and/or facial edema from superior vena cava (SVC) compression. Pain in the neck, jaw, back, shoulders, or abdomen can also be present. Additionally, new-onset heart failure symptoms may occur as aortic enlargement, which results in progressive AI (**Figure 9.1**).

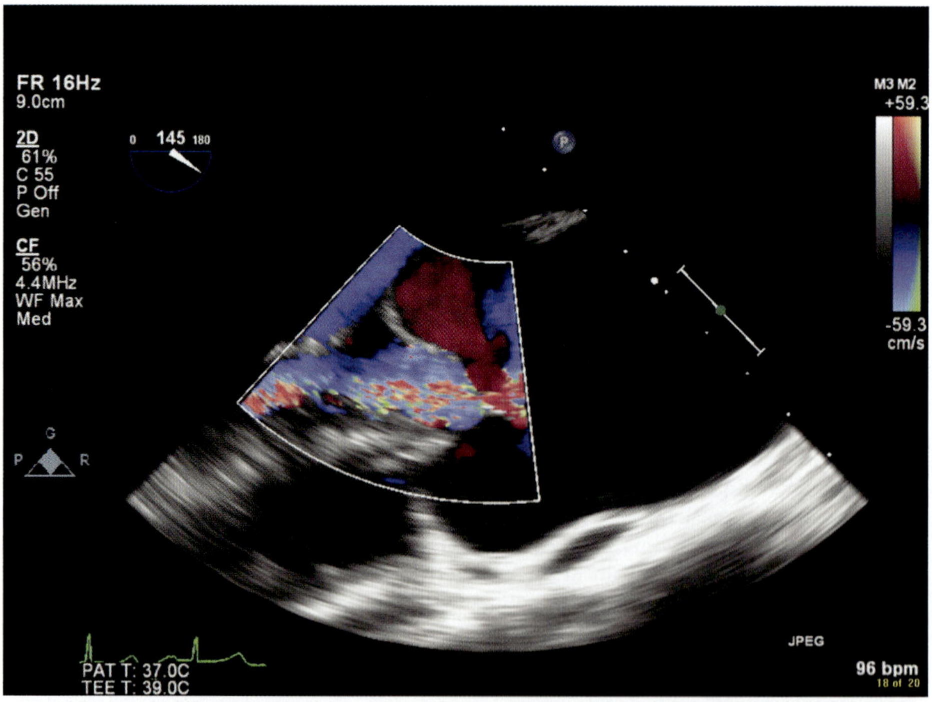

FIGURE 9.1. Midesophageal aortic valve long-axis view on transesophageal echocardiography demonstrating moderate central aortic insufficiency secondary to aortic root and ascending aortic dilatation in a young female with Turner syndrome.

CT angiography (**Figure 9.2**) is the first-line imaging modality that can provide accurate measurement of the maximal diameter of the aneurysm, delineate the extent of the aneurysm, and detect branch vessel involvement and acute aortic syndromes (AASs), such as aortic dissection, intramural hematoma (IMH), or penetrating aortic ulcer. Magnetic resonance angiography (MRA) also provides high-resolution three-dimensional aortic assessment but is considered a second-line modality due to longer scan times, higher costs, and limited availability. Transthoracic echocardiography (TTE) and transesophageal echocardiography (TEE) provide assessment of aortic pathology, valvular disease, and cardiac function; TEE has a limited role in the primary assessment of TAA unless concurrent structural cardiac disease or AASs are suspected (**Figure 9.3**).

Isselbacher EM. Thoracic and abdominal aortic aneurysms. *Circulation*. 2005;111:816-828.

Isselbacher EM, Preventza O, Hamilton Black J 3rd, et al; Peer Review Committee Members. 2022 ACC/AHA guideline for the diagnosis and management of aortic disease: a report of the American Heart Association/American College of Cardiology Joint Committee on clinical practice guidelines. *Circulation*. 2022;146:e334-e482.

Wang TKM, Desai MY. Thoracic aortic aneurysm: optimal surveillance and treatment. *Cleve Clin J Med*. 2020;87:557-568.

A.2. How are TAAs and thoracoabdominal aneurysms (TAAAs) classified?

TAAs do not follow a specific classification system but are described by the extent of the aorta that is involved, including the aortic root, ascending aorta, aortic arch, and descending thoracic aorta. TAAAs are described using the modified Crawford classification, which subdivides TAAAs into five types according to the extent of the surgical repair required (**Figure 9.4**).

- *Type I* begins distal to the left subclavian artery (LSCA) and extends down below the diaphragm to above the renal arteries.
- *Type II* begins distal to the left subclavian above the sixth intercostal space. It extends through the diaphragm and ends below the renal arteries.

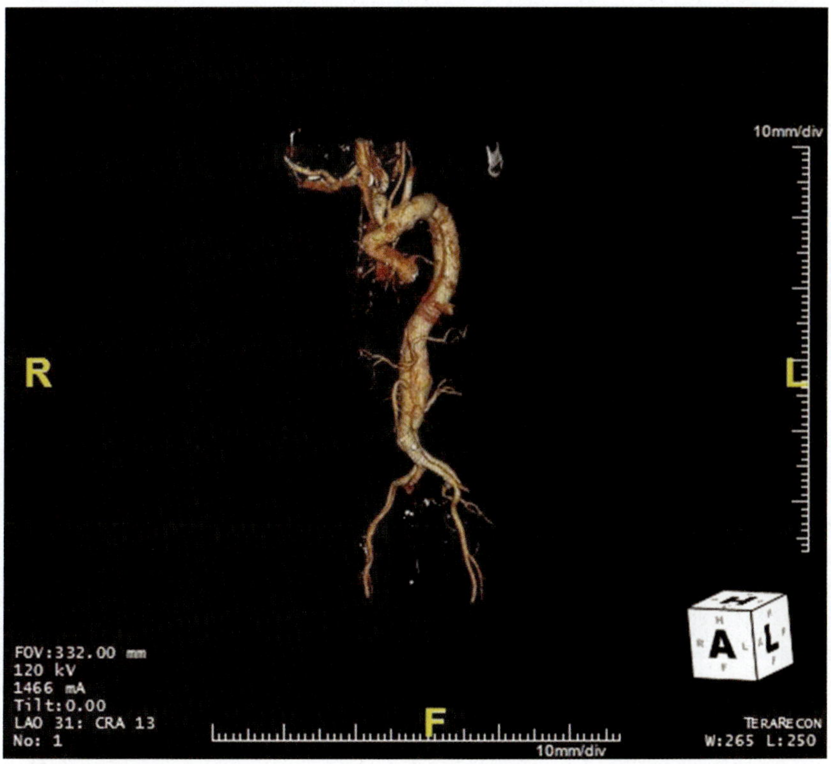

FIGURE 9.2. Three-dimensional (3D) compute tomography reconstruction demonstrating a thoracoabdominal aneurysm that begins in the descending thoracic aorta and extends to the infrarenal aorta, above the bifurcation into the iliac arteries. Also seen is a chronic type B aortic dissection.

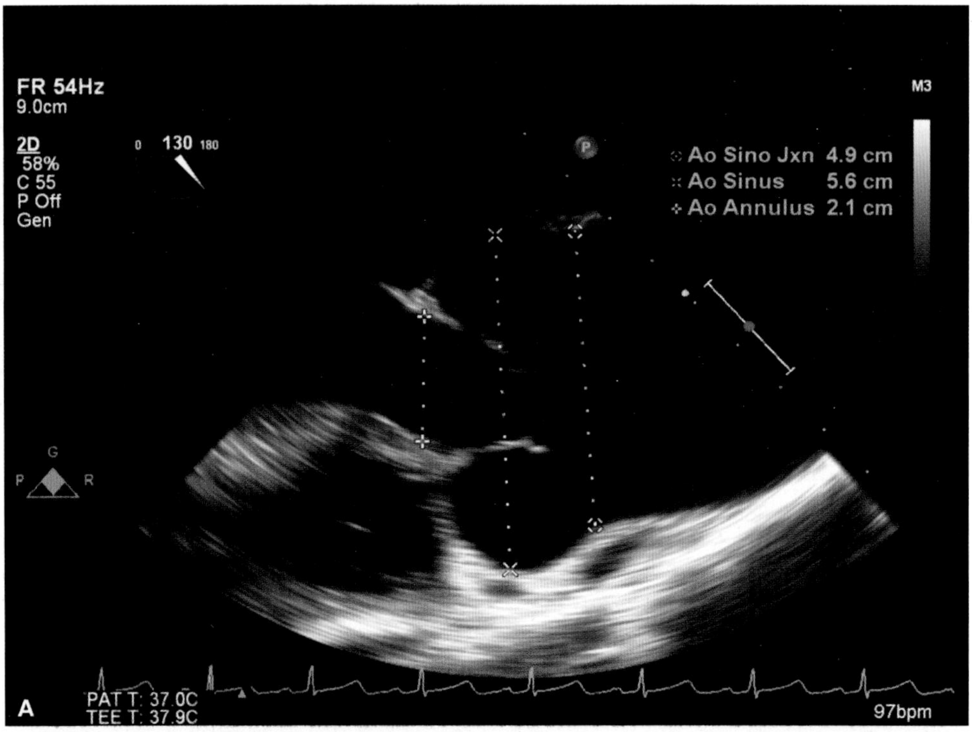

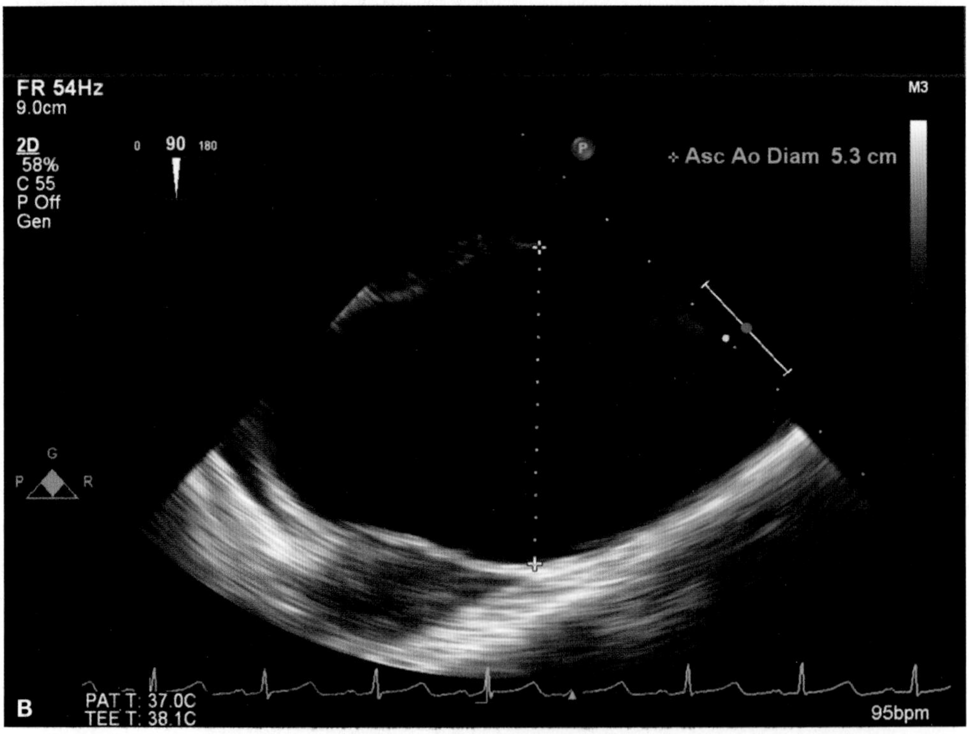

FIGURE 9.3. A. Midesophageal aortic valve long-axis view on transesophageal echocardiography demonstrating the aortic valve annulus, sinus, and sinotubular junction dimensions at mid-systole. **B.** Ascending aorta in short axis demonstrating aneurysmal enlargement with a diameter of 5.3 cm in a young female with Turner syndrome.

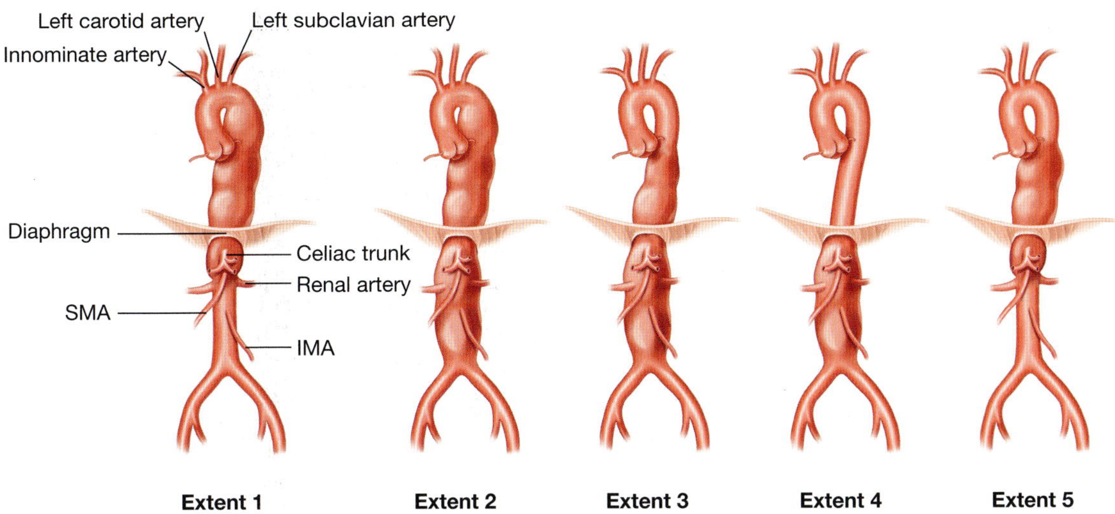

FIGURE 9.4. The modified Crawford classification of thoracoabdominal aortic aneurysms. (Reprinted with permission from Bolman R, Kaneko T. Open thoracoabdominal aneurysm repair. In: Darling RC, Ozaki CK, eds. *Vascular Surgery: Arterial Procedures.* Wolters Kluwer; 2016:74.)

- *Type III* begins below the sixth intercostal space but above the diaphragm. It extends below the renal arteries.
- *Type IV* begins below the diaphragm but above the renal arteries, with extension to below the renal arteries.
- *Type V* begins above the diaphragm and ends above the renal arteries.

Crawford ES, Crawford JL, Safi HJ, et al. Thoracoabdominal aortic aneurysms: preoperative and intraoperative factors determining immediate and long-term results of operations in 605 patients. *J Vasc Surg*. 1986;3:389-404.

Frederick JR, Woo YJ. Thoracoabdominal aortic aneurysm. *Ann Cardiothorac Surg*. 2012;1:277-285.

Hoel AW. Aneurysmal disease: thoracic aorta. *Surg Clin North Am*. 2013;93:893-910.

A.3. What is the pathogenesis of aortic aneurysms and what genetic conditions predispose to their formation?

TAAs primarily arise from cystic medial degeneration of the elastic and muscular tissue of the aortic wall. The resulting tissue weakness predisposes the wall to dilate under the stress of high pressures within the aorta. The dilation of the aorta is associated with decreased vessel wall compliance, increased wall stress, and a propensity for subsequent rupture of the aneurysm. Patients who develop TAAs are also predisposed to developing AAAs and cerebral aneurysms. Cystic medial degeneration occurs with aging but can be accelerated in male and in the presence of certain acquired risk factors, such as hypertension, smoking, atherosclerosis, and trauma, in addition to genetic, congenital, infectious, and autoimmune disease processes that are associated with aneurysm formation.

The presence of TAA in younger patients is often attributed to heritable causes, some of which are limited to the aorta while others have systemic features.

Marfan syndrome (MFS) is an autosomal dominant disorder caused by a mutation in the fibrillin-1 gene, which provides a framework for the stability and elasticity of the aorta. Patients with MFS have a characteristic overgrowth of the long bones of the arms and legs, increased finger length named arachnodactyly, and joint laxity. They can also demonstrate ocular abnormalities, most commonly lens dislocation. In addition, patients are at increased risk of aortic root dilation, ascending and descending aortic aneurysms, and aortic dissection. Atrioventricular valvular disease may occur, most commonly due to prolapse and regurgitation. Dilated cardiomyopathy and pulmonary hypertension associated with mitral regurgitation are thought to be the leading cause of MFS-related death in infancy. In addition to the 1847 fibrillin-1 mutations linked to MFS, increased transforming growth factor-β (TGF-β) signaling contributes to the increased risk of TAAs and dissections in MFS patients. Fibrillin-1 sequesters TGF-β within the walls of the aorta and therefore, fibrillin-1 mutations have been implicated in impaired TGF-β sequestering and homeostasis.

Vascular Ehlers-Danlos syndrome (vEDS), also known as Ehler-Danlos syndrome type IV, has an autosomal dominant inheritance and results from mutations in the collagen type III α 1 gene (*COL3A1*). Patients are predisposed to translucent and fragile skin, varicose veins, atrophic scars, fistula formation, and organ rupture, such as spontaneous intestinal or uterine perforation, in addition to the development of aneurysms and vessel dissections. Children can also present with an inguinal hernia, pneumothorax, or recurrent joint dislocations. Although diagnosis is often made clinically, many patients are only diagnosed after a major arterial or gastrointestinal event. In all, 80% of patients with vEDS experience a major complication prior to the age of 40 years. Clear genotype-phenotype associations are hindered by significant heterogeneity between patients with identical mutations.

Loeys-Dietz syndrome (LDS) is an autosomal dominant disease that has been linked with numerous mutations, such as TGFBR1, TGFBR2, SMAD3, and TGFB2, which correspond to LDS1-4 subtypes, respectively. Excessive collagen deposition in arterial walls due to increased TGFβ signaling results in dysfunctional elastogenesis, which leads to aortic and branch vessel aneurysms and dissections, arterial tortuosity, and intracranial aneurysms. LDS also manifests with characteristic hypertelorism, skeletal and craniofacial abnormalities, and translucent skin. There is substantial clinical variability within and between individuals with all four LDS subtypes, though LDS4 likely represents the mildest disease. Relative to patients with MFS, the clinical course of LDS1/2 patients appears to be more severe. Diagnosis is often made after a significant aortic event.

Bicuspid aortic valve (BAV) is the most common congenital cardiac abnormality and has an autosomal dominant inheritance. Accelerated aortic dilatation, which prevails in 50% of patients with BAV, commonly involves the aortic root and ascending aorta (**Figure 9.5**). Patients with BAV are 8 times more likely to have aortic dissections relative to the general population. The genetic basis for BAV aortopathy is complex and thought to be related to the loss of a dynamic balance between the expression of matrix metalloproteinases (MMPs) and endogenous inhibitors (matrix metalloproteinase organization inhibitors, TIMPs). For instance, mutations in TIMP3 are associated with a greater incidence of BAV and TAA in *Turner syndrome*. Turner syndrome is a genetic disorder characterized by the lack of an X-chromosome in a female patient (45, X). Females with Turner syndrome are often short in stature, have dysfunctional ovaries, and are at increased risk of cardiovascular disease. BAV disease is present in between 10% and 25% of females with Turner syndrome, and approximately 8% have coarctation of the aorta. To date, variants in 37 genes have been associated with TAA and dissection, yet up to 80% of familial TAAs have an unknown molecular etiology. Advances in genomic sequencing and bioinformatics tools will accelerate progress with the ultimate goal of providing personalized aortic care and tailoring surgical recommendations to individual genetic profiles.

There are additional rheumatologic, infectious, and traumatic etiologies for TAA that merit consideration. Giant cell arteritis and Takayasu arteritis are the most common causes of aortitis. Aortic infections are most commonly caused by the spread of *Staphylococcus aureus*, Pneumococcus, *Escherichia coli*, and Salmonella via a vulnerable plaque or preexisting aneurysm. Syphilitic aortitis, which occurs 10 to 25 years after systemic *Treponema pallidum* infection, is rare with antibiotic treatment. Fungal aortitis from Candida or Aspergillus and tuberculous aortitis may be seen in immunocompromised patients. HIV infection is associated with an increased risk of TAA formation. Furthermore, trauma from deceleration injuries can also lead to TAAs, typically at the aortic isthmus.

Faggion Vinholo T, Brownstein AJ, Ziganshin BA, et al. Genes associated with thoracic aortic aneurysm and dissection: 2019 update and clinical implications. *Aorta (Stamford)*. 2019;7:99-107.

Huguenard AL, Gupta VP, Braverman AC, Dacey RG. Genetic and heritable considerations in patients or families with both intracranial and extracranial aneurysms. *J Neurosurg*. 2021;134:1999-2006.

Isselbacher EM, Preventza O, Hamilton Black J 3rd, et al; Peer Review Committee Members. 2022 ACC/AHA guideline for the diagnosis and management of aortic disease: a report of the American Heart Association/American College of Cardiology Joint Committee on clinical practice guidelines. *Circulation*. 2022;146:e334-e482.

Jones JA, Ikonomidis JS. The pathogenesis of aortopathy in Marfan syndrome and related diseases. *Curr Cardiol Rep. 2010*;12:99-107.

Ostberg NP, Zafar MA, Ziganshin BA, Elefteriades JA. The genetics of thoracic aortic aneurysms and dissection: a clinical perspective. *Biomolecules*. 2020;10:182.

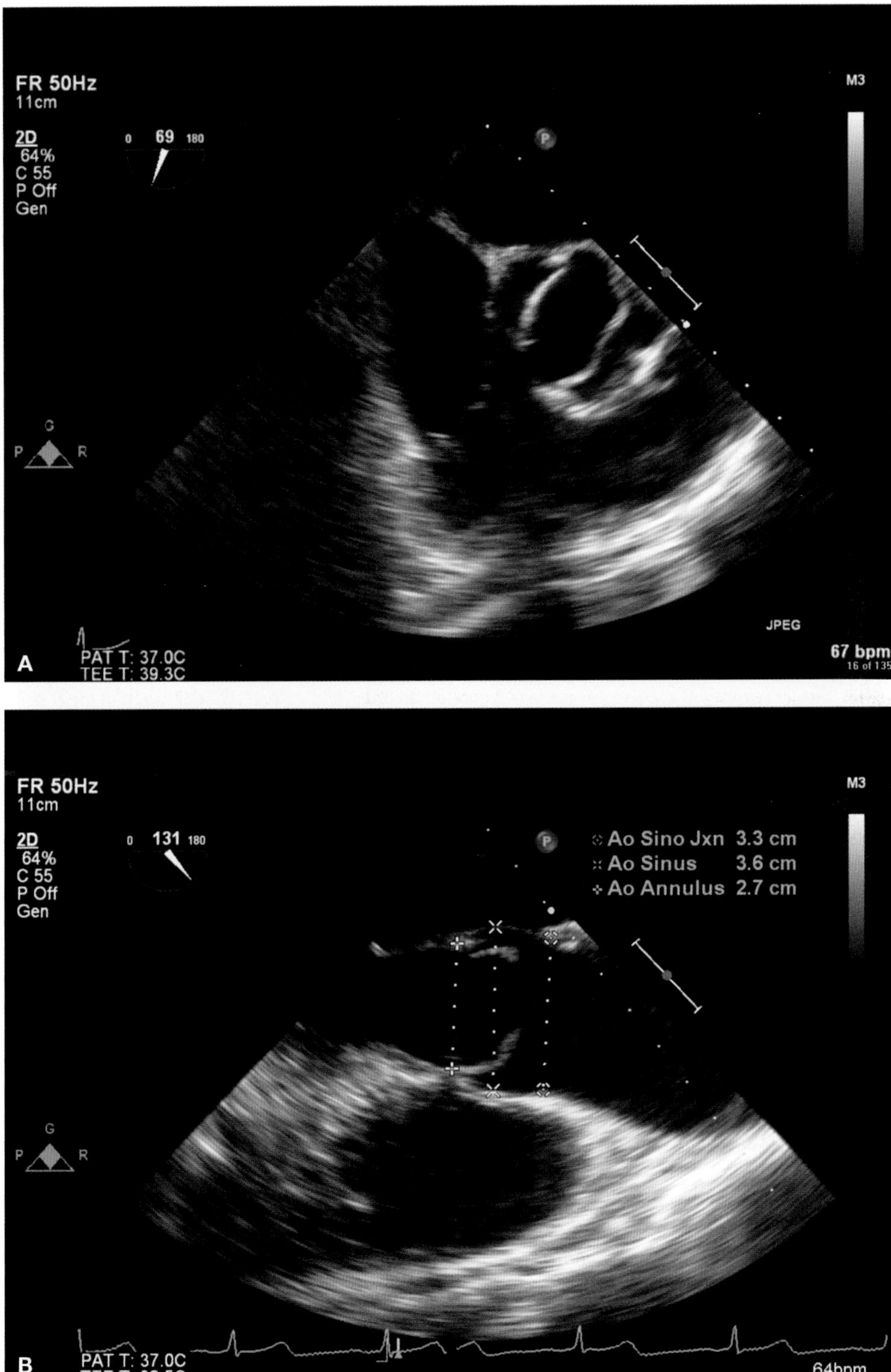

FIGURE 9.5. A. Midesophageal aortic valve (AV) short-axis view on transesophageal echocardiography showing a bicuspid valve, with the fusion of the left and right coronary cusps. **B.** Midesophageal aortic valve long-axis view on transesophageal echocardiography demonstrating the characteristic doming of a stenotic bicuspid AV and blunting of the sinotubular junction due to aortic root (ascending aortic) dilatation.

A.4. What is the natural history and medical management of thoracic aneurysms?

Mean growth rates for ascending and aortic arch aneurysms range from 0.2 to 2.8 mm/y, while those for descending and TAAs range from 1.9 to 3.4 mm/y. Accelerated TAA growth is associated with large aneurysm size, distal aneurysm locations, Marfan syndrome, BAV, chronic aortic dissection, and COPD. The goal of medical therapy in TAA disease is to reduce aneurysm growth rates, the risk of aortic (dissection or rupture) and nonaortic cardiovascular events, and the need for aortic repair. However, evidence for such practices remains limited. Lifestyle modifications include smoking cessation and avoidance of intense isometric exercises, as well as collision sports, to avoid increases in systolic blood pressure that pose a risk for aortic growth and rupture.

Pharmacotherapy for the treatment of aortic disease includes the use of select antihypertensive agents, such as β-blockers, angiotensin converting enzyme (ACE) inhibitors, and angiotensin receptor blockers (ARBs), to mitigate medial degeneration and reduce aortic wall stress, as well as statins to modulate inflammatory and atherosclerotic pathways. There are class I recommendations for treatment with either a β-blocker or an ARB in patients with MFS; class II recommendations exist for patients with LDS and sporadic or degenerative TAA disease. There is insufficient data to recommend pharmacotherapy in vEDS. The American College of Cardiology Joint Committee (ACC) and American Heart Association (AHA) recommended targets of systolic blood pressure (SBP) less than 130 mm Hg and/or diastolic blood pressure (DBP) less than 80 mm Hg in patients with cardiovascular disease, although the optimal threshold in patients with TAA has not been evaluated in randomized clinical trials. It is also reasonable to administer low-dose aspirin to patients with atherosclerotic TAA and concomitant aortic atheroma.

Isselbacher EM, Preventza O, Hamilton Black J 3rd, et al; Peer Review Committee Members. 2022 ACC/AHA guideline for the diagnosis and management of aortic disease: a report of the American Heart Association/American College of Cardiology Joint Committee on Clinical Practice Guidelines. *Circulation*. 2022;146:e334-e482.

Oladokun D, Patterson BO, Sobocinski J, et al. Systematic review of the growth rates and influencing factors in thoracic aortic aneurysms. *Eur J Vasc Endovasc Surg*. 2016;51:674-681.

Sharples L, Sastry P, Freeman C, et al. Aneurysm growth, survival, and quality of life in untreated thoracic aortic aneurysms: the effective treatments for thoracic aortic aneurysms study. *Eur Heart J*. 2022;43:2356-2369.

A.5. What are the risk factors for TAA-associated mortality?

Older age, female sex, New York Heart Association (NYHA) class, and baseline maximum aneurysm size (**Table 9.1**) have independent associations with aneurysm-related and all-cause mortality, while frailty, previous cardiac interventions, COPD, and lower body mass index (BMI) are additional risk factors. Each 1-cm increase in the maximal diameter more than doubles the risk of death. The hinge points for increased risk of aortic aneurysm rupture or dissection are 6.0 cm for the ascending aorta and 7.0 cm for the descending aorta, such that 31% and 43% of patients, respectively, will have experienced aneurysm-related complications at these stages of aneurysm growth.

Chau KH, Elefteriades JA. Natural history of thoracic aortic aneurysms: size matters, plus moving beyond size. *Prog Cardiovasc Dis*. 2013;56:74-80.

Elefteriades JA. Natural history of thoracic aortic aneurysms: indications for surgery, and surgical versus nonsurgical risks. *Ann Thorac Surg*. 2002;74:S1877-S1880; discussion S1892-S1898.

Sharples L, Sastry P, Freeman C, et al. Aneurysm growth, survival, and quality of life in untreated thoracic aortic aneurysms: the effective treatments for thoracic aortic aneurysms study. *Eur Heart J*. 2022;43:2356-2369.

A.6. What is a thoracic aortic dissection? How does it typically present? How is it diagnosed?

AAS can present as an aortic dissection, IMH, and penetrating atherosclerotic ulcer (PAU). The most common AAS is aortic dissection. An aortic dissection occurs when a tear in the aortic intima allows

TABLE 9.1 Annual Mortality Due to Aneurysm-Related Events (Rupture or Dissection) for Thoracic Aneurysms

Maximum Baseline Size of Aneurysm (cm)	Aneurysm-Related Mortality (%)
4-6	<10
7	12.4
8	22.2

blood to enter the aortic media, which creates a dissection flap that separates the true from the false lumen. The dissection flap can have anterograde or retrograde propagation, resulting in life-threatening complications, such as acute aortic regurgitation (AR), myocardial ischemia, cardiac tamponade with possible cardiogenic shock, acute stroke, or malperfusion syndromes (**Figures 9.6** and **9.7**). Blood in the false lumen can create a reentry tear back through the intima into the true lumen, or it can tear through the outer media and adventitia, resulting in aortic rupture. The relative risk of aortic dissection increases dramatically at a diameter greater than or equal to 4.5 cm. When blood infiltrates the aortic media, an IMH forms when the outer wall of the aorta is pushed outward or a PAU forms when blood is confined by the atherosclerotic scarring of the aorta, resulting in a localized dissection or pseudoaneurysm. Up to 47% of IMH can progress to aortic dissection while PAUs have up to a 40% risk of rupture.

Hypertension is the most common comorbid disease in patients with AAD, while hyperlipidemia, tobacco use, and cocaine use are other risk factors. Pregnancy can also increase the risk of AAD, with most females typically presenting during their third trimester or in the early postpartum period. Genetic conditions that increase the risk of AAD are discussed in the previous section. AAD can also occur iatrogenically during cardiac surgery, cardiac catheterization, and insertion of an intra-aortic balloon pump.

Patients with AAS classically report severe "sharp" or "stabbing" pain in the chest or back. Depending on the extent of aortic involvement, other signs and symptoms include diastolic murmur of AI (present in 44% of cases), gastrointestinal bleeding, bowel ischemia, dysphagia, dyspnea, hemoptysis, hoarseness, Horner syndrome, paraplegia, shock, SVC syndrome, and syncope. In roughly 6% of cases, the aortic dissection is painless and presents as new-onset heart failure, stroke, or syncope. These patients tend to have diabetes mellitus, a history of aortic aneurysm, or a history of prior cardiac surgery.

CT is the preferred diagnostic imaging modality, although TEE and MRI are also highly sensitive and specific for diagnosis. TEE may be preferred in unstable patients or those with a history of an iodinated contrast reaction. If left untreated, AAD of the ascending aorta has a high mortality of 1% to 2% per hour after symptom onset, which increases in the presence of complications. In contrast, patients with uncomplicated acute type B aortic dissection (TBAD) have a 30-day mortality rate of 10%, which rises considerably if malperfusion of aortic branch vessels occurs.

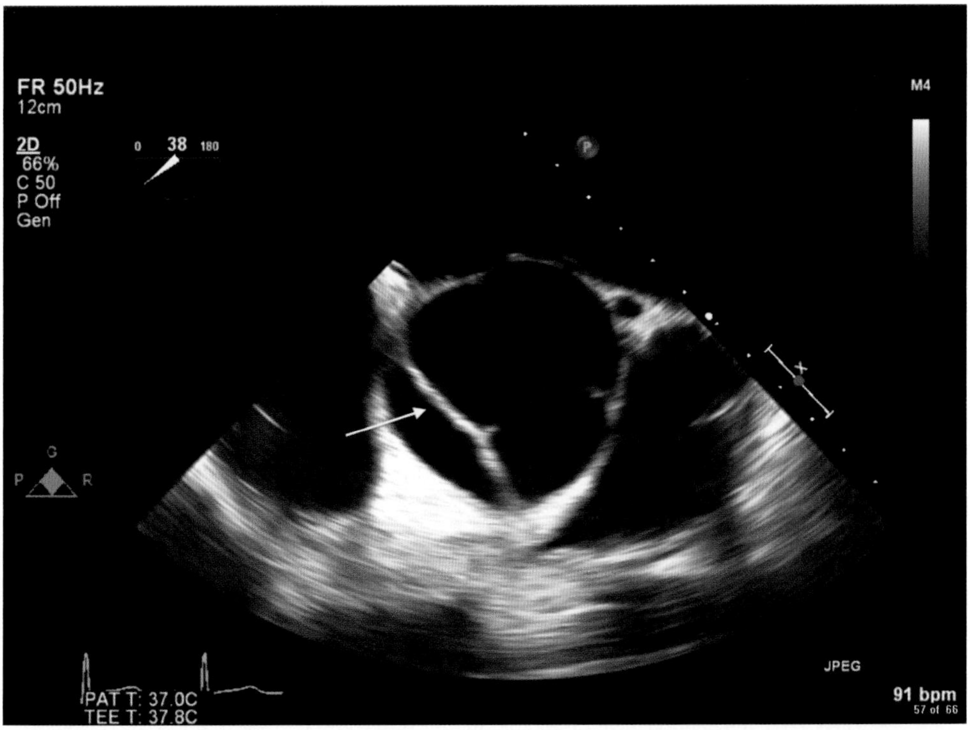

FIGURE 9.6. Midesophageal aortic valve short-axis view on transesophageal echocardiography demonstrating an acute aortic dissection (*arrow*) that extends proximally to the aortic valve in a young patient with Marfan syndrome.

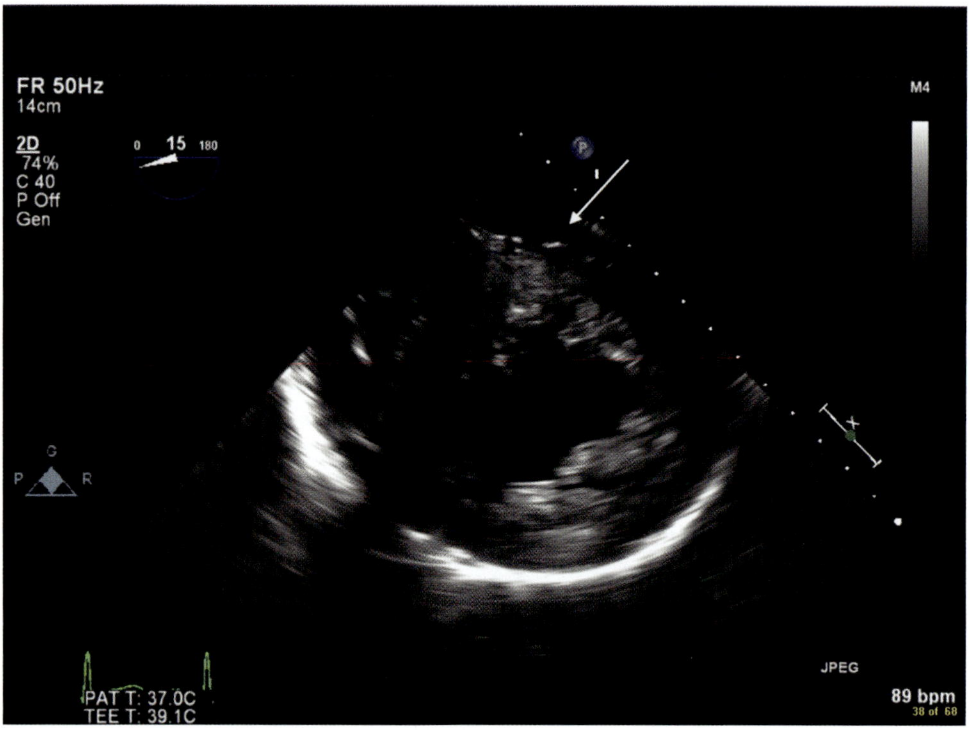

FIGURE 9.7. Transgastric midpapillary view on transesophageal echocardiography demonstrating accumulation of blood in the posterior pericardial space (*arrow*) after acute aortic dissection.

Isselbacher EM, Preventza O, Hamilton Black J 3rd, et al; Peer Review Committee Members. 2022 ACC/AHA guideline for the diagnosis and management of aortic disease: a report of the American Heart Association/American College of Cardiology Joint Committee on clinical practice guidelines. *Circulation*. 2022;146:e334-e482.

Ivascu NS, Skubas NJ. Aortic intramural hematoma: echocardiographic characteristics. *Anesth Analg*. 2012;114:286-288.

Ramanath VS, Oh JK, Sundt TM III, et al. Acute aortic syndromes and thoracic aortic aneurysm. *Mayo Clin Proc*. 2009;84:465-481.

Tsai TT, Trimarchi S, Nienaber CA. Acute aortic dissection: perspectives from the International Registry of Acute Aortic Dissection (IRAD). *Eur J Vasc Endovasc Surg*. 2009;37:149-159.

A.7. How are thoracic aortic dissections classified?

The most commonly used systems to classify aortic dissections focus on anatomic detail while others additionally consider whether malperfusion and associated symptoms are present (**Figure 9.8**).

DeBakey Classification

The DeBakey system categorizes dissections based on the origin of the intimal tear and the degree of distal extension. Type I and type II dissections are almost always treated surgically, while type III dissections are often managed medically.

- Type I: Dissection tear originates in the ascending aorta and propagates distally to include the aortic arch and typically the descending aorta.
- Type II: Dissection tear is confined only to the ascending aorta.
- Type III: Dissection tear originates in the descending thoracic aorta and propagates most often distally.
    - Type IIIA: Dissection tear is confined only to the descending thoracic aorta.
    - Type IIIB: Dissection tear originates in the descending thoracic aorta and extends below the diaphragm.

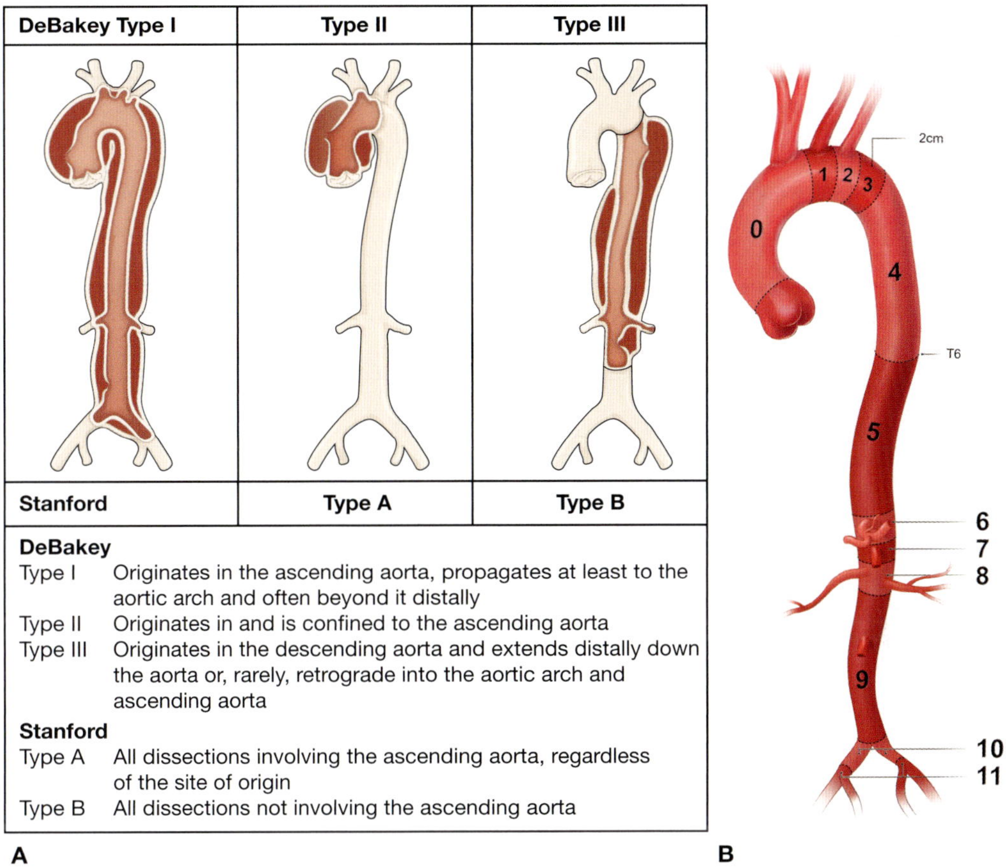

FIGURE 9.8. A. The Stanford and DeBakey classifications of aortic dissections. (Reprinted with permission from Nienaber CA, Eagle KA. Aortic dissection: new frontiers in diagnosis and management: part I: from etiology to diagnostic strategies. *Circulation.* 2003;108:628-635.) **B.** Classification of Aortic Anatomic Segments by 11 Landing Zones. Zone 0 (involves the ascending to the distal end of the origin of the innominate artery); Zone 1 (involves the origin of the left common carotid; between the innominate and the left carotid); Zone 2 (involves the origin of the left subclavian; between the left carotid and the left subclavian); Zone 3 (involves the proximal descending thoracic aorta down to the T4 vertebral body; the first 2 cm distal to the left subclavian); Zone 4 (the end of zone 3 to the mid-descending aorta—T6); Zone 5 (the mid-descending aorta to the celiac); Zone 6 (involves the origin of the celiac; the celiac to the superior mesenteric); Zone 7 (involves the origin of the SMA; the superior mesenteric to the renals); Zone 8 (involves the origin of the renal arteries; the renal to the infrarenal abdominal aorta); Zone 9 (the infrarenal abdominal aorta to the level of aortic bifurcation); Zone 10 (the common iliac); Zone 11 (involves the origin of the external iliac arteries). (From Czerny M, Schmidli J, Adler S, et al. Current options and recommendations for the treatment of thoracic aortic pathologies involving the aortic arch: an expert consensus document of the European Association for Cardio-Thoracic surgery [EACTS] and the European Society for Vascular Surgery [ESVS]. *Eur J Cardiothorac Surg.* 2019;55:133-162 by permission of Oxford University.)

Stanford Classification

The Stanford classification system is simpler and divides dissections according to whether the ascending aorta is involved or not, irrespective of the site of origin. It highlights the need for surgical repair to improve survival in the setting of Stanford type A dissections, in contrast to Stanford type B dissections that demonstrate survival benefit in response to medical therapy.

- Type A: All dissections involving the ascending aorta, irrespective of the site of the intimal tear
- Type B: All dissections that do not involve the ascending aorta (including dissections that involve the aortic arch but spare the ascending aorta)

Society for Vascular Surgery/Society of Thoracic Surgeons (SVS/STS) Classification

The DeBakey and Stanford criteria are limited by their inability to classify dissections originating in the aortic arch. Thus, after the introduction of a third category of non-A-non-B dissections for proximal dissection flaps that begin in the aortic arch, the SVS and STS introduced a new classification scheme in 2020 that subdivides aortic anatomy into 11 zones to allow for more granular reporting of aortic dissections.

- A_D denotes a type A dissection with an entry tear in zone 0 and extends distally to the zone designated by the subscript D (0-11).
- B_{PD} indicates a type B dissection with an entry tear in zone 1 or beyond with the proximal and distal extents of the dissection denoted by subscripts P and D, respectively.
- I_D indicates a dissection that begins in zone 0 but has an unidentified entry tear with the distal extent denoted by the subscript D.

Penn Classification of Malperfusion Syndromes

The Penn classification system was developed to better predict perioperative mortality among patients with acute Stanford type A dissections subcategorized according to ischemic symptoms from malperfusion on presentation.

- Class Aa patients are hemodynamically stable and present without ischemia, branch vessel malperfusion, or circulatory collapse.
- Class Ab patients present with branch vessel malperfusion that manifests as stroke, paraplegia, renal dysfunction, mesenteric malperfusion, or ischemic extremities.
- Class Ac patients experience circulatory collapse with or without cardiac involvement, such as cardiac tamponade, coronary dissection, myocardial infarction, new-onset left or right ventricular dysfunction, AR, or aortic rupture.
- Class Abc patients present with local ischemia from branch vessel malperfusion and generalized ischemia from circulatory collapse.

Prognosis is best for class Aa patients with a hospital mortality of only 3.1% and worst for class Abc patients with a hospital mortality of 40%. Class Ab and Ac patients had similar intermediate hospital mortalities (25.6% and 17.6%, respectively). The Penn classification system for predicting perioperative mortality may also be applicable to patients with type B dissections who undergo surgical or medical management.

Classification Based on Malperfusion Syndromes

Due to the substantial effects of malperfusion syndromes on patient outcomes, new classification systems have been proposed that integrate clinical evidence with symptoms and etiologies of malperfusion syndromes into the therapeutic approach for types A, B, non-A-non-B dissections. These systems may lead to a push for earlier, more aggressive open surgical or endovascular procedural management. The introduction of the first web-based score that predicts 30-day mortality in acute TAAD appears to be promising and can help refine disease process-oriented treatment strategies for patients.

Aortic dissections were historically regarded as acute or chronic if they occurred within or beyond 2 weeks of symptom onset, respectively. More recently, the SVS and STS proposed a contemporary temporal classification system to guide prognostication and clinical decision-making about interventions. This classification system is subdivided into four temporal types: hyperacute (<24 hours), acute (1-14 days), subacute (15-90 days), and chronic (>90 days).

Augoustides JG, Geirsson A, Szeto WY, et al. Observational study of mortality risk stratification by ischemic presentation in patients with acute type A aortic dissection: the Penn classification. *Nat Clin Pract Cardiovasc Med.* 2009;6:140-146.

Czerny M, Rylski B. Acute type A aortic dissection reconsidered: it's all about the location of the primary entry tear and the presence or absence of malperfusion. *Eur Heart J.* 282021;43:53-55.

Hagan PG, Nienaber CA, Isselbacher EM, et al. The International Registry of Acute Aortic Dissection (IRAD): new insights into an old disease. *JAMA.* 2000;283:897-903.

Isselbacher EM, Preventza O, Hamilton Black J 3rd, et al; Peer Review Committee Members. 2022 ACC/AHA guideline for the diagnosis and management of aortic disease: a report of the American Heart Association/American College of Cardiology Joint Committee on clinical practice guidelines. *Circulation.* 2022;146:e334-e482.

Tien M, Ku A, Martinez-Acero N, Zvara J, Sun EC, Cheung AT. The Penn Classification predicts hospital mortality in acute Stanford type A and type B aortic dissections. *J Cardiothorac Vasc Anesth.* 2020;34:867-873.

B. Preoperative Evaluation and Preparation

B.1. What are the indications and timing of surgical intervention for TAAs?

Patients diagnosed with aneurysms of the thoracic aorta require frequent surveillance to assess for aneurysmal expansion. The goal is to facilitate surgical intervention prior to the onset of aortic dissection or aneurysm rupture. Important considerations include the appropriate interval for surveillance imaging and the diameter at which surgical intervention should be recommended.

TABLE 9.2 Guidelines for Elective Intervention in Selected Categories of Asymptomatic Patients With Ascending or Descending Thoracic Aneurysms

Associated Condition with Aneurysm	Diameter Size for Surgical Intervention
Sporadic	≥5.5 cm
Heritable without Genetic Identification	≥5.0 cm
Marfan Syndrome	≥5.0 cm ≥4.5 cm with features associated with increased risk of dissection present
Loeys-Dietz Syndrome	≥4.5 cm - 5.0 cm, dependent on specific pathogenic variant, phenotypic features, patient age, aortic growth rates, and family history
BAV Aortopathy	≥5.5 cm 5.0 - 5.4 cm with additional risk factors for aortic dissection ≥4.5 cm with concomitant surgical aortic valve repair or replacement

BAV, bicuspid aortic valve; TAA, thoracic aortic aneurysm.

Patients diagnosed with TAAs and TAAAs should undergo initial CT or MRI to define the size and extent of the aneurysm. Follow-up surveillance imaging is typically performed 6 months after diagnosis, with continued follow-up imaging at an interval determined by the rate of growth. These aneurysms tend to grow slowly, with arch and ascending aneurysms growing 0.1 cm/y and descending aneurysms growing 0.3 cm/y.

Determining when to intervene depends on the underlying pathology, size, rate of expansion, and presence or absence of symptoms (**Table 9.2**). In patients without known connective tissue disease, surgical repair is recommended at 5.5 cm. In patients with concomitant aortic valve (AV) disease who are scheduled to undergo AV replacement, an aneurysm should be repaired if it is greater than or equal to 4.5 cm in diameter. Patients with symptomatic aneurysms of any size should be considered for surgical intervention. Very large and very small patients may be better managed by indexing aortic diameter to body size to determine the appropriate timing of repair.

Special recommendations exist for patients with underlying connective tissue disorders because these patients tend to suffer significant aortic events at smaller aortic diameters. Patients with MFS and LDS require frequent surveillance, with CT imaging 6 months after initial diagnosis followed by surveillance frequency depending on size and rate of growth. Earlier repair is acceptable and recommended in MFS and LDS, and the timing of a surgical intervention can be based on the presence of associated risk factors for aortic dissection, such as a family history of aortic dissection, accelerated growth rate, and aortic coarctation. Aneurysm repair for patients with BAV presenting for AV repair or replacement should be performed at a diameter of greater than or equal to 4.5 cm. Females with aortic aneurysms contemplating pregnancy might be candidates for prophylactic intervention at smaller aneurysm diameters in the context of connective tissue disorders and other risk factors for aortic dissection.

Overall, surgical decision-making in patients with TAAs, thoracoabdominal aneurysms, and combined aneurysmal and AV disease requires a careful comparison of operative risk with the risk of a significant aortic event. Consideration of medical comorbidities and the underlying pathology adds additional nuance to the decision of whether to undertake a surgical repair, and when that repair is recommended, what surgical technique should be utilized.

Harik L, Lau C. Open and endovascular repair of thoracoabdominal aortic aneurysm-a narrative review. *J Thorac Dis.* 2023;15:3984-3997.

Isselbacher EM, Preventza O, Hamilton Black J 3rd, et al; Peer Review Committee Members. 2022 ACC/AHA guideline for the diagnosis and management of aortic disease: a report of the American Heart Association/American College of Cardiology Joint Committee on clinical practice guidelines. *Circulation.* 2022;146:e334-e482.

B.2. Which patients are candidates for endovascular aortic repair, and what are the major advantages and disadvantages of this approach?

Thoracic endovascular aortic repair (TEVAR) is an alternative to open repair for patients with suitable anatomy offering a less invasive approach that has short- and intermediate-term benefits including decreased mortality, freedom from aneurysm-related morbidity, and hospital length of stay. After 5 years, however, the survival advantage with TEVAR is no longer demonstrated. Candidates for endovascular repair are patients who meet the criteria for intervention, have anatomy suitable for endovascular repair, have comorbidities associated with increased morbidity and mortality, and lack aortopathy related to connective tissue disorders. In recent years, aortic stent grafting has undergone a significant liberalization in its use for many aortic pathologies. In addition to the repair of TAAs, many centers are now treating complicated TBADs, traumatic aortic injuries, IMHs, and penetrating aortic ulcers via the endovascular approach.

The goal of endovascular aortic repair is to affix the stent graft to nonaneurysmal aortic or iliac segments, excluding blood flow to the aneurysm sac. TEVAR is currently only approved by the U.S. Food and Drug Administration (FDA) for interventions involving the descending thoracic, juxtarenal, and infrarenal aortic segments. The application of endovascular stenting to the ascending arch or thoracoabdominal aortic segments is not currently approved due to the increased risk of aneurysmal sac enlargement. Application of endovascular stenting to these segments may be performed as an investigational device exemption or expanded access.

Patient characteristics associated with increased morbidity and mortality following open TAAA repair include advanced age, CKD greater than or equal to Stage 3, COPD with FEV_1 less than or equal to 50%, and those with a history of a cerebral vascular event. TEVAR may be considered in these patients as an alternative to open repair despite suboptimal anatomy for endovascular repair. Relative contraindications to TEVAR include mycotic aneurysms, aneurysms secondary to connective tissue disease (MFS, Ehlers-Danlos syndrome [EDS], etc), and aneurysms extending proximal to the LSCA. Connective tissue disease also presents a relative contraindication due to concern for the longevity of the endovascular repair in this patient population. In certain instances, "hybrid" procedures, which consist of debranching of the visceral arterial supply followed by endovascular repair of the aneurysm, can also be considered.

The major advantages of endovascular repair include short- and intermediate-term reduced morbidity and mortality and hospital length of stay. Additionally, the outcome benefits of open repair are limited to high-volume centers, so TEVAR offers increased access and feasibility for aortic repair at low-volume centers. The major disadvantages of TEVAR include loss of survival advantage after 5 years and a significantly higher reintervention rate compared to open repair.

Harik L, Lau C. Open and endovascular repair of thoracoabdominal aortic aneurysm-a narrative review. *J Thorac Dis*. 2023;15:3984-3997.

Isselbacher EM, Preventza O, Hamilton Black J 3rd, et al; Peer Review Committee Members. 2022 ACC/AHA guideline for the diagnosis and management of aortic disease: a report of the American Heart Association/American College of Cardiology Joint Committee on Clinical Practice Guidelines. *Circulation*. 2022;146:e334-e482.

Lau C, Soletti GJ, Lawrence KM, et al. Contemporary outcomes of open repair of acute complicated type B aortic dissection. *J Vasc Surg*. 2023;78:593-601.e4.

B.3. What are the preoperative considerations for the anesthesiologist before TAA repair?

Surgery for TAA repair involves the potential for significant morbidity and mortality. A thorough preoperative workup is important to define the patient's risk of postoperative complications and to facilitate a coordinated anesthetic and surgical plan that provides the greatest likelihood of a good clinical outcome. Particular attention should be given to cardiac, respiratory, renal, and neurologic function because threats to these systems present the greatest risk of increased morbidity and mortality. Although thoracic and thoracoabdominal aneurysm repairs represent high-risk surgical procedures at baseline, patients presenting for urgent or emergent intervention are at the greatest risk of postoperative complications. Unfortunately, these patients may also be clinically unstable, and thorough preoperative workup might not be feasible.

Cardiovascular

Detailed evaluation of the cardiovascular system is essential prior to undertaking complex aortic repair. Major fluid shifts, aortic cross-clamping, and the physiologic stress of intraoperative and postoperative blood loss represent a significant threat to the cardiovascular system. Major thoracic aortic surgery falls into the highest risk group for perioperative cardiac morbidity. Up to two-thirds of patients demonstrate diastolic dysfunction with aortic cross-clamping, and 30% of patients manifest some degree of cardiac dysfunction postoperatively. Hypertension is a common comorbidity, and older patients may also have coexisting coronary artery disease (CAD). Evidence of congestive heart failure may also be present as a result of progressive AI due to aneurysm enlargement.

Cardiac workup should at least include an electrocardiogram (ECG) and TTE, although stress testing and/or coronary angiography are routinely performed at many centers. Patients who are found to have unstable CAD, left main stenosis, or three-vessel disease are typically revascularized prior to or during the repair of the aneurysm. There is debate about whether or not to perform percutaneous coronary intervention (PCI) on less complex lesions because the antiplatelet therapy that accompanies PCI may complicate surgical hemostasis. Occasionally, aneurysmal expansion can result in ischemia from compression of the coronary arteries. Patients taking antihypertensive and antianginal drugs should continue these until the time of surgery, and titrated preoperative anxiolysis medication is important to prevent stress-induced hypertension and tachycardia, which could precipitate aneurysm rupture. Therapeutic anticoagulation or antiplatelet agents should be discontinued or bridged with short-acting alternatives prior to surgical intervention.

Respiratory

The respiratory system also deserves special attention in the preoperative evaluation of patients undergoing thoracic aneurysm repair. Perioperative respiratory failure is the most common serious complication of thoracic and thoracoabdominal aneurysm repair, and patients with a history of smoking or COPD are at especially high risk. Pulmonary function testing and a room air arterial blood gas analysis should be obtained preoperatively because one-lung ventilation (OLV) is important for open surgical repair of Crawford type I, II, III, and V aneurysms. Patients with very poor pulmonary reserve may require cardiopulmonary bypass (CPB) because of an inability to tolerate OLV. Preoperative smoking cessation should be encouraged.

In addition to the evaluation of pulmonary mechanics, history should include consideration of positional dyspnea or stridor, which may indicate aneurysmal compression of the trachea or, more commonly, the left mainstem bronchus. A review of the CT or MRI is important to determine whether significant bronchial compression is present because this may complicate airway management and double-lumen endotracheal tube placement. Finally, patients with significant preoperative respiratory dysfunction should be counseled about the possible need for prolonged postoperative mechanical ventilation, including tracheostomy placement.

Renal

Many patients also have baseline renal insufficiency, which places them at risk for subsequent postoperative renal failure. There is a high incidence of postoperative acute kidney injury following TAAA, with series reporting 1% to 17% of patients requiring hemodialysis and 6% with chronic renal failure. Although evidence for preoperative hydration is minimal, at many centers, it is common practice to admit patients the night before surgery for intravenous (IV) hydration.

Neurologic

The neurologic system deserves special consideration, given the risk to both the brain and spinal cord during aneurysm repair. In an effort to minimize stroke risk, carotid and brachiocephalic angiography are often performed preoperatively, especially in patients with a prior history of stroke or transient ischemic attack. Patients should also be counseled about the risk of possible postoperative paralysis from spinal cord ischemia. Although the risk was historically much higher, the current incidence of postoperative spinal cord injury is between 2% and 15%, depending on the anatomy of the aneurysm, urgency of the repair, patient comorbidities, and surgeon and center experience. Onset can either be immediate or delayed up to 2 weeks, in both open and endovascular repairs.

In summary, preoperative assessment prior to thoracic aneurysm repair is important for both anesthetic and surgical planning. Although aortic surgery represents a high-risk procedure, evaluation of clinical risk factors, multisystem assessment, thoughtful preoperative testing, and, when appropriate, referral to subspecialists for medical optimization can improve perioperative outcome.

Anton JM, Herald KJ. Anesthetic management of open thoracoabdominal aortic aneurysm repair. *Int Anesthesiol Clin*. 2016;54:76-101.

Chatterjee S, Casar JG, LeMaire SA, Preventza O, Coselli JS. Perioperative care after thoracoabdominal aortic aneurysm repair: The Baylor College of Medicine experience. Part 1: preoperative considerations. *J Thorac Cardiovasc Surg*. 2021;161:693-698.

Isselbacher EM, Preventza O, Hamilton Black J 3rd, et al; Peer Review Committee Members. 2022 ACC/AHA guideline for the diagnosis and management of aortic disease: a report of the American Heart Association/American College of Cardiology Joint Committee on clinical practice guidelines. *Circulation*. 2022;146:e334-e482.

B.4. What is the preoperative management of a patient presenting with an acute aortic dissection (AAD)?

Patients presenting with an AAD will either be admitted to the ICU or progress immediately from the emergency department to the operating room. Invasive monitoring of blood pressure, large-bore IV access, and aggressive control of blood pressure and heart rate are priorities. Patients can experience pain if uncontrolled blood pressure and heart rate cause an extension of the dissection, and symptoms are often mitigated with hemodynamic management. Opioids should be utilized sparingly and with caution.

Blood pressure reduction is typically accomplished with β-blockers and vasodilators aiming to reduce myocardial contractility and minimize further extension of the dissection. The goal systolic blood pressure and heart rate are 100 to 120 mm Hg and less than 60 beats/min, respectively. If heart rate and blood pressure control remain inadequate after initializing β-blocker and vasodilator therapy, calcium channel blockers provide an adjunct. Hydralazine is typically not used because it can precipitate reflex tachycardia, which can worsen the dissection. Conversely, patients who are hypotensive on presentation should be treated aggressively with vasopressors and fluid resuscitation in an effort to maintain end-organ perfusion until the patient can undergo definitive operative repair.

A Stanford TAAD is typically treated as a surgical emergency because it is a highly lethal condition with a mortality of 1% per hour after onset. After 24 hours, 20% of patients will die without surgical intervention. Surgery for patients presenting with Stanford TAAD who are hemodynamically stable may be delayed for optimal resource availability or transfer to a high-volume center. Conversely, patients with a Stanford TBAD that is not complicated by limb ischemia, malperfusion, or rupture may be managed medically with aggressive blood pressure and heart rate reduction.

Isselbacher EM, Preventza O, Hamilton Black J 3rd, et al; Peer Review Committee Members. 2022 ACC/AHA guideline for the diagnosis and management of aortic disease: a report of the American Heart Association/American College of Cardiology Joint Committee on clinical practice guidelines. *Circulation*. 2022;146:e334-e482.

B.5. What is the spinal cord blood supply?

The spinal cord blood supply consists of both longitudinal and segmental components (**Figure 9.9**). The longitudinal arteries include the anterior and paired posterior spinal arteries. The anterior spinal artery (ASA) arises from paired feeding vessels that originate in the vertebral arteries near the foramen magnum. It extends the length of the spinal cord and is situated in the anterior spinal sulcus. The ASA is fed

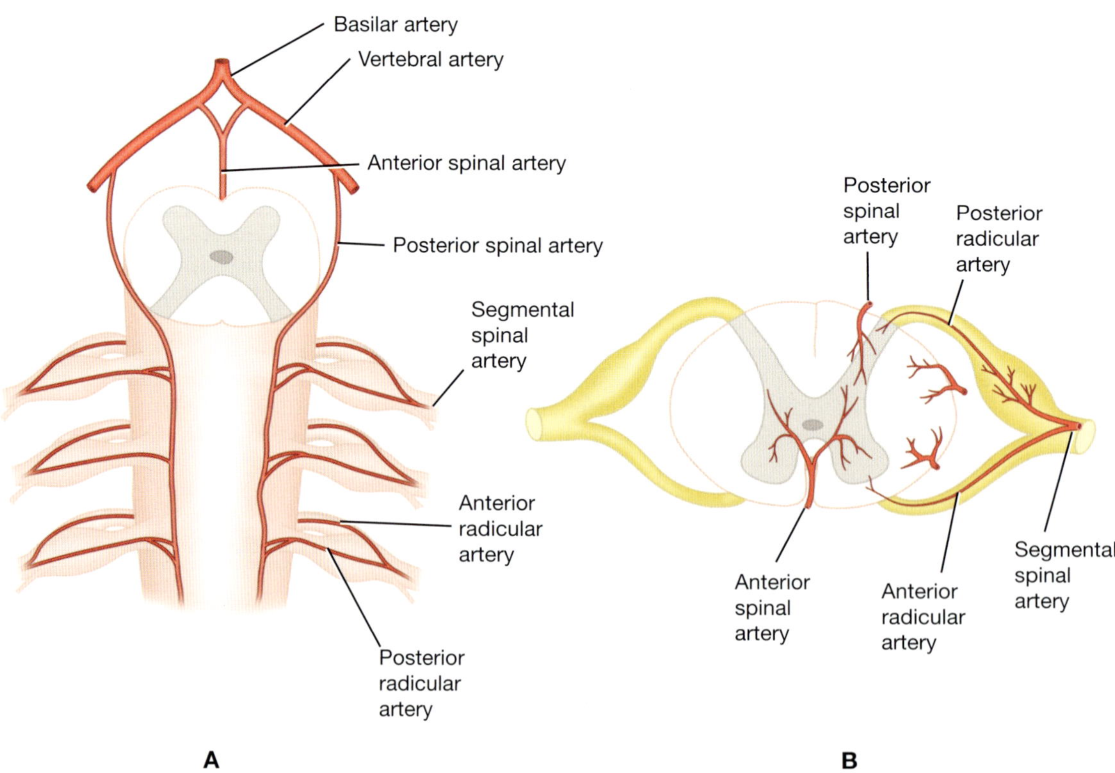

FIGURE 9.9. Spinal cord blood supply. A. Longitudinal spinal cord blood supply. **B.** Spinal and radiculary artery distributions. (Reprinted with permission from Splittgerber R. Blood supply of the brain and spinal cord. In: Snell's Clinical Neuroanatomy. 8th ed. Wolters Kluwer; 2018:471.)

by a series of radicular arteries, and the areas between these radicular contributions are watershed areas that are at the greatest risk of ischemia. The most significant of these radicular arteries is the artery of Adamkiewicz. It is a large radicular contribution that most commonly arises between T8 and L2, although it can originate as high as T5 and as low as L4. The artery of Adamkiewicz is critical to the maintenance of adequate collateral blood supply to the lower two-thirds of the spinal cord. The ASA supplies the anterior two-thirds of the spinal cord, including the corticospinal and spinothalamic tracts, and is dependent on a robust collateral circulation, making it particularly susceptible to ischemic injury.

There are two paired posterior spinal arteries that originate as branches of either the vertebral or posterior inferior cerebellar arteries and descend along the posterolateral portion of the spinal cord. The posterior spinal arteries are also fed by numerous radicular arteries. The anterior and posterior spinal arteries are connected to each other via a circular anastomosis known as the vasocorona medullaris.

In addition to the longitudinal arteries, there are multiple segmental branches that arise from the posterior portion of the aorta. These include the intercostal, subcostal, and lumbar segmental arteries. These arteries travel posteriorly and branch to supply the vertebral bodies, muscle and cutaneous structures, and spinal cord. The spinal division enters through the intervertebral foramen and subdivides to supply either the vertebral and ligamentous structures or the nerve roots and dura. At some levels, the arteries supplying the nerve roots and dura also supply the spinal cord. These vessels are termed radiculomedullary arteries and play an important role in supplying accessory flow to both the anterior and posterior spinal arteries.

Santillan A, Nacarino V, Greenberg E, et al. Vascular anatomy of the spinal cord. *J Neurointerv Surg*. 2012;4:67-74.

Ullery BW, Wang GJ, Low D, et al. Neurological complications of thoracic endovascular aortic repair. *Semin Cardiothorac Vasc Anesth*. 2011;15:123-140.

C. Intraoperative Management

C.1. What are the surgical approaches to thoracic aneurysm repair?

Ascending Aortic Aneurysms

Proximal ascending aneurysms not only cause aortic rupture and dissection but can also alter the three-dimensional conformation of the aortic root and/or AV, leading to AI (**Figure 9.1**). The extent of aortic root involvement determines the surgical procedure necessary for repair (**Table 9.3**). Repair with a supracoronary tube graft is indicated for patients who have ascending aortic aneurysms distal to the aortic root. The Wheat procedure is performed when the AV and proximal aorta are diseased without dilatation of the aortic root. It involves AV and supracoronary tube graft replacement, but spares the aortic root and, therefore, does not require reimplantation of the coronary arteries. When an ascending aortic repair involves the aortic root, various procedures can be performed depending on whether the architecture of the AV is preserved. If the AV is diseased, the Bentall procedure is performed to replace both the AV

TABLE 9.3 Types of Thoracic Ascending Aorta Aneurysm Repairs

Aortic Valve	Root	Ascending Aorta	Surgical Approach	Name of Procedure
Normal	Normal	Aneurysmal	Supracoronary tube graft	
Diseased	Normal	Aneurysmal	AVR + supracoronary tube graft	Wheat procedure
Diseased	Aneurysmal	Aneurysmal	AVR + replacement of aortic root and reimplantation of coronary arteries	Bentall
Normal	Aneurysmal	Aneurysmal	Valve-sparing root replacement; reimplantation of the AV into the graft	David procedure
Normal	Aneurysmal	Aneurysmal	Valve-sparing root replacement; remodeling of the AV into the graft via the creation of pseudo-sinuses	Yacoub procedure

AVR, aortic valve replacement.

and root as well as reimplant the coronary arteries with a collar of the normal surrounding aorta, termed coronary buttons, onto the neoaorta. If atherosclerosis or dissection preclude proximal coronary arteries or aorta from being suitable for creating an anastomosis, the Cabrol technique can be used to fashion a conduit that typically extends the anastomoses to more distal portions of the coronary arteries. However, if the AV is not diseased, valve-sparing modifications of the Bentall technique can be performed to preserve the flow dynamics of the native AV and avoid the need for anticoagulation. David repairs, the most common type of valve-sparing procedures, entail replacement of excised native aorta with a graft in which the native AV is resuspended; the aortic graft used in David repairs is typically sutured below the AV insertion site, thus preventing further dilatation of the aortic root and thereby decreasing AI. An older valve-sparing technique, known as the Yacoub repair, aims to reconstruct the aorta with a scalloped graft that recreates neo-sinuses of Valsalva and attaches above the AV plane.

Surgery for the proximal ascending aorta, including Bentall, Wheat, David, and Yacoub procedures, is performed through a median sternotomy with CPB.

Arch Aortic Aneurysms

Surgical options for aortic arch aneurysms include hemiarch replacement, total arch replacement with or without a distal elephant trunk, and hybrid techniques that combine open surgical techniques to create endograft landing zones with TEVAR to exclude diseased aorta from circulation (Figure 9.10). A hemiarch replacement is performed in patients whose aneurysm extends to the lesser curvature of the aortic

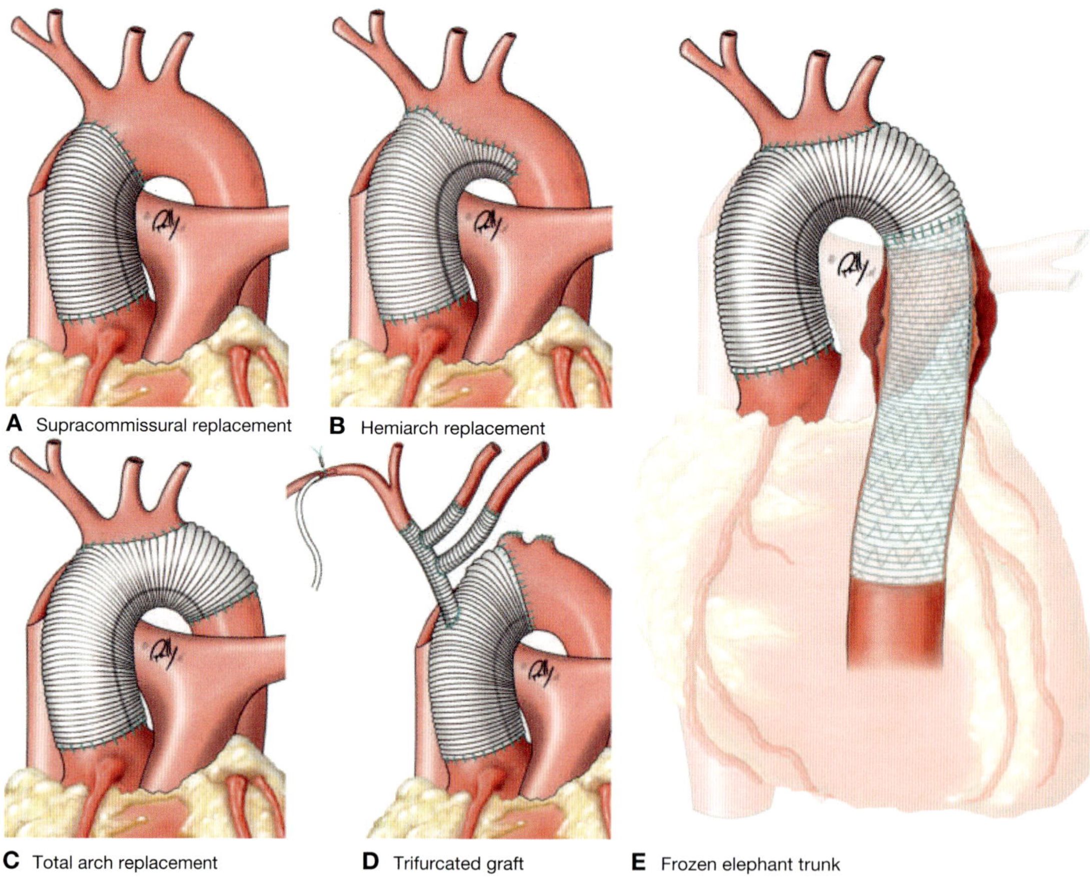

FIGURE 9.10. Surgical options for thoracic aortic aneurysms and dissections. A. Supracommissural replacement of the ascending aorta. **B.** Hemiarch replacement, aortic resection is extended to the lesser curvature (inferior portion) of the aortic arch. Reimplantation of the arch branches is not necessary. **C.** Total arch replacement, the aortic arch is resected, and the arch branches are reimplanted either as a button or with a composite graft. **D.** Trifurcated graft. **E.** Frozen elephant trunk (FET) procedure. (From Krüger T, Conzelmann IO, Bonser RS, et al. Acute aortic dissection type A. *Br J Surg.* 2012;99:1331-1344. Copyright © 2012 British Journal of Surgery Society Ltd. Reprinted by permission of John Wiley & Sons, Inc.)

arch. In patients whose aneurysm extends to the proximal descending aorta, either a total arch replacement with reimplantation of the great vessels separately or as a button can be performed, or the elephant trunk procedure can be performed (**Figure 9.10**). The elephant trunk procedure includes an aortic arch graft and reimplantation of the great vessels to the prosthetic graft, in addition to either a distal 5- to 7-cm "trunk" that dangles in the proximal descending aorta (classic elephant trunk) or a distal covered stent (frozen elephant trunk; **Figure 9.11**). Aortic arch procedures are performed through a median sternotomy with CPB and deep hypothermic circulatory arrest (DHCA) or alternative methods that incorporate neuroprotection, which will be discussed in detail in a later section.

The hybrid approach to aortic arch aneurysm repair provides an alternative option for patients at prohibitive surgical risk for morbidity and mortality with conventional aortic arch reconstruction. A hybrid procedure creates an adequate proximal landing zone (PLZ) during open aortic reconstruction to set the stage for a distal aortic operation to be performed using a TEVAR rather than an open thoracoabdominal aneurysm repair (**Figures 9.12** and **9.13**). TEVAR requires planning for the proximal and distal landing zones to be at least 2 cm to ensure optimal fixation and seal. First-stage repairs can entail (1) debranching of arch vessels using a multibranched Dacron graft (type I), (2) replacement of the ascending aorta and

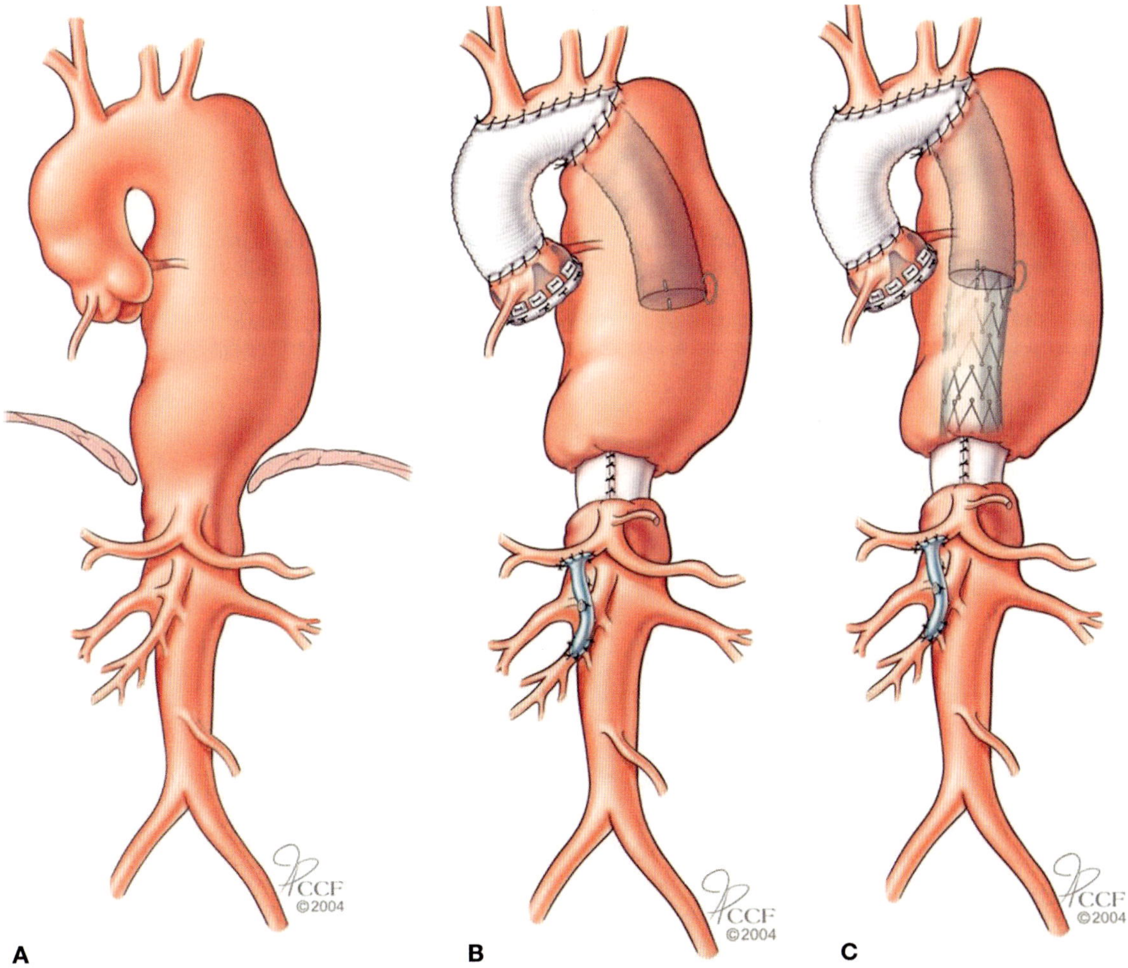

FIGURE 9.11. Elephant trunk procedure. A. Preoperative disease. **B.** Stage I with replacement of the ascending aorta and arch with a Dacron graft, with the distal graft sutured circumferentially to the aorta distal to the LSCA and the free end of the graft ("elephant trunk") within the descending aneurysm. **C.** Completion of the procedure using an endovascular stent graft attached proximally to the "elephant trunk" and the distal end secured to a Dacron graft cuff. (Reprinted from Hiratzka LF, Bakris GL, Beckman JA, et al. 2010 ACCF/AHA/AATS/ACR/ASA/SCA/SCAI/SIR/STS/SVM guidelines for the diagnosis and management of patients with thoracic aortic disease. *J Am Coll Cardiol.* 2010;55:e27-e129.)

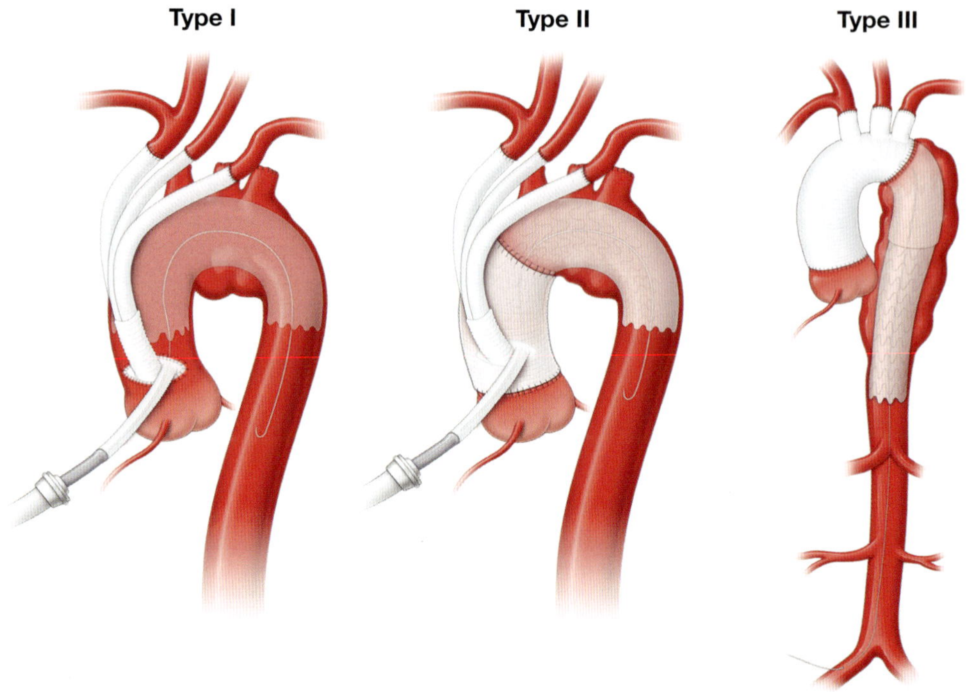

FIGURE 9.12. Surgical strategies for aortic arch debranching and thoracic endovascular aortic repair (TEVAR) for aortic arch aneurysms. A. Reimplantation of great vessels to the proximal ascending aorta to create a landing zone for TEVAR. **B.** Replacement of the ascending aorta with reimplantation of great vessels to the proximal ascending aortic graft. **C.** Total arch replacement, reimplantation of great vessels, and elephant trunk procedure. (Used with permission of AME Publishing Company, from Vallabhajosyula P, Szeto WY, Desai N, et al. Type II arch debranching procedure. *Ann Cardiothorac Surg*. 2013;2:378-386; permission conveyed through Copyright Clearance Center, Inc.)

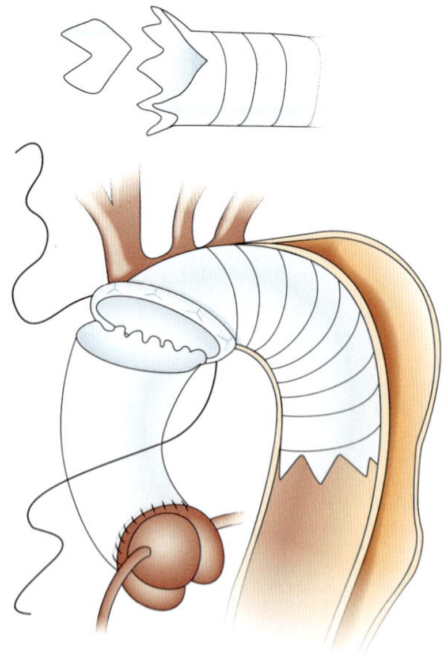

FIGURE 9.13. Illustration demonstrating a hybrid aortic arch repair, where an endograft is placed in the aortic arch and the proximal descending aorta to facilitate aortic remodeling and create the landing zone for future reinterventions. (Used with permission of AME Publishing Company, from Roselli EE. We should replace the aortic arch and more in DeBakey type I dissection—a perspective from the Cleveland Clinic. *Ann Cardiothorac Surg*. 2013;2:216-221; permission conveyed through Copyright Clearance Center, Inc.)

zones 1 or 2 of the aortic arch, along with debranching of the arch vessels (type II), or (3) replacement of the ascending aorta and aortic arch with an elephant trunk (type III). Approaches to creating a PLZ without the use of sternotomy and CPB have also been described and involve the creation of a right common carotid-left common carotid-LSCA bypass (cervical arch debranching) via neck incisions.

Thoracoabdominal Aneurysms

Open TAAA repair is the treatment of choice for appropriate surgical candidates but remains a challenging procedure complicated by the involvement of vital aortic branch vessels in the diseased aortic lesion. TEVAR has emerged as an alternative treatment for patients undergoing TAAA with complex aneurysms, chronic dissection, or failed aortic repair (**Figure 9.14**). Favorable anatomy, which includes adequate iliofemoral and brachial access, as well as suitable branch target vessels with no early bifurcation or occlusive disease, is critical for the success of the procedure. TEVARs can be performed using custom patient-specific fenestrated and branched stent grafts, though these bespoke devices are not yet readily available in many countries and cannot be utilized in more urgent clinical scenarios because they require 6 to 8 weeks to manufacture. When custom devices are not available, TEVARs can be performed with standardized multibranched stent grafts whose position is suitable for at least 50% of TAAAs treated with a patient-specific endograft; in addition, off-the-shelf devices, such as endografts with visceral parallel, that

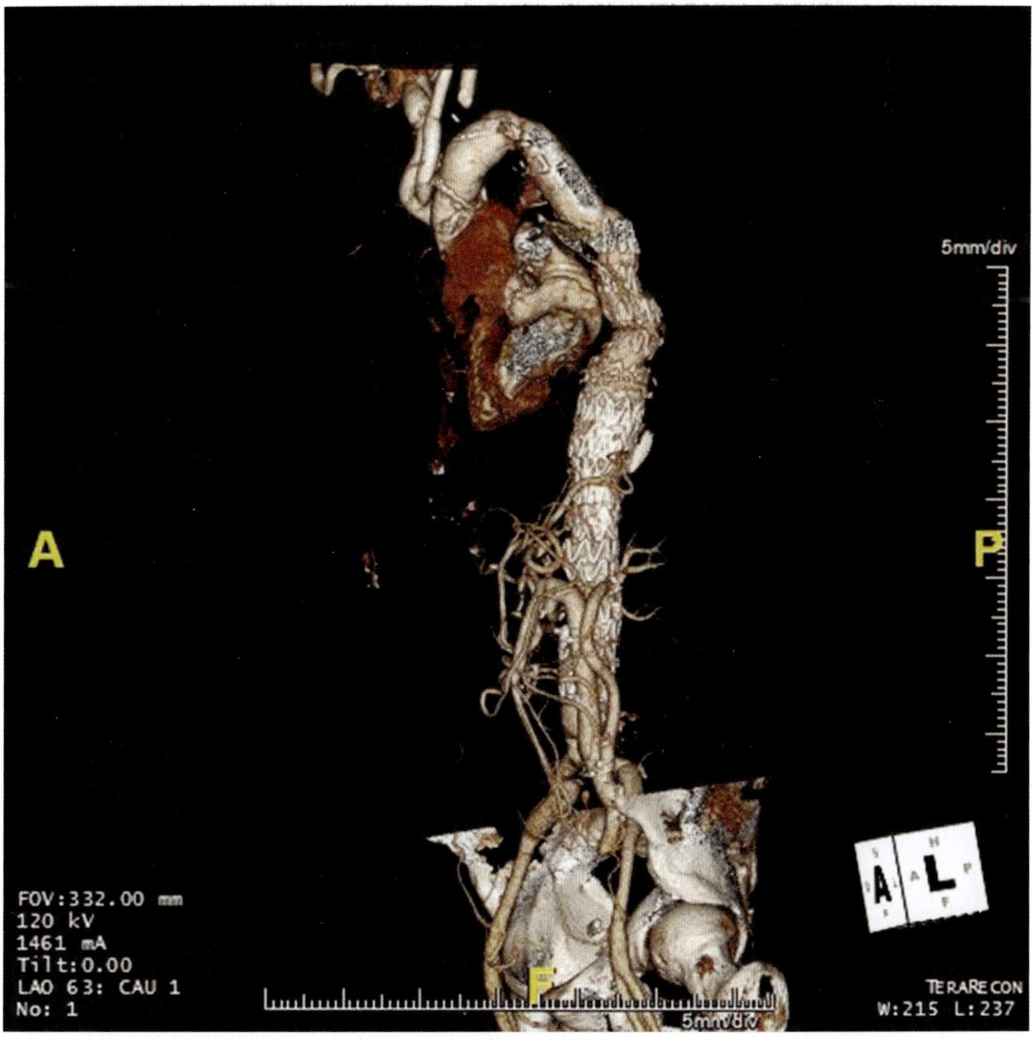

FIGURE 9.14. Three-dimensional (3D) computed tomography reconstruction demonstrating endovascular exclusion of the descending thoracic aorta aneurysm after abdominal and arch debranching.

is, chimney and snorkel, grafts, can be used. Chimney/snorkel techniques involve the placement of a stent or stent graft parallel to the main aortic stent graft to extend the proximal or distal sealing zone while maintaining perfusion to the visceral and renal vessels. The concern with chimney/snorkel techniques is the potential for gutter leaks, which occur due to incomplete apposition of chimney grafts and the main body graft. It is not yet widely known whether chimney/snorkel techniques are sufficient to treat extensive TAAAs or dissections; they are also not suitable for patients with significant aortic arch atherosclerosis because they require bilateral femoral access for delivery of the main body stent and axillary/subclavian artery approaches for branch access.

Furthermore, the hybrid TAAA repair was introduced to lessen the adverse effects associated with traditional open TAAA repair through avoidance of thoracotomy, extracorporeal perfusion, single-lung ventilation, and supraceliac aortic cross-clamping, which can lead to prolonged end-organ ischemia (**Figure 9.15**). It also avoids the dangers of occluding vital visceral vessels. Hybrid TAAA repair starts with total abdominal debranching using retrograde extra-anatomic bypass grafts via laparotomy to reroute the visceral and renal branches from the aneurysmal segment. The debranching procedure is followed by the exclusion of the aneurysm with stent grafting. Hybrid repairs still require laparotomy and long operative times; outcomes of hybrid procedures remain controversial as they reportedly carry high 30-day mortality ranging from 10% to 26% and high complication rates for spinal cord ischemia (7%),

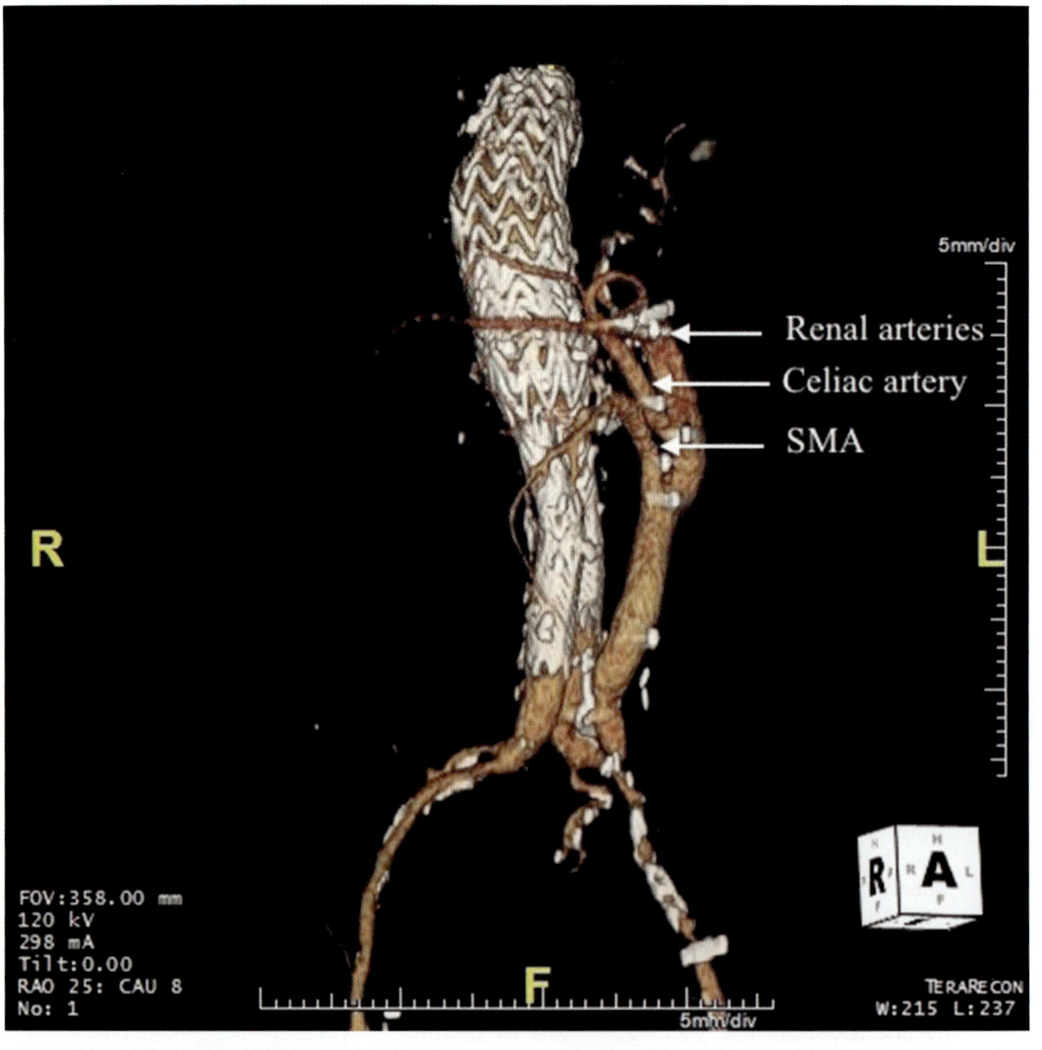

FIGURE 9.15. Three-dimensional (3D) computed tomography reconstruction after abdominal debranching. The superior mesenteric artery (SMA), celiac artery, and renal arteries arise from a left iliac artery graft.

4.5% for mesenteric ischemia (4.5%-18%), renal failure (7%-21%), and respiratory failure (28%-30%). In lieu of debranching, a more contemporary approach involves the performance of a less extensive open Crawford extent III or IV TAAA repair to reimplant the visceral arteries onto a short section of aortic graft, followed by interval extension of the repair with a stent graft. This contemporary hybrid repair is associated with a lower risk of renal failure, spinal cord deficits, and operative mortality.

Bisdas T, Donas KP, Bosiers MJ, Torsello G, Austermann M. Custom-made versus off-the-shelf multibranched endografts for endovascular repair of thoracoabdominal aortic aneurysms. *J Vasc Surg*. 2014;60:1186-1195.

Hughes GC, Vekstein A. Current state of hybrid solutions for aortic arch aneurysms. *Ann Cardiothorac Surg*. 2021;10:731-743.

Kothari R, Weldon SA, Koksoy C, Coselli JS. Narrative review: open surgery for thoracoabdominal aortic aneurysm—is it still a horrible surgery? *J Vis Surg*. 2022;8:4.

Marquis KM, Naeem M, Rajput MZ, et al. CT of postoperative repair of the ascending aorta and aortic arch. *Radiographics*. 2021;41:1300-1320.

Orozco-Sevilla V, Weldon SA, Coselli JS. Hybrid thoracoabdominal aortic aneurysm repair: is the future here? *J Vis Surg*. 2018;4:61.

Tanaka A, Oderich GS, Estrera AL. Total abdominal debranching hybrid thoracoabdominal aortic aneurysm repair versus chimneys and snorkels. *JTCVS Tech*. 2021;10:28-33.

C.2. How is open repair of thoracic aneurysms performed?

Ascending and Arch Aortic Aneurysms

Position: The surgical approach is through a median sternotomy with the patient positioned supine.

Cannulation for CPB: The CPB circuit requires a venous cannula that provides blood to the CPB pump and an arterial cannula that provides blood from the CPB pump to the patient. For aortic surgery, the arterial cannula can reside in any large artery, including the femoral, axillary, innominate, or carotid artery. Direct aortic cannulation can also be performed away from the site of the aneurysm if the anatomy allows it. Arterial cannulation can be accomplished either directly or with the use of a graft anastomosis to the target artery. Direct aortic and femoral cannulations are used less frequently because they carry a risk of embolization or malperfusion in patients with aortic dissection or atherosclerosis. Commonly, the axillary or innominate arteries are used for cannulation sites because they can provide adequate arterial flow during CPB and antegrade cerebral perfusion (ACP) during DHCA. Cannulation of these smaller arteries is achieved with end-to-side anastomosis with a synthetic graft. The venous cannula for CPB is commonly inserted into the right atrium or femoral vein.

Hypothermic circulatory arrest: Neurologic injury remains a major cause of morbidity and mortality after open aortic arch repair. Cerebral protection depends on decreasing metabolic demand and providing metabolic supply with adequate cerebral perfusion while excluding blood flow through the great vessels. Although DHCA improves ischemic tolerance of the brain considerably by suppressing metabolic demand, a major disadvantage of this technique is a limited "safe" time period of arrest before the risk of neurologic injury rises. Some authors have suggested that the "safe" time period of DHCA spans 45 to 60 minutes at 18 °C, while others have shown an increased risk of neurologic deficits with DHCA times that exceed 20 to 30 minutes. The incidence of postoperative stroke increases with greater than 40 minutes of DHCA. Another disadvantage of DHCA is the prolonged time needed to cool and rewarm patients on CPB, which predisposes patients to coagulopathy, systematic inflammatory response, organ ischemia reperfusion injury, or secondary cerebral damage from the release of free radicals. Moderate hypothermic circulatory arrest (MHCA) at 20 °C to 28 °C has been advocated for in recent years over DHCA, as it reduces bypass and cross-clamp times, efficiently prevents permanent neurologic deficits, and may be associated with decreased early in-hospital mortality relative to DHCA. Furthermore, MHCA provides comparable or superior visceral organ protection as it is associated with a lower incidence of renal failure when hypothermic circulatory arrest (HCA) was less than 30 minutes, whereas the risk is commensurate when HCA is greater than 30 minutes.

Adjunctive retrograde cerebral perfusion (RCP) and ACP techniques have been introduced to extend the "safe" time period of HCA, though the optimal temperature and duration of safe cerebral perfusion during arrest for arch reconstructive surgery still remain debatable. Direct delivery of oxygenated blood to the brain via ACP, which can be unilateral or bilateral, can be accomplished through cannulation of the brachiocephalic artery, the right axillary artery with snaring of the brachiocephalic artery to provide perfusion of the right common carotid artery, or the carotid artery; cannulation can increase the risk of thromboembolic events and air embolism. Unilateral and bilateral ACP permits tolerance of less than

50 minutes and up to 160 minutes of DHCA, respectively. Cerebral delivery of oxygenated blood through the venous system via RCP can be achieved by SVC cannulation with snaring above the right atrium. RCP allows for uniform cerebral cooling, decreased gaseous or particulate embolic events, flushing of accumulated toxins to limit acidosis, and deairing of arch vessels, though there is a potential increased risk of neurologic dysfunction. Outcomes data are inconclusive, and numerous variables affect the quality of cerebral protection, including flow rate, temperature, perfusion site(s), use of unilateral or bilateral perfusion, variable circle of Willis anatomy, embolization risk, and trauma to cranial vessels. RCP may be more likely utilized during short periods of HCA while bilateral ACP may be selected when longer periods are anticipated. There is no definitive recommendation for one method of cerebral protection and the choice of technique appears to be dictated by regional preferences as well as institutional practices.

Other neuroprotective strategies lack high-quality evidence to support their routine use. Topical head cooling is used to supplement cold perfusion to promote and sustain deeper hypothermia as well as to prevent rapid rewarming during emersion from HCA; concerns about this strategy include pressure on the eyes from the application of ice as well as interference with monitors such as electroencephalogram (EEG) and cerebral saturation probes. Barbiturates provide modest neuroprotection, but their true efficacy has been questioned. Corticosteroids have not been shown to be beneficial in stroke or in cardiac surgery. The antiapoptotic, osmotic, and free radical scavenging effects of mannitol are favorable, but no neuroprotective effects have been ascertained. Lidocaine and nimodipine are not associated with neuroprotection, although magnesium sulfate was associated with a lower incidence of new postoperative neurologic deficit.

Thoracoabdominal Aneurysms

Open TAAA repair remains the gold standard surgical approach, with long-term outcomes dependent on balancing the need for extensive aortic replacement with modulation of ischemia-related risk to the spinal cord and visceral organs.

Positioning: The surgical approach is typically through the left chest, with the patient positioned in a partial right lateral decubitus position, with the shoulders at 60° and the hips at 30°. The patient is supported with the use of a bean bag and an axillary roll placed under the patient's right axilla to minimize the chances of developing a brachial plexopathy.

Incision: A thoracoabdominal incision is the preferred approach for the majority of aneurysms. The proximal extent of the incision is dictated by the patient's body habitus and the aortic pathology. Typically, if the distal aortic arch and proximal descending aorta are to be exposed (Crawford types I and II), an incision to the fifth intercostal space is necessary. If the proximal extent of the aneurysm involves the distal thoracic aorta (Crawford types III and V), an incision to the 7th or 8th intercostal space is required. If the aneurysm is localized to the abdominal aorta (Crawford type IV), the proximal incision is made at the 9th or 10th intercostal space. The abdominal portion of the incision is typically limited to the retroperitoneum. Diaphragm preservation, defined as division only of the muscular portion of the diaphragm with preservation of the central tendinous portion, is performed to help improve postoperative respiratory mechanics.

Cannulation for and initiation of left-heart bypass: Open TAAA repair requires a period of ischemia to the lower portion of the body, including the spinal cord, viscera, and kidneys, while the aorta is cross-clamped. Left heart bypass (LHB) is utilized for patients with Crawford extent II aneurysms, extent I aneurysms due to dissection, and acute type B dissections. LHB provides isothermic oxygenated blood to the distal aorta to reduce the risk of spinal cord and visceral organ ischemia, permit longer cross-clamp times to complete the proximal anastomosis, and mitigate the acidosis that ensues after cross-clamp release. The pericardium is reflected or opened near the pulmonary veins, away from the phrenic nerve. The left atrium or pulmonary vein is cannulated, and blood is directed to the femoral artery via a centrifugal pump (**Figure 9.16**). Alternatively, passive axillary artery to femoral artery bypass can be used, which is dependent on the mean arterial blood pressure (MAP) proximal to the cross-clamp. In addition to the benefit of distal aortic perfusion, atrial-femoral bypass reduces preload to the left ventricle, reducing myocardial stress during cross-clamping. The use of LHB requires less systemic heparinization (100 units/kg given 5 minutes prior to cannulation) than CPB. Target activated clotting time (ACT) may vary from 200 to 300 seconds according to institutional preferences. Once LHB is initiated, the proximal aortic cross-clamp is applied to the aorta with careful attention to the preservation of the left recurrent laryngeal nerve. When possible, the proximal clamp is placed distal to the LSCA to preserve its contribution to spinal cord blood flow, though it may be positioned between the left common carotid artery and the LSCA if there is a large distal arch aneurysm. The distal clamp site is most commonly at the junction of

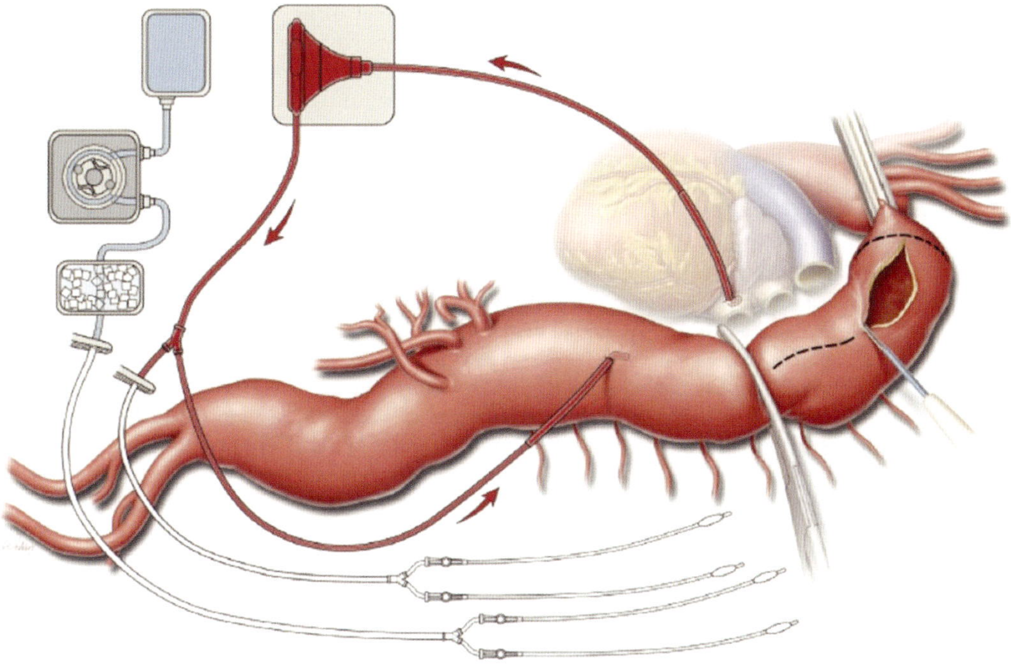

FIGURE 9.16. Left heart bypass is utilized for distal perfusion during thoracoabdominal aneurysm repair. The drainage cannula is placed in the left atrium, and the outflow cannula is placed in the thoracic aorta distal to the site of aortic cross-clamping. Additional catheters are available for selective perfusion of visceral arteries with blood during operative repair. A separate line may be set up to provide cold lactated Ringer solution through the renal arteries for renal protection. (Used with permission of AME Publishing Company, from de la Cruz KI, LeMaire SA, Weldon SA, et al. Thoracoabdominal aortic aneurysm repair with a branched graft. *Ann Cardiothorac Surg.* 2012;1:381-393; permission conveyed through Copyright Clearance Center, Inc.)

the upper and middle thirds of the descending thoracic aorta anterior to the hemiazygos and intercostal veins. Once the aorta is clamped, the LHB flows are increased to a target of 1.5 to 2.5 L/min.

Construction of anastomoses and preservation of mesenteric and visceral organs: The proximal aorta is opened between the two cross-clamps, and the proximal anastomosis is constructed in an end-to-end fashion; when an elephant trunk is present, a graft-to-graft anastomosis is performed. Intercostal arteries in the T4 to T8 region are oversewn if they exhibit excessive retrograde bleeding indicative of good collateral flow to improve visualization, minimize hemorrhage, and to prevent a steal phenomenon of shunting blood away from the spinal cord. When feasible, patent intercostal and lumbar arteries between T7 and L2 are reattached to the graft if they have marginal back-bleeding to decrease the incidence of paralysis due to spinal cord ischemia. LHB is weaned and discontinued once the proximal anastomosis is complete. The distal clamp is removed to prepare the distal aorta for replacement and reapplied just distal to the intercostal anastomoses. Shed blood is collected by a cell saver system and rapidly auto-transfused back into the patient.

Visceral and renal perfusion is utilized to limit ischemic time. Selective visceral perfusion with isothermic blood is given at a rate of 500 mL/min using catheters inserted into the celiac axis and the superior mesenteric artery (SMA), which are connected to the LHB circuit. Cold renal perfusion with mannitol and methylprednisolone in crystalloid solution extending from a separate cooling circuit is delivered using catheters in the renal arteries approximately every 6 minutes at a rate of 300 mL/min for 1 to 2 minutes.

The configuration of visceral artery reimplantation is variable and determined by the age of the patient, the presence of connective tissue disease, the quality of the aortic tissue, and the distance between the ostia of the arteries. In older patients with degenerative aortic disease, the four arteries can be reattached as one patch if they are close to one another. Alternatively, each vessel can be reimplanted individually into a four-vessel branch graft in younger patients with connective tissue disease or those whose arterial origins are significantly separated. When using a multibranched graft, the distal aortic anastomosis can be completed prior to reattachment of the visceral branches in order to restore blood flow to the iliac arteries that provide collateral perfusion to the spinal cord. Depending on the degree of aneurysmal dilatation of the distal aorta, iliac, and femoral vessels, an end-to-end anastomosis can be sewn proximal to the bifurcation or distal to using a bifurcated abdominal aortic graft. Once the aortic cross-clamp is released after the completion of the distal aortic anastomosis, individual clamps remain on each of the four branches of the visceral graft while the right renal, SMA, celiac, and left renal artery anastomoses are completed, respectively. The inferior mesenteric artery is usually oversewn, but reimplantation may be necessary if the patient has bilateral hypogastric artery occlusions, previous colectomy, or a diseased SMA. Protamine and dye, such as indigo carmine or methylene blue, are subsequently administered to reverse the effect of heparin and assess the adequacy of renal perfusion.

Cannulation for CPB with or without HCA: If the proximal extent of TAAA aneurysm involves the arch, CPB and HCA ± ACP/RCP can be used in lieu of proximal aortic cross-clamping, which reduces the potential for spinal cord injury and preserves end-organ function. Typically, a venous cannula is placed via the femoral vein prior to or after the right lateral positioning of the patient. Arterial cannulation can reside in the distal aortic arch, proximal descending aorta, axillary artery, or femoral artery.

Clamp and sew technique: The "clamp and sew" technique involves cross-clamping the proximal aorta and replacing the aneurysmal aorta with a graft without the use of LHB or HCA. The technique poses a time limit to the surgeon as the patient's organs are not being supported during cross-clamp. This technique is typically inadequate for difficult repairs and is preferred for patients presenting with isolated descending thoracic aneurysms, aortic rupture, and hemodynamic instability.

Outcomes: Experienced centers have reported acceptable outcomes, such as an early mortality rate of less than 8% with a nadir of 5.6%. The largest published series of 3,309 open TAAA repairs observed an incidence of permanent paraplegia of 2.9%, paraparesis of 2.4%, postoperative stroke of 2.2%, chronic renal failure of 5.7%, and gastrointestinal ischemia of 0.9%. Octogenarians were not at higher risk for operative mortality or postoperative complications, although survival was significantly reduced relative to younger patients. Patients with heritable thoracic aortic disease and chronic aortic dissection (rather than degenerative aneurysms) had more favorable outcomes. Patients with preoperative renal failure or pulmonary disease as well as those who underwent emergent or complex Crawford extent II repairs were at higher risk for adverse events. Open TAAA repairs tend to be durable, such that 94% of patients did not require reinterventions at 15 years from their index procedures.

Bilotta F, Gelb AW, Stazi E, Titi L, Paoloni FP, Rosa G. Pharmacological perioperative brain neuroprotection: a qualitative review of randomized clinical trials. *Br J Anaesth*. 2013;110:I113-I120.

Cao L, Guo X, Jia Y, Yang L, Wang H, Yuan S. Effect of deep hypothermic circulatory arrest versus moderate hypothermic circulatory arrest in aortic arch surgery on postoperative renal function: a systematic review and meta-analysis. *J Am Heart Assoc*. 2020;9:e017939.

Di Marco L, Murana G, Leone A, Pacini D. Con-debate: short circulatory arrest times in arch reconstructive surgery: is simple retrograde cerebral perfusion or hypothermic circulatory arrest as good or better than complex antegrade cerebral perfusion for open distal involvement or hemi-arch? *J Vis Surg*. 2018;4:46.

Fernandez Suarez FE, Fernandez Del Valle D, Gonzalez Alvarez A, Perez-Lozano B. Intraoperative care for aortic surgery using circulatory arrest. *J Thorac Dis*. 2017;9:S508-S520.

Girardi LN, Lau C, Munjal M, et al. Impact of preoperative pulmonary function on outcomes after open repair of descending and thoracoabdominal aortic aneurysms. *J Thorac Cardiovasc Surg*. 2017;153:S22-S29.e2.

Girardi LN, Ohmes LB, Lau C, et al. Open repair of descending thoracic and thoracoabdominal aortic aneurysms in patients with preoperative renal failure. *Eur J Cardiothorac Surg*. 2017;51:971-977.

Hong JC, Coselli JS. Open repair for thoracoabdominal aortic aneurysms precipitated by chronic aortic dissection. *Vessel Plus*. 2022;6:4.

Kothari R, Weldon SA, Koksoy C, Coselli JS. Narrative review: open surgery for thoracoabdominal aortic aneurysm—is it still a horrible surgery? *J Vis Surg*. 2022;8:4.

Malvindi PG, Scrascia G, Vitale N. Is unilateral antegrade cerebral perfusion equivalent to bilateral cerebral perfusion for patients undergoing aortic arch surgery? *Interact Cardiovasc Thorac Surg*. 2008;7:891-897.

Ouzounian M, LeMaire SA, Weldon S, Coselli JS. Open repair of thoracoabdominal aortic aneurysm: step-by-step. *Oper Tech Thorac Cardiovasc Surg*. 2018;23:2-20.

Reed H, Berg KB, Janelle GM. Aortic surgery and deep-hypothermic circulatory arrest: anesthetic update. *Semin Cardiothorac Vasc Anesth*. 2014;18:137-145.

C.3. What are the specific considerations for anesthetic management and monitoring of the patient presenting for open TAAA repair?

Patients presenting for TAAA repair typically have multiple preexisting comorbid conditions that require careful attention and evaluation, given that open TAAA repair poses a direct and immediate threat to the cardiac, pulmonary, renal, gastrointestinal, and neurologic systems.

Induction: Mitigating aortic wall stress is paramount during induction of anesthesia for patients presenting prior to rupture. A smooth and hemodynamically stable induction of general anesthesia with adequate depth of anesthesia and analgesia prevents hypertension, tachycardia, and increased stress on the aneurysm caused by stimulation during intubation. An awake arterial catheter should be placed for close continuous monitoring of arterial blood pressure with right radial access preferred in the event that the aortic cross-clamp is placed proximal to the LSCA.

Short-acting antihypertensive agents, such as nitroglycerin, nicardipine, esmolol, and labetalol, are useful for maintaining hemodynamic stability. When patients present for an emergent case with possible rupture, the risk of hypotension and malperfusion from bleeding must be balanced with the need to avoid hypertension. Hemodynamic collapse can occur after induction since the tamponade effect is lessened by the relaxation of abdominal vasculature, venous return is decreased with the onset of positive pressure ventilation, and sympathetic tone may be reduced by anesthetic agents. As surgical dissection exposes the aorta, the counterforce to the systemic blood pressure on the aneurysm wall is decreased, increasing the risk of aneurysm rupture. Prior to cross-clamp removal and reperfusion of the visceral organs and lower extremities, systemic blood pressure should be increased because removal of the cross-clamp and reperfusion can lead to profound hypotension.

Airway: Repair of type I, II, and some type III TAAAs requires lung isolation for adequate visualization, which can be accomplished with a double-lumen tube (DLT) or a bronchial blocker. A DLT provides access to the nonventilated lung for suctioning and the addition of continuous positive airway pressure (CPAP) when oxygenation is inadequate. Patients require intubation and mechanical ventilation in the intensive care unit postoperatively due to the need for large-volume resuscitation, correction of coagulopathy, and concern for pulmonary dysfunction, which can result from pulmonary edema, left lung trauma from retraction, diaphragmatic dysfunction, as well as possible phrenic and recurrent laryngeal nerve damage. The use of a bronchial blocker obviates the need to exchange the DLT for a single-lumen endotracheal tube at the conclusion of the procedure in a potentially edematous airway. Also, it can be simpler to place a larger single-lumen tube with a blocker than a DLT. A bronchial blocker is easier to position when large thoracic aneurysms displace or compress the left mainstem bronchus; alternatively, a right-sided DLT might be required since left-sided DLTs may be difficult to place in this circumstance. Lung-protective ventilation should be used regardless of airway technique.

Access: Central venous access with multiple 8.5F or 9F introducers should be obtained with consideration for additional large-bore peripheral access with 8.5F rapid infusion catheter or 14-gauge catheters in anticipation of the need for rapid resuscitation and vasoactive medication delivery. A rapid infusion system, such as the Belmont Rapid Infuser, is used to reinfuse shed blood and ensure timely resuscitation; the rate of flow should be confirmed both before and after positioning. The placement of a pulmonary artery catheter (PAC) can be useful for the optimization of volume status and mitigation of left and/or right heart dysfunction during aortic clamping/unclamping in centers that have expertise in PAC-guided management.

In addition to right radial arterial access, some centers consider simultaneous femoral arterial cannulation to assess perfusion distal to supraceliac cross-clamps and titrate LHB flow rates to optimize visceral, renal, spinal cord, and lower extremity perfusion.

Spinal cord protection: Spinal cord injury with resultant paraplegia remains one of the most serious complications of TAAA repair despite major advances in surgical technique. Temporary occlusion of the aorta with a cross-clamp, sacrificed intercostal arteries, and embolization of air or particulate matter to the aorta may contribute to the development of spinal cord injury. Enhancement of spinal cord perfusion by maximizing oxygen-carrying and delivery capacity with more liberal transfusion triggers (hemoglobin <10 g/dL) is thought to mitigate spinal cord injury, in addition to other techniques described in the sections that follow.

Hypothermia

Mild hypothermia to 32 °C might provide neuronal protection by reducing excitatory neurotransmitter release, decreasing free oxygen radical production, decreasing postischemic edema, and stabilizing central nervous system (CNS) blood flow. A core temperature of 32 °C to 34 °C is achieved via passive heat loss for cases not involving HCA, although active cooling can also be facilitated by heat exchangers on bypass circuits. It is also reasonable to use moderate hypothermia to protect the spinal cord from ischemic injury.

Some centers implement regional hypothermia of the spinal cord using epidural infusion of crystalloid solution at 4 °C in anticipation of aortic cross-clamping. Regional hypothermia might help avoid the detrimental effects of systemic hypothermia on the coagulation system. Epidural cooling can be instituted with the insertion of a T12-L1 epidural catheter and an L3-L4 intrathecal thermistor catheter, selectively cooling the spinal cord after aortic cross-clamp. The spinal cord is cooled at the T8-L1 region, a watershed area with variation in collateral blood supply most susceptible to ischemic injury. The thermistor catheter allows the measurement of temperature and cerebrospinal fluid (CSF) pressure. After full TAAA reconstruction is completed, epidural cooling is stopped. However, there is currently no data to support superior outcomes with regional hypothermia as compared to systemic hypothermia.

Cerebrospinal Drainage

CSF drainage in the perioperative period is the only technique with strong evidence to support a reduction in spinal cord injury in open and endovascular thoracic aortic repairs. During aortic cross-clamp and surgical retraction, CSF pressure can acutely increase due to a rise in venous pressure and a corresponding CSF pressure rise, which causes a decrease in spinal cord perfusion pressure (SCPP). Furthermore, the spinal cord can become edematous due to reperfusion injury. Lumbar drains are placed into the intrathecal space below the L2-L3 level preoperatively in hemodynamically stable patients and at the completion of the procedure in unstable patients to mitigate the rise in CSF pressure. CSF is drained to maintain a CSF pressure less than 10 to 15 mm Hg, without exceeding a maximal drainage rate of 10 to 15 mL/h. Careful titration may be necessary to permit more drainage if perfusion pressure drops, but at an elevated risk of subdural hematoma from tearing of bridging dural veins, especially when CSF pressure is less than 5 mm Hg. SCPP is estimated as the difference between the MAP and the CSF pressure. Therefore, measures that increase MAP and decrease CSF pressure result in improved spinal cord perfusion. It is reasonable to target a MAP of 85 to 100 mm Hg and an SCPP greater than or equal to 70 mm Hg.

Other pharmacologic strategies to decrease the risk of paraplegia and enhance spinal cord protection have been trialed without evidence to support improved outcomes. Such interventions include intrathecal papaverine, naloxone to reduce excitatory neurotransmitter release, and steroids to mitigate neuronal excitotoxicity, stabilize neuronal membranes, and decrease edema.

Neuromonitoring

Neuromonitoring of somatosensory evoked potential (SSEP) and motor evoked potential (MEP) can be utilized for timely diagnosis of ischemia and modification of surgical technique when ischemia occurs. SSEPs monitor the integrity of the dorsal column of the spinal cord while MEPs monitor the function of the corticospinal tract and anterior horn motor neurons. Use of MEPs necessitates the use of a total IV anesthetic, in addition to avoidance of paralysis, while the use of SSEP requires limitation of volatile anesthetic concentration to 0.5 minimum alveolar concentration (MAC). Although SSEPs are less sensitive to anesthetics and paralytics compared with MEPs, their utility is limited since revascularization of segments with associated SSEP changes ultimately did not affect the incidence of postoperative neurologic injury. Increased latency or decreased amplitude of MEPs is associated with paraplegia, which should prompt a higher MAP goal, increased CSF drainage, movement of the cross-clamp to improve perfusion of the intercostal arteries, and reimplantation of critical intercostal arteries. The use of neuromonitoring is supported by some institutions but is not a standard, widespread practice. Some institutions will institute a wake-up test prior to transportation to the ICU, during which the patient is asked to move their lower extremities. After completion of the wake-up test, the patient is reanesthetized.

The use of near-infrared spectroscopy (NIRS) along the paravertebral muscles for noninvasive surveillance of real-time spinal oxygenation and perfusion has been introduced but requires further investigation in human studies prior to routine clinical implementation. A pilot study validated the association between regional hemoglobin oxygen saturation using NIRS and MEP monitoring, in addition to demonstrating the feasibility of NIRS to surveil the hemodynamic changes in oxygenation of the paraspinal region during and after TAAA repair.

Left-Heart Bypass

LHB is commonly used to provide distal aortic perfusion during the period of aortic cross-clamp, as described in the previous sections (**Figure 9.14**).

Hemodynamic considerations for left-heart bypass and aortic cross-clamping: In anticipation of proximal aortic cross-clamping, LHB flow is initiated at 0.5 L/min and then gradually increased to 1 to 2.5 L/min once the cross-clamp is in place to maintain a MAP of 85 to 100 mm Hg. Careful assessment of arterial pressure is crucial as flow via the LHB circuit is increased since flow and perfusion can simultaneously be decreased to organs above the cross-clamp. The more proximal the aortic clamp, the more extreme the augmentation of blood pressure can be due to an increase in afterload. Nicardipine, nitroglycerin, nitroprusside, and the vasodilating properties of inhaled volatile can be used to help offset the increase in afterload seen with aortic cross-clamping. An increase in preload or central hypervolemia, manifested by increases in filling pressures, is also seen due to a decrease in venous capacitance that shifts blood away from vascular beds below the cross-clamp and toward the vasculature proximal to cross-clamp. Nitroglycerin-mediated venodilation helps mitigate the amplification in blood pressure that results from a reduction in venous capacity and permits volume expansion in anticipation of the central hypovolemia that will ensue with cross-clamp removal.

Once the distal anastomosis is completed, the aortic cross-clamp is slowly removed to reestablish blood flow to the lower body. The hypotension that ensues with cross-clamp release requires treatment with infusion of vasopressor medications and sodium bicarbonate to counteract the metabolic acidosis that results from the accumulation of vasoactive and myocardial-depressant metabolites in hypoperfused tissues that become released upon cross-clamp removal. Sodium bicarbonate can be administered as an infusion at 1 to 2 mg/kg/h during the cross-clamp period. The hypotension can also be combated with volume loading. Intermittent partial reapplication of the cross-clamp may be necessary to provide time for pharmacologic elevation of systemic vascular resistance (SVR), volume replacement, and reversal of metabolic acidosis with sodium bicarbonate.

A higher blood pressure than normal (MAP > 85 mm Hg) is typically maintained after cross-clamp release to ensure adequate renal and spinal cord perfusion. However, the blood pressure goal might be dependent on the complexity of the repair, as there are multiple suture lines prone to bleeding, as well as the fragility of aortic tissue in patients with heritable pathology.

Boezeman RP, van Dongen EP, Morshuis WJ, et al. Spinal near-infrared spectroscopy measurements during and after thoracoabdominal aortic aneurysm repair: a pilot study. *Ann Thorac Surg*. 2015;99:1267-1274.

Cambria RP, Davison JK, Carter C, et al. Epidural cooling for spinal cord protection during thoracoabdominal aneurysm repair: a five-year experience. *J Vasc Surg*. 2000;31:1093-1102.

Chatterjee S, Preventza O, Orozco-Sevilla V, Coselli JS. Perioperative management of patients undergoing thoracic endovascular repair. *Ann Cardiothorac Surg*. 2021;10:768-777.

Gelman S. The pathophysiology of aortic cross-clamping and unclamping. *Anesthesiology*. 1995;82:1026-1060.

Lester LC, Kostibas MP. Anesthetic management for open thoracoabdominal and abdominal aortic aneurysm repair. *Anesthesiol Clin*. 2022;40:705-718.

C.4. What is the pathophysiology of aortic clamping and unclamping?

Aortic Clamping

Hemodynamic response: Hypertension is the primary hemodynamic response typically seen with aortic cross-clamp application that results from an increase in afterload. Blood volume redistributes after aortic cross-clamping such that venous capacitance decreases below the clamp, expelling blood from the splanchnic and nonsplanchnic vascular beds, and increases above the clamp. The increase in upper body blood volume results in increased central venous pressure (CVP), pulmonary capillary wedge pressure (PCWP), and left ventricular end-diastolic pressure (LVEDP). Differences in hemodynamic responses are observed with occlusion at different levels of the aorta and can be the result of different patterns of blood volume distribution. Supraceliac cross-clamp application results in the most consistent redistribution of blood flow as described in the previous section(s). With infraceliac aortic cross-clamping, blood volume shifts into the splanchnic system and reduces preload if the splanchnic venous tone is low or, alternatively, it can be expelled into the vasculature of other tissues proximal to the clamp to increase preload. Variability in blood volume redistribution and splanchnic vascular tone also result from differences in fluid loading, depth of anesthesia, or anesthetic pharmacodynamics.

Oxygen consumption: Oxygen consumption decreases both proximal and distal to the aortic occlusion. The reason for the paradoxical decrease in oxygen consumption above the cross-clamp is unknown but might be related to sympathetic discharge from the adrenal glands that decreases capillary flow, increased arteriovenous shunting, or microcirculatory disturbances that compromise oxygen exchange due to proximal hypervolemia. Mixed venous oxygen saturation increases during aortic cross-clamp, indicating decreased extraction. A reduction in oxygen consumption and cardiac output reflects reduced global oxygen uptake and perfusion.

Coronary blood flow and contractility: Aortic cross-clamping results in increased myocardial oxygen demand. In an intact coronary blood supply, an increase in demand would lead to coronary artery vasodilation and a concomitant increase in oxygen supply. When coronary blood flow increases, the subendocardium is perfused and contractility will increase in response to aortic cross-clamping, which is also known as the Anrep effect. In the presence of inadequate coronary blood flow, the LVEDP increases and an increase in contractility does not manifest since the subendocardium is not perfused, thereby leading to decreased cardiac output. The beneficial effect of vasodilators on myocardial function during aortic cross-clamping is attributable to a decrease in preload resulting from an increase in venous capacitance, a decrease in afterload resulting from vasodilation, dilation of the coronary arteries with an increase in coronary blood flow, and facilitation of the Anrep effect.

Level and duration of aortic cross-clamp: As discussed in the previous section(s), the level of the aortic cross-clamp affects the hemodynamic response observed. Changes in MAP, filling pressures, ejection fraction, and wall motion are minimal during infrarenal aortic cross-clamping but exaggerated during supraceliac aortic cross-clamping. With increased duration of aortic cross-clamping, SVR increases and cardiac output decreases, which remains incompletely understood. Elevated proximal aortic pressure may ultimately increase fluid extravasation into the interstitial space, resulting in a decrease in circulating blood volume and a compensatory increase in SVR.

Renal effects: Cross-clamping of both the suprarenal and infrarenal aorta results in an increase in renin and angiotensin, which contributes to hypertension. Cross-clamping of the thoracic aorta is associated with severe decreases in renal blood flow, glomerular filtration rate, and urine output. Ischemia-reperfusion injury to the kidneys plays a central role in renal dysfunction after aortic surgery and is also present after infrarenal cross-clamping. Although mannitol is still often used to help maintain renal perfusion, it has not been consistently shown to reduce the incidence of renal failure. The use of dopamine, furosemide, and fenoldopam has also not been found to preserve renal function.

Effects on spinal cord: Cross-clamping of the aorta is associated with a decrease in distal aortic pressure and possibly ASA pressure, depending on the anatomy and presence of collateral blood supply, as well as an increase in CSF pressure and a decrease in the compliance of the spinal fluid space. Vasodilators used to decrease proximal aortic pressure should ideally possess minimal cerebral vasodilating properties that would decrease SCPP by decreasing distal aortic pressure and increasing CSF pressure. Sodium nitroprusside, which decreases distal aortic pressure and increases CSF pressure, and nitroglycerin, which predominantly decreases distal aortic pressure, can both decrease SCPP. However, unlike nitroglycerin, nitroprusside has the undesirable effect of causing vascular steal, which has the potential to worsen both spinal cord and myocardial ischemia during cross-clamping by diverting flow from maximally vasodilated ischemic regions to nonischemic regions.

Aortic Unclamping

Hemodynamic response: Unclamping of the thoracic aorta leads to a sudden decrease in SVR with a resultant decrease in arterial blood pressure. Cardiac output can increase, decrease, or remain the same. Myocardial blood flow increases and LVEDP decreases. Hypotension results from central hypovolemia that develops due to pooling of blood into reperfused tissues distal to the aortic occlusion, as well as hypoxia-mediated vasodilation and accumulation of myocardial-depressant metabolites. The metabolism of oxygen free radicals can also lead to an increase in microvascular permeability and loss of intravascular volume that lead to central hypovolemia, arterial hypotension, and ischemia-reperfusion injury.

Acidosis: Hypoperfusion of tissues distal to the aortic cross-clamp leads to the accumulation of vasoactive and myocardial-depressant metabolites, such as lactate, which contribute to metabolic acidosis after release of the aortic cross-clamp. The degree of acidosis present depends on the underlying pathology. Aortic cross-clamping in patients with aneurysmal disease was associated with more dramatic increases in lactate concentration and lactate-pyruvate ratio relative to patients with concomitant occlusive aortic disease, presumably due to the presence of collateral vessels and better tissue perfusion distal to the cross-clamp. Cross-clamp removal is also associated with a transient increase in carbon dioxide release and oxygen consumption.

Renal effects: Unclamping of the aorta results in a significant increase in renin and angiotensin that lasts for 6 hours but is unrelated to hypertension. Maldistribution of renal blood flow is seen, with a decrease in renal cortical blood flow. Glomerular filtration rate and renal plasma flow can remain at decreased values even 6 months following surgery. Optimization of circulating blood volume is thought to be protective from renal complications associated with aortic cross-clamp-induced ischemic insult, possibly due to inhibition of the production of certain vasoconstrictive compounds by volume loading.

Gelman S. The pathophysiology of aortic cross-clamping and unclamping. *Anesthesiology*. 1995;82:1026-1060.

Lester LC, Kostibas MP. Anesthetic management for open thoracoabdominal and abdominal aortic aneurysm repair. *Anesthesiol Clin*. 2022;40:705-718.

Vaughn SB, LeMaire SA, Collard CD. Case scenario: anesthetic considerations for thoracoabdominal aortic aneurysm repair. *Anesthesiology*. 2011;115:1093-1102.

C.5. How are endovascular repairs of TAAAs performed?

A purely endovascular approach to TAAA repair can reduce the physiologic stress response to surgery, end-organ ischemia, and blood loss. However, these procedures require extensive preoperative planning and a thorough understanding of associated shortcomings and anatomical constraints. The introduction of low-profile devices in the past decade has allowed patients with smaller iliofemoral or brachial vasculature to be candidates for endovascular interventions and preloaded systems. Preloaded systems (wires and catheters) can shorten procedural times by providing direct access to branches and fenestrations.

As part of preoperative planning, three-dimensional CT angiography is utilized to assess proximal and distal landing zones, the anatomy of the aorta and target vessels, and patency of target vessels and spinal collateral networks; the anatomy of access vessels, including common femoral, iliac and brachial arteries, is also evaluated. Approved thoracic stent grafts require greater than or equal to 2 cm proximal seal zones. Three-dimensional workstations and imaging are also utilized intraoperatively in dedicated hybrid operating rooms to ensure accurate deployment of the aortic stent graft and its side branches while minimizing radiation exposure.

Paraplegia is a feared complication of both open and endovascular TAAA repairs. Hemodynamic instability that results in spinal cord infarction secondary to loss of intercostal arteries coupled with insufficient collateral network, microembolization from catheter or device manipulations, reperfusion injury, and spinal cord edema may be contributory. Although patent segmental arteries can be reimplanted during open surgical repair, these vessels are often too small to accommodate bridging stents. Staged segmental arterial occlusion is thought to allow rapid recruitment of the spinal collateral networks, which is the mainstay of strategies to reduce spinal cord ischemia in endovascular approaches. Staging can be performed using embolization of intercostal and lumbar arteries, temporary aneurysm sac perfusion, or the performance of TEVAR above the celiac artery for coverage of proximal intercostal arteries.

Position: Patients are supine with both arms raised overhead and the right axilla prepped in the event that brachial access is needed.

Surgical exposure and technique: Bilateral percutaneous femoral access is obtained. Open surgical exposure of the femoral arteries might be necessary if there is a high femoral bifurcation or the femoral arteries are small and calcified. Before the graft introducer is inserted into the arterial system, systemic anticoagulation with 100 U/kg of heparin is typically administered for a goal ACT greater than 200 seconds, although the goal may vary across institutions. Temporary iliac or femoral conduits can be used to facilitate early pelvic and lower limb perfusion in longer, complex cases. Most endovascular TAAA cases are performed using a total transfemoral approach, though some centers use brachial access to facilitate the procedure and minimize lower extremity ischemia. Fenestrated-branched endovascular stent grafts and off-the-shelf, multibranched devices, which are designed with four downgoing branches to incorporate the celiac axis, SMA, and renal arteries, are deployed in a staggered fashion. Precise graft positioning is facilitated by angiography in the setting of apnea. Once the stent grafts are deployed via the femoral approach, the target vessels are catheterized and stented, and the distal bifurcated device and iliac limb extensions are placed. Balloon dilation at seal zones and overlap zones between multiple grafts may be performed to ensure an adequate seal to the aortic wall. The LSCA may need to be covered by the endograft in order to achieve an adequate PLZ with the distal subclavian artery gaining perfusion from collateral vessels, including the left internal mammary artery and vertebral artery. If occlusion is not tolerated, a left carotid to subclavian bypass is performed.

Once the procedure is complete, contrast angiography is also used to evaluate for endoleaks and assess the integrity of the arterial system from the aorta to the iliac artery.

Limitations: Endovascular approaches have a steep learning curve for both physicians and centers. Proper development of technical strategies requires accurate measurements to ensure that the graft is an optimal fit, in addition to clinical experience to determine feasibility. Although intercostal arteries can be reimplanted during open surgical repair, they are often too small to be reconstructed endovascularly, which raises concern that extensive aortic coverage may increase the risk of spinal cord ischemia. In addition, extensive catheter and wire manipulations may lead to embolization of atheromatous debris and end-organ damage.

It is common for patients, especially females, to be ineligible for endovascular interventions based on anatomic criteria specific to devices. Use of endovascular devices outside of the manufacturer's instructions for use has been reported, though outcomes are controversial with evidence to suggest that nonadherence to these instructions is associated with higher rates of complications. Furthermore, custom-made branched and fenestrated devices are not available to patients in need of urgent or emergent interventions.

Although chimney/snorkel grafts and standardized multibranched devices are options when TAAA repair is imminent, they may not be suitable for the repair of complex aneurysms extending above the visceral branches.

The need for relatively frequent reinterventions with total endovascular approaches, especially in patients with heritable thoracic aortic disease, is another shortcoming of TEVAR. This is, at least in part, why patients who undergo endovascular procedures require meticulous longitudinal annual surveillance. Imaging with CT angiography or duplex ultrasound is recommended annually after CT angiography is performed 1-month postoperatively; surveillance is indicated more frequently at 6-month intervals for patients with known type II endoleaks. Although many secondary procedures can also be performed using endovascular techniques, serious complications, such as expanding aneurysms, infection, fistula formulation, and aneurysm rupture, require open repair.

Outcomes

Few studies directly assess the efficacy of endovascular relative to open surgical TAAA repairs, and high-quality evidence is lacking. Clinical equipoise appears to persist with regard to the superiority of one technique over the other. TEVAR was associated with higher rates of spinal cord injury (13.5%) relative to open repair (7.4%), although rates of permanent paralysis were similar. TEVAR was also associated with lower rates of postoperative dialysis (6.4%) in comparison to open repair (12.0%), but rates of discharge on permanent dialysis were similar. There were no significant differences in the risks of perioperative mortality or stroke between the two techniques, even though TEVAR might be associated with 60% fewer complications overall and a shorter though more expensive length of stay. There is also insufficient data to determine which endovascular technique is preferable. Small studies on fenestrated and branched endografts have reported low rates of mortality (4%), new-onset dialysis (1%), paraplegia, stroke, and bowel ischemia (each ≤3%), although there was a high rate of acute kidney injury (22%). Outcomes from chimney/snorkel repairs performed in experienced centers are highly variable with regard to operative mortality and acute kidney injury (AKI), although the rates of spinal cord injury and bowel ischemia are low.

Furthermore, serious concerns remain about the durability of endovascular repairs, given the high rates of reintervention, which could explain why open repair is associated with similar and sometimes higher rates of long-term survival and adverse events relative to TEVAR. Endoleaks, which occur when there is persistent blood flow into the aneurysm sac, are major sources of complications unique to endovascular approaches. Endoleaks that originate from the proximal or distal landing zones, fenestrations, or branch point ends (type I) or those that result from failed apposition or fabric tears (type III) are most dangerous and require immediate treatment. Another rare but often fatal complication of TEVAR is retrograde TAAD, which is more common in patients who undergo TEVAR for treatment of dissection and can be associated with a mortality rate of 37%.

Kothari R, Weldon SA, Koksoy C, Coselli JS. Narrative review: open surgery for thoracoabdominal aortic aneurysm—is it still a horrible surgery? *J Vis Surg*. 2022;8:4.

Oderich GS, Ribeiro M, Reis de Souza L, Hofer J, Wigham J, Cha S. Endovascular repair of thoracoabdominal aortic aneurysms using fenestrated and branched endografts. *J Thorac Cardiovasc Surg*. 2017;153:S32-S41.e7.

Swerdlow NJ, Wu WW, Schermerhorn ML. Open and endovascular management of aortic aneurysms. *Circ Res*. 2019;124:647-661.

Tanaka A, Oderich GS, Estrera AL. Total abdominal debranching hybrid thoracoabdominal aortic aneurysm repair versus chimneys and snorkels. *JTCVS Tech*. 2021;10:28-33.

Tenorio ER, Dias-Neto MF, Lima GBB, Estrera AL, Oderich GS. Endovascular repair for thoracoabdominal aortic aneurysms: current status and future challenges. *Ann Cardiothorac Surg*. 2021;10:744-767.

C.6. What are the specific considerations for anesthetic management and monitoring of the patient presenting for endovascular TAAA repair?

Although endovascular treatment of thoracic aneurysms is typically less invasive than open surgical repair, preparation for possible open repair must be undertaken in longer, complex cases with more bleeding. General and regional anesthetic techniques have been described, but general anesthesia remains the most popular anesthetic technique for TEVAR. General anesthesia facilitates neuromonitoring and, if need be, TEE monitoring, as well as immobility to improve intraoperative angiographic imaging and provide stability during endograft deployment.

Induction: As for open repair, avoidance of hypertension, tachycardia, and increased stress on the aneurysm is key.

IV Access: Routine use of central venous access is recommended to facilitate the rapid transfusion of IV fluids and blood products, as well as the use of vasoactive medications. As for open repair, placement of a preinduction arterial catheter is necessary for close continuous monitoring of arterial blood pressure. The location of the arterial line should be discussed with the vascular surgeon, as it may vary depending on the surgical approach and landing zones of the TEVAR. For example, coverage of the left subclavian arterial takeoff by the endograft or surgical placement of an angiography catheter into the left brachial artery can necessitate right radial arterial cannulation. If monitoring of arterial pressure distal to the endograft is necessary, femoral arterial access may be established and transduced simultaneously with the radial arterial line for a comparison of pressures.

Spinal cord protection: The risk of spinal cord ischemia can be mitigated with the placement of CSF drains in high-risk patients, such as those with a history of aortic repair and extent I to III thoracoabdominal aneurysms, as well as those who require graft coverage of extensive portions of the aorta. Prophylactic placement of CSF drains in lower-risk elective TEVARs remains controversial and, thus, requires consideration of whether the benefits outweigh the risks. CSF is drained to typically maintain a CSF pressure less than 10 to 15 mm Hg, without exceeding a maximal drainage rate of 20 to 25 mL/h, as well as an SCPP greater than or equal to 70 mm Hg.

Neuromonitoring with SSEPs and MEPs may be used to assess the integrity of spinal cord pathways and global spinal cord perfusion. For instance, a reduction in 50% to 75% from baseline amplitude merits further augmentation of SCPP by raising MAP to greater than 90 to 100 mm Hg and reducing CSF pressure to 5 mm Hg, according to a protocol from the Mayo Clinic. If signals do not normalize, flow to the pelvis and lower extremities should be restored and a decision is made either to place an arterial conduit prior to proceeding or to perform the procedure in stages.

Hemodynamic considerations: It is reasonable to maintain the MAP close to baseline for elective TEVARs while a lower blood pressure goal may be sought when there is a concern for aneurysm rupture or extension of an acute dissection. Vasoconstrictors and vasodilators should be readily available to allow precise titration of blood pressure. Immediately before endograft deployment, migration of the graft should be minimized using techniques such as induced hypotension, rapid ventricular pacing, adenosine-induced cardiac arrest, and right atrial-inferior vena cava balloon occlusion. This results in significant transient hemodynamic instability, particularly if the patient has poor cardiac function. Transient balloon occlusion of the aorta during deployment can have a similar effect. After deployment, it is reasonable to target a MAP of 85 to 100 mm Hg to achieve an SCPP greater than or equal to 70 mm Hg. The indication for TEVAR helps determine the precise blood pressure target; hypertension is well tolerated after repair of degenerative aneurysms, but it can lead to exacerbation of residual dissection after repair of TBADs.

TEE: TEE can be used to guide vascular access by visualizing the placement of wires and to ensure the exclusion of aortic pathology by the endograft. Once the endograft is deployed, TEE can be used to evaluate for endoleaks and rule out the occurrence of retrograde dissection.

Chatterjee S, Preventza O, Orozco-Sevilla V, Coselli JS. Perioperative management of patients undergoing thoracic endovascular repair. *Ann Cardiothorac Surg*. 2021;10:768-777.

Cheruku S, Huang N, Meinhardt K, Aguirre M. Anesthetic management for endovascular repair of the thoracic aorta. *Anesthesiol Clin*. 2019;37:593-607.

Isselbacher EM, Preventza O, Hamilton Black J 3rd, et al; Peer Review Committee Members. 2022 ACC/AHA guideline for the diagnosis and management of aortic disease: a report of the American Heart Association/American College of Cardiology Joint Committee on clinical practice guidelines. *Circulation*. 2022;146:e334-e482.

Nation DA, Wang GJ. TEVAR: endovascular repair of the thoracic aorta. *Semin Intervent Radiol*. 2015;32:265-271.

Pulido JN, Wittwer ED, Baker AC, Oderich GS. Anesthetic considerations for complex endovascular aortic repair. In: Oderich GS, *ed. Endovascular Aortic Repair: Current Techniques with Fenestrated, Branched and Parallel Stent-Grafts*. Springer International Publishing; 2017.

C.7. What are the surgical approaches to aortic dissections?

Type A Aortic Dissection

Unlike elective surgery for TAAs, TAAD repair is generally an emergency procedure, and the real-time operative approach can deviate from the original plan. As the extent of surgical repair is dictated primarily by the location(s) of the intimal entry tear(s), intraoperative decision-making is critical.

A median sternotomy is performed for exposure, preceded or followed by arterial and venous cannulation, initiation of CPB, and cooling to the desired temperature for hypothermic cardiac arrest (HCA). The choice of cannulation site is dictated by the extent of dissection, hemodynamic stability, and patient-specific factors. Femoral artery cannulation can be performed when prompt initiation of CPB is desired, although right axillary artery cannulation might be preferable because it facilitates ACP during HCA and can be associated with superior outcomes relative to femoral artery cannulation. Central cannulation of the true lumen of the ascending aorta can also be performed under the guidance of TEE or epiaortic ultrasound. Placement of a left ventricular vent and a retrograde cardioplegia cannula is usually necessary in the setting of AR. Surgical goals include excision of the primary intimal tear, obliteration of the false lumen, resumption of forward blood flow through the true lumen, and correction of associated pathologic conditions, such as AR and malperfusion.

The standard TAAD repair entails a supracoronary hemiarch replacement with the distal anastomosis performed under HCA, which facilitates direct inspection of the aortic arch to ensure the absence of distal tears. When an intimal tear extends into the aortic root, a composite graft or a valve-sparing Bentall procedure may be necessary when the left and right coronary sinuses are involved. If involvement is limited to the noncoronary sinus, limited repair of the aortic root may be performed without the need for coronary artery reimplantation. Dissections involving a coronary ostium may require ligation of the affected ostium in combination bypass grafts. Surgical approaches to repair the distal extent of the TAAD vary from an ascending aorta replacement to a hemi- or total-aortic arch replacement with or without an elephant trunk procedure that can be classic or frozen (FET) (**Figures 9.10** and **9.11**). The choice of technique requires weighing the risk of late reintervention against the operative risk of a more complex distal repair.

Approximately 20% to 30% of patients who survive the initial surgery for aortic dissections extending into the abdominal aorta (DeBakey type I) require future reinterventions on the distal aorta. The FET procedure has shown promise as an adjunct to standard surgical repair. It not only facilitates false-lumen thrombosis and aortic remodeling but also expedites the second-stage surgery for the downstream aorta; the hybrid stent-graft prosthesis can also serve as the extended landing zone for future endovascular repair. Concerns about potential increases in spinal cord ischemia associated with the procedure have prompted the use of short endografts (10-15 cm in length). Other modified approaches to hybrid aortic arch repair have been discussed in a previous section (**Figures 9.12** and **9.13**).

Type B Aortic Dissection

TBAD is managed medically unless complications have developed or are impending. TEVAR has become a popular intervention in the current era due to the high mortality and considerable morbidity associated with open repair. The goal of TEVAR for TBAD is to obliterate the blood flow into the false lumen by covering the intimal entry tear, thereby promoting expansion of the true lumen. Although the benefits of TEVAR for complicated TBAD are well known, there remains great interest in exploring whether earlier TEVAR might improve outcomes in uncomplicated TBAD, especially in patients with high-risk imaging and clinical features. Prophylactic TEVAR in conjunction with medical therapy was associated with less incomplete or no false-lumen thrombosis, aortic dilation, and rupture in the ADSORB (Acute Dissection: Stent graft OR Best medical therapy) trial, as well as improved 5-year aorta-specific survival and delayed disease progression in the INSTEAD-XL (Investigation of Stent Grafts in Patients with Type B Aortic Dissection) trial. Larger trials with longer-term data are still needed to determine precisely when TEVAR should be performed in uncomplicated TBAD and how it influences patient outcomes. The technical considerations and limitations of TEVAR are discussed in previous sections.

El-Hamamsy I, Ouzounian M, Demers P, et al. State-of-the-art surgical management of acute type A aortic dissection. *Can J Cardiol.* 2016;32:100-109.

Hanif H, Dubois L, Ouzounian M, et al; Canadian Thoracic Aortic Collaborative (CTAC) Investigators. Aortic arch reconstructive surgery with conventional techniques vs frozen elephant trunk: a systematic review and meta-analysis. *Can J Cardiol.* 2018;34:262-273.

Isselbacher EM, Preventza O, Hamilton Black J 3rd, et al; Peer Review Committee Members. 2022 ACC/AHA guideline for the diagnosis and management of aortic disease: a report of the American Heart Association/American College of Cardiology Joint Committee on Clinical Practice Guidelines. *Circulation.* 2022;146:e334-e482.

Waterford SD, Gardner RL, Moon MR. Extent of aortic replacement in type A dissection: current answers for an endless debate. *Ann Thorac Surg.* 2018;106:1246-1250.

C.8. Why does a coagulopathy ensue and how is it prevented/treated?

TAA or TAAA repair is associated with significant hemorrhage from multiple causes, including surgical dissection, hypothermia, CPB, fibrinolysis, dilution or consumption of coagulation factors, anticoagulant therapy, preoperative antithrombotic therapy, and congenital or acquired coagulopathies. About 5 to 10 units of packed red blood cells (pRBCs) should be immediately available in the operating room, with a similar number of units available in the blood bank. About 5 to 10 units of fresh frozen plasma, typically given in a ratio of 1:1 or 1:2 pRBCs transfused, should be readily available. Thrombocytopenia and platelet dysfunction develop secondary to hypothermia and the use of extracorporeal mechanical support, and the need for platelet transfusion is common.

The use of prothrombin complex concentrates (PCCs) is useful in cases with refractory international normalized ratio (INR) elevation as the cause of coagulopathy or in patients with depressed cardiac or renal function. PCCs offer the advantage of rapid correction of INR with a minimal volume load without the need for crossmatching. Caution must be exercised, given the possibility of thrombosis. In patients with heparin-induced thrombocytopenia (HIT), PCCs should not be administered because most contain heparin.

Fibrinolysis develops not only from the use of CPB but also from supraceliac aortic cross-clamping and peripheral ischemia, which can be attenuated by the use of selective SMA perfusion. Supraceliac cross-clamping and peripheral ischemia promote activation of tissue-type plasminogen activator and decrease plasminogen activator inhibitor. The use of lysine analogues ε-aminocaproic acid and tranexamic acid is common in TAA repairs, but its use has been derived from studies in other cardiac surgeries. There is currently no literature to support prophylactic use of antifibrinolytic medications in TAA repair.

The use of a blood-salvaging device ("cell saver") is essential to decreasing allogeneic red blood cell transfusions. Unfortunately, the use of a cell saver is associated with the loss of platelets, plasma proteins, and coagulation factors. In heparinized patients, the use of cardiotomy suction permits the autotransfusion of filtered unwashed whole blood, which preserves platelets and coagulation factors.

Ferraris VA, Brown JR, Despotis GJ, et al. 2011 update to the Society of Thoracic Surgeons and the Society of Cardiovascular Anesthesiologists blood conservation clinical practice guidelines. *Ann Thorac Surg*. 2011;91:944-982.

Ghadimi K, Levy JH, Welsby IJ. Prothrombin complex concentrates for bleeding in the perioperative setting. *Anesth Analg*. 2016;122:1287-1300.

Levine WC, Lee JJ, Black JH, et al. Thoracoabdominal aneurysm repair: anesthetic management. *Int Anesthesiol Clin*. 2005;43:39-60.

D. Postoperative Anesthetic Management

D.1. What are the goals of immediate postoperative care following TAAA repair?

Continued from the operating room, the immediate focus of postoperative management centers on hemodynamic management and major volume resuscitation guided by PAC monitoring, ideally with continuous cardiac output and continuous mixed venous capability. Coagulation management should continue with consideration that as the patient is actively warmed, decreased venous return from vasodilation can contribute to lower cardiac output and MAP. Surgical trauma, fluid and coagulation resuscitation, and postoperative third-spacing contribute to challenges with oxygenation and ventilation for which inhaled nitric oxide may be considered. Serial arterial blood gas analysis for lactate, pH, and hemoglobin levels at least every hour is useful to monitor and guide resuscitation.

Chatterjee S, Casar JG, LeMaire SA, Preventza O, Coselli JS. Perioperative care after thoracoabdominal aortic aneurysm repair: The Baylor College of Medicine experience. Part 2: Postoperative management. *J Thorac Cardiovasc Surg*. 2021;161:699-705.

Khan FM, Naik A, Hameed I, et al. Open repair of descending thoracic and thoracoabdominal aortic aneurysms: a meta-analysis. *Ann Thorac Surg*. 2020;110:1941-1949.

D.2. Two hours following arrival in the ICU, the patient is unable to move his lower extremities. How are symptoms of spinal cord compromise or ischemia managed?

Postoperative neurologic complications can contribute to significant morbidity following open TAAA repair. The incidence of perioperative stroke is 2% to 3%, and spinal cord injury is 3% to 10%. Neurologic assessment, especially of lower extremity movement, is paramount in the immediate postoperative period.

The degree of neuromuscular block should be noted upon exiting the operating room (OR), and reversal considered to facilitate a neurologic assessment. An effective sedation strategy can include liberal opioid administration and limited sedatives/ hypnotics.

Spinal cord injury can be immediate or delayed. Spinal cord injury occurs more often with type I and II TAAAs, emergent operations, intercostal sacrifice, and intraoperative hypotension. The majority of deficits are immediate; however, delayed deficits can occur hours to weeks postoperatively. Immediate-onset deficits are irreversible and portend a poor prognosis, whereas delayed-onset deficits typically have a better prognosis with partial and reversible deficits and acceptable functional outcomes. Management of immediate- and delayed-onset deficits focuses on CSF drainage to a CSF pressure of 12 mm Hg and limited to 20 mL/h, maintaining systemic blood pressure to a MAP of 85 to 95 mm Hg for improved spinal cord perfusion, and a hemoglobin threshold of 10 g/dL for oxygen delivery. Further increases in MAP or additional CSF drainage can be considered with continued evidence of spinal cord ischemia.

Chatterjee S, Casar JG, LeMaire SA, Preventza O, Coselli JS. Perioperative care after thoracoabdominal aortic aneurysm repair: The Baylor College of Medicine experience. Part 2: Postoperative management. *J Thorac Cardiovasc Surg.* 2021;161:699-705.

Coselli JS, LeMaire SA, Orozco-Sevilla V, Preventza O, Moon MR, Barron LM, Chatterjee S. Current approaches to spinal cord protection during open thoracoabdominal aortic aneurysm repair. *Ann Cardiothorac Surg.* 2023;12:429-437.

Khan FM, Naik A, Hameed I, et al. Open repair of descending thoracic and thoracoabdominal aortic aneurysms: a meta-analysis. *Ann Thorac Surg.* 2020;110:1941-1949.

D.3. For how long is postoperative mechanical ventilation required?

Mechanical ventilation can be anticipated for at least 12 to 48 hours postoperatively. Weaning can commence once relative hemodynamic stability can be maintained, coagulation status corrected, and the patient begins mobilizing interstitial fluid with reduced airway edema and improved oxygenation.

Respiratory failure after TAAA repair remains one of the most commonly reported complications, with reported rates of postoperative tracheostomy as high as 8.5%. The large thoracoabdominal incision, diaphragmatic incision, and need for lung isolation all predispose the patient to pulmonary dysfunction. The diaphragmatic incision may lead to hemidiaphragm dysfunction or paralysis. Preoperative pulmonary dysfunction, tobacco use, postoperative cardiac complications, and postoperative renal complications are independent risk factors for postoperative respiratory failure.

Chatterjee S, Casar JG, LeMaire SA, Preventza O, Coselli JS. Perioperative care after thoracoabdominal aortic aneurysm repair: The Baylor College of Medicine experience. Part 2: postoperative management. *J Thorac Cardiovasc Surg.* 2021;161:699-705.

Khan FM, Naik A, Hameed I, et al. Open repair of descending thoracic and thoracoabdominal aortic aneurysms: a meta-analysis. *Ann Thorac Surg.* 2020;110:1941-1949.

D.4. On postoperative day 2, the patient's creatinine approaches 2.5 mg/dL. What is the incidence of postoperative acute kidney injury and renal failure requiring chronic hemodialysis?

Postoperative renal dysfunction is a common postoperative complication, occurring in as many as 33% of patients and necessitating dialysis in as many as 8% of patients. Risk factors associated with postoperative renal failure include age older than 50 years, preexisting renal dysfunction, administration of greater than 5 units of either pRBCs or salvaged washed autologous blood, and aortic cross-clamp time of greater than 100 minutes. Postoperative renal dysfunction of any degree is associated with increased perioperative mortality.

Chatterjee S, Casar JG, LeMaire SA, Preventza O, Coselli JS. Perioperative care after thoracoabdominal aortic aneurysm repair: The Baylor College of Medicine experience. Part 2: Postoperative management. *J Thorac Cardiovasc Surg.* 2021;161:699-705.

Khan FM, Naik A, Hameed I, et al. *Ann Thorac Surg.* 2020;110:1941-1949.

D.5. What are the unique postoperative complications after endovascular TAAA repair?

Left Upper Extremity Ischemia

Aneurysms involving the aortic arch pose a significant risk to cerebral and upper extremity blood flow with endovascular repair. Intentional coverage of the LSCA with the endovascular graft can occur in approximately 50% of thoracic endograft implants. Most patients can tolerate LSCA coverage without left upper extremity ischemia. However, if the right subclavian and vertebral arteries are not patent, ischemia can ensue. Additionally, the patient can experience decreased blood flow to the left internal mammary artery, leading to significant myocardial ischemia to a prior coronary artery bypass graft. If left upper extremity ischemia occurs, an LSCA bypass should be performed postoperatively.

Stroke

Intravascular wires and endografts that are introduced into the atherosclerotic aorta can come in contact with mobile thrombi in the arch and brachiocephalic vessels, leading to cerebral ischemia. Iatrogenic dissection of the carotid or vertebral arteries and retrograde dissection of the aorta have been described as devastating complications. If the LSCA is covered during endograft deployment, cerebral ischemia can develop due to decreased flow from the left vertebral artery. A left carotid to left subclavian bypass graft should first be placed if the left subclavian will be covered by the graft. The incidence of stroke after TEVAR ranges from 2% to 8%. Risk factors for perioperative stroke include severe atheromatous aortic disease (grade IV or V aortic disease on TEE), endovascular coverage of aortic arch vessels, history of prior stroke, long extent of aortic coverage, preexisting CAD, longer procedure duration, and female sex.

Spinal Cord Ischemia

Spinal cord ischemia is also a possible complication of endovascular treatment of TAAAs, although with less incidence than after open repair. Intercostal arteries are intentionally covered during endovascular stent placement of a TAAA, possibly compromising spinal cord perfusion by obliterating the collateral circulation. Endovascular coverage of the LSCA can compromise spinal cord perfusion in patients with a left-dominant vertebral artery, solitary vertebral artery, carotid artery disease, or an incomplete circle of Willis. Spinal cord injury after TAAA repair is a heterogeneous syndrome manifesting as a spectrum of impairments that varies depending on the severity and extent of ischemia. Additionally, delayed-onset neurologic deficits, like those seen after open repair, can also be seen after endovascular treatment. Delayed-onset deficits are thought to be due to postoperative events such as hypotension, thrombosis, hematoma, embolization, and elevated CSF pressure. Injury to the spinal cord is directly related to the extent of the aorta that is involved and is highest with Crawford type II repairs. Risk factors for spinal cord injury after TEVAR include LSCA coverage without revascularization, concomitant open abdominal aortic surgery, and the use of three or more stent grafts.

Renal Failure

Similar to open repair of TAAAs, renal insufficiency can develop after endovascular repair with an incidence rate of 14%. Deployment of the endograft in a diseased, atherosclerotic aorta can lead to embolic showers and occlusion of mesenteric, splenic, or renal arteries. This phenomenon contributes to the development of renal insufficiency. Risk factors for postoperative renal dysfunction after TEVAR include preoperative chronic renal insufficiency, perioperative blood transfusions, and the thoracoabdominal extent of the aneurysm.

Postimplantation Syndrome

This commonly observed phenomenon consisting of fever, leukocytosis, and an elevation in inflammatory markers normally occurs in the early postoperative period, although it occasionally has a delayed presentation. It is usually mild and self-limiting, responding to conservative management with nonsteroidal anti-inflammatory drugs.

Endograft Collapse

Endograft collapse is a rare but serious complication after TEVAR, typically presenting in the first 3 months after endovascular repair. Endograft collapse can present asymptomatically or can present with diminished or absent femoral pulses, abdominal pain, or multiorgan failure. Excessive oversizing of the endograft and poor apposition of the proximal endograft to the aortic wall are the primary causes of endograft collapse. Maldeployment of the endograft and progression of the aortic disease are rare causes of endograft collapse.

Endoleaks

An endoleak is a leakage of blood into an aneurysm sac previously excluded during TEVAR. Endoleaks after TEVAR occur in 5% to 30% of patients. Endoleak is a complication unique to the endovascular approach to aortic repair, and there are four types:

- *Type I endoleak* is caused by incomplete seal at the end of the graft, leading to blood flow into the aneurysm sac.
- *Type II endoleak* is caused by leaking of blood into the aneurysm from collateral vessels excluded during the repair.

- *Type III endoleak* is caused by inadequate sealing of overlapping graft joints or rupture of graft fabric, leading to blood flow into the aneurysm sac.
- *Type IV endoleak* is caused by the direct leakage of blood through a porous graft.

Management includes aggressive endovascular repair of type I and III endoleaks, with observation of type II endoleaks. Type IV endoleaks are of historical interest because new graft material has virtually eliminated the incidence of this complication. Risk factors for the development of endoleaks include larger preoperative aneurysm sac diameter, greater length of stent coverage, and the use of multiple stent grafts.

Diamond KR, Simons JP, et al. Effect of thoracoabdominal aortic aneurysm extent on outcomes in patients undergoing fenestrated/branched endovascular aneurysm repair. *J Vasc Surg*. 2021;74:833-842.e2.

Harik L, Lau C. Open and endovascular repair of thoracoabdominal aortic aneurysm-a narrative review. *J Thorac Dis*. 2023;15:3984-3997.

Isselbacher EM, Preventza O, Hamilton Black J 3rd, et al; Peer Review Committee Members. 2022 ACC/AHA guideline for the diagnosis and management of aortic disease: a report of the American Heart Association/American College of Cardiology Joint Committee on clinical practice guidelines. *Circulation*. 2022;146:e334-e482.

10

Abdominal Aortic Aneurysm Repair

Anup Pamnani and Shreyajit R. Kumar

A 79-year-old female with a 6-cm infrarenal aortic aneurysm discovered on routine physical examination and confirmed by abdominal computed tomography (CT) scan is referred for abdominal aortic aneurysm repair. She is a former smoker with a 40 pack-year history and complains of dyspnea on exertion and claudication. Her electrocardiogram (ECG) shows normal sinus rhythm; chest radiography shows mild hyperinflation of the lung fields. Her hematocrit is 39%. The rest of her laboratory studies are normal except for a serum creatinine of 1.7.

A. Medical Disease and Differential Diagnosis

1. What risk factors are associated with an abdominal aortic aneurysm (AAA)?
2. What comorbid diseases are commonly found in patients with AAAs?
3. What is the incidence of morbidity and mortality in these patients if they undergo elective open surgical repair? What is the natural history of the disease without surgical repair?
4. What should be done for smaller AAAs that are found in patients?
5. What are the risk factors for perioperative myocardial infarction (MI) in patients with ischemic heart disease? What can be done to reduce the risk of ischemic events in these patients?
6. Does the morbidity and mortality of elective repair of an AAA differ significantly from that of an emergency repair?

B. Preoperative Evaluation and Preparation

1. Which preoperative laboratory tests would you require for this patient?
2. What is the significance of the preoperative ECG? Would you wish to pursue a preoperative cardiac workup? What tests would you request, and what would they tell you?
3. How do you evaluate this patient's pulmonary status?
4. Preoperative arterial blood gas (ABG) analysis shows pH, 7.35; $Paco_2$, 50 mm Hg; and Pao_2, 68 mm Hg on room air. What is the significance of this result?
5. How would you measure creatinine clearance in this patient, and what is its value in this case?
6. What are the various surgical approaches to repair an AAA?
7. How does the choice of surgical technique affect anesthetic management?
8. How would you premedicate this patient?

C. Intraoperative Management

1. Would you use an arterial catheter? What are the complications of arterial catheter placement?
2. What various monitors are available for myocardial ischemia? Is a pulmonary artery catheter (PAC) helpful in determining the occurrence of ischemia?
3. What additional monitors would you employ?
4. How would you anesthetize this patient for an open repair of the aneurysm? What techniques could be used for an endovascular AAA repair? Discuss the various anesthetic techniques that can be employed for this surgery.
5. This patient is to be heparinized intraoperatively, and anticoagulation might be continued postoperatively. Is this a contraindication to the preoperative placement of either an epidural or intrathecal catheter? What if the patient is receiving anticoagulants in the preoperative period?
6. What are your plans for fluid and blood replacement during surgery?

7. What are the hemodynamic changes of aortic cross-clamp placement? What efforts can be made to minimize these changes both before and during cross-clamping? If the patient develops ST-segment depressions with a rising pulmonary capillary wedge pressure (PCWP) during cross-clamp, what maneuvers should be taken?
8. Because this case involves an infrarenal aneurysm, is renal blood flow affected with the placement of the cross-clamp? If an endovascular repair is chosen, what are the risks to the kidneys? Are there any treatment maneuvers that can be taken to minimize these risks in either repair?
9. What are the hemodynamic consequences of aortic cross-clamp placement and removal? What can be done to minimize the effects of the aortic cross-clamp?

D. Postoperative Management

1. What are the parameters used for tracheal extubation of this patient?
2. What are the anticipated changes in postoperative pulmonary function in these patients? How does the surgical technique affect postoperative pulmonary function? Are there any postoperative maneuvers that can improve respiratory parameters?
3. How would you control postoperative pain? What are the alternatives in the management of this patient's postoperative pain?

A. Medical Disease and Differential Diagnosis

A.1. What risk factors are associated with an abdominal aortic aneurysm (AAA)?

An AAA is a full-thickness dilatation of a segment of the abdominal aorta located between the diaphragm and the bifurcation of the aorta to the common iliac arteries. Risk factors for AAA include older age, male sex, family history of AAA, smoking, hypertension, hyperlipidemia, atherosclerotic occlusive disease, and obesity. Lifestyle factors reducing risk for AAA include regular exercise, smoking cessation, and improvements in diet. Interestingly, diabetes mellitus is associated with *decreased* risk of AAA. The prevalence of AAA is lower in African American, Hispanic, and Asian populations in comparison to White and Native American populations.

Haque K, Bhargava P. Abdominal aortic aneurysm. *Am Fam Physician*. 2022;106:165-172.

Kent KC, Zwolak RM, Egorova NN, et al. Analysis of risk factors for abdominal aortic aneurysm in a cohort of more than 3 million individuals. *J Vasc Surg*. 2010;52:539-548.

A.2. What comorbid diseases are commonly found in patients with AAAs?

The major pathologic cause of aneurysmal disease is atherosclerosis. In addition, hypertension (55%), heart disease (73.5%), peripheral vascular disease (21%), stroke and transient ischemic attacks (22%), diabetes mellitus (7%), and renal insufficiency (10%) are the most common comorbid illnesses. Smoking history has been reported in as many as 80% of patients presenting for AAA repair.

Haque K, Bhargava P. Abdominal aortic aneurysm. *Am Fam Physician*. 2022;106:165-172.

Howard DP, Banerjee A, Fairhead JF, et al. Age-specific incidence, risk factors and outcome of acute abdominal aortic aneurysms in a defined population. *Br J Surg*. 2015;102:907-915.

A.3. What is the incidence of morbidity and mortality in these patients if they undergo elective open surgical repair? What is the natural history of the disease without surgical repair?

Morbidity in this patient group is most commonly due to cardiovascular, pulmonary, and renal complications. Perioperative mortality for elective open AAA repair is 2% to 5%. Increased postoperative mortality was associated with older age, elevated serum creatinine, lower forced expiratory volume in 1 second (FEV_1), and sex. One retrospective study demonstrated higher mortality in females than males: 7% versus 5% for open repair and 2% versus 1% for endovascular repair. Despite the increasing fraction of patients undergoing endovascular repair, numerous large studies have not shown significant long-term differences in mortality between open and endovascular repair.

The major cause of death in the nonsurgically treated patient is rupture, which is associated with mortality of up to 80%. Ruptured AAAs account for ~9,000 deaths per year in the United States. One study demonstrated a doubling of expectancy after repair of AAA. The incidence of rupture within 5 years of diagnosis of AAA is 80%. The incidence of rupture increases with aneurysmal size: 25% for lesions of 4 to 7 cm in diameter, 45% for lesions 7 to 10 cm, and 60% for lesions larger than 10 cm. Repairing aneurysms smaller than 5.5 cm has not been shown to improve survival. Thus, only patients with aneurysms 5.5 cm or larger should be considered for surgical intervention.

Ketelsen D, Thomas C, Schmehl J, et al. Endovascular aneurysm repair of abdominal aortic aneurysms: standards, technical options and advanced indications. *Rofo*. 2014;186:337-347.

LeFevre ML; U.S. Preventive Services Task Force. Screening for abdominal aortic aneurysm: U.S. Preventive Services Task Force recommendation statement. *JAMA*. 2019;322:2211-2218.

Reimerink JJ, van der Laan MJ, Koelemay MJ, et al. Systematic review and meta-analysis of population-based mortality from ruptured abdominal aortic aneurysm. *Br J Surg*. 2013;100:1405-1413.

A.4. What should be done for smaller AAAs that are found in patients?

The U.S. Preventive Services Task Force (USPSTF) 2019 update on screening recommendations for AAA reinforces that early surgical intervention of smaller AAAs smaller than 5.5 cm (open or endovascular) does not reduce mortality. In addition, smaller AAAs (3-4 cm) can be reimaged with ultrasound once a year depending on the patient's other medical conditions. Patients with AAAs with a diameter of 4 to 5 cm should undergo repeat imaging every 6 months because it is not possible to predict which AAAs will enlarge more than 0.1 to 0.2 cm/y. Those AAAs that do enlarge by more than 0.5 cm within 6 months are considered at high risk for rupture and should be promptly repaired.

LeFevre ML; U.S. Preventive Services Task Force. Screening for abdominal aortic aneurysm: U.S. Preventive Services Task Force recommendation statement. *JAMA*. 2019;322:2211-2218.

A.5. What are the risk factors for perioperative myocardial infarction (MI) in patients with ischemic heart disease? What can be done to reduce the risk of ischemic events in these patients?

Morbidity and mortality are high for patients who undergo vascular surgery and experience postoperative myocardial ischemia. Key factors that determine perioperative morbidity and mortality rates include the stress of surgery (aortic, peripheral vascular, emergency surgery), increased blood loss, poor preoperative cardiac functional status, history of congestive heart failure (CHF), low ejection fraction, known coronary artery disease (CAD), and preoperative history of coronary artery bypass grafting.

Special consideration needs to be given to patients who have recently undergone percutaneous coronary intervention procedures for coronary revascularization and are maintained on antiplatelet therapy. This is due to the significant risk of acute stent restenosis or thrombosis if antiplatelet therapy is prematurely terminated. Management of the dual antiplatelet therapy regimen should be customized to each patient depending on the type and urgency of surgery, type of coronary stent, time since the coronary intervention, and complexity of the coronary intervention. Current recommendations for perioperative management of patients with drug-eluting stent (DES) are shown in **Figure 10.1**. For patients identified at high risk for stent thrombosis, surgery should be planned in a hospital with cardiac catheterization facilities. Postoperatively, these patients require a monitored setting and immediate resumption of antiplatelet therapy. Signs and symptoms of stent thrombosis should be promptly recognized and aggressively treated with percutaneous coronary intervention.

The 2016 American College of Cardiology (ACC)/American Heart Association (AHA) guideline focused update on duration of dual antiplatelet therapy in patients with CAD recommended the following:

- Elective noncardiac surgery should be delayed 30 days after bare metal stent (BMS) implantation and optimally 6 months after DES implantation.
- In patients who must undergo surgical procedures that mandate discontinuation of $P2Y_{12}$ inhibitor therapy, aspirin be continued if possible and $P2Y_{12}$ platelet receptor inhibitors be restarted as soon as possible after surgery.
- When noncardiac surgery is required in patients currently taking a $P2Y_{12}$ inhibitor, a consensus decision among treating clinicians as to the relative risks of surgery and discontinuation or continuation of antiplatelet therapy can be useful.
- Elective noncardiac surgery after DES implantation in patients for whom $P2Y_{12}$ inhibitor therapy will need to be discontinued can be considered after 3 months if the risk of further delay of surgery is greater than the expected risks of stent thrombosis.

Prevention of perioperative myocardial ischemia is the goal of the anesthesiologist in patients with preoperative cardiac risk factors regardless of the anesthetic technique chosen. This entails reduction of myocardial oxygen demand (avoid tachycardia and hypertension), while increasing oxygen supply (prevent hypotension and anemia). Oxygen demand of the left ventricle is dependent on heart rate, contractility, and ventricular loading conditions. Of the three, increase in heart rate

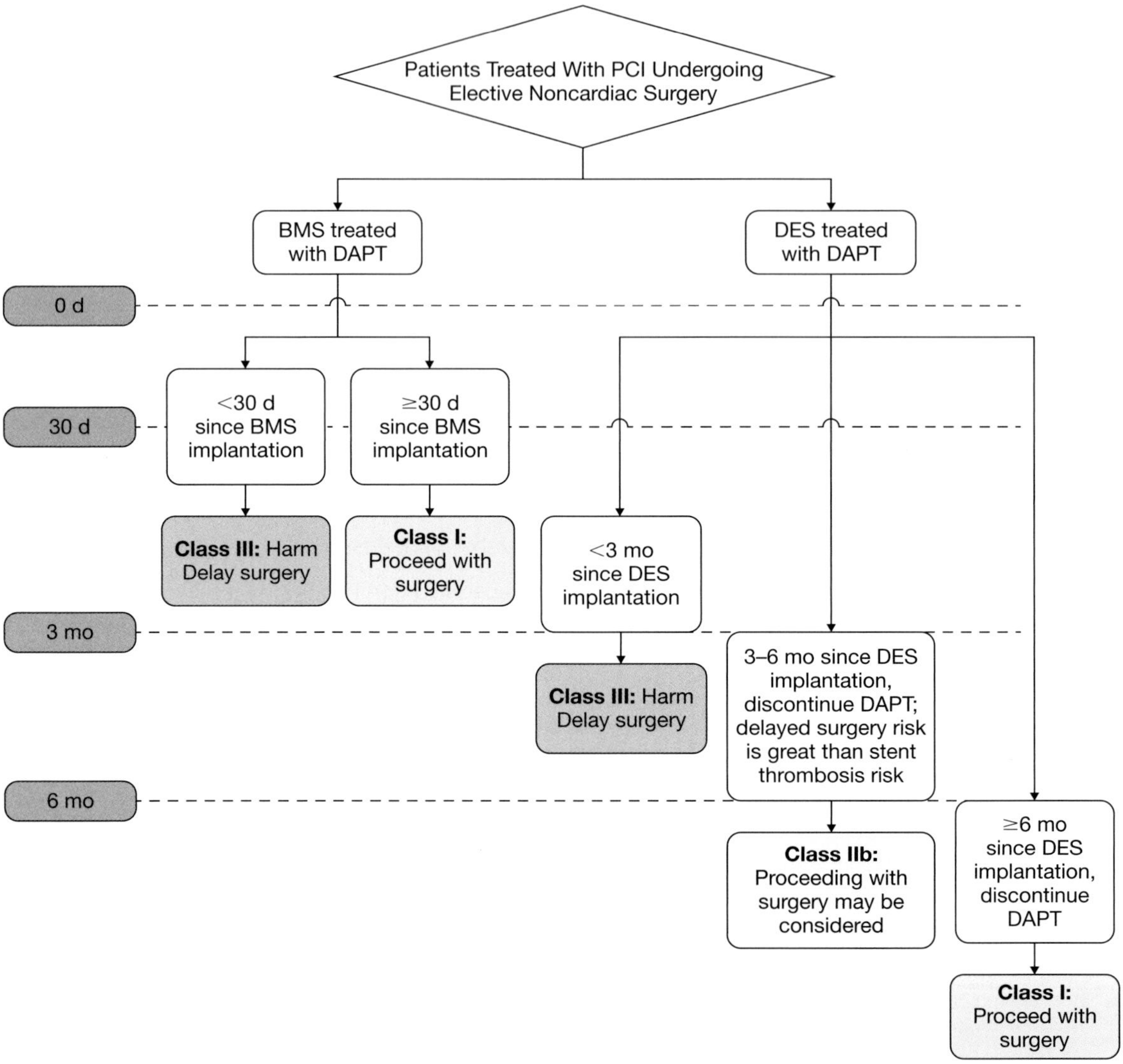

FIGURE 10.1. Treatment algorithm for timing of elective noncardiac surgery in patients with coronary stents. BMS, bare metal stent; DAPT, dual antiplatelet therapy; DES, drug-eluting stent; PCI, percutaneous coronary intervention. (Reprinted with permission from Levine GN, Bates ER, Bittl JA, et al. 2016 ACC/AHA guideline focused update on duration of dual antiplatelet therapy in patients with coronary artery disease: a report of the American College of Cardiology/American Heart Association Task Force on clinical practice guidelines. *Circulation.* 2016;134:e123-e155.)

imposes the greatest demand and should be readily controlled by the anesthesiologist. Left ventricular preload and afterload also affect oxygen demand by end-diastolic and systolic wall tension. Other factors, such as coronary collateral blood flow, hemoglobin, and blood rheology can also influence myocardial ischemia.

β-blockers are a well-established class of drugs effective in reducing myocardial oxygen consumption. Randomized controlled trials have yielded conflicting results regarding the ability of β-blockers to influence perioperative cardiovascular morbidity and mortality. Thus, routine prescription of these drugs in unselected patients remains controversial. In noncardiac surgery, evidence shows an association of β-blockers with increased all-cause mortality. Data from low risk-of-bias trials further suggest an increase in stroke rate with initiation of β-blockers at the time of surgery. As the quality of evidence is still low to moderate, more evidence is needed before a definitive conclusion can be drawn. The substantial reduction in supraventricular arrhythmias and acute myocardial infarction (AMI) in this setting may be offset by the potential increase in mortality and stroke.

Nitrates can also reduce myocardial oxygen demand by decreasing preload and by dilating large epicardial coronary arteries and collateral conduit vessels. However, the benefit of perioperative nitroglycerin prophylaxis has not been proven.

Use of statins in patients with cardiovascular disease is increasingly supported by multiple studies that display a reduction in the risk of MI, stroke, and mortality. Accumulating data suggest that continuation of statin therapy in the preoperative period reduces the risk of postoperative death and acute coronary syndromes.

Beaulieu RJ, Sutzko DC, Albright J, Jeruzal E, Osborne NH, Henke PK. Association of high mortality with postoperative myocardial infarction after major vascular surgery despite use of evidence-based therapies. *JAMA Surg*. 2020;155:131-137.

Cao D, Chandiramani R, Capodanno D, et al. Non-cardiac surgery in patients with coronary artery disease: risk evaluation and periprocedural management. *Nat Rev Cardiol*. 2021;18:37-57.

Chan WW, Wong GT, Irwin MG. Perioperative statin therapy. *Expert Opin Pharmacother*. 2013;14:831-842.

Hajibandeh S, Hajibandeh S, Antoniou SA, Torella F, Antoniou GA. Effect of beta-blockers on perioperative outcomes in vascular and endovascular surgery: a systematic review and meta-analysis. *Br J Anaesth*. 2017;118:11-21.

Levin GN, Bates ER, Bittl JA, et al. 2016 ACC/AHA guideline focused update on duration of dual antiplatelet therapy in patients with coronary artery disease: a report of the American College of Cardiology/American Heart Association Task Force on Clinical Practice Guidelines: an update of the 2011 ACCF/AHA/SCAI guideline for percutaneous coronary intervention, 2011 ACCF/AHA guideline for coronary artery bypass graft surgery, 2012 ACC/AHA/ACP/AATS/PCNA/SCAI/STS guideline for the diagnosis and management of patients with stable ischemic heart disease, 2013 ACCF/AHA guideline for the management of ST-elevation myocardial infarction, 2014 AHA/ACC guideline for the management of patients with non-ST-elevation acute coronary syndromes, and 2014 ACC/AHA guideline on perioperative cardiovascular evaluation and management of patients undergoing noncardiac surgery. *Circulation*. 2016;134:e123-e155.

Wijeysundera DN, Duncan D, Nkonde-Price C, et al. Perioperative beta blockade in noncardiac surgery: a systematic review for the 2014 ACC/AHA guideline on perioperative cardiovascular evaluation and management of patients undergoing noncardiac surgery: a report of the American College of Cardiology/American Heart Association Task Force on Practice Guidelines. *Circulation*. 2014;130:2246-2264.

A.6. Does the morbidity and mortality of elective repair of an AAA differ significantly from that of an emergency repair?

The overall mortality for a ruptured AAA is greater than 50%. One study showed an overall survival rate of 19.8% as compared with an elective surgical survival rate of 95%. The worst prognosis occurred in patients older than 80 years; a systolic blood pressure of less than 80 mm Hg on admission; a prior history of hypertension, angina, or previous MI; and an operating time of greater than 4 hours. Other risk factors include a systolic blood pressure less than 100 mm Hg at the end of surgery and blood loss greater than 11,000 mL. Retroperitoneal rupture was associated with a higher rate of survival. Elective surgical intervention should be considered if the size of the aneurysm changes rapidly or if its diameter is greater than 5.5 cm.

AlOthman O, Bobat S. Comparison of the short and long-term outcomes of endovascular repair and open surgical repair in the treatment of unruptured abdominal aortic aneurysms: meta-analysis and systematic review. *Cureus*. 2020;12:e9683.

Eefting D, Ultee KH, Von Meijenfeldt GC, et al. Ruptured AAA: state of the art management. *J Cardiovasc Surg (Torino)*. 2013;54:47-53.

B. Preoperative Evaluation and Preparation

B.1. Which preoperative laboratory tests would you require for this patient?

The patient should have the following laboratory tests as part of the preoperative evaluation: complete blood count and platelet count, serum electrolytes, blood urea nitrogen (BUN), creatinine, and coagulation profile. A chest radiograph will help ascertain whether signs of heart failure, pulmonary disease, or acute pneumonia are present. Spirometry should be considered in the patient with significant pulmonary disease and those in whom an adequate medical history is not available. In addition, spirometric data may be useful in assessing the effects of inhaler therapy.

An ECG should be obtained because this patient displays multiple risk factors for ischemic disease. The ECG is a sensitive and simple screening test for active cardiac conditions, such as unstable coronary syndromes and significant arrhythmias, which necessitate further management prior to proceeding to surgery. Additionally, preoperative laboratory tests should be defined by positive findings on history and physical exam.

Edwards AF, Forest DJ. Preoperative laboratory testing. *Anesthesiol Clin*. 2018;36:493-507.

B.2. What is the significance of the preoperative ECG? Would you wish to pursue a preoperative cardiac workup? What tests would you request, and what would they tell you?

The patient's preoperative ECG is consistent with a prior inferior wall MI. Patients with a history of a prior MI or angina in conjunction with an abnormal ECG have a 5-fold increase in postoperative mortality when compared with those with no clinical indication of CAD. This patient's history of claudication suggests peripheral vascular disease. Peripheral artery disease is associated with a 4-fold increase in risk for MI and a 2-fold to 3-fold increase in risk of stroke. In selected patients with severe or unstable cardiac ischemia, evaluation is needed to assess if prior myocardial revascularization is indicated.

When coronary angiography was performed on 1,000 patients undergoing elective peripheral vascular surgery, over half of the patients had significant CAD (>50% stenosis), and 33% had severe stenosis (>70%). Of the asymptomatic patients with no history or electrocardiographic evidence of ischemic heart disease, 15% had severe CAD and 22% of these seemingly normal patients had impaired left ventricular function. Hertzer et al found that only 8% of patients undergoing elective vascular surgery had normal coronary arteries.

A comparison of this patient's current ECG with a prior ECG can aid in assessing the timing of the previous infarction if the history alone is not helpful. The last update to the joint AHA/ACC guidelines concerning perioperative cardiovascular assessment in 2014 suggests incorporating clinical risk factors, exercise tolerance, and surgical risk when determining whether further testing is necessary. Vascular surgeries, such as AAA repair, are categorized as high-risk procedures. In addition, clinical risk factors include a history of ischemic disease, compensated or prior heart failure, cerebrovascular disease, diabetes mellitus, and renal insufficiency. The algorithm for the cardiac assessment of patients undergoing surgical procedures associated with a high perioperative cardiac risk is shown in **Figure 10.2**.

Many vascular surgery patients are unable to undergo exercise stress testing because of limitations presented by their cardiac, pulmonary, or peripheral vascular disease. A dipyridamole-thallium stress test or a dobutamine stress echocardiogram is a pharmacologic test to assess ischemic potential. Dipyridamole causes vasodilation of normal coronary arteries. This results in steal of blood flow from the area beyond a coronary stenosis. Blood flow redistributes as the drug dissipates.

Positive results on preoperative stress testing do not always necessitate revascularization. There is evidence to suggest that vascular patients who undergo coronary revascularization have an increased risk of periprocedural and long-term complications. The decision to perform coronary revascularization procedures, rather than employ medical management, should be undertaken in close consultation with a cardiologist and a cardiac surgeon. Recent evidence also suggests that patients at significant risk for ischemic heart disease can benefit from an endovascular approach, if anatomically feasible.

Perioperative cardiovascular care for noncardiac surgery is clearly evolving with the publication of large-scale clinical trials, and the focus on determining the value of different assessment and treatment strategies to clinical outcome and long-term improvement in quality of life can be better determined. Although there is a growing trend to move from extensive preoperative testing to more targeted surveillance and treatment, the key question will be ensuring that patients make the most informed decision regarding the indication for surgery given the patient's trajectory for recovery, including returning to baseline or improved functional status and health.

Fleisher LA. The value of preoperative assessment before noncardiac surgery in the era of value-based care. *Circulation.* 2017;136:1769-1771.

Glance LG, Faden E, Dutton RP, et al. Impact of the choice of risk model for identifying low-risk patients using the 2014 American College of Cardiology/American Heart Association perioperative guidelines. *Anesthesiology.* 2018;129:889-900.

Hertzer NR, Beven EG, Young JR et al. Coronary artery disease in peripheral vascular patients. A classification of 1000 coronary angiograms and results of surgical management. *Annals of Surgery.* 1984;199:223-33.

Shamaki GR, Markson F, Soji-Ayoade D, Agwuegbo CC, Bamgbose MO, Tamunoinemi BM. Peripheral artery disease: a comprehensive updated review. *Curr Probl Cardiol.* 2022;47:101082.

Smilowitz NR, Berger JS. Perioperative cardiovascular risk assessment and management for noncardiac surgery: a review. *JAMA.* 2020;324:279-290.

Thompson A, Fleishmann KE, Smilowitz N et al. 2024 AHA/ACC/ASNC/HRS/SCA/SCCT/SCMR/SVM Guideline for Perioperative Cardiovascular Management for Noncardiac Surgery: A Report of the American College of Cardiology/American Heart Association Joint Committee on Clinical Practice Guidelines. *Circulation.* 2024;150:e351.

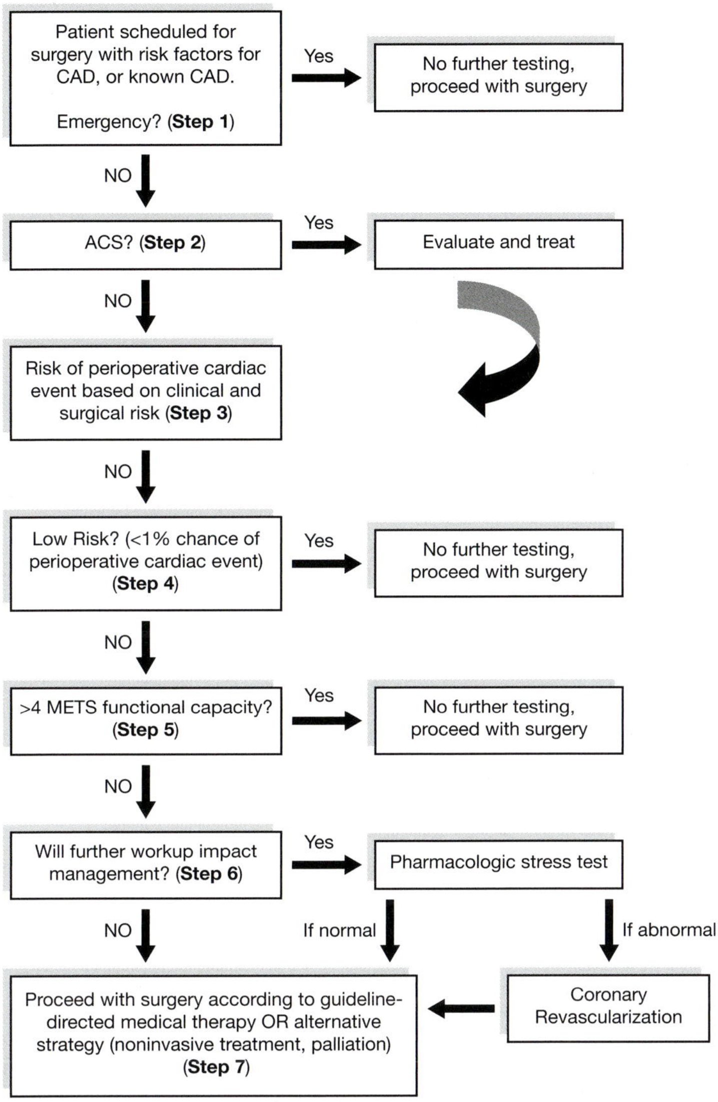

FIGURE 10.2. Stepwise algorithm for preoperative assessment for patients with coronary artery disease (CAD) undergoing noncardiac surgery. ACS, acute coronary syndrome; METS, metabolic equivalents. (Reprinted with permission from Fleisher LA, Fleischmann KE, Auerbach AD, et al. 2014 ACC/AHA guidelines on perioperative cardiovascular evaluation and management of patients undergoing noncardiac surgery: executive summary: a report of the American College of Cardiology/American Heart Association Task Force on Practice Guidelines. *Circulation*. 2014;130:2215-2245. Copyright © 2014 American Heart Association, Inc.)

B.3. How do you evaluate this patient's pulmonary status?

The patient's smoking history and the chronic changes present on her chest radiograph are evidence of chronic obstructive pulmonary disease (COPD). Provided the patient is minimally symptomatic and has good functional status, a detailed history and thorough physical exam can provide significant information regarding pulmonary status. A chest radiograph can be particularly useful at detecting underlying lung infection. If the radiograph displays the absence of acute pulmonary processes, as in this patient, further pulmonary testing might not be indicated. In the patient with severe signs and symptoms of COPD, ABG analysis can evaluate the patient's ability to oxygenate and ventilate. Patients with severe COPD can be chronically hypercarbic and hypoxaemic. Preoperative ABG analysis can guide perioperative ventilatory management and predicting the likelihood of postoperative mechanical ventilation.

In those patients with severe disease, particularly those with poor functional status and significant findings on physical exam and chest radiograph, pulmonary function testing might be indicated. Preoperative pulmonary function testing evaluates baseline forced vital capacity (VC) and FEV_1. Maximum mid-expiratory flow rate (MMEFR) is an effort-independent value that is a sensitive index of small airway obstruction. Peak expiratory flow rate is related to the FEV_1 and MMEFR, although it is less reproducible. These tests should be performed before and after bronchodilator therapy to assess reversibility of airway obstruction. A 15% improvement is considered a positive response.

This patient is a 2-pack-per-day smoker with dyspnea on exertion, and the anticipated surgery requires an upper abdominal incision. These factors likely affect her baseline pulmonary function and presage postoperative ventilatory problems. Relative to lifetime non-smokers, ex-smokers have an increased risk of developing postoperative pulmonary complications, which is related to the total pack-years of smoking.

Current evidence suggests that smokers should always strive to stop smoking pre-operatively, and that the longer the period of cessation, the greater will be the benefit in terms of reducing pulmonary complications.

Lumb BA. Pre-operative respiratory optimisation: an expert review. *Anaesthesia*. 2019;74:43-48.

Riley CM, Sciurba FC. Diagnosis and outpatient management of chronic obstructive pulmonary disease: a review. *JAMA*. 2019;321:786-797.

B.4. Preoperative arterial blood gas (ABG) analysis shows pH, 7.35; $Paco_2$, 50 mm Hg; and Pao_2, 68 mm Hg on room air. What is the significance of this result?

The assessment of this patient's blood gas analysis reveals moderate hypoxemia with a mildly elevated CO_2 tension. The pH is consistent with mild respiratory acidosis. The main causes of arterial hypoxemia are hypoventilation, diffusion impairment, shunting, and ventilation/perfusion ($\dot{V}/\dot{Q}$) mismatch. The major causes of hypercarbia or carbon dioxide retention are hypoventilation and $\dot{V}/\dot{Q}$ mismatch. Mild $\dot{V}/\dot{Q}$ mismatch does not necessarily cause an increase in arterial CO_2. This is due to the fact that CO_2 is a highly diffusible gas and central chemoreceptors compensate for increasing CO_2 tension by causing an increase in ventilation. The same is not true of arterial oxygenation, however, as even mild degrees of $\dot{V}/\dot{Q}$ mismatch can lead to hypoxemia.

West JB. Physiological effects of chronic hypoxia. *N Engl J Med*. 2017;376:1965-1971.

B.5. How would you measure creatinine clearance in this patient, and what is its value in this case?

Preoperative renal dysfunction indicates potential postoperative impairment. Despite maximal medical management, including hemodialysis, acute renal failure (ARF) after aortic reconstruction carries a mortality of less than 30% postoperatively. Maintenance of intravascular volume and adequate blood pressure are the best means of avoiding postoperative renal failure. This complication is more likely in patients requiring a suprarenal cross-clamp but also occurs with infrarenal clamping.

The most direct measurement of glomerular filtration rate (GFR) is the measurement of creatinine clearance. Although BUN and serum creatinine are related to renal function, they are altered by such nonrenal factors as protein metabolism, diet, liver dysfunction, or skeletal muscle mass. A 24-hour collection of urine is measured, and the following equation is used to calculate GFR: $GFR = U \times V / P$. U, urine concentration of creatinine (milligrams per deciliter); V, volume of urine measured (milliliter per minute); P, plasma concentration of creatinine (milligrams per deciliter). A 2-hour sample collected through a Foley catheter has been shown to correlate well with a 24-hour sample collection.

Despite the widespread use of creatinine clearance to detect renal impairment, as much as 50% of functional nephron mass can be lost before changes in creatinine concentration become apparent. As a result, patients with lower baseline creatinine concentration can have acute kidney injury (AKI) despite normal creatinine clearance. Several novel biomarkers are being studied that might be able to detect AKI earlier than traditional markers such as urinary output and serum creatinine. Neutrophil gelatinase-associated lipocalin (NGAL) is a protein found in excess in urine and plasma in patients with AKI as many as 48 hours prior to increase in serum concentration. Serum cystatin C, a protease inhibitor that is less affected by sex, age, muscle mass, and diet than creatinine, also allows earlier detection of AKI.

Gumbert SD, Kork F, Jackson ML, et al. Perioperative acute kidney injury. *Anesthesiology*. 2020;132:180-204.

Zarbock A, Koyner JL, Hoste EAJ, Kellum JA. Update on perioperative acute kidney injury. *Anesth Analg*. 2018;127:1236-1245.

B.6. What are the various surgical approaches to repair an AAA?

The classical approach to the abdominal aorta is through a vertical anterior midline incision with a transperitoneal approach to the retroperitoneal space. This gives access to all major arteries in the abdomen and pelvis. A transverse abdominal incision (supraumbilical) is also adequate for a transperitoneal approach. Although the entry is slower, there is less pain and pulmonary impairment postoperatively. The transperitoneal approach, with the necessary exposure of the abdominal organs, causes major heat and fluid loss and prolonged postoperative ileus.

The retroperitoneal approach is performed through a left flank incision with the patient in the right lateral decubitus position. In some studies, this approach led to less respiratory and wound complications, less postoperative ileus, less blood loss, lower fluid requirements, and earlier discharge from the hospital. Monitoring and line placement must take the lateral position into consideration.

A less invasive approach to AAA repair is endovascular aneurysm repair (EVAR) surgery. The EVAR technique has the advantage of a shorter length of stay (LOS) relative to open repair and a shortened recovery period. Due to the cost of the stent grafts and imaging equipment, this does not necessarily translate to overall cost reduction. Anatomic issues can significantly complicate stent placement. A common problem is iliac and common femoral arteries that are of insufficient caliber. Problems of the procedure include vessel perforation, inability to seal the aneurysm (endoleaks), and inability to advance the device past the iliac artery, ultimately necessitating the conversion to an open repair. In general, compared to open surgery, EVAR results in better outcome during the first 6 months but carries an increased risk of aneurysm-related mortality after 8 years.

In the EVAR-1 and Dutch Randomized Endovascular Aneurysm Management (DREAM) randomized clinical trials, reinterventions were required in 2 to 3 times as many patients in the endovascular group as in those who had open repair. Endovascular leaks are one of the leading causes of postoperative complications necessitating reintervention in up to 15% of patients. The various types of endovascular leaks are shown in **Figure 10.3**. In the EVAR-1 trial, postoperative complications were 5 times more

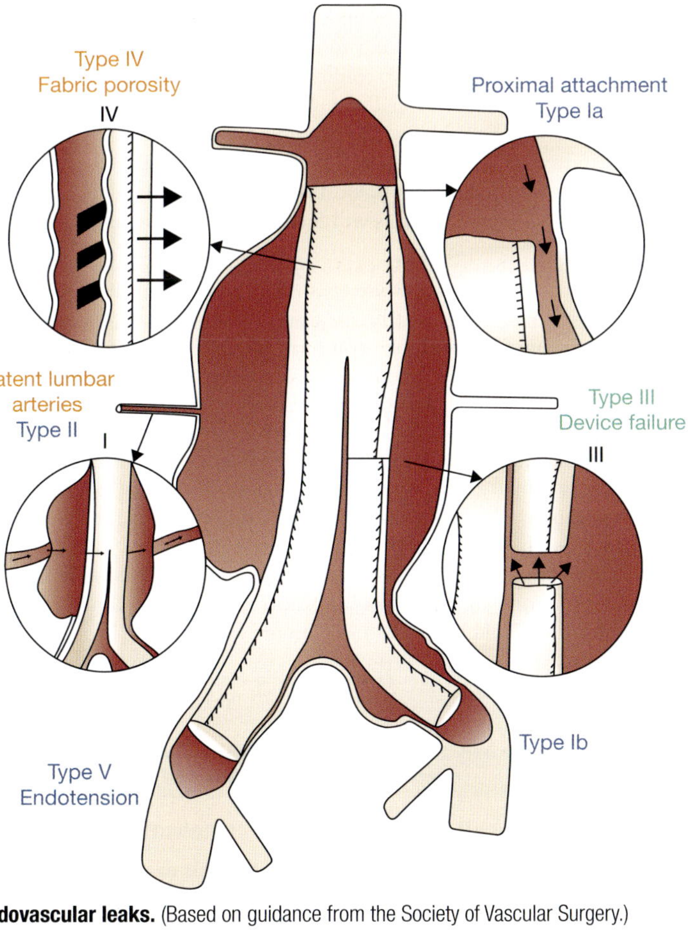

FIGURE 10.3. Types of endovascular leaks. (Based on guidance from the Society of Vascular Surgery.)

frequent with endovascular repair when compared to the open repair group. This highlights the importance of close follow-up in these patients and necessitates periodic reimaging. Endovascular repair has not been shown to improve survival in patients who have medical contraindication to open repair.

In contrast, when compared with open abdominal repair in the perioperative period, endovascular surgery is associated with 60% less blood loss, and decreased ventilator days, decreased LOS in intensive care unit (ICU) and decreased hospital LOS. Currently, overall mortality of the procedures appears similar, with a slight decrease in morbid cardiac events (6% in the open repair group vs 4.8% in the endovascular group).

Antoniou GA, Antoniou SA, Torella F. Editor's choice—Endovascular vs. open repair for abdominal aortic aneurysm: systematic review and meta-analysis of updated peri-operative and long term data of randomised controlled trials. *Eur J Vasc Endovasc Surg*. 2020;59:385-397.

Endovascular Aneurysm Repair (EVAR) Trial Participants. Comparison endovascular aneurysm repair versus open repair in patients with abdominal aortic aneurysm (EVAR trial 1), 30-day operative mortality results: randomized controlled trial. *Lancet*. 2004;364:843-848.

Endovascular Aneurysm Repair (EVAR) Trial Participants. Endovascular aneurysm repair and outcome in patients unfit for open repair of abdominal aortic aneurysms (EVAR trial 2): randomized controlled trial. *Lancet*. 2005;365:2179-2186.

Huang Y, Gloviczki P, Oderich GS, et al. Outcome after open and endovascular repairs of abdominal aortic aneurysms in matched cohorts using propensity score modeling. *J Vasc Surg*. 2015;62:304-311.e2.

B.7. How does the choice of surgical technique affect anesthetic management?

Debate exists over the advantages of general anesthesia compared with locoregional anesthesia or combined approaches in the management of patients with CAD. Meticulous control of heart rate and blood pressure should be the goals regardless of technique. Regional anesthesia blunts sympathetic tone, potentially decreasing coronary perfusion pressure; general anesthesia increases in sympathetic stimulation with tracheal intubation and emergence. Regional anesthesia can decrease hypercoagulability and thrombotic events in patients undergoing vascular surgery and confers significant postoperative pain control. While locoregional anesthesia might be associated with decreased morbidity and mortality during endovascular repair techniques compared to general anesthesia, more data are needed to confirm a benefit associated with a particular anesthetic technique.

The goals for the management of patients with CAD include prevention and mitigation of sympathetic stimulation. This can be achieved by using β-receptor antagonists, opioids, or volatile anesthetics during the perioperative period. Coronary perfusion pressure, defined as aortic diastolic pressure minus left ventricular end-diastolic pressure, should be meticulously maintained. Myocardial contractility and heart rate should not be increased, as this will increase oxygen demand.

Ruetzler K, Khanna AK, Sessler DI. Myocardial injury after noncardiac surgery: preoperative, intraoperative, and postoperative aspects, implications, and directions. *Anesth Analg*. 2020;131:173-186.

Zottola ZR, Kruger JL, Kong DS, et al. Locoregional anesthesia is associated with reduced hospital stay and need for intensive care unit care of elective endovascular aneurysm repair patients in the vascular quality initiative. *J Vasc Surg*. 2023;77:1061-1069.

B.8. How would you premedicate this patient?

Typically, a low-dose anxiolytic is likely to be sufficient premedication for most patients. Any other preoperative medications can be given intravenously upon arrival to the operating room. If oral medications are used, then they can be taken with a sip of water 1 hour prior to the procedure.

Additional specific pharmacologic regimens should be tailored to individual patient needs. Various medications and combinations have been used, including opioids, anticholinergics, barbiturates, and benzodiazepines. No single agent or combination has been demonstrated to be superior to others. Respiratory depressants should be avoided in patients with chronic hypercapnia.

Valentine EA, Ochroch EA. Anesthesia for vascular and endovascular surgery. In: Cullen BF, Stock MC, Ortega R, et al, eds. *Barash, Cullen, and Stoelting's Clinical Anesthesia*. 9th ed. Wolters Kluwer; 2024:1083-1112.

C. Intraoperative Management

C.1. Would you use an arterial catheter? What are the complications of arterial catheter placement?

Arterial pressure monitoring is exceedingly important in this case, from induction of anesthesia through emergence. Continuous arterial blood pressure monitoring allows for more accurate titration of blood pressure and for frequent sampling of blood for analysis during the case.

Vascular insufficiency and infection are the two major complications of arterial line placement. Catheter size and duration of cannulation are implicated in vascular occlusion. The causes of most vascular injuries are embolic. Radial artery cannulation is a low-risk, high-benefit method that can be used to closely monitor blood pressure in this patient. Whenever feasible, ultrasound should be used to guide placement as it might be associated with fewer complications.

Open AAA repair is frequently associated with blood pressure lability, particularly on clamping and unclamping, and arterial blood pressure monitoring is particularly helpful in this situation. In addition, frequent ABG sampling to assess hematocrit, ventilation, perfusion, electrolyte levels, glucose, and level of anticoagulation can be necessary. If a radial artery catheter cannot be placed, cannulation attempts can be made at the brachial or axillary arteries. Concerns have been raised that brachial artery cannulation might be inadvisable given the lack of adequate collateral supply to the forearm and hand. In practice, complications from brachial artery cannulation have been reported rarely and the risk of vascular insufficiency appears to be no different from that of radial artery cannulation. Axillary artery cannulation, however, might carry an added risk of vascular insufficiency and nerve injury from thrombosis and hematoma formation. This added risk is likely since the axillary neurovascular bundle travels in the confined space of the axillary sheath.

Fatima H, Chaudhary O, Krumm S, et al. Workflow of ultrasound-guided arterial access. *J Cardiothorac Vasc Anesth*. 2021;35:1611-1617.

Handlogten KS, Wilson GA, Clifford L, et al. Brachial artery catheterization: an assessment of use patterns and associated complications. *Anesth Analg*. 2014;118;288-295.

C.2. What various monitors are available for myocardial ischemia? Is a pulmonary artery catheter (PAC) helpful in determining the occurrence of ischemia?

Monitoring of the patient undergoing aortic reconstruction surgery should be aimed at preserving myocardial, pulmonary, and renal function as well as maintaining intravascular volume. Therefore, it is mandatory, particularly in this patient with known CAD, to monitor for myocardial ischemia and maintain volume status in the face of fluid shifts. Monitoring of the ST segments of the V_5 and II leads of the ECG is the most common method used to assess for intraoperative myocardial ischemia. However, in some studies, this alone was insufficient to recognize from 40% to 75% of intraoperative ischemic events detected by wall-motion abnormalities seen with a two-dimensional transesophageal echocardiogram.

Monitoring the pulmonary artery (PA) pressure tracing for the appearance of V waves and increasing PCWP with decreasing cardiac output are other methods of detecting intraoperative myocardial ischemia. Unfortunately, the PAC is not a particularly sensitive technique for detecting ischemic events. Wall-motion abnormalities, detected by transesophageal echocardiography (TEE), are highly sensitive markers of myocardial ischemia and appear earlier than either ST segment or PAC waveform changes.

A microcomputer-based ECG reader (ST-segment trend monitor) has also been advocated as a monitor of myocardial ischemia. These systems can pick up more subtle changes in ST segments than by simple observation. Multilead ECG systems are most helpful. The most sensitive means for monitoring patients to determine the development of myocardial ischemia at its earliest presentation is, in fact, wall-motion abnormalities demonstrated by two-dimensional TEE. As yet, no improvement in outcome has been demonstrated by the use of any of these monitors.

American Society of Anesthesiologists Task Force on Pulmonary Artery Catheterization. Practice guidelines for pulmonary artery catheterization: an updated report by the American Society of Anesthesiologists Task Force on Pulmonary Artery Catheterization. *Anesthesiology*. 2003;99:998-1014.

Nicoara A, Skubas N, Ad N, et al. Guidelines for the Use of Transesophageal Echocardiography to Assist with Surgical Decision-Making in the Operating Room: A Surgery-Based Approach From the American Society of Echocardiography in Collaboration with the Society of Cardiovascular Anesthesiologists and the Society of Thoracic Surgeons. *J Am Soc Echocardiogr*. 2020;33:692-734.

C.3. What additional monitors would you employ?

An invasive monitor of volume status is recommended in patients undergoing open AAA repair. The choice of invasive monitoring, central venous pressure (CVP) or PAC can be based on the level of aortic cross-clamping and the severity of the patient's underlying cardiac disease. The CVP is informative at low and high extremes. As the right side of the heart is usually a compliant system, large shifts of intravascular volume can occur without significant CVP alteration. The PCWP, obtained by a PAC, can be more accurate in determining intravascular volume status. In addition, the PAC allows measurement of cardiac output, helpful during aortic cross-clamping in the patient with left ventricular dysfunction.

In this situation, CVP might not accurately represent left-sided pressures reflected by the PCWP. This is also true of the patient with significant pulmonary disease. The decision to place a PAC can also be influenced by the level at which the cross-clamp is applied. Suprarenal and supraceliac cross-clamping are associated with greater hemodynamic lability than infrarenal clamp application. Thus, PAC insertion can be of greater utility during proximal procedures, particularly if cardiac dysfunction is also present.

The American Society of Anesthesiologists (ASA) practice guidelines support the prudent use of a PAC in select situations. A PAC should be employed in high-risk procedures (cardiac, aortic reconstruction, anticipated hemodynamic instability, and large-volume fluid shifts) and used in patients with a minimal risk of complication from catheter placement. Furthermore, when PAC monitoring is employed, it should only be utilized by those who are trained to appropriately interpret and intervene based on the data.

TEE is another monitoring modality that is being increasingly utilized in aortic reconstruction procedures. TEE has several potential benefits over invasive monitors such as the PAC. It is the most sensitive modality for detecting myocardial ischemia. Regional wall-motion abnormalities appear on TEE well before changes appear on other heart monitors such as the ECG or PAC. In addition, TEE allows for detailed analysis of valvular dysfunction, which may significantly alter perioperative anesthetic management. The ASA practice guidelines state that use of perioperative TEE can be appropriate when the nature of the planned surgery or the patient's cardiovascular pathology might result in severe hemodynamic, pulmonary, or neurologic compromise. In addition, TEE should be used when unexplained life-threatening circulatory instability persists despite corrective therapy.

Another useful measure of intravascular volume status is the collection of urine through a Foley catheter. Urine output will diminish with decreasing glomerular filtration caused by decreased renal blood flow. Assessment of urine output, provided kidney function is unimpaired, can be an accurate and cost-effective measure of volume status.

Temperature monitoring should also be employed as with any case under general anesthesia. Body temperature should be closely monitored and aggressively maintained. These patients can undergo tremendous heat and insensible fluid loss as a result of the enormous incisional surface area exposed to room air. If forced hot air thermal blankets are used, they are contraindicated on the lower extremities when an aortic cross-clamp is applied. They can be used on the upper body throughout the procedure, along with fluid warmers, to maintain temperature.

Pulse oximetry, capnography, and mass spectral analysis of inhaled agents should also be utilized. Combined with ABG analysis, they permit efficient ventilatory management and accurate delivery of anesthetic gases.

American Society of Anesthesiologists and Society of Cardiovascular Anesthesiologists Task Force on Transesophageal Echocardiography. Practice guidelines for perioperative transesophageal echocardiography. An updated report by the American Society of Anesthesiologists and the Society of Cardiovascular Anesthesiologists Task Force on Transesophageal Echocardiography. *Anesthesiology*. 2010;112:1084-1096.

American Society of Anesthesiologists Task Force on Pulmonary Artery Catheterization. Practice guidelines for pulmonary artery catheterization: an updated report by the American Society of Anesthesiologists Task Force on Pulmonary Artery Catheterization. *Anesthesiology*. 2003;99:998-1014.

C.4. How would you anesthetize this patient for an open repair of the aneurysm? What techniques could be used for an endovascular AAA repair? Discuss the various anesthetic techniques that can be employed for this surgery.

All anesthetic techniques have been used and advocated for abdominal aortic surgery. General anesthesia, regional blockade, or combined general and regional techniques, have all have been described. Outcome studies are equivocal among the various techniques, affording flexibility in the anesthetic approach to these patients. Tailoring this plan to each patient's medical condition is the most effective strategy. The primary goals in the anesthetic management of patients undergoing aortic reconstruction include protection of myocardial, neurologic, and renal function.

When combined regional (epidural) and general anesthesia techniques are employed, fluid requirements can be increased to maintain hemodynamic stability. In addition, neuraxial sympathectomy can predispose to hypotension upon clamp removal. However, placement of an epidural catheter will afford optimal postoperative pain management.

Anesthesia for endoluminal repair has ranges from general, general combined with epidural anesthesia, lumbar epidural with sedation, or sedation with local anesthesia. Considerations for choice of anesthesia include the need for patient immobility, the need for systemic anticoagulation (heparin), the possibility of exsanguination, and prevention of heat loss. Blood pressure stability is imperative during aortic balloon occlusion, to prevent distal migration of the stent. If neuraxial techniques are used, coagulation status must be carefully monitored in the perioperative period. There are some data to suggest locoregional anesthesia techniques offer improved morbidity and mortality during endoluminal repair techniques. However, more data are needed before a conclusive recommendation can be made.

Bardia A, Sood A, Mahmood F, et al. Combined epidural-general anesthesia vs general anesthesia alone for elective abdominal aortic aneurysm repair. *JAMA Surg*. 2016;151:1116-1123.

Faizer R, Weinhandl E, El Hag S, et al. Decreased mortality with local versus general anesthesia in endovascular aneurysm repair for ruptured abdominal aortic aneurysm in the Vascular Quality Initiative database. *J Vasc Surg*. 2019;70:92-101.e1.

Van Orden K, Farber A, Schermerhorn ML, et al. Local anesthesia for percutaneous endovascular abdominal aortic aneurysm repair is associated with fewer pulmonary complications. *J Vasc Surg*. 2018;68:1023-1029.e2.

C.5. This patient is to be heparinized intraoperatively, and anticoagulation might be continued postoperatively. Is this a contraindication to the preoperative placement of either an epidural or intrathecal catheter? What if the patient is receiving anticoagulants in the preoperative period?

Epidural catheter placement in the setting of anticoagulation increases the risk of epidural hematoma and subsequent neurologic deficit. Procedural risk of spinal cord ischemia confounds the diagnosis of neuraxial hematoma and usually precludes placement of an epidural catheter. However, an epidural catheter can be placed with a relative degree of confidence in patients who are not anticoagulated at the time of the puncture but who will receive anticoagulation later. Current guidelines suggest administration of intravenous heparin at least 1 hour after neuraxial catheter placement. In patients who have undergone systemic heparinization, heparin should be discontinued for at least 2 to 4 hours prior to epidural catheter removal. Coagulation status must be assessed prior to catheter manipulation, and frequent lower extremity neurologic assessment must continue for at least 12 hours after catheter removal.

Low-molecular-weight heparins (LMWHs), which are increasingly being employed for thromboprophylaxis, pose a significant potential for increased risk of neuraxial hematoma. In patients receiving these drugs, needle placement should occur at least 12 hours after the last dose. If higher doses have been used (eg, enoxaparin 1 mg/kg twice daily), needle placement should be delayed at least 24 hours. It is currently recommended that indwelling catheters be removed prior to initiation of LMWH thromboprophylaxis, and the first dose should be administered at least 2 hours after catheter removal.

In patients on chronic anticoagulation with oral warfarin, several recommendations are applicable regarding perioperative management of neuraxial anesthesia. Oral warfarin should be discontinued at least 4 to 5 days prior to surgery. International normalized ratio (INR) should be measured at least 24 hours prior to the procedure. Neuraxial manipulation must commence only when INR has normalized. Neurologic testing of sensory and motor function should be performed routinely during epidural analgesia for patients on warfarin therapy. The type of analgesic solution should also be tailored to minimize the degree of sensory and motor blockade to allow frequent neurologic monitoring. As thromboprophylaxis with warfarin is reinitiated in the postsurgical period, neuraxial catheters should be removed while the INR is less than 1.5.

Fibrinolytic and thrombolytic drugs predispose to a high risk of hematoma formation in conjunction with neuraxial techniques. Recent American Society of Regional Anesthesia and Pain Medicine (ASRA) practice guidelines addressing regional anesthesia in anticoagulated patients recommend avoidance of all neuraxial manipulation in patients who have received thrombolytic or fibrinolytic therapy. There are no clear data detailing the length of time neuraxial puncture should be avoided after discontinuation of these drugs.

Although use of antiplatelet agents such as aspirin and nonsteroidal anti-inflammatory drugs (NSAIDs) do not contraindicate the use of neuraxial techniques, care should be exercised when combinations of anticoagulants and antiplatelet drugs are used. Such combinations increase the risk of hemorrhagic complications in the perioperative period. Neurologic testing of sensory and motor function should be routinely performed on patients with indwelling catheters undergoing simultaneous anticoagulation.

Horlocker TT, Vandermeulen E, Rowlingson JC, et al. Regional anesthesia in the patient receiving antithrombotic or thrombolytic therapy: American Society of Regional Anesthesia and Pain Medicine Evidence-Based Guidelines (Fourth Edition). *Reg Anesth Pain Med*. 2018;43:566.

Kaushal M, Rubin RE, Kaye AD, Gritsenko K. Anticoagulation and neuraxial/peripheral anesthesia. *Anesthesiol Clin*. 2017;35:e21-e39.

C.6. What are your plans for fluid and blood replacement during surgery?

Fluid replacement should maintain intravascular filling pressures. Isotonic crystalloid should be used, as there is little evidence to suggest that colloid administration poses any advantage over crystalloid administration.

There has been much controversy in recent literature regarding the use of "liberal" versus "restrictive" fluid protocols during open abdominal procedures. Most data have been gathered on patients undergoing bowel procedures but are applicable to patients undergoing open AAA repair. There is a lack of consensus regarding the optimal fluid management protocol. What has emerged is use of fluid therapy to optimize tissue perfusion rather than predefined volume replacement.

Current approaches shift away from the classic model of calculation of the nothing by mouth (NPO) fluid deficit, intraoperative insensible losses, and third-space losses. Increasingly, most clinicians are employing "demand-related" regimens with the goal of maximizing tissue blood flow while minimizing interstitial edema. Surrogates for estimated intravascular losses include vital signs, urinary output, hematocrit, acid-base status, invasive and noninvasive hemodynamic measurements, and echocardiography. The traditional concept of a third-space compartment is increasingly being abandoned. Instead, it is now recognized that fluid shift into the interstitium is a function of crystalloid overload and deterioration of vascular integrity.

Concurrent use of cell salvage and autotransfusion decreases the need for exogenous blood transfusions. Liberal blood product administration should be avoided due to increased risk of immune suppression, hemolytic transfusion reactions, infectious disease transmission, and lung injury.

Heming N, Moine P, Coscas R, Annane D. Perioperative fluid management for major elective surgery. *Br J Surg*. 2020;107:e56-e62.

C.7. What are the hemodynamic changes of aortic cross-clamp placement? What efforts can be made to minimize these changes both before and during cross-clamping? If the patient develops ST-segment depressions with a rising pulmonary capillary wedge pressure (PCWP) during cross-clamp, what maneuvers should be taken?

The systemic hemodynamic response to aortic cross-clamping is shown in Figure 10.4.

Arterial hypertension is the most dramatic and consistent result of the application of an aortic cross-clamp. This is the result of a sudden increase in afterload and left ventricular end-diastolic wall stress. Usually, these changes are accompanied by decreased cardiac output. Some of these changes can also be due to redistribution of blood volume from the venous vasculature to the upper part of the body. All the previously stated factors are more profound in the case of supraceliac or thoracic cross-clamp placement.

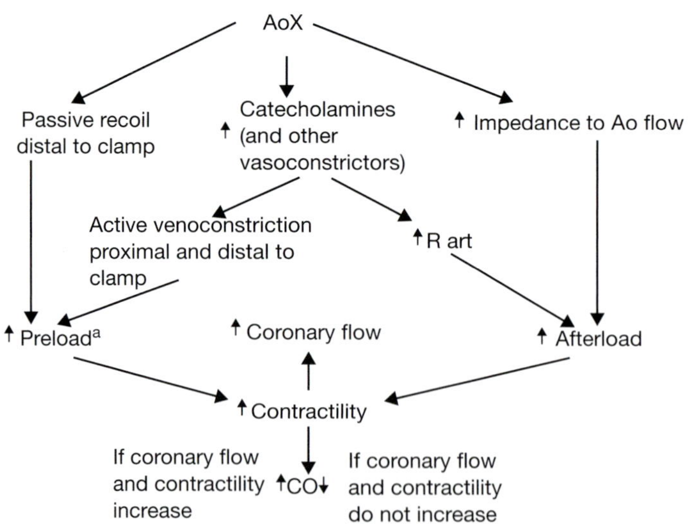

FIGURE 10.4. Systemic hemodynamic response to aortic cross-clamping (AoX). Ao, aortic; R art, arterial resistance; ↑ and ↓, increase and decrease, respectively. [a]Different patterns are possible. (Reprinted with permission from Gelman S. The pathophysiology of aortic cross-clamping and unclamping. *Anesthesiology*. 1995;82:1026-1060.)

Variations in blood volume status or splanchnic vascular tone are affected by anesthetic depth, anesthesia technique, and intravascular volume status. These factors all determine the pattern of blood volume redistribution.

A sudden increase in afterload can lead to left ventricular failure, particularly in the patient with a noncompliant left ventricle. Ideally, the patient should have lower filling pressures for the half hour prior to cross-clamp placement. This mitigates the adverse response to sudden increased afterload. A PAC is helpful in accurately assessing and maintaining preclamp values for the left side of the heart. A potent anesthetic agent and/or a vasodilator such as nicardipine is used to revert afterload to near normal. This also helps increase the cardiac output and decrease stress on the left ventricle. If this is insufficient to reverse left ventricular failure, then addition of an inotrope may be necessary.

The increase in afterload following cross-clamp placement can also result in myocardial ischemia. Ischemia, reflected as a rising PCWP and ST-segment depressions, can be managed with intravenous nitroglycerin, a potent dilator of the capacitance vessels. This drug is used to decrease left ventricular end-diastolic volume and left ventricular end-diastolic pressure. Decreasing left ventricular end-diastolic pressure also decreases the transluminal pressure across the coronary vasculature and augments blood flow to the myocardium.

Zammert M, Gelman S. The pathophysiology of aortic cross-clamping. *Best Pract Res Clin Anaesthesiol.* 2016;30:257-269.

C.8. Because this case involves an infrarenal aneurysm, is renal blood flow affected with placement of the cross-clamp? If an endovascular repair is chosen, what are the risks to the kidneys? Are there any treatment maneuvers that can be taken to minimize these risks in either repair?

ARF after AAA repair is associated with a mortality greater than 30%. Decreased renal function is observed in many patients after aortic cross-clamping, even when the clamp is placed distal to the renal arteries. Although a suprarenal cross-clamp will decrease renal blood flow by up to 80%, an infrarenal cross-clamp also causes a decrease in renal cortical blood flow with an associated decrease in GFR. The degree of decrease in urine output does not correlate with the decrease in GFR nor does it predict postoperative renal failure. The most dangerous complication of alteration in renal blood flow is acute tubular necrosis and ARF.

Maintenance of cardiac output and adequate circulating blood volume is of cardinal importance in sustaining renal blood flow and in the prevention of renal failure. Low-dose dopamine (2-3 µg/kg/min) increases renal blood flow and can improve urine output, although reduced incidence of postoperative renal failure has not been proven. Use of mannitol attenuates the reduction of renal cortical blood flow before, during, and after renal ischemia, increases glomerular ultrafiltration flow, and is a hydroxyl free radical scavenger. Fenoldopam and furosemide can also be utilized during aortic reconstruction procedures to minimize nephrotoxicity. Unfortunately, strong clinical evidence is currently lacking for any of these measures.

During endovascular repair, radiocontrast dye can cause further damage to the kidneys. There is some suggestion that use of a bicarbonate infusion or pretreatment with *N*-acetyl cysteine may be protective. It is prudent to minimize exposure to nonionic contrast or replace with gadolinium dimeglumine.

Radak D, Neskovic M, Otasevic P, Isenovic ER. Renal dysfunction following elective endovascular aortic aneurysm repair. *Curr Vasc Pharmacol.* 2019;17:133-140.

Yeung KK, Groeneveld M, Lu JJ, van Diemen P, Jongkind V, Wisselink W. Organ protection during aortic cross-clamping. *Best Pract Res Clin Anaesthesiol.* 2016;30:305-315.

Zhang F, Lu Z, Wang F. Advances in the pathogenesis and prevention of contrast-induced nephropathy. *Life Sci.* 2020;259:118379.

C.9. What are the hemodynamic consequences of aortic cross-clamp placement and removal? What can be done to minimize the effects of the aortic cross-clamp?

During cross-clamping, blood flow to the lower extremities is grossly decreased. Metabolism switches from aerobic to anaerobic as ischemia develops. This results in maximal vasodilation and lactic acid production. When the cross-clamp is released, systemic vascular resistance and arterial blood pressure decreases abruptly. Peripheral vasodilation can result in relative volume depletion and hypotension. Vasodilation can become systemic as the lactic acid is washed out of the extremities into the central circulation. This condition is sometimes known as "declamping shock."

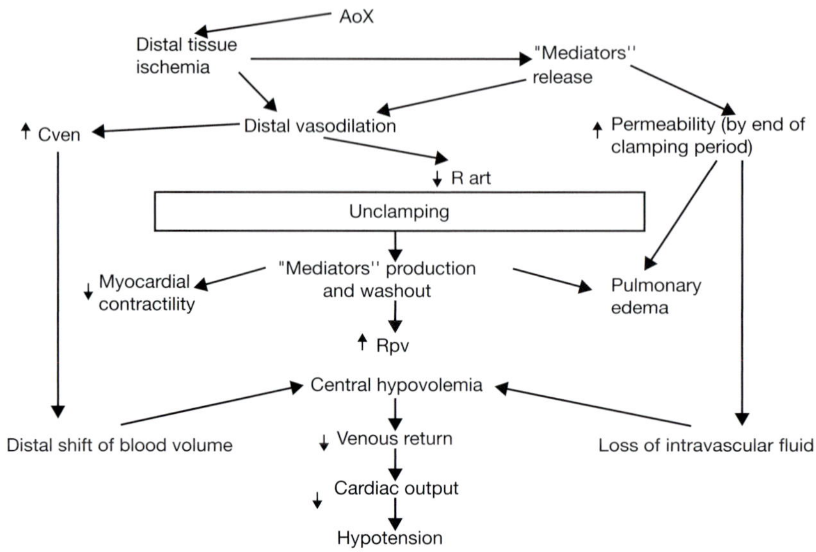

FIGURE 10.5. Systemic hemodynamic response to aortic unclamping. AoX, aortic cross-clamping; Cven, venous capacitance; R art, arterial resistance; Rpv, pulmonary vascular resistance; ↑ and ↓, increase and decrease, respectively. (Reprinted with permission from Gelman S. The pathophysiology of aortic cross-clamping and unclamping. *Anesthesiology.* 1995;82:1026-1060.)

To minimize the hypotensive response, volume loading in the period prior to cross-clamp release is suggested to raise filling pressures to slightly above normal. Gentle titration of vasodilators such as nicardipine and/or nitroglycerin during this period allows additional volume loading with maintenance of filling pressures. In addition, gradual release of the clamp allows time for adjustments in volume, pressure, and correction of acidosis.

Sometimes, even in the face of adequate volume loading, the blood pressure remains low following cross-clamp removal. Proximal cross-clamping is associated with a higher incidence of hypotension. In this situation, it is advisable to ask the surgeon to reapply the aortic cross-clamp to a varying degree depending on the severity of hypotension. Such maneuvers allow more time for correction of blood volume or acidosis.

Other causes of sustained hypotension in the face of adequate management include a continued site of hemorrhage and myocardial ischemia and/or failure. Measurement of filling pressures or use of TEE can particularly help in the differentiation of the etiology of sustained hypotension. Cardiac ischemia can be detected by wall-motion abnormalities or elevated filling pressures accompanying systemic hypotension. In contrast, hemorrhage is diagnosed by low filling pressures and increased systemic vascular resistance (due to reflex vasoconstriction).

The hemodynamic response to aortic unclamping is shown in **Figure 10.5**.

Yeung KK, Groeneveld M, Lu JJ, van Diemen P, Jongkind V, Wisselink W. Organ protection during aortic cross-clamping. *Best Pract Res Clin Anaesthesiol.* 2016;30:305-315.

Zammert M, Gelman S. The pathophysiology of aortic cross-clamping. *Best Pract Res Clin Anaesthesiol.* 2016;30:257-269.

D. Postoperative Management

D.1. What are the parameters used for tracheal extubation of this patient?

The following ventilatory criteria can be used to assess suitability for tracheal extubation: the patient is awake and alert, has an adequate gag reflex, displays signs of adequate reversal of neuromuscular block, and meets minimum respiratory parameters for extubation. The typical respiratory parameters used to assess suitability for extubation are shown in **Table 10.1**.

These parameters should serve merely as a guide in the clinical assessment of suitability for extubation. The decision to extubate should be ultimately guided by assessment of the patient's overall

TABLE 10.1 Typical Respiratory Parameters Used to Determine Suitability for Tracheal Extubation

Vital capacity >15 mL/kg
pH >7.30
Pa_{O_2} >60 mm Hg at F_{IO_2} <50%
Pa_{CO_2} <50 mm Hg
Maximal negative inspiratory force > −20 cm H_2O
Stable hemodynamic status
Respiratory rate <30 breaths per minute

F_{IO_2}, fraction of inspired oxygen.

status and clinical judgment. Extubation might need to be delayed in patients who display labored breathing on physical exam, inadequate pain control, residual neuromuscular block or hemodynamic instability.

Perioperative fluid management also should be carefully considered when assessing a patient's suitability for extubation. For shorter cases with minimal anticipated fluid shifts, the patient can be extubated in the immediate postoperative period. For longer cases, instances of large volumes of fluid replacement and significant blood product administration, extubation should be delayed until the hemodynamics are stabilized and the patient no longer requires vasopressors. Body temperature should also be within normal limits.

In cases where significant fluids or blood products have been administered, airway swelling can be a significant concern and could lead to ventilatory failure in the postoperative period. A "cuff leak" test can help in assessment of the degree of airway edema. It is performed by occluding the endotracheal tube of a spontaneously breathing patient and auscultating for breath sounds with the cuff deflated.

Wong TH, Weber G, Abramowicz AE. Smooth extubation and smooth emergence techniques: a narrative review. *Anesthesiol Res Pract*. 2021;2021:8883257.

D.2. What are the anticipated changes in postoperative pulmonary function in these patients? How does the surgical technique affect postoperative pulmonary function? Are there any postoperative maneuvers that can improve respiratory parameters?

The transabdominal approach to the aorta involves an upper abdominal incision. Total lung capacity and its subdivisions decrease after upper abdominal surgery. VC decreases and takes 1 to 2 weeks to normalize. Residual volume also decreases slightly. Functional residual capacity declines as well, and takes a few days to recover. Expiratory reserve volume declines after lower abdominal surgery and considerably after upper abdominal and thoracic incisions. The retroperitoneal approach to the aorta involves a flank incision, which leads to far less respiratory compromise.

In a series of adult males undergoing abdominal surgery, postoperative pulmonary complications occurred more frequently than cardiac complications (9.6% vs 5.7%) and were associated with significantly greater length of hospitalization. The effects of surgical trauma are most pronounced after upper abdominal surgery; lower abdominal and thoracic incisions impact the respiratory muscles to a lesser degree. This occurs through surgical disruption of the respiratory muscles and postoperative pain, preventing normal diaphragm excursion. The patient follows a rapid shallow breathing pattern without sighs.

The overall effect of postoperative regional analgesia on breathing mechanics is complex, but epidural analgesia might decrease the risk for postoperative pulmonary complications. Ambulation and control of postoperative pain diminish splinting and help maximize respiratory parameters. Maneuvers to encourage deep breathing are of proven benefit.

Miskovic A, Lumb AB. Postoperative pulmonary complications. *Br J Anaesth*. 2017;118:317-334.

D.3. How would you control postoperative pain? What are the alternatives in the management of this patient's postoperative pain?

The goal of effective postoperative pain relief is to produce a high quality of pain control with the fewest number of side effects and complications. Neuraxial analgesia in the immediate postoperative period is the preferred method of pain management in this high-risk patient population. The ideal opioid, its concentration, and combination with local anesthetic have yet to be defined. (For suggested protocols, see **Table 10.2**.)

Complications of the epidural route of analgesia include dural puncture, epidural hematoma, and epidural abscess. The risk of epidural hematoma is small in patients receiving appropriate doses of anticoagulation postoperatively but is prohibitively high in patients receiving thrombolytic treatment or LMWH. Careful consideration should be given to the timing of insertion and removal of the catheter. The risk of complications is similar whether the catheter is placed at the thoracic or lumbar level. Other complications include pruritus, nausea, urinary retention, delayed respiratory depression, and potentially increased transfusion requirements. Difficulty ambulating and orthostatic hypotension are minimized when catheters are placed in the thoracic region with low infusion rates and bupivacaine concentrations less than 0.08%. There is some evidence to suggest that combined epidural/general anesthesia is associated with improved survival and lower mortality and morbidity in patients undergoing elective AAA repair.

Systemic opioid analgesia can be used to provide effective postoperative pain control. Intravenous opioids are commonly administered by a patient-controlled analgesia (PCA) pump after this type of procedure, thereby allowing the patient to titrate the dose to achieve adequate pain control.

TABLE 10.2 Epidural Opioid/Bupivacaine Combinations Administered by Continuous Infusion[a]

Drug Combinations	Solution[b]	Bolus Dose of Bupivacaine	Basal Infusion[c]	Breakthrough Doses	Increments in Breakthrough[d]
Morphine	0.01%		6-8 mL/h	1-2 mL every 10-15 min	1 mL of the solution
Bupivacaine[e]	0.05%-0.1%	0.5%-0.25%			
Hydromorphone	0.0025%-0.005%		6-8 mL/h	1-3 mL every 10-15 min	1 mL of the solution
Bupivacaine[f]	0.05%-0.1%	0.5%-0.25%			
Fentanyl	0.001%		0.1-0.15 mL/kg/h	1-1.5 mL every 10-15 min	1 mL of the solution
Bupivacaine[g]	0.05%-0.1%	0.5%-0.25%			
Sufentanil	0.0001%		0.1-0.2 mL/kg/h	1-1.5 mL every 10-15 min	1 mL of the solution
Bupivacaine[h]	0.05%-0.1%	0.5%-0.25%			

[a]Catheter insertion site is the dermatome corresponding to the middle of the surgical incision. Administer a bolus dose of 0.5% bupivacaine or 2% lidocaine to establish surgical anesthesia or 0.25% bupivacaine to induce postoperative analgesia in 5-mL aliquots.

[b]Due to infectious control, a total volume of 150 mL is recommended.

[c]Initial basal infusion rates will depend on the age, general condition, and weight of the patient.

[d]If analgesia is inadequate after 1 hour, then increase the breakthrough dose by the recommended amount. If analgesia is inadequate after one additional hour, then decrease the lockout interval by 5 minutes.

[e]Prepare this solution by mixing 75 to 150 mg of bupivacaine with 15 mg of preservative-free morphine in a total volume of 150 mL of preservative-free normal saline.

[f]Prepare this solution by mixing 75 to 150 mg of bupivacaine with 3.75 to 7.5 mg of hydromorphone in a total volume of 150 mL of preservative-free normal saline.

[g]Prepare this solution by mixing 75 to 150 mg of bupivacaine with 1,500 μg of fentanyl in a total volume of 150 mL of preservative-free normal saline.

[h]Prepare this solution by mixing 75 to 150 mg of bupivacaine with 150 to 300 μg of sufentanil in a total volume of 150 mL of preservative-free normal saline.

Reprinted with permission from de Leon-Casasola OA, Lema MJ. Postoperative epidural opioid analgesia: what are the choices? *Anesth Analg.* 1996;83:867-875.

These modified infusion pumps can administer infusions of opioids, preprogrammed small bolus doses on patient demand, and larger bolus doses by clinician intervention. The PCA technique allows patients to self-titrate opioid doses to achieve optimal analgesic doses while avoiding the toxic side effects that result from high peak serum levels.

Bardia A, Sood A, Mahmood F, et al. Combined epidural-general anesthesia vs general anesthesia alone for elective abdominal aortic aneurysm repair. *JAMA Surg*. 2016;151:1116-1123.

Greco KJ, Brovman EY, Nguyen LL, Urman RD. The impact of epidural analgesia on perioperative morbidity or mortality after open abdominal aortic aneurysm repair. *Ann Vasc Surg*. 2020;66:44-53.

Mann C, Pouzeratte Y, Boccara G, et al. Comparison of intravenous or epidural patient-controlled analgesia in the elderly after major abdominal surgery. *Anesthesiology*. 2000;92:433-441.

11

Hypertension

Liang Shen and Natalia Ivascu Girardi

A 70-year-old male with cholelithiasis is scheduled for a cholecystectomy. His blood pressure (BP) is 230/120 mm Hg; pulse, 60 beats per minute. Hemoglobin is 12.5 g/dL, hematocrit 38%; serum sodium, 140 mEq/L; and serum potassium, 2.7 mEq/L. His medications include metoprolol, aspirin, atorvastatin (Lipitor), and hydrochlorothiazide.

A. Medical Disease and Differential Diagnosis

1. Define hypertension and categorize its severity.
2. What is the prevalence of hypertension?
3. What is the general classification of hypertension? Enumerate the causes of each type of hypertension.
4. What are the clinical patterns of hypertension encountered?
5. What is the pathophysiology of essential hypertension?
6. What is the pathophysiology of isolated systolic hypertension (ISH) and of pulse pressure hypertension (PPH)?
7. What end-organ damage can be caused by long-standing hypertension?
8. Are patients with hypertension at an increased risk for perioperative cardiac morbidity?
9. Perioperative cerebral and renal complications are mostly associated with which subtype of hypertension?
10. Would you employ a controlled-hypotensive technique for patients with hypertension?
11. How much could you safely lower the BP?
12. Can you determine the patient's cerebral autoregulatory range?
13. What are the BP goals for patients with hypertension and when should antihypertensive drugs be initiated?
14. What is the mechanism of action of the major antihypertensive drugs?
15. Does the choice of antihypertensive therapy influence hemodynamic responses to induction, laryngoscopy, and tracheal intubation?
16. Does chronic angiotensin-converting enzyme (ACE) inhibition influence anesthetic induction?

B. Preoperative Evaluation and Preparation

1. How would you evaluate this patient preoperatively?
2. Would you postpone the surgery? Why? What baseline BP would you like the patient to achieve before surgery?
3. Should all or any of the chronic medications be discontinued before the operation?
4. Should hypokalemia be treated before anesthesia? Why?
5. Should hypomagnesemia be treated before anesthesia? Why?
6. The surgery was postponed for 6 weeks. The patient presents for surgery again, currently on a regimen of metoprolol, aspirin, atorvastatin, captopril, hydrochlorothiazide, and potassium chloride. Their BP is 160/60 mm Hg and potassium 4.0 mEq/L. Would you premedicate this patient?

C. Intraoperative Management

1. How would you monitor this patient?
2. What are the anesthetic goals for patients with hypertension?
3. How would you induce anesthesia for the patient with hypertension?
4. How does tracheal intubation produce hypertension?

5. What happens to left ventricular ejection fraction (LVEF) during and immediately following tracheal intubation?
6. What other measures can prevent hypertension and tachycardia at the time of tracheal intubation?
7. After induction and intubation, the BP decreases to 70/40 mm Hg. What would you do?
8. What is your choice of agents for maintenance of anesthesia? Why?
9. How would you manage fluid therapy for patients with hypertension?
10. During the surgery, the BP increases to 220/120 mm Hg. How would you treat the hypertension?
11. What could you do to prevent hypertension during tracheal extubation and emergence?
12. Would you consider regional anesthesia for this patient?

D. Postoperative Management

1. The patient developed hypertension, BP 210/110 mm Hg, in the postanesthesia care unit. What would you do?

A. Medical Disease and Differential Diagnosis

A.1. Define hypertension and categorize its severity

Systemic hypertension is consistently a leading contributor to cardiovascular death in the United States. Uncontrolled hypertension is the most important modifiable risk factor for stroke, all common forms of heart failure, renal failure, and memory loss. According to the seventh report on classification and characterization of BP by the Joint National Committee (JNC) on Evaluation, Detection, and Prevention of High Blood Pressure in 2003, hypertension is defined as an average systolic BP greater than 120 mm Hg and a diastolic pressure greater than 80 mm Hg. The classification stages of hypertension have been updated since 2003 with tightened guidelines for diagnosis of hypertension. According to the American College of Cardiology (ACC)/American Heart Association (AHA) recommendations from 2017, hypertension is classified as normal, elevated, stage 1 hypertension, and stage 2 hypertension. The term "pre-hypertension" as seen in the JNC 7 report has been replaced by "elevated blood pressure" in the current guidelines. The current recommended BP ranges for each category are shown in **Table 11.1**. The tightened BP classification is expected to increase the prevalence of hypertension by 14% in the USA and about 2% increase in antihypertensive therapy usage.

The definition of hypertension in children and adolescents has also been updated by the American Academy of Pediatrics in 2017. Similar to the adult recommendations, the pediatric definition for hypertension has also been tightened in the most current updated guidelines. According to American Association of Pediatrics (AAP), pediatric hypertension is classified as normal, elevated, stage 1 hypertension, and stage 2 hypertension. As in the adult update, the term "pre-hypertension" has been replaced by "elevated blood pressure" in the current guidelines. The current recommended BP ranges are shown in **Table 11.2**.

Uncontrolled hypertension can escalate to a hypertensive crisis defined as systolic BP greater than 180 mm Hg or diastolic BP greater than 120 mm Hg and categorized as urgent and emergent. According to the ACC/AHA guidelines 2017, hypertensive emergency is defined as elevated BP (usually >180/120 mm Hg) complicated by evidence of impending or progressive end-organ damage, whereas hypertensive urgency is severe elevation of BP without progressive end-organ damage.

TABLE 11.1 Categories of Blood Pressure in Adults

BP Category	Systolic Blood Pressure	Diastolic Blood Pressure
Normal	<120 mm Hg	<80 mm Hg
Elevated	120-129 mm Hg	<80 mm Hg
Hypertension		
Stage 1	130-139 mm Hg	80-89 mm Hg
Stage 2	≥140 mm Hg	≥90 mm Hg

BP, blood pressure.
Reprinted with permission from Whelton PK, Carey RM, Aronow WS, et al. 2017 ACC/AHA/AAPA/ABC/ACPM/AGS/APhA/ASH/ASPC/NMA/PCNA guideline for the prevention, detection, evaluation, and management of high blood pressure in adults: a report of the American College of Cardiology/American Heart Association Task Force on Clinical Practice Guidelines. *Hypertension.* 2018;71:e13-e115. Copyright © 2018 American Heart Association, Inc.

TABLE 11.2 Categories of Blood Pressure in Pediatrics

BP Category	Children Aged 1 to <13 Y	Children Aged ≥13 Y
Normal	<90th percentile	<120/<80 mm Hg
Elevated	≥90th percentile to <95th percentile or 120/80 mm Hg to <95th percentile (whichever is lower)	120/<80 to 129/<80 mm Hg
Stage 1 hypertension	≥95th percentile to <95 percentile + 12 mm Hg or 130/80 to 139/89 mm Hg (whichever is lower)	130/80 to 139/89 mm Hg
Stage 2 hypertension	≥95th percentile + 12 mm Hg or ≥140/90 mm Hg (whichever is lower)	≥140/90 mm Hg

Reproduced with permission from Flynn JT, Kaelber DC, Baker-Smith CM, et al. Clinical practice guideline for screening and management of high blood pressure in children and adolescents. *Pediatrics.* 2017;140:e20171904. Copyright © 2017 by the American Academy of Pediatrics.

Bakris GL, Sorrentino MJ. Systemic hypertension: mechanisms, diagnosis, and treatment. In: Libby P, Bonow RO, Mann DL, et al, eds. *Braunwald's Heart Disease.* 12th ed. Elsevier; 2022:471-501.

Flynn JT, Kaelber DC, Baker-Smith CM, et al. Clinical practice guideline for screening and management of high blood pressure in children and adolescents. *Pediatrics.* 2017;140:e20171904.

Whelton PK, Carey RM, Aronow WS, et al. 2017 ACC/AHA/AAPA/ABC/ACPM/AGS/APhA/ASH/ASPC/NMA/PCNA guideline for the prevention, detection, evaluation, and management of high blood pressure in adults: a report of the American College of Cardiology/American Heart Association Task Force on Clinical Practice Guidelines. *Circulation.* 2018;138:e484-e594.

A.2. What is the prevalence of hypertension?

The prevalence of hypertension depends on both the racial composition of the population and the criteria used to define hypertension. In a white suburban population like that of the Framingham study, nearly one-fifth had a BP greater than 160/95 mm Hg and almost one-half had a BP greater than 140/90 mm Hg. A higher prevalence of hypertension has been found in the non-White population. The frequency increases with the age of the population, with nearly two-thirds of patients with hypertension being older than 50 years, and by the age of 75 years, almost 90% of patients have hypertension. In the United States, with the 2017 ACC/AHA definition of hypertension, the prevalence of hypertension was 46%. The highest prevalence is found in the non-Hispanic Black population with an overall prevalence of close to 60% with the current updated definition. However, the prevalence of pharmacologic therapy has not increased with this updated definition because for the percentage of population where patients are now considered hypertensive, the recommended therapy is conservative lifestyle changes. The number of hypertensive persons in the United States in 1983 was estimated to be 57.7 million, more than double the estimate made in 1960 to 1962. Currently, about 1 in 3 or 75 million Americans suffer from hypertension.

Franklin SS, Larson MG, Khan SA, et al. Does the relation of blood pressure to coronary heart disease risk change with aging? The Framingham Heart Study. *Circulation.* 2001;103:1245-1249.

Merai R, Siegel C, Rakotz M, et al. CDC grand rounds: a public health approach to detect and control hypertension. *MMWR Morb Mortal Wkly Rep.* 2016;65:1261-1264.

A.3. What is the general classification of hypertension? Enumerate the causes of each type of hypertension

Hypertension can be classified into primary, or "essential," hypertension, and secondary hypertension, in which the hypertension is caused by a specific other disorder. A categorization of various etiologies of hypertension, although not exhaustive, is shown in **Table 11.1**. Hypertension can also be thought of based on its separate components: systolic, diastolic, and pulse pressure. Average systolic blood pressure is typically higher for males than for females in early adulthood, although the age-related rate of rise is steeper for females. Diastolic blood pressure also increases progressively with age until about 55 years, and subsequently declines. Thus, in older individuals, the pulse pressure tends to be elevated. This phenomenon is thought to be at least partially explained by the decrease in arterial compliance, or increasing arterial stiffness, with advancing age. The ranges of systolic, diastolic, and pulse pressure that define each subtype of hypertension are presented in **Table 11.1**.

Etiologies of Hypertension

- *Primary "essential" hypertension.* Multifactorial, including genetics and environmental factors
- *Renal.* Acute and chronic glomerulonephritis, chronic pyelonephritis, polycystic kidney disease, diabetic nephropathy, hydronephrosis, renovascular stenosis, renin-producing tumors, primary sodium retention
- *Endocrine.* Cushing's syndrome, primary hyperaldosteronism, congenital adrenal hyperplasia, pheochromocytoma, acromegaly, hyperthyroidism, hypothyroidism, carcinoid, oral contraceptives, corticosteroids
- *Neurogenic.* Psychogenic, increased intracranial pressure, spinal cord injury, familial dysautonomia, lead poisoning, Guillain-Barré syndrome, sleep apnea
- *Miscellaneous.* Coarctation of aorta, increased intravascular volume, pregnancy-induced hypertension, polyarteritis nodosa, acute porphyria, hypercalcemia, alcohol and drug use, acute stress including surgery

Bakris GL, Sorrentino MJ. Systemic hypertension: mechanisms, diagnosis, and treatment. In: Libby P, Bonow RO, Mann DL, et al, eds. *Braunwald's Heart Disease.* 12th ed. Elsevier; 2022:471-501.

Kotchen TA. Hypertension. In: Loscalzo J, Fauci AS, Kasper DL, et al, eds. *Harrison's Principles of Internal Medicine.* 21st ed. McGraw-Hill; 2022:2072-2087.

A.4. What are the clinical patterns of hypertension encountered?

The common patterns of hypertension can be understood through the two main determinants of arterial blood pressure, which are cardiac output (the product of stroke volume and heart rate), and peripheral vascular resistance (with contributions from vascular structure and function).

- "Vasoconstricted" hypertension—commonly found in medical patients with chronic renovascular hypertension, characterized by diastolic hypertension and high systemic vascular resistance, with normal or even decreased cardiac output and heart rate
- "Hyperdynamic" hypertension—in postoperative surgical patients, characterized by systolic hypertension, widened pulse pressure, and increased cardiac output, heart rate, and systemic vascular resistance

Bakris GL, Sorrentino MJ. Systemic hypertension: mechanisms, diagnosis, and treatment. In: Libby P, Bonow RO, Mann DL, et al, eds. *Braunwald's Heart Disease.* 12th ed. Elsevier; 2022:471-501.

Kotchen TA. Hypertension. In: Loscalzo J, Fauci AS, Kasper DL, et al, eds. *Harrison's Principles of Internal Medicine.* 21st ed. McGraw-Hill; 2022:2072-2087.

Whelton PK, Carey RM, Aronow WS, et al. 2017 ACC/AHA/AAPA/ABC/ACPM/AGS/APhA/ASH/ASPC/NMA/PCNA guideline for the prevention, detection, evaluation, and management of high blood pressure in adults: a report of the American College of Cardiology/American Heart Association Task Force on Clinical Practice Guidelines. *Circulation.* 2018;138:e484-e594.

A.5. What is the pathophysiology of essential hypertension?

The underlying mechanisms of primary, or "essential" hypertension, is thought to be multifactorial, including genetic and environmental. A variety of abnormalities, including hereditary, fetal undernutrition, abnormal sympathetic nervous system activity, cell membrane defects, renal retention of excess salt, microcirculatory alterations, endothelial cell dysfunction, hyperinsulinemia secondary to insulin resistance, vascular hypertrophy, and altered renin-angiotensin system regulation are implicated. Thus, essential hypertension is likely a spectrum of disorders with different underlying pathophysiology. Common hemodynamic changes include:

- Increased systemic vascular resistance with normal cardiac output
- Exaggerated sympathetic response to stress such as tracheal intubation
- A greater increase in BP with vasoconstriction and a greater decrease in BP with vasodilation because of the increased thickening of arterial walls and a high ratio of wall thickness to internal luminal diameter

The higher a patient's BP is chronically, the more likely that patient will develop various cardiovascular diseases prematurely through acceleration of arteriosclerosis. If untreated, a significant proportion of patients with hypertension will die of coronary heart disease or congestive heart failure (CHF), stroke, or renal failure.

Bakris GL, Sorrentino MJ. Systemic hypertension: mechanisms, diagnosis, and treatment. In: Libby P, Bonow RO, Mann DL, et al, eds. *Braunwald's Heart Disease.* 12th ed. Elsevier; 2022:471-501.

Kotchen TA. Hypertension. In: Loscalzo J, Fauci AS, Kasper DL, et al, eds. *Harrison's Principles of Internal Medicine.* 21st ed. McGraw-Hill; 2022:2072-2087.

A.6. What is the pathophysiology of isolated systolic hypertension (ISH) and of pulse pressure hypertension (PPH)?

ISH is a manifestation of atherosclerotic disease involving predominantly the aorta and its major branches. Both ISH and PPH reflect arterial stiffening and represent the pulsatile component of BP, whereas the mean arterial pressure (MAP) represents the static state. Systole, then, is directly influenced by the ventricular contractile state, the ejected volume, heart rate, and, importantly, compliance of the aorta and pulse wave velocity. With increasing age and factors such as diabetes mellitus, smoking, and increased cholesterol as well as some genetic factors, compliance of the aorta markedly diminishes (**Figure 11.1**). The net result is stiffening of the arterial tree and inability to absorb the pulsatile load, thereby causing the systolic pressure to rise sharply. Pulse wave velocity has gained much attention lately because it provides a richer substrate for characterizing the physiology of blood flow and pressure. Under normal physiologic conditions, the ejected blood volume is transmitted peripherally as a propagated wave. After reaching the periphery, in particular, at sites of bifurcation, a reflected wave or a retrograde wave is generated from the encountered impedance. Under normal conditions, wave reflection arrival coincides with the beginning of diastole, thereby augmenting the diastolic pressure. However, with stiffening of the aorta as occurs with aging, both the propagated and the reflected waves travel much more rapidly, and early return of the reflected arterial wave during late systole augments the systolic component, effectively increasing afterload. The ensuing loss of diastolic augmentation results in a disproportionate increase in the systolic BP and lower diastolic BP, a hallmark of ISH and of PPH.

Mechanistically, pulse pressure is also an index of the stiffness of conduit vessels and the rate of pressure wave propagation and reflection within the arterial tree. About half of patients with ISH also have wide pulse pressure; however, both individuals who are normotensive (systolic BP <120 mm Hg) with a low diastolic pressure or persons with combined systolic and diastolic hypertension (systolic BP >130 mm Hg and diastolic BP >80 mm Hg) can have wide pulse pressure (normal being ≤40 mm Hg).

Dart AM, Kingwell BA. Pulse pressure—a review of mechanism and clinical relevance. *J Am Coll Cardiol.* 2001;37:975-984.

O'Rourke MF, Nichols WW. Aortic diameter, aortic stiffness, and wave reflection increase with age and isolated systolic hypertension. *Hypertension.* 2005;45:652-658.

Schiffrin EL. Vascular stiffening and arterial compliance. Implications for systolic blood pressure. *Am J Hypertens.* 2004;17:39S-48S.

A.7. What end-organ damage can be caused by long-standing hypertension?

End-organ damage caused by long-standing hypertension includes:

Cardiac

Left ventricular hypertrophy (LVH)
Angina or myocardial infarction (MI)

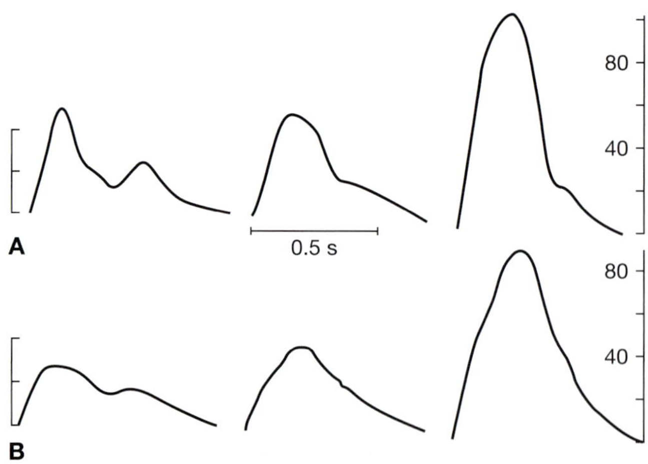

FIGURE 11.1. Change in amplitude and contour of the upper limb (A) and ascending aortic (B) pressure wave with age, as recorded in three female members of a family, at age 18 (left), at age 48 (center), and at age 97 years (right). Upper limb pulse pressure was just more than twice as high in the old compared with the young subject (102 vs 46 mm Hg), whereas aortic pulse pressure was more than 3 times higher (104 vs 27 mm Hg). (Reprinted with permission from O'Rourke MF, Nichols WW. Aortic diameter, aortic stiffness, and wave reflection increase with age and isolated systolic hypertension. *Hypertension.* 2005;45:652-658.)

Arrhythmias
Congestive failure

Ophthalmologic

Hypertensive retinopathy

Renal

Nephropathy

Cerebral

Cerebrovascular Accident (CVA) or Transient Ischemic Attack (TIA)

Complications of hypertension probably involve three interrelated vascular processes: pulsatile flow, endothelial cell dysfunction, and smooth muscle cell hypertrophy. These three processes likely contribute to arteriolar and arterial sclerosis in long-standing hypertension. Large vessels such as the aorta can be directly affected and be at risk for aneurysms and dissection. As discussed earlier, the consequences of long-standing hypertension need be addressed according to the subtypes of hypertension since the associated risks for cerebral, cardiac, and renal vascular complications differ according to systolic, diastolic, and PPH. For example, diastolic hypertension is a better predictor of coronary heart disease in younger patients, whereas systolic and PPH being associated with greater risk of stroke, coronary heart disease, and mortality in persons older than 60 years.

Aronson S, Fontes ML. Hypertension: a new look at an old problem. *Curr Opin Anaesthesiol.* 2006;19:59-64.

Bakris GL, Sorrentino MJ. Systemic hypertension: mechanisms, diagnosis, and treatment. In: Libby P, Bonow RO, Mann DL, et al, eds. *Braunwald's Heart Disease.* 12th ed. Elsevier; 2022:471-501.

A.8. Are patients with hypertension at an increased risk for perioperative cardiac morbidity?

Patients with hypertension are at increased risk for coronary artery disease, silent myocardial ischemia, CHF, and stroke. However, whether preoperative hypertension is predictive of perioperative major cardiac morbidity remains controversial. Some investigators have shown that patients with untreated, poorly controlled, or labile preoperative hypertension are at increased risk for perioperative BP lability, dysrhythmias, myocardial ischemia, and transient neurologic complications. Some suggest that preoperative hypertension predicts perioperative MI. However, recent accumulated evidence suggests that mild-to-moderate hypertension does not increase the risk of perioperative complications. Instead, preoperative hypertension predicts several intermediary outcomes, such as BP lability and myocardial ischemia. The controversy is possibly due to the wide variability in the hypertensive population. Hypertension might affect perioperative morbidity through the extent of end-organ damage and not the manifestation of the disease itself. LVH, which signifies long-standing poorly controlled hypertension, can increase the risk of myocardial ischemia from imbalances of myocardial oxygen (O_2) supply and demand, with or without coronary artery disease.

ISH (systolic BP >140 mm Hg and diastolic BP <90 mm Hg) has been identified as a risk factor for cardiovascular complications in the general population, and treatment reduces the future risk of stroke. Aronson et al and Fontes et al found that among the various components of BP, preoperative PPH was independently and significantly associated with postoperative stroke, renal failure, and mortality in patients undergoing coronary artery bypass. Neither ISH nor isolated diastolic hypertension was predictive of vascular complications. This finding is consistent with results of longitudinal studies finding that increase in pulse pressure is a better predictor of major vascular complications than increase in either systolic or diastolic BP. Interestingly, rises in pulse pressure as few as 10 mm Hg in both normotensive and hypertensive individuals are associated with 20% or more increase risk of renal, coronary, and cerebral events.

Aboyans V, Frank M, Nubret K, et al. Heart rate and pulse pressure at rest are major prognostic markers of early postoperative complications after coronary bypass surgery. *Eur J Cardiothorac Surg.* 2008;33:971-976.

Aronson S, Fontes ML, Miao Y, Mangano DT; Investigators of the Multicenter Study of Perioperative Ischemia Research Group and the Ischemia Research and Education Foundation. Risk index for perioperative renal dysfunction/failure: critical dependence on pulse pressure hypertension. *Circulation.* 2007;115:733-742.

Casadei B, Abuzeid H. Is there a strong rationale for deferring elective surgery in patients with poorly controlled hypertension? *J Hypertens.* 2005;23:19-22.

Fontes ML, Aronson S, Mathew JP, et al; Multicenter Study of Perioperative Ischemia (McSPI) Research Group and the Ischemia Research and Education Foundation (IREF) Investigators. Pulse pressure and risk of adverse outcome in coronary bypass surgery. *Anesth Analg.* 2008;107:1122-1129.

Howell SJ. Preoperative hypertension. *Curr Anesthesiol Rep.* 2018;8:25-31.

A.9. Perioperative cerebral and renal complications are mostly associated with which subtype of hypertension?

Both systolic hypertension and high pulse pressure are strongly associated with risk for perioperative CVA and acute renal failure. The brain, kidneys, and heart differ from most organs in that they receive high blood flow and have very low resistance. As such, the pulsatile load (pulse pressure) tends to be very high. Over years of poorly or untreated hypertension, endothelial injury and vascular remodeling changes can promote both arteriosclerosis and atherosclerosis, which are known risk factors for cerebral and renal vascular complications. The pulsatile stress can also cause dislodgment of plaques from the aorta and its major branches, resulting in embolic stroke.

In patients with hypertension, autoregulation of cerebral blood flow is reset to a higher range than normal; although this protects the brain from sudden increases in pressure, it makes it more vulnerable to hypotension. Therefore, when BP is lowered acutely, patients with hypertension show signs of cerebral ischemia at a higher BP than normotensive patients.

Hypertension can accelerate cognitive decline with age. Hypertension, particularly systolic, is a major risk factor for initial and recurrent stroke and for transient ischemia attacks caused by extracranial atherosclerosis.

Chronic renal insufficiency is a common sequela of hypertension. Patients with hypertension should have a measurement of baseline serum creatinine. In the Revised Cardiac Risk Index, a preoperative serum creatinine level more than 2.0 mg/dL (176.8 mmoL/L) is one of six independent factors that predicted increased cardiovascular risk.

Aronson S, Fontes ML, Miao Y; Investigators of the Multicenter Study of Perioperative Ischemia Research Group and the Ischemia Research and Education Foundation. Risk index for perioperative renal dysfunction/failure: critical dependence on pulse pressure hypertension. *Circulation*. 2007;115:733-742.

Benjo A, Thompson RE, Fine D, et al. Pulse pressure is an age-independent predictor of stroke development after cardiac surgery. *Hypertension*. 2007;50:630-635.

Finnerty FA Jr, Witkin L, Fazekas JF. Cerebral hemodynamics during cerebral ischemia induced by acute hypotension. *J Clin Invest*. 1954;33:1227-1232.

A.10. Would you employ a controlled-hypotensive technique for patients with hypertension?

Uncontrolled or untreated severe hypertension places patients at higher risk of organ malperfusion during periods of hypotension, and is a contraindication to controlled-hypotension techniques. In patients with treated hypertension, however, controlled-hypotension can be used with caution. The concern regarding hypotension in any patient is the potential for compromised perfusion to various end-organs, including the brain, heart, and kidneys. A number of studies in adults undergoing noncardiac surgery have demonstrated that intraoperative MAP less than 60 mm Hg is associated with myocardial injury, acute kidney injury, and death. Since the cerebral autoregulatory curve is shifted to the right with chronic hypertension, the lower BP limit during controlled-hypotension should be set higher for patients with hypertension. With long-term treatment, the autoregulation curve tends to shift leftward toward normal, although in many patients, the curve does not improve even after 12 months of treatment.

Saugel B, Sessler DI. Perioperative blood pressure management. *Anesthesiology*. 2021;134:250-261.

Strandgaard S. Autoregulation of cerebral blood flow in hypertensive patients. The modifying influence of prolonged antihypertensive treatment on the tolerance to acute, drug-induced hypotension. *Circulation*. 1976;53:720-727.

Wesselink EM, Kappen TH, Torn HM, Slooter AJC, van Klei WA. Intraoperative hypotension and the risk of postoperative adverse outcomes: a systematic review. *Br J Anaesth*. 2018;121:706-721.

A.11. How much could you safely lower the blood pressure?

Firm limits on minimally allowable BP have not been established for the perioperative period. Past studies have typically defined hypotension as either a reduction in BP of 20% from the patient's baseline or an absolute MAP less than 65 mm Hg. As mentioned above, intraoperative MAP less than 60 to 70 mm Hg is associated with organ injury in patients undergoing noncardiac surgery. The risk of organ injury appears to be proportional both to the magnitude and the cumulative duration of hypotension. A systematic review from 2018 noted that the risk of any organ injury slightly increased when MAP was sustained at less than 70 mm Hg for 10 minutes, moderately increased with MAP less than 60 to 65 mm Hg for 5 minutes, and greatly increased with MAP less than 50 mm Hg for 5 minutes. The association with acute kidney injury and myocardial injury (defined as postoperative troponin elevation, independent of clinical signs of myocardial ischemia) is strong when using both relative and absolute definitions of hypotension: a relative reduction of at 30% from baseline, or an absolute MAP less than 65 mm Hg. However, baseline BP can be difficult to determine with accuracy given evidence that immediate pre-induction BP poorly reflects ambulatory BP. Thus, for ease of applicability, an absolute low MAP threshold of 65 mm Hg is reasonable.

Importantly, currently available vasoactive agents are not selective in lowering or raising systolic and diastolic BP components without a concomitant increase or fall in the other component. In individuals with demonstrable coronary disease, namely, those with previous infarcts, coronary mortality was significantly related to diastolic pressure in a U-shaped configuration—occurring more frequently in those with very high or very low diastolic BP. This can be particularly concerning in patients with ISH and with very wide pulse pressure where the diastolic BP is already critically low. By reducing the systolic component, further lowering of the diastolic BP can result in ischemic complications in most sensitive vascular beds such as the brain, heart, and kidneys. Lastly, it is critical to recognize that peripheral arterial pressures do not necessarily reflect central pressures with exception of the MAP. In a subset of hypertensive individuals, both systolic and pulse pressures are grossly higher peripherally compared to central aortic pressures, such that lowering of the peripheral BP can result in critical reduction in perfusion pressure.

Fontes ML, Aronson S, Mathew JP, et al; Multicenter Study of Perioperative Ischemia (McSPI) Research Group and the Ischemia Research and Education Foundation (IREF) Investigators. Pulse pressure and risk of adverse outcome in coronary bypass surgery. *Anesth Analg.* 2008;107:1122-1129.

Saugel B, Reese PC, Sessler DI, et al. Automated ambulatory blood pressure measurements and intraoperative hypotension in patients having noncardiac surgery with general anesthesia: a prospective observational study. *Anesthesiology.* 2019;131:74-83.

Saugel B, Sessler DI. Perioperative blood pressure management. *Anesthesiology.* 2021;134:250-261.

Strandgaard S. Autoregulation of cerebral blood flow in hypertensive patients. The modifying influence of prolonged antihypertensive treatment on the tolerance to acute, drug-induced hypotension. *Circulation.* 1976;53:720-727.

Wesselink EM, Kappen TH, Torn HM, Slooter AJC, van Klei WA. Intraoperative hypotension and the risk of postoperative adverse outcomes: a systematic review. *Br J Anaesth.* 2018;121:706-721.

A.12. Can you determine the patient's cerebral autoregulatory range?

Since the cerebral autoregulatory curve of a patient with hypertension is variably shifted to the right, it would improve perioperative BP management to know their autoregulatory range. Noninvasive cerebral oximetry using near-infrared spectroscopy can be used to monitor O_2 saturation of hemoglobin in the cerebral cortex to determine the lower limit of cerebral autoregulation, and help ensure adequate cerebral oxygenation. The values of cerebral O_2 saturations correspond with those of a mixture of 85% jugular venous O_2 saturation and 15% arterial O_2 saturation. It reflects the balance between cerebral O_2 delivery and O_2 demand. At a steady state of anesthesia, cerebral O_2 demand does not change significantly. Therefore, cerebral O_2 saturations do not decrease until BP falls below its autoregulation range. Unfortunately, studies have demonstrated wide variability in measured cerebral saturations with some individual's baseline oximetric saturation values being near 50% at baseline. Furthermore, the measured value is reflective of regional saturation such that distant areas that may be ischemic are not detected. These technical limitations, as well as insufficient data for improved patient outcomes with its use, have curtailed widespread clinical adoption of this technology.

Hogue CW, Levine A, Hudson A, Lewis C. Clinical applications of near-infrared spectroscopy monitoring in cardiovascular surgery. *Anesthesiology.* 2021;134:784-791.

Yao FS, Tseng CC, Ho CY, et al. Cerebral oxygen desaturation is associated with early postoperative neuropsychological dysfunction in patients undergoing cardiac surgery. *J Cardiothorac Vasc Anesth.* 2004;18:552-558.

A.13. What are the blood pressure goals for patients with hypertension and when should antihypertensive drugs be initiated?

The current ACC/AHA guidelines outline the BP treatment goals based on systematic review of the literature. According to the current ACC/AHA guidelines from 2017, it is a class Ia recommendation to treat patients with antihypertensive drug therapy in addition to lifestyle modification as secondary prevention if patients currently have cardiovascular disease and an average systolic BP 130 mm Hg or more or diastolic BP 80 mm Hg or more or as primary prevention in patients with no history of cardiovascular disease but with an estimated 10-year cardiovascular disease risk of less than 10% and systolic BP 140 mm Hg or more or diastolic BP 90 mm Hg or more. Cardiovascular disease includes coronary heart disease, CHF, and stroke. For patients in the elevated BP category, lifestyle modification alone is the recommended treatment modality.

Whelton PK, Carey RM, Aronow WS, et al. 2017 ACC/AHA/AAPA/ABC/ACPM/AGS/APhA/ASH/ASPC/NMA/PCNA guideline for the prevention, detection, evaluation, and management of high blood pressure in adults: a report of the American College of Cardiology/American Heart Association Task Force on Clinical Practice Guidelines. *Circulation*. 2018;138:e484-e594.

A.14. What is the mechanism of action of the major antihypertensive drugs?

Antihypertensive drugs are categorized by their mechanism of action as follows:

Diuretics

This class includes thiazides (eg, hydrochlorothiazide, chlorthalidone), loop diuretics (eg, furosemide, ethacrynic acid), aldosterone antagonists (eg, spironolactone), and potassium sparing agents (eg, amiloride, triamterene). All diuretics initially lower the BP by increasing urinary sodium excretion and by reducing plasma volume, extracellular fluid volume, and cardiac output. Within 6 to 8 weeks, the cardiac output returns to normal. The lowered BP is related to a fall in peripheral resistance. Diuretics can cause hypokalemia, hypomagnesemia, hyperuricemia, hyperlipidemia, hypercalcemia, and hyperglycemia. For patients with ST-segment changes and evidence of pulmonary edema and hypertension or with increased intracranial cerebral pressure and hypertension, intravenous (IV) furosemide can be used.

Anti-adrenergic Agents

- *Centrally acting drugs*. Clonidine, dexmedetomidine. These drugs and their metabolites are primarily α_2-receptor agonists. Stimulation of α_2 receptors in the vasomotor centers of the brain reduces sympathetic outflow.
- *Peripherally acting drugs*
  - α-Receptor blockers

    α_1 and α_2 Receptors: phenoxybenzamine (Dibenzyline), phentolamine (Regitine)

    α_1 Receptor: prazosin (Minipress), doxazosin (Cardura)

    By blocking α-mediated vasoconstriction, these drugs induce a fall in peripheral resistance with both arteriolar and venous dilation.
  - β-Receptor blockers: atenolol (Tenormin), metoprolol (Lopressor), nadolol (Corgard), pindolol (Visken), propranolol (Inderal), esmolol (Brevibloc). These drugs lower BP by decreasing heart rate, contractility, cardiac output, and renin levels. BP is decreased without reflex tachycardia or widening of the pulse pressure. They also have antiarrhythmic activity and suppress both ventricular and supraventricular ectopic rhythms.
  - α- and β-Receptor blockers: labetalol (Tranadate), carvedilol (Coreg)

Direct Vasodilators

This class includes hydralazine, nitroprusside, nitroglycerin, and calcium channel blockers. These drugs directly relax the smooth muscle of resistance and capacitance vessels to different degrees.

Dopaminergic Agonists

Dopaminergic agonists (DAs) are classified into DA_1 and DA_2 subtypes. Stimulation of DA_1 receptors causes vasodilation, and inhibition of active sodium transport in the proximal tubule, thereby leading to natriuresis. Stimulation of DA_2 receptors inhibits norepinephrine release and promotes peripheral vasodilation.

Fenoldopam, a dopamine receptor (DA_1 selective) agonist and a systemic and renal vasodilator, is a unique, parenterally administered agent for management of hypertensive emergencies and in the perioperative setting. Parenteral fenoldopam has a rapid onset and offset of effect, with an elimination half-time of ~10 minutes. The drug is used as a titrated infusion and should not be administered in a bolus, as the incidence of reflex tachycardia is related to rapidity of upward titration. Unlike dopamine, it has no β- or α-adrenergic activity, and increasing doses result in increasing vasodilation without tachycardia or tachyarrhythmias.

Calcium Channel Blockers

The cardiovascular effects of calcium antagonists are listed in **Table 11.3**. These drugs decrease BP mainly by peripheral vasodilation. Renin and aldosterone secretion can be reduced as well.

TABLE 11.3 Cardiovascular Effects of Calcium Channel Blockers

	Verapamil	Diltiazem	Nifedipine	Nicardipine	Clevidipine
Heart rate	↓	↓	↓ or –	↑ or –	–
Nodal conduction	↓↓	↓	↓ or –	–	–
Myocardial depression	↑↑	↑	–	–	–
Vasodilation	↑	↑	↑↑	↑↑	↑↑

↑↑, more increase; ↓↓, more decrease; ↑, increase; ↓, decrease; –, no change.

Angiotensin-Converting Enzyme Inhibitors

This class includes captopril, enalapril, lisinopril, quinapril, and ramipril. The renin-angiotensin system can be inhibited in four ways as shown in **Figure 11.2**. These drugs inhibit the conversion of the inactive decapeptide angiotensin I to the active octapeptide angiotensin II. Lower levels of angiotensin II decrease BP by reducing angiotensin II-induced vasoconstriction and by decreasing aldosterone synthesis. ACE inhibitors also inhibit degradation of a potent vasodilator (bradykinin), alter prostaglandin production (most notably with captopril), and can modify the activity of the adrenergic nervous system.

ACE inhibitors provide predominantly arterial vasodilation and have become primary therapy for the treatment of CHF by afterload reduction. Cardiac output is increased without excessive decrease in preload, with a favorable effect on survival.

Angiotensin II Receptor Blockers

Angiotensin II receptor antagonists or blockers (ARBs) represent the third class that antagonizes the renin-angiotensin-aldosterone system. Blockade of the action of angiotensin II leads to elevations in plasma renin, angiotensin I, and angiotensin II. However, this buildup of precursors does not overwhelm the receptor blockade, as evidenced by a persistent fall in both BP and plasma aldosterone levels. There are several possible differences between ACE inhibitors and angiotensin II receptor antagonists. These include:

- ACE is a kininase. Inhibiting this enzyme, which normally degrades bradykinin, with an ACE inhibitor leads to increased kinin levels. This effect is not seen with an angiotensin II receptor antagonist. High bradykinin levels provide additional vasodilation and other benefits not observed with angiotensin II receptor antagonists.
- ACE inhibitors, by decreasing angiotensin II production, reduce the effect of both angiotensin II receptor type 1 (AT1) and type 2 (AT2); only the former is inhibited by ARBs. Chronic stimulation of the AT2 receptor may be beneficial.

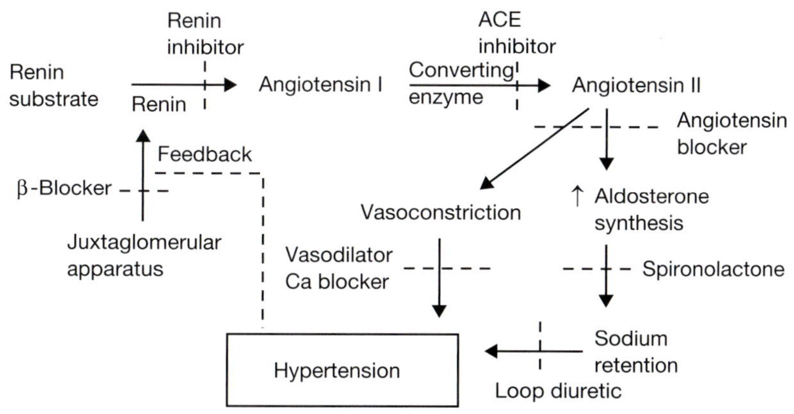

FIGURE 11.2. The renin-angiotensin system and the mechanism of action of antihypertensive drugs. ACE, angiotensin-converting enzyme.

- In the heart, kidney, and perhaps blood vessels, production of angiotensin II can be catalyzed by enzymes other than ACE, such as chymase. The effect of the angiotensin II produced by this reaction can be inhibited by the angiotensin II receptor antagonists but not by ACE inhibitors.

Other Vasodilators

These include brain natriuretic peptides such as nesiritide that is primarily used in acute exacerbation of heart failure to improve forward flow and reduce symptoms and signs of heart failure. There has been controversy about the clinical efficacy of these agents, and reports suggesting that renal outcomes are worsened in patients receiving nesiritide.

Bakris GL, Sorrentino MJ. Systemic hypertension: mechanisms, diagnosis, and treatment. In: Libby P, Bonow RO, Mann DL, et al, eds. *Braunwald's Heart Disease.* 12th ed. Elsevier; 2022:471-501.

Doerschug KC, Delsing AS, Schmidt GA, et al. Renin-angiotensin system activation correlates with microvascular dysfunction in a prospective cohort study of clinical sepsis. *Crit Care.* 2010;14:R24.

Ferrari R, Guardigli G, Ceconi C. Secondary prevention of CAD with ACE inhibitors: a struggle between life and death of the endothelium. *Cardiovasc Drugs Ther.* 2010;24:331-339.

Kotchen TA. Hypertension. In: Loscalzo J, Fauci AS, Kasper DL, et al, eds. *Harrison's Principles of Internal Medicine.* 21st ed. McGraw-Hill; 2022:2072-2087.

Spinler SA, Cziraky M, Miller A. ACE inhibitors versus ARBs: comparison of practice guidelines and treatment selection considerations. *Formulary.* 2006;41:274-284.

A.15. Does the choice of antihypertensive therapy influence hemodynamic responses to induction, laryngoscopy, and tracheal intubation?

The vasopressor responses to induction, laryngoscopy, and intubation differ little whether patients with mild-to-moderate hypertension receive a β-blocker, a calcium channel blocker, an ACE inhibitor, or a diuretic. Changes of a similar magnitude are also observed in untreated patients with hypertension. On the contrary, hypotensive responses can be magnified in patients with poorly controlled hypertension following induction, generally due to a reduced intravascular volume in the face of increased vascular sympathetic tone. Attention should be directed not only to the systolic but also to pulse and diastolic pressures.

Sear JW, Jewkes C, Tellez JC, et al. Does the choice of antihypertensive therapy influence haemodynamic responses to induction, laryngoscopy and intubation? *Br J Anaesth.* 1994;73:303-308.

A.16. Does chronic angiotensin-converting enzyme (ACE) inhibition influence anesthetic induction?

Numerous studies have noted that patients who take ACE inhibitors up until the day of surgery are more likely to experience an exaggerated hypotensive response to anesthetic induction. These studies showed inconsistent effects on postoperative morbidity and mortality, including possibly an association with increased death, stroke, and myocardial injury in those continuing the medications up through the morning of surgery. In 2018, a meta-analysis found that taking ACE inhibitors and ARBs on the morning of surgery was associated with an increased incidence of intraoperative hypotension, but without an increased risk of perioperative death or major cardiac events, compared to patients who withheld the medications on the morning of surgery. The 2024 ACC/AHA guideline on perioperative cardiovascular evaluation and management of patients undergoing noncardiac surgery states that "in select patients on chronic renin-angiotensin-aldosterone system inhibitors (RAASi) for hypertension undergoing elevated-risk noncardiac surgery, omission 24 hours before surgery may be beneficial to limit intraoperative hypotension" with a class IIb recommendation. The "select" patients referenced here refer to those with controlled BP and undergoing elevated-risk surgical procedures. The guideline concludes that "larger RCTs [**randomized controlled trial**] are still needed before recommending routine interruption of RAASi in all patients" and "an individualized approach ... is warranted."

Benedetto U, Sciarretta S, Roscitano A, et al. Preoperative angiotensin-converting enzyme inhibitors and acute kidney injury after coronary artery bypass grafting. *Ann Thorac Surg.* 2008;86:1160-1165.

Coriat P, Richer C, Douraki T, et al. Influence of chronic angiotensin-converting enzyme inhibition on anesthetic induction. *Anesthesiology.* 1994;81:299-307.

Hollmann C, Fernandes NL, Biccard BM. A systematic review of outcomes associated with withholding or continuing angiotensin-converting enzyme inhibitors and angiotensin receptor blockers before noncardiac surgery. *Anesth Analg.* 2018;127:678-687.

Kwapisz MM, Müller M, Schindler E, et al. The effect of intravenous quinaprilat on plasma cytokines and hemodynamic variables during cardiac surgery. *J Cardiothorac Vasc Anesth.* 2004;18:53-58.

Thompson A, Fleishmann KE, Smilowitz N et al. 2024 AHA/ACC/ASNC/HRS/SCA/SCCT/SCMR/SVM Guideline for Perioperative Cardiovascular Management for Noncardiac Surgery: A Report of the American College of Cardiology/American Heart Association Joint Committee on Clinical Practice Guidelines. *Circulation.* 2024;150:e351-e442.

B. Preoperative Evaluation and Preparation

B.1. How would you evaluate this patient preoperatively?

In addition to the routine systemic preoperative physical and history, special attention should be paid to the following: etiology and severity of hypertension, subtype of hypertension, current therapy, and end-organ damage from chronic hypertension.

The underlying cause of hypertension should be clear. Surgical mortality is relatively high in patients with renovascular hypertension. Moreover, failure to diagnose a pheochromocytoma preoperatively, albeit a rare finding, can prove fatal because anesthetic agents are well known to precipitate a crisis in such patients. Meanwhile, the severity of hypertension alters anesthetic risk.

Antihypertensive drugs have different anesthetic implications. Diuretics frequently cause chronic hypokalemia and hypomagnesemia, which increase the risk of arrhythmia. Therefore, serum electrolytes should be checked preoperatively.

The presence of end-organ damage in the brain, heart, and kidney signifies long-standing, poorly controlled hypertension. Unfortunately, markers of organ dysfunction become demonstrable only after significant damage has occurred.

For cardiac evaluation, an electrocardiogram (ECG) is indicated to identify arrhythmias, LVH, or active myocardial ischemia. An echocardiogram can also be helpful to identify LVH and regional wall motion abnormalities suggestive of ischemic heart disease. LVH can increase the risk of perioperative myocardial ischemia from imbalances of myocardial O_2 supply and demand regardless of the presence of coronary artery disease. There is a high correlation between LVH, ISH, and PPH; it is uncertain which comes first. Some authorities believe that patients with hypertension without evidence of LVH or other risk factors are at a lower perioperative cardiac risk and do not require further evaluation for most operations. Patients with severe hypertension are also at an increased risk for diastolic dysfunction causing heart failure with preserved ejection fraction (HFpEF). If acute heart failure exacerbation is suspected in this patient, for example, with the finding of crackles on chest auscultation or significant peripheral edema, then a chest radiograph can be helpful to confirm the diagnosis of pulmonary edema.

For renal evaluation, urinalysis and a basic metabolic panel including serum creatinine and blood urea nitrogen should be obtained to define the presence and extent of renal parenchymal disease. If chronic kidney disease exists, then hyperkalemia and hypervolemia can be of concern.

For cerebrovascular evaluation, a thorough history to investigate CVAs and TIAs and the presence of hypertensive retinopathy should be performed.

Fleisher LA. Preoperative evaluation of the patient with hypertension. *JAMA*. 2002;287:2043-2046.

Hata TM, Licina LK, Wyler DJ. Preoperative patient assessment and management. In: Cullen BF, Stock MC, Ortega R, et al, eds. *Barash, Cullen, and Stoelting's Clinical Anesthesia*. 9th ed. Wolters Kluwer; 2024:551-576.

Selzer A, Fontes M, Heerdt PM. Systemic and pulmonary arterial hypertension. In: Hines RL, Jones SB, eds. *Stoelting's Anesthesia and Co-Existing Disease*. 8th ed. Elsevier; 2022:187-202.

B.2. Would you postpone the surgery? Why? What baseline blood pressure would you like the patient to achieve before surgery?

It is prudent to postpone elective surgery with a BP of 230/120 mm Hg. This patient should be considered to have hypertensive emergency if additional end-organ sequelae are present, in which case they need to be admitted for IV control of BP. Otherwise, for hypertensive urgency, it is recommended that the patient be placed in a quiet environment and managed with rest and oral antihypertensives. The patient should be discharged and instructed to follow up with their primary care provider for management and control of hypertension. Prior to rescheduling for surgery, if time permits, then the BP should be gradually lowered over 6 to 8 weeks to less than 140/90 mm Hg. Acute BP control within several hours is inadvisable before elective surgery because this practice can put the brain and other organs at risk for ischemia.

In patients with moderate hypertension with severe end-organ involvement, preoperative BP should be normalized as much as possible, although in asymptomatic patients with mild-to-moderate hypertension (systolic BP <180 mm Hg, diastolic BP <110 mm Hg), elective surgery can proceed, as these patients do not appear to be at increased risk of cardiovascular complications provided they have no other risk factors for coronary heart disease. The thresholds recommended apply only in part to today's surgical population. Most patients with hypertension presenting for surgery are older patients who suffer almost exclusively from ISH and PPH. It is uncertain what acute changes in BP preoperatively will have on outcome given that the pathologic changes are chronic and unlikely to normalize with treatment.

Fleisher LA. Preoperative evaluation of the patient with hypertension. *JAMA*. 2002;287:2043-2046.

Goldman L. Cardiac risk in noncardiac surgery: an update. *Anesth Analg*. 1995;80:810-820.

Nikolov NM, Fontes ML, White WD, et al. Pulse pressure and long-term survival after coronary artery bypass graft surgery. *Anesth Analg*. 2010;110:335-340.

Selzer A, Fontes M, Heerdt PM. Systemic and pulmonary arterial hypertension. In: Hines RL, Jones SB, eds. *Stoelting's Anesthesia and Co-Existing Disease*. 8th ed. Elsevier; 2022:187-202.

B.3. Should all or any of the chronic medications be discontinued before the operation?

Current opinion generally favors continuation of antihypertensive medications, especially β-blockers, up to the time of surgery. The safety of β-blockers and their benefits (prevention of hypertensive responses, dysrhythmias, and myocardial ischemia) have been established. There is additional concern that acute withdrawal of these medications can precipitate ischemic myocardial events. The withdrawal syndrome is characterized by enhanced sensitivity to sympathetic stimulation and has been attributed to various factors including sympathetic overactivity, increased triiodothyronine levels, and increased β-receptor density. Continuing β-blockade does not appear to impair the hemodynamic response to hemorrhage and does not adversely affect responses to hypoxemia. Similarly, treatment with calcium channel blockers, ACE inhibitors, statins, and diuretics can be maintained, particularly if they are prescribed for heart failure. Withdrawal of clonidine has been associated with rebound hypertension.

Of note, as ACE inhibitors and ARBs have been associated with intraoperative hypotension, although without clearly increased risk of mortality or major cardiac events, some would advocate for withholding these medications on the morning of surgery, and restarting them as soon as clinically feasible postoperatively.

Fleisher LA. Preoperative evaluation of the patient with hypertension. *JAMA*. 2002;287:2043-2046.

Hata TM, Licina LK, Wyler DJ. Preoperative patient assessment and management. In: Cullen BF, Stock MC, Ortega R, et al, eds. *Barash, Cullen, and Stoelting's Clinical Anesthesia*. 9th ed. Wolters Kluwer; 2024:551-576.

Hollmann C, Fernandes NL, Biccard BM. A systematic review of outcomes associated with withholding or continuing angiotensin-converting enzyme inhibitors and angiotensin receptor blockers before noncardiac surgery. *Anesth Analg*. 2018;127:678-687.

B.4. Should hypokalemia be treated before anesthesia? Why?

Hypokalemia is a frequent finding in patients with hypertension treated with thiazide diuretics. Vitez et al concluded that chronic hypokalemia per se is not associated with a higher incidence of intraoperative arrhythmia, although it is important to maintain normal electrolyte balance in patients with cardiac or coronary artery disease. A low value of potassium (3.0-3.5 mEq/L) in these patients can cause arrhythmias, increase sensitivity to digoxin, and depress neuromuscular function. In patients without risk of cardiac complications from surgery and anesthesia, this modest reduction (3.0-3.5 mEq/L) should not prompt postponement of surgery or immediate potassium replacement. Patients with more severe potassium depletion (≤2.9 mEq/L) should be treated and/or undergo workup for such profound hypokalemia. For those patients, at least 1 week before surgery, supplemental potassium should be given if renal function is not impaired. In surgical emergencies, potassium can be given IV at a rate not to exceed 0.5 mEq/kg of body weight per hour. Administration should be stopped during surgery and restarted postoperatively, depending on serial potassium determinations.

Archibald T, Peramunage DS, Barnes CR. Acid-base, fluids, and electrolytes. In: Cullen BF, Stock MC, Ortega R, et al, eds. *Barash, Cullen, and Stoelting's Clinical Anesthesia*. 9th ed. Wolters Kluwer; 2024:362-397.

Schonberger RB. Fluid, electrolyte, and acid-base disorders. In: Hines RL, Jones SB, eds. *Stoelting's Anesthesia and Co-Existing Disease*. 8th ed. Elsevier; 2022:397-414.

Vitez TS, Soper LE, Wong KC, et al. Chronic hypokalemia and intraoperative dysrhythmias. *Anesthesiology*. 1985;63:130-133.

B.5. Should hypomagnesemia be treated before anesthesia? Why?

The normal level of magnesium is 1.5 to 2.5 mEq/L. Magnesium ion is essential for the proper function of most enzyme systems. Depletion is characterized by neuromuscular and central nervous system hyperexcitability. These signs are similar to those of calcium deficiency. Cardiovascular abnormalities include coronary artery spasm, cardiac failure, and dysrhythmias. When severe, hypomagnesemia can induce seizures, confusion, and coma. Decisions about treatment should be based on severity of symptoms. Hypomagnesemia can also potentiate hypokalemia, and for potassium repletion to be effective, it might be necessary to administer magnesium simultaneously. Magnesium, being renally excreted, should be administered cautiously to patients with renal failure. In that case, smaller IV doses should be used, with careful observation for toxicity (lethargy, weakness, and loss of deep tendon reflexes).

Archibald T, Peramunage DS, Barnes CR. Acid-base, fluids, and electrolytes. In: Cullen BF, Stock MC, Ortega R, et al, eds. *Barash, Cullen, and Stoelting's Clinical Anesthesia*. 9th ed. Wolters Kluwer; 2024:362-397.

Schonberger RB. Fluid, electrolyte, and acid-base disorders. In: Hines RL, Jones SB, eds. *Stoelting's Anesthesia and Co-Existing Disease*. 8th ed. Elsevier; 2022:397-414.

B.6. The surgery was postponed for 6 weeks. The patient presents for surgery again, currently on a regimen of metoprolol, aspirin, atorvastatin, captopril, hydrochlorothiazide, and potassium chloride. Their BP is 160/60 mm Hg and potassium 4.0 mEq/L. Would you premedicate this patient?

Because half or more of patients with hypertension still have elevated BP despite treatment, the anesthesiologist should determine whether other contributing factors play a role, such as patient anxiety. If the patient is severely anxious, then premedication with a benzodiazepine such as diazepam, lorazepam, or midazolam can be titrated with the aim of the patient arriving in the operating room sedated. However, large observational trials have demonstrated a strong association with perioperative benzodiazepine use and postoperative delirium, particularly in older patients. As a result, in older patients routine premedication with such agents has declined, and the decision to use them should be individualized.

Jin Z, Hu J, Ma D. Postoperative delirium: perioperative assessment, risk reduction, and management. *Br J Anaesth*. 2020;125:492-504.

C. Intraoperative Management

C.1. How would you monitor this patient?

Standard basic anesthetic monitoring as prescribed by the American Society of Anesthesiologists is indicated for this patient, with particular attention to, and addition of, the following:

- *Electrocardiogram*. Simultaneous leads V_5 and II, multiple-lead ST-segment analysis, if possible, are essential because patients with hypertension are at increased risk for myocardial ischemia regardless of the presence of coronary disease.
- *BP*. Continuous monitoring of BP is essential because of lability of BP in these patients. Direct arterial catheter measurement of BP permits beat-to-beat observation. However, noninvasive automatic oscillometric techniques are typically sufficient.
- *Pulse oximeter*. This should be used to monitor peripheral blood flow and oxygenation.
- *End-tidal CO_2 analyzer*. This monitor will help maintain normocarbia.
- *Pulmonary artery catheter (PAC)*. Only for those patients with hypertension with a history of CHF or a recent MI, a PAC can be helpful in managing fluid replacement and monitoring ventricular function. Of note, there is a strong correlation between hypertension and LVH, which results in poor ventricular compliance reflected by elevated pulmonary artery occlusion pressure in the face of low or normal ventricular volumes and normal contractility. Patients with hypertension tend to manifest HFpEF, rather than heart failure with reduced ejection fraction (HFrEF).

Committee on Standards and Practice Parameters of the American Society of Anesthesiologists. Standards for basic anesthetic monitoring. December 13, 2020. Accessed March 23, 2023. https://www.asahq.org/standards-and-guidelines/standards-for-basic-anesthetic-monitoring

C.2. What are the anesthetic goals for patients with hypertension?

One anesthetic goal is to minimize wide lability of BP in response to anesthetic and surgical stimuli to prevent organ injury, including the following:

- Myocardial ischemia from tachycardia or less commonly from either hypertension or hypotension
- Cerebral hypoperfusion from hypotension
- Cerebral hemorrhage and hypertensive encephalopathy resulting from hypertension, or embolic stroke from rupture of plaques either locally or from the aorta and neck vessels
- Renal injury from renal hypoperfusion

Particular attention to diastolic BP is recommended while attempting to reduce systolic BP. Careful control of the hemodynamic responses to noxious stimuli such as tracheal intubation, surgical incision and manipulation, and emergence from anesthesia is essential in the patient with hypertension.

Selzer A, Fontes M, Heerdt PM. Systemic and pulmonary arterial hypertension. In: Hines RL, Jones SB, eds. *Stoelting's Anesthesia and Co-Existing Disease*. 8th ed. Elsevier; 2022:187-202.

C.3. How would you induce anesthesia for the patient with hypertension?

While the patient is being preoxygenated, fentanyl, 1 to 2 μg/kg, is given slowly to achieve drowsiness and to blunt the imminent sympathetic surge from laryngoscopy. Propofol in 30 to 50 mg increments is then titrated to produce unconsciousness while maintaining normal BP, followed by paralysis with succinylcholine, 1 mg/kg, or a nondepolarizing neuromuscular blocker to facilitate tracheal intubation.

All anesthetic agents are acceptable with the possible exception of ketamine, which can produce significant hypertension and tachycardia. However, deep anesthesia with volatile anesthetic agents should be performed with caution because of a higher incidence of hypotension arising from both vasodilation and cardiac depression. A slow induction is important in patients with severe hypertension because of the risk of significant hypotension with most induction agents.

Martin DE, Rosenberg H, Aukburg SJ, et al. Low-dose fentanyl blunts circulatory responses to tracheal intubation. *Anesth Analg*. 1982;61:680-684.

Selzer A, Fontes M, Heerdt PM. Systemic and pulmonary arterial hypertension. In: Hines RL, Jones SB, eds. *Stoelting's Anesthesia and Co-Existing Disease*. 8th ed. Elsevier; 2022:187-202.

C.4. How does tracheal intubation produce hypertension?

Translaryngeal intubation of the trachea stimulates laryngeal and tracheal receptors, resulting in marked increase in the elaboration of sympathomimetic amines. This sympathetic stimulation results in tachycardia and a rise in BP. In normotensive patients, this rise is 20 to 25 mm Hg; it can be much greater in patients with hypertension.

Prys-Roberts C, Greene LT, Meloche R, et al. Studies of anaesthesia in relation to hypertension. II. Haemodynamic consequences of induction and endotracheal intubation. *Br J Anaesth*. 1971;43:531-547.

C.5. What happens to left ventricular ejection fraction (LVEF) during and immediately following tracheal intubation?

During and immediately following intubation associated with tachycardia and hypertension, there is a decrease in the LVEF. This is particularly marked in patients with coronary artery disease. Such hemodynamic perturbations can be anticipated and treated accordingly with β-blockade, opioid, and titration of hypnotic and/or inhalation agents.

Giles RW, Berger JH, Barash PG, et al. Continuous monitoring of left ventricular performance with the computerized nuclear probe during laryngoscopy and intubation before coronary artery bypass surgery. *Am J Cardiol*. 1982; 50:735-741.

C.6. What other measures can prevent hypertension and tachycardia at the time of tracheal intubation?

The rise in BP and heart rate occurs ~14 seconds after the start of laryngoscopy and becomes maximal after 30 to 45 seconds of direct laryngoscopy. If possible, laryngoscopy time should be 15 seconds or less to minimize BP elevation. Simultaneous administration of fentanyl with the induction dose of propofol can blunt the cardiovascular response to tracheal intubation. Other potential strategies include:

- Lidocaine, 1.5 mg/kg, given 2 minutes before intubation.
- Esmolol, up to 2 mg/kg, appears to be especially effective in providing consistent and reliable protection against hypertension and tachycardia with intubation. It is easy to titrate and does not exacerbate postintubation hypotension because of its short half-life of 9 minutes.
- Labetalol, 0.15 to 0.45 mg/kg, is comparable to esmolol, 1.5 to 4.5 mg/kg, in attenuating hemodynamic effects. However, the half-life of IV labetalol is 5 hours, limiting its utility for such a brief stimulus. Additionally, labetalol has minimal effects on heart rate.
- Nicardipine, 1 mg IV, 2 minutes before tracheal intubation. Both doses of 0.015 and 0.03 mg/kg can attenuate BP but not heart rate responses during emergence and extubation.

It is important to remember that these doses are for use as a single agent only. If a combination of different agents or anesthetics is used, then doses should be decreased accordingly. Otherwise, severe hypotension can ensue.

Gold MI, Sacks DJ, Grosnoff DB, et al. Use of esmolol during anesthesia to treat tachycardia and hypertension. *Anesth Analg*. 1989;68:101-104.

Hata TM, Licina LK, Wyler DJ. Preoperative patient assessment and management. In: Cullen BF, Stock MC, Ortega R, et al, eds. *Barash, Cullen, and Stoelting's Clinical Anesthesia*. 9th ed. Wolters Kluwer; 2024:551-576.

Helfman SM, Gold MI, Delisser EA, et al. Which drug prevents tachycardia and hypertension associated with tracheal intubation: lidocaine, fentanyl, or esmolol? *Anesth Analg*. 1991;72:482-486.

Kapnoudhis P, Vaghadia H, Jenkins LC, et al. Esmolol versus fentanyl for preventing haemodynamic response to intubation in cardiovascular disease. *Can J Anaesth*. 1990;37:S145.

Kovac AL, McKinley C, Tebbe CJ, et al. Comparison of nicardipine versus placebo to control hemodynamic responses during emergence and extubation. *J Cardiothorac Vasc Anesth*. 2001;15:704-709.

C.7. After induction and intubation, the BP decreases to 70/40 mm Hg. What would you do?

Hypotension after induction of anesthesia is usually due to a combination of vasodilation, hypovolemia, and cardiac depression. Vasodilation can be caused by induction agents such as propofol; moderate-to-high doses of opioids; and potent inhalation agents. Patients with hypertension are relatively hypovolemic because of chronic vasoconstriction and/or diuretic therapy. Preoperative bowel preparation and nothing by mouth status further contribute to hypovolemia. Barbiturates, benzodiazepines, and inhalation agents can cause a mild-to-moderate degree of cardiac depression.

Hypotension after induction of anesthesia can usually be easily corrected by volume replacement and simultaneous titration of vasopressors such as phenylephrine in 80 to 100 μg increments or ephedrine 5 to 10 mg. Caution with ephedrine-induced tachycardia is warranted in patients at risk of myocardial ischemia.

Abola R, Geralemou S, Szafran M, Gan TJ. Intravenous anesthetics. In: Cullen BF, Stock MC, Ortega R, et al, eds. *Barash, Cullen, and Stoelting's Clinical Anesthesia*. 9th ed. Wolters Kluwer; 2024:463-481.

Coriat P, Richer C, Douraki T, et al. Influence of chronic angiotensin-converting enzyme inhibition on anesthetic induction. *Anesthesiology*. 1994;81:299-307.

C.8. What is your choice of agents for maintenance of anesthesia? Why?

No particular anesthetic technique or specific drug combination has been demonstrated to be superior to others in patients with hypertension. Potent inhalation anesthetics or opioids should be titrated to the desired level of central nervous system depression while BP is monitored continuously.

Opioids and nitrous oxide provide anesthesia with less overall BP lability, but commonly, intraoperative hypertension is difficult to control by moderate doses of opioids. High doses of opioids are not suitable for early extubation. Likewise, use of nitrous oxide is debatable in open cholecystectomy given its propensity to increase bowel distention; the severity is related to higher concentrations of nitrous oxide and to longer duration of use. This concern is less pertinent for laparoscopic cholecystectomy whereby insufflation of gas to pressurize the abdomen should counteract the distensible property of nitrous oxide.

Potent inhalation agents provide greater control of hypertension but seem to produce less stability. Isoflurane, desflurane, and sevoflurane possess the advantage of more peripheral vasodilation and less cardiac depression.

Akca O, Lenhardt R, Fleischmann E, et al. Nitrous oxide increases the incidence of bowel distension in patients undergoing elective colon resection. *Acta Anaesthesiol Scand*. 2004;48:894-898.

Taylor E, Feinstein R, White PF, et al. Anesthesia for laparoscopic cholecystectomy. Is nitrous oxide contraindicated? *Anesthesiology*. 1992;76:541-543.

C.9. How would you manage fluid therapy for patients with hypertension?

Patients with essential hypertension are often hypovolemic because of vasoconstriction and diuretic therapy. Hydration of patients with hypertension should be started before induction of anesthesia to minimize hemodynamic changes. However, overhydration should be avoided because it can contribute to postoperative hypertension when the vasodilating effects of anesthetics have dissipated. Therefore, careful estimation of fluid intake and output is essential. Insertion of a urine catheter is indicated for major surgery with extensive fluid shifts, and more invasive hemodynamic monitors of volume status, such as central venous pressure or pulmonary artery pressure, can be considered.

The presence of LVH in patients with hypertension shifts the left ventricular compliance curve upward and leftward such that for the same ventricular volume, higher left ventricular diastolic pressure is attained compared to a nonhypertrophied ventricle. When managing these patients with a PAC, higher pulmonary artery occlusion pressure (sometimes >20 mm Hg) is necessary to achieve normovolemia. Cardiac output should be checked before and after volume challenges to confirm increases in stroke volume.

Selzer A, Fontes M, Heerdt PM. Systemic and pulmonary arterial hypertension. In: Hines RL, Jones SB, eds. *Stoelting's Anesthesia and Co-Existing Disease.* 8th ed. Elsevier; 2022:187-202.

C.10. During the surgery, the blood pressure increases to 220/120 mm Hg. How would you treat the hypertension?

Medications used in the intraoperative control of hypertension are outlined in **Table 11.4**. Severe hypertension that occurs during a surgical procedure is most frequently due to inadequate anesthesia. Inadequate blockade of sensory input from the surgical procedure produces sympathetic nervous system stimulation, resulting in hypertension and tachycardia. If a potent inhalational anesthetic is being used, the level of anesthesia should be deepened by increasing the inspired concentration of the anesthetic.

Labetalol, in 5 to 10 mg increments, is useful in controlling hypertension and tachycardia. It makes sense to use β-blockers after a significant rise in BP and HR because these agents act directly to antagonize the effects of the catecholamines. Although other agents lower the BP, the excessive availability of both norepinephrine and epinephrine can continue to compromise tissue perfusion due to vasoconstriction. This might explain the broad anti-ischemic effects of perioperative β-blockers on the brain, heart, and kidneys.

Hydralazine, in 5 mg increments, can be titrated to decrease BP safely with little chance of excessive reduction. The onset of action is in 10 to 15 minutes with a duration of 1 to 2 hours. Reflex tachycardia can occur, and caution is warranted in patients at risk of myocardial ischemia who tolerate tachycardia poorly.

Continuous infusions of nicardipine, nitroglycerin, or nitroprusside, which are direct arteriolar vasodilators, can also be used to control hypertension during anesthesia. These agents have a short half-life, and are most helpful to treat transient hypertension.

Lindenauer PK, Pekow P, Wang K, et al. Perioperative beta-blocker therapy and mortality after major noncardiac surgery. *N Engl J Med.* 2005;353:349-361.

Selzer A, Fontes M, Heerdt PM. Systemic and pulmonary arterial hypertension. In: Hines RL, Jones SB, eds. *Stoelting's Anesthesia and Co-Existing Disease.* 8th ed. Elsevier; 2022:187-202.

TABLE 11.4 Intraoperative Control of Hypertension

Anesthetics
Opioids, inhalational agents, lidocaine
Antihypertensive drugs
Adrenergic blockers
α-Blocker: phentolamine
β-Blocker: esmolol, metoprolol, propranolol
α- and β-Blocker: labetalol
Calcium channel blockers
Diltiazem, nicardipine, verapamil
ACE inhibitors
Enalapril
Direct vasodilators
Hydralazine, nitroglycerin, nitroprusside
Dopaminergic agonists
Fenoldopam

ACE, angiotensin-converting enzyme.

C.11. What could you do to prevent hypertension during tracheal extubation and emergence?

Many drugs or combinations are effective in treating hypertension due to extubation and emergence, including IV lidocaine, esmolol, labetalol, verapamil, or diltiazem given 2 minutes before extubation. If BP rises above desired levels after extubation, then additional doses can be titrated to control BP.

Emergence hypertension is also frequently related to coughing because of the tracheal tube. A recent systematic review and meta-analysis concluded that effective medications to decrease the incidence of emergence coughing include dexmedetomidine, remifentanil, fentanyl, or lidocaine.

Mikawa K, Nishina K, Maekawa N, et al. Attenuation of cardiovascular responses to tracheal extubation: verapamil versus diltiazem. *Anesth Analg*. 1996;82:1205-1210.

Tung A, Fergusson NA, Ng N, et al. Medications to reduce emergence coughing after general anaesthesia with tracheal intubation: a systematic review and network meta-analysis. *Br J Anaesth*. 2020;124:480-495.

C.12. Would you consider regional anesthesia for this patient?

Use of a regional anesthetic technique without tracheal intubation can avoid the marked increases in sympathetic tone and hemodynamic changes that occur with intubation and extubation. Spinal or epidural anesthesia can be used for lower abdominal surgery. For cholecystectomy, higher dermatomal levels of neuraxial anesthesia are needed that can compromise respiratory function or unmask hypovolemia. In addition, prolonged surgery in a nonsedated patient can cause anxiety that can induce hypertension and tachycardia.

Brull R, Macfarlane AJ, Chan VW. Spinal, epidural, and caudal anesthesia. In: Gropper MA, Cohen LI, Fleisher LA, Leslie K, Wiener-Kronish JP, eds. *Miller's Anesthesia*. 9th ed. Elsevier; 2020:1413-1449.

Selzer A, Fontes M, Heerdt PM. Systemic and pulmonary arterial hypertension. In: Hines RL, Jones SB, eds. *Stoelting's Anesthesia and Co-Existing Disease*. 8th ed. Elsevier; 2022:187-202.

D. Postoperative Management

D.1. The patient developed hypertension, BP 210/110 mm Hg, in the postanesthesia care unit. What would you do?

Management of postoperative hypertension depends on the etiology of the hypertension, the clinical scenario, and the degree of hypertension. First, the cause of hypertension should be determined. The causes of postoperative hypertension include pain, emergence excitement, hypoxemia, hypercarbia, reaction to endotracheal tube, full bladder, hypothermia, relative hypervolemia from excess intraoperative fluid administration, and chronic medication and withdrawal. The most common cause of postoperative hypertension is incisional pain. As the patient awakens, pain triggers catecholamine release. The extreme lability of BP in many patients with hypertension makes this rapid increase in BP critical to control. Depending on the cause of hypertension, IV analgesics, antihypertensives, or diuretics should be titrated to control the hypertension. If both tachycardia and hypertension occur postoperatively, then calcium channel blockers such as verapamil, diltiazem, or nicardipine and β-blocking agents such as propranolol, esmolol, labetalol, or metoprolol, are preferred agents. Hypertension resulting from incisional pain can be prevented or attenuated by using a long-lasting local anesthetic along the incision or use of a local field nerve block.

Macres SM, Saldanha U, Zhou JY, Bishop R, Chen A. Acute pain management. In: Cullen BF, Stock MC, Ortega R, et al, eds. *Barash, Cullen, and Stoelting's Clinical Anesthesia*. 9th ed. Wolters Kluwer; 2024:1479-1513.

12 Cardiac Tamponade

James A. Osorio and June M. Chan

Four days after a two-vessel coronary artery bypass graft procedure with a mitral valve replacement, a 69-year-old, 90-kg, 167-cm tall female presents with shortness of breath, orthopnea, oliguria, and overt weakness. On examination, she is sitting fully upright and appears anxious; her skin is cold and clammy. Her vital signs are: heart rate (HR), 120 beats per minute (sinus tachycardia); respiratory rate, 38 breaths per minute; and systemic arterial pressure, 115/66 mm Hg. A pulmonary artery catheter (PAC) is inserted and reveals: pulmonary artery (PA) pressure, 55/21 mm Hg; pulmonary artery occlusion pressure (PAOP), 14 mm Hg; central venous pressure (CVP), 23 mm Hg; and cardiac output (CO), 2.7 L/min.

A. Medical Disease and Differential Diagnosis

1. What is the differential diagnosis of low CO following cardiac surgery?
2. Describe the pathophysiology of cardiac tamponade.
3. What are the common etiologies of cardiac tamponade?
4. What is the difference between acute and delayed cardiac tamponade?
5. What is regional cardiac tamponade?
6. Describe the ventricular interaction in cardiac tamponade.
7. How is coronary blood flow affected by cardiac tamponade?
8. What is the Beck triad? Describe the typical signs and symptoms of cardiac tamponade.
9. Define pulsus paradoxus, and describe its pathophysiology.
10. What is the Kussmaul sign? Is this finding consistent with cardiac tamponade physiology?
11. Which medical conditions mimic cardiac tamponade?

B. Preoperative Evaluation and Preparation

1. Interpret and explain the pathophysiologic basis for this patient's hemodynamic findings.
2. How would you optimize this patient's cardiovascular status before definitive diagnosis and treatment?
3. What are the chest radiographic findings in cardiac tamponade?
4. A limited bedside transthoracic echocardiogram is performed, demonstrating a layer of clotted blood anterior to the right atrium (RA) and ventricle. What echocardiographic findings support the diagnosis of cardiac tamponade?
5. What additional information should be obtained from a limited echocardiographic study?
6. Describe the procedures for treating cardiac tamponade. What are the clinical indications for each approach?
7. Having made the diagnosis of cardiac tamponade, what additional investigations are required before surgery?
8. Explain the technical and physiologic principles behind rotational thromboelastometry.
9. A rotational thromboelastometry was performed, and a 10-minute analysis reveals the following results (see **Figure 12.9** and **Table 12.8**). How do you interpret this information?
10. Given the thromboelastometry findings and high clinical suspicion for occult postsurgical bleeding, what hemostatic products would you arrange to have in the operating room?
11. How would you organize and conduct the transport of this patient to the operating room?

C. Intraoperative Management

1. What are the cardiovascular effects of commonly used intravenous anesthetic and coinduction agents?
2. What is the effect of supine positioning and positive pressure ventilation on the hemodynamics of a patient with cardiac tamponade?
3. Describe the anesthetic induction process for cardiac tamponade.
4. Following anesthetic induction and tracheal intubation, the systemic blood pressure decreases to 55/30 mm Hg. Describe your management.
5. What hemodynamic changes are frequently associated with opening the pericardial space?
6. Following removal of approximately 500 mL of dark blood and clots from the mediastinum, the patient's CO remains low. What are your differential diagnoses?
7. What is pericardial decompression syndrome (PDS)?

D. Postoperative Management

1. A pericardial drain is placed following mediastinal decompression. How should this drainage tube be managed?
2. How would you manage hypertension in the intensive care unit?

A. Medical Disease and Differential Diagnosis

A.1. What is the differential diagnosis of low CO following cardiac surgery?

CO is the product of stroke volume (SV) and HR:

$$CO = HR \times SV$$

According to this relationship, low SV and/or low HR result in a low CO state. However, rapid HR of either ventricular or atrial origin (ie, atrial fibrillation) can also cause a low CO state because diastolic filling time is decreased or the atrial contribution to ventricular filling is reduced. Preload, afterload, and contractility all contribute to SV and their alteration can also reduce CO (Table 12.1). A decrease in preload will decrease SV if the ventricle is underfilled. An increase in preload can also decrease SV if it

TABLE 12.1 Differential Diagnoses of a Low Cardiac Output

Parameter	Change	Examples
Heart rate	Decrease	Bradycardia
		Heart block causing loss of AV synchrony
	Increase	Atrial fibrillation
		Ventricular tachyarrhythmias
Preload	Decrease	Hypovolemia
		Mitral stenosis
	Increase	Ventricular overdistension and systolic dysfunction
		Mitral regurgitation
Afterload	Increase	Embolism
		Outflow tract obstruction
Contractility	Direct decrease	Right and/or left ventricle • Ischemia/infarction • Stunning/hibernation
	Indirect decrease	Cardiac tamponade
		Embolism
		Negative inotropic agents
		Toxins (endotoxin, inflammatory cytokines)

AV, atrioventricular.

causes ventricular overdistension, thereby stretching ventricular myocytes beyond the working limits of the length–tension relationship. A decrease in myocardial contractility can compromise CO. Finally, in a ventricle with systolic dysfunction, an increase in afterload can further impair ventricular ejection and SV. A combination of these hemodynamic disturbances can coexist in the same patient. For example, a patient can have both a decrease in contractility and reduced preload, thereby resulting in low CO. Therefore, correcting one problem alone might not optimize hemodynamic conditions.

Levy JH, et al. Postoperative Cardiovascular Management. In: Kaplan JA, et al., eds. *Kaplan's Cardiac Anesthesia*. 8th ed. Elsevier; 2023:1094-1123.

Kaufmann J, Kung E. Factors affecting cardiovascular physiology in cardiothoracic surgery: implications for lumped-parameter modeling. *Front Surg*. 2019;6:62.

A.2. Describe the pathophysiology of cardiac tamponade.

The pericardium is a two-layered blind sac surrounding the atria, ventricles, proximal great vessels, venae cava, and pulmonary veins. Normally, 10 to 50 mL of fluid exists within the pericardial space. This plasma-like fluid is produced by the serous pericardium and is drained by the lymphatic system. The serous pericardium consists of a visceral portion, which is adherent to the epicardium, and a parietal layer, which is adherent to the outer, fibrous pericardium. The relatively noncompliant fibrous pericardium constrains the heart within the thoracic cavity. The normal physiologic functions of this pericardial constraint include limiting acute ventricular dilatation with increases in preload, preserving the "optimal" ventricular shape for mechanical efficiency, and maintaining the normal coupling of right ventricular (RV) and left ventricular (LV) function.

Cardiac tamponade is defined as a pathologic increase in intrapericardial pressure causing a decrease in CO. In normal conditions, intrapericardial pressure is very close to intrathoracic pressure, being slightly negative relative to atmosphere at rest. In cardiac tamponade, intrapericardial pressure increases and approaches atrial and ventricular diastolic pressures. This forms a Starling resistor system that progressively impairs diastolic cardiac filling and SV, eventually causing hypotension and shock depending on the rate of pericardial pressure increase relative to intracardiac filling pressures and the compliance of the pericardial sac (**Table 12.2**).

In defining cardiac tamponade as a state where intrapericardial pressure approaches cardiac diastolic pressures, it is important to note that cardiac tamponade can result from a decrease in cardiac filling pressures in the presence of a modest elevation in intrapericardial pressure. This has been described as "low-pressure cardiac tamponade."

Ariyarajah Y, Spodick DH. Cardiac tamponade revisited: a postmortem look at a cautionary case. *Tex Heart Inst J*. 2007;34:347-351.

Imazio M, De Ferrari GM. Cardiac tamponade: an educational review. *Eur Heart J Acute Cardiovasc Care*. 2020;10:102-109.

Saito Y, Donohue A, Attai S, et al. The syndrome of cardiac tamponade with "small" pericardial effusion. *Echocardiography*. 2008;25:321-327.

A.3. What are the common etiologies of cardiac tamponade?

Common causes of increased intrapericardial pressure include blood, exudate, transudate, and air (**Table 12.3**). In the United States, the most common cause of pericardial effusions complicated by cardiac tamponade is malignancy, followed by iatrogenic from interventional cardiologic procedures and surgical cardiotomy.

TABLE 12.2 Three Phases of Cardiac Tamponade

Phase	Pathophysiologic Events	Pressure Relationship
I	Pericardial fluid increases ventricular stiffness, increasing filling pressures.	LVEDP > RVEDP > IPP
II	Pericardial pressure approaches right-sided filling pressures, exerts Starling resistor forces on RV filling. Respirophasic variation in stroke volume appears.	LVEDP > IPP = RVEDP
III	Pericardial pressure approaches left-sided filling pressures. Hemodynamic instability is prominent.	IPP = LVEDP = RVEDP

IPP, intrapericardial pressures; LVEDP, left ventricular end-diastolic pressure; RV, right ventricular; RVEDP, right ventricular end-diastolic pressure.

TABLE 12.3 Causes of Cardiac Tamponade

Category	Differential Diagnoses
Blood	• Iatrogenic/postcardiotomy • Trauma • Aortic dissection • Anticoagulation

Exudate	• Locoregional inflammation
	  • Infectious: viral, bacterial, tuberculous
	  • Postmyocardial infarction
	  • Dressler syndrome
	• Systemic inflammation
	  • Systemic lupus erythematosus
	  • Rheumatoid arthritis
	  • Sarcoidosis
	  • Malignancy

Transudate	• Congestive heart failure • Uremia • Hypothyroidism • Radiation • Pulmonary hypertension • Hypoalbuminemia
Air	• Iatrogenic/postsurgical • Trauma • Mechanical ventilation

Adler Y, Charron P, Imazio M, et al. 2015 ESC guidelines for the diagnosis and management of pericardial diseases: the Task Force for the Diagnosis and Management of Pericardial Diseases of the European Society of Cardiology (ESC) endorsed by: the European Association for Cardio-Thoracic Surgery (EACTS). *Eur Heart J.* 2015;36:2921-2964.

Imazio M, De Ferrari GM. Cardiac tamponade: an educational review. *Eur Heart J Acute Cardiovasc Care.* 2021;10:102-109.

Lazaros G, Vlachopoulos C, Lazarou E, Tsioufis K. New approaches to management of pericardial effusions. *Curr Cardiol Rep.* 2021;23:106.

Spodick DH. Pathophysiology of cardiac tamponade. *Chest.* 1998;113:1372-1378.

A.4. What is the difference between acute and delayed cardiac tamponade?

Normal adult pericardial reserve is limited to acute increases in volume of 150 to 250 mL. Further acute increases in pericardial volume will cause dramatic changes in intrapericardial pressure. In slowly accumulating effusions, the pericardium can remodel and stretch, thereby increasing its capacitance (**Figure 12.1**). Massive, slowly accumulating pericardial effusions therefore can exist with little to no clinical evidence of cardiac tamponade.

Imazio M, Adler Y. Management of pericardial effusion. *Eur Heart J.* 2013;34:1186-1197.

Leiva EH, Carreño M, Bucheli FR, Bonfanti AC, Umaña JP, Dennis RJ. Factors associated with delayed cardiac tamponade after cardiac surgery. *Ann Card Anaesth.* 2018;21:158-166.

LeWinter MM. Pericardiectomy to treat heart failure with preserved ejection fraction: unrestrained enthusiasm? *Circ Heart Fail.* 2017;10:e003971.

A.5. What is regional cardiac tamponade?

In contrast to typical cardiac tamponade, where pericardial volume and pressure are evenly distributed around the heart, regional tamponade describes localized cardiac compression due to a loculated intrapericardial collection. This can occur as a result of hematoma formation postcardiotomy or subacutely from effusions developing around adhesions and septation of the pericardial space (**Figures 12.2** and **12.3**).

The low-pressure RA, right ventricle, and left atrium (LA) are most susceptible to postcardiotomy regional cardiac tamponade. Clot arising from right atrial bleeding typically localizes anteriorly and along the right lateral pericardial recess. Clot can also settle posteriorly behind the LA within the oblique sinus. Following cardiac surgery, the majority of effusions are anterior (especially after coronary artery bypass surgery), whereas posterolateral effusions are more commonly seen following valve replacement.

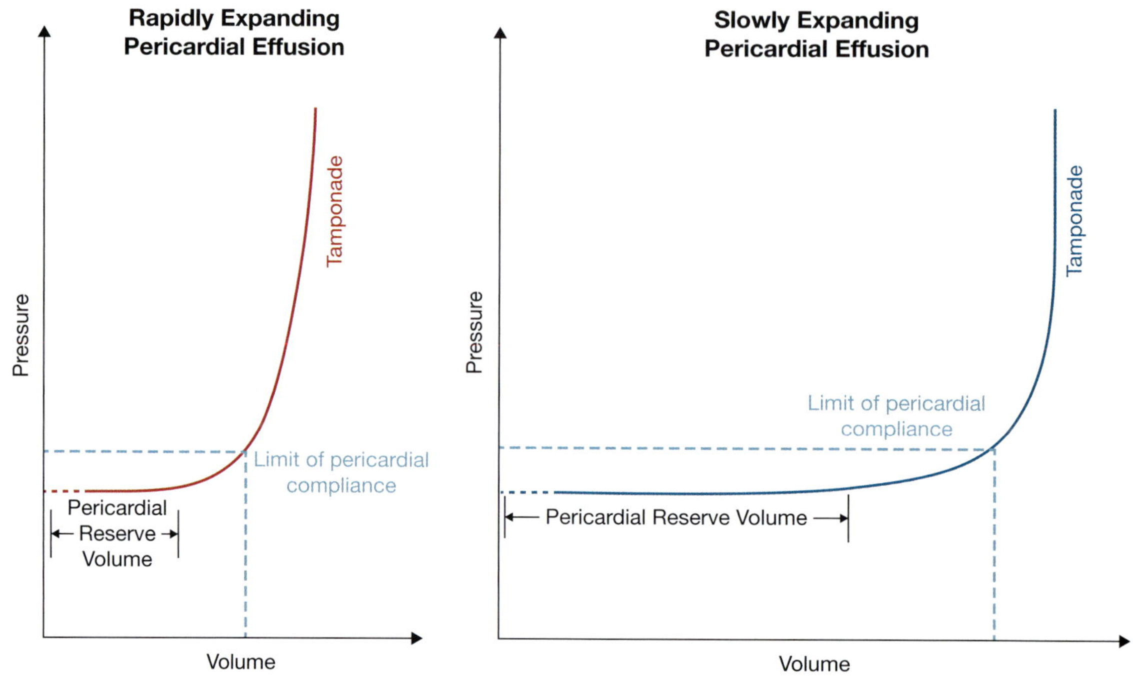

FIGURE 12.1. Acute versus delayed cardiac tamponade. In acute effusions, normal pericardium has a reserve volume of 150 to 250 mL. Until this volume is exceeded, intrapericardial pressure remains relatively low. Beyond this reserve, pericardial pressure rises until the limit of pericardial compliance is met. Once this inflection point is reached, pericardial pressure rises rapidly, which clinically corresponds to cardiac tamponade as cardiac structures become compressed. In slowly accumulating effusions, the pericardium remodels and increases its mass and surface area, thereby increasing its overall compliance. This increases pericardial reserve volume relative to rapidly growing effusions. (From Imazio M, Adler Y. Management of pericardial effusion. *Eur Heart J.* 2013;34:1186-1197. Copyright © 2012 The Author. Adapted by permission of Oxford University Press.)

Clinical signs and symptoms in regional cardiac tamponade can be subtle and atypical, corresponding to the discontinuous compression of cardiac chambers. Regional cardiac tamponade has been mistaken for congestive heart failure, acute ventricular dysfunction, septic shock, or pulmonary embolism.

Fowler NO, Gabel M, Buncher CR. Cardiac tamponade: a comparison of right versus left heart compression. *J Am Coll Cardiol.* 1988;12:187-193.

Ionescu A, Wilde P, Karsch KR. Localized pericardial tamponade: difficult echocardiographic diagnosis of a rare complication after cardiac surgery. *J Am Soc Echocardiogr.* 2001;14:1220-1223.

Russo AM, O'Connor WH, Waxman HL. Atypical presentations and echocardiographic findings in patients with cardiac tamponade occurring early and late after cardiac surgery. *Chest.* 1993;104:71-78.

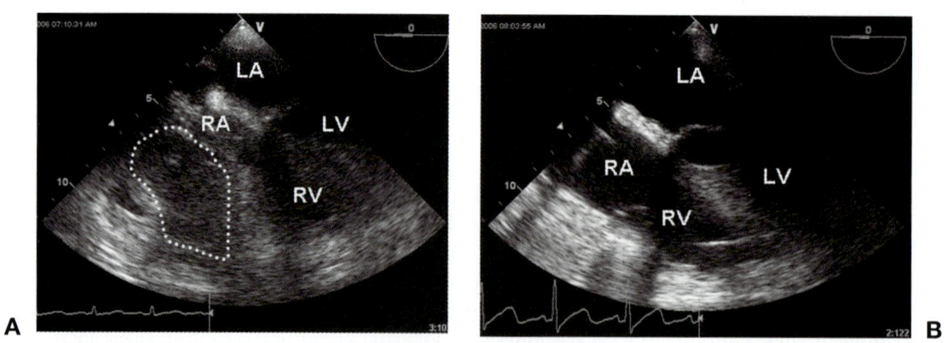

FIGURE 12.2. Acute regional pericardial effusion: right atrial compression. The heart is viewed in the midesophageal four-chamber view. **A.** A loculated pericardial clot (*dotted line*) is seen around the right atrium (RA), almost obliterating its cavity and partially compressing the right ventricle (RV). **B.** The same heart following decompression is seen. LA, left atrium; LV, left ventricle.

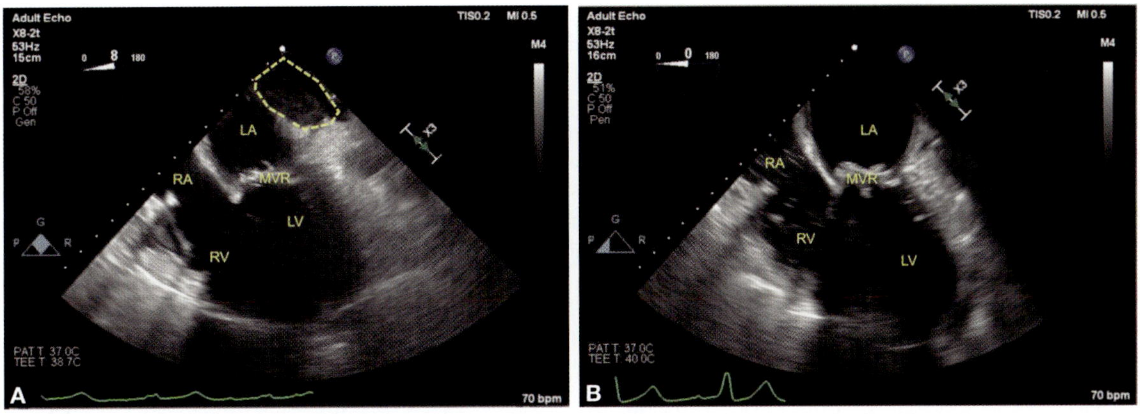

FIGURE 12.3. Acute regional pericardial effusion: left atrial compression. A and **B** show an example of regional pericardial effusion posterior to the heart, compressing the left atrium (LA), is shown. The heart is shown in a midesophageal four-chamber view, with (**A**) rotated leftward to center the view on the localized pericardial effusion (*dotted line*). In both views, the left ventricle (LV) is partially obscured by shadowing artifact from a bioprosthetic mitral valve replacement (MVR). **A.** The LA is partially compressed by the effusion. **B.** The same heart following decompression, showing restoration of LA size, is seen. Agitated blood can be seen in the right atrium (RA) and right ventricle (RV) during intravenous fluid administration.

A.6. Describe the ventricular interaction in cardiac tamponade.

RV and LV function are interdependent due to their shared septum and pericardial constraint, sometimes termed *parallel ventricular interdependence*. Under normal conditions, there is sufficient compliance in the cardiac chambers and pericardium to accommodate distension from diastolic filling of one ventricle with minimal effect on the function of the other. In cardiac tamponade, this shared septum impairs optimal diastolic filling with increasing pericardial constraint. Pericardial fluid competes with the cardiac chambers for a portion of a fixed cardiac volume. Increasing pericardial pressure increases filling pressures of all the cardiac chambers. Under these conditions, instead of free wall distension, RV filling during inspiration shifts the interventricular septum toward the left ventricle; this accommodates the diastolic volume augmented by negative pressure inspiration at the expense of LV cavity size and compliance (**Figure 12.4**).

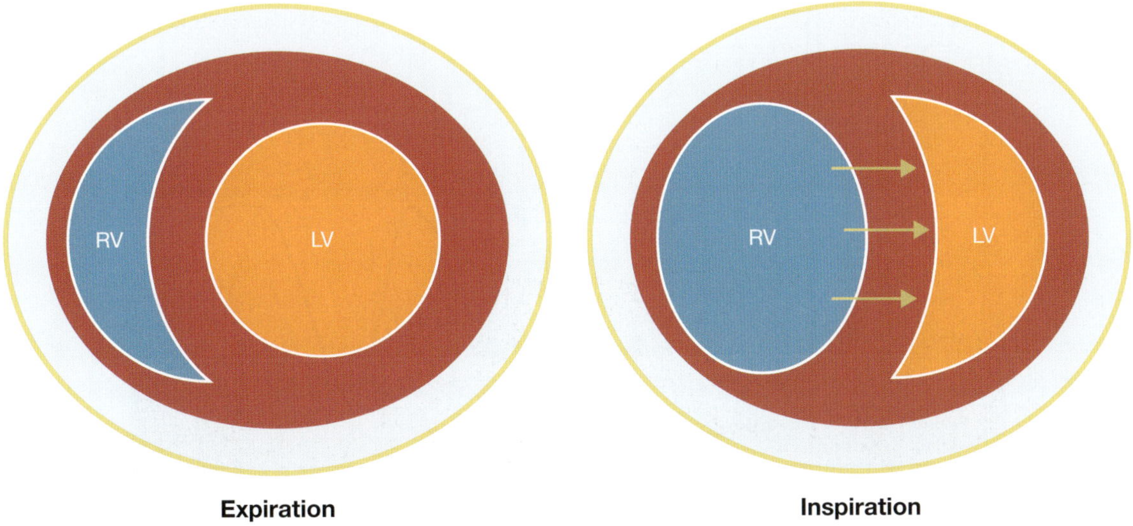

FIGURE 12.4. Parallel ventricular interdependence. In cardiac tamponade, diastolic ventricular filling is constrained by increased pericardial pressure. To accommodate increased right ventricular diastolic volume during inspiration, the interventricular septum shifts toward the left ventricle (LV). This alters LV compliance and mechanics, leading to a decrease in LV stroke volume during inspiration. RV, right ventricle.

Series ventricular interdependence refers to the dependence of LV filling on RV output. Changes in RV SV affect LV diastolic volume, albeit with a delay of several seconds as it crosses the pulmonary circulation to the left heart. This pulmonary transit time is highly variable, lasting 5 to 10 seconds in normal subjects at rest. In cardiac tamponade, the increasing dependence of RV filling on intrathoracic pressure results in similar phasic changes in pulmonary venous return and LV SV.

Taken together, cardiac tamponade exaggerates both parallel and series ventricular interdependence: to fill the right ventricle, LV filling and SV becomes compromised, and LV filling is reduced if RV SV is impaired. This augmented variability in ventricular filling can be measured with Doppler echocardiography of the transmitral and transtricuspid inflow velocities, demonstrating an increase while simultaneously reducing the other.

Depending on chronicity, size, and etiology of the cardiac tamponade (ie, fluid vs clot, regional vs global cardiac tamponade), exaggerated *atrioventricular interdependence* can develop as they become subject to worsening pericardial constraint and pressure. Normally, venous return to the atria is maximal during ventricular systole and early diastole (corresponding to the *x*-descent, *v*-wave, and *y*-descent). With cardiac tamponade, the atria fill more readily when the ventricles are small (ie, during ventricular systole) and passive atrioventricular filling becomes increasingly influenced by intrapericardial pressure as a Starling resistor. This leads to a deep *x*-descent as atrial filling occurs almost solely during ventricular systole and the loss of the early diastolic *y*-descent, both characteristic findings in cardiac tamponade (Figure 12.5). Eventually, pericardial pressure increases sharply as pericardial compliance is exhausted. This pressure first compresses the thin-walled atria, followed by the low-pressure RV, and finally the left ventricle.

Buckberg G, Hoffman JIE. Right ventricular architecture responsible for mechanical performance: unifying role of ventricular septum. *J Thorac Cardiovasc Surg*. 2014;148:3166.e4-3171.e4.

Hamzaoui O, Monnet X, Teboul JL. Pulsus paradoxus. *Eur Respir J*. 2013;42:1696-1705.

Hoit BD. Pathophysiology of the pericardium. *Prog Cardiovasc Dis*. 2017;59:341-348.

Spodick DH. Pathophysiology of cardiac tamponade. *Chest*. 1998;113:1372-1378.

A.7. How is coronary blood flow affected by cardiac tamponade?

In the absence of coronary artery disease, coronary blood flow can be reduced in cardiac tamponade due to the direct effect of pericardial pressure on the epicardium and extracardiac epicardial vessels.

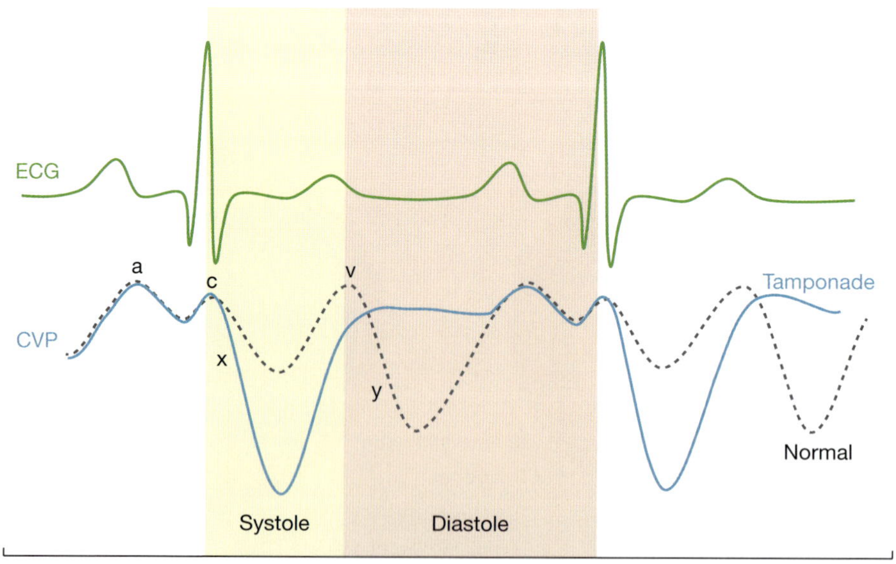

FIGURE 12.5. Central venous pressure (CVP) waveform abnormalities in cardiac tamponade. Compared with normal conditions, the CVP trace in cardiac tamponade is characterized by a deep *x*-descent, signaling increased atrial filling during ventricular systole (ie, when the ventricles are small) and a loss of the *y*-descent. The *y*-descent normally coincides with opening of the tricuspid and mitral valves. During this period of diastole, the atrium acts as a conduit between the large central veins and the ventricle with venous return following the hydrostatic pressure gradient to the ventricle. In cardiac tamponade, pericardial pressure acts as a Starling resistor to venous return on the atrium, dampening and eventually eliminating the *y*-descent as a result. ECG, electrocardiogram.

Although it has been argued that this reduction is not sufficient to cause myocardial ischemia because of a proportionate decrease in ventricular preload, the compensatory sympathetic outflow leading to tachycardia and increased contractility shifts the balance toward increasing myocardial oxygen demand. More recent reports have demonstrated a marked decline in coronary blood flow due to increased coronary vascular resistance with increasing pericardial pressures, with direct coronary arterial flow studies demonstrating decreased diastolic coronary blood flow and increased retrograde flow in systole.

Abusaid GH, Khalife WI. Reduced coronary blood flow in cardiac tamponade: mystery solved. *J Invasive Cardiol.* 2012;24:E328-E329.

Skalidis EI, Kochiadakis GE, Chrysostomakis SI, et al. Effect of pericardial pressure on human coronary circulation. *Chest.* 2000;117:910-912.

A.8. What is the Beck triad? Describe the typical signs and symptoms of cardiac tamponade.

The Beck triad, described in 1935 by Claude Beck, includes two characteristic triads for acute and chronic cardiac compression. In acute cardiac tamponade, the presence of the full triad of distended neck veins, diminished heart sounds, and hypotension is uncommon, occurring in only 10% to 40% of patients. Hypotension is present in 14% to 35% of patients, diminished heart sounds in 24% to 34%, and elevated jugular venous pressure in 53% to 88%. The most common presenting symptom in patients with symptomatic pericardial effusion requiring drainage is dyspnea (87%-88% sensitive), and the most sensitive and specific physical finding is pulsus paradoxus (98% sensitive, 83% specific with a >12 mm Hg change in pressure). Other signs and symptoms are listed in **Table 12.4**. Patients with loculated effusions or regional cardiac tamponade can present with very few or with an atypical constellation of these signs and symptoms.

The chronic cardiac compression triad consists of elevated jugular venous pressure, ascites, and diminished heart sounds. Beck described these signs in patients with tuberculous, idiopathic pericarditis, or constrictive pericarditis without effusion. The shift from hypotension to ascites reflects the longer-term restriction of venous return to the RA and RV, thereby leading to chronic passive hepatic congestion.

Hypertensive cardiac tamponade is an unusual variant thought to result from the sympathetic response to impaired cardiac filling in patients who develop cardiac tamponade over days to weeks. These patients challenge the classic aphorism of cardiac tamponade being a clinical diagnosis, with average systolic pressures of between 127 and 144 mm Hg at presentation based on six retrospective reviews including 239 patients. These patients all had echocardiographic criteria consistent with cardiac tamponade, including right atrial and RV collapse and exaggerated respiratory variation of RV and LV inflow velocities. Draining the effusion leads to normalization of blood pressure.

TABLE 12.4 Signs and Symptoms of Cardiac Tamponade

Symptoms	Dyspnea
	Fatigue
	Weakness
	Palpitations
	Orthopnea
Signs	Tachycardia
	Tachypnea
	Hypotension
	Diminished heart sounds
	Jugular venous distension
	Narrow pulse pressure
	Pulsus paradoxus
	"Unable to lie flat"

Argulian E, Herzog E, Halpern DG, et al. Paradoxical hypertension with cardiac tamponade. *Am J Cardiol.* 2012;110:1066-1069.

Argulian E, Messerli F. Misconceptions and facts about pericardial effusion and tamponade. *Am J Med.* 2013;126:858-861.

Jacob S, Sebastian JC, Cherian PK, et al. Pericardial effusion impending tamponade: a look beyond Beck's triad. *Am J Emerg Med.* 2009;27:216-219.

Roy CL, Minor MA, Brookhart MA, et al. Does this patient with a pericardial effusion have cardiac tamponade? *JAMA.* 2007;297:1810-1818.

A.9. Define pulsus paradoxus, and describe its pathophysiology.

Pulsus paradoxus describes an abnormal, exaggerated fall in arterial pressure during inspiration, conventionally defined as a fall in systolic pressure more than 10 mm Hg. Pulsus paradoxus was first described in 1873 by Adolf Kussmaul, the German pathologist who saw a "paradox" in three patients with constrictive pericarditis; their palpated pulse would disappear during inspiration and reappear during expiration, despite the uninterrupted presence of a precordial cardiac impulse.

In healthy individuals, quiet inspiration decreases intrathoracic pressure by 5 to 10 mm Hg, which is transmitted to the atria and ventricles. This augments venous return to the right heart, leading to maximal RV SV during inspiration. LV SV respiratory variation also occurs, influenced by both the lungs and the RV. During inspiration, lung expansion exerts radial traction on the pulmonary vasculature and increases its capacitance. This decreases LV filling and SV, with the reverse occurring in expiration. Changes in RV SV affect LV filling with a delay of several seconds as blood crosses the pulmonary circulation to the left heart. If both ventricles are "out of phase" with respect to pulmonary transit time, the effect of inspiration-augmented RV SV on LV filling is increased, increasing LV SV and systemic arterial pressure respiratory variation. The opposite can occur if the two ventricles are "in phase." This accounts for the respiratory variation in arterial pressure in healthy individuals with fluctuations in systolic arterial pressure of 10 mm Hg or less. This is more prominent when both ventricles are preload sensitive (ie, on the steep part of the Starling curve when the LV is constrained and made small by cardiac tamponade).

In cardiac tamponade, elevated pericardial pressure is transmitted to all cardiac chambers, increasing their filling pressures relative to extrapericardial structures including the vena cava. Furthermore, increasing pericardial constraint on the cardiac chambers exaggerates parallel and series ventricular interdependence. Both factors lead to an augmentation of the phasic rise and fall in LV SV.

Pulsus paradoxus is not a sensitive or specific sign of cardiac tamponade. It can also be seen in patients with respiratory distress due to increased negative intrathoracic pressures during inspiration, constrictive pericarditis, and RV failure. It can be absent, even in cardiac tamponade, in patients who cannot generate negative intrathoracic pressure (eg, neuromuscular disease, chest wall trauma) or in patients with aortic regurgitation or an atrial septal defect. Patients who are ventilated with positive pressure can display a "reversed" pulsus paradoxus, that is, an exaggerated increase in systolic arterial pressure with inspiration due to increased RV afterload causing a leftward septal shift during positive inspiratory pressure.

Ramachandran D, Luo C, Ma TS, Clark JW Jr. Using a human cardiovascular-respiratory model to characterize cardiac tamponade and pulsus paradoxus. *Theor Biol Med Model.* 2009 6;6:15.

Swami A, Spodick DH. Pulsus paradoxus in cardiac tamponade: a pathophysiologic continuum. *Clin Cardiol.* 2003;26:215-217.

Wong FW. Pulsus paradoxus in ventilated and non-ventilated patients. *Dynamics.* 2007;18:16-18.

A.10. What is the Kussmaul sign? Is this finding consistent with cardiac tamponade physiology?

The Kussmaul sign describes an abnormal rise or absence of a fall in jugular venous pressure with negative pressure inspiration. It is typically quantified as a less than 5 mm Hg fall in inspiratory right atrial pressure. It is classically associated with constrictive pericarditis, but can be seen in conditions associated with restricted right-sided filling including tricuspid stenosis and RV dysfunction.

Some controversy exists as to whether Kussmaul sign can be present in cardiac tamponade. If defined solely as a pathologic *rise* in jugular venous pressure with negative pressure inspiration, then Kussmaul sign cannot be present in cardiac tamponade unless there is concurrent constriction from an abnormal pericardium, pericardial clot, or adhesions. The difference between cardiac tamponade (assuming free-flowing intrapericardial fluid) and constrictive physiology is the influence of intrathoracic pressure on the intracardiac filling pressures. In constrictive pericarditis, changes in intrathoracic pressure are not well transmitted through the abnormally thickened pericardium. This effectively disassociates the cardiac chamber pressures from intrathoracic pressure changes. The RA and RV, invested within a constrictive pericardium, have abnormally high filling pressures with little to no respirophasic variation. During the rapid filling phase of diastole, right atrial and RV pressures equalize rapidly as they encounter pericardial constraint, and venous return from the inferior vena cava (IVC) and superior vena cava (SVC) compete for entry into the high-pressure RA. Because IVC inflow is favored over that from the SVC due to augmentation by transdiaphragmatic pressure, jugular venous pressure rises due to constricted SVC inflow. This causes the characteristic, paradoxical rise in jugular venous pressure of the Kussmaul sign.

In cardiac tamponade, respiratory changes in intrathoracic pressure are transmitted to the intrapericardial fluid. Right atrial and RV pressures fall together with intrathoracic pressure during spontaneous inspiration despite the presence of cardiac tamponade, thereby augmenting the gradient for venous return from both the SVC and IVC. This results in a fall in jugular venous pressure with inspiration.

Johnson SK, Naidu RK, Ostopowicz RC, et al. Adolf Kussmaul: distinguished clinician and medical pioneer. *Clin Med Res*. 2009;7:107-112.

Talreja DR, Nishimura RA, Oh JK, et al. Constrictive pericarditis in the modern era: novel criteria for diagnosis in the cardiac catheterization laboratory. *J Am Coll Cardiol*. 2008;51:315-319.

A.11. Which medical conditions mimic cardiac tamponade?

Cardiac tamponade is the pathologic increase in intrapericardial volume and pressure that impairs diastolic filling and CO. It is often classified as a form of "obstructive shock," which is clinically characterized by hemodynamic compromise with signs of elevated filling pressures and other evidence of great vessel obstruction or cardiac compression. Other causes of obstructive shock include pulmonary embolism, tension pneumothorax, dynamic ventricular inflow or outflow obstruction (eg, from asymmetrical septal hypertrophy, hyperdynamic mid-cavitary ventricular obstruction, or cardiac myxoma), and effusive constrictive pericarditis. An unusual cause of cardiac tamponade is a large pleural effusion, which can cause clinical and echocardiographic findings of cardiac tamponade in the presence of a small "low-pressure" pericardial effusion. Animal studies show that increasing intrapleural fluid and pleural pressure is transmitted to the pericardial sac, which then compresses the heart. In this situation, only thoracentesis will relieve cardiac tamponade.

Cardiogenic shock, and RV failure in particular, can have similar signs and symptoms to cardiac tamponade, including jugular venous distension, pulsus paradoxus, dyspnea, and hypotension. The presence of fever, especially in inflammatory pericarditis and cardiac tamponade, can confound the diagnosis. However, sepsis typically presents as hyperdynamic, vasodilatory shock, whereas cardiac tamponade is notable for low SV and vasoconstriction.

Saito Y, Donohue A, Attai S, et al. The syndrome of cardiac tamponade with "small" pericardial effusion. *Echocardiography*. 2008;25:321-327.

Traylor JJ, Chan K, Wong I, et al. Large pleural effusions producing signs of cardiac tamponade resolved by thoracentesis. *Am J Cardiol*. 2002;89:106-108.

Vaska K, Wann LS, Sagar K, et al. Pleural effusion as a cause of right ventricular diastolic collapse. *Circulation*. 1992;86:609-617.

B. Preoperative Evaluation and Preparation

B.1. Interpret and explain the pathophysiologic basis for this patient's hemodynamic findings.

This patient is normotensive but tachycardic, which together with her physical findings suggests a compensated shock state. This is confirmed by her low CO and high calculated systemic vascular resistance (SVR) (**Table 12.5**). The differential diagnoses for low SV include hypovolemia, impaired LV systolic and diastolic function and/or RV contractility, and obstruction of the heart or great vessels by pericardial fluid or embolism. PAC data can assist in narrowing the diagnosis, although changes in measured pressures do not always translate to changes in intracardiac volume.

The patient's CVP is markedly elevated, which can be a result of potential intracardiac or extracardiac pathology. In the absence of significant tricuspid valve stenosis or regurgitation, intracardiac causes include hypervolemia (unlikely, given this patient's clinical presentation) and RV dysfunction from ischemia or outflow obstruction. This dysfunction increases RV end-diastolic pressure (EDP) and leads to a corresponding rise in venous filling pressures. Extracardiac causes of elevated CVP include extrinsic cardiac compression by pericardial or intrapleural conditions, including cardiac tamponade, large pleural effusion(s) and tension pneumothorax. It is important to note that in cases of extrinsic compression, the

TABLE 12.5 Measured and Calculated Hemodynamic Parameters

Measured Parameters	Patient Data	
Heart rate (HR, bpm)	120	
Systemic arterial pressure (BP, mm Hg)	115/66	
Pulmonary arterial pressure (mm Hg)	55/21	
Central venous pressure (CVP, mm Hg)	23	
Pulmonary artery occlusion pressure (PAOP, mm Hg)	14	
CO (L/min)	2.7	
Calculated Parameters	**Patient Data**	**Equation**
Stroke volume (SV, mL)	22.5	SV = CO/HR
Mean arterial pressure (MAP, mm Hg)	82.3	MAP = dBP + 1/3 PP
Systemic vascular resistance (SVR, dynes/sec/cm^5)	1,758	SVR = ([MAP − CVP]/CO) × 80
Pulmonary vascular resistance (PVR, dynes/sec/cm^5)	543	PVR = ([mPAP − PAOP]/CO) × 80

CO, cardiac output; dBP, diastolic systemic blood pressure; mPAP, mean pulmonary arterial pressure; PP, systemic pulse pressure.

CVP is measuring the intracardiac pressure *and* the pressure applied to the RA (eg, a hypovolemic patient with a transmural right atrial pressure of 3 mm Hg can have a measured CVP of 23 mm Hg once 20 mm Hg of pressure is applied to the RA, creating a false impression of the patient's true filling pressures).

The patient's PA pressure is elevated. A PAOP less than 15 mm Hg and elevated diastolic pulmonary gradient points to a precapillary cause, and is confirmed by the elevated calculated pulmonary vascular resistance (PVR) (**Table 12.5**). In this patient, the most likely causes are long-standing pulmonary vascular remodeling from chronic mitral disease and pulmonary atelectasis from dyspnea and altered respiratory mechanics.

The PAOP is a surrogate measure for left atrial pressure (LAP) and can inform about LV filling as well as LV and mitral valve function. This patient's PAOP is normal and makes prosthetic mitral valve dysfunction from obstruction or regurgitation unlikely. As with CVP, caveats apply in the interpretation of PAOP and LAP concerning LV volume status. Furthermore, any alteration in the thick-walled LV compliance will affect the degree to which LAP represents LV preload, which is ultimately represented by LV end-diastolic volume (EDV). For example, acute ischemia will decrease LV compliance, which would result in a higher EDV for the same EDP.

Taken together, the patient's clinical and hemodynamic findings suggest a low CO state due to cardiac tamponade and/or RV dysfunction from ischemia or increased RV afterload due to embolism. Concurrent LV dysfunction cannot be excluded based on PAC data alone. Echocardiography can assist with further refinement of the differential diagnoses by defining RV and LV function, relative atrial pressures, and the presence of pericardial fluid.

Note the absence of "equalization of pressures" in this patient, that is CVP, PA diastolic, and PAOP are not within 5 mm Hg of each other. This does not exclude a diagnosis of cardiac tamponade, as the pericardium is often left open in cardiac surgery patients. Equalization of pressures presumes that intrapericardial pressure is equally distributed through the pericardial sac. This is usually a late finding when compensatory mechanisms are almost exhausted in patients with an intact pericardium, and might not be seen at all in patients where the pericardium is not intact.

Goldstein JA. Introduction to Pericardial Disease. In: Kern MJ, Lim MJ, Goldstein JA, eds. *Hemodynamic Rounds: Interpretation of Cardiac Physiology From Pressure Waveform Analysis*. 4th ed. Wiley-Blackwell; 2018:269.

Magder S. Invasive hemodynamic monitoring. *Crit Care Clin*. 2015;31:67-87.

Opitz CF, Hoeper MM, Gibbs SR, et al. Pre-capillary, combined, and post-capillary pulmonary hypertension: a pathophysiological continuum. *J Am Coll Cardiol*. 2016;68:368-378.

B.2. How would you optimize this patient's cardiovascular status before definitive diagnosis and treatment?

The key resuscitation goals before definitive management are:

- Optimize CO (which is determined by HR and SV), and
- Maintain adequate perfusion pressure to critical organs (ie, heart, brain, kidneys).

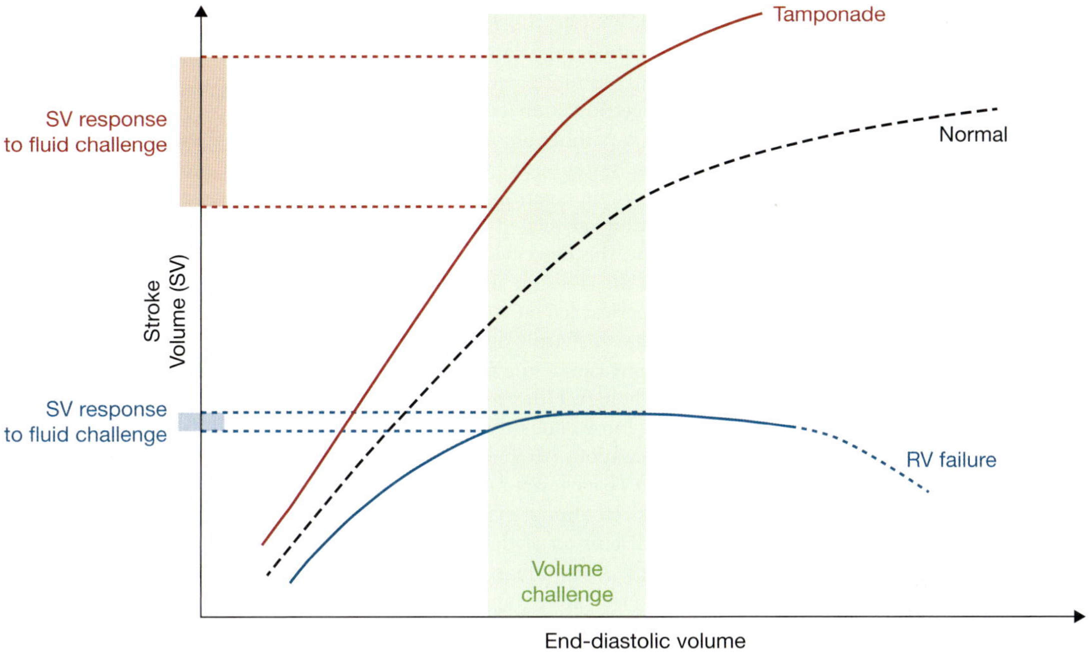

FIGURE 12.6. Predicted response to volume challenge in cardiac tamponade compared with right ventricular (RV) dysfunction. This figure shows two different Frank-Starling curves referenced to a hypothetical normal curve. In cardiac tamponade, the right ventricle is underfilled and hyperdynamic. This is in contrast to the curve in RV dysfunction, where the decreased slope and early plateau reflects its depressed inotropic state. Applying the same volume to these two models leads to a large SV response in cardiac tamponade, but a minimal change in RV dysfunction, and, in this example, pushes the right ventricle into failure.

Broadly, the hemodynamic goals for this patient are "full, tight and fast." This patient requires SV correction to increase CO; however, without a clear etiology for her low CO state, this should be approached cautiously. This high CVP is due to either cardiac tamponade or RV dysfunction; the effect of aggressive volume administration can either improve SV or precipitate RV failure because both conditions exist on different points of the Frank-Starling curve (**Figure 12.6**).

The distinction between cardiac tamponade from RV failure can be made with echocardiography to immediately and safely administer volume to maintain adequate cardiac preload.

A vasoconstrictor or a positive inotrope with vasoconstrictor properties should be initiated to maintain afterload (**Figure 12.6**). The choice of vasoactive agent should take into account the patient's clinical trajectory as well. Norepinephrine and epinephrine are titratable, maintain or increase HR and have short half-lives. Dopamine, however, is associated with severe arrhythmias and increased mortality when used in cardiogenic shock at higher doses (>2 µg/kg/min). The inodilators dobutamine and milrinone decrease SVR and PVR and can improve myocardial performance in a failing ventricle, but can also compromise organ perfusion. Titrating norepinephrine infusion (0.05-0.5 µg/kg/min) or low-dose infusion of epinephrine (0.02-0.05 µg/kg/min) might confer the greatest benefit, while minimizing unexpected afterload reduction and dose-related tachyarrhythmia from dobutamine.

Together with preload optimization, a systemic mean arterial pressure (MAP) of at least 60 to 65 mm Hg should be targeted to maintain adequate cerebral and renal perfusion. Myocardial perfusion in this patient is compromised due to depressed coronary blood flow, preexisting tachycardia, and potential cardiac tamponade. Any attempts to lower HR in an effort to reduce myocardial oxygen demand without correcting preload will risk a further decline in CO that will correspondingly lower all organ blood flow, including the heart.

Carmona P, Mateo E, Casanovas I, et al. Management of cardiac tamponade after cardiac surgery. *J Cardiothorac Vasc Anesth*. 2012;26:302-311.

De Backer D, Biston P, Devriendt J, et al. Comparison of dopamine and norepinephrine in the treatment of shock. *New Engl J Med*. 2010;362:779-789.

Grocott HP, Gulati H, Sadeesh S, Mackensen, GB. Anesthesia and the patient with pericardial disease. *Can J Anaesth*. 2011; 58:952-966.

Kline JA, Hall CL, Jones AE, et al. Randomized trial of inhaled nitric oxide to treat acute pulmonary embolism: the iNOPE trial. *Am Heart J*. 2017;186:100-110.

B.3. What are the chest radiographic findings in cardiac tamponade?

On standard posteroanterior chest radiography, cardiomegaly is a common finding in patients with pericardial effusion, especially of 200 mL or more; overall sensitivity is 89%. Evolving cardiomegaly in the absence of pulmonary vascular congestion supports the diagnosis of effusion over cardiomyopathy and associated congestive heart failure. A pathognomonic finding on an erect chest radiograph for massive effusions, often more than 1 L, is the "water bottle" heart. This reflects the dependent distribution of fluid within the pericardial space when upright, tapering up toward the pericardial reflection at the level of the proximal great vessels. Another finding associated with pericardial effusion is the "Oreo cookie" or "fat pad" sign on lateral chest radiography. This describes a vertical radiopaque line sandwiched by two vertical radiolucent stripes located between the sternum and RV border. The opaque line represents pericardial fluid separating epicardial fat from pericardial fat within the pericardial space. In tension pneumopericardium, air surrounding the heart creates a sharply delineated air pericardiogram.

Cardiac computerized tomography can define not just the presence of a pericardial effusion but also cardiac anatomy and pericardial pathology. However, its utility in a patient with unstable hemodynamics is limited and usually not practical. Intravenous contrast enhances pericardial inflammation and hemopericardium including active extravasation. Attenuation values of pericardial fluid can aid in characterizing the type of effusion. Transudates have lower radiodensity than exudates, which in turn are less dense than blood or clots. Other computerized tomography findings consistent with cardiac tamponade include compression of cardiac chambers, distension of the venae cavae, and reflux of contrast into the IVC or azygos vein suggesting impaired right-sided filling.

Two-dimensional and Doppler echocardiography are considered first-line imaging for cardiac tamponade. Advantages include a high sensitivity for detecting pericardial fluid and any related mass effect, the ability to assess cardiac function and filling patterns, portability, and the lack of ionizing radiation. However, the utility of transthoracic echocardiography is limited in postcardiac surgery patients due to sonographic artifact from sternal wires, chest tubes, and surgical dressings.

Bogaert J, Francone M. Pericardial disease: value of CT and MR imaging. *Radiology*. 2013;267:340-356.

Kearns MJ, Walley KR. Tamponade: hemodynamic and echocardiographic diagnosis. *Chest*. 2018;153:1266-1275.

Restrepo CS, Lemos DF, Lemos JA, et al. Imaging findings in cardiac tamponade with emphasis on CT. *Radiographics*. 2007;27:1595-1610.

B.4. A limited bedside transthoracic echocardiogram is performed, demonstrating a layer of clotted blood anterior to the right atrium (RA) and ventricle. What echocardiographic findings support the diagnosis of cardiac tamponade?

It is important to emphasize that cardiac tamponade is a *clinical diagnosis,* characterized by clinical deterioration (shortness of breath in the supine or even sitting position, worsening shock with low SV) and supported by echocardiographic findings.

A key concept when interpreting imaging in a patient with suspected cardiac tamponade is that the size of a pericardial effusion does not correspond to the severity of clinical symptoms; a small acute pericardial effusion can cause life-threatening cardiac tamponade but remain occult on imaging. For example, the presence of mediastinal clot is an anatomical finding that might simply reflect a postsurgical state. Echocardiographic findings that correspond to the pathophysiology of cardiac tamponade in this patient include the following:

a. *Increased intrapericardial pressures causing diastolic collapse of the atria and/or right ventricle.* The RA is most sensitive to compression just after the atrial kick (ie, P wave on electrocardiogram [ECG]), when atrial pressure is lowest (**Figure 12.7**). The period of collapse extends further through the cardiac cycle with increasing pericardial pressures, so that right atrial collapse exceeding one-third of the cardiac cycle is nearly 100% sensitive and specific for cardiac tamponade. The RV, with a higher chamber pressure than the atria, is less susceptible to compression, but the finding of RV diastolic collapse remains a highly specific sign of cardiac tamponade. The RV is most sensitive to compression in early diastole (ie, after T wave on ECG), when its chamber pressure is lowest.
b. *Exaggerated ventricular interdependence.* Doppler interrogation of mitral and tricuspid inflow velocities demonstrates increased RV filling and decreased LV filling during spontaneous inspiration. This increased RV filling causes a ventricular septal "bounce" toward the LV as RV free wall expansion meets pericardial constraint. Pulsed-wave Doppler of tricuspid inflow shows an increase in peak E-wave velocity by 40% compared with expiration, whereas mitral inflow shows a 25% inspiratory decrease in peak E-wave velocity (**Figure 12.8**). Venous inflow to the RA can also be interrogated via pulsed-wave Doppler of the hepatic vein, which initially shows systolic blunting of systolic velocities, with increased respiratory variation in diastolic velocity best seen by transesophageal echocardiography

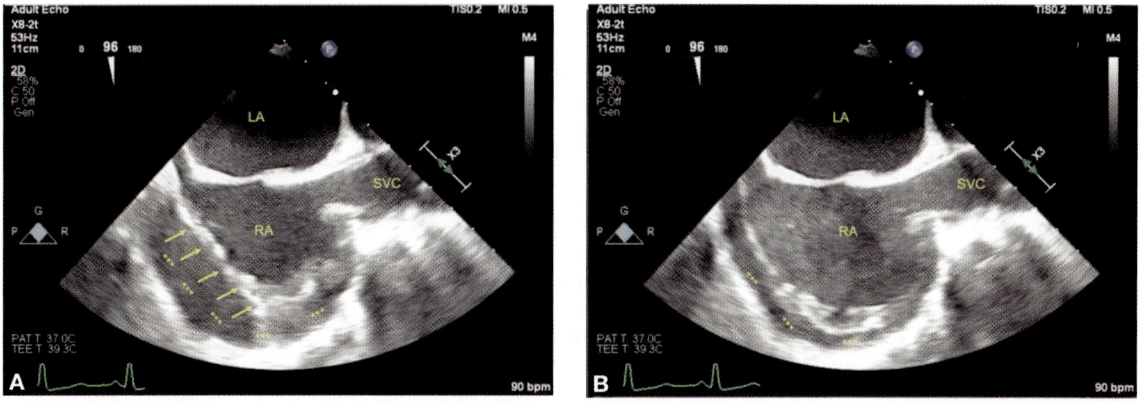

FIGURE 12.7. Right atrium (RA) collapse from early cardiac tamponade. The figures show the RA in the midesophageal bicaval view in the same patient with an acute pericardial effusion (labeled with *asterisks*). **A.** The RA is compressed by the effusion (*arrows*) in early ventricular systole as denoted by the ECG, corresponding approximately to the *x*-descent on a CVP waveform when the RA is most susceptible to compression. **B.** The RA in late ventricular systole is seen, corresponding to a point just before the V-wave, when the atrium is at its fullest just before tricuspid valve opening. LA, left atrium; SVC, superior vena cava.

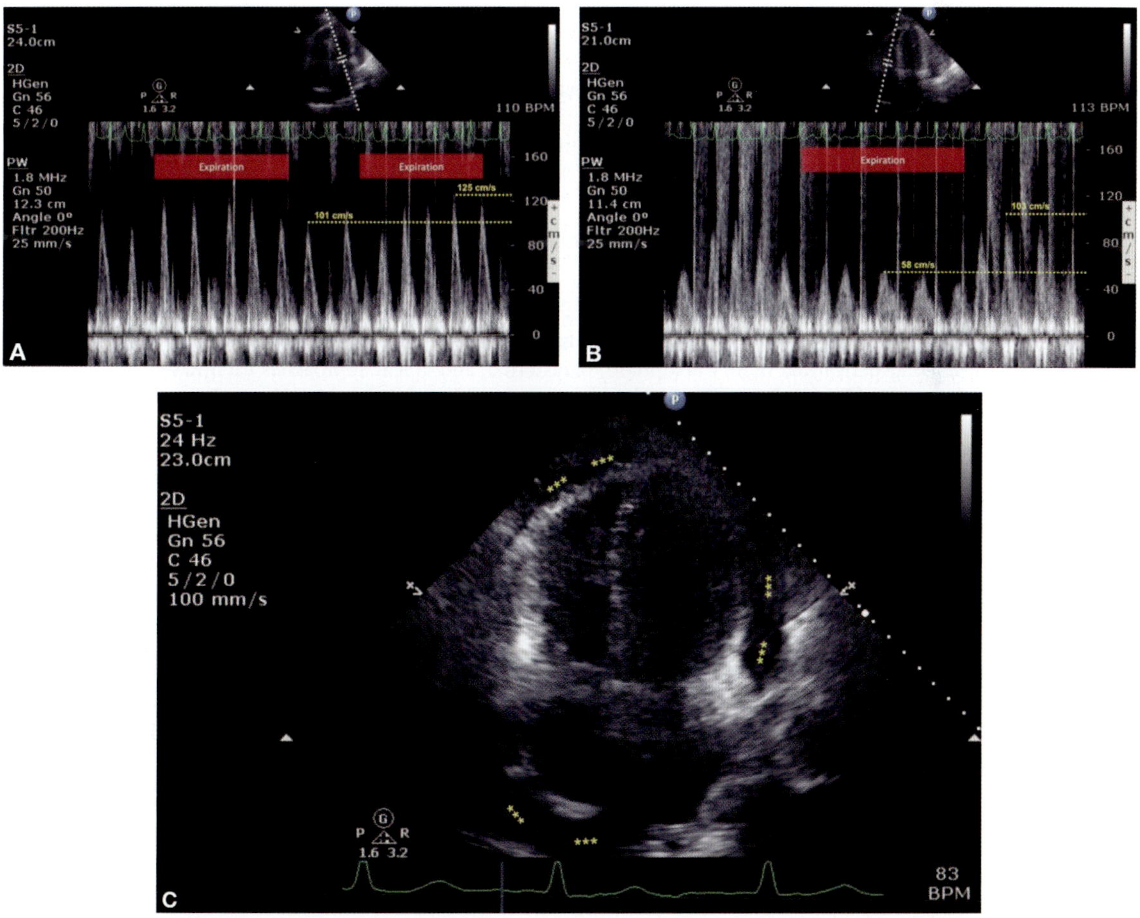

FIGURE 12.8. Exaggerated ventricular interdependence. A and **B** show pulsed-wave Doppler interrogation of transmitral and transtricuspid velocities obtained during a transthoracic echocardiographic study in a patient with suspected cardiac tamponade. The patient is breathing spontaneously; although there is no respirogram on the original images, the patient's marked sinus arrhythmia clearly defines inspiratory and expiratory phases. During negative pressure inspiration, **A** demonstrates a 25% decrease in transmitral E-wave velocities, whereas **B** shows a more than 45% increase in transtricuspid E-wave velocities. This exaggerated, reciprocal change in ventricular filling is a hallmark of cardiac tamponade and constrictive physiology. **C** shows an apical four-chamber view of this patient's heart, demonstrating a large effusion outside the right and left ventricles as well as a deep pool surrounding the right atrium (RA) (*labeled by asterisks*). Although not evident on this still image, interventricular septal "bounce" was prominent.

(TEE) or CVP tracing (**Figure 12.5**). In critical cardiac tamponade, diastolic velocities can be near-absent except during spontaneous inspiration or mechanical expiration.

c. *Decreased volume within cardiac chambers*. This is suggested by decreased LV cavity size and exaggerated interatrial septal motion (in the presence of a high measured CVP) reflecting low transmural LA and RA pressures and abnormal ventricular filling patterns due to increased interdependence. The IVC can be distended due to obstructed venous return.

Carmona P, Mateo E, Casanovas I, et al. Management of cardiac tamponade after cardiac surgery. *J Cardiothorac Vasc Anesth*. 2012;26:302-311.

Ellenbroek DFJ, van Kessel L, Compagner W, et al. Diagnostic performance of echocardiography to predict cardiac tamponade after cardiac surgery. *Eur J Cardiothorac Surg*. 2022;62:ezab468.

Gillam LD, Guyer DE, Gibson TC, et al. Hydrodynamic compression of the right atrium: a new echocardiographic sign of cardiac tamponade. *Circulation*. 1983;68:294-301.

B.5. What additional information should be obtained from a limited echocardiographic study?

Once the diagnosis of cardiac tamponade is established, a focused assessment of concurrent conditions by an appropriately trained echocardiographer is indicated as long as it does not delay clinical stabilization and definitive management. The RV and LV should be assessed for size and systolic function. A distended RV with or without worsening tricuspid regurgitation raises concern for outflow obstruction or systolic dysfunction. Regional wall motion abnormalities might be apparent if there is active myocardial ischemia. The mitral valve prosthesis should be evaluated for malfunction using color flow Doppler, which might reveal stenosis or intravalvular regurgitation from leaflet dysfunction or paravalvular leak from suture line dehiscence.

Carmona P, Mateo E, Casanovas I, et al. Management of cardiac tamponade after cardiac surgery. *J Cardiothorac Vasc Anesth*. 2012;26:302-311.

Labovitz AJ, Noble VE, Bierig M, et al. Focused cardiac ultrasound in the emergent setting: a consensus statement of the American Society of Echocardiography and American College of Emergency Physicians. *J Am Soc Echocardiogr*. 2010;23:1225-1230.

B.6. Describe the procedures for treating cardiac tamponade. What are the clinical indications for each approach?

Pericardial decompression can be performed percutaneously or surgically. Percutaneous echocardiographically guided catheter decompression is the treatment of choice in patients with nonloculated, free-flowing pericardial fluid. Subxiphoid, parasternal, and apical approaches each have advantages and disadvantages (**Table 12.6**). Existing literature and guidelines advocate taking the approach with the maximal effusion depth on ultrasound to minimize the risk of cardiac puncture. Percutaneous options are more likely to be appropriate in delayed cardiac tamponade, several days or weeks after cardiac surgery when pericardial blood has liquefied. It is unlikely to be appropriate for this patient because there is a high likelihood of compression from clotted blood on imaging.

In patients with an intact pericardium and free-flowing pericardial fluid, surgical decompression can be performed in conjunction with a limited pericardiectomy, opening a drainage "window" to the pleural space to prevent recurrence. Minor pericardial adhesions can be manually divided and loculated effusions drained. Subxiphoid, transthoracic via anterior mini-thoracotomy, and thoracoscopic approaches have been described. The subxiphoid approach does not technically create a "pericardial window"; rather, it

TABLE 12.6 Approaches to Pericardiocentesis

Approach	Insertion Site	Approach-Specific Complications
Subxiphoid	Between xiphoid process and left costal margin	Peritoneal injury
Apical	Near apex beat, at fifth to seventh intercostal space in the anterior axillary line	Left pneumothorax
Parasternal	Fifth intercostal space, left sternal margin	Pneumothorax Internal mammary artery injury

Adapted from De Carlini CC, Maggiolini S. Pericardiocentesis in cardiac tamponade: indications and practical aspects. *e-J Cardiol Pract*. 2017;15. https://www.escardio.org/Journals/E-Journal-of-Cardiology-Practice/Volume-15/Pericardiocentesis-in-cardiac-tamponade-indications-and-practical-aspects provokes inflammatory fusion of the pericardium to the epicardium, thereby obliterating the potential space for recurrence. In unstable patients, only subxiphoid and anterior thoracotomy approaches are suitable. An important advantage of the subxiphoid approach is that it can be performed under local anesthesia and conscious sedation in anatomically suitable patients (eg, not obese, absence of ascites) who are otherwise too unstable for induction of general anesthesia. Local anesthesia for the anterior thoracotomy approach has also been described but might be poorly tolerated because it requires dissection through the pectoralis muscles and intercostal spaces. After cardiac surgery, a limited sternal reopening under local anesthesia and conscious sedation might be tolerated and can confer some physiologic benefit prior to definitive exploration. However, most patients within this population are typically not candidates for limited rescue techniques and will require full sternotomy to evacuate clotted blood, drain residual fluid, and identify the source of ongoing bleeding.

Adler Y, Charron P, Imazio M, et al. 2015 ESC guidelines for the diagnosis and management of pericardial diseases: the Task Force for the Diagnosis and Management of Pericardial Diseases of the European Society of Cardiology (ESC) endorsed by: the European Association for Cardio-Thoracic Surgery (EACTS). *Eur Heart J*. 2015;36:2921-2964.

De Carlini CC, Maggiolini S. Pericardiocentesis in cardiac tamponade: indications and practical aspects. *e-J Cardiol Pract*. 2017;15.

Langdon SE, Seery K, Kulik A. Contemporary outcomes after pericardial window surgery: impact of operative technique. *J Cardiothorac Surg*. 2016;11:73.

Sugimoto JT, Little AG, Ferguson MK, et al. Pericardial window: mechanisms of efficacy. *Ann Thorac Surg*. 1990;50:442-445.

B.7. Having made the diagnosis of cardiac tamponade, what additional investigations are required before surgery?

This patient has cardiac tamponade likely arising from postcardiac surgery bleeding. Although her vital signs are adequate, she is at risk for decompensation and should undergo a focused, expedited workup so that surgical treatment is not delayed. Point-of-care blood tests such as arterial blood gas (ABG) analysis and rotational thromboelastometry (ROTEM) or thromboelastography (TEG) can provide rapid, relevant information to guide preoperative preparation. An ABG can reveal a low pH and/or elevated lactate from hypoperfusion, gas exchange abnormalities, electrolyte derangements, and anemia. ROTEM or TEG provides real-time information on coagulation factor activity and clotting kinetics. Formal laboratory investigations should include a complete blood count, coagulation profile, and blood type and cross-match. The presence of anemia, thrombocytopenia, or coagulation abnormalities guides the type and amount of blood products required, and should be immediately available in the operating room before surgery. A baseline ECG can provide additional information if the suspicion for ischemia is high and provide supportive information such as low-voltage QRS complexes, electrical alternans, and RV strain. Although radiographic findings were discussed earlier, a chest radiograph or computed tomography (CT) is unlikely to add diagnostic value in this patient and should not delay surgery unless there is a strong clinical indication.

Carmona P, Mateo E, Casanovas I, et al. Management of cardiac tamponade after cardiac surgery. *J Cardiothorac Vasc Anesth*. 2012;26:302-311.

B.8. Explain the technical and physiologic principles behind rotational thromboelastometry.

Rotational thromboelastometry measures the viscoelastic properties of blood. Citrated blood is introduced into a cuvette together with an activator, which is heated to 30 °C to 40 °C. A pin with a rotating axis is suspended into the cuvette during the test, and as the blood becomes more viscous, pin rotation is impeded. This impedance is detected by an optical detector system. The time course of changing viscoelasticity is plotted graphically and numerically. The parameters defining a typical assay correlate to the events of coagulation as described by the cell-based model of hemostasis as summarized in **Table 12.7**.

ROTEM *delta* (Werfen North America) and ROTEM *sigma coagulation testing* (Instrumentation Laboratories) are two commercially available devices that can perform up to four tests concurrently. ROTEM *delta* requires manual pipetting of blood samples and test reagents, whereas ROTEM *sigma* is a fully automated point-of-care system that uses a cartridge with integrated freeze-dried reagents. Depending on the activator reagents used, assays targeting specific components of the coagulation cascade can be performed. The INTEM reagent contains ellagic acid and phospholipid, which produces contact activation of the intrinsic pathway. EXTEM contains tissue factor and preferentially activates

TABLE 12.7 Rotational Thromboelastometry Numerical Parameters

Parameter	Definition	Physiologic Correlate
Clotting time (CT)	Time for trace to reach 2 mm amplitude	Clot initiation phase
Clot formation time (CFT)	Time for trace to increase from 2 to 20 mm	Clot amplification and propagation phase
Amplitude 10 min (A10)	Trace amplitude 10 min after CT	Fibrin-platelet interaction via glycoprotein IIb/IIIA receptors
Maximum clot firmness (MCF)	Maximum amplitude (MA) of the trace, when test is run for 20 min	
Lysis Index 30 (LI30)	Percentage reduction in amplitude 30 min after MA is reached	Plasmin, thrombin-activatable fibrinolysis inhibitor (TAFI) and plasminogen activator inhibitor (PAI) activity

the extrinsic pathway. FIBTEM also activates the extrinsic pathway but contains cytochalasin D, which blocks platelet contribution to clot formation, thus isolating the fibrinogen contribution to clot formation. APTEM contains aprotinin, an antifibrinolytic, and will "correct" an EXTEM assay in the presence of hyperfibrinolysis.

Dias JD, Haney EI, Mathew BA, et al. New-generation thromboelastography: comprehensive evaluation of citrated and heparinized blood sample storage effect on clot-forming variables. *Arch Pathol Lab Med.* 2017;141:569-577.

Erdoes G, Koster A, Levy JH. Viscoelastic coagulation testing: use and current limitations in perioperative decision-making. *Anesthesiology.* 2021;135:342-349.

Schenk B, Görlinger K, Treml B, et al. A comparison of the new ROTEM® sigma with its predecessor, the ROTEMdelta. *Anaesthesia.* 2019;74:348-356.

Whiting D, DiNardo JA. TEG and ROTEM: technology and clinical applications. *Am J Hematol.* 2014;89:228-232.

B.9. A rotational thromboelastometry was performed, and a 10-minute analysis reveals the following results (see Figure 12.9 and Table 12.8). How do you interpret this information?

There are significant derangements across the EXTEM, INTEM, FIBTEM, and APTEM assays. The EXTEM and INTEM clotting time are prolonged, which occurs in the presence of low coagulation factors (ie, usually <30% of normal levels). The EXTEM and INTEM A10 are decreased, indicating inadequate clot firmness. This can be due to a lack of platelets or fibrinogen. Because the FIBTEM A10 is also decreased, fibrinogen deficiency is implicated. Platelet deficiency or dysfunction might coexist, as the EXTEM and INTEM A10 are below the lower reference range, and platelet function contributes ~80% of clot amplitude. The APTEM does not significantly differ from EXTEM, which suggests that hyperfibrinolysis is unlikely. However, fibrinolysis might not be apparent at 10 minutes. The assays should continue running for at least 30 minutes to more fully assess hyperfibrinolysis.

Selby R. "TEG talk": expanding clinical roles for thromboelastography and rotational thromboelastometry. *Hematology Am Soc Hematol Educ Program.* 2020;2020:67-75.

Whiting D, DiNardo JA. TEG and ROTEM: technology and clinical applications. *Am J Hematol.* 2014;89:228-232.

B.10. Given the thromboelastometry findings and high clinical suspicion for occult postsurgical bleeding, what hemostatic products would you arrange to have in the operating room?

Clinical coagulopathy usually occurs when coagulation factor levels are below 30% of normal levels, fibrinogen levels are below ~70 mg/dL, and platelet count is 100,000/mL or below. By thromboelastometry, there is evidence of coagulation factor, fibrinogen, and possibly platelet deficiency. Therefore, sufficient plasma, cryoprecipitate, and platelets to normalize coagulation function should be arranged before the start of surgery.

Plasma, whether fresh frozen (ie, fresh frozen plasma, frozen within 8 hours of phlebotomy) or frozen within 24 hours of phlebotomy (FP24), differ slightly in their levels of the labile factors, factors VIII and V, but are dosed the same. A 15 mL/kg infusion of plasma will increase most coagulation factors by 25%. Therefore, it is reasonable to have 15 mL/kg of plasma available. In this patient, using her ideal or adjusted body weight of 60 to 70 kg, this corresponds to 4 units.

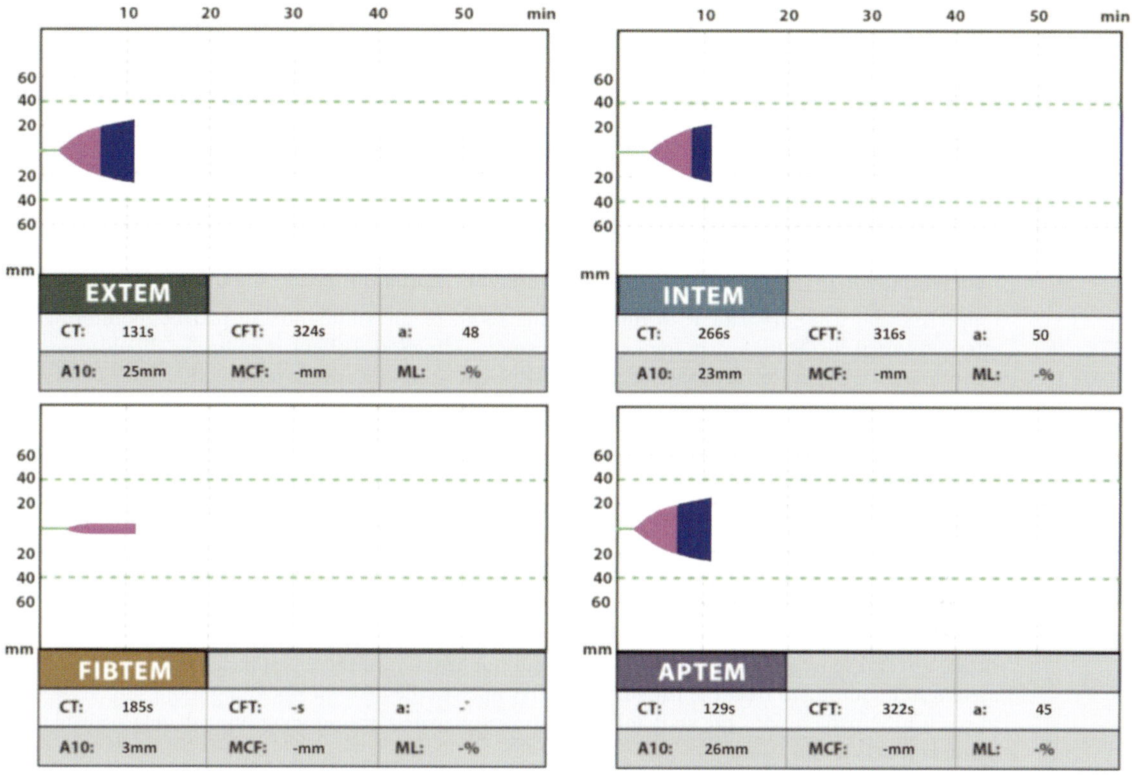

FIGURE 12.9. Rotational thromboelastometry viscoelastic assay data. See Section B.9.

Cryoprecipitate is a concentrated blood component made from frozen plasma thawed to 1 °C to 6 °C. At this temperature, residues that constitute cryoprecipitate appear in plasma and are separated from the supernatant. One unit of cryoprecipitate is prepared from 1 unit of plasma and contains approximately 10 to 15 mL plasma, 150 to 250 mg fibrinogen (ie, 300-3,000 mg/dL, 32% of original plasma content), and factors VIII and XIII. This is often pooled into a single bag containing 5 to 10 units from multiple donors. One unit of cryoprecipitate increases plasma fibrinogen by 10 mg/dL; therefore, the equivalent of 5 to 10 units should be available.

TABLE 12.8 Rotational Thromboelastometry Data for Section B.9

Parameters	Patient Data	Reference Range	Parameters	Patient Data	Reference Range
EXTEM			**INTEM**		
CT (s)	131	38-79	CT (s)	266	100-240
CFT (s)	324	34-159	CFT (s)	316	30-110
α (degrees)	48	63-83	α (degrees)	50	70-83
A10 (mm)	25	43-65	A10 (mm)	23	44-66
FIBTEM			**APTEM**		
CT (s)	185	N/A	CT (s)	129	38-79
A10 (mm)	3	7-23	CFT (s)	322	34-159
			α (degrees)	45	63-83
			A10 (mm)	26	43-65

References ranges are for ROTEM delta assays performed in European clinical reference laboratories in healthy adult population samples.
A10, amplitude 10 min; CFT, clot formation time; CT, clotting time; N/A, not available.

Platelets may be separated by apheresis directly from the donor, or separated from whole blood. The volume of one apheresed unit of platelets is 200 to 400 mL, whereas 4 to 6 units of platelets spun from whole blood will need to be pooled to produce the equivalent volume. A dose of 10 mL/kg will increase platelet count by 30,000 to 50,000/mL. For an ideal or adjusted body weight of 60 to 70 kg, 1 to 2 units of apheresed or pooled platelets should be available.

Nagrebetsky A, Al-Samkari H, Davis NM, et al. Perioperative thrombocytopenia: evidence, evaluation, and emerging therapies. *Br J Anaesth.* 2019;122:19-31.

Nascimento B, Goodnough LT, Levy JH. Cryoprecipitate therapy. *Br J Anaesth.* 2014;113:922-934.

B.11. How would you organize and conduct the transport of this patient to the operating room?

Proper transport of this patient to the operating room requires attention to patient monitoring and safety, essential medications, equipment, and team coordination. Patient monitoring should consist of a continuous ECG trace for arrhythmia and HR monitoring, invasive arterial catheter for continuous blood pressure monitoring, and audible pulse oximetry. The transport monitor should be confirmed to be functional, positioned so that the vital signs are clearly displayed, and the battery fully charged. An adequate oxygen supply and an effective oxygen delivery device should be initiated before transport. Emergency airway equipment and a defibrillator should accompany the patient. Intravenous access should be functional and secured with clearly identified injection ports for medication administration. Vasoactive infusions initiated by the treatment team should be verified and infusion pump settings confirmed. Syringes of vasopressors and inotropes, including phenylephrine, epinephrine, norepinephrine, calcium, and in-line intravenous fluid for volume resuscitation should be available for transport.

Given her respiratory distress, this patient should be transported in her position of comfort, likely sitting up. Transport to the operating room should not begin until there is sufficient transport personnel present to monitor and treat the patient, and safely operate the bed; the operating room should be ready to receive the patient with the staff and perfusionists prepared, the surgeon immediately available, and blood products in the room.

Fanara B, Manzon C, Barbot O, et al. Recommendations for the intra-hospital transport of critically ill patients. *Crit Care.* 2010;14:R87.

C. Intraoperative Management

C.1. What are the cardiovascular effects of commonly used intravenous anesthetic and coinduction agents?

Propofol

Propofol is a potent sympatholytic and vascular smooth muscle dilator. This results in hypotension from vasodilation, preload reduction from venodilation, and myocardial depression. It blunts the baroreceptor reflex while preserving vagal tone, and bradycardia can ensue. The overall effect is a decrease in venous return, CO, and systemic arterial pressure, which would hasten cardiovascular collapse in this patient if given in standard induction doses.

Etomidate

Etomidate is characterized by its stable hemodynamic profile when used for induction of anesthesia. Its imidazole-based structure bears structural similarities to α_2-agonists and is thought to be responsible for peripheral vasoconstriction and the occasional hypertensive response when injected rapidly as the sole agent. Minor decreases in SVR, much less than with propofol or thiopental, can occur in conjunction with a volatile agent. Baroreceptor and sympathetic reflexes are preserved, and there is minimal effect on myocardial contractility. Because hemodynamic responses to laryngoscopy are not affected by etomidate, a significant increase in HR and BP should be expected when given as a sole induction agent. The primary disadvantage of etomidate is the adrenocortical suppression with its use, which can occur after a single dose. However, this has not translated into increased postoperative hypotension, morbidity, or mortality in cardiac surgery patients. Taken together, etomidate is the most cardiostable intravenous anesthetic and is the drug of choice in patients with impending hemodynamic collapse.

Ketamine

Ketamine is associated with an increase in norepinephrine release that increases sympathetic outflow and is largely responsible for its stable hemodynamic profile. The mechanism by which it causes this norepinephrine release is unclear, but a direct central effect and reuptake inhibition has been postulated. An induction dose of ketamine increases blood pressure, HR, CO, and myocardial oxygen consumption. Ketamine should be used with caution in patients with depleted endogenous catecholamine levels, such as those who are critically ill, because this can unmask its direct negative inotropic effects. This patient's sympathetic outflow appears intact, as evidenced by her tachycardia and increased SVR. In the absence of myocardial ischemia, ketamine is a reasonable choice for induction.

Thiopental

Thiopental is included here for historical interest. It is a direct myocardial depressant and also has indirect negative inotropic effects through the suppression of sympathetic outflow. It also causes vascular dilation, but because the baroreceptor reflex is preserved, there is less hypotension when compared with an equivalent dose of propofol, and the subsequent tachycardia minimizes the decrease in CO from venodilation. In a patient with cardiac tamponade, however, the hypotensive effects are exaggerated, and its use is not recommended.

Fentanyl

The hallmark of fentanyl is that it causes minimal to no myocardial depression. However, its strong vagotonic effect leads to a decrease in HR, which can lead to a decrease in CO. It preserves coronary autoregulation and has no histaminergic effects. When given in combination with midazolam or other sedatives, however, fentanyl can produce more clinically significant hypotension.

Midazolam

Midazolam exerts a dose-related venous and arterial vasodilatory effect. When given in typical anxiolytic doses, it can decrease SV and SVR by 10%, but because the baroreceptor reflex is preserved, CO is maintained. Hypotension can become marked if it is used in higher doses or in combination with fentanyl. It suppresses sympathetic outflow and decreases myocardial oxygen consumption. Because of its rapid onset and MAC-sparing effect, midazolam can be a useful coinduction agent in this patient. Some hypotension should be expected because of her dependence on sympathetic tone to compensate for her shock state.

Carmona P, Mateo E, Casanovas I, et al. Management of cardiac tamponade after cardiac surgery. *J Cardiothorac Vasc Anesth*. 2012;26:302-311.

Wagner CE, Bick JS, Johnson D, et al. Etomidate use and postoperative outcomes among cardiac surgery patients. *Anesthesiology*. 2014;120:579-589.

C.2. What is the effect of supine positioning and positive pressure ventilation on the hemodynamics of a patient with cardiac tamponade?

Instituting positive pressure ventilation in a patient with cardiac tamponade can result in cardiovascular collapse due to the critical impedance of cardiac filling. The increase in intrathoracic pressure is added to intrapericardial pressure, which worsens the Starling resistor pathophysiology of cardiac tamponade. Supine positioning, with or without positive pressure, can further impede filling. An anterior clot or effusion can, with gravity, worsen right atrial and RV compression when the patient is supine. Increased diaphragmatic splinting in a patient already in respiratory distress will limit the negative intrathoracic pressure generated in spontaneous ventilation; this further compromises the gradient for venous return to the RA.

Carmona P, Mateo E, Casanovas I, et al. Management of cardiac tamponade after cardiac surgery. *J Cardiothorac Vasc Anesth*. 2012;26:302-311.

Faehnrich JA, Noone RB Jr, White WD, et al. Effects of positive-pressure ventilation, pericardial effusion, and cardiac tamponade on respiratory variation in transmitral flow velocities. *J Cardiothorac Vasc Anesth*. 2003;17:45-50.

O'Connor CJ, Tuman KJ. The intraoperative management of patients with pericardial tamponade. *Anesthesiol Clin*. 2010;28:87-96.

C.3. Describe the anesthetic induction process for cardiac tamponade.

Standard monitoring, secure intravenous access, functional equipment, and skilled assistance should be prepared. Intravenous fluids, vasopressors, positive inotropes, and blood products should be immediately available. Preinduction invasive arterial pressure monitoring is required due to expected hemodynamic instability during the procedure. Although PAC data can be useful for intra- and postoperative optimization, a PAC is not essential for safe induction. TEE is a useful adjunct and should be utilized postinduction if a skilled operator is available. A rapid sequence induction with etomidate or ketamine as the induction agent; a rapid-acting neuromuscular blocking agent; and additional modifiers, such as midazolam, lidocaine, and an opioid, to ensure amnesia and to blunt the hemodynamic responses to tracheal intubation, should be the primary induction plan. During the preoxygenation process, the patient should be positioned in a way that considers the patient's comfort (eg, sitting upright) while allowing for quick conversion to a more favorable intubating stance following induction of anesthesia. Because of the potential for hemodynamic collapse with general anesthesia and positive pressure ventilation, it is imperative that induction only takes place once the patient is surgically draped and the surgeons are gowned and gloved ready for immediate chest decompression.

Carmona P, Mateo E, Casanovas I, et al. Management of cardiac tamponade after cardiac surgery. *J Cardiothorac Vasc Anesth.* 2012;26:302-311.

Morozowich ST, et al. Uncommon Cardiac Diseases. In: Kaplan JA, et al., eds. *Kaplan's Cardiac Anesthesia.* 8th ed. Elsevier; 2023:698-759.

O'Connor CJ, Tuman KJ. The intraoperative management of patients with pericardial tamponade. *Anesthesiol Clin.* 2010;28:87-96.

C.4. Following anesthetic induction and tracheal intubation, the systemic blood pressure decreases to 55/30 mm Hg. Describe your management.

This is likely due to the anticipated effects of anesthetic agents, the supine position, and positive pressure ventilation. Pericardial decompression is the definitive treatment; the surgeons should be informed immediately to begin without delay while resuscitative efforts continue. Preload should be maximized with fluid bolus and minimization of positive pressure ventilation using a combination of hand ventilation with low tidal volumes and limited apnea with 100% inspired oxygen. Contractility should be maintained with boluses of epinephrine and calcium if deficient, and anesthetic agents should be titrated to ensure amnesia without excessive negative inotropy. Afterload should be maintained by titrating norepinephrine to achieve a MAP of 60 to 65 mm Hg to preserve critical organ perfusion. In the event of worsening CO, cardiac massage might be required. It should be noted that external cardiac massage has reduced efficacy in cardiac tamponade due to the elevated cardiac filling pressures, which continue to impede venous return during the relaxation phase of chest compressions. In a situation where chest compressions are being considered, opening the pericardium should occur immediately instead.

Carmona P, Mateo E, Casanovas I, et al. Management of cardiac tamponade after cardiac surgery. *J Cardiothorac Vasc Anesth.* 2012;26:302-311.

Morozowich ST, et al. Uncommon Cardiac Diseases. In: Kaplan JA, et al., eds. *Kaplan's Cardiac Anesthesia.* 8th ed. Elsevier; 2023:698-759.

C.5. What hemodynamic changes are frequently associated with opening the pericardial space?

When opened, the pericardial space is exposed to atmospheric pressure. For free-flowing pericardial effusions, this will immediately decompress the cardiac chambers, thereby leading to a rapid rise in preload, SV, and CO. This can often be seen on hemodynamic monitoring as a dramatic rise in systemic blood pressure, a reduction in pulmonary artery pressure (PAP) and CVP, and normalization of tachycardia (**Figure 12.10**). In a patient receiving high doses of vasopressors to maintain perfusion prior to pericardiotomy, this can result in severe hypertension. In patients who have had overly aggressive fluid resuscitation, the sudden release of cardiac constraint can lead to acute pulmonary edema as well as RV dysfunction. For this reason, it is important to be aware of surgical progress to properly anticipate the effects of pericardial opening. Should extremes of hypertension occur, it is effectively treated with rapid weaning of vasopressors, deepening the level of anesthesia, administering analgesia, and titrating short-acting vasodilators until blood pressure is normalized.

Carmona P, Mateo E, Casanovas I, et al. Management of cardiac tamponade after cardiac surgery. *J Cardiothorac Vasc Anesth.* 2012;26:302-311.

O'Connor CJ, Tuman KJ. The intraoperative management of patients with pericardial tamponade. *Anesthesiol Clin.* 2010;28:87-96.

C.6. Following removal of approximately 500 mL of dark blood and clots from the mediastinum, the patient's CO remains low. What are your differential diagnoses?

Persistent hypotension following pericardial decompression results from insufficient preload, afterload, and/or contractility. If there is surgical evidence of ongoing hemorrhage, then treating hypovolemia should be a priority. Because this patient has a PAC, a review of CVP and diastolic PAP trends can be helpful in assessing ventricular filling pressures and optimizing fluid resuscitation. Residual clot and regional cardiac tamponade should be evaluated with TEE and careful surgical exploration; in particular,

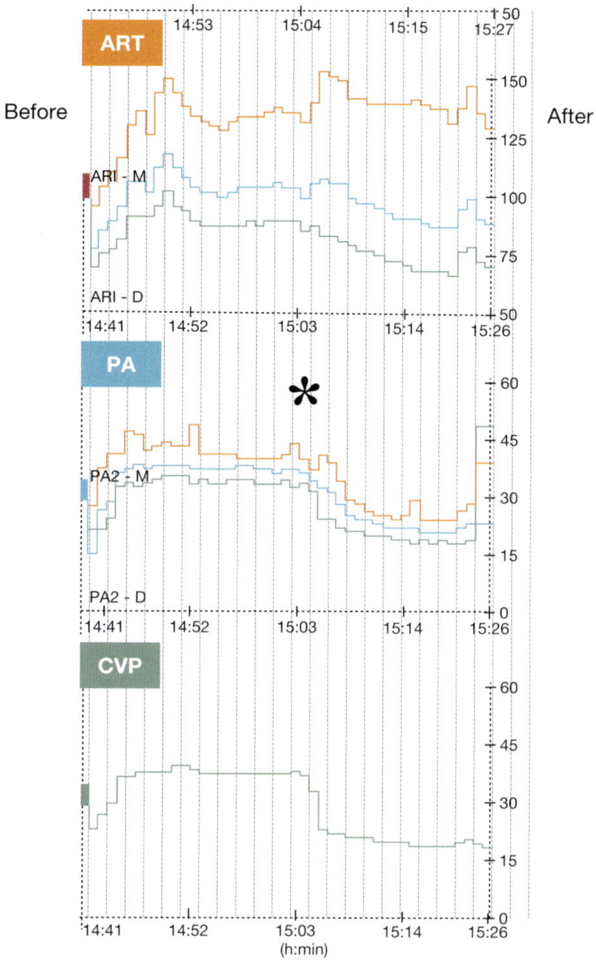

FIGURE 12.10. Intraoperative hemodynamics before and after pericardial decompression. Arterial blood pressure (ART), pulmonary artery pressure (PAP), and central venous pressure (CVP) are shown during mediastinal exploration for cardiac tamponade. The moment of pericardial decompression is marked by the *asterisk*. Note the elevated CVP, PA diastolic pressure, as well as the narrow systemic pulse pressure before decompression, demonstrating extrinsic pericardial pressure on the right atrium (RA) and left atrium (LA) and its effect on decreasing left ventricle (LV) stroke volume. Shortly following pericardial decompression, CVP and PA pressures decrease accompanied by an increase in systemic arterial pressure. Systemic pulse pressure continues to increase, reflecting the recovery of SV and presumably CO.

clot located posteriorly within the oblique sinus can continue to compress the LA (**Figure 12.3**) and might not be immediately apparent on initial surgical exploration.

TEE is invaluable in evaluating myocardial contractility. Ventricular function can be impaired from coronary insufficiency and active ischemia which can persist even after restoring adequate coronary perfusion (ie, "myocardial stunning"). Both conditions can present as cardiogenic shock and manifest wall motion abnormalities on TEE, and should be managed by optimizing myocardial oxygen supply and demand while preserving critical organ perfusion with careful use of inotropic support if required.

A low SVR state can result from vasodilatory medications, including anesthetics and inotropes (eg, milrinone, dobutamine, low-dose epinephrine). Isolated vasoplegia, although not typically associated with this procedure, can occur in the presence of a major surgical inflammatory response, stress-related depletion of endogenous vasopressin, and acquired catecholamine resistance. Norepinephrine is recommended as a first-line agent for treating vasoplegia, although this is largely extrapolated from septic shock study data. If high doses of norepinephrine are required to maintain adequate perfusion pressures, then the addition of vasopressin can be useful to overcome catecholamine resistance, limit catecholamine doses, and possibly reduce the incidence of postoperative renal failure.

Geffroy A, Beloeil H, Bouvier E, et al. Prolonged right ventricular failure after relief of cardiac tamponade. *Can J Anaesth.* 2004;51:482-485.

Lambden S, Creagh-Brown BC, Hunt J, et al. Definitions and pathophysiology of vasoplegic shock. *Crit Care.* 2018;22:174.

Shaefi S, Mittel A, Klick J, et al. Vasoplegia after cardiovascular procedure—pathophysiology and targeted therapy. *J Cardiothorac Vasc Anesth.* 2018;32:1013-1022.

C.7. What is pericardial decompression syndrome (PDS)?

PDS describes the cardiogenic shock and pulmonary edema following drainage of pericardial effusions. It can present immediately following percutaneous or surgical drainage but can be delayed by up to 24 to 48 hours. The etiology of PDS is unclear but has been attributed to many causes including myocardial stunning from impaired epicardial perfusion, acute RV failure from volume overload with decompression, acute septal shift from RV filling causing LV dysfunction, stress cardiomyopathy from post-drainage neurohormonal alterations, acute severe post-drainage hypertension, and abrupt catecholamine withdrawal after the restoration of normal cardiac filling dynamics. In a retrospective review of 35 cases, almost all of the patients presented with cardiac tamponade (94%) with normal pre-drainage ventricular function and large pericardial effusions, although PDS occurring after drainage of effusions as small 250 mL has been described. The majority of patients presented with LV or biventricular failure (60%), followed by isolated cardiogenic pulmonary edema (29%) and RV failure (9%). There is a paucity of information regarding preventive measures apart from slow, rather than rapid, pericardial decompression, and treatment is supportive. The timeline for myocardial recovery is variable.

Chung J, Ocken L, Wolo E, et al. Acute right ventricular failure after surgical drainage of pericardial tamponade: a case report of pericardial decompression syndrome and review of the literature. *J Cardiothorac Vasc Anesth.* 2019;33:768-771.

Geffroy A, Beloeil H, Bouvier E, et al. Prolonged right ventricular failure after relief of cardiac tamponade. *Can J Anaesth.* 2004;51:482-485.

Pradhan R, Okabe T, Yoshida K, et al. Patient characteristics and predictors of mortality associated with pericardial decompression syndrome: a comprehensive analysis of published cases. *Eur Heart J Acute Cardiovasc Care.* 2015;4:113-120.

Sobieski C, Herner M, Goyal N, Khor LL, Chang L, Bieging E, McGarry TJ. Pericardial decompression syndrome after drainage of chronic pericardial effusions. *JACC Case Rep.* 2022;4:1515-1521.

D. Postoperative Management

D.1. A pericardial drain is placed following mediastinal decompression. How should this drainage tube be managed?

Following open surgical drainage, a pericardial drain is connected to a closed, underwater seal system to prevent air entry into the mediastinum during negative pressure inspiration. Low-pressure suction (−15 to −25 cm H_2O) is typically applied to facilitate clearance of effusions and air, but clots can still form within the tubing leading to a recurrence of cardiac tamponade if not cleared. Although a small respiratory "swing" might be present in drain tubing fluid or the water seal, "bubbling" is not typical unless there is a concurrent pneumomediastinum or a pneumothorax in direct connection to the drain. For percutaneous drainage, a pigtail catheter is typically connected to a closed drainage system for gravity drainage with a stopcock for aspiration and flushing to maintain catheter patency. Some percutaneous drain care protocols advocate regular aspiration every 4 to 6 hours with instillation of heparinized saline after each aspiration attempt. Regardless of the type of drainage tube, all patients should be monitored closely for re-accumulation of pericardial fluid from catheter malfunction. The dwell time for the catheter should be minimized to prevent infection. Drains are typically removed when there is less than 30 to 50 mL drainage over a 24-hour period, or after 24 to 72 hours (**Figure 12.11**).

De Carlini CC, Maggiolini S. Pericardiocentesis in cardiac tamponade: indications and practical aspects. *e-J Cardiol Pract.* 2017;15.

Zisis C, Tsirgogianni T, Lazaridis G, et al. Chest drainage systems in use. *Ann Transl Med.* 2015;3:43.

D.2. How would you manage hypertension in the intensive care unit?

Hypertension following resolution of cardiac tamponade is common. The etiology can be directly related to the postcardiac tamponade state, a postprocedural complication, or from issues that are generally applicable to any postsurgical patient. In postcardiac tamponade patients, hypertension is typically due to ongoing sympathetic activation and relative baroreceptor insensitivity, although residual consequences of cardiac tamponade such as acidosis, hypervolemia or hypovolemia, and/or systemic inflammatory response can also be responsible. Serious complications that present with hypertension such as heart failure with pulmonary edema, stroke, hemorrhage, and myocardial ischemia should be ruled out. More general

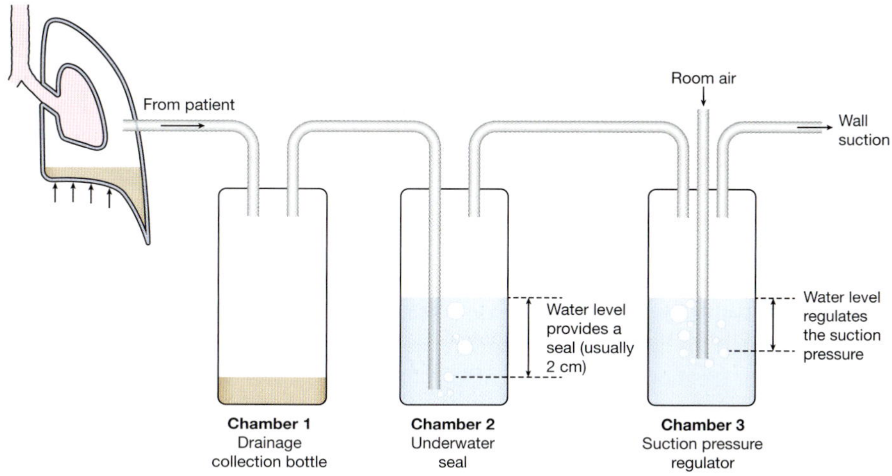

FIGURE 12.11. Basic three-bottle suction drainage system diagram. First bottle: drainage bottle; second bottle: water seal bottle; third bottle: negative pressure regulator bottle.

causes of postoperative hypertension including pain, anxiety, cold, hypoxemia, hypercarbia, and delirium should be individually addressed with specific pharmacologic and nonpharmacologic therapies.

Controlling hypertension is important not only to prevent myocardial strain and end-organ damage but also to limit direct complications including surgical bleeding and worsening reperfusion injury. The basis for maintaining MAP within 20% of baseline values comes from clinical data showing an increased risk of end-organ hyperperfusion and damage with sustained blood pressures (ie, >10 minutes) beyond this range. By targeting the patient's baseline MAP, organ perfusion pressures are maintained within the individual's autoregulatory range.

Assuming reversible causes of hypertension are corrected, the ideal antihypertensive agent for acute control should be short-acting and titratable. Clevidipine has a rapid onset–offset profile due to its metabolism by tissue and blood esterases, resulting in a half-life of approximately 1 minute and is an ideal agent for acutely controlling hypertension. Nicardipine, by contrast, has a rapid distributive α half-life of 2.7 minutes, which increases to 44.8 minutes and 14.4 hours for its intermediate β and γ half-lives, respectively. The dihydropyridine calcium channel blockers play an adjunctive role for chronic maintenance therapy in patients with ischemic heart disease and are not recommended in patients with heart failure with reduced ejection fraction.

Labetalol is a useful agent, especially in the presence of tachycardia. Given intravenously, it has an approximately 7:1 nonselective β- to α_1-antagonist effect with an onset of effect in 2 to 5 minutes. Its peak hypotensive effect occurs within 10 minutes, and its elimination half-life is 3 to 5 hours. If warranted, maintenance β-blocker therapy, with carvedilol, the nonselective β- and α_1-blocker or cardioselective agents such as metoprolol, confers additional survival benefit in this patient with ischemic heart disease and is a first-line therapy for chronic treatment.

Aronson S, Dyke CM, Stierer KA, et al. The ECLIPSE trials: comparative studies of clevidipine to nitroglycerin, sodium nitroprusside, and nicardipine for acute hypertension treatment in cardiac surgery patients. *Anesth Analg.* 2008;107:1110-1121.

Cheung AT. Exploring an optimum intra/postoperative management strategy for acute hypertension in the cardiac surgery patient. *J Card Surg.* 2006;21:S8-S14.

Espinosa A, Ripollés-Melchor J, Casans-Francés R, et al; Evidence Anesthesia Review Group. Perioperative use of clevidipine: a systematic review and meta-analysis. *PLoS One.* 2016;11:e0150625.

Whelton PK, Carey RM, Aronow WS, et al. 2017 ACC/AHA/AAPA/ABC/ACPM/AGS/APhA/ASH/ASPC/NMA/PCNA guideline for the prevention, detection, evaluation, and management of high blood pressure in adults: a report of the American College of Cardiology/American Heart Association Task Force on Clinical Practice Guidelines. *J Am Coll Cardiol.* 2018;71:e127-e248.

13 Heart Transplantation and Subsequent Noncardiac Surgery

Louise Y. Sun and Davy Cheng

A 27-year-old male with a history of viral myocarditis is urgently transferred to a quaternary cardiac center to be evaluated for heart transplantation. He has severe biventricular systolic dysfunction, with a left ventricular ejection fraction (EF) of less than 10% and a right ventricular fractional area change (FAC) of 5%. His pulmonary vascular resistance (PVR) is 3 Wood units. He was recently hospitalized with decompensated heart failure, acute kidney injury, and liver congestion with elevated international normalized ratio (INR) and liver enzymes. He is currently on intravenous (IV) inotropic and diuretic agents. A ventricular assist device (VAD) was inserted to provide temporary mechanical circulatory support (MCS) while waiting for a donor heart to become available.

A. Medical Disease and Differential Diagnosis

1. What are the common diagnoses requiring heart transplantation in adults?
2. What are the indications and relative contraindications for recipient selection?
3. What are the criteria for donor heart selection?
4. What is the role of donation after circulatory death (DCD) for heart transplantation?
5. What are the principles of perioperative donor management?
6. What are the risk factors associated with posttransplant mortality?
7. What is the difference between the biatrial and bicaval surgical techniques of heart transplantation?
8. When is a combined heart-lung transplant indicated? What are the important differences?
9. What are the medical and surgical alternatives to cardiac transplantation?
10. What is the role of VADs in this type of patient?
11. What are the considerations in anesthetizing patients for left ventricular assist device (LVAD) insertion?

B. Preoperative Management

Three weeks after insertion of an Impella VAD, a donor heart becomes available.

1. How would you assess this patient preoperatively?
2. How would you premedicate this patient? Why?

C. Intraoperative Management

1. What anesthetic equipment and monitors would you set up? Why?
2. What is the role of transesophageal echocardiography (TEE)?
3. Describe the induction and maintenance of anesthesia.
4. How would you manage this patient during cardiopulmonary bypass (CPB)?

D. Postoperative Management

1. What are the early postoperative complications?
2. What are the mechanisms of early right ventricular failure (RVF)?
3. How would you treat RVF following heart transplantation?
4. How does inhaled nitric oxide (NO) work as a selective pulmonary vasodilator?
5. What is the pathophysiology of the denervated heart?
6. What are the common cardiac dysrhythmias following heart transplantation?
7. What are the causes of posttransplant bleeding?
8. How would you treat posttransplant bleeding?
9. What are the causes of early graft failure?
10. How would you manage this patient in the intensive care unit?

E. Subsequent Noncardiac Surgery

The patient recovers successfully following heart transplantation. However, 2 years postoperatively, he fractures his left radius after a fall and presents for open reduction and internal fixation of the fracture.

1. How would you monitor this patient?
2. What type of anesthetic is best for heart transplant recipients?
3. What anesthetic technique would you choose for this patient?
4. Do you need to use a muscarinic antagonist with cholinesterase inhibitors to reverse the neuromuscular block in heart transplant patients?
5. What are the anesthetic considerations for heart transplant patients?
6. What are the significant implications of the denervated heart?
7. What is the significance of allograft rejection?
8. What is the significance of infection in these patients?
9. What are the significant implications of drug interactions?
10. What is cardiac allograft vasculopathy? Why is this important?
11. What are the significant implications of posttransplant hypertension?
12. What are the significant implications of renal dysfunction?
13. What types of malignancy are common in heart transplant recipients?
14. Is ambulatory surgery appropriate for heart transplant recipients?

A. Medical Disease and Differential Diagnosis

A.1. What are the common diagnoses requiring heart transplantation in adults?

Heart transplantation is a treatment option for selected patients with end-stage heart disease. According to the United Network for Organ Sharing, 7,152 heart transplants were performed worldwide in 2022. The indications for adult heart transplantation, as reported to the Registry of the International Society for Heart and Lung Transplantation between 2010 and 2018, are shown in **Figure 13.1**. Nonischemic cardiomyopathy (51.4%) and ischemic coronary artery disease (32.4%) represent the most frequent diagnoses leading to transplantation.

A.2. What are the indications and relative contraindications for recipient selection?

Indications and contraindications for heart transplantation can be flexible and may vary between transplant centers.

Criteria for selection include the following:

- End-stage heart disease with poor quality of life or poor survivability
- Refractory arrhythmias or angina despite optimal medical and surgical care

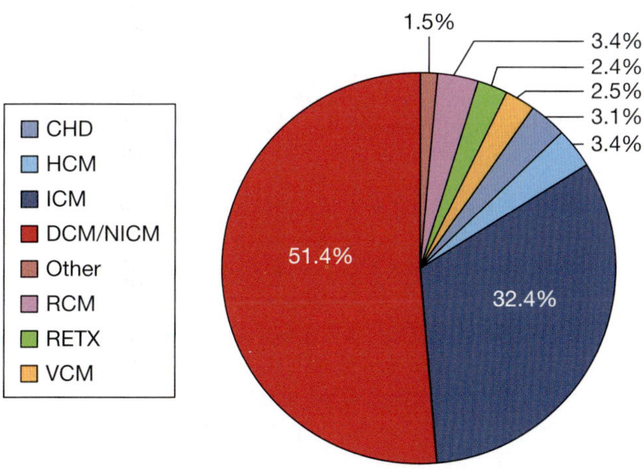

FIGURE 13.1. International Society for Heart and Lung Transplantation: Adult Heart Transplant Diagnosis for transplants performed between 2010 and 2018. CHD, congenital heart disease; DCM, dilated cardiomyopathy; HCM, hypertrophic cardiomyopathy; ICM, ischemic cardiomyopathy; NICM, nonischemic cardiomyopathy; RCM, restrictive cardiomyopathy; RETX, retransplant; VCM, valvular cardiomyopathy. (Data from International Society for Heart and Lung Transplantation; Slide11, ISHLT registry slides. *J Heart Lung Transplant.* 2022;41:1335-1375.)

- Physiologic age younger than 70 years. Some patients with chronologic age older than 70 years are deemed eligible for receiving a heart transplant. Notably, in 2016, more than 13% of heart transplant recipients were 65 years of age or older.
- Peak oxygen consumption (Vo_2) during cardiopulmonary exercise testing is considered. According to the International Society for Heart and Lung Transplantation (ISHLT) guidelines, patients with Vo_2 less than 14 mL/kg/min in the absence of a β-blocker or Vo_2 less than 12 mL/kg/min in the presence of a β-blocker are acceptable for transplantation.
- A heart failure survival score can also be used to guide listing for transplantation for ambulatory patients.

Relative Contraindications

- Neoplasm with a significant chance of recurrence
- Obesity (body mass index [BMI] >30 kg/m^2)
- Fixed (nonresponsive) pulmonary hypertension: PVR greater than 6 Wood units or pulmonary artery transpulmonary gradient greater than 15 mm Hg
- Irreversible renal dysfunction with eGFR less than 30 mL/min/1.73 m^2
- Physiologic age greater than 70 years
- Frailty (three of five of the following: unintentional weight loss of ≥10 lb in 1 year, muscle loss, fatigue, slow walking speed, low levels of physical activity)
- Clinically severe symptomatic cerebrovascular disease
- Diabetes with end-organ damage other than nonproliferative retinopathy or persistent poor glycemic control (HbA_{1c} >7.5%)
- Tobacco use, substance abuse, psychosocial impairments that will limit compliance with postoperative care, or history of noncompliance
- Other diseases that can limit survival (HIV, severe pulmonary disease, hepatitis, etc)

Chan WX, Ross H. Who needs a transplant and when? *Curr Opin Organ Transplant.* 2012;17:531-539.

Hsich E, Singh TP, Cherikh WS, et al. International Society for Heart and Lung Transplantation. The International Thoracic Organ Transplant Registry of the International Society for Heart and Lung Transplantation: thirty-ninth adult heart transplantation report—2022; focus on transplant for restrictive heart disease. *J Heart Lung Transplant.* 2022;41:1366-1375.

Merha MR, Canter CE, Hannan MM, et al. The 2016 International Society for Heart Lung Transplantation listing criteria for heart transplantation: a 10-year update. *J Heart Lung Transplant.* 2016;35:1-23.

United Network for Organ Sharing. Organ transplant trends. More transplants than ever. Accessed March 21, 2023. https://unos.org/data/

A.3. What are the criteria for donor heart selection?

The limiting factor in heart transplantation is the shortage of donor organs. In Canada, there were 142 heart transplants performed in 2021, with 135 people on the waiting list at the end of that year. In the United States, 4,111 heart transplants were performed in 2022. Following the diagnosis of brain death, organ procurement can be considered for the purpose of donation. Preferably, the donor should not have sustained prolonged cardiac arrest, severe chest trauma, intracardiac injections, septicemia, or excessive inotropic support and should be younger than 55 years of age. Careful clinical examination of the potential donor is undertaken to rule out coronary artery atherosclerosis and contractile dysfunction; investigations can include angiography and echocardiography. The use of coronary angiography would be dictated by the patient's age, sex, and risk factors. In general, a contrast left ventriculogram is avoided to reduce the risk of nephrotoxicity.

Poor EF, despite optimization of physiologic variables, excludes a potential donation. However, donor hearts with initial low EF that improves are associated with similar short- and long-term survival compared with those with normal initial EF. The use of donor hearts with mild left ventricular hypertrophy (LVH) has yielded mixed results; however, wall thickness greater than 13 mm or electrocardiographic (ECG) criteria for LVH make transplantation unadvisable. In general, severe congenital or valvular abnormalities preclude donation, except abnormalities in which "bench" repair can be undertaken before transplant.

Blood group ABO compatibility is important because mismatch can result in hyperacute rejection. The donor's body weight should be within 20% of that of the recipient. However, in the case of a small donor, using BMI or height is more accurate than using weight. Undersized transplanted hearts require a higher heart rate to maintain adequate cardiac output due to smaller stroke volume. Oversized donor hearts are preferred in high-risk recipients such as those with pulmonary hypertension. Prolonged ischemic time can contribute to early allograft failure. A recent analysis using ISHLT data found that donor heart ischemic time less than 4 hours was associated with better 30-day and 5-year survival compared to longer ischemic times.

The use of "extended-donor criteria" is increasing, and outcomes are favorable. At times, donor hearts are considered for transplant with one or more of the following: size mismatch, ischemic time greater than 4 hours, LVH, donor age greater than 55 years, malignant brain tumors, long-standing death by poisoning, and significant inotropic requirements. Reviewing the wide variety of traditional reasons for not accepting a donor heart, only donor age and diabetes were found to be predictive of 1-year mortality in a recipient, leading to concerns that many viable, albeit "less than perfect," potential donor hearts are not being used for transplant.

Canadian Institute for Health Information. Organ transplants in Canada: donations and need. Accessed March 21, 2023. https://www.cihi.ca/en/organ-transplants-in-canada-donations-and-need

Copeland H, Knezevic I, Baran DA, et al. Donor heart selection: evidence-based guidelines for providers. *J Heart Lung Transplant*. 2023;42:7-29.

Tong CK, Khush KK. New approaches to donor selection and preparation in heart transplantation. *Curr Treat Options Cardiovasc Med*. 2021;23:1-14.

United Network for Organ Sharing. 2022 Organ transplants again set annual records. Accessed March 21, 2022. https://unos.org/news/2022-organ-transplants-again-set-annual-records

Velleca A, Shullo MA, Dhital K, et al. The International Society for Heart and Lung Transplantation (ISHLT) guidelines for the care of heart transplant recipients. *J Heart Lung Transplant*. 2023;42:e1-e141.

A.4. What is the role of donation after circulatory death (DCD) for heart transplantation?

Cardiac transplantation is limited by a critical shortage of suitable organs. DCD was introduced to clinical practice in 2014 and has since opened a significant new donor pool for patients with end-stage heart failure. Hearts from DCD donors suffer considerable ischemic injury prior to organ procurement such that the traditional approach to the transplantation of hearts from brain-dead donors is not applicable for DCD. Advances in the understanding of ischemic postconditioning have facilitated the development of DCD heart resuscitation strategies that can be used to minimize ischemia-reperfusion injury at the time of organ procurement. Clinically approved ex situ heart perfusion devices allow for DCD heart preservation in a normothermic beating state and minimize exposure to cold ischemia. Organ viability can then be assessed prior to transplantation, thereby minimizing the risk of primary graft dysfunction. A study of 28 DCD heart transplants showed comparable short-term outcomes to traditional donation before cardiac death (DBD) heart transplants with respect to hospital length of stay, treated rejection episodes, allograft function, and 1-year survival (DCD 86%; DBD 88%; $P = .98$). Limited available data suggest that 29% of DCD heart transplant recipients will require temporary MCS at the time of transplantation. However, all patients were successfully weaned from support, and the majority exhibited normal biventricular function on follow-up echocardiogram. The Donors after Circulatory Death Heart Trial (NCT03831048) has recruited over 270 DCD heart transplants so far; DCD hearts were noninferior to the standard of care heart donation after brain death. Further investigation into optimizing resuscitation, preservation, and long-term outcomes is vital to ensure a broader application of DCD heart transplantation in the future.

Beaupré RA, Morgan JA. Donation after cardiac death: a necessary expansion for heart transplantation. *Semin Thorac Cardiovasc Surg*. 2019;31:721-725.

Jawitz OK, Bryner BS, Schroder JN, DeVore AD. Donation after circulatory death heart transplantation in the United States: an early report of donor characteristics. *JTCVS Tech*. 2022;12:104-107.

Messer S, Page A, Axell R, et al. Outcome after heart transplantation from donation after circulatory-determined death donors. *J Heart Lung Transplant*. 2017;36:1311-1318.

Niederberger P, Farine E, Raillard M, et al. Heart transplantation with donation after circulatory death. *Circ Heart Fail*. 2019;12:e005517.

Scheuer SE, Jansz PC, Macdonald PS. Heart transplantation following donation after circulatory death: expanding the donor pool. *J Heart Lung Transplant*. 2021;40:882-889.

A.5. What are the principles of perioperative donor management?

The goals of management are to maintain euvolemia, achieve relatively normal afterload, and optimize cardiac output (CO) without excessive use of inotropic medications, in particular β-agonists. Donors after brain death often can become hemodynamically unstable and challenging to manage, and the treatment goals to support different end organs before donation are often conflicting. The onset of diabetes insipidus needs to be considered when excessive urine output (>300 mL/h) is observed and must be treated promptly with desmopressin (1-deamino-8-D-arginine vasopressin [DDAVP]). As a result of dysfunction of the hypothalamic-pituitary system, hormonal replacement therapy should be undertaken, including the use of IV thyroxine, arginine vasopressin, and methylprednisolone, along with glycemic control.

Souter MJ, Eidbo E, Findlay JY, et al. Organ donor management: part 1. Toward a consensus to guide anesthesia services during donation after brain death. *Semin Cardiothorac Vasc Anesth*. 2018;22:211-222.

Velleca A, Shullo MA, Dhital K, et al. The International Society for Heart and Lung Transplantation (ISHLT) guidelines for the care of heart transplant recipients. *J Heart Lung Transplant*. 2023;42:e1-e141.

A.6. What are the risk factors associated with posttransplant mortality?

Heart transplant outcomes have progressively improved over the past three decades, despite the increasing use of higher-risk donors and the increasing medical complexity of recipients. According to the ISHLT, 1-year survival in those who received a heart transplant between 2012 and 2017 is nearly 90% in North America and nearly 80% in Europe and other regions and is higher in younger recipients. One-year survival and 5-year survival in those who were transplanted between 2008 and 2013 was higher in Europe (89%) than in North America (87%) and other regions (85%). Interestingly, younger patients (ages 18-39 years) in North America had the lowest 5-year survival, possibly due to the lack of universal health care and poorer compliance to medications and follow-up.

Factors associated with increased 1-year mortality are mostly recipient-based and include valvular, ischemic and restrictive cardiomyopathy, congenital heart disease, repeat transplantation and/or sternotomy, use of MCS, hospitalization and mechanical ventilation prior to transplant; older donor age, donor-recipient sex mismatch (specifically, male donor and female recipient), higher recipient BMI, PVR, and panel reactive antibody (PRA), younger or older recipient age, longer ischemic time, worse recipient kidney and liver function, and lower transplant center volume. Risk factors for mortality at 5 years are similar to those at 1 year, with the exception of hypertrophic cardiomyopathy and congenital heart disease being associated with a lower risk of 5-year mortality and diabetes being a risk factor for death at 5 years. Factors associated with early mortality (ie, recipient PRA and ischemic time) are not significantly associated with 5-year mortality.

The most common causes of death are the following:

Within 30 days after transplant:

- Graft failure, multiorgan failure, opportunistic infection

From 31 to 365 days after transplant:

- Opportunistic infection, graft failure, acute rejection

After 5 years:

- Allograft vasculopathy, late graft failure, malignancy, opportunistic infection

Alvarez PA, Briasoulis A, Malik AH. Trends, risk factors, and mortality of unplanned 30-day readmission after heart transplantation. *Am J Cardiol*. 2021;154:130-133.

Khush KK, Hsich E, Potena L, et al. The International Thoracic Organ Transplant Registry of the International Society for Heart and Lung Transplantation: thirty-eighth adult heart transplantation report—2021; focus on recipient characteristics. *J Heart Lung Transplant*. 2021;40:1035.

Prieto D, Correia PM, Batista M, Antunes MJ. Primary graft failure after cardiac transplantation: prevalence, prognosis and risk factors. *Interact Cardiovasc Thorac Surg*. 2018;27:765-772.

A.7. What is the difference between the biatrial and bicaval surgical techniques of heart transplantation?

The older biatrial technique involves anastomoses of the recipient and donor atrial cuffs. The bicaval technique maintains the aforementioned left atrial anastomoses and attempts to maintain cardiac anatomy with separate recipient bicaval anastomoses to the donor right atrium. There might be an advantage in reduced need for pacing, lower incidence of tricuspid and mitral regurgitation, and improved survival with the bicaval technique.

Davies RR, Russo MJ, Morgan JA, et al. Standard versus bicaval techniques for orthotopic heart transplantation: an analysis of the United Network for Organ Sharing database. *J Thorac Cardiovasc Surg*. 2010;140:700-708.

Hwang NC, Sivathasan C. Review of postoperative care for heart transplant recipients. *J Cardiothorac Vasc Anesth*. 2023;37:112-126.

Morgan JA, Edwards NM. Orthotopic cardiac transplantation: comparison of outcome using biatrial, bicaval, and total techniques. *J Card Surg*. 2005;20:102-106.

Zijderhand CF, Veen KM, Caliskan K, et al. Biatrial versus bicaval orthotopic heart transplantation: a systematic review and meta-analysis. *Ann Thorac Surg*. 2020;110:684-691.

A.8. When is a combined heart-lung transplant indicated? What are the important differences?

Concomitant severe left or RVF and end-stage pulmonary disease (eg, idiopathic pulmonary hypertension or cystic fibrosis) and congenital heart disease with Eisenmenger syndrome are the most common indications for a combined heart-lung transplant. Other indications include cystic fibrosis, α_1-antitrypsin deficiency, and other forms of lung disease, such as emphysema and idiopathic pulmonary fibrosis. The procedure is performed through a transverse thoracotomy incision, and the donor heart/lungs are transplanted en bloc. Heart-lung transplantation carries a high rate of early mortality. Despite improvement in survival over time, survival rates in those transplanted between 1992 and 2017 are 74% at 90 days, 66% at 1 year, 49% at 5 years, and 36% at 10 years. Important postoperative problems include bleeding and reperfusion lung injury, which can require inhaled NO or extracorporeal membrane oxygenation (ECMO).

Chambers DC, Cherikh WS, Harhay MO, et al; International Society for Heart and Lung Transplantation. The International Thoracic Organ Transplant Registry of the International Society for Heart and Lung Transplantation: thirty-sixth adult lung and heart-lung transplantation report—2019; focus theme: donor and recipient size match. *J Heart Lung Transplant*. 2019;38:1042-1055.

Le Pavec J, Hascoët S, Fadel E. Heart-lung transplantation: current indications, prognosis and specific considerations. *J Thorac Dis*. 2018;10:5946.

Weill D, Benden C, Corris PA, et al. A consensus document for the selection of lung transplant candidates: 2014—an update from the Pulmonary Transplantation Council of the International Society for Heart and Lung Transplantation. *J Heart Lung Transplant*. 2015;34:1.

A.9. What are the medical and surgical alternatives to cardiac transplantation?

An ongoing worldwide shortage of donor hearts has put ongoing pressure to medically or surgically manage patients with end-stage cardiac failure. Patients need to adhere to strict lifestyle and diet modifications, as well as optimal medical therapy. Angiotensin converting enzyme (ACE) inhibitors improve symptoms and decrease mortality in patients with heart failure. Angiotensin II receptor blockers can be considered for patients who cannot tolerate ACE inhibitors. Patients with severe forms of heart failure can also benefit from a low-dose aldosterone antagonist (spironolactone), with attention paid to the potential for hyperkalemia. Tailored diuretic therapy can offer symptomatic relief. β-Blockade with carvedilol, sustained-release metoprolol, or bisoprolol reduces the risk of sudden cardiac death. Therapy to maintain sinus rhythm is recommended. The risk of sudden cardiac death in patients with advanced heart failure can be reduced by inserting an internal cardiac defibrillator (ICD). Cardiac resynchronization therapy, with or without an ICD, can improve functional class and survival in medically optimized advanced heart failure patients. Intra-aortic balloon pump (IABP) and VAD implantation or semi-implantable paracorporeal devices are finding a role in the management of patients as a bridge to transplant, particularly for those presenting in acute decompensated heart failure.

Hunt SA, Abraham WT, Chin MH, et al. ACC/AHA 2005 guideline update for the diagnosis and management of chronic heart failure in the adult-summary article. *Circulation*. 2005;112:1825-1852.

Ramani GV, Uber PA, Mehra MP. Chronic heart failure: contemporary diagnosis and management. *Mayo Clin Proc*. 2010;85:180-195.

Yancy CW, Jessup M, Bozkurt B, et al. 2013 ACCF/AHA guideline for the management of heart failure. *J Am Coll Cardiol*. 2013;62:e147-e239.

A.10. What is the role of VADs in this type of patient?

The Interagency Registry for Mechanically Assisted Circulatory Support (INTERMACS) database has tracked over 15,000 patients, with total annual implants approaching 2,500. The indications for LVAD insertion have been changing since 2006 when 40.8% were due to life-threatening cardiogenic shock. In 2018, only 15.3% of the patients had cardiogenic shock, and progressive decline of cardiac function (37%) remains the largest single indication. Of those who received an LVAD, 46.0% were listed or were being considered for a heart transplant in 2014. The three major categories of patients considered for VAD include (1) temporary insertion while cardiac function recovers from a (usually surgical) insult (bridge to recovery), (2) insertion while awaiting transplant or transplant assessment (bridge to transplant), or

(3) need for long-term support but are not transplant candidates (destination therapy). Interestingly, in 2018, the INTERMACS registry found that in 81.1% of patients, LVAD insertion was considered destination therapy. The vast majority of VADs are continuous-flow pumps instead of pulsatile flow. A variety of composite risk scores have been developed to help guide patient selection for LVAD implantation. LVADs are inserted to improve end-organ function ahead of a heart transplant. Issues such as aortic valve incompetence and the presence of intracardiac shunts need to be investigated because these make LVAD insertion unadvisable without repair. Right ventricle (RV) function needs to be carefully assessed before and after LVAD insertion because it can preclude the insertion of an LVAD or require a biventricular device.

Birks EJ. Left ventricular assist devices. *Heart*. 2010;96:63-71.

Miller LW, Guglin M. Patient selection for ventricular assist devices: a moving target. *J Am Coll Cardiol*. 2013;61:1209-1221.

Wilson SR, Mudge GH Jr, Stewart GC, et al. Evaluation for a ventricular assist device: selecting the appropriate candidate. *Circulation*. 2009;119:2225-2232.

Yuzefpolskaya M, Schroeder SE, Houston BA, et al. The Society of Thoracic Surgeons Intermacs 2022 Annual Report: focus on the 2018 heart transplant allocation system. *Ann Thorac Surg*. 2023;115:311-327.

A.11. What are the considerations in anesthetizing patients for left ventricular assist device (LVAD) insertion?

Significant cardiac abnormalities that could interfere with LVAD function (eg, aortic insufficiency, patent foramen ovale) should be identified preoperatively and, if possible, addressed at the time of surgery. The choice and dose of agents for induction and maintenance of general anesthesia should be cautiously considered in the context of frailty, end-stage heart failure, and/or cardiogenic shock. These patients often have ICDs in place, which, if deactivated, warrant the placement of external defibrillator pads. The Impella is a percutaneous LVAD that is intended for temporary MCS for up to 14 days, whereas the HeartMate III is a permanent LVAD. HeartWare is a smaller permanent LVAD that was discontinued in June 2021 due to thrombotic complications. As LVAD placement can be associated with significant perioperative blood loss, large-bore IV access is essential, and antifibrinolytic agents are routinely administered. TEE plays an essential role in ruling out cardiac anomalies that impair LVAD function (eg, patent foramen ovale, aortic insufficiency), confirming proper position and assessing flows in the inflow and outflow cannulae, and continuous monitoring of RV size, function, and the degree of LV decompression to optimize LVAD flow and fluid management. RVF is a frequent complication of LVAD insertion and can be treated with phosphodiesterase inhibitors, dobutamine, epinephrine, and/or inhaled NO. Norepinephrine and/or vasopressin are often needed to maintain adequate systemic vascular resistance following CPB, while carefully balancing device flow and end-organ perfusion.

Broussard D, Donaldson E, Falterman J, et al. Anesthesia for left ventricular assist device insertion: a case series and review. *Ochsner J*. 2011;11:70-77.

Feussner M, Mukherjee C, Garbade J, et al. Anaesthesia for patients undergoing ventricular assist-device implantation. *Best Pract Res Clin Anaesthesiol*. 2012;26:167-177.

Ma W, Suhitharan T, Shah S, Kothandan H. Anesthesia for left ventricular assisted device insertion in a patient with multiple organ failure. *Saudi J Anaesth*. 2021;15:210.

US Food and Drug Administration. Stop new implants of the Medtronic HVAD System—letter to health care providers. Accessed January 3, 2025. https://public4.pagefreezer.com/content/FDA/21-02-2024T12:58/https://www.fda.gov/medical-devices/letters-health-care-providers/stop-new-implants-medtronic-hvad-system-letter-health-care-providers

B. Preoperative Management

Three weeks after the insertion of an Impella VAD, a donor heart becomes available.

B.1. How would you assess this patient preoperatively?

Patients presenting for heart transplantation can be phenotyped into three categories. In the first category, patients are relatively compensated and are either ambulatory or stabilized with IV inotropic support. The second category involves stable, ambulatory patients with an LVAD in place. This category is expanding due to increasing numbers of patients having LVADs as a bridge to transplant. In the third category, patients are moribund and decompensated, requiring MCS. Based on INTERMACS data from

2009 to 2017, 39.7% of patients presented for heart transplant while on IV inotropes, 41.7% with an LVAD, 7.0% with an IABP, and 1.9% were mechanically ventilated.

Prospective transplant candidates are usually evaluated by a multidisciplinary team, including transplant cardiologists, pulmonologists, cardiac surgeons, and cardiac anesthesiologists. The anesthesiologist should make a detailed assessment of the recipient's current cardiac status, including functional capacity, recent decompensation, medications, and level of inotropic and MCS, with particular attention to hemodynamic parameters derived from right heart catheterization and reversibility of elevated PVR. It is important to note baseline and recent deterioration in kidney and liver function, frailty, and nutritional status, and rule out active infection. In addition to routine anesthetic history, including concomitant diseases and fasting status, workup includes complete blood count (CBC), electrolytes, urea, creatinine, liver function tests, glycemic control, INR/prothrombin time (PT), type, and screen. Specific investigations need to be reviewed, including echocardiogram, right heart catheterization, pulmonary function tests, ECG, and chest radiograph. A plan also needs to be devised regarding the management of an ICD if present. The anticoagulant effect of warfarin should be reversed with vitamin K preoperatively and vitamin K–dependent clotting factors (either fresh frozen plasma or prothrombin complex concentrate) intraoperatively at separation from cardiopulmonary bypass. A previous sternotomy increases the risk of major bleeding and coagulopathy and requires crossmatched blood to be checked and readily available in the operating room before sternotomy.

Chambers DC, Cherikh WS, Goldfarb SB, et al. The International Thoracic Organ Transplant Registry of the International Society for Heart and Lung Transplantation: thirty-fifth adult lung and heart-lung transplantation report—2018; focus theme: multiorgan transplantation. *J Heart Lung Transplant*. 2018;37:1169-1183.

Pal N, Gay SH, Boland CG, Lim AC. Heart transplantation after ventricular assist device therapy: benefits, risks, and outcomes. *Semin Cardiothorac Vasc Anesth*. 2020;24:9-23.

B.2. How would you premedicate this patient? Why?

Patients should be transported to the operating room with oxygen supplementation. Caution should be exercised with sedative or opioid premedication. Sedation can blunt respiratory and sympathetic drive, leading to hypoxemia, hypercapnia, and hypotension. Antibiotic prophylaxis is often with cefazolin or vancomycin.

Jhaveri R, Tardiff B, Stanley TE III. Anesthesia for heart and lung transplantation. *Anesthesiol Clin North Am*. 1994;12:729-747.

C. Intraoperative Management

C.1. What anesthetic equipment and monitors would you set up? Why?

Equipment setup should include a ventilator, anesthesia machine, airway, fluid warmer, forced air warming blanket, ultrasonography for central line insertion, CO and pressure monitoring systems, TEE, and defibrillator. Ultrasonography can also be useful for arterial line insertion in this patient group due to poor peripheral circulation and nonpulsatile flow in the case of LVAD. All invasive lines are placed with a sterile technique, with judicious sedation and supplemental oxygen. Routine monitors include five-lead ECG, pulse oximeter, noninvasive and arterial blood pressure, central venous pressure (CVP), pulmonary artery catheter for continuous CO and mixed venous saturation, TEE, depth of anesthesia monitor, capnography, urinary catheter, and temperature. In some centers, cerebral oximetry is used as a monitor of cerebral oxygen delivery. Large-bore peripheral and central IV access and antifibrinolytic agents are a routine part of management, and crossed-matched blood should be readily available.

Neethling E, Garijo JM, Mangalam TK, et al. Intraoperative and early postoperative management of heart transplantation: anesthetic implications. *J Cardiothorac Vascu Anesth*. 2020;34:2189-2206.

C.2. What is the role of transesophageal echocardiography (TEE)?

The echocardiographer can provide feedback to the surgeon regarding the overall function of the transplanted heart. In particular, ventricular size, systolic function, valvular function, and anomalies such as patent foramen ovale. Of particular interest is RV function assessment, which includes RV size, function, ventricular interdependence, and features of RV pressure and volume overload. TEE can also be useful in assessing the patency of the surgical anastomosis: the venae cavae and main PA anastomoses should be evaluated for stenosis, and pulmonary vein flows should be documented. The long-axis view of the left atrium is composed of recipient and donor tissue and can appear large. If excessive tissue is present, an acquired cor triatriatum can develop. Stored images of the baseline function of the transplanted heart can serve as a useful comparison after transplantation.

Denault AY, Couture P, Vegas A, Buithieu J, Tardif JC. Transesophageal echocardiography: a perioperative transdisciplinary approach. *Transesophageal Echocardiography Multimedia Manual.* 2nd ed. Taylor & Francis Group; 2011:547-560.

Orihashi K. The history of transesophageal echocardiography: the role of inspiration, innovation, and applications. *J Anesth.* 2020;34:86-94.

Romano P, Mangion JM. The role of intraoperative transesophageal echocardiography in heart transplantation. *Echocardiography.* 2002;19:599-604.

Suriani RJ. Transesophageal echocardiography during organ transplantation. *J Cardiothorac Vasc Anesth.* 1998;12:686-694.

C.3. Describe the induction and maintenance of anesthesia.

It is important to time the induction of anesthesia carefully so that CPB could be established at the time of donor heart arrival. Patients requiring resternotomy will have more adhesions to dissect with a risk of laceration of the heart. Defibrillator pads should be applied prior to induction. Securing the airway quickly might be required if the patient is not fasted; however, a rapid sequence induction needs to be balanced against the risk of hemodynamic compromise. Induction can be achieved through titration of agents such as midazolam, ketamine, and fentanyl, keeping in mind that those with pulmonary hypertension are sensitive to the effects of hypercapnia and hypoxemia secondary to hypoventilation. Neuromuscular block can be achieved with a nondepolarizing agent. Anesthesia is maintained with a balanced technique, using a combination of volatile agents, opioids, and additional boluses of neuromuscular blocking agents as needed. Massive hemorrhage can occur with resternotomy, warranting immediate availability of blood products in the operating room prior to sternotomy. Antifibrinolytic agents are routinely used for heart transplant surgery. The pulmonary artery catheter should be retracted to the proximal superior vena cava (SVC) prior to initiation of cardiopulmonary bypass.

Edwards S, Allen S, Sidebotham D. Anaesthesia for heart transplantation. *BJA Educ.* 2021;21:284-291.

C.4. How would you manage this patient during cardiopulmonary bypass (CPB)?

The anesthetic management of CPB is similar to that in other cardiac surgeries, except for prolonged reperfusion to compensate for the long ischemic time on the donor heart. Anesthesia is often maintained with an infusion of propofol, opioid supplementation, and delivery of volatile anesthetic through the CPB circuit. Care includes maintaining the hematocrit, electrolyte and acid-base balance, and correction of hyperglycemia with an insulin infusion. Once the anastomosis of the pulmonary artery is completed, the patient is placed in the head-down position to facilitate deairing. The heart is often paced via epicardial leads, and inotropic agents such as milrinone and dobutamine are often needed for RV support during CPB wean. In those with preexisting pulmonary hypertension, inhaled nitric oxide might be needed to reduce RV afterload. Blood products and clotting factors should be readily available to treat coagulopathy, especially when LVAD explant precedes heart transplantation.

D. Postoperative Management

D.1. What are the early postoperative complications?

Early postoperative complications include:

- Early graft dysfunction
- RVF
- Vasoplegia
- Coagulopathy
- Acute kidney injury
- Infection

D.2. What are the mechanisms of early right ventricular failure (RVF)?

RVF is frequent after transplant and is a major cause of morbidity and mortality. It has a diverse number of etiologies related to increased flow or resistance across the pulmonary vascular bed. An important cause of posttransplant RVF is a long-standing elevation in left ventricular end-diastolic pressure of the recipient heart, which leads to elevated PVR, a known risk factor for RVF after transplant, as the transplanted RV is not pressure adapted. A normal preoperative PVR does preclude the potential for RVF posttransplant. Poor organ preservation, long ischemic time, and fluid overload can have deleterious effects on graft RV function.

Arrigo M, Huber LC, Winnik S, et al. Right ventricular failure: pathophysiology, diagnosis and treatment. *Card Fail Rev*. 2019;5:140.

Iyer A, Kumarasinghe G, Hicks M, et al. Primary graft failure after heart transplantation. *J Transplant*. 2011;2011:175768.

Stobierska-Dzierzek B, Awad H, Michler RE. The evolving management of acute right-sided heart failure in cardiac transplant recipients. *J Am Coll Cardiol*. 2001;38:923-931.

Wagner F. Monitoring and management of right ventricular function following cardiac transplantation. *Appl Cardiopulm Pathophysiol*. 2011;15:220-229.

D.3. How would you treat RVF following heart transplantation?

RVF is associated with reduced CO and reduced left ventricle (LV) filling due to ventricular interdependence. Basic therapeutic goals are to increase heart rate through atrial epicardial pacing, maintain adequate coronary and systemic perfusion, optimize oxygen delivery, prevent further distension of the RV by judicious use and removal of fluids, and reduce RV afterload using agents that decrease PVR.

Phosphodiesterase inhibitors, such as milrinone, have systemic and pulmonary vasodilatory effects in addition to inotropic and lusitropic effects and are particularly useful. Prostacyclin (PGI_2), isoproterenol (1-5 μg/min), dobutamine, epinephrine, and nitrates can also be used to treat RVF. However, vasodilator use can cause arterial hypotension, requiring high-dose vasopressors to maintain adequate coronary and end-organ perfusion. Inhaled NO is widely used as a selective pulmonary vasodilator in refractory RVF. Avoiding hypoxia and hypercarbia will also mitigate elevated PVR. In severe cases of refractory RVF, posttransplant mechanical support should be considered, including IABP, right VAD (RVAD), or ECMO.

Arrigo M, Huber LC, Winnik S, et al. Right ventricular failure: pathophysiology, diagnosis and treatment. *Card Fail Rev*. 2019;5:140.

Costanzo MR, Dipchand A, Starling R, et al. The International Society of Heart and Lung Transplantation guidelines for the care of heart transplant recipients. *J Heart Lung Transplant*. 2010;29:914-956.

Granton J, Moric J. Pulmonary vasodilators—treating the right ventricle. *Anesthesiol Clin*. 2008;26:337-353.

Stobierska-Dzierzek B, Awad H, Michler RE. The evolving management of acute right-sided heart failure in cardiac transplant recipients. *J Am Coll Cardiol*. 2001;38:923-931.

Wagner F. Monitoring and management of right ventricular function following cardiac transplantation. *Appl Cardiopulm Pathophysiol*. 2011;15:220-229.

D.4. How does inhaled nitric oxide (NO) work as a selective pulmonary vasodilator?

The advantage of inhaled NO as a pulmonary vasodilator is mainly due to its selective pulmonary vascular smooth muscle relaxation. The in vivo half-life of inhaled NO is only a few seconds. Therefore, it has little effect on the systemic circulation, unlike IV vasodilators such as nitroprusside, nitroglycerin, prostaglandins, and calcium channel blockers. Furthermore, inhaled NO selectively causes vasodilation in ventilated lung units, thus decreasing $\dot{V}/\dot{Q}$ mismatch and shunt. Inhaled NO at 1 to 20 ppm can significantly reduce PA pressure, PVR, and CVP while increasing mean arterial pressure, CO, and arterial oxygenation by restoration of RV size and function.

Girard C, Durand PG, Vedrinne C, et al. Inhaled nitric oxide for right ventricular failure after heart transplantation. *J Cardiothorac Vasc Anesth*. 1993;7:481-485.

Haddad H, Isaac D, Legare JF, et al. Canadian Cardiovascular Society Consensus Conference update on cardiac transplantation 2008: executive summary. *Can J Cardiol*. 2009;25:197-205.

Konstadt S. Nitric oxide: has it progressed from molecule of the year to wonder drug of the decade? *J Cardiothorac Vasc Anesth*. 1995;9:625-626.

Yu B, Ichinose F, Bloch DB, Zapol WM. Inhaled nitric oxide. *Br J Pharmacol*. 2019;176:246-255.

D.5. What is the pathophysiology of the denervated heart?

Following cardiac transplantation, the cardiac plexus is interrupted, and the heart is denervated. The recipient atrium remains innervated but hemodynamically unimportant, whereas the donor atrium is denervated and responsible for the electrophysiologic responses of the transplanted heart. The ECG often contains two P waves. The denervated heart retains its intrinsic control mechanisms, including the Frank-Starling mechanism and intact α- and β-adrenoreceptor responses to circulating catecholamines. However, the denervated heart lacks the ability to respond acutely to hypovolemia or hypotension with reflex tachycardia and responds to stress primarily by an increase in stroke volume. This reflects the dependence of the donor heart sinus node on direct stimulation by endogenously released catecholamines and the absence of control by neural mechanisms. Interestingly, some studies have reported reinnervation within a year after transplantation, which has led to angina pectoris when ischemia develops in the transplanted heart.

Cheng DC, Ong DD. Anaesthesia for non-cardiac surgery in heart-transplanted patients. *Can J Anaesth.* 1993;40:981-986.

Kobashigawa JA. Postoperative management following heart transplantation. *Transplant Proc.* 1999;31:2038-2046.

D.6. What are the common cardiac dysrhythmias following heart transplantation?

A wide variety of arrhythmias can occur in the heart transplant recipient. Early after the transplant, bradyarrhythmia is common and often self-limited. Patients are often paced using epicardial wires in the early postoperative period. The spectrum of other arrhythmias includes premature ventricular complexes, atrioventricular (AV) block, right bundle branch block, and supraventricular tachycardia. In fact, 5% to 24% of heart transplant recipients suffer from atrial fibrillation. The causes of arrhythmia include surgical disruption of normal conduction pathways and the sinus node, denervation, rejection, and coronary allograft vasculopathy. About 5% to 10% of patients require permanent pacemaker insertion after a heart transplant due to sinus node dysfunction or AV block. Persistent arrhythmias, in particular ventricular, are associated with increased long-term morbidity and mortality.

Chang HY, Lo LW, Feng AN, et al. Long-term follow-up of arrhythmia characteristics and clinical outcomes in heart transplant patients. *Transplant Proc.* 2013;45:369-375.

Hwang NC, Sivathasan C. Review of postoperative care for heart transplant recipients. *J Cardiothorac Vasc Anesth.* 2023;37:112-126.

Isath A, Sherif AA, Siroky GP, et al. Trends, burden, and impact of arrhythmias on cardiac transplant recipients: a 16-year nationwide study: arrhythmias in cardiac transplant recipients. *Curr Probl Cardiol.* 2022;48:101504.

Joglar JA, Wan EY, Chung MK, et al. Management of arrhythmias after heart transplant: current state and considerations for future research. *Circ Arrhythmia Electrophysiol.* 2021;14:e007954.

Stecker EC, Sterlich KR, Chugh SS, et al. Arrhythmias after orthotopic heart transplantation. *J Card Fail.* 2005;11:464-472.

D.7. What are the causes of posttransplant bleeding?

Perioperative bleeding is a significant contributor to mortality following heart transplantation. The causes of bleeding are anastomotic leaks and coagulopathy. Immediately before weaning from CPB with the heart filled, the posterior anastomosis is carefully inspected by the surgeon for "water tightness" because leaks in this area are more difficult and riskier to repair. Coagulopathy often results from a combination of mechanisms, including inadequate heparin reversal, dilution of platelets and coagulation factors, hypothermia, and CPB effects on fibrinolysis, platelet function, and factor activation. Patients with a VAD in place before transplant are at particular risk for perioperative hemorrhage, possibly exacerbated by the presence of acquired von Willebrand syndrome.

Bourge RC, Naftel DC, Costanzo-Nordin MR, et al. Pretransplantation risk factors for death after heart transplantation: a multi-institutional study. *J Heart Lung Transplant.* 1993;12:549-562.

Diaz-Martin A, Escoresca-Ortega AM, Hernandez-Caballero C, et al. Considerations regarding major bleeding after cardiac transplantation. *Transplant Proc.* 2010;42:3204-3205.

Uriel N, Pak SW, Jorde UP, et al. Acquired von Willebrand syndrome after continuous-flow mechanical device support contributes to a high prevalence of bleeding during long-term support and at the time of transplantation. *J Am Coll Cardiol.* 2010;56:1207-1213.

Wegner JA, DiNardo JA, Arabia FA, et al. Blood loss and transfusion requirements in patients implanted with a mechanical circulatory support device undergoing cardiac transplantation. *J Heart Lung Transplant.* 2000;19:504-506.

D.8. How would you treat posttransplant bleeding?

Prevention is key and can be accomplished with meticulous surgical technique, use of antifibrinolytic agents, avoidance of excessive hemodilution, maintaining normothermia, and proactive point-of-care coagulation testing prior to separation from CPB, ensuring coagulation factors are readily available. Treatment of coagulopathy needs to be carefully balanced with the need to avoid fluid overload, which is detrimental to RV function. In patients who are anticoagulated with warfarin, prothrombin complex concentrates should be considered as low-volume alternatives. Although not routine, desmopressin (0.3 μg/kg) also has a role in refractory cases. Finally, recombinant factor VIIa has been used to treat hemorrhage in cardiac transplant patients. When using recombinant factor IIa, the risk of thrombosis needs to be weighed against that of ongoing bleeding, and consultation with a hematologist is advisable before administration. Bleeding that is excessive and not clearly secondary to coagulopathy warrants surgical reexploration.

Costanzo MR, Dipchand A, Starling R, et al. The International Society of Heart and Lung Transplantation guidelines for the care of heart transplant recipients. *J Heart Lung Transplant*. 2010;29:914-956.

Kogan A, Berman M, Kassif Y, et al. Use of recombinant factor VII to control bleeding in a patient supported by right ventricular assist device after heart transplantation. *J Heart Lung Transplant*. 2005;24:347-349.

Lindauer KE, Ingemi AI, McMahon MR, et al. The utilization and safety of apixaban for therapeutic anticoagulation in heart transplant population requiring routine endomyocardial biopsies. *Clin Transplant*. 2022;36:e14828.

D.9. What are the causes of early graft failure?

Graft failure, primary and secondary, is the most common cause of death in the first 30 days after a heart transplant. Primary graft failure can result from biventricular failure or isolated LV or RVF and is often due to ischemia-reperfusion injury, myocardial edema, and/or preexisting disease of the donor heart such as unrecognized coronary artery disease and hypertrophy. Allografts from donors older than 55 years of age who suffered from intracranial hemorrhage, and who required high doses of inotropic support to maintain cardiac function after brainstem death, are especially susceptible to ischemic injury. Recipient-specific risk factors for primary graft failure are older age, amiodarone therapy, diminished renal function, longer time on the wait list, previous cardiac surgery, pulmonary hypertension, and ECMO or LVAD prior to transplant surgery. Secondary graft failure can also be due to hyperacute rejection, restrictive anastomosis, or RVF from elevated PVR or volume overload.

Hwang NC, Sivathasan C. Review of postoperative care for heart transplant recipients. *J Cardiothorac Vasc Anesth*. 2023;37:112-126.

Luckraz H, Goddard M, Charman SC, et al. Early mortality after cardiac transplantation: should we do better? *J Heart Lung Transplant*. 2005;24:401-405.

Lund LH, Edwards LB, Kucheryavaya AY, et al. The registry of the International Society for Heart and Lung Transplantation: thirty-first official adult heart transplant report—2014. *J Heart Lung Transplant*. 2014;33:996-1008.

Prieto D, Correia PM, Batista M, Antunes MJ. Primary graft failure after cardiac transplantation: prevalence, prognosis and risk actors. *Interact Cardiovasc Thorac Surg*. 2018;27:765-772.

Singh SSA, Dalzell JR, Berry C, Al-Attar N. Primary graft dysfunction after heart transplantation: a thorn amongst the roses. *Heart Fail Rev*. 2019;24:805-820.

D.10. How would you manage this patient in the intensive care unit?

Within the first 30 days, posttransplant graft failure (primary and secondary), multiorgan failure, and infection are the most common causes of death at 39%, 18%, and 12.7%, respectively. Early management goals include prevention of infection and rejection, treatment of coagulopathy and dysrhythmias, inotropic support, and avoidance of RV pressure or volume overload. If possible, the patient is weaned from the ventilator and extubated within 24 hours. In order to facilitate oxygenation and weaning, strict supervision of fluid balance and body weight is required. Close monitoring of mediastinal drainage is needed, with prompt treatment of excessive drainage due to surgical bleeding or coagulopathy. Sudden decreases in mediastinal drainage can be due to the accumulation of fluid in the pericardial space. This is especially relevant as heart transplant recipients are often adapted to cardiomegaly, which leaves a large pericardial space that allows hemodynamic stability until pericardial effusions become large. The incidence of large pericardial effusions is up to 30% in transplant recipients.

Vasoplegia is a known complication after a heart transplant; it occurs in up to 58% of transplant recipients, typically within 6 hours after bypass separation. Norepinephrine and vasopressin are typical first-line agents. Although methylene blue and hydroxocobalamin have been used to treat catecholamine-resistant vasoplegia with some success, caution should be exercised when administering NO synthase inhibitors due to side effects and lack of efficacy in randomized controlled trials.

Immunosuppression often is achieved with a number of medications, including corticosteroids (methylprednisolone followed by prednisone), calcineurin inhibitors (eg, tacrolimus), or antiproliferative agents (eg, mycophenolate mofetil). Some patients benefit from induction therapy using interleukin-2 (IL-2) antagonists and/or polyclonal antibodies, for example, highly sensitized patients, those with reactive donor-specific antigens, or those with renal dysfunction on tacrolimus-delaying immunosuppression strategies. A significant number of centers no longer routinely administer induction immunosuppression with good results. Secondary to immunosuppression, patients are sometimes treated with ganciclovir for cytomegalovirus (CMV) prophylaxis.

Blasco LM, Parameshwar J, Vuylsteke A. Anaesthesia for noncardiac surgery in the heart transplant recipient. *Curr Opin Anaesthesiol.* 2009;22:109-113.

Costanzo MR, Dipchand A, Starling R, et al. The International Society of Heart and Lung Transplantation guidelines for the care of heart transplant recipients. *J Heart Lung Transplant.* 2010;29:914-956.

Hwang NC, Sivathasan C. Review of postoperative care for heart transplant recipients. *J Cardiothorac Vasc Anesth.* 2023;37:112-126.

Lund LH, Edwards LB, Kucheryavaya AY, et al. The registry of the International Society for Heart and Lung Transplantation: thirty-first official adult heart transplant report—2014. *J Heart Lung Transplant.* 2014;33:996-1008.

Subramani S, Aldrich A, Dwarakanath S, Sugawara A, Hanada S. Early graft dysfunction following heart transplant: prevention and management. *Semin Cardiothorac Vasc Anesth.* 2020;24:24-33. .

E. Subsequent Noncardiac Surgery

The patient recovers following heart transplant. However, 2 years postoperatively, he fractures his left radius after a fall and presents for open reduction and internal fixation of the fracture.

E.1. How would you monitor this patient?

This patient should be monitored as for other patients undergoing similar procedures. Safe anesthesia is contingent upon careful preoperative assessment, which can reduce the need for invasive monitoring with its attendant risks. Adequate preload must be attained preoperatively and intravascular volume status maintained intraoperatively because the transplanted heart is preload dependent. Monitors in this case should include 5-lead ECG, noninvasive blood pressure, capnometry, and peripheral oximetry; if general anesthesia is used, temperature, inhaled gas, and neuromuscular function should be monitored. For surgeries with the potential for blood loss and fluid shifts, additional intraoperative monitors including invasive arterial and central venous pressure monitoring and TEE could be considered. Postoperatively, increased attention should be paid to preload status, renal function, and prevention of infection. Immunosuppressants should be continued postoperatively, and blood levels should be monitored.

Cheng DC, Ong DD. Anaesthesia for non-cardiac surgery in heart-transplanted patients. *Can J Anaesth.* 1993;40:981-986.

Choudury M. Post-cardiac transplant recipient: implications for anaesthesia. *Indian J Anaesth.* 2017;61:768-774.

E.2. What type of anesthetic is best for heart transplant recipients?

In a series of 86 heart transplant recipients, 18 returned for 32 noncardiac surgical procedures. Anesthesia included 18 neurolept-anesthesia cases, 12 general anesthesia cases with a combination of N_2O/O_2/opioid/neuromuscular blocker and low doses of volatile agents, and two spinal anesthesia cases. The patients had normal requirements for IV and inhalational agents, neuromuscular blocking drugs, and local anesthetics, without prolonged action of any anesthetic agents. Generally, the choice of general or regional anesthesia does not affect postoperative outcome in heart transplant recipients undergoing subsequent noncardiac surgery. However, neuraxial anesthesia can result in profound hypotension with a lack of compensatory tachycardia to restore CO.

Blasco LM, Parameshwar J, Vuylsteke A. Anaesthesia for noncardiac surgery in the heart transplant recipient. *Curr Opin Anaesthesiol.* 2009;22:109-113.

Cheng DC, Ong DD. Anaesthesia for non-cardiac surgery in heart-transplanted patients. *Can J Anaesth.* 1993;40:981-986.

Navas-Blanco JR, Modak RK. Perioperative care of heart transplant recipients undergoing non-cardiac surgery. *Ann Card Anaesth.* 2021;24:140-148.

Šoltés J, Říha H, Bruthans J, Kramář P, Ročeň M. Anaesthesia for non-cardiac surgical procedures in patients after heart transplantation. *Cas Lek Cesk.* 2022;161:139-143.

E.3. What anesthetic technique would you choose for this patient?

This patient could safely receive general anesthesia or a regional block of his brachial plexus. No anesthetic technique has been shown to be superior as long as preload is maintained.

Brusich KT, Acan I. Anesthetic considerations in transplant recipients for nontransplant surgery. In: Tsoulfas G, ed. *Organ Donation and Transplantation—Current Status and Future Challenges*. IntechOpen; 2018:229-257.

Cheng DC, Ong DD. Anaesthesia for non-cardiac surgery in heart-transplanted patients. *Can J Anaesth*. 1993;40:981-986.

Choudhury M. Post-cardiac transplant recipient: implications for anaesthesia. *Indian J Anaesth*. 2017;61:768.

Navas-Blanco JR, Modak RK. Perioperative care of heart transplant recipients undergoing non-cardiac surgery. *Ann Card Anaesth*. 2021;24:140-148.

E.4. Do you need to use a muscarinic antagonist with cholinesterase inhibitors to reverse the neuromuscular block in heart transplant patients?

Neostigmine produces dose-dependent bradycardia in heart transplant patients. Patients should be closely monitored and treated with a direct-acting chronotropic agent if needed. A muscarinic antagonist should be administered simultaneously with cholinesterase inhibitors.

Ashary N, Kaye AD, Hegazi AR, et al. Anesthetic considerations in the patient with a heart transplant. *Heart Dis*. 2002;4:191-198.

Backman SB, Fox GS, Stein RD, et al. Neostigmine decreases heart rate in heart transplant patients. *Can J Anaesth*. 1996;43:373-378.

Bjerke RJ, Mangione MP. Asystole after intravenous neostigmine in a heart transplant recipient. *Can J Anaesth*. 2001;48:305-307.

Wilson RF, Christensen BV, Olivari MT, et al. Evidence for structural sympathetic reinnervation after orthotopic cardiac transplantation in humans. *Circulation*. 1991;83:1210-1221.

E.5. What are the anesthetic considerations for heart transplant patients?

Anesthetic considerations for heart transplant patients include:

- Denervated heart
- Allograft rejection
- Infection due to immunosuppression
- Drug interactions
- Allograft coronary artery disease
- Hypertension
- Renal and hepatic dysfunction
- Immunosuppression-related malignancy
- Adrenal suppression

Ashary N, Kaye AD, Hegazi AR, et al. Anesthetic considerations in the patient with a heart transplant. *Heart Dis*. 2002;4:191-198.

Cheng DC, Ong DD. Anaesthesia for non-cardiac surgery in heart-transplanted patients. *Can J Anaesth*. 1993;40:981-986.

Choudhury M. Post-cardiac transplant recipient: implications for anaesthesia. *Indian J Anaesth*. 2017;61:768.

Ejtehadi F, Carter S, Evans L, et al. General anaesthesia and emergency surgery in heart transplant recipient. *Case Rep Surg*. 2015;2015:256465.

Neethling E, Garijo JM, Mangalam TK, et al. Intraoperative and early postoperative management of heart transplantation: anesthetic implications. *J Cardiothorac Vasc Anesth*. 2020;34:2189-2206.

E.6. What are the significant implications of the denervated heart?

The denervated heart retains its intrinsic control mechanisms such as the Frank-Starling mechanism, impulse formation and conduction, and responsiveness to circulating catecholamines in the form of increased heart rate and contractility. However, normal respiratory variation or response to carotid sinus massage or Valsalva maneuver is absent, and baroreceptor reflexes are lost. At rest, heart rate reflects the intrinsic rate of depolarization of the donor sinoatrial node and, in the absence of vagal tone, is faster than normal at about 90 to 110 beats per minute. The denervated heart responds to direct-acting vasoactive medications such as phenylephrine, vasopressin, isoproterenol, epinephrine, and dobutamine, whereas indirect agents such as ephedrine and anticholinergic agents such as atropine are ineffective. Additionally, exaggerated response to vasodilators (eg, nitroglycerin, nitroprusside, hydralazine) can occur.

Cardiac dysrhythmias can occur in heart transplant patients. Atrial, and less frequently ventricular, tachyarrhythmias are common. Bradyarrhythmia therapy should be with a direct β-adrenergic stimulating agent (epinephrine, isoproterenol). Medications used to treat tachyarrhythmias (calcium channel blockers, β-blockers) need to be used with caution due to their negative inotropic effects.

Ashary N, Kaye AD, Hegazi AR, et al. Anesthetic considerations in the patient with a heart transplant. *Heart Dis.* 2002;4:191-198.

Blasco LM, Parameshwar J, Vuylsteke A. Anaesthesia for noncardiac surgery in the heart transplant recipient. *Curr Opin Anaesthesiol.* 2009;22:109-113.

Chang HY, Lo LW, Feng AN, et al. Long-term follow-up of arrhythmia characteristics and clinical outcomes in heart transplant patients. *Transplant Proc.* 2013;45:369-375.

Jurgens PT, Aquilante CL, Page RL II, et al. Perioperative management of cardiac transplant recipients undergoing noncardiac surgery: unique challenges created by advancements in care. *Semin Cardiothorac Vasc Anesth.* 2017;21:235-244.

Stein KL, Darby JM, Grenvik A. Intensive care of the cardiac transplant recipient. *J Cardiothorac Anesth.* 1988;2:543-553.

E.7. What is the significance of allograft rejection?

Most rejection episodes occur in the first 6 months after transplantation. Patients can present with fever, malaise, arrhythmias, and shortness of breath. Hemodynamic compromise is considered a late sign of rejection. The gold standard for diagnosis is endomyocardial biopsy. Rejection episodes are treated primarily with steroids; however, more severe forms require aggressive immunosuppression with antithymocyte antibodies or plasmapheresis. The type of therapy is guided by symptom severity and type of rejection (cell mediated vs antibody mediated).

Costanzo MR, Dipchand A, Starling R, et al. The International Society of Heart and Lung Transplantation guidelines for the care of heart transplant recipients. *J Heart Lung Transplant.* 2010;29:914-956.

Kobashigawa JA. Postoperative management following heart transplantation. *Transplant Proc.* 1999;31:2038-2046.

Zhao K, Wang R, Kamoun M, et al. Incidence of acute rejection and patient survival in combined heart–liver transplantation. *Liver Transplant.* 2022;28:1500-1508.

E.8. What is the significance of infection in these patients?

Immunosuppressive drugs are continued indefinitely in heart transplant patients, and infection remains a major cause of death, with 10% of mortality at 5 years after transplant secondary to non-CMV infections. Early postoperative bacterial and opportunistic infections (eg, CMV, *Pneumocystis jirovecii*, *Toxoplasma*) are of great concern. Typical early postoperative infections include sternal wound infection, pneumonia, and urinary tract infection. Invasive monitoring techniques and all forms of instrumentation should be kept to a minimum, consistent with safe anesthesia. Attention to sterile technique is paramount. Orotracheal intubation is preferable to nasotracheal intubation because the latter is associated with infection by diphtheroids and staphylococci from the nasopharynx and skin.

Blasco LM, Parameshwar J, Vuylsteke A. Anaesthesia for noncardiac surgery in the heart transplant recipient. *Curr Opin Anaesthesiol.* 2009;22:109-113.

Lund LH, Edwards LB, Kucheryavaya AY, et al. The registry of the International Society for Heart and Lung Transplantation: thirty-first official adult heart transplant report—2014. *J Heart Lung Transplant.* 2014;33:996-1008.

Morrissey CO. Unraveling the relationship between rejection and infection. *J Heart Lung Transplant.* 2019;38:1233-1234.

Shaw IH, Kirk AJB, Conacher ID. Anaesthesia for patients with transplanted hearts and lungs undergoing non-cardiac surgery. *Br J Anaesth.* 1991;67:772-778.

Taylor DO, Stehlik J, Edwards LB, et al. Registry of the International Society for Heart and Lung Transplantation: twenty-sixth official adult heart transplant report—2009. *J Heart Lung Transplant.* 2009;28:1007-1022.

E.9. What are the significant implications of drug interactions?

Chronic steroid treatment is associated with relative adrenal insufficiency, and corticosteroids should be administered in accordance with the expected magnitude of surgical stress. Azathioprine has been reported to antagonize competitive neuromuscular blocking drugs due to its phosphodiesterase-inhibiting properties; therefore, larger doses might be required. In animals, cyclosporine infusion potentiates the neuromuscular blocking effects of atracurium and vecuronium. A single dose of cyclosporine can also result in a prolonged duration of both barbiturates and opioids.

Ashary N, Kaye AD, Hegazi AR, et al. Anesthetic considerations in the patient with a heart transplant. *Heart Dis.* 2002;4:191-198.

Cirella VN, Pantuck CB, Lee YJ, et al. Effects of cyclosporine on anesthetic action. *Anesth Analg.* 1987;66:703-706.

Gago-Sánchez AI, Font P, Cárdenas M, Aumente MD, Del Prado JR, Calleja MÁ. Real clinical impact of drug–drug interactions of immunosuppressants in transplant patients. *Pharmacol Res Perspect.* 2021;9:e00892.

Rančić NK, Vavić NN, Kovačević AM, et al. Drug-drug interactions of tacrolimus. *Hosp Pharmacol.* 2015;2:291-296.

E.10. What is cardiac allograft vasculopathy? Why is this important?

The transplanted heart is vulnerable to accelerated atherosclerosis (ie, cardiac allograft vasculopathy [CAV]). By 10 years after transplant, over 40% of patients develop CAV. CAV is characterized by concentric intimal hyperplasia and diffuse narrowing of coronary arteries and is the primary risk factor for graft rejection and dysfunction. The etiology is multifactorial with both immunologic and nonimmunologic factors. Traditional risk factors, such as pretransplant coronary artery disease, diabetes, and hyperlipidemia, are risk factors for CAV. Donor characteristics, such as advanced donor age and mechanism of donor death, are also risk factors. The type of immunosuppression regime, CMV infection, and episodes of rejection also impact CAV development.

Blasco LM, Parameshwar J, Vuylsteke A. Anaesthesia for noncardiac surgery in the heart transplant recipient. *Curr Opin Anaesthesiol.* 2009;22:109-113.

Laks JA, Dipchand AI. Cardiac allograft vasculopathy: a review. *Pediatr Transplant.* 2022;26:e14218.

Lund LH, Edwards LB, Kucheryavaya AY, et al. The registry of the International Society for Heart and Lung Transplantation: thirty-first official adult heart transplant report—2014. *J Heart Lung Transplant.* 2014;33:996-1008.

Pober JS, Chih S, Kobashigawa J, Madsen JC, Tellides G. Cardiac allograft vasculopathy: current review and future research directions. *Cardiovas Res.* 2021;117:2624-2638.

Spartalis M, Spartalis E, Siasos G. Cardiac allograft vasculopathy after heart transplantation: pathophysiology, detection approaches, prevention, and treatment management. *Trends Cardiovasc Med.* 2022;32:333-338.

E.11. What are the significant implications of posttransplant hypertension?

After 5 years, 91% of surviving patients have developed hypertension. Calcineurin inhibitors often are cited as a causative factor. Current therapy consists of a calcium channel blocker such as diltiazem. However, care must be taken because diltiazem can increase cyclosporine serum levels. Nifedipine tends to cause significant vasodilatation and might be poorly tolerated. When necessary, an ACE inhibitor can be added. Because cardiac responsiveness during exercise is dependent on circulating catecholamines, β-blockers are often avoided after heart transplantation.

Bennett AL, Ventura HO. Hypertension in patients with cardiac transplantation. *Med Clin.* 2017;101:53-64.

Costanzo MR, Dipchand A, Starling R, et al. The International Society of Heart and Lung Transplantation guidelines for the care of heart transplant recipients. *J Heart Lung Transplant.* 2010;29:914-956.

Lund LH, Edwards LB, Kucheryavaya AY, et al. The registry of the International Society for Heart and Lung Transplantation: thirty-first official adult heart transplant report—2014. *J Heart Lung Transplant.* 2014;33:996-1008.

Valerio R Jr, Durra O, Gold ME. Anesthetic considerations for an adult heart transplant recipient undergoing noncardiac surgery: a case report. *AANA J.* 2014;82:293-299.

E.12. What are the significant implications of renal dysfunction?

Renal dysfunction is found in 51.1% of recipients at 5 years. Due to the nephrotoxic effects of calcineurin inhibitors, serum creatinine concentrations often gradually increase after cardiac transplantation, with 6.7% of recipients requiring dialysis after 10 years. Repeated contrast exposure with cardiac catheterizations is another contributing factor. Anesthetic drugs that are excreted mainly by renal clearance should be minimized or avoided if renal function is severely reduced. Also, one needs to be mindful of medications that can further compromise renal function, such as nonsteroidal anti-inflammatory drugs (NSAIDs).

Bianco JC, Stang MV, Denault AY, Marenchino RG, Belziti CA, Musso CG. Acute kidney injury after heart transplant: the importance of pulmonary hypertension. *J Cardiothorac Vasc Anesth.* 2021;35:2052-2062.

Jiang Y-Y, Kong X-R, Xue F-L, et al. Incidence, risk factors and clinical outcomes of acute kidney injury after heart transplantation: a retrospective single center study. *J Cardiothorac Surg.* 2020;15:1-10.

Lindenfeld JA, Page RL II, Zolty R, et al. Drug therapy in the heart transplant recipient: part III: common medical problems. *Circulation*. 2005;111:113-117.

Lund LH, Khush KK, Cherikh WS, et al. The registry of the International Society for Heart and Lung Transplantation: thirty-fourth adult heart transplantation report—2017; focus theme: allograft ischemic time. *J Heart Lung Transplant*. 2017;36:1037-1046.

Roest S, Hesselink DA, Klimczak-Tomaniak D, et al. Incidence of end-stage renal disease after heart transplantation and effect of its treatment on survival. *ESC Heart Fail*. 2020;7:533-541.

E.13. What types of malignancy are common in heart transplant recipients?

Chronic immunosuppression puts patients at risk for cancer. After 10 years, 27.7% of survivors have some form of malignancy. The vast majority are skin cancers, whereas a much smaller percentage suffers from posttransplant lymphoproliferative disorders. Malignancies account for 23% of deaths 5 years after transplant.

Haddad H, Isaac D, Legare JF, et al. Canadian Cardiovascular Society Consensus Conference update on cardiac transplantation 2008: executive summary. *Can J Cardiol*. 2009;25:197-205.

Jäämaa-Holmberg S, Salmela B, Lemström K, Pukkala E, Lommi J. Cancer incidence and mortality after heart transplantation—a population-based national cohort study. *Acta Oncol*. 2019;58:859-863.

Lund LH, Khush KK, Cherikh WS, et al. The registry of the International Society for Heart and Lung Transplantation: thirty-fourth adult heart transplantation report—2017; focus theme: allograft ischemic time. *J Heart Lung Transplant*. 2017;36:1037-1046.

Mancini D, Rakita V. Malignancy post heart transplantation: no free lunch. *J Am Coll Cardiol*. 2018;71:50-52.

Mudigonda P, Berardi C, Chetram V, Barac A, Cheng R. Implications of cancer prior to and after heart transplantation. *Heart*. 2022;108:414-421.

E.14. Is ambulatory surgery appropriate for heart transplant recipients?

There is a paucity of information about ambulatory surgery in heart transplant recipients. Choice of anesthetic technique seems to have no influence on the outcome. Regardless, these patients should be seen in preadmission clinics before the day of surgery and have appropriate screening tests done preoperatively, including CBC, electrolytes, renal function tests, ECG, and accurate blood pressure measurement. They also should be evaluated by the cardiac transplant service, and if any concern is raised, further testing such as echocardiography, coronary angiography, or endomyocardial biopsy might be suggested. Recommendations also should be obtained from the cardiac transplant service regarding perioperative antibiotic prophylaxis and immunosuppression.

Blasco LM, Parameshwar J, Vuylsteke A. Anaesthesia for noncardiac surgery in the heart transplant recipient. *Curr Opin Anaesthesiol*. 2009;22:109-113.

Bryson GL, Chung F, Finegan BA, et al. Patient selection in ambulatory anesthesia—an evidence-based review: part I. *Can J Anaesth*. 2004;51:768-781.

14 Ischemic Heart Disease and Noncardiac Surgery

Sagar Navare and June M. Chan

A 72-year-old male is scheduled for a pancreaticoduodenectomy for pancreatic cancer. His history is significant for an ST-elevation myocardial infarction (STEMI) 5 months ago, treated with a bifurcating drug-eluting stent (DES) in the distal left main coronary artery. He also has hypertension, type 2 diabetes, and chronic renal impairment (estimated glomerular filtration rate [GFR] = 35 mL/min/1.73 m^2). His medications include aspirin, ticagrelor, atenolol, sacubitril/valsartan, empagliflozin, and occasional sublingual nitroglycerin (NTG).

A. Medical Disease and Differential Diagnosis

1. What are the preoperative predictors for perioperative major adverse cardiac events (MACE)?
2. What are the determinants of myocardial oxygen demand? How are they measured clinically?
3. What factors determine myocardial oxygen supply?
4. What are the mechanisms of perioperative myocardial injury and ischemia?
5. What is the incidence of perioperative myocardial injury, infarction, and MACE in patients with coronary artery disease (CAD) undergoing noncardiac surgery?
6. Which perioperative medical therapies would you employ to reduce the incidence of myocardial ischemia?
7. Based on his history, would you recommend that this patient's surgery be postponed for a certain period? If so, why?

B. Preoperative Evaluation and Preparation

1. How would you evaluate this patient's cardiac condition? What laboratory tests would you order?
2. What is the role of cardiac stress testing and noninvasive coronary imaging for this patient?
3. What is the role of coronary revascularization before surgery?
4. How would you classify this patient's surgery-specific MACE risk?
5. How should this patient's antiplatelet therapy be managed perioperatively?
6. How should the patient's other medications be managed before surgery?
7. What is the role of cardiac prehabilitation in optimizing this patient's postoperative outcome?

C. Intraoperative Management

1. What are the intraoperative predictors for perioperative MACE?
2. How would you monitor the patient in the operating room?
3. What electrocardiogram (ECG) leads would you monitor? Which leads are the most sensitive for monitoring myocardial ischemia?
4. Would you place invasive monitors such as a central venous catheter (CVC), pulmonary artery catheter (PAC), and/or an intra-arterial catheter?
5. Would you use transesophageal echocardiography (TEE) as a monitor?
6. Is regional anesthesia better than general anesthesia for patients with cardiac disease?
7. How will you induce general anesthesia?
8. What is the best choice of anesthetic agents for the maintenance of anesthesia? Why?
9. You notice a new 3-mm ST-segment depression in lead V_5. How would you treat it?
10. What is the significance of tight control of the heart rate intraoperatively?
11. When would you extubate the trachea in this patient? What could you do to prevent hypertension and tachycardia during extubation and emergence?

D. Postoperative Management

1. What are the postoperative predictors of perioperative MACE?
2. How would you control postoperative pain?
3. Is postoperative anemia associated with adverse cardiac outcomes?
4. Is postoperative hypothermia associated with postoperative myocardial ischemia?
5. How would you make a diagnosis of perioperative myocardial infarction (PMI)?
6. How would you manage a patient with a suspected PMI?

A. Medical Disease and Differential Diagnosis

A.1. What are the preoperative predictors for perioperative major adverse cardiac events (MACE)?

MACE are composite outcomes for death, nonfatal myocardial infarction (MI), and nonfatal stroke, typically within 30 days of an intervention. Although MACE is one of the most commonly used outcome measures in cardiovascular research, its definition varies between studies, with many expanding MACE to include heart failure (HF) hospitalization and/or the need for coronary revascularization (so-called 3-, 4-, and 5-point MACE definitions).

The 2024 American College of Cardiology (ACC)/American Heart Association (AHA) guidelines categorize patients undergoing noncardiac surgery into two groups: *low risk* and *elevated risk* based on the presence of clinical risk factors and risk of surgical procedures. Patients with less than 1% chance of MACE are categorized as low risk, whereas patients with a cumulative risk of MACE of more than 1% are categorized as elevated risk.

Numerous risk indices and predictors for MACE have been published over the last 40 years, but the development of risk stratification tools powered by data from vast perioperative patient registries has significantly improved the degree to which perioperative risk discussions may be personalized.

The Revised Cardiac Risk Index (RCRI), first developed in 1979 and revised in 1999, describes six independent predictors of cardiac risk (see **Table 14.1**). Although it is referenced in the ACC/AHA and European guidelines, recent validation studies suggest that the RCRI underperformed for low-risk patients, same-day surgery patients, and those with severe chronic renal impairment. This likely reflects the

TABLE 14.1 Risk Indices for Predicting Perioperative MACE

	Demographic Data	Comorbidities	Surgical Factors
RCRI	N/A	Ischemic heart disease Congestive heart failure Cerebrovascular disease Preoperative insulin therapy Preoperative creatinine >2 mg/dL	Elevated risk surgery
MICA	Age	ASA physical status Functional dependence Creatinine level	Procedure type (by organ/organ system)
ACS	Age Body mass index Sex	ASA physical status Functional dependence Hypertension requiring medication Congestive heart failure within 30 d Presence of dyspnea within 30 d Smoker within 1 y Chronic obstructive pulmonary disease Ventilator dependence Chronic steroid therapy Dialysis dependence Acute renal failure Ascites within 30 d Systemic sepsis within 48 h Disseminated cancer	Procedure/CPT code Emergency surgery

ACS, American College of Surgeons Surgical Risk Calculator; ASA, American Society of Anesthesiologists; CPT, current procedural terminology; MICA, Gupta perioperative risk for myocardial infarction or cardiac arrest calculator; RCRI, Revised Cardiac Risk Index.

TABLE 14.2 Specific Conditions Associated With Increased Perioperative MACE Risk

Unstable Coronary Syndromes	Acute MI (Within 7 d) or Recent MI (Within 1 mo)
Severe angina	Canadian Class III and IV
Severe valvular disease	Severe aortic stenosis (<1 cm^2) or symptomatic
High-risk arrhythmias	High-grade atrioventricular (AV) block Mobitz type II AV block Third-degree heart block Symptomatic supraventricular and ventricular arrhythmias
Pulmonary hypertension	Right atrial pressure >7 mm Hg Decreased 6-min walking distance History of pulmonary embolism Right-axis deviation on electrocardiography Right ventricular: Systemic systolic pressure >0.66 Brain natriuretic peptide >300 pg/mL
Cerebrovascular disease	Stroke within 3 mo of surgery

MACE, major adverse cardiac events; MI, myocardial infarction.

dataset upon which the RCRI was based, which was from a single center, limited to patients 50 years of age or older who were undergoing nonambulatory surgery between 1989 and 1994.

The Gupta Myocardial Infarction and Cardiac Arrest (MICA) score and the American College of Surgeons National Surgical Quality Improvement Program (ACS NSQIP) Surgical Risk Calculator (http://riskcalculator.facs.org) are modeled after data from the ACS NSQIP database. Although the MICA score appears to be more predictive for perioperative MACE, the ACS Surgical Risk Calculator predicts MACE and 17 other perioperative outcomes based on specific surgery and patient characteristics including age, body mass index, and comorbidities (see **Table 14.1**). It should be noted that the MICA score was derived from a single year's NSQIP dataset from 2007, which contains just more than 200,000 operations. By contrast, the Surgical Risk Calculator is derived from multiyear datasets containing over 5 million operations from more than 800 participating sites globally and continues to be updated with new data.

Prior iterations of the ACC/AHA guidelines specified conditions that are associated with a significantly increased risk of perioperative MACE. These are summarized in **Table 14.2**.

Fleisher LA. The value of preoperative assessment before noncardiac surgery in the era of value-based care. *Circulation*. 2017;136:1769-1771.

Glance LG, Faden E, Dutton RP, et al. Impact of the choice of risk model for identifying low-risk patients using the 2014 American College of Cardiology/American Heart Association Perioperative Guidelines. *Anesthesiology*. 2018;129:889-900.

Halvorsen S, Mehilli J, et al. 2022 ESC Guidelines on cardiovascular assessment and management of patients undergoing non-cardiac surgery. *Eur Heart J*. 2022;43:3826-3924. Erratum in: *Eur Heart J*. 2023;44:4421.

Harrison TG, Hemmelgarn BR, James MT, et al. Using the revised cardiac risk index to predict major postoperative events for people with kidney failure: an external validation and update. *CJC Open*. 2022;4:905-912.

Rajagopal S, Ruetzler K, Ghadimi K, et al; American Heart Association Council on Cardiopulmonary, Critical Care, Perioperative and Resuscitation, and the Council on Cardiovascular and Stroke Nursing. Evaluation and management of pulmonary hypertension in noncardiac surgery: a scientific statement from the American Heart Association. *Circulation*. 2023;147:1317-1343.

Thompson A, Fleischmann KE, et al. AHA/ACC/ACS/ASNC/HRS/SCA/SCCT/SCMR/SVM Guideline for Perioperative Cardiovascular Management for Noncardiac Surgery: a report of the American College of Cardiology/American Heart Association Joint Committee on Clinical Practice Guidelines. *Circulation*. 2024;150:e351-e442. Erratum in: *Circulation*. 2024;150:e466.

Vascular Events in Noncardiac Surgery Patients Cohort Evaluation (VISION) Study Investigators. Association between complications and death within 30 days after noncardiac surgery. *CMAJ*. 2019;191:E830-E837.

A.2. What are the determinants of myocardial oxygen demand? How are they measured clinically?

The three major determinants of myocardial oxygen demand are (1) myocardial left ventricular (LV) wall tension, (2) cardiac contractility, and (3) heart rate.

Mechanical work accounts for 80% of myocardial oxygen demand (60% used for systole, 15%-20% for diastole), with the remaining contributing to electrical activity and cellular maintenance. The myocardium extracts approximately 75% of coronary blood oxygen content at rest, which is near-maximal: increasing oxygen demand can only be met by increasing coronary blood flow.

LV preload and afterload both affect wall tension and can be described by Laplace Law:

$$\text{Wall tension} = \frac{\text{Internal pressure} \times \text{Radius}}{2\,(\text{Thickness})}.$$

Myocardial oxygen consumption has a linear relationship with LV mass and peak wall tension. Resting myocardial oxygen consumption is 8 to 13 mL/100 g/min; doubling wall tension doubles oxygen consumption. Increasing afterload imposes greater wall tension than a proportionate increase in preload due to the cube root relationship between radius and volume:

$$\text{Volume} = \frac{4}{3}\pi \times \text{Radius}^3.$$

Of the three factors, tachycardia can substantially increase myocardial oxygen demand by increasing the frequency of wall tension cycling per minute, and to a lesser extent by increasing contractility through the Bowditch effect.

Clinical measures of preload include vital signs, assessment of hydration status, pulmonary and peripheral venous congestion, and point-of-care ultrasound (POCUS) evaluation of LV end-diastolic volume. Contractility, defined as the force of myocardial shortening at a given preload and afterload, is rarely measured outside of laboratory settings. Practical surrogates for measuring contractility include echocardiographic assessment of ejection fraction (EF) and myocardial strain.

Amzulescu MS, De Craene M, Langet H, et al. Myocardial strain imaging: review of general principles, validation, and sources of discrepancies. *Eur Heart J Cardiovasc Imaging*. 2019;20:605-619.

Hoffman JI, Buckberg GD. The myocardial oxygen supply:demand index revisited. *J Am Heart Assoc*. 2014;3:e000285.

A.3. What factors determine myocardial oxygen supply?

Arterial oxygen content and coronary blood flow are the primary determinants of myocardial oxygen supply. Heart rate is also an important factor.

Normal coronary blood flow in adults is approximately 250 mL/min, or 3% to 5% of cardiac output. It is subject to autoregulation through local and neurohumoral alterations in coronary vascular resistance. Coronary perfusion is governed by aortic root pressure (from which the coronary arteries originate) and intracavitary pressure.

$$\text{Coronary blood flow} = \frac{\text{Aortic root pressure - Intracavitary pressure}}{\text{Coronary vascular resistance}}.$$

The LV is primarily perfused during diastole when aortic root pressure consistently exceeds intracavitary pressure. This stands in contrast to the normal right ventricle (RV), which is perfused throughout the cardiac cycle, but predominantly in systole. It is important to note that in patients with severe pulmonary hypertension, RV perfusion can become increasingly reliant on diastolic time, taking on LV perfusion characteristics as pulmonary arterial pressures approach near-systemic levels.

Coronary autoregulation occurs through myogenic, metabolic, endothelial, and neurohumoral pathways, which may be disrupted pharmacologically or by ischemia. In healthy hearts, coronary blood flow is stable between coronary perfusion pressures (CPPs) between 40 and 110 mm Hg. Regional wall motion abnormalities occur at CPP below 40 mm Hg and below 20 mm Hg ischemic injury occurs.

Johnson NP, Gould KL, De Bruyne B. Autoregulation of coronary blood supply in response to demand: JACC review topic of the week. *J Am Coll Cardiol*. 2021;77:2335-2345.

A.4. What are the mechanisms of perioperative myocardial injury and ischemia?

Myocardial ischemia occurs whenever myocardial oxygen supply does not match myocardial oxygen demand. The term myocardial injury after noncardiac surgery (MINS) was devised in 2014 to address acute isolated postoperative cardiac troponin elevations, absent other evidence of ischemia. The presence of clinical ischemia with elevated troponins is diagnostic of a PMI.

Recent studies suggest Type 2 PMI accounts for 40% to 80% of all PMI after noncardiac surgery. Type 2 PMI, which occurs in the absence of an acute coronary plaque event, can be precipitated by increases in myocardial oxygen demand caused by tachycardia, hypertension, anemia, hypothermia, pain, surgical stress, sympathomimetic drugs, or discontinuation of β-blockers. Causes of decreased supply include hypotension, bradycardia or tachycardia, increased cardiac filling pressures, and hypoxemia. The Vascular Events in Noncardiac Surgery Patients Cohort Evaluation (VISION) study identified strong associations between PMI, intraoperative tachycardia and, to a lesser extent, hypertension. Isolated tachycardia, systolic hypotension, and the two factors combined were strongly associated with MINS.

In patients with coronary atherosclerosis, perioperative hypercoagulability and inflammation may precipitate plaque erosion, rupture, and thrombosis (termed Type 1 MI). This mechanism accounts for approximately 20% to 60% of all PMIs, but the interaction between anatomic findings and functional factors is unpredictable. Postmortem analyses found plaque rupture in approximately 50% of PMI cases. However, the timing of death and the presence of plaque rupture appear to be inversely related. Newer analysis suggests that myocardial oxygen supply/demand imbalance predominates in the first 3 to 4 postoperative days (PODs) and patients primarily suffer fatal PMI in this early postoperative period from demand ischemia (~70% without histologic plaque rupture). Conversely, PMI more than 7 days postoperatively becomes increasingly associated with acute plaque rupture. In PMI, the severity of underlying coronary artery stenosis does not necessarily predict the infarct territory; however, upward of 90% fatal perioperative myocardial events occur in patients with established coronary artery disease.

Patients with Type 2 PMI are typically older, female patients, are less likely to receive invasive management (including angiography and surgery), and have reduced mortality rates compared with patients who had Type 1 PMI (12.1% vs 17.4%). However, mortality was still significantly increased compared with those without PMI (1.2%).

Abbott TEF, Pearse RM, Archbold RA, et al. A prospective international multicentre cohort study of intraoperative heart rate and systolic blood pressure and myocardial injury after noncardiac surgery: results of the VISION study. *Anesth Analg*. 2018;126:1936-1945.

Cheung C, Martyn A, Campbell N, et al. Predictors of intraoperative hypotension and bradycardia. *Am J Med*. 2015;128:532-538.

Helwani MH, Amin A, Lavigne P, et al. Etiology of acute coronary syndrome after noncardiac surgery. *Anesthesiology*. 2018;128:1084-1091.

Raphael CE, Roger VL, Sandoval Y, et al. Incidence, trends, and outcomes of type 2 myocardial infarction in a community cohort. *Circulation*. 2020;141:454-463.

Ruetzler K, Smilowitz NR, Berger JS, et al. Diagnosis and management of patients with myocardial injury after noncardiac surgery: a scientific statement from the American Heart Association. *Circulation*. 2021;144:e287-e305.

Smilowitz NR, Shah B, Ruetzler K, et al. Characteristics and outcomes of type 1 versus type 2 perioperative myocardial infarction after noncardiac surgery. *Am J Med*. 2022;135:202-210.e3.

Smit M, Coetzee AR, Lochner A. The pathophysiology of myocardial ischemia and perioperative myocardial infarction. *J Cardiothorac Vasc Anesth*. 2020;34:2501-2512.

Thompson A, Fleischmann KE, et al. AHA/ACC/ACS/ASNC/HRS/SCA/SCCT/SCMR/SVM Guideline for Perioperative Cardiovascular Management for Noncardiac Surgery: a report of the American College of Cardiology/American Heart Association Joint Committee on Clinical Practice Guidelines. *Circulation*. 2024;150:e351-e442. Erratum in: *Circulation*. 2024;150:e466.

Thygesen K, Alpert JS, Jaffe AS, et al; Executive Group on behalf of the Joint European Society of Cardiology (ESC)/American College of Cardiology (ACC)/American Heart Association (AHA)/World Heart Federation (WHF) Task Force for the Universal Definition of Myocardial Infarction. Fourth universal definition of myocardial infarction (2018) [published correction appears in *Circulation*. 2018;138:e652]. *Circulation*. 2018;138:e618-e651.

A.5. What is the incidence of perioperative myocardial injury, infarction, and MACE in patients with coronary artery disease (CAD) undergoing noncardiac surgery?

Evolving diagnostic criteria for PMI and MINS have complicated the description of their incidence. PMI occurs in approximately 1% to 13% of patients undergoing noncardiac surgery, with most occurring within the first 24 to 48 hours postoperatively. The incidence of myocardial events increases with routine postoperative biomarker surveillance and the use of high-sensitivity troponin T assays. MINS is seen in 18% to 25% of patients aged 45 years of age and above. About 78% of MINS were diagnosed within the first POD and 94% within the second POD. A meta-analysis of 169 studies found that in patients with prior MI, the relative risk of MINS is 1.92 (95% CI 1.19-3.12, $P < .001$). Patients who develop MINS and PMI have an increased 30-day mortality and are at elevated risk of MACE for up to 1 to 2 years following surgery.

The overall incidence of MACE after noncardiac surgery has dramatically decreased in the past two decades. Landesberg et al reported that early mortality after PMI ranges from 3.5% to 25% and is higher among patients with marked troponin elevation compared with patients with minor troponin elevation (0%-7%). This contrasts with older data that reported a very high incidence of mortality, which reflects improvements in the management of this patient cohort. A 2016 study, using a large administrative database of US hospital admissions (2004-2013), found a 3% incidence of major adverse cardiovascular and cerebrovascular events (in-hospital, all-cause death, acute MI, or acute ischemic stroke). These events were most common after vascular, thoracic, and transplant surgery.

Landesberg G, Beattie WS, Mosseri M, et al. Perioperative myocardial infarction. *Circulation*. 2009;119:2936-2944.

Livhits M, Ko CY, Leonardi MJ, et al. Risk of surgery following recent myocardial infarction. *Ann Surg*. 2011;253:857-864.

Puelacher C, Gualandro DM, Glarner N, et al; BASEL-PMI Investigators. Long-term outcomes of perioperative myocardial infarction/injury after non-cardiac surgery. *Eur Heart J*. 2023;44:1690-1701.

Ruetzler K, Smilowitz NR, Berger JS, et al. Diagnosis and management of patients with myocardial injury after non-cardiac surgery: a scientific statement from the American Heart Association. *Circulation*. 2021;144:e287-e305.

Smilowitz NR, Gupta N, Ramakrishna H, et al. Perioperative major adverse cardiovascular and cerebrovascular events associated with noncardiac surgery. *JAMA Cardiol*. 2017;2:181-187.

Smilowitz NR, Redel-Traub G, Hausvater A, et al. Myocardial injury after noncardiac surgery: a systematic review and meta-analysis. *Cardiol Rev*. 2019;27:267-273.

Thygesen K, Alpert JS, Jaffe AS, et al; Executive Group on behalf of the Joint European Society of Cardiology (ESC)/American College of Cardiology (ACC)/American Heart Association (AHA)/World Heart Federation (WHF) Task Force for the Universal Definition of Myocardial Infarction. Fourth universal definition of myocardial infarction (2018). *Circulation*. 2018;138:e618-e651.

A.6. Which perioperative medical therapies would you employ to reduce the incidence of myocardial ischemia?

β-Adrenergic Antagonists (Esmolol, Atenolol, Metoprolol, Bisoprolol)

β-Blockers reduce myocardial oxygen consumption, improve coronary blood flow by prolonging the diastolic perfusion period, improve the supply:demand ratio, and inhibit platelet aggregation. The influential PeriOperative Ischemic Evaluation (POISE) study identified an association between stable preoperative use of β-blockers and a reduction in cardiac events, but also an increase in mortality, bradycardia, and stroke. However, more recent data suggest that while there is an association between preoperative β-blocker use and perioperative stroke, in a cohort of patients undergoing major abdominal surgery, there was no difference in stroke rates between patients started on β-blockers less than 60 days prior to surgery and those on the medications chronically.

Likewise, the timing of β-blocker initiation is a matter of ongoing study. Initiation less than 7 days before noncardiac surgery has been repeatedly associated with increased mortality and poorer outcomes; however, a large cohort of patients with diabetes initiated on β-blocker at least 30 days prior to their operation showed improved mortality. Currently, the only class I recommendation for perioperative β-blocker use is to continue their use in the patients who are already on β-blockers (class I, level of evidence B). β-Blockers can be used in patients with elevated risk, such as ischemia during preoperative stress testing, or in patients with elevated risk (class IIb, level of evidence B). Although there are some differences between the European Society of Cardiology (ESC) and the AHA guidelines, both recommend that if β-blockers are used for prophylactic purposes, they should be slowly titrated (2-7 days before elective surgery), and acute administration of high-dose β-blockers in high-risk patients undergoing low-risk surgery is not recommended (class III, level of evidence B).

α_2-Adrenergic Agonist (Clonidine)

α_2-Agonists (eg clonidine) decrease sympathetic outflow, blood pressure, and heart rate. Although older studies suggested a possible beneficial effect of α_2-agonists, the POISE-2 trial did not show any statistically beneficial effect of clonidine. Clonidine did not reduce the rate of 30-day risk of all-cause death or nonfatal MI in patients with or at risk of atherosclerotic disease who were undergoing noncardiac surgery.

Clonidine did increase the rate of nonfatal cardiac arrest and clinically important hypotension. Follow-up of these patients at 1 year demonstrated no significant differences in mortality or the development of chronic pain between those given clonidine and those who did not. Based on both the ACC/AHA and ESC guidelines, α_2-agonists for prevention of cardiac events are not recommended in patients who are undergoing noncardiac surgery (class III recommendation).

Nitrovasodilators (Nitroglycerin, Isosorbide Dinitrate)

Nitrates improve myocardial oxygen balance by decreasing preload and afterload while improving coronary circulation through coronary arterial dilation. NTG, one of the oldest antianginal therapies, has had very few trials in noncardiac surgery to evaluate its role in perioperative ischemia reduction. However, there have been no significant studies within the past 10 years examining the effect of prophylactic NTG on perioperative myocardial ischemia. Prior studies yielded conflicting results, were small (<50 patients), and were not blinded. A recent meta-analysis by Zhao et al further strengthened the position of not using prophylactic nitrates for noncardiac surgery.

The current guidelines do not recommend the use of prophylactic intravenous NTG to reduce myocardial ischemia undergoing noncardiac surgery.

Calcium Channel Blockers (Verapamil, Diltiazem, Nifedipine, Nicardipine)

Calcium channel blockers reduce myocardial oxygen demand by depressing myocardial contractility and dilating coronary and collateral vessels, which improves blood flow. However, the most important effect may be the prevention of sympathetically mediated coronary vasoconstriction.

A meta-analysis of perioperative calcium channel blockers in noncardiac surgery (11 studies involving 1,007 patients) showed significantly reduced ischemia and postoperative supraventricular tachycardia. The beneficial effects were mostly due to the use of diltiazem, whereas the use of a 1,4-dihydropyridine (DHP) derivative, nifedipine, was associated with ischemia. Another study in 1,000 patients having acute or elective aortic aneurysm surgery showed that DHP calcium channel blocker use was independently associated with an increased incidence of perioperative mortality. The use of short-acting DHP, in particular nifedipine capsules, should be avoided. The AHA makes no specific recommendations for the prophylactic use of calcium channel blockers. Routine use of calcium channel blockers to reduce the risk of perioperative cardiovascular complications is not recommended (class III recommendation).

Aspirin

Aspirin (acetylsalicylic acid) inhibits platelet aggregation by blocking the production of thromboxane A_2. Observational data suggest that preoperative withdrawal of aspirin increases thrombotic complications. However, the value of aspirin use in unstented patients to prevent ischemic complications is uncertain. The Pulmonary Embolism Prevention (PEP) trial, which randomized 13,356 patients undergoing hip surgery to 160 mg of aspirin or placebo, did not show any benefit with aspirin. The POISE-2 trial randomized 10,010 patients who were undergoing noncardiac surgery to 200 mg of aspirin or placebo. Aspirin did not have a protective effect for MACE or death in all patients either continuing aspirin or starting aspirin. However, aspirin did show a reduction in nonfatal MI and death in subgroup analyses of patients with prior percutaneous coronary intervention (PCI). The risk of major bleeding, especially in the first 5 days after surgery, was notably higher in patients taking aspirin. This is supported by a previous large meta-analysis, including 41 studies in 49,590 patients, which compared periprocedural withdrawal versus bleeding risks of aspirin and concluded that the risk of bleeding complications was increased by 1.5 but that aspirin did not lead to higher severity levels of bleeding complications. The 1-year follow-up of POISE-2 confirmed these prior findings, and subgroup analyses continued to show a reduction in MI and death in only those patients with prior PCI. Initiation of aspirin is not beneficial in patients undergoing elective noncardiac, noncarotid surgery who have not had previous coronary stenting, unless the risk of ischemic events outweighs the risk of surgical bleeding.

Statins

Statins are primarily used for their lipid-lowering effects and are widely prescribed in patients with or at risk for IHD. Statins also induce coronary plaque stabilization by decreasing lipid oxidation, inflammation, matrix metalloproteinase, and cell death. These nonlipid or pleiotropic effects may prevent plaque rupture and subsequent MI in the perioperative period. A meta-analysis of 223,010 patients from 12 retrospective and 3 prospective trials showed that statins reduced mortality significantly by 44% in noncardiac surgery and by 59% in vascular surgery. The accumulated evidence to date suggests a protective effect of perioperative statin use on cardiac complications during noncardiac surgery. Most of the data come from observational studies. The time of initiation of statin therapy and the duration of therapy are often unclear in the observational trials. Randomized clinical trials are limited in patient numbers and types of noncardiac surgery. Both the AHA and ESC guidelines recommend continuing statin therapy for patients currently taking statins and scheduled for noncardiac surgery (class I recommendation). ESC recommends that preoperative statin therapy should be considered in patients undergoing vascular surgery and initiated at least 2 weeks before surgery.

Chen RJ, Chu H, Tsai LW. Impact of beta-blocker initiation timing on mortality risk in patients with diabetes mellitus undergoing noncardiac surgery: a nationwide population-based cohort study. *J Am Heart Assoc.* 2017;6:e004392.

Devereaux PJ, Mrkobrada M, Sessler DI, et al. Aspirin in patients undergoing noncardiac surgery. *N Engl J Med.* 2014;370:1494-1503.

Devereaux PJ, Sessler DI, Leslie K, et al. Clonidine in patients undergoing noncardiac surgery. *N Engl J Med.* 2014;370:1504-1513.

Devereaux PJ, Yang H, Yusuf S, et al. Effects of extended-release metoprolol succinate in patients undergoing non-cardiac surgery (POISE trial): a randomised controlled trial. *Lancet.* 2008;371:1839-1847.

Halvorsen S, Mehilli J, et al. 2022 ESC Guidelines on cardiovascular assessment and management of patients undergoing non-cardiac surgery. *Eur Heart J.* 2022;43:3826-3924. Erratum in: *Eur Heart J.* 2023;44:4421.

McKenzie NL, Ward RP, Nagele P, et al. Preoperative β-blocker therapy and stroke or major adverse cardiac events in major abdominal surgery: a retrospective cohort study. *Anesthesiology.* 2023;138:42-54.

Roth S, Torregroza C, Huhn R, et al. Perioperative cardioprotection: clinical implications. *Anesth Analg.* 2020;131:1751-1764.

Schouten O, Boersma E, Hoeks SE, et al. Fluvastatin and perioperative events in patients undergoing vascular surgery. *N Engl J Med.* 2009;361:980-989.

Sessler DI, Conen D, Leslie K, et al. One-year results of a factorial randomized trial of aspirin versus placebo and clonidine versus placebo in patients having noncardiac surgery. *Anesthesiology.* 2020;132:692-701.

Thompson A, Fleischmann KE, et al. AHA/ACC/ACS/ASNC/HRS/SCA/SCCT/SCMR/SVM Guideline for Perioperative Cardiovascular Management for Noncardiac Surgery: a report of the American College of Cardiology/American Heart Association Joint Committee on Clinical Practice Guidelines. *Circulation.* 2024;150:e351-e442. Erratum in: *Circulation.* 2024;150:e466.

Wang X, Fernandez Robles C, Kertai MD. Perioperative β-blocker use: what is new in 2020? *Curr Opin Anaesthesiol.* 2020;33:417-422.

Zhao N, Xu J, Singh B, et al. Nitrates for the prevention of cardiac morbidity and mortality in patients undergoing non-cardiac surgery. *Cochrane Database Syst Rev.* 2016:CD010726.

A.7. Based on his history, would you recommend that this patient's surgery be postponed for a certain period? If so, why?

The arbitrary delaying of a surgical procedure is not supported by the ACC/AHA or ESC guidelines. In a patient with a DES placed 5 months before surgery in the setting of ACS, the discontinuation of dual-antiplatelet therapy (DAPT) increases the risk of stent thrombosis. This history warrants individualized, shared decision-making with the patient, anesthesiologist, surgeon, and treating cardiologist. Key considerations for this patient include the indication for surgery, duration since his MI, and the acceptable interval for interruption of DAPT after cardiac stenting that balances the risks of surgical bleeding and stent complications.

Cancer surgery is considered a time-sensitive procedure, in which a delay of more than 1 to 6 weeks can negatively affect the outcome. Any delay in surgery requires justification of benefit over the risk of cancer spread. A strong risk factor for PMI and MINS is the duration between MI and subsequent surgery. A discharge database of more than 5,000,000 patients undergoing surgery between 1999 and 2004 demonstrated that the PMI rate for the recent MI cohort decreased substantially as the length of time from MI to operation increased (0-30 days = 32.8%; 31-60 days = 18.7%; 61-90 days = 8.4%; and 91-180 days = 5.9%), as did 30-day mortality (0-30 days = 14.2%; 31-60 days = 11.5%; 61-90 days = 10.5%; and 91-180 days = 9.9%). The rates do not reach parity with non-MI controls until 1 year after MI.

In patients continuing DAPT perioperatively, surgical blood loss is increased by 30% to 50% by aspirin and clopidogrel, but there is no increased risk of stroke, MI, or mortality, except during intracranial surgery. For aspirin alone, a large meta-analysis concluded that although the risk of bleeding complications was increased by 50%, it did not lead to greater severity of bleeding complications. Even in subjects at risk of, or with proven, ischemic heart disease (IHD), nonadherence/withdrawal of aspirin tripled the risk of MACE.

Acute stent thrombosis increases when DAPT is discontinued within 6 months of stent implantation and is associated with mortality rates of up to 20%. High-risk features for stent thrombosis include diabetes, complex bifurcating stents, stents in the left main coronary artery, and stents placed for the management of acute coronary syndrome. Current ACC/AHA and ESC recommendations for DAPT after cardiac stenting include both aspirin and another $P2Y_{12}$ platelet inhibitor (clopidogrel, prasugrel, or ticagrelor) for a minimum of 30 to 45 days to prevent restenosis and allow reendothelialization of the stent to be completed. The recommendations for the earliest, acceptable time for DAPT interruption vary depending on the original indication for stenting and between society guidelines (See Section B.4).

Taken together, evidence suggests that it be prudent to delay time-sensitive, nonurgent surgery for a minimum of 30 days and for up to 3 months after stent implantation for stable IHD, and for a minimum of 3 months and preferably 6 months after ACS. A careful case-by-case approach is recommended.

Kristensen SD, Knuuti J, Saraste A, et al. 2014 ESC/ESA guidelines on non-cardiac surgery: cardiovascular assessment and management: the joint task force on non-cardiac surgery: cardiovascular assessment and management of the European Society of Cardiology (ESC) and the European Society of Anaesthesiology (ESA). *Eur Heart J.* 2014;35:2383-2431.

Oprea AD, Popescu WM. Perioperative management of antiplatelet therapy. *Br J Anaesth.* 2013;111:i3-i17.

Stefanini GG, Holmes DR Jr. Drug-eluting coronary-artery stents. *N Engl J Med.* 2013;368:254-265.

Thompson A, Fleischmann KE, et al. AHA/ACC/ACS/ASNC/HRS/SCA/SCCT/SCMR/SVM Guideline for Perioperative Cardiovascular Management for Noncardiac Surgery: a report of the American College of Cardiology/American Heart Association Joint Committee on Clinical Practice Guidelines. *Circulation.* 2024;150:e351-e442. Erratum in: *Circulation.* 2024;150:e466.

Vetter TR, Hunter JM Jr, Boudreaux AM. Preoperative management of antiplatelet drugs for a coronary artery stent: how can we hit a moving target? *BMC Anesthesiol.* 2014;14:73.

Vetter TR, Short RT III, Hawn MT, et al. Perioperative management of the patient with a coronary artery stent. *Anesthesiology.* 2014;121:1093-1098.

Wolf AM, Pucci MJ, Gabale SD, et al. Safety of perioperative aspirin therapy in pancreatic operations. *Surgery.* 2014;155:39-46.

B. Preoperative Evaluation and Preparation

B.1. How would you evaluate this patient's cardiac condition? What laboratory tests would you order?

Preoperative testing should be limited to circumstances in which the results will affect patient treatment and outcomes. The initial history and physical examination should focus on defining the severity, stability, and treatment history of his preexisting heart disease, and exclude the presence of concurrent high-risk conditions or decompensation.

Functional capacity is a cornerstone of preoperative evaluation. The self-reported inability to walk four blocks on level ground or two flights of stairs is associated with postoperative cardiovascular complications in noncardiac surgery (adjusted hazard ratio 1.63; CI 1.23-2.15). A prospective cohort study in 1,401 patients demonstrated the predictive value of the Duke Activity Status Index (DASI), in which patients with a DASI score of less than 25 were at increased risk of 30-day death or MI (adjusted OR 1.49; CI 1.01-2.20) and moderate-to-severe postoperative complications (adjusted OR 1.29; CI 1.07-1.57).

Other conditions that warrant attention in this patient include diabetes and frailty. The risk of an MI in patients with diabetes and no evidence of CAD match that of patients without diabetes who have had a previous MI. Patients with CAD and diabetes tend to have a worse outcome for any adverse coronary event, and the mortality rate can be up to 70% in 10 years. Although there are multisystem benefits to long-term diabetic control, evidence suggests that preoperative hyperglycemia is more predictive of MINS than preoperative hemoglobin A_{1c} levels.

Perioperative frailty is associated with increased morbidity and mortality, even after minor surgical procedures. A variety of frailty assessment instruments are available but do not appear to differ in their predictive values. Patients with medium and high hospital frailty risk scores are at an increased risk of perioperative MACE following noncardiac surgery, with the highest odds seen in patients between 45 and 64 years of age.

Preoperative laboratory tests should include hemoglobin for anemia assessment, creatinine and fasting glucose for perioperative risk stratification, and a blood group typing and antibody screen. Preoperative cardiac biomarkers, including natriuretic peptides and troponins, show promise in predicting postoperative MACE in patients at high risk of HF and coronary artery disease and may assist in the interpretation of postoperative surveillance values. However, the paucity of high-quality evidence has limited the application of these biomarkers to a case-by-case basis, in consultation with expert advice.

De Hert SG, Lurati Buse GA. Cardiac biomarkers for the prediction and detection of adverse cardiac events after noncardiac surgery: a narrative review. *Anesth Analg*. 2020;131:187-195.

Hanley C, Wijeysundera DN. Perioperative risk assessment—focus on functional capacity. *Curr Opin Anaesthesiol.* 2021;34:309-316.

McIsaac DI, MacDonald DB, Aucoin SD. Frailty for perioperative clinicians: a narrative review. *Anesth Analg*. 2020;130:1450-1460.

Park J, Oh AR, Lee SH, et al. Associations between preoperative glucose and hemoglobin A1c level and myocardial injury after noncardiac surgery. *J Am Heart Assoc*. 2021;10:e019216.

Siddiqui E, Banco D, Berger JS, Smilowitz NR. Frailty assessment and perioperative major adverse cardiovascular events after noncardiac surgery. *Am J Med*. 2023;136:372-379.e5.

B.2. What is the role of cardiac stress testing and noninvasive coronary imaging for this patient?

The ACC/AHA and ESC guidelines have suggested that a stepwise approach to the assessment of CAD is both efficacious and cost-effective. This patient sustained MI 5 months ago and was managed with a complex DES and is scheduled for pancreaticoduodenectomy, which is considered an intermediate-risk procedure. If the patient can perform more than four metabolic equivalents (METs) of physical activity (eg, washing dishes, climbing one flight of stairs with a bag of groceries, walking on level ground at 4 miles/h) without chest pain or shortness of breath, if no new cardiac symptoms are present since his stent implantation, and if the resting ECG showed no new changes compared to 5 months ago, the patient can undergo anesthesia and surgery without further testing.

If any one of the above criteria is absent, stress testing is recommended. In patients with recent MI, stress testing is also used to stratify the risk of reinfarction. If a stress test does not indicate residual myocardium at risk, the likelihood of reinfarction after noncardiac surgery is low. If the ischemic area is small, surgery is permissible with optimized medical management. If the ischemic area is moderate to large, with suspicion of new or severe coronary stenosis, cardiac catheterization is recommended before the planned surgery. Also see Chapter 10: Abdominal Aortic Aneurysm Repair, Section B.2, **Figure 10.2**.

Noninvasive tests of myocardial perfusion are classified by the type of stress applied to elicit transient and reversible ischemia or by the mode of detecting the ischemic area. Myocardial stress can be induced by exercise, by a pharmacologic agent that increases heart rate and contractility (eg, dobutamine, atropine), or by agents that redistribute coronary blood flow (eg, dipyridamole, regadenoson).

Physiologic exercise provides an estimate of functional capacity, provides blood pressure and heart rate response, and detects myocardial ischemia through ECG ST-segment or other imaging technique changes. The accuracy of exercise ECG varies significantly among studies. Preexisting ST-segment abnormalities at rest, especially in precordial leads V_5 and V_6, hamper reliable ST-segment analysis. However, most of these studies do not reflect current protocols and contemporary practice. Meta-analysis of studies using treadmill testing in vascular surgery patients showed a rather low sensitivity (74%) and specificity (69%) to detect myocardium at risk, comparable with daily clinical practice.

Pharmacologic stress testing with dobutamine stress echocardiography (DSE), dipyridamole/adenosine/regadenoson myocardial perfusion imaging with thallium-201, and/or technetium-99m and rubidium-82 can be used in patients undergoing noncardiac surgery who cannot perform exercise to detect stress-induced myocardial ischemia and CAD. Reversible wall motion abnormalities on echocardiography or reversible perfusion defects on radionuclide imaging suggest reversible ischemia.

The myocardial perfusion imaging and DSE before vascular surgery predict PMI or death, with a positive predictive value of only 12% to 14% and a negative predictive value of 88% and 94%, respectively. However, the large majority of the thallium studies involved older planar imaging technology that is no longer used. The newer nuclear imaging studies have higher sensitivity for detecting myocardial ischemia, and patients with normal scans have an excellent prognosis.

Cardiovascular magnetic resonance (CMR) imaging is also used for the detection of myocardial ischemia. Although it is accurate for detecting myocardial ischemia, there is practically no data in the setting of preoperative risk stratification. Computed tomography is used to detect coronary calcium, which reflects coronary atherosclerosis; however, currently, there is no evidence to support its use in preoperative risk stratification.

Selection of the noninvasive stress test should be based primarily on patient characteristics, local availability, and expertise in interpretation. DSE is the preferred test if there is an additional question regarding valvular function or LV dysfunction.

Akhtar S. Ischemic heart disease. In: Hines RL, Marschall K, eds. *Stoelting's Anesthesia and Co-Existing Disease*. 8th ed. Elsevier; 2021:85-114.

Thompson A, Fleischmann KE, et al. AHA/ACC/ACS/ASNC/HRS/SCA/SCCT/SCMR/SVM Guideline for Perioperative Cardiovascular Management for Noncardiac Surgery: a report of the American College of Cardiology/American Heart Association Joint Committee on Clinical Practice Guidelines. *Circulation*. 2024;150:e351-e442. Erratum in: *Circulation*. 2024;150:e466.

B.3. What is the role of coronary revascularization before surgery?

The ACC/AHA guidelines do not recommend routine coronary revascularization before noncardiac surgery to reduce perioperative cardiac events (class III, level of evidence B). However, in a high-risk subset of patients, such as those with left main or severe multivessel disease, severe AS, and EF less than 20%, revascularization or valve replacement may be indicated. A discharge database analysis showed that patients with a recent MI who were revascularized before surgery had an approximately 50% decreased rate of reinfarction (5.1% vs 10.0%). Thirty-day (5.2% vs 11.3%) and 1-year mortality (18.3% vs 35.8%) were also decreased in the revascularized patients.

There is overwhelming agreement that aggressive medical management to provide myocardial protection during the perioperative period is a very important element in the reduction of perioperative cardiovascular complications.

McFalls EO, Ward HB, Moritz TE, et al. Coronary-artery revascularization before elective major vascular surgery. *N Engl J Med*. 2004;351:2795-2804.

Thompson A, Fleischmann KE, et al. AHA/ACC/ACS/ASNC/HRS/SCA/SCCT/SCMR/SVM Guideline for Perioperative Cardiovascular Management for Noncardiac Surgery: a report of the American College of Cardiology/American Heart Association Joint Committee on Clinical Practice Guidelines. *Circulation*. 2024;150:e351-e442. Erratum in: *Circulation*. 2024;150:e466.

B.4. How would you classify this patient's surgery-specific MACE risk?

Surgery-specific cardiac risk of noncardiac surgery is related to two factors: the type of surgery and the degree of hemodynamic stress associated with the procedure(s). The duration and intensity of coronary and myocardial stressors can help estimate the likelihood of perioperative cardiac events and guide preoperative risk modification.

The 2014 and 2024 ACC/AHA guidelines featured the concept of combined clinical/surgical risk in the preoperative assessment, which relies on validated risk prediction indices such as the RCRI, MICA, and ACS risk calculator to individualize the risk of MACE. ESC guidelines continue to define individual surgical procedures as low- (<1%), intermediate- (1%-5%), and high-risk procedures (>5%):

- *High-risk* surgery (cardiac risk >5%) includes major emergency surgery, particularly in older adults; aortic and other major vascular surgery; peripheral vascular surgery; and anticipated prolonged procedures associated with large fluid shifts and/or blood loss.
- *Intermediate-risk* procedures (cardiac risk <5%) include carotid endarterectomy, head and neck surgery, intraperitoneal and intrathoracic, orthopedic, and prostate surgery. Endovascular aortic stent procedures are also included in this category.
- *Low-risk* procedures (cardiac risk <1%) include endoscopic and superficial procedures, cataract surgery, and breast surgery.

According to the ACC guideline criteria, this patient is considered elevated risk, for an intermediate-risk procedure (by ESC guidelines).

Thompson A, Fleischmann KE, et al. AHA/ACC/ACS/ASNC/HRS/SCA/SCCT/SCMR/SVM Guideline for Perioperative Cardiovascular Management for Noncardiac Surgery: a report of the American College of Cardiology/American Heart Association Joint Committee on Clinical Practice Guidelines. *Circulation*. 2024;150:e351-e442. Erratum in: *Circulation*. 2024;150:e466.

B.5. How should this patient's antiplatelet therapy be managed perioperatively?

Coronary stents are particularly predisposed to stent thrombosis, a complication that is dramatically reduced by DAPT. Both bare metal stents (BMS) and DES are predisposed to stent thrombosis and require prolonged DAPT after stent placement (see **Figure 14.1**).

The interruption of DAPT in a patient with recent coronary stents requires a careful balance of surgical bleeding risk and the risk of stent thrombosis causing myocardial ischemia. This patient has multiple features that increase the risk of a stent complication including diabetes and a bifurcating stent within the left main coronary artery, placed 5 months before surgery for ACS.

The 2024 ACC/AHA guidelines recommend that patients with DES placed for ACS maintain DAPT for at least 12 months and lifelong low-dose aspirin (Class I recommendation), but it may be reasonable to consider P2Y12 inhibitor cessation in patients requiring elective surgery after 6 months (Class IIb recommendation). This recommendation is based on several observational studies that reported stabilization of MACE in patients undergoing noncardiac surgery 6 months after stent implantation, regardless of stent type.

The 2022 ESC guidelines, and more recently, the 2024 ACC/AHA guidelines, has shortened the period for time-sensitive surgery to 3 months following stent placement for ACS (Class IIb recommendation). The guidelines diverge for time-sensitive surgery after elective PCI for chronic coronary disease: the 2022 ESC recommends 1 month minimum of DAPT, whereas the 2024 ACC/AHA guidelines maintain a minimum of 3 months DAPT. A cohort registry study conducted from a Veteran's Administration hospital compared the MACE rate in 9,391 patients treated with stents between 2000 and 2010 undergoing noncardiac surgery against 18,782 matched unstented controls. Notably, 62.5% of the stent cohort were treated for ACS. This study identified the highest MACE rates for surgery performed within the first 6 weeks of PCI for BMS and DES (see **Table 14.3**), although stented patients do not approach parity with the nonstent cohort until a post-PCI surgical delay of 12 months.

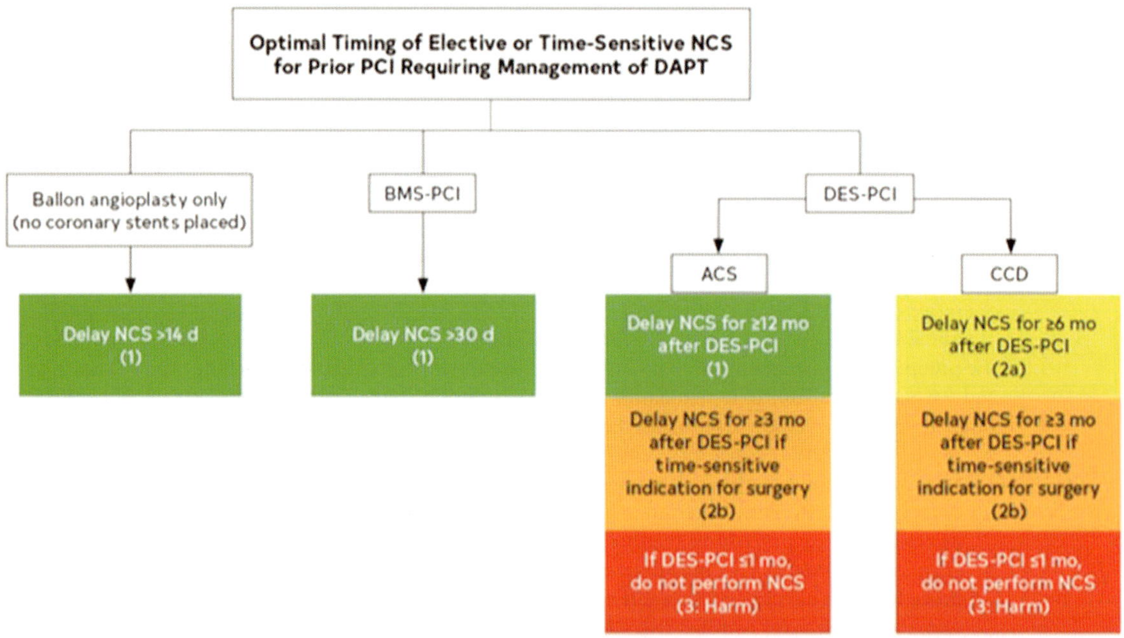

FIGURE 14.1. Treatment algorithm for the timing of elective or time-sensitive non cardiac surgery in patients with prior PCI requiring management of DAPT. BMS, bare metal stents; DAPT, dual-antiplatelet therapy; DES, drug-eluting stent; PCI, percutaneous coronary intervention. (Reprinted with permission from Thompson A, Fleischmann KE, et al. AHA/ACC/ACS/ASNC/HRS/SCA/SCCT/SCMR/SVM Guideline for Perioperative Cardiovascular Management for Noncardiac Surgery: A Report of the American College of Cardiology/American Heart Association Joint Committee on Clinical Practice Guidelines. *Circulation.* 2024;150:e351-e442. Erratum in: *Circulation.* 2024;150:e466.)

TABLE 14.3 Incremental Risk of Noncardiac Surgery After Stent Placement

	<6 wk of Stent Implant (%)	6 wk to 6 mo (%)	>6 mo to 24 mo (%)
Postoperative acute MI and/or revascularization	9.0	4.6	2.3
All-cause mortality	3.2	2.1	1.1

MI, myocardial infarction.
Data were derived from Holcomb CN, Graham LA, Richman JS, et al. The incremental risk of noncardiac surgery on adverse cardiac events following coronary stenting. *J Am Coll Cardiol*. 2014;64:2730-2739.

For patients with stable IHD, a similar Danish registry study matched 4,303 patients treated with DES between 2005 and 2012 with 20,232 control patients and showed an increased risk of MI (1.6% vs 0.2%, OR 4.82) and cardiac death (1.0% vs 0.2%, OR 5.87) relative to those without IHD. This difference was attributable almost entirely to surgeries performed within the first month after PCI.

Ticagrelor therapy warrants additional consideration. It is a noncompetitive, reversible P2Y12 receptor inhibitor that has more predictable pharmacokinetics compared with clopidogrel. Evidence that it may improve outcomes after PCI for patients with ACS compared with clopidogrel is evolving, but there is a definite association with increased spontaneous and procedure-related bleeding. The US Food and Drug Administration (FDA) and ACC/AHA guidelines recommend its cessation 3 to 5 days before elective surgery. Given the risk of stent thrombosis, the time sensitivity of cancer surgery, and the not-insignificant risk of surgical bleeding, it would be reasonable to continue low-dose aspirin throughout the perioperative period. Ticagrelor should be stopped 5 days before surgery and resumed as soon as possible postoperatively. For patients deemed to be at a very elevated risk of stent thrombosis with DAPT interruption, antiplatelet bridging with cangrelor (an intravenous, reversible P2Y12 inhibitor with a plasma half-life of 3-6 minutes) may be considered, starting 48 hours after cessation of ticagrelor and stopping 1 to 2 hours before surgery.

Childers CP, Maggard-Gibbons M, Ulloa JG, et al. Perioperative management of antiplatelet therapy in patients undergoing non-cardiac surgery following coronary stent placement: a systematic review. *Syst Rev*. 2018;7:4.

Egholm G, Kristensen SD, Thim T, et al. Risk associated with surgery within 12 months after coronary drug-eluting stent implantation. *J Am Coll Cardiol*. 2016;68:2622-2632.

Halvorsen S, Mehilli J, Cassese S, et al. 2022 ESC guidelines on cardiovascular assessment and management of patients undergoing non-cardiac surgery. *Eur Heart J*. 2022;43:3826-3924.

Holcomb CN, Graham LA, Richman JS, et al. The incremental risk of noncardiac surgery on adverse cardiac events following coronary stenting. *J Am Coll Cardiol*. 2014;64:2730-2739.

Sullivan AE, Nanna MG, Wang TY, et al. Bridging antiplatelet therapy after percutaneous coronary intervention: JACC review topic of the week. *J Am Coll Cardiol*. 2021;78:1550-1563.

Thompson A, Fleischmann KE, et al. AHA/ACC/ACS/ASNC/HRS/SCA/SCCT/SCMR/SVM Guideline for Perioperative Cardiovascular Management for Noncardiac Surgery: A Report of the American College of Cardiology/American Heart Association Joint Committee on Clinical Practice Guidelines. Circulation. 2024;150:e351-e442. Erratum in: *Circulation*. 2024;150:e466.

B.6. How should the patient's other medications be managed before surgery?

All antianginal drugs, especially β-blockers and statins, should be continued up to the time of surgery. Sudden withdrawal of antianginal drugs may produce rebound tachycardia and hypertension that may precipitate acute myocardial ischemia or infarction.

Current management of hypertensive patients suggests the continuation of antihypertensive therapy up to the day of surgery. There is continued controversy about withholding angiotensin converting enzyme (ACE) inhibitors and angiotensin-2 receptor blockers (ARBs) 24 hours before surgery. Prolonged hypotension has been observed in patients who are undergoing general anesthesia and who have chronically been treated with ACE inhibitors. A meta-analysis demonstrated a 30% increase in relative risk for severe hypotension in patients taking ACE inhibitors or ARBs on the day of surgery but no difference in MACE, stroke, acute renal injury, or death compared with those who held their medication. A subset analysis of the VISION prospective cohort study demonstrated that patients who stopped their ACE inhibitor or ARB in the 24 hours before surgery had a 20% adjusted relative risk reduction in clinically important intraoperative hypotension, and an 18% reduction in composite 30-day all-cause death, stroke, and myocardial injury.

In light of this evidence, it is prudent to withhold ACE inhibitors and ARBs for 24 hours prior to surgical procedures involving major body fluid shifts and significant blood loss. If ACE inhibitors are withheld, it is important to restart them as soon as possible. Hypotension attributed to ACE inhibitors is frequently responsive to fluid and/or administration of vasopressors, such as phenylephrine, ephedrine, and norepinephrine. If hypotension is refractory to these measures, treatment with vasopressin or its long-acting analogue, terlipressin, may be effective.

Sacubitril-valsartan is an angiotensin receptor and neprilysin inhibitor (ANRI) that is primarily used in the treatment of patients with HF with reduced EF but has a newer indication for treating patients with HF with preserved EF. The ACC/AHA guidelines do not specify recommendations for the management of ANRIs, although the European guidelines recommend continuing ARBs when used to manage HF.

Hollmann C, Fernandes NL, Biccard BM. A systematic review of outcomes associated with withholding or continuing angiotensin-converting enzyme inhibitors and angiotensin receptor blockers before noncardiac surgery. *Anesth Analg*. 2018;127:678-687.

Roshanov PS, Rochwerg B, Patel A, et al. Withholding versus continuing angiotensin-converting enzyme inhibitors or angiotensin II receptor blockers before noncardiac surgery: an analysis of the Vascular events In noncardiac Surgery patIents cOhort evaluatioN Prospective Cohort. *Anesthesiology*. 2017;126:16-27.

Turan A, You J, Shiba A, et al. Angiotensin converting enzyme inhibitors are not associated with respiratory complications or mortality after noncardiac surgery. *Anesth Analg*. 2012;114:552-560.

B.7. What is the role of cardiac prehabilitation in optimizing this patient's postoperative outcome?

Prehabilitation entails a preoperative regimen to improve functional capacity and address modifiable risk factors to improve perioperative outcomes. There is controversy surrounding the scope, optimal methods, goals, and effect of prehabilitation before major surgery. There is weak evidence that prehabilitation improves outcomes in cardiac patients undergoing noncardiac surgery. Among patients undergoing cardiac surgery, a preoperative exercise program is associated with reducing hospital length of stay, postoperative atrial fibrillation, and pulmonary complications. In diverse samples of patients undergoing major abdominal cancer surgery, there is equivocal evidence that it improves the length of stay or pulmonary complication rates.

Barakat HM, Shahin Y, Khan JA, et al. Preoperative supervised exercise improves outcomes after elective abdominal aortic aneurysm repair: a randomized controlled trial. *Ann Surg*. 2016;264:47-53.

Fleisher LA. The value of preoperative assessment before noncardiac surgery in the era of value-based care. *Circulation*. 2017;136:1769-1771.

Hughes MJ, Hackney RJ, Lamb PJ, et al. Prehabilitation before major abdominal surgery: a systematic review and meta-analysis. *World J Surg*. 2019;43:1661-1668.

Steinmetz C, Bjarnason-Wehrens B, Walther T, et al. Efficacy of prehabilitation before cardiac surgery: a systematic review and meta-analysis. *Am J Phys Med Rehabil*. 2023;102:323-330.

C. Intraoperative Management

C.1. What are the intraoperative predictors for perioperative MACE?

Intraoperative Predictors

Classic intraoperative predictors for perioperative MACE include emergency surgery, major vascular surgery, and prolonged (>3 hours) thoracic or upper abdominal surgery. Intraoperative predictors include hypotension, tachycardia, a fall in mean arterial blood pressure (MAP) greater than 20 mm Hg for more than 60 minutes, an increase in baseline systolic pressure greater than 30%, or tachycardia in the recovery room (>30 beats per minute from baseline) for more than 5 minutes. However, these associations have not been consistent, and recent data suggest that even targeting a higher MAP greater than 75 does not significantly change rates of MACE. Intraoperative blood transfusion is independently associated with MACE, which likely reflects significant intraoperative hemorrhage. Most MIs occur early after surgery and are commonly associated with ST-segment depression. Prolonged myocardial ischemia (>20-30 minutes or cumulative duration of >1-2 hours) seems to be the key factor associated with adverse cardiac outcomes.

Biccard BM, Rodseth RN. What evidence is there for intraoperative predictors of perioperative cardiac outcomes? A systematic review. *Perioper Med (Lond)*. 2013;2:14.

Grocott MP, Dushianthan A, Hamilton MA, et al. Perioperative increase in global blood flow to explicit defined goals and outcomes following surgery. *Cochrane Database Syst Rev*. 2012:CD004082.

Kheterpal S, O'Reilly M, Englesbe MJ, et al. Preoperative and intraoperative predictors of cardiac adverse events after general, vascular, and urological surgery. *Anesthesiology*. 2009;110:58-66.

Priebe HJ. Perioperative myocardial infarction—aetiology and prevention. *Br J Anaesth*. 2005;95:3-19.

Sprung J, Abdelmalak B, Gottlieb A, et al. Analysis of risk factors for myocardial infarction and cardiac mortality after major vascular surgery. *Anesthesiology*. 2000;93:129-140.

Wanner PM, Wulff DU, Djurdjevic M, et al. Targeting higher intraoperative blood pressures does not reduce adverse cardiovascular events following noncardiac surgery. *J Am Coll Cardiol*. 2021;78:1753-1764.

C.2. How would you monitor the patient in the operating room?

The patient should be monitored according to the American Society of Anesthesiologists guidelines. In this case, that would include the following:

- *ECG*—simultaneous leads V_5 and II
- *Blood pressure*—noninvasive automatic Doppler sphygmomanometer and an invasive arterial catheter
- *End-tidal carbon dioxide*—continuous expired CO_2 levels
- *Pulse oximetry*—arterial oxygenation level
- *Fractional inspired oxygen concentration*—to determine the inspired fraction of oxygen
- *Respiratory rate*—which is determined by multiple monitors
- *Availability of esophageal/bladder temperature probe*—to determine temperature changes

In addition to these monitors, this patient will require the monitoring of urine output with a Foley catheter.

American Society of Anesthesiologists. *Standards for Basic Anesthetic Monitoring*. American Society of Anesthesiologists; 2020.

C.3. What electrocardiogram (ECG) leads would you monitor? Which leads are the most sensitive for monitoring myocardial ischemia?

ECG ST-segment changes are commonly used for the detection of intraoperative myocardial ischemia. Multiple-lead ECG monitoring provides the best clinically available method of detecting perioperative ischemia, primarily by combining leads II, V_3, V_4, and V_5 (detection of ischemia is 80% with leads II/V_5 and 96% with leads II/V_4 and V_5).

Landesberg et al were able to correlate the duration of ischemia observed in the ST-segment analysis of a continuously monitored 12-lead ECG throughout the perioperative period with the incidence of PMI. They also found that ischemia is transient even in patients who will develop an infarct.

Certain prerequisites must be met to use the ECG effectively:

- The diagnostic mode allows the detection of ST-segment changes that are filtered out by the monitoring mode.
- The number of ECG leads and their location affect the detection of ischemic events.
- Immediate availability of a hard copy of the ECG leads for more detailed analysis
- Studies have reported that even trained observers recognize only 15% to 40% of electrocardiographic ischemic events displayed on the monitor.
- ST-segment trending helps as an early warning detection system but should not replace the examination of the ECG waveform.

In the context of suspected acute coronary syndrome without obvious ST elevations, alternative 12-lead ECG placement can be of benefit, as left circumflex (LCx) and right coronary artery (RCA) lesions may be missed with conventional ECG. In these cases, posterior V4-5-6 (LCx) or right V3-4 (RCA) leads can help assess those areas. ECG analysis can also be repeated every 15 to 30 minutes in the acute context if concern for ischemia persists and the patient is clinically deteriorating. Regardless, the utilization of cardiac troponins and other testing modalities should not be delayed for these ECG data.

Gulati M, Levy PD, et al. 2021 AHA/ACC/ASE/CHEST/SAEM/SCCT/SCMR Guideline for the Evaluation and Diagnosis of Chest Pain: A Report of the American College of Cardiology/American Heart Association Joint Committee on Clinical Practice Guidelines. Circulation. 2021;144:e368-e454. Published online October 28, 2021. Erratum in: *Circulation*. 2021;144:e455. Erratum in: *Circulation*. 2023;148:e281.

Landesberg G, Beattie WS, Mosseri M, et al. Perioperative myocardial infarction. *Circulation*. 2009;119:2936-2944.

Landesberg G, Mosseri M, Wolf Y, et al. Perioperative myocardial ischemia and infarction: identification by continuous 12-lead electrocardiogram with online ST-segment monitoring. *Anesthesiology*. 2002;96:264-270.

London MJ, Hollenberg M, Wong MG, et al. Intraoperative myocardial ischemia: localization by continuous 12-lead electrocardiography. *Anesthesiology*. 1988;69:232-241.

C.4. Would you place invasive monitors such as a central venous catheter (CVC), pulmonary artery catheter (PAC), and/or an intra-arterial catheter?

Routine utilization of invasive monitors is not recommended and should always be placed, reevaluated, and removed in the clinical context of the patient's state.

CVCs facilitate the monitoring of central venous pressures (CVPs) and assessment of central venous oxygen saturations ($Scvo_2$). The routine utilization of CVP to guide resuscitation is not recommended, given its inconsistent relationship with fluid responsiveness. Likewise, while $Scvo_2$ serves as a proxy for global oxygen delivery and the adequacy of cardiac output, the absolute value of the test is not as useful as its trend over time. This need for frequent resampling makes $Scvo_2$ less beneficial in the intraoperative context. Nonetheless, a CVC provides additional utility by securing venous access for resuscitation and allowing the administration of vasoactive agents that require central venous delivery.

Multiple studies have evaluated the risks and benefits of the utilization of PACs. Notably, there has been no significant impact on survival and hospital length of stay associated with PAC utilization in the general patient population. Several studies report that PAC is an insensitive monitor for myocardial ischemia and should not be inserted with this as a primary indication. Expert consensus suggests that the utilization of PACs should be contextualized to the patient and remains a valuable tool, especially if HF may be at least in part responsible for hemodynamic compromise. The PAC is a diagnostic hemodynamic monitoring tool and not a therapeutic intervention.

An intra-arterial catheter provides the benefit of continuous blood pressure monitoring in addition to sampling arterial blood for gas analysis or lactate measurement. Continuous blood pressure measurements inherently minimize the amount of time hypotension remains untreated (in comparison to intermittent measurement). As MAPs less than 65 mm Hg are strongly correlated with adverse outcomes, blood pressure remains one of the most actionable clinical data in the operating room. However, optimized blood pressure targets for a particular patient remain difficult to define, and maintaining higher blood pressures (MAP >75 mm Hg) does not appear to change rates of postoperative cardiac events. Arterial lactate elevation has been extensively proven to correlate with poor clinical outcomes and may be of utility in guiding resuscitation. More recently, proprietary analyses of arterial waveforms have been reliably used as a proxy for cardiac output, but the association becomes weaker at extremes of cardiac output when compared to PAC-derived measurements. Newer technologies such as continuous noninvasive blood pressure monitors are promising but appear to lose correlation with invasive blood pressure measurements in the older adults and may not be reliable in those with cardiovascular disease. Machine learning technologies applied to arterial waveform patterns are hoping to provide the means to accurately predict hypotension but have yet to prove clinical reliability in nonstandardized contexts.

Castro R, Kattan E, Ferri G, et al. Effects of capillary refill time-vs. lactate-targeted fluid resuscitation on regional, microcirculatory and hypoxia-related perfusion parameters in septic shock: a randomized controlled trial. *Ann Intensive Care*. 2020;10:150.

Khanna AK, Nosow L, Sands L, et al. Agreement between cardiac output estimation by multi-beat analysis of arterial blood pressure waveforms and continuous thermodilution in post cardiac surgery intensive care unit patients. *J Clin Monit Comput*. 2023;37:559-565.

Monge García MI, García-López D, Gayat É, et al. Hypotension prediction index software to prevent intraoperative hypotension during major non-cardiac surgery: protocol for a European Multicenter Prospective Observational Registry (EU-HYPROTECT). *J Clin Med*. 2022;11:5585.

Pinsky MR, Cecconi M, Chew MS, et al. Effective hemodynamic monitoring. *Crit Care*. 2022;26:294.

Rajaram SS, Desai NK, Kalra A, et al. Pulmonary artery catheters for adult patients in intensive care. *Cochrane Database Syst Rev*. 2013:CD003408.

Thompson A, Fleischmann KE, et al. AHA/ACC/ACS/ASNC/HRS/SCA/SCCT/SCMR/SVM Guideline for Perioperative Cardiovascular Management for Noncardiac Surgery: a report of the American College of Cardiology/American Heart Association Joint Committee on Clinical Practice Guidelines. *Circulation*. 2024;150:e351-e442. Erratum in: *Circulation*. 2024;150:e466.

Wu J, Liang Q, Hu H, et al. Early pulmonary artery catheterization is not associated with survival benefits in critically ill patients with cardiac disease: an analysis of the MIMIC-IV database. *Surgery*. 2022;172:1285-1290.

Xu Z, Chen H, Zhou H, et al. Comparison of noninvasive continuous arterial blood pressure measured by NICAP with arterial line in elderly patients [published correction appears in *BMC Geriatr*. 2022;22:164]. *BMC Geriatr*. 2022;22:108.

C.5. Would you use transesophageal echocardiography (TEE) as a monitor?

TEE is a sensitive diagnostic method to detect new-onset myocardial ischemia. The echocardiographic diagnosis of myocardial ischemia is based on the development of new regional wall motion abnormalities, decreased systolic wall thickening, and ventricular dilation. Usually, a cross-sectional view (transgastric short axis) of the LV is imaged because this view displays the myocardial perfusion territories of the three major coronary arteries. TEE was found to be twice as predictive as ECG in identifying coronary artery bypass graft (CABG) patients who have an MI. In CABG patients, postbypass regional wall motion abnormalities were related to adverse clinical outcomes.

The key risks and limitations of TEE relate to potential trauma with probe placement (eg, risk for esophageal or gastric injury), probe overheating leading to esophageal injury, and the need for specialized training to appropriately acquire and interpret images.

Notwithstanding its limitations, ESC and the AHA guidelines recommend the use of TEE intraoperatively or perioperatively to determine the cause of an acute, persistent, and life-threatening hemodynamic abnormality (class IIa recommendation). However, its use as an ischemia monitor in noncardiac surgery is less validated and may only be considered in patients at high risk for developing myocardial ischemia who undergo major noncardiac surgery (class IIb recommendation by ESC). The routine use of intraoperative TEE during noncardiac surgery to screen for cardiac abnormalities or to monitor for myocardial ischemia is *not* recommended in patients without significant patient or procedural risk factors.

American Society of Anesthesiologists and Society of Cardiovascular Anesthesiologists Task Force on Transesophageal Echocardiography. Practice guidelines for perioperative transesophageal echocardiography. An updated report by the American Society of Anesthesiologists and the Society of Cardiovascular Anesthesiologists Task Force on Transesophageal Echocardiography. *Anesthesiology*. 2010;112:1084-1096.

Porter TR, Shillcutt SK, Adams MS, et al. Guidelines for the use of echocardiography as a monitor for therapeutic intervention in adults: a report from the American Society of Echocardiography. *J Am Soc Echocardiogr*. 2015;28:40-56.

C.6. Is regional anesthesia better than general anesthesia for patients with cardiac disease?

Multiple studies have compared the effects of regional versus general anesthetics on the incidence of perioperative cardiac events. No distinct advantage is apparent between them when considering cardiac outcomes and mortality in patients undergoing peripheral vascular surgery. There is evidence to support regional anesthesia over general anesthesia to optimize graft patency if the technique is extended into the postoperative period to provide neuraxial analgesia. Meta-analyses of patients undergoing vascular surgery have found comparable rates of PMI and death when comparing regional (neuraxial and/or peripheral nerve block) with general anesthesia. However, data from a 2022 systematic review of patients undergoing amputation did show reduced rates of respiratory failure when a regional technique is employed.

The Multicenter Australian Study of Epidural Anesthesia (MASTER) trial randomized 915 patients undergoing major abdominal surgery to receive either combined general and epidural anesthesia/epidural analgesia or general anesthesia with opioid analgesia. Epidural anesthesia/analgesia did not decrease death or cardiovascular outcomes, but modestly improved pulmonary outcomes compared with the general anesthesia group.

A retrospective analysis, published in 2013, of approximately 400,000 patients undergoing total hip or knee arthroplasty, observed a significantly lower incidence of major morbidity and mortality in patients receiving neuraxial anesthesia. A meta-analysis in patients undergoing total hip replacement showed significant improvements in rates of deep venous thrombosis (DVT)/pulmonary emboli (PE), intraoperative blood loss, and operative time when a neuraxial technique was utilized.

Current guidelines recommend that the choice of anesthesia is best left to the discretion of the anesthesia care team, which will consider the need for postoperative ventilation; pulmonary/neuromuscular comorbidities; cardiovascular effects, including myocardial depression; sympathetic blockade consequences; and dermatomal level of the procedure.

Barbosa FT, Jucá MJ, Castro AA, et al. Neuraxial anaesthesia for lower-limb revascularization. *Cochrane Database Syst Rev*. 2013:CD007083.

Gogarten W, Vandermeulen E, Van Aken H, et al. Regional anaesthesia and antithrombotic agents: recommendations of the European Society of Anaesthesiology. *Eur J Anaesthesiol*. 2010;27:999-1015.

Mauermann WJ, Shilling AM, Zuo Z. A comparison of neuraxial block versus general anesthesia for elective total hip replacement: a meta-analysis. *Anesth Analg*. 2006;103:1018-1025.

Memtsoudis SG, Sun X, Chiu YL, et al. Perioperative comparative effectiveness of anesthetic technique in orthopedic patients. *Anesthesiology*. 2013;118:1046-1058.

Mufarrih SH, Qureshi NQ, Yunus RA, et al. A systematic review and meta-analysis of general versus regional anesthesia for lower extremity amputation. *J Vasc Surg*. 2022;S0741-521402338-2.

C.7. How will you induce general anesthesia?

It is essential to prevent hypotension, hypertension, and tachycardia, which can precipitate myocardial ischemia in patients at risk. Fentanyl (up to 5 μg/kg) can be given slowly to achieve drowsiness and to attenuate the sympathetic response to direct laryngoscopy and intubation of the trachea. Higher-dose opioid regimens were once popular but have been associated with prolonged mechanical ventilation postoperatively. As an anesthetic adjunct with propofol, lidocaine (1 mg/kg) appears to provide better hemodynamics postinduction when compared to fentanyl (1 μg/kg). Etomidate has a more stable hemodynamic profile when compared to propofol for induction of general anesthesia and is commonly utilized in patients with cardiac disease. In patients undergoing cardiac surgery, volatile anesthetics have been shown to decrease troponin release and maintain LV function compared with propofol, midazolam, or a balanced anesthesia technique with opioids. However, no real difference between volatile inhalational anesthesia and intravenous anesthesia has been shown in randomized controlled trials or meta-analyses. A meta-analysis of over 6,000 patients undergoing noncardiac surgery failed to show a difference in MI rates between patients who received volatile and total intravenous anesthesia (TIVA). The current AHA guidelines state that "use of either a volatile anesthetic agent or total intravenous anesthesia is reasonable for patients undergoing noncardiac surgery, and the choice is determined by factors other than the prevention of myocardial ischemia and MI."

Amin SM, Hasanin A, ElSayed OS, et al. Comparison of the hemodynamic effects of opioid-based versus lidocaine-based induction of anesthesia with propofol in older adults: a randomized controlled trial [published online ahead of print, 2023 Apr 6]. *Anaesth Crit Care Pain Med*. 2023;42:101225.

Bignami E, Greco T, Barile L, et al. The effect of isoflurane on survival and myocardial infarction: a meta-analysis of randomized controlled studies. *J Cardiothorac Vasc Anesth*. 2013;27:50-58.

Haessler R, Madler C, Klasing S, et al. Propofol/fentanyl versus etomidate/fentanyl for the induction of anesthesia in patients with aortic insufficiency and coronary artery disease. *J Cardiothorac Vasc Anesth*. 1992;6:173-180.

Martin DE, Rosenberg H, Aukburg SJ, et al. Low-dose fentanyl blunts circulatory responses to tracheal intubation. *Anesth Analg*. 1982;61:680-684.

Sprung J, Ogletree-Hughes ML, Moravec CS, et al. The effects of etomidate on the contractility of failing and nonfailing human heart muscle. *Anesth Analg*. 2000;91:68-75.

Thompson A, Fleischmann KE, et al. AHA/ACC/ACS/ASNC/HRS/SCA/SCCT/SCMR/SVM Guideline for Perioperative Cardiovascular Management for Noncardiac Surgery: a report of the American College of Cardiology/American Heart Association Joint Committee on Clinical Practice Guidelines. *Circulation*. 2024;150:e351-e442. Erratum in: *Circulation*. 2024;150:e466.

C.8. What is the best choice of anesthetic agents for the maintenance of anesthesia? Why?

There does not appear to be a single best myocardial protective agent or technique. Knowledge of the physiologic and pharmacologic effects of anesthetic agents in patients with cardiac disease will allow flexibility in their selection. The use of inhalation versus TIVA in patients with cardiac disease is still debated, although the cardiovascular effects of both techniques and the physiologic differences between them are well-documented. However, most outcome studies have not demonstrated a difference between the techniques. Studies of more than 3,000 noncardiac surgical patients with CAD have concluded that anesthetic type does not affect outcomes.

Volatile anesthetics are thought to possess ischemic preconditioning properties. Most investigations of anesthetic ischemic preconditioning have been done in patients undergoing cardiac surgery where there may be some advantages to the utilization of inhalational agents. By extension, there may be beneficial effects of volatile inhalational agents in high-risk cardiac patients undergoing noncardiac surgery. The current consensus is that the use of either a volatile anesthetic agent or TIVA is reasonable for patients undergoing noncardiac surgery.

The use of nitrous oxide in patients with a history of CAD has been questioned since the early 1990s when animal and human studies showed an increase in peripheral vascular resistance, diastolic dysfunction, and subsequently myocardial ischemia. Badner et al demonstrated the increase in homocysteine plasma levels of patients during carotid endarterectomy when nitrous oxide was administered and the correlation of those levels with increased incidence of myocardial ischemia. However, the Evaluation of Nitrous Oxide in the Gas Mixture for Anaesthesia (ENIGMA-II) trial, which enrolled 7,110 patients, showed that nitrous oxide did not increase the risk of death, cardiovascular complications, or surgical site infection.

Badner NH, Beattie WS, Freeman D, et al. Nitrous oxide-induced increased homocysteine concentrations are associated with increased postoperative myocardial ischemia in patients undergoing carotid endarterectomy. *Anesth Analg*. 2000;91:1073-1079.

Imberger G, Orr A, Thorlund K, et al. Does anaesthesia with nitrous oxide affect mortality or cardiovascular morbidity? A systematic review with meta-analysis and trial sequential analysis. *Br J Anaesth*. 2014;112:410-426.

Ko H, Kaye AD, Urman RD. Nitrous oxide and perioperative outcomes. *J Anesth*. 2014;28:420-428.

Landoni G, Greco T, Biondi-Zoccai G, et al. Anaesthetic drugs and survival: a Bayesian network meta-analysis of randomized trials in cardiac surgery. *Br J Anaesth*. 2013;111:886-896.

Leslie K, Myles P, Devereaux PJ, et al. Nitrous oxide and serious morbidity and mortality in the POISE trial. *Anesth Analg*. 2013;116:1034-1040.

Myles PS, Leslie K, Chan MT, et al. The safety of addition of nitrous oxide to general anaesthesia in at-risk patients having major non-cardiac surgery (ENIGMA-II): a randomised, single-blind trial. *Lancet*. 2014;384:1446-1454.

Nigro Neto C, Landoni G, Cassarà L, et al. Use of volatile anesthetics during cardiopulmonary bypass: a systematic review of adverse events. *J Cardiothorac Vasc Anesth*. 2014;28:84-89.

Sanders RD, Graham C, Lewis SC, et al. Nitrous oxide exposure does not seem to be associated with increased mortality, stroke, and myocardial infarction: a non-randomized subgroup analysis of the general anaesthesia compared with local anaesthesia for carotid surgery (GALA) trial. *Br J Anaesth*. 2012;109:361-367.

C.9. You notice a new 3-mm ST-segment depression in lead V_5. How would you treat it?

ST-segment depression can be an indicator of myocardial ischemia. Initial efforts should be focused on determining its etiology. Management of ischemia should include pharmacologic manipulation of the determinants of myocardial oxygen supply and demand. Most intraoperative myocardial infarctions are Type II MIs secondary to global hypoperfusion and demand ischemia.

The crucial aspect of such management includes the following:

- Heart rate control and adequate CPP. If ST-segment depression is associated with tachycardia and hypertension, the most common cause during surgery is inadequate anesthesia. Therefore, adequate levels of anesthesia and analgesia should be achieved first. Heart rate control can also be achieved using β-blockers, which will reduce myocardial oxygen demands. Caution should be exercised in patients with known contraindications and acute hemodynamic instability.
- Avoidance of hypotension and use of vasopressors to sustain CPP
- Oxygen delivery should be increased by correcting significant anemia (<7 g/dL) and increasing the fraction of inspired oxygen.
- Oxygen demand could also be reduced by correction of hypothermia and/or shivering, if present.
- In the context of ST-segment elevation and concerns for acute coronary syndrome, nitrates and antiplatelet agents may be utilized.
- The procedure should be terminated or completed as soon as feasible to facilitate further evaluation and definitive treatment.

Thompson A, Fleischmann KE, et al. AHA/ACC/ACS/ASNC/HRS/SCA/SCCT/SCMR/SVM Guideline for Perioperative Cardiovascular Management for Noncardiac Surgery: a report of the American College of Cardiology/American Heart Association Joint Committee on Clinical Practice Guidelines. *Circulation*. 2024;150:e351-e442. Erratum in: *Circulation*. 2024;150:e466.

C.10. What is the significance of tight control of the heart rate intraoperatively?

Numerous studies have shown that intraoperative tachycardia and the duration of tachycardia could cause myocardial ischemia. Therefore, control of heart rate intraoperatively could significantly reduce the risk of perioperative myocardial events. However, the optimal heart rate for all patients has not been determined. Tachycardia is associated with intraoperative myocardial ischemia. Raby et al demonstrated that in high-risk patients with signs of ischemia on preoperative Holter tracing, controlling the heart rate 20% below the ischemia threshold (or 60 beats per minute) with esmolol reduced the risk of perioperative myocardial ischemia. Feringa et al also demonstrated that tight heart rate control reduced perioperative myocardial ischemia and improved long-term outcomes in vascular surgery patients.

Biccard BM, Sear JW, Foëx P. Meta-analysis of the effect of heart rate achieved by perioperative beta-adrenergic blockade on cardiovascular outcomes. *Br J Anaesth*. 2008;100:23-28.

Feringa H, Bax J, Boersma E, et al. High-dose beta-blockers and tight heart rate control reduce myocardial ischemia and troponin T release in vascular surgery patients. *Circulation*. 2006;114:I344-I349.

Landesberg G, Beattie WS, Mosseri M, et al. Perioperative myocardial infarction. *Circulation*. 2009;119:2936-2944.

Raby KE, Brull SJ, Timimi F, et al. The effect of heart rate control on myocardial ischemia among high-risk patients after vascular surgery. *Anesth Analg*. 1999;88:477-482.

Slogoff S, Keats AS. Myocardial ischemia revisited. *Anesthesiology*. 2006;105:214-216.

C.11. When would you extubate the trachea in this patient? What could you do to prevent hypertension and tachycardia during extubation and emergence?

At the end of the surgery, assuming no intraoperative complications, the trachea would be extubated when the patient is fully awake, breathing adequately, and neuromuscular blockade is fully reversed. To mitigate the tachycardia and hypertension associated with extubation and emergence, low doses of medications such as lidocaine, esmolol, nicardipine, or labetalol can be administered.

Atlee JL, Dhamee MS, Olund TL, et al. The use of esmolol, nicardipine, or their combination to blunt hemodynamic changes after laryngoscopy and tracheal intubation. *Anesth Analg*. 2000;90:280-285.

Halvorsen S, Mehilli J, et al. 2022 ESC Guidelines on cardiovascular assessment and management of patients undergoing non-cardiac surgery. *Eur Heart J*. 2022;43:3826-3924. Erratum in: *Eur Heart J*. 2023;44:4421.

Mikawa K, Nishina K, Maekawa N, et al. Attenuation of cardiovascular responses to tracheal extubation: verapamil versus diltiazem. *Anesth Analg*. 1996;82:1205-1210.

D. Postoperative Management

D.1. What are the postoperative predictors of perioperative MACE?

In noncardiac surgical patients, the highest risk of cardiac morbidity is in the postoperative period, when up to 67% of perioperative ischemic events occur. This period is characterized by an increase in heart rate, blood pressure, sympathetic discharge, and hypercoagulability. Heart rate commonly increases postoperatively by 25% to 50% over intraoperative values, and tachycardia occurs in 10% to 25% of patients. Likewise, hypotension, hemorrhage, and the need for blood transfusion are associated with worse cardiac outcomes. Postoperative myocardial ischemia occurs in 27% to 41% of high-risk patients, with most events without angina. PMI is usually preceded by prolonged ST-segment depression. However, routine continuous postoperative ECG monitoring is not recommended, and even routine daily ECG for 3 days is no longer advocated. In a study involving 337 vascular surgery patients in whom troponin I levels were collected within 48 hours of surgery and 12-lead ECGs were performed daily for three PODs, 40% of the patients had elevated troponin levels, but only 6% of patients had ischemic changes on the ECG. PMI may be associated with tachycardia and pain.

The highest incidence of troponin elevation, a biochemical marker of ischemia, frequently occurs 8 to 24 hours after the surgical procedure. Even mild elevations in troponin are associated with postoperative cardiac ischemia and are independent predictors of mortality. PMI has also been associated with other clinical conditions such as postoperative hypothermia, hypercoagulability, postoperative pain, and anemia. Postoperative ischemia is the most important marker of immediate and long-term adverse cardiovascular events. It is associated with a 2.8-fold increase in the odds of all adverse cardiac outcomes.

Garcia S, Marston N, Sandoval Y, et al. Prognostic value of 12-lead electrocardiogram and peak troponin I level after vascular surgery. *J Vasc Surg*. 2013;57:166-172.

Le Manach Y, Perel A, Coriat P, et al. Early and delayed myocardial infarction after abdominal aortic surgery. *Anesthesiology*. 2005;102:885-891.

Nagele P, Brown F, Gage BF, et al. High-sensitivity cardiac troponin T in prediction and diagnosis of myocardial infarction and long-term mortality after noncardiac surgery. *Am Heart J*. 2013;166:325-332.

D.2. How would you control postoperative pain?

The postoperative period can be stressful due to the onset of pain during emergence from anesthesia, fluid shifts, temperature changes, and alteration of respiratory function. Marked changes occur in plasma catecholamine concentration, hemodynamics, ventricular function, and coagulation following noncardiac surgery, particularly in patients with preexisting cardiac disease. These stressors place the patient at increased risk for the development of adverse cardiac outcomes. Severe postoperative pain was reported in 5% to 10% of patients. Effective pain management is essential to prevent adverse outcomes and promote early recovery. Intravenous patient-controlled analgesia and/or patient-controlled epidural analgesia are popular methods for reducing postoperative pain. Several studies suggest that effective pain management leads to a reduction in postoperative catecholamine surges and hypercoagulability. A meta-analysis published in 2013, which analyzed the impact of epidural analgesia versus systemic analgesia, concluded that epidural analgesia was associated with a 40% decrease in mortality and a significant decrease in the risk of atrial fibrillation, supraventricular tachycardia, deep vein thrombosis, respiratory depression, atelectasis, pneumonia, ileus, and postoperative nausea and vomiting, and also improved recovery of bowel function. Within a thoracic surgery population, epidural analgesia was associated with significantly reduced postoperative pulmonary complications. However, epidural analgesia also significantly increases the risk of arterial hypotension, pruritus, urinary retention, and motor blockade, and exposes the patient to risks related to catheter placement and removal (nerve injury, trauma, hematoma, etc). Hence, while attentive pain control is important in the postoperative period, the method employed should always consider patient and procedure-related needs and risks.

Baar W, Semmelmann A, Knoerlein J, et al. Risk factors for postoperative pulmonary complications leading to increased in-hospital mortality in patients undergoing thoracotomy for primary lung cancer resection: a multicentre retrospective cohort study of the German Thorax Registry. *J Clin Med*. 2022;11:5774.

Norris EJ, Beattie C, Perler BA, et al. Double-masked randomized trial comparing alternate combinations of intraoperative anesthesia and postoperative analgesia in abdominal aortic surgery. *Anesthesiology*. 2001;95:1054-1067.

Pöpping DM, Elia N, Van Aken HK, et al. Impact of epidural analgesia on mortality and morbidity after surgery: systematic review and meta-analysis of randomized controlled trials. *Ann Surg*. 2014;259:1056-1067.

D.3. Is postoperative anemia associated with adverse cardiac outcomes?

Patients with cardiac disease may be adversely affected by anemia. Based on existing literature, the evidence is sufficient to state that transfusions are rarely beneficial if the hemoglobin (Hgb) level exceeds 10 g/dL (hematocrit >30%) in the absence of acute blood loss. It is also reasonable to state that the patient may benefit from a transfusion if the Hgb level falls below 7 g/dL. The controversy remains between Hgb concentrations of 8.0 and 10.0 g/dL. The 2016 American Association of Blood Banks Guideline, which is based on expert opinion and studies, recommends a restricted transfusion strategy (Hgb <7 g/dL) in asymptomatic, hemodynamically stable patients without CAD. The guideline also recommends adherence to a restrictive transfusion strategy in hospitalized patients with cardiovascular disease and consideration of transfusion for patients with symptoms (eg, chest pain, orthostasis, CHF) or Hgb less than 8 g/dL. In postoperative patients, the recommended maintenance Hgb concentration is 8 g/dL or more, unless the patient exhibits symptoms. There were no specific recommendations for hemodynamically stable patients with ACS because of the lack of high-quality evidence for either a liberal or a restrictive transfusion strategy in these patients. The consensus of those experts recommended a symptom-guided approach to evaluating an Hgb level to determine whether to transfuse a patient with anemia.

Beattie WS, Karkouti K, Wijeysundera DN, et al. Risk associated with preoperative anemia in noncardiac surgery: a single-center cohort study. *Anesthesiology*. 2009;110:574-581.

Carson JL, Guyatt G, Heddle NM, et al. Clinical practice guidelines from the AABB: red blood cell transfusion thresholds and storage. *JAMA*. 2016;316:2025-2035.

Qaseem A, Humphrey LL, Fitterman N, et al. Treatment of anemia in patients with heart disease: a clinical practice guideline from the American College of Physicians. *Ann Intern Med*. 2013;159:770-779.

Simmons JW, Pittet JF. Revealing the real risks of perioperative transfusion: rise of the machines! *Anesthesiology*. 2015;122:1-2.

D.4. Is postoperative hypothermia associated with postoperative myocardial ischemia?

Hypothermia is common during anesthesia and surgery owing to anesthetic-induced inhibition of thermoregulatory control. The principal initial cause of hypothermia is core-to-peripheral redistribution of body heat.

Perioperative hypothermia triples the incidence of adverse myocardial outcomes in high-risk patients. Core hypothermia may increase circulating catecholamine levels, leading to tachycardia, hypertension, systemic vasoconstriction, and an imbalance between oxygen demand and supply. Frank et al studied 100 patients undergoing lower extremity vascular surgery. They found that unintentional hypothermia (sublingual temperature <35 °C [95 °F]) on arrival to postoperative ICU is associated with a significantly higher incidence of myocardial ischemia (36% vs 13%), angina (18% vs 15%), and Pao_2 less than 80 mm Hg (52% vs 30%) during the early postoperative period. However, a subsequent trial involving 1,000 patients with subarachnoid hemorrhage, randomized to perioperative hypothermia or normothermia, did not show a difference in perioperative cardiac events. Maintenance of normothermia may be a reasonable strategy to reduce perioperative cardiac events in patients undergoing noncardiac surgery.

Frank SM, Beattie C, Christopherson R, et al. Unintentional hypothermia is associated with postoperative myocardial ischemia. *Anesthesiology*. 1993;78:468-476.

Todd MM, Hindman BJ, Clarke WR, et al. Mild intraoperative hypothermia during surgery for intracranial aneurysm. *N Engl J Med*. 2005;352:135-145.

D.5. How would you make a diagnosis of perioperative myocardial infarction (PMI)?

The definition of myocardial infarction, according to the fourth universal definition of MI, is the presence of myocardial injury detected by abnormal cardiac biomarkers in the setting of acute myocardial ischemia.

Most ischemic episodes occur after and not during the operation. Several studies have examined the optimal method for diagnosing a PMI, as most patients do not complain of chest pain and the value of routine serial postoperative ECG is limited. Cardiac-specific enzyme elevations such as troponin I (cTnI) and troponin T (cTnT) are currently the standard of care for the biochemical diagnosis of a PMI because they demonstrate sensitivity and tissue specificity superior to other available biomarkers; however, cTnT elevations have also been noted in the context of skeletal muscle injury. Newer, high-sensitivity cardiac troponin assays are the preferred diagnostic test, and elevations in any cardiac troponin above the 99th percentile upper reference limit (URL) confirm a diagnosis of MINS.

In the purest physiologic sense, any detectable necrosis is an acute MI; however, troponin elevation can be observed in many other conditions in which the heart is stressed. Even small elevations of specific markers of myocardial damage, such as cardiac troponins, should be acknowledged as indicative of myocardial injury. While any cardiac troponin elevation greater than the 99th URL indicates myocardial injury, the etiology remains to be determined. Anemia, hypoxemia, hypotension, arrhythmia, critical illness, stress, sepsis, cardiotoxins, chronic kidney disease, cardiac trauma, and cardiovascular procedures can all produce significant perioperative troponin elevations. Most PMIs in the first 7 days after an operation tend to be myocardial injury related to demand (type II), and PMI related to plaque rupture (type I) predominates more than 7 days postoperatively. From a clinical perspective, there is clear evidence that any amount of detectable cardiac troponin release is associated with an increased risk of new adverse cardiac events and poorer long-term outcomes.

Clinicians need to be sensitive to redundancy in testing. Some authors have demonstrated that routine cardiac troponin monitoring is an easy, effective, and inexpensive way to detect postoperative myocardial injury. However, the ACC/AHA guidelines reserve the use of these biomarkers for patients at high risk and those with clinical, ECG, or hemodynamic evidence of cardiovascular dysfunction. Routine measurement of postoperative troponins in asymptomatic or low-risk patients undergoing low-risk procedures is not warranted.

Landesberg G, Shatz V, Akopnik I, et al. Association of cardiac troponin, CK-MB, and postoperative myocardial ischemia with long-term survival after major vascular surgery. *J Am Coll Cardiol*. 2003;42:1547-1554.

Lopez-Jimenez F, Goldman L, Sacks DB, et al. Prognostic value of cardiac troponin T after noncardiac surgery: 6-month follow-up data. *J Am Coll Cardiol*. 1997;29:1241-1245.

Thompson A, Fleischmann KE, et al. AHA/ACC/ACS/ASNC/HRS/SCA/SCCT/SCMR/SVM Guideline for Perioperative Cardiovascular Management for Noncardiac Surgery: a report of the American College of Cardiology/American Heart Association Joint Committee on Clinical Practice Guidelines. *Circulation*. 2024;150:e351-e442. Erratum in: *Circulation*. 2024;150:e466.

Thygesen K, Alpert JS, Jaffe AS, et al. Fourth universal definition of myocardial infarction (2018) [published correction appears in *Circulation*. 2018;138:e652]. *Circulation*. 2018;138:e618-e651.

White HD, Thygesen K, Alpert JS, et al. Clinical implications of the third universal definition of myocardial infarction. *Heart*. 2014;100:424-432.

D.6. How would you manage a patient with a suspected PMI?

There is a lack of evidence regarding the management of PMI in the postsurgical patient. PMI could include three different clinical presentations: unstable angina (UA), non–ST-elevation MI (NSTEMI), and STEMI.

The initial management should focus on the following diagnostics:

- Clinical evaluation of chest pain, or angina-equivalent symptoms (dyspnea, diaphoresis, etc)
- 12-Lead ECG and determination of changes

- Serial measurement of biomarkers of cardiac injury. A cardiac-specific high-sensitivity troponin is the preferred marker.
- Transthoracic echocardiography
- Immediate consultation with a cardiologist and risk stratification to determine high-risk patients

It is important to consider the recent surgical procedure and consultation with the surgical team regarding the impact of aspirin and anticoagulant therapy.

Unless a contraindication exists, patients with UA or NSTEMI should be treated with oxygen, aspirin (acetylene salicylic acid), sublingual/intravenous NTG for chest pain relief, a β-blocker (assuming appropriate hemodynamics), and unfractionated heparin or low-molecular-weight heparin.

The cardiology consultant should guide further management:

- Option 1 is a routine angiographic approach, in which coronary angiography and revascularization are performed unless a contraindication exists. Within this approach, the most common strategy advocates for a period of medical stabilization. A more aggressive approach calls for coronary angiography and revascularization performed within 24 hours of the onset of symptoms or diagnosis; the rationale for the more aggressive approach is the protective effect of carefully administered anticoagulant and antiplatelet therapy on the outcome of reperfusion procedures.
- The alternative approach, commonly referred to as the initially conservative strategy, is guided by ischemia, with angiography reserved for patients with recurrent ischemia despite medical therapy.

Regardless of the angiographic strategy, an assessment of LV function (echocardiography, ventriculogram, or nuclear ventriculography) should be strongly considered because of the importance of treating patients who have impaired LV function with ACE inhibitors, β-blockers, and surgical revascularization (CABG) when appropriate (eg, three-vessel disease or equivalent).

If the patient presents with a STEMI, recognized based on the 12-lead ECG, the management will be initially similar to UA/NSTEMI (oxygen, acetylene salicylic acid, NTG, β-blockers), followed by an attempt to restore flow in the infarct artery by PCI (balloon angioplasty with or without deployment of an intracoronary stent under the support of pharmacologic measures to prevent thrombosis), or surgical revascularization (CABG).

Evidence supports the expeditious restoration of flow in the obstructed infarct artery after the onset of symptoms in patients with STEMI as a key determinant of short- and long-term outcomes. Early reperfusion of ischemic myocardium within the risk region of an occluded infarct-related artery interrupts the occurring necrosis, reduces ultimate infarct size, preserves regional and global ventricular function, and improves survival. A subset of patients will have severe three-vessel or left main disease or anatomic features unfavorable for PCI and may be candidates for urgent or emergency CABG.

Thompson A, Fleischmann KE, et al. AHA/ACC/ACS/ASNC/HRS/SCA/SCCT/SCMR/SVM Guideline for Perioperative Cardiovascular Management for Noncardiac Surgery: a report of the American College of Cardiology/American Heart Association Joint Committee on Clinical Practice Guidelines. *Circulation.* 2024;150:e351-e442. Erratum in: *Circulation.* 2024;150:e466.

Thygesen K, Alpert JS, Jaffe AS, et al. Fourth universal definition of myocardial infarction (2018) [published correction appears in *Circulation.* 2018;138:e652]. *Circulation.* 2018;138:e618-e651.

15 Intestinal Obstruction and Enhanced Recovery After Surgery

Shaker J. Morcous, Leif Ericksen, and Tong J. Gan

A 73-year-old woman with an acute abdomen was scheduled to undergo an emergency exploratory laparotomy. She complained of severe abdominal pain with periodic bouts of bilious vomiting. Her past surgical history included a right hemicolectomy for colon cancer. She had a blood pressure (BP) of 85/60 mm Hg, pulse of 115 beats per minute, and hematocrit of 45%.

A. Medical Disease and Differential Diagnosis

1. What is the differential diagnosis of the acute abdomen?
2. What are the causes of intestinal obstruction of the small bowel and of the large bowel?
3. Differentiate between simple and strangulated bowel obstruction.
4. Is it important to differentiate whether the bowel obstruction is in the small bowel or large bowel? Why? How might the distinction be made?
5. What are the causes and effects of bowel distension?
6. Describe the fluid shifts during small bowel intestinal obstruction.
7. Discuss the systemic derangements that occur with intestinal obstruction.
8. What is an ileus? Discuss its causes and pathophysiology.

B. Preoperative Evaluation and Preparation

1. What is an Enhanced Recovery After Surgery (ERAS) program? What are the core tenets of these programs?
2. Can ERAS be used in this case?
3. What components of ERAS are applied in the preoperative phase of the care of patients undergoing colorectal surgery (CRS)?
4. Is it important to decompress the abdomen before induction of anesthesia? Why?
5. Describe the respiratory implications.
6. What are the implications of a tense abdominal wall?
7. Outline the methods of abdominal decompression.
8. Discuss the goals of fluid management.
9. What would you use as a guide to fluid volume replacement?

C. Intraoperative Management

1. What dangers are present during induction? How are they planned for?
2. Does the administration of antacids and/or histamine-2 (H_2) blockers before the induction of anesthesia have a significant value in patients with small bowel obstruction?
3. In what position would you intubate this patient?
4. What is the best neuromuscular blocking drug to use for rapid-sequence induction?
5. Would you remove or leave the nasogastric tube (NGT) in place before inducing anesthesia?
6. Would you use nitrous oxide in this patient?

7. Are there any benefits to using a high concentration of inspired oxygen (FIO_2)?
8. What components of ERAS are applied in the intraoperative phase of the care of patients undergoing CRS?
9. What are the strengths, weaknesses, benefits, and challenges of ERAS?
10. What are the indications for ERAS?

D. Postoperative Management

1. What are the principles of postoperative care in this patient?
2. Are there any postoperative respiratory problems associated with factors other than aspiration?
3. If the patient aspirates gastric contents, what are the possible sequelae? What is the treatment?
4. What is gram-negative sepsis? Describe the clinical picture and treatment.
5. What components of ERAS are applied in the postoperative phase of the care of patients following CRS?

A. Medical Disease and Differential Diagnosis

A.1. What is the differential diagnosis of the acute abdomen?

An acute abdomen refers to a number of conditions, with the most prominent feature being severe abdominal pain of abrupt onset that can necessitate urgent surgical intervention. The differential is challenging because there are a number of etiologies. The most common diagnoses vary by age; many organ systems may cause an acute abdomen, and the presenting symptom is often nonspecific. Some of the most common causes are listed in **Table 15.1**. Visceral and somatic afferents are the two systems that transmit abdominal pain. Visceral pain is dull, deep, poorly localized, and transmitted by C fibers in the mucosa, muscularis, and visceral peritoneum. Visceral pain is generated by nerve endings without specialized structures that are primarily sensitive to tissue tension typically caused by distension, spasm, and ischemia. Somatic pain is sharp, well localized, and transmitted by chemical (inflammation), thermal, or mechanical irritation of the Aδ fibers of the parietal peritoneum. These fibers are derived from the same origin as those innervating muscle and skin, which cause the guarding and cutaneous sensitivity that can accompany an acute abdomen. Abdominal pathology frequently has a mixed picture of visceral and somatic pain.

The two processes typically implicated in an acute abdomen are inflammation and obstruction. The inflammatory milieu causes a direct chemical irritation and causes the tissue to become edematous and distended. Impeded flow through a hollow organ causes smooth muscle to contract in an attempt to overcome the obstruction, resulting in increased tension and dilation. Both of these processes can contribute to ischemia and perforation, which can in turn also cause pain.

Etiologies of an acute abdomen vary and require either medical and/or surgical treatment, be intra- and/or extra-abdominal, and be associated with almost any organ system. Characteristics such as intensity, chronology, location, diffuse or localized, radiation, and comorbidities in addition to testing help to construct a differential diagnosis.

Feldmen M, Friedman LS, Brandt LJ, eds. Pancreatic physiology and functional assessment. In: *Sleisenger and Fordtran's Gastrointestinal and Liver Disease: Pathophysiology, Diagnosis, Management*. 10th ed. Elsevier Saunders; 2016:161-174.

Garden JO, Parks RW, Wigmore SJ, eds. Preoperative considerations, anaesthesia and analgesia. In: *Principles and Practice of Surgery*. 8th ed. Elsevier; 2022:162-179.

A.2. What are the causes of intestinal obstruction of the small bowel and of the large bowel?

Obstruction occurs due to either an inhibition of physiologic peristalsis (ileus) or mechanical obstruction. Mechanical obstructions are broadly divided into extrinsic, intramural, and intraluminal categories.

Adhesions resulting from the inflammation and healing process of prior surgery account for the vast majority (>70%) of small bowel obstructions and are followed in order by hernias, malignancy, and then inflammatory bowel disease. Diagnoses of volvulus and hernia strangulation are less common but are surgical emergencies. Large bowel obstructions occur less frequently; the most common etiologies are adenocarcinoma, volvulus, and sequelae from diverticulitis. Adenocarcinoma causes more than 50% of all large bowel obstructions.

Bower KL, Lollar DI, Williams SL, et al. Small bowel obstruction. *Surg Clin North Am*. 2018;98:945-971.

Feldmen M, Friedman LS, Brandt LJ, eds. Tropical diarrhea and malabsorption. In: *Sleisenger and Fordtran's Gastrointestinal and Liver Disease: Pathophysiology, Diagnosis, Management*. 11th ed. Elsevier Saunders; 2020:2021-2059.

Yeo CJ, ed. Gastric cancer. In: *Shackelford's Surgery of the Alimentary Tract*. 8th ed. Elsevier; 2019:842-850.

TABLE 15.1 Acute Abdomen Differential

Surgical	Medical	Gynecologic
Inflammation	Cardiovascular	Ectopic pregnancy
Inflammatory bowel disease	Myocardial ischemia	Ovarian cyst
Acute appendicitis	Myocardial infarction (inferior)	Torsion
Acute diverticulitis	Gastrointestinal	Rupture
Acute pancreatitis	Gastritis	Hemorrhage
Acute cholecystitis	Gastroenteritis	Infarction
Acute cholangitis	Mesenteric adenitis	Infection
Meckel diverticulitis	Hepatitis	Pelvic inflammatory disease
Obstruction	Hepatic abscess	Fibroid degeneration
Intestinal obstruction	Fitz-Hugh-Curtis syndrome	Salpingitis
Biliary colic	Primary peritonitis	Mittelschmerz
Ureteric colic	Abdominal wall conditions	Endometriosis
Acute retention of urine	Rectus sheath hematoma	
Ischemia	Genitourinary	
Mesenteric ischemia	Urinary tract infection	
Torsion of a viscus	Pyelonephritis	
Perforation	Neurologic	
Perforated peptic ulcer disease	Tabes dorsalis	
Perforated small bowel (salmonella, cytomegalovirus, and tuberculosis infection)	Hematologic	
Perforated diverticular disease	Sickle cell disease	
Perforated appendix	Malaria	
Toxic megacolon with perforation	Hereditary spherocytosis	
Acute cholecystitis and perforation	Endocrine	
Perforated esophagus	Diabetes	
Perforated bladder	Thyrotoxicosis	
Perforation of a length of strangulated bowel	Addison disease	
Ruptured abdominal aortic aneurysm	Metabolic	
	Uremia	
	Hypercalcemia	
	Porphyria	
	Infective	
	Herpes zoster	

The colored cells represent pathophysiologies. Noncolored cells represent specific diagnoses. The table is presented in the context of forming a differential diagnosis for an acute abdomen. The table presents categories that become more specific (eg, surgical/medical/gynecologic, then pathophysiology, then specific diagnoses) that can be matched to a patient's presenting symptoms and history. Reprinted from Garden JO, Parks RW, eds. The acute abdomen and intestinal obstruction. In: *Principles and Practice of Surgery*. 7th ed. Elsevier; 2018:159. Copyright © 2018 Elsevier. With permission.

A.3. Differentiate between simple and strangulated bowel obstruction.

A simple bowel obstruction refers to a single section of occlusion, whereas a strangulated obstruction refers to an area of compromised perfusion. It is important to recognize bowel strangulation because it increases mortality 2- to 10-fold from generally less than 5% to 25%, depending on comorbid conditions. Strangulation is typically discussed in concert with an incarcerated segment of the bowel (eg, a hernia or hole in the omentum) but can also be due to inadequate perfusion pressure secondary to increased intraluminal or intramural pressure. As venous outflow decreases, the bowel wall becomes edematous, obstruction worsens, pressure increases, and eventually arterial inflow is compromised. Affected sections become ischemic, infarct, and perforate, after which peritonitis ensues.

The classic signs of strangulation are constant (as opposed to intermittent) pain, fever, tachycardia, leukocytosis, and peritonitic signs (eg, guarding and rebound tenderness). However, no clinical parameter reliably rules strangulation in or out, so a thorough history and physical examination and a high index of suspicion must guide the decision to operate. Risk factors for bowel strangulation include female sex, femoral hernia, and history of hospitalization related to groin hernia.

Doherty GM, ed. Breast disorders. In: *Current: Diagnosis & Treatment: Surgery*. 14th ed. McGraw-Hill; 2015:660-663.

Doherty GM, ed. Endocrine tumors of the pancreas. In: *Current: Diagnosis & Treatment: Surgery*. 14th ed. McGraw-Hill; 2015:692-695.

Garden JO, Parks RW, Wigmore SJ, eds. Preoperative considerations, anaesthesia and analgesia. In: *Principles and Practice of Surgery*. 8th ed. Elsevier; 2022:78-99.

Garden JO, Parks RW, Wigmore SJ, eds. Principles of the surgical management of cancer. In: *Principles and Practice of Surgery*. 8th ed. Elsevier; 2022:100-110.

Harken AH, Moore EE, eds. Breast disorders. In: *Abernathy's Surgical Secrets*. 7th ed. Elsevier: 2018;215-218.

HerniaSurge Group. International guidelines for groin hernia management. *Hernia*. 2018;22:1-165.

Sutton JM, Beckwith MA, Johnson BL, et al, eds. Intestinal obstruction. In: *The Mont Reid Surgical Handbook*. 7th ed. Elsevier; 2018:331-344.

Townsend CM, Beauchamp RD, Evers BM, et al, eds. Stomach. In: *Sabiston Textbook of Surgery: The Biological Basis of Modern Surgical Practice*. 20th ed. Elsevier; 2017:1237-1295.

A.4. Is it important to differentiate whether the bowel obstruction is in the small bowel or large bowel? Why? How might the distinction be made?

Yes, it is important not only to differentiate between large and small bowel obstruction but also to determine the position of the obstruction within those sections of the bowel. Both small and large bowel obstructions can present with colicky abdominal pain, nausea and vomiting, distension, and obstipation. The location, however, differentiates between the etiologies of the obstruction, which will dictate management strategy, systemic consequences, and possible special considerations. Prognosis can also vary widely. For instance, a large bowel obstruction presenting with the clinical features of a small bowel obstruction can have a mortality rate 4 times greater than from other causes.

Small bowel obstruction is associated with more bilious vomiting sooner after the obstruction occurs. Patients continue to have bowel movements as the distal bowel continues to function. Time intervals between bouts of abdominal pain are shorter, the more proximal the obstruction is. The majority of small bowel obstructions are thought to be caused by adhesive disease, which typically resolve with nonoperative management, including decompression using an NGT and fluid resuscitation. The small bowel is involved in a number of secretory and absorptive processes. During a trial of conservative management, a stable patient must be monitored for indications to proceed to surgery because altered function can lead to accumulation of air and fluid, bowel distension, increased intraluminal pressure according to the law of Laplace, and possible bowel infarction and rupture. Small bowel obstruction also alters gut flora balance, leading to translocation of bacteria. Vomiting occurs earlier and more frequently with a small bowel obstruction, which contributes to anesthetic concerns including decreased intravascular volume, metabolic alkalosis, and airway management. Crohn disease, irradiated bowel, and Richter hernias require additional considerations based on location and level of involvement.

Large bowel obstructions are usually slower in onset, more frequently associated with distension and lower abdominal pain, and caused most frequently by adenocarcinoma. Surgical intervention is typically required before infarction and perforation occur. Fewer fluid shifts occur in the large bowel, and vomiting occurs later in the disease process if at all, so less resuscitation and electrolyte correction are required. Plain film upright and supine x-rays are less accurate than computed tomography (CT) but are faster and might provide other indications to proceed directly to surgery, such as free air. Depending on the location, surgical interventions can include resection, anastomoses, and/or ostomy, all of which have varying risks of leak and infection. Adjuvant radiation and chemotherapy can be part of the perioperative planning process. Stable patients with a sigmoid volvulus might undergo an attempt to relieve the torsion with flexible sigmoidoscopy.

Cameron JL, Cameron AM, eds. *Current Surgical Therapy*. 12th ed. Elsevier; 2017:109-113, 180-183.

Hines RL, Jones SB, eds. Diseases of the liver, biliary tract, and pancreas. In: *Stoelting's Anesthesia and Co-existing Disease*. 8th ed. Elsevier; 2021:347-365.

Kelley SR, Larson DW. Colonic emergencies. In: Paterson-Brown S, Paterson HM, eds. *Core Topics in General and Emergency Surgery*. 6th ed. Elsevier; 2019:193-215.

Weaver JL, Barnett RE, Patterson DE, et al. Large-bowel disease presenting as small-bowel obstruction is associated with a poor prognosis. *Am J Emerg Med*. 2016;34:477-479.

A.5. What are the causes and effects of bowel distension?

In a simple obstruction, the primary contributors to bowel distension are swallowed air and secretions from proximal sections of the gastrointestinal (GI) tract. Bacterial overgrowth also contributes in the form of carbon dioxide and fermentation products that accumulate more rapidly due to an impaired ability to diffuse out of the bowel. Endotoxin-stimulated chemoreceptors and mechanoreceptors activated by distension activate autocrine, luminal, paracrine, and immune neuroendocrine systems (ALPINES) to attract neutrophils and macrophages. Prostaglandins and inflammatory mediators directly alter the activity of ion transporters (and therefore affect the flow of fluid) and the barrier function of the gut. The net result is increased secretion into the lumen of the intestine, decreased absorption, and further distension forming a feedback loop unless decompressed (**Figure 15.1**). Interestingly, this effect is seen both proximally and distally to an obstruction and can lead to bowel movements even during a complete obstruction. Decreased intravascular volume and electrolyte imbalances are common, which may present as hypotension and lactic acidosis. According to Laplace Law, as the lumen of the bowel grows larger, the pressure increases. Lymphatic drainage is impaired first, further increasing pressure, which then impedes venous drainage and compromises perfusion. Ischemia, infarction, and perforation soon follow. Septic shock ensues if it has not already been initiated by translocated bacteria.

Closed-loop obstructions result from volvulus, herniation, or a large bowel obstruction with a competent ileocecal valve. The same pathology applies but has an accelerated course due to an inability of the obstruction to be relieved proximally. Urgent operative management is typically required.

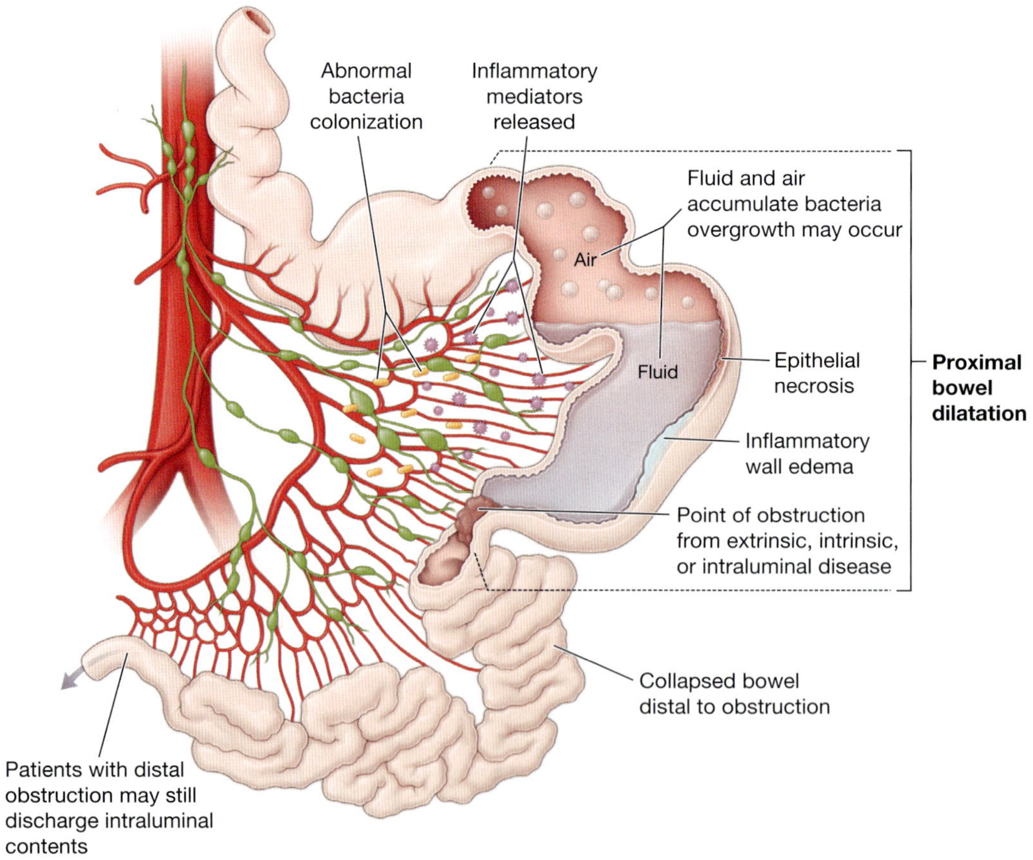

FIGURE 15.1. Pathophysiologic changes of intestinal obstruction. Note: Intraluminal obstruction is displayed. (Derived from Jameson JL, Fauci AS, Kasper DL, et al, eds. *Harrison's Principles of Internal Medicine*. 20th ed. McGraw-Hill Education; 2018:2296.)

Feldmen M, Friedman LS, Brandt LJ, eds. Tropical sprue and other tropical enteropathies. In: *Sleisenger and Fordtran's Gastrointestinal and Liver Disease: Pathophysiology, Diagnosis, Management*. 11th ed. Elsevier Saunders; 2020:2021-2059.

Jameson JL, Fauci AS, Kasper DL, Hauser SL, Longo DL, Loscalzo J, eds. Disorders of the sense of smell and taste. In: *Harrison's Principles of Internal Medicine*. 20th ed. McGraw-Hill; 2018:2294-2298.

A.6. Describe the fluid shifts during small bowel intestinal obstruction.

A normal physiologic small bowel fluid load is 8 to 9 L/d (**Figure 15.2**). Obstruction causing distension increases the secretory activity of the bowel and decreases absorptive capacity, leading to fluid sequestration in the lumen of the bowel. The more proximal the obstruction is, the more severe the fluid loss is. Bowel wall edema, vomiting, NGT suctioning, and transudative fluid loss into the peritoneum can all contribute to the decrease in intravascular fluid. In general, vomiting occurs when 3 L of fluid has been sequestered. Hemodynamic parameters, such as heart rate (HR) and BP, become abnormal at greater than or equal to 6 L of sequestered fluid.

Boron WF, Boulpaep EL, eds. Gastrointestinal motility. In: *Medical Physiology*. 3rd ed. Elsevier; 2017:899-913.

Costanzo LS, ed. Acid-base physiology. In: *Physiology*. 7th ed. Elsevier; 2021:339-394.

Freeman B, Berger J, eds. Organ-based advanced sciences: Cardiovascular physiology and anesthesia. In: *Anesthesiology Core Review: Part Two ADVANCED Exam*. McGraw-Hill; 2016:323-327.

A.7. Discuss the systemic derangements that occur with intestinal obstruction.

Systemic derangements in intestinal obstruction can be severe and even fatal if left unchecked. Hypotension results from hypovolemia secondary to fluid sequestration in the bowel lumen and wall as well as loss from vomiting and gastric suctioning. When the bowel is distended and intra-abdominal pressure is high, venous return is impaired and hypotension worsens. Other mechanical consequences of a distended abdomen include reduced functional residual capacity (FRC) and increased work of breathing.

The proximal bowel secretes a great deal of potassium, sodium, and chlorine. A very proximal obstruction can result in hypochloremic, hypokalemic, metabolic alkalosis. A more common finding is metabolic acidosis related to compromised perfusion. Hyponatremia can further contribute to intravascular fluid loss.

Normal bowel functions as a barrier, keeping bacterial flora intraluminal if any exist (many are sterile). In obstruction, intestinal flora such as *Escherichia coli*, *Enterococcus faecalis*, and *Klebsiella* increase in count profoundly. Advanced stages can lead to translocation from the gut and contribute to gram-negative sepsis, shock, and death even in the absence of perforation. Finally, inflammatory mediators and relative hypovolemia can also cause damage to remote organs.

Yeo CJ, ed. Gastric cancer. In: *Shackelford's Surgery of the Alimentary Tract*. 8th ed. Elsevier; 2019:842-850.

A.8. What is an ileus? Discuss its causes and pathophysiology.

Ileus describes a lack of physiologic peristalsis in the absence of a mechanical obstruction. Different etiologies exist, including spastic and disorganized motility, but the cause is most germane to the perioperative world, and this case study is the adynamic ileus from the inhibition of intestinal myocytes. The most frequent cause is surgical abdominal manipulation. However, a number of other factors including inflammation, iatrogenic drugs, electrolyte imbalances, excessive crystalloid administration, and trauma can also contribute.

Two mechanisms contribute to postsurgical adynamic ileus. The first is a short-lived neurogenic phase. Incision of the peritoneum activates adrenergic afferents linked to an inhibitory spinal reflex. Subsequent, more intense manipulation of the bowel activates higher-order supraspinal pathways, which then stimulate both adrenergic and vagal pathways to release motility-impairing neurohumoral substances, such as norepinephrine and nitric oxide (NO), and vasoactive intestinal peptide (VIP), respectively. Corticotropin-releasing factor (CRF) has been implicated in the coordination of this pathway.

A longer-lasting inflammatory phase causes uncomplicated postoperative (3-5 days) ileus. Surgical manipulation activates macrophages residing in the myenteric plexus, stimulating the innate immune response. An inflammatory milieu is generated within 3 to 4 hours after surgery. Cytokines alter the release of enteric neurotransmitters. Prostaglandins generated by cyclooxygenase-2 (COX-2) can activate many of the splanchnic afferents and cause reflex spinal inhibition, as discussed in the neurogenic phase. NO also continues to be generated by recruited monocytes and neutrophils.

Infection, sepsis, peritonitis, and trauma cause or contribute to an inflammatory state that can cause an ileus or independently prolong a postoperative ileus (POI). Opioid administration, hypomagnesemia, hyponatremia, and hypercalcemia can also contribute and must be monitored in the perioperative period.

Chapman SJ, Pericleous A, Downey C, et al. Postoperative ileus following major colorectal surgery. *Br J Surg*. 2018;105:797-810.

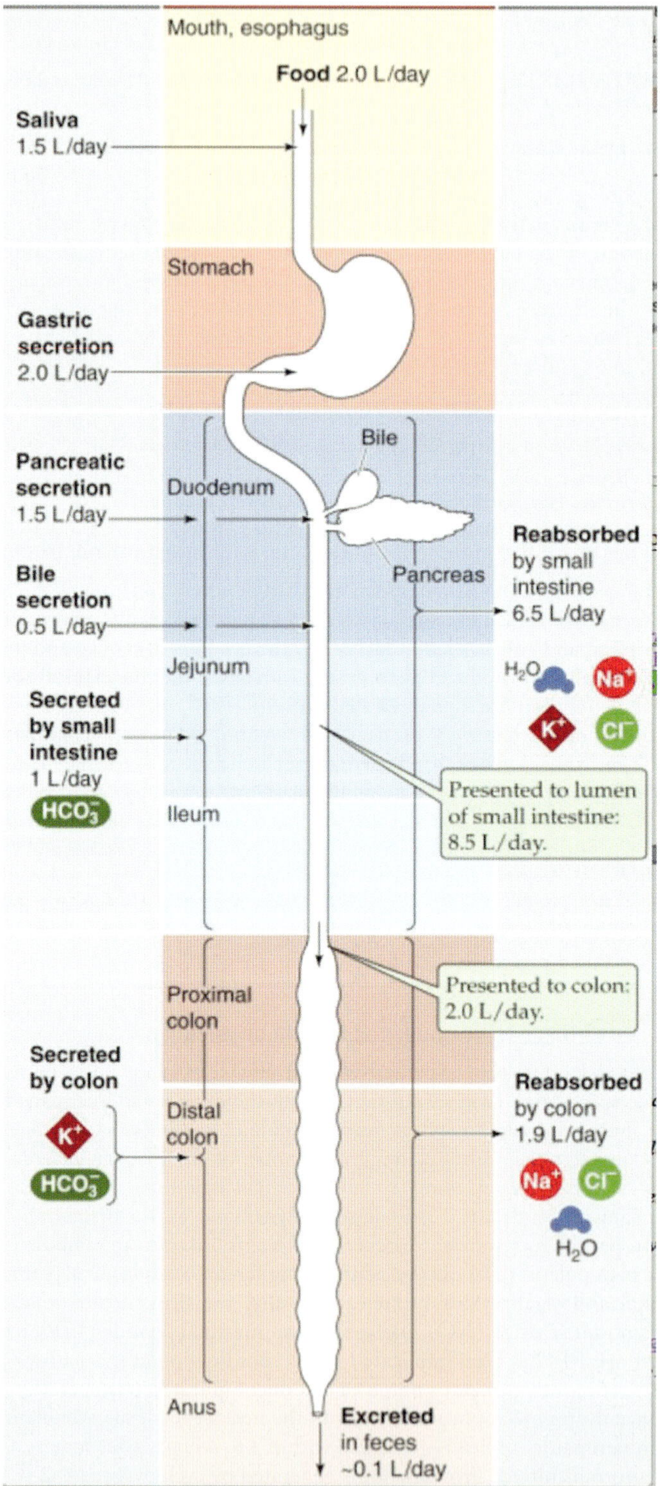

FIGURE 15.2. Gastrointestinal fluids. Fluid balance in the gastrointestinal tract. For each segment of the GI tract, the figure shows substances flowing into the lumen on the left and substances flowing out of the lumen on the right. Of the ~8.5 L/d that is presented to the small intestine, the small intestine removes ~6.5 L/d, delivering ~2 L/d to the colon. The large intestine removes ~1.9 L/d, leaving ~0.1 L/d in the feces. GI, gastrointestinal. (Reprinted from Boron WF, Boulpaep EL, eds. Gastrointestinal motility. In: *Medical Physiology*. 3rd ed. Elsevier; 2017:899-913.. Copyright © 2017 Elsevier. With permission.)

B. Preoperative Evaluation and Preparation

B.1. What is an enhanced recovery after surgery (ERAS) program? What are the core tenets of these programs?

ERAS is a bundle of evidence-based interdisciplinary practices emphasizing early return to functional status. Some of the main tenets include attenuating the physiologic stress response to surgery, improving metabolic responses, and preventing perioperative organ damage. Common strategies include "optimal analgesia," encouraging metabolic optimization, aggressive postoperative nausea and vomiting (PONV) prophylaxis and treatment, goal-directed fluid therapy (GDFT), minimally invasive surgical techniques, avoidance of postoperative NGTs and peritoneal drains, and early enteral feeding and ambulation. ERAS programs have demonstrated accelerated recovery, reduced complication rate, reduction in length of stay, reduced readmission rate, and increased health care value by increasing quality while decreasing cost.

Gan TJ, Thacker JK, Miller TE, et al, eds. Foreword and Preface. In: *Enhanced Recovery for Major Abdominopelvic Surgery*. Professional Communications; 2016:xvi-xxii.

Gan TJ, Thacker JK, Miller TE, et al, eds. Preoperative optimization. In: *Enhanced Recovery for Major Abdominopelvic Surgery*. Professional Communications; 2016:39-48.

Gan TJ, Thacker JK, Miller TE, et al, eds. Intraoperative fluid management. In: *Enhanced Recovery for Major Abdominopelvic Surgery*. Professional Communications; 2016:105-109.

Gan TJ, Thacker JK, Miller TE, et al, eds. Postoperative analgesia. In: *Enhanced Recovery for Major Abdominopelvic Surgery*. Professional Communications; 2016:151-160.

Gan TJ, Thacker JK, Miller TE, et al, eds. Early mobilization. In: *Enhanced Recovery for Major Abdominopelvic Surgery*. Professional Communications; 2016:191-194.

Gan TJ, Thacker JK, Miller TE, et al, eds. Enhanced recovery in colorectal surgery. In: *Enhanced Recovery for Major Abdominopelvic Surgery*. Professional Communications; 2016:199-212.

Gan TJ, Thacker JK, Miller TE, et al, eds. Enhanced recovery in gynecologic surgery. In: *Enhanced Recovery for Major Abdominopelvic Surgery*. Professional Communications; 2016:215-223.

Gan TJ, Thacker JK, Miller TE, et al, eds. Enhanced recovery in liver surgery. In: *Enhanced Recovery for Major Abdominopelvic Surgery*. Professional Communications; 2016:227-233.

Gan TJ, Thacker JK, Miller TE, et al, eds. Enhanced recovery in pancreatic surgery. In: *Enhanced Recovery for Major Abdominopelvic Surgery*. Professional Communications; 2016:237-247.

Gan TJ, Thacker JK, Miller TE, et al, eds. Overcoming challenges: anesthesiologists. In: *Enhanced Recovery for Major Abdominopelvic Surgery*. Professional Communications; 2016:263-275.

B.2. Can ERAS be used in this case?

ERAS protocols are designed to minimize the physiologic impact and stress response of the surgical insult. For patients who require emergency laparotomy, the insult and physiologic disturbance resulting from inflammation, surgical stress, and decompensation are already present prior to the surgery. Many of the ERAS principles can be applied to urgent and emergent procedures as well, especially after patient optimization.

Gan TJ, Thacker JK, Miller TE, et al, eds. Early mobilization. In: *Enhanced Recovery for Major Abdominopelvic Surgery*. Professional Communications; 2016:189, 199.

Peden CJ, Aggarwal G, Aitken RJ, et al. Guidelines for perioperative care for emergency laparotomy enhanced recovery after surgery (ERAS) society recommendations: part 1-preoperative: diagnosis, rapid assessment and optimization. *World J Surg*. 2021;45:1272-1290.

B.3. What components of ERAS are applied in the preoperative phase of the care of patients undergoing colorectal surgery (CRS)?

Multimodal analgesia helps prevent ileus through an opioid-sparing strategy. Preoperative nonsteroidal anti-inflammatory drugs (NSAIDs) and intravenous (IV) acetaminophen have opioid-sparing effects. Thoracic epidural analgesia (TEA) (typically placed in the preoperative period) for open procedures is associated with earlier return of bowel function, superior postoperative analgesia, and decreased cardiopulmonary morbidity. Improved GI outcomes may be due to the combination of reflex sympathetic inhibition of gut function and opioid sparing. Hypotension is a relative contraindication for TEA. The global benefit of TEA is not as clear in laparoscopic procedures. Single-shot spinal can reduce pain scores and reduce opioid consumption. A number of peripheral blocks have demonstrated improved pain scores and decreased opioid use. The most well-studied, transversus abdominal plane (TAP) blocks or catheters have improved early postoperative pain scores, opioid consumption, and length of stay.

The role of gabapentinoids is controversial, as two large database studies reported that gabapentinoid use after colorectal or orthopedic surgery was associated with increased postoperative pulmonary complications and no reduction in postoperative opioid consumption. A meta-analysis evaluating the perioperative use of gabapentinoids also reported no clinically significant analgesic effect from gabapentinoid use and did not recommend their routine use.

Preoperative nutritional optimization improves functional recovery by encouraging an anabolic, rather than catabolic, state. Patients should be screened for malnutrition, and when present should receive protein-rich nutritional supplementation for at least 7 days. Screening and correction of anemia improves oxygen delivery and end-organ function. Those without specific risk for aspiration can ingest solids up to 8 hours before induction. Clear fluids are given, preferably with at least 45 g of carbohydrates, to reduce insulin resistance the evening before surgery and up to 2 hours before induction of anesthesia. Metabolic conditioning can also include prehabilitation programs aimed at improving functional capacity and immunonutrition, both of which have demonstrated improved clinical outcomes.

Bowel preparation in elective CRS has been studied for more than 50 years, and a number of differing opinions still exist. The most current consensus guideline from the American Society for Enhanced Recovery (ASER) and the Perioperative Quality Initiative (POQI) endorses combined isosmotic mechanical bowel preparation with oral antibiotics (MBP-OAB). MBP-OAB has been shown to lower surgical-site infections and is associated with decreased rates of postoperative gastric dysfunction.

Nausea and vomiting prophylaxis is routinely used in ERAS even in low-risk patients because it is difficult to predict who is likely to develop symptoms. Managing modifiable risk factors preoperatively and planning an anesthetic that reduces baseline risk are encouraged. Strategies include the use of propofol for induction and maintenance, avoiding nitrous oxide and inhalational agents, minimizing opioid use, and adequate hydration while avoiding excessive fluid administration.

Maintenance of normothermia improves surgical outcomes and is affected by preoperative interventions. Ambient temperature maintained above 26 °C, dry surgical garments, and warming blankets help ensure that the initial redistribution of blood at induction does not drop a patient's core temperature. Care must be taken not to overheat a patient, which can lead to evaporative heat loss.

Favuzza J, Delaney CP. Outcomes of discharge after elective laparoscopic colorectal surgery with transversus abdominis plane blocks and enhanced recovery pathway. *J Am Coll Surg*. 2013;217:503-506.

Gan TJ, Thacker JK, Miller TE, et al, eds. Preoperative optimization. In: *Enhanced Recovery for Major Abdominopelvic Surgery*. Professional Communications; 2016:39-49.

Gan TJ, Thacker JK, Miller TE, et al, eds. Preoperative carbohydrate loading. In: *Enhanced Recovery for Major Abdominopelvic Surgery*. Professional Communications; 2016:53-63.

Gan TJ, Thacker JK, Miller TE, et al, eds. Intraoperative fluid management. In: *Enhanced Recovery for Major Abdominopelvic Surgery*. Professional Communications; 2016:105-109.

Guay J, Nishimori M, Kopp S. Epidural local anaesthetics versus opioid-based analgesic regimens for postoperative gastrointestinal paralysis, vomiting and pain after abdominal surgery. *Cochrane Database Syst Rev*. 2016:CD001893.

Hedrick TL, McEvoy MD, Mythen MMG, et al. American Society for Enhanced Recovery and Perioperative Quality Initiative Joint consensus statement on postoperative gastrointestinal dysfunction within an enhanced recovery pathway for elective colorectal surgery. *Anesth Analg*. 2018;126:1896-1907.

Irani JL, Hedrick TL, Miller TE, et al. Clinical practice guidelines for enhanced recovery after colon and rectal surgery from the American Society of Colon and Rectal Surgeons and the Society of American Gastrointestinal and Endoscopic Surgeons. *Surg Endosc*. 2023;37:5-30.

McEvoy MD, Scott MJ, Gordon DB, et al. American Society for Enhanced Recovery (ASER) and Perioperative Quality Initiative (POQI) joint consensus statement on optimal analgesia within an enhanced recovery pathway for colorectal surgery: part 1-from the preoperative period to PACU. *Perioper Med (Lond)*. 2017;6:8.

Ohnuma T, Krishnamoorthy V, Ellis AR, et al. Association between gabapentinoids on the day of colorectal surgery and adverse postoperative respiratory outcomes. *Ann Surg*. 2019;270:e65-e67.

Peden CJ, Aggarwal G, Aitken RJ, et al. Guidelines for perioperative care for emergency laparotomy enhanced recovery after surgery (ERAS) society recommendations: part 1-preoperative: diagnosis, rapid assessment and optimization. *World J Surg*. 2021;45:1272-1290.

Pöpping DM, Elia N, Van Aken HK, et al. Impact of epidural analgesia on mortality and morbidity after surgery: systematic review and meta-analysis of randomized controlled trials. *Ann Surg*. 2014;259:1056-1067.

Wischmeyer PE, Carli F, Evans DC, et al. American Society for Enhanced Recovery and Perioperative Quality Initiative Joint consensus statement on nutrition screening and therapy within a surgical enhanced recovery pathway. *Anesth Analg*. 2018;126:1883-1895.

B.4. Is it important to decompress the abdomen before induction of anesthesia? Why?

Yes. The most important reason for preinduction nasogastric suctioning in obstructed and distended patients is to prevent aspiration of gastric contents. These patients are high risk, particularly for postoperative ventilatory support, which dramatically increases morbidity from 5% to 80%. Therefore, it is desirable to decompress the stomach while the patient has intact upper airway reflexes. NGTs have been shown not to interfere with the function of the lower esophageal sphincter (LES) and do not reduce the efficacy of cricoid pressure (CP), but they might not be effective in removing particulate matter and all gastric contents. In fact, it has been shown that when fully decompressed, the stomach can refill by reverse peristalsis during intestinal obstruction. However, the volume of aspirate is one of the main determinants of morbidity, and nasogastric suctioning has been shown to decrease residual volume in the stomach.

Hagberg CA, Artime CA, Aziz MF, eds. Algorithms for management of the difficult airway. In: *Hagberg and Benumof's Airway Management*. 4th ed. Elsevier; 2022:229-242.

Peden CJ, Aggarwal G, Aitken RJ, et al. Guidelines for perioperative care for emergency laparotomy enhanced recovery after surgery (ERAS) society recommendations: part 1-preoperative: diagnosis, rapid assessment and optimization. *World J Surg*. 2021;45:1272-1290.

B.5. Describe the respiratory implications.

In addition to the increased risk of pulmonary aspiration, a distended abdomen can transmit pressure via the diaphragm to reduce the compliance of the respiratory system; decrease FRC and minute ventilation; and increase the work of breathing, atelectasis, shunt fraction, dead space, and airway pressures. Hypoxemia, hypercapnia, and respiratory failure can result.

Bersten AD. Respiratory monitoring. In: Bersten AD, Handy JM, eds. *Oh's Intensive Care Manual*. 8th ed. Elsevier; 2019:492-501.

Davis PJ. Wilms tumor. In: Fleisher LA, Roizen MF, Roizen J, eds. *Essence of Anesthesia Practice*. 4th ed. Elsevier; 2018:600.

B.6. What are the implications of a tense abdominal wall?

A tense abdominal wall can have significant hemodynamic implications. Increased abdominal pressure in both spontaneously and mechanically ventilated patients will increase inspiratory intrathoracic pressure and decrease venous return. High abdominal pressure will also cause vena caval compression, which decreases venous return and contributes to hypotension. Deep abdominal muscle relaxation should be targeted to optimize the surgical conditions.

Hines RL, Marschall KE, eds. Critical illness. In: *Stoelting's Anesthesia and Co-existing Disease*. 7th ed. Elsevier; 2018:53-78.

Townsend CM, Beauchamp RD, Evers BM, Mattox KL, eds. *Sabiston Textbook of Surgery: The Biological Basis of Modern Surgical Practice*. 20th ed. Elsevier; 2017:1120-1138.

B.7. Outline the methods of abdominal decompression.

A sumping NGT with a lumen for suctioning and a lumen for allowing air to be drawn into the stomach helps prevent the tube from sticking to the mucosa during suctioning. An NGT is advanced 50 to 60 cm for intragastric placement. The location of the tip of the tube should be confirmed before use. Inadvertent laryngeal placement can occur and is associated with morbidity and mortality. Imaging is the gold standard, but other reassuring signs include auscultation of the stomach while insufflating air, absence of coughing and gagging during placement, lack of resistance on placement, and commercial electromagnetic sensors. Once positioning has been confirmed, the tube must be secured (avoid the tube pressing forward on the nares causing ischemia and possibly erosion) and can then be set to gravity or suction. Tracking the output of the NGT can help demonstrate the resolution of obstruction over time.

Fleisher LA, Gaiser R, Kofke WA. Nasogastric tube placement. *ProceduresConsult*. Elsevier; 2018. Accessed October 26, 2018. https://www.clinicalkey.com/#!/content/medical_procedure/19-s2.0-mp_AN-006

Yeo CJ, ed. Diaphragmatic relaxing incisions for crural tension during hiatal hernia repair. In: *Shackelford's Surgery of the Alimentary Tract*. 8th ed. Elsevier; 2019:663-672.

B.8. Discuss the goals of fluid management.

The goals of fluid management include maintaining an effective circulating volume to support O_2 delivery and avoid organ hypoperfusion. Adverse effects of fluids, such as nonphysiologic electrolyte levels,

TABLE 15.2 Transcellular Fluid Composition

Daily Volume (L)	Daily Volume (L)	Cations				Anions		pH
Fluid		Na^+	K^+	Ca^{2+}	Mg^{2+}	Cl^-	HCO_3^-	
Gastrointestinal tract								
Saliva	1-1.5	30-90	20-40	2.5	0.6	15-35	10-40	6-7
Gastric	1.5-2.5	20-60	10-20			20-160	0	1-3.5
Bile	0.7-1.2	130-150	5-12	10-50		25-100	10-45	7-8
Pancreatic	1-1.5	125-150	5-10			30-110	40-115	8-8.3
Small bowel (concentration from proximal to distal)	1.8	140-125	5-9			110-60	100-75	7-8
Large bowel	0.2 (lost in feces)	20-40	30-90			0-15	40	7-8

Reprinted from Miller RD, Cohen NH, Eriksson LI, et al, eds. Anesthesia for cardiac surgical procedures. In: *Miller's Anesthesia*. 8th ed. Elsevier Saunders; 2015:1769. Copyright © 2015 Elsevier. With permission.

toxicities, and excessive volume administration, must be avoided. Care is taken to treat specific pathologic insults. For example, active bleeding decreases intravascular volume; gastric losses deplete Na^+, K^+, and Cl^-; small bowel losses deplete K^+, Cl^-, and HCO_3^-; and large bowel losses deplete K^+ (**Table 15.2**). Sequestered fluid has a composition similar to plasma. Inflammation results in the redistribution of fluid from the intravascular into the extracellular compartment.

Both the volume and composition of resuscitative fluids must be considered. Hypovolemia predisposes to hypotension. Hypervolemia induces the release of natriuretic peptides that degrade the endothelial glycocalyx, which can contribute to capillary leakage, decreased oncotic pressure, and tissue edema. Pulmonary edema predisposes to pulmonary infection, and edematous bowel can contribute to postoperative bowel dysfunction. Other consequences of hypervolemia include impaired healing due to decreased oxygenation and increased myocardial work due to supraoptimal ventricular filling on the Frank-Starling curve.

Administration of different fluids with varying compositions can lead to metabolic acidosis, renal dysfunction, and abnormalities in hemostasis. Clinical trials evaluating fluid administration yield differing results between healthy and critically ill patients and those with various pathologic processes. Interpatient responsiveness can also vary.

Cameron JL, Cameron AM, eds. *Current Surgical Therapy*. 14th ed. Elsevier; 2023:1502-1510.

Edwards MR, Grocott MPW. Perioperative fluid and electrolyte therapy. In: Gropper MA, Cohen NH, Eriksson LI, Fleisher LA, Leslie K, Johnson-Akeju O, eds. *Miller's Anesthesia*. 10th ed. Elsevier; 2024:1331–1373.

B.9. What would you use as a guide to fluid volume replacement?

For this patient undergoing emergency major abdominal surgery with possible sepsis and vascular compromise, reasonable choices to guide fluid volume replacement include dynamic physiologic variables such as cardiac output (CO), stroke volume variation (SVV), or pulse pressure variation (PPV) coupled with a marker of global perfusion like successive lactate levels.

Approaches to fluid therapy involving prescriptive fluid administration based on a weight-based formula and estimations of the deficit and maintenance requirements lead to increased complications when more than 3.5 to 5 L are given in the perioperative period. Current data suggest that tailoring fluid therapy to physiologic endpoints results in better outcomes. There is increasing evidence that traditional markers such as HR, BP, urine output, and central venous pressure (CVP) are nonspecific and should not be used as the sole endpoints for resuscitation. GDFT is a strategy to optimize flow-related hemodynamic variables and end-organ function by guiding the use of fluids, vasopressors, and inotropes. Numerous studies have shown that mortality can be improved by targeting CO or end-organ O_2 delivery, and patients with the highest mortality risk benefit the most. A number of minimally invasive CO monitors are available to measure physiologic variables including esophageal Doppler, arterial waveform analysis, bioimpedance and bioreactance, and a host of other increasingly less invasive devices. Recent meta-analyses evaluating all perioperative time frames and GDFT tools have demonstrated decreased morbidity and hospital length of stay. Common algorithms involve constant assessment of the chosen variable coupled with suggested hemodynamic interventions as in this sample (**Figure 15.3**). Heterogeneity in prospective studies and meta-analyses has prevented researchers from

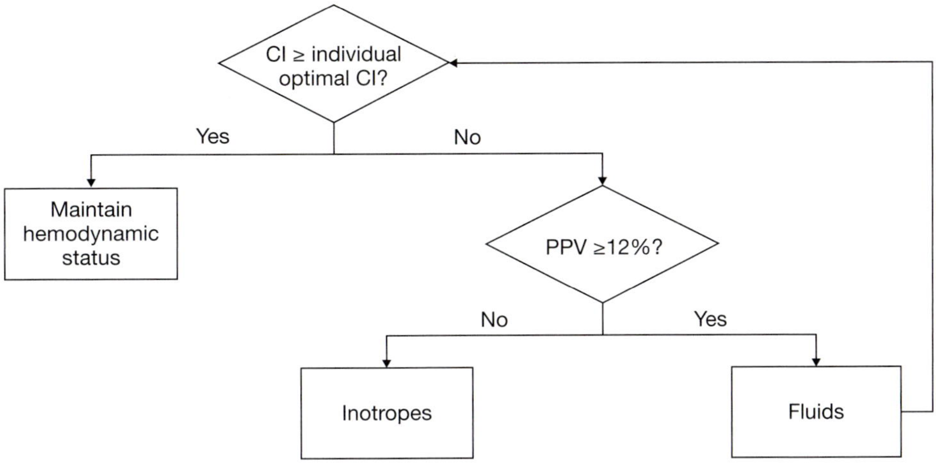

FIGURE 15.3. Sample GDFT algorithm. Intervention algorithm during mechanical ventilation. CI, cardiac index; GDFT, goal-directed fluid therapy; PPV, pulse pressure variation. (From Funcke S, Saugel B, Koch C, et al. Individualized, perioperative, hemodynamic goal-directed therapy in major abdominal surgery [iPEGASUS trial]: study protocol for a randomized controlled trial. *Trials.* 2018;19:273. http://creativecommons.org/licenses/by/4.0/. Copyright © The Author(s). 2018 Open Access.)

determining the best hemodynamic targets, monitoring tools, and interventions. However, a few key points are evident.

- Fluid therapy produces better outcomes when tailored to the patient's physiologic state.
- Dynamic- and flow-related indicators of hemodynamic status perform better than static variables.
- Timing of fluid intervention appears to affect outcomes.
- Consider early administration of vasopressors in fluid nonresponders with signs of hypoperfusion.
- As newer technology is developed, its utility in GDFT must be evaluated. New monitoring tools are valuable because they trigger intervention at critical times. The manipulation of physiologic variables is what improves outcomes, not so much the specific monitor used. This may explain why newer devices might not demonstrate a substantial benefit over existing monitors.
- Hypotension should be avoided, as even short durations (5 min) of mean arterial pressure (MAP) less than 65 mm Hg can be associated an increase risk of acute kidney injury.

Abbott TEF, Pearse RM, Archbold RA, et al. A prospective international multicentre cohort study of intraoperative heart rate and systolic blood pressure and myocardial injury after noncardiac surgery: results of the VISION study. *Anesth Analg*. 2018;126:1936-1945.

Carsetti A, Amici M, Bernacconi T, et al. Estimated oxygen extraction versus dynamic parameters of fluid-responsiveness for perioperative hemodynamic optimization of patients undergoing non-cardiac surgery: a non-inferiority randomized controlled trial. *BMC Anesthesiol.* 2020;20:87.

Edwards MR, Grocott MPW. Perioperative fluid and electrolyte therapy. In: Gropper MA, Cohen NH, Eriksson LI, Fleisher LA, Leslie K, Johnson-Akeju O, eds. *Miller's Anesthesia*. 10th ed. Elsevier; 2024:1331–1373.

Funcke S, Saugel B, Koch C, et al. Individualized, perioperative, hemodynamic goal-directed therapy in major abdominal surgery (iPEGASUS trial): study protocol for a randomized controlled trial. *Trials*. 2018;19:273.

Irani JL, Hedrick TL, Miller TE, et al. Clinical practice guidelines for enhanced recovery after colon and rectal surgery from the American Society of Colon and Rectal Surgeons and the Society of American Gastrointestinal and Endoscopic Surgeons. *Surg Endosc*. 2023;37:5-30.

Maheshwari K, Turan A, Mao G, et al. The association of hypotension during non-cardiac surgery, before and after skin incision, with postoperative acute kidney injury: a retrospective cohort analysis. *Anaesthesia*. 2018;73:1223-1228.

Pisano A, Oppizzi M, Turi S, Landoni G. Reducing major adverse cardiac events and all-cause mortality in non-cardiac surgery: perioperative strategies. In: Kaplan JA, Cronin B, Maus TM, eds. *Kaplan's Essentials of Cardiac Anesthesia for Noncardiac Surgery*. Elsevier; 2019:538-577.

C. Intraoperative Management

C.1. What dangers are present during induction? How are they planned for?

Aspiration of gastric contents and hypotension are the biggest dangers of induction. Mortality from aspiration ranges widely from 5% to 80%. Patients scheduled for emergency surgery are at high risk for aspiration, and intestinal obstruction is the most common predisposing condition in patients who do aspirate.

If the airway does not appear difficult, rapid-sequence induction and intubation (RSII) is used to shorten the time between loss of airway reflexes and placement of a cuffed endotracheal tube to minimize the chance of pulmonary aspiration. Common components of RSII are CP (controversial), administration of an IV anesthetic followed immediately by a rapid-acting neuromuscular blocker, avoidance of preinduction sedation, and foregoing (at least initially) positive pressure mask ventilation.

CP has been widely adopted in RSII, but there are no prospective randomized control data to rate its effectiveness. Different aspects of CP have been the focus of intense study and are well summarized in the literature. The 2015 Difficult Airway Society guidelines for unanticipated difficult intubation in adults recommend CP be applied, the release of CP if laryngoscopy is difficult, and reapplication in the event of vomiting. The goal is that CP prevents regurgitated contents from reaching the oropharynx. A modified RSII uses CP to prevent air from entering the stomach, allowing for gentle positive pressure ventilation during induction, which might be helpful in patients with sepsis. Patients regurgitate when barrier pressure (LES pressure – gastric pressure) is reduced below zero (**Table 15.3**). Opioids and sedatives can negatively affect barrier pressure and are avoided.

If the airway appears difficult or the patient has a history of difficult intubation, an awake intubation must be considered. The lips, tongue, and pharynx can be anesthetized, but the larynx's innervation should be kept intact in order to maintain protective reflexes.

Hemodynamics typically dictates the choice of induction agent. Propofol is the most popular induction agent. Ketamine and etomidate, however, are first-line agents when a patient is already hypotensive. Both agents produce similar intubating conditions, but even one intubating dose of etomidate has been shown to cause adrenal insufficiency in acutely ill patients. Ketamine might be the best choice for patients with sepsis.

Frerk C, Mitchell VS, McNarry AF, et al. Difficult airway society 2015 guidelines for management of unanticipated difficult intubation in adults. *Br J Anaesth*. 2015;115:827-848.

Hagberg CA, Artime CA, Aziz MF, eds. Video-assisted laryngoscopy. In: *Hagberg and Benumof's Airway Management*. 5th ed. Elsevier; 2022:242-261.

Jabre P, Combes X, Lapostolle F, et al. Etomidate versus ketamine for rapid sequence intubation in acutely ill patients: a multicentre randomised controlled trial. *Lancet*. 2009;374:293-300.

Mosier JM, Sakles JC, Law JA, Brown CA 3rd, Brindley PG. Tracheal Intubation in the critically Ill. Where we came from and where we should go. *Am J Respir Crit Care Med*. 2020;201:775-788.

Warner MA, Warner ME, Weber JG. Clinical significance of pulmonary aspiration during the perioperative period. *Anesthesiology*. 1993;78:56-62.

TABLE 15.3 Factors That Increase Intragastric Volume and Pressure

Increased gastric filling
Air insufflation during mask ventilation
Increased gastric acid production
Gastrin
Histamine-2 (H_2) receptor stimulation
Recent ethanol ingestion
Recent hypoglycemic episode
Decreased gastric emptying
Intestinal obstruction
Diabetic gastroparesis
Opioids
Anticholinergics
Sympathetic stimulation (pain and anxiety)

Reprinted from Hagberg CA, Artime CA, Aziz MF, eds. Preparation of the patient for awake intubation. In: *Hagberg and Benumof's Airway Management*. 4th ed. Elsevier; 2018:237. Copyright © 2018 Elsevier. With permission.

C.2. Does the administration of antacids and/or histamine-2 (H_2) blockers before the induction of anesthesia have a significant value in patients with small bowel obstruction?

Histamine H_2 blockers have a low value in small bowel obstruction and even less value in emergency surgery. Acidic pH is one of the main determinants of morbidity in aspiration. H_2 blockers are used in patients at high risk for aspiration to increase gastric pH by blocking the ability of histamine to induce secretion of gastric fluid with high H^+ concentration. In patients with a high GI obstruction, however, a significant amount of acidic fluid is already present. Administration of an H_2 blocker has no immediate effect on the pH of this fluid. In studies evaluating the effect of H_2 blockers, they are typically administered more than 1 hour before surgery. The largest benefit is from a multidose regimen starting the night before, making this prophylaxis less valuable before induction of an emergency case. Some benefits might be derived, however, during extubation.

Hagberg CA, Artime CA, Aziz MF, eds. Flexible scope intubation techniques. In: *Hagberg and Benumof's Airway Management*. 5th ed. Elsevier; 2022: 261-275.

Hata TM, Licina LK, Wyler DJ. Preoperative patient assessment and management. In: Cullen BF, Stock MC, Ortega R, et al, eds. *Barash, Cullen, and Stoelting's Clinical Anesthesia*. 9th ed. Wolters Kluwer; 2024:551-576.

C.3. In what position would you intubate this patient?

This patient is at high risk for aspiration, is hypotensive, and has a clinical picture of sepsis. Positioning the patient with 25° to 30° of head elevation, her head and neck in the sniffing position, and her legs up making her into a "V" shape might be most beneficial. This combination should improve upper airway patency and access, increase FRC, and reduce aspiration risk; the legs up position might help prevent hypotension on induction if her body habitus does not increase gastric pressure.

Higgs A, McGrath BA, Goddard C, et al. Guidelines for the management of tracheal intubation in critically ill adults. *Br J Anaesth*. 2018;120:323-352.

Mosier JM, Sakles JC, Law JA, Brown CA 3rd, Brindley PG. Tracheal Intubation in the critically Ill. Where we came from and where we should go. *Am J Respir Crit Care Med*. 2020;201:775-788.

C.4. What is the best neuromuscular blocking drug to use for rapid-sequence induction?

A rapid-sequence dose of rocuronium, assuming the availability of sugammadex, may be the best option for intubation. Succinylcholine had been the preferred agent, in spite of its side effects, because of its fast offset, should a difficult airway be encountered. Both produce similar intubating conditions. An emergency dose of sugammadex (16 mg/kg), however, is capable of a more rapid return of spontaneous ventilation than succinylcholine when reversed with sugammadex. However, spontaneous ventilation is not guaranteed because the hypnotic agent can still interfere with the patient's respiratory effort. Succinylcholine-induced fasciculations also increase O_2 consumption, which might be significant in the setting of a difficult airway.

Frerk C, Mitchell VS, McNarry AF, et al. Difficult airway society 2015 guidelines for management of unanticipated difficult intubation in adults. *Br J Anaesth*. 2015;115:827-848.

Hagberg CA, Artime CA, Aziz MF, eds. Airway management education. In: *Hagberg and Benumof's Airway Management*. 5th ed. Elsevier; 2022:556-567.

Higgs A, McGrath BA, Goddard C, et al. Guidelines for the management of tracheal intubation in critically ill adults. *Br J Anaesth*. 2018;120:323-352.

Mosier JM, Sakles JC, Law JA, Brown CA 3rd, Brindley PG. Tracheal intubation in the critically ill. Where we came from and where we should go. *Am J Respir Crit Care Med*. 2020;201:775-788.

C.5. Would you remove or leave the nasogastric tube (NGT) in place before inducing anesthesia?

A strong case can be made for leaving an NGT in place for induction of anesthesia and tracheal intubation of this patient. They are indicated for patients with obstruction and distended abdomens, and NGTs in place on arrival to the operating room (OR) should be used to decompress the stomach before induction. Modern guidelines recommend against routine postoperative NGTs unless there is a specific indication. The decision then becomes the timing of removal of the NGT. One can leave an NGT in place during induction to act as a release for gastric pressure during induction when paralysis reduces muscle tone; removal preinduction might induce vomiting and can be very stimulating and uncomfortable to an awake patient. Advocates for NGT removal point to decreased LES tone and obscured laryngoscopy from a foreign body in the airway. However, studies have shown that neither the presence nor size of an NGT has an effect on gastric reflux, and effective CP can be maintained with an NGT in place. If an NGT is obstructing laryngoscopy, it can always be removed. Of course, the presence of an NGT does not guarantee an empty stomach, and particulate matter is difficult to remove. Proper airway planning is always paramount.

Hagberg CA, Artime CA, Aziz MF, eds. Flexible scope intubation techniques. In: *Hagberg and Benumof's Airway Management*. 4th ed. Elsevier; 2018:235-248.

Hagberg CA, Artime CA, Aziz MF, eds. Lung isolation techniques. In: *Hagberg and Benumof's Airway Management*. 4th ed. Elsevier; 2018:235-248.

Mosier JM, Sakles JC, Law JA, Brown CA 3rd, Brindley PG. Tracheal Intubation in the critically Ill. Where we came from and where we should go. *Am J Respir Crit Care Med*. 2020;201:775-788.

Peden CJ, Aggarwal G, Aitken RJ, et al. Guidelines for perioperative care for emergency laparotomy enhanced recovery after surgery (ERAS) society recommendations: part 1-preoperative: diagnosis, rapid assessment and optimization. *World J Surg*. 2021;45:1272-1290.

C.6. Would you use nitrous oxide in this patient?

No. Nitrous oxide is relatively contraindicated in patients with an intestinal obstruction. Nitrous oxide can diffuse into gas-filled spaces more than 30 times faster than nitrogen can diffuse out. The increased gas and intraluminal pressure already present in the bowel during intestinal obstruction combined with the nitrous could cause ischemia and necrosis.

Zafirova Z, Sheehan C, Hosseinian L. Update on nitrous oxide and its use in anesthesia practice. *Best Pract Res Clin Anaesthesiol*. 2018;32:113-123.

C.7. Are there any benefits to using a high concentration of inspired oxygen (FIO_2)?

No. A high inspired concentration of O_2 does not prevent infection or healing complications after major intestinal surgery. The dose-response curve for oxidative killing of bacteria is nonlinear. In the context of wound healing, O_2 is used as a cofactor for oxidant production rather than the energy-producing oxidative phosphorylation of aerobic respiration. Rate constants for collagen synthesis, angiogenesis, and epithelialization all fall within a physiologic range that is normally achieved with an FIO_2 of 30% to 40%. Normothermia, euvolemia, and appropriate prophylactic antibiotics are important determinants of infection and wound healing outcomes.

Typically, hemoglobin and CO are considered the main determinants of O_2 delivery, which holds true in highly metabolically active tissue that is one cell away from a capillary. In subcutaneous tissue, the capillary distance is farther, O_2 consumption is lower, and the O_2 is consumed during healing and immune function. The main determinant of oxygenation in these environments is PaO_2. PaO_2 drives the diffusion of O_2, especially where microvasculature has been damaged by surgical incisions. Vasoconstriction to the subcutaneous tissue will limit the O_2 delivered and diffused. Normothermia and avoidance of hypovolemia then become pillars of wound healing and immune function.

Hyperoxia can have deleterious effects. Even breathing 28% FIO_2 for 1 hour increases reactive O_2 species (ROS) in exhaled gas, which can damage DNA and cause lung injury. Supplemental O_2 impairs mucociliary function, leading to plugging, atelectasis, and secondary infection; causes edema in large airways; and creates absorption atelectasis in healthy volunteers. There is also evidence that some specific populations can be harmed by hyperoxia, specifically patients with chronic obstructive pulmonary disease (COPD), postcardiac arrest, postmyocardial infarction (MI), stroke, and traumatic brain injury (TBI). ROS can also reduce $PaCO_2$ by acting at respiratory centers in the brainstem, which can lead to vasoconstriction and decreased delivery of O_2.

Ball J, Ranzani OT. Hyperoxia following cardiac arrest. *Intensive Care Med*. 2015;41:534-536.

Brown DI, Griendling KK. Regulation of signal transduction by reactive oxygen species in the cardiovascular system. *Circ Res*. 2015;116:531-549.

El Maleh Y, Fasquel C, Quesnel C, Garnier M. Updated meta-analysis on intraoperative inspired fraction of oxygen and the risk of surgical site infection in adults undergoing general and regional anesthesia. *Sci Rep*. 2023;13:2465.

Hopf HW, Cochran A, Ueno CM, Morrissey CK. Inflammation, wound healing, and infection. In: Cullen BF, Stock MC, Ortega R, et al, eds. *Barash, Cullen, and Stoelting's Clinical Anesthesia*. 9th ed. Wolters Kluwer; 2024:169-187.

Kurz A, Kopyeva T, Suliman I, et al. Supplemental oxygen and surgical-site infections: an alternating intervention controlled trial. *Br J Anaesth*. 2018;120:117-126.

Reiterer C, Fleischmann E, Taschner A, et al. Perioperative supplemental oxygen and oxidative stress in patients undergoing moderate- to high-risk major abdominal surgery–A subanalysis of randomized clinical trial. *J Clin Anesth*. 2022;77:110614.

van Ooij PJ, Hollmann MW, van Hulst RA, et al. Assessment of pulmonary oxygen toxicity: relevance to professional diving; a review. *Respir Physiol Neurobiol*. 2013;189:117-128.

C.8. What components of ERAS are applied in the intraoperative phase of the care of patients undergoing CRS?

Intraoperative components of ERAS pathways focus on the maintenance of euvolemia, the optimal analgesia paradigm for pain control, surgical stress response attenuation, PONV prophylaxis, optimal depth of anesthesia, and maintenance of normothermia. Both excessive and inadequate intravascular volumes are associated with poor surgical outcomes. Hypovolemia predisposes to renal injury and end-organ damage, whereas hypervolemia can lead to delayed return of gut function, decreased oxygenation, and increased myocardial work. GDFT has been shown to improve outcomes in high-risk patients and moderate-risk patients undergoing major abdominal surgery. Risk factors may include ischemic heart disease, heart failure, cerebrovascular disease, diabetes requiring insulin, and pre-op creatinine levels greater than 2.0 mg/dL. Patient and procedure risk factors may be used to help guide the use of advanced hemodynamic monitors (Figure 15.4). Patients are euvolemic at the level portion of the Frank-Starling Curve. These protocols have reduced the variability with which fluid is administered. Some recent trials have suggested that GDFT may not show improved outcomes in the context of enhanced recovery pathways. This is likely due to redundant ERAS components that restrict fluid administration while avoiding

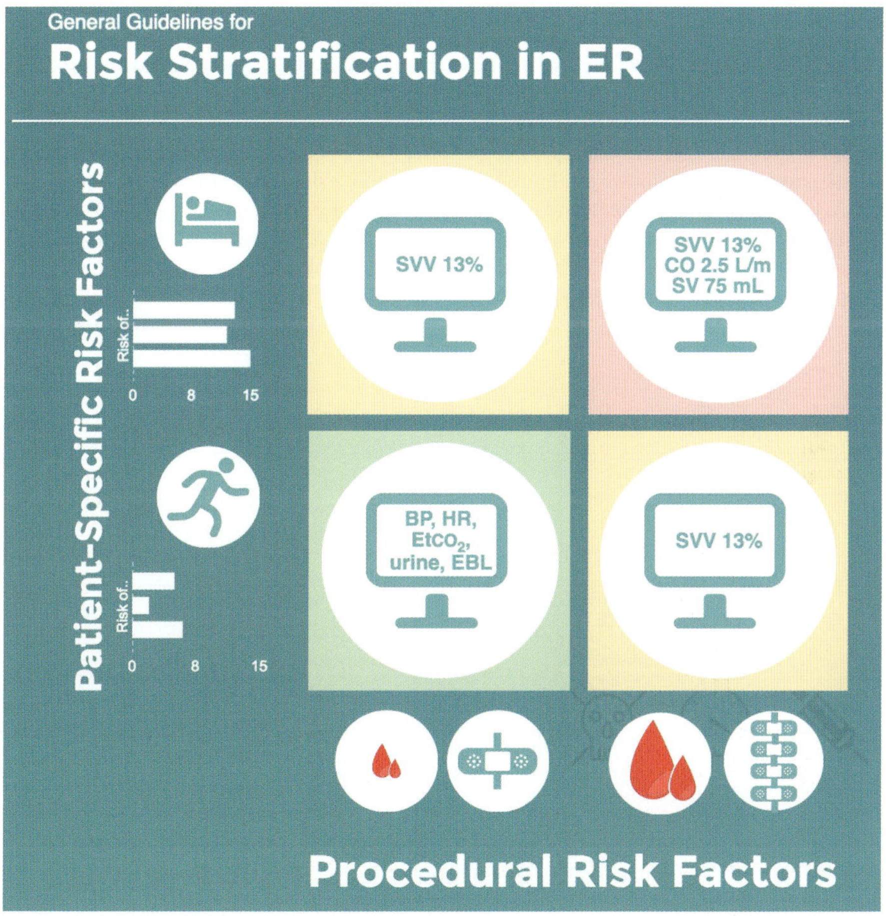

FIGURE 15.4. Perioperative quality initiative (POQI) risk stratification for monitoring in enhanced recovery protocol. Proposed risk stratification scheme for patients undergoing colorectal surgical procedures in the context of an enhanced recovery protocol. Patient-specific risk factors: poor functional status and elevated cardiac risk **(top)** and good functional status and low cardiac risk **(bottom)**. Procedural risk factors: minimally invasive and small fluid shifts **(left)** and maximally invasive and large fluid shifts **(right)**. BP, blood pressure; CO, cardiac output; EBL, estimated blood loss; $EtCo_2$, end-tidal carbon dioxide; HR, heart rate; SV, stroke volume; SVV, stroke volume variation. (From Thiele R, Raghunathan K, Brudney CS, et al. American Society for Enhanced Recovery (ASER) and Perioperative Quality Initiative (POQI) joint consensus statement on perioperative fluid management within an enhanced recovery pathway for colorectal surgery. *Perioper Med [Lond]*. 2016;5:24. https://creativecommons.org/licenses/by/4.0/. Copyright © 2016 The Author[s].)

hypovolemia within those pathways. The guiding principle of fluid therapy remains titration to dynamic physiologic endpoints rather than the application of a particular GDFT tool.

Analgesia strategies intraoperatively continue to revolve around the paradigm of optimal analgesia by balancing comfort, early functional recovery, and minimizing side effects. A number of multimodal nonopioid adjuncts are efficacious and recommended in the ASER and POQI consensus statement (**Figure 15.5**). They include NSAIDs, acetaminophen, single-shot and continuous nerve blocks, infusions of lidocaine, low-dose ketamine, and dexamethasone. The routine use of gabapentinoids is controversial, with recent evidence suggesting an increase in respiratory depression events, especially in the older adult population. The key point is that the combination of agents selected is not as important so long as they are effective. It is also important to note that ERAS programs focus on minimizing opioid use. Pain is not perceived during general anesthesia (GA), and hemodynamic consequences of surgery can be controlled with β-blockers, calcium channel blockers, and lidocaine without increased opioid consumption postoperatively.

Minimizing the harmful effects of the surgical stress response is a cornerstone of enhanced recovery. Patients experience stress if their typical homeostatic mechanisms are insufficient, and they must alter their basic physiology. For instance, during hypoglycemia, neurohumoral mediators promote gluconeogenesis and insulin resistance in order to deliver the valuable but scarce glucose to glucose-dependent end organs. Mediators of the stress response like cortisol, glucagon, catecholamines, antidiuretic hormone (ADH), and cytokines affect multiple-organ systems and can lead to undesirable surgical outcomes including myocardial ischemia, large fluid shifts, breakdown of lean muscle, poor wound healing, and impaired immune function. Some of the challenges of perioperative homeostasis and its management are listed in **Table 15.4**. Oxygenation, perfusion, fluids, and nutrition can be artificially supported in the perioperative period. ERAS pathways to minimize components of the stress response focused on these variables. The most effective interventions are the ones that directly reduce a physiologic challenge, such as a laparoscopic rather than an open surgical approach. A conceptual framework for the stress response is shown in **Figure 15.6**. Interventions shown to improve outcomes after surgery include TEA, high-dose corticosteroids, and intensive insulin therapy.

Patients in ERAS protocols are risk stratified for PONV, and prophylaxis is tailored to risk level. A simplified Apfel risk score identifies female sex, nonsmoker, history of PONV, and postoperative opioids as factors increasing the risk of PONV. Intraoperative strategies to decrease the risk of PONV include the use of regional over GA, propofol used as induction and maintenance agent, avoidance of

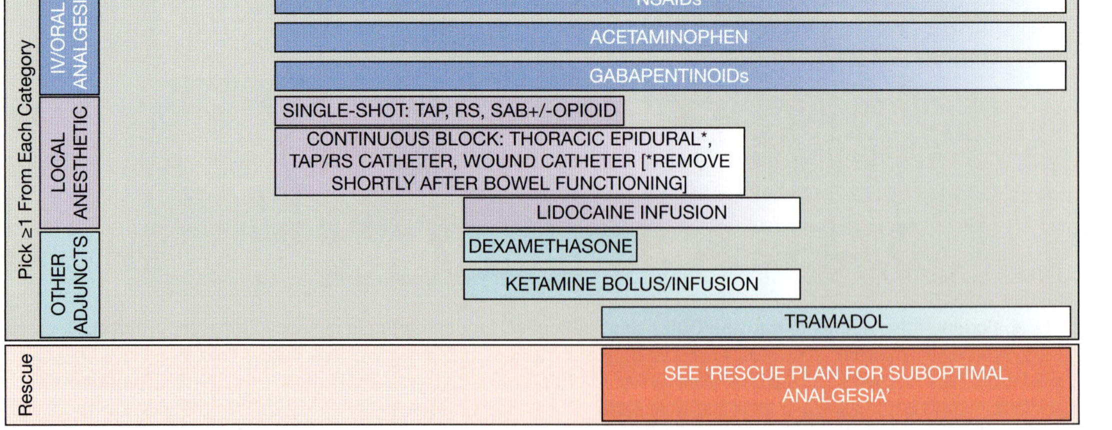

FIGURE 15.5. Treatment algorithm for achieving optimal analgesia after colorectal surgery. NSAIDs, nonsteroidal anti-inflammatory drugs; PACU, postanesthesia care unit. (From McEvoy MD, Scott MJ, Gordon DB, et al. American Society for Enhanced Recovery (ASER) and Perioperative Quality Initiative (POQI) joint consensus statement on optimal analgesia within an enhanced recovery pathway for colorectal surgery: part 1-from the preoperative period to PACU. *Perioper Med (Lond).* 2017;6:8. http://creativecommons.org/licenses/by/4.0/. Copyright © The Author(s). 2017 Open Access.)

TABLE 15.4 Physiologic Challenges to Homeostasis

Perioperative Physiologic Challenge	Management
Anxiety	Preoperative patient education
	Same-day admission
Preoperative dehydration	Adherence to modern preoperative fasting guidelines
	Avoidance of hyperosmolar oral bowel preparation
Preoperative fasting	Preoperative oral carbohydrate treatment
Preoperative transfusion	Preoperative iron infusion
Tissue injury and contamination	Minimally invasive surgical approaches
	Short incisions
	Atraumatic technique
Nociception and pain	Effective analgesia
	Regional analgesia
	Multimodal analgesia
Hypothermia	Active and passive warming
Intravenous fluid loading	Protocol-driven, balanced fluid therapy
Intra- and postoperative transfusion	Red-cell saving techniques
	Strict transfusion triggers
Postoperative fasting	Early oral diet
	Techniques to avoid or minimize ileus
Postoperative lack of physical activity	Protocol-driven postoperative mobilization

From Gan TJ, Thacker JK, Miller TE, et al. *Enhanced Recovery for Major Abdominopelvic Surgery.* 1st ed. Professional Communications, Inc.; 2016:203. With permission.

nitrous oxide and volatile anesthetics, minimal opioid administration, adequate but not excessive fluid hydration, and administration of a number of antiemetic pharmacologic agents. ERAS pathways encourage multimodal antiemetic prophylaxis, even for low-risk patients (Figure 15.7). If prophylaxis fails, a different pharmacologic class of antiemetic should be used. Dexamethasone and transdermal scopolamine need not be redosed within 24 to 48 hours. Other antiemetics, for example, 5HT-3 antagonists, readministered within 6 hours are ineffective (Table 15.5).

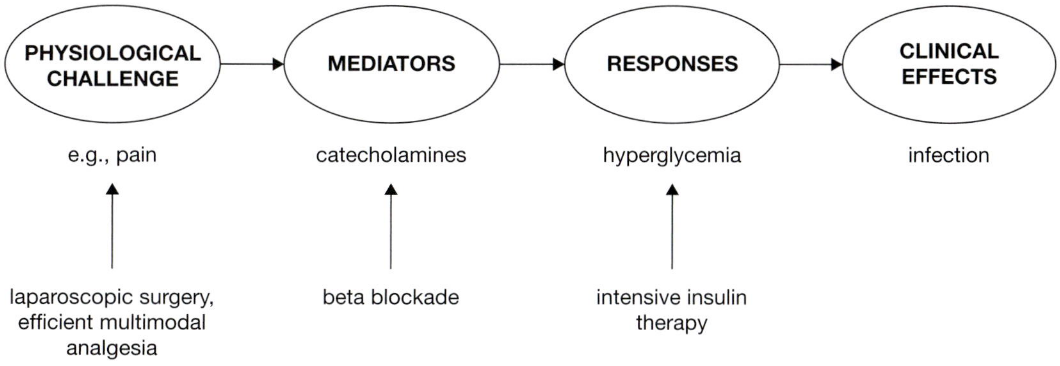

FIGURE 15.6. Conceptual framework of mechanisms of the surgical stress response. Conceptual framework of the surgical stress responses, showing potential opportunities for intervention for the example of pain, catecholamines, and hyperglycemia. Experience has shown that the most successful and feasible interventions aim to blunt the physiologic challenge in the first place (eg, nociception), rather than blunt the release of the mediators (eg, β-adrenergic receptor blockade) or the response itself (eg, hyperglycemia). Successful enhanced recovery protocols (ERPs) consist of a series of interventions that target mainly the physiologic challenges. (From Gan TJ, Thacker JK, Miller TE, et al. Enhanced recovery in colorectal surgery. In: *Enhanced Recovery for Major Abdominopelvic Surgery.* Professional Communications, Inc.; 2016:201. With permission.)

SECTION 3

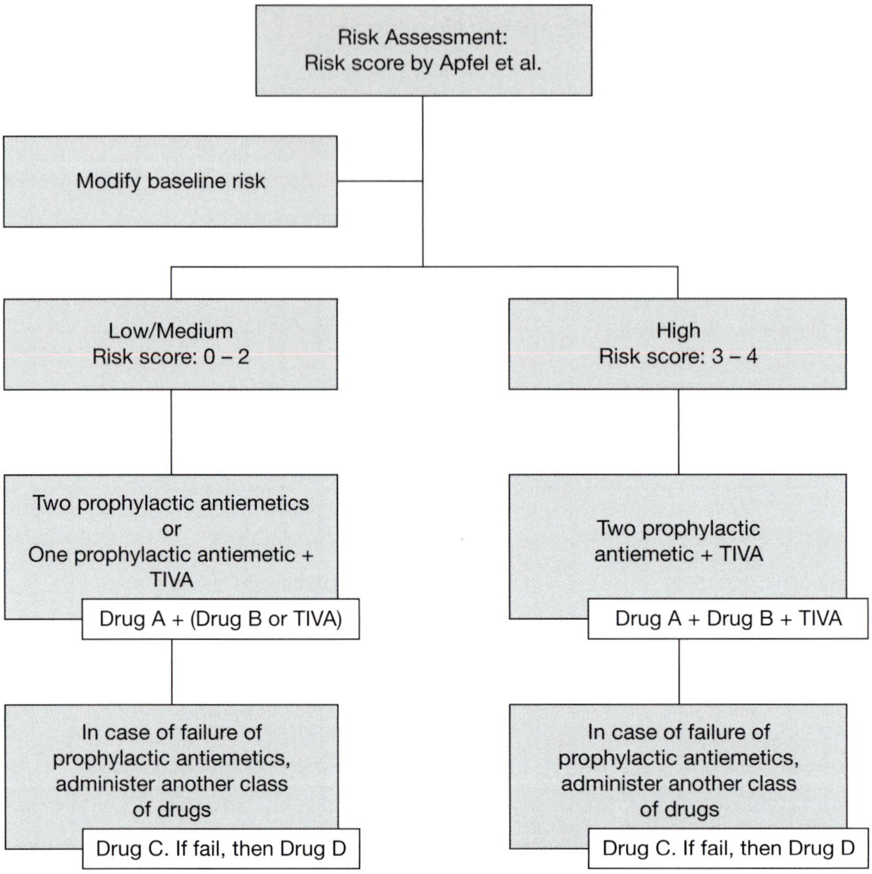

FIGURE 15.7. Flow chart for management of postoperative nausea and vomiting in the context of enhanced recovery. Example interventions: drug A = dexamethasone 4 mg in adults or 0.15 mg/kg of body weight in children; drug B = ondansetron 4 mg in adults or 0.1 mg/kg of body weight in children; drug C = promethazine 6.25 mg in adults; drug D = dimenhydrinate 1 mg/kg of body weight in adults or 0.5 to 1.0 mg/kg of body weight in children. The given drug examples are used to illustrate how the algorithm may be actually implemented but may not represent the most favorable approach. The latter may be context sensitive (children, adults, or other issues). In the event of treatment failure, timely assessment is essential and an alternate antiemetic agent should be used. A multimodal treatment approach may be appropriate to increase the likelihood of success. The Apfel Simplified Risk Score is a widely used tool for predicting the likelihood of postoperative nausea and vomiting (PONV). It assesses four independent risk factors: female gender, non-smoking status, history of PONV or motion sickness, and anticipated use of postoperative opioids. Each factor contributes one point to the score, resulting in a total score ranging from 0 to 4. The corresponding risk of experiencing PONV increases with the number of risk factors present: 0 factors: ~10% risk, 1 factor: ~20% risk, 2 factors: ~40% risk, factors: ~60% risk, and 4 factors: ~80% risk. This scoring system aids clinicians in identifying patients at higher risk for PONV, allowing for the implementation of appropriate prophylactic measures. https://pubmed.ncbi.nlm.nih.gov/33721198/; https://pmc.ncbi.nlm.nih.gov/articles/PMC10661641/TIVA, total intravenous anesthesia, that is, propofol induction and maintenance, no nitrous oxide. (From Gan TJ, Diemunsch P, Habib AS, et al. Consensus guidelines for the management of postoperative nausea and vomiting. *Anesth Analg.* 2014;118:85-113.)

Postoperative delirium and perioperative neurocognitive dysfunction (PND) impair a patient's mental and motor functions, preventing them from participating in their recovery, postponing their discharge, and increasing their risk of mortality. The pathophysiology is not yet well understood, but high-dose anesthetics, inflammation, stress response hormones, and other perioperative insults might contribute to neurologic dysfunction in the postoperative period. Inadequate anesthesia also prevents patients from gaining the neuroprotective benefits of anesthesia. In many situations, hemodynamic values alone are inadequate to reflect anesthetic depth. Methods to detect an optimal depth of anesthesia using electroencephalography (EEG), electromyography (EMG), and auditory evoked potential (AEP) monitoring have been shown to improve neurocognitive outcomes in older high-risk patients, probably by optimizing the depth of anesthesia.

Normothermia is crucial because even mild hypothermia can increase rates of infection, platelet dysfunction, and protein catabolism; decrease drug metabolism, renal function, and wound healing; and have major cardiovascular implications such as arrhythmias, left shift of hemoglobin-O_2 saturation curve, and

TABLE 15.5 Choices of Antiemetic Agents in Adults: Dosage and Timing

Drugs	Dose	Evidence	Timing	Evidence
Amisulpride	5 mg	A2	At induction	A2
Aprepitant	40 mg PO	A1	At induction	A2
Casopitant	150 mg PO	A1	At induction	
Dexamethasone	4-8 mg IV	A1	At induction	A1
Dimenhydrinate	1 mg/kg IV	A1		
Dolasetron	12.5 mg IV	A2	End of surgery; timing may not affect the efficacy.	A2
Droperidol[a]	0.625 mg IV	A1	End of surgery	A1
Ephedrine	0.5 mg/kg IM	A2		
Granisetron	0.35-3 mg IV	A1	End of surgery	A1
Haloperidol	0.5 to <2 mg IM/IV	A1		
Methylprednisolone	40 mg IV	A2		
Metoclopramide	10 mg	A1		
Ondansetron	4 mg IV 8 mg PO or ODT	A1	End of surgery	A1
Palonosetron	0.075 mg IV	A1		
Perphenazine	5 mg IV	A1		
Promethazine[a]	6.25 mg	A2		
Ramosetron	0.3 mg IV	A1	End of surgery	A2
Rolapitant	70-200 mg PO	A3	At induction	
Scopolamine	Transdermal patch	A1	Prior evening or 2 h before surgery	A1
Tropisetron	2 mg IV	A1	End of surgery	

Category A: Supportive literature.
Randomized controlled trials report statistically significant differences between clinical interventions for a specified clinical outcome.
Level 1: The literature contains multiple randomized controlled trials, and aggregated findings are supported by meta-analysis.
Level 2: The literature contains multiple randomized controlled trials, but the number of studies is insufficient to conduct a viable meta-analysis for the purpose of these guidelines.
Level 3: The literature contains a single randomized controlled trial.
These recommendations are evidence based, and not all the drugs have a US Food and Drug Administration (FDA) indication for postoperative nausea and vomiting (PONV). Drugs are listed alphabetically.
IM, intramuscular; IV, intravenous; ODT, orally disintegrating tablet; PO, per os.
[a]See FDA black box warning.
Reprinted with permission from Gan TJ, Belani KG, Bergese S, et al. Fourth consensus guidelines for the management of postoperative nausea and vomiting. *Anesth Analg* 2020;131:411-448.

increased peripheral vascular resistance. Core temperature monitoring is recommended in all patients undergoing anesthesia. Interventions recommended for maintaining normothermia include warming the periphery prior to surgery to avoid the initial drop in core temperature on induction, maintaining an OR temperature above 21 °C and possibly even at 26 °C until the prep solution is dry and the patient is draped, limiting areas of exposed skin, fluid warmers for boluses above 500 mL, heated and humidified gases, and forced air warmers over the largest available surface area.

Cameron JL, Cameron AM, eds. *Current Surgical Therapy*. 14th ed. Elsevier; 2023:303-314.

Gan TJ, Diemunsch P, Habib AS, et al. Consensus guidelines for the management of postoperative nausea and vomiting. *Anesth Analg*. 2014;118:85-113.

Gan TJ, Thacker JK, Miller TE, et al. Postoperative gastrointestinal care. In: *Enhanced Recovery for Major Abdominopelvic Surgery*. Professional Communications; 2016:133-146.

Gan TJ, Thacker JK, Miller TE, et al. Postoperative mobilization. In: *Enhanced Recovery for Major Abdominopelvic Surgery*. Professional Communications; 2016:165-186.

Gan TJ, Thacker JK, Miller TE, et al. Enhanced recovery in colorectal surgery. In: *Enhanced Recovery for Major Abdominopelvic Surgery*. Professional Communications; 2016:190-212.

Gan TJ, Thacker JK, Miller TE, et al. Appendix—sample order sets. In: *Enhanced Recovery for Major Abdominopelvic Surgery*. Professional Communications; 2016:360.

SECTION 3

Apfel CC, Laara E, Koivuranta M, Greim CA, Roewer N. A simplified risk score for predicting postoperative nausea and vomiting: conclusions from cross-validations between two centers. *Anesthesiology*. 1999;91:693-700.

Edwards MR, Grocott MPW. Perioperative fluid and electrolyte therapy. In: Gropper MA, Cohen NH, Eriksson LI, Fleisher LA, Leslie K, Johnson-Akeju O, eds. *Miller's Anesthesia*. 10th ed. Elsevier; 2024:1331–1373.

Hedrick TL, McEvoy MD, Mythen MMG, et al. American Society for Enhanced Recovery and Perioperative Quality Initiative joint consensus statement on postoperative gastrointestinal dysfunction within an enhanced recovery pathway for elective colorectal surgery. *Anesth Analg*. 2018;126:1896-1907.

McEvoy MD, Scott MJ, Gordon DB, et al. American Society for Enhanced Recovery (ASER) and Perioperative Quality Initiative (POQI) joint consensus statement on optimal analgesia within an enhanced recovery pathway for colorectal surgery: part 1-from the preoperative period to PACU. *Perioper Med (Lond)*. 2017;6:8.

Ohnuma T, Krishnamoorthy V, Ellis AR, et al. Association between gabapentinoids on the day of colorectal surgery and adverse postoperative respiratory outcomes. *Ann Surg*. 2019;270:e65-e67.

Punjasawadwong Y, Chau-In W, Laopaiboon M, et al. Processed electroencephalogram and evoked potential techniques for amelioration of postoperative delirium and cognitive dysfunction following non-cardiac and non-neurosurgical procedures in adults. *Cochrane Database Syst Rev*. 2018:CD011283.

Srinivasa S, Kahokehr AA, Yu TC, et al. Preoperative glucocorticoid use in major abdominal surgery: systematic review and meta-analysis of randomized trials. *Ann Surg*. 2011;254:183-191.

van den Berghe G, Wouters P, Weekers F, et al. Intensive insulin therapy in critically ill patients. *N Engl J Med*. 2001;345:1359-1367.

Wischmeyer PE, Carli F, Evans DC, et al. American Society for Enhanced Recovery and Perioperative Quality Initiative joint consensus statement on nutrition screening and therapy within a surgical enhanced recovery pathway. *Anesth Analg*. 2018;126:1883-1895.

C.9. What are the strengths, weaknesses, benefits, and challenges of ERAS?

Strengths

ERAS uses evidence-based interventions that are customized to the patient and the resources of the institution. Protocols reduce the variability in care and outcomes, which help to continually evaluate and improve the pathway. Multidisciplinary care allows each member of the team to focus on what they do best.

Weakness

Individual interventions included in ERAS pathways show benefits in a general population but may be redundant with other components. Attributing a benefit to a specific intervention is difficult, and only the bundled program can be credited. Also, many benefits come from suppressing the surgical stress response in elective major abdominal surgeries and older patients with comorbid disease. Cardiovascular, pulmonary, and infectious complications show improvement. Advantages are not as clear-cut in surgical complications. Therefore, ERAS might not offer a marked improvement in the uncomplicated laparoscopic procedure in an otherwise healthy young patient.

Benefits

ERAS programs consistently demonstrate accelerated recovery, reduced complication rate, reduced length of stay, reduced readmission rate, increased value by improving quality while decreasing cost, and improved patient satisfaction.

Challenges

The biggest challenges in ERAS come in implementation and maintenance. Input and consensus from members of surgery, anesthesia, nursing, and a host of other services can be difficult on an organizational level. Additional resources, such as a program coordinator or patient education materials, order sets, and data tracking systems, can be extremely useful but take time to develop and implement. Sustaining improvements can also be challenging. Outcomes can initially improve but later decline, and the reason is not always clear. Documentation might not accurately reflect clinical activities, new staff might not be oriented to the pathway, or experienced providers might not realize how their contributions affect downstream portions of care. Mechanisms for regularly scheduled auditing and frequent opportunities for education have to be devised for sustained improvement.

Current ERAS protocols can be optimized by further clinical investigation. Optimization of perioperative pain management should include improved study designs to be procedure and patient specific. Additional clinical trials are needed to determine the role of goal-directed fluid and hemodynamic therapy in high-risk versus low-risk patients. The choice of fluid, for example, the use of crystalloid versus colloid, and the use of vasopressors and inotropes should be studied. Orthostatic intolerance represents a specific stress response to major surgical trauma, and additional research should focus on clarifying the mechanisms and preventive interventions, as early postoperative mobilization is an important part of ERAS protocol.

Cameron JL, Cameron AM, eds. *Current Surgical Therapy*. 12th ed. Elsevier; 2017:325-334.

Kehlet H. Enhanced postoperative recovery: good from afar, but far from good? *Anaesthesia*. 2020;75(Suppl 1):e54-e61.

Kehlet H. Postoperative recovery: DrEaMing as a wake-up call? *Br J Anaesth*. 2022;129:1-3.

Ljungqvist O, Hubner M. Enhanced recovery after surgery-ERAS-principles, practice and feasibility in the elderly. *Aging Clin Exp Res*. 2018;30:249-252.

Orringer MB, Chang A. Gastric adenocarcinoma. In: Cameron JL, Cameron AM, eds. *Current Surgical Therapy*. 12th ed. Elsevier; 2017:325-334.

C.10. What are the indications for ERAS?

Any patient may benefit from ERAS pathway elements implemented at their institution, provided they do not have a contraindication to any of the components (eg, anaphylactic acetaminophen allergy, antiplatelet therapy that cannot be interrupted for neuraxial analgesia). Larger, more invasive cases, patients with more comorbidities, and more prolonged length of hospital stay may see the biggest benefit.

Bloomstone J. Overcoming challenges—anesthesiologists. In: Gan TJ, Thacker JK, Miller TE, Scott MJ, Holubar SD, eds. *Enhanced Recovery for Major Abdominopelvic Surgery*. 1st ed. Professional Communications; 2016.

SECTION 3

D. Postoperative Management

D.1. What are the principles of postoperative care in this patient?

The ultimate goal of postoperative care is the recovery of bowel function to the point where the patient can resume oral hydration and take in sufficient nutrition on their own. Many principles of postoperative care are the same as preoperative concerns including maintenance of euvolemia, correction of electrolyte and acid-base imbalances, nutritional support, avoiding bowel distension, and pain management. There are additional considerations of anastomotic leak, perforation, infection, bleeding, thrombosis, and wound complications that need to be guarded against.

Tissue injury and inflammation continue after surgery, which present a challenge to maintaining euvolemia. Increased endothelial permeability and damage to the glycocalyx are a result of systemic inflammation. Fluids are frequently required postoperatively. However, hypervolemia can cause the release of cardiac natriuretic peptides, which degrade the glycocalyx. Water and electrolytes are lost to the interstitium, which compromises gut perfusion. When the systemic inflammatory response decreases, fluids mobilize back into the intravascular space and fluid administration must be decreased. Urine output is a poor indicator of volume status, as sympathetic stimulation and increases in the renin-angiotensin-aldosterone system cause fluid retention despite the adequate intravascular volume.

Bowel function must be monitored postoperatively, and physiologic POI must be differentiated from pathologic ileus. In general, gastric and small intestinal mobility occurs within hours of surgery and colonic activity returns within 72 hours. Sections of the bowel that were directly manipulated will take longer to recover and extend to areas not directly manipulated. If the ileus is prolonged, metabolic derangements like hypokalemia, hyponatremia, and uremia can occur; iatrogenic medications, ischemia, hemorrhage, and sepsis should all be considered as contributing factors. Laparoscopic surgery can be associated with hernias, and an obstructive point seen on imaging should prompt surgical reintervention.

Edwards MR, Grocott MPW. Perioperative fluid and electrolyte therapy. In: Gropper MA, Cohen NH, Eriksson LI, Fleisher LA, Leslie K, Johnson-Akeju O, eds. *Miller's Anesthesia*. 10th ed. Elsevier; 2024:1331–1373.

Irani JL, Hedrick TL, Miller TE, et al. Clinical practice guidelines for enhanced recovery after colon and rectal surgery from the American Society of Colon and Rectal Surgeons and the Society of American Gastrointestinal and Endoscopic Surgeons. *Surg Endosc*. 2023;37:5-30.

Townsend CM Jr, Beauchamp RD, Evers BM, Mattox KL, eds. Urologic surgery. In: *Sabiston Textbook of Surgery: The Biological Basis of Modern Surgical Practice*. 20th ed. Elsevier; 2017:1320-1400.

D.2. Are there any postoperative respiratory problems associated with factors other than aspiration?

Yes. Respiratory challenges exist in the immediate postoperative period as well as during the inpatient recovery phase. As with all general anesthetics, there is a decreased respiratory drive, increased airway resistance, and neuromuscular impairment caused by residual anesthetics. Immediately after surgery, the bowel can be edematous, which increases the diaphragmatic work of breathing and shunt while decreasing FRC. As recovery continues, if fluids are not carefully managed, pulmonary edema can impair gas exchange and further increase the work of breathing. Carbon dioxide production can increase beyond ventilatory capacity in the face of parenteral nutrition and infection.

Fowler MA, Howell KA. Postanesthesia recovery. In: Cullen BF, Stock MC, Ortega R, et al, eds. *Barash, Cullen, and Stoelting's Clinical Anesthesia*. 9th ed. Wolters Kluwer; 2024:1455-1478.

D.3. If the patient aspirates gastric contents, what are the possible sequelae? What is the treatment?

Aspiration of gastric contents causes a chemical pneumonitis initially characterized by hypoxemia, bronchospasm, and atelectasis. Morbidity is increased with larger volumes of aspirate and/or a low pH aspirate. Particulate matter can also be more damaging because it can obstruct the airway, cause distal atelectasis, and act as a nidus for infection, resulting in a superimposed pneumonia. If pneumocytes are injured and the surfactant is washed away, the clinical picture can resemble acute respiratory distress syndrome (ARDS) (**Table 15.6**). Pulmonary edema, decreased pulmonary compliance, increased pulmonary vascular resistance, and $\dot{V}/\dot{Q}$ mismatching are seen in severe cases. Radiographic evidence might not develop until 6 to 12 hours after the event.

If a patient begins to vomit, their head should be placed in a lateral position with the head down if possible. Treatment is similar to ARDS, mainly supportive with supplemental O_2. Intubation frequently has to be continued with mechanical ventilation and positive end-expiratory pressure (PEEP) to keep O_2 levels acceptable. If the particulate matter was aspirated, lavage or bronchoscopy can be considered, but neither will be helpful if the aspirate was purely an acidic fluid because it is quickly distributed, diluted, and neutralized. If bronchospasm is present, pharmacologic bronchodilation is indicated. A superimposed infection does not always occur, and no evidence exists to support prophylactic antibiotics. If an infection does occur, treatment should start with broad-spectrum antibiotics covering gram-negative rods and anaerobes including *Bacteroides fragilis,* and then narrowed to the appropriate antibiotics based on culture sensitivities. Steroids do not improve the clinical picture and may increase the incidence of bacterial infection. Pulmonary edema should not be treated with diuretics unless high filling pressures or hypervolemia exist.

Fowler MA, Howell KA. Postanesthesia recovery. In: Cullen BF, Stock MC, Ortega R, et al, eds. *Barash, Cullen, and Stoelting's Clinical Anesthesia*. 9th ed. Wolters Kluwer; 2024:1455-1478.

Hagberg CA, Artime CA, Aziz MF. Human factors in airway management. In: Hagberg CA, Artime CA, Aziz MF, eds. *Hagberg and Benumof's Airway Management*. 5th ed. Elsevier; 2022:242-261.

Hines RL, Marschall KE, eds. Obstructive respiratory diseases. In: *Stoelting's Anesthesia and Co-existing Disease*. 7th ed. Elsevier; 2018:33-52.

D.4. What is gram-negative sepsis? Describe the clinical picture and treatment.

Sepsis is a clinical syndrome resulting from a dysregulated inflammatory response to infection. This response is aimed at eliminating a threat through the generation of noxious O_2 metabolites and cytokines. When inflammation is systemic and long lasting, it can cause end-organ damage that may trigger further inflammation, leading to a destructive positive feedback loop. Gram-negative sepsis causes the inflammatory response to certain highly conserved microbial molecules such as the lipid A moiety of lipopolysaccharides (LPSs, also called endotoxin). About 20% to 50% of patients can progress to hypotension and shock.

Early signs of gram-negative sepsis include an abrupt onset of fever and chills, hyperventilation with respiratory alkalosis, and mental status changes. Neutropenia with increased immature polymorphonuclear leukocytes is the most common lab abnormality. Thrombocytopenia and coagulation abnormalities can also be present.

As the condition progresses to septic shock, vascular endothelial damage from NO causes systemic vasodilation and fluid extravasation, leading to a relative hypovolemia. Early shock is characterized by an increased CO, decreased systemic vascular resistance (SVR), hypotension, and warm extremities (warm

TABLE 15.6 Pathophysiology of Aspiration

Particulate aspiration → Airway obstruction →
Granulomatous inflammation → Acid aspiration →
Neutrophilic inflammation → Hemorrhagic pulmonary edema →
Destruction of airway epithelium → Loss of type 1 alveolar cells →
Loss of surfactant → Alveolar instability and collapse →
Disruption of alveolar-capillary membrane → Plasma leakage from pulmonary capillaries →
Noncardiogenic pulmonary edema → Hypovolemia

Reprinted from Hagberg CA, Artime CA, Aziz MF, eds. Preparation of the patient for awake intubation. In: *Hagberg and Benumof's Airway Management*. 4th ed. Elsevier; 2018:238.

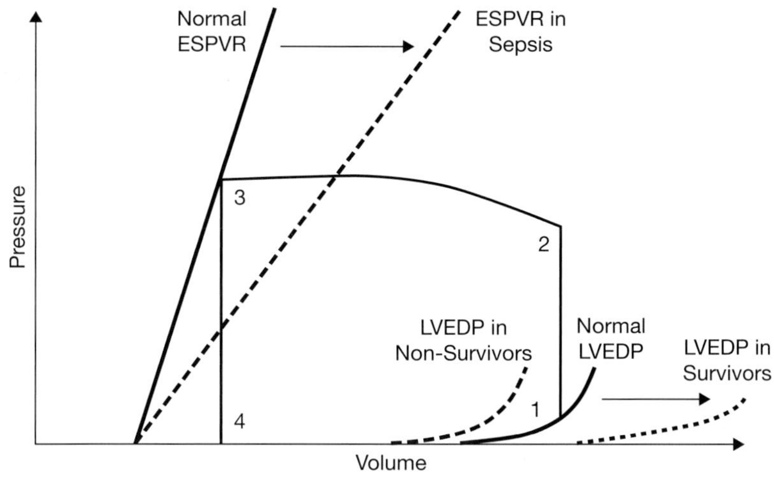

FIGURE 15.8. Myocardial dysfunction in sepsis. Left ventricular pressure-volume relationships. The *bold straight line* shows the normal end-systolic pressure-volume relationship (ESPVR), defining ventricular contraction. ESPVR is independent of changes in preload and afterload. The slope is maximal at end systole and has the units of elastance, $E = \Delta P/\Delta V$. It has therefore been designated E_{max}. The *bold curved line* shows normal end-diastolic pressure-volume relationship (EDPVR). The straight section of the line represents the addition of the initial volume. Whereas ventricular volume increases from 0 to approximately 50 mL, transmural pressure remains at 0. Left ventricular end-diastolic pressure (LVEDP) then increases in a curvilinear manner during the addition of further volume. The pressure-volume loop (1-4) represents one cardiac cycle (1-2, isovolumetric contraction; 2-3, stroke volume; 3-4, isovolumetric relaxation). The interrupted *straight line* represents E_{max} in sepsis, with depressed contractility indicated by a downward and right shift of the ESPVR. In survivors of septic shock, this is accompanied by a right shift of the EDPVR (*interrupted curved line*) caused by ventricular dilatation, enabling an increase in stroke volume. In nonsurvivors, diastolic stiffness develops, represented by an upward and left shift of the EDPVR (*bold, interrupted curved line*), leading to impaired diastolic filling and a reduction in stroke volume. *Arrows* represent possible contribution of nitric oxide (NO) to the pressure-volume relationships in sepsis. Although NO may be responsible for the reduction in systolic contractility, the patient with sepsis is able to maintain end-systolic volume because of a reduction in SVR; therefore, the overriding hemodynamic effect of NO in sepsis may facilitate ventricular dilatation, which acts to further stroke volume and maintain CO. Potentially, NO blockade in sepsis may convert the EDPVR of a surviving patient with sepsis to a nonsurvivor. (Reproduced from Belcher E, Mitchell J, Evans T. Myocardial dysfunction in sepsis: no role for NO? *Heart.* 2002;87:508; with permission from BMJ Publishing Group Ltd.)

phase). If the relative hypovolemia persists without adequate resuscitation, the resulting "cold phase" is characterized by an increased SVR and a low CO because blood flow is directed back to vital organs, and ultimately death. Both phases experience myocardial dysfunction due to circulating cytokines as evidenced by the left ventricular end-systolic pressure-volume relationship (**Figure 15.8**). Patients who survived were given fluid and were then able to maintain an adequate stroke volume through ventricular dilation without increases in pressure via the Frank-Starling mechanism. Nonsurvivors instead developed a diastolic dysfunction and were unable to maintain an adequate cardiac index. Fluid extravasation also leads to pulmonary edema, and as many as 40% of patients may progress to ARDS. Adrenal insufficiency, disseminated intravascular coagulation, and immunosuppression are also recognized complications of sepsis.

Treatment guidelines are summarized in the "Surviving Sepsis" campaign bundles. Mechanical ventilation with lung protective strategies, such as tidal volumes less than 6 mL/kg predicted body weight and plateau pressures less than 30 cm H_2O, are frequently required because acute lung injury is the most common complication. Circulatory support should be given in the form of an initial fluid bolus and then vasopressors. First line is usually norepinephrine, and if a goal of mean arterial pressure (MAP) greater than 65 mm Hg is not met, second- and third-line agents, usually vasopressin and epinephrine, can be added. Angiotensin II receptor agonists have also recently shown promise in the treatment of catecholamine-resistant shock with a mechanism different from norepinephrine and vasopressin. Tissue oxygenation is not impaired in septic shock. The ability of mitochondria to use O_2 becomes impaired by bacterial endotoxins and results in lactate production. Therefore, efforts to improve tissue oxygenation with transfusions are not indicated. Broad-spectrum antibiotics should be administered within 1 hour of identifying a patient in septic shock and then be narrowed and targeted as soon as culture results are available. Corticosteroid administration has been controversial, but current guidelines recommend it be used in patients poorly responsive to vasopressors.

Belcher E, Mitchell J, Evans T. Myocardial dysfunction in sepsis: no role for NO? *Heart.* 2002;87:507-509.

Jameson JL, Fauci AS, Kasper DL, et al, eds. *Harrison's Principles of Internal Medicine.* 20th ed. McGraw-Hill; 2018.

Khanna A, English SW, Wang XS, et al. Angiotensin II for the treatment of vasodilatory shock. *N Engl J Med.* 2017;377:419-430.

Marino PL, ed. Inflammatory shock syndromes. In: *Marino's The ICU Book.* 5th ed. Wolters Kluwer; 2025:271-287.

Papadakis MA, McPhee SJ, Rabow MW, McQuaid KR, eds. Mycobacterial infections. In: *Current Medical Diagnosis & Treatment* 2023. 62nd ed. McGraw Hill; 2023:1448-1492.

Rhodes A, Evans LE, Alhazzani W, et al. Surviving sepsis campaign: international guidelines for management of sepsis and septic shock: 2016. *Crit Care Med.* 2017;45:486-552.

D.5. What components of ERAS are applied in the postoperative phase of the care of patients following CRS?

Postoperative components of ERAS include early oral feeding, ileus prevention, restrictive use of NGTs/lines/drains, early mobilization, and optimal analgesia. These components were developed for elective procedures, but many of the concepts may still be applied to urgent/emergent procedures.

Traditional dogma of postoperative care restricted oral intake in order to protect patients from aspiration, anastomotic leak, and wound dehiscence. Contemporary practice shows early postoperative nutrition is associated with reductions in mortality, complications, anastomotic dehiscence, hyperglycemia, length of stay, and time to return of bowel function. The benefits of parenteral and enteral feeding have been well described in the literature, but oral feeding is the only form of nutritional intake that elicits all of the gut's stimulating reflexes and most closely aligns with the theme of functional recovery. Early oral nutrition in an ERAS pathway has also been shown to decrease complications and hospital length of stay even if the duration of ileus was not reduced significantly. We also now know that the presence of fluid and some semidigested material in the gut does not threaten fresh anastomoses any more than natural content such as enzymes, bile juice, and stomach acids. Oral feeding is tolerated within 24 hours by 80% to 90% of CRS patients and is an inexpensive intervention not shown to be associated with adverse events. Oral intake has to be adapted to individual tolerance, surgery, and risk factors, but general recommendations for postoperative care of uncomplicated cases include encouraging drinking as soon as they are fully awake, resumption of normal diet when tolerating fluids, nutritional supplement beverages, glucose monitoring and treatment, and gum chewing.

Ileus, as described in the pathophysiology section earlier, refers to abnormal GI motility. POI is a significant challenge in ERAS pathways because it is a major factor in determining hospital length of stay, inhibits functional recovery, and causes discomfort to patients. We do not know the exact causes of ileus because it represents complex interactions between a number of processes (**Figure 15.9**), but treatment involves managing inflammation, autonomic dysfunction and the stress response to surgery, intestinal opioid receptors, GI hormones, electrolyte imbalances, and impaired gut contractility. Many of the recommendations to limit POI are interventions already suggested for other indications but include minimal preoperative fasting; preoperative optimization including correction of electrolyte abnormalities and anemia; minimizing insulin resistance with a carbohydrate drink 2 hours before surgery and treatment of abnormal glucose levels; minimizing fluid shifts due to iso-osmolar bowel prep by only doing it when indicated; standardized protocols for fluid management; and multimodal pain management with a thoracic epidural for open cases, minimizing systemic opioid use, and use of alvimopan when postoperative opioids are used. Other interventions that have limited evidence of decreased POI and are not yet included in consensus statements include nicotine gum chewing, magnesium, coffee, Dai-Kenchu-To (DKT), and polyunsaturated fats.

NGTs traditionally were maintained into the postoperative period until evidence of bowel function returned. The goal was to avoid an early gastric challenge and protect anastomoses by preventing distension. This practice was not evidence based. We now have good evidence that selective versus routine use of NGTs is associated with a decreased incidence of ileus, a shorter duration of ileus when it does occur, fewer fevers, less atelectasis, and decreased incidence of pneumonia. We also know that tubes and drains are an obstacle to independent ambulation, are uncomfortable, and do not provide a benefit with regard to leaks or infections. Similarly, several reviews and meta-analyses now tell us that routine abdominal drains do not help detect leaks. Urinary catheters prevent ambulation and are not necessary to quantitate urine output. Reasonable policies in an ERAS pathway for colon surgery recommend against the routine continuation of NGTs, drains, and urinary catheters postoperatively. This recommendation refers to routine uncomplicated colon surgeries. Individual patients may have indications not present in a routine case. For instance, patients that received GA with epidural analgesia can be at increased risk for urinary retention, and the catheter can be removed on postoperative day (POD) 1. Some hepatic and pancreatic procedures require the use of early postoperative abdominal drains.

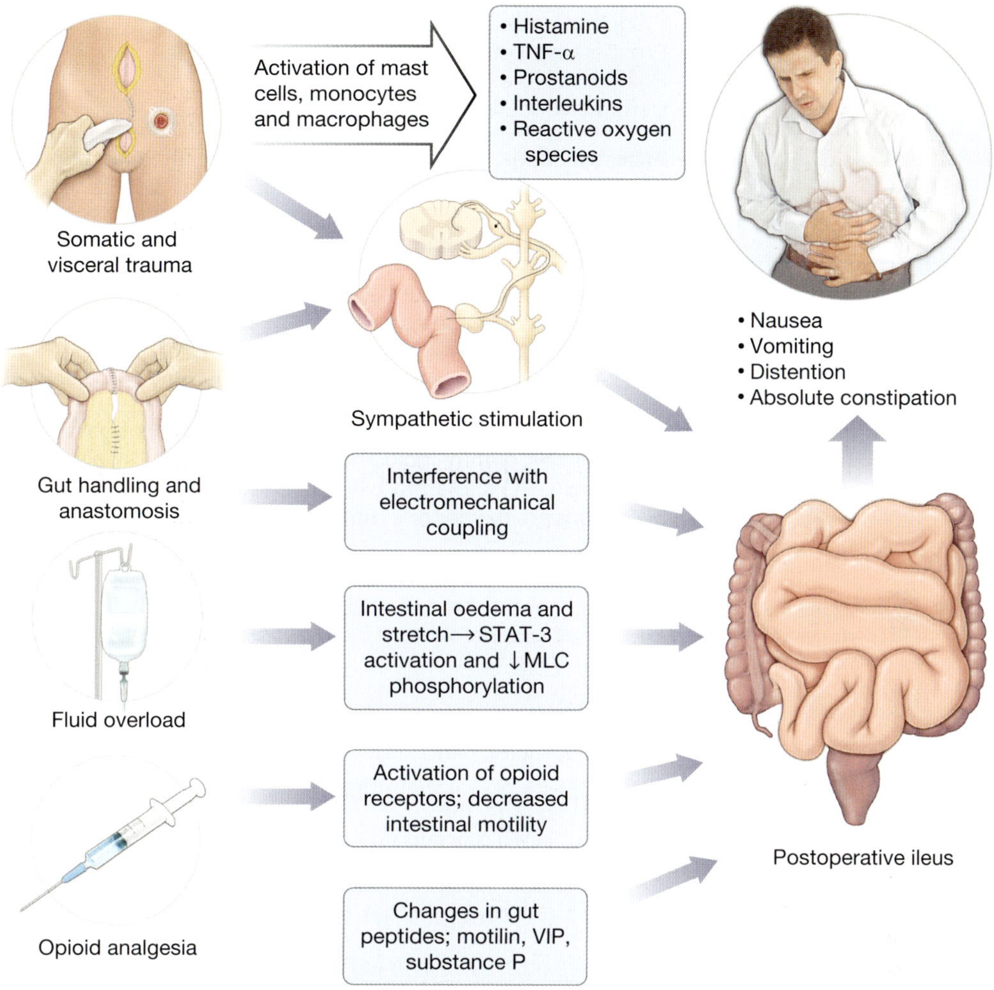

FIGURE 15.9. Schematic diagram showing proposed mechanisms for the pathogenesis of postoperative ileus. MLC, myosin light chain; STAT, signal transducer and activator of transcription; TNF, tumor necrosis factor; VIP, vasoactive intestinal polypeptide. (Reprinted from Bragg D, El-Sharkawy AM, Psaltis E, et al. Postoperative ileus: recent developments in pathophysiology and management. *Clin Nutr.* 2015;34:367-376. Copyright © 2015 Elsevier. With permission.)

Early mobilization best exemplifies functional recovery in ERAS. Lack of physical activity suppresses cardiopulmonary and musculoskeletal systems after a short period of time. Early mobility is also correlated with a decreased incidence of atelectasis, pneumonia, thromboembolism, delirium, hospital length of stay, and an increase in muscle strength and tissue oxygenation. The amount of mobilization for each patient needs to be individualized, and the extent of mobility required to see a beneficial effect is unclear. Studies that have shown benefit have had the goals of 15 minutes of mobilization on the day of surgery and 3 hours on POD 1.

Postoperative optimal analgesia involves many of the same principles as other phases of the pathway, including multimodal analgesia and minimizing opioid use. TEA is recommended for open abdominal surgery, and ideally, the infusion is started before the procedure. Laparoscopic surgery is typically associated with a shorter duration of postoperative pain; routine TEA is not recommended. However, comorbid pulmonary disease or chronic opioid therapy with tolerance can be indications for TEA in laparoscopic surgery. If TEA is not used, paravertebral blocks, peripheral catheters, and TAP blocks can be helpful. IV lidocaine infusion administered in the postanesthesia care unit (PACU) (or upon removal of catheter for patients receiving TEA) can lower opioid consumption, reduce nausea and vomiting, and decrease time to resumption of diet. Acetaminophen and NSAIDs are the mainstay of postoperative pain

STEP 1	Perform Focused H&P	- Preoperative analgesia use - Preoperative pain baseline - Postoperative exam - Determine location & etiology of pain
STEP 2	Assess Pain SEVERITY	- Assess location, severity, duration, & aggravating factors - Limitations due to pain? (i.e., drinking, eating, mobilizing, sleeping) - Any adverse drug events due to current pain regimen?
STEP 3	Determine Pain TYPE	- Determine the pain type: neuropathic, inflammatory, visceral, or somatic in nature? - Consider the combination of multiple pain generators (EXCLUDE surgical/medical complications prior to treating)
STEP 4	Administer Rescue TREATMENT	- Confirm use of all appropriate non-opioid options from Treatment Algorithm, including tramadol.* - Add opioid. PO if tolerated, IV if needed (e.g., hydrocodone, oxycodone, morphine, hydromorphone)

*Table 4: Treatment Algorithm for Achieving Optimal Analgesia After Colorectal Surgery

FIGURE 15.10. Rescue plan for suboptimal analgesia. (From Scott MJ, McEvoy MD, Gordon DB, et al. American Society for Enhanced Recovery [ASER] and Perioperative Quality Initiative [POQI] joint consensus statement on optimal analgesia within an enhanced recovery pathway for colorectal surgery: part 2-from PACU to the transition home. *Perioper Med [Lond].* 2017;6:7. http://creativecommons.org/licenses/by/4.0/. Copyright © The Author[s]. 2017 Open Access.)

control and are recommended to be scheduled, rather than ordered on as needed (PRN) basis along with the other adjuncts (**Figure 15.5**). Patients still experiencing breakthrough pain *after* these interventions may be given a short-acting opioid (**Figure 15.10**).

Early discharge prior to return of bowel function may be feasible in low-risk patients undergoing minimally invasive colectomy when there is optimal communication, support system, and close follow-up.

Bragg D, El-Sharkawy AM, Psaltis E, et al. Postoperative ileus: recent developments in pathophysiology and management. *Clin Nutr.* 2015;34:367-376.

Cameron JL, Cameron AM, eds. *Current Surgical Therapy.* 14th ed. Elsevier; 2023:303-314.

Gan TJ, Thacker JK, Miller TE, et al. *Enhanced Recovery for Major Abdominopelvic Surgery.* Professional Communications; 2016:215-259.

Irani JL, Hedrick TL, Miller TE, et al. Clinical practice guidelines for enhanced recovery after colon and rectal surgery from the American Society of Colon and Rectal Surgeons and the Society of American Gastrointestinal and Endoscopic Surgeons. *Surg Endosc.* 2023;37:5-30.

Scott MJ, McEvoy MD, Gordon DB, et al. American Society for Enhanced Recovery (ASER) and Perioperative Quality Initiative (POQI) joint consensus statement on optimal analgesia within an enhanced recovery pathway for colorectal surgery: part 2-from PACU to the transition home. *Perioper Med (Lond).* 2017;6:7.

Venara A, Neunlist M, Slim K, et al. Postoperative ileus: pathophysiology, incidence, and prevention. *J Visc Surg.* 2016;153:439-446.

Ventham NT, Kennedy ED, Brady RR, et al. Efficacy of intravenous lidocaine for postoperative analgesia following laparoscopic surgery: a meta-analysis. *World J Surg.* 2015;39:2220-2234.

Weimann A, Braga M, Carli F, et al. ESPEN guideline: clinical nutrition in surgery. *Clin Nutr.* 2017;36:623-650.

16

Liver Transplantation

Christine M. Lennon and Vivek K. Moitra

A 66-year-old female with a history of alcoholic cirrhosis and portal hypertension is admitted to the intensive care unit with altered mental status and low urine output. She has ascites and encephalopathy. Her kidney injury is acute with a creatinine clearance of 30 mL/min. Her international normalized ratio (INR) is 3.0. Her hemoglobin is 10.2 g/dL. She has a model for end-stage liver disease (MELD) score of 28 points. Her respiratory rate is 30 breaths per minute. She is scheduled for orthotopic liver transplantation.

A. Medical Disease and Differential Diagnosis

1. What are the potential graft options for liver transplantation?
2. What are the indications and contraindications for liver transplantation?
3. What is acute liver failure (ALF)?
4. What is the model for end-stage liver disease (MELD) score and how is it used in liver transplantation evaluation?
5. What is portal hypertension? What are the sequelae of portal hypertension?
6. Describe the cardiovascular physiology of patients with end-stage liver disease (ESLD).
7. What causes acute kidney injury (AKI) in patients with cirrhosis?
8. What causes hyponatremia in patients with cirrhosis?
9. Discuss the neurologic manifestations of acute and chronic liver disease.
10. Why do patients with ESLD have abnormalities of hemostasis?
11. What is the differential diagnosis for hypoxemia in patients with cirrhosis?
12. What are the risk factors and treatment guidelines for spontaneous bacterial peritonitis (SBP)?

B. Preoperative Evaluation and Preparation

1. What preoperative workup is desirable?
2. How is ascites managed preoperatively?
3. How is hyponatremia managed preoperatively?
4. What is a transjugular intrahepatic portosystemic shunt (TIPS) procedure? What is the role of TIPS in the management of patients with ESLD?
5. How are hepatic encephalopathy and elevated intracranial pressure (ICP) treated?
6. Should this patient be transfused with fresh frozen plasma (FFP) prior to surgery?

C. Intraoperative Management

1. What monitors would you use? Why?
2. What are the considerations for induction of anesthesia?
3. How does the liver disease affect intraoperative medication management?
4. What happens during the first stage (pre-anhepatic phase) of liver transplantation?
5. What happens during the second stage (anhepatic phase) of the liver transplantation?
6. What physiologic disturbances should be anticipated during the second stage (anhepatic phase) of liver transplantation?
7. What is venovenous bypass? What are the potential advantages and disadvantages of this procedure?
8. What surgical techniques anastomose the donor and recipient inferior vena cava (IVC)?
9. What are the potential advantages of "piggyback" (vena cava preservation) technique?
10. What hemodynamic changes are expected after removal of vascular clamps? What is postreperfusion syndrome?

11. How would you treat hyperkalemia?
12. Why should you anticipate hypocalcemia?
13. What happens during the third stage of liver transplantation?
14. What causes intraoperative bleeding during each phase of liver transplantation? How is coagulopathy monitored and treated? What are thromboelastography (TEG) and rotational thromboelastography (ROTEM)?
15. What are the complications of massive transfusion?
16. How are the complications of massive transfusion prevented?
17. How is hyperfibrinolysis managed?
18. When is intraoperative renal replacement therapy (RRT) indicated?
19. What intraoperative signs suggest that the hepatic graft is working?

D. Postoperative Management

1. What are the goals of immediate postoperative care of the liver transplant patient?
2. What postoperative findings suggest that the hepatic graft is functioning?
3. What coagulation disturbances should be anticipated in the postoperative period?
4. Can renal function change after liver transplantation?
5. What vascular and biliary complications can occur after liver transplantation?
6. What immunosuppressive agents will be given after liver transplantation? What are the major side effects?

A. Medical Disease and Differential Diagnosis

A.1. What are the potential graft options for liver transplantation?

Liver grafts are procured from deceased or living donors. Cadaveric livers are procured after brain or cardiac death. Because of the increasing number of patients who die waiting for a transplant, efforts to expand the donor pool have focused on donation after cardiac death (DCD), extending donor criteria, and partial grafts from live donors. DCD is the fastest growing source of transplant organs in the United States. Upon cardiac death (defined as the irreversible cessation of circulatory and respiratory function) and after a mandatory waiting period of 1 to 5 minutes, the liver is procured. Warm ischemic time begins when the waiting period starts and ends when the liver is flushed with cold preservative solution. Transplantation of a DCD liver that has been exposed to a longer warm ischemic time than a graft from a brain-dead donor may be associated with ischemia-reperfusion injury leading to early graft dysfunction and potential graft loss. Newly emerging alternatives to standard cold preservation of a DCD liver include hypothermic or normothermic machine perfusion of the explanted organ as well as normothermic regional perfusion, which involves placement of cannulae and initiation of machine perfusion to the graft immediately after declaration of donor death. These techniques are increasingly utilized to reduce graft ischemia and improve liver quality and outcomes. Ideal organs have shorter warm and cold ischemic times and are harvested from hemodynamically stable donors, younger than 50 years of age, who are free of hepatobiliary or renal disease, infection, and cancer.

Extending donor criteria (age >65 years; positive viral serology; hypernatremia; prior carcinoma, steatosis, or high-risk behaviors; split livers) to use organs with poor initial function or primary nonfunction also expands the donor pool. Split liver transplantation creates two transplants from one allograft. This is especially important in pediatric patients, where size-matched whole liver allografts are scarce, resulting in increased waiting list mortality.

A related or unrelated healthy individual can donate a portion of their liver for transplantation. Usually, the right hepatic lobe is removed and transplanted into an adult recipient. Transplantation of the smaller left hepatic lobe into a pediatric patient or small adult can decrease the incidence of complications in the donor. This chapter focuses on cadaveric liver transplantation into adult recipients.

Halazun KJ, Quillin RC, Rosenblatt R, et al. Expanding the margins: high volume utilization of marginal liver grafts among >2000 liver transplants at a single institution. *Ann Surg*. 2017;266:441-449.

Jackson WE, Malamon JS, Kaplan B, et al. Survival benefit of living-donor liver transplant. *JAMA Surg*. 2022;157:926-932.

Sellers MT, Nassar A, Alebrahim M, et al. Early United States experience with liver donation after circulatory determination of death using thoraco-abdominal normothermic regional perfusion: a multi-institutional observational study. *Clin Transplant*. 2022;36:e14659.

Wray CL, Klinck JR, Steadman RH. Anesthesia for abdominal organ transplantation. In: Gropper MA, Miller RD, Cohen NH, et al, eds. *Miller's Anesthesia*. 9th ed. Elsevier; 2020:1960-1992.

A.2. What are the indications and contraindications for liver transplantation?

Patients with ALF, decompensated cirrhosis, or hepatocellular carcinoma are candidates for liver transplantation. In the United States, alcoholic liver disease is the most common cause of ESLD and is the most common indication for orthotopic liver transplantation. Fatty liver disease or nonalcoholic steatohepatitis (NASH) is the second most common indication for liver transplantation. Other indications for transplantation include hepatocellular carcinoma (HCC), recurrent cholangitis in patients with primary sclerosing cholangitis, or intractable pruritus in patients with primary biliary cirrhosis. The proportion of patients being listed and receiving liver transplants for cirrhosis from hepatitis C (HCV) has decreased in recent years because of advances in viral therapeutics. Uncommon indications for liver transplantation include hepatic tumors such as carcinoid tumors and hepatic adenoma, genetic disorders such as α_1-antitrypsin deficiency, vascular disorders such as Budd-Chiari syndrome, cystic fibrosis, hemochromatosis, amyloidosis, sarcoidosis, hyperoxaluria, and adult polycystic liver disease. Biliary atresia is the most common indication for pediatric liver transplantation.

SECTION 3

Most centers do not offer transplantation to patients with severe cardiopulmonary or neurologic disease, significant hemodynamic instability, sepsis, extrahepatic malignancy, active alcohol or drug use, or unfavorable psychosocial circumstances. The decision to offer transplantation considers age and infection with human immunodeficiency virus.

Kwong AJ, Ebel NH, Kim WR, et al. OPTN/SRTR 2020 annual data report: liver. *Am J Transplant*. 2022;22:204-309.

Martin P, DiMartini A, Feng S, et al. Evaluation for liver transplantation in adults: 2013 practice guidelines by the American Association for the Study of Liver Diseases and the American Society of Transplantation. *Hepatology*. 2014;59:1144-1165.

Philip G, Hookey L, Richardson H, Flemming JA. Alcohol-associated liver disease is now the most common indication for liver transplant waitlisting among young American adults. *Transplantation*. 2022;106:2000-2005.

Wray CL, Klinck JR, Steadman RH. Anesthesia for abdominal organ transplantation. In: Gropper MA, Miller RD, Cohen NH, et al, eds. *Miller's Anesthesia*. 9th ed. Elsevier; 2020:1960-1992.

Younossi ZM, Stepanova M, Ong J, et al. Nonalcoholic steatohepatosis is the most rapidly increasing indication for liver transplantation in the United States. *Clin Gastroenterol Hepatol*. 2021;19:580-589.

A.3. What is acute liver failure (ALF)?

ALF is a rare and serious disorder that can lead to death without liver transplantation. ALF is defined by the absence of chronic liver disease, acute hepatitis (elevation in transaminases with an elevation in INR), encephalopathy, and illness less than 26 weeks. The most common causes of ALF in developed countries are acetaminophen toxicity, ischemia, drug-induced liver injury, hepatitis B virus, and autoimmunity. In developing countries, the most common causes of ALF are viral hepatitis A, B, and E. Less common causes of ALF include Wilson disease, Budd-Chiari syndrome, pregnancy, and indeterminate.

Shingina A, Mukhtar N, Wakim-Fleming J, et al. Acute liver failure guidelines. *Am J Gastroenterol*. 2023;118:1128-1153.

Stravitz RT, Lee WM. Acute liver failure. *Lancet*. 2019;394:869-881.

A.4. What is the model for end-stage liver disease (MELD) score and how is it used in liver transplantation evaluation?

Grafts from deceased donors are offered to patients with the highest risk of death. The MELD is a validated and widely used prognostic tool to prioritize organ allocation that estimates disease severity and 3-month survival in patients with chronic liver disease. Patients with a high score rank high on the transplant list and have a greater short-term risk of dying from liver disease than patients with lower scores. The MELD score ranges from 6 to 40 points and is calculated from the patient's serum bilirubin, serum creatinine, and INR. In 2016, the MELD score was modified to include sodium (MELD-Na) since hyponatremia is an important prognostic factor in patients with cirrhosis. After this change, waitlist mortality has decreased and transplant probability has increased (**Figure 16.1**). In 2020, the United Network for Organ Sharing (UNOS) adopted a new policy of liver allocation to reduce waitlist mortality and reduce geographic disparities in medical acuity at the time of transplant. This policy, based on acuity

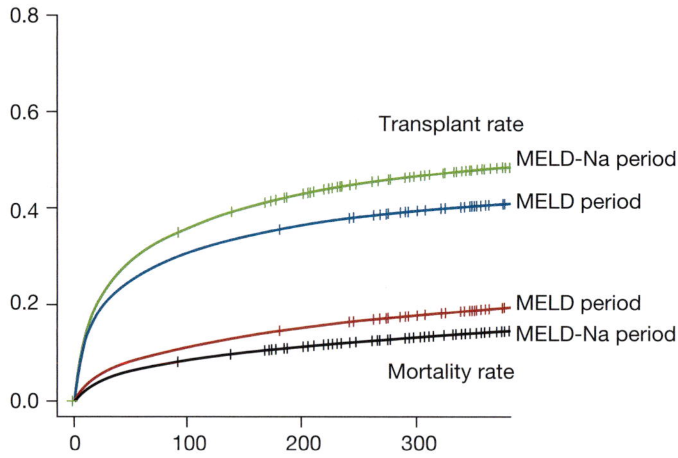

FIGURE 16.1. Comparison of waitlist mortality and transplantation rate between model for end-stage liver disease (MELD) and MELD-sodium (Na) scores in patients with cirrhotic liver disease. (Reprinted from Nagai S, Chau LC, Schilke RE, et al. Effects of allocating livers for transplantation based on model for end-stage liver disease-sodium scores on patient outcomes. *Gasteroenterology.* 2018; 155:1451-1462, with permission from Elsevier.)

circles, prioritizes allocation in candidates based on the MELD score and distance from the donor hospital rather than prioritizing allocation within the fixed boundaries of a donation service area or region.

Equation 1

MELD Score = 11.2 × ln (INR) + 9.57 × ln (creatinine, milligrams per deciliter) + 3.78 × ln (bilirubin, milligrams per deciliter) + 6.43 (an intercept), rounded to the nearest whole number.

Equation 2

$$\text{MELD-Na} = \text{MELD} + 1.32 \times (137 - \text{Na}) - [0.033 \times \text{MELD} \times (137 - \text{Na})],$$
rounded to the nearest whole number.

There is a lower limit of 1 for all variables. The maximum creatinine value is 4 mg/dL. For patients who receive dialysis, creatinine is set to 4 mg/dL.

Exceptions to the MELD classification exist for patients with fulminant hepatic failure and life expectancy of less than 7 days without a liver transplant. These patients are classified as *status 1* and ranked highest on the waiting list. This group includes patients who develop ALF without a history of liver disease, suffer from primary graft nonfunction or hepatic artery thrombosis within 7 days of a liver transplant, or have acutely decompensated Wilson disease. Special case exceptions also exist for patients with hepatocellular carcinoma, hepatopulmonary syndrome, portopulmonary hypertension, familial amyloidosis, primary oxaluria, cystic fibrosis, and cholangiocarcinoma.

Pediatric patients less than 12 years of age are ranked on the transplant waiting list according to the pediatric end-stage liver disease (PELD) model. The PELD score is similar in derivation to the MELD but does not consider creatinine and incorporates bilirubin, INR, albumin, age, and growth failure into the formula.

Choi C, Manecke GR, Lindberg S, Steadman RH. Transplant anesthesia. In: Cullen BF, Stock MC, Ortega R, et al, eds. *Barash, Cullen, and Stoelting's Clinical Anesthesia*. 9th ed. Wolters Kluwer; 2024:1407-1435.

Krowka M, Wiesner R, Heimbach J. Pulmonary contraindications, indications and MELD exceptions for liver transplantation: a contemporary view and look forward. *J Hepatol.* 2013;59:367-374.

Martin P, DiMartini A, Feng S, et al. Evaluation for liver transplantation in adults: 2013 practice guidelines by the American Association for the Study of Liver Diseases and the American Society of Transplantation. *Hepatology*. 2014;59:1144-1165.

Nagai S, Chau LC, Schilke RE, et al. Effects of allocating livers for transplantation based on model for end-stage liver disease-sodium scores on patient outcomes. *Gastroenterology*. 2018;155:1451-1462.

United Network for Organ Sharing. System notice: liver and intestinal organ distribution based on acuity circles implemented Feb. 4. Published February 4, 2020. Accessed January 25, 2023. https://unos.org/news/system-implementation-notice-liver-and-intestinal-organ-distribution-based-on-acuity-circles-implemented-feb-4/

A.5. What is portal hypertension? What are the sequelae of portal hypertension?

The normal portosystemic gradient between the portal vein and hepatic vein is less than 5 mm Hg. Greater intrahepatic vascular resistance and portal venous blood flow increase this gradient, which characterizes portal hypertension. Liver fibrosis, regenerative nodules, collagen deposition in the space of Disse, endothelial dysfunction, and an imbalance between endogenous vasoconstrictors, such as norepinephrine, thromboxane A, endothelin I, angiotensin II, leukotrienes, and vasodilators, such as nitric oxide, increase vascular resistance in the liver. As the pressure gradient between the portal vein and the hepatic vein increases, collaterals such as gastroesophageal and hemorrhoidal varices develop to decompress the portal system. Portal hypertension causes shear stress in the splanchnic vessels, which along with translocation of bacterial lipopolysaccharides increase endogenous vasodilators that cause vasodilation. Splanchnic vasodilation in turn increases portal blood flow and exacerbates portal hypertension.

Complications of portal hypertension include gastrointestinal bleeding from expansion and rupture of varices, intraoperative bleeding from intra-abdominal collaterals, and formation of ascites and pleural effusions.

Bloom S, Kemp W, Lubel J. Portal hypertension: pathophysiology, diagnosis and management. *Intern Med J.* 2015:45:16-26.

A.6. Describe the cardiovascular physiology of patients with end-stage liver disease (ESLD).

The cardiovascular system of patients with ESLD mimics the hyperdynamic circulatory changes of patients with sepsis, including tachycardia, elevated cardiac output, low arterial blood pressure, and low systemic vascular resistance. Enhanced endogenous production or diminished hepatic clearance of vasodilating substances, such as nitric oxide, carbon monoxide, and endogenous cannabinoids, and the inflammatory response to bacterial translocation cause splanchnic arterial vasodilation. Increased venous capacitance from formation of portosystemic shunts because of portal hypertension increases venous capacitance and contributes to hyperdynamic circulation. Cirrhotic cardiomyopathy is characterized by impaired systolic and diastolic function, resistance to β-adrenergic stimulation, and QTc prolongation. In the perioperative period, the circulatory system can be challenged with surgical stress, changes in preload and afterload from fluid shifts, placement of clamps across great vessels, and/or shunt insertion; these physiologic changes can unmask underlying cardiomyopathy and potentially lead to acute cardiac decompensation and heart failure.

Systemic conditions such as hemochromatosis (ventricular hypertrophy with increased end-diastolic and end-systolic volumes), amyloidosis (restrictive cardiomyopathy), Wilson disease (supraventricular extrasystolic beats), and alcoholism (systolic and diastolic dysfunction) can affect liver and cardiac function. Patients with portal hypertension can develop portopulmonary hypertension, leading to right ventricular dysfunction. Mean pulmonary artery pressure greater than 25 mm Hg at rest, mean pulmonary capillary wedge pressure less than 15 mm Hg, and pulmonary vascular resistance (PVR) greater than 240 dynes/sec/cm^{-5} define portopulmonary hypertension. The mechanism is not fully understood, and histologically, there are no clear distinguishable features from idiopathic pulmonary arterial hypertension. A mean pulmonary artery pressure greater than 50 mm Hg and/or PVR greater than 250 dynes/sec/cm^{-5} are contradictions for liver transplantation due to risk of fulminant right heart failure.

Fritz JS, Fallon MB, Kawut SM. Pulmonary vascular complications of liver disease. *Am J Respir Crit Care Med.* 2013;187:133-143.

Krowka MJ, Fallon MB, Kawut SM, et al. International Liver Transplant Society practice guidelines: diagnosis and management of hepatopulmonary syndrome and portopulmonary hypertension. *Transplantation.* 2016;100:1440-1452.

Rahman S, Mallett SV. Cirrhotic cardiomyopathy: implications for the perioperative management of liver transplant patients. *World J Hepatol.* 2015;7:507-520.

A.7. What causes acute kidney injury (AKI) in patients with cirrhosis?

Patients with AKI and cirrhosis have more complications and increased risk of mortality after liver transplantation than those without renal failure. Gastrointestinal bleeding, diarrhea from infection or lactulose administration, and diuretic medications impair circulatory function via hypovolemia and can cause renal injury. As cirrhosis progresses, there is compensatory activation of renin-angiotensin and sympathetic nervous systems, which leads to ascites, severe renal vasoconstriction, and, ultimately, renal hypoperfusion. This in turn leads to electrolyte abnormalities including hyponatremia and hypokalemia.

Hepatorenal syndrome (HRS) is caused by functional renal vasoconstriction in response to splanchnic arterial vasodilation; it does not have clear histologic findings. HRS-AKI (formerly known as type 1 HRS) is a type of AKI, usually caused by an acute insult such as SBP or large volume paracentesis, resulting in rapid and progressive loss of renal function. Diagnostic criteria for HRS-AKI include (1) cirrhosis with ascites, (2) increase in serum creatinine greater than 0.3 mg/dL from baseline within 48 hours or greater than or equal to 50% increase in serum creatinine within 7 days, (3) no improvement of creatinine after 2 days of diuretic withdrawal and plasma volume expansion with albumin, (4) absence of shock, (5) no current or recent exposure to nephrotoxic drugs, and (6) absence of parenchymal kidney disease. The prognosis of HRS-AKI is poor, with a median survival of less than or equal to 3 months. Patients with HRS-CKD (chronic kidney disease) (formerly known as type 2 HRS) have serum creatinine greater than 1.5 mg/dL with reduction in eGFR less than 60 mL/1.73 m^2/min for at least 3 months, and does not meet the criteria for HRS-AKI; median survival in these patients is 4 to 6 months. Distinguishing between HRS and acute tubular necrosis is difficult. Fractional excretion of sodium less than 1% suggests tubular function and favors a diagnosis of HRS. The presence of renal tubular epithelial cells in urinary sediment favors a diagnosis of acute tubular necrosis.

The administration of vasopressors (particularly terlipressin, a vasopressin analogue) with intravenous albumin is effective in patients with type HRS-AKI. The magnitude of blood pressure increase, rather than a specific vasopressor type, is best correlated with renal recovery. Medical management of HRS is marginally effective, but liver transplantation can reverse HRS. Kidneys transplanted from patients with HRS function normally in new hosts, suggesting the essential role of hepatic disease in the pathogenesis. Up to 40% of patients with HRS do not recover kidney function after transplantation. In these cases, systemic inflammation with hyperbilirubinemia might contribute to irreversible structural renal damage.

Biggins SW, Angeli P, Garcia-Tsao G, et al. Diagnosis, evaluation, and management of ascites, spontaneous bacterial peritonitis and hepatorenal syndrome: 2021 practice guidance by the American Association for the Study of Liver Diseases. *Hepatology*. 2021;74:1014-1048.

Bonavia A, Singbartl K. Kidney injury and electrolyte abnormalities in liver failure. *Semin Respir Crit Care*. 2018;39:556-565.

Ginès P, Solà E, Angeli P, Wong F, Nadim MK, Kamath PS. Hepatorenal syndrome. *Nat Rev Dis Primers*. 2018;4:23. Erratum in: *Nat Rev Dis Primers*. 2018;4:33.

A.8. What causes hyponatremia in patients with cirrhosis?

Patients with advanced cirrhosis have decreased effective blood volume with circulatory dysfunction. They develop hypervolemic hyponatremia from increased secretion of antidiuretic hormone, which acts on the vasopressin-2 receptors of the renal tubular collecting duct to impair excretion of solute-free water leading to expanded extracellular volume, ascites, and edema.

Patients who develop hypovolemic hyponatermia via loss of extracellular fluid from the kidneys (overdiuresis) or gastrointestinal tract rarely have ascites or edema. These patients can have prerenal failure from low plasma volume and dehydration or hepatic encephalopathy from a rapid reduction in serum osmolality.

Alukal JJ, John S, Thuluvath PJ. Hyponatremia in cirrhosis: an update. *Am J Gastroenterol*. 2020;115:1775-1785.

Leise M, Cárdenas A. Hyponatremia in cirrhosis: implications for liver transplantation. *Liver Transpl*. 2018;24:1612-1621.

A.9. Discuss the neurologic manifestations of acute and chronic liver disease.

Hepatic encephalopathy is a neuropsychiatric complication of acute and chronic liver disease that causes disturbances in consciousness, cognitive abilities, behavior, and motor function. Features range from subclinical alterations or mild confusion to intracranial hypertension, cerebral edema, and coma. The pathogenesis of hepatic encephalopathy is not understood, but elevated levels of ammonia, a neurotoxin produced by bacteria in the gut, shunted from the portal system to the systemic circulation has been implicated. Ammonia crosses the blood-brain barrier into astrocytes, where it is detoxified to glutamine. The increased concentration of intracellular glutamine causes swelling of astrocytes and impaired neurotransmission. High serum ammonia levels are common among patients with hepatic encephalopathy, even though the degree of elevation of ammonia does not correlate with severity of neurologic symptoms. This observation suggests that other factors such as hyponatremia, gastrointestinal bleeding, and infection contribute to development of hepatic encephalopathy. Left untreated, cerebral edema can progress to intracranial hypertension and uncal herniation. Multiple grading scales assess the severity of hepatic encephalopathy. The most common scales are the West Haven Criteria (Conn Score) and the Glasgow Coma Scale (GCS).

It is important to rule out other underlying causes of altered mental status in patients with cirrhosis, including metabolic causes such as uremia, sepsis, glucose and electrolyte abnormalities; endocrinopathies; infections; and impaired hepatic or renal metabolism of sedative medications.

Vilstrup H, Amodio P, Bajaj J, et al. Hepatic encephalopathy in chronic liver disease: 2014 practice guideline by the American Association for the Study of Liver Diseases and the European Association for the Study of the Liver. *Hepatology*. 2014;60:715-735.

Wray C, Andreatta B, Adelmann D. Anesthesia for abdominal organ transplantation. In: Gropper MA, Cohen NH, Eriksson LI, Fleisher LA, Leslie K, Johnson-Akeju O, eds. *Miller's Anesthesia*. 10th ed. Elsevier; 2025:1833-1870.

A.10. Why do patients with ESLD have abnormalities of hemostasis?

Patients with ESLD have hemostatic derangements that promote both bleeding and thrombosis (**Figure 16.2**). Inadequate synthesis of coagulation factors (except for von Willebrand factor and factor VIII), thrombocytopenia, platelet function defects, dysfibrinogenemia, and elevated tissue plasminogen activator (tPA) levels cause bleeding. Elevations of von Willebrand factor and factor VIII and decreased levels of a disintegrin and metalloproteinase with a thrombospondin type 1 motif, member 13 (ADAMTS-13), protein C, protein S, antithrombin, α_2-macroglobulin, plasminogen, and heparin cofactor II favor thrombosis.

Factors VII, X, V, II (prothrombin), and I (fibrinogen) have a short half-life (hours to days) and are synthesized solely by hepatocytes making possible evaluation of hepatic synthetic function. Although patients with liver disease can have abnormal prothrombin time (PT) from decreased production of procoagulant factors, the rebalanced state of pro- and anticoagulants in patients with liver disease makes the PT an unreliable tool for evaluating tendency to bleed or clot; viscoelastic testing such as TEG (thromboelastography) and ROTEM (rotational thromboelastometry) in patients with liver disease provide a more accurate representation of the dynamics of clot formation and lysis.

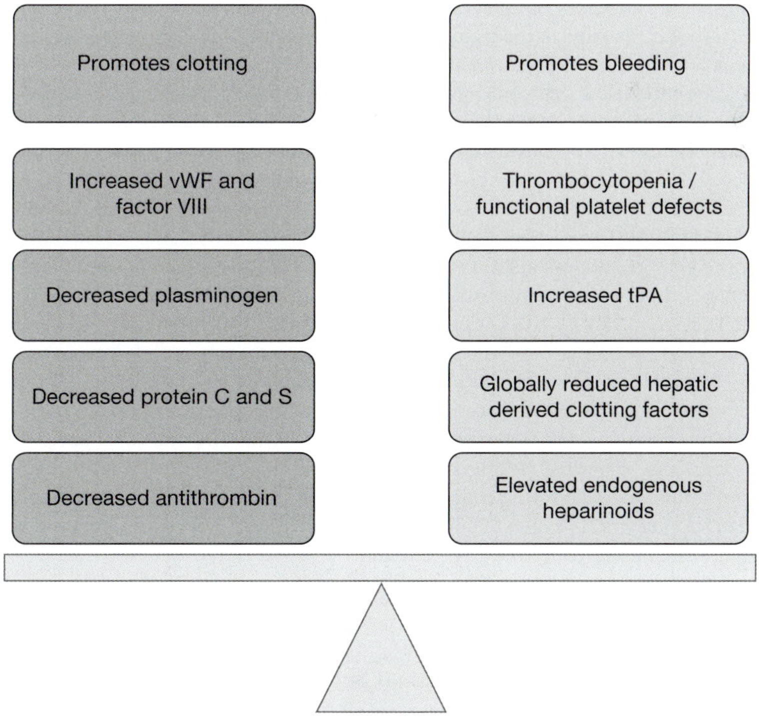

FIGURE 16.2. Changes of the coagulation and fibrinolytic system in end-stage liver disease. tpa, tissue plasminogen activator. (Modified from Intagliata NM, Davis J, Caldwell SH. Coagulation pathways, hemostasis, and thrombosis in liver failure. *Semin Respir Crit Care Med.* 2018;39:598-608. © Georg Thieme Verlag KG.)

Levels of fibrinogen, an acute phase reactant, are normal or increased in liver disease. Patients with severe hepatic dysfunction, however, synthesize fibrinogen poorly, which increases the risk of bleeding. Although high concentrations of fibrinogen are found in patients with chronic hepatitis, cholestatic jaundice, and hepatocellular carcinoma, clot formation is not enhanced because the fibrinogen is dysfunctional. Hyperfibrinolysis (from increased levels of tPA and reduced levels of thrombin-activatable fibrinolysis inhibitor [TAFI] and plasmin inhibitor) has been observed in cirrhotic patients, but its association with bleeding is unclear. Hypofibrinolysis (from increased levels of plasminogen activator inhibitor [PAI] and reduced levels of plasminogen) may restore the balance of fibrinolysis.

Thrombocytopenia and platelet dysfunction are also characteristics of ESLD. Thrombocytopenia results from several factors: hypersplenism, which sequesters platelets; consumption of platelets during systemic intravascular coagulation; and impaired hepatic synthesis of thrombopoietin, which produces platelets in the bone marrow. Defective signal transduction; uremia from AKI; and intrinsic defects of responses to adenosine diphosphate (ADP), arachidonic acid, collagen, and thrombin prevent platelet aggregation.

There can be little evidence of deranged coagulation when normal hepatic parenchyma is preserved, such as in an isolated hepatoma.

Lisman T, Hernandez-Gea V, Magnusson M, et al. The concept of rebalanced hemostasis in patients with liver disease: communication from the ISTH SSC working group on hemostatic management of patients with liver disease. *J Thromb Haemost*. 2021;19:1116-1122.

Northup PG, Garcia-Pagan JC, Garcia-Tsao G, et al. Vascular liver disorders, portal vein thrombosis, and procedural bleeding in patients with liver disease: 2020 practice guidance by the American Association for the Study of Liver Diseases. *Hepatology*. 2021;73:366-413.

Tripodi A, Mannucci PM. The coagulopathy of chronic liver disease. *N Engl J Med*. 2011;365:147-156.

A.11. What is the differential diagnosis for hypoxemia in patients with cirrhosis?

Potential causes of preoperative hypoxemia and respiratory failure in patients with cirrhosis include atelectasis from the compressive effects of ascites, hepatic hydrothorax, hepatopulmonary syndrome (HPS), and underlying chronic pulmonary disease. Muscle wasting and intra-abdominal hypertension from ascites increase the work of breathing.

Ascites fluid can enter the pleural space through small channels in the diaphragm to cause a hepatic hydrothorax (usually on the right side). Negative intrathoracic pressure during inspiration facilitates movement of fluid from the peritoneum to the pleural space to minimize ascites. A pleural fluid culture with polymorphonuclear cell count greater than 250 cells/μL or isolated polymorphonuclear cell count greater than 500 cells/μL diagnose spontaneous bacterial empyema.

A diagnosis of HPS is considered in patients without cardiopulmonary disease who have a Pao_2 less than or equal to 70 mm Hg in any position. The triad of liver disease and/or portal hypertension, widened age-corrected alveolar-arterial oxygen gradient (>15 or 20 mm Hg) while breathing room air, and documented intrapulmonary vascular dilation (IPVD) define HPS. Enhanced production or impaired hepatic clearance of endogenous vasodilators (ie, nitric oxide, carbon monoxide, vasodilator prostaglandins, substance P) or inhibition of vasoconstrictors (ie, tyrosine, serotonin, and endothelin) by a damaged liver might contribute to IPVD. IPVD causes hypoxemia via $\dot{V}/\dot{Q}$ mismatching, intrapulmonary shunt physiology, and diffusion limitation. Patients with HPS often complain of dyspnea and fatigue; they can have clubbing and spider angiomata on physical examination. Patients can experience platypnea (dyspnea in the upright position relieved by recumbency) or have orthodeoxia (arterial oxyhemoglobin desaturation in the upright position) due to preferential perfusion (while the patient is upright). Contrast-enhanced echocardiography or perfusion lung scanning with technetium-99m-labeled macroaggregated albumin detects intrapulmonary shunting suggestive of IPVD. There is no established medical therapy for HPS other than supplemental oxygen to correct hypoxemia. The only known treatment for HPS is liver transplantation, which usually improves oxygenation.

Fritz JS, Fallon MB, Kawut SM. Pulmonary vascular complications of liver disease. *Am J Respir Crit Care Med*. 2013;187:133-143.

Hemprich U, Papadakos PJ, Lachmann B. Respiratory failure and hypoxemia in the cirrhotic patient including hepatopulmonary syndrome. *Curr Opin Anaesthesiol*. 2010;23:133-138.

Krowka MJ, Fallon MB, Kawut SM, et al. International Liver Transplant Society practice guidelines: diagnosis and management of hepatopulmonary syndrome and portopulmonary hypertension. *Transplantation*. 2016;100:1440-1452.

Rodríguez-Roisin R, Krowka MJ. Hepatopulmonary syndrome–a liver-induced lung vascular disorder. *N Engl J Med*. 2008;358:2378-2387.

A.12. What are the risk factors and treatment guidelines for spontaneous bacterial peritonitis (SBP)?

The American Association for the Study of Liver Diseases recommends paracentesis for all hospitalized patients with ascites because infections of ascitic fluid are common. Delaying paracentesis and initiation of antibiotics is associated with higher in-hospital and three-month mortality (each hour delay increases in-hospital mortality by 3.3%). SBP is diagnosed by polymorphonuclear cell counts greater than 250 cells/μL without evidence of an intra-abdominal surgically treatable source of infection.

Cirrhotic patients have a disproportionate growth of pathogenic bacteria for numerous reasons. They have a smaller bile pool and less conversion of primary to secondary bile acids, which have bactericidal properties. This causes dysbiosis from an overgrowth of Enterobacteriaceae. Reduced gut motility and proton pump inhibitor use stimulates small intestinal overgrowth and may increase intestinal permeability and rate of bacterial translocation.

A minimum of 5 days of empiric treatment with a third-generation cephalosporin is usually an adequate coverage for the typical organisms known to cause SBP (ie, *Escherichia coli*, *Klebsiella*). There are a few data to support the use of large volume paracentesis for SBP. Administration of intravenous albumin as part of the routine treatment for SBP can decrease overall mortality and incidence of HRS. Repeat paracentesis should be considered with ascitic fluid analysis in patients with inadequate response to treatment, an atypical organism on culture, or suspected secondary peritonitis.

Biggins SW, Angeli P, Garcia-Tsao G, et al. Diagnosis, evaluation, and management of ascites, spontaneous bacterial peritonitis and hepatorenal syndrome: 2021 practice guidance by the American Association for the Study of Liver Diseases. *Hepatology*. 2021;74:1014-1048.

Cheung A, Tanna S, Ison MG. Infectious complications in critically ill liver failure patients. *Semin Respir Crit Care Med*. 2018;39:578-587.

Pericleous M, Sarnowski A, Moore A, et al. The clinical management of abdominal ascites, spontaneous bacterial peritonitis and hepatorenal syndrome: a review of current guidelines and recommendations. *Eur J Gastroenterol Hepatol*. 2016;28:e10-e18.

B. Preoperative Evaluation and Preparation

B.1. What preoperative workup is desirable?

Anesthesiologists face several preoperative challenges when patients with ESLD need surgery. Surgical and anesthetic management is complicated for patients who often have preoperative encephalopathy, AKI, electrolyte abnormalities, ascites, myocardial and pulmonary dysfunction, or coagulopathy. To anticipate and prevent complications from transplantation, underlying conditions should be thoroughly evaluated before surgery. A multidisciplinary team including an anesthesiologist, hepatologist, psychologist, and surgeon should be involved in preoperative preparation. Cardiology, pulmonology, infectious diseases, and nephrology consultations can be requested for patients with comorbidities.

Electrolyte, blood urea nitrogen, creatinine, albumin, bilirubin, and transaminase levels, complete blood count, coagulation studies, and glucose values should be obtained. An electrocardiogram and chest radiograph to rule out pulmonary edema and cardiomegaly should also be obtained. Blood group and antibody screening in advance is necessary for crossmatching large amounts of blood products, especially in patients who have received prior transfusions. Echocardiography should be obtained to evaluate cardiac function and determine right ventricular systolic pressure (RVSP), which is a marker for pulmonary hypertension. If RVSP is elevated, pretransplant right heart catheterization is warranted. In patients with coronary artery disease risk factors (hyperlipidemia, hypertension, diabetes mellitus, cigarette consumption, age >60 years), functional testing such as exercise or dobutamine stress echocardiography is recommended. A vasodilatory (eg, adenosine, persantine) myocardial stress test is less useful in patients with ESLD because resting vascular tone is so low that provoking further vasodilation with drugs is difficult.

In cases of altered mental status, a head computed tomography (CT) scan often is indicated to evaluate intracranial bleeding, uncal herniation, and/or the extent of cerebral edema. Pulmonary function studies may be indicated in smokers or patients with pre-existing pulmonary disease. If intraoperative RRT (continuous venovenous hemofiltration) is a consideration, a nephrologist should be consulted.

Barman PM, VanWagner LB. Cardiac risk assessment in liver transplant candidates: current controversies and future directions. *Hepatology*. 2020;73:2564-2576.

SECTION 3

Martin P, DiMartini A, Feng S, Brown R, Fallon M. Evaluation for liver transplantation in adults: 2014 practice guideline by the American Association for the Study of Liver Diseases and the American Society of Transplantation. *Hepatology*. 2014;59:1144-1165.

Wray C, Andreatta B, Adelmann D. Anesthesia for abdominal organ transplantation. In: Gropper MA, Cohen NH, Eriksson LI, Fleisher LA, Leslie K, Johnson-Akeju O, eds. *Miller's Anesthesia*. 10th ed. Elsevier; 2025:1833-1870.

B.2. How is ascites managed preoperatively?

Ascites is initially managed with a low-sodium diet (<2 g/d) and diuretic therapy. Spironolactone as a sole agent or in combination with furosemide is typically used. Patients with ascites refractory to treatment with diuretics can require large volume paracentesis. If more than 5 L of ascites are drained, albumin is replaced to prevent hypotension and HRS. Patients with ascites should avoid nephrotoxic agents such as nonsteroidal anti-inflammatory drugs (NSAIDs), aminoglycosides, angiotensin-converting enzyme (ACE) inhibitors, and α_1-blockers. Patients can be treated by transjugular intrahepatic portosystemic shunting (TIPS) in refractory cases of ascites or hepatic hydrothorax.

Liou I. Management of end-stage liver disease. *Med Clin North Am*. 2014;98:119-152.

Pericleous M, Sarnowski A, Moore A, et al. The clinical management of abdominal ascites, spontaneous bacterial peritonitis and hepatorenal syndrome: a review of current guidelines and recommendations. *Eur J Gastroenterol Hepatol*. 2016;28:e10-e18.

B.3. How is hyponatremia managed preoperatively?

Hyponatremia (serum sodium <130 mEq/L in patients with cirrhosis) is an important prognostic indicator in the peri-transplant period. In 2016, UNOS incorporated serum sodium into the MELD score after it was demonstrated that MELD-Na helps predict waitlist mortality more accurately than MELD alone. Cirrhotic patients typically have hypervolemic hyponatremia due to splanchnic vasodilation and reduced effective arterial blood volume, resulting in increased antidiuretic hormone (ADH) production and stimulation of the renin-angiotensin-aldosterone and sympathetic nervous systems. A minority of hyponatremia cases are from hypovolemia due to excessive diuretic use or gastrointestinal losses such as diarrhea or vomiting.

Hypervolemic hyponatremia is managed with fluid restriction (1-1.5 L/d), temporary withholding of diuretics and correction of hypokalemia, and albumin infusion. Vaptans are medications that block the vasopressin-2 receptor and increase solute-free water excretion. These medications are reserved for severe episodes of hyponatremia. Hypertonic saline can be cautiously used in cases of symptomatic or profound hyponatremia (Na <110 mEq/L), to raise serum sodium not more than 8 mEq in 24 hours to avoid osmotic demyelination syndrome (ODS), a neurologic condition characterized by myelinolysis or destruction of astrocytes in the pons and other brain areas. Hypovolemic hyponatremia is treated with discontinuation of diuretics and expansion of plasma volume with intravenous saline. Preoperative correction of hyponatremia can prevent a rapid rise in serum sodium intraoperatively and postoperatively. During intraoperative fluid replacement, high sodium loads cause rapid swings in serum sodium, or even hypernatremia. Sodium bicarbonate should be administered cautiously because it has a high concentration of sodium. Tris-hydroxymethyl aminomethane (THAM), although a weaker base, is an alternative because of its lower sodium content.

Alukal JJ, John S, Thuluvath PJ. Hyponatremia in cirrhosis: an update. *Am J Gastroenterol*. 2020;115:1775-1785.

Leise M, Cárdenas A. Hyponatremia in cirrhosis: implications for liver transplantation. *Liver Transpl*. 2018;24:1612-1621.

B.4. What is a transjugular intrahepatic portosystemic shunt (TIPS) procedure? What is the role of TIPS in the management of patients with ESLD?

During a TIPS procedure, an expandable stent is deployed into the liver parenchyma to bridge the hepatic and portal vein to reduce the portosystemic pressure gradient and decrease portal hypertension. Unlike older, surgically created portosystemic and peritoneovenous shunts, a TIPS does not require an abdominal operation or vascular diversion, both of which impose technical hazards to future liver transplantation. Early TIPS intervention after an episode of esophageal variceal bleeding is associated with decreased risk of rebleeding and reduced mortality. The procedure can be performed under local or general anesthesia as a bridge to liver transplantation in patients with severe liver disease. General anesthesia is preferred because of the duration of the procedure and the potential for life-threatening events such as bleeding, aspiration, hemobilia, arrhythmias, liver ischemia, and stent migration. Preoperative evaluation of cardiac function (particularly right ventricular function and presence of pulmonary hypertension) is essential because stent placement can rapidly increase venous return to unmask an underlying cardiomyopathy. Encephalopathy can worsen in some patients because there is an increased systemic delivery of biogenic amines normally cleared by the liver. The long-term patency of a TIPS is poor, especially prior to the introduction of polytetrafluoroethylene-covered stents, and multiple revisions can be required.

Njei B, McCarty TR, Laine L. Early transjugular intrahepatic portosystemic shunt in US patients hospitalized with acute esophageal variceal bleeding. *J Gastroenterol Hepatol.* 2017;32:852-858.

Wray C, Andreatta B, Adelmann D. Anesthesia for abdominal organ transplantation. In: Gropper MA, Cohen NH, Eriksson LI, Fleisher LA, Leslie K, Johnson-Akeju O, eds. *Miller's Anesthesia.* 10th ed. Elsevier; 2025:1833-1870.

B.5. How are hepatic encephalopathy and elevated intracranial pressure (ICP) treated?

Initial therapy for hepatic encephalopathy includes identification and treatment of reversible triggers (ie, gastrointestinal bleeding, infection, metabolic disturbances, or medication side effects). Nonabsorbable disaccharides such as lactulose and lactitol decrease absorption of ammonia from the gut via a variety of mechanisms; however, excessive dosing of these drugs can cause dehydration. Oral antibiotics such as rifaximin reduce ammonia-producing enteric bacteria. Patients are often maintained on a combination of lactulose and rifaximin to prevent recurrent episodes of hepatic encephalopathy. L-ornithine L-aspartate (LOLA) is used outside the United States to decrease ammonia levels by enhancing metabolism of ammonia. Malnutrition is often present in patients with hepatic encephalopathy and should be treated; there is consensus that low-protein nutrition should be avoided in these patients.

Patients who develop fulminant hepatic failure are at risk for hepatic encephalopathy, cerebral edema with increased ICP, and herniation. In cases of altered mental status, a head CT or MR scan is often indicated to evaluate for intracranial bleeding and the extent of cerebral edema and/or herniation. There is an ongoing debate as to whether ICP monitoring should be performed for these patients with severe encephalopathy, given the bleeding risks associated with invasive monitors. Epidural transducers can be preferable to intradural monitors to minimize bleeding risk. Consideration should be given to correction of coagulopathy prior to placement of invasive ICP monitors. Alternate noninvasive ultrasonographic modalities such as transcranial Doppler and optic nerve sheath diameter measurements can be used to estimate ICP.

Sustained ICP elevations greater than 20 mm Hg should be treated with mannitol or hypertonic saline to achieve hyperosmolarity. Preoperative hyperventilation has not been shown to improve outcome, and corticosteroids are not indicated. A medically induced coma can be used for patients unresponsive to mannitol, but coma can worsen cerebral hypoperfusion because sedatives cause systemic hypotension and confound the neurologic exam. Many centers consider sustained cerebral hypoperfusion (cerebral perfusion pressure <40 mm Hg) a contraindication to transplant because of the high risk for brain death. During anesthesia, drugs or conditions that exacerbate elevations in ICP should be avoided.

Jinadasa SP, Ruan QZ, Bayoumi AB, et al. Hemorrhagic complications of invasive intracranial pressure monitor placement in acute liver failure: outcomes of a single-center protocol and comprehensive literature review. *Neurocrit Care.* 2021;35:87-102.

Vilstrup H, Amodio P, Bajaj J, et al. Hepatic encephalopathy in chronic liver disease: 2014 practice guideline by the American Association for the Study of Liver Diseases and the European Association for the Study of the Liver. *Hepatology.* 2014;60:715-735.

Wijdicks EFM. Hepatic encephalopathy. *N Engl J Med.* 2016;375:1660-1670.

B.6. Should this patient be transfused with fresh frozen plasma (FFP) prior to surgery?

Management of coagulopathy is challenging because conventional blood tests such as PT and activated partial thromboplastin time (aPTT) are not predictive of transfusion requirements during liver transplantation.

Patients who need an orthotopic liver transplant usually have severe perturbations in coagulation, but it is neither necessary nor possible to correct them preoperatively. In patients with active sites of bleeding, it is reasonable to administer FFP, packed red blood cells, cryoprecipitate, or platelets as dictated by clinical assessment and laboratory tests, including viscoelastic testing. Desmopressin (1-deamino-8-D-arginine vasopressin [DDAVP]) can be considered for patients with concomitant renal dysfunction and uremic bleeding. Potentially curative transplant surgery should not be postponed to correct coagulation defects.

Pillai AA, Kriss M, Al-Adra DP, et al. Coagulopathy and hemostasis management in patients undergoing liver transplantation: Defining a dynamic spectrum across phases of care. *Liver Transpl.* 2022;28:1651-1663.

Wray C, Andreatta B, Adelmann D. Anesthesia for abdominal organ transplantation. In: Gropper MA, Cohen NH, Eriksson LI, Fleisher LA, Leslie K, Johnson-Akeju O, eds. *Miller's Anesthesia.* 10th ed. Elsevier; 2025:1833-1870..

C. Intraoperative Management

C.1. What monitors would you use? Why?

In addition to the standard monitors recommended by the American Society of Anesthesiologists (electrocardiogram, pulse oximetry, capnography, temperature, and noninvasive blood pressure), placement of additional invasive monitors should be guided by the degree of cardiovascular and pulmonary disease as well as surgical considerations and local institutional practice. A radial arterial catheter is placed for beat-to-beat blood pressure monitoring and frequent sampling of blood. Pulse pressure variation, calculated from the invasive arterial tracing, assesses fluid responsiveness. A second arterial catheter can be placed in the femoral artery to measure central aortic blood pressure. Peripheral arterial pressures can be unreliable in a patient with vasoconstriction, vasodilation, or compression of the subclavian artery with rib retraction.

Central venous access is established to measure right atrial pressure and to administer drugs. Central venous pressure monitoring does not reliably measure blood volume or change in blood volume. Use of a pulmonary artery catheter depends on local practice and the physiologic state of the patient. Thermodilution measurements for cardiac output can be inaccurate with large volume administration of intravenous fluids and the rapid return of cooled blood during reperfusion. Mixed venous oxygen saturation values can aid in the assessment of cardiac output, but these measurements also are influenced by changes in oxygen-carrying capacity and oxygen consumption.

Transesophageal echocardiography (TEE) assesses ventricular filling, contractility, and function in real time. Numerous case reports have reported its usefulness in diagnosing portopulmonary hypertension, ischemic heart disease, cirrhotic cardiomyopathy, and intraoperative thromboembolic events. While grade 4 varices may be a contraindication, risk of rupture of grade 1 and 2 esophageal varices with TEE is rare.

Rudnick MR, March LD, Plotkin JS, et al. Hemodynamic monitoring during liver transplantation: a state of the art review. *World J Hepat.* 2015;7:1302-1311.

Sakai T. Liver transplantation anesthesiology. In: Subramaniam K, Sakai T, eds. *Anesthesia and Perioperative Care for Organ Transplantation.* Springer Science+Business Media; 2017:353-364.

Schumann R, Mandell MS, Mercaldo N, et al. Anesthesia for liver transplantation in United States academic centers: intraoperative practice. *J Clin Anesth.* 2013;25:542-550.

Wray C, Andreatta B, Adelmann D. Anesthesia for abdominal organ transplantation. In: Gropper MA, Cohen NH, Eriksson LI, Fleisher LA, Leslie K, Johnson-Akeju O, eds. *Miller's Anesthesia.* 10th ed. Elsevier; 2025:1833-1870.

C.2. What are the considerations for induction of anesthesia?

If there is evidence of tense ascites, recent food ingestion, or a propensity for delayed gastric emptying, a rapid sequence induction of general endotracheal anesthesia is performed. AKI with elevated potassium levels or prolonged immobilization can preclude the use of succinylcholine. Compressive atelectasis from ascites and pleural effusions reduces functional residual capacity and decrease the time to hemoglobin desaturation. Vasodilating anesthetic agents cause hypotension if intravascular volume is depleted (eg, overdiuresis or gastrointestinal losses).

Wray C, Andreatta B, Adelmann D. Anesthesia for abdominal organ transplantation. In: Gropper MA, Cohen NH, Eriksson LI, Fleisher LA, Leslie K, Johnson-Akeju O, eds. *Miller's Anesthesia.* 10th ed. Elsevier; 2025:1833-1870.

C.3. How does the liver disease affect intraoperative medication management?

The metabolic activity and clearance of anesthetic medications is impaired in patients with liver disease. Without adjusted doses of medications, duration of drug actions is extended and toxic levels result. Emergence from anesthesia can be prolonged.

Hepatic metabolism takes place via two pathways: biotransformation via the cytochrome P450 system (which requires delivery of oxygen via hepatic perfusion) and glucuronide conjugation. The first is decreased in liver disease; the second is relatively spared when dysfunction begins. Many anesthetic drugs (ie, opioids, barbiturates) bind to plasma albumin. Low albumin levels increase the free fraction of drug and can exaggerate its effects. ESLD alters many other aspects of normal pharmacokinetics such as drug volume of distribution, hepatic extraction and metabolism, renal excretion, and levels of serum proteins other than albumin. The net effect of these changes is unpredictable, making general recommendations for drug administration difficult. A safe approach is to titrate the drug to the desired effect.

Patients with hepatic dysfunction can be more sensitive to sedatives such as midazolam and diazepam. In contrast, lorazepam, which undergoes glucuronidation, is less likely to be affected by liver disease. Benzodiazepines can precipitate hepatic encephalopathy, and flumazenil can reverse this condition. Conversely, patients who have a history of alcohol misuse might require large doses of benzodiazepines. Rapid redistribution of propofol determines its duration of action following bolus injection; this is not affected by impaired liver metabolism.

The adverse effects of morphine can be more pronounced in patients with severe liver disease. Morphine is metabolized by glucuronidation in the liver, and its intermediate metabolites are eliminated renally. Although the pharmacokinetics of morphine can be unaltered in patients with mild hepatic disease, prolonged half-life is associated with more advanced disease. The elimination of morphine's metabolites, some of which are active, can also be prolonged in patients with HRS. Metabolism of fentanyl, sufentanil, and morphine, which have a high hepatic extraction ratio, is slowed by impaired hepatic blood flow.

In patients with liver disease and edema, doses of neuromuscular blocking agents must be increased because fluid retention increases volume of distribution. The duration of action of agents metabolized by the liver (ie, vecuronium and rocuronium) is prolonged. Liver disease reduces plasma cholinesterase activity, and prolonged neuromuscular blockade after succinylcholine has been reported.

Vasodilating anesthetic agents such as propofol and volatile anesthetics cause hypotension if intravascular volume is depleted (eg, overdiuresis or gastrointestinal losses) and reduce liver perfusion. In addition to perioperative hemorrhage and hypotension, volatile anesthetics can reduce hepatic blood flow and hepatic oxygen uptake.

Patients with ESLD often exhibit coagulation disorders. The presence of a coagulopathy is a contraindication to regional anesthesia, particularly epidural anesthesia.

Kiamanesh D, Rumley J, Moitra VK. Monitoring and managing hepatic disease in anaesthesia. *Br J Anaesth.* 2013;111:i50-i61.

C.4. What happens during the first stage (pre-anhepatic phase) of liver transplantation?

The pre-anhepatic phase begins with induction of anesthesia and ends with clamping of the hepatic artery. The diseased liver is mobilized; the suprahepatic and infrahepatic vena cava, portal vein, and hepatic artery are isolated; and the bile duct is divided. The anesthesia team manages disorders of coagulation and hemodynamic disturbances. Large losses of ascites cause hypotension and require early fluid resuscitation. Albumin solution and FFP are often used to replete intravascular volume.

Sakai T. Liver transplantation anesthesiology. In: Subramaniam K, Sakai T, eds. *Anesthesia and Perioperative Care for Organ Transplantation*. Springer Science+Business Media; 2017:353-364.

Wray C, Andreatta B, Adelmann D. Anesthesia for abdominal organ transplantation. In: Gropper MA, Cohen NH, Eriksson LI, Fleisher LA, Leslie K, Johnson-Akeju O, eds. *Miller's Anesthesia*. 10th ed. Elsevier; 2025:1833-1870.

C.5. What happens during the second stage (anhepatic phase) of the liver transplantation?

The second stage of liver transplantation, the anhepatic phase, begins after removal of the diseased liver and ends with reperfusion of the new liver. If the IVC and portal vein are clamped, venous return to the heart and cardiac output decreases. In preparation for clamping and dividing the IVC, a test clamp maneuver (occlusion of the suprahepatic IVC) is performed to assess the resilience of the circulatory system. Hypotension is managed with vasoactive medications, fluid repletion, adjustment of anesthetic agents, correction of hypocalcemia, and venovenous bypass. Anastomoses between the recipient and donor liver are performed in the following order: caval, portal, hepatic artery, and biliary.

Sakai T. Liver transplantation anesthesiology. In: Subramaniam K, Sakai T, eds. *Anesthesia and Perioperative Care for Organ Transplantation*. Springer Science+Business Media; 2017:353-364.

Wray C, Andreatta B, Adelmann D. Anesthesia for abdominal organ transplantation. In: Gropper MA, Cohen NH, Eriksson LI, Fleisher LA, Leslie K, Johnson-Akeju O, eds. *Miller's Anesthesia*. 10th ed. Elsevier; 2025:1833-1870.

C.6. What physiologic disturbances should be anticipated during the second stage (anhepatic phase) of liver transplantation?

Without a liver, the patient can develop acidosis and hypocalcemia due to lack of lactate and citrate metabolism. Acidemia as well as reduced urine output lead to hyperkalemia. In the anhepatic phase, hepatic gluconeogenesis is absent; therefore, blood glucose levels are monitored regularly for both hyperglycemia and hypoglycemia. Decreased clearance of tissue plasminogen activator (tPA) and endogenous heparinoids causes coagulopathy. If possible, aggressive correction of coagulopathy should be avoided during this phase because these changes are temporary and are expected to resolve with graft reperfusion.

Sakai T. Liver transplantation anesthesiology. In: Subramaniam K, Sakai T, eds. *Anesthesia and Perioperative Care for Organ Transplantation*. Springer Science+Business Media; 2017:353-364.

Wray C, Andreatta B, Adelmann D. Anesthesia for abdominal organ transplantation. In: Gropper MA, Cohen NH, Eriksson LI, Fleisher LA, Leslie K, Johnson-Akeju O, eds. *Miller's Anesthesia*. 10th ed. Elsevier; 2025:1833-1870.

C.7. What is venovenous bypass? What are the potential advantages and disadvantages of this procedure?

Some centers routinely use venovenous bypass to divert blood flow from the portal circulation and IVC to the right atrium. Standard venovenous bypass uses a Y-shaped tubing. One limb of the tubing is inserted into the recipient's portal vein to drain the splanchnic beds. Another limb of the tubing is placed, through a groin cut, down into a femoral or iliac vein or the distal IVC. The outflow tubing passes through a pump. Blood returns to the patient through a cut down access to an axillary vein or through percutaneous access to an internal jugular or subclavian vein (**Figure 16.3**).

Venovenous bypass can decompress the portal circulation and reduce congestion of the gut, decrease hemodynamic instability during clamping of the IVC, maintain normothermia via continuous warming of the bypass circuit, manage blood volume overload, preserve renal perfusion pressure, and improve surgical exposure during dissection. Disadvantages include the complications of venous cannula placement

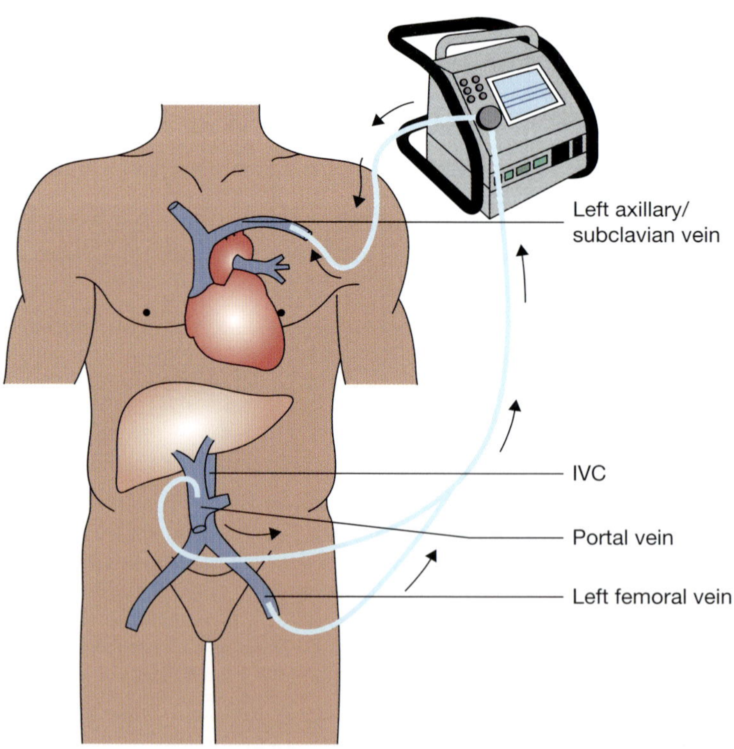

FIGURE 16.3. Schematic diagram of venovenous bypass circuit during liver transplantation. Venous return comes from the femoral and portal veins connected with the tubing connected together into a single venous return line. The centrifugal pump returns the blood into the axillary or subclavian vein. IVC, inferior vena cava.

(bleeding, air, thrombotic embolism); release of proinflammatory mediators; activation of complement, which can contribute to tissue injury and organ failure; and the time and cost of an expensive procedure.

The efficacy and benefits of routine use of venovenous bypass remain controversial. However, portal decompression clearly improves surgical visualization in certain circumstances. Other centers reserve venovenous bypass for situations in which interrupted venous return through the IVC depresses the recipient's circulation; with the increase in popularity of the piggyback anastomosis technique, this indication is less common. Budd-Chiari syndrome is a contraindication for bypass, because there is an increased risk of pulmonary embolism and poor shunt flow rates.

Sakai T. Liver transplantation anesthesiology. In: Subramaniam K, Sakai T, eds. *Anesthesia and Perioperative Care for Organ Transplantation*. Springer Science+Business Media; 2017:353-364.

Sakai T, Gligor S, Diulus J, McAffee R, Wallis Marsh J, Planinsic RM. Insertion and management of percutaneous veno-venous bypass cannula for liver transplantation: a reference for transplant anesthesiologists. *Clin Transplant*. 2010;24:585-591.

C.8. What surgical techniques anastomose the donor and recipient inferior vena cava (IVC)?

There are several techniques to anastomose the donor and recipient IVC. Conventionally, blood flow through the IVC is completely interrupted and a cylinder of the recipient's IVC is removed with the diseased liver. An end-to-end anastomosis is created between the donor and the recipient IVC (**Figure 16.4A**). In the piggyback method, the diseased liver is dissected off the IVC. The recipient IVC is preserved, and blood flow is not completely interrupted. One end of the graft's segment of IVC is oversewn, and the orifice of the hepatic veins (the liver's venous outflow) is anastomosed to the preserved recipient suprahepatic IVC (**Figure 16.4B**). A third technique creates a side-to-side cavo-caval anastomosis (**Figure 16.4C**).

Lam H, Humar A. Anatomy and surgical procedures of liver transplantation. In: Subramaniam K, Sakai T, eds. *Anesthesia and Perioperative Care for Organ Transplantation*. Springer; 2017:345-352.

C.9. What are the potential advantages of "piggyback" (vena cava preservation) technique?

Potential advantages of the piggyback technique for vascular reconstruction include hemodynamic stability because cardiac filling is preserved; protected perfusion pressure; no need for the surgical interventions associated with venovenous bypass; reduced need for retrocaval dissection, which lessens the likelihood of damage to the adrenal vein; and shorter anhepatic and warm ischemia time. A disadvantage of the technique is that outflow obstruction results in hepatic congestion. Unfavorable anatomy in the recipient can preclude the piggyback technique.

Lam H, Humar A. Anatomy and surgical procedures of liver transplantation. In: Subramaniam K, Sakai T, eds. *Anesthesia and Perioperative Care for Organ Transplantation*. Springer; 2017:345-352.

Sakai T. Liver transplantation anesthesiology. In: Subramaniam K, Sakai T, eds. *Anesthesia and Perioperative Care for Organ Transplantation*. Springer; 2017:353-364.

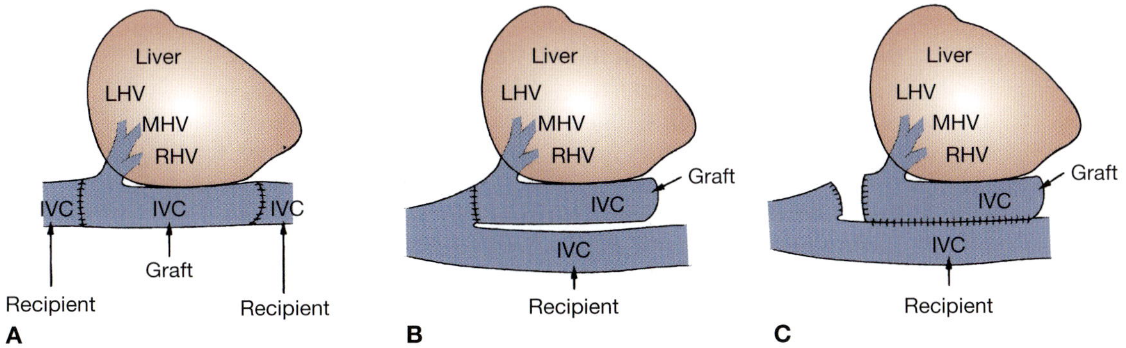

FIGURE 16.4. Three techniques to reconstruct the hepatovenous outflow. A. End-to-end interposition of the donor vena cava to the recipient vena cava. **B.** End-to-end anastomosis of the vena cava to the hepatic veins. **C.** Side-to-side cavo-cavostomy. IVC, inferior vena cava; LHV, left hepatic vein; MHV, middle hepatic vein; RHV, right hepatic vein. (Modified from Hesse UJ, Berrevoet F, Troisi R, et al. Hepatovenous reconstruction in orthotopic liver transplantation with preservation of the recipients' inferior vena cava and veno-venous bypass. *Langenbecks Arch Surg*. 2000;385:350-356.)

C.10. What hemodynamic changes are expected after removal of vascular clamps? What is postreperfusion syndrome?

Removal of the suprahepatic IVC clamp is not associated with hemodynamic changes. Unclamping the infrahepatic IVC restores venous return. After unclamping of the portal vein, desaturated blood from the obstructed portal circulation, inflammatory mediators such as interleukin-6 (IL-6) and tumor necrosis factor-α (TNF-α), potassium, protons, and cold components are released into the systemic circulation. Hemodynamic instability, characterized by a decrease in blood pressure, heart rate, systemic vascular resistance, stroke volume index, and an increase in pulmonary arterial pressures, can follow unclamping of the portal vein and reperfusion of the liver. After reperfusion, an increase in plasma potassium and a decrease in calcium are seen. A sustained 30% decrease in mean arterial blood pressure for more than 1 minute during the first 5 minutes after reperfusion defines postreperfusion syndrome (PRS). A prolonged cold ischemic time, age of the donor, and mismatch in size between the recipient and grafted organ are associated with development of PRS. Careful flushing of the graft just before completion of the anastomoses attenuates reperfusion disturbances by removing the cold hyperkalemic preservative solution as well as mediators of ischemia-reperfusion injury. Although venovenous bypass provides improved hemodynamic stability, it is not protective for PRS.

Before reperfusing the new graft, the following measures should be considered: (1) preemptive administration of calcium to correct hypocalcemia; (2) sodium bicarbonate, dichloroacetate, or THAM to adjust pH; and (3) inotropes or vasopressors for circulatory support. The surgical and anesthesia teams must be prepared to diagnose and treat dysrhythmias or cardiac arrest.

Siniscalchi A, Gamberini L, Laici C, et al. Post reperfusion syndrome during liver transplantation: from pathophysiology to therapy and preventive strategies. *World J Gastroenterol.* 2016;22:1551-1569.

C.11. How would you treat hyperkalemia?

Hyperkalemia is treated with diuretics, aldosterone agonists, β-adrenergic agonists, insulin in combination with glucose, and alkalinization via hyperventilation. Calcium should be administered to temporarily stabilize the myocardium and prevent arrhythmias. Rarely, when hyperkalemia is refractory to the preceding treatments, dialysis with continuous venovenous hemofiltration may reduce the elevated serum potassium level.

Wray C, Andreatta B, Adelmann D. Anesthesia for abdominal organ transplantation. In: Gropper MA, Cohen NH, Eriksson LI, Fleisher LA, Leslie K, Johnson-Akeju O, eds. *Miller's Anesthesia.* 10th ed. Elsevier; 2025:1833-1870.

C.12. Why should you anticipate hypocalcemia?

The principal reason to anticipate hypocalcemia is a failure to clear citrate, which normally is metabolized by the liver. This calcium-chelating agent accumulates in patients who receive transfusion of citrated blood products.

Wray C, Andreatta B, Adelmann D. Anesthesia for abdominal organ transplantation. In: Gropper MA, Cohen NH, Eriksson LI, Fleisher LA, Leslie K, Johnson-Akeju O, eds. *Miller's Anesthesia.* 10th ed. Elsevier; 2025:1833-1870.

C.13. What happens during the third stage of liver transplantation?

The third stage of the liver transplantation, the neohepatic phase, follows reperfusion of the new liver. After stable hemodynamic status is achieved following reperfusion, the remaining inflow vessels are anastomosed and the biliary drainage system is constructed. Reconstruction can be straightforward, with an anastomosis between the graft's common bile duct and the biliary stump of the recipient. More complex reconstructions are sometimes required, such as creation of a choledochojejunostomy. A donor cholecystectomy is generally performed. A T-tube is placed in the reconstructed biliary outflow system, with external drainage. The third stage ends with closure of all incisions and transport to the intensive care unit.

During the third stage of the procedure, it is important to monitor the coagulation status to ensure hemostasis before proceeding to biliary reconstruction. Coagulation status reflected by viscoelastic testing 30 minutes after graft reperfusion can guide further coagulation management and assessment of hepatic function because a reasonable improvement in the coagulation profile is expected at this stage.

Sakai T. Liver transplantation anesthesiology. In: Subramaniam K, Sakai T, eds. *Anesthesia and Perioperative Care for Organ Transplantation.* Springer; 2017:353-364.

C.14. What causes intraoperative bleeding during each phase of liver transplantation? How is coagulopathy monitored and treated? What are thromboelastography (TEG) and rotational thromboelastography (ROTEM)?

The etiology of intraoperative bleeding during liver transplantation is multifactorial. Patients with ESLD have serious hemostatic defects, and coagulation is also affected by alterations in body temperature, tissue perfusion, acid-base balance, and fluid balance.

During the pre-anhepatic phase, bleeding from the surgical dissection is influenced by the patient's underlying coagulopathy. Excessive fluid administration can produce dilutional coagulopathy and increase venous congestion of the splanchnic area, leading to more bleeding at the surgical site. Bleeding can be minimal in a hypercoagulable state such as hepatocellular carcinoma or cholestatic cirrhosis.

During the anhepatic phase, there is a net increase in systemic tPA derived from endothelial cells, which is normally cleared by the liver. Although PT and aPTT values might not change, hyperfibrinolysis is possible.

During reperfusion, bleeding from the surgical anastomotic sites and insidious bleeding can be profound. Disseminated intravascular coagulation, increased fibrinolysis, release of heparin or heparin-like substances, and platelets trapped in the graft cause coagulopathy. After reperfusion, platelet counts drop due to sinusoidal obstruction and entrapment by the new liver, generalized platelet aggregation, and a consumptive disseminated intravascular coagulation-like process.

Coagulation status should be monitored by inspection of the surgical field. Routine laboratory tests (PT, aPTT, platelet count, fibrinogen level) are used in some centers for evaluating the coagulation status and directing treatment. Multiple studies have shown that routine laboratory tests have limited utility in the ESLD population because of complex changes in hemostasis. Viscoelastic tests (TEG or ROTEM) assess the viscoelastic properties of a whole blood sample as a function of time to reflect the global function and interaction of the plasma, blood cells, and platelets. These measurements detect hypercoagulability and distinguish hyperfibrinolysis from other causes of coagulopathy, such as factor depletion or thrombocytopenia, to offer a dynamic and rapid composite picture of the entire clotting cascade. Heparinase can be used to help diagnose coagulopathy resulting from the presence of heparinoids (see Chapter 12: Cardiac Tamponade, Section A.11 and Chapter 57: Trauma, Section C.13).

Over-transfusion of procoagulant blood products and factors should be avoided to minimize thrombotic complications. Platelet transfusion has been associated with mortality and graft survival in liver transplants. Cryoprecipitate administration is associated with major thrombotic complications in liver transplant. Occasionally, prothrombin complex concentrate can be used to correct refractory coagulopathy or to counteract the effects of oral anticoagulant medication that was not discontinued prior to surgery.

Bezinover D, Dirkmann D, Findlay J, et al. Perioperative coagulation management in liver transplant recipients. *Transplantation*. 2018;102:578-591.

Clevenger B, Mallett SV. Transfusion and coagulation management in liver transplantation. *World J Gastroenterol*. 2014;20:6146-6158.

Nguyen-Buckley C, Gao W, Agopian V, Wray C, Steadman RH, Xia VW. Major thromboembolic complications in liver transplantation: the role of rotational thromboelastometry and cryoprecipitate infusion. *Transplantation*. 2021;105:1771-1777.

Pillai AA, Kriss M, Al-Adra DP, et al. Coagulopathy and hemostasis management in patients undergoing liver transplantation: defining a dynamic spectrum across phases of care. *Liver Transpl*. 2022;28:1651-1663.

C.15. What are the complications of massive transfusion?

Uncontrolled hemorrhage and massive transfusion can lead to the lethal triad of acidosis, coagulopathy, and hypothermia. Left uncorrected, each of these abnormalities can exacerbate the other, creating a "blood vicious cycle." Additional early complications of massive transfusion include (1) acute hemolytic transfusion reactions, (2) febrile nonhemolytic transfusion reactions, (3) transfusion-related acute lung injury, (4) transfusion-associated circulatory overload, (5) allergic reactions, (6) bacterial sepsis, (7) hypocalcemia, (8) hyperkalemia, and (9) transfusion-related immunomodulation.

Sihler KC, Napolitano LM. Complications of massive transfusion. *Chest*. 2010;137:209-220.

C.16. How are the complications of massive transfusion prevented?

Warming the room, applying forced warming systems, administering blood products and fluids through a fluid warmer, and heating and humidifying inspired gases help reduce the risk of hypothermia. Dilutional coagulopathy and thrombocytopenia were previously prevented by transfusing packed red blood cells, FFP, and platelets in a 1:1:1 ratio. Because of increased morbidity and mortality with blood product transfusion in liver transplantation, bedside-guided transfusion with TEG or ROTEM is encouraged. Potassium, magnesium, and calcium levels are frequently monitored and corrected. Metabolic acidosis is managed by improving hemodynamic parameters, adjusting minute ventilation, and administering sodium bicarbonate or tromethamine for severe metabolic acidosis. The risk of transfusion-related acute lung injury (TRALI) can be reduced by minimizing transfusions and transfusing packed red blood cells with a short storage time and FFP from male or nulliparous female donors.

Hartmann M, Szalai C, Saner FH. Hemostasis in liver transplantation: pathophysiology, monitoring, and treatment. *World J Gastroenterol.* 2016;22:1541-1550.

Pillai AA, Kriss M, Al-Adra DP, et al. Coagulopathy and hemostasis management in patients undergoing liver transplantation: defining a dynamic spectrum across phases of care. *Liver Transpl.* 2022;28:1651-1663.

Sihler KC, Napolitano LM. Complications of massive transfusion. *Chest.* 2010;137:209-220.

C.17. How is hyperfibrinolysis managed?

tPA has been implicated as causal in hyperfibrinolysis. A functioning graft liver will eventually clear excess tPA from the circulation; however, levels seem to peak at reperfusion and are associated with greater intraoperative blood loss. Pharmacologic therapy with antifibrinolytic agents (tranexamic acid, ε-aminocaproic acid) blocks fibrin degradation by plasmin, but the full spectrum of their actions remains incompletely defined. The use of prophylactic antifibrinolytic agents in liver transplant surgery can reduce transfusion requirements, but this remains controversial because of concern for development of thromboses that can be catastrophic.

Badenoch A, Sharma A, Gower S, et al. The effectiveness and safety of tranexamic acid in orthotopic liver transplantation clinical practice: a propensity score matched cohort study. *Transplantation.* 2017;101:1658-1665.

Kim E, Ko JS, Gwak M, et al. Incidence and clinical significance of hyperfibrinolysis during living donor liver transplantation. *Blood Coagul Fibrinolysis.* 2018;29:322-326.

Pillai AA, Kriss M, Al-Adra DP, et al. Coagulopathy and hemostasis management in patients undergoing liver transplantation: defining a dynamic spectrum across phases of care. *Liver Transpl.* 2022;28:1651-1663.

C.18. When is intraoperative renal replacement therapy (RRT) indicated?

Managing patients with low urine output, renal dysfunction, or preoperative hyperkalemia who undergo liver transplantation is challenging. Continuous RRT can be used intraoperatively to manage volume shifts, acid-base balance, and electrolyte disturbances. There are no guidelines governing the decision to utilize intraoperative RRT; however, patients with underlying renal dysfunction, higher MELD scores, and worse illness severity can benefit from RRT.

Huang H, Xu Y, Zhou H, Zhu Y, Qin J. Intraoperative continuous renal replacement therapy during liver transplantation: a meta-analysis. *Liver Transpl.* 2020;26:1010-1018.

Townsend DR, Bagshaw SM, Jacka MJ, et al. Intraoperative renal support during liver transplantation. *Liver Transpl.* 2009;15:73-78.

C.19. What intraoperative signs suggest that the hepatic graft is working?

Good texture and color of the graft, evidence of bile production, and hemodynamic stability are signs that the graft is working. Hypocalcemia often resolves quickly, even with rapid FFP administration. Metabolic alkalemia can develop as a result of citrate metabolism. Potassium levels tend to normalize with the onset of hepatocyte function. A number of recipients exhibit hyperglycemia resistant to insulin.

Choi C, Manecke GR, Lindberg S, Steadman RH. Transplant anesthesia. In: Cullen BF, Stock MC, Ortega R, et al, eds. *Barash, Cullen, and Stoelting's Clinical Anesthesia.* 9th ed. Wolters Kluwer; 2024:1407-1435.

D. Postoperative Management

D.1. What are the goals of immediate postoperative care of the liver transplant patient?

After liver transplantation, patients are admitted to the intensive care unit for monitoring of organ function, management of intraoperative complications, correction of coagulopathy, evaluation of graft function, and initiation of immunosuppression. Although many patients remain on mechanical ventilation for 24 hours or more, there is a growing trend toward early extubation, especially in patients with low baseline mortality, low intraoperative blood product transfusion requirement, and low vasopressor requirement at the end of the case.

Haque ME, Badenoch AD, Orlov D, Selzner M, McCluskey SA. Predicting early extubation after liver transplantation: external validation and improved generalizability of a proposed fast-track score. *Transplantation*. 2021;105:2029-2036.

Wray C, Andreatta B, Adelmann D. Anesthesia for abdominal organ transplantation. In: Gropper MA, Cohen NH, Eriksson LI, Fleisher LA, Leslie K, Johnson-Akeju O, eds. *Miller's Anesthesia*. 10th ed. Elsevier; 2025:1833-1870.

D.2. What postoperative findings suggest that the hepatic graft is functioning?

Clearance of lactic acid, production of glucose, resolution of encephalopathy, normothermia, normalization of coagulopathy, decreasing total bilirubin levels, production of bile (through the biliary tube), and adequate urine output suggest a functioning graft. Preservation injury causes transaminases to rise immediately after surgery, but enzyme levels usually fall within 24 to 48 hours. New synthesis of coagulation factors will not correct factor depletion for hours to days after the transplant.

Wray C, Andreatta B, Adelmann D. Anesthesia for abdominal organ transplantation. In: Gropper MA, Cohen NH, Eriksson LI, Fleisher LA, Leslie K, Johnson-Akeju O, eds. *Miller's Anesthesia*. 10th ed. Elsevier; 2025:1833-1870.

D.3. What coagulation disturbances should be anticipated in the postoperative period?

Typically, heparin effects, disseminated intravascular coagulation, or hyperfibrinolysis have been resolved in the operating room. However, dilutional coagulopathy, along with ongoing platelet and factor consumption in the early postoperative phase and poor graft function, contribute to clinical bleeding. Postoperative uremia also compromises platelet function. A functioning graft liver does not produce substantial levels of clotting factors for several days. Therefore, fresh or frozen plasma, cryoprecipitate, and/or platelets might be needed in the early postoperative period.

Wray C, Andreatta B, Adelmann D. Anesthesia for abdominal organ transplantation. In: Gropper MA, Cohen NH, Eriksson LI, Fleisher LA, Leslie K, Johnson-Akeju O, eds. *Miller's Anesthesia*. 10th ed. Elsevier; 2025:1833-1870.

D.4. Can renal function change after liver transplantation?

Postoperative renal function is correlated with preoperative glomerular filtration rate, and about 10% of liver transplant patients require postoperative dialysis. For patients on RRT prior to surgery, rate of renal recovery is negatively associated with increasing age, presence of diabetes mellitus, and duration of RRT for more than 8 weeks. An expedited liver transplant for patients with high MELD scores on preoperative RRT is likely to reduce the need for postoperative RRT and future kidney transplant. For patients with cirrhosis who have HRS resistant to diuretics, renal function can improve after transplantation. Postoperatively, sepsis and the nephrotoxic calcineurin inhibitors such as cyclosporin A and FK-506 (tacrolimus) contribute to renal dysfunction. A balanced immunosuppression regimen can minimize posttransplant renal dysfunction. Chronic allograft nephropathy in patients who have received liver, heart, lung, or kidney transplants is now the third most common reason for patients to be on the waiting list for a kidney transplant.

Ali B, Gadiparthi C, Cholankeril G, Satapathy SK, Eason J, Nair S. Expedited liver transplant enables recovery of renal function in patients with high MELD (MELD≥35) on renal replacement therapy at the time of isolated liver transplant. *Gastroenterology*. 2017;152:S1125-S1126.

Trotter J, Kahn B. Renal dysfunction and the liver transplant recipient; novel strategies for determination of reversibility and renal protective therapies pretransplant and posttransplant. *Curr Opin Organ Transplant*. 2012;17:225-229.

D.5. What vascular and biliary complications can occur after liver transplantation?

Arterial and venous vascular complications include anastomotic bleeding leading to hypovolemia, acute stenosis or occlusion from thrombosis or kinking of the graft vessels, and development of an aneurysm or pseudoaneurysm. Thrombosis of the portal vein or hepatic artery compromises viability of the graft. Abdominal Doppler ultrasound is used to assess the hepatic vessels. Hepatic artery thrombosis, which is more common than portal vein thrombosis, can cause severe liver failure from necrosis. Portal vein thrombosis can cause liver dysfunction, tense ascites, and variceal bleeding.

Biliary complications include bile leak, bile duct stricture, ductal stones, and sphincter of Oddi dysfunction, and are associated with the use of T-tubes, Roux-en-Y anastomoses, ischemia-reperfusion injury, cytomegalovirus infection, and hepatic artery thrombosis (leading to duct ischemia). Patients with bile leaks experience fever, abdominal pain, and peritoneal irritation. Bile leaks develop early in the postoperative course and can be identified by ultrasonography showing abdominal fluid collections or cholangiography. Bile leaks are managed with endoscopic placement of a biliary stent or relaparotomy.

TABLE 16.1 Adverse Effects of Immunosuppressant Medications

Medication	Adverse Effects
FK-506 (tacrolimus)	Nephrotoxicity Hypertension Neurotoxicity (tremors, seizures, posterior leukoencephalopathy)
Cyclosporine	Nephrotoxicity Hypertension
Mycophenolate mofetil	Hypertension Bone marrow suppression Abdominal pain Diarrhea Vomiting
Azathioprine	Leukopenia Anemia Thrombocytopenia
Glucocorticoid	Glucose intolerance Osteoporosis Peptic ulcer disease Adrenal suppression
OKT3	Symptoms of cytokine release (fever, chills, dyspnea, wheezing, chest pain) Leukopenia
Basiliximab	Gastrointestinal upset
Daclizumab	Gastrointestinal upset

Kochhar G, Parungao JM, Hanouneh IA, et al. Biliary complications following liver transplantation. *World J Gastroenterol.* 2013;19:2841-2846.

Lam H, Humar A. Anatomy and surgical procedures of liver transplantation. In: Subramaniam K, Sakai T, eds. *Anesthesia and Perioperative Care for Organ Transplantation.* Springer; 2017:345-352.

D.6. What immunosuppressive agents will be given after liver transplantation? What are the major side effects?

Immunosuppression after liver transplantation is divided into the induction and maintenance phases. The risk of organ rejection is balanced against the adverse side effects of immunosuppressive medications (ie, neurotoxicity, nephrotoxicity, infection, metabolic abnormalities, malignancy, and recurrence of pretransplant conditions such as hepatitis C, hepatocellular carcinoma, and sclerosing cholangitis). Although protocols vary, newer regimens have reduced the degree of immunosuppression. Induction therapy usually consists of intravenous corticosteroids immediately posttransplant for several days until oral corticosteroids can be initiated. Use of IL-2 receptor antibodies (eg, basiliximab) or antibodies directed against T-cell lymphocytes (eg, antithymocyte globulin) is increasing because these are often used to delay introduction of calcineurin inhibitor (CNI) therapy (eg, cyclosporine or FK-506 [tacrolimus]) in patients with kidney dysfunction. CNIs are the mainstay of maintenance therapy. Antiproliferative agents, such as mycophenolic acid and azathioprine, and mammalian target of rapamycin (mTOR) inhibitors can be used to lower the toxicity of CNI therapy or for those at higher risk of rejection, usually in combination with lower dose CNI therapy. The adverse effects of these medications are listed in **Table 16.1**.

Charlton M, Levitsky J, Aqel B, et al. International liver transplantation society consensus statement on immunosuppression in liver transplant recipients. *Transplantation.* 2018;102:727-743.

Moser MA. Options for induction immunosuppression in liver transplant recipients. *Drugs.* 2002;62:995-1011.

Acknowledgment

We gratefully acknowledge the contributions of previous edition author, Christopher H. Choi, as portions of those chapters have been retained in this revision.

17

Robotic-Assisted Laparoscopic Surgery

Seema Brar and Peter A. Goldstein

A 74-year-old female with biopsy-proven colon cancer (localized, not metastatic) has chosen to pursue surgical treatment, specifically robotic laparoscopic resection of the colon. Her comorbidities include hypertension and atrial fibrillation, for which she takes apixaban, but otherwise negative cardiac workup, and her exercise tolerance is more than four metabolic equivalents (METs). She has a 50 pack-year smoking history (former smoker), has controlled chronic obstructive pulmonary disease (COPD), and her body mass index (BMI) is 40. She has an unremarkable personal and family history of adverse events with anesthesia.

A. Medical Disease and Differential Diagnosis

1. What is the incidence of colorectal cancer?
2. How is colorectal cancer diagnosed?
3. How is colorectal cancer treated?
4. Define laparoscopy.
5. Describe the development of robotic-assisted laparoscopy.
6. What are the advantages and disadvantages of minimally invasive surgery over open surgery?
7. What are the contraindications to laparoscopic or robotic-assisted laparoscopic surgery? Is pregnancy a contraindication to robotic surgery?
8. What other specialties commonly perform robotic surgery?
9. Why is carbon dioxide (CO_2) the gas of choice for robotic laparoscopy? What are its disadvantages?
10. How much endogenous CO_2 is produced at the basal level and at maximal exercise?
11. How much CO_2 is stored in the body? Where is it stored? Of what significance is this to laparoscopy?
12. Describe the diffusion and solubility properties of CO_2 and their significance in laparoscopy.
13. Is CO_2 soluble in water or plasma? Is it soluble in blood? Why?

B. Preoperative Evaluation and Preparation

1. What do you want to know about this patient's history and physical condition that might affect whether she is cleared for robotic surgery?
2. What factors increase this patient's risk of pulmonary complications?
3. What laboratory tests should be performed preoperatively?
4. What specific information should the patient be given about robotic surgery before obtaining informed consent?
5. What additional procedures should be done before surgery?
6. What are the three major forces that uniquely alter physiology during robotic laparoscopy?

C. Intraoperative Management

1. What is the anesthetic technique of choice for robotic-assisted laparoscopy? Why?
2. Can a laryngeal mask airway (LMA) be used?
3. What anesthetic agents or adjuvant drugs are recommended for laparoscopy? Are any anesthetic agents contraindicated?
4. Should nitrous oxide (N_2O) be used during laparoscopy? What are the pros and cons? Does N_2O cause bowel distension during laparoscopy? Does N_2O cause nausea and vomiting after laparoscopy?
5. Can laparoscopy be performed under local or regional anesthesia?
6. What monitors and devices would you apply to the patient? Why?

7. How is the patient to be positioned? What special precautions are required for robotic laparoscopy?
8. How will you ventilate the patient? What are the respiratory and circulatory effects of the Trendelenburg position during laparoscopy?
9. What techniques are available for initial access to the peritoneal cavity? What anesthetic problems can arise during insufflation?
10. What intravenous (IV) solution and how much fluid volume do you plan to infuse?
11. Under what circumstances should laparoscopy be converted to laparotomy?
12. What is the arterial to end-tidal CO_2 gradient ($Paco_2$-$Etco_2$) in the normal awake patient? What is the cause of the gradient? Does the gradient change during laparoscopy? Why?
13. Is an arterial catheter necessary? Why? Does end-tidal CO_2 ($Etco_2$) tension accurately reflect arterial CO_2 tension? Under what circumstances can the $Etco_2$ exceed the $Paco_2$? Why?
14. What are the possible causes of hypercarbia?
15. What factors play a role in the unusually rapid and marked elevation of CO_2 that is sometimes seen in laparoscopy?
16. How rapidly does the $Paco_2$ rise in a patient with apnea (endogenous CO_2)? How rapidly does the $Paco_2$ rise if 5% CO_2 gas is inhaled (exogenous)? How rapidly can the CO_2 rise during laparoscopy? What factors explain the differences?
17. What is the net effect of pneumoperitoneum, hypercarbia, and steep Trendelenburg on the cardiovascular system?
18. What is the net effect of pneumoperitoneum, hypercarbia, and steep Trendelenburg on the respiratory system?
19. What is the net effect of pneumoperitoneum, hypercarbia, and steep Trendelenburg on the central nervous system?
20. What are the neuroendocrine changes that occur during laparoscopy?
21. What is the net effect of pneumoperitoneum, hypercarbia, and steep Trendelenburg on the renal system?
22. What is the net effect of pneumoperitoneum, hypercarbia, and steep Trendelenburg on the bowel and gastrointestinal system?
23. How would you recognize a CO_2 embolism during laparoscopy? How does this differ from an air embolism? Why should N_2O be discontinued during suspected embolization? Will N_2O increase the size of CO_2 emboli?
24. What is the mechanism of increased shunting resulting from embolization?
25. How is a gas embolism (CO_2 or air) treated?
26. What are the causes of pneumothorax or pneumomediastinum during laparoscopy? How would you diagnose it? How would you treat it?
27. How would you decide when to extubate the trachea?

D. Postoperative Management

1. What are some of the unique complications of laparoscopy?
2. In the postanesthesia care unit (PACU), the patient complains of numbness and weakness of the lower extremities after 6 hours of anesthesia for robotic prostatectomy. What tests will you order? When would you remove the Foley catheter and arterial line? Under what circumstances would you order a chest radiograph?
3. What is the incidence of postoperative nausea and vomiting (PONV)?

A. Medical Disease and Differential Diagnosis

A.1. What is the incidence of colorectal cancer?

Colorectal cancer is the third most common type of cancer diagnosed in males and females in the United States (excluding skin cancer). The American Cancer Society estimated that in 2023, there will be over 100,000 new cases of colon cancer and over 40,000 new cases of rectal cancer in the United States. The lifetime risk for colorectal cancer is 1 in 23 for males and 1 in 26 for females. Over the past few decades, the rate of new colorectal cancer diagnosis has declined. This is likely related to a modification in lifestyle risk factors and an increase in screening programs. In the previous decade (2011-2019), incidence rates decreased by 1% each year, but this decline was most prominent in older adults. In adults younger than 50 years old, incidence rates have increased by 1% to 2% each year. In the United States, American

Indians and Alaskan natives have the highest rates of colorectal cancer, while African Americans have the second highest rate. The Ashkenazi Jewish ethnic group has the highest risk of colorectal cancer in the world.

In both males and females in the United States, colorectal cancer is the third leading cause of cancer-related death. Combining males and females, it becomes the second leading cause of cancer death. In 2023, it is estimated that colorectal cancer will lead to over 50,000 deaths. However, death from colorectal cancer has declined over the past few decades, likely due to improved screening and improvements in treatment.

American Cancer Society. Colorectal cancer facts and figures. 2020-2022. Accessed March 2023. https://www.cancer.org/cancer/colon-rectal-cancer/about/key-statistics.html

Zavala VA, Bracci PM, Carethers JM, et al. Cancer Health disparities in racial/ethnic minorities in the United States. *Br J Cancer*. 2021;124:315-332.

A.2. How is colorectal cancer diagnosed?

Screening is a very important tool for early detection and diagnosis of colorectal cancer. This is particularly true for people with a personal or family history of colorectal cancer (or adenomatous polyps), inflammatory bowel disease, an inherited disorder (Lynch syndrome or familial adenomatous polyposis), or with other risk factors (such as older age, smoking, heavy alcohol use, obesity, and inactivity). Those with a personal history of adenomatous polyps are at increased risk of developing colorectal cancer (particularly if dysplasia is detected), and those with a personal history of colorectal cancer, even if treated, are more likely to develop a secondary colorectal cancer. There are two main types of screening tools: stool-based tests (fecal immunochemical test or guaiac-based fecal occult blood test) and colonoscopy/flexible sigmoidoscopy or virtual colonoscopy. If polyps are detected on colonoscopy, they can be biopsied and sent to pathology (and also removed at an early stage before developing into advanced cancer). If colorectal cancer is detected, further computed tomography (CT)/magnetic resonance imaging (MRI) and positron emission tomography (PET) scanning are done to stage the cancer. Stages can be classified as localized, regional (spread to adjacent structures/lymph nodes), or distant (metastatic). The American Joint Committee on Cancer (AJCC) also stages colorectal cancer based on the TNM (tumor extent, lymph nodes, metastasis) classification.

American Cancer Society. Colorectal cancer facts and figures. 2020-2022. Accessed March 31, 2023. https://www.cancer.org/cancer/colon-rectal-cancer/about/key-statistics.html

A.3. How is colorectal cancer treated?

Treatment choices for colorectal cancer depend on the stage of the disease and patient factors such as age, associated medical conditions, and life expectancy. Local treatments include surgery, ablation and embolization, and radiation therapy (alone or in combination). Surgical options include polypectomy and local excision (performed during colonoscopy) for early colorectal cancers. More advanced colon cancers require colectomy with lymph node dissection; this can range from a hemicolectomy, partial colectomy, segmental resection, to total colectomy. Rectal cancers can require a transanal excision, low anterior resection, proctectomy, or abdominoperineal resection. Some patients require colostomy or ileostomy. The surgical approach can be open or a minimally invasive approach, including laparoscopic and robotic techniques. Systemic treatments include chemotherapy, targeted drug therapy, and immunotherapy; these can be combined with a surgical approach.

American Cancer Society. Colorectal cancer facts and figures. 2020-2022. Accessed March 31, 2023. https://www.cancer.org/cancer/colon-rectal-cancer/about/key-statistics.html

Huynh C, Minkova S, Kim D, Stuart H, Hamilton TD. Laparoscopic versus open resection in patients with locally advanced colon cancer. *Surgery*. 2021;170:1610-1615.

A.4. Define laparoscopy.

Laparoscopy is a minimally invasive procedure, allowing endoscopic access to the peritoneal cavity after insufflation of a gas (CO_2) to create space between the anterior abdominal wall and the viscera. The space is necessary for the safe manipulation of instruments and organs. Laparoscopic surgery can also be extraperitoneal. It can also be gasless with abdominal wall retraction, and more recently, it can be hand-assisted or robotically assisted.

A.5. Describe the development of robotic-assisted laparoscopy.

Minimally invasive surgery involves using laparoscopes (cameras) that can be inserted through small ports in the abdomen and insufflation of the abdomen. However, conventional laparoscopy is limited by poor depth perception (visualization on a two-dimensional monitor) and the use of long, straight instruments with limited mobility and dexterity.

Robotic devices were initially designed by the National Aeronautics and Space Administration (NASA). This technology was adapted for surgery as the da Vinci computer-assisted robotic system (Intuitive Surgical Inc). In robotic surgery, the surgeon sits at a remote control console near the patient and operating room table and views the operative field as a high-resolution, magnified, three-dimensional image transmitted from a video camera. Using hand-and-finger control devices, the surgeon can precisely manipulate the mechanical arms of the robot to achieve wrist-like motion. Foot pedals also allow more precise control of the robot, camera, and cautery.

Awad H, Walker CM, Shaikh M, et al. Anesthetic considerations for robotic prostatectomy: a review of the literature. *J Clin Anesth*. 2012;24:494-504.

A.6. What are the advantages and disadvantages of minimally invasive surgery over open surgery?

Advantages of a minimally invasive approach include smaller incision sites, decreased blood loss, less postoperative pain and ileus, shorter hospitalization stays, and ultimately lower cost. Postoperative respiratory muscle function returns to baseline more quickly than in open surgery, especially in upper abdominal procedures. Wound complications such as infection and dehiscence are less frequent than in open procedures.

The disadvantages include the significant learning curve for the surgeon, the narrowed two-dimensional visual field on video in conventional laparoscopy, the need for general anesthesia with muscle paralysis, and potentially longer operative time.

In contrast to nonrobotic procedures, robotic-assisted laparoscopy provides high-resolution three-dimensional visualization and greater precision, offers a greater likelihood of nerve sparing in prostatectomy and, therefore, retention of continence and sexual potency. The disadvantages of robotic surgery include added operative time, the high cost of equipment (capital cost for the robot [millions of dollars] and nonreusable consumables [thousands of dollars]), and the need for a dedicated operating room location for the large equipment.

Soto E, Lo Y, Friedman K, et al. Total laparoscopic hysterectomy versus da Vinci robotic hysterectomy: is using the robot beneficial? *J Gynecol Oncol*. 2011;22:253-259.

Wilson T, Torrey R. Open versus robotic-assisted radical prostatectomy: which is better? *Curr Opin Urol*. 2011;21:200-205.

A.7. What are the contraindications to laparoscopic or robotic-assisted laparoscopic surgery? Is pregnancy a contraindication to robotic surgery?

Most contraindications to laparoscopic surgery are relative, rather than absolute. Most of the contraindications involve patients who are unable to tolerate extremes of position, pneumoperitoneum, and/or hypercarbia. Relative contraindications include severe cardiovascular or pulmonary disease (including bullae), morbid obesity, increased intracranial pressure or space-occupying masses, coagulopathy, diaphragmatic hernia, retinal detachment, acute glaucoma, renal dysfunction, a history of extensive surgery or adhesions, sickle cell disease, peritonitis, a large intra-abdominal mass, a tumor of the abdominal wall, or hypovolemic shock. Patients with ventriculoperitoneal shunts are at higher risk for gas emboli, shunt obstruction, and intracranial hypertension. These adverse events can occur during laparoscopy and can require intracranial pressure monitoring and ventricular drainage. The decision to proceed with laparoscopic or robotic-assisted surgery requires clinician judgment, the relative risk or tolerance of the patient, and the benefit of having minimally invasive surgery for the patient. Pregnancy is no longer considered a contraindication to robotic surgery; however, consultation with the obstetrician concerning the need for preoperative and postoperative fetal and uterine monitoring is required.

Chohan L, Kilpatrick CC. Laparoscopy in pregnancy: a literature review. *Clin Obstet Gynecol*. 2009;52:557-569.

Ravaoherisoa J, Meyer P, Afriat R, et al. Laparoscopic surgery in a patient with ventriculoperitoneal shunt: monitoring of shunt function with transcranial Doppler. *Br J Anaesth*. 2004;92:434-437.

Steinbrook RA, Bhavani-Shankar K. Hemodynamics during laparoscopic surgery in pregnancy. *Anesth Analg*. 2001;93:1570-1571.

A.8. What other specialties commonly perform robotic surgery?

Robotic procedures in urology have become standard, especially for prostatectomy, uncomplicated adrenalectomy, and nephrectomy. Robotic gynecologic surgery includes tubal surgery, cystectomies, hysterectomies, and ablations (eg, for endometriosis). Robotic surgery can be performed in pregnancy and also in pediatrics. Robotic general surgery routinely includes cholecystectomy, hernia repair, antireflux procedures, splenectomy, appendectomy, bowel surgery including bariatric procedures (see Chapter 63: Morbid Obesity, Obstructive Sleep Apnea, and Bariatric Anesthesia), and various abdominal procedures. As presented in this case, robot-assisted surgery can be used in procedures on the colon and rectum (for colorectal cancer).

Robotic surgery is also used in thoracoscopic, cardiovascular, and neurosurgical intracranial surgery, using modified laparoscopic instruments without the need for gas insufflation. Lumbar discectomies and other types of spinal surgery have also been done laparoscopically through an anterior approach.

Muñoz CJ, Nguyen HT, Houck CS. Robotic surgery and anesthesia for pediatric urologic procedures. *Curr Opin Anaesthesiol.* 2016;29:337-344.

Rodrigues ES, Lynch JJ, Suri RM, et al. Robotic mitral valve repair: a review of anesthetic management of the first 200 patients. *J Cardiothorac Vasc Anesth.* 2014;28:64-68.

A.9. Why is carbon dioxide (CO_2) the gas of choice for robotic laparoscopy? What are its disadvantages?

CO_2 is used for insufflation as it is nonflammable, does not support combustion, readily diffuses across membranes, is rapidly eliminated by the lungs, and is highly soluble (buffered in whole blood). The risk of CO_2 embolization is small (compared to air embolism). It is easy to measure CO_2 levels in blood and expired air. As long as oxygen requirements are met, a high concentration of blood CO_2 can be tolerated. CO_2 elimination is easy to facilitate by increasing minute ventilation. Lastly, medical grade CO_2 is readily available and inexpensive.

These gases are unsatisfactory for pneumoperitoneum: N_2O (does not cause pain intra-abdominally but does not suppress combustion); oxygen (facilitates combustion); helium, air, and nitrogen (each has no hemodynamic or acid-base sequelae but can cause gas emboli); and argon (adverse effect on hepatic blood flow, emboli).

The disadvantages of CO_2 are that it is not inert. Changes in its concentration and tension have significant biochemical and physiologic consequences. It causes direct peritoneal irritation and pain during laparoscopy (under local anesthesia and postoperatively). In addition, CO_2 is not very soluble in blood in the absence of red blood cells; it can remain in gaseous form intraperitoneally (subhepatic) after laparoscopy, causing referred shoulder pain. Hypercarbia and respiratory acidosis occur when the buffering capacity of blood is exceeded. In addition, CO_2 exerts systemic effects, resulting in hypertension, tachycardia, cerebral vasodilation, hypercarbia, and respiratory acidosis.

Menes T, Spivak H. Laparoscopy: searching for the proper insufflation gas. *Surg Endosc.* 2000;14:1050-1056.

Tsereteli Z, Terry ML, Bowers SP, et al. Prospective randomized clinical trial comparing nitrous oxide and carbon dioxide pneumoperitoneum for laparoscopic surgery. *J Am Coll Surg.* 2002;195:173-180.

A.10. How much endogenous CO_2 is produced at the basal level and at maximal exercise?

CO_2 and water are the major end products of aerobic metabolism in the mitochondria of cells. CO_2 and water react to create carbonic acid (H_2CO_3), which is catalyzed by carbonic anhydrase. Carbonic acid readily dissociates into bicarbonate (HCO_3^-) and H^+ ions, and HCO_3^- is renally excreted. CO_2 is cleared through the lungs.

The average adult creates approximately 200 mL of CO_2 per minute (while consuming 250 mL of oxygen) or 12 L of CO_2 (35 g) per hour. At maximal metabolic rate, it is estimated that the body can produce, transport, and excrete 90 to 100 L of CO_2 per hour, an 800% increase over the basal rate.

Lumb AB, Thomas CR. Carbon dioxide. In: Lumb AB, Thomas CR, eds. *Nunn and Lumb's Applied Respiratory Physiology*. 9th ed. Elsevier; 2021:122-135.

A.11. How much CO_2 is stored in the body? Where is it stored? Of what significance is this to laparoscopy?

The body contains approximately 120 L of stored CO_2, with most of it in the form of carbonate ion in bone. CO_2 in the blood is in equilibrium with CO_2 in various tissues. The rate of uptake and distribution of CO_2 from the blood (where it exists as a bicarbonate ion) depends on the perfusion and storage capacity of those tissues. The well-perfused tissues, including brain, kidney, and blood, come to rapid equilibrium. The medium-perfused compartment consists mainly of resting skeletal muscle. The slowly perfused compartment, mainly fat and bone (where it exists as carbonate ion), has the largest CO_2 storage capacity. In contrast to rapidly changing oxygen levels, CO_2 levels reach equilibrium more slowly.

These storage sites serve to buffer and stabilize blood CO_2 levels because they provide a place for excess CO_2 to remain until ventilation can catch up and restore equilibrium. The increase in CO_2 storage during laparoscopy is illustrated clinically by the decelerating rate of rise in end-tidal CO_2 ($Etco_2$) despite continuing insufflation. Blood or $Etco_2$ levels increase rapidly at first and plateau after 15 to 35 minutes despite continuing low-flow insufflation. At constant ventilation, CO_2 levels increase but not as much as if no simultaneous storage processes were occurring. But if ventilation is increased to keep CO_2 constant, the increase needed is only approximately 40% of the predicted volume of ventilation because of the uptake of CO_2 into the storage sites.

Lumb AB, Thomas CR. Carbon dioxide. In: Lumb AB, Thomas CR, eds. *Nunn and Lumb's Applied Respiratory Physiology*. 9th ed. Elsevier; 2021:122-135.

Seed RF, Shakespeare TF, Muldoon MJ. Carbon dioxide homeostasis during anaesthesia for laparoscopy. *Anaesthesia*. 1970;25:223-231.

A.12. Describe the diffusion and solubility properties of CO_2 and their significance in laparoscopy.

Diffusion is the process by which gases diffuse from an area of higher partial pressure to one of lower partial pressure. The rate of diffusion of a gas is inversely proportional to the square root of its density (Graham law). When that same gas molecule arrives at an aqueous membrane (eg, a gas-liquid interface), the solubility of that gas in water becomes the major factor in determining its diffusing capacity (**Table 17.1**). The water solubility of CO_2 is 24 times that of oxygen, whereas the diffusion capacity of CO_2 is 20.5 times that of oxygen. The capacity of a gas to diffuse across an aqueous membrane is directly proportional to its solubility in water and inversely proportional to its molecular weight. However, the actual movement of a gas across an aqueous membrane depends not only on its diffusing capacity but also more importantly on the pressure gradient across that membrane (**Table 17.1**).

The fate of CO_2 gas insufflated into the peritoneal cavity is the same as that would occur in any closed but distensible cavity. The pressure obtained within the cavity varies directly with the volume of gas insufflated and indirectly with the compliance of the closed cavity. Therefore, the ability of CO_2 to move from the closed peritoneal cavity to the lungs for excretion depends on its intrinsic diffusion and solubility properties, the rate of continuing CO_2 insufflation, the surface area of the cavity, and the partial pressure difference across membranes.

Lumb AB, Thomas CR. Diffusion of respiratory gases. In: Lumb AB, Thomas CR, eds. *Nunn and Lumb's Applied Respiratory Physiology*. 9th Ed. Elsevier; 2021:111-121.

McHoney M, Corizia L, Eaton S, et al. Carbon dioxide elimination during laparoscopy in children is age dependent. *J Pediatr Surg*. 2003;38:105-110.

A.13. Is CO_2 soluble in water or plasma? Is it soluble in blood? Why?

CO_2 is relatively insoluble in plasma, interstitial fluid, and water. The solubility of CO_2 in water at 37 °C (98.6 °F) is only 0.03 mmol/L/mm Hg. This must be contrasted to the very high solubility of CO_2 in

TABLE 17.1 Influence of Physical Properties on the Diffusion of Gas Through a Gas-Liquid Interface

Gas	Molecular Weight	Density Relative to O_2	Solubility Relative to O_2	Water Diffusion Capacity Relative to O_2
O_2	32	1.0	1.0	1.0
N_2	28	0.88	0.515	0.55
CO_2	44	1.37	24.0	20.5
N_2O	44	1.37	16.3	14.0
He	4	0.125	0.37	1.05

CO_2, carbon dioxide; He, helium; N_2, nitrogen; N_2O; nitrous oxide; O_2, oxygen.

whole blood. This is an important distinction because of a zinc-containing enzyme, carbonic anhydrase, that exists within the erythrocyte but is absent from plasma.

$$H_2O + CO_2 \xrightarrow{\text{carbonic anhydrase}} H_2CO_3 \rightarrow H^+ + HCO_3^-$$

In the equation shown, carbonic anhydrase catalyzes the left side of the equation (ie, the hydration of CO_2 to $H_2CO_3^-$). Once formed, carbonic acid is unstable and immediately dissociates into H^+ and HCO_3. Because blood travels through the pulmonary capillaries in less than 1 second, carbonic anhydrase speeds up the reaction by a factor of 7,500. Carbonic anhydrase, therefore, allows the insufflated CO_2 gas to be dissolved and carried as bicarbonate in the blood. The process is reversed in the lungs, and the reconstituted CO_2 gas is exhaled during respiration.

Christian G, Greene NM. Blood carbonic anhydrase activity in anesthetized man. *Anesthesiology*. 1962;23:179-186.

Lumb AB, Thomas CR. Carbon dioxide. In: Lumb AB, Thomas CR, eds. *Nunn and Lumb's Applied Respiratory Physiology*. 9th ed. Elsevier; 2021:122-135.

B. Preoperative Evaluation and Preparation

B.1. What do you want to know about this patient's history and physical condition that might affect whether she is cleared for robotic surgery?

A thorough medical history and physical exam must be obtained preoperatively in order to determine whether a patient is a suitable candidate for robotic surgery. This patient is of advanced age, so we must also assess her level of frailty. Her cardiac status is stable, but she is anticoagulated for her atrial fibrillation, so we must ensure this was stopped with apixaban at an appropriate time. She has a smoking history and COPD, which make her at higher risk of perioperative pulmonary complications (especially in robotic surgery). She is morbidly obese (BMI of 40, see Chapter 63: Morbid Obesity, Obstructive Sleep Apnea, and Bariatric Anesthesia), so we must assess for associated obstructive sleep apnea, potential for difficult intubation, and potential difficulties in positioning and vascular access. We must determine whether we would like any additional cardiac or pulmonary testing such as echocardiography, cardiac stress test, or pulmonary function testing (as suggested by history, physical exam, or both).

B.2. What factors increase this patient's risk of pulmonary complications?

- *The robotic procedure itself*: The steep Trendelenburg position and the increased intraperitoneal volumes and pressures in a paralyzed mechanically ventilated patient can cause respiratory dysfunction. Insufflation pressures should not exceed 12 to 15 mm Hg. Lower peak airway pressures are especially advantageous in American Society of Anesthesiologists (ASA) physical status 3 and 4 patients with diminished cardiopulmonary reserve. In addition, hypercarbia might require increased minute ventilation, which could further cardiopulmonary compromise. The robotic procedure itself, including docking and undocking, adds additional immobile time under anesthesia.
- *Age*: Pulmonary function declines with age, especially in a patient over 70 years.
- *Smoking/COPD*: Smokers have increased tracheobronchial secretions with decreased ciliary transport function. They can already have significant pulmonary dysfunction, which might be manifested as diminished exercise tolerance. Forced vital capacity can be diminished in restrictive pulmonary disease, whereas forced expired volume in 1 second is likely to be decreased in obstructive pulmonary disease.
- *Obesity*: Obesity compounds the problems of immobility and increased intra-abdominal pressure in the Trendelenburg position, possibly for many hours. Excessive weight and pressure on the diaphragm and lung bases can lead to marked ventilation and perfusion abnormalities, difficulty in inserting trocars, upward displacement of the carina (leading to possible endobronchial intubation), and barotrauma.
- *Overhydration*: Patients often experience oliguria during laparoscopy. This might be interpreted as insufficient hydration, and a relative overhydration with IV fluids can ensue. Unless pulmonary edema occurs, this cause of mild or moderate respiratory distress in the PACU might not be recognized without a chest radiograph.

Kendall AP, Bhatt S, Oh TE. Pulmonary consequences of carbon dioxide insufflation for laparoscopic cholecystectomies. *Anaesthesia*. 1995;50:286-289.

B.3. What laboratory tests should be performed preoperatively?

Basic tests should include complete blood count, urinalysis, clotting tests, electrocardiogram (ECG), and blood typing and screening. In addition, baseline electrolytes, chemistries, and renal function tests (blood urea nitrogen, creatinine) should be obtained because of the possibility of oliguria during a long laparoscopy. Baseline pulmonary function tests, arterial blood gas measurement, and oxygen saturation values on room air would provide valuable information. Markedly abnormal values might suggest the need for bronchodilators, antibiotics, postural drainage, and a delay in surgery until pulmonary function is optimal for this particular patient. Baseline chest radiography is necessary not only to rule out active disease but also for postoperative comparison of acute changes such as subcutaneous or mediastinal emphysema, pneumothorax, or interstitial or pulmonary edema. The presence of bullae on preoperative chest radiography can represent a contraindication to laparoscopic surgery because of the accompanying large tidal volumes and high intrathoracic pressures.

In a patient with cardiac disease, additional preoperative cardiovascular testing should adhere to published guidelines on the evaluation and management of patients undergoing noncardiac surgery.

Fleisher LA, Fleischmann KE, Auerbach AD, et al. 2014 ACC/AHA guideline on perioperative cardiovascular evaluation and management of patients undergoing noncardiac surgery: a report of the American College of Cardiology/American Heart Association Task Force on Practice Guidelines. *Circulation*. 2014;130:e278-e333.

Wijeysundera DN, Finlayson E. Preoperative evaluation. In: Gropper MA, Cohen NH, Erkisson LI, Fleisher LA, Johnson-Akeju S, eds. *Miller's Anesthesia*. 10th ed. Elsevier; 2025:808-872.

Halvorsen S, Mehilli J, Cassese S, et al. 2022 ESC guidelines on cardiovascular assessment and management of patients undergoing non-cardiac surgery. *Eur Heart J*. 2022;43:3826-3924.

B.4. What specific information should the patient be given about robotic surgery before obtaining informed consent?

In addition to the usual general complications of the planned surgery and general anesthesia, the patient must be told of the complications unique to robotic laparoscopy, and consent for possible open laparotomy must be obtained. Emergency laparotomy can be required in the event of complications such as hemorrhage, organ perforation, or anatomic or technical difficulties.

B.5. What additional procedures should be done before surgery?

Although the surgery is described as minimally invasive, the patient must be ready for maximally invasive surgery if necessary. Therefore, the patient must comply with preoperative orders regarding the following:

- *Diet*: clear liquids up to 2 hours before procedures requiring general anesthesia, regional anesthesia, or procedural sedation and anesthesia. A light meal can be ingested up to 6 hours before elective procedures requiring anesthesia. Additional fasting time, up to 8 hours or more, can be needed for fried foods, fatty foods, or meat.
- A complete bowel preparation is necessary.
- Preoperative antibiotics.

American Society of Anesthesiologists Practice guidelines for preoperative fasting and the use of pharmacologic agents to reduce the risk of pulmonary aspiration: application to healthy patients undergoing elective procedures: an updated report by the American Society of Anesthesiologists Task Force on preoperative fasting and the use of pharmacologic agents to reduce the risk of pulmonary aspiration. *Anesthesiology*. 2017;126:376-393.

B.6. What are the three major forces that uniquely alter physiology during robotic laparoscopy?

- *Pneumoperitoneum* and problems related to the creation, maintenance, and consequences of the increase in intra-abdominal pressure and volume
- *CO_2*, including its chemical and physical properties and its local and systemic effects
- Extremes of patient *positioning* on the operating table, which in this case will be steep Trendelenburg with total immobility and inaccessibility of the patient's limbs

It is important that the anesthesiologist appreciates the physiologic consequences of changes in these three forces. Separately or in combination, they have profound effects on hemodynamic, respiratory, and metabolic functions. Early gynecologic laparoscopies were usually brief, and they were performed on young, healthy females who tolerated these physiologic trespasses with nearly insignificant changes. These same forces, however, can produce significant physiologic changes in long, complex procedures in older, sicker patients who likely have less physiologic reserve.

Henny CP, Hofland J. Laparoscopic surgery: pitfalls due to anesthesia, positioning, and pneumoperitoneum. *Surg Endosc.* 2005;19:1163-1171.

O'Malley C, Cunningham AJ. Physiologic changes during laparoscopy. *Anesthesiol Clin North Am.* 2001;19:1-19.

Ost MC, Tan BJ, Lee BR. Urological laparoscopy: basic physiological considerations and immunological consequences. *J Urol.* 2005;174:1183-1188.

C. Intraoperative Management

C.1. What is the anesthetic technique of choice for robotic-assisted laparoscopy? Why?

The technique of choice for robotic-assisted laparoscopy is general anesthesia with a cuffed tracheal tube and controlled positive pressure ventilation for the following reasons:

- The duration of the procedure can be long.
- The Trendelenburg position can cause respiratory compromise and dyspnea in the awake or in the spontaneously breathing patient with abdominal contents under pressure. The patient with obesity can be especially uncomfortable in this position.
- A nasogastric or orogastric tube, which can be difficult to insert in a conscious patient, is necessary to decompress the stomach and minimize the risk of aspiration or perforation by trocars. CO_2, as well as N_2O, diffuses into the stomach.
- The patient requires neuromuscular block. This is because the increase in intra-abdominal pressure and upward displacement of the diaphragm make spontaneous breathing difficult. It provides a quieter surgical field and better surgical exposure. "Bucking" increases negative pressure in the chest, which increases the risk of pneumothorax or gas dissection. Coughing can further increase pressure in the abdomen and cause movement of, and perforation by, intra-abdominal instruments. Any movement of the patient while robotic instruments are docked can lead to devastating injuries. Moreover, neuromuscular block is necessary to control and augment ventilation to compensate for the hypercarbia and respiratory acidosis that result from absorption of CO_2.

Whalley DG, Berrigan MJ. Anesthesia for radical prostatectomy, cystectomy, nephrectomy, pheochromocytoma, and laparoscopic procedures. *Anesthesiol Clin North Am.* 2000;18:899-917.

C.2. Can a laryngeal mask airway (LMA) be used?

The use of an LMA is generally contraindicated in laparoscopic and robotic procedures of long duration. Their use is limited by concerns that peak airway pressures required to maintain adequate mechanical ventilation can often exceed that of lower esophageal sphincter pressure (15 mm Hg at end expiration), particularly in the setting of steep Trendelenburg positioning, which could result in gastric distension and potentially alveolar hypoventilation. Further limiting its utility is the fact that an LMA does not adequately secure the airway against the risk of aspiration and might interfere with proper placement of an orogastric tube.

Bapat PP, Verghese C. Laryngeal mask airway and the incidence of regurgitation during gynecological laparoscopies. *Anesth Analg.* 1997;85:139-143.

Pandolfino JE, Kahrilas PJ, American Gastroenterological Association. AGA technical review on the clinical use of esophageal manometry. *Gastroenterology.* 2005;128:209-224.

C.3. What anesthetic agents or adjuvant drugs are recommended for laparoscopy? Are any anesthetic agents contraindicated?

Almost any drug combination that provides amnesia, analgesia, and paralysis is suitable.

Use of an antiemetic is recommended to counteract nausea that results from peritoneal stimulation and bowel distension (secondary to diffusion of CO_2 into the bowel). Pharmacologic approaches to reducing PONV are reviewed in Chapter 61: Ambulatory Surgery.

Propofol reportedly has antiemetic properties, which might arise from antagonism of serotonergic receptors. However, a propofol-based maintenance anesthetic, when combined with neuromuscular block, might not adequately prevent patient awareness. A processed electroencephalogram (EEG) monitor such as the Sedline (Masimo) or Bispectral Index (BIS) Monitoring System (Medtronic) can be helpful in that situation.

A vagolytic drug should be at hand because acute stretching of the peritoneum can cause reflex bradycardia. This is more likely to occur in young females than in older adults.

SECTION 3

Sedatives such as benzodiazepines should be used cautiously, if at all, in older adults because their duration can be prolonged and contribute to postoperative delirium.

Gan TJ, Belani KG, Bergese S, et al. Fourth consensus guidelines for the management of postoperative nausea and vomiting. *Anesth Analg* 2020;131:411-448.

Scuderi PE, D'Angelo R, Harris L, et al. Small-dose propofol by continuous infusion does not prevent postoperative vomiting in females undergoing outpatient laparoscopy. *Anesth Analg*. 1997;84:71-75.

Seed RF, Shakespeare TF, Muldoon MJ. Carbon dioxide homeostasis during anaesthesia for laparoscopy. *Anaesthesia*. 1970;25:223-231.

C.4. Should nitrous oxide (N_2O) be used during laparoscopy? What are the pros and cons? Does N_2O cause bowel distension during laparoscopy? Does N_2O cause nausea and vomiting after laparoscopy?

The use of N_2O in laparoscopy is controversial because of its effects on bowel distension during surgery and on nausea and vomiting postoperatively.

In examining the issue of bowel distension with N_2O, note that the diffusion capacity of N_2O is approximately 14 times that of oxygen and 28 times that of nitrogen (see **Table 17.1**). Therefore, in a closed space that contains air, N_2O enters faster than N_2 can leave, thereby increasing the size of a closed space. If the walls of that space cannot expand, then the pressure within that space will rise. When N_2O is limited to 50%, volume increases no more than 50%. A much more rapid increase in gas volume occurs in the pleural space, where volume can double in 10 minutes, triple in 45 minutes, and quadruple in 2 hours. The faster rate of pleural gas expansion compared to bowel gas expansion might in part be due to the greater blood flow to the pleura and possibly due to direct diffusion of N_2O from the alveoli adjacent to the pleura.

For laparoscopy, we are concerned about CO_2 pockets and not air pockets. N_2O, which has a diffusion capacity almost as great as CO_2, will diffuse from the bloodstream into the intraperitoneal pocket of 100% CO_2 at a rate determined by its solubility in water, its diffusing capacity through an aqueous membrane, and its pressure gradient (Section A.12). Similarly, CO_2 will leave the peritoneal cavity according to its pressure gradients and solubility and diffusion characteristics. Eventually, the amount of N_2O found in the peritoneal cavity can be significant, and theoretically, it can form a combustion hazard.

In the situation of an air pocket in the bowel, it is well known that N_2O will diffuse in according to its gradients, thereby enlarging the pocket. However, even in the absence of N_2O, CO_2 will diffuse into this pocket and expand it in a manner that is clinically indistinguishable from N_2O.

N_2O is often blamed for a distended bowel during laparoscopy; however, CO_2 is equally capable of diffusing into and distending the bowel. In addition, PONV is independent of the use of N_2O if exposure time is less than 1 hour. Because of these issues, it is recommended that N_2O, if used at all, be limited to less than 50% of the inspired mixture. Alternatively, a mixture of 75% air and 25% oxygen (fraction of inspired oxygen [F_{IO_2}] = 40%) might be a wiser choice.

Arellano RJ, Pole ML, Rafuse SE, et al. Omission of nitrous oxide from a propofol-based anesthetic does not affect the recovery of women undergoing outpatient gynecologic surgery. *Anesthesiology*. 2000;93:332-339.

Diemunsch PA, Torp KD, Van Dorsselaer T, et al. Nitrous oxide fraction in the carbon dioxide pneumoperitoneum during laparoscopy under general inhaled anesthesia in pigs. *Anesth Analg*. 2000;90:951-953.

Diemunsch PA, Van Dorsselaer T, Torp KD, et al. Calibrated pneumoperitoneal venting to prevent N_2O accumulation in the CO_2 pneumoperitoneum during laparoscopy with inhaled anesthesia: an experimental study in pigs. *Anesth Analg*. 2002;94:1014-1018.

Eger EI II, Saidman LJ. Hazards of nitrous oxide anesthesia in bowel obstruction and pneumothorax. *Anesthesiology*. 1965;26:61-66.

Hunter JG, Staheli J, Oddsdotti M, et al. Nitrous oxide pneumoperitoneum revisited. Is there a risk of combustion? *Surg Endosc*. 1995;9:501-504.

Munson ES. Transfer of nitrous oxide into body air cavities. *Br J Anaesth*. 1974;46:202-209.

Sukhani R, Lurie J, Jabamoni R. Propofol for ambulatory gynecologic laparoscopy: does omission of nitrous oxide alter postoperative emetic sequelae and recovery? *Anesth Analg*. 1994;78:831-835.

C.5. Can laparoscopy be performed under local or regional anesthesia?

Yes. Although unsuitable for robotic procedures, use of local or regional anesthesia for very brief diagnostic laparoscopic procedures has been reported. However, under local anesthesia, CO_2 can cause pain intraperitoneally that is referred to the shoulder. Rapid peritoneal distension causes nausea that can be exacerbated without a nasogastric tube. Because of patient discomfort, the surgeon might not obtain optimal visualization of the surgical field due to the need to use low insufflation pressure. Also, the possibility of converting to laparotomy favors the use of general anesthesia.

Regional anesthesia can be used for laparoscopy. However, it too has serious drawbacks. It requires a high level of sensory block, possibly causing dyspnea in the Trendelenburg position. A nasogastric tube might not be tolerated. Hyperventilation in response to hypercarbia can cause excessive movement of the surgical field, and spontaneous ventilation might be inadequate to compensate for hypercarbia in the Trendelenburg position.

Regional anesthesia can also be combined with general anesthesia. Because the systemic response to hypercarbia is mediated primarily through sympathetic stimulation, the sympathetic block resulting from high regional anesthesia results in hypotension and decreased cardiac output rather than the hypertension and increased cardiac output usually seen with general anesthesia.

Use of IV analgesics or propofol during regional anesthesia can result in respiratory depression or obstruction, especially in steep Trendelenburg position. Hypoxemia in the presence of hypercarbia can have serious cardiovascular consequences.

Collins LM, Vaghadia H. Regional anesthesia for laparoscopy. *Anesthesiol Clin North Am*. 2001;19:43-55.

Vaghadia H, Solylo MA, Henderson CL, et al. Selective spinal anesthesia for outpatient laparoscopy. II: epinephrine and spinal cord function. *Can J Anaesth*. 2001;48:261-266.

C.6. What monitors and devices would you apply to the patient? Why?

The usual intraoperative monitors, including standard five-lead ECG with ST trending, systemic arterial blood pressure (BP) using automated oscillometry, pulse oximetry, capnography, a peripheral nerve stimulator, indicators of inspired oxygen fraction, minute ventilation, and peak airway pressures, are necessary, as is temperature monitoring. Body temperature should be maintained with a forced warm air heating blanket, warmed IV fluids, or other means. An arterial catheter is suggested for longer, more complex procedures in sicker (ASA physical status 3 and 4) patients. Rarely, central venous pressure (CVP), pulmonary artery pressure, pulmonary artery occlusion pressure (PAOP), and cardiac output measurements are needed in patients with severe cardiac or pulmonary disease. A processed EEG monitor is optional. Other possibilities include Doppler, transesophageal echocardiography, and noninvasive assessment of cardiac output by thoracic bioimpedance or thoracic ultrasound. All monitors must be placed and checked before the patient becomes secured to the table and inaccessible once the robot is docked into position.

Intermittent sequential compression stockings should be applied for thromboembolism prophylaxis. Shoulder braces or adhesive taping are used for support in the Trendelenburg position. After induction of anesthesia, a nasogastric or orogastric tube and a Foley catheter are inserted for decompression of the stomach and bladder. In addition to the danger of regurgitation from the increased abdominal pressure, there are reports of stomach perforation by trocars. The orogastric tube should not be clamped after initial placement, and intermittent suctioning should continue because CO_2 continues to diffuse into the stomach, causing distension.

In addition to mechanical monitoring, visual and tactile monitoring should be attempted if the position of the robotic arms allows it. Skin color, skin turgor, and capillary refill should be monitored because they can change abruptly. The head, neck, and upper chest can assume a purplish color in the dependent position, especially during hypercarbia and steep Trendelenburg. The upper chest wall might not be readily accessible to check for subcutaneous emphysema. The cornea and conjunctiva should be checked periodically for edema, especially in the Trendelenburg position, and whenever oliguria occurs because the extent of the edema can influence the decision on when to extubate.

It is important to maintain accurate data recording with respect to the volume (and type) of fluids infused, along with urine output, blood loss, and other potential sources of volume losses. Despite adequate hydration, oliguria frequently occurs during pneumoperitoneum due to a decrease in renal blood flow resulting from renal compression, especially at intra-abdominal pressures approaching or exceeding 15 mm Hg. The acute increase in intra-abdominal pressure is transmitted to the kidneys and is believed to cause shunting from the cortex to the medulla of the kidney, resulting in decreased urine output. Diuresis usually occurs rapidly on release of intra-abdominal pressure.

Jacobs VR, Morrison JE Jr, Mettler L, et al. Measurement of CO_2 hypothermia during laparoscopy and pelviscopy: how cold it gets and how to prevent it? *J Am Assoc Gynecol Laparosc*. 1999;6:289-295.

SECTION 3

Ogunnaike BO, Jones SB, Jones DB, et al. Anesthetic considerations for bariatric surgery. *Anesth Analg.* 2002;95:1793-1805.

Tournadre JP, Chassard D, Berrada KR, et al. Effect of pneumoperitoneum and Trendelenburg position on gastro-oesophageal reflux and lower oesophageal sphincter pressure. *Br J Anaesth.* 1996;76:130-132.

C.7. How is the patient to be positioned? What special precautions are required for robotic laparoscopy?

Often in abdominal surgeries, the operative side is elevated, enabling gravity to assist in separating the organs and allowing blood to pool away from the operative field. For other laparoscopic procedures, the patient is supine, in the Trendelenburg position for urologic procedures, in dorsal lithotomy for gynecologic procedures, in the head-up position for upper gastrointestinal and biliary tract surgery, and in the lateral decubitus position for thoracoscopy, nephrectomy, and adrenalectomy. For standard conventional laparoscopy, it might be possible to keep one or both arms out on boards.

Robotically assisted laparoscopy requires careful attention to detail before the robot is docked; there should be no unintentional patient movement. Thus, it is especially important to check that any IV or arterial lines, as well as BP, ECG, and pulse oximetry monitors, are functioning properly after the arms have been carefully padded and tucked. Once the robot is locked into position, there is limited access to check the arms or look under the drapes.

After induction of general endotracheal anesthesia, the surgeons must secure the patient on the table so there is no slippage when placed in extreme Trendelenburg position. Shoulder braces can be used instead of tape to secure the patient, but be mindful of potential brachial plexus injury.

With the knees flexed in padded leg holders, the patient is now carefully lowered into steep Trendelenburg position. Robotic laparoscopy frequently requires steeper Trendelenburg positioning than conventional laparoscopy, resulting in more positioning injuries. Care must also be taken to ensure that movements of the large bulky robotic arms do not come in contact with the patient.

Kalmar AF, Foubert L, Hendrickx JF, et al. Influence of steep Trendelenburg position and CO_2 pneumoperitoneum on cardiovascular, cerebrovascular, and respiratory homeostasis during robotic prostatectomy. *Br J Anaesth.* 2010;104:433-439.

Klauschie J, Wechter ME, Jacob K, et al. Use of anti-skid material and patient-positioning to prevent patient shifting during robotic-assisted gynecologic procedures. *J Minim Invasive Gynecol.* 2010;17:504-507.

Phong SV, Koh LK. Anaesthesia for robotic-assisted radical prostatectomy: considerations for laparoscopy in the Trendelenburg position. *Anaesth Intensive Care.* 2007;35:281-285.

C.8. How will you ventilate the patient? What are the respiratory and circulatory effects of the Trendelenburg position during laparoscopy?

Respiratory

Vital capacity and functional residual capacity (FRC) are reduced. The abdominal contents restrict movement of the diaphragm, especially in those who are obese and in older adults. Decreased compliance, increased $\dot{V}/\dot{Q}$ abnormalities, and cephalad displacement of the mediastinum commonly occur. Upper airway edema and displacement of the endotracheal tube can occur.

Circulatory

In healthy patients, the Trendelenburg position results in minimal circulatory changes. Venous return and cardiac output are increased, whereas CVP, PAOP, systemic vascular resistance (SVR), and heart rate are essentially unchanged. In patients with cardiovascular disease, the Trendelenburg position can result in increased CVP, PAOP, and decreased cardiac output. The increase in venous return and myocardial oxygen demand that occurs in severe cardiovascular disease can precipitate acute heart failure.

These respiratory and circulatory changes caused by the Trendelenburg position are further augmented following CO_2 insufflation. Ventilation can become difficult, especially in patients with obesity. Use of positive end-expiratory pressure (PEEP) is advised to prevent atelectasis. To prevent peak inspiratory pressures from becoming excessive, switching from volume-controlled to pressure-controlled ventilation can be useful.

Choi EM, Na S, Choi SH, et al. Comparison of volume-controlled and pressure-controlled ventilation in steep Trendelenburg position for robot-assisted laparoscopic radical prostatectomy. *J Clin Anesth.* 2011;23:183-188.

Kim JY, Shin CS, Kim HS, et al. Positive end-expiratory pressure in pressure-controlled ventilation improves ventilatory and oxygenation parameters during laparoscopic cholecystectomy. *Surg Endosc.* 2010;24:1099-1103.

Kim MS, Kim NY, Lee KY, et al. The impact of two different inspiratory to expiratory ratios (1:1 and 1:2) on respiratory mechanics and oxygenation during volume-controlled ventilation in robot-assisted laparoscopic radical prostatectomy: a randomized controlled trial. *Can J Anaesth*. 2015;62:979-987.

Kim WH, Hahm TS, Kim JA, et al. Prolonged inspiratory time produces better gas exchange in patients undergoing laparoscopic surgery: a randomised trial. *Acta Anaesthesiol Scand*. 2013;57:613-622.

Lestar M, Gunnarsson L, Lagerstrand L, et al. Hemodynamic perturbations during robot-assisted laparoscopic radical prostatectomy in 45° Trendelenburg position. *Anesth Analg*. 2011;113:1069-1075.

Oğurlu M, Küçük M, Bilgin F, et al. Pressure-controlled vs volume-controlled ventilation during laparoscopic gynecologic surgery. *J Minim Invasive Gynecol*. 2010;17:295-300.

Russo A, Di Stasio E, Scagliusi A, et al. Positive end-expiratory pressure during laparoscopy: cardiac and respiratory effects. *J Clin Anesth*. 2013;25:314-320.

Tyagi A, Kumar R, Sethi AK, et al. A comparison of pressure-controlled and volume-controlled ventilation for laparoscopic cholecystectomy. *Anaesthesia*. 2011;66:503-508.

C.9. What techniques are available for initial access to the peritoneal cavity? What anesthetic problems can arise during insufflation?

Pneumoperitoneum can be achieved by a blind or closed technique of percutaneous insertion of the 2-mm diameter hollow Veress needle, which after verification of correct positioning is connected to the CO_2 insufflator. Alternatively, if previous surgery or adhesions are to be avoided, an open approach or periumbilical mini-incision is created, and the blunt-tipped Hasson cannula is inserted without prior pneumoperitoneum. The laparoscope is then inserted through the trocar to verify the intra-abdominal position before insufflation begins.

Before either technique is attempted, the stomach must be decompressed with an orogastric tube and the bladder drained with a Foley catheter. During insufflation, abdominal distension should be evenly distributed in all four quadrants. CO_2 is insufflated slowly until a pressure of 10 to 15 cm H_2O is reached. Respiratory variations in intraperitoneal pressure should be visible, and peak inspiratory pressures gradually increase as the abdomen distends. At this time, the anesthesiologist should be alert to the possibility of vagally mediated reflexes. Bronchospasm, bradycardia, and even sinus arrest have been reported, especially in young females. Visceral and vascular perforations are also reported complications, especially with the blind technique. Cardiovascular collapse and gas emboli have been reported when CO_2 is inadvertently injected into a blood vessel.

Merlin TL, Hiller JE, Maddern GJ, et al. Systematic review of the safety and effectiveness of methods used to establish pneumoperitoneum in laparoscopic surgery. *Br J Surg*. 2003;90:688-679.

Teoh B, Sen R, Abbott J. An evaluation of four tests used to ascertain Veres needle placement at closed laparoscopy. *J Minim Invasive Gynecol*. 2005;12:153-158.

Vilos GA, Vilos AG. Safe laparoscopic entry guided by Veress needle CO_2 insufflation pressure. *J Am Assoc Gynecol Laparosc*. 2003;10:415-420.

C.10. What intravenous (IV) solution and how much fluid volume do you plan to infuse?

Large-bore IV catheters should be placed because of the possibility of major hemorrhage. Transient oliguria during laparoscopy is common. In calculating fluid requirements during laparoscopy, it is important to remember that much less third space distribution occurs than in open surgery, fluid loss by evaporation is minimal, and the volume of retained (after suctioning) intraperitoneal saline used for irrigation by the surgeon should be added to the final total volume of infused IV fluids. In addition, intra-abdominal humidification of the insufflated anhydrous CO_2 gas minimizes insensible water loss. Unlike open intraperitoneal cases, starting fluid replacement is approximately 4 mL/kg/h of a balanced crystalloid solution; additional fluid is given based on the patient's preoperative hemodynamic status, intraoperative blood loss, and the volume of residual intraperitoneal irrigation fluid used by the surgeon. Urine output per se is not a reliable indicator of intravascular volume due to insufflation-induced oliguria. After the pneumoperitoneum is released, diuresis occurs and renal function quickly returns to normal (see Section C.22).

For robotic laparoscopy, surgeons prefer that IV fluids are minimized until the anastomoses are completed. This helps prevent edema of the face, eyes, and larynx while in the steep Trendelenburg position. After the anastomoses are complete, IV infusion can be increased; average blood loss is less than 250 mL, and total fluid replacement is 3 to 3.5 L.

Concha MR, Mertz VF, Cortínez LI, et al. The volume of lactated Ringer's solution required to maintain preload and cardiac index during open and laparoscopic surgery. *Anesth Analg*. 2009;108:616-622.

London ET, Ho HS, Neuhaus AM, et al. Effect of intravascular volume expansion on renal function during prolonged CO_2 pneumoperitoneum. *Ann Surg*. 2000;231:195-201.

Olsson J, Svensén CH, Hahn RG. The volume kinetics of acetated Ringer's solution during laparoscopic cholecystectomy. *Anesth Analg*. 2004;99:1854-1860.

C.11. Under what circumstances should laparoscopy be converted to laparotomy?

Laparotomy should be performed immediately for major bleeding or organ damage. Other circumstances include persistent problems with inadequate exposure, a technically challenging procedure, a procedure taking too long, inability to create or maintain pneumoperitoneum, patient deterioration, equipment failure, and discovery of other unsuspected disease.

Tabboush ZS. When hypotension during laparoscopic cholecystectomy indicates termination of the laparoscopy. *Anesth Analg*. 1994;79:195-196.

C.12. What is the arterial to end-tidal CO_2 gradient ($Paco_2$-$Etco_2$) in the normal awake patient? What is the cause of the gradient? Does the gradient change during laparoscopy? Why?

In the awake person at rest, the normal arterial to end-tidal CO_2 gradient is 2 to 6 mm Hg. The gradient and its variations are measures of the alveolar dead space. The gradient is the sum of the difference between the arterial CO_2 ($Paco_2$) and alveolar CO_2 ($Paco_2$) plus the difference between the alveolar CO_2 ($Paco_2$) and $Etco_2$. It is often increased in emphysema. The difference is increased when underperfused alveoli are ventilated, as often occurs during hyperventilation in laparoscopy.

The total physiologic dead space consists of the anatomic dead space (airways that do not participate in gas exchange, ~150 mL) and the alveolar dead space (ie, underperfused alveoli). The alveolar dead space gas is expired at the same time as the alveolar ideal gas from well-perfused alveoli in equilibrium with pulmonary capillary blood. The dilution of the ideal alveolar gas by the alveolar dead space gas is represented by $Etco_2$.

Some of the factors resulting in a relative increase in $\dot{V}/\dot{Q}$ ratio include mechanical ventilation, hyperventilation, rapid or shallow ventilation, and the Trendelenburg or lateral decubitus position.

Some of the factors resulting in a relative decrease in $\dot{V}/\dot{Q}$ ratio include hypotension, decreased cardiac output, myocardial depression from inhalational anesthetics, pulmonary embolus, high positive airway pressure, and ablation of the hypoxic pulmonary vasoconstriction reflex.

Christensen MA, Bloom J, Sutton KR. Comparing arterial and end-tidal carbon dioxide values in hyperventilated neurosurgical patients. *Am J Crit Care*. 1995;4:116-121.

Lumb AB, Thomas CR. Anaesthesia. In: Lumb AB, Thomas CR, eds. *Nunn and Lumb's Applied Respiratory Physiology*. 9th ed. Elsevier; 2021:244-267.

C.13. Is an arterial catheter necessary? Why? Does end-tidal CO_2 ($Etco_2$) tension accurately reflect arterial CO_2 tension? Under what circumstances can the $Etco_2$ exceed the $Paco_2$? Why?

An arterial catheter is recommended whenever the laparoscopic procedure is unusually complex or long or when the patient has significant cardiopulmonary disease. In such cases, $\dot{V}/\dot{Q}$ abnormalities, intraoperative hypoxemia, marked hypercarbia, or high airway pressures can be expected. During these situations, and possibly in all laparoscopies, the assumption that $Etco_2$ accurately reflects a predictable relationship to $Paco_2$ is not valid.

$Etco_2$ tension can accurately estimate $Paco_2$, frequently underestimate $Paco_2$, or infrequently overestimate $Paco_2$. Furthermore, the values for these two measurements do not always change proportionally or in the same direction. The relationship between $Etco_2$ and $Paco_2$ varies during the course of the procedure. At the beginning of insufflation, $Etco_2$ can be used as a rough estimate of $Paco_2$. However, when redistribution of excess CO_2 from the well-perfused tissues to the less well-perfused tissues begins, $Etco_2$ begins to underestimate the $Paco_2$. Characteristically, the arterial to end-tidal CO_2 difference progressively increases as hyperventilation (and dead space) increases.

Bhavani-Shankar K, Steinbrook RA, Brooks DC, et al. Arterial to end-tidal carbon dioxide pressure difference during laparoscopic surgery in pregnancy. *Anesthesiology*. 2000;93:370-373.

Lumb AB, Thomas CR. Anaesthesia. In: Lumb AB, Thomas CR, eds. *Nunn and Lumb's Applied Respiratory Physiology*. 9th ed. Elsevier; 2021:244-267.

Scheid P, Meyer M, Piiper J. Arterial-expired Pco_2 differences in the dog during acute hypercapnia. *J Appl Physiol Respir Environ Exerc Physiol*. 1979;47:1074-1078.

Strang CM, Hachenberg T, Fredén F, et al. Development of atelectasis and arterial to end-tidal Pco_2 difference in a porcine model of pneumoperitoneum. *Br J Anaesth*. 2009;103:298-303.

Wulkan ML, Vasudevan SA. Is end-tidal CO_2 an accurate measure of arterial CO_2 during laparoscopic procedures in children and neonates with cyanotic congenital heart disease? *J Pediatr Surg*. 2001;36:1234-1236.

C.14. What are the possible causes of hypercarbia?

- Hypoventilation
- CO_2 in the inspired gas: rebreathing endogenous CO_2 will increase $Paco_2$ by 3 to 6 mm Hg/min.
- Increased endogenous CO_2 production or exogenous CO_2 supply, occurring in the hypermetabolic states of malignant hyperthermia, fever, and hyperthyroidism, or following administration of bicarbonate or lactate
- Increased dead space (rare) as in pulmonary embolism, ventilation of a lung cyst, or advanced COPD

Lumb AB, Thomas CR. Changes in the carbon dioxide partial pressure. In: Lumb AB, Thomas CR, eds. *Nunn and Lumb's Applied Respiratory Physiology*. 9th ed. Elsevier; 2021:268-272.

Wolf JS Jr, Clayman RV, Monk TG, et al. Carbon dioxide absorption during laparoscopic pelvic operation. *J Am Coll Surg*. 1995;180:555-560.

C.15. What factors play a role in the unusually rapid and marked elevation of CO_2 that is sometimes seen in laparoscopy?

- Patients with significant cardiopulmonary disease
- Intra-abdominal pressure greater than 15 mm Hg
- Presence of subcutaneous emphysema
- Retroperitoneal rather than intraperitoneal approach
- Long duration of laparoscopy

Bozkurt P, Kaya G, Yeker Y, et al. Arterial carbon dioxide markedly increases during diagnostic laparoscopy in portal hypertensive children. *Anesth Analg*. 2002;95:1236-1240.

Liem MS, Kallewaard JW, de Smet AM, et al. Does hypercarbia develop faster during laparoscopic herniorrhaphy than during laparoscopic cholecystectomy? Assessment with continuous blood gas monitoring. *Anesth Analg*. 1995;81:1243-1249.

C.16. How rapidly does the $Paco_2$ rise in a patient with apnea (endogenous CO_2)? How rapidly does the $Paco_2$ rise if 5% CO_2 gas is inhaled (exogenous)? How rapidly can the CO_2 rise during laparoscopy? What factors explain the differences?

In the patient with apnea, $Paco_2$ increases rapidly by 12 to 13 mm Hg during the first minute; thereafter, it increases by approximately 3 to 5 mm Hg/min. Rebreathing, or inhalation of 5% CO_2 in oxygen, causes a much more rapid rise in $Paco_2$, up to 8 to 10 mm Hg/min. The difference in the rate of rise between endogenous and exogenous CO_2 is explained by the presence of large body stores of CO_2. There is approximately 120 L of CO_2 stored in the body (100 times the amount of oxygen), distributed among well-perfused tissues (eg, blood, brain), moderately perfused tissues (eg, muscle), and poorly perfused tissues (eg, fat, bone). These tissues adjust slowly to acute changes in CO_2. In the steady state, the amount of CO_2 produced metabolically in the body is equal to the amount expired from the lungs, and there is no change in body stores of CO_2. During laparoscopy, a steady state does not exist, with the rate of rise of Pco_2 being greatest during the first 20 to 30 minutes. After that time, a new equilibrium is reached between the different compartments, and the Pco_2 rate of rise is slower.

Lumb AB, Thomas CR. Changes in the carbon dioxide partial pressure. In: Lumb AB, Thomas CR, eds. *Nunn and Lumb's Applied Respiratory Physiology*. 9th ed. Elsevier; 2021:268-272.

Riva T, Greif R, Kaiser H, et al. Carbon dioxide changes during high-flow nasal oxygenation in apneic patients: a single-center randomized controlled noninferiority trial. *Anesthesiology*. 2022;136:82-92.

C.17. What is the net effect of pneumoperitoneum, hypercarbia, and steep Trendelenburg on the cardiovascular system?

The effects of hypercarbia on the circulatory system are complex. At the cellular level, hypercarbia is a direct depressor of myocardial contractility and rate of contraction; it is also a direct stimulant of myocardial irritability and arrhythmicity. These effects can be enhanced by acidosis.

The direct effect of hypercarbia on isolated or denervated blood vessels is a diminished responsiveness to catecholamines and vasodilation, especially on the venous side, leading to peripheral pooling, decreased venous return, and decreased cardiac output. The exception to the dilatory effect of hypercarbia and acidosis on blood vessels exists in the pulmonary vessels, which vasoconstrict. It appears that the effects on the pulmonary vessels are due to acidosis rather than hypercarbia: if pH is kept constant while P_{CO_2} rises, pulmonary vascular resistance (PVR) does not change.

However, the direct or local effects of CO_2 can be overshadowed by the systemic effects of CO_2. Simultaneous with these local or direct effects, hypercarbia causes profound systemic changes secondary to stimulation of the central nervous system and the sympathoadrenal system. The net effect usually includes an increase in cardiac output, heart rate, force of myocardial contraction, BP, and CVP, vasoconstriction in the pulmonary (capacitance) vessels, and a decrease in peripheral resistance. The increase in cardiac output of up to 50% exceeds the rise in BP because of the drop in peripheral resistance and increase in blood flow primarily in the cerebral and coronary circulations. This net stimulatory effect accompanies the elevation of Pa_{CO_2} up to approximately 90 mm Hg. Above this level, further increases in CO_2 markedly reduce the response.

Hypercarbia can cause arrhythmias during epinephrine administration or in the presence of halothane but not other volatile anesthetics. Other than in these two circumstances, hypercarbia is not arrhythmogenic unless hypoxemia also is present.

The full range of possible effects of hypercarbia on the cardiovascular system is subject to many influences. Healthy (ASA physical status 1) patients are less likely than ASA three patients to undergo extreme changes. Similarly, short surgical duration, head-up positioning, low intra-abdominal pressure, and intraperitoneal (rather than extraperitoneal) surgery can limit the range of physiologic and metabolic responses to near normal.

In patients with marginal cardiovascular function, peritoneal insufflation can result in a significant increase in cardiac workload. In this situation, transesophageal echocardiography can be a useful method to assess left ventricular function.

Arrhythmias such as bradycardia, nodal rhythm, or even asystole can follow rapid peritoneal distension and vagal stimulation. In general, BP, pulse, cardiac output, and CVP increase up to an intra-abdominal pressure of 15 mm Hg. At insufflation pressures of 20 to 30 mm Hg, a decrease in BP, cardiac output, and CVP occurs due to reduced venous return. Pneumoperitoneum can also induce changes in the cardiac electrical axis, which can affect the interpretation of the ECG.

With regard to the use of steep Trendelenburg positioning during robot-assisted pelvic surgery (RAPS), a recent meta-analysis of 10 randomized controlled trials (RCTs) and 47 nonrandomized controlled studies with a total of 380,125 patients found that RAPS was associated with a decreased risk of venous thromboembolism and cardiac complications compared to laparoscopic/open pelvic surgery in nonrandomized controlled studies (risk ratio [RR] 0.59, 95% CI 0.51-0.72, $P < .001$; and RR 0.93, 95% CI 0.58-1.50, $P = .78$, respectively), but these differences were not confirmed in RCTs (RR 0.92, 95% CI 0.52-1.62, $P = .77$; and RR 0.93, 95% CI 0.58-1.50, $P = .78$, respectively).

Ekici Y, Bozbas H, Karakayali F, et al. Effect of different intra-abdominal pressure levels on QT dispersion in patients undergoing laparoscopic cholecystectomy. *Surg Endosc.* 2009;23:2543-2549.

Falabella A, Moore-Jeffries E, Sullivan MJ, et al. Cardiac function during steep Trendelenburg position and CO_2 pneumoperitoneum for robotic-assisted prostatectomy: a trans-oesophageal Doppler probe study. *Int J Med Robot.* 2007;3:312-315.

Hofer CK, Zalunardo MP, Klaghofer R, et al. Changes in intrathoracic blood volume associated with pneumoperitoneum and positioning. *Acta Anaesthesiol Scand.* 2002;46:303-308.

Joshi GP, Hein HA, Mascarenhas WL, et al. Continuous transesophageal echo-Doppler assessment of hemodynamic function during laparoscopic cholecystectomy. *J Clin Anesth.* 2005;17:117-121.

Katayama S, Mori K, Pradere B, et al. Influence of steep Trendelenburg position on postoperative complications: a systematic review and meta-analysis. *J Robot Surg.* 2022;16:1233-1247.

Lumb AB, Thomas CR. Changes in the carbon dioxide partial pressure. In: Lumb AB, Thomas CR, eds. *Nunn and Lumb's Applied Respiratory Physiology.* 9th ed. Elsevier; 2021:268-272.

Rist M, Hemmerling TM, Rauh R, et al. Influence of pneumoperitoneum and patient positioning on preload and splanchnic blood volume in laparoscopic surgery of the lower abdomen. *J Clin Anesth.* 2001;13:244-249.

Russo A, Marana E, Viviani D, et al. Diastolic function: the influence of pneumoperitoneum and Trendelenburg positioning during laparoscopic hysterectomy. *Eur J Anaesthesiol.* 2009;26:923-927.

C.18. What is the net effect of pneumoperitoneum, hypercarbia, and steep Trendelenburg on the respiratory system?

Hypercarbia and acidosis stimulate the respiratory center both directly and indirectly through chemoreceptors, hormones, and autonomic innervation. In the conscious patient breathing oxygen, the maximal respiratory stimulating effect occurs at 100 to 150 mm Hg, producing minute volumes of up to 75 L.

Above these levels, CO_2 becomes a respiratory depressant. Current anesthetics blunt the stimulatory respiratory response to CO_2.

In the awake patient, each mm Hg increase in $Paco_2$ increases ventilation by 2 to 3 L/min (if Pao_2 is constant). This response is diminished by anesthesia. Hypercarbia also produces bronchodilatation; acidosis, rather than hypercarbia per se, causes pulmonary vascular constriction.

General anesthesia with tracheal intubation and mechanical ventilation results in a decrease in FRC, which is caused by loss of muscle tone, diaphragmatic displacement, and loss of thoracic volume. Lung compliance drops, airway pressure increases, and $\dot{V}/\dot{Q}$ mismatch occurs. However, most patients have no difficulty tolerating these changes. These changes are exaggerated in the Trendelenburg position, especially in older adults, those with obesity, and those with preexisting cardiopulmonary disease. Intrathoracic, peak inspiratory, and plateau pressures increase, and increase even further when pneumoperitoneum creates an increase in pressure and volume by pushing abdominal contents cephalad. Endobronchial intubation can occur as a result of cephalad movement of the carina, and it should be ruled out if hypoxemia occurs.

Andersson LE, Bååth M, Thörne A, et al. Effect of carbon dioxide pneumoperitoneum on development of atelectasis during anesthesia, examined by spiral computed tomography. *Anesthesiology*. 2005;102:293-299.

Kendall AP, Bhatt S, Oh TE. Pulmonary consequences of carbon dioxide insufflation for laparoscopic cholecystectomies. *Anaesthesia*. 1995;50:286-289.

Lobato EB, Paige GB, Brown MM, et al. Pneumoperitoneum as a risk factor for endobronchial intubation during laparoscopic gynecologic surgery. *Anesth Analg*. 1998;86:301-303.

Lumb AB, Thomas CR. Anaesthesia. In: Lumb AB, Thomas CR, eds. *Nunn and Lumb's Applied Respiratory Physiology*. 9th ed. Elsevier; 2021:244-267.

Rauh R, Hemmerling TM, Rist M, et al. Influence of pneumoperitoneum and patient positioning on respiratory system compliance. *J Clin Anesth*. 2001;13:361-365.

Sprung J, Whalley DG, Falcone T, et al. The effects of tidal volume and respiratory rate on oxygenation and respiratory mechanics during laparoscopy in morbidly obese patients. *Anesth Analg*. 2003;97:268-274.

Whalen FX, Gajic O, Thompson GB, et al. The effects of the alveolar recruitment maneuver and positive end-expiratory pressure on arterial oxygenation during laparoscopic bariatric surgery. *Anesth Analg*. 2006;102:298-305.

C.19. What is the net effect of pneumoperitoneum, hypercarbia, and steep Trendelenburg on the central nervous system?

The brain is particularly sensitive to changes in $Paco_2$. Slight elevations of CO_2 cause direct cortical depression and increase the threshold for seizures. Higher levels of CO_2 (25%-30% increase) stimulate subcortical hypothalamic centers, resulting in increased cortical excitability and seizures. This hyperexcitability is enhanced by adrenal cortical and medullary hormones released secondary to hypercarbia-induced stimulation of the hypothalamus. Further elevations of CO_2 cause an anesthetic-like state of cortical and subcortical depression.

CO_2, not H^+, crosses the blood-brain barrier. Therefore, a change in $Paco_2$ also causes a rapid change in cerebrospinal fluid (CSF) pH. CO_2 is the most important factor in regulating cerebral blood flow (CBF). The relation between CBF and $Paco_2$ is essentially linear from 20 to 100 mm Hg, with maximal vasodilatation occurring at approximately 120 mm Hg. Normal CBF is approximately 12% to 15% of cardiac output or 50 mL/100 g/min. For each 1 mm Hg increase in $Paco_2$ between 20 and 80 mm Hg, CBF increases by 2% to 4%. Hypercarbia decreases cerebral vascular resistance, causing CBF to increase.

Hypercarbia increases intracranial pressure, probably secondary to cerebral vasodilation. In the Trendelenburg position, venous congestion of the head and neck occurs. Additional increases in intra-abdominal and intrathoracic pressures contribute to further increases in intracranial and CSF pressures. However, steep Trendelenburg does not appear to be associated with an increase in postoperative cerebrovascular complications.

Therefore, an acute rise in intra-abdominal pressure (pneumoperitoneum) causes an immediate rise in intracranial pressure. This occurs through compression of the inferior vena cava (resulting in decreased drainage in the lumbar plexus), increased CVP, increased mean arterial pressure, increased intrathoracic pressure, increased venous stasis, increased pressure in the sagittal sinus, and decreased resorption of CSF. Hypercarbia contributes to the increased intracranial pressure, but hyperventilation will not decrease the elevated intracranial pressure until the elevated intra-abdominal pressure is released. Intraocular pressure is also increased during Trendelenburg position with pneumoperitoneum; postoperative visual loss has been reported, but is exceedingly rare.

Awad H, Santilli S, Ohr M, et al. The effects of steep Trendelenburg positioning on intraocular pressure during robotic radical prostatectomy. *Anesth Analg*. 2009;109:473-478.

Hoshikawa Y, Tsutsumi N, Ohkoshi K, et al. The effect of steep Trendelenburg positioning on intraocular pressure and visual function during robotic-assisted radical prostatectomy. *Br J Ophthalmol.* 2014;98:305-308.

Irgau I, Koyfman Y, Tikellis JI. Elective intraoperative intracranial pressure monitoring during laparoscopic cholecystectomy. *Arch Surg.* 1995;130:1011-1013.

Kalmar AF, Dewaele F, Foubert L, et al. Cerebral haemodynamic physiology during steep Trendelenburg position and CO_2 pneumoperitoneum. *Br J Anaesth.* 2012;108:478-484.

Kim MS, Bai SJ, Lee JR, et al. Increase in intracranial pressure during carbon dioxide pneumoperitoneum with steep Trendelenburg positioning proven by ultrasonographic measurement of optic nerve sheath diameter. *J Endourol.* 2014;28:801-806.

Lumb AB, Thomas CR. Anaesthesia. In: Lumb AB, Thomas CR, eds. *Nunn and Lumb's Applied Respiratory Physiology.* 9th ed. Elsevier; 2021:244-267.

Park EY, Koo BN, Min KT, et al. The effect of pneumoperitoneum in the steep Trendelenburg position on cerebral oxygenation. *Acta Anaesthesiol Scand.* 2009;53:895-899.

Ripa M, Schipa C, Kopsacheilis N, et al. The impact of steep Trendelenburg position on intraocular pressure. *J Clin Med.* 2022;11:2844.

Schramm P, Treiber AH, Berres M, et al. Time course of cerebrovascular autoregulation during extreme Trendelenburg position for robotic-assisted prostatic surgery. *Anaesthesia.* 2014;69:58-63.

C.20. What are the neuroendocrine changes that occur during laparoscopy?

Excessive intra-abdominal pressure and hypercarbia activate the sympathoadrenal axis, resulting in increased plasma epinephrine and norepinephrine. Renin, cortisol, aldosterone, antidiuretic hormone, and atrial natriuretic peptide levels are also increased. In awake patients in the Trendelenburg position, increased secretion of atrial natriuretic peptide occurs, probably in response to increased atrial stretching. During pneumoperitoneum, secretion of atrial natriuretic peptide diminishes, suggesting interference with venous return.

Mann C, Boccara G, Pouzeratte Y, et al. The relationship among carbon dioxide pneumoperitoneum, vasopressin release, and hemodynamic changes. *Anesth Analg.* 1999;89:278-283.

Marana E, Colicci S, Meo F, et al. Neuroendocrine stress response in gynecological laparoscopy: TIVA with propofol versus sevoflurane anesthesia. *J Clin Anesth.* 2010;22:250-255.

Mikami O, Fujise K, Matsumoto S, et al. High intra-abdominal pressure increases plasma catecholamine concentrations during pneumoperitoneum for laparoscopic procedures. *Arch Surg.* 1998;133:39-43.

C.21. What is the net effect of pneumoperitoneum, hypercarbia, and steep Trendelenburg on the renal system?

Oliguria is frequently observed during laparoscopy despite adequate hydration. Although prerenal causes such as hypovolemia, positive pressure ventilation, and PEEP can contribute to oliguria, it is believed that neurohumoral changes (eg, antidiuretic hormone secretion) secondary to hypercarbia and increased intra-abdominal pressure secondary to insufflation are responsible for the oliguria that occurs during laparoscopy. Sympathetic stimulation causes a release of catecholamines, resulting in decreased renal cortical blood flow with shunting of blood to the renal medulla, constriction of glomerular afferent arterioles, and decreased glomerular filtration rate. When intraperitoneal insufflation reaches a pressure of 15 mm Hg, renal cortical blood flow decreases by 60% and a reversible 50% drop in urine volume occurs. Pneumoretroperitoneum, which causes a more gradual increase in intra-abdominal pressure, also causes a more gradual decrease in renal perfusion.

Cho JE, Shim JK, Chang JH, et al. Effect of nicardipine on renal function after robot-assisted laparoscopic radical prostatectomy. *Urology.* 2009;73:1056-1060.

Demyttenaere S, Feldman LS, Fried GM. Effect of pneumoperitoneum on renal perfusion and function: a systematic review. *Surg Endosc.* 2007;21:152-160.

Dunn MD, McDougall EM. Renal physiology. Laparoscopic considerations. *Urol Clin North Am.* 2000;27:609-614.

Hazebroek EJ, de Vos tot Nederveen Cappel R, Gommers D, et al. Antidiuretic hormone release during laparoscopic donor nephrectomy. *Arch Surg.* 2002;137:600-605.

Nguyen NT, Perez RV, Fleming N, et al. Effect of prolonged pneumoperitoneum on intraoperative urine output during laparoscopic gastric bypass. *J Am Coll Surg.* 2002;195:476-483.

Wiesenthal JD, Fazio LM, Perks AE, et al. Effect of pneumoperitoneum on renal tissue oxygenation and blood flow in a rat model. *Urology.* 2011;77:1508.e9-1508.e15.

C.22. What is the net effect of pneumoperitoneum, hypercarbia, and steep Trendelenburg on the bowel and gastrointestinal system?

Although CO_2 directly causes vasodilatation of the splanchnic capillary beds, the increased intra-abdominal pressure of laparoscopy decreases perfusion, increases SVR, impairs gastric submucosal perfusion and metabolism, and can cause bowel hypoxia at high pressures. On the release of the intra-abdominal pressure, residual CO_2 again causes vascular dilation, allowing additional CO_2 to enter the bloodstream. Myoelectric activity and recovery from ileus are faster after laparoscopic than after open surgery. The combined effect of the increase in abdominal pressure, stretching of the peritoneum by insufflation, and diffusion of CO_2 into the bowel can contribute to postoperative nausea.

Böhm B, Milsom JW, Fazio VW. Postoperative intestinal motility following conventional and laparoscopic intestinal surgery. *Arch Surg*. 1995;130:415-419.

Meierhenrich R, Gauss A, Vandenesch P, et al. The effects of intraabdominally insufflated carbon dioxide on hepatic blood flow during laparoscopic surgery assessed by transesophageal echocardiography. *Anesth Analg*. 2005;100:340-347.

Schwarte LA, Scheeren TW, Lorenz C, et al. Moderate increase in intraabdominal pressure attenuates gastric mucosal oxygen saturation in patients undergoing laparoscopy. *Anesthesiology*. 2004;100:1081-1087.

Takagi S. Hepatic and portal vein blood flow during carbon dioxide pneumoperitoneum for laparoscopic hepatectomy. *Surg Endosc*. 1998;12:427-431.

Trencheva K, Dhar P, Sonoda T, et al. Physiologic effects of simultaneous carbon dioxide insufflation by laparoscopy and colonoscopy: prospective evaluation. *Surg Endosc*. 2011;25:3279-3285.

C.23. How would you recognize a CO_2 embolism during laparoscopy? How does this differ from an air embolism? Why should N_2O be discontinued during suspected embolization? Will N_2O increase the size of CO_2 emboli?

The incidence of venous gas embolism is lower in robotic-assisted laparoscopic radical prostatectomy than in radical retropubic prostatectomy. It is more likely to occur during the transection of the deep dorsal venous plexus than during the initial insufflation.

Gas embolism can occur whenever the internal pressure of an open vessel is less than the external pressure. Gas embolism can increase ventilatory dead space, increase PVR, increase pulmonary artery pressure, and decrease cardiac output. Early signs include a rapid drop in $Etco_2$ and Pao_2 and an increase in $Paco_2$. During laparoscopy, insufflation of a large amount of CO_2 directly into a blood vessel can occur initially after blind Veress needle insertion, especially at high pressures. Hypotension, hypoxemia, cyanosis, and/or cardiac arrest can occur. If the gas volume is large enough, a "mill-wheel" murmur can be heard through a precordial or esophageal stethoscope. If ventilation is kept constant, a sudden decrease in $Etco_2$ occurs. The most sensitive means to detect gas emboli are precordial, transesophageal Doppler, and transesophageal echocardiography. Aspiration of foamy blood from a central venous catheter is also diagnostic.

CO_2 embolism must be distinguished from air embolism, which is far more serious, as shown in Table 17.2. CO_2, being extremely soluble in the presence of red blood cells, is much less life-threatening than an identically sized intravascular air embolism.

Air emboli can be entrained into open veins above the level of the heart (eg, head and neck surgery, neurosurgery, cesarean delivery). Other gases that are present, such as N_2O, diffuse into that air space according to their diffusion capacities and pressure gradients. Therefore, N_2O will diffuse into, oxygen will

TABLE 17.2 Differences Between Air and Carbon Dioxide Emboli

Embolism	Air	CO_2
Composition	79% N_2, 21% O_2	100% CO_2
Origin	Vein open to air	No contact with air
Pressure source	Hydrostatic	Insufflator
Solubility	Negligible	Large
Effect of N_2O	Enlarged	Not enlarged

CO_2, carbon dioxide; N_2, nitrogen; N_2O; nitrous oxide; O_2, oxygen.

be consumed and/or diffuse out, and the size or pressure of the bubble will increase in proportion to the concentration and duration of N_2O administered until equilibrium is reached. When N_2O is limited to 50, the size of the gas pocket will not be more than doubled at equilibrium.

A gas bubble composed of 100% CO_2 will not enlarge in a patient inhaling 50% or even 75% N_2O because more CO_2 will diffuse out, be absorbed, or be buffered (also more quickly) than N_2O diffuses in. CO_2 has caused fatal embolisms, and N_2O should be discontinued if embolism is suspected. Conditions for creating a CO_2 embolism differ from the conditions required for an air embolism. Other than during direct insufflation of CO_2 into a vein, as during Veress needle insufflation, capillaries and veins within the abdomen are collapsed by the positive pressure within the abdomen, thereby minimizing the chance for CO_2 to enter open vessels.

Fong J, Gadalla F, Pierri MK, et al. Are Doppler-detected venous emboli during cesarean section air emboli? *Anesth Analg*. 1990;71:254-257.

Hong JY, Kim WO, Kil HK. Detection of subclinical CO_2 embolism by transesophageal echocardiography during laparoscopic radical prostatectomy. *Urology*. 2010;75:581-584.

Ishiyama T, Hanagata K, Kashimoto S, et al. Pulmonary carbon dioxide embolism during laparoscopic cholecystectomy. *Can J Anaesth*. 2001;48:319-320.

Jayaraman S, Khakhar A, Yang H, et al. The association between central venous pressure, pneumoperitoneum, and venous carbon dioxide embolism in laparoscopic hepatectomy. *Surg Endosc*. 2009;23:2369-2373.

Kim CS, Kim JY, Kwon JY, et al. Venous air embolism during total laparoscopic hysterectomy: comparison to total abdominal hysterectomy. *Anesthesiology*. 2009;111:50-54.

C.24. What is the mechanism of increased shunting resulting from embolization?

Emboli in the pulmonary capillaries cause an increase in PVR (ie, vasoconstriction), which leads to increased pulmonary artery, right ventricular, and right atrial pressures and an opening of pulmonary precapillary arteriovenous anastomoses, resulting in shunt and hypoxemia.

Lumb AB, Thomas CR. Distribution of pulmonary ventilation and perfusion. In: Lumb AB, Thomas CR, eds. *Nunn and Lumb's Applied Respiratory Physiology*. 9th ed. Elsevier; 2021:88-103.

C.25. How is a gas embolism (CO_2 or air) treated?

- N_2O should be discontinued, and FIO_2 increased to 100%.
- Identify and occlude the site of air entrainment. Insufflation (in the case of CO_2) should be halted, and pneumoperitoneum should be released immediately.
- An increase in the rate and volume of controlled ventilation with PEEP has been suggested as a method of minimizing air entrainment. However, this can reduce cardiac output and increase airway pressure and PVR, and can lead to paradoxical air embolization.
- If possible, the patient should be placed in a steep left lateral decubitus Trendelenburg position to prevent obstruction of the pulmonary outflow tract and right ventricular failure. However, during robotic surgery, the movement of the patient is prevented until the robot is undocked.
- A multi-orifice CVP catheter can be useful for diagnosis and for therapeutic aspiration of air. Radial artery cannulation can be useful to track the improvement or deterioration of BP and arterial blood gases (ABGs).
- Therapy is essentially supportive and includes fluids, vasopressors, and pulmonary arterial catheterization. A large bolus of gas can form a gas lock in the right atrium, decreasing cardiac output. Smaller bubbles can lodge in the lungs, causing pulmonary hypertension, right ventricular failure, and pulmonary edema. Venous gas emboli can also enter the arterial circulation through an atrial septal defect or patent foramen ovale, a condition that exists in 20% of patients.

Gutsche JT, Hanson W III. Pulmonary embolism. In: Lobato EB, Gravenstein N, Kirby RR, eds. *Complications in Anesthesiology*. 3rd ed. Lippincott Williams & Wilkins; 2008:198-200.

Hong JY, Kim JY, Choi YD, et al. Incidence of venous gas embolism during robotic-assisted laparoscopic radical prostatectomy is lower than during radical retropubic prostatectomy. *Br J Anaesth*. 2010;105:777-781.

C.26. What are the causes of pneumothorax or pneumomediastinum during laparoscopy? How would you diagnose it? How would you treat it?

Pneumothorax can result from the migration of laparoscopic gas under pressure or from direct pulmonary barotrauma. CO_2 gas insufflated retroperitoneally gains rapid direct access to a vast space and can result in widespread subcutaneous emphysema and a pneumomediastinum. During laparoscopy, CO_2 under pressure can pass from the abdominal cavity into the pleural and pericardial spaces through anatomic or congenital paths (eg, the hiatus around the esophagus) or through acquired defects in the diaphragm.

Pneumothorax can be diagnosed by a sudden decrease in pulmonary compliance, increase in airway pressure, increase in $Etco_2$ and $Paco_2$, unchanged or decreased Pao_2, unchanged or decreased BP, abnormal motion of the involved hemidiaphragm, and absence of breath sounds without wheezing on the affected side. The shape of the capnogram usually is unchanged. Fiberoptic bronchoscopy can rule out endobronchial intubation, and intraoperative chest fluoroscopy or radiography confirms the diagnosis.

Pneumothorax caused by laparoscopic gas is easily treated, or it can resolve spontaneously. Intraoperative treatment consists of PEEP and increased minute ventilation to reinflate the lung, and increased pressure to decrease the gradient from the abdomen to the pleural cavity and possibly to seal the tear.

Alternatively, pneumothorax can be undetected until the patient regains consciousness and exhibits respiratory distress and restlessness, which can be misinterpreted as pain or inadequate reversal of neuromuscular blockade. Treatment consists of 100% oxygen by mask. CO_2 quickly diffuses out, as can be seen by serial ABGs and chest radiograms; invasive treatment might not be required if the patient is hemodynamically stable.

Subcutaneous emphysema is usually identified by crepitus on physical examination; it can also be seen on a radiograph. A pneumomediastinum is diagnosed with a chest radiograph; treatment usually consists of oxygen and supportive measures. However, tension pneumomediastinum and compartment syndrome due to severe subcutaneous emphysema require surgical intervention.

Because of the increased lung volumes and pressures during laparoscopy, pneumothorax, pneumomediastinum, and subcutaneous emphysema can also result from barotrauma. This cause of pneumothorax is far more serious and can require tube thoracostomy. Attempts at hyperventilating to decrease $Etco_2$ can result in overdistension and rupture of alveoli, with subsequent dissection of the anesthetic gases into the perivascular sheaths, mediastinum, pleura, and fascial planes of the head and neck. Large tidal volumes and rapid ventilator rates can be especially dangerous in patients with COPD or bullae because insufficient emptying time may increase air trapping.

Bartelmaos T, Blanc R, De Claviere G, et al. Delayed pneumomediastinum and pneumothorax complicating laparoscopic extraperitoneal inguinal hernia repair. *J Clin Anesth*. 2005;17:209-212.

Joris JL, Chiche JD, Lamy ML. Pneumothorax during laparoscopic fundoplication: diagnosis and treatment with positive end-expiratory pressure. *Anesth Analg*. 1995;81:993-1000.

C.27. How would you decide when to extubate the trachea?

In addition to the usual criteria for tracheal extubation, prolonged laparoscopy in the Trendelenburg position requires that the following problems are resolved before the trachea is extubated. If significant subcutaneous emphysema has occurred (diagnosed by crepitus and persistent hypercarbia), continue mechanical ventilation with oxygen. A significant amount of CO_2 can be held in the vast retroperitoneal space. Delay extubation if the patient has facial edema, venous congestion, or discoloration of the head and neck. Check the tongue for edema and the eyes for periorbital, conjunctival, or eyelid edema. The cuff of the endotracheal tube should be deflated to make sure that a gas leak exists. If it does not, the patient should remain intubated. Keep the patient in a head-up position until conjunctival edema resolves; laryngeal edema will also be diminished by the head-up position.

Causes of edema include dependent stasis while in Trendelenburg position, resistance from elevated abdominal and thoracic pressures, and temporary fluid overload after intraoperative oliguria or anuria. In some cases, it is best to leave the trachea intubated and a Foley catheter in place until diuresis has begun.

D. Postoperative Management

D.1. What are some of the unique complications of laparoscopy?

Injuries From Instruments

Improper placement of Veress needle or trocars can cause abdominal wall bleeding, blood vessel or visceral puncture, subcutaneous emphysema, peritonitis, wound infection, hernia at the trocar site, and hemorrhage. Thermal injuries can occur from cautery or laser use. Staples and clips can cause nerve entrapment.

Complications of Pneumoperitoneum

Increased intra-abdominal pressure can result in bowel ischemia, omental or bowel herniation, gastric regurgitation, excessive compression of vena cava, decreased venous return, venous stasis in the legs, hypotension, increased intrathoracic pressure, mediastinal and subcutaneous emphysema, pneumothorax, barotrauma, CO_2 gas embolism, atelectasis, bradyarrhythmia from vagal stimulation in response to trocar insertion and peritoneal distension, dysfunction of ventriculoperitoneal shunts, referred shoulder pain from CO_2 gas retained under the diaphragm, and nausea and vomiting.

Systemic Effects of CO_2 Absorption

Among the systemic effects of CO_2 absorptions are hypercarbia, acidosis, increased sympathoadrenal stimulation, hypertension, tachycardia, increased intracranial pressure, subcutaneous emphysema, embolization, and sickle cell crisis. Arrhythmias can occur from hypercarbia, hypoxemia, and increased catecholamine release.

Trendelenburg Position

Venous congestion of head and neck, increased venous pressure, increased intracranial pressure, retinal hemorrhage, retinal detachment, increased intraocular pressure and glaucoma attack, corneal and conjunctival edema, endobronchial intubation and hypoxemia, $\dot{V}/\dot{Q}$ mismatch and hypoxemia, edema of airway including the larynx, airway obstruction and closure, brachial plexus injury from shoulder braces, femoral nerve, peroneal, and other neuropathies, and various respiratory complications have been reported with use of the Trendelenburg position.

Late Complications

Among the late complications are bowel obstruction from injury, cautery burn, intestine or omental herniation through the trocar site, adhesions, deep vein thrombosis, and nerve injury resulting from improper padding. Fever can indicate infection from bowel necrosis. Cutaneous metastases can occur at the port site.

Awad H, Santilli S, Ohr M, et al. The effects of steep Trendelenburg positioning on intraocular pressure during robotic radical prostatectomy. *Anesth Analg*. 2009;109:473-478.

Fahlenkamp D, Rassweiler J, Fornara P, et al. Complications of laparoscopic procedures in urology: experience with 2,407 procedures at 4 German centers. *J Urol*. 1999;162:765-771.

Fuller J, Ashar BS, Carey-Corrado J. Trocar-associated injuries and fatalities: an analysis of 1399 reports to the FDA. *J Minim Invasive Gynecol*. 2005;12:302-307.

Gkegkes ID, Karydis A, Tyritzis SI, et al. Ocular complications in robotic surgery. *Int J Med Robot*. 2015;11:269-274.

Joshi GP. Complications of laparoscopy. *Anesthesiol Clin North Am*. 2001;19:89-105.

Koç G, Tazeh NN, Joudi FN, et al. Lower extremity neuropathies after robot-assisted laparoscopic prostatectomy on a split-leg table. *J Endourol*. 2012;26:1026-1029.

Miele VJ, Bendok B, Bloomfield SM, et al. Ventriculoperitoneal shunt dysfunction in adults secondary to conditions causing a transient increase in intra-abdominal pressure: report of three cases. *Neurosurgery*. 2004;55:434.

Mills JT, Burris MB, Warburton DJ, et al. Positioning injuries associated with robotic assisted urological surgery. *J Urol*. 2013;190:580-584.

Nishikawa K, Nagashima C, Shimodate Y, et al. Migration of the endotracheal tube during laparoscopy-assisted abdominal surgery in young and elderly patients. *Can J Anaesth*. 2004;51:1053-1054.

Pridgeon S, Bishop CV, Adshead J. Lower limb compartment syndrome as a complication of robot-assisted radical prostatectomy: the UK experience. *BJU Int*. 2013;112:485-488.

Sharma A, Berkeley A. Intraoperative drug-eluting stent thrombosis in a patient undergoing robotic prostatectomy. *J Clin Anesth*. 2009;21:517-520.

D.2. In the postanesthesia care unit (PACU), the patient complains of numbness and weakness of the lower extremities after 6 hours of anesthesia for robotic prostatectomy. What tests will you order? When would you remove the Foley catheter and arterial line? Under what circumstances would you order a chest radiograph?

Rhabdomyolysis and compartment syndrome must be ruled out because both occur more frequently in patients with obesity undergoing long immobilizing procedures. Serial monitoring should be begun for creatine phosphokinase, lactate dehydrogenase, creatinine, electrolytes including potassium and calcium, and urinalysis for the presence of myoglobin and casts. Treatment should include diuretics and alkalinization of the urine to increase urine output.

Immediate chest radiography is ordered if respiratory distress, subcutaneous emphysema, and actual or suspected pneumothorax are present.

Do not remove the arterial line until the patient is stable and arterial blood gas values are normal. For patients with uneventful recovery, expect an immediate diuresis. Do not remove the Foley catheter until the patient is stable with fluid intake and volume output that are stable. Check voiding after the catheter is removed. Appropriate medications for nausea and pain control must be written. Ketorolac can be given if there is no contraindication. Prophylactic antimuscarinic belladonna and opium suppositories can be given to reduce the pain from bladder spasms. Patient-controlled analgesia usually is not necessary. For ambulatory patients, an adult escort must be available. Most patients, however, stay overnight.

Karaoren G, Bakan N, Kucuk EV, et al. Is rhabdomyolysis an anaesthetic complication in patients undergoing robot-assisted radical prostatectomy? *J Minim Access Surg*. 2017;13:29-36.

Keene R, Froelich JM, Milbrandt JC, et al. Bilateral gluteal compartment syndrome following robotic-assisted prostatectomy. *Orthopedics*. 2010;33:852.

Scavonetto F, Lamborn DR, McCaffrey JM, et al. Prophylactic belladonna suppositories on anesthetic recovery after robotic assisted laparoscopic prostatectomy. *Can J Urol*. 2013;20:6799-6804.

D.3. What is the incidence of postoperative nausea and vomiting (PONV)?

The incidence of nausea and vomiting after laparoscopy has been reported to be as high as 42%. It is the most important factor in causing overnight admission after ambulatory surgery. The major cause of nausea and vomiting is believed to be rapid peritoneal distension. Neurogenic pathways are activated by traction reflexes and by splanchnic pressure and manipulation. PONV prophylaxis and treatment should follow recent consensus guidelines.

McKeen DM, Arellano R, O'Connell C. Supplemental oxygen does not prevent postoperative nausea and vomiting after gynecological laparoscopy. *Can J Anaesth*. 2009;56:651-657.

Wilson EB, Bass CS, Abrameit W, et al. Metoclopramide versus ondansetron in prophylaxis of nausea and vomiting for laparoscopic cholecystectomy. *Am J Surg*. 2001;181:138-141.

SECTION 4 The Nervous System

18 Brain Tumor and Craniotomy

Philip C. Kuo, June M. Chan, and Kane O. Pryor

A 47-year-old female who was previously healthy presents with a 4-month history of headache, with intermittent diplopia and gait disturbance developing over the last month. She is admitted after her family witnesses an acute episode of profound lethargy, altered cognition, and vomiting. Neurologic examination is remarkable for abnormal right-sided cranial nerve V, VII, and VIII function; nystagmus; and ataxic gait. Magnetic resonance imaging (MRI) shows a large, right posterior fossa mass that is only slightly hyperintense on T2-weighted images but is clearly demarcated after the intravenous injection of gadolinium contrast. The impression is of a petroclival meningioma, with a mass effect on the pons and fourth ventricle. Magnetic resonance angiogram shows a highly vascular tumor drawing principal blood supply from the ascending pharyngeal branch of the ipsilateral external carotid artery. The patient improves clinically following the administration of dexamethasone and mannitol and the infusion of 2% sodium chloride and is monitored in the neurosurgical intensive care unit (NSICU). The day after admission, the patient undergoes uneventful cerebral angiography and partial embolization of the tumor under general anesthesia. She is now scheduled for posterior fossa craniotomy and resection of the tumor.

A. Medical Disease and Differential Diagnosis

1. How are central nervous system (CNS) tumors classified?
2. What is intracranial pressure (ICP), and what are its determinants?
3. How does the presence of a mass alter the ICP in this patient, and what are the clinical manifestations of these alterations?
4. What is cerebral blood flow (CBF), and what are its determinants?
5. What are cerebral steal syndromes?
6. Are there any issues specific to posterior cranial fossa pathology?
7. What is the role of preoperative embolization therapy?

B. Preoperative Evaluation and Preparation

1. What are the special considerations in the preoperative evaluation of the patient scheduled for posterior fossa craniotomy?
2. In a patient who presents with intracranial hypertension, what management might have already been initiated preoperatively, and what are the implications for anesthetic management?
3. What are the types of intraoperative neurophysiologic monitoring (IOM) that would likely be used for this procedure, and how will they affect the anesthetic management plan?
4. What are the options for patient positioning during posterior fossa surgery?
5. What are the principal disadvantages associated with the common posterior fossa craniotomy positions?
6. How does the sitting position affect your preoperative assessment and planning?
7. How should the patient's position ultimately be determined?
8. Should this patient receive premedication?

C. Intraoperative Management

1. What are the anesthetic goals for craniotomy?
2. What monitors should be used during craniotomy?
3. Would you monitor for venous air embolism (VAE)? What are the monitoring options?
4. What specific risks are associated with the induction of anesthesia?
5. How would you induce anesthesia?
6. What are the effects of anesthetics on the cerebral metabolic rate of oxygen ($CMRO_2$), CBF, and ICP? With this in mind, how would you maintain anesthesia?
7. How would you manage ventilation and maintain arterial carbon dioxide (CO_2)?
8. How would you approach diuretic therapy?
9. How would you manage serum glucose?
10. How would you approach fluid management?
11. Once the bone plate is removed and the dura retracted, the surgeon reports that the brain is still "tight." What would be your response?
12. If deliberate hypotension is indicated, how will you achieve it?
13. While the surgeon is resecting a tumor from near the brainstem, the patient's heart rate suddenly drops to 20 beats per minute. What is your assessment and management?
14. Are there any measures you can take to prevent VAE?
15. During the procedure, the precordial Doppler becomes loud and turbulent. The end-tidal CO_2 ($Etco_2$) drops from 31 to 13 mm Hg, and the systemic pressure from 121/63 to 64/32 mm Hg. What is your assessment and management plan?
16. What is your approach to emergence? What if the patient does not regain consciousness?

D. Postoperative Management

1. What postoperative complications are of greatest concern? What level of monitoring is required?
2. What is your approach to postoperative pain control?
3. In the ICU, the patient's neurologic status deteriorates and ICP monitoring is instituted. What are the different methods of monitoring ICP, and what are their limitations?

SECTION 4

A. Medical Disease and Differential Diagnosis

A.1. How are central nervous system (CNS) tumors classified?

Pathologic description and classification of CNS tumors is constantly evolving, as an increased molecular and genetic understanding of tumor origin is added to the established classification systems based on histology and immunohistochemistry. The international standard is the World Health Organization Classification of Tumors of the Central Nervous System (WHO CNS5), updated in 2021 (**Table 18.1**). Primary malignant CNS tumors are the most common solid organ malignancy in children and the second overall after hematologic malignancy. In adults, CNS tumors are the eighth most common cancer, with nonmalignant tumors approximately 2.5× more common than malignant tumors. The most common form of malignant tumor in adults is glioma, with meningioma being the most common form of nonmalignant tumor.

Diagnostic genes, molecules, and pathways are associated with over 40 forms of CNS tumors. Most of this science lies beyond the required knowledge of the anesthesiologist; however, the anesthesiologist should be aware of relatively common genetic conditions linked to CNS tumor development that are also associated with extra-tumor manifestations. For instance, there is a clear association between meningiomas and neurofibromatosis type 2. Other conditions linked with the development of brain tumors include neurofibromatosis types 1 and 2, von Hippel-Lindau syndrome, tuberous sclerosis, Li-Fraumeni syndrome, and Turcot syndrome (**Table 18.2**). The preoperative assessment should be informed by an appreciation of the multiorgan nature of these genetic conditions.

Louis DN, Perry A, Wesseling P, et al. The 2021 WHO classification of tumors of the central nervous system: a summary. *Neuro Oncol.* 2021;23:1231-1251.

Nolan C, DeAngelis LM. Primary neoplasms of the central nervous system in adults. In: Hong WK, Bast RC, Hait WN, et al, eds. *Holland-Frei Cancer Medicine.* 8th ed. PMPH-USA; 2010.

Ostrom QT, Francis SS, Barnholtz-Sloan JS. Epidemiology of brain and other CNS tumors. *Curr Neurol Neurosci Rep.* 2021;21:68.

TABLE 18.1 Key Divisions of the WHO CNS5 Classification of CNS Tumors

Gliomas, glioneuronal tumors, and neuronal tumors
- *Adult-type diffuse gliomas*
- *Pediatric-type diffuse low-grade gliomas*
- *Pediatric-type diffuse high-grade gliomas*
- *Circumscribed astrocytic gliomas*
- *Glioneuronal and neuronal tumors*
- *Ependymal tumors*

Choroid plexus tumors
Embryonal tumors
- *Medulloblastoma*
- *Other CNS embryonal tumors*

Pineal tumors
Cranial and paraspinal nerve tumors
Meningiomas
Mesenchymal, nonmeningothelial tumors
- *Soft tissue tumors*
- *Chondro-osseous tumors*

Melanocytic tumors
Hematolymphoid tumors
- *Lymphomas*
- *Histiocytic tumors*

Germ cell tumors
Tumors of the sellar region
Metastases to the CNS

CNS, central nervous system; WHO CNS5, World Health Organization Classification of Tumors of the Central Nervous System.

A.2. What is intracranial pressure (ICP), and what are its determinants?

Normal ICP ranges from 5 to 15 mm Hg (6-20 cm H_2O). This pressure results from the physiologic interactions of intracranial structures within the rigid skull. Anatomically, these structures are enclosed within a cranial vault that is partitioned by rigid dural folds, the falx cerebri, falx cerebelli, and tentorium cerebelli. Functionally, intracranial structures can be conceptualized as three compartments within a minimally compliant space:

TABLE 18.2 Genetic Conditions Associated With Intracranial Tumors

Syndrome	Chromosome	Characteristic Tumor	Other Pathognomic Lesions
NF-1	17q11	Optic glioma Brainstem glioma	Café-au-lait spots, Lisch nodules
NF-2	22q12	Bilateral acoustic neuromas Multiple meningiomas	Subcutaneous schwannomas
Retinoblastoma	13q14	Trilateral retinoblastoma	
von Hippel-Lindau	3p25	Cerebellar, retinal, and spinal hemangioblastoma	
Tuberous sclerosis	9q34	Subependymal astrocytoma Retinal astrocytoma	Ash-leaf spots Shagreen patch Adenoma sebaceum
Sturge-Weber	9q21	Leptomeningeal angiomatosis Choroidal hemangioma	Port-wine nevus Glaucoma
Turcot	5q21	Glioblastoma Medulloblastoma	
Li-Fraumeni	17q	Malignant glioma PNET	

NF-1, neurofibromatosis type 1; NF-2, neurofibromatosis type 2; PNET, primitive neuroectodermal tumor.

- *Parenchyma*, consisting of cellular, extracellular, and intracellular fluid components, occupying 80% to 85% of total intracranial volume (~1,400 mL in the average adult)
- *Cerebrospinal fluid (CSF)*, occupying 10% of total intracranial volume (~75 mL in the cisterns, 50 mL in the subarachnoid space, and 25 mL in the ventricles)
- *Intracranial blood volume*, consisting of both arterial and venous blood, which occupies 5% to 10% of total intracranial volume (averaging 150 mL in the adult)

Without compensation, alterations in any one of these compartments will eventually lead to increases in ICP, which may impede blood flow and result in ischemia. Monro (1783) and Kellie (1824) first hypothesized that an increase in the volume of one compartment results in a compensatory decrease in the other compartments, thereby preserving normal ICP. Initially, CSF can drain to the spinal CSF reservoir, while venous blood flows into the extracranial veins. This minimizes the change in ICP during the early phases of intracranial volume expansion; however, this compensation is limited, especially if the expansion is rapid. At a critical point, these compensatory mechanisms are exhausted, and even small increases in intracranial volumes will result in significant increases in ICP. Although this phenomenon is frequently described as reflecting *decreased compliance* ($\Delta V/\Delta P$), this is a longstanding error in nomenclature; the correct description is that it reflects *increased elastance* ($\Delta P/\Delta V$).

Early signs of increased ICP include headache (classically occipital), vomiting, behavioral changes, sedation, and cognitive slowing. Papilledema on fundoscopy is an important sign that is often missed on examination. Further increases in ICP can eventually lead to compressive cranial neuropathies (typically cranial nerve VI, causing unilateral mydriasis) and herniation of brain tissue through a noncompliant partition—rapidly resulting in irreversible regional and global neuronal injuries.

Kasprowicz M, Lalou DA, Czosnyka M, et al. Intracranial pressure, its components and cerebrospinal fluid pressure-volume compensation. *Acta Neurol Scand.* 2016;134:168-180.

Kellie G. An account of the appearances observed in the dissection of two of three individuals presumed to have perished in the storm of the 3rd, and whose bodies were discovered in the vicinity of Leith on the morning of the 4th November 1821 with some reflections on the pathology of the brain. *Trans Med Chir Sci Edinburgh.* 1824;1:84-169.

Lanier WL, Warner DO. Intracranial elastance versus intracranial compliance: terminology should agree with that of other disciplines. *Anesthesiology.* 1992;77:403-404.

Lemkuil BP, Drummond JC, Patel PM, Lam AM. Anesthesia for neurologic surgery and neurointerventions. In: Gropper MA, Eriksson LI, Fleisher LA, Cohen NH, Leslie K, Johnson-Akeju O, eds. *Miller's Anesthesia.* 10th ed. Elsevier; 2025:1740–1783.

Monro A. *Observations on the Structure and Functions of the Nervous System: Illustrated with Tables.* Creech and Johnson; 1783.

A.3. How does the presence of a mass alter the ICP in this patient, and what are the clinical manifestations of these alterations?

Within the constraints of the intracranial elastance model outlined earlier, there are certain characteristics of an intracranial mass that influence the degree of ICP alteration:

- *Size*: An intracranial mass exerts effects through its intrinsic volume and any surrounding edema. Any space-occupying lesion within a relatively fixed intracranial compartment is compensated for by decreases in the volume of other intracranial contents.
- *Rate of growth*: A rapidly expanding mass outpaces the rate at which compensatory volume shifts can occur, which leads to an increase in ICP.
- *Anatomic location*: The infratentorial space is notable for being highly susceptible to mass-related alterations in ICP. The area bound by the tentorium cerebelli and occiput is much lower in volume and elastance when compared with the supratentorial space. It also contains vital structures involved in CSF bulk flow between different compartments: the fourth ventricle, which communicates with the supratentorial ventricles and subarachnoid cisterns, and the foramen magnum, which communicates with the spinal column. Any volume shift within the infratentorial space may therefore precipitate a noncommunicating hydrocephalus, which further compromises compensatory mechanisms for intracranial hypertension.
- *Local tissue dysfunction*: The presence of an intracranial tumor causes local effects on surrounding tissue through invasive destruction, induction of neoangiogenesis through the release of oncogenic factors, or compression with ischemic cellular disruption. This results in an inflammatory response that causes further tissue edema and increases in ICP.

Taken together, these considerations account for the differences in the clinical presentation of intracranial masses. A slow-growing mass, particularly in the peripheral supratentorial space, can become sizable over a period of years with minimal symptoms due to compensatory volume remodeling, whereas

SECTION 4

a small infratentorial lesion can obstruct the fourth ventricle and rapidly cause significant intracranial hypertension.

In this patient, a slow-growing meningioma has been able to attain a large size before becoming symptomatic. The patient's earliest signs and symptoms were most likely due to a localized mass effect. The more acute decompensation, with rapidly developing signs and symptoms of elevated ICP, probably represents the added component of CSF outflow obstruction at the fourth ventricle. Even with the clinical improvement achieved by steroid therapy and osmotic diuresis, this patient has very little volume reserve and intracranial elastance, so even small increases in volume—such as an increase in cerebral blood volume (CBV) precipitated by hypercapnia or a minimum alveolar concentration (MAC) of volatile anesthetic—have the potential to cause a precipitous spike in ICP.

Ropper AH. Lateral displacement of the brain and level of consciousness in patients with an acute hemispheral mass. *N Engl J Med.* 1986;314:953-958.

Ropper AH. A preliminary MRI study of the geometry of brain displacement and level of consciousness with acute intracranial masses. *Neurology.* 1989;39:622-627.

Schaller B, Graf R. Different compartments of intracranial pressure and its relationship to cerebral blood flow. *J Trauma.* 2005;59:1521-1531.

A.4. What is cerebral blood flow (CBF), and what are its determinants?

Despite only constituting about 2% of total body weight, the brain receives approximately 15% to 20% of resting cardiac output as CBF via the carotid and vertebral arteries. This disproportionately high blood flow is due to the brain's high metabolic requirement for oxygen (MRO_2)—approximately 3.5 mL O_2/min/100 g brain tissue, totaling 20% of total body MRO_2. CBF is approximately 750 mL/min in the adult or 50 mL/min/100 g averaged across gray and white matter. Gray matter, which contains neuronal nuclei, is metabolically more active than white matter and consumes 75 versus 45 mL O_2/min/100 g of tissue.

CBF is determined by cerebral perfusion pressure (CPP), which describes the pressure gradient for blood flow across the cerebral vascular bed, and cerebral vascular resistance (CVR):

$$\text{CBF} = \text{CPP/CVR}.$$

On a global level, CPP is the difference between the inflow and outflow pressures of the brain's blood supply. However, the cerebral circulation behaves as a Starling resistor: Its enclosure within the rigid cranial vault allows extravascular pressure (ICP) to compress and compromise venous outflow. Hence, CBF can be expressed as:

$$\text{CBF} = (\text{mean arterial pressure [MAP]} - \text{outflow pressure})/\text{CVR}.$$

Where outflow pressure = CVP or ICP, whichever is higher.

CBF is highly regulated to ensure substrate delivery matches the metabolic demands of neural tissue in a phenomenon known as *flow-metabolism coupling*. Depending on neuronal activation and metabolic demands, regions of the brain may be either hypoperfused or hyperperfused. A sudden decrease in CBF (such as during the occlusion of a cerebral artery) results in an ischemic injury with neurologic deficits and potentially irreversible tissue damage. An excess of blood flow leads to hyperemia and potential increases in ICP that can cause tissue compression and damage. Therefore, it is essential to maintain brain homeostasis; this is achieved through alterations in CVR via four overlapping mechanisms occurring on a regional and global cerebral level:

- *Vascular myogenic autoregulation*
  - Classical teaching is that CBF is maintained constant across MAPs of approximately 50 to 150 mm Hg. Based on recent studies in humans, the extremes of this range should be approached with caution, especially the lower boundary; CBF can decrease at MAPs of 60 or even 70 mm Hg. Chronic hypertension causes a rightward shift in the CBF-MAP relationship. Hypocapnia has been demonstrated to broaden the autoregulatory range, whereas hypercapnia and elevated ICP decrease the responsiveness of pressure autoregulation.
- *Metabolic autoregulation*
  - CO_2: CO_2 is a potent cerebral vasodilator. It exerts its effects on the cerebral vasculature primarily by altering CSF pH, although there is evidence that CSF P_{CO_2} also has a direct effect on cerebral vascular smooth muscle. At normotensive ranges, CBF has a linear relationship with acute changes in Pa_{CO_2} between 20 and 80 mm Hg, with CBF changing by 2% to 4% for every mm Hg change in Pa_{CO_2}. Beyond this range, further changes are limited by extremes in vascular diameter. This response is blunted

by systemic hypotension and volatile anesthesia. It is important to note that prolonged hypocarbia or hypercarbia (beyond 6-8 hours) will ultimately have little effect on CVR, as CSF pH normalizes with active transport of bicarbonate over the blood-brain barrier (BBB). Furthermore, subsequent correction of $Paco_2$ would likely result in rebound cerebral hyper- or hypoperfusion.

  - Oxygen (O_2): Acute exposure to hypoxia causes an immediate increase in CBF in a curvilinear relation with respect to arterial Po_2 and linear with respect to hemoglobin saturation. Acute hypoxemia below 50 mm Hg causes cerebral vasodilation, rapidly reaching maximal response at approximately 30 mm Hg. The exact mechanism of how this occurs is unclear, but it likely involves the direct effects of by-products from anaerobic metabolism and cellular ischemia, such as lactic acid and adenosine. This mechanism is also impaired in the presence of volatile anesthetics.
- *Neurogenic autoregulation*
  - Compared with myogenic and metabolic mechanisms, the autonomic nervous system plays a minor role in cerebral autoregulation. Both sympathetic innervation of cerebral arterioles and circulating sympathomimetics attenuate increases in CBF during severe hypertension, hypoxia, and hypercapnia.

As stated earlier, the presence of an intracranial mass induces dysfunction in surrounding neural tissue, resulting in ischemia and inflammation. This acidic microenvironment promotes local vasodilatation and vasoplegia, with subsequent narrowing of the pressure autoregulatory range. Regional CBF becomes dependent on MAP and ICP, with little ability to compensate for changes in systemic blood pressure. Mass effect alone can increase ICP enough to critically compromise CPP with apparently normal MAP.

A conservative approach to the management of CPP would suggest that it should not be allowed to fall below 70 mm Hg for any extended period in the baseline normotensive patient. Although a more moderate approach targeting CPPs in the 60- to 70-mm Hg range is commonly used, most neuroanesthesiologists agree that sustained CPP values under 60 mm Hg place the brain at risk, despite the possible neuroprotection afforded by the presence of a γ-aminobutyric acid (GABA)ergic anesthetic agent.

Lemkuil BP, Drummond JC, Patel PM. Central nervous system physiology: cerebrovascular. In: Hemmings HC, Egan TD, eds. *Pharmacology and Physiology for Anesthesia: Foundations and Clinical Application*. 2nd ed. Elsevier; 2019:174-192.

Sharma D, Bithal PK, Dash HH, et al. Cerebral autoregulation and CO_2 reactivity before and after elective supratentorial tumor resection. *J Neurosurg Anesthesiol.* 2010;22:132-137.

ter Laan M, van Dijk JM, Elting JW, et al. Sympathetic regulation of cerebral blood flow in humans: a review. *Br J Anaesth.* 2013;111:361-367.

Venkat P, Chopp M, Chen J. New insights into coupling and uncoupling of cerebral blood flow and metabolism in the brain. *Croat Med J.* 2016;57:223-228.

Yoon S, Zuccarello M, Rapoport RM. pCO(2) and pH regulation of cerebral blood flow. *Front Physiol.* 2012;3:365.

A.5. What are cerebral steal syndromes?

Any intracranial pathology, including marginal ischemia and inflammation surrounding a mass lesion, can cause localized dysfunction of normal cerebral autoregulation and an impaired response to vasoactive agents. The microvasculature in the pathologic region can have an essentially fixed resistance. In this case, if vasodilation occurs in other normal regions of the brain, the decreased vascular resistance in the normal tissue can theoretically shunt blood flow away from the pathologic regions, which are already the most vulnerable. This phenomenon is known as *cerebral steal.*

In anesthesia management, cerebral steal is most relevant in the context of hypercapnia and the use of volatile anesthetics. Both cause vasodilation of normal vasculature and potentially decrease regional CBF in pathologic areas. For volatile anesthetics, cerebral vasodilatation is usually considered to be significant when given in doses of 1 MAC or greater, but as a dose-dependent effect, it may be clinically apparent at 0.5 MAC. During hypocapnia, when there is vasoconstriction in normal tissue, the opposite may occur. In this case, blood flow to pathologic regions can actually increase. This phenomenon is known as *inverse steal* or the *Robin Hood effect*. Although both steal effects have been well reported in human literature, the clinical relevance of steal and inverse steal phenomena remains unclear. Nonetheless, it is prudent to consider them in anesthetic management.

Alexandrov AV, Sharma VK, Lao AY, et al. Reversed Robin Hood syndrome in acute ischemic stroke patients. *Stroke.* 2007;38:3045-3048.

Darby JM, Yonas H, Marion DW, et al. Local "inverse steal" induced by hyperventilation in head injury. *Neurosurgery.* 1988;23:84-88.

Lemkuil BP, Drummond JC, Patel PM. Central nervous system physiology: cerebrovascular. In: Hemmings HC, Egan TD, eds. *Pharmacology and Physiology for Anesthesia: Foundations and Clinical Application*. 2nd ed. Elsevier; 2019:174-192.

McCulloch TJ, Thompson CL, Turner MJ. A randomized crossover comparison of the effects of propofol and sevoflurane on cerebral hemodynamics during carotid endarterectomy. *Anesthesiology.* 2007;106:56-64.

Patel PM, Drummond JC, Lemkuil BP. Cerebral physiology and the effects of anesthetic drugs. In: Gropper MA, Eriksson LI, Fleisher LA, Cohen NH, Leslie K, Johnson-Akeju O, eds. *Miller's Anesthesia.* 10th ed. Elsevier; 2025:180–224.

A.6. Are there any issues specific to posterior cranial fossa pathology?

Surgery for tumors in the posterior fossa presents several challenges not seen with supratentorial surgery (**Table 18.3**). The posterior fossa extends from tentorium cerebelli superiorly to foramen magnum inferiorly, housing the cerebellum and most of the brainstem—specifically the pons and medulla. The posterior fossa is a tightly enclosed space in which tumors are often in direct contact with critical brainstem structures, including the cranial nerves and brainstem nuclei. The smaller volume of the posterior fossa means that less mass effect is needed to produce symptoms from compression of the cerebellum, brainstem, or fourth ventricle, with the potential risk of superior vermian or inferior tonsillar herniation. The patient with a posterior fossa tumor, especially one close to the brainstem, can worsen neurologically in the hours following surgery as a result of postsurgical inflammation and edema.

In addition to the risk of neuronal damage, surgery in proximity to brainstem nuclei can trigger significant intraoperative autonomic and collateral hemodynamic instability, which can be extremely challenging to manage. The most common autonomic event is an acute increase in vagal tone, which can result in pronounced bradycardia (and possibly asystole), and can be immediately followed by a reflexive surge in sympathetic tone. Furthermore, the risk to cranial nerves and other structures often demands IOM—such as somatosensory evoked potentials (SSEPs), brainstem auditory evoked potentials, or electromyography (EMG)—all of which can substantially restrict and dictate anesthetic management.

Finally, the posterior fossa cannot be accessed with the patient in the conventional supine position. In the past, the sitting position was highly favored by neurosurgeons and presented marked anesthetic challenges because of the increased risk of VAE. Although still used in some centers, the sitting position has fallen out of favor; nonetheless, all of the positions that permit access to the posterior fossa pose management difficulties that must be considered. The risk of VAE, although reduced, often still exists. Other considerations include loss of jugular outflow, deterioration of pulmonary compliance, strain on the cervical spine and brachial plexus, and a lack of access to central venous lines and the airway. In patients who are critically ill or otherwise at risk for life-threatening intraoperative events, it must be remembered that cardiopulmonary resuscitation will always require that the patient be rapidly returned to the supine position.

Bullock MR, Chesnut R, Ghajar J, et al. Surgical management of posterior fossa mass lesions. *Neurosurgery.* 2006;58:S47-S55.

Gale T, Leslie K. Anaesthesia for neurosurgery in the sitting position. *J Clin Neurosci.* 2004;11:693-696.

Gurol ME, St Louis EK. Treatment of cerebellar masses. *Curr Treat Options Neurol.* 2008;10:138-150.

Kan P, Couldwell WT. Posterior fossa brain tumors and arterial hypertension. *Neurosurg Rev.* 2006;29:265-269.

Shih RY, Smirniotopoulos JG. Posterior fossa tumors in adult patients. *Neuroimaging Clin N Am.* 2016;26:493-510.

TABLE 18.3 Specific Anesthetic Considerations in Posterior Fossa Craniotomy

Specific Challenges	Management Considerations

Need for adequate surgical access	• High likelihood of nonsupine positioning
	  • Sitting position
	  • Prone/semiprone position
	• Reduced access to airway and precordium in case of emergency
	• Risk of disrupting airway, vascular access, and monitors during position changes
	• Specific hemodynamic effects of nonsupine positioning
	  • Venous air embolism risk
	  • Venous pooling in sitting position
	  • External abdominal compression in prone position
	• Positioning-related nerve and soft tissue injury

Brainstem dysfunction	• Intraoperative autonomic instability • Postoperative central respiratory failure
Intraoperative neuromonitoring	• Limitations in the administration of volatile agents and neuromuscular blockade • Need to understand the implications of pathologic alterations in intraoperative monitoring signals and the appropriate management response

A.7. What is the role of preoperative embolization therapy?

Highly vascular tumors, especially those that are anatomically difficult to access, present a high risk for substantial intraoperative bleeding. In addition to the systemic risks associated with gross blood loss, peri-tumor bleeding can severely compromise surgical exposure and exacerbate neuronal and neurovascular inflammation.

To reduce this risk, patients often undergo embolization of the vessels feeding the tumor in the days immediately before surgery. An appropriately sized neuroangiography catheter is inserted—frequently in the femoral artery, although newer techniques permit radial access—and fluoroscopically guided until it sits in a vessel that has evolved to supply only the tumor and not the normal brain. Low-dose systemic heparinization (~50-60 units heparin per kg) to achieve activated clotting times of 200 to 300 seconds is required to prevent the formation of microthrombi. At this point, an embolic agent is slowly delivered to occlude the vessel, reducing the tumor's vascular supply and thus the degree of bleeding during subsequent operative resection. A variety of embolic agents can potentially be used and can be classified into two groups: particulate (using a variety of substances such as coils, gelatin sponges, fibrin glue, and polyvinyl alcohol) and liquid (ethylene vinyl alcohol, hyperosmolar mannitol). The choice of agent is determined by angiographic anatomy, tumor vascularity, and tumor histology (if known). Because of collateralization and reestablishment of blood supply, embolization is effective for only a short period and is usually performed within 48 hours of the intracranial resection.

SECTION 4

Tumor embolization comes with its own risks and challenges: Vascular anatomy might not always permit embolization, and the embolization itself can precipitate peri-tumor edema and hyperemic changes in blood flow dynamics. These changes are particularly relevant in this patient with a posterior fossa tumor proximate to the brainstem. Deposition of the embolic agent into vessels supplying the normal brain amounts to an embolic stroke and can have catastrophic consequences. Catheter-related complications, including vessel dissection and rupture, and access site hematomas are well described. Furthermore, embolization frequently requires general anesthesia and thus assumes all of the associated risks. Current literature reports embolization-related complication rates for meningiomas between 2.9% and 4.6%, but with significant decreases in intraoperative blood loss.

Ashour R, Aziz-Sultan A. Preoperative tumor embolization. *Neurosurg Clin N Am.* 2014;25:607-617.

Carli DF, Sluzewski M, Beute GN, et al. Complications of particle embolization of meningiomas: frequency, risk factors, and outcome. *Am J Neuroradiol.* 2010;31:152-154.

Raper DM, Starke RM, Henderson F Jr, et al. Preoperative embolization of intracranial meningiomas: efficacy, technical considerations, and complications. *Am J Neuroradiol.* 2014;35:1798-1804.

Young WL. Anesthesia for endovascular neurosurgery and interventional neuroradiology. *Anesthesiol Clin.* 2007;25:391-412.

B. Preoperative Evaluation and Preparation

B.1. What are the special considerations in the preoperative evaluation of the patient scheduled for posterior fossa craniotomy?

In addition to the routine thorough preoperative evaluation, the evaluation of the patient for craniotomy should answer several questions that critically influence anesthesia management:

- What is the ICP? If ICP is still in the normal range, how much intracranial compliance reserve is likely to exist?
- How is autoregulation likely to be affected by the pathology and chronic changes in blood pressure? What range of arterial pressures will be required to preserve adequate CPP and CBF?
- Does the patient have any of the electrolyte and endocrine abnormalities associated with intracranial pathology or treatment, such as neurogenic diabetes insipidus, or hypernatremia resulting from hypertonic saline therapy?
- Is the lesion highly vascular, difficult to access, or situated proximate to one of the large draining veins—all of which increase the probability of significant bleeding?
- What is the likely positioning, and does it incur a risk of VAE, obstruction of jugular venous outflow, or neck hyperrotation? Are there preoperative patient conditions that would significantly increase the risk of or preclude certain positions, such as patent foramen ovale and right-to-left intracardiac shunts?
- Is the tumor located in a position close to the brainstem such that severe autonomic dysfunction is likely?

- Will the baseline neurologic status affect the ability to extubate or establish an early neurologic assessment after general anesthesia?
- Will the anesthetic technique need to accommodate specific monitoring requirements, such as electroencephalography (EEG), electrocorticography, brainstem auditory evoked responses (BAERs), or SSEPs?

Fischer SP. Preoperative evaluation of the adult neurosurgical patient. *Int Anesthesiol Clin.* 1996;34:21-32.

Jellish WS, Murdoch J, Leonetti JP. Perioperative management of complex skull base surgery: the anesthesiologist's point of view. *Neurosurg Focus.* 2002;12:E5.

Lemkuil BP, Drummond JC, Patel PM, Lam AM. Anesthesia for neurologic surgery and neurointerventions. In: Gropper MA, Eriksson LI, Fleisher LA, Cohen NH, Leslie K, Johnson-Akeju O, eds. *Miller's Anesthesia.* 10th ed. Elsevier; 2025:1740–1783.

Lieb K, Selim M. Preoperative evaluation of patients with neurological disease. *Semin Neurol.* 2008;28:603-610.

B.2. In a patient who presents with intracranial hypertension, what management might have already been initiated preoperatively, and what are the implications for anesthetic management?

A patient with evidence of intracranial hypertension will be aggressively monitored and treated preoperatively; the preoperative assessment will likely occur in an intensive care setting. The anesthesiologist must be familiar with the management of intracranial hypertension, as various therapies will likely need to be initiated or continued in the operating room. Furthermore, the anesthesiologist must be mindful of potential sequelae that can arise from various perioperative therapies and interventions such as:

- *Corticosteroids*: Treatment can lead to hyperglycemia, which should be aggressively treated to maintain plasma glucose at less than 200 mg/dL while taking care to avoid hypoglycemia.
- *Head elevation*: Care should be taken to maintain 30° head elevation, where possible, and to avoid rapidly lowering the head during transport.
- *Diuretics (mannitol, furosemide)*: These can result in electrolyte or acid-base abnormalities. Decreased preload can increase the risk of hypotension in the peri-induction period.
- *Isotonic or hypertonic saline therapy*: This can result in hypernatremia or a hyperchloremic, non–anion gap metabolic acidosis.
- *Intubation and institution of hyperventilation*: If prolonged, the CBF response to CO_2 can become diminished or absent, with a risk for dangerous increases in CBF and ICP if hyperventilation is rapidly ceased. It can also lead to a compensatory loss of bicarbonate and other basic metabolic buffers, leading to the development of acidosis if ventilation was normalized. Care should be taken to avoid hypoventilation during transport.
- *Ventriculostomy*: This is usually clamped during transport to or from the ICU, as the level of the drain relative to the head is critical, and accidental changes in position can result in excessive draining of CSF. It should be attended to on arrival to the operating room because even relatively short periods of clamping can result in elevations in ICP.
- *Manipulation of systemic pressures to optimize CPP*: Care should be taken to ensure drug infusions are maintained during transport to avoid rebound hypertension or hypotension.
- *Drug-induced cerebral vasoconstriction and coma*: Propofol is the typical first-line agent currently used in the United States for sedation, with pentobarbital used only in critical refractory situations. This signifies a critical neurologic status. The therapy is often continued as the primary anesthetic.
- *Deliberate hypothermia*: This signifies a critical neurologic status and requires a discussion of intraoperative temperature management goals with the neurosurgeon and neurointensivist because the neuroprotective benefits may be countered by hypothermia-induced coagulopathy.

Li LM, Timofeev I, Czosnyka M, et al. Review article: the surgical approach to the management of increased intracranial pressure after traumatic brain injury. *Anesth Analg.* 2010;111:736-748.

Perez-Barcena J, Llompart-Pou JA, O'Phelan KH. Intracranial pressure monitoring and management of intracranial hypertension. *Crit Care Clin.* 2014;30:735-750.

Stevens RD, Bhardwaj A. Evolving paradigms in the management of severe traumatic brain injury. *Crit Care Med.* 2005;33:2415-2417.

Vincent JL, Berré J. Primer on medical management of severe brain injury. *Crit Care Med.* 2005;33:1392-1399.

B.3. What are the types of intraoperative neurophysiologic monitoring (IOM) that would likely be used for this procedure, and how will they affect the anesthetic management plan?

IOM uses a combination of stimulators and sensing electrodes to assess the functional integrity of sensory, motor, and cranial nerves and their associated nerve tracts and/or muscles. The primary monitoring modalities are EMG, evoked potentials (EPs), and EEG. EEG is rarely used for craniotomies for tumor resection and will not be considered in detail in this chapter.

EMG records the electrical activity within muscles in response to stimulation of their innervating cranial or peripheral nerves. The most common EMG monitoring during posterior fossa surgery is for cranial nerve VII, although monitoring of cranial nerves V, IX, X, and XI is frequently encountered. Usually, the surgeon will deliver a very low current to a structure they believe could be the cranial nerve of interest, and motor activity is monitored in the distribution of the nerve through small needles placed in the appropriate muscle body. Mechanical manipulation of a nerve will often also cause muscular activity, which may herald potential inadvertent injury. EMG is relatively unaffected by volatile and intravenous anesthetic agents but requires intact functioning of the neuromuscular junction. Therefore, neuromuscular blockers cannot be used in the setting of EMG monitoring beyond anesthetic induction. Some anesthesiologists advocate the use of succinylcholine for intubation; however, monitoring usually only commences after a substantial time following induction, and the use of a short-acting agent is rarely obligatory. An intubating dose of a medium-duration nondepolarizing agent such as rocuronium or vecuronium is appropriate; with sugammadex now widely available, the neuromuscular blockade can be quickly reversed if needed at the time monitoring is required. The use of a remifentanil infusion is common to secure motionlessness during periods when the neuromuscular blockade is not present.

SECTION 4

EPs assess sensory pathways by measuring electrical activity generated within the nervous system in response to a stimulus. The most common EP monitoring encountered during resection of posterior fossa tumors is the BAER, which monitors cranial nerve VIII and auditory pathway function (including portions of the brainstem, midbrain, and the primary auditory cortex) in response to sounds generated in the auditory canal. SSEPs can also be used to monitor dorsal column-medial lemniscus tract integrity, which is useful for posterior fossa surgery, given the superficial location of the medial lemniscus in the brainstem and pons. These are elicited via electrical stimulation of peripheral sensory nerves (most commonly median and posterior tibial nerves) and recorded via scalp needle electrodes directed over the somatosensory cortex. Similarly, motor evoked potentials (MEPs) are obtained through transcranial stimulation of cortical pyramidal cells and recorded distally along the spinal cord, motor nerves, and muscle.

EPs are recorded as positive and negative deflections from baseline. The time delay from stimulus to the first recorded deflection is termed the *latency*, and the maximal deflection from baseline is the *amplitude*. A significant increase in latency or decrease in amplitude of EPs can reflect injury along the nerve tract or dysfunction due to physiologic or pharmacologic factors. Anesthetic agents can dramatically alter EPs in the absence of other abnormalities (**Table 18.4**). Although BAERs are reasonably robust, MEPs (and SSEPs to a lesser but still significant degree) are exquisitely sensitive to volatile anesthetics, which cause decreases in amplitude and increases in latency in a dose-dependent manner. Furthermore, neuromuscular blockers cannot be used if MEPs are proposed. When SSEPs are being monitored, volatile agents should be kept at less than 0.5 MAC, and nitrous oxide (N_2O) should not be used; when MEPs

TABLE 18.4 Anesthetic Effects on Intraoperative Neuromonitoring

	Affected by	Resistant to
SSEP	Volatile agents (goal <0.5 MAC) Nitrous oxide Intravenous agents	Muscle relaxants Opioids
BAER		Volatile agents Nitrous oxide Muscle relaxants Intravenous agents Opioids
MEP	Muscle relaxants Volatile agents (avoid; use TIVA)	Opioids
EMG	Muscle relaxants	Volatile agents Propofol Nitrous oxide Opioids

BAEP, brainstem auditory evoked response; EMG, electromyography; MAC, minimum alveolar concentration; MEP, motor evoked potential; SSEP, somatosensory evoked potential; TIVA, total intravenous anesthetic.

are monitored, a propofol-based total intravenous anesthetic (TIVA) is indicated. The anesthetic plan will often rely heavily on opioids; dexmedetomidine infusions are also often incorporated, which may also offer improvements in overall hemodynamic stability. Low doses of ketamine are sometimes used to augment MEP and SSEP monitoring, but evidence supporting this is conflicting. Perhaps more important than the specific anesthetic regimen is that a maintenance equilibrium is established for the baseline neurophysiology measurements and is then kept constant throughout the procedure. Pseudo-equilibrated steady-state continuous infusions are key to this strategy.

Although anesthetic agents are major influences on the accuracy of IOM, it should be remembered that physiologic factors such as hypothermia, acidosis, excessive hemodilution, and hypotension can also influence EPs as well as neuronal integrity, and should be avoided (**Table 18.5**).

Andleeb R, Agrawal S, Gupta P. Evaluation of the effect of continuous infusion of dexmedetomidine or a subanesthetic dose ketamine on transcranial electrical motor evoked potentials in adult patients undergoing elective spine surgery under total intravenous anesthesia: a randomized controlled exploratory study. *Asian Spine J.* 2022;16:221-230.

Bala E, Sessler DI, Nair DR, et al. Motor and somatosensory evoked potentials are well maintained in patients given dexmedetomidine during spine surgery. *Anesthesiology.* 2008;109:417-425.

Banoub M, Tetzlaff JE, Schubert A. Pharmacologic and physiologic influences affecting sensory evoked potentials: implications for perioperative monitoring. *Anesthesiology.* 2003;99:716-737.

Deiner S. Highlights of anesthetic considerations for intraoperative neuromonitoring. *Semin Cardiothorac Vasc Anesth.* 2010;14:51-53.

Lotto ML, Banoub M, Schubert A. Effects of anesthetic agents and physiologic changes on intraoperative motor evoked potentials. *J Neurosurg Anesthesiol.* 2004;16:32-42.

B.4. What are the options for patient positioning during posterior fossa surgery?

- *Sitting position*: Although used far less often now than two decades ago, it is critically important for the anesthesiologist to understand the sitting position partly because it could still have specific surgical advantages in some situations and partly because it provides the archetype for the risks and management of VAE. The patient is in a reclined sitting posture such that the feet are at or near the level of the heart. The head is held in a flexed position with a skull fixation device, and the arms are crossed over the chest.
- *Modified sitting position*: Due to concerns about the sitting position, a modified sitting position has been described. It involves the same reclining position as described earlier but with careful positioning of the hips and legs so that the feet and knees are above the level of the heart. The head is anteriorly flexed and held in place with a fixation device, and the arms are padded and placed on arm boards by the patient's side.

TABLE 18.5 Physiologic Effects on Intraoperative Neuromonitoring

	Effects
Temperature	• Progressive hypothermia predictably increases latency in SSEPs but has variable effects on amplitude (can increase in mild hypothermia and decrease with moderate hypothermia). • VEPs are completely lost at 25 °C-27 °C. • BAERs are more resistant to hypothermia, but changes reflect those of SSEPs at lower temperature thresholds. • Hyperthermia to 40 °C decreases latency but with further increases slowing occurs, likely reflecting neuronal injury.
Hematocrit	• Changes similar to ischemia in SSEPs and VEPs are seen with acute isovolemic hemodilution to hematocrit of 10%-15% in animals, with resolution when hematocrit was increased to 20%-22%.
Oxygen	• Mild hypoxemia has minimal effects on SSEPs and BAERs. • Severe ischemia increases latency and decreases the amplitude of SSEPs, with cortical responses being more sensitive than spinal responses. BAERs are similarly affected.
Carbon dioxide	• Hypocarbia ($Paco_2$ 20-25 mm Hg) decreases latency in SSEPs. • Hypercarbia (to $Paco_2$ 55 mm Hg) has minimal effects on SSEPs.

BAERs, brainstem auditory evoked responses; SSEPs, somatosensory evoked potentials; VEPs, visually evoked potentials.

- *Prone position*: This is especially suitable for lesions in the midline but can be adapted for more lateral approaches by having the head slightly rotated. Depending on body habitus, supporting rolls are placed horizontally across the chest and hips or in parallel along the longitudinal axis of the body. The head is held with a skull fixation device with the neck in a neutral to flexed position.
- *Lateral decubitus position*: This position is suited to cerebellopontine angle tumors and cerebellar hemispheric lesions.
- *Park bench (semiprone) position*: The patient is turned toward a more prone position, moving the upper shoulder out of the surgeon's view and permitting better access to midline lesions.
- *Supine position*: This can sometimes be used with the patient's head rotated. To reduce the amount of rotation of the neck, which can obstruct venous outflow, a supporting roll can be placed under the ipsilateral shoulder and the whole bed rotated away from the surgeon.

Jadik S, Wissing H, Friedrich K, et al. A standardized protocol for the prevention of clinically relevant venous air embolism during neurosurgical interventions in the semisitting position. *Neurosurgery.* 2009;64:533-538.

Lemkuil BP, Drummond JC, Patel PM, Lam AM. Anesthesia for neurologic surgery and neurointerventions. In: Gropper MA, Eriksson LI, Fleisher LA, Cohen NH, Leslie K, Johnson-Akeju O, eds. *Miller's Anesthesia.* 10th ed. Elsevier; 2025:1740–1783.

Rozet I, Vavilala MS. Risks and benefits of patient positioning during neurosurgical care. *Anesthesiol Clin.* 2007;25:631-653.

B.5. What are the principal disadvantages associated with the common posterior fossa craniotomy positions?

The greatest concern for the sitting position is the increased risk of VAE. In this position, the head is elevated above the right atrium and beyond the height of the central venous fluid column. This reduces venous bleeding but also enables large volumes of air to be entrained into the central venous circulation, especially through the large dural sinuses, which are tented open. When propagated to the right heart and pulmonary circulation, VAE can range in severity from subclinical to severe, precipitating acute hemodynamic collapse and in rare cases death. In a patient with a patent foramen ovale—which is present in 25% of the general population and often undetected—air can traverse to the arterial circulation, causing embolic stroke. Although VAE can occur with other positions, the risk and severity are substantially higher in the sitting position, with recent reported incidences detected by precordial Doppler as high as 50% for minor and major VAE, and significant VAE causing hypotension at 2% to 6%; other literature using transesophageal echocardiography (TEE) for detection has reported even higher rates. Furthermore, the sitting position complicates the effective treatment of VAE, as it is difficult to rapidly lower the patient's head below heart level, and easy access for airway manipulation and cardiopulmonary resuscitation maneuvers is precluded. The sitting position is also associated with a greater degree of hypotension (thus compromising CPP), an increased risk of pneumocephalus causing postoperative drowsiness, and compression of vulnerable structures, including the cervical spinal cord from neck flexion causing quadriplegia, oropharyngeal structures causing macroglossia, and peripheral nerves, causing nerve palsies and pressure sores.

In the prone position, the head is usually slightly elevated above the heart; therefore, the risk of VAE remains present, although the risk of massive entrainment is reduced. Prone positioning can cause a significant decrease in pulmonary compliance and will increase $\dot{V}/\dot{Q}$ mismatch, leading to atelectasis, venous admixture, and shunting. Virtually no access is available to the airway, chest, or limbs, and in the event of an airway, pulmonary, or cardiovascular emergency, the prone position places the anesthesiologist in a substantially compromised position.

The supine position alleviates many of these issues. Nevertheless, to access even the lateral posterior fossa from the supine position usually requires substantial rotation of the neck. This can cause obstruction of jugular venous outflow, leading to cerebral venous engorgement, with potentially undesirable effects on ICP, CPP, surgical exposure, and bleeding. Neck rotation can also cause brachial plexus injury as well as significant pressure on laryngeal structures with potential vocal cord injury. Placing supports to elevate the ipsilateral shoulder can reduce rotation at the neck.

Fathi AR, Eshtehardi P, Meier B. Patent foramen ovale and neurosurgery in sitting position: a systematic review. *Br J Anaesth.* 2009;102:588-596.

Feigl GC, Decker K, Wurms M, et al. Neurosurgical procedures in the semisitting position: evaluation of the risk of paradoxical venous air embolism in patients with a patent foramen ovale. *World Neurosurg.* 2014;81:159-164.

Ganslandt O, Merkel A, Schmitt H, et al. The sitting position in neurosurgery: indications, complications and results. A single institution experience of 600 cases. *Acta Neurochir.* 2013;155:1887-1893.

Lindroos AC, Niiya T, Silvasti-Lundell M, et al. Stroke volume-directed administration of hydroxyethyl starch or Ringer's acetate in sitting position during craniotomy. *Acta Anaesthesiol Scand.* 2013;57:729-736.

Rath GP, Bithal PK, Chaturvedi A, et al. Complications related to positioning in posterior fossa craniectomy. *J Clin Neurosci.* 2007;14:520-525.

B.6. How does the sitting position affect your preoperative assessment and planning?

In addition to the standard preanesthetic and neurologic assessment, preoperative evaluation should focus on the following:

- *Presence of intracardiac shunts*: The presence of a patent foramen ovale, right-to-left intracardiac shunts, and pulmonary arteriovenous malformations are generally considered absolute contraindications to the sitting position due to the risk of VAE and subsequent paradoxical air embolism (PAE), which can have disastrous clinical consequences. Preoperative contrast echocardiography with Valsalva has become part of the routine workup for those considered for elective sitting position craniotomy. However, there is a significant drop-off between the incidences of diagnosed VAE, PAE, and subsequent neurologic sequelae. Therefore, in the rare patient with a demonstrated shunt who still requires sitting position craniotomy, it is not routine to proceed to percutaneous shunt closure. Rather, it serves to heighten the surgeon's awareness for absolute, meticulous control of venous bleeding because it is the presence of open entraining vessels that ultimately determines the risk of VAE.
- *Other complications of the sitting position and their impact on the patient*: General anesthesia in the sitting position is associated with a greater degree of hypotension compared with other positions. This is in large part due to venous pooling in the dependent portions of the body causing a fall in preload, coupled with anesthetic depressant effects on systemic vascular resistance and inotropy. This results in a fall in stroke volume and cardiac output, which is compensated in otherwise healthy patients with increases in heart rate and vasoconstriction. Conditions that exaggerate this fall in MAP include hypovolemia and preoperative diuresis, cachexia, advanced age, and therapeutic β-blockade, all of which can blunt compensatory autonomic responses. The concern with aggressive fluid loading intraoperatively is that it could run counter to the therapeutic goals of diuresis and ICP reduction, and the subsequent redistribution when returned to the supine position can cause an exaggerated increase in cardiac filling pressures. Furthermore, the use of vasoconstrictors to maintain adequate MAP in the face of a preload deficit increases the risk of end-organ hypoperfusion and dysfunction, particularly in the kidneys. This is particularly relevant if electrolyte derangements coexist because they may worsen with perioperative renal injury.
- *Invasive monitoring*: This involves planning for the detection and management of potential VAE as well as routine invasive arterial pressure monitoring. Patients with neck pathology, scarring from prior central access or irradiation, and morbid obesity can present a challenge with respect to central venous or right atrial catheter placement, conditions that may render emergency placement impossible. This may influence the decision to place a central line preoperatively under radiologic guidance. Collateral flow for arterial catheterization should also be assessed, and the patient interviewed for contraindications for TEE if it is a part of the management plan.

The additional hydrostatic gradient between the heart and cerebral vasculature in the sitting position places the brain at a greater risk of hypoperfusion, particularly in patients who have underlying carotid or vertebrobasilar atherosclerosis. This history should be actively sought because these patients may require higher MAPs intraoperatively to maintain adequate CPP, and intraoperative MAP measurements should be made at the level of the circle of Willis. There is also a hydrostatic gradient in lung perfusion when under positive pressure ventilation, with the lung apices being susceptible to hypoperfusion. Functionally termed West Zone 1, after physician and physiologist John West, this area becomes alveolar dead space. A hallmark of increasing alveolar dead space is a broadening arterial–$Etco_2$ gap, which places the patient at risk of hypercarbia and increased ICP if $Etco_2$ is used as a surrogate for $Paco_2$ monitoring. Increases in alveolar dead space also place a greater ventilatory burden on the rest of the lung, which may be of particular concern in patients with obstructive airway disease, despite the gains in functional residual capacity and $\dot{V}/\dot{Q}$ matching in the dependent portions of the lung in the upright position.

Patients with cervical spinal stenosis and occult atlantoaxial instability are at an increased risk of cervical spinal cord ischemia from compression in the anterior flexed neck position and cord hypoperfusion for the reasons discussed earlier. Quadriplegia is a rare but well-documented complication of the sitting position. The patient should be carefully examined for motion that elicits neurologic symptoms, and these findings discussed with the neurosurgeon. Similarly, patients with macroglossia and obstructive sleep apnea should be identified because they are at risk of further airway swelling and potential obstruction postextubation due to direct compression and potential decrease in venous drainage. Finally, the presence of pressure sores and preexisting peripheral neuropathies should be evaluated because these can potentially worsen even with careful padding in the sitting position.

Gale T, Leslie K. Anaesthesia for neurosurgery in the sitting position. *J Clin Neurosci.* 2004;11:693-696.

Gracia I, Fabregas N. Craniotomy in sitting position: anesthesiology management. *Curr Opin Anaesthesiol.* 2014;27:474-483.

Kwapisz MM, Deinsberger W, Müller M, et al. Transesophageal echocardiography as a guide for patient positioning before neurosurgical procedures in semi-sitting position. *J Neurosurg Anesthesiol.* 2004;16:277-281.

Stendel R, Gramm HJ, Schröder K, et al. Transcranial Doppler ultrasonography as a screening technique for detection of a patent foramen ovale before surgery in the sitting position. *Anesthesiology.* 2000;93:971-975.

B.7. How should the patient's position ultimately be determined?

This requires careful patient evaluation and clear communication between the surgeon and anesthesiologist. Surgical exposure should be a primary determinant for patient positioning; however, the vigilant anesthesiologist should be aware of specific patient conditions that may preclude certain positions, anticipate any physiologic insult that may result, and ensure adequate access and planning to treat these occurrences. If there are significant safety concerns, the anesthesiologist is obliged to discuss these with the neurosurgeon and advocate for alternative positioning if appropriate. One such safety concern is the presence of a patent foramen ovale or right-to-left intracardiac shunt. Other conditions may be amenable to a trial of positioning prior to anesthetic induction or surgery. For example, a patient with cervical spinal canal stenosis should be evaluated for neck and shoulder positions that may precipitate neurologic symptoms. A patient with compromised pulmonary compliance or reserve can be positioned prone and monitored during other preparations, with alternative positioning sought if the trial fails.

It bears repeating that the risk of VAE is such that we are very reluctant to use the sitting position except where there are overwhelming surgical exposure considerations.

Lemkuil BP, Drummond JC, Patel PM, Lam AM. Anesthesia for neurologic surgery and neurointerventions. In: Gropper MA, Eriksson LI, Fleisher LA, Cohen NH, Leslie K, Johnson-Akeju O, eds. *Miller's Anesthesia.* 10th ed. Elsevier; 2025:1740–1783.

B.8. Should this patient receive premedication?

Although preoperative anxiety is common among neurosurgical patients, pharmacologic premedication in patients with intracranial mass lesions presents risks that can result in neurologic decompensation. It is prudent, therefore, to avoid sedative premedication in low-monitored settings outside of the operating room in these patients. Emphasis should instead be placed on nonpharmacologic methods to address anxiety, including a professional, empathetic preoperative visit from the neuroanesthesiologist. Psychoactive medications can unmask subclinical neurologic symptoms and can have lingering effects at the end of surgery, which at best confuses the postoperative neurologic examination and at worst contributes to a failure to emerge from anesthesia. Opioids can cause sedation, partial upper-airway obstruction, and hypoventilation, all of which lead to hypercarbia and increases in intracranial blood volume. In patients with limited intracranial elastance reserve, this small degree of hypoventilation can lead to dangerous increases in ICP. For these reasons, it is imperative that sedating premedication only be administered in a fully monitored setting and under the direct supervision of an anesthesiologist who is able to rapidly intervene and control ventilation if necessary. Once the patient is transferred to the operating room and monitored, small doses of short-acting analgesics and/or anxiolytics may be administered as needed to facilitate the placement of invasive monitors prior to induction.

Oral dosing of gabapentin and clonidine will attenuate the hyperdynamic hemodynamic response resulting from laryngoscopy and head pinning when given before anesthetic induction and potentially decrease postoperative pain and nausea. The effects of clonidine can likely be mimicked by starting an infusion of dexmedetomidine—also an α_2-adrenergic agonist—as soon as the patient arrives in the operating room.

Misra S, Koshy T, Suneel PR. Oral clonidine attenuates the fall in mean arterial pressure due to scalp infiltration with epinephrine-lidocaine solution in patients undergoing craniotomy: a prospective, randomized, double-blind, and placebo-controlled trial. *J Neurosurg Anesthesiol.* 2009;21:297-301.

Misra S, Koshy T, Unnikrishnan KP, et al. Gabapentin premedication decreases the hemodynamic response to skull pin insertion in patients undergoing craniotomy. *J Neurosurg Anesthesiol.* 2011;23:110-117.

Misra S, Parthasarathi G, Vilanilam GC. The effect of gabapentin premedication on postoperative nausea, vomiting, and pain in patients on preoperative dexamethasone undergoing craniotomy for intracranial tumors. *J Neurosurg Anesthesiol.* 2013;25:386-391.

SECTION 4

C. Intraoperative Management

C.1. What are the anesthetic goals for craniotomy?

It goes without saying that the anesthetic goals for craniotomy include the basic principles of physiologic stability that are common to all anesthetic management. Additionally, craniotomy incurs several specific goals that follow from the effects—both helpful and unhelpful—of anesthetic drugs on the brain. In short, the anesthetic goals specific to craniotomy are to protect the brain from injury resulting from mechanical or physiologic insult during the perioperative period. *Direct* protection (often referred to simply as *neuroprotection*) can be conceptualized as actions that facilitate the ability of neural tissue to withstand ischemic episodes without inflammation or activation of the apoptotic cascade leading to infarction. Less discrete is the concept of *indirect* protection, which aims to minimize the anteceding ischemic episodes. The principal elements are as follows:

- Management of CBF and CPP
- Management of ICP while the skull is intact
- The provision of a "relaxed" brain. This optimizes surgical exposure, which is critically important in many cases because the field of view available to the surgeon in many craniotomy approaches can be extremely narrow. Furthermore, relaxation reduces the parenchymal pressure exerted by the retraction devices on underlying brain tissue.
- Implementation and timing of pharmacologic measures specifically intended to effect direct neuroprotection, traditionally involving induction of an anesthetic-induced burst-suppression pattern on the EEG (although it must be noted that experimental evidence on the protective effects of anesthetic agents is complex and inconsistent)
- Strict management of physiologic parameters that may contribute to brain injury, such as serum glucose, osmolarity, and acid-base balance
- Minimize the effects of anesthetic pharmacology, cerebral perfusion, and temperature on neurophysiologic monitoring, such as EEG, BAERs, or SSEPs.
- Facilitate early neurologic assessment.

Chui J, Mariappan R, Mehta J, et al. Comparison of propofol and volatile agents for maintenance of anesthesia during elective craniotomy procedures: systematic review and meta-analysis. *Can J Anesth.* 2014;61:347-356.

Mantz J, Degos V, Laigle C. Recent advances in pharmacologic neuroprotection. *Eur J Anaesthesiol.* 2010;27:6-10.

Miura Y, Kamiya K, Kanazawa K, et al. Superior recovery profiles of propofol-based regimen as compared to isoflurane-based regimen in patients undergoing craniotomy for primary brain tumor excision: a retrospective study. *J Anesth.* 2012;26:721-727.

Pasternak JJ, Lanier WL. Neuroanesthesiology update. *J Neurosurg Anesthesiol.* 2010;22:86-109.

Schifilliti D, Grasso G, Conti A, et al. Anaesthetic-related neuroprotection: intravenous or inhalational agents? *CNS Drugs.* 2010;24:893-907.

C.2. What monitors should be used during craniotomy?

In addition to electrocardiography (ECG), noninvasive blood pressure, pulse oximetry, temperature, and capnography monitoring, an arterial line is considered mandatory for all except the most superficial and nonvascular supratentorial tumors, even in those without significant comorbidity. The real-time dynamic assessment of arterial pressure is of paramount importance in patients with intracranial pathology and impaired autoregulation, as CPP and CBF become entirely dependent on MAP. There are multiple occasions of high hemodynamic stress that require rapid measurement and management of blood pressure, such as induction, intubation, head pinning, epinephrine infiltration of the scalp, and emergence (intraoperative emergencies notwithstanding). It also allows for repeated arterial blood monitoring of CO_2, glucose, acid-base physiology, hematocrit, and electrolytes, all of which critically affect patient management. A key concept in neuroanesthesia practice is to ensure the measured arterial blood pressure reflects cerebral inflow pressure. In the prone or sitting position, the head may be significantly higher than the level of the heart, so care must be taken to position the arterial pressure transducer at the level of the circle of Willis, which corresponds approximately to the level of the tragus.

The use of central venous and right heart catheters is less common in craniotomies, except in cases where the sitting position is planned or where preexisting comorbidity or therapies require it. A central venous catheter allows the safe infusion of hypertonic saline and allows for air aspiration in the event of VAE, although its performance is variable. Beyond these reasons, there is little additional advantage in patient management. Because of this and the potential for complications in its placement, the placement of central lines is not routine in our practice.

If surgical access permits, depth of anesthesia monitors incorporating quantitative EEG (qEEG) is frequently used in some institutions to allow for titration of anesthetic agents and possible induction of burst suppression. Although the use of proprietary qEEG measures such as the bispectral index (BIS) or patient state index (PSI) is common, intraoperative neurophysiology monitoring such as EEG, EMG, BAERs, or SSEPs may provide raw data that can be similarly used to guide anesthetic management and may be the only source of data in surgical approaches that preclude the placement of a qEEG monitor. Although these methods are often performed by neurophysiologists, the anesthesiologist must understand the principles behind them and be aware of the effects of anesthetics, other drugs, and physiologic variables on their integrity. Evidence from the awareness literature means that the use of some form of EEG monitoring is strongly advised in TIVA cases.

Lemkuil BP, Drummond JC, Patel PM, Lam AM. Anesthesia for neurologic surgery and neurointerventions. In: Gropper MA, Eriksson LI, Fleisher LA, Cohen NH, Leslie K, Johnson-Akeju O, eds. *Miller's Anesthesia*. 10th ed. Elsevier; 2025:1740–1783.

C.3. Would you monitor for venous air embolism (VAE)? What are the monitoring options?

VAE can potentially occur whenever there is an open venous channel beyond the venous fluid column to the heart. The sitting position confers the highest risk of VAE, although it is also been described in prone and lateral position craniotomies where the head is typically slightly elevated above the heart. An additional consideration is that the posterior fossa contains several major dural venous sinuses and their confluences, which are noncollapsible and drain into the internal jugular vein. For these reasons, any posterior fossa craniotomy, regardless of position, should be considered for VAE monitoring.

- *TEE* is the most sensitive monitor for VAE and PAE, able to detect volumes of 0.02 mL/kg in both the right and left heart but is invasive and requires expertise in interpretation. Furthermore, it requires constant vigilance and can divert attention from other essential monitoring.
- *Precordial Doppler ultrasound* is noninvasive, highly sensitive (able to detect air volumes of 0.05 mL/kg), and is a part of our routine monitoring for posterior fossa craniotomies. However, the requirement for precise placement of the Doppler probe over the right heart becomes challenging when the variety of surgical positioning is considered and is particularly difficult in the prone position. This limits its sensitivity when applied in real-world scenarios. We find that a rapid intravenous injection of 5 to 10 mL of saline is useful to ensure adequate detection of turbulent flow, which causes a characteristic coarse change in the basal "swishing" sound of normal pulsatile blood flow.
- *Pulmonary artery catheters* are less sensitive detectors of VAE (0.25 mL/kg air), and invasiveness generally limits use in patients with no other indication for right heart monitoring. Characteristically, a sudden increase in pulmonary artery pressures occurs with VAE, first from reflex pulmonary vasoconstriction and later from the air lock formed by the embolus at the right ventricular outflow tract.
- *End-tidal nitrogen (N_2) monitoring* is not routinely available on anesthesia gas monitors but is noninvasive and highly specific for air embolism. It is superior to $Etco_2$ despite the latter's ubiquity, being more sensitive, specific, and rapidly responsive to air in the pulmonary circulation, but it can be difficult to interpret when using air-oxygen carrier gas mixtures. Both end-tidal N_2 and CO_2 can be affected by pulmonary hypoperfusion.
- *Esophageal stethoscope* is discussed here for its historical interest in producing a characteristic "mill wheel" murmur but is too low in sensitivity (1.7 mL air per kg) and of limited use in detecting late, large VAE.

In our experience, the combination of precordial Doppler, $Etco_2$, and arterial pressure monitoring is minimally invasive and extremely effective at detecting clinically significant VAE.

The use of a right atrial catheter as a means to aspirate air should be considered in any situation when the risk of VAE is high, although in practice it is infrequently used. Catheter tip position, type, and size have been extensively studied, but consensus on the ideal approach remains disputed. Large-bore (14 gauge), single-lumen, multiorifice catheters have performed best in animal and human studies. Traditionally, the ideal catheter tip position is 2 cm distal to the superior vena cava–right atrial junction. This can be established through TEE, radiographic, or intravascular ECG guidance. In the last method, the patient is attached to a standard three-lead ECG, and the catheter is inserted in the usual manner. The lumen is then flushed with sodium bicarbonate ($NaHCO_3$) to reduce electrical impedance along the catheter, and the right-arm ECG lead is attached to a conductive connector placed on the line. The catheter should then be advanced into the right ventricle, which can be detected by transducing the pressure waveform. It should then be drawn back until the P wave on the catheter lead is biphasic (mid-atrium) and then back further to the point at which the P wave and QRS complex are of equal amplitude. The catheter is then pulled back another centimeter and secured. The right atrial catheter can confirm the presence of

VAE through the aspiration of air, but its principal utility is therapeutic: it enables significant volumes of air to be rapidly extracted from the right atrium, thus breaking the "air lock" that causes the loss of cardiac output. Nonetheless, even under controlled conditions using ideal equipment, the success rate of air aspiration is 30% to 60% at best, and the catheter is liable to migrate as the patient position is changed.

Brull SJ, Prielipp RC. Vascular air embolism: a silent hazard to patient safety. *J Crit Care.* 2017;42:255-263.

Jadik S, Wissing H, Friedrich K, et al. A standardized protocol for the prevention of clinically relevant venous air embolism during neurosurgical interventions in the semisitting position. *Neurosurgery.* 2009;64:533-538.

Schubert A, Deogaonkar A, Drummond JC. Precordial Doppler probe placement for optimal detection of venous air embolism during craniotomy. *Anesth Analg.* 2006;102:1543-1547.

C.4. What specific risks are associated with the induction of anesthesia?

The key considerations for anesthetic induction in a patient with marginal intracranial reserve include the onset of apnea and the hemodynamic effects of anesthetic agents and intubation. With prolonged apnea and hypercarbia, CBV and CBF increase, worsening ICP. Hypoxemia also has similar effects on ICP, although unless it is in the extremes, hypoxemia causes more deleterious effects by impacting oxygen delivery to the brain.

Hypotension from induction agents compromises CPP, whereas hypertension with laryngoscopy and coughing from inadequate neuromuscular blockade abruptly increases CBF and CBV further. The end point of all these events is a tendency to increase ICP and reduce CPP, leading to decreased cerebral oxygen delivery, ischemia, and potentially herniation in a patient with poor intracranial elastance.

Lemkuil BP, Drummond JC, Patel PM, Lam AM. Anesthesia for neurologic surgery and neurointerventions. In: Gropper MA, Eriksson LI, Fleisher LA, Cohen NH, Leslie K, Johnson-Akeju O, eds. *Miller's Anesthesia.* 10th ed. Elsevier; 2025:1740–1783.

Sharma D, Brown MJ, Curry P, et al. Prevalence and risk factors for intraoperative hypotension during craniotomy for traumatic brain injury. *J Neurosurg Anesthesiol.* 2012;24:178-184.

C.5. How would you induce anesthesia?

In the absence of potential airway difficulty, the most common choice of anesthetic agents typically involves an opioid, intravenous induction agent, and neuromuscular blocker. Benzodiazepines are infrequently recommended due to their prolonged elimination and disinhibiting effects, especially in the older adults, and can delay awakening and cloud the postoperative neurologic examination. If preinduction anxiolysis is required, dexmedetomidine can be given as a preinduction infusion in the operating room during monitor placement and invasive monitoring access. It has advantages over benzodiazepines, including preservation of respiratory effort, minimal disinhibition, and reduced interference with EP monitoring. The infusion can be continued throughout the case, with the additional benefits of MAC reduction and improved intraoperative and postoperative hemodynamic stability.

A common induction technique is to coadminister large doses of opioids. This reduces the ED_{50} of intravenous anesthetic dosing (thereby limiting postinduction hypotension), blunts the responses to intubation, and diminishes the hypertensive spike seen with head pinning. Fentanyl (slowly titrated to a total dose of 5-10 μg/kg), remifentanil bolus and infusion (1 μg/kg bolus, followed by infusion at 0.1 μg/kg/min or a target effect site concentration of 3 ng/mL), and alfentanil (30 μg/kg bolus) are all effective regimens. Fentanyl has the advantage of achieving these characteristics without the inconvenience and technical risks of a continuous infusion but at the expense of titratability. All contribute to a relatively hemodynamically stable induction (especially with an appropriately decreased dose of the intravenous anesthetic agent) and steady maintenance levels, thereby extending MAC- and ED_{50}-sparing effects throughout the procedure. If volatile agents are used, this allows us to run at less than 1 MAC (and typically at 0.5-0.6 MAC) with greater confidence in adequate anesthesia while limiting deleterious effects on ICP. Despite these advantages, high-dose opioids can cause significant sympatholysis, particularly in patients with a dominant sympathetic tone (such as the older adults), necessitating small doses of phenylephrine (either as a bolus or infusion) or ephedrine (5-10 mg) to support vascular tone and/or cardiac output. All opioids given in high doses, particularly the more potent drugs such as remifentanil and alfentanil, can produce chest wall rigidity, which can compromise ventilation and increase ICP. Finally, it should be reiterated that this technique is only safe if there is certainty that immediate control of ventilation can be achieved.

Propofol is the induction agent of choice, given its favorable effects on CBF, $CMRO_2$, and ICP. However, its vasodilating and negative inotropic effects can cause significant hypotension even in the dose-sparing presence of opioids. Etomidate should be considered in patients where the cardiodepressant effects of propofol are considered unacceptable. Ketamine is inappropriate at induction doses in patients with marginal intracranial compliance due to increases in CBF, $CMRO_2$, and ICP, despite promising data regarding potential protective effects in the neurotrauma literature. An alternative is to add lidocaine 1.5 mg/kg to a high-dose opioid induction, which can further reduce the ED_{50} of the induction agent.

Although succinylcholine is not contraindicated in patients with increased ICP, the risks and benefits should be assessed prior to its use. It is preferred in situations where a rapid-sequence induction is required and IOM is proposed. However, because fasciculations can transiently increase ICP, it is recommended to administer a defasciculating dose of a nondepolarizing neuromuscular blocker (typically 10% of the ED_{95} for single twitch suppression) or lidocaine 1.5 mg/kg prior to the administration of succinylcholine. In recent years, with the increased availability of sugammadex, it would also be acceptable to consider using a rapid-sequence induction dose of rocuronium and reversing it before acquiring IOM signals. Sugammadex at a dose of 16 mg/kg can be used for the reversal of neuromuscular block as early as 3 minutes after rocuronium administration, allowing for adequate IOM. In most other situations, the use of nondepolarizing neuromuscular blockers is generally preferred.

Bekker AY, Mistry A, Ritter AA, et al. Computer simulation of intracranial pressure changes during induction of anesthesia: comparison of thiopental, propofol, and etomidate. *J Neurosurg Anesthesiol.* 1999;11:69-80.

Bekker A, Sturaitis M, Bloom M, et al. The effect of dexmedetomidine on perioperative hemodynamics in patients undergoing craniotomy. *Anesth Analg.* 2008;107:1340-1347.

Bozeman WP, Idris AH. Intracranial pressure changes during rapid sequence intubation: a swine model. *J Trauma.* 2005;58:278-283.

Lemkuil BP, Drummond JC, Patel PM. Central nervous system physiology: cerebrovascular. In: Hemmings HC, Egan TD, eds. *Pharmacology and Physiology for Anesthesia: Foundations and Clinical Application.* 2nd ed. Elsevier; 2019:174-192

Marsch SC, Steiner L, Bucher E, et al. Succinylcholine versus rocuronium for rapid sequence intubation in intensive care: a prospective, randomized controlled trial. *Crit Care.* 2011;15:R199.

Schreiber JU, Lysakowski C, Fuchs-Buder T, Tramér. Prevention of succinylcholine-induced fasciculation and myalgia: a meta-analysis of randomized trials. *Anesthesiology.* 2005;103:877-884.

C.6. What are the effects of anesthetics on the cerebral metabolic rate of oxygen ($CMRO_2$), CBF, and ICP? With this in mind, how would you maintain anesthesia?

Volatile Anesthetics

Volatile anesthetics have the characteristic of being direct cerebral vasodilators while concurrently reducing $CMRO_2$ in a dose-related fashion. This has been described as an "uncoupling" of the flow-metabolism relationship; however, autoregulation remains largely intact at doses up to 1 MAC. It is more accurate to say that it is a balance between the reduction in $CMRO_2$, which leads to a decrease in CBF, and the direct vasodilator effect that causes an increase in CBF. At 1 MAC or greater, the vasodilating effect becomes dominant. In most patients, this increased CBF would be potentially beneficial to the extent that it improves the supply-demand balance (termed *luxury perfusion*), with minor, compensated effects on ICP. In patients with intracranial pathology, however, this increase in CBF causes an increase in CBV and can potentially elevate ICP while the cranium is intact or impede surgical exposure once the cranial bone plate is removed. At doses below 1 MAC in the normal brain, this increase in CBV and ICP can potentially be reversed by hypocapnia, as cerebrovascular CO_2 reactivity is preserved. However, as previously discussed, this is impaired or absent in pathologic states.

At equivalent doses, isoflurane causes the greatest decrease in $CMRO_2$, which mitigates some of its direct cerebral vasodilator effect, leading to a proportionately modest increase in CBF and ICP. Desflurane exhibits effects similar to isoflurane but appears to cause greater increases in ICP in normocapnic patients and in those with intracranial mass lesions. Sevoflurane causes minimal or slight changes in CBF and ICP despite dose-related decreases in $CMRO_2$ and appears to have the most favorable characteristics in patients with raised ICP.

Nitrous Oxide

Despite conflicting studies, N_2O is generally agreed to increase CBF, $CMRO_2$, and ICP. The difficulty with interpreting data on the cerebrovascular effects of N_2O is the heterogeneity of existing literature, with large variations in the anesthetic regimens. When given as a sole agent or with minimal adjuvant anesthesia, N_2O markedly increases global CBF, $CMRO_2$, and ICP. This effect is preserved when N_2O is given together with volatile anesthetics but attenuated when intravenous anesthetics are administered. As an *N*-methyl-D-aspartic acid (NMDA) receptor antagonist, N_2O has been associated with both neuroprotective and neurotoxic effects due to its modulation of glutamate-mediated excitotoxicity. N_2O has also been shown to induce neuronal apoptosis via its effects on homocysteine and the formation of reactive oxygen species.

In the absence of high levels of evidence deriving from human studies, synthesizing the neuroprotection/neurotoxicity literature into practice guidance is challenging; however, we would argue that at best, N_2O offers no meaningful neuroprotection, and at worst, its effects might be neurotoxic and counterproductive to surgical exposure. When considered together with other detrimental effects seen with prolonged use, including the increased risk of vascular thrombosis, postoperative nausea and vomiting (when administered for periods longer than one hour), and the potential expansion of air in the cranium and vasculature, N_2O should not be used as a maintenance anesthetic in craniotomies, and any exposure should be limited.

Intravenous Anesthetics

Intravenous anesthetics that act through GABAergic mechanisms (eg, barbiturates, propofol, etomidate) cause a dose-dependent reduction in $CMRO_2$, CBF, CBV, and ICP. In contrast to volatile anesthetics, CBF-$CMRO_2$ coupling is preserved in the basal state, with no added vasodilatory effect. Thus, the direct effect of a drug such as propofol is to cause a reduction in $CMRO_2$, and the decreases in CBF, CBV, and ICP follow from intact normal physiologic responses. CO_2 reactivity is preserved. $CMRO_2$ can be reduced to as low as 40% of resting values in the presence of an isoelectric EEG. The preservation of CBF-$CMRO_2$ coupling affords many benefits but also carries an underappreciated risk: If hyperventilation is instituted, it will have an additive effect on the decrease in CBF caused by an intravenous anesthetic. The result is an appreciable risk of inadequate CBF and hypoperfusion ischemia. It must be remembered that the mantra of "*craniotomy → hyperventilation*" owes its legacy to a time when most neuroanesthetics involved the use of MAC equivalents of vasodilating volatile agents. Etomidate impairs collateral perfusion of ischemic brain in animal experiments through the inhibition of nitric oxide synthase and is, therefore, relatively contraindicated in cerebral ischemia.

The NMDA receptor antagonist ketamine can increase $CMRO_2$, CBF, and ICP. However, concerns regarding these effects are likely overstated when using low doses. In fact, although ketamine may negatively impact the oxygen supply-demand relationship, some recent literature suggests the possibility of direct neuroprotective effects, especially when combined with GABAergic agents. We emphasize that there is not yet any high-level evidence for this in clinical settings; our position is that any use of ketamine should be judicious, but that it may be used when there are compelling appropriate indications.

Opioids

Broadly speaking, synthetic opioids such as fentanyl, alfentanil, and remifentanil have minimal effects on or slightly decrease $CMRO_2$, CBF, and ICP. In human and animal studies, opioids appear to complement the cerebrovascular effects of the background anesthetic, displaying vasoconstrictor effects in the presence of vasodilating agents and minimal effects when used with vasoconstricting anesthetics. In the spontaneously breathing patient, however, it must be remembered that opioids cause hypoventilation and hypercarbia in the patient breathing spontaneously, leading to increases in CBF, CBV, and ICP.

Many neuroanesthesiologists favor a maintenance strategy of TIVA in an oxygen and air mixture, which is difficult to fault, provided that hyperventilation is not excessive. A TIVA approach maximizes the ability to reduce $CMRO_2$ without impairing surgical exposure through increased CBF or causing cerebral steal, but it incurs the disadvantage of complex pharmacokinetics. Other neuroanesthesiologists (including the authors) favor a mixed volatile-intravenous regimen as a primary strategy in most patients. We typically use 0.3 to 0.5 MAC equivalent of a volatile agent, with propofol titrated to the EEG as a goal-directed end point. Dexmedetomidine and opioids (fentanyl or remifentanil) are added to blunt hemodynamic responses and confer hemodynamic stability. This strategy causes a reduction in $CMRO_2$ but with minimal impairment of surgical exposure. Unless precluded by monitoring, a nondepolarizing muscle relaxant is added to ensure that the patient does not move while the head is fixed. We revert to TIVA if there is inadequate brain relaxation or if monitoring dictates.

The effects of various anesthetics on $CMRO_2$, CBF, and ICP are shown in **Table 18.6**.

Choudhury D, Autry AE, Tolias KF, et al. Ketamine: neuroprotective or neurotoxic? *Front Neurosci.* 2021;15:672526.

Fraga M, Rama-Maceiras P, Rodiño S, et al. The effects of isoflurane and desflurane on intracranial pressure, cerebral perfusion pressure, and cerebral arteriovenous oxygen content difference in normocapnic patients with supratentorial brain tumors. *Anesthesiology.* 2003;98:1085-1090.

Neag MA, Mitre AO, Catinean A, et al. An overview on the mechanisms of neuroprotection and neurotoxicity of isoflurane and sevoflurane in experimental studies. *Brain Res Bull.* 2020;165:281-289.

Petersen KD, Landsfeldt U, Cold GE, et al. Intracranial pressure and cerebral hemodynamic in patients with cerebral tumors: a randomized prospective study of patients subjected to craniotomy in propofol-fentanyl, isoflurane-fentanyl, or sevoflurane-fentanyl anesthesia. *Anesthesiology.* 2003;98:329-336.

Savage S, Ma D. The neurotoxicity of nitrous oxide: the facts and "putative" mechanisms. *Brain Sci.* 2014;4:73-90.

TABLE 18.6 The Effects of Anesthetic Agents on Cerebral Blood Flow, Metabolism, and Intracranial Pressure

	CBF	$CMRO_2$	ICP
Nitrous oxide	↑↑	↑ or =	↑↑
Halothane (1 MAC)	↑↑↑	↓↓	↑↑
Isoflurane (1 MAC)	↑ or =	↓↓↓	↑ or =
Sevoflurane (1 MAC)	↓ or =	↓↓	↑ or =
Desflurane (1 MAC)	↑	↓↓	↑
Propofol	↓↓↓	↓↓	↓↓
Thiopental	↓↓↓	↓↓↓	↓↓
Ketamine	↑↑	=	↑ or =
Etomidate	↓↓	↓↓	↓
Fentanyl	= or ↓	= or ↓	=
Lidocaine	↓↓	↓↓	
Dexmedetomidine	= or ↓	= or ↓	=

CBF, cerebral blood flow; $CMRO_2$, cerebral metabolic rate of oxygen; ICP, intracranial pressure; MAC, minimum alveolar concentration.

SECTION 4

C.7. How would you manage ventilation and maintain arterial carbon dioxide (CO_2)?

A reduction in $Paco_2$ decreases CBF and CBV within minutes. Therefore, hyperventilation is a rapidly effective measure that can be implemented to decrease ICP and undoubtedly improve surgical exposure. Nevertheless, hyperventilation has substantial limitations. At $Paco_2$ values less than 25 mm Hg, cerebral ischemia can result from a critical reduction in CBF combined with impaired oxygen unloading caused by a large left shift of the oxyhemoglobin dissociation curve due to respiratory alkalosis. Prolonged hyperventilation leads to a compensatory loss of serum bicarbonate and can result in rebound acidosis if hyperventilation is abruptly terminated. Furthermore, hyperventilation-induced alkalosis decreases ionized Ca^{2+}, leading to hemodynamic difficulties and prolonged emergence from effects on synaptic function.

It is important to remember that the difference between $Paco_2$ and $Etco_2$ can vary greatly. Therefore, arterial blood gas analysis should be performed as soon as possible after induction to establish the arterial–end-tidal gradient in CO_2 partial pressure. A $Paco_2$ of approximately 35 to 38 mm Hg is reasonable unless ICP is elevated. If, once the bone plate is removed, the surgeons determine that exposure is suboptimal, hyperventilation to a $Paco_2$ of 30 mm Hg for a limited period is helpful for temporizing while other methods to improve brain relaxation are implemented. Further hyperventilation is reserved for situations in which establishing adequate exposure is extremely difficult. To avoid postoperative acid-base instability, hyperventilation can be gradually reduced throughout the closure, permitting the reestablishment of bicarbonate and Ca^{2+} equilibrium.

Curley G, Kavanagh BP, Laffey JG. Hypocapnia and the injured brain: more harm than benefit. *Crit Care Med.* 2010;38:1348-1359.

Gelb AW, Craen RA, Rao GS, et al. Does hyperventilation improve operating condition during supratentorial craniotomy? A multicenter randomized crossover trial. *Anesth Analg.* 2008;106:585-594.

Meyer MJ, Megyesi J, Meythaler J, et al. Acute management of acquired brain injury part I: an evidence-based review of non-pharmacological interventions. *Brain Inj.* 2010;24:694-705.

C.8. How would you approach diuretic therapy?

The purpose of diuretic therapy in intracranial procedures is to dehydrate the brain, thereby leading to a reduction in the volume of the parenchymal compartment. This facilitates surgical exposure and reduces the pressure exerted by retraction. Similarly, mannitol is used as therapy for elevated ICP states when the cranium is closed.

Mannitol, an osmotic diuretic, is typically prepared in a 20% solution (20 g/100 mL). It should initially be given in a dose of 0.5 to 1 g/kg; the total dose can be increased to 1.5 g/kg if initial efforts are ineffective. Higher doses have been reported to lead to cardiac arrest from disruption of cardiac cellular function. Because mannitol initially draws water into the vascular space before it is excreted, rapid dosing can cause a transient increase in ICP, so it should be infused over 20 to 30 minutes. If there is very little intracranial elastance reserve, aggressive dosing should be synchronized with the removal of the bone plate. Caution should be used, however, in patients with pronounced diastolic dysfunction, as rapid expansion in intravascular volume may precipitate congestive heart failure.

If mannitol alone does not provide adequate surgical conditions, the loop diuretic furosemide can be used. In a diuretic-naive adult patient, a dose as low as 5 mg may be sufficient. Furosemide does not cause an initial increase in vascular volume and so is preferred in patients with marginal cardiac function who could develop congestive heart failure due to a large mannitol load. The combination of mannitol and furosemide can lead to electrolyte abnormalities and severe systemic dehydration, placing the patient at risk for hemodynamic instability and cardiac arrhythmias. Point-of-care testing for electrolyte derangements is extremely useful in correcting acute changes in serum sodium and potassium levels. Because mannitol therapy alone is often adequate, we do not routinely administer furosemide, instead reserving its use for situations when surgical exposure is suboptimal. There is evidence in the neurocritical care setting that substituting loop diuretics with an aldosterone antagonist (which is potassium sparing) may reduce the severity of potassium flux and arrhythmias; however, this is infrequently used in the perioperative arena.

Although not diuretic therapy per se, it is worth noting here that in cases of extreme cerebral edema, hypertonic saline in concentrations of up to 20% can be used, although 2% or 3% concentrations are most common. This can be effective in refractory intracranial hypertension and may even be superior to mannitol for routine diuresis, particularly in patients with preexisting hypovolemia. Its use requires caution because of the risk of severe hypernatremia, and central access is required. Patients already receiving hypertonic saline should typically have the infusion maintained during the operative period.

Bebawy JF, Ramaiah VK, Zeeni C, et al. The effect of furosemide on intravascular volume status and electrolytes in patients receiving mannitol: an intraoperative safety analysis. *J Neurosurg Anesthesiol.* 2013;25:51-54.

Bilotta F, Giovannini F, Aghilone F, et al. Potassium sparing diuretics as an adjunct to mannitol therapy in neurocritical care patients with cerebral edema: effects on potassium homeostasis and cardiac arrhythmias. *Neurocrit Care.* 2012;16:280-285.

Fang J, Yang Y, Wang W, et al. Comparison of equiosmolar hypertonic saline and mannitol for brain relaxation during craniotomies: a meta-analysis of randomized controlled trials. *Neurosurg Rev.* 2018;41:945-956.

Thenuwara K, Todd MM, Brian JE Jr. Effect of mannitol and furosemide on plasma osmolality and brain water. *Anesthesiology.* 2002;96:416-421.

C.9. How would you manage serum glucose?

Serum glucose control and its impact on critical care outcomes have been exhaustively studied in the last two decades. However, there is a paucity of literature specific to neurosurgical patients, and fewer yet focusing on the influence of intraoperative glucose control on morbidity and mortality. To date, no study has definitively recommended one strategy over another for neurosurgical patients—much of the neuroanesthesiologist's practice is guided by the medical and general surgical critical care experience.

The relationship between glucose control and morbidity can be described as a U-shaped curve, with worsened outcomes seen with both hypo- and hyperglycemia. Hyperglycemia in neuroanesthesia is common due to the surgical stress response and perioperative administration of corticosteroids. It is associated with increased rates of infection and sepsis, renal insufficiency, and longer duration of intensive care admission. On the other hand, hypoglycemia is particularly detrimental to the brain, which relies on glucose as a major metabolic substrate.

The two primary treatment strategies are intensive insulin therapy (IIT) to maintain serum glucose between 80 and 100 mg/dL, and standard therapy (ST) to maintain serum glucose below 180 mg/dL. Neurologic subgroup analyses of the landmark study by Van Den Berghe et al suggested that IIT was associated with a reduction in ICP, seizures, critical illness polyneuropathy, and diabetes insipidus. However, subsequent data from the Normoglycemia in Intensive Care Evaluation-Surviving Using Glucose Algorithm Regulation (NICE-SUGAR) study investigators did not demonstrate a benefit in IIT over ST and actually suggested IIT might be harmful due to higher rates of severe hypoglycemia. This is supported by microdialysis studies in patients with traumatic brain injury showing that IIT can cause precipitous neuroglycopenia and increase neuronal injury. It should be noted that follow-up from the NICE-SUGAR study did not demonstrate differences in long-term outcomes in patients with traumatic brain injury. Nonetheless, with the current state of evidence, it would be prudent to aim for serum glucose levels between 110 and 180 mg/dL in the intraoperative setting while taking meticulous care to avoid hypoglycemia.

Finfer S, Chittock D, Li Y, et al; The NICE-SUGAR Study Investigators for the Australian and New Zealand Intensive Care Society Clinical Trials Group and the Canadian Critical Care Trials Group. Intensive versus conventional glucose control in critically ill patients with traumatic brain injury: long-term follow-up of a subgroup of patients from the NICE-SUGAR study. *Intensive Care Med.* 2015;41:1037-1047.

Finfer S, Chittock DR, Su SY, et al; for NICE-SUGAR Study Investigators. Intensive versus conventional glucose control in critically ill patients. *N Engl J Med.* 2009;360:1283-1297.

Lipshutz AK, Gropper MA. Perioperative glycemic control: an evidence-based review. *Anesthesiology.* 2009;110:408-421.

Rice MJ, Pitkin AD, Coursin DB. Review article: glucose measurement in the operating room: more complicated than it seems. *Anesth Analg.* 2010;110:1056-1065.

Van den Berghe G, Schoonheydt K, Becx P, et al. Insulin therapy protects the central and peripheral nervous system of intensive care patients. *Neurology.* 2005;64:1348-1353.

C.10. How would you approach fluid management?

If the BBB is intact, the principal determinant of brain tissue water is the osmotic gradient across the BBB. The importance of this osmotic gradient guides the use of hypertonic solutions such as mannitol or hypertonic saline to reduce interstitial water and decrease ICP or to optimize surgical exposure. By the same principle, hypotonic solutions are rarely used because they favor the transport of water into the brain interstitium, thereby promoting the development of edema.

In regions where the BBB is not intact because of pathology or surgical tissue injury, osmotic particles can cross from the capillaries into the interstitial tissue. Consequently, the benefits of hypertonic solutions are lost in these areas. It follows that the benefits obtained from the use of hypertonic solutions result from an *overall* effect on the brain, not from a *specific* effect in localized regions of brain injury.

These considerations favor the use of isotonic fluids as maintenance fluid in craniotomies. Conventionally, normal saline has been the preferred crystalloid solution; however, concerns over the risk of developing a non–anion gap and hyperchloremic metabolic acidosis have led to the use of other isotonic crystalloids, such as Plasma-Lyte (**Table 18.7**). More controversial is the approach to volume management. Historically, craniotomy patients have been kept deliberately hypovolemic in the belief that this would increase the passage of free water from the brain in situations involving a disrupted BBB. Relatively recent evidence suggests that there is, in fact, very little reduction in interstitial water, and it comes at the cost of significant systemic hypoperfusion and hypotension. However, there are also some data to support that an intraoperative goal-directed fluid restriction strategy may reduce ICU length of stay. On balance, the favored approach to fluid management is now the maintenance of isovolemia with isotonic fluids. Dextrose-containing solutions should never be used except to treat hypoglycemia. Colloids, such as 5% albumin, can be used when volume expansion is required. Albumin has a plasma half-life of 16 hours, and little is known about how the passage of albumin across a damaged BBB influences interstitial water movement over this time period. Therefore, its routine use is not recommended.

Lemkuil BP, Drummond JC, Patel PM, Lam AM. Anesthesia for neurologic surgery and neurointerventions. In: Gropper MA, Eriksson LI, Fleisher LA, Cohen NH, Leslie K, Johnson-Akeju O, eds. *Miller's Anesthesia.* 10th ed. Elsevier; 2025:1740–1783.

Luo J, Xue J, Liu J, et al. Goal-directed fluid restriction during brain surgery: a prospective randomized controlled trial. *Ann Intensive Care.* 2017;7:16.

Tommasino C. Fluids and the neurosurgical patient. *Anesthesiol Clin North America.* 2002;20:329-346.

C.11. Once the bone plate is removed and the dura retracted, the surgeon reports that the brain is still "tight." What would be your response?

In almost all cases, the most effective initial response is to transiently increase hyperventilation to a $Paco_2$ of approximately 27 to 30 mm Hg. If mannitol 1 g/kg has already been administered, small doses of intravenous furosemide can be given until diuresis is established. If a volatile agent is being used, it should

TABLE 18.7 The Osmolarity and Composition of Commonly Used Crystalloid Solutions

	Osmolarity (mOsm/L)	Sodium Concentration (mmol/L)	Chloride Concentration (mmol/L)
Plasma	280-300	140	100
0.9% Saline	308	154	154
Lactated Ringer's	273	130	109
Plasma-Lyte	294	140	98
5% Albumin	290	145	0

SECTION 4

be discontinued and the maintenance strategy converted to TIVA. If the patient has a CSF drain, it can be opened and CSF removed in no greater than 10- to 20-mL aliquots, with reassessment in between. Hypertension should be addressed and treated, and the patient should be well anesthetized to attenuate CBF responses to surgical stimulation. Positioning should be reassessed to eliminate any obstruction to jugular venous outflow and the head elevated if possible. Deliberate hypotension can reduce swelling but carries the risk of inadequate CPP and hypoperfusion ischemia; thus, it is implemented sparingly.

C.12. If deliberate hypotension is indicated, how will you achieve it?

Although sodium nitroprusside and volatile anesthetics were historically the most commonly used drugs to achieve sustained decreases in blood pressure, both are far from ideal. Nitroprusside is highly effective and titratable over extremely short periods, but since it causes cerebral vasodilation, it can actually increase vascular engorgement. Nitroglycerin is also a potent cerebral venous vasodilator and has the same limitation. Similarly, high levels of volatile anesthetics have direct cerebral vasodilatory effects. Furthermore, the uncoupled cerebral vasodilation caused by nitrates and volatile anesthetics can theoretically produce cerebral steal. Both of these approaches are now used rarely.

In most cases, the required level of blood pressure reduction can be achieved with the use of high-dose remifentanil (or other opioids) and propofol, possibly with the addition of a β-adrenergic blocker. Remifentanil enables a profound but rapidly reversible opioid level without unfavorable effects on CBF or vasodilation. Similarly, propofol can produce hypotension through systemic vasodilation but does not cause cerebral vasodilation and is rapidly reversible. The mixed adrenergic receptor blocker labetalol is often effective as an adjunctive agent. However, the calcium channel blocker nicardipine is probably the most versatile drug for blood pressure control: It is titratable over relatively short periods and is an excellent choice if hypotension is required in situations where opioids and anesthetic agents are not appropriate—such as during emergence or in the ICU—although it might impair autoregulation. Esmolol infusions can be utilized for a rapidly titratable β_1-adrenergic blockade but are not especially effective if the problem is refractory hypertension.

Degoute CS. Controlled hypotension: a guide to drug choice. *Drugs.* 2007;67:1053-1076.

Hoffman WE, Edelman G, Ripper R, et al. Sodium nitroprusside compared with isoflurane-induced hypotension: the effects on brain oxygenation and arteriovenous shunting. *Anesth Analg.* 2001;93:166-170.

Narotam PK, Puri V, Roberts JM, et al. Management of hypertensive emergencies in acute brain disease: evaluation of the treatment effects of intravenous nicardipine on cerebral oxygenation. *J Neurosurg.* 2008;109:1065-1074.

C.13. While the surgeon is resecting a tumor from near the brainstem, the patient's heart rate suddenly drops to 20 beats per minute. What is your assessment and management?

Surgery near the brainstem nuclei can result in dramatic autonomic disturbances. Profound vagal reflexes can be alarming, sometimes leading to a period of asystole. These are often followed by a compensatory parasympatholytic-sympathetic reflex. Under such circumstances, the hemodynamics can shift from extreme bradycardia and hypotension to tachycardia and hypertension in a matter of seconds.

The first step is to alert the surgeon to stop operating, which almost always alleviates the problem. Once the hemodynamic status has stabilized, an "autonomic blunting" prophylactic regimen can be given. Glycopyrrolate should be titrated until a 15% to 20% increase in heart rate is observed; if sympathetic reflexes are also involved, β-adrenergic blockade can be added. This approach is usually effective in attenuating the reflexes. In surgeries with an elevated risk of autonomic instability, the implementation of parasympatholytic prophylaxis should be strongly considered from the outset.

The sudden development of bradycardia should always alert the anesthesiologist to the possibility of a sudden increase in ICP, leading to the Cushing reflex. In this case, hypertension would also be seen, and the surgeon should be immediately notified.

Acioly MA, Carvalho CH, Koerbel A, et al. The role of the trigeminocardiac reflex in postoperative hearing function in non-vestibular schwannoma cerebellopontine angle tumors. *J Clin Neurosci.* 2011;18:237-240.

Koerbel A, Gharabaghi A, Samii A, et al. Trigeminocardiac reflex during skull base surgery: mechanism and management. *Acta Neurochir. (Wien).* 2005;147:727-733.

Schaller B, Probst R, Strebel S, et al. Trigeminocardiac reflex during surgery in the cerebellopontine angle. *J Neurosurg.* 1999;90:215-220.

C.14. Are there any measures you can take to prevent VAE?

Prevention is the cornerstone of VAE management, as current treatment methods for established VAE have limited efficacy. The best prevention of VAE is the neurosurgeon's meticulous control of venous bleeding and the tolerance of lower head positions. Extra vigilance on the part of the neuroanesthesiologist also plays an important role—observing a lack of bleeding on the cut edge of bone during removal of the craniotomy bone flap is an early sign of negative venous pressure and an increased likelihood of VAE. Active measures to reduce VAE include ensuring adequate hydration to raise the venous fluid column and minimizing venous capacitance through the use of pneumatic calf compression devices and avoidance of venodilators such as nitroglycerin; bone wax can be applied to cut bone edges to further minimize air entrainment.

The use of positive end-expiratory pressure (PEEP) is controversial: PEEP increases cerebral venous pressure and can reduce the risk of entrainment, but it also increases surgical bleeding and can potentially impede CPP. It promotes right-to-left intracardiac shunting, which increases the risk of VAE in susceptible patients, and sudden releases of PEEP (such as ventilator adjustments or a recruitment maneuver performed during craniotomy) can increase air entrainment as well as the propagation of PAE. We recommend limiting the PEEP to less than or equal to 5 cm H_2O and using it only as a means to optimize patient oxygenation. Monitoring of jugular bulb pressure may predict the occurrence of VAE, but catheterization of the jugular vein is excessively invasive to suggest routine use.

The use of N_2O has clear theoretical disadvantages in posterior fossa craniotomy, not only in the risk of expanding subclinical intravascular air but also in postoperative tension pneumocephalus. Although there are no clear clinical data to demonstrate these associations, its additional adverse effects on CBF and metabolism, ICP, and neurotoxicity make it difficult to justify its use, particularly with the easy availability of excellent alternatives.

SECTION 4

Giebler R, Kollenberg B, Pohlen G, et al. Effect of positive end-expiratory pressure on the incidence of venous air embolism and on the cardiovascular response to the sitting position during neurosurgery. *Br J Anaesth.* 1998;80:30-35.

Pasternak JJ, Lanier WL. Is nitrous oxide use appropriate in neurosurgical and neurologically at-risk patients? *Curr Opin Anaesthesiol.* 2010;23:544-550.

Schmitt HJ, Hemmerling TM. Venous air emboli occur during release of positive end-expiratory pressure and repositioning after sitting position surgery. *Anesth Analg.* 2002;94:400-403.

Wang X, Li M, Liang J, et al. Monitoring of intracranial venous sinus pressure and prevention for venous air embolism during operation with semi-sitting position. *J Clin Neurosci.* 2020;81:220-226.

C.15. During the procedure, the precordial Doppler becomes loud and turbulent. The end-tidal CO_2 ($Etco_2$) drops from 31 to 13 mm Hg and the systemic pressure from 121/63 to 64/32 mm Hg. What is your assessment and management plan?

This is a classic presentation of VAE. Immediately inform the surgeon, administer 100% oxygen, and call for skilled assistance. The surgeon should flood the field with saline and urgently prepare the field for lowering the head (eg, placement of a protective drape over the operative site and adjusting the head fixation device to allow for position change). If possible, an assistant should reach under the drapes and apply pressure to the jugular veins to prevent further entrainment (but not enough to occlude carotid flow), although this should be only a temporary measure. If a right atrial catheter is in place, an attempt should be made to aspirate air with a large syringe (enough to accommodate 15-20 mL of air). Intravenous fluids should be opened to full flow, and inotropes and vasopressors should be titrated to support the altered hemodynamics. The head should then be lowered to a level below the heart, or as much as possible. The left lateral decubitus position has been advocated but is probably of little benefit.

If the VAE is detected early, the episode will usually resolve. In most cases, it is appropriate to resume and complete the surgery, although placement of additional monitors before resumption might be warranted. Undetected, massive, or prolonged entrainment of air can lead to cardiac arrest. If cardiac arrest is present or imminent, and the patient is in a prone or semiprone position, the anesthesiologist must prepare the surgeon and others in the room for an emergent move to the supine position to enable resuscitation. For this reason, a stretcher must always be available outside the operating room when patients are in a prone position.

Kerr RH, Applegate RL II. Accurate placement of the right atrial air aspiration catheter: a descriptive study and prospective trial of intravascular electrocardiography. *Anesth Analg.* 2006;103:435-438.

Mirski MA, Lele AV, Fitzsimmons L, et al. Diagnosis and treatment of vascular air embolism. *Anesthesiology.* 2007;106:164-177.

C.16. What is your approach to emergence? What if the patient does not regain consciousness?

Providing an early neurologic assessment is one of the most valuable contributions of the anesthesiologist to the outcome in neurosurgical patients. As such, it is crucial to ensure patients emerge quickly, even after prolonged surgery. At the same time, emergence from anesthesia involves substantial changes in blood pressure, $Paco_2$, CBF, and autonomic activity and therefore must be carefully planned. The transition from hyperventilation should be gradual to prevent rebound acidosis. Adrenergic blocking agents should be administered to attenuate the sympathetic effects often seen during and following emergence in these patients. Nicardipine or labetalol can be considered if the patient exhibits refractory hypertension or hyperreactivity. Reversal of neuromuscular blockade should be carefully timed and executed to ensure that the patient does not move while their head is fixed in pins. Antiemetic therapy should be aggressive, as the elevation in ICP caused by retching and vomiting is particularly undesirable in craniotomy patients.

Coughing or "bucking" during emergence causes dramatic spikes in ICP and must be avoided. Several approaches can be used to prevent this, including intravenous lidocaine, an opioid-based anesthetic, or a deep extubation. In the case of deep extubation, it must be kept in mind that an intraoperative neurologic event might cause delayed or failed emergence. A strategy of converting the final phase of the anesthetic to a high-dose remifentanil infusion (0.2-0.4 µg/kg/min) can be highly effective and enables the volatile agent to be eliminated without the patient reacting. Once the remifentanil infusion is discontinued, the reliable pharmacokinetics lead to emergence conditions in most patients after approximately 10 minutes.

Failure to emerge can represent a neurologic event resulting from the surgery (such as an intracranial bleed, vessel occlusion, embolic event, or seizure), metabolic derangements, or a pharmacologic effect. In such cases, the time to diagnosis is a critical determinant of the outcome. The anesthesiologist must be able to state with confidence that the delayed emergence is unlikely to be pharmacologic. A rapid assessment can be made in the operating room to exclude nonneurologic causes of failure to emerge (**Table 18.8**); unless there is a clear cause found, a computed tomography (CT) scan should be performed immediately. Should this be necessary, the operating room should be kept available in case an emergent return is required.

In some posterior fossa procedures—especially when near the brainstem—postoperative edema can lead to an anticipated worsening of neurologic status before subsequent improvement on the first or second postoperative day, necessitating prolonged intubation. In these cases, the patient can be awakened at the conclusion of the surgery, and once a neurologic assessment is obtained, re-sedated for transport to the ICU. A remifentanil infusion of approximately 0.05 to 0.1 µg/kg/min usually enables an intubated patient to perform a cognitive examination while still tolerating the presence of the endotracheal tube.

TABLE 18.8 Rapid Assessment of Persistent Coma Immediately Postcraniotomy

Intervention	Assess the Cause of Coma
Pupillary exam	• New anisocoria suggesting herniation • Pinpoint pupils suggesting narcotic overdose • Dilated reactive pupils suggesting central anticholinergic syndrome
Arterial blood gas with electrolyte and glucose analysis	• Hypoxia • Hypercarbia • Acidosis • Hypoglycemia/hyperglycemia • Hyponatremia/hypernatremia
Processed electroencephalogram (eg, BIS monitor, IOM)	• Assess the depth of anesthesia • Seizure activity
Nerve stimulator	• Deep neuromuscular blockade
Core temperature	• Hypothermia

Review medication syringes, infusions, vaporizer	• Inadvertent overdose
	• Medication swap
	• Consider reversal agents:
	  • Naloxone in 40 µg aliquots, up to 400 µg
	  • Flumazenil 200 µg aliquots, up to 1 µg
	  • Physostigmine 1.25 mg, if centrally acting anticholinergics administered

CT scan	• Hemorrhage • Thrombosis (consider basilar artery thrombosis) • Pneumocephalus • Cerebral edema
Other considerations	• Hypothyroidism • Addisonian crisis

BIS, bispectral index; CT, computed tomography; IOM, intraoperative neurophysiologic monitoring.

Bilotta F, Lam AM, Doronzio A, et al. Esmolol blunts postoperative hemodynamic changes after propofol-remifentanil total intravenous fast-track neuroanesthesia for intracranial surgery. *J Clin Anesth.* 2008;20:426-430.

Lauta E, Abbinante C, Del Gaudio A, et al. Emergence times are similar with sevoflurane and total intravenous anesthesia: results of a multicenter RCT of patients scheduled for elective supratentorial craniotomy. *J Neurosurg Anesthesiol.* 2010;22:110-118.

D. Postoperative Management

D.1. What postoperative complications are of greatest concern? What level of monitoring is required?

Part of the neurologic assessment conducted immediately upon emergence should include an evaluation of the lower cranial nerves. Damage to these nerves or their nuclei can result in difficulty swallowing and protecting the airway. The principal concern is the development of edema or hematoma, causing compression of the brainstem or midbrain structures. The brainstem sits in an anatomic location with very low compliance; even small degrees of edema that would be well tolerated following supratentorial procedures can lead to catastrophic neurologic compromise. It is crucial to understand that edema and hematoma can develop over several hours following the procedure; a patient who had a satisfactory emergence might deteriorate neurologically in the middle of the night. In certain circumstances, the risk of postoperative edema is so high that the patient is left intubated prophylactically, as discussed earlier. Deterioration cannot always be anticipated, and these patients should be initially monitored in an intensive care setting in all cases.

Dubey A, Sung WS, Shaya M, et al. Complications of posterior cranial fossa surgery: an institutional experience of 500 patients. *Surg Neurol.* 2009;72:369-375.

Sughrue ME, Rutkowski MJ, Shangari G, et al. Risk factors for the development of serious medical complications after resection of meningiomas. Clinical article. *J Neurosurg.* 2011;114:697-704.

Wong JM, Panchmatia JR, Ziewacz JE, et al. Patterns in neurosurgical adverse events: intracranial neoplasm surgery. *Neurosurg Focus.* 2012;33:E16.

D.2. What is your approach to postoperative pain control?

Optimal pain control after craniotomy has traditionally faced several challenges. One misconception is that craniotomy and tumor resection cause minimal pain, despite the rich nociceptive afferents to the meninges, dura, falx, and calvarial periosteum. Using traditional analgesic approaches, nearly 70% of postcraniotomy patients experience moderate to severe pain on the first postoperative day, and just under half continue to do so on the second postoperative day.

Another persistent dogma is that most analgesics are dangerous for postcraniotomy patients and should be dosed sparingly. There is concern that opioids have the potential to cause sedation and respiratory depression in neurologically vulnerable patients. However, patient-controlled analgesia (PCA) opioid regimens have been used safely in both supra- and infratentorial postcraniotomy patients, improving pain control and patient satisfaction.

In addition to opioid PCAs, we suggest a multimodal approach to minimize opioid use and its side effects. Acetaminophen is nonsedating and safe in recommended doses in the absence of liver disease. Neurosurgeons have traditionally avoided nonsteroidal anti-inflammatory drugs (NSAIDs) in the perioperative period due to the risk of postoperative hematoma, although the available evidence is not robust. Nonetheless, it behooves the neuroanesthesiologist to discuss the use of NSAIDs with the surgeon before prescribing. Scalp blocks or scalp infiltration performed at the end of surgery have low morbidity and improve pain control in the early postoperative period. Although this effect is not sustained beyond the first postoperative day, there is evidence to suggest that this technique reduces the development of chronic postcraniotomy pain. An alternative option involves regional blockade of the lesser and greater occipital nerves by the anesthesiologist. Ideally, these would be performed immediately prior to surgery, as anatomy may be altered by the surgical procedure. These have proven to be an effective alternative to scalp blocks for craniotomy and have a longer duration of analgesia. Preinduction gabapentin, in addition to its beneficial effects on minimizing the hemodynamic response to laryngoscopy and head pinning, decreases postoperative pain and opioid requirements, although it may result in increased sedation and slow emergence. Tramadol has been used successfully for postcraniotomy pain; however, due to its increased risk of nausea and vomiting and the lowering of the seizure threshold, we do not recommend it as part of a first-line analgesic regimen.

Dunn LK, Naik BI, Nemergut EC, et al. Post-craniotomy pain management: beyond opioids. *Curr Neurol Neurosci Rep.* 2016;16:93.

Jayaram K, Srilata M, Kulkarni D, et al. Regional anesthesia to scalp for craniotomy: innovation with innervation. *J Neurosurg Anesthesiol.* 2016;28:32-37.

SECTION 4

Morad A, Winters B, Stevens R, et al. The efficacy of intravenous patient-controlled analgesia after intracranial surgery of the posterior fossa: a prospective, randomized controlled trial. *Anesth Analg.* 2012;114:416-423.

Rahimi SY, Alleyne CH, Vernier E, et al. Postoperative pain management with tramadol after craniotomy: evaluation and cost analysis. *J Neurosurg.* 2010;112:268-272.

Tsaousi GG, Logan SW, Bilotta F. Postoperative pain control following craniotomy: a systematic review of recent clinical literature. *Pain Pract.* 2017;17:968-981.

Türe H, Sayin M, Karlikaya G, et al. The analgesic effect of gabapentin as a prophylactic anticonvulsant drug on postcraniotomy pain: a prospective randomized study. *Anesth Analg.* 2009;109:1625-1631.

D.3. In the ICU, the patient's neurologic status deteriorates and ICP monitoring is instituted. What are the different methods of monitoring ICP, and what are their limitations?

ICP monitoring is commonly used in neurosurgical critical care as a marker of intracranial compliance and to allow a more objective calculation of CPP. Typically, an ICP monitor is placed at a discrete anatomic point of measurement, and data from this monitor are extrapolated to the whole brain. It is important to remember, however, that significant differences in regional ICP can exist, particularly in patients with a pathologic disruption of normal CSF circulation. In the case of this patient, for instance, an ICP monitor positioned in the supratentorial region may not accurately represent the pressure in the posterior fossa.

Various methods of ICP monitoring are available, differing in invasiveness, site of measurement, and degree of validation. An external ventricular drain (EVD) is considered the gold standard and allows for both ICP measurement and CSF drainage to treat intracranial hypertension (although not simultaneously). The catheter tip is introduced into one of the lateral ventricles either through a blind technique or with imaging guidance and connected to a fluid column with a pressure transducer and drainage system. It is the most invasive method of ICP monitoring and is associated with significant rates of intracranial infection and bleeding during placement. Other limitations of the EVD include difficult placement in patients with midline shift, catheter malfunction, and potential CSF overdrainage. An alternative method for measuring ICP is through the use of microtransducers. These devices transduce an external force (eg, applied by edematous brain tissue) into an alteration in the electrical or light signal. Fiberoptic devices transmit light to a flexible reflective tip that is displaced by an external force, and the change in light reflection is extrapolated into a change in ICP. Similarly, electronic strain gauge devices are deformed by external pressure, thereby inducing a change in electrical resistance. These devices are miniaturized to the extent that their placement into brain parenchyma causes minimal damage and are typically secured to the skull with a bone bolt. Depending on the manufacturer, microtransducers may also be introduced into the subarachnoid, epidural, or subdural spaces, with some reduction in accuracy. The primary advantages of microtransducers are the decreased rate of intracranial infection, the absence of catheter-related malfunction, and the stability of the fixation bolt. However, these devices are prone to zero drift over time and cannot be rezeroed without removing the device entirely. Further limitations include a local sampling of parenchymal pressure and significantly higher cost compared to catheter systems.

In recent years, noninvasive methods, such as transcranial Doppler (TCD) and optic nerve sheath diameter (ONSD) measurements, have shown promise for assessing ICP and CPP. TCD analyzes middle cerebral artery flow characteristics and utilizes derived parameters, including the Pulsatility Index (PI), as surrogate measurements for various neurovascular parameters, such as cerebrovascular resistance, vasospasm, and CPP. However, the clinical utility of the PI has been questioned due to its sensitivity to changes in arterial blood pressure and carbon dioxide levels. Other formulas, such as one based on diastolic flow velocity, have shown better sensitivity for detecting increased ICP in pilot studies.

ONSD measurements are another ultrasound-based technique that has gained attention for noninvasive ICP assessment. The optic nerve sheath is continuous with the dura mater of the brain and surrounds the subarachnoid space containing CSF. When there is an increase in CSF pressure, the distensible optic nerve sheath expands, causing the ONSD to enlarge. This method has demonstrated promising results in predicting increased ICP, showing a strong correlation with invasive ICP measurements.

Although both TCD and ONSD have shown encouraging results in noninvasive ICP assessment, further investigations are needed to establish their consistency and reliability compared to invasive methods of ICP measurement.

Hawryluk GWJ, Citerio G, Hutchinson P, et al. Intracranial pressure: current perspectives on physiology and monitoring. *Intensive Care Med.* 2022;48:1471-1481.

Raboel PH, Bartek J Jr, Andresen M, et al. Intracranial pressure monitoring: invasive versus non-invasive methods—a review. *Crit Care Res Pract.* 2012;2012:950393.

Steiner LA, Andrews PJD. Monitoring the injured brain: ICP and CBF. *Br J Anaesth.* 2006;97:26-38.

Zweifel C, Czosnyka M, Carrera E, et al. Reliability of the blood flow velocity pulsatility index for assessment of intracranial and cerebral perfusion pressures in head-injured patients. *Neurosurgery.* 2012;7:853-861.

19

Carotid Artery Disease

Maria Bustillo

A 76-year-old male is scheduled for a right carotid endarterectomy (CEA) for asymptomatic left carotid stenosis. He has 90% occlusion of his right carotid artery and 60% occlusion of the left carotid artery. His past medical history is remarkable for hypertension, insulin-dependent diabetes mellitus, and coronary artery disease. He had cardiac stents placed 4 years ago. His blood pressure is 180/78 mm Hg, and his pulse is 59 beats per minute and regular.

A. Medical Disease and Differential Diagnosis

1. What are the presenting symptoms of carotid stenosis?
2. What is the prevalence of carotid artery disease?
3. What is the natural course of carotid artery disease as it relates to stroke?
4. What in the patient's history puts them at higher risk for having carotid atherosclerosis?
5. Do we screen patients for asymptomatic carotid stenosis?
6. What is the risk of stroke and cardiovascular events in asymptomatic carotid atherosclerosis?
7. What are the current medical options that the patient has for treating carotid atherosclerosis?
8. What are the indications for CEA and carotid artery stenting (CAS) in asymptomatic carotid atherosclerotic disease?
9. What are the indications for performing a CEA in symptomatic carotid stenosis?
10. Is there any role for CAS in symptomatic patients?
11. Discuss the anatomy of the cerebral vasculature, including the carotid artery and the circle of Willis.
12. Discuss cerebral blood flow (CBF) in the presence of carotid artery disease.
13. Discuss the different surgical approaches to carotid revascularization.
14. Discuss the endovascular approaches to carotid stenting.
15. What is normal CBF?
16. What is critically low CBF as measured by the electroencephalogram (EEG)?
17. What is cerebral autoregulation?
18. How does $Paco_2$ affect CBF?
19. What are the principal determinants of CBF?
20. What is meant by the term *luxury perfusion*?
21. What is meant by the term *intracerebral steal*?

B. Preoperative Evaluation and Preparation

1. What will you look for in your preoperative evaluation of this patient?
2. Is this patient's blood pressure too high for elective surgery?
3. What laboratory data are required preoperatively?
4. Will you treat this patient's blood glucose?
5. Will you premedicate this patient?

C. Intraoperative Management

1. How will you monitor this patient?
2. How will you know that the patient's cerebral perfusion is adequate during surgery?
3. Discuss the differences and relative advantages and disadvantages of unprocessed EEG and processed EEG monitoring.

4. How will you measure CBF intraoperatively? What are the relative advantages and disadvantages of each technique?
5. Describe the use of stump pressure and its limitations.
6. Describe the use of transcranial Doppler (TCD) and its limitations.
7. Describe the use of jugular venous oxygen saturation ($Sjvo_2$) and its limitations.
8. Describe the use of cerebral oximetry and its limitations.
9. Discuss somatosensory evoked potentials (SSEPs) as a monitor of CBF during CEA.
10. What type of anesthesia will you choose for this patient if she chose to have an endarterectomy?
11. What type of anesthesia will you choose for this patient if she chose to have a carotid stent?
12. How will you induce and maintain general anesthesia in this patient for CEA?
13. How would you proceed if the patient were to receive regional anesthesia?
14. Discuss the effects of anesthetics on CBF.
15. Discuss the protective effects of anesthetic agents on cerebral function.
16. How will you manage this patient's ventilation under general anesthesia?
17. How will you manage this patient's blood pressure intraoperatively?
18. Discuss reperfusion injury following CEA and CAS.
19. What intravenous fluids will you give this patient intraoperatively?

D. Postoperative Management

1. The patient does not "wake up" from general anesthesia. Why?
2. Postoperatively, the patient's blood pressure is 170/96 mm Hg. Will you treat this?
3. What immediate postoperative complications might you expect after a CEA?
4. What postoperative complications might you expect after a CAS?
5. Discuss postoperative neurocognitive dysfunction following uncomplicated carotid intervention.

A. Medical Disease and Differential Diagnosis

A.1. What are the presenting symptoms of carotid stenosis?

Carotid stenosis is often asymptomatic, only to be discovered on physical exam as a carotid bruit or incidentally on imaging.

- Symptomatic carotid stenosis presents with focal neurologic deficits in the corresponding carotid artery territory. These focal neurologic deficits can be characterized as a transient ischemic attack (TIA) or ischemic stroke. A TIA is a transient focal neurologic deficit attributable to a vascular cause **without** corresponding appropriate lesions on imaging.
- An ischemic stroke is characterized by an acute onset of focal neurologic symptoms that leaves permanent injury, either seen clinically or by appropriate corresponding lesions on imaging. Ischemic symptoms from carotid stenosis originate from the vascular distribution supplied by the internal or external carotid artery. The symptoms can be from artery-to-artery embolization of the plaque or from cerebral hypoperfusion caused by the stenotic lesion.
- Ischemic symptoms can be divided into three main categories: (1) ocular ischemia or infarction, (2) ipsilateral hemispheric signs, and (3) atypical symptoms. Ocular ischemia or infarction symptoms include partial or complete blindness in one eye. Ipsilateral hemispheric signs include contralateral homonymous hemianopsia, hemiparesis, or hemisensory loss. Specific ischemic signs associated most commonly with left-side lesions include aphasia, whereas right hemispheric symptoms can include visuospatial neglect. Atypical symptoms include unilateral limb shaking and transient monocular vision loss when exposed to bright light, which can also occur from ischemia downstream to the embolus.

Javaid A, Alfishawy M. Internal carotid artery stenosis presenting with limb shaking TIA. *Case Rep Neurol Med.* 2016;2016:3656859.

Kernan WN, Ovbiagele B, Black HR, et al. Guidelines for the prevention of stroke in patients with stroke and transient ischemic attack: a guideline for healthcare professionals from the American Heart Association/American Stroke Association. *Stroke.* 2014;45:2160-2236.

Liberman AL, Zandieh A, Loomis C, et al. Symptomatic carotid occlusion is frequently associated with microembolization. *Stroke.* 2017;48:394-399.

Pickett CA, Jackson JL, Hemann BA, et al. Carotid bruits and cerebrovascular disease risk: a meta-analysis. *Stroke.* 2010;41:2295-2302.

A.2. What is the prevalence of carotid artery disease?

Carotid artery disease is a marker of generalized arteriosclerosis. The prevalence of asymptomatic carotid disease, which is defined as stenosis greater than 50%, ranges from 4% to 8%. In a meta-analysis of 40 studies, the prevalence of moderate stenosis increased with age in both males and females. Males at all ages have the highest prevalence estimates. Carotid artery disease accounts for 10% to 20% of all strokes in the United States (~200,000 strokes per year).

Adams HP Jr, Bendixen BH, Kappelle LJ, et al. Classification of subtype of acute ischemic stroke. Definitions for use in a multicenter clinical trial. TOAST. Trial of Org 10172 in acute stroke treatment. *Stroke*. 1993;24:35-41.

de Weerd M, Greving JP, de Jong AW, et al. Prevalence of asymptomatic carotid artery stenosis according to age and sex: systematic review and metaregression analysis. *Stroke*. 2009;40:1105-1113.

Nelson P, Bustillo M. Anesthesia for carotid endarterectomy, angioplasty, and stent. *Anesthesiol Clin*. 2021;39:37-51.

Pujia A, Rubba P, Spencer MP. Prevalence of extracranial carotid artery disease detectable by echo-Doppler in an elderly population. *Stroke*. 1992;23:818-822.

Safian RD. Carotid artery revascularization: the known knowns and the known unknowns. *J Am Coll Cardiol*. 2017;69:2276-2278.

A.3. What is the natural course of carotid artery disease as it relates to stroke?

Carotid artery disease carries a typical natural course of plaque development, which is cumulative. Continued development leads to possible stenosis or the possibility of plaque rupture. Atherosclerosis in the extracranial carotid arteries is usually most severe within 2 cm of the bifurcation of the internal and external carotid arteries. Atherosclerotic lesions are predominantly found in the posterior wall of the internal carotid artery. Over time, the plaque extends proximally into the common carotid artery, and the stenotic lesion takes on an hourglass shape. Extracranial carotid atherosclerotic disease can lead to stroke by embolism of cholesterol crystals or debris, artery-to-artery embolism, dissection or disintegration of the arterial wall, and decreased cerebral perfusion because of the stenosis caused by plaque buildup. Emboli from carotid artery disease usually lodge in the middle cerebral artery; however, depending on the anatomy of the circle of Willis, they can also settle in the anterior and posterior cerebral arteries. Although the risk of stroke has historically been correlated to the degree of carotid stenosis, new markers for plaque vulnerability as it relates to disease severity are emerging. They include plaque progression, ulcerations seen on plaques, echo-lucency, intraplaque hemorrhage, and high lipid content of the stenotic lesion. The risk factors for the development of carotid artery disease are similar to those causing atherosclerotic occlusive disease in other vascular beds, namely, increasing age, male gender, hypertension, tobacco smoking, diabetes, homocysteinemia, and hyperlipidemia.

Fisher M, Paganini-Hill A, Martin A, et al. Carotid plaque pathology: thrombosis, ulceration, and stroke pathogenesis. *Stroke*. 2005;36:253-257.

Furie KL. Pathophysiology of symptoms from carotid atherosclerosis. Accessed October 19, 2018. https://www.uptodate.com/contents/pathophysiology-of-symptoms-from-carotid-atherosclerosis

Grotta JC. Clinical practice. Carotid stenosis. *N Engl J Med*. 2013;369:1143-1150.

Nelson P, Bustillo M. Anesthesia for carotid endarterectomy, angioplasty, and stent. *Anesthesiol Clin*. 2021;39:37-51.

Ooi YC, Gonzalez NR. Management of extracranial carotid artery disease. *Cardiol Clin*. 2015;33:1-35.

Valentine EA, Ochroch EA. Anesthesia for vascular and endovascular surgery. In: Cullen BF, Stock MC, Ortega R, et al, eds. *Barash, Cullen, and Stoelting's Clinical Anesthesia*. 9th ed. Wolters Kluwer; 2024:1083-1112.

A.4. What in the patient's history puts them at higher risk for having carotid atherosclerosis?

Hypertension, hyperlipidemia, obesity, smoking, diabetes, and physical inactivity put one at high risk for carotid atherosclerosis. These risk factors also increase the risk of coronary artery disease.

Conrad MF, Boulom V, Mukhopadhyay S, et al. Progression of asymptomatic carotid stenosis despite optimal medical therapy. *J Vasc Surg*. 2013;58:128-135.e121.

Mathiesen EB, Joakimsen O, Bønaa KH. Prevalence of and risk factors associated with carotid artery stenosis: the Tromso Study. *Cerebrovasc Dis*. 2001;12:44-51.

A.5. Do we screen patients for asymptomatic carotid stenosis?

The prevalence of asymptomatic carotid atherosclerosis in the general population is approximately 3%. The U.S. Preventive Services Task Force (USPSTF), American College of Cardiology and American

Heart Association (AHA), and American Stroke Association (ASA) recommend against routine screening of asymptomatic patients who have no clinical manifestations of or risk factors for atherosclerosis. In asymptomatic patients with known or suspected carotid stenosis, duplex ultrasonography, performed by a qualified technologist in a certified laboratory, is recommended as the initial diagnostic test to detect hemodynamically significant carotid stenosis (Level of Evidence: C).

Brott TG, Halperin JL, Abbara S, et al. 2011 ASA/ACCF/AHA/AANN/AANS/ACR/ASNR/CNS/SAIP/SCAI/SIR/SNIS/SVM/SVS guideline on the management of patients with extracranial carotid and vertebral artery disease: executive summary. *Circulation.* 2011;124:489-532.

de Weerd M, Greving JP, de Jong AW, et al. Prevalence of asymptomatic carotid artery stenosis according to age and sex: systematic review and meta regression analysis. *Stroke.* 2009;40:1105-1113.

de Weerd M, Greving JP, Hedblad B, et al. Prevalence of asymptomatic carotid artery stenosis in the general population: an individual participant data meta-analysis. *Stroke.* 2010;41:1294-1297.

Meschia JF, Bushnell C, Boden-Albala B, et al. Guidelines for the primary prevention of stroke: a statement for healthcare professionals from the American Heart Association/American Stroke Association. *Stroke.* 2014;45: 3754-3832.

Wolff T, Guirguis-Blake J, Miller T, et al. Screening for carotid artery stenosis: an update of the evidence for the U.S. Preventive Services Task Force. *Ann Intern Med.* 2007;147:860-870.

A.6. What is the risk of stroke and cardiovascular events in asymptomatic carotid atherosclerosis?

Although ischemic stroke is the most feared event with carotid atherosclerosis, the estimated risk is 0.5% to 1% per year ipsilaterally in patients with more than 50% stenosis. Asymptomatic carotid stenosis is considered a risk equivalent for coronary artery disease and is a marker for increased risk of myocardial infarction (MI) and death.

Goessens BM, Visseren FL, Kappelle LJ, et al. Asymptomatic carotid artery stenosis and the risk of new vascular events in patients with manifest arterial disease: the SMART study. *Stroke.* 2007;38:1470-1475.

Spence JD. Management of asymptomatic carotid stenosis. *Neurol Clin.* 2015;33:443-457.

A.7. What are the current medical options that the patient has for treating carotid atherosclerosis?

Best medical therapy was outlined by the Asymptomatic Carotid Surgery Trial (ACST) and includes the use of a 3-hydroxy-3-methylglutaryl-coenzyme (HMG-CoA) reductase inhibitor (statin), aggressive blood pressure control with antihypertensive drugs, strict glycemic control for patients with diabetes, smoking cessation, weight reduction, and of antiplatelet drugs.

Meschia JF, Bushnell C, Boden-Albala B, et al. Guidelines for the primary prevention of stroke: a statement for healthcare professionals from the American Heart Association/American Stroke Association. *Stroke.* 2014;45:3754-3832.

Nelson P, Bustillo M. Anesthesia for carotid endarterectomy, angioplasty, and stent. *Anesthesiol Clin.* 2021;39:37-51.

A.8. What are the indications for CEA and carotid artery stenting (CAS) in asymptomatic carotid atherosclerotic disease?

The recommendation for surgical treatment by many societies is based on three major trials that took place in patients with asymptomatic carotid stenosis: the Veterans Administration (VA) trial, the Asymptomatic Carotid Atherosclerosis Study (ACAS) trial, and the ACST trial.

The indications differ by society. The AHA and the ASA note the following with respect to CEA: If the risks of perioperative stroke, MI, and death are low (<3%), it may be reasonable to consider CEA in asymptomatic patients with more than 70% stenosis. AHA/ASA with respect to CAS: In asymptomatic patients with more than 60% stenosis by angiography or more than 70% by duplex ultrasound, prophylactic CAS might be considered, but its effectiveness compared to medical therapy is not well established.

The Society for Vascular Surgery notes the following: Asymptomatic patients with 70% to 90% diameter stenosis CEA should be considered if the perioperative and death rates are less than 3%. They do not recommend CAS for asymptomatic patients because there are insufficient data.

Three main trials examined carotid stenting versus endarterectomy for asymptomatic stenosis. They include the ACST 1 trial, the Carotid Revascularization Endarterectomy Versus Stenting (CREST) trial, and the Stenting and Angioplasty with Protection in Patients at High Risk for Endarterectomy (SAPPHIRE) trial. A meta-analysis of these trials indicated that both endarterectomy and CAS are viable long-term options for patients with carotid atherosclerosis. The evidence suggests that the 30-day risk of stroke or death is higher with CAS compared to CEA, but after 30 days, the risks of stroke and death are similar. Patients older than 70 years of age had poorer outcomes with stenting than endarterectomy.

Significant progress has been made since the late 1980s and early 1990s when the major CEA trials were underway. At that time, the best medical treatment was antiplatelet therapy with aspirin. Since then, the utility of statins, antihypertensive drugs, smoking cessation, and lifestyle modification has been shown. This change in medical therapy and its effect on carotid stenosis became apparent from the ACST-1. Over the 10-year course, statin usage became more prevalent, from 17% in 1993 to 1996 to 58% from 2000 to 2003. With this modern multimodal approach to medical therapy, many experts argue that the gap between medical and surgical treatment of carotid disease has narrowed for reducing the risk of stroke.

If a surgical option is chosen, keep in mind that it is a long-term investment and that the benefit may not be apparent until 2 years or more. Also, trials show that there was a trend toward CEA being less effective in females and older individuals and that these procedures should be performed at institutions where the perioperative stroke and death rates are less than 3%. Contralateral stenosis also matters when considering a surgical option. When a subgroup analysis was performed, CEA with contralateral total occlusion provided no long-term benefit.

AbuRahma AF, Avgerinos ED, Chang RW, et al. Society for vascular surgery clinical practice guidelines for management of extracranial cerebrovascular disease. *J Vasc Surg*. 2022;75:4S-22S.

Baker WH, Howard VJ, Howard G, et al. Effect of contralateral occlusion on long-term efficacy of endarterectomy in the asymptomatic carotid atherosclerosis study (ACAS). ACAS investigators. *Stroke*. 2000;31:2330-2334.

Brett AS, Levine JD. The case against identifying carotid stenosis in asymptomatic patients. *JAMA Intern Med*. 2014;174:2004-2008.

Brott TG, Hobson RW II, Howard G, et al. Stenting versus endarterectomy for treatment of carotid-artery stenosis. *N Engl J Med*. 2010;363:11-23.

Brott TG, Howard G, Roubin GS, et al. Long-term results of stenting versus endarterectomy for carotid-artery stenosis. *N Engl J Med*. 2016;374:1021-1031.

Halliday A, Harrison M, Hayter E, et al. 10-Year stroke prevention after successful carotid endarterectomy for asymptomatic stenosis (ACST-1): a multicenter randomized trial. *Lancet*. 2010;376:1074-1084.

Halliday A, Mansfield A, Marro J, et al. Prevention of disabling and fatal strokes by successful carotid endarterectomy in patients without recent neurological symptoms: randomized control trial. *Lancet* 2004;363:1491-1502.

Hobson RW II, Weiss DG, Fields WS, et al. Efficacy of carotid endarterectomy for asymptomatic carotid stenosis. The veterans affairs cooperative study group. *N Engl J Med*. 1993;328:221-227.

Moresoli P, Habib B, Reynier P, et al. Carotid stenting versus endarterectomy for asymptomatic carotid artery stenosis: a systematic review and meta-analysis. *Stroke*. 2017;48:2150-2157.

Müller MD, Lyrer P, Brown MM, Bonati LH. Carotid artery stenting versus endarterectomy for treatment of carotid artery stenosis. *Cochrane Database Syst Rev*. 2020;2:CD000515.

Rosenfield K, Matsumura JS, Chaturvedi S, et al. Randomized trial of stent versus surgery for asymptomatic carotid stenosis. *N Engl J Med*. 2016;374:1011-1020.

Sardar P, Chatterjee S, Aronow HD, et al. Carotid artery stenting versus endarterectomy for stroke prevention: a meta-analysis of clinical trials. *J Am Coll Cardiol*. 2017;69:2266-2275.

Spence JD. Asymptomatic carotid stenosis. *Circulation*. 2013;127:739-742.

Voeks JH, Howard G, Roubin GS, et al. Age and outcomes after carotid stenting and endarterectomy: the carotid revascularization endarterectomy versus stenting trial. *Stroke*. 2011;42:3484-3490.

Yadav JS, Wholey MH, Kuntz RE, et al. Protected carotid-artery stenting versus endarterectomy in high-risk patients. *N Engl J Med*. 2004;351:1493-1501.

A.9. What are the indications for performing a CEA in symptomatic carotid stenosis?

Symptomatic carotid stenosis is defined as focal neurologic symptoms, attributable to the appropriate carotid distribution, that have occurred within the past 6 months. Decisions for care in symptomatic disease come from three main trials, which include the North American Symptomatic Carotid Endarterectomy (NASCET) trial, the European Carotid Surgery Trial (ECST), and the VA trials.

Guidelines issued in 2014 by the AHA/ASA make the following recommendations with respect to CEA:

CEA is recommended for severe symptomatic stenosis (70%-99%) as long as the perioperative morbidity and mortality risk is estimated to be less than 6%. The number needed to treat (NNT) to prevent one stroke at 5 years is 6.3.

CEA is also recommended for moderate symptomatic patients (50%-69% stenosis) depending on patient characteristics if the perioperative morbidity and mortality risk is estimated to be less than 6%. The NNT to prevent one stroke over 5 years is 22 in moderate symptomatic stenosis.

CEA or stenting (CAS) is not recommended for less than 50% stenosis. Carotid revascularization was found to be harmful for symptomatic patients with less than 30% stenosis.

In studies leading to these recommendations, surgeries were performed at high-volume centers where the combined morbidity and mortality did not exceed 6%. Although it may be difficult to decipher one surgeon or institution's morbidity or mortality rate, a rate over 6% can negate the benefit gained from a CEA. Other factors that may impact the benefit gained from CEA include the timing of surgery, age, sex, presenting symptoms, and plaque morphology. There is evidence that performing CEA within 2 weeks of a nondisabling TIA or stroke improves outcomes compared with later surgery, but that performing it within 48 hours of a stroke or TIA leads to an elevated risk of stroke. This decline in benefits with time was more rapid with females than males. It was also noted that females who did not have their CEA within 2 weeks did not gain any benefit from the procedure irrespective of the degree of stenosis. Best medical therapy has also improved significantly from when the first CEA trials in the 1980s were started. As such, the NNT may be higher to prevent one stroke today with current medical therapy.

Meschia JF, Bushnell C, Boden-Albala B, et al. Guidelines for the primary prevention of stroke: a statement for healthcare professionals from the American Heart Association/American Stroke Association. *Stroke.* 2014;45:3754-3832.

MRC European Carotid Surgery Trial: interim results for symptomatic patients with severe (70-99%) or with mild (0-29%) carotid stenosis. European Carotid Surgery Trialists' Collaborative Group. *Lancet.* 1991;337:1235-1243.

Rerkasem K, Rothwell PM. Carotid endarterectomy for symptomatic carotid stenosis. *Cochrane Database Syst Rev.* 2011:CD001081.

Rothwell PM, Eliasziw M, Gutnikov SA, et al. Analysis of pooled data from the randomised controlled trials of endarterectomy for symptomatic carotid stenosis. *Lancet.* 2003;361:107-116.

A.10. Is there any role for CAS in symptomatic patients?

CAS and CEA achieve similar long-term outcomes for symptomatic disease, but the periprocedural stroke or death rate was greater with CAS than with CEA. The increased risk of stroke was only found in patients over 70 years of age. Although old age was originally proposed to be a high risk for surgery and therefore an indication for stenting, studies have shown that older adults have worse outcomes with CAS. Age above 70 years linearly correlated with the risk of stroke during CAS. The CAS group had a lower rate of MI, cranial nerve palsy, or access site hematoma.

The guidelines issued in 2014 by the AHA/ASA make the following recommendations with respect to CAS.

CAS is indicated as an alternative to CEA for symptomatic patients at average or low risk of complications associated with endovascular intervention for stenosis more than 70% by noninvasive imaging or more than 50% with angiography as long as the anticipated perioperative morbidity and mortality is less than 6%.

Consider the patient's age when choosing between CEA and CAS, as patients older than 70 years of age might have improved outcomes with CEA. For patients younger than 70 years, CAS is equivalent to CEA with respect to periprocedural complications, namely stroke, MI, and death.

CAS is reasonable for patients with symptomatic severe stenosis who have anatomic or medical conditions that greatly increase the risk of surgery.

Carotid revascularization is not recommended for patients with severe disability caused by cerebral infarction that precludes useful function or for patients with chronic total occlusion of the targeted artery. Conditions thought to increase the risk for surgery include radiation-induced stenosis, contralateral vocal cord paralysis, and tracheostomy.

Bonati LH, Lyrer P, Ederle J, et al. Percutaneous transluminal balloon angioplasty and stenting for carotid artery stenosis. *Cochrane Database Syst Rev.* 2012:CD000515.

Brott TG, Hobson RW II, Howard G, et al. Stenting versus endarterectomy for treatment of carotid-artery stenosis. *N Engl J Med.* 2010;363:11-23.

Meschia JF, Bushnell C, Boden-Albala B, et al. Guidelines for the primary prevention of stroke: a statement for healthcare professionals from the American Heart Association/American Stroke Association. *Stroke.* 2014;45:3754-3832.

Müller MD, Lyrer P, Brown MM, et al. Carotid artery stenting versus endarterectomy for the treatment of carotid artery stenosis. *Cochrane Database Syst Rev.* 2020;2:CD000515.

A.11. Discuss the anatomy of the cerebral vasculature, including the carotid artery and the circle of Willis.

The common carotid arteries originate in the thorax. The right common carotid artery originates at the bifurcation of the brachiocephalic trunk, and the left originates from the aortic arch. In the neck, the common carotid arteries travel within the carotid sheath. At the level of the thyroid cartilage, each common carotid artery bifurcates into the internal and external carotid arteries.

Branches of the external carotid artery include the superior thyroid, lingual, facial, ascending pharyngeal, occipital, posterior auricular, maxillary, and superficial temporal arteries.

The internal carotid artery passes through the neck without branching to enter the middle cranial fossa. It enters the middle cranial fossa through the carotid canal of the temporal bone, adjacent to the sphenoid bone. It supplies the hypophysis cerebri, the orbit, and the major portion of the supratentorial region of the brain. The cerebral arteries are derived from the internal carotid and vertebral arteries. The anastomosis they form at the base of the brain is known as the *circle of Willis* (**Figure 19.1**). The two anterior cerebral arteries form the circle anteriorly. They are connected through the anterior communicating artery. The two posterior cerebral arteries form the circle posteriorly, which then ends at the junction of the basilar artery. The posterior cerebral arteries are connected to the internal carotid arteries by the two posterior communicating arteries. The middle cerebral artery primarily supplies the lateral surface of each cerebral hemisphere. The anterior cerebral and posterior cerebral arteries supply the medial and inferior surfaces of the cerebral hemisphere.

Dalley AF II, Agur AMR. *Moore's Clinically Oriented Anatomy*. 9th ed. Wolters Kluwer; 2023:855-996.

SECTION 4

A.12. Discuss cerebral blood flow (CBF) in the presence of carotid artery disease.

Stable CBF is maintained within a given range of systemic blood pressure through autoregulation and collateral flow. Whereas most studies focus on the degree of carotid stenosis and the risk of stroke, emerging evidence indicates that downstream hemodynamic effects distal to the stenosis also play an important role in stroke risk classification.

Cerebrovascular reserve is the capacity of the brain to increase cerebral blood volume through vasodilation to maintain a constant regional CBF in the face of low cerebral perfusion pressure (CPP). When CPP is reduced, the cerebral vasculature autoregulates by dilation of cerebral arterioles to maintain CBF. With severe carotid stenosis, vasodilatory capacity is maximally exhausted, and a further decrease in CPP, such as with induction of anesthesia, can also decrease CBF and increase the risk of stroke.

The hemodynamic intracerebral effects of carotid stenosis also depend on collateral flow. The circle of Willis is the primary collateral circulation of cerebral arteries, followed by the ophthalmic artery, leptomeningeal vessels, and anastomoses among the perforating cortical arteries.

Current understanding of CBF is incomplete, as most of our knowledge of cerebral hemodynamics comes from changes that occur in the large vessels. Flow in the large cerebral vessels may not correlate to flow in the capillary network, which limits our current knowledge of microvascular perfusion.

Edvinsson L, Krause D. *Cerebral Blood Flow and Metabolism*. 2nd ed. Lippincott Williams & Wilkins; 2002.

Ellis JA, Joshi S. Cerebral and spinal blood flow. In: Cottrell JE, Patel PM, Soriano SG, eds. *Neuroanesthesia*. 7th ed. Elsevier; 2024:22-26.

Gupta A, Chazen JL, Hartman M, et al. Cerebrovascular reserve and stroke risk in patients with carotid stenosis or occlusion: a systematic review and meta-analysis. *Stroke*. 2012;43:2884-2891.

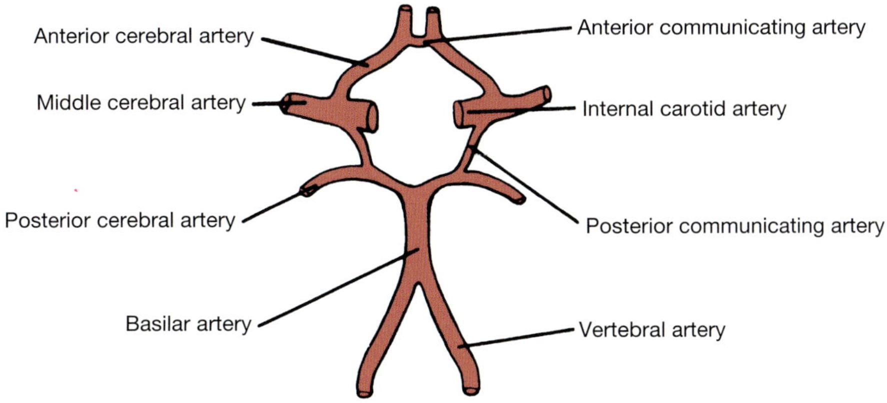

FIGURE 19.1. Arterial circle of Willis.

Gur AY, Bova I, Bornstein NM. Is impaired cerebral vasomotor reactivity a predictive factor of stroke in asymptomatic patients? *Stroke.* 1996;27:2188-2190.

Hedera P, Bujdáková J, Traubner P. Effect of collateral flow patterns on outcome of carotid occlusion. *Eur Neurol.* 1995;35:212-216.

Markus H, Cullinane M. Severely impaired cerebrovascular reactivity predicts stroke and TIA risk in patients with carotid artery stenosis and occlusion. *Brain.* 2001;124:457-467.

Silvestrini M, Vernieri F, Pasqualetti P, et al. Impaired cerebral vasoreactivity and risk of stroke in patients with asymptomatic carotid artery stenosis. *JAMA.* 2000;283:2122-2127.

Tsivgoulis G, Alexandrov AV. Cerebral hemodynamics in acute stroke: pathophysiology and clinical implications. *J Vasc Interv Neurol.* 2008;1:65-69.

Vernieri F, Pasqualetti P, Matteis M, et al. Effect of collateral blood flow and cerebral vasomotor reactivity on the outcome of carotid artery occlusion. *Stroke.* 2001;32:1552-1558.

Zhou H, Sun J, Ji X, et al. Correlation between the integrity of the circle of Willis and the severity of initial noncardiac cerebral infarction and clinical prognosis. *Medicine (Baltimore).* 2016;95:e2892.

A.13. Discuss the different surgical approaches to carotid revascularization.

CEA is performed through either a transverse incision or an incision bordering the sternocleidomastoid muscle (also known as a carotid incision). The subcutaneous tissue and platysma muscle are divided, and the carotid sheath is exposed. Usually, dissection is performed by exposing the common carotid artery to a point distal to the bifurcation of the internal carotid artery and external carotid artery. Next, in this order, the internal, common, and external arteries are sequentially clamped, and the patient is given a heparin bolus. Depending on the institution and surgeon's preference, carotid stump pressures can be obtained by attaching a transducer into the common carotid artery after clamping the proximal common and external carotid arteries. A mean pressure of 40 to 50 mm Hg suggests adequate collateralization through the circle of Willis from the contralateral carotid artery. Some use lower stump pressures, as an indication for shunt placement manipulation of the carotid bulb can result in hemodynamic instability (eg, bradycardia) due to the carotid sinus reflex. Typically, reducing direct surgical pressure will allow for the return of normal sinus rhythm. Pharmacologic therapy can involve direct injection of lidocaine into the sinus or intravenous administration of atropine, both of which can lead to cessation of the reflex.

To remove the lesion, a longitudinal arteriotomy is performed below the level of the bifurcation and extended both proximally and distally. At this point, some surgeons routinely place shunts, others choose to do so only if there are signs of cerebral ischemia, and others opt to not place shunts altogether and decrease the cerebral metabolic rate by requesting an increase in anesthetic depth to achieve EEG burst suppression; the true utility of shunt placement is uncertain. If a shunt is placed, it is done after the vessel is open but before the plaque is removed. The plaque is dissected and freed from the deep layers of the media, after which the arteriotomy is repaired. Some surgeons do a primary repair while others patch the artery with a synthetic or biologic patch. The clamps are sequentially released to back bleed the external and internal carotid arteries and forward flush the common carotid artery. After the suture line is completed, flow is restored in the external carotid artery and then internal carotid artery. A Jackson-Pratt drain can be placed to prevent incisional hematoma. A completion study to assess the integrity of the repair is usually performed using a duplex ultrasound or contrast angiogram. Another variation of the conventional CEA is eversion endarterectomy. Here, the carotid is transected horizontally at the carotid bulb, and the artery is turned inside out or everted, although this variation is infrequently performed. There is no evidence indicating one technique is superior to the other; the surgical method is usually chosen because of institution and surgeon preference.

Calligaro KD, Dougherty MJ. Correlation of carotid artery stump pressure and neurologic changes during 474 carotid endarterectomies performed in awake patients. *J Vasc Surg.* 2005;42:684-689.

Cao P, Giordano G, De Rango P, et al. A randomized study on eversion versus standard carotid endarterectomy: study design and preliminary results: the Everest Trial. *J Vasc Surg.* 1998;27:595-605.

Chuatrakoon B, Nantakool S, Rerkasem A, Orrapin S, Howard DP, Rerkasem K. Routine or selective carotid artery shunting for carotid endarterectomy (and different methods of monitoring in selective shunting). *Cochrane Database Syst Rev.* 2022;6:CD000190.

Jacob T, Hingorani A, Ascher E. Carotid artery stump pressure (CASP) in 1135 consecutive endarterectomies under general anesthesia: an old method that survived the test of times. *J Cardiovasc Surg.* 2007;48:677-681.

Kumar S, Lombardi JV, Alexander JB, et al. Modified eversion carotid endarterectomy. *Ann Vasc Surg.* 2013;27:178-185.

Rerkasem K, Rothwell PM. Routine or selective carotid artery shunting for carotid endarterectomy (and different methods of monitoring in selective shunting). *Cochrane Database Syst Rev.* 2009:CD000190.

A.14. Discuss the endovascular approaches to carotid stenting.

Access to the carotid artery is usually obtained through the common femoral artery or transradial approach. Transcervical (through a cutdown or percutaneously) via the common carotid approach has also been used. If the transfemoral or transradial approach is chosen, an angiogram is performed to identify the aortic arch anatomy to safely maneuver the catheter, wires, and embolic protection device up to the internal carotid artery. If the transcervical route is chosen, the arch is bypassed. This approach is appealing, but currently, only a handful of centers are adept with this technique.

The patient is heparinized prior to manipulating guidewires and catheters. The goal is to maintain an activated clotting time (ACT) of 250 to 300 seconds. The common steps for stenting are (1) advancement of a guidewire, (2) sheath placement, (3) embolic protection device placement, (4) carotid lesion predilation (if needed), (5) stent positioning, (6) stent deployment, and (7) stent expansion with poststent angioplasty to ensure good apposition against the arterial wall. As it can be difficult to get the wire and embolic protection device across a stenotic lesion, predilation may be needed. Predilation is recognized as a risk factor for perioperative stroke and vasospasm. During dilation, stenting, and angioplasty, bradycardia and hypotension due to baroreceptor activation can occur and are usually treated with vagolytic drugs such as atropine or glycopyrrolate; glycopyrrolate has the advantage of not crossing the blood-brain barrier, and as such, adverse central side effects (at low doses: headache, impaired memory, reduced cognitive function, behavioral disturbances, anxiety, and insomnia; at higher doses: agitation, confusion, delirium, and seizures) associated with anticholinergic administration are avoided. The carotid baroreceptors are located within the adventitia of the origin of the internal carotid artery and innervated by a branch of the glossopharyngeal nerve called the sinus of Hering. The baroreceptors are stretch-sensitive mechanoreceptors that respond to alterations in blood pressure.

The two main considerations in the stent procedure are the type of stent utilized and the type of embolic protection device that is used. The two types of bare-metal carotid stents that are commonly placed are open and closed architecture stents. Open stents are typically more flexible and are used for complex angulated carotid lesions. Closed stents cover more surface area and are commonly used in straighter less complex carotid lesions. Randomized clinical trials have failed to show any relationship between the type of stent used and complications that stem from CAS.

Embolic protection device technology is evolving but in general falls into three main types: (1) distal filters, (2) distal occlusion devices, and (3) proximal protection devices. The filter design allows for antegrade flow through the internal carotid artery during stent placement and is commonly used. The main limitation of distal filter devices is that they need to cross the lesion, which in and of itself can lead to embolism. Distal occlusion devices have a low profile and require a short landing zone. This is advantageous for tortuous vessels. The lesion is crossed with a wire, the balloon inflated, and angiography used to confirm that there are no leaks. After the stent is deployed, an aspiration catheter is advanced to the occlusion device to remove all debris, after which the balloon is deflated. The main concerns are intolerance to occlusion of the artery and embolism. Careful preoperative assessment of collaterals (ie, via the circle of Willis) is important. Retrograde flow devices are the newest advancement in embolic protection devices and are designed to promote flow and debris away from the internal carotid artery. Balloons are deployed in the common carotid and external carotid arteries, causing flow stasis or reversal. With these devices, there is no interaction with the plaque until reversal or stasis of flow is achieved. Some patients may not tolerate occlusion or flow reversal in the internal carotid artery. Evidence of which embolic protection device to use and whether they decrease the rate of periprocedural stroke and death is conflicting, although the studies trend toward a decrease in the risk of perioperative stroke.

Alvarez B, Matas M, Ribo M, et al. Transcervical carotid stenting with flow reversal is a safe technique for high-risk patients older than 70 years. *J Vasc Surg*. 2012;55:978-984.

Etxegoien N, Rhyne D, Kedev S, et al. The transradial approach for carotid artery stenting. *Catheter Cardiovasc Interv*. 2012;80:1081-1087.

Garg N, Karagiorgos N, Pisimisis GT, et al. Cerebral protection devices reduce periprocedural strokes during carotid angioplasty and stenting: a systematic review of the current literature. *J Endovasc Ther*. 2009;16:412-427.

Giri J, Kennedy KF, Weinberg I, et al. Comparative effectiveness of commonly used devices for carotid artery stenting: an NCDR analysis (National Cardiovascular Data Registry). *JACC Cardiovasc Interv*. 2014;7:171-177.

Knappich C, Kuehnl A, Tsantilas P, et al. The use of embolic protection devices is associated with a lower stroke and death rate after carotid stenting. *JACC Cardiovasc Interv*. 2017;10:1257-1265.

Kwolek CJ, Jaff MR, Leal JI, et al. Results of the ROADSTER multicenter trial of transcarotid stenting with dynamic flow reversal. *J Vasc Surg*. 2015;62:1227-1234.

SECTION 4

Lin PH, Zhou W, Kougias P, et al. Factors associated with hypotension and bradycardia after carotid angioplasty and stenting. *J Vasc Surg*. 2007;46:846-853; discussion 853-854.

Macdonald S. New embolic protection devices: a review. *J Cardiovasc Surg (Torino)*. 2011;52:821-827.

Mousa AY, Campbell JE, Aburahma AF, et al. Current update of cerebral embolic protection devices. *J Vasc Surg*. 2012;56:1429-1437.

Mylonas SN, Moulakakis KG, Antonopoulos CN, et al. Carotid artery stenting-induced hemodynamic instability. *J Endovasc Ther*. 2013;20:48-60.

Timaran CH, Rosero EB, Higuera A, et al. Randomized clinical trial of open-cell vs closed-cell stents for carotid stenting and effects of stent design on cerebral embolization. *J Vasc Surg*. 2011;54:1310-1316.e1311; discussion e1316.

White CJ. Carotid artery stenting. *J Am Coll Cardiol*. 2014;64:722-731.

A.15. What is normal CBF?

Normal CBF is approximately 50 mL/100 g/min for the entire brain. Blood flow is about 4 times higher in gray matter than in white matter, or 80 and 20 mL/100 g/min, respectively.

Kety SS, Schmidt CF. The nitrous oxide method for the quantitative determination of cerebral blood flow in man: theory, procedure and normal values. *J Clin Invest*. 1948;27:476-483.

Lassen NA, Munck O. The cerebral blood flow in man determined by the use of radioactive krypton. *Acta Physiol Scand*. 1955;33:30-49.

Patel PM, Drummond JC, Lemkuil BP. Cerebral physiology and the effects of anesthetic drugs. In: Gropper MA, Eriksson LI, Fleisher LA, Cohen NH, Leslie K, Johnson-Akeju O, eds. *Miller's Anesthesia*. 10th ed. Elsevier; 2024:180-224.

A.16. What is critically low CBF as measured by the electroencephalogram (EEG)?

Assuming normal temperature and hematocrit, 100 mL of blood contains approximately 20 mL of oxygen. Normal global CBF of 50 mL/100 g/min delivers oxygen to the brain at a rate of 10 mL/100 g/min. This is more than the high metabolic requirements of the brain for oxygen (3-5 mL/100 g/min), which affords a relative margin of safety. The CBF at which ischemia becomes apparent in the EEG is approximately 20 mL/100 g/min. Changes in EEG may be delayed for up to 150 seconds following the onset of ischemia. It is currently not possible to define the specific changes that represent irreversible ischemia. In the setting of an isoelectric EEG, oxygen delivery to the brain can be adequate to keep neurons alive but can provide insufficient energy for neuronal function.

The development of cerebral infarction depends on both the degree and duration of ischemia. Jones et al showed in an animal model of reversible ischemia that with CBF of 18 to 23 mL/100 g/min, animals recovered from impaired neurologic function when blood flow was returned to normal levels, regardless of the duration of the ischemic period. Infarction development at lower flows depends on both the degree of regional CBF reduction and the duration of ischemia. Neurons that are nonfunctional but will recover fully with the restoration of adequate flow are said to be in an ischemic penumbra. Neuronal death occurs with CBF less than 10 mL/100 g/min.

Bebawy JPF, Hemmer LB, Pasternak JJ. Anesthesia for neurosurgery. In: Cullen BF, Stock MC, Ortega R, et al, eds. *Barash, Cullen, and Stoelting's Clinical Anesthesia*. 9th ed. Wolters Kluwer; 2024:979-1002.

Boysen G, Engell HC, Pitolese GR, et al. On the critical level of cerebral blood flow in man with particular reference to carotid surgery. *Circulation*. 1974;49:1023-1025.

Jones TH, Morawetz RB, Crowell RM, et al. Threshold of focal cerebral ischemia in awake monkeys. *J Neurosurg*. 1981;54:773-782.

A.17. What is cerebral autoregulation?

Cerebral autoregulation is the tendency of the brain to match cerebral oxygen delivery with metabolic oxygen requirements despite variations in blood pressure. In normotensive individuals, CBF is relatively constant between mean arterial pressures of 70 and 150 mm Hg. It is generally considered that the lower limit of autoregulation is a mean arterial pressure of 50 mm Hg based on animal studies. Above and below the plateau phase, CBF is dependent on pressure and varies linearly with CPP. Note that the limits of autoregulation are a conceptual construct and not an "all-or-none" phenomenon and can vary between individuals and with comorbidities such as hypertension. In addition, autoregulation is affected by the underlying level of vasodilation or vasoconstriction that depends on the $Paco_2$ or anesthetic conditions, among other things.

In hypertensive patients, the upper and lower limits of the autoregulatory curve are shifted to the right, to higher arterial pressures (**Figure 19.2**). What this means is that a mean arterial pressure of 60 mm Hg, which would be well tolerated in a normotensive individual, could be below the lower limit of autoregulation in the hypertensive individual, resulting in cerebral hypoperfusion. Conversely, hypertensive

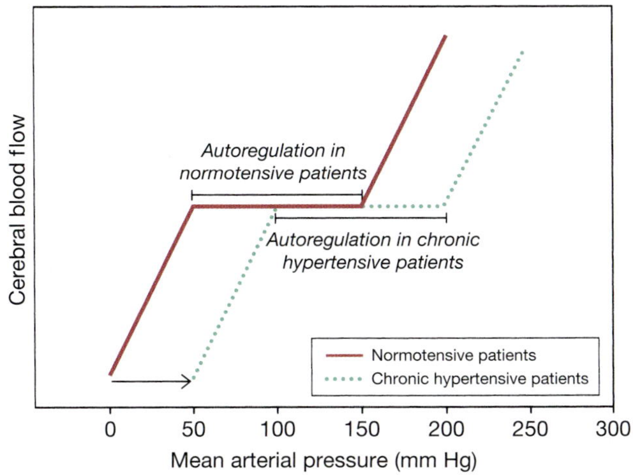

FIGURE 19.2. Cerebral autoregulatory curves in normotensive and chronically hypertensive patients. A shift in the autoregulation curve occurs with chronic hypertension. The curve shifts back to a normotensive range over time once hypertension is well controlled.

patients tolerate marked increases in mean arterial pressure better than their normotensive counterparts. In treated hypertensive patients, the limits of autoregulation are shifted with time toward normal.

Patel PM, Drummond JC, Lemkuil BP. Cerebral physiology and the effects of anesthetic drugs. In: Gropper MA, Eriksson LI, Fleisher LA, Cohen NH, Leslie K, Johnson-Akeju O, eds. *Miller's Anesthesia*. 10th ed. Elsevier; 2024:180-224.

Paulson OB, Strandgaard S, Edvinsson L. Cerebral autoregulation. *Cerebrovasc Brain Metab Rev*. 1990;2:161-192.

A.18. How does $Paco_2$ affect CBF?

Hypercarbia results in cerebral vasodilation and increased blood flow, and hypocarbia causes cerebral vasoconstriction and a decrease in cerebral blood flow. CBF changes about 4% for each mm Hg increase or decrease in arterial $Paco_2$ for partial pressures between 20 and 80 mm Hg. The appropriate level of $Paco_2$ during carotid revascularization has not been established, and because there are no clear clinical benefits to either hypercapnia or hypocapnia, it is recommended to maintain normocapnia.

Ellis JA, Joshi S. Cerebral and spinal blood flow. In: Cottrell JE, Patel PM, Soriano SG, eds. *Neuroanesthesia*. 7th ed. Elsevier; 2024:22-26.

Patel PM, Drummond JC, Lemkuil BP. Cerebral physiology and the effects of anesthetic drugs. In: Gropper MA, Eriksson LI, Fleisher LA, Cohen NH, Leslie K, Johnson-Akeju O, eds. *Miller's Anesthesia*. 10th ed. Elsevier; 2024:180-224.

A.19. What are the principal determinants of CBF?

The principal determinants of CBF are neuronal activity, CPP, blood viscosity, $Paco_2$, pH of brain extracellular fluid, Pao_2, and neurogenic influences.

Ellis JA, Joshi S. Cerebral and spinal blood flow. In: Cottrell JE, Patel PM, Soriano SG, eds. *Neuroanesthesia*. 7th ed. Elsevier; 2024:22-26.

Patel PM, Drummond JC, Lemkuil BP. Cerebral physiology and the effects of anesthetic drugs. In: Gropper MA, Eriksson LI, Fleisher LA, Cohen NH, Leslie K, Johnson-Akeju O, eds. *Miller's Anesthesia*. 10th ed. Elsevier; 2024:180-224.

Schaeffer S, Iadecola C. Revisiting the neurovascular unit. *Nat Neurosci*. 2021;24:1198-1209.

A.20. What is meant by the term *luxury perfusion*?

Luxury perfusion is the blood flow that is in excess of metabolic need (increased CBF relative to the cerebral metabolic rate for oxygen). It is most frequently observed in tissues surrounding tumors or areas of infarction. It has also been described in tissues that have been manipulated during surgery.

Ellis JA, Joshi S. Cerebral and spinal blood flow. In: Cottrell JE, Patel PM, Soriano SG, eds. *Neuroanesthesia*. 7th ed. Elsevier; 2024:22-26.

A.21. What is meant by the term *intracerebral steal*?

Intracerebral steal is a paradoxical response to carbon dioxide in which hypercapnia decreases blood flow to an ischemic area. With hypercapnia, normally perfused arterioles vasodilate, and this shunts blood from the ischemic lesion. This occurs because, at baseline, hypoperfused regions in the brain are maximally dilated and cannot dilate further to hypercapnia. As a result, it is common practice to maintain normocapnia during carotid surgery.

Ellis JA, Joshi S. Cerebral and spinal blood flow. In: Cottrell JE, Patel PM, Soriano SG, eds. *Neuroanesthesia*. 7th ed. Elsevier; 2024:22-26.

Paulson OB. Cerebral apoplexy (stroke): pathogenesis, pathophysiology and therapy as illustrated by regional blood flow measurements in the brain. *Stroke*. 1971;2:327-360.

B. Preoperative Evaluation and Preparation

B.1. What will you look for in your preoperative evaluation of this patient?

Once the presence of a carotid lesion amenable to surgical treatment has been documented by Doppler ultrasonography or angiographic studies, the anesthesiologist will be asked to evaluate the patient regarding readiness for surgery. Because most patients who have carotid disease also have coexisting cardiac atherosclerosis, the main focus of the preoperative evaluation will be to optimize cardiac function. Evidence of medical conditions associated with arteriosclerosis, such as coronary artery disease, hypertension, renal disease, obesity, diabetes, and pulmonary disease secondary to cigarette smoking, should be sought.

The patient's neurologic status also needs to be evaluated preoperatively. Although it would be preferable to medically optimize the patient with uncontrolled hypertension or untreated metabolic disease, or if possible, delay surgery in the patient with a recent MI, the presence of symptomatic carotid disease may not allow that option. This is because there is good evidence that surgical intervention should take place within 2 weeks of symptoms in order to reap the benefits of surgery.

The patient's airway needs to be assessed for ease of ventilation and intubation. A patient who is difficult to ventilate may become hypercarbic during induction, and the increase in $Paco_2$ can have adverse effects on regional CBF. As part of the airway evaluation, the range of motion of the patient's neck that is tolerated without evidence of cerebral ischemia needs to be determined so that relative extremes of extension and lateral rotation of the neck during ventilation, intubation, and patient positioning can be avoided. Extreme extension and rotation of the neck can occlude the vertebral artery and contribute to postoperative neurologic deficits.

Bebawy JPF, Hemmer LB, Pasternak JJ. Anesthesia for neurosurgery. In: Cullen BF, Stock MC, Ortega R, et al, eds. *Barash, Cullen, and Stoelting's Clinical Anesthesia*. 9th ed. Wolters Kluwer; 2024:979-1002.

Thompson A, Fleischmann KE, Smilowitz NR, et al. 2024 ACC/AHA guideline on perioperative cardiovascular evaluation and management of patients undergoing noncardiac surgery: A report of the American College of Cardiology/American Heart Association Joint Committee on Practice Guidelines. *Circulation*. 2024;150:e351-e441.

B.2. Is this patient's blood pressure too high for elective surgery?

Although hypertension is present in most patients presenting for CEA, its rapid correction is not recommended because this may exacerbate cerebral ischemia. If this patient had evidence of myocardial ischemia at this blood pressure and was stable from a neurologic standpoint, blood pressure could be gradually decreased with antihypertensive medications.

Normal myocardial and cerebral functions need to be preserved. These goals are not necessarily at odds with each other. To decrease myocardial oxygen consumption, one would want to decrease heart rate, blood pressure, and myocardial contractility. In this patient population, decreasing heart rate can decrease myocardial work, whereas CPP is maintained with adequate mean arterial pressure. If a hypertensive patient presents with an unstable neurologic status, it may be necessary to control blood pressure only once the obstruction to CBF has been relieved.

A single blood pressure measurement is of little use in the preoperative assessment of the patient. It is the range of the blood pressures normally tolerated by the patient that will guide perioperative blood pressure management. For example, if the patient's blood pressure is measured at 80/50 mm Hg and at 170/100 mm Hg preoperatively, and at these blood pressures, she does not develop any new neurologic deficits or myocardial ischemia, the clinician will be inclined to treat blood pressures only beyond these two extremes.

Because this patient is hypertensive, one can expect that wide swings in blood pressure will occur while she is receiving anesthesia. Variations in blood pressure should be minimized because these have been related to increased cardiac and neurologic morbidity. The anesthesiologist must be prepared for blood pressure variations by having both vasopressors and vasodilators readily available. Total fluid administration should be limited to no more than 10 mL/kg for a typical 2-hour procedure.

Bebawy JPF, Hemmer LB, Pasternak JJ. Anesthesia for neurosurgery. In: Cullen BF, Stock MC, Ortega R, et al, eds. *Barash, Cullen, and Stoelting's Clinical Anesthesia*. 9th ed. Wolters Kluwer; 2024:979-1002.

Smith JS, Roizen MF, Cahalan MK, et al. Does anesthetic technique make a difference? Augmentation of systolic blood pressure during carotid endarterectomy: effects of phenylephrine versus light anesthesia and of isoflurane versus halothane on the incidence of myocardial ischemia. *Anesthesiology*. 1988;69:846-853.

B.3. What laboratory data are required preoperatively?

Laboratory tests should be ordered based on the patient's cardiac, respiratory, and metabolic status. Hemoglobin and hematocrit should be determined preoperatively because values may be abnormal in a patient with advanced age, renal, or pulmonary disease. A type and screen while routinely performed at most institutions is rarely needed, as transfusion after CEA or stenting is rare. A baseline basic metabolic panel is useful to determine the electrolyte status. Blood urea nitrogen and creatinine help to determine baseline renal status.

An electrocardiogram (ECG) should be examined preoperatively to look for arrhythmias, evidence of ischemia, previous MIs, or left ventricular hypertrophy. Where appropriate, the preoperative ECG should be compared with earlier studies to determine whether interval changes have occurred. An echocardiogram is part of the workup and can help guide anesthetic therapy as well as blood pressure management during the carotid cross-clamp.

If present, the chest radiograph should be examined to look for cardiomegaly, evidence of pulmonary edema, chronic obstructive pulmonary disease, or pneumonia. If the patient has a history of chronic obstructive pulmonary disease, a preoperative arterial blood gas reading should be obtained once the arterial line is placed to identify the baseline $Paco_2$. In patients who are chronically hypercarbic, rapid adjustment to normocarbia intraoperatively will result in relative hypocarbia and CBF will be reduced accordingly. Management of intraoperative ventilation should be aimed at maintaining normal $Paco_2$.

Bebawy JPF, Hemmer LB, Pasternak JJ. Anesthesia for neurosurgery. In: Cullen BF, Stock MC, Ortega R, et al, eds. *Barash, Cullen, and Stoelting's Clinical Anesthesia*. 9th ed. Wolters Kluwer; 2024:979-1002.

Nelson P, Bustillo M. Anesthesia for carotid endarterectomy, angioplasty, and stent. *Anesthesiol Clin*. 2021;39:37-51.

Stangenberg L, Curran T, Shuja F, et al. Development of a risk prediction model for transfusion in carotid endarterectomy and demonstration of cost-saving potential by avoidance of "type and screen." *J Vasc Surg*. 2016;64:1711-1718.

B.4. Will you treat this patient's blood glucose?

Hyperglycemia lowers the ischemic threshold in clinical and experimental models. Poorly controlled diabetes is a marker for vascular disease, and preoperative optimization, if time allows, might improve perioperative outcome.

McGirt MJ, Woodworth GF, Brooke BS, et al. Hyperglycemia independently increases the risk of perioperative stroke, myocardial infarction, and death after carotid endarterectomy. *Neurosurgery*. 2006;58:1066-1073.

B.5. Will you premedicate this patient?

Ideally, the patient should present to the operating room calm and awake. Preoperative anxiety should be alleviated in these patients because it can lead to hypertension, which has been associated with adverse neurologic outcome. Increases in heart rate in the anxious patient lead to increased myocardial oxygen consumption and, potentially, ischemia, ventricular dysfunction, and arrhythmias.

Premedication, however, can lead to ventilatory depression, with resultant hypercarbia and alterations in CBF that can exacerbate cerebral ischemia. Sedation can also interfere with the immediate postoperative neurologic assessment of the patient because it may cause delayed awakening from anesthesia. One of the anesthetic goals for CEA under general anesthesia is prompt emergence from anesthesia so the patient is able to cooperate with a basic neurologic evaluation.

To achieve these goals, a thorough and reassuring preoperative visit alone may provide sufficient anxiolysis. The anesthesiologist should explain the preoperative procedure and what can be expected in the postoperative period, answering any questions that the patient has. If an anxiolytic is chosen, a short-acting agent should be used after documentation of the patient's neurologic exam.

Bebawy JPF, Hemmer LB, Pasternak JJ. Anesthesia for neurosurgery. In: Cullen BF, Stock MC, Ortega R, et al, eds. *Barash, Cullen, and Stoelting's Clinical Anesthesia*. 9th ed. Wolters Kluwer; 2024:979-1002.

C. Intraoperative Management

C.1. How will you monitor this patient?

Regardless of whether the patient has an awake CEA or a carotid stent, routine monitoring of cardiovascular, pulmonary, and metabolic function is important. ECG leads II and V_5, noninvasive blood pressure monitor, pulse oximetry, end-tidal capnometry, and temperature are monitored (the role of neurophysiologic monitoring is discussed in Section C.3). An arterial catheter should be used to monitor arterial blood pressure closely. Its presence will permit immediate identification of blood pressure changes and allow for repetitive sampling of arterial blood gases.

Rarely is a central venous catheter or a pulmonary artery catheter required to monitor cardiac function. Large fluid shifts or major blood loss is not anticipated.

Bebawy JPF, Hemmer LB, Pasternak JJ. Anesthesia for neurosurgery. In: Cullen BF, Stock MC, Ortega R, et al, eds. *Barash, Cullen, and Stoelting's Clinical Anesthesia*. 9th ed. Wolters Kluwer; 2024:979-1002.

C.2. How will you know that the patient's cerebral perfusion is adequate during surgery?

In the awake patient undergoing CEA or stent under local anesthesia, repeated neurologic examinations can be done to assess the adequacy of cerebral perfusion. This is the most sensitive and specific way to detect intraoperative cerebral ischemia.

If the patient receives general anesthesia, neuromonitoring is generally employed in order to detect and treat ischemia in a timely fashion. Various neuromonitoring modalities exist, which are classified into the categories such as brain activity monitoring, cerebral perfusion monitoring, and brain oxygen saturation monitoring. These include the EEG, SSEPs, TCD, internal carotid stump pressure, $Sjvo_2$, and near-infrared spectroscopy (NIRS). No one monitor is routinely used, and each modality has its specific indications, strengths, and weaknesses. Therefore, the simultaneous application of more than one monitoring device is recommended.

Bebawy JPF, Hemmer LB, Pasternak JJ. Anesthesia for neurosurgery. In: Cullen BF, Stock MC, Ortega R, et al, eds. *Barash, Cullen, and Stoelting's Clinical Anesthesia*. 9th ed. Wolters Kluwer; 2024:979-1002.

Bozzani A, Arici V, Ticozzelli G, et al. Intraoperative cerebral monitoring during carotid surgery: a narrative review. *Ann Vasc Surg*. 2022;78:36-44.

Pennekamp CW, Moll FL, de Borst GJ. The potential benefits and the role of cerebral monitoring in carotid endarterectomy. *Curr Opin Anaesthesiol*. 2011;24:693-697.

C.3. Discuss the differences and relative advantages and disadvantages of unprocessed EEG and processed EEG monitoring.

The 16-channel EEG is a sensitive indicator of cerebral ischemia. Intraoperative changes in EEG related to ischemia are classified as mild, moderate, or severe. Severe EEG changes (>50% decrease in waveform amplitude in a generalized or lateralized distribution) suggest a need for blood pressure augmentation by the anesthesiologist or shunt placement by the surgeon. The EEG is neither a measure of CBF nor a way to determine whether irreversible neuronal damage has occurred. Rather, it is an indicator that areas of the brain might be at risk for infarction. Changes that occur in the EEG with hypothermia, hypocarbia, hypoxemia, and deep anesthesia mimic those of ischemia. In patients who have had a cerebrovascular accident, the processed EEG does not predict cerebral ischemia.

Problems associated with intraoperative monitoring of the 16-lead EEG have detracted from its popularity. These include difficulty in obtaining a meaningful recording in the electrically noisy environment of the operating room, the bulk of the equipment required, and the need for specially trained personnel for interpretation.

The processed EEG has eliminated many of the problems associated with the 16-channel EEG. The equipment is generally compact, and the data display allows for ease of interpretation. One commonly used processed encephalogram is power spectrum analysis. For this analysis, the EEG is studied in short time intervals of 2 to 16 minutes, called *epochs*. Each epoch then is subjected to a fast Fourier transform analysis, during which the complex waveform of the unprocessed EEG is broken down into its component sine waves of varying amplitudes and frequencies. The power spectrum is calculated by squaring the amplitude of the individual frequency components. The power spectrum can then be displayed in various forms, two of which are the compressed spectral array and the density-modulated spectral array. Data are displayed in these two forms as relative power versus frequency (**Figure 19.3**).

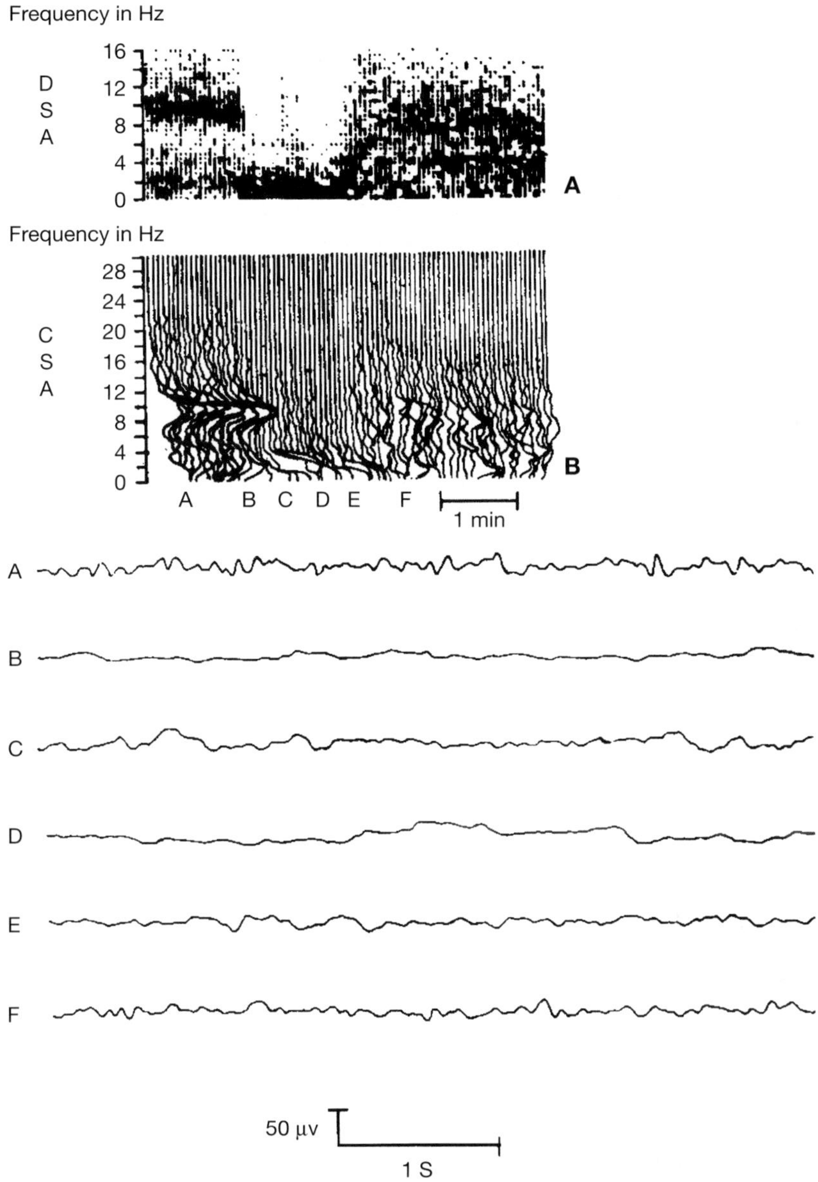

FIGURE 19.3. An example of density spectral array (A) and compressed spectral array (B) for processed EEG during a period of marked hypotension during initiation of carotid artery bypass. Slowing waveform activity in the unprocessed electroencephalogram (EEG) (B-E) is also evident in the density-modulated spectral array (DSA) and compressed spectral array (CSA). Points A-F are samples of unprocessed EEG. Slowing waveform activity is evident in B-E. (Reprinted with permission from Levy WJ, Shapiro HM, Maruchak G, et al. Automated EEG processing for intraoperative monitoring. *Anesthesiology.* 1980;53:223.)

The processed EEG is only as good as the original signals from which it was obtained. Therefore, meticulous recording techniques are required even when monitoring a processed EEG. During CEA, generally, two or four channels of the EEG are monitored to determine right and left symmetry in neuronal activity during interruption of CBF.

The bispectral index (BIS) is another commonly used processed EEG parameter that involves a proprietary methodology to calculate indices of the EEG power spectrum, burst synchronization, and phase coupling. It is primarily used as a monitor to assess the depth of anesthesia. Although the BIS might have some utility as a marker of global cerebral ischemia, it is unreliable as an indicator of hemispheric cerebral ischemia during carotid cross-clamping.

At present, there are insufficient data to recommend one form of neuromonitoring over another, and the choice is one of local preference.

Deogaonkar A, Vivar R, Bullock RE, et al. Bispectral index monitoring may not reliably indicate cerebral ischaemia during awake carotid endarterectomy. *Br J Anaesth*. 2005;94:800-804.

Kearse LA, Martin D, McPeck K, et al. Computer-derived density spectral array in detection of mild analog electroencephalographic ischemic pattern changes during carotid endarterectomy. *J Neurosurg*. 1993;78:884-890.

Rampil IJ, Holzer JA, Quest DO, et al. Prognostic value of computerized EEG analysis during carotid endarterectomy. *Anesth Analg*. 1983;62:186-192.

Seubert CN, Ok MSJ. Neurophysiologic monitoring. In: Gropper MA, Eriksson LI, Fleisher LA, Cohen NH, Leslie K, Johnson-Akeju O, eds. *Miller's Anesthesia*. 10th ed. Elsevier; 2025:1099-1132.

Sundt TM Jr, Sharbrough FW, Piepgras DG, et al. Correlation of cerebral blood flow and electroencephalographic changes during carotid endarterectomy: with results of surgery and hemodynamics of cerebral ischemia. *Mayo Clin Proc*. 1981;56:533-543.

C.4. How will you measure CBF intraoperatively? What are the relative advantages and disadvantages of each technique?

CBF can be indirectly measured by neurophysiologic monitoring. Monitoring techniques can be broken down into techniques that assess the overall integrity of cerebral function, cerebral flow, and cerebral metabolism. EEG, SSEPs, and motor evoked potentials (MEPs) assess the integrity of cerebral function. Cerebral perfusion monitoring can be done indirectly with internal carotid artery stump pressures or directly with TCD, which assesses flow in large intracranial vessels. Brain oxygen saturation monitoring can be done with jugular venous bulb monitoring ($Sjvo_2$) or cerebral oximetry by NIRS, and they assess overall cerebral metabolism.

Bebawy JPF, Hemmer LB, Pasternak JJ. Anesthesia for neurosurgery. In: Cullen BF, Stock MC, Ortega R, et al, eds. *Barash, Cullen, and Stoelting's Clinical Anesthesia*. 9th ed. Wolters Kluwer; 2024:979-1002.

C.5. Describe the use of stump pressure and its limitations.

Internal carotid artery stump pressure is one way to assess cerebral perfusion; however, this is indirect because it measures perfusion pressure and not flow per se. Typically, the stump pressure is obtained after the initial clamping of the internal carotid artery. The stump pressure presumably reflects pressure transmitted through collateral vessels. Maintaining stump pressures from 25 to 70 mm Hg has been described as necessary to avoid neurologic injury. Nevertheless, this range of stump pressures may not reliably represent the adequacy of collateral CBF because it does not correlate consistently with changes in the EEG, regional CBF, or changes in the neurologic status of the awake patient. Furthermore, anesthetic agents can alter carotid stump pressure without changing regional CBF. Inadequate stump pressures have been shown when measured regional CBF was adequate. If shunting during CEA were to be done only on the basis of stump pressures, some patients would unnecessarily receive shunts. Finally, because stump pressure is not continuously monitored, it only gives a snapshot of the time of cerebral perfusion and therefore this technique is less commonly used.

Bebawy JPF, Hemmer LB, Pasternak JJ. Anesthesia for neurosurgery. In: Cullen BF, Stock MC, Ortega R, et al, eds. *Barash, Cullen, and Stoelting's Clinical Anesthesia*. 9th ed. Wolters Kluwer; 2024:979-1002.

Harada RN, Comerota AJ, Good GM, et al. Stump pressure, electroencephalographic changes, and the contralateral carotid artery: another look at selective shunting. *Am J Surg*. 1995;170:148-153.

C.6. Describe the use of transcranial Doppler (TCD) and its limitations.

Another technique that can be used to assess CBF is TCD ultrasonography, which uses pulse wave Doppler ultrasound to measure flow in the ipsilateral middle cerebral artery. It can aid in determining the need for a shunt by detecting a decrease in the middle cerebral artery blood flow velocity with placement of the carotid cross-clamp. It allows for continuous assessment of shunt function. It can be used to assess the adequacy of pharmacologically induced intraoperative hypertensive therapy. TCD also allows the detection of air or particulate embolization with endarterectomy or stenting. A higher embolic burden has been associated with stroke. The disadvantage of TCD is that it is technically demanding and not obtainable in about 20% of patients. As changes in flow velocity can be due to changes in arterial diameter or low perfusion, it is not very sensitive or specific for assessing cerebral perfusion.

Bebawy JPF, Hemmer LB, Pasternak JJ. Anesthesia for neurosurgery. In: Cullen BF, Stock MC, Ortega R, et al, eds. *Barash, Cullen, and Stoelting's Clinical Anesthesia*. 9th ed. Wolters Kluwer; 2024:979-1002.

C.7. Describe the use of jugular venous oxygen saturation ($Sjvo_2$) and its limitations.

$Sjvo_2$ follows oxygen saturation obtained from a catheter that is inserted into the internal jugular vein of the carotid surgical site. The major disadvantage of $Sjvo_2$ monitoring is that it is a global and not a regional monitor for ischemia. $SjvO_2$ also has a wide range of normal values, and there is a possibility of extracranial blood sampling. This technique has not been shown to improve outcomes with CAS or CEA.

Bebawy JPF, Hemmer LB, Pasternak JJ. Anesthesia for neurosurgery. In: Cullen BF, Stock MC, Ortega R, et al, eds. *Barash, Cullen, and Stoelting's Clinical Anesthesia*. 9th ed. Wolters Kluwer; 2024:979-1002.

C.8. Describe the use of cerebral oximetry and its limitations.

Cerebral oximetry uses NIRS to detect regional cerebral oxygen saturation. This is done by applying small adhesive monitoring pads to the forehead. The major limitations to NIRS are the wide variations in baseline readings in a single individual and the lack of agreement as to what constitutes ischemic changes to warrant interventions like shunt placement. The ability to detect ischemia is limited to the region in the frontal cortex and limited by the sampling window.

Bebawy JPF, Hemmer LB, Pasternak JJ. Anesthesia for neurosurgery. In: Cullen BF, Stock MC, Ortega R, et al, eds. *Barash, Cullen, and Stoelting's Clinical Anesthesia*. 9th ed. Wolters Kluwer; 2024:979-1002.

Grubhofer G, Plöchl W, Skolka M, et al. Comparing Doppler ultrasonography and cerebral oximetry as indicators for shunting in carotid endarterectomy. *Anesth Analg*. 2000;91:1339-1344.

C.9. Discuss somatosensory evoked potentials (SSEPs) as a monitor of CBF during CEA.

SSEPs are a specialized form of electrophysiologic monitoring that reflects the presence of intact sensory pathways from a stimulated peripheral nerve to the cerebral cortex, where electrical activity is monitored. Distortion of certain waveforms is associated with ischemia. These SSEP changes are not consistently associated with changes in the EEG. Questions have been raised regarding whether SSEPs can overpredict the presence of ischemia and the need for shunting. If SSEPs are a useful indicator of ischemia, they can be used when ischemia cannot be detected on an EEG tracing, such as during barbiturate anesthesia (which is rarely used), where the isoelectric EEG can only indicate that neurons are quiet and cannot indicate whether these neurons are ischemic. The SSEP tracing remains intact with barbiturate anesthesia and, therefore, would potentially be more useful as a clinical monitor. Patients who have had strokes have some asymmetry in baseline SSEP waveforms. This asymmetry does not appear to affect the SSEP as an effective clinical monitor, which can also be a relative advantage over the EEG in patients with prior stroke.

Manninen PH, Tan TK, Sarjeant RM. Somatosensory evoked potential monitoring during carotid endarterectomy in patients with a stroke. *Anesth Analg*. 2001;93:39-44.

Seubert CN, Ok MSJ. Neurophysiologic monitoring. In: Gropper MA, Eriksson LI, Fleisher LA, Cohen NH, Leslie K, Johnson-Akeju O, eds. *Miller's Anesthesia*. 10th ed. Elsevier; 2025:1099-1132.

C.10. What type of anesthesia will you choose for this patient if she chose to have an endarterectomy?

Regional or general anesthesia can be used for patients undergoing CEA. Each type of anesthesia has advantages and disadvantages that must be considered when choosing the optimal anesthetic for each patient. Benefits of general anesthesia include a still patient and a quiet operative field; early control of the airway and ventilation; and the ability to protect the brain should ischemia, which cannot be eliminated, develop. A disadvantage of general anesthesia is the inability to perform repeated neurologic evaluations requiring patient responses during surgery. Therefore, patients receiving general anesthesia should have their CBF or neurologic function monitored as previously discussed.

The primary advantage of a regional anesthetic technique is that the patient remains responsive, allowing for repeated neurologic evaluations. Although anecdotal reports support that regional anesthesia allows for greater stability of blood pressure, decreased requirement for vasoactive medications to support blood pressure, and decreased incidence of perioperative MI, further outcome studies are needed. Potential complications associated with regional anesthesia include seizures, alteration of mental status with cerebral ischemia, and loss of patient cooperation associated with cerebral hypoperfusion, inadequate ventilation, and sedation.

Early analyses of mainly nonrandomized trials comparing regional and general anesthesia for CEA initially suggested a reduced risk of morbidity and mortality with regional anesthesia. However, subsequent analyses of larger, randomized trials have generally refuted this finding. The general anesthesia *versus* local anesthesia for carotid surgery (GALA) trial was a multicenter, randomized controlled trial that included 3,526 patients with symptomatic or asymptomatic carotid stenosis who were randomly assigned to surgery under general anesthesia or regional anesthesia. This study showed no differences in the primary study outcome (stroke, MI, or death within 30 days), quality of life, or length of hospital stay. However, there was a nonsignificant trend toward a higher rate of MI in the regional anesthesia group as well as a nonsignificant trend toward a higher rate of stroke among patients with bilateral carotid disease in the general anesthesia group.

A meta-analysis of 14 randomized trials involving 4,596 procedures (the majority of which came from the GALA study) found that there was no statistically significant difference between general and regional anesthesia groups in the proportion of patients who had a stroke or died within 30 days of surgery. In this meta-analysis, there was a nonsignificant trend toward lower operative mortality with regional anesthetic; however, none of the individual studies or the meta-analysis were adequately powered to reliably detect an effect on mortality. Therefore, evidence suggests that patients and surgeons can choose either anesthetic technique, depending on the clinical situation and individual preference.

Bebawy JPF, Hemmer LB, Pasternak JJ. Anesthesia for neurosurgery. In: Cullen BF, Stock MC, Ortega R, et al, eds. *Barash, Cullen, and Stoelting's Clinical Anesthesia*. 9th ed. Wolters Kluwer; 2024:979-1002.

Nelson P, Bustillo M. Anesthesia for carotid endarterectomy, angioplasty, and stent. *Anesthesiol Clin*. 2021;39:37-51.

Unic-Stojanovic D, Babic S, Neskovic V. General versus regional anesthesia for carotid endarterectomy. *J Cardiothorac Vasc Anesth*. 2013;27:1379-1383.

Vaniyapong T, Chongruksut W, Rerkasem K. Local versus general anaesthesia for carotid endarterectomy. *Cochrane Database Syst Rev*. 2013:CD000126.

C.11. What type of anesthesia will you choose for this patient if she chose to have a carotid stent?

Carotid stents are usually performed under local anesthesia. Patients get minimal to no sedation so that a continuous neurologic assessment can be performed. An arterial line is placed in addition to standard monitoring, as hemodynamic instability is common during and after stenting is performed. During the angioplasty and stent placement, studies have reported bradycardia, hypotension, and asystole. Bradycardia and hypotension are seen more often when angioplasty is performed prior to stenting. The interventionalist will usually ask for prophylactic atropine or glycopyrrolate before balloon angioplasty and stent deployment. Satya et al reported about 5% incidence of asystole after stenting and found a higher association with right-sided stents in patients with reduced left ventricular ejection fraction and significant contralateral stenosis.

Bussière M, Lownie SP, Lee D, et al. Hemodynamic instability during carotid artery stenting: the relative contribution of stent deployment versus balloon dilation. *J Neurosurg*. 2009;110:905-912.

Cayne NS, Faries PL, Trocciola SM, et al. Carotid angioplasty and stent-induced bradycardia and hypotension: impact of prophylactic atropine administration and prior carotid endarterectomy. *J Vasc Surg*. 2005;41:956-961.

Satya K, Dougherty K, Lee W. Determinants and outcomes of asystole during carotid artery stenting. *J Endovasc Ther*. 2011;18:513-517.

Shalabi A, Chang J. Anesthesia for vascular surgery. In: Gropper MA, Eriksson LI, Fleisher LA, Cohen NH, Leslie K, Johnson-Akeju O, eds. *Miller's Anesthesia*. 10th ed. Elsevier; 2025:1696-1732.

C.12. How will you induce and maintain general anesthesia in this patient for CEA?

Any anesthetic regimen is suitable if it provides hemodynamic stability, does not exacerbate cerebral ischemia, and allows for prompt emergence from anesthesia at the end of surgery. Premedication with midazolam has the potential to compromise early neurologic assessment and is usually avoided. Following preoxygenation, anesthetics should be titrated slowly with special attention to their effect on blood pressure. Control of the airway should be taken as soon as the patient is no longer able to breathe adequately to maintain normocarbia. While breathing oxygen, short-acting opioids are administered until the patient is comfortably sedated. Lidocaine 1 mg/kg is administered intravenously at least 2 minutes before laryngoscopy and intubation to blunt the hemodynamic response to airway manipulation. Following administration of propofol or etomidate, controlled ventilation is instituted with 100% oxygen to avoid hypoxemia and hypercarbia. A neuromuscular blocker is administered to facilitate tracheal intubation. Succinylcholine should be avoided in hemiparetic patients because of the possibility of a hyperkalemic response. Nondepolarizing neuromuscular blocking agents with significant hemodynamic effects, such as sympathomimetic activity, vagolysis, or histamine release, should be avoided. Once the patient is relaxed, expeditious laryngoscopy and intubation are performed. Atomized lidocaine can be used prior to intubation to minimize stimulation by the endotracheal tube during surgery and prevent coughing on emergence.

During the induction and intubation sequence, blood pressure is kept in the patient's normal range using vasopressors or vasodilators as indicated. Short-acting and easily titratable vasoactive medications should be chosen to facilitate blood pressure control.

Anesthesia can be maintained with volatile anesthetics or intravenous agents. The addition of short-acting opioids to a volatile or intravenous anesthetic will decrease heart rate and, when properly dosed, allow for a prompt, smooth emergence from general anesthesia. Maintenance of a light anesthetic appears to have several advantages over deep anesthesia. It allows ischemic patterns on the EEG to be recognized easily. It also facilitates the maintenance of blood pressure. In addition, administration of a light anesthetic, compared to deep anesthesia using phenylephrine to maintain blood pressure, results in a lower incidence of perioperative MI. Arterial blood pressure should be maintained in the high normal range throughout the procedure. When the carotid artery is clamped, induced hypertension (10%-20% above baseline) is often requested by the surgeon to increase contralateral flow and prevent ischemia. During surgical manipulation of the carotid sinus, sudden bradycardia and hypotension can occur. Alerting the surgeon and asking them to stop manipulating the area usually restores hemodynamics.

Bebawy JPF, Hemmer LB, Pasternak JJ. Anesthesia for neurosurgery. In: Cullen BF, Stock MC, Ortega R, et al, eds. *Barash, Cullen, and Stoelting's Clinical Anesthesia*. 9th ed. Wolters Kluwer; 2024:979-1002.

Jellish WS, Sheikh T, Baker WH, et al. Hemodynamic stability, myocardial ischemia, and perioperative outcome after carotid surgery with remifentanil/propofol or isoflurane/fentanyl anesthesia. *J Neurosurg Anesthesiol.* 2003;15:176-184.

Mutch WA, White IW, Donen N, et al. Haemodynamic instability and myocardial ischaemia during carotid endarterectomy: a comparison of propofol and isoflurane. *Can J Anaesth.* 1995;42:577-587.

Shalabi A, Chang J. Anesthesia for vascular surgery. In: Gropper MA, Eriksson LI, Fleisher LA, Cohen NH, Leslie K, Johnson-Akeju O, eds. *Miller's Anesthesia*. 10th ed. Elsevier; 2025:1696-1732.

Umbrain V, Keeris J, D'Haese J, et al. Isoflurane, desflurane and sevoflurane for carotid endarterectomy. *Anaesthesia.* 2000;55:1052-1057.

C.13. How would you proceed if the patient were to receive regional anesthesia?

Patient cooperation is essential for regional anesthesia to proceed successfully. For a patient to be adequately anesthetized, a sensory blockade is required in the C2 to C4 dermatomes. This can be accomplished with either deep or superficial cervical plexus blocks. In doing the blocks, care must be taken not to excessively palpate the neck because part of the plaque in the carotid artery might dislodge and embolize.

Superficial cervical plexus block is performed by infiltrating along with the middle third of the posterior border of the sternocleidomastoid muscle with local anesthetics. Deep cervical plexus block is performed with three injections along a line drawn from the Chassaignac tubercle (C6) to the mastoid process. The C4 nerve root is located at the intersection of that line with one drawn horizontally from the lower border of the mandible. C2 and C3 are located by dividing the distance between the mastoid process and the horizontal line into thirds. Alternatively, a single injection of local anesthetic can be made on the line between the mastoid process and Chassaignac tubercle at the level of C4 with the needle directed medially and slightly caudad.

Patients receiving regional anesthesia must be both cooperative and not overly sedated with intravenous medications. If they are unable to cooperate and become obtunded, the primary advantage of regional anesthesia (continuous neurologic evaluation) is lost. Intravenous sedation, therefore, must be given judiciously, if at all, to these patients.

Shalabi A, Chang J. Anesthesia for vascular surgery. In: Gropper MA, Eriksson LI, Fleisher LA, Cohen NH, Leslie K, Johnson-Akeju O, eds. *Miller's Anesthesia*. 10th ed. Elsevier; 2025:1696-1732.

Unic-Stojanovic D, Babic S, Neskovic V. General versus regional anesthesia for carotid endarterectomy. *J Cardiothorac Vasc Anesth.* 2013;27:1379-1383.

C.14. Discuss the effects of anesthetics on CBF.

General anesthetics affect CBF and cerebral oxygen consumption. This can be used to advantage when the decrease in oxygen consumption is greater than the decrease in CBF.

In general, volatile anesthetics are cerebral vasodilators, and intravenous anesthetics are cerebral vasoconstrictors. Ketamine is an exception because it can increase both CBF and cerebral metabolic rate. Volatile anesthetics produce a dose-dependent increase in CBF. The magnitude of vasodilation depends on the balance between vasodilation and vasoconstriction secondary to the reduction in cerebral metabolic rate.

SECTION 4

Studies suggest that anesthetic agents only affect the blood flow in normally perfused areas of the brain. If this is the case, volatile anesthetics could cause a steal phenomenon, in which the blood vessels in the normal brain dilate and steal blood flow away from ischemic areas of the brain that are both already maximally vasodilated and unresponsive to further vasodilating effects of the anesthetics.

Bebawy JPF, Hemmer LB, Pasternak JJ. Anesthesia for neurosurgery. In: Cullen BF, Stock MC, Ortega R, et al, eds. *Barash, Cullen, and Stoelting's Clinical Anesthesia*. 9th ed. Wolters Kluwer; 2024:979-1002.

Patel PM, Drummond JC, Lemkuil BP. Cerebral physiology and the effects of anesthetic drugs. In: Gropper MA, Eriksson LI, Fleisher LA, Cohen NH, Leslie K, Johnson-Akeju O, eds. *Miller's Anesthesia*. 10th ed. Elsevier; 2025:180-224.

C.15. Discuss the protective effects of anesthetic agents on cerebral function.

Although it has not been proven that general anesthetics afford brain protection, agents that cause the greatest decrease in cerebral metabolic oxygen consumption should lessen the risk of cerebral ischemia. Whether a particular anesthetic is optimal for these patients is an area of discussion. Avoiding or eliminating ischemia is preferable to protecting against it.

Messick et al examined the effects of volatile anesthetics on critical regional CBF, that is, the regional CBF at which EEG evidence of cerebral ischemia became apparent. Critical regional CBF in patients receiving isoflurane was less than 10 mL/100 g/min, and in patients receiving halothane was 18 to 20 mL/100 g/min. This decrease in critical CBF suggests that isoflurane might offer some protective effect. Because of its potential to cause a decrease in blood pressure and a reflex increase in heart rate, it probably should not be used at high concentrations as the sole anesthetic. A significant proportion of patients with carotid artery disease also have coronary artery disease and might not tolerate the hypotension and tachycardia associated with the use of high-dose isoflurane. By using this anesthetic in low concentrations in combination with other anesthetic agents, one can better maintain hemodynamic stability while perhaps providing for an increased tolerance of cerebral hypoperfusion. Other evidence suggests that isoflurane does not offer protection during regional cerebral ischemia.

Both sevoflurane and desflurane have also been examined for their possible role in neuroanesthesia. Compared to isoflurane, desflurane has no significant difference in its effects on decreasing cerebral glucose utilization, increasing blood flow, and maintaining coupling between local CBF and local cerebral glucose utilization. Although sevoflurane showed no significant difference in its effects on decreasing cerebral glucose utilization and coupling between local CBF and local cerebral glucose utilization at one minimum alveolar concentration (MAC), it did show less of an increase in CBF. This difference between isoflurane and sevoflurane was independent of their effects on systemic blood flow and cardiac output. Hence, desflurane and sevoflurane might have similar neuroprotective effects as isoflurane and, with their lower blood gas solubility coefficients, promote a more rapid recovery from anesthesia, allowing faster evaluation of neurologic status. Due to adverse environmental effects, however, the routine use of desflurane is rapidly diminishing.

Thiopental (currently not available in the United States) affords cerebral protection against focal or incomplete global cerebral ischemia. It is a cerebral vasoconstrictor, as are most other intravenous anesthetics. It will also transiently decrease cerebral metabolism to up to 50% of baseline. The combined effect is that cerebral metabolic oxygen consumption is decreased more than oxygen delivery. The reduction in oxygen demand is the result of inhibition of functioning neurons, which can be observed as a quiet or isoelectric EEG. When dosing barbiturates for cerebral protection, the EEG should be monitored and repeated doses should be given to achieve and then maintain a burst suppression pattern. Once the EEG is isoelectric, indicating a lack of neuronal function, further doses of thiopental do not provide additional protection. It is generally not recommended that thiopental be used for cerebral protection during CEA. As mentioned previously, avoidance of ischemia is preferable to its treatment. If thiopental is used, burst suppression can develop or the EEG can become isoelectric; at that point, the EEG becomes useless as a monitor of cerebral ischemia. This is especially problematic if selective shunting is to be used. Furthermore, the doses of thiopental required to suppress the EEG cause hypotension and a delayed emergence from anesthesia. Barbiturate use to minimize the possibility of cerebral ischemia has been advocated for patients undergoing carotid bypass procedures in which temporary occlusion of the recipient vessel is required. Whether the treatment of patients with a 3 to 5 mg/kg dose of thiopental affects their outcome in terms of neurologic deficit is not known, although it has been shown to be efficacious in animal models.

Like barbiturates, the intravenous anesthetics propofol and etomidate decrease brain electrical activity and cellular oxygen requirements while preserving cerebral autoregulation of blood flow. Although the available evidence for the protective effects of etomidate and propofol during CEA is inconclusive, these agents reduce brain infarction and prolong tolerable ischemia time in patients undergoing temporary ischemia for intracranial aneurysm clipping. Additionally, animal studies suggest a degree of neuroprotection with propofol.

Dexmedetomidine is a selective α_2-adrenergic agonist with sedative, analgesic, and anxiolytic properties. It does not cause respiratory depression. In animal studies, dexmedetomidine reduces ischemic damage after transient and permanent ischemia. Its mechanism of neuroprotection is unclear. One hypothesis suggests that with the onset of cerebral ischemia, one of the initial responses in the central nervous system is the excessive release of norepinephrine and glutamate during energy failure. If the increase in norepinephrine release is a causative component of injury, an α_2-adrenergic agonist may decrease the damage afforded by cerebral ischemia. Dexmedetomidine has been shown to reduce arousal and decrease CBF in volunteers.

Bebawy JPF, Hemmer LB, Pasternak JJ. Anesthesia for neurosurgery. In: Cullen BF, Stock MC, Ortega R, et al, eds. *Barash, Cullen, and Stoelting's Clinical Anesthesia*. 9th ed. Wolters Kluwer; 2024:979-1002.

Hendrickx JFA, Nielsen OJ, De Hert S, De Wolf AM. The science behind banning desflurane: a narrative review. *Eur J Anaesthesiol*. 2022;39:818-824.

Hicks RG, Kerr DR, Horton DA. Thiopentone cerebral protection under EEG control during carotid endarterectomy. *Anaesth Intensive Care*. 1986;14:22-28.

Holzer A, Greher M, Hetz H, et al. Influence of aortic blood flow velocity on changes of middle cerebral artery blood flow velocity during isoflurane and sevoflurane anaesthesia. *Eur J Anaesthesiol*. 2001;18:238-244.

Kuhmonen J, Pokorný J, Miettinen R, et al. Neuroprotective effects of dexmedetomidine in the gerbil hippocampus after transient global ischemia. *Anesthesiology*. 1997;87:371-377.

Matta BF, Heath KJ, Tipping K, et al. Direct cerebral vasodilatory effects of sevoflurane and isoflurane. *Anesthesiology*. 1999;91:677-680.

Messick JM Jr, Casement B, Sharbrough FW, et al. Correlation of regional cerebral blood flow (rCBF) with EEG changes during isoflurane anesthesia for carotid endarterectomy: critical rCBF. *Anesthesiology*. 1987;66:344-349.

Michenfelder JD, Sundt TM, Fode N, et al. Isoflurane when compared to enflurane and halothane decreases the frequency of cerebral ischemia during carotid endarterectomy. *Anesthesiology*. 1987;67:336-340.

Nehls DG, Todd MM, Spetzler RF, et al. A comparison of the cerebral protective effects of isoflurane and barbiturates during temporary focal ischemia in primates. *Anesthesiology*. 1987;66:453-464.

C.16. How will you manage this patient's ventilation under general anesthesia?

Because carbon dioxide is a potent cerebral vasodilator, patients undergoing CEA historically were hypoventilated intraoperatively to achieve hypercarbia and cerebral vasodilation. However, it is now accepted that hypercapnia should be avoided in patients with carotid artery disease. Carbon dioxide causes vasodilation in normally reactive, nonischemic, vascular beds. In patients with carotid artery disease, this means that blood flow is diverted away from the already maximally dilated vessels in the territory of the occluded carotid and toward normal areas of the brain. This decrease in regional CBF in ischemic areas of the brain with increased CBF in normal areas of the brain is known as *intracerebral steal*.

Other authors have recommended extreme hypocapnia during CEA, reasoning that this would result in an "inverse steal" or a "Robin Hood" phenomenon. Hypocapnia will cause constriction of cerebral vessels in normally perfused areas of the brain, possibly diverting blood flow into the maximally vasodilated, unreactive, hypoperfused regions of the brain. Clinical trials have been unable to demonstrate any benefit from hypocapnia, and animal studies have shown that it might, in fact, exacerbate ischemia. This most likely happens not only because of intense vasoconstriction but also because of a leftward shift of the oxyhemoglobin dissociation curve so that hemoglobin is less able to transfer oxygen to tissues.

The general recommendation for patients with cerebrovascular disease is that normocarbia or mild hypocarbia be maintained. After repair of their carotid stenosis, some patients will have a marked hyperemia with CBF of 100 mL/100 g/min. In these patients, decreasing both blood pressure and arterial carbon dioxide tension to decrease their CBF is indicated. Without a decrease in CBF, these patients are at risk for postoperative intracerebral hemorrhage.

Baker WH, Rodman JA, Barnes RW, et al. An evaluation of hypocarbia and hypercarbia during carotid endarterectomy. *Stroke*. 1976;7:451-454.

Bebawy JPF, Hemmer LB, Pasternak JJ. Anesthesia for neurosurgery. In: Cullen BF, Stock MC, Ortega R, et al, eds. *Barash, Cullen, and Stoelting's Clinical Anesthesia*. 9th ed. Wolters Kluwer; 2024:979-1002.

Nelson P, Bustillo M. Anesthesia for carotid endarterectomy, angioplasty, and stent. *Anesthesiol Clin*. 2021;39:37-51.

Shalabi A, Chang J. Anesthesia for vascular surgery. In: Gropper MA, Eriksson LI, Fleisher LA, Cohen NH, Leslie K, Johnson-Akeju O, eds. *Miller's Anesthesia*. 10th ed. Elsevier; 2025:1696-1732.

C.17. How will you manage this patient's blood pressure intraoperatively?

Various factors need to be considered in the blood pressure management of patients undergoing CEA. In the patients with carotid artery disease, a loss of autoregulation occurs in ischemic areas of the brain. In areas of chronic hypoperfusion, vessels are maximally vasodilated and unresponsive to vasomotor stimuli. Perfusion in these ischemic areas is pressure dependent.

During cerebral arterial occlusion, systemic blood pressure may need to be increased to augment collateral blood flow. The primary collateral pathways include the Willisian channels. If Willisian channels are not available, either because of the patient's anatomy or a therapeutic intervention, secondary collateral channels are available that bridge adjacent major vascular territories. These pathways are known as the *pial-to-pial collateral* or *leptomeningeal* pathways.

Because of the adjustment of the autoregulatory limits in hypertensive patients and because of a lack of autoregulation in ischemic areas of the brain, hypotension should be avoided. Blood pressure should be maintained in its high normal range. During arterial occlusion, the only practical way to increase collateral blood flow might be by increasing the collateral perfusion pressure by raising systemic blood pressure. The extent to which blood pressure should be raised depends on the nature of the disease. During deliberate hypertension, systemic blood pressure is raised by 30% to 40% above baseline or until ischemic symptoms resolve. Both maintenance of and increases in blood pressure can be accomplished with light anesthesia and, when necessary, infusion of the α-agonist phenylephrine. Phenylephrine has no direct effect on the cerebral vasculature; therefore, cerebral perfusion is increased by an elevation in the CPP. Phenylephrine increases blood pressure, CPP, stump pressure, and regional CBF. It also increases myocardial oxygen consumption. Because it increases afterload, care must be taken when it is used in patients with coronary artery disease, and it can exacerbate myocardial ischemia and congestive heart failure. In patients with coronary artery disease, blood pressure should not be increased above baseline unless evidence of cerebral ischemia develops. Extreme increases in blood pressure can and should be managed with easily titratable intravenous vasodilators.

Once the stenosis has been relieved and the carotid cross-clamp removed, the patient's blood pressure should be maintained in a low normal range. Lowering blood pressure offers several advantages. It decreases myocardial oxygen consumption by decreasing the work of the heart, decreases the amount of stress on the suture line in the carotid artery, and minimizes the possibility of reperfusion hemorrhage.

Aaslid R, Lindegaard KF, Sorteberg W, et al. Cerebral autoregulation dynamics in humans. *Stroke*. 1989;20:45-52.

Bebawy JPF, Hemmer LB, Pasternak JJ. Anesthesia for neurosurgery. In: Cullen BF, Stock MC, Ortega R, et al, eds. *Barash, Cullen, and Stoelting's Clinical Anesthesia*. 9th ed. Wolters Kluwer; 2024:979-1002.

Shalabi A, Chang J. Anesthesia for vascular surgery. In: Gropper MA, Eriksson LI, Fleisher LA, Cohen NH, Leslie K, Johnson-Akeju O, eds. *Miller's Anesthesia*. 10th ed. Elsevier; 2025:1696-1732.

Smith JS, Roizen MF, Cahalan MK, et al. Does anesthetic technique make a difference? Augmentation of systolic blood pressure during carotid endarterectomy: effects of phenylephrine versus light anesthesia and of isoflurane versus halothane on the incidence of myocardial ischemia. *Anesthesiology*. 1988;69:846-853.

C.18. Discuss reperfusion injury following CEA and CAS.

Blood pressure can be labile after carotid manipulation and must be an area of focus as the case concludes. The systolic blood pressure should be maintained between 100 and 150 mm Hg, using short-acting vasoactive agents, as needed. Reperfusion injury involves cerebral hemorrhage or the development of cerebral edema after obstruction to flow through the carotid artery has been relieved. Although rare, it can be a fatal complication of CEA. Patients present with headache, seizure, focal neurologic signs, brain edema, and intracerebral bleeds. The incidence of intracerebral hemorrhage after CEA ranges from 0.4% to 2.0% and usually occurs 1 to 5 days after surgery. Patients with a previous stroke are most likely to suffer reperfusion hemorrhage, but it can occur in otherwise normal brain tissue. Poorly controlled blood pressure after the carotid cross-clamp has been removed contributes to this complication. One proposed mechanism for this injury is that once flow is returned to normal, vascular beds in previously hypoperfused areas of the brain are unable to respond properly with vasoconstriction. They are unable to maintain normal flow with increased perfusion. Because hypoperfusion distal to the carotid stenosis has been long-standing, these vessels have lost their ability to autoregulate. Once the carotid stenosis is eliminated, the perfusion pressure distal to the former site of the stenosis is markedly increased. Because of the lack of autoregulation in this area, CBF increases with increasing perfusion pressure. The patients at the highest risk for reperfusion injury have the greatest degree of stenosis and the greatest pressure drop across the carotid lesion.

Bebawy JPF, Hemmer LB, Pasternak JJ. Anesthesia for neurosurgery. In: Cullen BF, Stock MC, Ortega R, et al, eds. *Barash, Cullen, and Stoelting's Clinical Anesthesia*. 9th ed. Wolters Kluwer; 2024:979-1002.

Breen JC, Caplan LF, DeWitt LD, et al. Brain edema after carotid surgery. *Neurology*. 1996;46:175-181.

Nelson P, Bustillo M. Anesthesia for carotid endarterectomy, angioplasty, and stent. *Anesthesiol Clin*. 2021;39:37-51.

Shalabi A, Chang J. Anesthesia for vascular surgery. In: Gropper MA, Eriksson LI, Fleisher LA, Cohen NH, Leslie K, Johnson-Akeju O, eds. *Miller's Anesthesia*. 10th ed. Elsevier; 2025:1696-1732.

Solomon RA, Loftus CM, Quest DO, et al. Incidence and etiology of intracerebral hemorrhage following carotid endarterectomy. *J Neurosurg*. 1986;64:29-34.

C.19. What intravenous fluids will you give this patient intraoperatively?

Because moderate hyperglycemia has been shown to worsen neurologic outcome after ischemia, care must be taken to avoid increasing glucose by exogenous administration. Balanced intravenous fluids such as PlasmaLyte, lactated Ringer solution, or another buffered crystalloid solution would be appropriate choices for patients undergoing CEA.

These patients should not be vigorously hydrated intraoperatively. It is best to limit their intraoperative fluids to what is required for maintenance, with additional colloid and blood replacement being given as needed. Intraoperative overhydration can contribute to the frequently observed postoperative hypertension and in patients with myocardial disease can exacerbate congestive heart failure.

Bebawy JPF, Hemmer LB, Pasternak JJ. Anesthesia for neurosurgery. In: Cullen BF, Stock MC, Ortega R, et al, eds. *Barash, Cullen, and Stoelting's Clinical Anesthesia*. 9th ed. Wolters Kluwer; 2024:979-1002.

Li PA, Siesjö BK. Role of hyperglycaemia-related acidosis in ischaemic brain damage. *Acta Physiol Scand*. 1997; 161:567-580.

McGrit MJ, Woodworth GF, Brooke BS, et al. Hyperglycemia independently increases the risk of perioperative stroke, myocardial infarction, and death after carotid endarterectomy. *Neurosurgery*. 2006;58:1066-1073.

Shalabi A, Chang J. Anesthesia for vascular surgery. In: Gropper MA, Eriksson LI, Fleisher LA, Cohen NH, Leslie K, Johnson-Akeju O, eds. *Miller's Anesthesia*. 10th ed. Elsevier; 2025:1696-1732.

D. Postoperative Management

D.1. The patient does not "wake up" from general anesthesia. Why?

Once other causes of slow emergence from general anesthesia (eg, hyperglycemia or hypoglycemia, hypothermia, anesthetic overdose, hypercarbia, and hypoxemia) have been ruled out, the possibility of an adverse intraoperative event needs to be considered. Patency of the carotid artery should be evaluated. This can be done by Doppler studies while the patient is still in the operating room. If no blood flow is seen in the carotid artery, the incision can be reexplored immediately. If Doppler studies are normal, the possibility of a cerebral infarction from prolonged hypoperfusion or from emboli must be considered. The patient should remain intubated while further studies, including a computed tomography (CT) scan and cerebral angiography, are done expeditiously. The incidence of new perioperative neurologic deficits is 3% or less in centers where the operation is done commonly.

Graber JN, Vollman RW, Johnson WC, et al. Stroke after carotid endarterectomy: risk as predicted by preoperative computerized tomography. *Am J Surg*. 1984;147:492-497.

Paciaroni M, Eliasziw M, Kappelle LJ, et al. Medical complications associated with carotid endarterectomy. *Stroke*. 1999;30:1759-1763.

Shalabi A, Chang J. Anesthesia for vascular surgery. In: Gropper MA, Eriksson LI, Fleisher LA, Cohen NH, Leslie K, Johnson-Akeju O, eds. *Miller's Anesthesia*. 10th ed. Elsevier; 2025:1696-1732.

D.2. Postoperatively, the patient's blood pressure is 170/96 mm Hg. Will you treat this?

This patient's blood pressure needs to be carefully controlled because postoperative hypertension is associated with bleeding at the operative site, myocardial ischemia, arrhythmias, intracerebral hemorrhage, and cerebral edema.

Hypertension is observed more commonly than hypotension after CEA. Causes of hypertension include hypoxemia, hypercarbia, pain, and a full bladder. If any or all of these causes are present, they need to be dealt with promptly. Another common cause of postoperative hypertension and tachycardia is blunting of the carotid baroreceptor mechanism secondary to carotid sinus dysfunction caused by surgical trauma. If this is the cause of hypertension, therapy with antihypertensive agents should be started.

This patient's systolic blood pressure should be maintained between 100 and 150 mm Hg. Elevated blood pressure can be treated with short-acting vasoactive agents like nicardipine infusion, hydralazine in 5-mg increments, or labetalol in 5- to 10-mg increments. β-Blockade with metoprolol or an infusion of esmolol can be added to this regimen to treat tachycardia and hypertension if present.

Bebawy JPF, Hemmer LB, Pasternak JJ. Anesthesia for neurosurgery. In: Cullen BF, Stock MC, Ortega R, et al, eds. *Barash, Cullen, and Stoelting's Clinical Anesthesia*. 9th ed. Wolters Kluwer; 2024:979-1002.

Shalabi A, Chang J. Anesthesia for vascular surgery. In: Gropper MA, Eriksson LI, Fleisher LA, Cohen NH, Leslie K, Johnson-Akeju O, eds. *Miller's Anesthesia*. 10th ed. Elsevier; 2025:1696-1732.

D.3. What immediate postoperative complications might you expect after a CEA?

Immediate postoperative complications include neurologic deficits, hemodynamic instability, and respiratory insufficiency. Evaluation of the NASCET showed that 8.1% of patients had medical complications: 1% with MIs, 7.1% with other cardiovascular disorders such as arrhythmias and congestive heart failure, 0.8% with respiratory complications, 0.4% with transient confusion, and 0.7% with other complications. CEA is 1.5 times more likely to be associated with complications in patients with a history of cardiac disease or hypertension.

Postoperative neurologic complications are usually embolic in nature, occurring during surgery. Other neurologic complications result from reperfusion injury and intracranial hemorrhage.

Circulatory instability is common after CEA, with either hypotension or hypertension observed. Hypotension can have any of several causes, as does hypertension, as noted previously. These include hypovolemia, depression of the circulation by residual anesthetics, prolonged effect of intraoperatively administered antihypertensives, dysrhythmias, and myocardial ischemia. Each of these causes needs to be sought and, if present, treated. Another possible cause of hypotension is an excessive reflex response because of increased sensitivity of the carotid sinus after exposure of the baroreceptor mechanism to a higher pressure with the removal of the plaque. If this is the cause, therapy needs to be instituted with fluids and vasopressors.

Postoperative respiratory insufficiency is a rare but potentially life-threatening complication. This can be due to vocal cord paralysis from intraoperative traction on the laryngeal nerves. Should this present with an inability to protect the airway, the patient should be reintubated immediately. A prospective trial found that 12.5% of patients had nerve injuries after CEA, but all were transient, lasting from 1 week to 37 months. No patient had life-threatening respiratory insufficiency from the nerve injuries. The most commonly injured nerves were the hypoglossal, recurrent laryngeal, superior laryngeal, and greater auricular nerves.

Airway obstruction can also occur from hematoma formation at the operative site, from either arterial or venous bleeding. The hematoma needs to be evacuated as quickly as possible, and depending on the ventilatory status, reintubation might be necessary. This is most easily done after evacuation of the hematoma if the clinical condition allows. Supraglottic edema is a rare cause of postoperative upper airway obstruction after CEA. CT analysis of airways postoperatively showed a reduction in the volume of the airway in all patients, with a greater reduction seen in intubated patients (63% ± 9%) than in nonintubated patients (32% ± 7%).

Tension pneumothorax can result from air dissecting through the wound and the mediastinum to the pleura. This diagnosis should be considered in all patients after CEA who seem to have respiratory distress and no evidence of upper airway obstruction. Absence of breath sounds over half of the chest and hemodynamic instability would support this diagnosis.

Chemoreceptor function is impaired in most patients after CEA for up to 10 months. Lack of chemoreceptor function means that there is a loss of circulatory response to hypoxemia and an increase in resting $Paco_2$ of approximately 6 mm Hg. This complication is potentially very serious, and one needs to be most concerned about its development in patients who have had a previous contralateral CEA, where function can be lost bilaterally. In all patients after CEA, supplemental oxygen should be provided and opioids administered cautiously.

Ballotta E, Da Giau G, Renon L, et al. Cranial and cervical nerve injuries after carotid endarterectomy: a prospective study. *Surgery*. 1999;125:85-91.

Bebawy JPF, Hemmer LB, Pasternak JJ. Anesthesia for neurosurgery. In: Cullen BF, Stock MC, Ortega R, et al, eds. *Barash, Cullen, and Stoelting's Clinical Anesthesia*. 9th ed. Wolters Kluwer; 2024:979-1002.

Carmichael FJ, McGuire GP, Wong DT, et al. Computed tomographic analysis of airway dimensions after carotid endarterectomy. *Anesth Analg*. 1996;83:12-17.

Nelson P, Bustillo M. Anesthesia for carotid endarterectomy, angioplasty, and stent. *Anesthesiol Clin*. 2021;39:37-51.

Paciaroni M, Eliasziw M, Kappelle LJ, et al. Medical complications associated with carotid endarterectomy. *Stroke*. 1999;30:1759-1763.

Shalabi A, Chang J. Anesthesia for vascular surgery. In: Gropper MA, Eriksson LI, Fleisher LA, Cohen NH, Leslie K, Johnson-Akeju O, eds. *Miller's Anesthesia*. 10th ed. Elsevier; 2025:1696-1732.

Wade JG, Larson CP Jr, Hickey RF, et al. Effects of carotid endarterectomy on carotid chemoreceptor and baroreceptor function in man. *N Engl J Med*. 1970;282:823-829.

D.4. What postoperative complications might you expect after a CAS?

Complications after CAS include hemodynamic instability, stroke, MI, renal failure, and access-related problems. In a pooled analysis of 27 studies, Mylonas et al found that about 39% of patients experienced some degree of hemodynamic instability (bradycardia or hypotension) after CAS, but in a majority of patients, it resolved in 8 to 10 hours. Stroke following CAS could be secondary to thromboembolism, hypoperfusion, stent thrombosis, intracranial hemorrhage, or cerebral hyperperfusion. In several pooled meta-analysis studies, the periprocedural risk of stroke following stenting appears to be higher than CEA, but this is debated as stroke rates have improved since the introduction of CAS. The risk of MI in CAS ranges from 1% to 4%. Renal dysfunction following CAS is attributed to contrast-induced nephropathy, atheroembolism from instrumentation of the aorta, or hypoperfusion from hemodynamic instability. Access-related problems are related to pseudoaneurysm formation, bleeding, and atheroembolism to the lower extremities.

SECTION 4

Economopoulos KP, Sergentanis TN, Tsivgoulis G, et al. Carotid artery stenting versus carotid endarterectomy: a comprehensive meta-analysis of short-term and long-term outcomes. *Stroke*. 2011;42:687-692.

Kim LK, Yang DC, Swaminathan RV, et al. Comparison of trends and outcomes of carotid artery stenting and endarterectomy in the United States, 2001 to 2010. *Circ Cardiovasc Interv*. 2014;7:692-700.

Moulakakis KG, Mylonas SN, Lazaris A, et al. Acute carotid stent thrombosis: a comprehensive review. *Vasc Endovascular Surg*. 2016;50:511-521.

Mylonas SN, Moulakakis KG, Antonopoulos CN, et al. Carotid artery stenting-induced hemodynamic instability. *J Endovasc Ther*. 2013;20:48-60.

Qureshi AI, Luft AR, Sharma M, et al. Frequency and determinants of postprocedural hemodynamic instability after carotid angioplasty and stenting. *Stroke*. 1999;30:2086-2093.

Vincent S, Eberg M, Eisenberg MJ, et al. Meta-analysis of randomized controlled trials comparing the long-term outcomes of carotid artery stenting versus endarterectomy. *Circ Cardiovasc Qual Outcomes*. 2015;8:S99-S108.

D.5. Discuss postoperative neurocognitive dysfunction following uncomplicated carotid intervention.

CEA can reduce the incidence of stroke in patients with high-grade carotid artery stenosis. Increasing evidence suggests that as many as 28% of surgical patients have significant neuropsychological dysfunction 1 day after carotid artery surgery. Between 9% and 23% of these patients continue to exhibit cognitive decline 1 month after surgery.

The apolipoprotein E (APOE)-ε4 allele has been associated with worse outcome following stroke. One month after CEA, APOE-ε4-positive patients were more likely to have suffered a neurocognitive injury (42%) than APOE-ε4-negative patients (5%). The presence of the APOE-ε4 allele increases the risk of neurocognitive dysfunction 62-fold 1 month after surgery. Diabetes and obesity also predispose to injury.

Evidence also indicates increased cognitive dysfunction in patients with carotid stenosis treated with stenting performed under cerebral embolic protection. In a prospective case-control study, 41% of patients undergoing carotid stenting developed moderate-to-severe cognitive dysfunction compared to a matched control group. The average deficit score was significantly higher in the CAS group at 1 day. These differences were independent of age and history of stroke or TIA. The absence of oral statin medication might increase the probability of cognitive dysfunction.

The influence of regional or general anesthesia on postoperative subclinical cognitive dysfunction remains unclear, although a study by Heyer et al showed no difference in the incidence of cognitive dysfunction in patients who underwent CEA under general or regional anesthesia. Most concur that multiple factors, including surgical technique, anesthetic technique, and patient status, influence postoperative outcome.

Gaudet JG, Meyers PM, McKinsey JF, et al. Incidence of moderate to severe cognitive dysfunction in patients treated with carotid artery stenting. *Neurosurgery*. 2009;65:325-329.

Heyer EJ, Gold MI, Kirby EW, et al. A study of cognitive dysfunction in patients having carotid endarterectomy performed with regional anesthesia. *Anesth Analg*. 2008;107:636-642.

Heyer EJ, Wilson DA, Sahlein DH, et al. APOE-epsilon4 predisposes to cognitive dysfunction following uncomplicated carotid endarterectomy. *Neurology*. 2005;65:1759-1763.

Mazul-Sunko B, Hromatko I, Tadinac M, et al. Subclinical neurocognitive dysfunction after carotid endarterectomy–the impact of shunting. *J Neurosurg Anesthesiol*. 2010;22:195-201.

20 Awake Craniotomy for Surgery in the Eloquent Cortex

Thomas A. Moore II and Kenneth G. Smithson

A 30-year-old right-handed male presented with increased seizure frequency and tumor progression following two prior awake craniotomies. The initial pathology was reported as a World Health Organization (WHO) grade II oligodendroglioma. Following the second awake craniotomy, the tumor had undergone malignant transformation to a WHO grade IV glioblastoma multiforme (isocitrate dehydrogenase [IDH] mutated). Magnetic resonance imaging (MRI) revealed a 5.6 × 2.9 × 3.6 cm heterogeneously enhancing lesion with associated marked vasogenic edema in the right frontoparietal and temporoparietal white matter, with effacement of the right lateral ventricle (Figure 20.1A). His anticonvulsant medications were increased, and he was given a short course of a corticosteroid with symptom improvement. He underwent functional MRI (fMRI) that revealed asymmetric cortical activation in the right motor cortex when compared to the left side. The primary descending fibers of the corticospinal tract (CST) were intimately associated with the medial enhancing margin of the tumor (Figure 20.1B). He underwent a third uncomplicated awake craniotomy with motor and sensory mapping. He was discharged to home on postoperative day 2. Final pathology revealed a WHO grade IV glioblastoma multiforme (IDH mutated).

A. Medical Disease and Differential Diagnosis

1. What is the eloquent cortex?
2. What is the underlying pathology?
3. What determines intracranial pressure (ICP)?
4. How does a space-occupying mass alter ICP?
5. What is autoregulation, and why is it important?
6. How is cerebral blood flow (CBF) regulated?
7. What drug therapies can be associated with this pathology?

B. Preoperative Evaluation and Preparation

1. Why is the craniotomy performed awake?
2. What neurologic symptoms of the patient are important?
3. What is the status of their other comorbid conditions?
4. Are there anesthetic implications from current treatment drugs?
5. What laboratory data are required?
6. What radiology data should be reviewed?
7. How do you prepare the patient for an awake craniotomy?
8. Should this patient receive premedication?
9. What precautions should be taken for airway management?

C. Intraoperative Management

1. How should this patient be monitored?
2. Does this patient require invasive monitoring?
3. Can current drug therapy alter eloquent cortex mapping?
4. Why are hypertonic fluids used during a craniotomy?
5. What intravenous fluids (IVFs) are recommended?
6. Would a lumbar drain for cerebrospinal fluid (CSF) removal benefit this patient?
7. Is venous air embolism (VAE) a concern in this case?

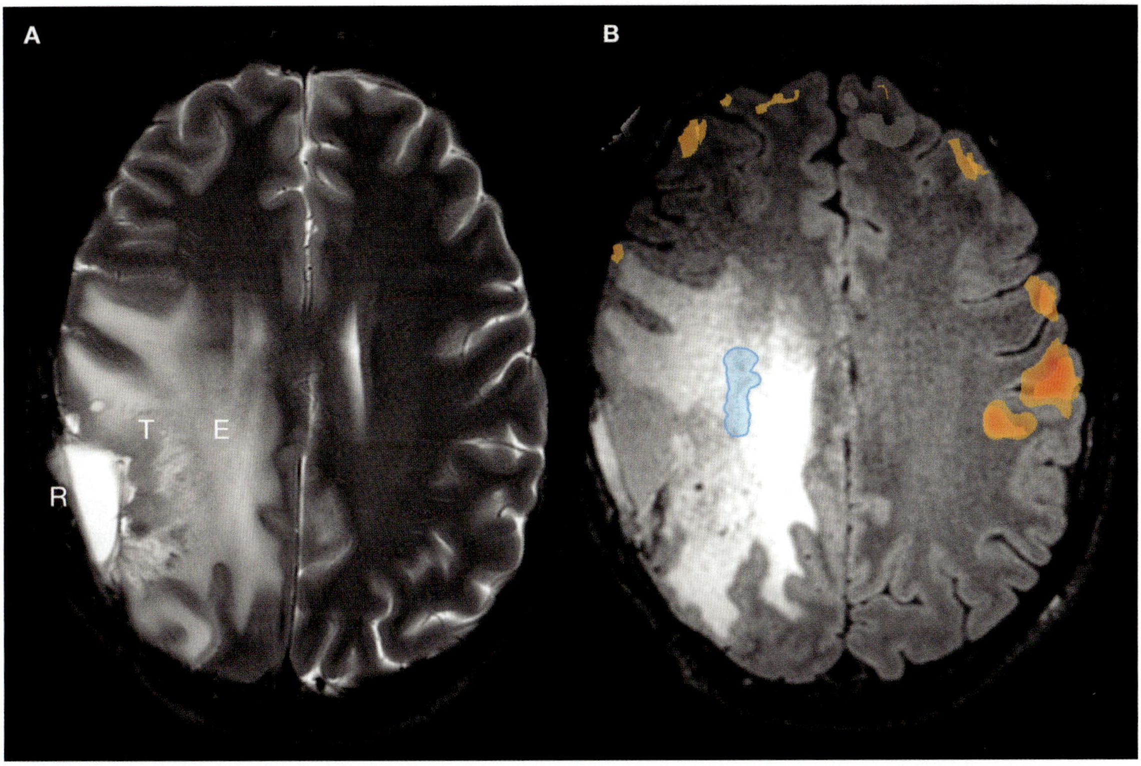

FIGURE 20.1. A. A 30-year-old male with a glioblastoma presents with increasing seizure frequency and tumor progression in follow-up studies. Note the remarkable level of vasogenic edema (E) surrounding the tumor (T) and extensive effacement of the right lateral ventricle. He underwent an uncomplicated repeat awake craniotomy with motor and sensory mapping. Final pathology was World Health Organization (WHO) grade IV glioblastoma multiforme. R, prior resection cavity. **B.** Functional magnetic resonance imaging (fMRI) demonstrates asymmetric cortical activity from bilateral and right-hand tapping in orange color. The intimate proximity of the corticospinal tract (CST), in blue, to the medial enhancing margin of the tumor is evident. Juxtaposition of new tumor growth, edema, and the CST proximity made simple resection via stereotactic methods virtually impossible. Only an awake patient who is actively involved in cortical mapping via task performance could minimize damage to the corticospinal tract.

8. How is the eloquent cortex mapped?
9. How are intraoperative seizures treated?
10. How will you conduct this anesthetic?

D. Postoperative Management

1. What are the major concerns following craniotomy?

A. Medical Disease and Differential Diagnosis

A.1. What is the eloquent cortex?

The *eloquent cortex* is a term used to describe functional areas of the cerebral cortex associated with motor, language, and sensory activity. Traditionally, tumors or epileptic foci within or near these areas have been considered *inoperable* because of the likely devastating consequences to the patient caused by iatrogenic injury to these critical brain regions.

De Benedictis A, Moritz-Gasser S, Duffau H. Awake mapping optimizes the extent of resection for low-grade gliomas in eloquent areas. *Neurosurgery*. 2010;66:1074-1084.

A.2. What is the underlying pathology?

The underlying pathology requiring an awake craniotomy for mapping and resection within the eloquent cortex can be either a space-occupying lesion or an epileptic focus. Mapping of the cortical and subcortical structures with an awake and cooperative patient is necessary to minimize neurologic injury and maximize lesion resection. Mapping of the motor cortex is often done under general anesthesia, usually total intravenous anesthesia (TIVA), typically using combined propofol and remifentanil infusions, after reversal of any residual neuromuscular block because the stimulated area(s) can usually be seen by an observer. Additionally, motor responses are directly measured electrophysiologically as muscle motor evoked potentials (mMEPs). Intraoperatively, somatosensory evoked potential (SEP) phase reversal can also be used to precisely define the extent of the central sulcus; using a strip electrode positioned across the central sulcus, phase reversal is demonstrated when an evoked somatosensory potential is recorded from the sensory cortex, and its mirror image is recorded from the motor cortex. The risk of seizure with this approach is low, and if a seizure occurs, irrigation with ice-cold Ringer lactate solution can quickly stop the seizure. These same techniques can also be used in the awake patient. Nevertheless, there are potential problems. For a space-occupying lesion, the neuronal pathways can become distorted secondary to the expanding mass and mislead the surgeon who is searching not only for the functional area but also a "quiet" area of the cortex through which to do the resection. In addition, patients are frequently in a lateral decubitus position, with the side to be observed in the down position, obscuring small motor responses. Visualization of the patient can be further obstructed with sheets, blankets, forced warm-air blankets, and other patient-positioning devices. Hence, the motor cortex is usually mapped during an awake craniotomy whenever possible, and mMEPs are monitored simultaneously. In cases involving complex sensory or motor activities such as language comprehension or speech production, current electrophysiologic and imaging techniques remain limited compared to the awake and interactive patient.

Supratentorial brain tumors are about 31% gliomas, 15% meningiomas, 12% metastatic lesions, and 8% pituitary tumors (**Figure 20.1**). Metastatic lesions are most frequently lung, breast, or gastrointestinal tract tumors. Additional space-occupying lesions include blood and blood vessels, infections, hydrocephalus, cerebral infarctions, radiation necrosis, arachnoid cysts, and cerebral edema. Several of these often coexist depending on the primary pathology of the lesion.

The most common presentations for brain tumors are a progressive neurologic deficit (68%), usually motor weakness (45%), headache (54%), and seizures (26%). Others present as progressive focal deficits resulting from infiltration of tumor cells and destruction of normal brain cytoarchitecture or compression or displacement of normal brain structures by the mass itself or peritumoral edema. Additional presentations include nausea, vomiting, vertigo, lethargy, apathy, and changes in mental status.

In addition to these presenting signs and symptoms, asymmetric supratentorial tumors can enlarge to the point of causing a midline shift of the intracranial contents, possibly leading to brain herniation. The brain can be displaced across the midline beneath the falx or compressed through the tentorial incisura into the posterior fossa. As the brain is compressed against these dense fibrous structures, stretching and shearing of penetrating arteries can result in devastating neurologic injuries.

An area of cerebral edema surrounds most intracranial masses secondary to the disruption of the blood-brain barrier (BBB) and is usually associated with localized acidosis. Vasogenic edema reflects a shift of fluid from the intravascular to the extravascular space, which is the interstitial space of the brain. Cytotoxic edema represents a shift of fluid from the extracellular to the intracellular space. Vasogenic edema responds very well to corticosteroid treatment, usually dexamethasone. This area of cerebral edema is known as the penumbral area and represents areas of autoregulatory dysfunction as well as BBB breakdown. The vasculature in this area of the brain is usually maximally vasodilated. Hypercapnia in the surrounding normal brain causes vasodilation in the normal vasculature and could result in decreased flow to the ischemic area due to a steal phenomenon. Hypocapnia, on the other hand, causes vasoconstriction of the normal adjacent vascular beds, with the resultant redistribution of blood to the ischemic area, referred to as the "Robin Hood" phenomenon or "inverse steal." The formation of peritumoral edema increases the overall size of the tumor, which can lead to or exacerbate the signs and symptoms noted earlier. Such was the case in our patient (**Figure 20.1**), who had a tumor with much vasogenic edema and who had a dramatic improvement in symptoms after dexamethasone therapy.

Patients presenting for awake craniotomy for excision of epileptic foci have usually had a seizure disorder for many years and have been on numerous antiepileptic drugs (AEDs) in an attempt to control their seizures. Many of these patients develop adverse reactions or cannot tolerate the side effects of the AEDs and become medication failures. **Table 20.1** lists the more common AEDs and the types of seizure disorders they are used to treat.

Only patients with seizures in whom the foci are localized in an area of the eloquent cortex require an awake craniotomy. Temporal lobe and hippocampal foci are usually resected under general anesthesia

TABLE 20.1 Commonly Used Drugs in Seizure Control

Type of Seizure	First-Line Drug	Second-Line Drug
Generalized tonic-clonic	Carbamazepine Phenytoin Valproate Levetiracetam	Clobazam Clonazepam Lamotrigine Phenobarbital Vigabatrin Felbamate Acetazolamide
Generalized absence	Valproate Ethosuximide	Clonazepam Lamotrigine Acetazolamide
Tonic, atonic, atypical absences	Valproate Clobazam Clonazepam Lamotrigine Phenytoin	Carbamazepine Phenobarbital Felbamate Acetazolamide
Myoclonic seizures	Valproate Clonazepam	Phenobarbital Acetazolamide Levetiracetam
Simple partial, complex partial, secondarily generalized	Carbamazepine Valproate Phenytoin Levetiracetam	Clobazam Lamotrigine Gabapentin Vigabatrin Phenobarbital Felbamate Acetazolamide

SECTION 4

with intraoperative electrocorticography. Most of these patients have had preceding intracranial strips, grids, or electrodes placed to help localize the seizure foci.

Cedzich C, Taniguchi M, Schafer S, Schramm J. Somatosensory evoked potential phase reversal and direct motor cortex stimulation during surgery in and around the central region. *Neurosurgery* 1996;38:962-970.

Fishman RA. Brain edema. *N Engl J Med.* 1975;293:706-711.

Greenburg MS. Tumors of the Nervous and Related Systems. In: Greenburg MS ed. Greenburg's *Handbook of Neurosurgery*. 10th ed. Thieme; 2023.

Kawaguchi M, Iida H, Tanaka S, et al. A practical guide for anesthetic management during intraoperative motor evoked potential monitoring. *J Anesth* 2020;34:5-28.

O'Rourke DK, Oldfield EH. Supratentorial masses: surgical considerations. In: Cottrell JE, Patel P, eds. *Cottrell and Patel's Neuroanesthesia*. 6th ed. Elsevier; 2017:298-316.

A.3. What determines intracranial pressure (ICP)?

The adult skull is a rigid bony structure with a fixed volume. Neonatal and infant skulls have several noncalcified portions, called fontanels, which allow the skull to deform during passage through the birth canal. These noncalcified areas also allow the volume of the skull to increase in the presence of increased ICP such as in congenital hydrocephalus. Once these areas have calcified, the pediatric skull is also a rigid, fixed-volume structure.

The intracranial constituents are intravascular blood, CSF, and the brain. As liquids, the blood and CSF are noncompressible but can be redistributed outside of the intracranial space. Although water can be extracted from the brain using osmotic diuretics and other hypertonic fluids, this does not result in much change in brain volume, which is also virtually incompressible, yet both movable and deformable, often resulting in irreversible damage. The brain can also be redistributed pathologically outside the intracranial vault by uncal herniation.

ICP reflects the balance of the noncompressible cranial contents within a fixed-volume container, the skull. The normal value is 10 to 15 mm Hg. In the early 19th century, the Monro-Kellie hypothesis was the first attempt to describe this relationship. Although several modifications have been made, the basic principle still holds: Because the intact skull is unyielding, an increase in the volume of any one of the normal contents or the addition of a space-occupying lesion must be accompanied by a reduction in one or more of the normal constituents to maintain normal ICP.

Matsumoto M, Yamashita A. Effects of Anesthetic Agents and other Drugs on Cerebral Blood Flow, Metabolism, and Intracranial Pressure. In: Cottrell JE, Patel PM, Soriano S eds. *Cottrell and Patel's Neuroanesthesia*, 7th ed. Elsevier; 2024.

Mokri B. The Monro-Kellie hypothesis: applications in CSF volume depletion. *Neurology*. 2001;56:1746-1748.

A.4. How does a space-occupying mass alter ICP?

There are limits to the balanced relationship described by the Monro-Kellie hypothesis. Figure 20.2 represents an idealized ICP-volume curve that diagrams these limitations.

The flat portion of the curve represents increasing volume with no increase in ICP. Several compensatory mechanisms are at work to keep the ICP stable. The most effective of these mechanisms is the dynamic nature of CSF. The rate of absorption increases or the rate of production decreases in light of an increase in ICP. Cerebral blood volume (CBV) is decreased by a redistribution primarily of intracranial venous blood volume. These mechanisms work to keep ICP in its normal range of 10 to 15 mm Hg. As volume continues to increase, these compensatory mechanisms become exhausted, and ICP starts to rise as represented by the "knee" of the graph. In this area of the curve, small increases in volume give rise to a much larger increase in ICP. The sharp rise demonstrates rapidly increasing ICP with even smaller increases in volume. As volume continues to rise and ICP continues to increase, the risk of cerebral herniation also increases. An acute rise in ICP is often a localized increase in intracranial volume associated with the underlying pathologic process with a corresponding localized increase in ICP producing a vectorial force and resulting in movement of the brain. Cerebral perfusion pressure (CPP) is also adversely affected by a rise in ICP. CPP is defined as CPP = MAP − ICP (or CVP, depending on which is higher), where MAP = mean arterial pressure and CVP = central venous pressure. MAP, for the purposes of calculating CPP, is measured at the tragus. Implicit in this measurement is that the position of the head relative to the heart can dramatically affect these estimates. This equation also shows that an increase in ICP leads to a decrease in CPP if MAP does not increase to maintain CPP. However, an increase in MAP is one of the normal physiologic compensatory mechanisms to maintain CPP and hence brain perfusion. Yet, there are many common clinical situations where this compensatory response has been blunted by preexisting comorbid conditions, acute injury, or drugs (eg, large doses of propofol).

Figure 20.3 shows that CBF is *independent* of MAP over a range of pressures from 50 to 150 mm Hg. CBF is determined by the metabolic demands of the brain. Here, the CBF is dynamically increased or decreased to accommodate the changing electrical activity of the brain and the associated metabolic processes. Some have advocated that the lower threshold for autoregulation should be shifted toward 70 mm Hg and the upper threshold shifted toward 180 mm Hg. In the supine position, ICP is effectively zero when the dura is opened, making CPP directly related to MAP (at least for structures adjacent to the open dura).

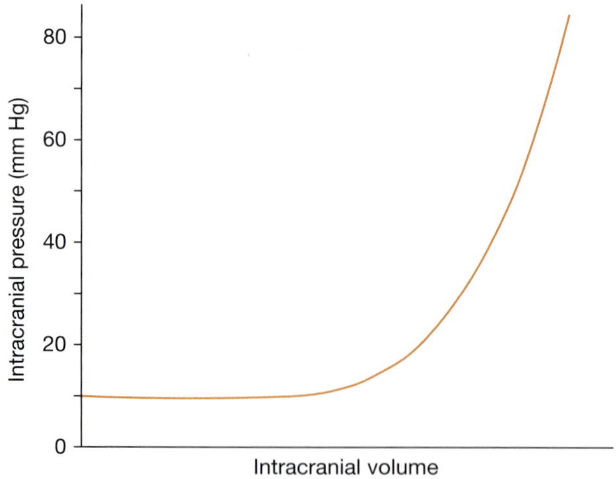

FIGURE 20.2. Idealized intracranial pressure-volume curve. (Reprinted with permission from Hou YJ, Kass IS. Physiology and metabolism of the brain and spinal cord. In: Newfield P, Cottrell JE, eds. *Handbook of Neuroanesthesia*. 5th ed. Wolters Kluwer; 2012:16.)

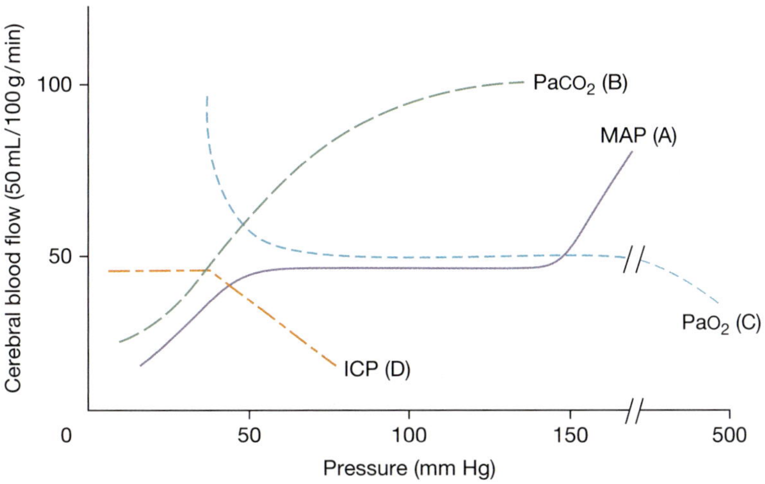

FIGURE 20.3. Pressure-cerebral blood flow relationships. A. Cerebral blood flow (CBF) autoregulation. CBF is maintained at 50 mL/100 g/min for mean arterial pressure (MAP)/cerebral perfusion pressure (CPP) = 50 to 150 mm Hg; **B.** Linear relationship between $Paco_2$ and CBF for $Paco_2$ = 20 to 80 mm Hg; **C.** Pao_2, and CBF; **D.** Intracranial pressure (ICP) and CBF. (Reprinted with permission from Hou YJ, Ravussin PA. Anesthesia for supratentorial tumors. In: Newfield P, Cottrell JE, eds. *Handbook of Neuroanesthesia.* 5th ed. Wolters Kluwer; 2012:118.)

A.5. What is autoregulation, and why is it important?

Autoregulation is a dynamic myogenic response of the vascular smooth muscle of the intracranial cerebral arterioles to maintain a nearly constant CBF in the face of changing CPP. Not all of the mechanisms controlling this action are fully understood.

When MAP is less than 50 mm Hg or greater than 150 mm Hg, CBF becomes pressure passive. This response is important to keep in mind when considering the use of deliberate hypotension. MAP of less than 50 mm Hg could theoretically cause a decrease in CPP and thereby decrease CBF to the point of causing cerebral ischemia. On the other hand, MAP of greater than 150 mm Hg can cause disruption of the BBB and vasogenic edema of the brain, not only in the area of vasogenic edema surrounding the tumor.

The autoregulation curve is shifted to the right in the presence of chronic uncontrolled hypertension, as shown in Figure 20.4. This is important because now the lower threshold for cerebral ischemia is higher than in the normal state. Although there is not a direct correlation between the degree of hypertension and

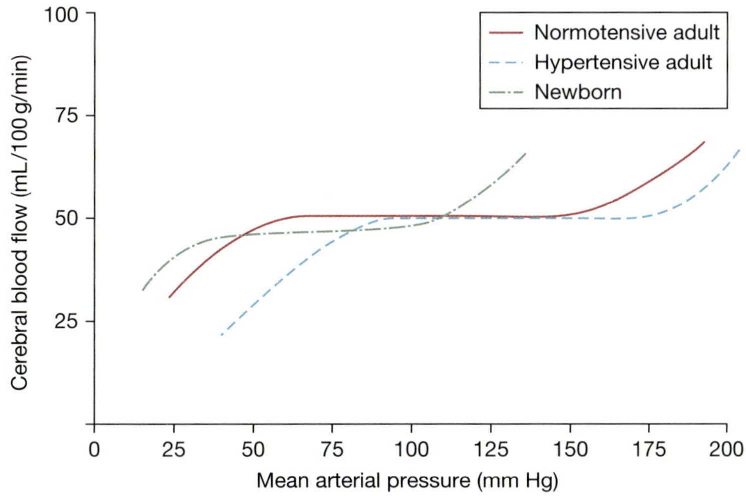

FIGURE 20.4. Autoregulatory curve of the cerebral vasculature in the normotensive adult, hypertensive adult, and newborn. (Reprinted with permission from Hou YJ, Ravussin PA. Anesthesia for supratentorial tumors. In: Newfield P, Cottrell JE, eds. *Handbook of Neuroanesthesia.* 5th ed. Wolters Kluwer; 2012:15.)

a rightward shift of the autoregulatory curve, it is possible that where signs of cerebral ischemia might not have become obvious until the CPP was 30 to 40 mm Hg in a normotensive person, these signs now occur with a CPP of 80 to 90 mm Hg, usually a normal CPP. Therefore, great care must be taken to keep MAP near the patient's usual range in uncontrolled or poorly controlled hypertensive patients. On the other end of the curve, it is possible that the rightward shift adds some form of cerebral protection against perfusion breakthrough at the higher CPPs. Chronic treatment with antihypertensive drugs modifies this rightward shift back toward the normal range. The degree to which this occurs depends both on the length of time the hypertension has been treated and the resultant decrease in blood pressure.

The type of drug used to treat hypertension can also determine the effect on autoregulation. Systemic direct-acting vasodilators without action on cerebrovascular smooth muscle and α-adrenergic and ganglionic blocking drugs should have no effect on cerebrovascular autoregulation. Systemic direct-acting vasodilators that also have an action on the cerebrovascular smooth muscle, such as hydralazine, sodium nitroprusside, nitroglycerin, and calcium channel blockers, can influence autoregulation. Treating congestive heart failure might also improve CPP by lowering CVP, thereby decreasing cerebral venous outflow pressure.

Drummond JC. The lower limit of autoregulation: time to revise our thinking? *Anesthesiology*. 1997;86:1431-1433.

Ellis JA, Joshi S. Cerebral and Spinal Cord Blood Flow. In: Cottrell JE, Patel PM, Soriano S eds. *Cottrell and Patel's Neuroanesthesia*, 7th ed. Elsevier; 2024.

Hoiland RL, Fisher JA, Ainslie PN. Regulation of the cerebral circulation by arterial carbon dioxide. *Compr Physiol.* 2019;9:1101-1154.

Lemkuil BP, Drummond JC, Patel PM, et al. Anesthesia for Neurologic Surgery and Neurointerventions. In: Gropper MA, Miller RD, eds. *Miller's Anesthesia*, 10th ed. Elsevier; 2025.

Paulson OB, Strandgaard S, Edvinsson L. Cerebral autoregulation. *Cerebrovasc Brain Metab Rev*. 1990;2:161-192.

A.6. How is cerebral blood flow (CBF) regulated?

In addition to metabolic demand, CBF responds to modulation by dissolved gases. **Figure 20.3** demonstrates these relationships in arterial carbon dioxide partial pressure ($Paco_2$) and arterial oxygen partial pressure (Pao_2) curves. Carbon dioxide (CO_2) concentration is the most potent modulator of CBF. Insonating the middle cerebral artery of a volunteer by means of a transcranial Doppler device and asking the subject to hyperventilate will show an increase in cerebral blood velocity, reflecting a decrease in CBF secondary to cerebral vascular constriction, usually within 3 to 4 breaths. This principle is utilized to treat increased ICP by decreasing CBV secondary to hyperventilation. However, this mechanism is self-limited after 6 to 10 hours and will no longer reduce ICP.

As shown in **Figure 20.3**, there is a near-linear response in CBF at a $Paco_2$ between 20 and 80 mm Hg, with CBF increasing about 2% to 4% for each mm Hg change in $Paco_2$. In general, doubling $Paco_2$ from 40 to 80 mm Hg doubles CBF and likewise halving $Paco_2$ from 40 to 20 mm Hg halves CBF. This represents maximal vasodilation at extreme hypercapnia and maximal vasoconstriction at extreme hypocapnia, respectively.

CBF also responds to Pao_2. As shown in **Figure 20.3**, when Pao_2 reaches approximately 50 mm Hg, a steep increase in CBF occurs as Pao_2 continues to fall. At normal Pao_2 levels, CBF is not affected. Hyperoxia can actually cause a 10% to 15% decrease in CBF at 1 atm. Temperature can also affect CBF: for each 1 °C decrease in body temperature, the cerebral metabolic rate for oxygen consumption ($CMRO_2$) decreases by approximately 7%. The regulation of CBF is closely coupled to the cerebral metabolism and is reflected by a parallel decrease. These changes are not homogeneous, with more changes seen in the cerebral and cerebellar cortices, less so in the thalamus, and no difference in the hypothalamus and brainstem. During hypothermic cardiopulmonary bypass, lowering body temperature to 26 °C results in a 56% calculated reduction in $CMRO_2$ and a 55% reduction in CBF.

The potent inhalational anesthetics can also increase CBF in the presence of decreasing $CMRO_2$, thus uncoupling their relationship. Increasing doses can also blunt the CO_2 response or render CBF pressure passive. CO_2 reactivity is preserved during intraoperative use of opioids including fentanyl and remifentanil.

Cottrell JE, Patel PM. Brain Metabolism, Pathophysiology, and Potential Beneficial Agents. In: Cottrell JE, Patel PM eds. *Cottrell and Patel's Neuroanesthesia*, 7th ed; Elsevier. 2024.

Govier AV, Reves JG, McKay RD, et al. Factors and their influence on regional cerebral blood flow during nonpulsatile cardiopulmonary bypass. *Ann Thorac Surg*. 1984;38:592-600.

A.7. What drug therapies can be associated with this pathology?

Patients can present with intracranial pathology at any age. Patients with comorbidities can be taking medications for hypertension, diabetes, congestive heart failure, atrial fibrillation, prior myocardial infarction (MI), and reactive airway disease with and without chronic obstructive pulmonary disease (COPD) as examples. It is not uncommon today for many patients with cardiac comorbidities to be on anticoagulation and also some form of antiplatelet drug, whether they have suffered an MI or not. These chronic comorbid conditions should be well treated and relatively stable, with the coagulation system reconstituted prior to undertaking an awake procedure. The success of the procedure is critically dependent on a compensated and stable cardiopulmonary system and an expectation of relatively small blood loss (<500 mL). The effects of some of these drugs can be reversed, whereas others are not immediately reversible and need 7 to 10 days before their effect is gone.

Patients with epilepsy can be on several medications in an attempt to control their seizures. These drugs are listed in **Table 20.1**. Presenting signs and symptoms have been described earlier. AEDs are indicated in 26% of patients presenting with seizures who are later diagnosed with a brain tumor.

Another 20% to 45% of patients with brain tumors will eventually develop a seizure after diagnosis. The current standard is that prophylactic AEDs should not be started in this group of patients. In patients with brain tumors undergoing craniotomy, prophylactic AEDs can be used, and if there is no seizure activity, they can be tapered, starting 1 week postoperatively. If initiated at the time of surgery, they should be administered early in the procedure because they often have sedating properties and can delay awakening.

As previously discussed, most intracranial mass lesions are surrounded by an area of vasogenic edema to varying extents. Steroids, in particular dexamethasone, are commonly used to treat this. Dexamethasone is more beneficial, and the effect of reducing the area of edema is often much more dramatic in metastatic tumors than in primary tumors. The usual dosage in the corticosteroid-naive patient is a loading dose of 10 mg IV and then 4 to 6 mg by mouth or IV every 6 hours. Doses of up to 10 mg every 4 hours have been given for severe vasogenic edema. For the patient previously diagnosed and on corticosteroids, the current dose is doubled for acute deterioration.

Greenberg MS. General information, classification and tumor markers. In: Greenberg MS, ed. *Handbook of Neurosurgery*. 9th ed. Thieme; 2020:1113-1164.

Kanner AM, Ashman E, Gloss D, et al. Practice guideline update summary: efficacy and tolerability of the new antiepileptic drugs II: treatment-resistant epilepsy: report of the American Epilepsy Society and the Guideline Development, Dissemination, and Implementation Subcommittee of the American Academy of Neurology. *Epilepsy Curr.* 2018;18:269-278.

B. Preoperative Evaluation and Preparation

B.1. Why is the craniotomy performed awake?

Awake craniotomy is performed when the pathologic lesion, be it a tumor or an epileptic focus, is in or near an area of eloquent cortex, as defined earlier, in an effort to preserve neurologic function. Awake craniotomies are associated with improved survival, a greater extent of tumor resection, and fewer postoperative complications compared to those done under general anesthesia.

The extent of the craniotomy is variable. Some neurosurgeons advocate a carefully planned, limited-exposure craniotomy defined with neuronavigational devices to encompass primarily the area of the lesion and immediate surrounding brain. Others advocate a large craniotomy exposing a wide cortical area for mapping. In either case, the primary goal of the surgical procedure is to obtain the greatest degree of tumor resection with as little damage to the eloquent cortex as possible and hence the least postoperative neurologic deficit.

Even with the cortex exposed, there are many challenges in identifying the areas of eloquent cortex that demand an awake and cooperative patient. As a tumor within or near the eloquent cortex grows and expands, various neuronal pathways can become distorted from their normal anatomic locations. Ultrasonography can assist the neurosurgeon in identifying the lesion borders so testing can proceed in the surrounding areas of the cortex. Areas that do not elicit a response are also identified as areas of negative mapping and can serve as an entrance site for both cortical and subcortical resection as needed. Several studies have indicated that surgery through these areas of absolute negative mapping has a lower incidence of both intraoperative and postoperative neurologic deficits. There is also an increasing realization that there are more cortical areas that relate to an acceptable quality of life other than the areas of eloquent cortex. Nonlanguage areas that have to do with visual and vestibular functions, spatial awareness, cognitive function, understanding and judgment, memory, calculation, and emotion can be mapped both cortically and subcortically to help prevent postoperative complications that are usually not discussed or described.

De Benedictis A, Moritz-Gasser S, Duffau H. Awake mapping optimizes the extent of resection for low-grade gliomas in eloquent areas. *Neurosurgery*. 2010;66:1074-1084.

Duffau H. Awake surgery for nonlanguage mapping. *Neurosurgery*. 2010;66:523-529.

Gerritsen JKW, Zwarthoed RH, Kilgallon JL, et al. Effect of awake craniotomy in glioblastoma in eloquent areas (GLIOMAP): a propensity score-matched analysis of an international, multicentre, cohort study. *Lancet Oncol.* 2022;23:802-817.

Kim SS, McCutcheon IE, Suki D, et al. Awake craniotomy for brain tumors near eloquent cortex: correlation of intraoperative cortical mapping with neurological outcomes in 309 consecutive patients. *Neurosurgery*. 2009;64:836-846.

Sewell D, Smith M. Awake craniotomy: anesthetic considerations based on outcome evidence. *Curr Opin Anaesthesiol.* 2019;32:546-552.

B.2. What neurologic symptoms of the patient are important?

In order to complete an awake craniotomy, the patient must be motivated to undergo the demanding procedure and able to communicate effectively with the neurosurgeon, the neurologist or the speech pathologist, and the neuroanesthesiologist. The patient's ability to understand and execute a myriad of tasks, depending on the tumor's location, remains of paramount importance. In many cases, the patient must also be able to read short phrases, identify various objects, and describe pictures.

A patient who presents with some form of dysphasia might not be able to participate at all. Expressive dysphasia and global dysphasia are extreme examples but not uncommon presentations. At times, a short course of corticosteroids will decrease the penumbral area enough that verbal testing is practical. Some patients will present greatly agitated. Although this is usually their presenting symptom, they cannot cooperate in any fashion, even with minimal commands, and other means are necessary to care for these patients.

Areas of muscular weakness or paralysis, either from the current problem or past injury, must be identified preoperatively to differentiate between postoperative worsening and new neurologic deficits. Rarely will the patient show improvement in the immediate postoperative period; however, preexisting problems can actually be accentuated in the postoperative period. Overall, patients who cannot communicate effectively or cooperate are not appropriate candidates for an awake craniotomy.

In those patients with an ongoing seizure disorder associated with their tumor or epilepsy, the frequency and character of their ictal and postictal periods should be well understood. Limited seizures during mapping procedures are usually well tolerated if treated promptly. Patients with worsening seizures or generalized tonic-clonic seizures that are frequent are not ideal candidates for an awake procedure. The movements of the body while fixed in a rigid Mayfield frame, hemodynamic derangements, and altered control of the upper airway and ventilation associated with tonic-clonic seizures are potentially life-threatening. Failed awake procedures are associated with increased postoperative morbidity and reduction of gross total resection. Thus, the success of these procedures is critically dependent on appropriate patient selection and the experience of the anesthesia and surgical teams with the nuances of these procedures.

Kutteruf R, Yang JT, Hecker JG, Kinney GA, Furman MA, Sharma D. Incidence and risk factors for intraoperative seizures during elective craniotomy. *J Neurosurg Anesthesiol.* 2019;31:234-240.

Nossek E, Matot I, Shahar T, et al. Failed awake craniotomy: a retrospective analysis in 424 patients undergoing craniotomy for brain tumor. *J Neurosurg* 2013;118:243-249.

B.3. What is the status of their other comorbid conditions?

Aside from the symptoms associated with their neurologic condition, those associated with the patient's other comorbid conditions can limit the potential success of, and are a relative contraindication to, an awake procedure. This procedure requires the patient to lie in one position with little ability to move and "get comfortable" for a period of wakefulness of 2 to 4 hours and to remain "motionless" for the remainder of the procedure, typically requiring about 6 to 8 hours of stable hemodynamics and adequate ventilation with an unsecured airway. This represents both psychological stress and physiologic stress. There are five common areas of comorbidity to consider when evaluating the fitness of a patient for this procedure: morbid obesity, pulmonary, cardiac, chronic pain, and psychiatric disorders. Patient who is morbidly obese with a body mass index (BMI) greater than 40 presents significant challenges in positioning without incurring skin breakdown and maintenance of upper airway patency with functional obstructive sleep apnea or hypoventilation syndromes. Poor upper airway control, rocking-shaking ventilatory effort, and inability to maintain normocarbia all pose significant challenges. Much of this can be ameliorated with the use of airway adjuncts such as a nasal trumpet. Similarly, COPD, particularly with CO_2 retention, complicates CO_2 management. Together, these conditions lead to cerebral vasodilation and increased CBV. Elevations of CO_2 are particularly detrimental for patients with pulmonary hypertension, especially those with right heart strain. Thus, monitoring end-tidal CO_2 to help ensure the adequacy of ventilation and minimize CO_2 rebreathing during the initial stages of the procedure is important.

Cardiac arrhythmias such as atrial fibrillation with poor ventricular rate control and poorly or uncontrolled hypertension both place the patient at increased risk for untoward hypotension or hypertension, respectively. Exacerbations of congestive heart failure or ischemic heart disease require further treatment prior to the procedure. Patients with chronic pain pose a special dilemma, especially those on chronic opioid therapy. The short-term management of their chronic pain during the procedure remains problematic because opioids are usually spared to avoid oversedation and hypoventilation. However, this can be addressed with low-dose remifentanil infusion. Paramount to the success of the procedure is the awake and communicative patient; preexisting psychiatric conditions that impair calm and focused attention will not improve under the conditions of this procedure.

B.4. Are there anesthetic implications from current treatment drugs?

AEDs currently available for treating patients with seizure disorders or those secondary to a brain tumor are listed in **Table 20.1**. Many of these drugs, such as benzodiazepines, hydantoin analogues, and phenytoin, can interfere with hepatic drug metabolism, requiring increased dosages of IV anesthetic agents and opioids.

Potential side effects associated with corticosteroid use include increased white blood cell count, glucose intolerance, corticosteroid "stress ulcers," corticosteroid-induced psychosis, hypertension, water and electrolyte imbalance, suppression of the hypothalamic-pituitary-adrenal axis, weight gain, infection, and impaired wound healing.

B.5. What laboratory data are required?

Although the current practice is to minimize the number of preoperative laboratory tests obtained, several are necessary for the patient undergoing a craniotomy, awake or under general anesthesia, for tumor or epileptic foci resection.

Coagulation studies are required. Although some tumors can have a significant amount of blood loss associated with their resection (meningioma), bleeding from an abnormal coagulation system into a tumor bed can pose serious and life-threatening problems. Partial thromboplastin time, prothrombin time, international normalized ratio, fibrinogen level, and platelet count are routinely obtained. If patients have been on novel oral anticoagulant therapy (eg, dabigatran, rivaroxaban, apixaban), there are no routine standardized laboratory studies to quantify the drug effect. Institution-specific approaches to monitoring anticoagulation with these drugs should be available in consultation with a hematologist. In patients who are or have recently taken clopidogrel or other antiplatelet adenosine diphosphate inhibitors, a platelet activity test is beneficial. This test requires specialized equipment and might be done only at certain times of the day or require prenotification to the laboratory. Some AEDs can cause thrombocytopenia, but leukopenia is more common.

Electrolyte studies are necessary. This patient population can have imbalances from substances secreted by the tumor, such as atrial natriuretic factor, or secondary to drug effects, such as hyponatremia or hypokalemia. Blood glucose levels should ideally be controlled to 120 to 180 mg/dL, and hypoglycemia (<55 mg/dL) should be avoided. Complete blood count with differential will give information about the hematocrit and white blood cell count. The differential will be normal if the white blood cell count is elevated from degranulation caused by preoperative corticosteroids. If not, an infection might be present and must be addressed. A routine urinalysis will rule out asymptomatic urinary tract infection.

Blood type, antibody screen, and crossmatch are also required. In the case of a positive antibody screen, at least 4 units of crossmatched blood are recommended to be available before starting the procedure. Transfusion during awake craniotomy is uncommon because these lesions are usually small. Nevertheless, if it becomes necessary, the need will be immediate. For a negative antibody screen, 2 units of blood readily available is acceptable.

Depending on comorbidities, an electrocardiogram (ECG) can be obtained.

B.6. What radiology data should be reviewed?

Reviewing the most recently obtained MRI or computed tomography (CT) scans can provide a great deal of insight into intracranial pathology. Characteristics of the tumor, such as ring enhancement, cystic or lobulated nature, or variously weighted CT studies, give the neuroradiologist and neurosurgeon some insight into the diagnosis of the tumor as well as the location of the lesion. The location of the lesion might correlate with the presenting symptoms. Vasogenic edema is readily seen, and the progress of resolution with corticosteroids is possible by reviewing a series of CT scans since presentation. Additional information can be gained but is not always present for the smaller lesions usually associated with awake craniotomy. A midline shift would be evidence of increased ICP, as would the loss of sulci and gyri, not to mention the presence of uncal or subfalcine herniation (**Figure 20.5**). The presence of hydrocephalus from blockage of CSF pathways is also readily seen and could be a source of increased ICP. Previous areas of stroke are usually easily visualized and need to be noted. There should be no hesitation in calling on the neuroradiologist or neurosurgeon to point out the pathology and their major concerns. Important considerations are lesion size and how much work needs to be done to provide safe and effective brain relaxation. The neuroanesthesiologist can never overcommunicate with the neurosurgeon.

B.7. How do you prepare the patient for an awake craniotomy?

The most important preparation is proper patient selection, as alluded to earlier. A patient who cannot effectively communicate and cooperate will not do well with this procedure, regardless of how well everything else is done.

The need for an awake craniotomy is usually first broached by the neurosurgeon during the workup. It is not unusual then to have a rather concerned and anxious patient arrive in the preanesthetic clinic. Ideally, the neuroanesthesiologist who will provide intraoperative care will conduct the interview, although this is not always possible. The neuroanesthesiologist must make every effort to see the patient well before the patient arrives in the operating room. In either case, a direct and detailed explanation of what will happen should be provided. Assure the patient that adequate means will be taken to control pain and that they can ask for more medications if needed, given the limitation of needing to remain awake and cooperative. Also discuss additional IV lines, invasive monitors if necessary and why they are used, and when they will be placed.

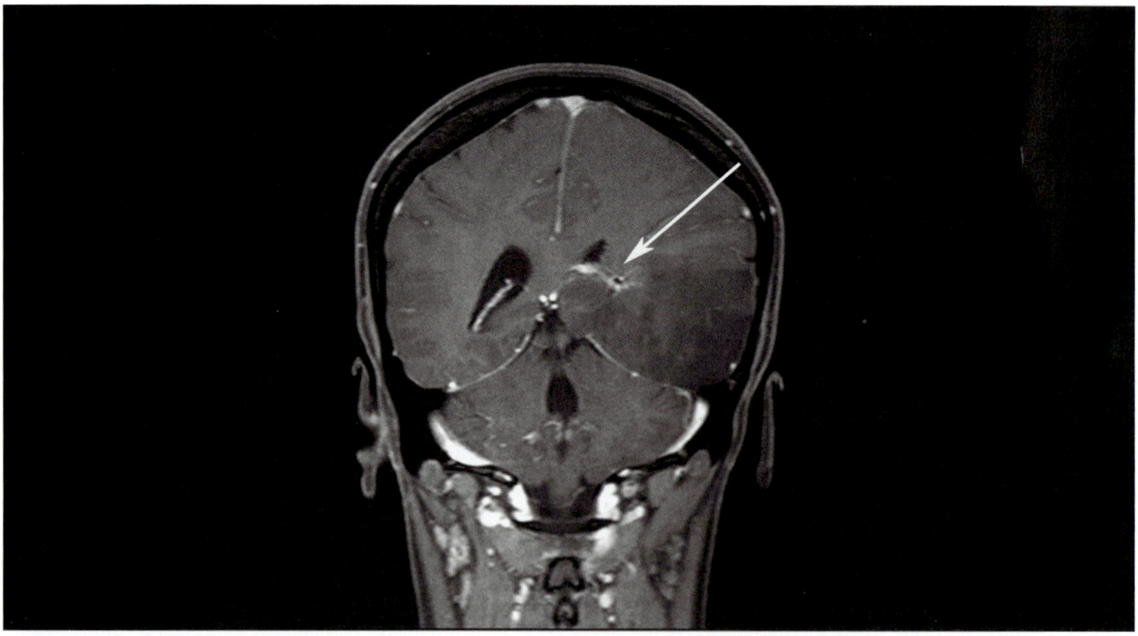

FIGURE 20.5. MRI scan of a 29-year-old female with a 2-week history of word-finding difficulty and no other symptoms. Note the significant uncal herniation (*arrow*). The patient underwent an uneventful left awake craniotomy with language area mapping and was discharged home the next day. Final pathology revealed WHO grade III anaplastic oligoastrocytoma. MRI, magnetic resonance imaging; WHO, World Health Organization.

A discussion about the anesthetic itself is essential. Usually, if patients have a good understanding of the sequence of the procedure and that they may not be exactly fully awake for the entire time they are in the operating room, they are more at ease. Describe everything in detail. This may be the first surgical procedure they have had.

B.8. Should this patient receive premedication?

Any premedication that might affect the ability to map the cortex intraoperatively is contraindicated. This includes medications that might cause prolonged sedation, and in the case of epilepsy, surgery can interfere with intraoperative intracranial electrocorticography to define epileptic foci. Benzodiazepines and barbiturates should be avoided for these reasons. A calm and reassuring neuroanesthesiologist is usually the best "premedication." The placement of invasive monitors, when necessary, is covered in Section C.2, paragraph 7.

Other premedications are those taken for preexisting conditions, including antihypertensives, antiarrhythmics, bronchodilators, and so on, as would be standard practice at the institution, with the exception of anxiolytics, short- and long-acting opioids, aspirin, and nonsteroidal anti-inflammatory drugs. Patients on AEDs for tumor-related seizures should take their AED prior to the procedure. Patients with epilepsy as their primary diagnosis should follow the neurosurgeon's instruction on taking their AED. Often, these medications are held prior to surgery to help with intraoperative electrocorticography.

B.9. What precautions should be taken for airway management?

Airway evaluation is extremely important in this patient population. The head will most likely be fixed in a three-pronged device, making the ability to intubate the trachea by direct laryngoscopy virtually impossible. Further limitations include the surgical drapes and the instrument table, which often extend over the patient completely. The patient is often positioned in the lateral decubitus position, making moving the patient to a flat position time-consuming, if possible, at all. Patient's body habitus can also make tracheal intubation challenging in the nonsupine position. Patients who are obese and those who are morbidly obese also present challenges; edentulous patients have bone erosion of both the maxilla and mandible that could make mask ventilation difficult in any position. Patients on phenytoin can have rather impressive gingival hypertrophy and associated bleeding that can interfere with intubation; teeth can be loose and easily displaced. These problems can make the placement of an airway or laryngeal mask airway (LMA) difficult or impossible. The use of an LMA or endotracheal intubation for these cases is for some the preferred method.

Having an airway cart immediately available and prepared for a fiberoptic intubation with an assorted and readily available selection of LMAs is recommended. At baseline, a nasal cannula for oxygen delivery and CO_2 measurement should be placed before starting sedation. The maintenance of a patent airway is often facilitated by the placement of a nasal trumpet after sedation and can be removed while the patient is awake for testing.

C. Intraoperative Management

C.1. How should this patient be monitored?

Monitoring should be in accordance with the guidelines of the American Society of Anesthesiologists, including pulse oximetry, electrocardiography, noninvasive blood pressure monitoring, capnography, and temperature measurement as a minimum.

American Society of Anesthesiologists. Standards for basic anesthetic monitoring. Accessed January 21 , 2025. https://www.asahq.org/standards-and-practice- parameters/standards-for-basic-anesthetic-monitoring

C.2. Does this patient require invasive monitoring?

For awake craniotomy, invasive blood pressure monitoring is not an absolute requirement, but should be placed in patients with comorbid conditions who would regularly receive invasive arterial monitoring. Such monitoring might be considered a local "standard of care" as a matter of institutional preference; however, its use intraoperatively can facilitate postoperative management. Blood pressure measurement with an oscillometric device can be problematic in patients with atrial fibrillation; it also overestimates both systolic and diastolic blood pressure readings in patients with stiff arteries, such as in diabetes. Patients with diabetes might also require frequent blood glucose measurements, and the presence of an arterial line facilitates this. In several of the comorbid diseases of particular concern (eg, obesity, COPD, pulmonary hypertension), the objective data of interest is $Paco_2$, and arterial sampling offers the most reliable method, although this could be accomplished with the measurement of venous CO_2. Lastly, an arterial line can be placed for comfort, as a regular inflation of a blood pressure cuff can be distracting to some patients. In this case, a radial arterial line can be placed in the arm that will not be involved in testing. A central venous line (CVL) for pressure measurement is not required in the awake patient, but venous access can be so poor that one needs to be placed for that purpose. The best monitoring system for this case is the awake, cooperative patient.

Lemkuil BP, Drummond JC, Patel PM, et al. Anesthesia for Neurologic Surgery and Neurointerventions. In: Gropper MA, Miller RD, eds. *Miller's Anesthesia*, 10th ed. Elsevier; 2025.

van Popele NM, Bos WJ, de Beer NA, et al. Arterial stiffness as underlying mechanism of disagreement between an oscillometric blood pressure monitor and a sphygmomanometer. *Hypertension*. 2000;36:484-488.

C.3. Can current drug therapy alter eloquent cortex mapping?

For mapping of the language areas, any drug that causes long-lasting, deep sedation, as discussed earlier, would be contraindicated. Patients presenting with new onset of seizures associated with the new diagnosis of brain tumor might have been started on any one or several of the AEDs listed in **Table 20.1**. These drugs can interfere with the mapping of the eloquent cortex. In patients undergoing epilepsy surgery, these drugs are usually stopped several days in advance so as not to interfere with intraoperative electrocorticography or placing of electrodes directly on the surface of the exposed brain. Corticosteroids and opioids do not interfere, but propofol can produce a pattern of high-frequency, high-amplitude β activity on the electroencephalogram for at least 20 minutes, which can cloud the abnormal activity being sought and should be stopped appropriately.

C.4. Why are hypertonic fluids used during a craniotomy?

The intact brain, primarily the BBB, acts as an osmometer. Water can freely cross this semipermeable membrane in response to osmotic pressures created by dissolved solutes until there is equal osmotic pressure across the membrane. This is a function of the number of osmotically active, dissolved solutes present in a solution: the greater the number of osmotically active solutes, the greater the osmolarity or osmotic activity of the solution. *Osmolarity* is defined as osmoles per liter of fluid and is a calculated value. *Osmolality* is one of the four colligative properties of a solution, is defined as osmoles per kilogram of fluid, and is a measured value, usually by the freezing point depression method.

Table 20.2 lists several commonly used IVFs and compares their osmolarity and osmolality. The osmolality is lower secondary to the presence of undissociated solutes in the solution. When solutes are given intravenously, the intact BBB prevents polar solutes from crossing into the brain, thus sequestering them to the intracranial intravascular space and creating a high vascular osmotic pressure, with resultant movement of free water from the brain into the vascular space. This reduces brain bulk, which can provide better visualization of the tumor, and hopefully decreases the need to apply retractors to the brain surface to enhance visualization. This in turn minimizes ischemic injury to the brain directly under the retractors

TABLE 20.2 Osmotic Values of Common Intravenous Fluids

Fluid	Osmolarity (mOsm/L)	Osmolality (mOsm/kg)
Water	0	0
5% Dextrose (D_5W)	252	259
Normal saline	308	282
Lactated Ringer	273	250
3% Saline	1,027	921
6% Hetastarch	310	307
20% Mannitol	1,098	1,280
5% Albumin	290	283
Normosol-R	294	281
D_5W/0.2 NaCl	325	321

D_5W, 5% dextrose in water; D_5W/0.2 NaCl, 5% dextrose and 0.2% sodium chloride.

and decreases ICP in the intact brain. Intravascular proteins create a much smaller oncotic pressure in the intracranial vasculature than do the dissolved solutes, secondary to the intact BBB, and play a lesser role than they do in the peripheral circulation, where they are the primary determinant of fluid moving from extravascular to intravascular.

Biel S, Vagnerova K. Fluid Management During Craniotomy. In: Cottrell JE, Patel PM eds. *Cottrell and Patel's Neuroanesthesia*. 7th ed. Elsevier; 2024.

Cerebral Blood Flow, cerebrospinal fluid, and brain metabolism. In: Hall JE, Hall M, eds. *Guyton and Hall Textbook of Medical Physiology*. 14th ed. Elsevier; 2020.

C.5. What intravenous fluids (IVFs) are recommended?

Commonly used IVFs during craniotomy include 0.9% saline, 3% saline, 20% mannitol, and 5% albumin.

Normal plasma osmolality is 285 to 295 mOsm/kg. Therefore, any solution with a higher osmolality could act to extract water from the brain. The exception to this is any solution containing 5% dextrose. These solutions have an effective osmolality of 259 mOsm less than the measured osmolality because glucose (osmolality 259 mOsm/kg) is rapidly transported intracellularly into neurons and glia and subsequently metabolized, resulting in an effective osmolality of 0, and 5% *dextrose*/0.2 NaCl has an effective osmolality of 62 mOsm/kg for example. Dextrose-containing solutions represent a very high concentration of potential free water within the intracranial intravascular space and result in water movement into the brain, causing an increase in ICP or brain bulk.

Hyperglycemia before or during an episode of cerebral ischemia worsens outcomes, although the mechanism is not clear. One hypothesis is that during a hyperglycemic episode, increased intraparenchymal glucose leads to lactic acid production during ischemia, which is thought to enhance neuronal death. Thus, solutions containing dextrose are not routinely used during intracranial surgery.

Mannitol 20% is the most widely used IVF for the treatment of elevated ICP. It also acts to decrease CSF production and as a scavenger of oxygen-free radicals. Mannitol should be given intravenously over 10 to 15 minutes to prevent sudden exposure of the cerebral circulation to extreme hyperosmolality (mannitol has an osmolality of 1,280 mOsm/kg), which could lead to a vasodilatory effect with resultant increased CBV, possible brain engorgement, and increased ICP. Increased urine output secondary to osmotic diuresis should be replaced with normal saline. The usual mannitol dose is 0.25 to 1 g/kg. Mannitol use is contraindicated in renal failure because it can exacerbate renal insufficiency, and in cases of severe oliguric renal failure, it accumulates in the intravascular space, leading to volume overload and pulmonary edema.

Hypertonic saline comes in a range of concentrations, with 3% being the most commonly used during intracranial surgery. A recent study showed no difference between equiosmolar mannitol and hypertonic saline infusions for providing brain relaxation.

Normal saline is the fluid of choice for intracranial procedures to cover fluid requirements and replace blood loss until red blood cells are required. A hyperchloremic, hypokalemic non–anion gap metabolic acidosis can occur when large volumes are given. This can mask other forms of acidosis and cloud the diagnostic picture. Lactated Ringer solution (osmolality 250 mOsm/kg) would not be an ideal replacement for blood loss, insensible loss, or third-space losses due to its lower osmolality. Colloids, in the form of 5% or 25% albumin, are rarely, if ever, needed in awake craniotomy.

Biel S, Vagnerova K. Fluid Management During Craniotomy. In: Cottrell JE, Patel PM eds. *Cottrell and Patel's Neuroanesthesia*, 7th ed. Elsevier; 2024.

Fandino W. Understanding the physiological changes induced by mannitol: from the theory to the clinical practice in neuroanesthesia. *J Neuroanesthesiol Crit Care*. 2017;4:138-146.

Lemkuil BP, Drummond JC, Patel PM, et al. Anesthesia for Neurologic Surgery and Neurointerventions. In: Gropper MA, Miller RD, eds. *Miller's Anesthesia*. 10th ed. Elsevier; 2025.

Myburgh J, Cooper J, Finfer S, et al. Saline or albumin for fluid resuscitation in patients with traumatic brain injury. *N Engl J Med*. 2007;357:874-884.

Rozet I, Tontisirin N, Muangman S, et al. Effect of equiosmolar solutions of mannitol versus hypertonic saline on intraoperative brain relaxation and electrolyte balance. *Anesthesiology*. 2007;107:697-704.

Suarez JI, Shannon I, Zaidat OO, et al. Effect of human albumin administration on clinical outcome and hospital cost in patients with subarachnoid hemorrhage. *J Neurosurg*. 2004;100:585-590.

C.6. Would a lumbar drain for cerebrospinal fluid (CSF) removal benefit this patient?

Lesions in the eloquent cortex are usually small, so a lumbar drain is not indicated. Neurosurgeons place a lumbar drain before the start of the surgery to allow CSF to be drained slowly, usually 10 mL/h, to decrease brain bulk. The drain can be placed in an "open" position when the time comes to open the dura, allowing for maximal brain relaxation and visualization in addition to preventing any intracranial contents from herniating through the craniotomy site.

Kirkman MA, Kumaria A, Smith M. Multimodal Neurological Monitoring. In: Cottrell JE, Patel PM eds. *Cottrell and Patel's Neuroanesthesia*. 7th ed. Elsevier; 2024.

Lemkuil BP, Drummond JC, Patel PM, et al. Anesthesia for Neurologic Surgery and Neurointerventions. In: Gropper MA, Miller RD, eds. *Miller's Anesthesia*. 10th ed. Elsevier; 2025.

C.7. Is venous air embolism (VAE) a concern in this case?

VAE is the entrainment of air into open, noncollapsible vascular structures located above the level of the heart. Thus, it is a concern in this case because the level of the surgical site meets this definition. VAE is usually associated with posterior fossa craniotomies and cervical spine surgery in the sitting position. Fatal VAE has been described with as little as 3 to 5 cm of surgical site elevation above the heart during lumbar spinal surgery using a four-poster support device in the prone position.

In this case, tumors are usually small and within the cortex, and the patient is supine or in a nearly horizontal lateral decubitus position. Parasagittal and falcine meningiomas encroaching on the posterior portion of the sagittal sinus are the most common situations for VAE. Fortunately, the eloquent cortical areas are not in this location. Nonetheless, VAE has been reported after pin head holder placement and after craniotomy but before dural opening. This implies that free air can be entrained through the diploic space of the skull unless adequately sealed during the cranial opening. This is usually done with wax. Therefore, VAE is a possibility during awake craniotomy.

Although transesophageal echocardiography is the most sensitive means of detecting VAE, it is impractical in the setting of awake craniotomy. A precordial Doppler device is the monitor of choice if the head is elevated above the level of the heart. When placed in the right or left parasternal region between the third and fourth ribs, Doppler ultrasonography has a high detection rate for VAE. The awake patient can experience an episode of paroxysmal coughing with entrainment of air. The best chance of aspirating a VAE is through a properly placed, multi-orifice central line that is positioned 2 cm below the superior vena caval–atrial junction by using intravascular ECG. Lead II is observed while the electrode of the catheter is attached to the leg lead. An equi-biphasic P wave indicates that the tip of the catheter is in the mid-atrial position.

If VAE is suspected, the surgeon must be immediately informed and the surgical field flooded with saline to help prevent further air entrainment. Jugular compression and lowering the head are also maneuvers to help stop air entrainment. If it is present, an attempt should be made to aspirate air through the CVL simultaneously with the surgeon addressing the surgical field. Vasopressors or inotropes are given to support hemodynamics and cardiopulmonary resuscitation initiated for cardiac arrest.

Albin MS, Ritter RR, Pruett CE, et al. Venous air embolism during lumbar laminectomy in the prone position: report of three cases. *Anesth Analg*. 1991;73:346-349.

Lemkuil BP, Drummond JC, Patel PM, et al. Anesthesia for Neurologic Surgery and Neurointerventions. In: Gropper MA, Miller RD, eds. *Miller's Anesthesia*. 10th ed. Elsevier; 2025.

Jellish WS, Murdoch J, Leonetti JP. Perioperative management of complex skull base surgery: the anesthesiologist's point of view. *Neurosurg Focus*. 2002;12:e5.

C.8. How is the eloquent cortex mapped?

Before the start of the case, a neurologist and/or speech pathologist will go over the intraoperative testing procedure with the patient. This usually consists of confrontational-type testing in which the patient may be asked to count. At other times, the patient may be asked to name items on a card preceded with the phrase "that is a . . . ." Patients are sometimes asked to do simple math problems. A patient who speaks multiple languages might need to have each language tested separately since not all learned languages are localized to the same cortical area. This requires extensive preoperative planning to have interpreters available to help with this testing.

Once the craniotomy is completed, the dura opened, and the patient awakened, testing can begin. The tumor surface is often visible and helps guide the surgeon as to where to start the mapping. A handheld wand with two probes, separated by 5 mm, is gently placed on the brain surface about 2 cm from the tumor edge. This is connected to a constant-current, biphasic stimulator. Neurologists or speech pathologists usually stimulate for 2 to 5 seconds, with a frequency of 50 Hz and a pulse width of 200 ms. Responses are usually noted with a constant current range of 4 to 6 mA. After each test, the surgeon moves the wand freely to other areas of the cortex, repeating this procedure until satisfied that functional areas of the cortex have been localized and marked and that an area of negative mapping has been identified through which the tumor or epileptic foci can be resected.

For seizure focus resection, there are no visible signs to follow. Often, the areas of eloquent cortex in danger will have been mapped out by magnetoencephalography (MEG), a noninvasive technique for mapping brain activity by recording the magnetic fields produced by the electrical currents of the brain. These studies can then be overlaid onto an MRI study and appear as colored squares representing areas of the eloquent cortex tested, and used for tumor or epilepsy surgery to help identify the functional areas. Mapping can then start outside of these designated areas looking for a quiet area.

Moore TA II, Markert JM, Knowlton RC. Dexmedetomidine as a rescue drug during awake craniotomy for cortical mapping and tumor resection. *Anesth Analg*. 2006;102:1556-1558.

Pallud J, Rigaux-Viode O, Corns R, et al. Direct electrical bipolar electrostimulation for functional cortical and subcortical cerebral mapping in awake craniotomy. Practical considerations. *Neurochirurgie*. 2017;63:164-174.

C.9. How are intraoperative seizures treated?

Intraoperative seizures can be the type for which the patient presented or can be caused by the surface stimulation used to map the cortex. The surgeon usually does not stimulate the same area more than two consecutive times to avoid this complication. If a seizure should occur, it usually will take the form of the patient no longer answering questions, but maintaining their airway, and at times a moaning sound is made. This usually responds rapidly to the application of cold irrigation solution, usually lactated Ringer solution, to the cortex by the surgeon. If this fails, small doses of propofol, 10 to 20 mg, usually stop the seizure. An uncontrolled seizure that is not terminated with these measures can progress into a surgical emergency. The spreading electrical activity dramatically increases CBF and blood volume in the cortex exposed beneath the cranial defect. The rapid increase in blood volume pushes the exposed cortex up through the craniotomy, a process that can tear delicate cortical veins and result in a cortical venous infarction.

Cottrell JE, Patel PM. Brain Metabolism, Pathophysiology, and Potential Beneficial Agents. In: Cottrell JE, Patel PM eds. *Cottrell and Patel's Neuroanesthesia.* 7th ed. Elsevier; 2024.

Paquin-Lanthier G, Subramaniam S, Leong KW, et al. Risk factors and characteristics of intraoperative seizures during awake craniotomy: a retrospective cohort study of 562 consecutive patients with a space-occupying brain lesion. *J Neurosurg Anesthesiol.* 2023;35:194-200.

C.10. How will you conduct this anesthetic?

The patient must be very motivated for awake craniotomy to be successful. They must realize fully that this is a lengthy procedure, and 4 to 8 hours is not unusual. The patient's family must also be involved and have the same understanding. Most important is a motivated and experienced neurosurgeon, neurologist or speech pathologist, and neuroanesthesiologist. Each must realize that time is of the essence and the procedures must be completed as quickly as is safely possible.

The neurosurgeon will be the first person to suggest or inform the patient that this form of surgery is necessary to preserve language or motor-sensory function. Ideally, the neurosurgeon and the neuroanesthesiologist have developed a technique that allows them to have an awake, cooperative patient when the time comes for cortical or subcortical mapping and resection.

In the operating room, before the patient's arrival, several steps are taken to make the patient as comfortable as possible during this long and demanding procedure. A full-length gel pad is placed on the operating room table under the sheets, an underbody warmer is placed, and in some cases, the room temperature is set at 70 °F or higher. Additional gel pads and foam sheets are available as needed, as well as warm blankets.

Following the preoperative visit and IV catheter placement, the patient is brought to the operating room. Premedications that interfere with the ability to cooperate and follow instructions are avoided. Standard intraoperative monitors are placed, and a CO_2 monitoring nasal oxygen cannula is placed.

The various anesthetic techniques for awake craniotomy include a triphasic "asleep-awake-asleep" technique utilizing a combination of moderate reversible sedation and regional scalp blocks. Some of these techniques use intubation of the trachea and potent inhalational agents until approximately 20 to 30 minutes before cortex mapping when the anesthetic is discontinued and the trachea extubated. Others use a supraglottic airway in the same fashion. Use of propofol, fentanyl, remifentanil, dexmedetomidine, and combinations of these drugs is added to these approaches as a means of transitioning the patient from general anesthesia to the awake state for mapping and surgery within the eloquent cortex. Use of TIVA with the same drugs and a supraglottic airway or an unprotected airway (sometimes supported with a nasal trumpet) with spontaneous respiration is also used.

Similar, but not identical, approaches for mapping or other tasking have been successful for one group and not for another. This can lead to frustration in trying to decide on the anesthetic approach. Many times, the technique is institutionally defined and has worked well for many years. It is critical to fully understand the pharmacology of the anesthetic regimen chosen.

We use a triphasic TIVA technique with spontaneous breathing without a supraglottic airway or tracheal intubation. Two separate infusions are started. Dexmedetomidine is started at 1.0 μg/kg/h, continued for 10 minutes, and reduced to 0.5 to 0.75 μg/kg/h. Propofol is started at 50 to 100 μg/kg/min. These drugs are titrated as needed to achieve a sedated yet spontaneously breathing patient, corresponding to an Observer's Assessment of Alertness/Sedation scale (OAA/S) of 3 to 4 or a Richmond Agitation-Sedation Scale (RASS) of −2 to −3. Patients on multiple AEDs often require higher doses of sedatives for this procedure. When the patient no longer responds to name call, a urethral catheter, additional IV lines, and an arterial line, as deemed necessary, are placed. Small bolus doses of propofol, 10 to 20 mg, are given depending on the patient's response to these procedures. A loading dose of dexmedetomidine can be given: the recommended dose is 1 μg/kg over 10 minutes, followed by a maintenance infusion. Reports of persistent bradycardia and hypotension have been reported with this approach compared with starting the infusion without a loading dose. Bradycardia is treated with small doses (0.2-0.4 mg) of glycopyrrolate, and hypotension is treated with a low-dose (0.1-0.3 μg/kg/min) phenylephrine infusion. The dexmedetomidine and propofol combination provides good sedation, anxiolysis, and amnesia without causing significant respiratory depression.

The success of this procedure lies in the precision and adequacy of the scalp blocks performed by the anesthesiologist or neurosurgeon. No amount of sedation will compensate for poorly performed blocks. The scalp block addresses the supratrochlear, supraorbital, zygomaticotemporal, auriculotemporal, greater auricular, and the lesser and greater occipital nerves. A combination of equal volumes of 2% lidocaine with epinephrine 1:100,000 and 0.5% bupivacaine with epinephrine 1:200,000 provides a rapid onset and longer duration than either component separately, although no convincing data support this practice. Use of ropivacaine alone for the same purpose is also described. Following the individual nerve blocks, an intradermal ring of the local anesthetic solution is placed around the operative side of the scalp. Each pin site for the pin head holder device is injected. The surgical incision site is also infiltrated by the surgeon after the patient is prepped and draped.

Dexmedetomidine and propofol infusions are continued for cranial opening. When the surgeon has made the final burr hole, propofol infusion is terminated and dexmedetomidine dose is reduced to 0.2 μg/kg/h. Cranial opening continues, and 15 to 20 minutes later, the patient is awake and conversant. The neurosurgeon and neurologist or speech pathologist begin the mapping process, which can take several hours, but usually about 1 hour. Dexmedetomidine is continued at 0.2 μg/kg/h throughout the mapping process. When satisfied that areas of the eloquent cortex adjacent to the tumor have been localized and an area of negative mapping has been demonstrated, the surgeon proceeds with tumor resection. If the patient is resting comfortably, no changes in the anesthetic are necessary. For deeper sedation, dexmedetomidine is increased to 0.35 μg/kg/h; this usually keeps the patient comfortable for the remainder of the procedure. From time to time, the surgeon may ask to remap certain areas, and the dexmedetomidine is again lowered to 0.2 μg/kg/h. The dexmedetomidine is stopped at skin stapling. The pin head holder is removed, dressings are placed, and preparations are made for transfer to the neurosurgery intensive care unit. A transport monitor capable of providing pulse oximetry, blood pressure measurements, and ECG tracing is attached, and nasal cannula oxygen is continued during the transport.

Bustillo MA, Lazar RM, Finck AD, et al. Dexmedetomidine may impair cognitive testing during endovascular embolization of cerebral arteriovenous malformations: a retrospective case report series. *J Neurosurg Anesthesiol.* 2002;14:209-212.

Conte V, Magni L, Songa V, et al. Analysis of propofol/remifentanil infusion protocol for tumor surgery with intraoperative brain mapping. *J Neurosurg Anesthesiol.* 2010;22:119-127.

Ely EW, Truman B, Shintani A, et al. Monitoring sedation status overtime in ICU patients: reliability and validity of the Richmond agitation-sedation Scale (RASS). *JAMA.* 2003;289:1983-1991.

Höhener D, Blumenthal S, Borgeat A. Sedation and regional anaesthesia in the adult patient. *Br J Anaesth.* 2008;100:8-16.

Kim SS, McCutcheon IE, Suki D, et al. Awake craniotomy for brain tumors near eloquent cortex: correlation of intraoperative cortical mapping with neurological outcomes in 309 consecutive patients. *Neurosurgery.* 2009;64:836-846.

Mack PF, Perrine K, Kobylarz E, et al. Dexmedetomidine and neurocognitive testing in awake craniotomy. *J Neurosurg Anesthesiol.* 2004;16:20-25.

Moore TA II, Markert JM, Knowlton RC. Dexmedetomidine as a rescue drug during awake craniotomy for cortical mapping and tumor resection. *Anesth Analg.* 2006;102:1556-1558.

Salinas FV, Auyong DB. Local anesthetics. In: Evers AS, Maze M, Kharasch ED, eds. *Anesthetic Pharmacology: Basic Principles and Clinical Practice.* 2nd ed. Churchill Livingstone; 2011:574-588.

D. Postoperative Management

D.1. What are the major concerns following craniotomy?

The patient is transported to the neurosurgical intensive care unit and monitored as described. The head of the bed is usually elevated 20° to 30° to maximize cerebral venous drainage, with the care of the patient transferred to the neurointensivist and the neurosurgical service.

Several problems can occur in the immediate postoperative period following craniotomy. The key feature of a good anesthetic is the ability to quickly awaken the patient following the procedure so that a neurologic exam can be performed. Typically, the patient will awaken within 5 minutes after the end of the procedure. However, awakening in patients who have required larger doses of medication to achieve an adequate level of sedation (OAA/S 3-4) can take 10 to 20 minutes until a suitable neurologic exam can be obtained. Not infrequently, the patient has a subtle diminution of the neurologic exam compared to the end of the tumor resection. These small differences are likely due to residual anesthetics and progressive edema around the resection site. The former will usually improve over the next 1 to 2 hours, and the latter can take several days to resolve completely.

Emergence hypertension is common in the perioperative period: the incidence of postcraniotomy hypertension is about 57%. In a series of 11,214 craniotomies, perioperative systemic hypertension was associated with postoperative intracranial hematoma, with resultant increased mortality and increased length of hospital stay. Other possible causes are pain, hypercapnia, and shivering. Most (85%) postoperative intracranial hematomas become evident within 6 hours of surgery and usually present as a progressive decrease in level of consciousness. Up to 17% of these hematomas present at sites remote to the surgical site. Aggressive efforts at controlling hypertension are required to prevent devastating complications such as bleeding into the tumor bed, requiring a second surgical procedure to evacuate the clot.

Systolic blood pressure goals in a normotensive patient are 120 to 140 mm Hg and for a chronically poorly controlled hypertensive patient 140 to 160 mm Hg. In both cases, aggressive measures to maintain blood pressures at the lower end of the range are warranted if the resection site is large and/or hemostasis is difficult. Often, if not contraindicated, labetalol 5 to 10 mg IV (to a total of 60 mg) is effective. Persistent hypertension, without signs of intracranial hypertension, requires additional treatment. Given the strict blood pressure parameters, failing suitable control with labetalol or hydralazine 5 to 10 mg IV, patients are usually transferred to the intensive care unit on an infusion of nicardipine 5 to 15 mg/h or clevidipine 1 to 2 mg/h rapidly titrated up to 16 mg/h. Alternatively, depending on the patient's comorbid conditions, infusion of sodium nitroprusside or nitroglycerin is possible. A combination of enalapril and labetalol versus nicardipine alone has been reported, with little difference in the ability to control emergence hypertension. Rather than simply treating hypertension at the time of emergence, the use of a dexmedetomidine infusion during the procedure itself, as noted in Section C, reduces the need for the administration of antihypertensive medications (labetalol and hydralazine) at the time of emergence and reduces the incidence of hypertensive episodes immediately following surgery.

Acute pain control is essential in the postoperative period. Not only are patients more comfortable with adequate pain relief, but good analgesia helps control postoperative hypertension and decreases the possibility of intracranial hematoma. Pain following craniotomy has probably been vastly understated secondary to concern about respiratory depression and sedation as well as the traditional thought that craniotomies are less painful than other operations. The incidence of postcraniotomy pain may be as high as 70%. However, our experience is that pain following an awake procedure is much less common as the duration of the scalp blocks can extend well into the postoperative period. Another helpful adjunct is IV acetaminophen given either during or after the procedure.

In the immediate postoperative period, almost all analgesics are given intravenously. Morphine sulfate patient-controlled analgesia can produce good results without respiratory depression or the need for reintubation. One regimen consists of morphine 1.5 mg with a lockout period of 8 minutes and a total dose not to exceed 40 mg in 4 hours.

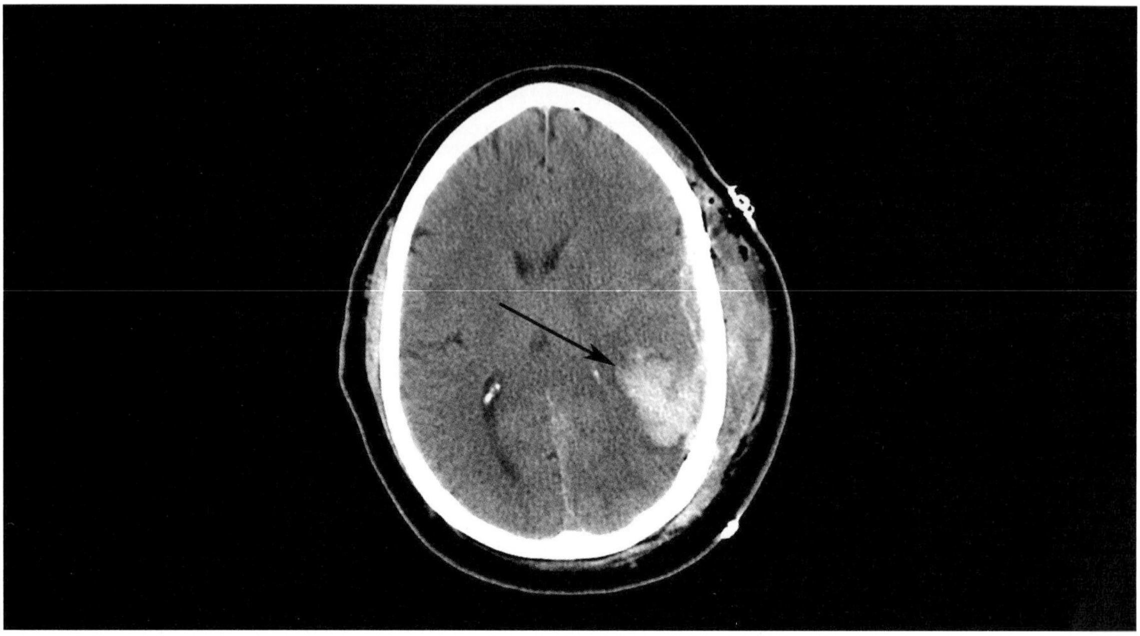

FIGURE 20.6. CT scan of a 73-year-old male who underwent an uneventful left awake craniotomy with motor and language area mapping. On postoperative day 2, he suffered a generalized tonic-clonic seizure and was extremely slow to awaken. CT scan revealed the presence of a large intracranial hematoma (*arrow*) in the operative site requiring return to the operating room for evacuation. Also note the small epidural and subgaleal hematomas. Coagulation studies were normal. The patient was placed on AEDs and did well on follow-up visits without further seizure activity. AEDs were successfully weaned over several weeks. Final pathology revealed glioblastoma multiforme. AEDs, antiepileptic drugs; CT, computed tomography.

Nonsteroidal anti-inflammatory drugs have been associated with postoperative intracranial hematoma. Administration of antiplatelet agents (aspirin and nonsteroidal anti-inflammatory drugs) was the most common risk factor. Therefore, this class of analgesics should be avoided in the immediate postoperative period.

Postoperative nausea and vomiting are common following craniotomy and can cause hypertension and increased ICP. Infratentorial surgery, female sex, and young age are associated risk factors. Ondansetron 4 to 8 mg IV can provide effective treatment.

Seizures can occur following intracranial tumor resections and can cause serious complications such as secondary intracranial bleeding, hypoxemia, and aspiration. An intracranial mass, such as a hematoma (**Figure 20.6**), should be suspected if the patient does not regain consciousness within a short period after the seizure has ceased. Small doses of midazolam, 1 to 2 mg, or other benzodiazepines can treat seizures effectively without compromising the airway.

Increased ICP commonly occurs after intracranial surgery, with the most common finding on CT scan being brain edema. Maximum pressures are usually recorded within 16 hours of surgery. Associated risk factors are glioblastoma resection and surgery lasting over 6 hours. Continuing corticosteroids, such as dexamethasone 4 to 10 mg every 6 hours, usually controls this problem.

Peripheral nerve injuries are uncommon after awake craniotomy because patient comfort or discomfort can easily be assessed, and minor movements are made if needed. Blister formation along the downside of the upper leg of patients who are morbidly obese can occur after about 5 hours in the lateral decubitus position despite gel pads beneath the thigh.

Aronson RV, Dyke CM, Stierer KA, et al. The ECLIPSE trials: comparative studies of clevidipine to nitroglycerin, sodium nitroprusside, and nicardipine for acute hypertension treatment in cardiac surgery patients. *Anesth Analg.* 2008;107:1110-1121.

Artime CA, Aijazi H, Zhang H, et al. Acetaminophen improves patient satisfaction with postcraniotomy pain management: a prospective, randomized, placebo-controlled, double-blind study. *J Neurosurg Anesthesiol.* 2018;30:231-236.

Basali A, Mascha EJ, Kalfas I, et al. Relation between perioperative hypertension and intracranial hemorrhage after craniotomy. *Anesthesiology*. 2000;93:48-54.

Bebawy JF, Houston CC, Kosky JL, et al. Nicardipine is superior to esmolol for the management of postcraniotomy emergence hypertension: a randomized open-label study. *Anesth Analg*. 2015;120:186-192.

Bekker A, Sturaitis M, Bloom M, et al. The effect of dexmedetomidine on perioperative hemodynamics in patients undergoing craniotomy. *Anesth Analg* 2008;107:1340-1347.

de Gray LC, Matta BF. Acute and chronic pain following craniotomy: a review. *Anaesthesia*. 2005;60:693-704.

Gottschalk A, Berkow LC, Stevens RD, et al. Prospective evaluation of pain and analgesic use following major elective intracranial surgery. *J Neurosurg*. 2007;106:210-216.

Immink RV, van de Born BJ, van Montfrans GA, et al. Cerebral hemodynamics during treatment with sodium nitroprusside versus labetalol in malignant hypertension. *Hypertension*. 2008;52:236-240.

Jellish WS, Murdoch J, Leonetti JP. Perioperative management of complex skull base surgery: the anesthesiologist's point of view. *Neurosurg Focus*. 2002;12:e5.

Kross RA, Ferri E, Leung D, et al. A comparative study between a calcium channel blocker (nicardipine) and a combined alpha-beta blocker (labetalol) for the control of emergence hypertension during craniotomy for tumor surgery. *Anesth Analg*. 2000;91:904-909.

Lemkuil BP, Drummond JC, Patel PM, et al. Anesthesia for Neurologic Surgery and Neurointerventions. In: Gropper MA, Miller RD, eds. *Miller's Anesthesia*. 10th ed. Elsevier; 2025.

Nemergut EC, Durieux ME, Missaghi NB, et al. Pain management after craniotomy. *Best Pract Res Clin Anaesthesiol*. 2007;21:557-573.

Parida S, Badhe AS. Emergence hypertension in patients undergoing intracranial surgery. *Int J Anesthesiol*. 2009;22:1-5.

Tsaousi GG, Logan SW, Bilotta F. Postoperative pain control following craniotomy: a systemic review of recent clinical literature. *Pain Pract*. 2017;17:968-981.

Acknowledgments

We would like to thank the following people for their assistance in making this endeavor possible: Mark R. Harrigan and James M. Markert, chairman, University of Alabama School of Medicine (UABSOM), Department of Neurosurgery, for their assistance in the acquisition and preparation of the radiographs used in this chapter; and David Miller and Richard C. Cross, UABSOM, Department of Anesthesiology and Perioperative Medicine, for their critical reading, suggestions, and encouragement.

21 Traumatic Brain Injury (TBI)

Chris C. Lee, Susan A. Ironstone, and M. Angele Theard

A 52-year-old female with an unknown past medical history was involved in a high-speed motorcycle collision and airlifted to a trauma center. On the scene, she was unresponsive and intubated. She was found to have a left small pneumothorax, rib fractures, and an open tibial/fibular fracture that was reduced and fixed with return of pulses after an initial pulseless left leg. She had a skull fracture extending to the left parietal bone, occipital bone, clivus sphenoid sinus, and temporal bone diagnosed at an outside hospital.

On admission, the patient had a Glasgow Coma Score (GCS) of 7T, and her vital signs were blood pressure (BP), 69/40 mm Hg; heart rate, 150 beats per minute; respiratory rate, 20 breaths per minute; and oxygen saturation, 100% on 60% fraction of inspired oxygen (FIO_2). The patient was aggressively resuscitated with packed red blood cell transfusions, 0.9% normal saline (NS), and norepinephrine infusion.

Head computed tomography (CT) scans showed bilateral traumatic subarachnoid hemorrhage (tSAH) and subdural hematoma (**Figures 21.1** and **21.2**). Her laboratory values were hemoglobin, 9.8 g/dL; hematocrit, 29.5%; platelets, 137,000/μL; lactate, 6.5 mM; international normalized ratio (INR), 1.73; troponin-I, 1.27 ng/mL; glucose, 418 mg/dL; sodium (Na), 141 mM; potassium (K), 3.6 mM; and creatinine, 1.36 mg/dL. Fresh frozen plasma (FFP) and prothrombin complex concentrate (PCC) were given immediately to treat the coagulopathy.

The GCS was 7T; therefore, a right frontal external ventriculostomy drain (EVD) was emergently placed for intracranial pressure (ICP) monitoring and cerebrospinal fluid (CSF) drainage because her CT scan showed tSAH and early signs of cerebral swelling. The patient was managed conservatively for her ICP but required increasing medical treatment, including maximal hyperosmolar therapy, pain control, sedation, and paralysis. Her ICP readings remained in the 30 mm Hg range after initially low ICP readings. The patient was taken to the operating room for a bifrontal craniectomy for emergency decompression secondary to severe bifrontal contusions with malignant cerebral edema (**Figures 21.3** and **21.4**).

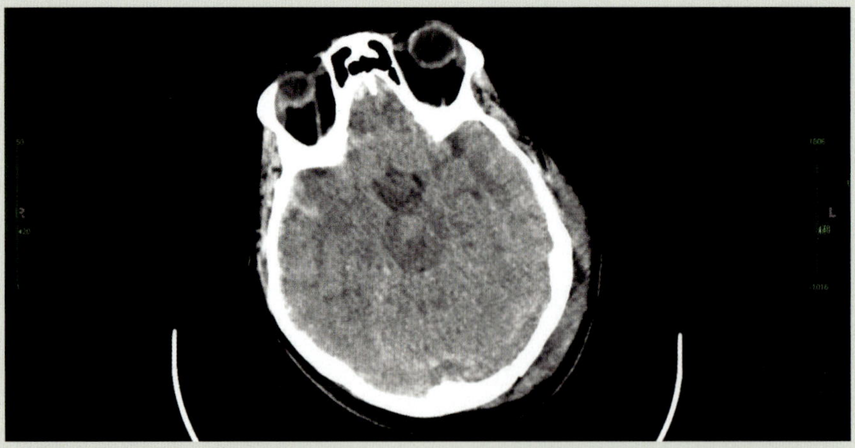

FIGURE 21.1. Initial head CT scan (basal): bilateral tSAH. CT, computed tomography; tSAH, traumatic subarachnoid hemorrhage.

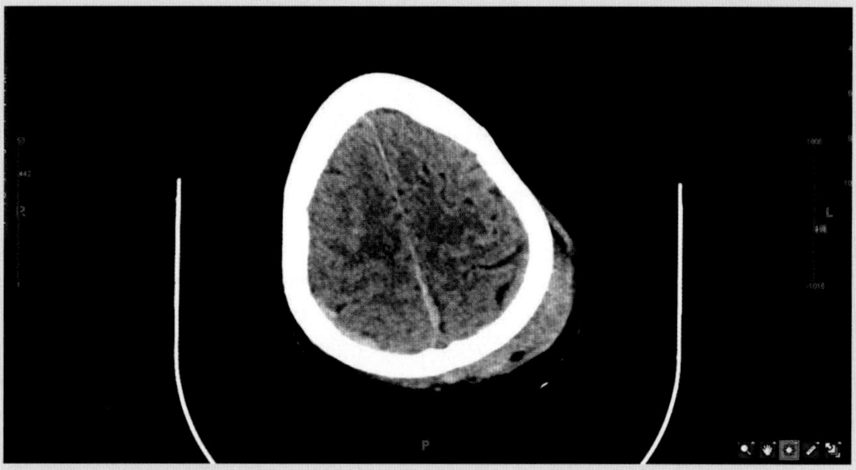

FIGURE 21.2. Initial head CT scan (vertex): bilateral tSAH. CT, computed tomography; tSAH, traumatic subarachnoid hemorrhage.

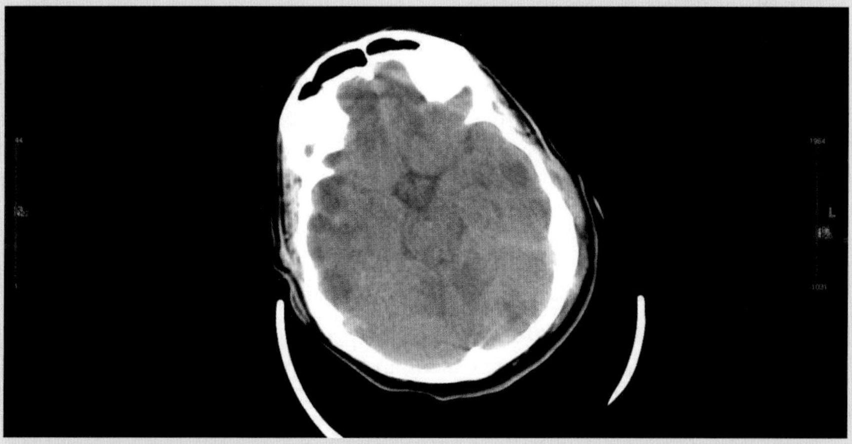

FIGURE 21.3. Follow-up head CT scan: contusions with malignant cerebral edema. CT, computed tomography.

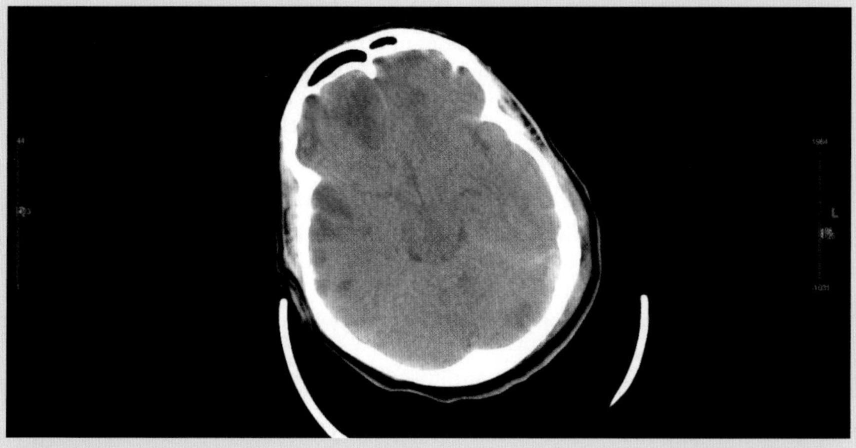

FIGURE 21.4. Follow-up head CT scan: contusions with brain swelling and effacement of sulci and basal cisterns.

A. Pathophysiology and Differential Diagnosis

1. What types of intracranial injuries are most likely to have occurred in this patient?
2. What is the difference between primary and secondary injury? What factors contribute to secondary injury?
3. What are the benefits and risks of administering mannitol?
4. What is the effect of hyperglycemia on neurologic outcome following head trauma?
5. What alterations in sodium and potassium balance can occur in patients with head injury?
6. In addition to sodium and potassium, what other electrolyte abnormalities can be present after head trauma?
7. What are the neuroprotective effects of administering magnesium (Mg)?
8. What role do sex and female sex hormones have in the pathophysiology of traumatic brain injury (TBI)?
9. What is the role of decompressive craniectomy as a treatment option for ICP control after head injury?
10. Do genetic factors play a role in outcomes after head injury?

B. Preoperative Evaluation and Preparation

1. What is GCS? What is the significance of a GCS of 7T in this patient?
2. In addition to the GCS, what other assessments can be done to evaluate neurologic function?
3. What is the role of CT scanning in the initial evaluation of the patient with head injury? What are the management options for patients whose neurologic condition is deteriorating before obtaining a CT scan?
4. What is the role of ICP monitoring in the management of head injury?
5. How can you clear this patient's cervical spine?
6. What are the advantages of early endotracheal intubation in this patient?
7. What is your plan for airway management in this patient? How would it change if the patient was responsive but combative? How would it change if the patient had facial fractures with significant swelling of the head and neck?
8. What are the effects of succinylcholine on ICP? What is the significance of the effect, if any?
9. What coagulation abnormalities are present after TBI? What modalities can be used to provide hemostasis and reduce intracranial hematoma expansion?

C. Intraoperative Management

1. What is appropriate hemodynamic monitoring during CT scanning and during craniotomy for evacuation of a subdural hematoma?
2. Should hyperventilation be used in this patient?
3. What are the implications of arterial hypertension in patients with head injury? How should BP be managed?
4. What should be done about intravenous (IV) fluid replacement? Should corticosteroids be given empirically?
5. Should hypertonic saline (HTS) be administered to this patient? How is HTS administered?
6. The patient underwent a craniectomy for evacuation of a frontal intracerebral hematoma. Which anesthetic agents should be avoided in this situation? What agents might be preferred in this situation?
7. Should hypothermia be employed in this patient?

D. Postoperative Neurointensive Care Management

1. What are the postoperative ventilation concerns in this patient?
2. What specific measure should be used to control the patient's ICP? What type of monitoring devices can be used to measure ICP?
3. What is neurogenic pulmonary edema? Would you avoid positive end-expiratory pressure (PEEP) in a patient with increased ICP?
4. What is the role of antiseizure prophylaxis in the perioperative management of head trauma?
5. How can cerebral oxygenation monitoring be used in the clinical management of TBI?
6. What methods can be used in the neurointensive care unit to prevent hyperthermia?

A. Pathophysiology and Differential Diagnosis

A.1. What types of intracranial injuries are most likely to have occurred in this patient?

The common causes of TBI include falls, motor vehicle accidents (MVAs), assaults, and gunshots. TBI is a leading cause of death and disability after injury in the United States. The following types of intracranial injuries are most likely to have occurred in this patient:

- **Concussion** is both the most common type of TBI and the least apparent on imaging. It is often completely invisible to any type of imaging and must be assessed and diagnosed clinically. It is also the most common type of TBI to result in long-term morbidity, causing decreased job and school performance from lasting cognitive symptoms. This is a very complex type of injury and is a big focus of professional sports team injury experts. There is currently a social movement to raise awareness of these injuries, particularly in young athletes.
- **Diffuse axonal injury (DAI)** is difficult to detect on CT of the brain, although small punctate hemorrhages in white matter tracts might be seen. Magnetic resonance imaging (MRI), particularly weighted imaging, is a more sensitive way to detect it. DAI can produce severe neurologic impairment with a poor prognosis.
- **tSAH** is the most common type of posttraumatic intracranial hemorrhage and the least severe indicator of injury. Although this finding often signals the presence of significant concussion injury, it does not require surgical intervention. tSAH resolves within days and carries a far lower risk of the secondary consequences than those associated with spontaneous aneurysmal subarachnoid hemorrhage (eg, hydrocephalus and stroke from intracerebral vasospasm). Follow-up CT scans are usually not necessary due to this low risk of secondary neurologic injury.
- **Epidural hematoma** (located between the skull and dura mater) is classically associated with displaced temporal bone skull fractures, causing a laceration of the middle meningeal artery. This arterial hemorrhage results in a rapidly expanding hematoma lateral to the temporal lobe, which can lead to death from brain herniation if it is not emergently surgically evacuated. Injury to large venous structures including dural sinuses or venous bleeding from fractured bone can lead to venous epidural hematoma. Due to the fact that these hemorrhages occur at venous pressure, they are thought to be less likely to expand to a dangerous volume, but sometimes surgical treatment is required. Patients with acute epidural hematoma often exhibit a lucid interval after the initial impact before deteriorating. The signs of this deterioration can include depressed mental status, an ipsilateral fixed and dilated pupil, contralateral hemiplegia, and imaging demonstrating uncal herniation due to the rapidly expanding hematoma. Arterial epidural hematomas are almost always a true neurosurgical emergency; rapid intervention makes the difference between a good prognosis and death.
- **Subdural hematoma** (located between the brain and dura) arises from a tear in the dural sinuses or bridging veins and accumulates more insidiously than an epidural hematoma. They are classified as acute (up to 48 hours), subacute (48 hours to 12 days), and chronic (>12 days) according to the interval of time between the TBI and the onset of symptoms. Subdural hematoma greater than 1 cm in thickness or causing more than 1 cm of midline shift is generally associated with significant lateralizing neurologic symptoms and often constitutes a surgical emergency. Small subdural hematomas can expand in volume, as they grow more chronic and can produce delays in the onset of significant neurologic signs and symptoms.
- **Intracerebral hematoma and hemorrhage** arise from the tearing of small vessels in the white matter and are due to penetrating head injury or caused by acceleration-deceleration injuries that involve laceration of cortical arteries. These hemorrhages and hematomas can often be managed medically with serial follow-up head CT scans. Surgical evacuation of intracerebral hematomas is rarely indicated due to the deep location of many of these hemorrhages. Although they can be associated with trauma, more common causes include hypertension, amyloid angiopathy, and/or profound coagulopathy.
- **Cerebral contusions** are superficial hemorrhages that occur mainly when the anterior temporal and frontal lobes strike the rough edges of the tentorium (contrecoup contusion). In a patient without focal neurologic deficits, the most probable intracranial injury is a cerebral contusion after ruling out other focal brain injuries. This type of injury is often associated with cerebral edema and can require aggressive management with hyperosmolar therapy or surgical craniectomy for decompression.

Faul M, Xu L, Wald MM, et al. *Traumatic Brain Injury in the United States: Emergency Department Visits, Hospitalizations and Deaths 2002–2006*. U.S. Department of Health and Human Services, Centers for Disease Control and Prevention, National Center for Injury Prevention and Control; 2010.

Ghajar J. Traumatic brain injury. *Lancet*. 2000;356:923-929.

Pan JZ, Meng LZ. Traumatic brain injury: risk assessment and perioperative management. In: Brambrink AM, Kirsch JR, eds. *Essentials of Neurosurgical Anesthesia & Critical Care: Strategies for Prevention, Early Detection, and Successful Management of Perioperative Complications*. 2nd ed. Springer; 2020:67-75.

Picetti E, Rossi S, Abu-Zidan FM, et al. WSES consensus conference guidelines: monitoring and management of severe adult traumatic brain injury patients with polytrauma in the first 24 hours. *World J Emerg Surg*. 2019;14:53.

Steinberg GK, Dodd RL, Chaudhary N, et al. Intracranial neurosurgery. In: Jaffe RA, Schmiesing CA, Golianu B, eds. *Anesthesiologist's Manual of Surgical Procedures*. 6th ed. Wolters Kluwer; 2019:3-72.

van den Bergh WM, Absalom AR, Cremer OL. Perioperative challenges during surgical evacuation of subdural and epidural hematomas. In: Brambrink AM, Kirsch JR, eds. *Essentials of Neurosurgical Anesthesia & Critical Care: Strategies for Prevention, Early Detection, and Successful*. 2nd ed. Springer; 2020:201-206.

A.2. What is the difference between primary and secondary injury? What factors contribute to secondary injury?

Primary injury refers to the direct injury of tissue at the moment of head trauma.

Secondary injury occurs minutes, hours, and even days after the initial head trauma and is the consequence of ischemic insults to the brain. The major goal of perioperative management of patients with TBI is to prevent secondary injury. The factors contributing to secondary injury include systemic causes (ie, hypoxia, hypotension, hypocarbia or hypercarbia, fever, and hypoglycemia or hyperglycemia) and intracranial causes (ie, intracranial hypertension, elevated ICP, and brain herniation). Systemic hypotension and intracranial hypertension are factors related to increased morbidity and mortality in patients with severe TBI. Mental status changes suggest inadequate cerebral perfusion, from either decreased systemic BP or elevated ICP. Cerebral perfusion pressure (CPP) is the mean arterial pressure (MAP) minus either ICP or central venous pressure (CVP), whichever is greater (CPP = MAP − ICP or CVP). Achieving a CPP between 60 and 70 mm Hg requires maintaining adequate BP, oxygenation, and a normal $Paco_2$ in order to decrease the chance of morbidity, mortality, or deleterious sequelae caused by secondary injury.

Algattas H, Huang JH. Traumatic brain injury pathophysiology and treatments: early, intermediate, and late phases post-injury. *Int J Mol Sci*. 2013;15:309-341.

Carney N, Totten AM, O'Reilly C, et al. Guidelines for the management of severe traumatic brain injury, fourth edition. *Neurosurgery*. 2017;80:6-15.

Lemkuil BP, Drummond JC, Patel PM, et al. Anesthesia for neurologic surgery and neurointerventions. In: Gropper MA, Cohen NH, Eriksson LI, et al, eds. *Miller's Anesthesia*. 9th ed. Elsevier; 2020:2680-2681.

A.3. What are the benefits and risks of administering mannitol?

Benefits

Mannitol (20%) 0.25 to 1.0 g/kg body weight is effective in acutely reducing cerebral edema, brain volume, and ICP by increasing serum osmolality to 305 to 320 mOsm/L and thereby improving CPP, which also facilitates surgical exposure and reduces tissue trauma from surgical retraction. Use of hyperosmolar agents is theoretically limited by an upper acceptable osmolality limit of about 320 mOsm/L. Onset of mannitol-induced osmotic diuresis is 5 to 15 minutes, with a peak effect in 30 minutes, and lasts for 2 to 3 hours. For decades, mannitol has been commonly accepted as an acute treatment for cerebral edema and raised ICP.

Risks

- After TBI, the possibility of loss of blood-brain barrier (BBB) integrity leading to leak of mannitol into cerebral interstitial tissue might actually worsen cerebral edema.
- Osmotic diuresis can cause hypovolemia, and the resultant hypotension can reduce CPP and aggravate cerebral ischemia.
- Mannitol can transiently cause hypervolemia and worsen or result in congestive heart failure and pulmonary edema in those patients who have borderline cardiopulmonary function.
- Electrolyte abnormalities (eg, hypernatremia) due to diuresis can occur.
- A serum osmolality above 320 mOsm/L can cause acute renal failure.
- Mannitol can cause intracranial rebleeding in patients with expanding hematoma by removing a tamponading effect on the hematoma if administered before the dura is opened.

Colton K, Yang S, Hu PF, et al. Responsiveness to therapy for increased intracranial pressure in traumatic brain injury is associated with neurological outcome. *Injury*. 2014;45:2084-2088.

Lemkuil BP, Drummond JC, Patel PM, et al. Anesthesia for neurological surgery and neurointerventions. In: Gropper MA, Cohen NH, Eriksson LI, et al, eds. *Miller's Anesthesia*. 9th ed. Elsevier; 2020:1870-1875.

A.4. What is the effect of hyperglycemia on neurologic outcome following head trauma?

Hyperglycemia resulting from the nervous system response to injury following moderate to severe head trauma is associated with an increased odds ratio for an unfavorable neurologic outcome and an increased risk of mortality. Additionally, persistent hyperglycemia is an independent predictor of an unfavorable outcome in patients with severe TBI. The degree of stress-induced hyperglycemia (SIH) corresponds to the severity of TBI.

Although there is a possibility that intensive glucose control with blood glucose targets of less than 126 mg/dL is associated with improved neurologic outcome, it has not been shown to reduce mortality and does increase the risk of severe hypoglycemia. In critically ill patients, hypoglycemia is strongly correlated with increased morbidity and mortality. Therefore, moderate glucose control targets with a range of 144 to 180 mg/dL are currently recommended so that hyperglycemia and hypoglycemia can be avoided.

Hermanides J, Plummer MP, Finnis M, et al. Glycaemic control targets after traumatic brain injury: a systematic review and meta-analysis. *Crit Care*. 2018;22:11.

Lemkuil BP, Drummond JC, Patel PM, et al. Anesthesia for neurological surgery and neurointerventions. In: Gropper MA, Cohen NH, Eriksson LI, et al, eds. *Miller's Anesthesia*. 9th ed. Elsevier; 2020:1884.

Muehlschlegel S, Carandang R, Ouillette C, et al. Frequency and impact of intensive care unit complications on moderate-severe traumatic brain injury: early results of the Outcome Prognostication in Traumatic Brain Injury (OPTIMISM) Study. *Neurocrit Care*. 2013;18:318-331.

A.5. What alterations in sodium and potassium balance can occur in patients with head injury?

Electrolyte abnormalities such as hyponatremia and hypokalemia are commonly seen following head trauma. Hyponatremia can result via several mechanisms, including hypothalamus-pituitary dysfunction, cerebral salt-wasting syndrome, and syndrome of inappropriate antidiuretic hormone (SIADH). Additionally, sodium loss can be exacerbated by medications used to treat cerebral edema. Hyponatremia is strongly correlated with poor outcomes. Severe hypokalemia is an independent mortality risk factor in patients with TBI and is likely related to trauma and stress-related catecholamine surge. Hypernatremia resulting from mannitol use, HTS, or diabetes insipidus is also frequently seen in association with severe TBI. Hypernatremia itself is an independent risk factor for postoperative death in patients with severe TBI.

Hoffman H, Jalal MS, Chin LS. Effect of hypernatremia on outcomes after severe traumatic brain injury: a nationwide inpatient sample analysis. *World Neurosurg*. 2018;118:e880-e886.

Pin-On P, Saringkarinkul A, Punjasawadwong Y, et al. Serum electrolyte imbalance and prognostic factors of postoperative death in adult traumatic brain injury patients: a prospective cohort study. *Medicine (Baltimore)*. 2018;97:e13081.

Wu X, Lu X, Lu X, et al. Prevalence of severe hypokalemia in patients with traumatic brain injury. *Injury*. 2015;46:35-41.

Zhang W, Li S, Visocchi M, et al. Clinical analysis of hyponatremia in acute craniocerebral injury. *J Emerg Med*. 2010;39:151-157.

A.6. In addition to sodium and potassium, what other electrolyte abnormalities can be present after head trauma?

Multiple electrolyte abnormalities, including hypomagnesemia and hypophosphatemia, are often associated with TBI and can be challenging to treat.

Symptoms of hypomagnesemia include ventricular arrhythmias, widened QRS, prolonged PR interval, weakness, and seizures. Symptomatic hypomagnesemia, or magnesium (Mg) level of less than 0.8 mM, should be treated with IV Mg, although oral Mg should be used for asymptomatic patients. Mg repletion may also be required for successful correction of hypokalemia or hypocalcemia.

Patients with hypophosphatemia can present with hypotension, seizures, and cardiac or respiratory failure. Treatment of hypophosphatemia can result in severe hypocalcemia and so should only be considered in moderate to severe hypophosphatemia or symptomatic patients.

Ko NU, Engelhard K, Neurocritical care. In: Gropper MA, Cohen NH, Eriksson LI, et al, eds. *Miller's Anesthesia*. 10th ed. Elsevier; 2025:2571.

Steurer MP, Sikorski RA, Richards JE, et al. Anesthesia for trauma. In: Gropper MA, Cohen NH, Eriksson LI, et al, eds. *Miller's Anesthesia*. 10th ed. Elsevier; 2025:2000-2043.

Wu X, Lu X, Lu X, et al. Prevalence of severe hypokalemia in patients with traumatic brain injury. *Injury*. 2015;46:35-41.

A.7. What are the neuroprotective effects of administering magnesium (Mg)?

N-methyl-D-aspartate (NMDA) receptors (NMDARs) gate open in response to the excitatory amino acid glutamate, which increases in the central nervous system soon after primary TBI. Once stimulated, NMDARs facilitate calcium entry into the cell, which leads to mitochondrial damage. Damaged mitochondria and ischemia-induced depletion of adenosine triphosphate (ATP) contribute to early cytotoxic edema in patients with TBI. Mg, a noncompetitive inhibitor of NMDARs and an intracellular calcium antagonist, helps to limit the influx of calcium, thereby reducing cell death. Other effects of Mg include downregulation of the membrane protein aquaporin 4, which is known to increase cerebral edema, and decreased upregulation of the tumor suppressor gene *TP53*, which causes apoptosis. Other properties of Mg demonstrated in animal and in vitro models include vasodilation and BBB preservation, which can contribute to the decreased cortical damage noted in the rat brain after brain injury.

Human studies evaluating the effect of Mg in TBI suggest a beneficial effect on the Glasgow Outcome Score (GOS) and Glasgow Coma Score (GCS) and on the release of enzymes like neuron-specific enolase (NSE) released from neurons in response to neuronal damage and BBB disruption. The varied results of magnesium's effects on mortality and outcome after TBI might reflect the need for consideration of a more multifaceted approach. Ninety patients with severe TBI (GCS = 3) were randomly assigned to receive combination therapy with nimodipine, progesterone, and Mg (study group) or control. Although there was no difference in jugular venous oxygen saturation ($Sjvo_2$) between groups, GCS in the study group was significantly higher over the next four hospital days and at 3 months, and mortality was less in the study group compared to control (22% vs 42%; P = .42). Burgeoning interest in mitigating the impact of concussive injury or mild TBI has compelled evaluation of Mg in this group. In a small group of patients who presented 48 hours after concussion randomized to receive Mg PO or placebo, patients who received Mg had a statistically significant decrease in postconcussion severity score at 48 hours.

Abdoli A, Rahimi-Bashar F, Torabian S, et al. Efficacy of simultaneous administration of nimodipine, progesterone, and magnesium sulfate in patients with severe traumatic brain injury: a randomized controlled trial. *Bull Emerg Trauma*. 2019;7:124-129

Li W, Bai Y, Li Y, et al. Magnesium sulfate for acute traumatic brain injury. *J Craniofac Surg*. 2015;26:393-398

Sen AP, Gulati A. Use of magnesium in traumatic brain injury. *Neurotherapeutics*. 2010;7:91-99.

Standiford L, O'Daniel M, Hysell M, Trigger C. A randomized cohort study of the efficacy of PO magnesium in the treatment of acute concussions in adolescents. *Am J Emerg Med*. 2021;44:419-422.

Zhao L, Wang W, Zhong J, et al. The effects of magnesium sulfate therapy after severe diffuse axonal injury. *Ther Clin Risk Manag*. 2016;12:1481-1486.

A.8. What role do sex and female sex hormones have in the pathophysiology of traumatic brain injury (TBI)?

Estrogen and progesterone are known for their immunomodulating potential in neurotrauma. Neuroprotective effects of estradiol include antioxidant functions and prevention of mitochondrial damage. Estrogen might also be beneficial in the setting of cerebral ischemia by stabilizing the BBB and increasing blood flow during and after ischemia as well as improving regeneration and plasticity of new neurons. Progesterone promotes an anti-inflammatory action by reducing microglia activation and proinflammatory cytokines and by stimulation of postinjury remyelination and repair. These hormonal benefits support the evidence for improved functional outcome in females after TBI in preclinical studies. In other animal studies, however, female animals exhibited greater neurodegeneration after TBI compared to male animals, and in other work, estrogen resulted in no difference in neurodegeneration between female and male mice after TBI. Similar discrepancies in preclinical study outcomes are evident with progesterone.

Although some clinical trials suggest some benefits from hormones in outcomes after TBI, results of two multicenter clinical trials (SYNAPSE and PRoTECT III) failed to demonstrate an outcome benefit of progesterone administered to patients with moderate and severe TBI 6 months after injury. In a secondary analysis of serum biomarkers of glial and neuronal cell death (glial fibrillary acidic protein [GFAP]), ubiquitin carboxyterminal hydrolase, S100 calcium-binding protein, and α-II Spectrin

Breakdown Product 150 were examined (BIO-ProTECT study). Treatment with progesterone did not decrease levels of biomarkers of glial and neuronal cell death during the first 48 hours after injury, which may explain the lack of benefit of progesterone on mortality after TBI. In a recent systematic review of 156 published human studies and 46 animal studies examining sex differences in TBI, the authors concluded that overall, human studies report worse outcomes in females than in males, whereas animal studies tended to report better outcomes in females than in males. Conflicting results regarding outcome after TBI and sex in both preclinical and clinical research reflect in part the multifactorial nature of TBI: injury type and severity, genetics, hormonal fluctuations, and environmental factors all influence outcomes from TBI. Larger trials, validated TBI-specific biomarkers to better characterize outcomes, and increasing representation of females in studies will undoubtedly help elucidate the impact of sex on TBI outcomes.

Gupte R, Brooks W, Vukas R, Pierce J, Harris J. Sex differences in traumatic brain injury: what we know and what we should know. *J Neurotrauma*. 2019;36:3063-3091.

Korley F, Pauls Qi, Yeatts SD, et al. Progesterone treatment does not decrease serum levels of biomarkers of glial and neuronal cell injury in moderate and severe traumatic brain injury subjects: a secondary analysis of the progesterone for traumatic brain injury, experimental clinical treatment (ProTEXT) III Trial. *J Neurotrauma*. 2021;38:1953-1960.

Mollayeva T, Mollayeva S, Colantonio A. Traumatic brain injury: sex, gender and intersecting vulnerabilities. *Nat Rev Neurol*. 2018;14:711-722.

Nasre-Nasser RG, Severo MMR, Pires GN, Hort MA, Arbo BD. Effects of progesterone on preclinical animal models of traumatic brain injury: systematic review and meta-analysis. *Mol Neurobiol*. 2022;59:6341-6362.

Raghava N, Das BC, Ray SK. Neuroprotective effects of estrogen in CNS injuries: insights from animal models. *Neurosci Neuroecon*. 2017;6:15-29.

Skolnick BE, Maas AI, Narayan RK, et al. A clinical trial of progesterone for severe traumatic brain injury. *N Engl J Med*. 2014;371:2467-2476.

Wright DW, Yeatts SD, Silbergleit R, et al. Very early administration of progesterone for acute traumatic brain injury. *N Engl J Med*. 2014;371:2457-2466.

SECTION 4

A.9. What is the role of decompressive craniectomy as a treatment option for ICP control after head injury?

In TBI, decompressive craniectomy has been reserved for those patients with increasing ICP refractory to medical therapy (eg, sedation, hyperventilation, osmotic diuretics, HTS, paralysis, and/or ventriculostomy). A skull flap is removed to make space for the expanding traumatized brain, thereby decreasing ICP and improving cerebral blood flow (CBF). However, this procedure is associated with 26% mortality and is not without morbidity: contusion expansion, contralateral subdural hematoma or epidural hematoma, CSF leakage, herniation, and infection. Consequently, translating the benefits of decompressive craniectomy (ie, decreased ICP and increased cerebral perfusion) into better neurologic outcome in this patient population has been challenging.

Patients with TBI who underwent bifrontal craniectomy as an *early intervention* for increased ICP after failed medical therapy in the Decompressive Craniectomy (DECRA) trial had poorer outcomes (worse scores on the Extended GCS) compared to patients who received standard care. Rates of death at 6 months were similar between the decompressive craniectomy group and the standard care managed group. In a secondary analysis, outcomes (mortality, severe and moderate disability) at 12 months after injury were similar for patients medically managed and those managed with early decompressive craniectomy. While more patients treated with decompressive craniectomy as a *last tier* effort in the larger Randomized Evaluation of Surgery with Craniectomy for Uncontrollable Elevation of Intracranial Pressure (RESCUEicp) trial were in a vegetative state at 6 months after injury compared to patients medically managed, at 24 months follow-up, more patients treated surgically achieved some neurologic improvement (30.4%), defined by increased Glasgow Outcome Scale-Extended (GOS-E) grade, compared to patients medically managed (14.5%). The decision to perform decompressive craniectomy should be made in conjunction with the family to understand patient and family priorities.

Algattas H, Huang JH. Traumatic brain injury pathophysiology and treatments: early, intermediate, and late phases post-injury. *Int J Mol Sci*. 2014;15:309-341.

Cooper DJ, Rosenfeld JV, Murray L, et al. Patient outcomes at 12 months after early decompressive craniectomy for diffuse traumatic brain injury in the randomized DECRA clinical trial. *J Neurotrauma*. 2020;37:810-816.

Kolias AG, Adams H, Timofeev IS, et al. Evaluation of outcomes among patients with traumatic intracranial hypertension treated with decompressive craniectomy vs standard medical care at 24 months. A secondary analysis of the RESUCEicp randomized clinical trial. *JAMA Neurology*. 2023;797:664-671.

Shutter LA, Timmons SD. Intracranial pressure rescued by decompressive surgery after traumatic brain injury. *N Engl J Med*. 2016;375:1183-1184.

Soustiel JF, Sviri GE, Mahamid E, et al. Cerebral blood flow and metabolism following decompressive craniectomy for control of increased intracranial pressure. *Neurosurgery*. 2010;67:65-72.

A.10. Do genetic factors play a role in outcomes after head injury?

Age, preinjury health, and injury severity account for less than 35% of outcome variability after TBI. In genome-wide association studies (GWAS) of TBI outcome, the estimated heritability of the impact of genetic variation on outcome is 26%. Although no genetic variants reached genome-wide significance, the authors detected some variants associated with TBI outcome.

Polymorphism in *MBL*$_2$ demonstrated an association with TBI outcome, in addition to associations with *TNF.APOE*-ε4, a well-studied gene known for its association with Alzheimer disease and other dementias, has been implicated in less desirable outcomes in athletes and the general population after mild traumatic brain injury (MTBI), such as impaired neurocognitive scores and high-performance variability, and problems with cognitive processing. In this GWAS of TBI outcome, however, there was no association between *APOE*-ε4 and TBI outcomes in the overall cohort (N = 5,268). Caution is advised in interpreting these results, as this homogenous sample consisted of mostly individuals of European ancestry.

Other genes implicated in TBI include *p53*, the ACE (angiotensin-converting enzyme) gene (*17p23*), interleukins (IL), and TNF (tumor necrosis factor-α). The gene *p53*, a tumor suppressor gene, can cause apoptosis in response to cellular stress, thereby mitigating the chance of mutation and cancer. Given that the *p53 gene* is induced after TBI, a functional polymorphism of this gene was studied in a group of 90 patients with severe head injury. Patients with the Arg/Arg genotype of *p53* had a 2.9-fold increased risk of having a bad outcome at the time of discharge from the intensive care unit (ICU; GOS, 1-3) compared to other genotypes (Arg/Pro and Pro/Pro) (95% confidence interval, 1.05-8.31; P = .039). The absence of an association between *p53* polymorphisms and GOS at 6 months could indicate that other mechanisms are involved in longer term neurologic outcomes.

The ACE insertion/deletion (I/D) polymorphism influences TBI outcomes by altering ACE plasma levels and local tissue production. The worse neurologic outcomes (poor performance on attention tests and processing speed) noted in an investigation of 73 patients after moderate or severe TBI were attributed in part to being a *D* allele carrier (D/D) compared to having the I/I polymorphism of the ACE gene (circulating and tissue ACE concentrations are higher among D/D homozygous subjects).

Finally, polymorphism of the cytokine gene IL-1β has also been implicated in unfavorable outcomes in patients after TBI (Uzan et al 2005). In this small study of 69 patients admitted for head injury, more patients with IL-1β +3953 allele (56%) or IL-1β −511 (71%) allele had an unfavorable outcome (dead, vegetative state, or severe disability) compared to 18% without IL-1β +3953 (P = .0004) and 5% without IL-1β −511 (P = .005). In contrast, in a larger cohort ($N >$ 1,000) of patients with TBI, Waters and colleagues were not able to find an association between IL-1 single nucleotide polymorphisms and outcome at 6 months after TBI and a weak association between IL-1β +3953 and increased ICP. They did find an association between TNFA −308 SNP and an unfavorable outcome 6 months after TBI (as determined by GOS) in allele 2 carriers compared to noncarriers (39% vs 31%). Examining larger cohorts together with different combinations of alleles will further elucidate the associations between cytokines and TBI.

Ariza M, Matarin MD, Junqué C, et al. Influence of angiotensin-converting enzyme polymorphism on neuropsychological subacute performance in moderate and severe traumatic brain injury. *J Neuropsychiatry Clin Neurosci*. 2006;18:39-44.

Deng H, Ordaz A, Uadyhahula P, et al. Apolipoprotein E epsilon 4 genotype, mild traumatic brain injury and the development of chronic traumatic encephalopathy. *Med Sci*. 2018;6:1-21.

Honnalli NM, Adiga US, Kanchan SM, Association of Arg72Pro single nucleotide polymorphism of p53 Gene with functional outcome after TBI: a meta-analysis. *J Clinical Diagnostic Res*. 2019;13:1-4.

Kals M, Kunzmann K, Radmenesh F, et al. A genome-side association study of outcome from traumatic brain injury. *eBioMedicine*. 2022;77:103933.

Martínez-Lucas P, Moreno-Cuesta J, García-Olmo DC, et al. Relationship between the Arg72Pro polymorphism of p53 and outcome for patients with traumatic brain injury. *Intensive Care Med*. 2005;31:1168-1173.

Uzan M, Tanriverdi T, Baykara O, et al. Association between interleukin-1 beta (IL-1β) gene polymorphism and outcome after head injury: an early report. *Acta Neurochirurgica*. 2005;147:715-720.

Waters RJ, Murray GD, Teasdale GM, et al. Cytokine gene polymorphisms and outcome after traumatic brain injury. *J Neurotrauma*. 2013;30:1710-6.

B. Preoperative Evaluation and Preparation

B.1. What is GCS? What is the significance of a GCS of 7T in this patient?

GCS is an assessment tool in use since 1974 that uses eye-opening and verbal and motor responses to evaluate neurologic status and severity of TBI (**Table 21.1**); its range is 3 (worst possible score) to 15 (best possible score). It was initially developed to assess head trauma patients, although its use has expanded to many other patient populations. In this patient, a GCS of 7T signifies that she has severe TBI and is intubated (T).

Patients with a GCS score of 13 to 15 are considered to have mild TBI; moderate TBI is classified by a GCS score of 9 to 12, whereas a GCS score of 8 and below corresponds with severe TBI. Compared to patients with other types of traumatic injury, mortality risk is significantly increased with severe TBI. Even with isolated TBI, these patients are also at high risk of nonneurologic organ failure. Guidelines published for the management of severe head injury by the American Society of Neurological Surgeons (ASNS) and Brain Trauma Foundation (BTF) recommend early therapy directed toward avoiding hypotension and hypoxia as well as ICP monitoring in order to guide therapy for maintenance of cerebral perfusion. Adherence to these guidelines has been associated with improved survival following severe head injury.

Bratton SL, Chestnut RM, Ghajar J, et al. Guidelines for the management of severe traumatic brain injury. I. Blood pressure and oxygenation. *J Neurotrauma*. 2007;24:S7-S13.

Ko NU, Engelhard K, Neurocritical care. In: Gropper MA, Cohen NH, Eriksson LI, et al, eds. *Miller's Anesthesia*. 10th ed. Elsevier; 2025:2571.

Matis G, Birbilis T. The Glasgow Coma Scale–A brief review. Past, present, future. *Acta Neurol Belg*. 2008;108:75-89.

Steurer MP, Sikorski RA, Richards JE, et al. Anesthesia for trauma. In: Gropper MA, Cohen NH, Eriksson LI, et al, eds. *Miller's Anesthesia*. 10th ed. Elsevier; 2025:2000-2043.

Talving P, Karamanos E, Teixeira PG, et al. Intracranial pressure monitoring in severe head injury: compliance with Brain Trauma Foundation guidelines and effect on outcomes: a prospective study. *J Neurosurg*. 2013;119:1248-1254.

B.2. In addition to the GCS, what other assessments can be done to evaluate neurologic function?

Although the GCS is the most commonly used assessment tool, there are other methods available to assess neurologic function. Abnormalities in pupil size, symmetry, and light reflex can reveal conditions requiring immediate intervention such as uncal or cerebellar herniation. The World Federation of Neurological Surgeons (WFNS) scale is a modified GCS, which grades patients according to GCS score and the presence or absence of motor deficits. The Hunt and Hess (HH) scale is a grading system that predicts mortality in patients with subarachnoid hemorrhage based on clinical presentation and may also be useful for the evaluation of patients with TBI. The Abbreviated Injury Scale (AIS) is an anatomic

TABLE 21.1 Glasgow Coma Scale (GCS)

Eye opening	None	1
	To pain	2
	To verbal command	3
	Spontaneous	4
Best verbal response	No verbal response	1
	Incomprehensible sounds	2
	Inappropriate words	3
	Disoriented, conversing	4
	Oriented, conversing	5
Best motor response	No response (flaccid)	1
	Extension (decerebrate)	2
	Abnormal flexion (decorticate)	3
	Flexion/withdrawal	4
	Localizes to pain	5
	Obeys verbal commands	6

SECTION 4

scale for assessing the severity of traumatic injuries. It can be useful in conjunction with the GCS in more accurately evaluating TBI in older patients.

Ko NU, Engelhard K, Neurocritical care. In: Gropper MA, Cohen NH, Eriksson LI, et al, eds. *Miller's Anesthesia*. 10th ed. Elsevier; 2025:2579.

Rau CS, Wu SC, Chen YC, et al. Effect of age on Glasgow Coma Scale in patients with moderate and severe traumatic brain injury: an approach with propensity score-matched population. *Int J Environ Res Public Health*. 2017;14:1378.

Steurer MP, Sikorski RA, Richards JE, et al. Anesthesia for trauma. In: Gropper MA, Cohen NH, Eriksson LI, et al, eds. *Miller's Anesthesia*. 10th ed. Elsevier; 2025:2000-2043.

B.3. What is the role of CT scanning in the initial evaluation of the patient with head injury? What are the management options for patients whose neurologic condition is deteriorating before obtaining a CT scan?

Following head trauma, a CT scan can be very useful for revealing acute brain injury. An early CT scan is indicated for a GCS of 9 to 12 (moderate head injury) as well as severe head injury. Any patient with a deteriorating GCS score requires an immediate CT scan.

The Canadian CT Head Rule is a clinical decision-making tool that was developed to guide the use of CT scans in head injury because the vast majority of CT scans performed in the context of head trauma are negative for significant brain injury. The rule is used to assess risk level for neurosurgical intervention and brain injury on CT in patients with minor head injury and GCS of 13 to 15. Patients considered to be at high risk for neurologic intervention have any one of the following findings:

- GCS score less than 15 at 2 hours beyond the time of injury
- Any suspected open or depressed skull fracture
- Signs of basal skull fracture (hemotympanum, Battle sign, raccoon eyes, otorrhea, or CSF rhinorrhea)
- Two or more episodes of vomiting
- 65 Years of age or older

Patients with injury resulting from any dangerous mechanism, such as ejection from a motor vehicle, fall from a height of 3 feet or more, or any patient who exhibits retrograde amnesia of 30 minutes or more prior to injury are considered to be at medium risk for brain injury findings on CT.

It is important to note that the Canadian CT Head Rule does not apply to trauma patients with GCS less than 13, obvious open skull fracture, age less than 16 years, or in patients with a bleeding disorder or taking anticoagulant medications.

The airway should be secured with an endotracheal tube as soon as possible in patients with deterioration in neurologic function or in those who are likely to have such changes prior to obtaining a CT scan.

Steurer MP, Sikorski RA, Richards JE, et al. Anesthesia for trauma. In: Gropper MA, Cohen NH, Eriksson LI, et al, eds. *Miller's Anesthesia*. 10th ed. Elsevier; 2025:2026.

Stiell IG, Clement CM, Grimshaw JM, et al. A prospective cluster-randomized trial to implement the Canadian CT head rule in emergency departments. *CMAJ*. 2010;182:1527-1532.

Stiell IG, Wells GA, Vandemheen K, et al. The Canadian CT head rule for patients with minor head injury. *Lancet*. 2001;357:1391-1396.

B.4. What is the role of ICP monitoring in the management of head injury?

ASNS/BTF guidelines recommend early ICP monitoring and concomitant goal-directed therapy for maintenance of cerebral perfusion in patients with severe head injury. A recent analysis of outcomes in patients with penetrating brain injury indicates that ICP monitoring was associated with an increased likelihood of survival (along with an increase in ICU length of stay), but no clear impact on favorable discharge disposition. Adherence to these guidelines might improve outcome in this patient population, primarily through guiding therapy to minimize secondary insults following the initial injury.

Because of impaired CBF and autoregulation in the injured brain, cerebral perfusion is highly dependent on CPP for oxygen delivery and prevention of cerebral ischemia.

Systemic hypotension and intracranial hypertension are related to increased morbidity and mortality in severe TBI. Because CPP values of less than 50 mm Hg are correlated with poor outcomes, continuous monitoring of ICP should be used to guide therapy in patients with severe TBI. The target range for CPP is 60 to 70 mm Hg according to the most recent ASNS/BTF guidelines.

Currently, recommendations for ICP monitoring include (1) patients with GCS 3 to 8 following resuscitation and abnormal CT scan related to the injury (contusion, swelling, compressed basal cisterns, or hematoma on CT) and (2) patients with severe TBI if two or more of the following features are present:

age over 40 years, motor posturing, or systolic BP (SBP) less than 90 mm Hg, even if the CT scan is normal. Current recommendations include treating ICP greater than 22 mm Hg, although treatment decisions also depend on CT findings and clinical presentation.

ICP monitoring can be performed using ventricular catheters or intraparenchymal fiberoptic monitors. Ventricular catheters have the advantage of allowing CSF drainage, although they do carry a higher infection risk. In the setting of coagulopathy, placing an ICP monitor is contraindicated.

Carney N, Totten AM, O'Reilly C, et al. Guidelines for the management of severe traumatic brain injury, fourth edition. *Neurosurgery*. 2017;80:6-15.

Griesdale D, Ortenwall V, Norena M, et al. Adherence to guidelines for management of cerebral perfusion pressure and outcome in patients who have severe traumatic brain injury. *J Crit Care*. 2015;30:111-115.

Ko NU, Engelhard K, Neurocritical care. In: Gropper MA, Cohen NH, Eriksson LI, et al, eds. *Miller's Anesthesia*. 10th ed. Elsevier; 2025:2575.

Mansour A, Rowell S, Powla PP, Horowitz P, Goldenberg FD, Lazaridis C. Comparative effectiveness of intracranial pressure monitoring vs no monitoring in severe penetrating brain injury management. *JAMA Netw Open*. 2023;6:e231077.

Steurer MP, Sikorski RA, Richards JE, et al. Anesthesia for trauma. In: Gropper MA, Cohen NH, Eriksson LI, et al, eds. *Miller's Anesthesia*. 10th ed. Elsevier; 2025:2000-2043.

Talving P, Karamanos E, Teixeira PG, et al. Intracranial pressure monitoring in severe head injury: compliance with brain trauma foundation guidelines and effect on outcomes: a prospective study. *J Neurosurg*. 2013;119:1248-1254.

B.5. How can you clear this patient's cervical spine?

The National Emergency X-Radiography Utilization Study (NEXUS) low-risk criteria are commonly used to determine the need for radiographic imaging in the clinical evaluation of cervical spine injury. A patient is considered to be low risk for cervical spine injury if they meet *all* of the following criteria:

1. No posterior midline cervical spine tenderness
2. No evidence of intoxication
3. GCS score of 15—normal level of alertness
4. No focal neurologic deficit
5. No painful distracting other injuries

However, there is evidence that patients with clinically significant cervical spine injuries, such as ligamentous injury, cervical spine fracture, or dislocation, can be considered low risk according to the NEXUS criteria, particularly older patients. This may be a result of variation in determining the extent or presence of distracting injuries.

The Canadian C-spine Rule is another clinical decision-making tool that can be used in evaluating the need for further imaging in cervical spine injury. The criteria take into account the mechanism of injury, midline neck tenderness, and the ability to rotate the neck more than 45° without pain (if it is safe for the patient to do so). A recent comparison of the Canadian C-spine and NEXUS rules indicated that the Canadian C-spine Rule has greater reliability.

Nevertheless, CT evaluation is still recommended in the case of major trauma because of the possibility of misdiagnosis of a clinically significant cervical spine injury.

Collins NC, McKenzie JV. The NEXUS criteria: do they stand the test of time? *Eur J Emerg Med*. 2013;20:58-60.

Duane TM, Mayglothling J, Wilson SP, et al. National emergency x-radiography utilization study criteria is inadequate to rule out fracture after significant blunt trauma compared with computed tomography. *J Trauma*. 2011;70:829-831.

Ehrlich F, Wee C, Drongowski R, et al. Canadian C-spine rule and the national emergency x-radiography utilization low-risk criteria for C-spine radiography in young trauma patients. *J Pediatric Surg*. 2009;44:987-991.

Michaleff ZA, Maher CG, Verhagen AP, et al. Accuracy of the Canadian C-spine rule and NEXUS to screen for clinically important cervical spine injury in patients following blunt trauma: a systematic review. *CMAJ*. 2012;184:E867-E876.

B.6. What are the advantages of early endotracheal intubation in this patient?

Endotracheal intubation is indicated in this patient with a severe TBI and a strong probability of further neurologic deterioration. Choosing early endotracheal intubation provides the advantage of securing the airway under more controlled and optimized circumstances as well as providing safer conditions for further evaluation and treatment.

Guidelines published by the Eastern Association for the Surgery of Trauma recommend early endotracheal intubation for all patients with a GCS score of 8 or less (level 1 indication). Other level 1 indications include airway obstruction, persistent hypoxemia, hypoventilation, hemorrhagic shock, and cardiac arrest.

Mayglothling J, Duane TM, Gibbs M, et al. Emergency tracheal intubation immediately following traumatic injury: an Eastern Association for the Surgery of Trauma practice management guideline. *J Trauma Acute Care Surg*. 2012;73:S333-S340.

B.7. What is your plan for airway management in this patient? How would it change if the patient was responsive but combative? How would it change if the patient had facial fractures with significant swelling of the head and neck?

The practitioner considering airway management in a trauma patient should take into account their skill level and experience with different approaches to intubation. Although fiberoptic intubation could minimize manipulation of the cervical spine, difficulty is increased substantially under emergent conditions, especially in the presence of bleeding or secretions. Additionally, in a combative, uncooperative patient, attempting an awake or lightly sedated fiberoptic intubation would be inadvisable. Rapid sequence induction (RSI) can provide the best intubating conditions in the trauma patient, who should be considered a full stomach and at high risk for aspiration of gastric contents.

There is some controversy among practitioners regarding the use of both ventilatory breaths and cricoid pressure during RSI of the trauma patient. The risks of oxygen desaturation and hypercarbia must be taken into consideration when deciding whether ventilation should be used. If ventilatory breaths are necessary, cricoid pressure could limit gastric inflation caused by positive pressure ventilation, although it can also reduce tidal volumes. There is also evidence that cricoid pressure can degrade laryngoscopic view in up to 30% of patients and should therefore be discontinued if required to improve intubating conditions and expedite securing the airway.

A recent large study conducted in 10 academic centers suggests that the risk of pulmonary aspiration does not increase if cricoid pressure (the Sellick maneuver) is not applied during RSI induction of anesthesia. It is important to note, however, that this trial did not extend to patients outside of the operating room or to pregnant patients.

In-line stabilization (facilitated by removal of the front of the cervical collar if needed) is recommended in the setting of cervical spine injury. Assistance from one or more individuals will be required in this endeavor, particularly with a combative patient.

Videolaryngoscopy (as compared to the use of a video stylet) can be beneficial under these circumstances (depending on clinician experience) for the facilitation of intubation while reducing stress on the cervical spine. Difficult airway equipment should also be immediately accessible should the need to follow the difficult airway algorithm arise. If an extremely difficult airway is anticipated, very cautious use or avoidance of neuromuscular blocking drugs (NMBDs) should be exercised, and alternative methods for securing an airway, such as cricothyroidotomy, should be considered.

A primary concern in a patient with facial fractures is the ability to provide adequate ventilation and preoxygenation prior to induction. Additionally, there is a substantial probability that swelling, blood, and secretions will limit visibility and markedly increase difficulty in securing the airway. Light palpation of the facial bones can help ascertain the presence of facial fractures.

Oral intubation is highly preferred in traumatic situations. Nasal intubation should be avoided in head injury because of the possibility of fractures of the basilar skull and cribriform plate and concerns over entering the cranial vault as well as failed intubation.

Birenbaum A, Hajage D, Roche S, et al. Effect of cricoid pressure compared with a sham procedure in the rapid sequence induction of anesthesia: the IRIS randomized clinical trial. *JAMA Surg*. 2019;154:9-17.

Steurer MP, Sikorski RA, Richards JE, et al. Anesthesia for trauma. In: Gropper MA, Cohen NH, Eriksson LI, et al, eds. *Miller's Anesthesia*. 10th ed. Elsevier; 2025:2006-2010.

Yoon HK, Lee HC, Park JB, Oh H, Park HP. McGrath MAC videolaryngoscope versus optiscope video stylet for tracheal intubation in patients with manual inline cervical stabilization: a randomized Trial. *Anesth Analg*. 2020;130:870-878.

B.8. What are the effects of succinylcholine on ICP? What is the significance of the effect, if any?

The rapid onset and short duration of succinylcholine make it a suitable NMBD for facilitating intubation in trauma patients. Succinylcholine has been shown to transiently increase ICP, but this effect should be weighed against the potential detrimental effects of hypercarbia and hypoxia in patients with severe head injury and is not a contraindication to its use. The rise in ICP may be attenuated by pretreatment with a small dose of a nondepolarizing NMBD; however, the benefits of this practice have not been proven.

In cases where succinylcholine is not considered to be suitable, high-dose rocuronium (1.2 mg/kg) is an alternative for RSI, particularly when sugammadex is available.

The cyclodextrin sugammadex is a neuromuscular blockade reversal drug for use with the aminosteroid nondepolarizing agents, rocuronium and vecuronium. In high doses (16 mg/kg), sugammadex can be considered for emergency reversal of rocuronium when the post-tetanic count (PTC) is 0. It should be noted, however, that bradycardia and dose-dependent transient elevated activated partial thromboplastin time (aPPT) and prothrombin time (PT)/INR have been reported with sugammadex.

Steurer MP, Sikorski RA, Richards JE, et al. Anesthesia for trauma. In: Gropper MA, Cohen NH, Eriksson LI, et al, eds. *Miller's Anesthesia*. 10th ed. Elsevier; 2025:2010.

Lee IO, Kim YS, Chang HW, et al. In vitro investigation of the effects of exogenous sugammadex on coagulation in orthopedic surgical patients. *BMC Anesthesiol*. 2018;18:56.

Mayglothling J, Duane TM, Gibbs M, et al. Emergency tracheal intubation immediately following traumatic injury: an eastern association for the surgery of trauma practice management guideline. *J Trauma Acute Care Surg*. 2012;73:S333-S340.

Oliveira C, Marques C, Simões V, et al. Severe bradycardia and asystole associated with sugammadex: case report. *Rev Bras Anestesiol*. 2019;69:218-221.

B.9. What coagulation abnormalities are present after TBI? What modalities can be used to provide hemostasis and reduce intracranial hematoma expansion?

Coagulopathy, particularly in the first 24 to 72 hours following severe TBI, is associated with a high risk of mortality and can occur in greater than 60% of these patients. The risk of poor outcome is increased up to 30-fold in patients with TBI presenting to the emergency department with abnormal coagulation; consequently, the initiation of early coagulation monitoring is recommended.

Both hypo- and hypercoagulable states can be present and include disorders of coagulation enzymes, platelet function, thrombocytopenia, and hyperfibrinolysis. Although no specific mechanism has been established, release of tissue factor leading to a consumptive coagulopathy as well as hyperfibrinolysis and abnormal activation of the protein C pathway have been proposed.

Acute coagulopathy following severe head injury is complex and might not be distinguishable from coagulopathy associated with other types of trauma. Treatment should address the primary cause with correction of the coagulation abnormality and a focus on controlling bleeding. Although plasma could be useful when there is evidence of coagulopathy, prophylactic early use in head trauma has not proven to be beneficial and is related to adverse events. Conflicting information exists with respect to platelet administration. Goal-directed platelet use can be effective in reversing platelet dysfunction, particularly in reversal of aspirin therapy, but might not be as effective with other antiplatelet medications. Nevertheless, it is recommended that an INR above 1.4 and a platelet count at or below 75,000/μL be corrected.

Recombinant factor VIIa rapidly corrects INR and possibly allows earlier neurosurgical intervention, although a higher incidence of asymptomatic deep vein thrombosis has also been observed. Additionally, administration of recombinant factor VIIa has not been found to improve clinical outcomes and might be associated with lower GCS at discharge. Four-factor PCC has been recommended for vitamin K antagonist reversal, as well as for reversal of factor Xa inhibitors, in patients with TBI and ICH.

Tranexamic acid might show some benefit with reduction in intracranial hemorrhage progression, particularly in the first 1 to 3 hours following injury. Idarucizumab is a specific antibody now available for the reversal of dabigatran and can be considered for patients taking dabigatran who have hemorrhagic TBI.

de Oliveira Manoel AL, Neto AC, Veigas PV, et al. Traumatic brain injury associated coagulopathy. *Neurocrit Care*. 2015;22:34-44.

Furay E, Daley M, Teixeira PG, et al. Goal-directed platelet transfusions correct platelet dysfunction and may improve survival in patients with severe traumatic brain injury. *J Trauma Acute Care Surg*. 2018;85:881-887.

Lombardo S, Millar D, Jurkovich GJ, et al. Factor VIIa administration in traumatic brain injury: an AAST-MiTC propensity score analysis. *Trauma Surg Acute Care Open*. 2018;3:e000134.

Maegle M. Coagulopathy after traumatic brain injury: incidence, pathogenesis, and treatment options. *Transfusion*. 2013;53:28S-39S.

Medzon R, Bracken M, Rathlev NK, et al. Clinically suspected coagulopathy in blunt head trauma. *J Emerg Med*. 2010;39:399-405.

Qureshi H, Mithaiwala H, Ezell J, et al. Anesthetic management of traumatic brain injury. *Clin Med Rev Case Rep*. 2017;4:159.

Wiegele M, Schochi H, Haushofer A, et al. Diagnostic and therapeutic approach in adult patients with traumatic brain injury receiving oral anticoagulation therapy: an Austrian interdisciplinary consensus statement. *Crit Care*. 2019;23:62.

C. Intraoperative Management

C.1. What is appropriate hemodynamic monitoring during CT scanning and during craniotomy for evacuation of a subdural hematoma?

First, the patient should be stabilized prior to CT scanning or any other diagnostic studies. When a patient with TBI is uncooperative, combative, or comatose and requires airway control, emergent endotracheal intubation is necessary to protect the airway, facilitate diagnostic procedures, such as head CT scan or MRI, and prevent hypoxia and hypercarbia, which are two important secondary insults. Hemodynamic monitoring should include standard American Society of Anesthesiologists (ASA) monitors: noninvasive BP, electrocardiography (ECG), pulse oximetry, capnography (end-tidal carbon dioxide [$Etco_2$]), and temperature. Maintaining a patent airway, adequate ventilation, and stable hemodynamics are initial priorities.

If the patient with TBI shows signs of intracranial hypertension (defined as sustained ICP >20 mm Hg), such as headache, nausea/vomiting (N/V), papilledema, focal neurologic deficits, altered consciousness, neurogenic pulmonary edema, or Cushing triad (reflex arterial hypertension, bradycardia, and bradypnea), hyperosmolar therapy (eg, mannitol, HTS) should be started immediately to lower ICP without direct ICP measurement during CT scanning.

In addition to the aforementioned standard ASA monitors, during the craniotomy for evacuation of a subdural hematoma (which is much more common than epidural hematoma and carries a worse prognosis), an intra-arterial catheter for continuous BP monitoring and urine output monitoring is appropriate. Central line placement should be considered if the patient has difficult peripheral venous access, the injury is extensive or unknown, or the patient is hemodynamically unstable requiring infusion of vasopressor(s) other than phenylephrine. ICP monitoring is indicated in this patient because she has severe TBI and abnormal findings (eg, malignant cerebral edema) on head CT. Important objectives in the management of the patient with TBI are to maintain adequate MAP, keep ICP less than 20 mm Hg, prevent or reverse brain herniation, minimize retractor pressure, and facilitate surgical access. Additionally, CPP monitoring and novel techniques, such as $Sjvo_2$ for advanced cerebral monitoring (ACM), help guide management and improve outcome. Normal $Sjvo_2$ threshold is 55% to 75% (see Section D.5 for additional information). Medical treatment and surgical intervention decisions are ideally driven by multiple monitoring approaches and ongoing clinical assessments. In addition, monitoring for venous air embolism (VAE) is reasonable if the head is elevated above the heart during craniotomy.

Bendo A. Severe traumatic brain injury: how can we improve outcomes? *ASA Refresher Courses Anesthesiol.* 2018;111:1-6.

Carney N, Totten AM, O'Reilly C, et al. Guidelines for the management of severe traumatic brain injury, fourth edition. *Neurosurgery.* 2017;80:6-15.

Cooper DJ, Rosenfeld JV, Murray L, et al. Decompressive craniectomy in diffuse traumatic brain injury. *N Engl J Med.* 2011;364:1493-1502.

Lemkuil BP, Drummond JC, Patel PM, et al. Anesthesia for neurologic surgery. In: Gropper MA, Cohen NH, Eriksson LI, et al, eds. *Miller's Anesthesia.* 10th ed. Elsevier; 2025:1765-1767.

Steinberg GK, Dodd RL, Chaudhary N, et al. Intracranial neurosurgery. In: Jaffe RA, Schmiesing CA, Golianu B, eds. *Anesthesiologist's Manual of Surgical Procedures.* 6th ed. Wolters Kluwer; 2019:3-72.

C.2. Should hyperventilation be used in this patient?

The 2017 BTF guidelines recommend that hyperventilation be avoided during the first 24 hours after TBI when CBF is often critically reduced during the stage of primary brain injury. Hyperventilation is a quick way to reduce CBF and ICP through hypocarbia and cerebral vasoconstriction. Hyperventilation with maintenance of $Paco_2$ 30 to 35 mm Hg is an acceptable temporizing measure to reduce elevated ICP unresponsive to sedation, with a neutrally positioned head elevated to 15° to 30°, osmotic diuretics, and/or CSF drainage, but should be as brief as possible. Hyperventilation should be reserved for patients in whom herniation is suspected or imminent.

$Paco_2$ is a powerful determinant of CBF. The target $Paco_2$ is 35 to 45 mm Hg. Generally speaking, there is autoregulation of CBF when $Paco_2$ ranges from 20 to 80 mm Hg such that as $Paco_2$ decreases, there is a linear decrease in CBF and an accompanying decrease in ICP. Prolonged hyperventilation to $Paco_2$ less than 30 mm Hg should be avoided as it is associated with worse outcomes at 3 and 6 months (but not at 12 months). A modest decrease in $Paco_2$ is valuable to counteract the vasodilating effects of volatile anesthetics. However, hypocapnia with resultant vasoconstriction can cause cerebral ischemia, which can worsen cerebral injury in patients with focal ischemia, particularly in a recently injured brain and in the brain beneath a retractor. The most recent BTF and World Society of Emergency Surgery guidelines recommend that normal ventilation with $Paco_2$ of 35 to 45 mm Hg should be the goal for patients with TBI in the absence of cerebral herniation. Hyperventilation should be employed selectively and briefly rather than routinely in the management of patients with TBI. When prolonged hyperventilation is required, monitoring cerebral oxygenation with $Sjvo_2$ and CBF with transcranial Doppler ultrasonography should be considered.

Brain Trauma Foundation, American Association of Neurological Surgeons, Joint Section on Neurotrauma and Critical Care. Hyperventilation. *J Neurotrauma*. 2000;17:513-520.

Carney N, Totten AM, O'Reilly C, et al. Guidelines for the management of severe traumatic brain injury, fourth edition. *Neurosurgery*. 2017;80:6-15.

Lemkuil BP, Drummond JC, Patel PM, et al. Anesthesia for neurologic surgery. In: Gropper MA, Cohen NH, Eriksson LI, et al, eds. *Miller's Anesthesia*. 10th ed. Elsevier; 2025:1767.

Muizelaar JP, Marmarou A, Ward JD, et al. Adverse effects of prolonged hyperventilation in patients with severe head injury: a randomized clinical trial. *J Neurosurg*. 1991;75:731-739.

Picetti E, Rossi S, Abu-Zidan FM, et al. WSES consensus conference guidelines: monitoring and management of severe adult traumatic brain injury patients with polytrauma in the first 24 hours. *World J Emerg Surg*. 2019;14:53.

Steiner L, Andrews PJ. Monitoring the injured brain: ICP and CBF. *Br J Anaesth*. 2006; 97:26-38.

C.3. What are the implications of arterial hypertension in patients with head injury? How should BP be managed?

Hypertension is common in patients with head injury who do not have other injuries associated with massive blood loss. There are at least four important implications of arterial hypertension in patients with TBI: (1) Higher SBP might be required to achieve adequate CPP (CPP = MAP − ICP or CVP), particularly in patients with severely elevated ICP. MAP and CPP must be considered in addition to SBP. Efforts to optimize CPP should first lower ICP; (2) Because autoregulation of CBF is usually impaired in areas of brain injury, arterial hypertension can worsen cerebral edema, lead to secondary hemorrhage, and increase ICP because of the increased cerebral blood volume and hyperemia ("pressure passive" in patients with TBI with impaired cerebral autoregulation). Intra-arterial BP monitoring is necessary; (3) Cushing triad is reflex systemic hypertension, bradycardia, and bradypnea in association with elevated ICP. It is a late and unreliable sign that usually precedes brain herniation; (4) Other etiologies of arterial hypertension might be related to pain or catecholamine surge and can be treated with opioids and deepening anesthesia only after hypoxemia and hypercarbia are ruled out as causes.

It is ideal to maintain SBP greater than or equal to 100 mm Hg for patients 50 to 69 years old or greater than or equal to 110 mm Hg for patients 15 to 49 or over 70 years old. Recent guidelines recommend keeping CPP between 60 and 70 mm Hg for patients with severe TBI to ensure adequate brain perfusion and avoid secondary brain injury in order to improve outcomes. However, patients with TBI associated with multiple trauma injuries are at risk for arterial hypotension (SBP <90 mm Hg) related to bleeding and hypovolemia, especially when combined with tachycardia. Avoiding hypotension in patients with severe TBI is a primary perioperative goal. Hypotension can cause cerebral ischemia and is related to poor neurologic outcome in patients with TBI; treatment includes the judicious use of IV fluids, blood transfusion, and vasopressors. Interventions to stop bleeding and restore intravascular volume should precede surgical management of TBI. Attention to fluid resuscitation is critical because aggressive IV fluids to maintain CPP greater than 70 mm Hg could lead to acute respiratory failure.

Carey N, Totten AM, O'Reilly C, et al. Blood pressure thresholds. In: *Guidelines for the Management of Severe Traumatic Brain Injury*. 4th ed. Brain Trauma Foundation; 2016:164-172.

Carney N, Totten AM, O'Reilly C, et al. Guidelines for the management of severe traumatic brain injury, fourth edition. *Neurosurgery*. 2017;80:6-15.

Lemkuil BP, Drummond JC, Patel PM, et al. Anesthesia for neurologic surgery and neurointerventions. In: Gropper MA, Cohen NH, Eriksson LI, et al, eds. *Miller's Anesthesia*. 9th ed. Elsevier; 2020:2139-2140.

Rossi S, Picetti E, Zoerle T, et al. Fluid management in acute brain injury. *Curr Neurol Neurosci Rep*. 2018;18:74.

C.4. What should be done about intravenous (IV) fluid replacement? Should corticosteroids be given empirically?

This patient is presenting with multiple fractures, TBI, anemia, hypotension, and tachycardia secondary to hypovolemia. Hypotension (SBP <90 mm Hg) after head injury is associated with a greater than 70% increased incidence of morbidity and mortality when compared to patients with higher SBPs. Fluid resuscitation should be initiated prior to induction of anesthesia. A major concern during fluid resuscitation is the development of cerebral edema. Intravascular fluids are replaced in trauma patients to restore circulation secondary to blood loss and to maintain MAP and CPP. The important principles are that the chosen fluids should be able to prevent decreases in serum osmolality and colloid oncotic pressure. The choice of the best resuscitation fluids for patients with severe TBI is controversial. The Saline or Albumin for Fluid Resuscitation in Patients with Traumatic Brain Injury (SAFE-TBI) study (2007) indicated that resuscitation with 4% albumin (vs saline) might be linked with greater mortality in TBI; therefore, large-volume resuscitation with isotonic 0.9% NS is preferable in the presence of TBI because of the BBB's relatively impermeability to sodium. Lactated Ringer solution (LR) is mildly hypotonic (osmolality of 273 mOsm/kg) and exacerbates cerebral edema so should be avoided; it was associated with increased mortality compared with NS in patients with TBI. Therefore, isotonic fluids such as NS (0.9%) or PlasmaLyte are currently the commonly accepted choices for nonblood component volume resuscitation in patients with TBI.

Corticosteroids should not be given empirically in the operating room because there are no benefits in these patients. In patients with severe TBI, high-dose methylprednisolone was associated with increased mortality and is contraindicated; this is unlike the beneficial role they play in mitigating the swelling and edema that can occur with intracranial tumors, subdural hematomas, postoperative swelling, and acute spinal cord injury.

Bendo AA. Perioperative management of adult patients with severe head injury. In: Cottrell JE, Young WL, eds. *Cottrell and Young's Neuroanesthesia*. 5th ed. Elsevier Mosby; 2010:321.

Fuller G, Hasler RM, Mealing N, et al. The association between admission systolic blood pressure and mortality in significant traumatic brain injury: a multi-center cohort study. *Injury*. 2014;45:612-617.

Jungner M, Grände P, Mattiasson G, et al. Effects on brain edema of crystalloid and albumin fluid resuscitation after brain trauma and hemorrhage in the rat. *Anesthesiology*. 2010;112:1194-1203.

Myburgh J, Cooper DJ, Finfer S, et al. Saline or albumin for fluid evaluation (SAFE) in patients with traumatic brain injury. *N Engl J Med*. 2007;357:874-884.

Roswell SE, Fair KA, Barbosa RR, et al. The impact of pre-hospital administration of lactated Ringer's solution versus normal saline in patients with traumatic brain injury. *J Neurotrauma*. 2016;33:1054-1059.

Semler MW, Self WH, Wanderer JP, et al. Balanced crystalloids versus saline in critically ill adults. *N Engl J Med*. 2018;378:829-839.

C.5. Should hypertonic saline (HTS) be administered to this patient? How is HTS administered?

Hyperosmolar agents (mannitol and HTS) are widely used in neurosurgery to decrease the brain volume of the intra- and extracellular fluid compartments and to treat raised ICP after TBI. Mannitol (20%) is commonly used intraoperatively because of its rapid onset, efficacy in decreasing ICP, and improvements in CPP. Its use, however, raises concerns over diuresis-induced hypotension, especially in patients with hypovolemia, rebound cerebral edema, pulmonary edema, acute renal insufficiency, and renal damage due to increases in serum osmolarity. Mannitol—which can further worsen hypovolemia, exacerbate hypotension, and thus decrease in CPP—would not be the first choice in this patient.

HTS (3%, 5%, 7.5%, 15%, and 23.4%) has been used as an alternative agent for the treatment of elevated ICP based on the most recent clinical studies. It is a better choice to lower ICP in this hypotensive and hypovolemic patient because it will not exacerbate hypovolemia, thereby limiting a potential decrease in MAP and thus maintaining CPP. It can also be administered if this patient who was normotensive and normovolemic is refractory to mannitol or if repeated administration of mannitol results in adverse effects such as renal injury, hypovolemia, or electrolyte disturbances from profound diuresis.

HTS, like mannitol, creates a hyperosmotic state in the intravascular compartment but does not cross the intact BBB. Because of the osmotic gradient formed across the BBB, water flux from the extravascular to the intravascular compartment occurs, that is, HTS can reduce intracranial edema by osmotic water extraction across the BBB. The BTF guidelines, 4th edition, do not make specific recommendations on the use of HTS for the treatment of traumatic intracranial hypertension. Protocols recommended by clinical trials and clinical studies include (1) HTS concentrations of 3% to 23.4% with dose range from 1.0 to 4.0 mL/kg; (2) continuous IV infusion (central line recommended) of 3% HTS with 30 to 50 mL/h or 1.4 to 2.5 mL/kg given as a bolus; titrate to maintain serum sodium between 145 and 155 mM; and (3) intermittent bolus of 23.4% HTS (central line only) with 30 mL administered over 2 to 10 minutes as needed to treat herniation or acute ICP elevations. Low-volume HTS with slow administration is helpful in preventing significant hypernatremia and central pontine myelinolysis.

There are growing indications that HTS might be superior to mannitol in the management of TBI-associated elevated ICP. At this time, however, there is insufficient evidence to support the use of one rather than the other to improve outcomes such as mortality or functional recovery.

Ali A, Tetik A, Sabanci PA, et al. Comparison of 3% hypertonic saline and 20% mannitol for reducing intracranial pressure in patients undergoing supratentorial brain tumor surgery: a randomized, double-blind clinical Trial. *J Neurosurg Anesthesiol*. 2018;30:171-178.

Carney N, Totten AM, O'Reilly C, et al. Guidelines for the management of severe traumatic brain injury, fourth edition. *Neurosurgery*. 2017;80:6-15.

Lemkuil BP, Drummond JC, Patel PM, et al. Anesthesia for neurologic surgery and neurointerventions. In: Gropper MA, Cohen NH, Eriksson LI, et al, eds. *Miller's Anesthesia*. 9th ed. Elsevier; 2020:1870-1875.

Patil H, Gupta R. A comparative study of bolus dose of hypertonic saline, mannitol, and mannitol plus glycerol combination in patients with severe traumatic brain injury. *World Neurosurg.* 2019;125: e221-e228.

Shi J, Tan L, Ye J, et al. Hypertonic saline and mannitol in patients with traumatic brain injury: a systematic and meta-analysis. *Medicine (Baltimore)*. 2020;99:1-7.

Susanto M, Riantri I. Optimal dose and concentration of hypertonic saline in traumatic brain injury: a systematic review. *Medeni Med J*. 2022;37:203-211.

C.6. The patient underwent a craniectomy for evacuation of a frontal intracerebral hematoma. Which anesthetic agents should be avoided in this situation? What agents might be preferred in this situation?

The three important principles in providing anesthesia for craniectomy for evacuation of intracerebral hematoma in this patient are to maintain adequate MAP, control cerebral edema, and reduce ICP in order to maintain CPP and provide brain relaxation for surgical access. All inhaled anesthetics (both volatile anesthetics and nitrous oxide [N_2O]) have some cerebral vasodilatory effect. They increase CBF and ICP and are best avoided. Volatile anesthetics often uncouple CBF and cerebral metabolic rate for oxygen ($CMRO_2$); they produce a dose-dependent increase in CBF but decrease $CMRO_2$. However, all of the IV anesthetic agents, except ketamine, are cerebral vasoconstrictors and cause coupled decrease in CBF and $CMRO_2$ in a dose-dependent manner. IV anesthetic agents such as etomidate and opioids might be preferred in this patient. Even though propofol is most commonly used to reduce ICP, propofol at doses required for a surgical plane of anesthesia can produce significant hypotension and further impair CPP in this hypovolemic patient, and so should be administered with caution. It is critical to keep in mind that hemodynamic stability is essential before and during high-dose propofol. Like N_2O, ketamine increases both CBF and $CMRO_2$, but its use can be considered if necessary.

Carney N, Totten AM, O'Reilly C, et al. Guidelines for the management of severe traumatic brain injury, fourth edition. *Neurosurgery*. 2017;80:6-15.

Lemkuil BP, Drummond JC, Patel PM, et al. Anesthesia for neurologic surgery and neurointerventions. In: Gropper MA, Cohen NH, Eriksson LI, et al, eds. *Miller's Anesthesia*. 9th ed. Elsevier; 2020:1868-1908.

Zeiler FA, Teitelbaum J, West M, et al. The ketamine effect on ICP in traumatic brain injury. *Neurocrit Care*. 2014;21:163-173.

C.7. Should hypothermia be employed in this patient?

Moderate therapeutic hypothermia (34 °C-35 °C) is an effective method for reducing raised ICP and protecting the brain during focal and global ischemia. It can reduce both basal and electrical metabolic requirements throughout the brain. Induced hypothermia can be employed if this patient is at high risk of intraoperative ischemia and her elevated ICP is refractory to other therapies after discussion with her family or surrogates. However, early (within 2.5 hours), short-term (48 hours postinjury), and routine prophylactic hypothermia in neurosurgery is not recommended to improve clinical outcomes in patients with diffuse injuries.

Is there a role for induced hypothermia in patients with TBI? Following cardiac arrest, mild hypothermia (target temperature 32 °C-34 °C) improves neurologic outcome. In contrast, an international multicenter trial of mild hypothermia did not show neurologic improvement in patients with TBI. Clinicians should keep in mind that hypothermia can cause cardiac arrhythmias and coagulopathies (platelet dysfunction) and can worsen acidosis, which are deleterious to patients with TBI. Almost half of patients with severe TBI develop fever secondary to infection and/or hypothalamic dysfunction. Fever worsens clinical outcomes after severe TBI, presumably by aggravating secondary brain injury. Hyperthermia should be treated aggressively. Intraoperative normothermia is the goal for temperature management.

Arrich J, Schütz N, Oppenauer J, et al. Hypothermia for neuroprotection in adults after cardiac arrest. *Cochrane Database Syst Rev*. 2023;5:CD004128.

Bendo A. Severe traumatic brain injury: how can we improve outcomes? *ASA Refresher Courses Anesthesiol*. 2018;111:1-6.

Butterworth JF, Wasnick JD, Mackey DC, et al. Anesthesia for neurosurgery. In: Butterworth JF, Wasnick JD, Mackey DC, eds. *Morgan & Mikhail's Clinical Anesthesiology*. McGraw-Hill Education; 2018:601-620; 831.

Lemkuil BP, Drummond JC, Patel PM, et al. Anesthesia for neurologic surgery. In: Gropper MA, Cohen NH, Eriksson LI, et al, eds. *Miller's Anesthesia*. 10th ed. Elsevier; 2025:1756.

Madden LK, DeVon HA. A systematic review of the effects of body temperature on outcome after adult traumatic brain injury. *J Neurosci Nurs*. 2015;47:190-203.

Watson HI, Shepherd AA, Rhodes JK, et al. Revisited: a systemic review of therapeutic hypothermia for adult patients following traumatic brain injury. *Crit Care Med*. 2018;46:972-979.

D. Postoperative Neurointensive Care Management

D.1. What are the postoperative ventilation concerns in this patient?

This patient will undoubtedly remain intubated after decompressive craniectomy due to a presenting GCS of 7, acidosis, hyperglycemia, diabetes insipidus, probable lung injury, and pain due to rib fractures. Necessary fluid resuscitation can exacerbate respiratory failure in a patient who is at risk for cardiac dysfunction due to neurogenic pulmonary edema. ICP monitoring is helpful in managing ventilation in the postoperative period because controlling $Paco_2$ and ensuring adequate oxygenation are critical to limiting secondary brain injury. Additionally, CPP should be maintained between 60 and 70 mm Hg. To maintain a favorable balance between decreasing ICP and minimizing the decrease in CBF, hyperventilation to a $Paco_2$ 35 to 40 mm Hg is the goal. A low $Paco_2$ will result in low CBF and consequent cerebral ischemia, whereas high $Paco_2$ levels can result in cerebral hyperemia and high ICP. Prolonged prophylactic hyperventilation with $Paco_2$ less than or equal to 25 mm Hg is not recommended (level IIB evidence). An NMBD can be helpful in controlling ventilation and preventing unacceptable spontaneous increases in ICP (eg, during suctioning).

Avoiding high tidal volumes (V_T) and PEEP to avoid barotrauma while maintaining adequate oxygenation (Pao_2 >60 mm Hg) is important for limiting additional pulmonary damage. Secondary lung injury is the most common nonneurologic complication after TBI. In a randomized controlled study of 90 patients with TBI assigned to three intraoperative ventilatory strategies: A—conventional mechanical ventilation (V_T 10 mL/kg); B—V_T 8 mL/kg and PEEP of 5 cm H_2O; and C—V_T 8 mL/kg and PEEP 5 cm H_2O and recruitment maneuvers (Rms), Group C had decreased 30-day postoperative incidences of total pulmonary complications, hypoxemia, pulmonary infection, and atelectasis. Additional Rms should be performed with caution to avoid negatively impacting systemic and cerebral hemodynamics. Other ventilatory strategies may include high-frequency percussive ventilation (HFPV) and extracorporeal membrane oxygenation (ECMO) if oxygenation continues to be a problem.

Carney N, Totten AM, O'Reilly C, et al. Guidelines for the management of severe traumatic brain injury, fourth edition. *Neurosurgery*. 2017;80:6-15.

Jiang L, Wu Y, Zhang Y. et al. Effects of intraoperative lung-protective ventilation on clinical outcomes in patients with traumatic brain injury: a randomized controlled trial. *BMC Anesthesiol*. 2021;21:182.

Muizelaar JP, Marmarou A, Ward JD, et al. Adverse effects of prolonged hyperventilation in patients with severe head injury: a randomized clinical trial. *J Neurosurg*. 1991;75:731-739.

D.2. What specific measure should be used to control the patient's ICP? What type of monitoring devices can be used to measure ICP?

Controlling ICP (normal range: 7-15 mm Hg) is essential for maintaining cerebral perfusion and improving outcome after TBI. ICP should be monitored in patients with severe TBI (GCS 3-8) and a CT scan showing hematoma, contusion, swelling, herniation, or compressed basal cisterns. In the case of a normal CT scan, if that patient has two or more of the following features, ICP monitoring is indicated: more than 40 years of age, unilateral or bilateral motor posturing, and/or an SBP less than 90 mm Hg. Surgery is often required initially in order to evacuate a subdural or epidural hematoma causing increased ICP. A ventricular drain is often placed to drain CSF. The head of the bed is typically elevated 15° to promote venous drainage. Sedation, pain control, and avoiding hyperthermia also help to ensure decreased brain cerebral metabolic requirements for oxygen. Selective hyperventilation, as mentioned earlier, might be necessary to control ICP; however, this maneuver will also decrease CBF. Hyperventilation to a $Paco_2$ of less than 35 mm Hg as a temporizing measure is avoided unless transtentorial herniation is suspected. Assuming that the BBB is intact, hyperosmolar therapy with mannitol or HTS will increase serum osmolarity so that fluid is mobilized from the brain; serum osmolarity should not be allowed to be greater than 320 mOsm/L. Electrolyte abnormalities and changes in fluid status require regular blood sampling, close attention to fluid balance, hemodynamic monitoring, and the availability of vasoactive agents. Induction of a barbiturate coma to decrease cerebral metabolism in a patient whose ICP is refractory to treatment will require continued ventilator support, cardiovascular monitors, hemodynamic support, and electroencephalogram (EEG) monitoring. The decrease in ICP caused by mild hypothermia has not translated into improved outcomes in TBI.

An intraventricular catheter or ventriculostomy connected to a transducer is the most accurate, reliable, and low-cost method for monitoring ICP and guiding therapy. Intraparenchymal ICP monitors using microstrain pressure transducers have negligible drift but cannot be recalibrated in situ. Furthermore, unlike ventricular catheters, these catheters cannot be used for draining CSF to decrease ICP. Subdural, subarachnoid, and epidural monitors are less accurate than the aforementioned devices.

Carney N, Totten AM, O'Reilly C, et al. Guidelines for the management of severe traumatic brain injury, fourth edition. *Neurosurgery*. 2017;80:6-15.

Cooper DJ, Nichol AD, Bailey M, et al. Effect of early sustained prophylactic hypothermia on neurologic outcomes among patients with severe traumatic brain injury: the POLAR randomized clinical trial. *JAMA*. 2018;320:2211-2220.

Hawthorne C, Piper I. Monitoring of intracranial pressure in patients with traumatic brain injury. *Front Neurol.* 2014;5:121.

Maas AIR, Stocchetti N, Bullock R. Moderate and severe traumatic brain injury in adults. *Lancet Neurol.* 2008;7:728-741.

Stocchetti N, Maas A. Traumatic intracranial hypertension. *N Engl J Med.* 2014;370:2121-2130.

D.3. What is neurogenic pulmonary edema? Would you avoid positive end-expiratory pressure (PEEP) in a patient with increased ICP?

Neurogenic pulmonary edema occurs suddenly as a consequence of sympathetic nervous system stimulation from the hypothalamus and medulla after severe neurologic injury. Patients are dyspneic and tachypneic with pink, frothy sputum. They are often hypoxemic, tachycardic, and hypertensive. Crackles and rales can be heard on lung auscultation. The chest radiograph is often significant for bilateral infiltrates and Pao_2/Fio_2 ratio less than 200 (consistent with moderate to severe respiratory distress syndrome in adults).

The pathophysiology of this consequence of TBI is unclear. One theory is that myocardial injury from a surge in catecholamines causes pulmonary edema due to cardiac dysfunction, similar to that seen in Takotsubo cardiomyopathy. Neurohemodynamic neurogenic pulmonary edema occurs secondary to an acute rise in systemic and pulmonary pressures leading to left ventricular failure; fluid then shifts to the low-resistance pulmonary circulation causing pulmonary edema. Damage to the alveolar-capillary membrane from the rise in capillary pressure with a consequent transudative pulmonary edema is described as the "blast theory." Finally, trauma to the pulmonary capillary bed secondary to sympathetic discharge can occur without systemic changes according to the "pulmonary venule adrenergic hypersensitivity theory." After ruling out other causes of respiratory distress (ie, congestive heart failure, aspiration, acute respiratory distress syndrome, sepsis, and/or transfusion overload), treatment is supportive while addressing the underlying neurologic cause.

Adequate oxygenation is essential for ensuring cerebral perfusion. If ventilator support with an increased Fio_2 is not effective in maintaining a Pao_2 greater than 60 mm Hg, PEEP might help improve oxygenation. The unwanted consequences of PEEP can be successfully addressed by regular blood sampling and appropriate monitoring. Avoiding hypercarbia from overdistension of alveoli and increased dead space is essential to managing this patient. Elevation of the head of the bed helps to combat the transient increase in right atrial pressure from PEEP-induced impairment of cerebral venous drainage. Monitoring the central circulation to keep the patient euvolemic and close attention to cardiac function will help avoid decreases in venous return from high PEEP and maintain CPP.

Acosta P, Santisbon E, Varon J. The use of positive end-expiratory pressure in mechanical ventilation. *Crit Care Clin.* 2007;23:251-261.

Davison DL, Terek M, Chawla LS. Neurogenic pulmonary edema. *Crit Care.* 2012;16:212.

D.4. What is the role of antiseizure prophylaxis in the perioperative management of head trauma?

Between 4% and 25% of patients with TBI will develop posttraumatic seizures in the first 7 days after their trauma (early seizures). In all, 90% to 24% of patients with head injury are at risk for late seizures (7 days after TBI).

The risk of posttraumatic epilepsy increases with increasing severity of brain injury and can exacerbate the impact of TBI on the cerebrovascular system and BBB, memory and cognition. Prophylactic treatment with antiseizure drugs serves to decrease the risk of developing posttraumatic seizures after head injury. Guidelines from the BTF recommend seizure prophylaxis with phenytoin for prevention of early seizures. Other agents used for posttraumatic seizures prophylaxis include sodium valproate, phenobarbital, lamotrigine, oxcarbazepine, carbamazepine, and levetiracetam.

A systematic review and meta-analysis of 11 randomized controlled trials (RCTs) involving over 2,000 patients with TBI (mostly males over a wide range of ages) were treated with placebo, carbamazepine, phenytoin, levetiracetam, valproate, or magnesium sulfate. Overall, these anticonvulsants reduced early seizures but not late seizures compared to placebo. Phenytoin was more effective based on sensitivity analysis compared to placebo. In another meta-analysis, levetiracetam and phenytoin were comparable for prevention of early but not late seizures.

The consequential effects of phenytoin, including phlebitis with extravasation, hypotension or arrhythmias, its ability to induce the hepatic cytochrome system and its narrow therapeutic index, require close monitoring. Patients might benefit from levetiracetam's side-effect profile compared to phenytoin; however, levetiracetam's faster systemic clearance requires more frequent dosing.

Carney N, Totten AM, O'Reilly C, et al. Guidelines for the management of severe traumatic brain injury, fourth edition. *Neurosurgery*. 2017;80:6-15.

Huo X, Xu X, Li M, et al. Effectiveness of antiseizure medications therapy in preventing seizures in brain injury patients: aa network meta-analysis. *Front Pharmacol*. 2022;13:1001363.

Khan SA, Bhatti SN, Khan AA, et al. Comparison of the efficacy of phenytoin and levetiracetam for prevention of early post traumatic seizures. *J Ayub Med Coll Abottabad*. 2016;28:455-460.

Wang BC, Chiu HY, Luh HT, et al. Comparative efficacy of prophylactic anticonvulsant drugs following traumatic brain injury: a systematic review and network meta-analysis of randomized controlled trials. *PLoS One*. 2022;17:e0265932.

Wilson CD, Burks JD, Rodgers RB, et al. Early and late posttraumatic epilepsy in the setting of traumatic brain injury: a meta-analysis and review of antiepileptic management. *World Neurosurg*. 2018;110:e901-e906.

D.5. How can cerebral oxygenation monitoring be used in the clinical management of TBI?

Brain hypoxia from ischemia due to BBB disruption and cerebral edema, anemia, hypoxemia, and hyperventilation can worsen secondary brain injury. Monitoring of partial pressure of oxygen in brain tissue ($PbrO_2$) is appealing as a guide for managing TBI by helping determine optimal CPP for adequate brain tissue oxygenation. The monitor is inserted into the brain parenchyma typically at the time of ICP monitor placement and measures tissue oxygen in the immediate area. According to the BTF, evidence of a benefit in using this monitoring device to manage TBI is inconclusive. In a retrospective study, 123 patients with TBI who had ICP and $PbrO_2$ monitoring had a similar mortality rate to the other 506 patients whose treatment was guided by ICP monitoring only. Although hypoxia detected by brain tissue oxygen monitoring was associated with worse outcomes in this study, these researchers were unable to link treatment in response to $PbrO_2$ monitoring to outcome. Several class 3 studies (low-quality RCTs and noncomparative designs) examining $PbrO_2$ monitoring for patients with TBI revealed conflicting results regarding mortality and outcome, which has effectively removed the level III recommendation for this advanced monitor for the management of TBI.

Jugular bulb catheters for $Sjvo_2$ monitoring provide information regarding global cerebral oxygenation because arteriovenous difference of oxygen content ($AVDO_2$) is an indicator of cerebral oxygen extraction. A cervical spine radiograph is helpful in confirming placement into the dilated portion of the jugular vein just below the base of the skull. Like $PbrO_2$, there is insufficient evidence to support a level I or II recommendation for the use of $AVDO_2$ in managing TBI (level II evidence demonstrated no improvement in outcome for monitored patients). Nonrandomized, nonblinded observational studies suggest that jugular bulb monitoring in patients with TBI can result in reduced mortality and improved outcomes at 3 and 6 months postinjury (level III evidence).

Regarding threshold values to target or avoid for these advanced cerebral monitors, the BTF reports that there is insufficient evidence to inform level I or II recommendations. However, there is level III evidence to support a jugular venous saturation of less than 50% as a threshold to avoid in the management of TBI.

Carney N, Totten AM, O'Reilly C, et al. Guidelines for the management of severe traumatic brain injury, fourth edition. *Neurosurgery*. 2017;80:6-15.

Oddo M, Bösel J. Monitoring of brain and systemic oxygenation in neurocritical care patients. *Neurocrit Care*. 2014;21:S103-S120.

Schell RM, Cole DJ. Cerebral monitoring: jugular venous oximetry. *Anesth Anal*. 2000;90:559-566.

D.6. What methods can be used in the neurointensive care unit to prevent hyperthermia?

Fever (>38.3 °C) occurs in approximately 70% of patients with brain injury and can last weeks after injury. After ruling out infections, approximately one-third of patients require treatment for a central fever due to TBI. Damage to or irritation of the hypothalamus, the center for thermoregulation, and increased sympathetic tone are responsible for this elevation in temperature. The elevated temperature exacerbates secondary brain injury by increasing neurotransmitter release, oxygen-free radicals, high glutamate concentrations, ischemic damage in the penumbra, and BBB breakdown. Fever after TBI is associated with poor long-term outcome.

Antipyretic agents (eg, acetaminophen, aspirin, and nonsteroidal anti-inflammatory drugs) inhibit cyclooxygenase-mediated prostaglandin synthesis in the brain and lower the hypothalamic set point. The limited benefit of this mode of treatment relates to damage of the thermoregulatory center in head trauma patients.

Nonpharmacologic interventions include external and intravascular cooling. External cooling includes four modes of promoting heat loss: evaporation via sponge baths, conductive heat loss with water-circulating cooling blankets, convective heat loss using fans and air-circulating cooling blankets, and radiative by exposure of the patient's skin. Combining these modalities appears to be more effective than any single method for decreasing temperature in patients without brain injury. A new system of surface cooling includes tightly wrapped pads that circulate cold water to promote conductive heat loss. This mode of conductive heat loss reduces fever better and faster than the conventional water-circulating cooling blanket.

Intravascular cooling works by infusing cooled saline intravascularly. This method is more effective at cooling than other nonpharmacologic methods. The solution extracts heat from the blood, thereby lowering body temperature. Infusion of NS at 4 °C can decrease core temperature by 2.5 °C within an hour after the infusion is started with no untoward effects.

The hyperthermic patient must be continuously monitored for signs of infection and hypothermia. At temperatures less than 35 °C, the risk for dysrhythmias, coagulopathy, electrolyte abnormalities, and hypovolemia increase. Shivering and vasoconstriction (<36 °C) can complicate the cooling process with a significant increase in metabolic demand and unwanted tachycardia and hypertension. The injured hypothalamus can reset so that these effects can manifest at normothermia.

Badjatia N. Hyperthermia and fever control in brain injury. *Crit Care Med*. 2009;37:S250-S257.

Badjatia N, Bodock M, Guanci M, et al. Rapid infusion of cold saline (4 degrees C) as adjunctive treatment of fever in patients with brain injury. *Neurology*. 2006;66:1739-1741.

Mayer SA, Kowalski RG, Presciutti M, et al. Clinical trial of a novel surface cooling system for fever control in neurocritical care patients. *Crit Care Med*. 2004;32:2508-2515.

Meier K, Lee K. Neurogenic fever: review of pathophysiology, evaluation, and management. *J Intensive Care Med*. 2017;32:124-129.

22 Cerebral Aneurysm

Philip C. Kuo and Patricia Fogarty Mack

A 43-year-old female presented to the emergency room 2 days ago, complaining of severe headache, nausea, and vomiting, followed by a witnessed 3-minute loss of consciousness. On regaining consciousness, she was noted by her family to be confused. A computed tomography (CT) scan showed subarachnoid bleeding. You are called to the angiography suite because four-vessel angiography revealed an 18-mm basilar tip aneurysm and a 10-mm right middle cerebral artery aneurysm. The interventional neuroradiologist wishes to coil the basilar tip aneurysm but believes the middle cerebral artery aneurysm will require a craniotomy and clipping. At present, she is oriented only to person. She has no previous significant medical history; however, she has smoked one pack of cigarettes per day for the last 20 years. Her blood pressure is 130/80 mm Hg, pulse 90 beats per minute, and respiration 18 breaths per minute. She has no focal neurologic deficits. Laboratory examination revealed normal electrolytes and complete blood count but elevated creatine phosphokinase-myocardial band (CPK-MB) and troponin. Electrocardiogram (ECG) demonstrated normal sinus rhythm with flipped T waves throughout the precordium.

A. Medical Disease and Differential Diagnosis

1. What are the incidence, prevalence, and causes of subarachnoid hemorrhage (SAH), and what are the risk factors associated with the rupture of intracranial aneurysms?
2. What are the common sizes and locations of intracranial aneurysms?
3. What is the pathophysiology of aneurysmal rupture and SAH?
4. What are the symptoms and signs of SAH?
5. How does one assess the severity of SAH?
6. What are the cardiovascular effects of SAH?
7. How is the diagnosis of SAH made?
8. What is the risk for rebleeding for a patient with SAH?

B. Preoperative Evaluation and Preparation

1. What are some concerns in going to the interventional neuroradiology suite in the midst of an angiogram to be followed immediately with coiling of an aneurysm?
2. What type of anesthesia is required for coiling of an aneurysm?
3. Should one proceed with induction of general anesthesia under these circumstances?
4. What types of emergencies can occur during the coiling of an aneurysm, and how should they be managed?
5. What other modalities of endovascular therapy are available?
6. A craniotomy is planned for the following day to clip the middle cerebral artery aneurysm. Should surgery be postponed because of the patient's elevated troponin and CPK-MB fractions?
7. Would you premedicate this patient before craniotomy?

C. Intraoperative Management

1. What are the goals of the induction and maintenance of anesthesia for this patient?
2. Is the placement of an arterial catheter necessary for the induction of anesthesia in this patient in the interventional neuroradiology suite?
3. How would you assess fluid status in this patient?

4. Would monitoring central venous pressure (CVP) be useful for craniotomy and aneurysm clipping in this patient?
5. What other forms of monitoring would you consider?
6. What are your specific concerns during the induction of anesthesia in this patient?
7. How would you accomplish a smooth and safe induction of anesthesia and tracheal intubation in this patient?
8. Would you perform a rapid-sequence induction and tracheal intubation for this patient?
9. What are the effects of hypoxemia and hypercapnia, such as would be seen with loss of the airway on induction, on cerebral blood flow (CBF)?
10. What is optimal fluid management for aneurysm clipping? Would you use a dextrose-containing solution?
11. After the bone plate was removed and as the dura was being opened, the surgeon complained that the brain was "tight." What could you do to achieve better brain relaxation and facilitate surgical exposure?
12. How might transmural pressure be decreased to allow for aneurysm clip placement?
13. What is the purpose of controlled hypotension, and how is it achieved?
14. What are some of the drawbacks of controlled hypotension?
15. What methods of cerebral protection might you use during this operation?
16. Would you induce mild hypothermia as a means of cerebral protection?
17. What are the indications for deep hypothermic circulatory arrest?
18. What steps should be taken in the case of intraoperative rupture of an intracranial aneurysm?
19. How would you plan the emergence from anesthesia for aneurysm clipping?

D. Postoperative Management

1. Would you extubate the patient postoperatively?
2. What would be the differential diagnosis if the patient did not return to her preoperative neurologic condition?
3. On postoperative day 2, the patient became disoriented and developed hemiplegia. A CT scan was obtained, which showed no new intracranial bleeding. What other diagnostic studies should be performed?
4. What is cerebral vasospasm, and what causes it?
5. What are pathophysiologic changes seen in cerebral vasospasm?
6. How is the diagnosis of cerebral vasospasm made?
7. What steps can be taken to prevent cerebral vasospasm?
8. What treatments can be undertaken once a diagnosis of cerebral vasospasm is made?
9. What are other neurologic complications following SAH and aneurysm clipping?
10. What other organ systems can be affected postoperatively in patients following aneurysm clipping?

A. Medical Disease and Differential Diagnosis

A.1. What are the incidence, prevalence, and causes of subarachnoid hemorrhage (SAH), and what are the risk factors associated with the rupture of intracranial aneurysms?

The prevalence of SAH is 2% to 5%, with an incidence of 10 to 15 per 100,000 people. Each year, 25,000 cases of SAH occur in the United States, comprising 5% to 10% of all cases of stroke. In China and South America, the incidence is only 2 to 4 cases per 100,000 people, whereas higher rates of 19 to 23 per 100,000 are reported in Finland and Japan. In all, 60% of the cases occur in young individuals between the ages of 40 and 60. Therefore, a poor neurologic outcome is a devastating condition to be endured over a potentially long period.

Approximately one-quarter of patients die as a result of the acute bleed prior to hospitalization. Inpatient mortality rates range from 13% to 20%. Among those who survive, nearly 49% with good functional outcomes exhibit severe cognitive impairment. The predominant cognitive issues after SAH are mental slowness, memory lapses, and attention difficulties. Although many patients show improvement in these areas, around 50% continue to grapple with cognitive dysfunction for up to a year after the event.

Cerebral aneurysms account for 75% to 80% of SAH; arteriovenous malformations are the cause in 4% to 5%, whereas no specific cause can be found in 15% to 20% of SAH. Other causes of SAH include trauma, mycotic aneurysm, sickle cell disease, cocaine use, and coagulation disorders.

According to a Danish study of 250 patients with SAH compared to 250 control patients, the four strongest independent predictors of aneurysmal SAH are current smoking (odds ratio [OR] 5.9; 95%

confidence interval [CI] 4.1-8.6), family history of aneurysmal SAH (OR, 4.3; 95% CI 2.4-7.5), hypertension (OR, 2.3; 95% CI 1.5-3.7), and excessive alcohol use (≥18 units per week) (OR, 1.2; 95% CI 1.0-2.8). Other risk factors include pregnancy and vascular abnormalities (eg, type III collagen deficiency and elastase abnormalities). One-third of patients with polycystic kidney disease have been found to have intracranial aneurysms at autopsy. Genetic predisposition plays a role: Seven percent of berry aneurysms are familial, and 5% to 10% of patients with a ruptured aneurysm have a first-order relative with a ruptured aneurysm. The rupture rate for aneurysm has been estimated at 0.14% per year for a 5-mm lesion to 1.1% per year for a 10-mm lesion.

Smoking and alcohol abuse also appear to predispose to aneurysm formation and rupture. Smoking at any time and female sex are related to the presence of multiple intracranial aneurysms as well as accelerated aneurysm growth. Cocaine abuse and resultant episodic hypertension may predispose to aneurysmal rupture at an early age.

Death and disability are primarily due to the initial bleed, vasospasm, and rebleeding. Other causes include surgical complications, parenchymal hemorrhage, hydrocephalus, and complications of medical therapy.

Chang HS. Simulation of the natural history of cerebral aneurysms based on data from the International Study of Unruptured Intracranial Aneurysms. *J Neurosurg*. 2006;104:188-194.

de Rooij NK, Linn FH, van der Plas JA, et al. Incidence of subarachnoid haemorrhage: a systematic review with emphasis on region, age, gender and time trends. *J Neurol Neurosurg Psychiatry*. 2007;78:1365-1372.

Hoh BL, Ko NU, Amin-Hanjani S, et al. 2023 guideline for the management of patients with aneurysmal subarachnoid hemorrhage: a guideline from the American Heart Association/American Stroke Association. *Stroke*. 2023;54:e314-e370.

Pong RP, Lam AM. Anesthetic management of cerebral aneurysm surgery. In: Cottrell JE, Patel P, eds. *Cottrell and Patel's Neuroanesthesia*. 7th ed. Elsevier; 2024:244-271.

Vlak MH, Rinkel GJ, Greebe P, et al. Lifetime risks for aneurysmal subarachnoid haemorrhage: multivariable risk stratification. *J Neurol Neurosurg Psychiatry*. 2013;84:619-623.

Yoshimoto Y. A mathematical model of the natural history of intracranial aneurysm: quantification of the benefit of prophylactic treatment. *J Neurosurg*. 2006;104:195-200.

A.2. What are the common sizes and locations of intracranial aneurysms?

Small (<12 mm) aneurysms make up 78% of the total, whereas large (12-24 mm) are 20%, and giant (>24 mm) comprise 2%. Most aneurysms are located in the anterior circulation, with the junction of the anterior communicating and anterior cerebral arteries being the most common (39%). Thirty percent of aneurysms occur in the internal carotid artery, 22% in the middle cerebral artery, and 8% in the posterior circulation (posterior cerebral, basilar, and vertebral arteries).

Kassell NF, Torner JC, Haley EC Jr, et al. The international cooperative study on the timing of aneurysm surgery. Part 1: overall management results. *J Neurosurg*. 1990;73:18-32.

A.3. What is the pathophysiology of aneurysmal rupture and SAH?

On the basis of experimental models, aneurysmal rupture leads to the leakage of arterial blood and a rapid increase in intracranial pressure (ICP), approaching diastolic blood pressure in the proximal intracerebral arteries. This increase in ICP causes a decrease in cerebral perfusion pressure (CPP) and a fall in CBF, leading to a loss of consciousness. The decrease in CBF diminishes bleeding and expansion of the SAH. A gradual reduction in ICP and an increase in CBF indicate improved cerebral function and possibly a return to consciousness. A persistent increase in ICP (perhaps resulting from thrombi in the cranial cisterns), however, results in a persistent no-flow pattern with acute vasospasm, cell swelling, and death.

A.4. What are the symptoms and signs of SAH?

Severe headache, often described as "the worst headache of my life," occurs in 85% to 95% of patients. Often, a brief loss of consciousness occurs, followed by diminished mentation; consciousness may be impaired to any degree or may be unaffected at the time of presentation. Symptoms secondary to subarachnoid blood may be similar to those of infectious meningitis (nausea, vomiting, and photophobia). The patient may also experience motor and sensory deficits, visual field disturbances, and cranial nerve palsies. Finally, blood in the subarachnoid space may cause an elevated temperature.

Pong RP, Lam AM. Anesthetic management of cerebral aneurysm surgery. In: Cottrell JE, Patel P, eds. *Cottrell and Patel's Neuroanesthesia*. 7th ed. Elsevier; 2024:244-271.

TABLE 22.1 Modified Hunt and Hess Clinical Grades

Grade[a]	Criteria
0	Unruptured aneurysm
I	Asymptomatic or minimal headache and slight nuchal rigidity
II	Moderate to severe headache, nuchal rigidity, but no neurologic deficit other than cranial nerve palsy
III	Drowsiness, confusion, or mild focal deficit
IV	Stupor, mild to severe hemiparesis, possible early decerebrate rigidity, vegetative disturbance
V	Deep coma, decerebrate rigidity, moribund appearance

[a]Serious systemic diseases such as hypertension, diabetes, severe arteriosclerosis, chronic pulmonary disease, and severe vasospasm seen on arteriography result in placement of the patient in the next less favorable category.

From Hunt WE, Hess RM. Surgical risk as related to time of intervention in the repair of intracranial aneurysms. *J Neurosurg.* 1968;28:14-20, with permission.

A.5. How does one assess the severity of SAH?

Two grading scales are commonly used to assess neurologic status following SAH, the Hunt and Hess grade (**Table 22.1**) and the World Federation of Neurologic Surgeons' grade (**Table 22.2**), based on the Glasgow Coma Scale. The scales are useful in identifying a baseline neurologic status from which any acute changes should be assessed. In addition, the scales may correlate with physiologic status and patient morbidity and mortality risk. Patients who are Hunt and Hess grades I and II have near-normal cerebral autoregulation and ICP.

Drake CG. Report of World Federation of Neurological Surgeons Committee on a universal subarachnoid hemorrhage grading scale. *J Neurosurg*. 1988;68:985-986.

Hunt WE, Hess RM. Surgical risk as related to time of intervention in the repair of intracranial aneurysms. *J Neurosurg*. 1968;28:14-20.

A.6. What are the cardiovascular effects of SAH?

Injury to the posterior hypothalamus from SAH causes the release of norepinephrine from the adrenal medulla and cardiac sympathetic efferents. Norepinephrine can cause an increase in afterload and direct myocardial toxicity, leading to subendocardial ischemia. Pathologic analysis of the myocardium of patients who have died of acute SAH has revealed microscopic subendocardial hemorrhage and myocytolysis.

Electrocardiographic abnormalities are present in 50% to 80% of patients with SAH. Most commonly, these involve ST-segment changes and T-wave inversions but also include prolonged QT intervals, U waves, and P-wave changes. ST-T wave changes are usually scattered and not related to a particular distribution.

Dysrhythmias occur in 80% of patients, usually in the first 48 hours. Premature ventricular contractions are the most common abnormality, but any type of dysrhythmia is possible. They include severely prolonged QT interval, torsades de pointes, and ventricular fibrillation. In one series, 66% of arrhythmias were considered mild, 29% moderate, and 5% severe. In addition to increased catecholamine secretion, hypercortisolism and hypokalemia have been suggested as causes for the dysrhythmias seen with SAH.

TABLE 22.2 World Federation of Neurological Surgeons (WFNS) Grading Scale

WFNS Grade	Glasgow Coma Scale	Motor Deficit
I	15	Absent
II	14-13	Absent
III	14-13	Present
IV	12-7	Present or absent
V	6-3	Present or absent

From Drake CG. Report of World Federation of Neurological Surgeons Committee on a universal subarachnoid hemorrhage grading scale. *J Neurosurg.* 1988;68:985-986, with permission.

Ventricular dysfunction, possibly leading to pulmonary edema, is present in roughly 30% of patients with SAH.

Cardiac troponin I predicts myocardial dysfunction in SAH, with a sensitivity of 100% and a specificity of 91%. This compares with a sensitivity and specificity of 60% and 94% for CPK-MB in predicting myocardial dysfunction. For optimal anesthetic management, it is important to determine if any cardiac dysfunction is due to a myocardial infarction or reversible neurogenic left ventricular dysfunction. A retrospective study identified indicators suggestive of neurogenic stunned myocardium: absence of a history of heart disease, wall motion abnormalities discordant with ECG changes, and a comparatively modest release of cardiac troponin relative to the extent of left ventricular dysfunction. However, some patients might still require coronary angiography to differentiate between these two conditions.

Bulsara KR, McGirt MJ, Liao L, et al. Use of the peak troponin value to differentiate myocardial infarction from reversible neurogenic left ventricular dysfunction associated with aneurysmal subarachnoid hemorrhage. *J Neurosurg*. 2003;98:524-528.

Pong RP, Lam AM. Anesthetic management of cerebral aneurysm surgery. In: Cottrell JE, Patel P, eds. *Cottrell and Patel's Neuroanesthesia*. 7th ed. Elsevier; 2024:244-271.

A.7. How is the diagnosis of SAH made?

Noncontrast CT scan can determine the magnitude and location of the bleed. It may also be useful in assessing ventricular size and aneurysm location. High-resolution CT (CT angiogram) with contrast can more precisely determine the location of the aneurysm.

Lumbar puncture can be used to diagnose SAH if CT is negative, especially when the patient presents more than 1 week after an initial bleed. Xanthochromia, a yellow discoloration of the cerebrospinal fluid (CSF) after centrifugation, is present from 4 hours to 3 weeks after SAH. A lumbar puncture can cause herniation or rebleeding. Therefore, a CT scan should be performed first if the patient presents within 72 hours of suspected SAH.

Four-vessel angiography (right and left carotid and vertebral arteries) has been considered the gold standard in the diagnosis of an intracranial aneurysm; however, CT angiography has been used with increasing frequency and currently is used to determine whether an aneurysm is amenable to coiling or requires surgical clip placement. The goal is to visualize all of the intracranial vessels, to localize the source of bleeding, and to rule out multiple aneurysms (5%-33% of patients). Three-dimensional reconstructive angiograms and magnetic resonance angiography may also be used to further delineate the intracranial vasculature.

Guy J, McGrath BJ, Borel CO, et al. Perioperative management of aneurysmal subarachnoid hemorrhage: part 1. Operative management. *Anesth Analg*. 1995;81:1060-1072.

Lin A, Rawal R, Agid R, et al. Cerebrovascular imaging: which test is best? *Neurosurgery*. 2018;83:5-18.

Zhang LJ, Wu SY, Niu JB, et al. Dual-energy CT angiography in the evaluation of intracranial aneurysms: image quality, radiation dose, and comparison with 3D rotational digital subtraction angiography. *AJR Am J Roentgenol*. 2010;194:23-30.

A.8. What is the risk for rebleeding for a patient with SAH?

Absent treatment, the risk of rebleeding from a ruptured aneurysm is highest, 4%, in the first 24 hours after the initial bleed and 1.5% per day thereafter. The cumulative risk is 19% in 14 days and 50% in 6 months. After 6 months, the rebleeding risk is 3% per year.

Kassell NF, Torner JC. Aneurysmal rebleeding: a preliminary report from the cooperative aneurysm study. *Neurosurgery*. 1983;13:479-481.

B. Preoperative Evaluation and Preparation

B.1. What are some concerns in going to the interventional neuroradiology suite in the midst of an angiogram to be followed immediately with coiling of an aneurysm?

Whenever an anesthesiologist assumes care of a patient who is already sedated, it can be difficult, if not impossible, to obtain an accurate medical history. In addition, the physical examination will be limited by the patient's position for the diagnostic study. Finally, the patient's capacity to consent can also be impaired by previous sedation.

B.2. What type of anesthesia is required for coiling of an aneurysm?

Although there is a case series of aneurysm coiling under monitored anesthesia care with dexmedetomidine infusion without loading dose, in most institutions, general anesthesia is required for coiling of an intracranial aneurysm. First, intraoperative neurologic testing is generally not required. Second, immobility is critical, not only when the coils or stent are actually deployed but also while the interventionist is navigating the intracranial vessels to reach the aneurysm.

Lee H-H, Jung Y-J, Choi B-Y, et al. Usefulness of dexmedetomidine during intracerebral aneurysm coiling. *J Korean Neurosurg Soc*. 2014;55:185-189.

B.3. Should one proceed with induction of general anesthesia under these circumstances?

Obliteration of the aneurysm with coils has become the standard of care for basilar tip aneurysms, and it would be best for the patient to have this done in the same setting as the angiography. Additionally, general anesthesia is indicated if the patient is unable to follow commands and lie still for the procedure. Thus, it would be appropriate in this scenario to proceed with induction of general anesthesia, provided there were no other contraindications (eg, hemodynamic instability).

Lee CZ, Young WL. Anesthetic considerations for interventional neuroradiology. *ASA Refresher Course Anesthesiol*. 2005;33:145-154.

Pong RP, Lam AM. Anesthetic management of cerebral aneurysm surgery. In: Cottrell JE, Patel P, eds. *Cottrell and Patel's Neuroanesthesia*. 7th ed. Elsevier; 2024:244-271.

B.4. What types of emergencies can occur during the coiling of an aneurysm, and how should they be managed?

Intraoperative emergencies can be divided into two categories—hemorrhage and thrombosis. Appropriate management requires constant communication between the radiologist, surgeon, and anesthesiologist. If an intracranial hemorrhage occurs, the interventionalist may try to "glue" the hole in the aneurysm or embolize the parent vessel. If this is not possible, heparin should be rapidly reversed with protamine, and placement of a ventriculostomy by the surgical team considered. Management of arterial carbon dioxide partial pressure ($Paco_2$) can then be guided by the ICP.

As the technology of endovascular therapy has advanced to include balloon-assisted coiling (BAC) or stent-assisted coiling (SAC), the treatment of more complex aneurysms has increased. The rate of intraprocedural rupture (IPR) has increased as well. The rate of IPR may be as high as 7.5% in ruptured aneurysms and 2.5% in unruptured aneurysms. IPR may lead to significant clinical deterioration in previously unruptured aneurysms but does not appear to have a severe impact on patients undergoing endovascular treatment for SAH.

In the case of catheter-induced thrombosis, induced hypertension is usually desirable while tissue plasminogen activator or antiglycoprotein IIb/IIIa therapy is considered.

If a coil was malpositioned, anticoagulation would be continued while the interventional radiologist attempts to snare the coil. As with thrombosis, it might be desirable to augment the blood pressure.

Kocur D, Przybyłko N, Bażowski P, et al. Rupture during coiling of intracranial aneurysms: predictors and clinical outcome. *Clin Neurol Neurosurg*. 2018;165:81-87.

Park YK, Yi H-J, Choi K-S, et al. Intraprocedural rupture during endovascular treatment of intracranial aneurysm: clinical results and literature review. *World Neurosurg*. 2018;114:e605-e615.

Petr O, Brinjikji W, Cloft H, et al. Current trends and results of endovascular treatment of unruptured intracranial aneurysms at a single institution in the flow-diverter era. *AJNR Am J Neuroradiol*. 2016;37:1106-1113.

B.5. What other modalities of endovascular therapy are available?

Apart from traditional coiling methods, more advanced techniques such as SAC, BAC, and the use of closed-cell, open-cell, and braided stents have been utilized. SAC and BAC have shown potential in the treatment of wide-necked and large aneurysms, which are often not amenable to unassisted coiling. These methods aim to stabilize the coil mass inside the aneurysmal sac and prevent coil herniation into the parent artery.

Flow-diverting devices (stents) have been utilized for treating large, wide-necked, and fusiform aneurysms, which are otherwise not amenable to coiling. These devices aim to decrease blood flow within the aneurysm and redirect the blood to the parent vessel. Patients with flow diverters require dual antiplatelet therapy to prevent in-stent thrombosis. A recent meta-analysis found that the complication rate for flow-diverting stents is greater in ruptured versus unruptured aneurysms, with an overall complication rate of 17% and mortality of 2.8%.

Intrasaccular flow disruptors, such as the Woven EndoBridge (WEB) device, represent the latest developments in the field. These devices are specifically designed for overly wide-necked aneurysms and are deployed within the aneurysm sac, aiming to cause intra-aneurysmal thrombosis. The WEB device has shown promising results in terms of efficacy and complications.

Finally, in the case of cavernous carotid or otherwise nonclippable aneurysms without the possibility of traditional coil or stent embolization, the internal carotid artery might be occluded itself if sufficient collateral CBF can be maintained.

Adamou A, Alexandrou M, Roth C, Chatziioannou A, Papanagiotou P. Endovascular treatment of intracranial aneurysms. *Life (Basel)*. 2021;11:335.

Arthur AS, Molyneux A, Coon AL, et al; WEB-IT Study Investigators. The safety and effectiveness of the Woven EndoBridge (WEB) system for the treatment of wide-necked bifurcation aneurysms: final 12-month results of the pivotal WEB Intrasaccular Therapy (WEB-IT) Study. *J Neurointerv Surg*. 2019;11:924-930.

Bechan RS, Majoie CB, Sprengers ME, et al. Therapeutic internal carotid artery occlusion for large and giant aneurysms: a single center cohort of 146 patients. *AJNR Am J Neuroradiol*. 2016;37:125-129.

Srinivasan VM, Srivatsan A, Spiotta AM, et al. Early postmarket results with PulseRider for treatment of wide-necked intracranial aneurysms: a multicenter experience. *J Neurosurg*. 2019;133:1756-1765.

Zhou G, Su M, Yin YL, et al. Complications associated with the use of flow-diverting devices for cerebral aneurysms: a systematic review and meta-analysis. *Neurosurg Focus*. 2017;42:E17.

B.6. A craniotomy is planned for the following day to clip the middle cerebral artery aneurysm. Should surgery be postponed because of the patient's elevated troponin and CPK-MB fractions?

Fifty percent of patients will have an increase in CPK-MB fraction; however, CPK-MB per total CPK is usually not consistent with a transmural myocardial infarction. As discussed previously, troponin I levels are more sensitive. In addition, although some patients (0.7%) do sustain a myocardial infarction in the setting of SAH, little correlation is found between electrocardiographic abnormalities and myocardial ischemia in this population.

An echocardiogram may be useful in determining the severity of reversible neurogenic left ventricular dysfunction. If left ventricular function is found to be depressed, a pulmonary artery catheter, noninvasive cardiac output monitor, or intraoperative transesophageal echocardiography may be helpful for intraoperative management.

The desire to delay surgery because of cardiac abnormalities must be weighed against the risk of rebleeding and vasospasm. In most cases, the risk of recurrent hemorrhage outweighs the risk of perioperative myocardial infarction. Furthermore, even if coronary artery disease is present, these patients are not candidates for angioplasty or myocardial revascularization, which requires heparinization. If pulmonary edema or malignant dysrhythmias are present, it might be prudent to postpone surgery until such problems are controlled medically. However, if these problems are not present, clipping of the aneurysm might be indicated. In a study by Bulsara et al, 2.9% of patients had severe cardiac dysfunction, and neurogenic left ventricular dysfunction resolved over 4 to 5 days.

Bulsara KR, McGirt MJ, Liao L, et al. Use of the peak troponin value to differentiate myocardial infarction from reversible neurogenic left ventricular dysfunction associated with aneurysmal subarachnoid hemorrhage. *J Neurosurg*. 2003;98:524-528.

B.7. Would you premedicate this patient before craniotomy?

No. When the patient is in a Hunt and Hess grades III to V state, anxiety is unlikely. Furthermore, heavy sedation can decrease ventilation, raising $Paco_2$ and increasing CBF and ICP, which, at the very least, can hinder preoperative and postoperative neurologic evaluation. If patients are Hunt and Hess grades I to II and it appears that preoperative anxiety might lead to hemodynamic instability, a small dose of a benzodiazepine can be appropriate in a monitored setting.

Medications such as calcium channel blockers (nicardipine), anticonvulsants, and corticosteroids should be continued preoperatively on the day of surgery.

If the patient is at risk for aspiration, medications to decrease gastric acidity and volume are appropriate. Most patients will already be receiving a histamine-2 blocker or proton pump inhibitor if they are receiving a glucocorticoid.

Pong RP, Lam AM. Anesthetic management of cerebral aneurysm surgery. In: Cottrell JE, Patel P, eds. *Cottrell and Patel's Neuroanesthesia*. 7th ed. Elsevier; 2024:244-271.

C. Intraoperative Management

C.1. What are the goals of the induction and maintenance of anesthesia for this patient?

The primary goal is to prevent aneurysm rupture, either on induction or intraoperatively, while maintaining adequate CPP. The goal of matching anesthetic depth to surgical stimulation is more important than the specific drugs used. In general, the anesthesiologist should provide for rapid and reversible titration of blood pressure, maintain CPP, and protect against cerebral ischemia. An additional goal is to provide a "relaxed brain" for ease of surgical exposure with minimal brain retraction. Finally, the anesthetic should be planned to achieve a rapid, smooth emergence, allowing prompt neurologic assessment. This can be accomplished with a combination of balanced anesthesia, muscle relaxation, and sympathetic blockers as well as with total intravenous anesthesia. Dexmedetomidine has been shown to minimize the need for administration of antihypertensive medications during emergence from anesthesia and to decrease both the incidence of hypertensive events in the postanesthesia care unit (PACU) as well as PACU length of stay.

Bekker A, Sturaitis M, Bloom M, et al. The effect of dexmedetomidine on perioperative hemodynamics in patients undergoing craniotomy. *Anesth Analg*. 2008;107:1340-1347.

Bendo AA. Intracranial vascular surgery. *Anesthesiol Clin North Am*. 2002;20:377-388.

Pong RP, Lam AM. Anesthetic management of cerebral aneurysm surgery. In: Cottrell JE, Patel P, eds. *Cottrell and Patel's Neuroanesthesia*. 7th ed. Elsevier; 2024:244-271.

C.2. Is the placement of an arterial catheter necessary for the induction of anesthesia in this patient in the interventional neuroradiology suite?

In this case, because a femoral sheath is in place at the time that anesthesia is induced, one can transduce femoral arterial pressure during induction. However, because the patient has two aneurysms and because the sheath will be removed at the end of the procedure, an additional arterial catheter should be placed before the removal of the sheath. When a large coaxial catheter is placed through the femoral sheath, systolic pressure is underestimated, but mean pressure should be accurate. Studies suggest that for coiling an unruptured aneurysm, placing an arterial catheter prior to induction is not essential, provided hemodynamic stability can be reasonably assured with the use of opioids or antihypertensives.

Lai YC, Manninen PH. Anesthesia for cerebral aneurysms: a comparison between interventional neuroradiology and surgery. *Can J Anaesth*. 2001;48:391-395.

Pong RP, Lam AM. Anesthetic management of cerebral aneurysm surgery. In: Cottrell JE, Patel P, eds. Cottrell and Patel's Neuroanesthesia. 7th ed. Elsevier; 2024:244-271.

C.3. How would you assess fluid status in this patient?

Several issues in interventional radiology complicate fluid management. First, contrast material acts as an osmotic diuretic. Often, these patients have had a CT scan with contrast in addition to an angiogram and may become intravascularly depleted. Second, the femoral sheath and other catheters are constantly flushed with a heparinized saline solution. It is not uncommon for a patient to receive 1,000 mL or more of flush fluid during the case. This must be taken into account when calculating fluid balance.

C.4. Would monitoring central venous pressure (CVP) be useful for craniotomy and aneurysm clipping in this patient?

CVP monitoring can be helpful in assessing volume replacement needs because urine output will be affected by osmotic or loop diuretics administered to facilitate surgical exposure. In addition, should vasoactive medication become necessary, it can be effectively administered through a central venous catheter (assuming that it cannot be safely administered through a peripheral intravenous catheter).

One disadvantage of CVP monitoring in the neurosurgical patient is catheter placement. Some clinicians are concerned that placement of an internal jugular central venous catheter will compromise venous outflow from the head, thereby predisposing to bleeding or brain swelling, although this remains controversial. A "long-arm" or peripheral antecubital CVP catheter can be more difficult to insert and have a higher incidence of thrombophlebitis. Multiple studies have shown the complication rate of central catheter placement to be as high as 14%. When including failure to place the catheter, the complication rate rises to 54%. Nevertheless, the use of an ultrasound-guided approach to placement of central venous catheters reduces the complication rates to less than 2% to 5% and should be the standard of care whenever possible. Finally, a poor correlation between CVP and left ventricular end-diastolic pressure has been documented in SAH, so a pulmonary artery catheter can be more useful in assessing volume status as well as providing a monitor of cardiac output in those patients who have had preoperative cardiac problems. Central pressure monitoring is usually instituted after the patient is anesthetized to minimize patient stress. One should be careful to use the minimal degree of head-down tilt necessary to access the central circulation because the Trendelenburg position can increase ICP and thereby decrease CPP.

Based on the risks and benefits of central venous and pulmonary artery access, placement of CVP and pulmonary artery catheters is reserved for patients who have documented cardiac dysfunction, cerebral vasospasm, or poor peripheral intravenous access. Volume status can be assessed by noninvasive monitors that calculate stroke volume or by careful assessment of the arterial waveform utilizing calculated pulse pressure variation available on many monitoring systems.

Akmal AH, Hasan M, Mariam A. The incidence of complications of central venous catheters at an intensive care unit. *Ann Thorac Med.* 2007;2:61-63.

Eisen LA, Narasimhan M, Berger JS, et al. Mechanical complications of central venous catheters. *J Intensive Care Med.* 2006;21:40-46.

Marik PE, Cavallazzi R, Vasu T, et al. Dynamic changes in arterial waveform derived variables and fluid responsiveness in mechanically ventilated patients: a systematic review of the literature. *Crit Care Med.* 2009;37:2642-2647.

C.5. What other forms of monitoring would you consider?

Electroencephalography (EEG) and somatosensory evoked potentials (SSEPs) have been advocated by some, although they are not standard monitoring in most hospitals. Although EEG has been used to monitor cerebral ischemia, scalp electrodes might not reflect the activity of brain areas most at risk. Cortical electrodes, such as those used in epilepsy surgery, avoid the problem of attenuation of the scalp electroencephalographic signal by CSF drainage and air between the scalp electrodes and the brain surface during surgery. EEG is useful in titrating intravenous anesthetic infusion if burst suppression is desired during temporary clipping. In the absence of scalp or cortical electrodes, a frontal EEG monitor can be used instead.

SSEPs may detect reversible ischemia during temporary vessel occlusion, but they might not detect ischemia in subcortical structures and motor cortex. Furthermore, SSEPs have relatively high false-positive (38%-60%) and false-negative (5%-34%) rates. Brainstem auditory evoked responses can be useful for monitoring during posterior circulation aneurysm clipping. Motor evoked potentials may be superior in detecting subcortical ischemia. The use of SSEP and motor evoked potential monitoring usually warrants the use of total intravenous anesthesia and avoidance of neuromuscular blockers.

Microvascular Doppler ultrasound evaluation can detect inadvertent vessel occlusion, but it cannot assess the adequacy of collateral perfusion.

Monitoring of ICP is common, with the probability of increased ICP being greatest 24 to 48 hours after SAH. An intraventricular catheter allows for not only ICP monitoring but also CSF drainage to improve operating conditions. If an intraventricular catheter is not present, a lumbar spinal drain can be placed. One must be careful not to allow substantial CSF drainage before dural opening because this can decrease ICP, leading to an increase in transmural pressure and possible aneurysm rupture.

Intraoperative angiography is one means to assess complete obliteration of the aneurysm without clip occlusion of the parent artery or perforating branches. Its use has increased with the installation of hybrid operating rooms that are equipped with advanced angiography equipment.

Horiuchi K, Suzuki K, Sasaki T, et al. Intraoperative monitoring of blood flow insufficiency during surgery of middle cerebral artery aneurysms. *J Neurosurg.* 2005;103:275-283.

Neuloh G, Schramm J. Monitoring of motor evoked potentials compared with somatosensory evoked potentials and microvascular Doppler ultrasonography in cerebral aneurysm surgery. *J Neurosurg.* 2004;100;389-399.

Szelényi A, Langer D, Kothbauer K, et al. Monitoring of muscle motor evoked potentials during cerebral aneurysm surgery: intraoperative changes and postoperative outcome. *J Neurosurg.* 2006;105:675-681.

C.6. What are your specific concerns during the induction of anesthesia in this patient?

If an aneurysm ruptures during anesthetic induction, mortality is high (around 75%). Therefore, precise control of transmural pressure is important in preventing aneurysm rupture.

$$\text{Transmural pressure} = \text{CPP} = \text{MAP} - \text{ICP or CVP (whichever is greater)},$$
$$\text{where MAP} = \text{mean arterial pressure.}$$

On the other hand, one does not want CPP to be so low that ischemia develops, especially in areas of vasospasm.

Chowdhury T, Cappellani RB, Sandu N, et al. Perioperative variables contributing to the rupture of intracranial aneurysm: an update. *Sci World J*. 2013;2013:396404.

Tsementzis SA, Hitchcock ER. Outcome from "rescue clipping" of ruptured intracranial aneurysms during induction of anesthesia and endotracheal intubation. *J Neurol Neurosurg Psychiatry*. 1985;48:160-163.

C.7. How would you accomplish a smooth and safe induction of anesthesia and tracheal intubation in this patient?

Assuming that evaluation of the airway indicated that tracheal intubation is unlikely to be difficult, induction would begin with preoxygenation followed by propofol 1.5 to 2.5 mg/kg, thiopental 3 to 5 mg/kg, or etomidate 0.5 to 1 mg/kg, which have similar effects on CBF and cerebral metabolic rate. Given that this patient had no other medical problems, propofol is a reasonable choice. One may want to avoid ketamine for induction because of its potential to increase CBF and ICP. Thiopental is not presently available in North America but may be available elsewhere.

After loss of consciousness and apnea, care must be taken to maintain a normal $Paco_2$. Vigorous hyperventilation will lower $Paco_2$, decreasing CBF. This can lower ICP to such a degree that if MAP is maintained or increased, transmural pressure is increased, leading to aneurysm rupture.

A nondepolarizing neuromuscular blocking agent, which has no effect on ICP or CBF, should be given to facilitate tracheal intubation. Neuromuscular function should be monitored to ensure that the degree of paralysis is adequate to avoid coughing with intubation.

Fentanyl 3 to 5 μg/kg, sufentanil 0.5 to 1 μg/kg, or remifentanil 0.25 to 1 μg/kg can be given 3 to 5 minutes before laryngoscopy to blunt the hemodynamic response. Isoflurane, desflurane, or sevoflurane can be used to deepen anesthesia. Finally, about 90 seconds before laryngoscopy, lidocaine 1.5 to 2 mg/kg or esmolol 0.5 mg/kg can be given to blunt the hemodynamic response to intubation. Lidocaine decreases both CBF and cerebral metabolic rate for oxygen ($CMRO_2$), and at high concentrations can cause seizures. Esmolol and labetalol have no effect on CBF and ICP, even in brain areas where autoregulation is not intact. Extreme reductions in MAP (>35%) can compromise CPP in patients with increased ICP.

Pong RP, Lam AM. Anesthetic management of cerebral aneurysm surgery. In: Cottrell JE, Patel P, eds. *Cottrell and Patel's Neuroanesthesia*. 7th ed. Elsevier; 2024:244-271.

C.8. Would you perform a rapid-sequence induction and tracheal intubation for this patient?

There is no indication for rapid-sequence induction and intubation in this patient. The overall risk of aspiration during general anesthesia is about 0.05%; however, the risk of aneurysm rupture during induction is 1% to 2%. Therefore, unless a clear indication exists for rapid-sequence induction, it is best avoided.

If a rapid-sequence induction is indicated, one can consider using vecuronium 0.15 to 0.20 mg/kg or rocuronium 0.9 to 1.2 mg/kg rather than succinylcholine. Succinylcholine can increase ICP, although recent studies have noted no increase in ICP with the administration of succinylcholine, but rather with intubation. The increase in ICP can be attenuated or eliminated by deep anesthesia or prior defasciculation. Succinylcholine, more importantly, can lead to hyperkalemia and possibly ventricular fibrillation in patients presenting with motor deficits following SAH or in those who have been bedridden for some time.

In case of a full stomach or an anticipated difficult airway, awake fiberoptic intubation, with the use of appropriate sedation and topical application of local anesthesia, is an appropriate alternative. Under such circumstances, it is useful to have an assistant so that while one person is securing the airway, the other is solely focused on controlling the hemodynamics with titration of appropriate medication. Videolaryngoscopy can reduce the need for awake fiberoptic intubation. In addition, the use of supraglottic devices to maintain an airway during difficult intubation can be helpful in patients with an unanticipated difficult airway.

Guy J, McGrath BJ, Borel CO, et al. Perioperative management of aneurysmal subarachnoid hemorrhage: part 1. Operative management. *Anesth Analg*. 1995;81:1060-1072.

Pong RP, Lam AM. Anesthetic management of cerebral aneurysm surgery. In: Cottrell JE, Patel P, eds. *Cottrell and Patel's Neuroanesthesia*. 7th ed. Elsevier; 2024:244-271.

Zura A. Succinylcholine in the patient with increased intracranial pressure. In: Mashour GA, Farag E, eds. *Case Studies in Neuroanesthesia and Neurocritical Care*. Cambridge University Press; 2011:309-310.

C.9. What are the effects of hypoxemia and hypercapnia, such as would be seen with loss of the airway on induction, on cerebral blood flow (CBF)?

Each mm Hg increase in $Paco_2$ increases CBF 3% to 4% when $Paco_2$ is in the range of 20 to 80 mm Hg. In addition, hypoxemia will ensue if the airway is not secured in a timely manner and will also cause an increase in CBF once arterial oxygen partial pressure (Pao_2) is less than 60 mm Hg (**Figure 22.1**).

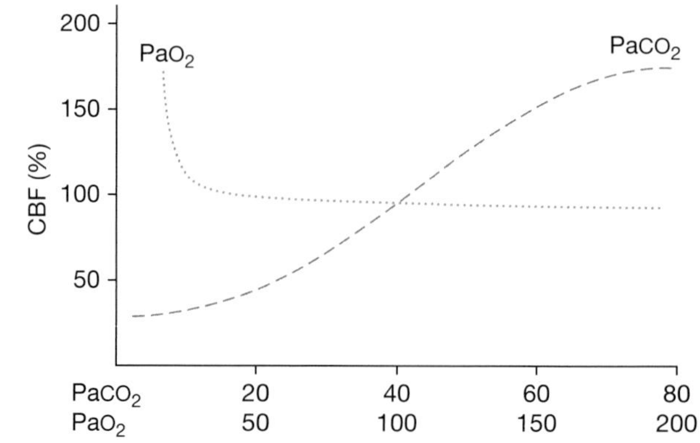

FIGURE 22.1. Change in CBF as a function of Pa_{CO_2} and Pa_{O_2}. (Derived from Albin MS, ed. *Textbook of Neuroanesthesia: With Neurosurgical and Neuroscience Perspectives.* 1st ed. McGraw-Hill; 1997:30.)

C.10. What is optimal fluid management for aneurysm clipping? Would you use a dextrose-containing solution?

Maintenance fluid requirements and blood loss should be replaced. One wants to avoid profound hypovolemia not only for its detrimental cardiovascular effects but also because it is associated with cerebral ischemia and perioperative neurologic deficits resulting from vasospasm. Some authors advocate mild hypervolemia to maximize cerebral CBF and minimize vasospasm; however, one must keep in mind the possibility of cerebral edema as well as acute congestive heart failure.

In general, dextrose-containing solutions should be avoided because an increased incidence of neurologic deficits associated with glucose administration has been found in experimental models of focal cerebral ischemia. Blood glucose should be maintained at less than 180 mg/dL.

The use of crystalloid versus colloid for fluid management and which type of crystalloid solution has long been a matter of controversy. Although some authors advocate colloid solutions to diminish the risk of brain swelling, evidence suggests that colloids can predispose to brain edema and contribute to hyponatremia, which might increase the incidence of delayed ischemic neurologic deficits. Hypotonic crystalloid solutions are avoided in neurosurgical patients; acceptable solutions include normal saline and balanced electrolyte solutions such as Normosol and PlasmaLyte.

A moderate degree of hemodilution to a hematocrit of 30% to 35% usually lowers blood viscosity, thereby increasing CBF. The goal is to increase oxygen delivery by increasing CBF, without allowing the hematocrit to decrease to a degree that reduction in oxygen content negates the increase in CBF. Hematocrit, serum sodium, and serum osmolality measurements can be used to guide fluid therapy. Serum sodium should be maintained within normal limits, both to maintain serum oncotic pressure and to avoid the hyponatremia associated with cerebral salt wasting.

Guy J, McGrath BJ, Borel CO, et al. Perioperative management of aneurysmal subarachnoid hemorrhage: part 1. Operative management. *Anesth Analg.* 1995;81:1060-1072.

Ibrahim GM, Macdonald RL. The effects of fluid balance and colloid administration on outcomes in patients with aneurysmal subarachnoid hemorrhage: a propensity score-matched analysis. *Neurocrit Care.* 2013;19:140-149.

Lanier WL, Stangland KJ, Scheithauer BW, et al. The effects of dextrose infusion and head position on neurologic outcome after complete cerebral ischemia in primates: examination of a model. *Anesthesiology.* 1987;66:39-48.

Perel P, Roberts I, Ker K. Colloids versus crystalloids for fluid resuscitation in critically ill patients. *Cochrane Database Syst Rev.* 2013:CD000567.

C.11. After the bone plate was removed and as the dura was being opened, the surgeon complained that the brain was "tight." What could you do to achieve better brain relaxation and facilitate surgical exposure?

Any method that rapidly decreases ICP before dural opening can increase transmural pressure and lead to aneurysm rupture. After dural opening, one of the fastest ways to decrease cerebral blood volume and improve exposure is through hyperventilation. Mild hypocarbia (Pa_{CO_2} = 30-35 mm Hg) can usually be established before dural opening, with moderate hypocarbia ($Paco_2$ = 25-30 mm Hg) after dural opening. Because of the risk of cerebral ischemia secondary to diminished CBF, normocarbia should be maintained whenever possible in patients with vasospasm.

Mannitol is the most frequently used diuretic to reduce brain swelling. It is given as an infusion to a total dose of 0.25 to 1 g/kg. Its immediate effect is a transient rise in intravascular volume, which can pose problems in patients with impaired ventricular function. In addition, too rapid infusion can lead to decreases in systemic vascular resistance. Its onset of diuretic action is in 10 to 15 minutes, with peak effect occurring at 30 to 45 minutes. If mannitol does not produce the desired brain relaxation and the serum osmolality is greater than 320 mOsm, additional mannitol is unlikely to produce an additional effect. In those patients who may not tolerate the initial effects of mannitol, intravenous furosemide 0.1 to 0.3 mg/kg can be substituted. Both medications can cause derangements in fluid status and serum electrolytes that require close monitoring.

Drainage of CSF from either a lumbar drain or an intraventricular catheter is usually effective in optimizing surgical exposure. One must be careful to avoid significant CSF drainage before dural opening to prevent either brainstem herniation or a sudden increase in transmural pressure. Similarly, hemodynamic instability can ensue if CSF is drained too rapidly at any point during the operation.

If a tight brain remains a problem, one must confirm that there is no hypoxemia or hypercarbia. In addition, one should consider eliminating nitrous oxide (N_2O) and reducing the amount of volatile anesthetic because all inhalational agents are cerebral vasodilators and potentially increase ICP. Of course, if inhaled agents are reduced, appropriate intravenous agents should be substituted to ensure adequate anesthesia. Total intravenous anesthesia can be useful in this situation.

One can give a bolus of propofol or thiopental to decrease $CMRO_2$ and CBF; nevertheless, one must maintain MAP to maintain CPP. At the time of patient positioning, one must ensure that no impediment exists to the venous outflow of the brain (ie, extreme flexion or rotation of the head should be avoided, and no monitor cables [ECG] should be draped across the neck). Even 10° of head-up positioning has been found to be effective at reducing ICP.

Pong RP, Lam AM. Anesthetic management of cerebral aneurysm surgery. In: Cottrell JE, Patel P, eds. *Cottrell and Patel's Neuroanesthesia*. 7th ed. Elsevier; 2024:244-271.

Sullivan HG, Keenan RL, Isrow L. The critical importance of $Paco_2$ during intracranial aneurysm surgery. Case report. *J Neurosurg*. 1980;52:426-430.

C.12. How might transmural pressure be decreased to allow for aneurysm clip placement?

The most widely accepted method for producing a slack aneurysm to allow for clip placement is the use of temporary clip occlusion of one or more parent vessels. For example, to place a permanent clip on an anterior communicating artery aneurysm, a temporary clip can be placed on either the right or left anterior cerebral artery or both. Advantages of temporary clip use include a greater reduction in transmural pressure, a greater ease in clipping, a decreased incidence of intraoperative rupture, and the avoidance of controlled hypotension.

The maximal duration of temporary clip application before a neurologic deficit occurs is unknown, but it is probably related to the location of the aneurysm and the distribution of perforating vessels distal to the temporary clip. White matter and major deep nuclei are likely to be more susceptible than gray matter to temporary ischemia. Risk factors for neurologic deficit following temporary clip placement include poor preoperative neurologic condition, age older than 61 years, and distribution of perforating arteries in distal basilar and horizontal segments of the middle cerebral artery. Recent studies suggest that there are regional differences in brain oxygenation during temporary clip occlusion, with the middle cerebral artery distribution being more susceptible to ischemia than the anterior cerebral artery distribution. In addition, patients who underwent multiple brief periods of temporary occlusion had less ischemia than those who underwent a single temporary artery occlusion of more than 10 minutes.

Adenosine-induced temporary flow arrest has also been reported as a mechanism to produce a slack aneurysm to facilitate clipping.

Bendok BR, Gupta DK, Rahme RJ, et al. Adenosine for temporary flow arrest during intracranial aneurysm surgery: a single-center retrospective review. *Neurosurgery*. 2011;69:815-821.

Ha SK, Lim DJ, Seok BG, et al. Risk of stroke with temporary arterial occlusion in patients undergoing craniotomy for cerebral aneurysm. *J Korean Neurosurg Soc*. 2009;46:31-37.

Silva PA, Cerejo A, Vilarinho A, et al. Regional variations in brain oxygenation during temporary clipping in aneurysm surgery. *Neurol Res*. 2012;34:971-976.

C.13. What is the purpose of controlled hypotension, and how is it achieved?

In the past, controlled hypotension was used to decrease transmural pressure, making the aneurysm neck slack enough to allow placement of a clip without vessel rupture. Various agents were used to achieve controlled hypotension, including volatile anesthetic, nitroprusside, esmolol, labetalol, nitroglycerin, and trimethaphan. Specific agents were selected based on the patient's preexisting medical conditions, especially coronary ischemia or poor ventricular function. In an otherwise healthy patient, sodium nitroprusside infusion can be used for its rapid onset, easy titratability, and quick offset. An esmolol infusion can be added to augment hypotension and counteract the reflex tachycardia; by decreasing the amount of nitroprusside needed to induce hypotension, the likelihood of cyanide toxicity diminishes. Side effects of nitroprusside include cyanide toxicity, rebound hypertension, and intrapulmonary shunting. Direct measurement of CVP is useful when planning to use controlled hypotension in these patients.

During controlled hypotension, MAP is usually maintained at a minimum of 50 mm Hg in previously normotensive individuals. Neurologic function monitors (EEG, SSEP, brainstem auditory evoked response, and cerebral oximetry) can be useful in guiding the target level of MAP.

Newfield P, Hamid RKA, Lam AM. Intracranial aneurysms and A-V malformations: anesthetic management. In: Albin MS, ed. *Textbook of Neuroanesthesia: With Neurosurgical and Neuroscience Perspectives*. McGraw-Hill; 1997:877-878.

Ornstein E, Young WL, Ostapkovich N, et al. Deliberate hypotension in patients with intracranial arteriovenous malformations: esmolol compared with isoflurane and sodium nitroprusside. *Anesth Analg*. 1991;72:639-644.

C.14. What are some of the drawbacks of controlled hypotension?

The main drawback of controlled hypotension is that it leads to a global decrease in CPP. CPP is then further diminished in the presence of vasospasm or in areas of brain retraction. In a retrospective study, multiple regression analysis indicated that patients who underwent even limited periods of controlled hypotension had worse outcomes, in terms of both the Glasgow Outcome Scale (multiple regression) and incidence and severity of vasospasm. Although further studies indicated that this effect was not seen when corrected for age, controlled hypotension is usually avoided in neurosurgery.

Connolly ES, Rabinstein AA, Carhuapoma JR, et al. Guidelines for the management of aneurysmal subarachnoid hemorrhage: a guideline for healthcare professionals from the American Heart Association/American Stroke Association. *Stroke*. 2012;43:11-37.

C.15. What methods of cerebral protection might you use during this operation?

Cerebral protection has long been a matter of much investigation and controversy. Barbiturate loading has been shown in animals to be protective against focal ischemia, although no controlled human studies have been performed. Barbiturates decrease cerebral metabolic rate for glucose and oxygen consumption and lower CBF and ICP. The dose is usually titrated to electroencephalographic silence or burst suppression. At doses used to suppress electroencephalographic activity, the patient can experience cardiovascular depression. The dose of barbiturate traditionally used for cerebral protection can also prolong emergence and hinder postoperative neurologic evaluation. Although barbiturates were originally thought to protect against ischemia through metabolic depression, other factors such as redistribution of blood flow to ischemic areas, blockade of sodium channels and glutamate receptors, and attenuation of *N*-methyl D-aspartate (NMDA) and α-amino-3-hydroxy-5-methyl-4-isoxazole propionic acid (AMPA) receptor–mediated glutamate toxicity all play a role.

Propofol has been used as an alternative to thiopental. Cerebral protection from propofol is thought to result from the scavenging of free radicals, inhibition of glutamate release, and prevention of lipid peroxidation. In studies involving both volatile anesthetics and propofol, apoptotic cell death was delayed, but not prevented, if the ischemic result was mild. Propofol can be titrated to burst suppression using EEG monitoring.

Etomidate decreases the cerebral metabolic rate at electroencephalographic burst suppression and prevents an increase in excitatory neurotransmitters during cerebral ischemia in animal models; nevertheless, it has been associated with a greater volume of the injured brain than thiopental and control groups in focal ischemia in hypertensive rats. The efficacy of burst suppression during aneurysm surgery, while commonly requested, has not been shown to change outcome.

Deliberate mild hypothermia (32.5 °C-35.5 °C), although promising in animal models, did not demonstrate efficacy with patients with good-grade aneurysms in the Intraoperative Hypothermia for Aneurysm Surgery Trial (IHAST) 2, although there was a suggestion of a trend toward benefit in subgroup analysis.

Although many pharmacologic targets for cerebral protection, including magnesium, lidocaine, and others, have shown promising results in laboratory analysis, none have been consistently proven effective in the clinical setting.

Engelhard K, Werner C, Eberspächer E, et al. Influence of propofol on neuronal damage and apoptotic factors after incomplete cerebral ischemia and reperfusion in rats: a long-term observation. *Anesthesiology*. 2004;101:912-917.

Guy J, McGrath BJ, Borel CO, et al. Perioperative management of aneurysmal subarachnoid hemorrhage: part 1. Operative management. *Anesth Analg*. 1995;81:1060-1072.

Hindman BJ, Bayman EO, Pfisterer WK, Torner JC, Todd MM, IHAST Investigators. No association between intraoperative hypothermia or supplemental protective drug and neurologic outcomes in patients undergoing temporary clipping during cerebral aneurysm surgery: findings from the intraoperative hypothermia for aneurysm surgery trial. *Anesthesiology*. 2010;112:86-101.

Kawaguchi M, Furuya H, Patel PM. Neuroprotective effects of anesthetic agents. *J Anesth*. 2005;19:150-156.

Todd MM, Hindman BJ, Clarke WR, et al. Intraoperative hypothermia for aneurysm surgery trial (IHAST) investigators. Mild intraoperative hypothermia during surgery for intracranial aneurysm. *N Engl J Med*. 2005;352:135-145.

C.16. Would you induce mild hypothermia as a means of cerebral protection?

Hypothermia causes a greater reduction in cerebral metabolic rate for glucose and oxygen than the level attained at electroencephalographic silence because its reduction of metabolism is caused by a reduction in both neuronal electrical activity and enzyme activity related to the maintenance of cellular function. Hypothermia also reduces the release of excitatory neurotransmitters. Significant reduction in infarct size after global and focal ischemia has been demonstrated in several animal studies. Unfortunately, these advantages have not been documented in clinical trials. The IHAST study showed no differences in the Glasgow Outcome Scale at 3 months in patients who present with good neurologic grade.

Disadvantages of unintentional hypothermia documented in the literature include an increased incidence of myocardial ischemia in peripheral vascular surgery, increased incidence of postoperative wound infection in abdominal surgery, coagulopathy, prolonged drug clearance, and hyperglycemia. In the IHAST study, the hypothermic group had a small increase in infection rate. The effect of hypothermia in poor clinical-grade patients is unknown.

Frank SM, Beattie C, Christopherson R, et al. Unintentional hypothermia is associated with postoperative myocardial ischemia. The perioperative ischemia randomized anesthesia trial study group. *Anesthesiology*. 1993;78:468-476.

Todd MM, Hindman BJ, Clarke WR, et al. Intraoperative hypothermia for aneurysm surgery trial (IHAST) investigators. Mild intraoperative hypothermia during surgery for intracranial aneurysm. *N Engl J Med*. 2005;352:135-145.

C.17. What are the indications for deep hypothermic circulatory arrest?

Hypothermic circulatory arrest at body temperature less than 22 °C (71.6 °F) is reserved for giant aneurysms, difficult basilar artery aneurysms, and anatomically complex aneurysms that are not clippable without a complete cessation of blood flow and are not amenable to the use of temporary clips. Deep hypothermic circulatory arrest requires cooperation between several services, including anesthesiology, neurosurgery, cardiac surgery, and perfusionists. In addition to the concerns mentioned regarding anesthesia for the person with an intracranial aneurysm and the need for prompt awakening for ease of neurologic assessment, deep hypothermic circulatory arrest adds concerns regarding the institution of and separation from cardiopulmonary bypass, systemic heparinization and protamine reversal, and, of course, rewarming from profound hypothermia. This is rarely performed now that coil embolization is possible for many of these aneurysms. Giant and complex aneurysms that are not amenable to coiling can be managed with flow diversion endovascular therapy.

Gross BA, Frerichs KU. Stent usage in the treatment of intracranial aneurysms: past, present and future. *J Neurol Neurosurg Psychiatry*. 2013;84:244-253.

Young WL, Lawton MI, Gupta DK, et al. Anesthetic management of deep hypothermic circulatory arrest for cerebral aneurysm clipping. *Anesthesiology*. 2002;96:497-503.

C.18. What steps should be taken in the case of intraoperative rupture of an intracranial aneurysm?

The incidence of intraoperative rupture is 2% to 19%. The stage of the operation at which rupture occurs affects outcome, with rupture at induction being the worst. After induction, the most common times for rupture are when the dura mater or arachnoid mater is being opened, during intracranial hematoma removal, or during dissection exposure of the aneurysm. At any point in the operation, a sudden sustained increase in blood pressure with or without bradycardia is suggestive of rupture. If rupture is suspected on induction, one must institute measures to control ICP while maintaining CPP.

If rupture occurs during surgical dissection, mortality is lower. The primary concern is to control bleeding while maintaining systemic perfusion. Bleeding is controlled by the placement of temporary clips or by clamping or compressing the ipsilateral carotid artery in the neck if the aneurysm is too proximal. If bleeding is not controlled in a timely manner and a significant amount of blood accumulates in the subarachnoid space, severe brain swelling that is refractory to all treatments can develop.

Houkin K, Kuroda S, Takahashi A, et al. Intra-operative premature rupture of the cerebral aneurysms. Analysis of the causes and management. *Acta Neurochir (Wien)*. 1999;141:1255-1263.

Lin BF, Kuo CY, Wu ZF. Review of aneurysmal subarachnoid hemorrhage—focus on treatment, anesthesia, cerebral vasospasm prophylaxis, and therapy. *Acta Anaesthesiol Taiwan*. 2014;52:77-84.

C.19. How would you plan the emergence from anesthesia for aneurysm clipping?

The goal is to have a patient comfortable and not coughing or straining or subject to hypercarbia or wide variations in blood pressure.

After discontinuing all anesthetic agents and reversing neuromuscular blockade, the use of lidocaine 1.5 mg/kg can minimize coughing and reaction to the endotracheal tube. Strict control of blood pressure must be observed, especially in the presence of ischemic heart disease or in patients suspected of having multiple aneurysms. One should keep the blood pressure within 20% of the patient's normal measurement.

D. Postoperative Management

D.1. Would you extubate the patient postoperatively?

Most patients who are in Hunt and Hess grades I and II can be extubated postoperatively with no need for airway support. Patients in grades IV and V usually require mechanical ventilation postoperatively, whereas grade III patients may or may not require intubation and mechanical ventilation. Patients with vertebral or basilar artery aneurysms may require airway protection secondary to cranial nerve damage and loss of protective reflexes.

If this patient is able to follow commands, is clinically recovered from the effects of muscle relaxants, and has established an adequate ventilatory pattern with the return of protective airway reflexes, extubation would be appropriate.

Bendo AA. Intracranial vascular surgery. *Anesthesiol Clin North Am*. 2002;20:377-388.

D.2. What would be the differential diagnosis if the patient did not return to her preoperative neurologic condition?

If the patient has a focal neurologic deficit on awakening in the operating room, the most likely cause would be a surgical one, although new-onset vasospasm is also a possibility.

If the patient fails to regain consciousness, the first step would be to ensure that all inhalational and infused anesthetics have been discontinued. Second, one should make sure that neuromuscular blockade is fully reversed. In addition, it is important to ensure that the patient is not hypothermic, as hypothermia can prolong the duration of action of intravenous medications. While considering the reversal of benzodiazepines and opioids, one should rule out other causes such as hypoxemia, hypercarbia, hyponatremia, and hypoglycemia. One should also consider the possibility of intraoperative seizure, with delayed emergence resulting from a postictal state. If after reversal of all anesthetic agents, the patient has not awakened, a CT scan should be obtained to rule out subdural hematoma, intracranial hemorrhage, hydrocephalus, and pneumocephalus. An angiogram may also be obtained to rule out vascular occlusion. An electroencephalogram might be appropriate to rule out subconvulsive status epilepticus.

Pong RP, Lam AM. Anesthetic management of cerebral aneurysm surgery. In: Cottrell JE, Patel P, eds. *Cottrell and Patel's Neuroanesthesia*. 7th ed. Elsevier; 2024:244-271.

D.3. On postoperative day 2, the patient became disoriented and developed hemiplegia. A CT scan was obtained, which showed no new intracranial bleeding. What other diagnostic studies should be performed?

If transcranial Doppler (TCD) is available, an increased value for cerebral arterial flow velocity would be suggestive of vasospasm, leading to delayed cerebral ischemia/infarction. Tissue oximetry can also be useful as a monitor for vasospasm. Angiography is the gold standard for the diagnosis of cerebral vasospasm and should be performed to confirm the diagnosis and characterize the number and location of the vessels involved.

Cerebral vasospasm can be localized to the area of aneurysm rupture or in an area of the brain remote from SAH. The worst prognosis is in those patients in whom vasospasm is diffuse. Of course, as these studies are being done, laboratory values should be checked to make sure no new or worsening metabolic derangement is contributing to the neurologic deterioration.

D.4. What is cerebral vasospasm, and what causes it?

Vasospasm is a segmental or diffuse narrowing of the lumen of one or more intracranial arteries, which occurs frequently after aneurysmal SAH. It was thought to be the leading cause of delayed cerebral ischemia/infarction (DCI); however, recent research suggests that vasospasm is just one of several factors contributing to DCI.

Mechanisms leading to cerebral vasospasm are multifaceted and not fully understood. Earlier hypotheses proposed that vasospasm results from the presence of blood breakdown products in the subarachnoid space, especially oxyhemoglobin, leading to the production of free radicals and the depletion of nitric oxide, a potent vasodilator. This results in the contraction of the arterial smooth muscle and subsequent vasospasm. However, recent insights highlight the role of inflammation and immune response in vasospasm. Particularly, activation of microglia, the primary immune cells in the brain, has been associated with the release of various inflammatory mediators contributing to vasospasm.

SECTION 4

It is important to note that vasospasm is not synonymous with DCI. Although vasospasm was once considered the primary cause of DCI, it is now understood that DCI is a multifactorial syndrome, with contributions from various factors. One significant contributing factor is the immediate brain damage that transpires after aneurysmal SAH, known as early brain injury (EBI). This encompasses a series of pathophysiologic events, including cerebral edema, disruption of the blood-brain barrier, global cerebral ischemia, and neuroinflammation.

Borsody M, Burke A, Coplin W, et al. Haptoglobin and the development of cerebral artery vasospasm after subarachnoid hemorrhage. *Neurology*. 2006;66:634-640.

Dodd WS, Laurent D, Dumont AS, et al. Pathophysiology of delayed cerebral ischemia after subarachnoid hemorrhage: a review. *J Am Heart Assoc*. 2021;10:e021845.

Kale SP, Edgell RC, Alshekhlee A, et al. Age-associated vasospasm in aneurysmal subarachnoid hemorrhage. *J Stroke Cerebrovasc Dis*. 2013;22:22-27.

D.5. What are pathophysiologic changes seen in cerebral vasospasm?

In cerebral vasospasm, structural and functional alterations occur within the cerebral vasculature. Structurally, leukocytes, erythrocytes, and macrophages infiltrate arterial walls. These infiltrating cells, along with resident microglia, contribute to a heightened inflammatory response, leading to increased levels of inflammatory mediators such as eicosanoids, interleukin-1, and immune complexes. The vessel wall thickens due to the proliferation of smooth muscle cells and the deposition of collagen. This thickening accompanies degenerative changes in the tunica intima and media. Functionally, carbon dioxide reactivity is impaired, and autoregulation is often impaired, perhaps correlating to the degree of DCI. CBF in some areas appears to be pressure dependent. Underlying these changes are several pathophysiologic processes, including vessel constriction, neuroinflammation, and the occurrence of spreading depolarization. Spreading depolarization evokes a hyperemic response in healthy tissue, which often leads to hypoperfusion in injured or compromised brain tissue, further contributing to vasospasm.

Dodd WS, Laurent D, Dumont AS, et al. Pathophysiology of delayed cerebral ischemia after subarachnoid hemorrhage: a review. *J Am Heart Assoc*. 2021;10:e021845.

Li K, Barras CD, Chandra RV, et al. A review of the management of cerebral vasospasm after aneurysmal subarachnoid hemorrhage. *World Neurosurg*. 2019;126:513-527.

Weyer GW, Nolan CP, Macdonald RL. Evidence-based cerebral vasospasm management. *Neurosurg Focus*. 2006;21:E8.

D.6. How is the diagnosis of cerebral vasospasm made?

The clinical diagnosis of cerebral vasospasm is made when the patient experiences an altered level of consciousness (drowsiness, disorientation) or a new focal neurologic deficit. These can be accompanied by increasing headache, meningismus, and fever. Vasospasm is rare in the first 3 days following SAH. It reaches peak incidence at 3 to 10 days and usually resolves by 10 to 14 days after SAH. In this patient, the new onset of hemiplegia suggests that the middle cerebral artery is involved. If vessels in the posterior fossa are involved, respiratory and hemodynamic abnormalities can develop.

The differential diagnosis includes rebleeding, hydrocephalus, seizure, hyponatremia, and drug effects. TCD CBF velocity greater than 120 cm/s in association with a new focal neurologic deficit is usually sufficient to make the diagnosis of cerebral vasospasm; however, a change in TCD values over time is more useful than an absolute value. CBF velocity greater than 200 cm/s is associated with a high risk of cerebral infarct, whereas a velocity less than 100 cm/s indicates that cerebral vasospasm is unlikely. Recent evidence shows that TCD had only 63% sensitivity in identifying DCI, with a positive predictive value of only 22% in grades II and III patients. Cerebral perfusion imaging might be necessary in patients of poor grade who are unable to participate in neurologic examination.

Angiographic cerebral vasospasm can be found in 60% of patients following SAH, but only 50% of these patients develop clinical focal neurologic deficits.

Hoh BL, Ko NU, Amin-Hanjani S, et al. 2023 guideline for the management of patients with aneurysmal subarachnoid hemorrhage: a guideline from the American Heart Association/American Stroke Association. *Stroke.* 2023;54:e314-e370.

Pong RP, Lam AM. Anesthetic management of cerebral aneurysm surgery. In: Cottrell JE, Patel P, eds. *Cottrell and Patel's Neuroanesthesia.* 7th ed. Elsevier; 2024:244-271.

D.7. What steps can be taken to prevent cerebral vasospasm?

Calcium channel blockers are standard prophylactic therapy to prevent vasospasm. The mechanism is unknown, but presumably, calcium channel blockers aid in maintaining cellular integrity by preventing calcium entry into ischemic cells. Nimodipine, taken orally, improves neurologic outcome. Patients given nimodipine have no change in the overall incidence of vasospasm, but they have a lower incidence of severe narrowing. In addition, although no improvement is found in mortality, there is improvement in outcome for survivors.

The use of nicardipine, an intravenous agent, showed a lower incidence of vasospasm, but no improvement in outcome versus a placebo group; both groups received hypertension, hypervolemia, and hemodilution (HHH) therapy. The main complication of calcium channel blocker therapy is hypotension (0%-8%), which can complicate this therapy.

Intravenous nimodipine is not available in the United States, although patients are given nimodipine orally or via nasogastric tube every 4 hours. The incidence of vasospasm does not differ significantly between open surgical repair and endovascular procedures. In addition, although calcium channel blockers cross the blood-brain barrier, the dose needed to achieve significant levels at the site necessary might be limited by systemic hypotension. Prolonged-release nicardipine implants placed at the time of surgical clipping have been shown to reduce the incidence of vasospasm, improving outcome. In order to deliver calcium channel blockade intrathecally, nicardipine nanoparticles can be administered through external ventricular drains. The microparticles appeared safe, and there was no significant hypotension. In addition, there was a reduction in DCI and an improvement in clinical outcome.

Hydroxymethylglutaryl coenzyme A reductase inhibitors (statins) have shown potential in reducing cerebral vasospasm through endothelial protection and anti-inflammatory effects. Some studies show that patients receiving statins have a reduced incidence of vasospasm and associated ischemic deficits.

Endothelin receptor antagonists, such as clazosentan, have been suggested as potential therapeutics, but the recently completed clinical Phase 3 REACT study demonstrated that clazosentan failed to prevent clinical deterioration resulting from delayed cerebral ischemia following aneurysmal SAH.

Sodium nitroprusside, a direct nitric oxide donor, has shown promising results in early studies with improvements in TCD velocities in patients with severe cerebral vasospasm.

Thrombolytic agents, such as tissue plasminogen activators, have been investigated for their potential role in augmenting blood clearance from the CSF following SAH, and some studies have shown significant reductions in severe vasospasm with their use.

Free radical scavengers, such as tirilazad and nicaraven, have been studied for their potential role in reducing vasospasm. Some studies have shown a reduction in symptomatic vasospasm and improved outcomes with the use of these agents.

Inflammatory response reduction methods, such as the use of steroids, have also been studied. Some studies have shown a nonsignificant decrease in symptomatic vasospasm and a significant increase in excellent outcomes with the use of steroids.

Barth M, Capelle HH, Weidauer S, et al. Effect of nicardipine prolonged-release implants on cerebral vasospasm and clinical outcome after severe aneurysmal subarachnoid hemorrhage: a prospective, randomized, double-blind phase IIa study. *Stroke.* 2007;38:330-336.

Dodd WS, Laurent D, Dumont AS, et al. Pathophysiology of delayed cerebral ischemia after subarachnoid hemorrhage: a review. *J Am Heart Assoc*. 2021;10:e021845.

Hänggi D, Etminan N, Aldrich F, et al; for NEWTON Investigators. Randomized, open-label, phase 1/2a study to determine the maximum tolerated dose of intraventricular sustained release nimodipine for subarachnoid hemorrhage (NEWTON [nimodipine microparticles to enhance recovery while reducing toxicity after subarachnoid hemorrhage]). *Stroke*. 2017;48:145-151.

Hoh BL, Ko NU, Amin-Hanjani S, et al. 2023 guideline for the management of patients with aneurysmal subarachnoid hemorrhage: a guideline from the American Heart Association/American Stroke Association. *Stroke*. 2023;54:e314-e370.

D.8. What treatments can be undertaken once a diagnosis of cerebral vasospasm is made?

Treatment for cerebral vasospasm is multifactorial and includes continuation of prophylactic measures. In the past, HHH therapy was used to augment CBF past stenotic areas. It begins with hypervolemic hypertension, with intravascular volume expansion with crystalloid or colloid to increase cardiac output. Some recommended target values are a CVP of 10 to 12 mm Hg, pulmonary artery occlusion pressure of 15 to 18 mm Hg, cardiac index of 3.0 to 3.5 L/min/m^2, and hematocrit of 30% to 35%. Various blood pressure targets have been reported, but a reasonable plan is the systolic blood pressure of 160 to 200 mm Hg if the aneurysm is clipped and 120 to 150 mm Hg if unclipped. Vasoactive infusions are added if hypervolemia alone is inadequate. Endpoints of therapy are resolution of neurologic deficits or occurrence of complications of therapy, such as pulmonary edema (26%), myocardial ischemia, and rebleeding or rupture of a secondary aneurysm. A pulmonary artery catheter is often indicated. The fluid used for HHH should be isotonic and have enough sodium to avoid hyponatremia. Vasopressin, fludrocortisone, or hydrocortisone can be administered to counteract excessive sodium and fluid loss. Recent literature has demonstrated the benefit of maintenance of euvolemia with induced hypertension in contrast to strict HHH.

Other treatments for vasospasm, including intracranial administration of intra-arterial vasodilators and angioplasty, are utilized if the patient does not demonstrate prompt improvement with hypertensive therapy.

An emerging intervention for vasospasm is cervical sympathetic block (CSB). This procedure involves injecting a local anesthetic at the level of the cervical sympathetic trunk, which temporarily blocks the innervation of the cerebral arteries, resulting in arterial vasodilation. CSB offers a minimally invasive, cost-effective, and safe approach that might act as a supplementary treatment alongside traditional neurointerventional methods. This technique has shown potential in reducing vasospasm, offering a new avenue for treatment.

In spite of all attempted therapy, the outcome in patients with significant vasospasm is often poor. Most medications investigated to ameliorate the devastating consequences of vasospasm have limited efficacy. Nimodipine has some efficacy in treating vasospasm and improving outcome. A recent target of pharmacologic therapy has been endothelin, a potent long-lasting vasoconstrictor. Clazosentan, an endothelin receptor antagonist, reduced angiographic vasospasm but did not improve clinical outcomes.

Bombardieri AM, Albers GW, Rodriguez S, Pileggi M, Steinberg GK, Heit JJ. Percutaneous cervical sympathetic block to treat cerebral vasospasm and delayed cerebral ischemia: a review of the evidence. *J Neurointerv Surg*. 2023;15:1212-1217.

Dorhout Mees SM, Rinkel GJE, Feigin VL, et al. Calcium antagonists for aneurysmal subarachnoid haemorrhage. *Cochrane Database Syst Rev*. 2007;2007:CD000277.

Hoh BL, Ko NU, Amin-Hanjani S, et al. 2023 guideline for the management of patients with aneurysmal subarachnoid hemorrhage: a guideline from the American Heart Association/American Stroke Association. *Stroke*. 2023;54:e314-e370.

Hoh BL, Ogilvy CS. Endovascular treatment of cerebral vasospasm: transluminal balloon angioplasty, intra-arterial papaverine, and intra-arterial nicardipine. *Neurosurg Clin N Am*. 2005;16:501-516.

Macdonald RL, Higashida RT, Keller E, et al. Randomized trial of clazosentan in patients with aneurysmal subarachnoid hemorrhage undergoing endovascular coiling. *Stroke*. 2012;43:1463-1469.

Macdonald RL, Higashida RT, Keller E, et al. Randomised trial of clazosentan, an endothelin receptor antagonist, in patients with aneurysmal subarachnoid hemorrhage undergoing surgical clipping (CONSCIOUS-2). *Acta Neurochir Suppl*. 2013;115:27-31.

Muench E, Horn P, Bauhuf C, et al. Effects of hypervolemia and hypertension on regional cerebral blood flow, intracranial pressure, and brain tissue oxygenation after subarachnoid hemorrhage. *Crit Care Med*. 2007;35:1844-1852.

Raabe A, Beck J, Keller M, et al. Relative importance of hypertension compared with hypervolemia for increasing cerebral oxygenation in patients with cerebral vasospasm after subarachnoid hemorrhage. *J Neurosurg*. 2005;103:974-981.

D.9. What are other neurologic complications following SAH and aneurysm clipping?

Hydrocephalus, manifesting with a gradual decrease in level of consciousness, occurs in 25% of patients surviving SAH. Diagnosis is confirmed by CT scan. Treatment is by ventricular drainage.

Seizures occur in 13% of patients with SAH and may herald rebleeding or vasospasm. Seizures can increase MAP, CBF, ICP, and lactate production. These changes can predispose patients with unclipped aneurysms to rebleeding and cause cerebral ischemia in those patients with vasospasm. Most patients receive prophylactic anticonvulsants.

Hyponatremia occurs in 10% to 34% of patients with SAH over a time course that parallels that of vasospasm. Causes include the syndrome of inappropriate antidiuretic hormone secretion, "cerebral salt wasting," or prolonged or excessive mannitol use. Cerebral salt wasting syndrome is thought to be mediated by the release of atrial natriuretic factor by the hypothalamus secondary to distension of the cerebral ventricles from hydrocephalus. After SAH, patients also have an increase in intravascular volume. In these patients, fluid restriction is not the treatment of choice because hypovolemia can predispose to vasospasm. Serum brain natriuretic peptide, which causes diuresis and natriuresis, is elevated after SAH, and patients may require treatment with an isotonic or hypertonic salt-containing fluid. In addition, treatment with hydrocortisone can be considered. Finally, patients can experience brain swelling or edema, which is treated with hypertonic saline, mannitol, and/or dexamethasone.

Pong RP, Lam AM. Anesthetic management of cerebral aneurysm surgery. In: Cottrell JE, Patel P, eds. *Cottrell and Patel's Neuroanesthesia*. 7th ed. Elsevier; 2024:244-271.

D.10. What other organ systems can be affected postoperatively in patients following aneurysm clipping?

Pulmonary complications include both pneumonia and neurogenic pulmonary edema, in which disruption of the pulmonary capillary membrane occurs secondary to increased sympathetic nervous system activity. Because of inactivity, patients are predisposed to developing deep venous thromboses (DVTs) and pulmonary embolism. About 5% of patients develop heparin-induced thrombocytopenia, possibly due to heparin exposure during angiography. These patients tend to have increased rates of both vasospasm and DVT. In general, heparin prophylaxis is avoided in patients after SAH due to concerns for aneurysmal rebleeding, surgical site bleeding, or new bleeding around a ventriculostomy catheter. The incidence of venous thromboembolism in neurocritical care patients is as high as 14%.

There appears to be a relationship between the use of hypertonic saline in patients with SAH and the incidence of acute kidney injury. Patients can have a fever secondary to subarachnoid blood, which makes the workup of postoperative infection more difficult. Finally, as in most patients with head injury, those with SAH may have an increased metabolic rate.

Hoh BL, Ko NU, Amin-Hanjani S, et al. 2023 guideline for the management of patients with aneurysmal subarachnoid hemorrhage: a guideline from the American Heart Association/American Stroke Association. *Stroke*. 2023;54:e314-e370.

Kshettry VR, Rosenbaum BP, Seicean A, et al. Incidence and risk factors associated with in-hospital venous thromboembolism after aneurysmal subarachnoid hemorrhage. *J Clin Neurosci*. 2014;21:282-286.

Kumar AB, Shi Y, Shotwell MS, et al. Hypernatremia is a significant risk factor for acute kidney injury after subarachnoid hemorrhage: a retrospective analysis. *Neurocrit Care*. 2015;22:184-191.

SECTION 5 The Endocrine System

23 Pheochromocytoma

Gunisha Kaur and Vinod Malhotra

A 39-year-old male has a history of paroxysmal headaches, diaphoresis, and palpitations for several weeks. During a physical examination, he was found to have an exceptionally high blood pressure (BP) of 230/150 mm Hg, with a heart rate of 112 beats per minute. Prior to this, the patient claims to have been in good health. Further studies were obtained to evaluate the etiology of his arterial hypertension, tachycardia, and headaches.

A. Medical Disease and Differential Diagnosis

1. What are some common etiologies of arterial hypertension?
2. What is a pheochromocytoma?
3. Describe the anatomy of the adrenal gland.
4. What substances does the adrenal medulla secrete?
5. What are the mechanisms of action of epinephrine and norepinephrine?
6. What is the pathway for the synthesis and breakdown of catecholamines?
7. What does the adrenal cortex secrete?
8. What are the metabolic actions of the glucocorticoids and the mineralocorticoids?
9. What are the clinical features associated with a pheochromocytoma?
10. What is the prevalence of pheochromocytomas and paragangliomas?

B. Preoperative Evaluation and Preparation

1. How can you diagnose and localize the tumor preoperatively?
2. How do you pharmacologically prepare the patient with a pheochromocytoma for surgery?
3. What other aspects of preoperative management are important?

C. Intraoperative Management

1. What drugs should be avoided during the operation?
2. How would you monitor this patient?
3. Describe the anesthetic management of the patient with pheochromocytoma.
4. What drugs are used to control the effects of catecholamine stimulation during surgery?
5. What are some management concerns after the tumor is removed?
6. What is another intraoperative concern associated with a laparoscopic approach?

D. Postoperative Management

1. What is the significance of postoperative hypotension? How is it treated?
2. What other problems can arise in the postoperative period?

A. Medical Disease and Differential Diagnosis

A.1. What are some common etiologies of arterial hypertension?

The following is a partial list of etiologies of hypertension:

- *Essential hypertension* of unknown etiology; primary hypertension
- *Primary renal disease*: glomerulonephritis, renal artery stenosis, renal infarction
- *Endocrine*: hypothyroidism, hyperthyroidism, pheochromocytoma, hyperparathyroidism
- *Sympathetic stimulation*: hypoxemia, hypercarbia, pain
- *Neurogenic*: seizure activity, elevated intracranial pressure, denervation of the carotid sinus
- *Miscellaneous*: malignant hyperthermia, neuroleptic malignant syndrome, carcinoid syndrome, and preeclampsia

Kotchen TA. Hypertension. In: Loscalzo J, Fauci A, Kasper D, Hauser S, Longo D, Jameson JL, eds. *Harrison's Principles of Internal Medicine*. 21st ed. McGraw Hill Education LLC; 2021.

A.2. What is a pheochromocytoma?

Pheochromocytomas are catecholamine-secreting tumors of chromaffin cells. The precise cause of these tumors is unknown. They are usually located in the adrenal medulla or sympathetic paraganglia but can be found anywhere chromaffin tissue exists. These locations extend from the base of the skull to the anus. Traditionally, it was thought that 90% of pheochromocytomas were found in the adrenal medulla and 10% occurred elsewhere. Prevalence of extra-adrenal tumors is now thought to be as high as 20%. These are commonly called *paragangliomas*.

Pheochromocytomas and paragangliomas account for less than 0.2% of all cases of arterial hypertension. When unsuspected or improperly managed during surgery, the hemodynamic effects of the released catecholamines can be profound.

Araujo-Castro M, Pascual-Corrales E, Nattero Chavez L, et al. Protocol for presurgical and anesthetic management of pheochromocytomas and sympathetic paragangliomas: a multidisciplinary approach. *J Endocrinol Invest*. 2021;44:2545-2555.

Chen H, Sippel RS, O'Dorisio MS, et al. The North American Neuroendocrine Tumor Society consensus guideline for the diagnosis and management of neuroendocrine tumors: pheochromocytoma, paraganglioma, and medullary thyroid cancer. *Pancreas*. 2010;39:775-783.

Hines RL, Jones SB, eds. *Stoelting's Anesthesia and Co-existing Disease*. Elsevier; 2021:439-464.

Naranjo J, Dodd S, Martin YN. Perioperative management of pheochromocytoma. *J Cardiothorac Vasc Anesth*. 2017;31:1427-1439.

A.3. Describe the anatomy of the adrenal gland.

The adrenal glands are paired, mustard-colored structures positioned superior and slightly medial to the kidneys in the retroperitoneal space. Each gland is supplied by three arteries: the superior suprarenal arteries derived from the inferior phrenic artery, the middle suprarenal arteries derived from the aorta, and the inferior suprarenal arteries derived from the renal artery. In contrast to the arterial supply, each adrenal gland usually is drained by a single, major adrenal vein. The right adrenal vein is usually short (<1 cm) and drains into the inferior vena cava (IVC), whereas the left adrenal vein is longer (2-3 cm) and empties into the left renal vein. Accessory veins occur in 5% to 10% of patients and are an important consideration during pheochromocytoma resection.

In most respects, the cortex and medulla of the adrenal gland can be considered as two completely distinct organs that happen to colocalize during development. They are of separate embryologic origin and develop between the fifth and sixth weeks of growth; the medullary portion is derived from the chromaffin ectodermal cells of the neural crest and develops in parallel with the sympathetic nervous system, and the cortex originates from mesodermal tissue near the gonads on the adrenogenital ridge.

The chromaffin cells become enclosed within the cortex to form the medulla. The organs of Zuckerkandl are paraganglia around the aorta at the level of the kidney anterior to the inferior aorta. Accessory areas for the occurrence of pheochromocytoma are in the mediastinum, in the bladder, occasionally in the neck, in the sacrococcygeal region, or in the anal or vaginal areas.

Lal G, Clark OH. Thyroid, parathyroid, and adrenal. In: Brunicardi FC, Andersen D, Billiar TR, et al, eds. *Schwartz's Principles of Surgery*. 11th ed. McGraw Hill Education; 2019.

Yeh MW, Livhits M, Duh Q-Y. The adrenal glands. In: Townsend CM, Beauchamp RD, Evers MB, et al, eds. *Sabiston Textbook of Surgery: The Biological Basis of Modern Surgical Practice*. Elsevier; 2021:964-997.

A.4. What substances does the adrenal medulla secrete?

The adrenal medulla primarily secretes three catecholamines: epinephrine, norepinephrine, and dopamine. These three compounds are found in all the chromaffin cells of the sympathetic nervous system, which includes the adrenal medulla, aberrant tissue along the sympathetic chain, and paraganglia. Both norepinephrine and dopamine are found at the endings of the postganglionic fibers of the sympathetic nervous system and in the central nervous system.

Laird AM, Libutti SK. The multiple endocrine neoplasia syndromes. In: Townsend CM, Beauchamp RD, Evers MB, et al, eds. *Sabiston Textbook of Surgery: The Biological Basis of Modern Surgical Practice*. Elsevier; 2021:998-1012.

Lal G, Clark OH. Thyroid, parathyroid, and adrenal. In: Brunicardi FC, Andersen D, Billiar TR, et al, eds. *Schwartz's Principles of Surgery*. 11th ed. McGraw Hill Education; 2019.

Yeh MW, Livhits M, Duh Q-Y. The adrenal glands. In: Townsend CM, Beauchamp RD, Evers MB, et al, eds. *Sabiston Textbook of Surgery: The Biological Basis of Modern Surgical Practice*. Elsevier; 2021:964-997.

A.5. What are the mechanisms of action of epinephrine and norepinephrine?

These catecholamines exert their effects by acting on β-adrenergic and α-adrenergic receptors. β-Receptor stimulation results in G protein–mediated activation of adenylyl cyclase, which increases cyclic adenosine monophosphate (cAMP) levels.

Stimulation of the α_1 subtype of the α-receptor results in G protein–mediated hydrolysis of phospholipid membranes, which causes an increase in cytoplasmic Ca^2+ levels and subsequent smooth muscle contraction. The stimulation of α_2 receptors, conversely, inhibits the action of adenylyl cyclase and decreases cAMP.

The pharmacologic response is dependent on the cellular location of the catecholamine receptors in the body. The distribution and density of the receptors will determine the predominant response to each catecholamine.

Ebert TJ. Autonomic nervous system pharmacology. In: Hemmings HC Jr, Egan TD, eds. *Pharmacology and Physiology for Anesthesia*. 2nd ed. Elsevier; 2018:282-299.

Tilley DG, Houser SR, Koch WJ. Adrenergic agonists and antagonists. In: Brunton LL, Knollmann BC, Dandan R, eds. *Goodman and Gillman's The Pharmacological Basis of Therapeutics*. 14th ed. McGraw Hill; 2022.

Zou L, Dillman D. Endocrine disease. In: Hines RL, Jones SB, eds. *Stoelting's Anesthesia and Co-existing Disease*. Elsevier; 2021:439-464.

A.6. What is the pathway for the synthesis and breakdown of catecholamines?

The synthesis of endogenous catecholamines begins with the active transport of the amino acid tyrosine from the circulation into postganglionic sympathetic nerve endings. The hydroxylation of tyrosine is regarded as the rate-limiting step of the pathway (**Figure 23.1**). The termination of the action of catecholamines occurs primarily through reuptake at nerve terminals. Diffusion and metabolism by the enzymes catechol-*O*-methyltransferase (COMT) and monoamine oxidase (MAO) also play a role in the termination of action.

Ebert TJ. Autonomic nervous system pharmacology. In: Hemmings HC Jr, Egan TD, eds. *Pharmacology and Physiology for Anesthesia*. 2nd ed. Elsevier; 2018:282-299.

A.7. What does the adrenal cortex secrete?

The adrenal cortex secretes more than 30 different corticosteroids. These can be divided into three major classes: mineralocorticoids, glucocorticoids, and sex steroids (the androgens and estrogen).

The precursor of all corticosteroids is cholesterol. Aldosterone is the most important mineralocorticoid secreted by the adrenal cortex, whereas cortisol is the most important glucocorticoid secreted. The adrenal cortex is also responsible for secreting sex steroids.

Each of these substances is secreted by different zones. The mineralocorticoids are secreted by the zona glomerulosa, glucocorticoids are secreted by the zona fasciculata, and sex steroids are secreted by the zona reticularis.

Hupfeld CJ, Iniguez-Lluhi JA. Adrenocorticotropic hormone, adrenal steroids, and the adrenal cortex. In: Brunton LL, Knollmann BC. eds. *Goodman & Gilman's: The Pharmacological Basis of Therapeutics*. 14th ed. McGraw Hill; 2023.

Zou L, Dillman D. Endocrine disease. In: Hines RL, Jones SB, eds. *Stoelting's Anesthesia and Co-existing Disease*. Elsevier; 2021:439-464.

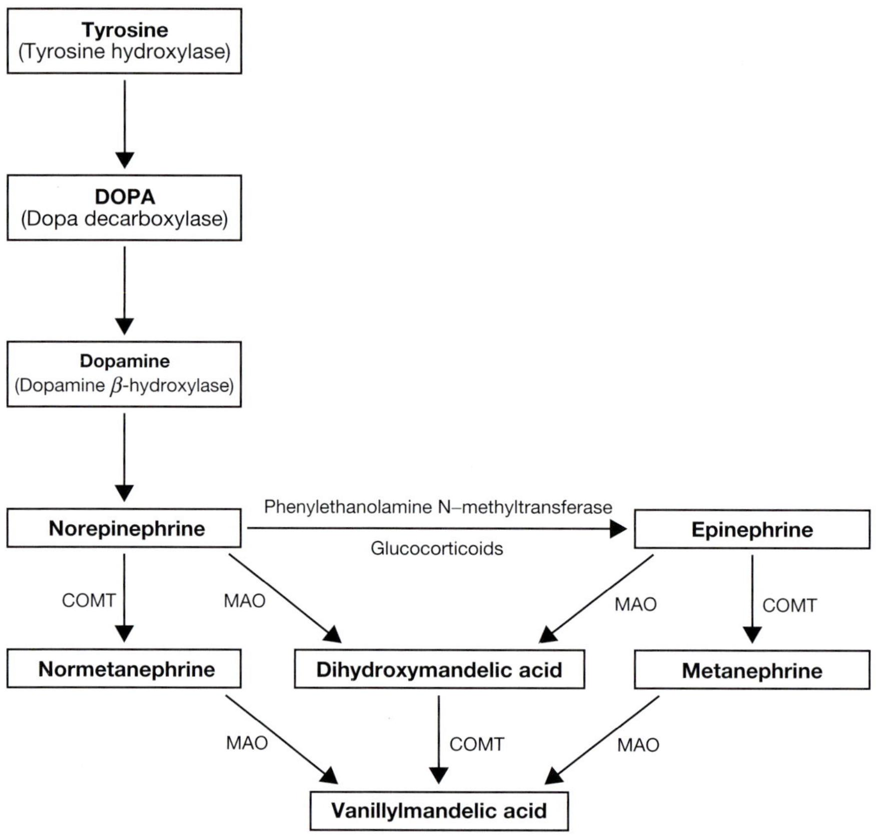

FIGURE 23.1. Synthesis and metabolism of endogenous catecholamine. COMT, catechol-*O*-methyltransferase; MAO, monoamine oxidase. (Reprinted by permission from Springer: Pullerits J, Ein S, Balfe JW. Anesthesia for phaeochromocytoma. *Can J Anesth.* 1988;35:526-534. Copyright © 1988 Canadian Anesthesiologists.)

A.8. What are the metabolic actions of the glucocorticoids and the mineralocorticoids?

The glucocorticoids have their predominant mechanism of action on intermediary metabolism. These effects include increased gluconeogenesis, fatty acid mobilization, protein catabolism, and anti-inflammatory effects. Cortisol can improve cardiac function by improving the responsiveness of β-adrenergic receptors. Approximately 95% of the glucocorticoid activity is from the secretion of cortisol.

The mineralocorticoids predominantly act on the body's minerals, such as sodium and potassium. By conserving sodium ions, they sustain extracellular fluid volume. They also help maintain normal potassium plasma concentrations.

Czock D, Keller F, Rasche FM, et al. Pharmacokinetics and pharmacodynamics of systemically administered glucocorticoids. *Clin Pharmacokinet.* 2005;44:61-98.

Hupfeld CJ, Iniguez-Lluhi JA. Adrenocorticotropic hormone, adrenal steroids, and the adrenal cortex. In: Brunton LL, Knollmann BC, eds. *Goodman & Gilman's: The Pharmacological Basis of Therapeutics.* 14th ed. McGraw Hill; 2023.

Zou L, Dillman D. Endocrine disease. In: Hines RL, Jones SB, eds. *Stoelting's Anesthesia and Co-existing Disease.* Elsevier; 2021:439-464.

A.9. What are the clinical features associated with a pheochromocytoma?

The classic triad is severe episodic headaches, diaphoresis, and palpitations. One or more of the following often signal the presence of a pheochromocytoma: sudden severe headaches, perspiration, weight loss, paroxysmal hypertension, pallor, palpitations, dyspnea, diabetes-like syndrome with elevated fasting blood sugar, nausea, vomiting, fever, encephalopathy, anxiety, myocardial infarction, stroke, or acute renal failure. The aforementioned symptoms are usually paroxysmal in nature. These "attacks" last from a few moments to hours.

A pressor response to particular drugs suggests the presence of this tumor. These drugs include histamine, glucagon, droperidol, tyramine, metoclopramide, saralasin, tricyclic antidepressants, and phenothiazines.

Laird AM, Libutti SK. The multiple endocrine neoplasia syndromes. In: Townsend CM, Beauchamp RD, Evers MB, et al, eds. *Sabiston Textbook of Surgery: The Biological Basis of Modern Surgical Practice*. Elsevier; 2021:998-1012.

Manger WM. An overview of pheochromocytoma: history, current concepts, vagaries, and diagnostic challenges. *Ann N Y Acad Sci*. 2006;1073:1-20.

Yeh MW, Livhits M, Duh Q-Y. The adrenal glands. In: Townsend CM, Beauchamp RD, Evers MB, et al, eds. *Sabiston Textbook of Surgery: The Biological Basis of Modern Surgical Practice*. Elsevier; 2021:964-997.

Zuber SM, Kantorovich V, Pacak K. Hypertension in pheochromocytoma: characteristics and treatment. *Endocrinol Metab Clin North Am*. 2011;40:295-311, vii.

A.10. What is the prevalence of pheochromocytomas and paragangliomas?

Pheochromocytomas occur in both sexes with peak incidence in the third to fifth decades of life. Advances in diagnosis and genetics now challenge the traditional "rule of 10" for pheochromocytomas (10% bilateral, 10% extra-adrenal, 10% familial, and 10% malignant). The prevalence of bilateral adrenal tumors is higher than 10% in some familial pheochromocytoma syndromes such as multiple endocrine neoplasia type 2 and von Hippel-Lindau syndrome (see **Table 23.1** for a complete list). The prevalence of extra-adrenal tumors (paragangliomas) is thought to reach as high as 20%. Between 30% and 50% of these tumors are thought to be hereditary.

Metastases are low for adrenal pheochromocytomas (~10%). The prevalence of malignant disease is 25% to 30% for extra-adrenal pheochromocytomas and even higher in patients with specific mutations such as those causing some forms of familial paragangliomas.

Kinney MA, Narr BJ, Warner MA. Perioperative management of pheochromocytoma. *J Cardiothorac Vasc Anesth*. 2002;16:359-369.

Lenders JW, Eisenhofer G, Mannelli M, Pacak K. Phaeochromocytoma. *Lancet*. 2005;366:665-675.

Naranjo J, Dodd S, Martin YN. Perioperative management of pheochromocytoma. *J Cardiothorac Vasc Anesth*. 2017;31:1427-1439.

Neumann HPH, Young WF Jr, Eng C. Pheochromocytoma and paraganglioma. *N Engl J Med*. 2019;381:552-565.

Parenti G, Zampetti B, Rapizzi E, Ercolino T, Giachè V, Mannelli M. Updated and new perspectives on diagnosis, prognosis, and therapy of malignant pheochromocytoma/paraganglioma. *J Oncol*. 2012;2012:872713.

Tanabe A, Naruse M. Recent advances in the management of pheochromocytoma and paraganglioma. *Hypertens Res*. 2020;43:1141-1151

TABLE 23.1 Syndromes Associated With Pheochromocytoma

Syndrome	Features
MEN type IIa (Sipple syndrome)	Parathyroid adenoma/hyperplasia Medullary carcinoma of the thyroid Pheochromocytoma
MEN type IIb	Medullary carcinoma of the thyroid Mucosal adenomas Marfanoid appearance Pheochromocytoma
von Hippel-Landau syndrome	Hemangioblastoma of the retina, cerebellum, or other parts of the CNS, pheochromocytoma
Neurofibromatosis	Neurofibromas, café-au-lait spots, axillary or inguinal freckling, optic nerve glioma, pheochromocytoma

CNS, central nervous system; MEN, multiple endocrine neoplasia.

SECTION 5

B. Preoperative Evaluation and Preparation

B.1. How can you diagnose and localize the tumor preoperatively?

Pheochromocytoma diagnosis is made by both biochemical analysis and imaging studies. The laboratory tests for pheochromocytoma are shown in **Table 23.2**. Biochemical diagnosis is based on the excess catecholamines and their metabolites released by the tumor.

The hydroxy-methoxy-mandelic acid (often misnamed as vanillylmandelic acid [VMA]) level should be the most reliable laboratory test because it is the final common product of both catecholamine metabolic pathways. In practice, however, the intermediate metanephrines have proved to be better discriminators of pheochromocytomas. Hydroxy-methoxy-mandelic acid can be used as an initial screening test because it has acceptable specificity and sensitivity and is relatively inexpensive.

Historically, 24-hour urine tests were generally considered superior to plasma tests in the diagnosis of pheochromocytomas because the tumor secretes catecholamines only intermittently and catecholamines have short half-lives. These factors could result in relatively normal plasma catecholamine levels in the presence of an active tumor.

Measurement of total metanephrines gives the highest true-positive results of 98% to 99%. Compelling evidence now indicates that initial screening for pheochromocytomas and paragangliomas can include measurements of plasma-fractionated metanephrines or urine-fractionated metanephrines. Despite its high sensitivity, the plasma test has a low specificity and can be difficult to implement under recommended conditions. As such, some guidelines suggest primarily utilizing the plasma test in cases where the suspicion of pheochromocytoma is high.

Computed tomography (CT) with or without iodine-131 (^{131}I)–labeled metaiodobenzylguanidine (MIBG) is extremely accurate in diagnosing and localizing these tumors. Low-osmolar contrast appears to be safe for patients with pheochromocytoma even prior to initiation of α- or β-adrenergic blocker treatment. CT scanning and magnetic resonance imaging (MRI) scanning can visualize normal adrenal glands when the diagnosis is equivocal. For extra-adrenal locations such as metastases and in pregnant patients or others for whom radiation exposure must be limited, MRI scanning might be preferred. If these imaging techniques do not demonstrate the presence of pheochromocytoma and the diagnosis is still clinically suspected, total body nuclear imaging might be warranted. This includes, for example, gallium-68 (Ga^{68}) DOTA-O-Phe1-Tyr-3 octreotate (gallium-68 DOTATATE) positron emission tomography (PET) scanning. The 2014 Endocrine Society clinical practice guidelines recommend considering genetic testing in all patients.

Baid SK, Lai EW, Wesley RA, et al. Brief communication: radiographic contrast infusion and catecholamine release in patients with pheochromocytoma. *Ann Intern Med.* 2009;150:27-32. Published correction appears in *Ann Intern Med.* 2009;150:292.

Lal G, Clark OH. Thyroid, parathyroid, and adrenal. In: Brunicardi FC, Andersen D, Billiar TR, et al, eds. *Schwartz's Principles of Surgery.* 11th ed. McGraw Hill Education; 2019.

TABLE 23.2 Biochemical Tests for Diagnosis of Pheochromocytoma

Urine Tests
Norepinephrine
Epinephrine
Dopamine
Total metanephrines
Fractionated metanephrines
Hydroxy-methoxy-mandelic acid (vanillylmandelic acid)
Plasma Tests
Norepinephrine
Epinephrine
Dopamine
Plasma-free metanephrines
Clonidine suppression of norepinephrine secretion

Chen H, Sippel RS, O'Dorisio MS, et al. The North American Neuroendocrine Tumor Society consensus guideline for the diagnosis and management of neuroendocrine tumors: pheochromocytoma, paraganglioma, and medullary thyroid cancer. *Pancreas*. 2010;39:775-783.

Lenders JW, Duh QY, Eisenhofer G, et al; Endocrine Society. Pheochromocytoma and paraganglioma: an endocrine society clinical practice guideline. *J Clin Endocrinol Metab*. 2014;99:1915-1942. Published correction appears in *J Clin Endocrinol Metab*. 2023;108:e200.

Neumann HPH, Young WF Jr, Eng C. Pheochromocytoma and Paraganglioma. *N Engl J Med*. 2019;381:552-565.

Tanabe A, Naruse M. Recent advances in the management of pheochromocytoma and paraganglioma. *Hypertens Res*. 2020;43:1141-1151.

B.2. How do you pharmacologically prepare the patient with a pheochromocytoma for surgery?

The major goals of pharmacologic therapy in the preoperative period are to control hypertension and tachycardia and to facilitate intravascular volume repletion.

Although the administration of α-adrenergic blocking drugs has been the cornerstone of preoperative management, there are several different approaches including combined α- and β-blockade, calcium channel blockade, and metyrosine inhibition of catecholamine synthesis. To facilitate preoperative α-blockade, phenoxybenzamine, prazosin, terazosin, and doxazosin can all be employed. Phenoxybenzamine is most commonly used due to its relatively long duration of action and ease of administration. It irreversibly and nonselectively alkylates α-adrenergic receptors, including α_1-receptors on vascular smooth muscle, rendering them nonfunctional. Selective α_1 blocking drugs such as prazosin, terazosin, or doxazosin have fewer side effects. Preoperative medical therapy is started 1 to 3 weeks prior to surgery, usually for a minimal duration of 7 to 10 days. Therapy is titrated to resolution of symptoms and decrease in BP to low normal values for age. During this period, the patient is encouraged to liberally take fluids and salt in order to facilitate volume replacement and minimize postural hypotension.

Reflex tachycardia is a frequent side effect of preoperative α-blockade. Tachycardia can be managed by subsequent addition of β-blocker therapy. However, β-blockade is best avoided in the initial phases of treatment. In the absence of adequate α-blockade, inhibition of β-receptor-mediated vasodilation can result in unopposed α-receptor-mediated vasoconstriction due to catecholamines secreted by the tumor. This can precipitate a hypertensive crisis, heart failure, and possibly end-organ damage. Chronic catecholamine elevation can also result in cardiomyopathy that is precipitated by β-blockade. Therefore, β-blockade should be initiated carefully and slowly.

Preoperative use of α-adrenergic blockers such as phenoxybenzamine can often be limited by frequent and sometimes severe side effects (postural hypotension, reflex tachycardia, nasal stuffiness, syncope, etc) as well as their uncommon use and high cost. Calcium channel blockers can be used as an alternative to α-blockade for preoperative management of pheochromocytoma. Nicardipine and amlodipine are the most commonly used calcium channel blockers in these cases. Oral therapy appears to be an equivalent alternative to phenoxybenzamine therapy and can be better tolerated, cheaper, and more accessible. This preoperative treatment can also be complemented by an intravenous (IV) infusion intraoperatively.

α-Methyl-para-tyrosine (α-metyrosine) is also an option for preoperative management of pheochromocytoma. This agent decreases the biosynthesis of catecholamines through competitive inhibition of the enzyme tyrosine hydroxylase. The significant depletion of catecholamine stores reduces hemodynamic fluctuations during tumor manipulation. For maximal effect, α-metyrosine must be administered a minimum of 2 to 3 days before surgery.

Brunaud L, Boutami M, Nguyen-Thi PL, et al. Both preoperative alpha and calcium channel blockade impact intraoperative hemodynamic stability similarly in the management of pheochromocytoma. *Surgery*. 2014;156:1410-1417.

Fagundes GFC, Almeida MQ. Perioperative management of pheochromocytomas and sympathetic paragangliomas. *J Endocr Soc*. 2022;6:bvac004.

Lenders JW, Duh QY, Eisenhofer G, et al. Pheochromocytoma and paraganglioma: an endocrine society clinical practice guideline. *J Clin Endocrinol Metab*. 2014;99:1915-1942.

Naranjo J, Dodd S, Martin YN. Perioperative management of pheochromocytoma. *J Cardiothorac Vasc Anesth*. 2017;31:1427-1439.

Wang J, Liu Q, Jiang S, et al. Preoperative α-blockade versus no blockade for pheochromocytoma-paraganglioma patients undergoing surgery: a systematic review and updated meta-analysis. *Int J Surg*. 2023;109:1470-1480.

Zou L, Dillman D. Endocrine disease. In: Hines RL, Jones SB, eds. *Stoelting's Anesthesia and Co-existing Disease*. Elsevier; 2021:439-464.

B.3. What other aspects of preoperative management are important?

The circulating blood volume is frequently decreased in these patients due to vasoconstriction from high levels of circulating catecholamines. Patients are encouraged to consume fluid and salt in order to facilitate volume expansion once α-blocker therapy is initiated. However, volume expansion should be undertaken with caution in those with decreased myocardial function to avoid precipitating congestive heart failure.

Sedation in the immediate preoperative period can be particularly helpful in attenuating catecholamine release secondary to anxiety. It can also help reduce vasodilator requirement subsequently in the intraoperative phase. Adequate sedation and analgesia should also be provided during invasive procedures such as arterial line access. Preoperative treatment of the airway with nebulized lidocaine or the use of less triggering techniques for tracheal intubation such as videolaryngoscopy can help attenuate the response to intubation.

Araujo-Castro M, Pascual-Corrales E, Nattero Chavez L, et al. Protocol for presurgical and anesthetic management of pheochromocytomas and sympathetic paragangliomas: a multidisciplinary approach. *J Endocrinol Invest.* 2021;44;2545-2555.

Fagundes GFC, Almeida MQ. Perioperative management of pheochromocytomas and sympathetic paragangliomas. *J Endocr Soc.* 2022;6:bvac004.

Lenders JW, Duh QY, Eisenhofer G, et al. Pheochromocytoma and paraganglioma: an Endocrine Society clinical practice guideline. *J Clin Endocrinol Metab.* 2014;99:1915-1942.

C. Intraoperative Management

C.1. What drugs should be avoided during the operation?

Some of the commonly administered drugs that should be avoided in patients with pheochromocytoma are listed in **Table 23.3**. Many of these agents release histamine (eg, morphine, atracurium), which is a potent activator of catecholamine release from the tumor. Agents that cause an indirect increase in catecholamine levels (eg, ketamine, ephedrine) should also be avoided. However, these are not absolute contraindications, and many of these agents can be used if clinically necessary, provided they are used judiciously with close monitoring.

Forkin KT, Huffmyer JL, Nemergut EC. Endocrine physiology. In: Hemmings HC Jr, Egan TD, eds. *Pharmacology and Physiology for Anesthesia.* 2nd ed. Elsevier; 2018:693-707.

Naranjo J, Dodd S, Martin YN. Perioperative management of pheochromocytoma. *J Cardiothorac Vasc Anesth.* 2017;31:1427-1439.

Zou L, Dillman D. Endocrine disease. In: Hines RL, Jones SB, eds. *Stoelting's Anesthesia and Co-existing Disease.* Elsevier; 2021:439-464.

C.2. How would you monitor this patient?

Monitoring in these patients generally includes an electrocardiogram with a V_5 lead, core temperature, pulse oximetry, and intra-arterial BP monitoring. It might also include central venous pressure monitoring and a urinary catheter. For patients with known or suspected myocardial dysfunction, a pulmonary artery catheter or transesophageal echocardiography should be considered. Devices that measure cardiac output and stroke volume variation noninvasively can be particularly helpful in titrating fluid therapy.

Most tumors are excised using laparoscopic techniques with minimal blood loss. With the increasing availability of noninvasive monitors of cardiac function, patients who are adequately optimized in the

TABLE 23.3 Suggested Drugs to Avoid in Patients With Pheochromocytoma
Droperidol
Morphine
Atracurium
Pancuronium
Ketamine
Ephedrine
Halothane
Cocaine
Metoclopramide

preoperative period and display minimal hemodynamic perturbation do not require central venous pressure monitoring.

Kinney MA, Narr BJ, Warner MA. Perioperative management of pheochromocytoma. *J Cardiothorac Vasc Anesth.* 2002;16:359-369.

Zou L, Dillman D. Endocrine disease. In: Hines RL, Jones SB, eds. *Stoelting's Anesthesia and Co-existing Disease.* Elsevier; 2021:439-464.

C.3. Describe the anesthetic management of the patient with pheochromocytoma.

General anesthesia is frequently employed for tumor resection because most resections are performed by laparoscopic technique. Neuromuscular block and controlled ventilation allow for adequate gas exchange during CO_2 insufflation for pneumoperitoneum.

The anesthetic induction technique should minimize hemodynamic changes and allow for adequate depth of anesthesia during tracheal intubation. Lidocaine 4% solution administered prior to intubation, via a mucosal atomizer device or 0.5 to 1.5 mg/kg IV 2 minutes before laryngoscopy, can significantly attenuate the response to tracheal intubation. Other measures to attenuate hemodynamic responses to intubation, such as the use of videolaryngoscopy, are described in Chapter 11: Hypertension, Sections C.4 and C.6. Most of the inhaled agents can be employed during the maintenance phase. However, caution should be used when desflurane is utilized because it can provoke sympathetic stimulation and subsequent catecholamine release. Halothane, now infrequently used in most clinical settings, should be avoided because it has the potential to incite arrhythmias in the presence of high levels of circulating catecholamines.

Zou L, Dillman D. Endocrine disease. In: Hines RL, Jones SB, eds. *Stoelting's Anesthesia and Co-existing Disease.* Elsevier; 2021:439-464.

SECTION 5

C.4. What drugs are used to control the effects of catecholamine stimulation during surgery?

Drugs frequently used to control intraoperative hypertension are listed in **Table 23.4**.

Nicardipine infusion can be easily titrated and is particularly effective at achieving systemic vasodilation. It is a good choice in patients that have already been started on oral nicardipine in the preoperative period. Sodium nitroprusside was used extensively previously, but concerns over toxic metabolites and handling precautions to prevent its degradation by light have largely resulted in nicardipine replacing it as a first-line agent. Phentolamine, a short-acting α-blocking agent, can also be given as a bolus medication or a continuous infusion to control BP.

Magnesium sulfate ($MgSO_4$) has been used in selected cases as an adjunct vasodilator. Data are still being gathered on its efficacy. Administration of $MgSO_4$ should be accompanied by close monitoring of plasma magnesium levels and other clinical signs of hypermagnesemia.

β-Blockers such as esmolol and labetalol can be a useful adjunct to control BP in the intraoperative phase, particularly if tachycardia is present. They should, however, not be used as the first-line agent for the treatment of intraoperative hypertension due to concerns about unopposed α-agonism.

Hodin R, Lubitz C, Phitayakorn R, et al. Diagnosis and management of pheochromocytoma. *Curr Probl Surg.* 2014;51:151-187.

Kinney MA, Narr BJ, Warner MA. Perioperative management of pheochromocytoma. *J Cardiothorac Vasc Anesth.* 2002;16:359-369.

Siddiqi HK, Yang HY, Laird AM, et al. Utility of oral nicardipine and magnesium sulfate infusion during preparation and resection of pheochromocytomas. *Surgery.* 2012;152:1027-1036.

TABLE 23.4 Intravenous Drugs to Control Intraoperative Hypertension

Drug	Dose
Nicardipine	Infusion of 5-15 mg/h. Increase by 2.5 mg/h every 15 min to effect.
Phentolamine	1-mg IV boluses every 5-10 min. Start infusion 0.1-2 mg/min and titrate to effect.
Nitroglycerin	20-40 μg boluses every 5-10 min to effect. Infusion 5-20 μg/min initial (maximum dose 400 μg/min)
Nitroprusside	Infuse initially with 0.5-1.5 μg/kg/min to a maximum of 8 μg/kg/min over 1-3 h.
Propranolol	1-mg boluses to total 10 mg
Esmolol	Load with 5- to 10-mg boluses and infuse at 0.25-0.5 μg/kg/min.
Labetalol	5- to 10-mg boluses every 20-30 min to a maximum dose of 150 mg

IV, intravenous.

C.5. What are some management concerns after the tumor is removed?

BP can decrease very quickly and profoundly within minutes after venous drainage of the tumor is interrupted. Any vasodilators being administered should be discontinued immediately prior to vein clipping. BP support can be provided by administering vasopressors, such as phenylephrine and norepinephrine, and by administering fluids. Vasopressor requirements can be substantial following tumor resection due to receptor insensitivity from chronic catecholamine exposure. Additional vasopressors, such as vasopressin or epinephrine, might need to be initiated.

Close communication between the anesthesia and surgical teams is essential during this period. Continued need for vasodilator support might indicate inadequate resection or previously undiagnosed extra-adrenal tumor.

Araujo-Castro M, Pascual-Corrales E, Nattero Chavez L, et al. Protocol for presurgical and anesthetic management of pheochromocytomas and sympathetic paragangliomas: a multidisciplinary approach. *J Endocrinol Invest.* 2021;44:2545-2555.

Zou L, Dillman D. Endocrine disease. In: Hines RL, Jones SB, eds. *Stoelting's Anesthesia and Co-existing Disease.* Elsevier; 2021:439-464.

C.6. What is another intraoperative concern associated with a laparoscopic approach?

Insufflation of CO_2, to facilitate pneumoperitoneum, is typically associated with an elevation in catecholamine levels in patients undergoing laparoscopic adrenalectomy, resulting in an associated increase in cardiac output and BP. Close monitoring of vital signs is essential once pneumoperitoneum is initiated. The use of lower intra-abdominal pressures during laparoscopy has been associated with decreased release of catecholamines and less hemodynamic fluctuation. If hemodynamic instability is sustained or refractory, insufflation should be terminated.

Fu SQ, Wang SY, Chen Q, Liu YT, Li ZL, Sun T. Laparoscopic versus open surgery for pheochromocytoma: a meta-analysis. *BMC Surg.* 2020;20:167.

Reijnders-Boerboom GTJA, Albers KI, Jacobs LMC, et al. Low intra-abdominal pressure in laparoscopic surgery: a systematic review and meta-analysis. *Int J Surg.* 2023;109:1400-1411.

D. Postoperative Management

D.1. What is the significance of postoperative hypotension? How is it treated?

Postoperative hypotension can be due to reduced circulating catecholamine levels following tumor resection, hypovolemia, or residual effects of phenoxybenzamine (which has a long half-life). In addition, the downregulation of catecholamine receptors, due to chronically elevated levels of catecholamines, renders administered catecholamines less effective. Hypotension should be treated with volume administration and, if needed, norepinephrine or another vasopressor. Vasopressin can be used to treat catecholamine-unresponsive hypotension. It is important that the clinician rule out other etiologies of hypotension, such as postoperative bleeding.

Zou L, Dillman D. Endocrine disease. In: Hines RL, Jones SB, eds. *Stoelting's Anesthesia and Co-existing Disease.* Elsevier; 2021:439-464.

D.2. What other problems can arise in the postoperative period?

Occasionally, patients are somnolent in the postoperative period. This is possibly due to the sudden removal of activating catecholamines. Opioid requirement might also be decreased.

Hypoglycemia is another significant concern. Severe hypoglycemia can cause loss of consciousness and respiratory arrest. Hypoglycemia is the result of decreased catecholamine levels (particularly when the tumor is epinephrine secreting). Neoglycogenesis and glycogenolysis, the result of chronic β-agonism, are no longer present, and chronically elevated insulin levels can decrease more gradually. Close monitoring of blood glucose levels is essential in the first 24 hours posttumor resection.

Persistent hypertension after removal of a pheochromocytoma occasionally signifies that a residual pheochromocytoma tumor is present. Also, plasma catecholamine levels may not decrease to normal levels for many days after removal of the tumor.

Chen Y, Hodin RA, Pandolfi C, Ruan DT, McKenzie TJ. Hypoglycemia after resection of pheochromocytoma. *Surgery.* 2014;156:1404-1408; discussion 1408-1409.

Zou L, Dillman D. Endocrine disease. In: Hines RL, Jones SB, eds. *Stoelting's Anesthesia and Co-existing Disease.* Elsevier; 2021:439-464.

24

Diabetes Mellitus

Justin C. De Biasio and Mark E. Nunnally

A 59-year-old female presents for vaginal hysterectomy for cervical cancer. She is obese (body mass index 32 kg/m^2) and has had diabetes mellitus (DM) type 2, hypertension, and dyslipidemia for 20 years. She takes enalapril, metoprolol, atorvastatin, metformin, sitagliptin, and recently, insulin glargine, 20 units subcutaneously daily for refractory hyperglycemia. She measures her serum glucose intermittently at home. Values are generally 150 to 220 mg/dL. She experiences an early and a prolonged sense of fullness after meals and an unpleasant sour taste at night 2 or 3 times per week. Laboratory values are notable for a serum creatinine of 2.2 mg/dL and a serum glucose of 206 mg/dL. She has not taken any medications today and has had nothing to eat since midnight.

A. Medical Disease and Differential Diagnosis

1. What is the epidemiology of DM in the general population?
2. What are the factors in the etiology of DM?
3. How is DM classified?
4. What are the complications of DM?
5. How are the different forms of DM treated?
6. How is control of DM adequately monitored?
7. What are some of the factors that alter insulin requirements?
8. What are the principles of management of diabetic ketoacidosis (DKA)?
9. What is a hyperglycemic hyperosmolar state?

B. Preoperative Evaluation and Preparation

1. How should this patient be evaluated?
2. How would the stiff joint syndrome affect her airway management?
3. What are the signs and implications of autonomic neuropathy in a patient with DM?
4. How should this patient be prepared for anesthesia and surgery?
5. For elective surgery, how are DM medications and glucose requirements managed in advance of surgery?
6. How should this patient be premedicated?

C. Intraoperative Management

1. What are the effects of anesthesia and surgery on insulin and glucose metabolism?
2. What anesthetic techniques should be considered?
3. How should this patient be monitored?
4. How is hyperglycemia treated intraoperatively?
5. How is hypoglycemic shock recognized and treated intraoperatively?

D. Postoperative Management

1. How is DM controlled in this patient postoperatively?
2. Does DM increase perioperative risk?
3. What are the common postoperative complications to be expected in a patient with DM?
4. Is it necessary to achieve tight perioperative control of glucose?

A. Medical Disease and Differential Diagnosis

A.1. What is the epidemiology of DM in the general population?

Diabetes mellitus, literally "sweet urine," is a group of metabolic disorders defined by elevated blood glucose. Data from the National Health and Nutrition Examination Survey suggest that the prevalence of DM has continued to increase from 1988 to 2020. Data from 2015 to 2018 suggest a prevalence of DM in the US adult population of 15.9%. DM prevalence increases with age: among patients 65 years or older, the prevalence is 29%. Although undiagnosed DM remains proportionally more common among patients with limited health care access, between 1988 and 2020, the estimated proportion of undiagnosed DM declined from about one-third to one-sixth of all those with the disease.

A substantial majority of adult patients with DM (~91%) have type 2 diabetes mellitus (DM2); a minority (~6%) have type 1 diabetes mellitus (DM1). The remainder of patients with DM have gestational diabetes or other specific types. Depending on the method of screening, about 5% to 11% of pregnant patients have gestational diabetes.

Bullard KM, Cowie CC, Lessem SE, et al. Prevalence of diagnosed diabetes in adults by diabetes type-United States, 2016. *MMWR Morb Mortal Wkly Rep*. 2018;67:359-361.

Centers for Disease Control and Prevention. Diabetes prevalence and glycemic control among adults aged 20 and over, by sex, age, and race and Hispanic origin: United States, selected years 1988-1994 through 2015-2018. Accessed January 3, 2023. https://www.cdc.gov/nchs/data/hus/2019/014-508.pdf

Fang M, Wang D, Coresh J, et al. Undiagnosed diabetes in U.S. adults: prevalence and trends. *Diabetes Care*. 2022;45:1994-2002.

Pillay J, Donovan L, Guitard S, et al. Screening for gestational diabetes: updated evidence report and systematic review for the US Preventive Services Task Force. *JAMA*. 2021;326:539-562.

A.2. What are the factors in the etiology of DM?

Because hyperglycemia defines DM, it is too easy to focus on elevations in serum glucose, ignoring other effects. Lipid and protein metabolism are generally deranged in DM. Tissue growth, signaling, and function are likewise impaired. Simple control of blood glucose might not adequately treat the complex hormonal and metabolic derangements of DM. Inflammation and immune dysfunction are often components of the disease. In both DM1 and DM2, genetic association is incomplete, and there is association with other diseases, including autoimmune disorders, hypertension, and dyslipidemias.

DM1 and DM2 are very different diseases. In DM1, exogenous insulin is essential for cellular metabolism. Untreated, DM1 is a wasting disease associated with ketoacidosis and severe cumulative organ failure. In DM1, there is usually autoimmune destruction of insulin-secreting pancreatic β cells. The diagnosis of DM1 is frequently made in childhood, although more gradual progression of disease can result in its diagnosis in adulthood.

DM2 is a metabolic disorder associated with resistance to insulin effects and sometimes inadequate insulin production. DM2 manifests in a variety of conditions that decrease the hypoglycemic effects of insulin. Among these are obesity and endocrine and inflammatory conditions. Because of the presence of circulating insulin, ketoacidosis is rare in DM2. A hyperglycemic hyperosmolar state is a more common risk in inadequately treated patients.

There are a range of other causes of DM that often manifest with substantial overlap with DM1 or DM2. Such causes include, but are not limited to, genetic defects, diseases affecting the exocrine pancreas, endocrinopathies, and medication effects. Gestational diabetes reflects insulin resistance exacerbated by the effects of pregnancy. It signals patients who are at increased risk of developing DM2.

Cowie CC, Rust KF, Byrd-Holt DD, et al. Prevalence of diabetes and impaired fasting glucose in adults in the U.S. population: national health and nutrition examination survey 1999-2002. *Diabetes Care*. 2006;29:1263-1268.

McDonald M, Hertz RP, Unger AN, et al. Prevalence, awareness, and management of hypertension, dyslipidemia, and diabetes among United States adults aged 65 and older. *J Gerontol Biol Sci Med Sci*. 2009;64:256-263.

A.3. How is DM classified?

Table 24.1 lists the criteria for the diagnosis of DM1, DM2, and gestational diabetes. Elevated (≥6.5%) hemoglobin A_{1c} (Hgb A_{1c}) or fasting hyperglycemia (≥126 mg/dL) are useful means to confirm metabolic derangement, but random hyperglycemia accompanied by classic symptoms (such as polyuria and polydipsia) or the inability to manage a glucose load is sufficient to make the diagnosis. Ketoacidosis and the need for insulin reflect DM1, whereas obesity, gradual symptom onset (usually at an older age),

TABLE 24.1 American Diabetes Association (ADA) Diagnostic Criteria for Diabetes Mellitus

1. Symptoms of diabetes mellitus plus random plasma glucose level greater than 200 mg/dL (11.1 mM)
2. Hemoglobin A_{1c} ≥6.5%
3. Fasting plasma glucose level ≥126 mg/dL (7.0 mM)
4. Two-hour plasma glucose level ≥200 mg/dL (11.1 mM) during oral glucose tolerance test

From American Diabetes Association. Classification and diagnosis of diabetes: standards of medical care in diabetes-2018. *Diabetes Care.* 2018;41:S13-S27.

and hyperosmolality without ketosis suggest DM2. Gestational diabetes resembles DM2 only in the setting of pregnancy.

Therapy for DM varies by type. Insulin is essential in DM1. In DM2 and gestational diabetes, diet, exercise, and drugs that modify insulin secretion or sensitivity can help correct hyperglycemia, although exogenous insulin may be necessary.

American Diabetes Association. 2. Classification and diagnosis of diabetes: standards of medical care in diabetes-2021. *Diabetes Care.* 2021;44:S15-S33.

A.4. What are the complications of DM?

Acute complications of DM include DKA and a hyperglycemic hyperosmolar state. Both are associated with severe systemic illness and a high mortality and will be discussed separately. Hypoglycemia is a serious risk of several therapies for DM.

Chronically, DM impacts virtually every organ system. Of most concern to the anesthetist are macrovascular disease, including accelerated atherosclerosis, and microvascular nephropathy, neuropathy, and cardiomyopathy. Tissues fail from a combination of advanced glycation end products, inflammation, connective tissue proliferation, and impaired perfusion. Renal failure, neuropathy, and accelerated coronary, cerebral, and peripheral vascular disease are common. Autonomic neuropathy and the stiff joint syndrome are both factors for preoperative evaluation (see Section B. 2. and B. 3.). Hypertension frequently accompanies DM, exacerbating organ failure. Impaired immune function predisposes to infection. Hypercoagulability exacerbates macrovascular disease. Dyslipidemias accelerate atherosclerotic lesions and may directly contribute to metabolic toxicities.

Cumulatively, the systemic lesions caused or exacerbated by DM reduce life expectancy. When diagnosed before the age of 35 years, DM causes an estimated mean of 25.9 years of lost life. Because complications worsen with time, this effect decreases as patients get older. About 50% of mortality in patients with DM comes from cardiovascular disease.

Although it would be helpful to stratify patients according to their risk of complications, the complexity of DM and its management makes risk stratification difficult. The safest assumption is that patients with DM are at high risk for coronary and other macrovascular disease, congestive heart failure, and renal insufficiency.

Ford ES, Zhao G, Li C. Pre-diabetes and the risk for cardiovascular disease: a systematic review of evidence. *J Am Coll Cardiol.* 2010;55:1310-1317.

Stolar M. Glycemic control and complications in type 2 diabetes mellitus. *Am J Med.* 2010;123:S3-S11.

A.5. How are the different forms of DM treated?

Diabetes care differs in chronic and acute settings. It is essential to differentiate between the agents used chronically and those used during acute perioperative stress.

Care of DM1 requires exogenous insulin therapy. Figure 24.1 illustrates the pharmacodynamics of several insulin preparations. A combination of a short- and a long-acting insulin preparation can help achieve the goals of resting and postprandial glycemic control. On an outpatient basis, these preparations are delivered either through multiple daily injections or continuous subcutaneous infusions (commonly referred to as insulin pump therapy).

In contrast to DM1, DM2 responds to insulin, oral insulin secretagogues, insulin sensitizers, glucose uptake inhibitors, gastrointestinal hormones, weight loss, dietary management, and exercise. Table 24.2 lists the major classes of drugs for the treatment of DM2, their mechanisms of action, pharmacokinetics, and particular concerns for the anesthetist.

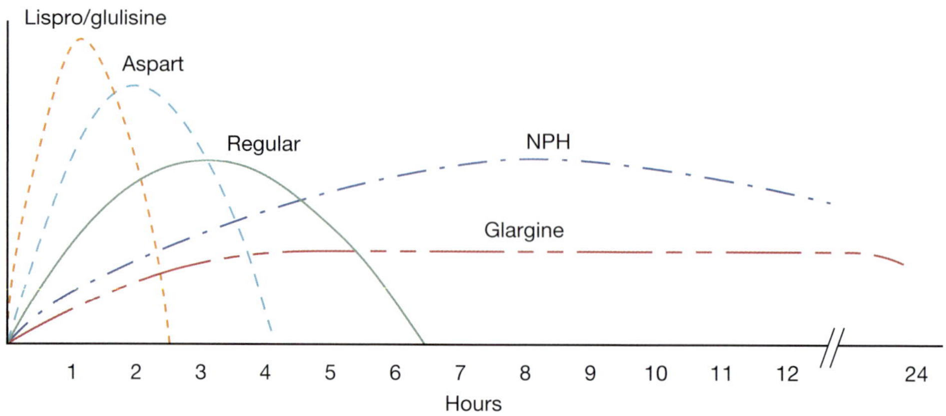

FIGURE 24.1. Onset and duration of action for common subcutaneous insulin preparations. Regular insulin given intravenously fits the best profile for a titratable drug in the operating room, as onset peak and offset all occur within 1 hour. NPH, neutral protamine Hagedorn.

Certain medications have adverse effects that deserve consideration. Metformin, the only available biguanide, increases peripheral glucose uptake but also predisposes patients to greater production of lactic acid and acidosis. Because of its long half-life, metformin can take up to 72 hours to clear, so discontinuation on the day of surgery does not minimize the risk of acidosis. Published guidelines vary with regard to the continuation of metformin during the perioperative period: it is reasonable to continue metformin in patients undergoing relatively minor procedures with short periods of starvation. On the other hand, metformin should be discontinued on the day of surgery for more major procedures, particularly those with the potential for major fluid losses as well as those that predispose to an increased risk of renal dysfunction such as the use of intravenous contrast. Thiazolidinediones have been associated with hepatic injury and congestive heart failure. Sulfonylureas can be associated with hypoglycemia, and this risk is increased when they are combined with other DM medications. Sodium-glucose transporter type 2 inhibitors, such as dapagliflozin, can be associated with urogenital infections and, especially during acute illness, euglycemic DKA. Glucagon-like peptide (GLP) agonists can be associated with delayed gastric emptying, particularly in the first several weeks after initiation of treatment, which could increase the risk of aspiration in the perioperative period. Exenatide is also associated with kidney dysfunction, which might be attributable to hypovolemia due to nausea and vomiting.

For these reasons, as well as unreliable pharmacokinetics, the best option for acute treatment of all types of diabetic hyperglycemia is insulin. Although subcutaneous dosing is often used in the hospital setting, intravenous insulin best meets the profile of an ideal titratable agent. It has a short time to onset (10-15 minutes), peak effect (<30 minutes), and duration of action (45 minutes). Frequent glucose monitoring is essential to titrate therapy.

Although serum glucose or other markers of chronic hyperglycemia, such as Hgb A_{1c}, are currently standard end points for chronic therapy, aggressive management of comorbid disease including coronary artery disease, obesity, hyperlipidemia, and hypertension can be just as important with regard to influencing many long-term DM-related complications. In addition to the reciprocal relationship of these disease processes, management decisions are often interconnected: for example, sodium-glucose cotransporter 2 inhibitors and GLP agonists are preferred medications for glycemic control in patients with coronary artery disease. Anesthesiologists should inquire about agents treating frequently coexisting conditions during preoperative evaluation.

Bagry HS, Raghavendran S, Carli F. Metabolic syndrome and insulin resistance: perioperative considerations. *Anesthesiology*. 2008;108:506-523.

Duggan EW, Carlson K, Umpierrez GE. Perioperative hyperglycemia management: an update. *Anesthesiology*. 2017;126:547-560.

Gourgari E, Wilhelm EE, Hassanzadeh H, et al. A comprehensive review of the FDA-approved labels of diabetes drugs: indications, safety, and emerging cardiovascular safety data. *J Diabetes Complications*. 2017;31:1719-1727.

Rottura M, Molonia A, Giorgi DA, et al. Pharmacological treatment of diabetic and non-diabetic patients with coronary artery disease in the real world of general practice. *Front Pharmacol*. 2022;13:858385.

Teck J. Diabetes-associated comorbidities. *Prim Care*. 2022;49:275-286.

TABLE 24.2 Therapies for Glycemic Control in Type 2 Diabetes Mellitus[a]

Drug Name/Class	Mechanism	Route	Onset	Duration	Important Considerations
Biguanide	↑ Peripheral glucose uptake in response to insulin	PO			Lactic acidosis risk may extend up to 72 h after administration.
Metformin (Glucophage)			1-3 h	17 h	
DPP-4 inhibitors (gliptins)	Inhibits incretin breakdown	PO			May be associated with increased risk of decompensated heart failure
Alogliptin (Nesina, Vipidia)			1-2 h	$T_{1/2}$ 21 h	
Linagliptin (Tradjenta)			1.5 h	$T_{1/2}$ 12 h	
Saxagliptin (Onglyza)			Hours	24 h	
Sitagliptin (Januvia)			Hours	Days	
GLP-1 agonists (Incretin-mimetics)	↑ Insulin, ↓ glucagon, hepatic glucose production, gastric emptying, and appetite	SC			Associated with delayed gastric emptying, weight loss, and gastrointestinal distress. Reports of gallbladder, biliary diseases, and pancreatitis
Dulaglutide (Trulicity)			Hours (48 h median)	$T_{1/2}$ 5 d	
Exenatide (Byetta, Bydureon)			10 min	6-8 h	
Liraglutide (Saxenda, Victoza)			Minutes	$T_{1/2}$ 13 h	
Lixisenatide (Adlyxin)			Hours	$T_{1/2}$ 3 h	
Semaglutide (Ozempic, Wegovy, Rybelsus)		SC or PO	Days or 1 h if PO	$T_{1/2}$ 1 wk	Semaglutide is currently the only available orally administered medication of this class.
GLP-1/GIP dual agonist	↑ Insulin, ↓ glucagon, hepatic glucose production, gastric emptying, and appetite	SC			Similar to GLP-1 agonists
Tirzepatide (Mounjaro)			Hours	$T_{1/2}$ 5 d	
SGLT-2 inhibitors (gliflozins)	Inhibit renal reabsorption of glucose	PO			High risk of diabetic ketoacidosis in the perioperative period; urinary tract infections; osmotic diuresis
Bexagliflozin (Brenzavvy)			Hours	$T_{1/2}$ 12 h	
Canagliflozin (Invokana)			Hours	$T_{1/2}$ 13 h	
Dapagliflozin (Farxiga)			Hours	$T_{1/2}$ 13 h	

(continued)

TABLE 24.2 Therapies for Glycemic Control in Type 2 Diabetes Mellitus[a] (*continued*)

Drug Name/Class	Mechanism	Route	Onset	Duration	Important Considerations
Empagliflozin (Jardiance)			Hours	$T_{1/2}$ 12 h	
Ertugliflozin (Steglatro)			1 h	$T_{1/2}$ 17 h	
Sulfonylureas	↑ β cell insulin secretion	PO			Hypoglycemia
Glimepiride (Amaryl)			2-3 h	24 h	
Glipizide ER (Glucotrol XL)			2-4 h	24 h	
Glipizide IR (Glucotrol)			30 min	24 h	
Glyburide (Micronase)			30 min	24 h	
Thiazolidinediones (glitazones)	↑ Peripheral glucose uptake	PO			Heart failure
Pioglitazone (Actos)			Hours	$T_{1/2}$ 3-7 h	Improves fibrosis and inflammation in non-alcoholic steatohepatitis
Rosiglitazone (Avandia)			Hours	$T_{1/2}$ 3-4 h	Rarely used because of increased risk of cardiovascular events
α-Glucosidase inhibitors	↓ Digestive carbohydrate breakdown	PO			Rarely used. Relatively poor efficacy and tolerability due to GI side effects
Acarbose (Precose)			2 h	NA	
Miglitol (Glyset)			2-3 h	NA	
Bile acid sequestrant	Binds bile acids in GI tract, preventing reabsorption. Mechanism for controlling blood sugar unknown	PO			Rarely used; may increase serum triglycerides and transaminases; GI side effects
Colesevelam (Welchol)			Minutes	Works concurrently with meals	
Dopamine-2 agonist	↓ Sympathetic tone, ↓ hepatic glucose production, ↓ postmeal free fatty acid levels	PO			Rarely used; poor efficacy and tolerability; hypotension
Bromocriptine (Cycloset)			Minutes	$T_{1/2}$ 6 h	
Meglitinides (glinides)	↑ β cell insulin secretion	PO			Hypoglycemia
Nateglinide (Starlix)			20 min	$T_{1/2}$ 1.5 h	
Repaglinide (Prandin)			15-60 min	4-6 h	
Amylin analogues	↑ Satiety, ↓ glucagon, and appetite, indication for DM1	SC			Rarely used; only approved in patients taking prandial insulin; hypoglycemia
Pramlintide (Symlin)			Minutes	Hours	

DM1, type 1 diabetes mellitus; DPP-4, dipeptidyl peptidase IV; ER, extended release; GI, gastrointestinal; GIP, glucose-dependent insulinotropic polypeptide; GLP-1, glucagon-like peptide-1; IR, immediate release; NA, not applicable; PO, per os (by mouth); SC, subcutaneous; SGLT-2, sodium-glucose transport protein 2; $T_{1/2}$, half-life.

[a]Onset and duration data are approximate only and subject to variability.

A.6. How is control of DM adequately monitored?

Self-monitoring of blood glucose is possible in all forms of DM, usually by using finger-stick blood samples and portable monitors. This method is the established standard of care in DM1 for carefully titrated control to prevent hypoglycemia and ketoacidosis. More recently, continuous glucose monitors have become common, providing improved accuracy and greater convenience compared to more traditional finger-stick sampling, which instead needs to be done only for calibration of the device. This method also allows for an integrated monitoring and treatment feedback loop within a single system. Many advocate self-monitoring for patients with DM2, especially if they take insulin, but compliance varies, and self-monitoring might not be beneficial in all patients. Hgb A_{1c}, the glycation product of Hgb exposure to hyperglycemic conditions, is a marker of long-term glycemic control. It can help identify subgroups of patients for whom the risk for complications is higher and can be a marker of disease control. The relationship between levels of glycemic control and Hgb A_{1c} is not linear, so a single laboratory value does not completely reveal the glycemic profile over time. Patients with DM have blood pressure and serum lipid profiles monitored as part of their long-term care because these factors increase the risk of lifetime complications.

In the operating room, serum glucose can be measured by pinprick or vascular blood sample. Use of continuous glucose monitoring devices in the acute setting represents an evolving area of interest that is not yet standard of care but will eventually allow for improved perioperative management of hypo- and hyperglycemic events through more frequent and less onerous assessment of blood glucose levels. Samples from a venous or arterial catheter offer greater reliability compared to pinprick samples during states of altered peripheral tissue perfusion. If insulin infusion is being used, monitoring is recommended hourly, and if subcutaneous insulin is used, monitoring is recommended at least every 2 hours.

SECTION 5

Duggan EW, Carlson K, Umpierrez GE. Perioperative hyperglycemia management: an update. *Anesthesiology*. 2017;126:547-560.

Inoue S, Egi M, Kotani J, et al. Accuracy of blood-glucose measurements using glucose meters and arterial blood gas analyzers in critically ill adult patients: systematic review. *Crit Care*. 2013;17:R48.

Kolb H, Kempf K, Martin S, et al. On what evidence-base do we recommend self-monitoring of blood glucose? *Diabetes Res Clin Pract*. 2010;87:150-156.

Price C, Ditton G, Russell GB, Aloi J. Reliability of inpatient CGM: comparison to standard of care. *J Diabetes Sci Technol*. 2023;17:329-335.

Vettoretti M, Facchinetti A. Combining continuous glucose monitoring and insulin pumps to automatically tune the basal insulin infusion in diabetes therapy: a review. *Biomed Eng Online*. 2019;18:37.

A.7. What are some of the factors that alter insulin requirements?

Insulin responsiveness is dynamic during stress or illness. Tissue injury from surgery, trauma, or inflammatory states, such as infection, decreases glycemic responsiveness to insulin as part of the stress response. These effects are maximal 2 to 3 days after injury and resolve over the course of a week, but there is substantial variability. Besides stress, other conditions that increase counter-regulatory hormones (glucagon, cortisol, and catecholamines) decrease insulin sensitivity and increase insulin requirements. Cushing disease and pheochromocytoma are examples of conditions that cause insulin resistance. Several medications administered in the perioperative period, including corticosteroids, β-adrenergic receptor agonists such as norepinephrine and epinephrine, and to a lesser extent inhaled volatile anesthetics, also increase insulin resistance. In solid organ transplant recipients, steroids and the calcineurin inhibitors tacrolimus and cyclosporine have been associated with insulin resistance or the onset of DM. Exercise and ethanol can decrease insulin requirements.

Shah T, Kasravi A, Huang E, et al. Risk factors for development of new-onset diabetes mellitus after kidney transplantation. *Transplantation*. 2006;82:1673-1676.

Tanaka T, Nabatame H, Tanifuji Y. Insulin secretion and glucose utilization are impaired under general anesthesia with sevoflurane as well as isoflurane in a concentration-independent manner. *J Anesth*. 2005;19:277-281.

Thorell A, Nygren J, Ljungqvist O. Insulin resistance: a marker of surgical stress. *Curr Opin Clin Nutr Metab Care*. 1999;2:69-78.

A.8. What are the principles of management of diabetic ketoacidosis (DKA)?

A hyperglycemic patient, especially those with DM1, should be assessed for DKA before surgery. Sodium-glucose cotransporter 2 inhibitors produce an elevated risk of euglycemic DKA (characterized by blood glucose <250 mg/dL) in patients with DM2. Because DKA is associated with higher perioperative mortality, patients should be monitored for intravascular volume and electrolyte abnormalities.

Withholding insulin contributes to DKA. Infection or tissue injury exacerbates DM and sets off a chain of events that can result in DKA. Because of increased risk to the patient, DKA should be corrected before surgery. When it is triggered by a surgical condition, time to correct it might be limited by the urgency of the surgery.

Patients with DKA have an anion gap metabolic acidosis in addition to hyperglycemia. Elevated serum ketone levels can help confirm the diagnosis, but urine ketones and serum anion gap are frequently easier to assay. Ketosis is corrected with insulin, which is best administered as an intravenous infusion. Because glucose levels frequently normalize before ketosis clears, insulin infusion is usually continued even after hyperglycemia corrects. Dextrose is administered simultaneously to avoid hypoglycemia.

Commonly, a patient will be hypovolemic from polyuria and incomplete hydration, and resuscitation with isotonic fluids is appropriate. Classically, normal saline has been used as the initial resuscitation fluid in DKA because of the in vivo conversion of lactate and acetate to glucose; however, more recent evidence indicates that the use of balanced crystalloids is likely associated with a shorter time to DKA resolution and less hyperchloremia.

During acidemia, hyperkalemia is common, resulting from shifts in body stores. However, patients frequently have a net potassium deficit. Hypokalemia during correction, which can reflect a deficit of up to 10 mEq potassium per kg body mass, should be treated aggressively. Likewise, hypocalcemia and hypomagnesemia should be anticipated and treated.

Alghamdi NA, Major P, Chaudhuri D, et al. Saline compared to balanced crystalloid in patients with diabetic ketoacidosis: a systematic review and meta-analysis of randomized controlled trials. *Crit Care Explor*. 2022;4:e0613.

Kitabchi AE, Murphy MB, Spencer J, et al. Is a priming dose of insulin necessary in a low-dose insulin protocol for the treatment of diabetic ketoacidosis? *Diabetes Care*. 2008;31:2081-2085.

Kitabchi AE, Nyenwe EA. Hyperglycemic crises in diabetes mellitus: diabetic ketoacidosis and hyperglycemic hyperosmolar state. *Endocrinol Metab Clin North Am*. 2006;35:725-751.

A.9. What is a hyperglycemic hyperosmolar state?

Any hyperglycemic patient should be evaluated for a hyperglycemic hyperosmolar state, another potentially fatal condition. The syndrome is more frequent in DM2. It includes hyperglycemia, hyperosmolarity, volume depletion, and changes in mental status. Adverse effects result from hyperosmolarity and hypovolemic shock. Glucose levels greater than 1,000 mg/dL have been described. Mortality can be high. Glycosuria and inadequate fluid intake contribute to the condition. Treatment consists of fluid resuscitation and intravenous insulin to correct the hyperglycemia. Sodium, potassium, calcium, and magnesium levels should be evaluated and normalized.

Kitabchi AE, Nyenwe EA. Hyperglycemic crises in diabetes mellitus: diabetic ketoacidosis and hyperglycemic hyperosmolar state. *Endocrinol Metab Clin North Am*. 2006;35:725-751.

B. Preoperative Evaluation and Preparation

B.1. How should this patient be evaluated?

The goals of preoperative evaluation are to stratify perioperative risk, ensure optimal management of concurrent illness, and screen for specific anesthetic-related problems. Patients are evaluated for cardiovascular disease, renal function, stiff joint syndrome, autonomic neuropathy, aspiration risk, and acute diabetic emergencies.

Both DM1 and DM2 increase the risk of coronary artery disease. The 2014 American College of Cardiology (ACC)/American Heart Association (AHA) Guideline on Perioperative Cardiovascular Evaluation and Care for Noncardiac Surgery recommends the use of the Revised Cardiac Risk Index (RCRI). This index uses a history of DM, ischemic heart disease, heart failure, cerebrovascular disease, and renal insufficiency to predict perioperative cardiovascular risk. According to the 2014 guidelines, patients are triaged based on risk for major adverse cardiac events (MACE). The RCRI, the American College of Surgeons National Surgical Quality Improvement Program (NSQIP) Surgical Risk Calculator, and the Myocardial Infarction and Cardiac Arrest (MICA) calculators are three tools to measure this risk. In the case of the RCRI, DM requiring insulin is one of six criteria used in the score. In the Surgical Risk Calculator, the risk is calculated from a larger group of factors, including surgery type and a diagnosis of DM. The MICA calculator risk is calculated based on surgery type, American Society of Anesthesiologists physical status classification, serum creatinine, and patient age. If MACE risk from these indices is greater than or equal to 1%, poor or unknown exercise tolerance and whether the results will change perioperative care determine the need for stress testing. A diagnosis of DM is thus a major factor for deciding whether to supplement a patient assessment preoperatively because of cardiovascular risk. According to the AHA, initiation of preoperative β-blocker therapy is reasonable (level of evidence: B) in patients with DM and three or more RCRI risk factors. The timing of initiation is likely to impact the potential for harm or benefit: β-blockers should not be initiated less than 1 day prior to surgery, and there is some evidence that starting therapy more than 30 days prior to surgery reduces the risk of morbidity and mortality.

Optimizing medical status is a consideration for all patients but particularly for patients with DM who have many comorbidities. Optimal management of coexisting hypertension and congestive heart failure can minimize perioperative risk. The decision to proceed with or delay a procedure for medical management depends on the urgency of the surgery and the potential for improving the patient's medical condition.

DM is a leading cause of renal insufficiency and failure. Because this patient already has an increased serum creatinine, she should be managed in the perioperative period with a presumptive diagnosis of renal insufficiency, and any fluid and metabolic derangements should be corrected. A metabolic panel, including serum creatinine, blood urea nitrogen, potassium, sodium, chloride, bicarbonate, and base deficit, can be useful, especially because angiotensin mediators, β-blockers, and insulin can affect serum potassium levels. Nephrotoxic medications should be administered cautiously or avoided entirely.

DM carries multiple considerations for decisions surrounding airway management. Joint stiffness is assessed with a comprehensive airway examination and the "prayer sign," in which a patient's hands are placed against each other at the palmar surface to see whether the fingers touch. Other considerations include the increased risk of aspiration due to gastroparesis in the setting of autonomic dysfunction as well as autonomic instability affecting hemodynamics. Although Hgb A_{1c} levels correlate with perioperative risk, the test does not add any information to the decision paradigm.

In addition to its chronic consequences, DM can produce a hyperglycemic hyperosmolar state and DKA. Both syndromes reflect severe metabolic abnormalities, most commonly resulting from infection. Because these syndromes can manifest as a result of a surgical emergency, patients with these conditions can present for perioperative management. Ideally, metabolic derangements should be corrected before anesthetic induction, but sometimes, patients must go to surgery urgently or emergently. Anesthesia providers should be prepared for hemodynamic instability, rapid fluid infusion, electrolyte repletion, and frequent monitoring of blood glucose and electrolytes. In both conditions, intravenous insulin infusion is indicated, titrated to normoglycemia in the hyperglycemic hyperosmolar state and to clearance of ketones in DKA. Supplemental dextrose is usually necessary to maintain insulin infusion in DKA.

Lee TH, Marcantonio ER, Mangione CM, et al. Derivation and prospective validation of a simple index for prediction of cardiac risk of major noncardiac surgery. *Circulation*. 1999;100:1043-1049.

Thompson A, Fleischmann KE, de las Fuentes L, et al. 2024 AHA/ACC/ACS/ASNC/HRS/SCA/SCCT/SCMR/SVM Guideline for Perioperative Cardiovascular Management for Noncardiac Surgery. *J Am Coll Cardiol*. 2024;84:1869-1969.

B.2. How would the stiff joint syndrome affect her airway management?

The stiff joint syndrome is thought to result from glycation of connective tissue with chronic exposure to hyperglycemia. This collagen glycation starts in the fourth and fifth interphalangeal joints, resulting in the patient not being able to completely appose the palms and fingers of the hands—the "prayer sign." The degree of interphalangeal involvement can also be assessed by scoring the ink impression made by the palm of the dominant hand "palm print (PP) sign." These are good screening tests for joint stiffness and indicate a reduced range of motion in the cervical spine, temporomandibular and arytenoid joints, and glottic structures, making endotracheal intubation more difficult. The PP and the prayer signs are sensitive and specific predictors of a difficult airway that might require a smaller endotracheal tube and difficult airway adjuncts.

Hashim KV, Thomas M. Sensitivity of palm print sign in prediction of difficult laryngoscopy in diabetes: a comparison with other airway indices. *Indian J Anaesth*. 2014;58:298-302.

Hogan K, Rusy D, Springman SR. Difficult laryngoscopy and diabetes mellitus. *Anesth Analg*. 1988;67:1162-1165.

Nadal JL, Fernandez BG, Escobar IC, et al. The palm print as a sensitive predictor of difficult laryngoscopy in diabetics. *Acta Anaesthesiol Scand*. 1998;42:199-203.

Salzarulo HH, Taylor LA. Diabetic "stiff joint syndrome" as a cause of difficult endotracheal intubation. *Anesthesiology*. 1986;64:366-368.

B.3. What are the signs and implications of autonomic neuropathy in a patient with DM?

Diabetic neuropathy involves both the peripheral and autonomic nervous systems. In the autonomic system, gastric motility, heart rate, and vasomotor tone can be impaired. Between 20% and 60% of asymptomatic patients with DM2 have coronary artery disease that does not present until overt myocardial infarction or sudden cardiac death because of the effects of diabetic neuropathy. This patient is at risk for pulmonary aspiration of gastric contents and hemodynamic instability. A history will elicit early satiety, prolonged postprandial fullness, and significant reflux symptoms. Potential difficulties with mask ventilation and intubation are assessed. Heart rate variability, best seen on an electrocardiogram (ECG) tracing in response to deep breathing, Valsalva maneuver, or position changes, identifies patients at risk for hemodynamic instability. Preparation is made to control hemodynamic instability, especially because this patient is taking an angiotensin converting enzyme inhibitor. Angiotensin receptor–blocking agents also increase the risk of postinduction hypotension. Because of a high likelihood of hemodynamic instability, the anesthesiologist should use slow titration of anesthetic agents, frequent blood pressure monitoring, and vasoactive agents, if necessary.

Baweja PS, Sandesara PB, Ashraf MJ. Asymptomatic coronary artery disease in type II diabetes. *Mo Med.* 2014;111:73-79.

Huang CJ, Kuok CH, Kuo TB, et al. Pre-operative measurement of heart rate variability predicts hypotension during general anesthesia. *Acta Anaesthesiol Scand.* 2006;50:542-548.

B.4. How should this patient be prepared for anesthesia and surgery?

This patient's cardiovascular risk is elevated. Her RCRI puts her risk for MACE at 10.1%, but the NSQIP Surgical Risk Calculator puts her cardiac complication risk at 0.2%. If her exercise tolerance is below 4 metabolic equivalents (METs), about the equivalent of climbing a flight of stairs with a bag of groceries or performing heavy work around the house, noninvasive stress testing can be considered if the results would change management. Insulin therapy is given for hyperglycemia. Because of her elevated serum glucose, she is asked about polyuria, a sign that she might be dehydrated from hyperglycemic diuresis. DKA is unlikely because she has DM2, but a metabolic panel is indicated to rule out electrolyte abnormalities. The presence of an elevated anion gap should provoke further investigation into the possibility of ketoacidosis. An ECG might be indicated based on her risk factors for cardiovascular disease.

Her symptoms, consistent with gastroparesis and gastroesophageal reflux, will influence premedication and airway management. Results from a comprehensive airway examination, including assessment of neck and jaw mobility and a check for the prayer sign, affect anesthetic management decisions. A rapid-sequence intubation could minimize aspiration risk but only if intubation is easy. If a difficult airway is suspected, awake intubation techniques should be considered.

Thompson A, Fleischmann KE, de las Fuentes L, et al. 2024 AHA/ACC/ACS/ASNC/HRS/SCA/SCCT/SCMR/SVM Guideline for Perioperative Cardiovascular Management for Noncardiac Surgery. *J Am Coll Cardiol.* 2024;84:1869-1969.

B.5. For elective surgery, how are DM medications and glucose requirements managed in advance of surgery?

The risk of hypoglycemia is balanced against the benefit of glycemic control. Anesthetized patients can have occult hypoglycemia, so blood glucose is checked frequently. During most procedures, intravenous insulin is titrated for glycemic control as needed. When administered intravenously, either as an infusion or as intermittent boluses, insulin has a fast onset and a short duration of action.

Subcutaneous insulin, with longer-lasting effects, is less predictable, especially during the hemodynamic changes of anesthesia and surgery. Those who are insulin dependent should remain on basal insulin (often at a dose reduced by 25%-50%) in order to mitigate the risk of DKA. Subcutaneous insulin pumps should be turned down or off for all but the most minor procedures.

Many noninsulin DM medications should be withheld at least on the day of surgery, except for minor procedures. Metformin should be withheld on the day of surgery to minimize the risk of lactic acidosis, although some advocate continued use through the perioperative period for minor procedures. Sodium-glucose cotransporter 2 inhibitors should be held 3 to 4 days prior to surgery to reduce the risk of likely underrecognized euglycemic DKA as well as preoperative hypovolemia. Injectable medications taken less often than daily, such as semaglutide, may be impractical to stop prior to surgery, and GLP agonists as well as dipeptidyl peptidase-4 inhibitors are less likely to result in hypoglycemia and can reasonably be continued on the day of surgery.

Initial enthusiasm for tight glycemic control in critically ill patients has given way to a much more cautious approach. Perioperatively, hyperglycemia is associated with worsened neurologic outcomes following craniotomy and subarachnoid hemorrhage, cardiac ischemia, and poor wound healing. The risk of surgical site infection is increased in the setting of perioperative hyperglycemia. Even though tight control of glucose has been associated with better outcomes in some settings, there is a risk associated with insulin therapy. Hypoglycemia is a serious risk, and insulin has multiple other effects that remain poorly described or difficult to appreciate in the context of perioperative care.

Evidence is limited to support glycemic control to a "normal" range of 80 to 110 mg/dL in the operating room. Higher targets minimize hypoglycemia. Levels higher than 180 mg/dL may cause protein glycation and osmotic diuresis. A range of 80 to 180 mg/dL is considered satisfactory in the perioperative period, and a more liberal range of 120 to 180 should typically be used as the target of insulin therapy if required.

Coursin DB, Connery LE, Ketzler JT. Perioperative diabetic and hyperglycemic management issues. *Crit Care Med.* 2004;32:S116-S125.

Duggan EW, Carlson K, Umpierrez GE. Perioperative hyperglycemia management: an update. *Anesthesiology.* 2017;126:547-560.

Lipshutz AK, Gropper MA. Perioperative glycemic control: an evidence-based review. *Anesthesiology.* 2009;110:408-421.

Martin ET, Kaye KS, Knott C, et al. Diabetes and risk of surgical site infection: a systematic review and meta-analysis. *Infect Control Hosp Epidemiol.* 2016;37:88-99.

Sharma D. Perioperative management of aneurysmal subarachnoid hemorrhage. *Anesthesiology.* 2020;133:1283-1305.

Zhang Y, Tan H, Jia L, et al. Association of preoperative glucose concentration with mortality in patients undergoing craniotomy for brain tumor. *J Neurosurg.* 2022;138:1254-1262.

B.6. How should this patient be premedicated?

Concerns with premedication include sensitivity to sedatives and aspiration risk. Preexisting cardiovascular, cerebrovascular, and renal diseases temper the administration of benzodiazepines and opioids. Because of the symptoms of gastroesophageal reflux and gastroparesis, histamine blockers, oral nonparticulate antacids, or prokinetic agents can be considered: metoclopramide, famotidine, and sodium citrate can reduce the risk of clinically significant pulmonary aspiration in this patient.

Additional concerns with regard to preoperative medications include the use of sodium-glucose transport protein 2 (SGLT2) inhibitors and GLP-1 agonists. SGLT2 inhibitors are US Food and Drug Administration (FDA) approved for use with diet and exercise to lower blood sugar in adults with MD2. SGLT2 inhibitors can lead to euglycemic ketoacidosis in fasted patients. In response to a published guideline, current recommendations at New York Presbyterian Weill Cornell Medical Center (NYP-WCMC) are to discontinue the following medications *3* days prior to the procedure: canagliflozin (Invokana), dapagliflozin (Farxiga), and empagliflozin (Jardiance), and to discontinue ertugliflozin (Steglatro) *4* days prior to the procedure.

GLP-1 agonists that are FDA approved for use in adults for the treatment of DM2 and obesity. These medications can delay gastric emptying and increase aspiration risk. In response to published guidelines, for patients taking a GLP-1 agonist, current recommendations at NYP-WCMC are to discontinue the following medications *1* day prior to the procedure: liraglutide (Victoza, Saxenda), exenatide (Byetta), and semaglutide oral tablet (Rybelsus), and to discontinue the following medications *1 week* prior to the procedure: dulaglutide (Trulicity), exenatide extended release (Bydureon BCise), semaglutide injection (Ozempic, Wegovy), and tirzepatide injection (Mounjaro).

FDA Drug Safety Communication. FDA revises labels of SGLT2 inhibitors for diabetes to include warnings about too much acid in the blood and serious urinary tract infections. Published March 2020. Accessed November 24, 2023. https://www.fda.gov/drugs/drug-safety-and-availability/fda-revises-labels-sglt2-inhibitors-diabetes-include-warnings-about-too-much-acid-blood-and-serious

Joshi GP, Abdelmalak BB, Weigel WA, et al; American Society of Anesthesiologist (ASA) Task Force on Perioperative Fasting. American Society of Anesthesiologists consensus-based guidance on preoperative management of patients (adults and children) on glucagon-like peptide-1 (GLP-1) receptor agonists. June 29, 2023. Accessed November 24, 2023. https://www.asahq.org/about-asa/newsroom/news-releases/2023/06/american-society-of-anesthesiologists-consensus-based-guidance-on-preoperative

C. Intraoperative Management

C.1. What are the effects of anesthesia and surgery on insulin and glucose metabolism?

As part of the stress response to surgery, metabolism increases and insulin resistance develops. This includes an increase in the mobilization of protein stores (mostly muscle), hepatic gluconeogenesis, and triglyceride metabolism. Hormones, including catecholamines, cortisol, glucagon, and even insulin, contribute to metabolic changes. Although glucose utilization increases, this effect is often outweighed by the increase in glucose production, adding to the risk of hyperglycemia. Administration of exogenous dextrose can exacerbate hyperglycemia in patients with DM.

Anesthetic techniques influence metabolism but generally to a lesser extent than the stress from surgical injury. Techniques that mitigate stress responses, such as neuraxial anesthesia, also can mitigate hyperglycemia. Some drugs affect regulatory hormones directly. Etomidate blocks cortisol synthesis due to inhibition of 11-β-hydroxylase. Benzodiazepines can decrease cortisol secretion. Halogenated anesthetic agents have effects on insulin secretion in vitro. However, these effects impact postoperative glycemic control less than the surgery itself.

American Diabetes Association Professional Practice Committee. 16. Diabetes care in the hospital: standards of medical care in diabetes-2022. *Diabetes Care.* 2022;45:S244-S253.

C.2. What anesthetic techniques should be considered?

Factors other than glycemic control influence the choice of anesthetic technique in patients with DM. Many patients with DM are at elevated risk for pulmonary aspiration. In general, the decision to deeply sedate a patient with DM without airway protection should take into account individual risk. If general anesthesia is indicated, rapid-sequence induction and tracheal intubation might be preferred. Assessment of gastric contents by ultrasound can aid in decision-making, although this is not currently considered standard practice.

Regional anesthesia techniques are chosen based on provider skill, patient and surgeon preferences, and postoperative pain control. Although still an unsettled question, the risk of significant neurologic dysfunction following peripheral nerve blocks might be elevated in patients with DM and underlying peripheral neuropathy. As such, peripheral neuropathy should be documented in a preoperative neurologic examination even though this is not a strict contraindication to regional techniques. Infection risk, particularly with the placement of a catheter, might be increased in patients with DM, and the duration of the effect of nerve blocks is prolonged.

Techniques that speed the time to oral intake by reducing nausea or minimizing ileus make glycemic management easier postoperatively. For this reason, antiemetics and the spare use of opioids can be beneficial.

Sedated or anesthetized patients cannot complain of hypoglycemic symptoms as unsedated patients can. Blood glucose is monitored regularly in all but the shortest cases.

In this patient, general endotracheal anesthesia with precautions to prevent aspiration, intravenous insulin titrated to blood glucose less than 180 mg/dL, and frequent blood glucose monitoring are reasonable.

Ljungqvist O, Nygren J, Soop M, et al. Metabolic perioperative management: novel concepts. *Curr Opin Crit Care.* 2005;11:295-299.

McAnulty GR, Robertshaw HJ, Hall GM. Anaesthetic management of patients with diabetes mellitus. *Br J Anaesth.* 2000;85:80-90.

Ten Hoope W, Looije M, Lirk P. Regional anesthesia in diabetic peripheral neuropathy. *Curr Opin Anaesthesiol.* 2017;30:627-631.

C.3. How should this patient be monitored?

If preoperative evaluation reveals a risk of hemodynamic instability, cardiac ischemia, or congestive heart failure, added cardiovascular monitoring should be considered, depending on the procedure. Peripheral vascular disease can complicate the placement of an arterial catheter but is not a contraindication because in patients who have cardiovascular comorbidities, the benefits of monitoring outweigh the risks.

Frequent glucose monitoring is recommended in cases lasting longer than an hour or when hypoglycemic agents are being used. Blood glucose by finger stick or, ideally, venous or arterial sample should be measured at least hourly when giving intravenous insulin.

In this patient, pulse oximetry, continuous ECG monitoring, end-tidal carbon dioxide and gas analysis, and noninvasive blood pressure monitoring are indicated if no further concerns arise from cardiovascular evaluation or surgical complexity.

Association of Anaesthetists of Great Britain and Ireland. Peri-operative management of the surgical patient with diabetes 2015: Association of Anaesthetists of Great Britain and Ireland. *Anaesthesia.* 2015;70:1427-1440.

McAnulty GR, Robertshaw HJ, Hall GM. Anaesthetic management of patients with diabetes mellitus. *Br J Anaesth.* 2000;85:80-90.

C.4. How is hyperglycemia treated intraoperatively?

The high end of a normal range for fasting serum glucose is 110 mg/dL; however, hyperglycemia in inpatients need not be treated until it reaches a higher level.

The best agent for treating intraoperative hyperglycemia is intravenous insulin. Onset takes minutes, peak effect is achieved in 15 to 30 minutes, and duration of effect is less than an hour, facilitating titration. Insulin can be administered by continuous infusion or as intermittent boluses; the bolus consumes less lead time and eliminates the risk of pump misprogramming or malfunction. Subcutaneous insulin can be used during short, outpatient procedures but is suboptimal for use during general anesthetics or complex procedures because variable peripheral blood flow can alter uptake and duration of action. Most other therapies for DM2 are not fit for intraoperative use. Oral agents cannot be easily administered, are not reliably absorbed, and have too long a duration of action to be practical perioperatively. They can be taken on the day of surgery before minor procedures.

In this case, sitagliptin can be continued because dipeptidyl peptidase-4 inhibitors do not carry a significantly increased risk of hypoglycemia in the perioperative period. Metformin increases the risk of lactic acidosis during periods of hypoperfusion and is discontinued for one or more days before extensive procedures when a large-volume blood loss is possible.

Duggan EW, Carlson K, Umpierrez GE. Perioperative hyperglycemia management: an update. *Anesthesiology.* 2017;126:547-560.

Smiley DD, Umpierrez GE. Perioperative glucose control in the diabetic or nondiabetic patient. *South Med J.* 2006;99:580-589.

C.5. How is hypoglycemic shock recognized and treated intraoperatively?

Hypoglycemia can lead to tissue energy failure and has been associated with hemodynamic collapse and brain injury. Any patient receiving insulin, pramlintide, sitagliptin (low risk), or sulfonylureas is at risk for hypoglycemia. Because risk is usually known beforehand, hourly or more frequent monitoring of glucose should detect hypoglycemia. If glucose levels are low or decrease rapidly, the fastest treatment is a bolus of intravenous dextrose 50%, administered slowly. In an emergency, one full ampoule is the starting dose. In less urgent settings when glucose is low but not critically so, smaller doses can be titrated to blood glucose values.

Dierdorf SF. Anesthesia for patients with diabetes mellitus. *Curr Opin Anaesthesiol.* 2002;15:351-357.

D. Postoperative Management

D.1. How is DM controlled in this patient postoperatively?

Unless there is a change in disease status as a consequence of surgery or preoperative care was inadequate, this patient should be transitioned back to her preoperative regimen. Before transitioning, she must recover from the stress response to the surgery. If this were a simple outpatient procedure, such as a cataract extraction, she could return home on her outpatient medication regimen. In this case, however, the effects of tissue injury might not peak for days; control of DM is thus a dynamic challenge. Regular monitoring of glucose is required (at a minimum, checks should be made every 2-4 hours).

She is monitored for hyperglycemia, and her nutrition regimen is adjusted to glucose measurements. Hourly glucose measurements and insulin infusion can control hyperglycemia. Most patients can be managed effectively with subcutaneous insulin and less frequent measurements. Insulin dose should take into account preoperative requirements, insulin resistance from the stress response, and caloric intake. Many patients receive intravenous dextrose postoperatively; if they are hyperglycemic on this regimen, dextrose is discontinued.

Oral medications can be reintroduced once the acute stress response begins to wane and the patient is cleared for a normal diet. Resumption of an oral diet can increase the risk of hyperglycemia, so ongoing monitoring is essential.

Smiley DD, Umpierrez GE. Perioperative glucose control in the diabetic or nondiabetic patient. *South Med J.* 2006;99:580-589.

D.2. Does DM increase perioperative risk?

Because patients with DM are at a greater risk of atherosclerosis, infection, autonomic and cardiovascular instability, and metabolic abnormalities than those without, perioperative risk is higher in this patient population. After surgery, the patient is monitored for hyperglycemia and hypoglycemia, ischemic complications, circulatory compromise, and wound and nosocomial infection. As a group, patients with DM have an increased risk for complications and poor outcomes from complications.

Lipshutz AK, Gropper MA. Perioperative glycemic control: an evidence-based review. *Anesthesiology.* 2009;110:408-421.

D.3. What are the common postoperative complications to be expected in a patient with DM?

Hyperglycemia and hypoglycemia, wound infections, and organ ischemia are the most common and worrisome postoperative complications in patients with DM. Following myocardial infarction or cerebrovascular accident, hyperglycemia is associated with a worse prognosis.

Smiley DD, Umpierrez GE. Perioperative glucose control in the diabetic or nondiabetic patient. *South Med J.* 2006;99:580-589.

D.4. Is it necessary to achieve tight perioperative control of glucose?

In the critical care setting, there is some evidence for improved outcomes with tight glycemic control, variably defined as glucose between 80 and 120 mg/dL or higher; other evidence has shown no benefit or even harm. Historic advocacy for tight glycemic control in cardiac and noncardiac surgery has tended to give way to more liberal targets as the risks of hypoglycemia appear to outweigh the benefits of tight control.

Potential benefits from tight glycemic control include improvement in metabolic, anti-inflammatory, organ, and circulatory function. Unfortunately, there is little evidence to suggest these benefits are substantial perioperatively, outside of the risk of surgical site infection. Unresolved details include the best timing for tight control, the goals of therapy, the effect of baseline glycemic control, the effect of nutrition, and the potential for significant hypoglycemia. The patient is transitioned to her preoperative level of control during recovery, and severe hyperglycemia is prevented by monitoring glucose closely. Glucose levels above 180 mg/dL increase the risk of protein glycation and osmotic diuresis; targeting serum glucose below this value makes physiologic sense.

Gandhi GY, Nuttall GA, Abel MD, et al. Intensive intraoperative insulin therapy versus conventional glucose management during cardiac surgery: a randomized trial. *Ann Intern Med.* 2007;146:233-243.

NICE-SUGAR Study Investigators. Intensive versus conventional glucose control in critically ill patients. *N Engl J Med.* 2009;360:1283-1297.

van den Berghe G, Wouters P, Weekers F, et al. Intensive insulin therapy in critically ill patients. *N Engl J Med.* 2001;345:1359-1367.

SECTION 6 The Genitourinary System

Transurethral Resection of the Prostate and Geriatric Anesthesia

25

Shelby Badani, Anuj Malhotra, Vinod Malhotra, and Fun-Sun F. Yao

A 79-year-old male with benign prostatic hypertrophy is scheduled for transurethral resection of the prostate (TURP). His past medical history includes myocardial infarction (MI) 7 months ago requiring drug-eluting stent (DES) placement and an implantable cardioverter-defibrillator (ICD) inserted for episodes of ventricular tachycardia. His current left ventricular ejection fraction is 45%. The patient has been taking diuretics, a β-blocker, clopidogrel, aspirin, and an angiotensin converting enzyme (ACE) inhibitor. However, clopidogrel was stopped 5 days before surgery.

A. Medical Disease and Differential Diagnosis

1. What comorbidities are common in patients undergoing TURP?
2. What are the normal physiologic consequences of aging for the various organ systems?
3. How should drug dosages be adjusted for older patients? Should any particular medications be avoided?
4. Does a history of prior MI increase the patient's risk of perioperative reinfarction or stent thrombosis?
5. In patients with a history of recent MI, would you recommend that the surgery be postponed for a certain period?

B. Preoperative Evaluation and Preparation

1. How would you evaluate the patient's cardiac condition? Is additional testing warranted?
2. Would you discontinue any antihypertensive drugs or any medications for angina?
3. For a patient with a cardiac implantable electronic device (CIED), what information should you know? What precautions should be taken?
4. What types of coronary stents are available? What is their perioperative relevance?
5. What is the conventional recommendation for dual antiplatelet therapy (DAPT) in a patient with previous percutaneous coronary intervention (PCI) undergoing elective noncardiac surgery?
6. What risk is associated with continuing perioperative antiplatelet therapy? What risk is there with stopping it?
7. How should patients with coronary stents undergoing noncardiac surgery be managed?
8. You are visiting the patient in the preoperative area before coming to the operating room. How would you discuss treatment options and obtain informed consent from this patient?
9. The patient and his family are worrying about memory loss from anesthesia. Would you discuss the periprocedural complications with the patient, and how would you do it?

C. Intraoperative Management

1. What monitors would you use for this patient?
2. Is there a preferred anesthetic technique for patients undergoing TURP, and why?
3. Does neuraxial anesthesia result in a lower incidence of perioperative mortality than general anesthesia?
4. What intravenous fluid would you use during TURP?
5. Forty minutes after a sensory level of T10 was established with spinal anesthesia, and monopolar TURP (M-TURP) resection was initiated with the use of glycine as the bladder-irrigating solution,

the patient becomes agitated and complains of nausea. Further sedation along with an antiemetic is administered. However, shortly thereafter, the patient becomes very restless, blood pressure rises, and heart rate decreases. The patient becomes cyanotic and obtunded, blood pressure precipitously falls, and pupils are dilated and unresponsive to light. What is the most likely cause of these signs and symptoms, and would these occur during bipolar TURP (B-TURP) or laser TURP (L-TURP) resection?

6. What are the important characteristics of irrigation solutions used during TURP?
7. What is the effect on body temperature of continuous bladder irrigation during TURP?
8. What is the definition of TURP syndrome? What are the signs and symptoms of the syndrome?
9. How does the patient absorb irrigation solution during TURP?
10. What factors increase the incidence of TURP syndrome?
11. What is the effect on cardiopulmonary, renal, and central nervous system (CNS) functions of excessive absorption of irrigation solution during TURP?
12. What causes CNS dysfunction in patients who have undergone M-TURP?
13. How does acute hyponatremia affect the cardiovascular system?
14. What prophylactic measures can reduce the incidence of TURP syndrome?
15. What therapeutic measures are recommended for patients with TURP syndrome?
16. Is hypertonic saline administration necessary to correct hyponatremia? Explain. What are the risks of rapidly correcting hyponatremia?
17. What are the toxic effects of glycine? Is there an antidote to glycine toxicity? What are the metabolic by-products of glycine?
18. What are the symptoms and clinical course of TURP-induced hyperammonemia?
19. What are the clinical characteristics, causes, and prognosis of TURP-related blindness?
20. What are the causes of excessive bleeding during TURP?
21. What are the causes, signs, symptoms, and treatment of bladder perforation during TURP?
22. What are the likely causes of hypotension during TURP?

D. Postoperative Management

1. What is the source of postoperative bacteremia in patients who have undergone TURP? What factors increase the incidence of bacteremia?
2. What are the signs of post-TURP septicemia? What preventive measures are generally recommended?
3. Is postoperative hypothermia a risk factor for myocardial ischemia?
4. What is postoperative cognitive dysfunction (POCD)? How does this differ from delirium, and what is the time course to resolution?
5. What are the mechanisms and risk factors for POCD? How would you mitigate the risk of POCD? Does the anesthetic technique influence the development of POCD?

E. Comparing M-TURP, B-TURP, and L-TURP

1. What differentiates M-TURP from B-TURP?
2. What differentiates the technologies for L-TURP?
3. Are there any alternatives to TURP for benign prostate hypertrophy (BPH)?

A. Medical Disease and Differential Diagnosis

A.1. What comorbidities are common in patients undergoing TURP?

Patients undergoing TURP are often advanced in age and have multiple comorbidities including cardiac, pulmonary, vascular, and endocrine disorders. The incidence of cardiac disease is 67%; vascular disease, 50%; chronic obstructive pulmonary disease, 29%; and diabetes, 8%.

Malhotra V. Transurethral resection of prostate. *Anesthesiol Clin North Am.* 2000;18:883-897.

Malhotra V, Malhotra A, Pamnani A. Anesthesia and the renal and genitourinary systems. In: Gropper MA, Cohen NH, Eriksson LI, et al, eds. *Miller's Anesthesia.* 9th ed. Elsevier; 2020:1929-1959.

A.2. What are the normal physiologic consequences of aging for the various organ systems?

- CNS changes include loss of brain volume through decreases in neuronal density, regional neurotransmitters, and neuroreceptors. Pharmacodynamic sensitivity increases with age for all intravenous agents (eg, propofol, fentanyl, and midazolam). The minimal alveolar concentration (MAC) of inhalational anesthetics decreases by approximately 6% per decade after age 40 years. Also, a decrease in cholinergic receptor activity may explain the aging patient's vulnerability to the anticholinergic side effects of medications such as diphenhydramine, meperidine, and scopolamine.

- In the cardiovascular system, loss of arterial compliance leads to an increase in afterload. The systolic function remains relatively preserved, but diastolic dysfunction is common, making patients dependent on adequate ventricular filling and atrial augmentation. Valvular dysfunction is common and aortic stenosis is particularly prevalent, occurring in more than 10% of patients older than 75 years.
- Total lung capacity remains unchanged, but residual volume increases, leading to an overall decrease in vital capacity. Closing capacity also increases with age and can exceed functional residual capacity, resulting in atelectasis. Decreased gas exchange and $\dot{V}/\dot{Q}$ mismatch also occur.
- The glomerular filtration rate (GFR) decreases by 1 mL/min/1.73 m^2/y starting at 40 years of age, which can slow clearance of renally excreted medications. Creatinine clearance is a reasonable estimate of GFR, whereas urine output is not.
- Hepatic blood flow also decreases, particularly affecting the metabolism of drugs, specifically phase I but not phase II metabolism.
- Lean muscle mass decreases, as does subcutaneous (but not total body) fat, predisposing to temperature dysregulation and hypothermia.

Cleeland C, Pipingas A, Scholey A, et al. Neurochemical changes in the aging brain: a systematic review. *Neurosci Biobehav Rev*. 2019;98:306-319.

Gabrielli EM, Schenning KJ, Deiner S. Geriatric Anesthesia. In: Gropper MA, Cohen NH, Eriksson LI, Fleisher LA, Johnson-Akeju S, Leslie K, eds. *Miller's Anesthesia*. 10th ed. Elsevier; 2025:1984-1999.

Nickalls RW, Mapleson WW. Age-related iso-MAC charts for isoflurane, sevoflurane and desflurane in man. *Br J Anaesth*. 2003;91:170-174.

Peters R. Ageing and the brain. *Postgrad Med J*. 2006;82:84-88.

A.3. How should drug dosages be adjusted for older patients? Should any particular medications be avoided?

Decreased GFR and decreased hepatic blood flow result in the prolonged effect of drugs metabolized and excreted through these pathways. It is important to note that normal creatinine or liver synthetic function alone is not indicative of GFR or hepatic blood flow because the former can reflect decreased muscle mass rather than preserved renal function and the latter is often preserved despite the significant decrease in liver mass with aging.

In general, older patients are more sensitive to the effects of all intravenous and inhalational anesthetics due to age-related physiologic changes in organ systems. Initial doses of intravenous anesthetic agents should be reduced, with a longer interval between repeat doses. It is safer to start with 50% of the regular doses and then titrate to the desired effect. The dose of all inhalational agents should also be reduced by approximately 6% per decade after age 40 years.

In addition, the American Geriatrics Society Beers Criteria for Potentially Inappropriate Medication Use in Older Adults identifies medications that are likely to cause cognitive issues for older patients, many of which are commonly used as part of an anesthetic (**Table 25.1**).

TABLE 25.1 Common Perioperative Medications With Potential Neurologic Effects

Drug	Rationale
Diphenhydramine	Highly anticholinergic; can increase confusion
Hydroxyzine	Highly anticholinergic; can increase confusion
Scopolamine	Highly anticholinergic
Amitriptyline	Highly anticholinergic; sedating
Antipsychotics	Increased risk of stroke and mortality in persons with dementia
Benzodiazepines	Older adults have increased sensitivity and decreased metabolism. Risk of cognitive impairment, delirium, and falls
Metoclopramide	Extrapyramidal side effects; risk increased in older adults
Pethidine	Not an effective analgesic; can cause neurotoxicity
Pentazocine	Can cause central nervous system adverse events, including confusion and hallucinations
Neuromuscular blocking drugs	Poorly tolerated by older adults, some with anticholinergic adverse effects

From American Geriatrics Society Expert Panel on Postoperative Delirium in Older Adults. American Geriatrics Society abstracted clinical practice guideline for postoperative delirium in older adults. *J Am Geriatr Soc.* 2015;63:142-150.

SECTION 6

Berger M, Schenning KJ, Brown CH IV, et al. Best practices for postoperative brain health: recommendations from the Fifth International Perioperative Neurotoxicity Working Group. *Anesth Analg*. 2018;127:1406-1413.

Nickalls RW, Mapleson WW. Age-related iso-MAC charts for isoflurane, sevoflurane and desflurane in man. *Br J Anaesth*. 2003;91:170-174.

Peters R. Ageing and the brain. *Postgrad Med J*. 2006;82:84-88.

A.4. Does a history of prior MI increase the patient's risk of perioperative reinfarction or stent thrombosis?

History of a prior MI or ischemic heart disease is considered an intermediate predictor of perioperative cardiac morbidity and is part of the revised cardiac risk index (RCRI). MI as the indication for initial stent placement also yields a higher risk for subsequent stent thrombosis.

Fleisher LA. The value of preoperative assessment before noncardiac surgery in the era of value-based care. *Circulation*. 2017;136:1769-1771.

Holcomb CN, Hollis RH, Graham LA, et al. Association of coronary stent indication with postoperative outcomes following noncardiac surgery. *JAMA Surg*. 2016;151:462-469.

Lee TH, Marcantonio ER, Mangione CM, et al. Derivation and prospective validation of a simple index for prediction of cardiac risk of major noncardiac surgery. *Circulation*. 1999;100:1043-1049.

Thompson A, Fleischmann KE, Smilowitz NR, et al. 2024 AHA/ACC/ACS/ASNC/HRS/SCA/SCCT/SCMR/SVM Guideline for Perioperative Cardiovascular Management of Noncardiac Surgery: A Report of the American College of Cardiology/American Heart Association Joint Committee on Clinical Practice Guidelines. *Circulation*. 2024;150:e351-e442.

A.5. In patients with a history of recent MI, would you recommend that the surgery be postponed for a certain period?

An acute MI (<7 days) or a recent MI (>7 days but <30 days) is considered an unstable coronary syndrome requiring additional evaluation and delay of elective noncardiac surgery. It is advised to wait for more than 60 days after an MI without revascularization before elective surgery is performed. Also see Chapter 14: Ischemic Heart Disease and Noncardiac Surgery.

Thompson A, Fleischmann KE, Smilowitz NR, et al. 2024 AHA/ACC/ACS/ASNC/HRS/SCA/SCCT/SCMR/SVM Guideline for Perioperative cardiovascular Management of Noncardiac Surgery: A Report of the American College of Cardiology/American Heart Association Joint Committee on Clinical Practice Guidelines. *Circulation*. 2024;150:e351-e442.

B. Preoperative Evaluation and Preparation

B.1. How would you evaluate the patient's cardiac condition? Is additional testing warranted?

The American College of Cardiology/American Heart Association guidelines suggest a stepwise approach that takes into account the clinical markers of cardiac risk, surgery risk, and functional capacity. The patient's medical history should focus on information about previous cardiac evaluations and interventions (coronary stent and automatic ICD [AICD] placement). Active cardiac conditions such as unstable coronary syndromes (recent MI or unstable angina), decompensated congestive heart failure (CHF), significant arrhythmias, or severe valvular disease warrant additional workup prior to surgery. If the patient has stable coronary artery disease (CAD), then the risk for the major adverse cardiac event (MACE) can be determined using a combined clinical/surgical risk score. If the risk for MACE is low (<1%), no additional information is required. If MACE risk is increased, the functional capacity of the patient is best evaluated by the activity history and assessment of metabolic equivalents (METs), with more than 4 METs being suggestive of sufficient cardiac reserve. Stress testing can be indicated for patients with poor exercise tolerance or unable to assess METs, if this would affect the decision to proceed with surgery. An electrocardiogram (ECG) is reasonable in a patient with a cardiac history undergoing greater than low-risk surgery but is not required. Assessment of left ventricular function is reserved for cases of active CHF or known history without reassessment within 1 year. Also see Chapter 14: Ischemic Heart Disease and Noncardiac Surgery.

Thompson A, Fleischmann KE, Smilowitz NR, et al. 2024 AHA/ACC/ACS/ASNC/HRS/SCA/SCCT/SCMR/SVM Guideline for Perioperative Cardiovascular Management of Noncardiac Surgery: A Report of the American College of Cardiology/American Heart Association Joint Committee on Clinical Practice Guidelines. *Circulation*. 2024;150:e351-e442.

B.2. Would you discontinue any antihypertensive drugs or any medications for angina?

Antianginal agents and β-blockers should be continued perioperatively, including the day of surgery, to prevent rebound hypertension and tachycardia that can result from sudden withdrawal of these drugs. Patients taking ACE inhibitors or angiotensin II receptor blockers (ARBs) can be predisposed to refractory intraoperative hypotension due to blunting of the sympathetic effect on vascular tone by anesthesia, increasing reliance on the renin-angiotensin-vasopressin system to maintain blood pressure and renal perfusion. It is recommended that these medications be held 24 hours before surgery.

Roshanov PS, Rochwerg B, Patel A, et al. Withholding versus continuing angiotensin-converting enzyme inhibitors or angiotensin II receptor blockers before noncardiac surgery: an analysis of the vascular events in noncardiac surgery patients cohort evaluation prospective cohort. *Anesthesiology*. 2017;126:16-27.

Thompson A, Fleischmann KE, Smilowitz NR, et al. 2024 AHA/ACC/ACS/ASNC/HRS/SCA/SCCT/SCMR/SVM Guideline for Perioperative cardiovascular Management of Noncardiac Surgery: A Report of the American College of Cardiology/American Heart Association Joint Committee on Clinical Practice Guidelines. *Circulation*. 2024;150:e351-e442.

B.3. For a patient with a cardiac implantable electronic device (CIED), what information should you know? What precautions should be taken?

Patients with a CIED undergoing surgery need to have the device interrogated prior to surgery to determine the device's features, settings, pacer function, pacing dependency, baseline rhythm and rate, ICD function, tachyarrhythmia history, effect of magnet, and battery status. Intraoperative management will be determined by risk for electromagnetic interference. Clear communication with the surgeon regarding electrocautery requirements and grounding for the case is essential. If there is a risk for interference, the pacer function can be programmed to asynchronous mode if pacemaker dependent, and the antitachycardia algorithm of the ICD should be turned off (via magnet or programming, depending on settings). If the ICD function is to be turned off, external cardioversion pads must be placed. Postoperatively, the device must be reprogrammed to the original settings if programming changes were made. Also see Chapter 8: Cardiac Implantable Electronic Device.

American Society of Anesthesiologists. Practice advisory for the perioperative management of patients with cardiac implantable electronic devices: pacemakers and implantable cardioverter-defibrillators: an updated report by the American Society of Anesthesiologists Task Force on Perioperative Management of Patients with Cardiac Implantable Electronic Devices. *Anesthesiology*. 2011;114:247-261.

B.4. What types of coronary stents are available? What is their perioperative relevance?

Coronary stent placement was introduced in order to reduce the risk of thrombosis, dissection, and restenosis after angioplasty. Two types of coronary stents have been used: bare metal stents (BMSs) and DESs. DESs have been used extensively to reduce the neointimal hyperplastic reaction seen with the use of BMS, which is the main cause of restenosis; however, by delaying endothelialization of coronary stent struts, DES predisposes to stent thrombosis if DAPT is stopped early. First-generation DES requires a minimum of 12 months of DAPT before cessation or interruption in therapy; however, second-generation DES endothelializes faster and can be safely stopped at 6 months. Also see Chapter 10: Abdominal Aortic Aneurysm Repair, Section A.5, **Figure 10.1**.

Levine GN, Bates ER, Bittl JA, et al. 2016 ACC/AHA guideline focused update on duration of dual antiplatelet therapy in patients with coronary artery disease: a report of the American College of Cardiology/American Heart Association Task Force on Clinical Practice Guidelines: an update of the 2011 ACCF/AHA/SCAI guideline for percutaneous coronary intervention, 2011 ACCF/AHA guideline for coronary artery bypass graft surgery, 2012 ACC/AHA/ACP/AATS/PCNA/SCAI/STS guideline for the diagnosis and management of patients with stable ischemic heart disease, 2013 ACCF/AHA Guideline for the Management of ST-Elevation Myocardial Infarction, 2014 AHA/ACC guideline for the management of patients with non-ST-elevation acute coronary syndromes, and 2014 ACC/AHA guideline on perioperative cardiovascular evaluation and management of patients undergoing noncardiac surgery [published correction appears in *Circulation*. 2016;134:e192-e194]. *Circulation*. 2016;134:e123-e155.

Thompson A, Fleischmann KE, Smilowitz NR, et al. 2024 AHA/ACC/ACS/ASNC/HRS/SCA/SCCT/SCMR/SVM Guideline for Perioperative Cardiovascular Management of Noncardiac Surgery: A Report of the American College of Cardiology/American Heart Association Joint Committee on Clinical Practice Guidelines. *Circulation*. 2024;150:e351-e442.

B.5. What is the conventional recommendation for dual antiplatelet therapy (DAPT) in a patient with previous percutaneous coronary intervention (PCI) undergoing elective noncardiac surgery?

Therapy with thienopyridines (ticlopidine or clopidogrel) and aspirin, known as DAPT, is recommended after PCI. However, due to the increased risk of bleeding, discontinuation is often required prior to surgery. DAPT is recommended for 2 to 4 weeks after dilatation without stenting (angioplasty); elective surgery should be postponed for 2 to 4 weeks. After BMS, antiplatelet therapy for 4 to 6 weeks is recommended; elective surgery should be postponed for 4 to 6 weeks, a minimum of 30 days. After implantation of newer generation DES, at least 6 months of antiplatelet therapy is required, although if the risk of delaying surgery would outweigh stent thrombosis, consideration can be given to proceeding at 3 months. In patients with an indication for PCI and a projected need for surgery within the next 6 months, balloon angioplasty or BMS can be considered. Daily aspirin should be continued during the perioperative period, and DAPT should be resumed as soon as possible postoperatively. A multidisciplinary plan should be agreed upon by the surgeon and cardiologist prior to an elective procedure. Also see Chapter 14: Ischemic Heart Disease and Noncardiac Surgery, **Figure 14.1**.

Levine GN, Bates ER, Bittl JA, et al. 2016 ACC/AHA guideline focused update on duration of dual antiplatelet therapy in patients with coronary artery disease: a report of the American College of Cardiology/American Heart Association Task Force on Clinical Practice Guidelines: an update of the 2011 ACCF/AHA/SCAI guideline for percutaneous coronary intervention, 2011 ACCF/AHA guideline for coronary artery bypass graft surgery, 2012 ACC/AHA/ACP/AATS/PCNA/SCAI/STS guideline for the diagnosis and management of patients with stable ischemic heart disease, 2013 ACCF/AHA guideline for the management of ST-elevation myocardial infarction, 2014 AHA/ACC guideline for the management of patients with non-ST-elevation acute coronary syndromes, and 2014 ACC/AHA guideline on perioperative cardiovascular evaluation and management of patients undergoing noncardiac surgery [published correction appears in *Circulation*. 2016;134:e192-e194]. *Circulation*. 2016;134:e123-e155.

B.6. What risk is associated with continuing perioperative antiplatelet therapy? What risk is there with stopping it?

In a meta-analysis of perioperative aspirin withdrawal versus low-dose aspirin, the aspirin group's relative risk of bleeding increased by a factor of 1.5, but there was no increase in bleeding complications or in perioperative mortality, with the possible exceptions of intracranial surgery and prostatectomy. Studies with ticlopidine or clopidogrel demonstrate a small increased risk of major perioperative bleeding with DAPT (0.4%-1%). The risk of stopping antiplatelet therapy is stent thrombosis with resultant acute MI, which carries a high mortality rate. Given the potentially lethal consequences, whether bleeding risks outweigh the benefit of protection from stent thrombosis must be carefully considered.

Burger W, Chemnitius JM, Kneissl GD, et al. Low-dose aspirin for secondary cardiovascular prevention—cardiovascular risks after its perioperative withdrawal versus bleeding risks with its continuation—review and meta-analysis. *J Intern Med*. 2005;257:399-414.

Oscarsson A, Gupta A, Fredrikson M, et al. To continue or discontinue aspirin in the perioperative period: a randomized, controlled clinical trial. *Br J Anaesth*. 2010;104:305-312.

B.7. How should patients with coronary stents undergoing noncardiac surgery be managed?

The preoperative evaluation of patients with coronary stents should include information regarding the date of stent placement, coronary anatomy, type of coronary stent, and antiplatelet strategy. Multidisciplinary discussions regarding how the risk of bleeding for the particular surgery compares with the risk of coronary stent thrombosis are strongly encouraged. When possible, continuing DAPT is recommended in patients with DES for surgery with minor or intermediate risk of perioperative bleeding. Discussion between the anesthesiologist, the surgeon, and the treating cardiologist is recommended.

Levine GN, Bates ER, Bittl JA, et al. 2016 ACC/AHA guideline focused update on duration of dual antiplatelet therapy in patients with coronary artery disease: a report of the American College of Cardiology/American Heart Association Task Force on Clinical Practice Guidelines: an update of the 2011 ACCF/AHA/SCAI guideline for percutaneous coronary intervention, 2011 ACCF/AHA guideline for coronary artery bypass graft surgery, 2012 ACC/AHA/ACP/AATS/PCNA/SCAI/STS guideline for the diagnosis and management of patients with stable ischemic heart disease, 2013 ACCF/AHA guideline for the management of ST-elevation myocardial infarction, 2014 AHA/ACC guideline for the management of patients with non-ST-elevation acute coronary syndromes, and 2014 ACC/AHA guideline on perioperative cardiovascular evaluation and management of patients undergoing noncardiac surgery [published correction appears in *Circulation*. 2016;134:e192-e194]. *Circulation*. 2016;134:e123-e155.

Thompson A, Fleischmann KE, Smilowitz NR, et al. 2024 AHA/ACC/ACS/ASNC/HRS/SCA/SCCT/SCMR/SVM Guideline for Perioperative Cardiovascular Management of Noncardiac Surgery: A Report of the American College of Cardiology/American Heart Association Joint Committee on Clinical Practice Guidelines. *Circulation*. 2024;150:e351-e442.

B.8. You are visiting the patient in the preoperative area before coming to the operating room. How would you discuss treatment options and obtain informed consent from this patient?

Discussing the patient's anesthetic options and obtaining consent should be interactive and include several key components. Although the patient's medical history will have been previously reviewed, important elements should be confirmed and any changes in health should be reviewed. Based on this information, you should explain your prescribed anesthetic plan as well as the risks and benefits of the anesthetic plan, including any involved procedures (tracheal intubation, arterial line, spinal anesthesia). Although it can be challenging to provide an exhaustive list of risks, including the most common and most serious risks associated with the anesthetic plan should be done alongside your plans to minimize the associated risk. Be sure to use simple language and avoid too many specific medical terms to improve comprehension. Allowing the patient opportunities for questions and clarification prior to affirming that they are amenable to the plan is essential to the consent process.

For example: *"For this procedure, I recommend spinal anesthesia. This involves placing a small amount of medication in to the fluid that surrounds your brain and spinal cord in order to make you numb where they will be operating. This option would mean that you would not need a breathing tube provided that the spinal medication has set up appropriately. Risks associated with spinal anesthesia include low blood pressure, which we treat, infection, bleeding, and very rare nerve injury. There is also the risk of a headache afterward, although you are at low risk for this side effect. After we confirm that you are numb for the procedure, we give you some sedation medication to make you comfortable during the procedure.*

The back-up method would be general anesthesia, which would involve placing a breathing tube during your procedure while you are completely asleep. This would only be done if needed for your safety or comfort.

Do you have any questions that I can answer for you about the anesthesia plan?"

King JS, Moulton BW. Rethinking informed consent: the case for Shared Medical Decision-Making. *American Journal of Law & Medicine*. 2006;32:429-501. doi:10.1177/009885880603200401

Sweitzer BJ, Pfeifer K. Preoperative evaluation for anesthesia for noncardiac surgery in adults. In: Connor RF, ed. *UpToDate*. Wolters Kluwer. Accessed July 24, 2023.

SECTION 6

B.9. The patient and his family are worrying about memory loss from anesthesia. Would you discuss the periprocedural complications with the patient, and how would you do it?

Discussing the risks and benefits associated with an anesthetic plan in the setting of specific patient risk factors is critical in the informed consent process. Given this patient's age and comorbidities, his risk for postoperative delirium and the potential for postoperative cognitive decline should be assessed and communicated. Eliciting a patient history of prior reactions to anesthesia as well as functional status and baseline concerns for cognitive decline will lay a foundation for an informed discussion of the likelihood for periprocedural cognitive concerns. Potential causes should be discussed in the context of surgical risk factors (eg duration of case, anticipated blood loss, surgical stress and extent, and anticipated postoperative course) as well as a plan to mitigate any harm from these factors. Patient and family members should be encouraged to voice questions and concerns as needed.

Cocanour CS. Informed consent—it's more than a signature on a piece of paper. *Am J Surg*. 2017;214:993-997.

C. Intraoperative Management

C.1. What monitors would you use for this patient?

The following monitors should be used for this patient:

American Society of Anesthesiologists standard monitors, including:

- EKG with ST-segment analysis
- Pulse oximetry
- Noninvasive blood pressure monitoring or invasive arterial blood pressure
- End-tidal carbon dioxide
- Temperature

C.2. Is there a preferred anesthetic technique for patients undergoing TURP, and why?

The choice of anesthetic technique should be guided by the requirements of the surgical procedure, coexisting diseases, the need to prevent postoperative complications, and patient preferences.

Neuraxial anesthesia has advantages for patients undergoing M-TURP for the following reasons:

- It allows monitoring of the patient's mental status, thereby facilitating early detection of signs of TURP syndrome.
- It can allow for earlier detection of prostate capsular tears or bladder perforation via patient reports of peritoneal or diaphragmatic (referred shoulder) pain.
- It promotes vasodilation and peripheral pooling of blood, thereby reducing the severity of circulatory overloading.
- It reduces blood loss by lowering arterial and venous blood pressure during surgery.
- Early postoperative analgesia improved with spinal anesthesia.
- Avoidance of tracheal intubation is preferred in patients with significant pulmonary pathology.
- However, less emphasis is placed on neuraxial anesthesia for TURP now because of the increased use of bipolar electrode and laser resection surgical techniques.

Gainsburg D, Pamnani A, Malhotra V. Anesthesia and the Renal and Genitourinary Systems. In: Gropper MA, Cohen NH, Eriksson LI, Fleisher LA, Johnson-Akeju S, Leslie K, eds. *Miller's Anesthesia*. 10th ed. Elsevier; 2025:1804-1832.

Malhotra V. Transurethral resection of prostate. *Anesthesiol Clin North Am*. 2000;18:883-897.

O'Donnell AM, Foo ITH. Anaesthesia for transurethral resection of the prostrate. *Contin Educ Anaesth Crit Care Pain*. 2009;9:92-96.

C.3. Does neuraxial anesthesia result in a lower incidence of perioperative mortality than general anesthesia?

Although spinal anesthesia offers distinct advantages over general anesthesia for TURP surgery, mortality and many markers of patient outcomes are similar for both groups, in large part because the safety of the procedure itself has advanced. The 30-day mortality associated with TURP has steadily declined from 2.5% in 1962 to current estimates of 0.2% to 0.8%. Mortality rates are similar in patients receiving regional anesthesia or general anesthesia. Increased morbidity is more associated with surgical and patient factors than anesthesia type and has been found in patients with resections exceeding 90 minutes, gland size greater than 45 g, acute urinary retention, and age older than 80 years. The incidence of postoperative complications, specifically MI, pulmonary embolism, cerebrovascular accidents, transient ischemic attacks, renal failure, hepatic insufficiency, and the need for prolonged ventilation, is similar in patients receiving regional anesthesia and those receiving general anesthesia. With the increased use of L-TURP resection surgical techniques, even less emphasis has been placed on regional anesthesia as the preferred anesthetic technique, given minimal absorption of irrigating fluid.

Gainsburg D, Pamnani A, Malhotra V. Anesthesia and the Renal and Genitourinary Systems. In: Gropper MA, Cohen NH, Eriksson LI, Fleisher LA, Johnson-Akeju S, Leslie K, eds. *Miller's Anesthesia*. 10th ed. Elsevier; 2025:1804-1832.

Gainsburg DM. Anesthesia for Urological Endoscopic Procedures. In: Gainsburg DM, Bryson EO, Frost EAM, eds. *Anesthesia for Urologic Surgery*. Springer; 2014:35-51.

Hanson RA, Zornow MH, Conlin MJ, et al. Laser resection of the prostate: implications for anesthesia. *Anesth Analg*. 2007;105:475-479.

Hawary A, Mukhtar K, Sinclair A, et al. Transurethral resection of the prostate syndrome: almost gone but not forgotten. *J Endourol*. 2009;23:2013-2020.

C.4. What intravenous fluid would you use during TURP?

Because dilutional hyponatremia commonly occurs in patients undergoing M-TURP, the intravenous fluid of choice perioperatively is normal saline that contains sodium, 154 mEq/L. Circulatory overloading from absorbed irrigant is common in patients undergoing M-TURP or B-TURP (but not L-TURP); therefore, the amount of intravenous fluid administered during surgery should be carefully monitored.

Gainsburg D, Pamnani A, Malhotra V. Anesthesia and the Renal and Genitourinary Systems. In: Gropper MA, Cohen NH, Eriksson LI, Fleisher LA, Johnson-Akeju S, Leslie K, eds. *Miller's Anesthesia*. 10th ed. Elsevier; 2025:1804-1832.

Gainsburg DM. Anesthesia for Urological Endoscopic Procedures. In: Gainsburg DM, Bryson EO, Frost EAM, eds. *Anesthesia for Urologic Surgery*. Springer; 2014:35-51.

C.5. A spinal anesthetic was performed and a sensory level of T10 was confirmed prior to the start of the procedure. About forty minutes after initiation of monopolar TURP (M-TURP) using glycine as the bladder-irrigating solution, the patient becomes agitated and complains of nausea. Further sedation along with an antiemetic is administered. However, shortly thereafter, the patient becomes very restless, blood pressure rises, and heart rate decreases. The patient becomes cyanotic and obtunded, blood pressure precipitously falls, and pupils are dilated and unresponsive to light. What is the most likely cause of these signs and symptoms, and would these occur during bipolar TURP (B-TURP) or laser TURP (L-TURP) resection?

Restlessness and incoherence during TURP are particularly ominous signs of TURP syndrome. These are caused by pulmonary edema, hypoxemia, and cerebral edema. These signs must not be misinterpreted as signs of inadequate anesthesia. Administration of sedatives or general anesthesia in the presence of TURP syndrome has been associated with severe complications including death. In B-TURP and L-TURP, normal saline can be used as the bladder-irrigating solution, and hyponatremia is not expected. In B-TURP, absorption of the intravascular bladder-irrigating solution can still occur via the prostatic venous sinuses, resulting in circulatory overload. This is not expected in L-TURP because the treatment zone is rapidly coagulated.

Chen Q, Zhang L, Fan QL, et al. Bipolar transurethral resection in saline vs traditional monopolar resection of the prostate: results of a randomized trial with a 2-year follow-up. *BJU Int.* 2010;106:1339-1343.

Geavlete B, Multescu R, Dragutescu M, et al. Transurethral resection (TUR) in saline plasma vaporization of the prostate vs standard TUR of the prostate: 'the better choice' in benign prostatic hyperplasia? *BJU Int.* 2010;106:1695-1699.

C.6. What are the important characteristics of irrigation solutions used during TURP?

Ideal TURP irrigation solutions would be either isotonic or nearly isotonic, electrically inert, nontoxic, and transparent. Electrolyte-containing solutions such as normal saline are avoided in M-TURP because they can conduct electrical current to surrounding tissues and cause burns. Instead, solutions with non-toxic solutes are used for M-TURP; however, the need for transparency necessitates a hypotonic solution. If intravascular hypotonic bladder-irrigating solution is absorbed, absorption can lead to hyponatremia, hyposmolality, and, in severe cases, hemolysis. These complications are avoided when normal saline is used with B-TURP and L-TURP resection.

Over the years, a number of irrigation solutions have been introduced. The most commonly used solution for M-TURP is glycine (1.2% and 1.5%). Mannitol (3%), glucose (2.5%-4%), Cytal (a mixture of sorbitol 2.7% and mannitol 0.54%), and urea (1%) solutions are also occasionally used.

Gainsburg D, Pamnani A, Malhotra V. Anesthesia and the Renal and Genitourinary Systems. In: Gropper MA, Cohen NH, Eriksson LI, Fleisher LA, Johnson-Akeju S, Leslie K, eds. *Miller's Anesthesia.* 10th ed. Elsevier; 2025:1804-1832.

Gainsburg DM. Anesthesia for Urological Endoscopic Procedures. In: Gainsburg DM, Bryson EO, Frost EAM, eds. *Anesthesia for Urologic Surgery.* Springer; 2014:35-51.

C.7. What is the effect on body temperature of continuous bladder irrigation during TURP?

Several liters of irrigation solution pass through the bladder during TURP. This can reduce body temperature at the rate of 1 °C per hour (**Figure 25.1**). About half of patients undergoing TURP become hypothermic and shiver at the conclusion of surgery.

Gainsburg D, Pamnani A, Malhotra V. Anesthesia and the Renal and Genitourinary Systems. In: Gropper MA, Cohen NH, Eriksson LI, Fleisher LA, Johnson-Akeju S, Leslie K, eds. *Miller's Anesthesia.* 10th ed. Elsevier; 2025:1804-1832.

Gainsburg DM. Anesthesia for Urological Endoscopic Procedures. In: Gainsburg DM, Bryson EO, Frost EAM, eds. *Anesthesia for Urologic Surgery.* Springer; 2014:35-51.

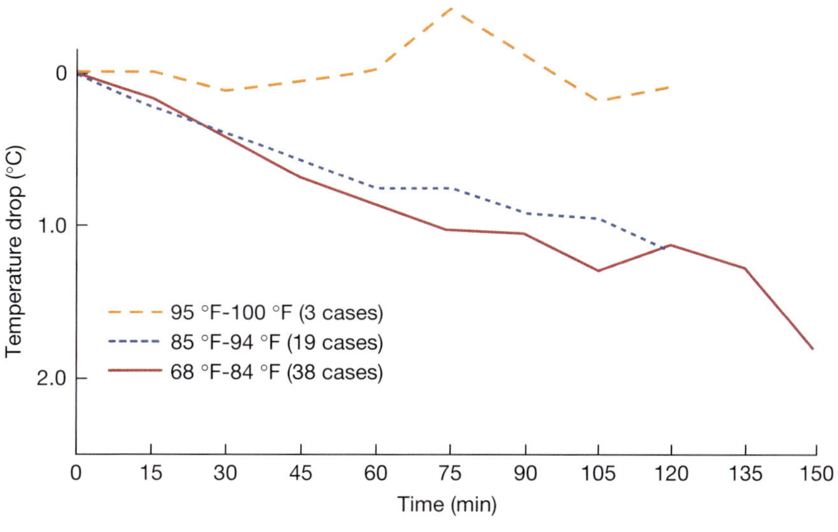

FIGURE 25.1. The reduction in body temperature during TURP is related to the temperature of the irrigating solution and the duration of surgery. TURP, transurethral resection of the prostate. (Modified with permission from Allen TD. Body temperature changes during prostatic resection as related to the temperature of the irrigating solution. *J Urol.* 1973;110:433-535.)

C.8. What is the definition of TURP syndrome? What are the signs and symptoms of the syndrome?

Rapid absorption of a large-volume, hypotonic bladder irrigation solution during TURP can lead to TURP syndrome. TURP syndrome is characterized by intravascular volume shifts and plasma-solute (osmolarity) effects. The signs and symptoms of TURP syndrome are as follows:

Cardiopulmonary
- Hypertension
- Bradycardia
- Dysrhythmia
- Respiratory distress
- Cyanosis
- Hypotension
- Shock
- Asystole

Hematologic and Renal
- Hyperglycinemia
- Hyperammonemia
- Hyponatremia
- Hyposmolality
- Hemolysis/anemia
- Acute renal failure

CNS
- Nausea/vomiting
- Confusion/restlessness
- Blindness
- Twitches/seizures
- Lethargy/paralysis
- Dilated/nonreactive pupils
- Coma
- Death

TURP syndrome can occur as early as 15 minutes after surgery has started and as late as 24 hours after surgery. Patient complaints of dizziness, headache, nausea, chest or throat tightness, and shortness of breath are often early clinical signs. Then the patient becomes restless, confused, and nauseated. Some patients complain of abdominal pain. Blood pressure often rises (both systolic and diastolic), and heart rate decreases (Figure 25.2). If not treated promptly, the patient becomes cyanotic and hypotensive, and ultimately this can lead to cardiac arrest.

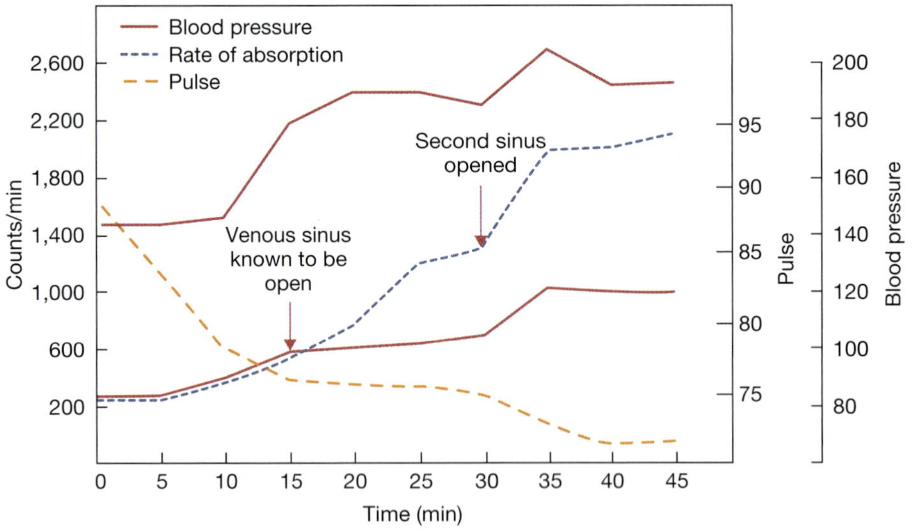

FIGURE 25.2. Blood pressure, heart rate, and absorption rate of radioactively tagged irrigation solution during TURP. TURP, transurethral resection of the prostate. (Modified with permission from Taylor RO, Maxson ES, Carter FH, et al. Volumetric gravimetric and radioisotopic determination of fluid transfer in transurethral prostatectomy. *J Urol.* 1958;79:490-499.)

Occasionally, TURP syndrome manifests with neurologic signs. The patient becomes lethargic and then unconscious, and pupils dilate, reacting sluggishly to light. These signs can be followed by short episodes of tonic-clonic seizures and then coma lasting minutes to hours.

If the patient is under general anesthesia, the presenting signs of TURP syndrome are typically a rise and then a fall in blood pressure, decreasing oxygen saturation, and severe refractory bradycardia. The ECG can show nodal rhythm, ST-segment changes, U waves, and widening of the QRS complex. Recovery from general anesthesia can be delayed.

Gainsburg D, Pamnani A, Malhotra V. Anesthesia and the Renal and Genitourinary Systems. In: Gropper MA, Cohen NH, Eriksson LI, Fleisher LA, Johnson-Akeju S, Leslie K, eds. *Miller's Anesthesia*. 10th ed. Elsevier; 2025:1804-1832.

Gainsburg DM. Anesthesia for Urological Endoscopic Procedures. In: Gainsburg DM, Bryson EO, Frost EAM, eds. *Anesthesia for Urologic Surgery*. Springer; 2014:35-51.

Gravenstein D. Transurethral resection of the prostate (TURP) syndrome: a review of the pathophysiology and management. *Anesth Analg*. 1997;84:438-446.

C.9. How does the patient absorb irrigation solution during TURP?

The bladder irrigation solution enters the bloodstream directly through open prostatic venous sinuses created during monopolar and bipolar resection techniques, particularly if the prostatic capsule is violated during surgery.

If bladder perforation occurs, accumulation of irrigating fluid in the intraperitoneal or retroperitoneal space can occur regardless of technique, resulting in significant intravascular absorption.

Gainsburg D, Pamnani A, Malhotra V. Anesthesia and the Renal and Genitourinary Systems. In: Gropper MA, Cohen NH, Eriksson LI, Fleisher LA, Johnson-Akeju S, Leslie K, eds. *Miller's Anesthesia*. 10th ed. Elsevier; 2025:1804-1832.

Gainsburg DM. Anesthesia for Urological Endoscopic Procedures. In: Gainsburg DM, Bryson EO, Frost EAM, eds. *Anesthesia for Urologic Surgery*. Springer; 2014:35-51.

Geavlete B, Multescu R, Dragutescu M, et al. Transurethral resection (TUR) in saline plasma vaporization of the prostate vs standard TUR of the prostate: 'the better choice' in benign prostatic hyperplasia? *BJU Int*. 2010;106:1695-1699.

SECTION 6

C.10. What factors increase the incidence of TURP syndrome?

TURP syndrome is more likely to occur if the prostatic gland is atypically large, the prostatic capsule is violated during surgery, or the hydrostatic pressure of the irrigation solution is excessively high. Large prostatic glands have rich venous networks that promote intravascular absorption of irrigation solution. Violation of the prostatic capsule during surgery promotes entry of irrigation solution into the periprostatic and retroperitoneal spaces. The hydrostatic pressure of the irrigation solution is an important determinant of the rate at which the patient will absorb the solution. This pressure depends primarily on the height of the irrigation solution pole. When the height of the pole exceeds 60 cm (~2 ft), absorption of irrigation solution is greatly enhanced. An excessively distended bladder during surgery also facilitates absorption.

Gainsburg D, Pamnani A, Malhotra V. Anesthesia and the Renal and Genitourinary Systems. In: Gropper MA, Cohen NH, Eriksson LI, Fleisher LA, Johnson-Akeju S, Leslie K, eds. *Miller's Anesthesia*. 10th ed. Elsevier; 2025:1804-1832.

Gainsburg DM. Anesthesia for Urological Endoscopic Procedures. In: Gainsburg DM, Bryson EO, Frost EAM, eds. *Anesthesia for Urologic Surgery*. Springer; 2014:35-51.

C.11. What is the effect on cardiopulmonary, renal, and central nervous system (CNS) functions of excessive absorption of irrigation solution during TURP?

Excessive absorption of irrigation solution during TURP causes hypervolemia and hypertension with bradycardia and can induce angina and pulmonary edema (**Figure 25.3**). It can also have an adverse effect on renal function. An inverse relation has been observed between the amount of irrigation solution absorbed during surgery and postoperative urinary output.

Some patients with TURP syndrome exhibit neurologic signs resulting from water intoxication if a hypotonic irrigating solution is used. Patients assume a decerebrate posture, exhibit clonus and positive Babinski reflex, and eventually convulse and lapse into coma. Examination of the eyes reveals papilledema and dilated and sluggishly reacting pupils. The electroencephalogram shows low voltage bilaterally. Patients can remain in a coma from a few hours to several days.

Gainsburg D, Pamnani A, Malhotra V. Anesthesia and the Renal and Genitourinary Systems. In: Gropper MA, Cohen NH, Eriksson LI, Fleisher LA, Johnson-Akeju S, Leslie K, eds. *Miller's Anesthesia*. 10th ed. Elsevier; 2025:1804-1832.

Gainsburg DM. Anesthesia for Urological Endoscopic Procedures. In: Gainsburg DM, Bryson EO, Frost EAM, eds. *Anesthesia for Urologic Surgery*. Springer; 2014:35-51.

C.12. What causes CNS dysfunction in patients who have undergone M-TURP?

The physiologic derangement of CNS function in TURP syndrome is not hyponatremia but acute hyposmolality, which is predictable because the blood-brain barrier is essentially impermeable to sodium but freely permeable to water, leading to cerebral edema. The primary factor governing the manifestations

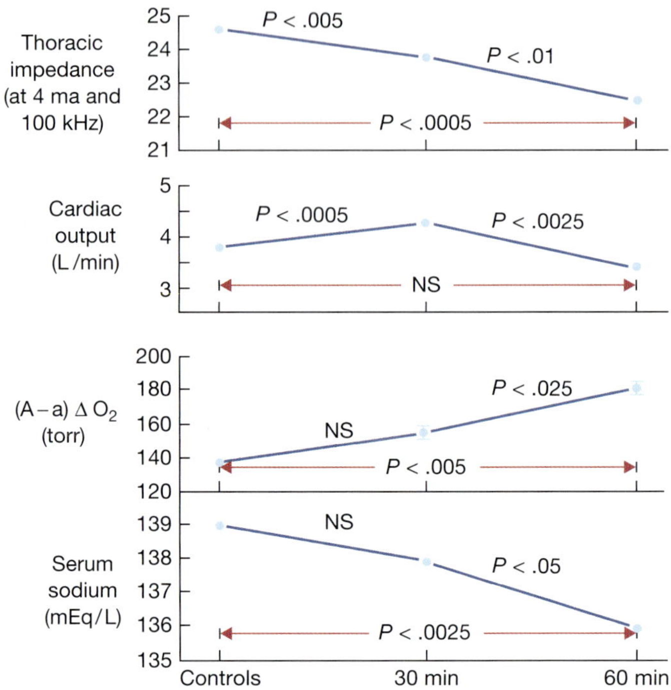

FIGURE 25.3. Mean changes in thoracic impedance, cardiac output, alveolar-arterial oxygen tension difference, and serum sodium concentration during TURP. NS, nonsignificant; TURP, transurethral resection of the prostate. (Modified with permission from Casthely P, Ramanathan S, Chalon J, et al. Decreases in electric thoracic impedance during transurethral resection of the prostate: an index of early water intoxication. *J Urol.* 1981;125:347-349.)

of symptoms is the rate at which serum sodium falls rather than the total fall itself; the faster the fall in serum sodium level, the greater the incidence of neurologic symptoms. However, below 120 mEq/L, all patients are symptomatic. Cerebral edema caused by acute hyposmolality can increase intracranial pressure, which results in bradycardia and hypertension by the Cushing reflex. The rise in intracranial pressure is directly correlated to the gain in body weight during TURP.

Fujiwara A, Nakahira J, Sawai T, et al. Prediction of clinical manifestations of transurethral resection syndrome by preoperative ultrasonographic estimation of prostate weight. *BMC Urol.* 2014;14:67.

Gainsburg D, Pamnani A, Malhotra V. Anesthesia and the Renal and Genitourinary Systems. In: Gropper MA, Cohen NH, Eriksson LI, Fleisher LA, Johnson-Akeju S, Leslie K, eds. *Miller's Anesthesia.* 10th ed. Elsevier; 2025:1804-1832.

Gainsburg DM. Anesthesia for Urological Endoscopic Procedures. In: Gainsburg DM, Bryson EO, Frost EAM, eds. *Anesthesia for Urologic Surgery.* Springer; 2014:35-51.

C.13. How does acute hyponatremia affect the cardiovascular system?

When serum sodium level falls below 120 mEq/L, signs of cardiovascular depression can occur. A decrease to less than 115 mEq/L causes bradycardia, widening of the QRS complex, ST-segment elevation, ventricular ectopic beats, and T-wave inversion. Patients with a serum sodium level below 110 mEq/L can develop respiratory and cardiac arrest.

Gainsburg D, Pamnani A, Malhotra V. Anesthesia and the Renal and Genitourinary Systems. In: Gropper MA, Cohen NH, Eriksson LI, Fleisher LA, Johnson-Akeju S, Leslie K, eds. *Miller's Anesthesia.* 10th ed. Elsevier; 2025:1804-1832.

Gainsburg DM. Anesthesia for Urological Endoscopic Procedures. In: Gainsburg DM, Bryson EO, Frost EAM, eds. *Anesthesia for Urologic Surgery.* Springer; 2014:35-51.

C.14. What prophylactic measures can reduce the incidence of TURP syndrome?

The most important preventive measure during surgery is the preservation of the prostatic capsule. Another preventive measure is restriction of the hydrostatic pressure of the irrigation solution to 60 cm H_2O. This can be accomplished by limiting the height of the irrigation pole to 60 cm (~2 ft) above patient level. Also, the bladder should not be allowed to overdistend, and the duration of surgery should be restricted.

Serial serum sodium and osmolality are advisable in order to detect a decreasing trend in M-TURP. If clinical signs of TURP syndrome are present, the surgeon should be informed and therapeutic measures immediately instituted. If serum sodium level approaches 120 mEq/L, surgery should be terminated as soon as possible.

Intravenous fluids should be cautiously administered during M-TURP and B-TURP. A microdrip is recommended, particularly for patients with cardiac or renal disease. If regional anesthesia causes hypotension, a small dose of a vasoconstrictor is recommended to raise the blood pressure rather than a rapid infusion of intravenous fluids.

Gainsburg D, Pamnani A, Malhotra V. Anesthesia and the Renal and Genitourinary Systems. In: Gropper MA, Cohen NH, Eriksson LI, Fleisher LA, Johnson-Akeju S, Leslie K, eds. *Miller's Anesthesia*. 10th ed. Elsevier; 2025:1804-1832.

Gainsburg DM. Anesthesia for Urological Endoscopic Procedures. In: Gainsburg DM, Bryson EO, Frost EAM, eds. *Anesthesia for Urologic Surgery*. Springer; 2014:35-51.

C.15. What therapeutic measures are recommended for patients with TURP syndrome?

When symptoms of TURP syndrome appear, the following therapeutic measures are recommended:

- Terminate surgery as soon as possible.
- Administer furosemide, 20 to 40 mg intravenously. Although furosemide results in natriuresis, this effect is negligible relative to the desired acute diuresis and loss of free water.
- Administer oxygen by nasal cannula or face mask to maintain oxygen saturation and consider intubation.
- Obtain arterial blood gas, serum osmolality, and sodium analysis.
- If serum sodium is abnormally low and clinical signs of hyponatremia are evident, intravenous administration of hypertonic saline (3%-5%) might be indicated. The hypertonic solution should be given at a rate no faster than 100 mL/h. In most cases, no more than 300 mL of hypertonic saline is needed to correct the hyponatremia.
- If the patient develops seizures, a short-acting anticonvulsant such as diazepam (5-20 mg) or midazolam (2-10 mg) can be administered intravenously. If these drugs do not arrest the seizures, a barbiturate or phenytoin can be added.
- If pulmonary edema or hypotension develops, invasive hemodynamic monitoring is recommended. This will serve as a guide for pharmacologic support and fluid administration.
- If significant blood loss is suspected, the administration of packed red blood cells should be considered. In general, intravenous fluids should be administered cautiously because of the propensity of these patients to develop pulmonary edema.

Gainsburg D, Pamnani A, Malhotra V. Anesthesia and the Renal and Genitourinary Systems. In: Gropper MA, Cohen NH, Eriksson LI, Fleisher LA, Johnson-Akeju S, Leslie K, eds. *Miller's Anesthesia*. 10th ed. Elsevier; 2025:1804-1832.

Gainsburg DM. Anesthesia for Urological Endoscopic Procedures. In: Gainsburg DM, Bryson EO, Frost EAM, eds. *Anesthesia for Urologic Surgery*. Springer; 2014:35-51.

C.16. Is hypertonic saline administration necessary to correct hyponatremia? Explain. What are the risks of rapidly correcting hyponatremia?

Administration of hypertonic saline to correct hyponatremia is rarely necessary and sometimes can be detrimental. Unless the patient develops severe clinical signs of hyponatremia, hypertonic saline administration is not recommended. Spontaneous or induced diuresis usually corrects the hyponatremia within a few hours.

Patients who have undergone TURP often sustain circulatory overload during surgery; consequently, hypertonic saline administration in these patients can induce pulmonary edema. In addition, rapid administration of hypertonic saline has been associated with central pontine myelinolysis (osmotic demyelination syndrome), a poorly understood and fatal neurologic complication.

To reduce the hazards of hypertonic saline administration, serum osmolarity should be monitored and corrected aggressively only until symptoms substantially subside and then hyponatremia should be corrected at a rate no faster than 1.5 mEq/L/h.

Gainsburg D, Pamnani A, Malhotra V. Anesthesia and the Renal and Genitourinary Systems. In: Gropper MA, Cohen NH, Eriksson LI, Fleisher LA, Johnson-Akeju S, Leslie K, eds. *Miller's Anesthesia*. 10th ed. Elsevier; 2025:1804-1832.

O'Donnell AM, Foo ITH. Anaesthesia for transurethral resection of the prostrate. *Contin Educ Anaesth Crit Care Pain*. 2009;9:92-96.

Sterns RH, Riggs JE, Schochet SS Jr. Osmotic demyelination syndrome following correction of hyponatremia. *N Engl J Med*. 1986;314:1535-1542.

C.17. What are the toxic effects of glycine? Is there an antidote to glycine toxicity? What are the metabolic by-products of glycine?

Glycine is an inhibitory neurotransmitter similar to γ-aminobutyric acid in the spinal cord and brain. When absorbed in large amounts, glycine has direct toxic effects on the heart and retina. In patients who have undergone M-TURP with glycine absorption, it has been shown to reduce cardiac output by almost

20%. In animal studies, administration of the amino acid arginine reversed the myocardial depressant effects of glycine. The mechanism by which glycine depresses cardiac function and the mechanism by which arginine protects the heart are unknown.

Hyperglycinemia can cause transient visual disturbance (blindness) during TURP. However, glycine toxicity in patients who have undergone TURP is uncommon, probably because most of the absorbed glycine is retained in the periprostatic and retroperitoneal spaces, where access to the circulation is limited.

The most common metabolites of glycine are ammonia, glyoxylic acid, and oxalic acid (**Figure 25.4**). Excessive absorption of glycine during TURP can lead to hyperammonemia. Hyperoxaluria could compromise renal function in patients with coexisting renal disease, which is often present in older patients undergoing TURP.

Gainsburg D, Pamnani A, Malhotra V. Anesthesia and the Renal and Genitourinary Systems. In: Gropper MA, Cohen NH, Eriksson LI, Fleisher LA, Johnson-Akeju S, Leslie K, eds. *Miller's Anesthesia*. 10th ed. Elsevier; 2025:1804-1832.

Gainsburg DM. Anesthesia for Urological Endoscopic Procedures. In: Gainsburg DM, Bryson EO, Frost EAM, eds. *Anesthesia for Urologic Surgery*. Springer; 2014:35-51.

Ovassapian A, Joshi CW, Brunner EA. Visual disturbances: an unusual symptom of transurethral prostatic resection reaction. *Anesthesiology*. 1982;57:332-334.

C.18. What are the symptoms and clinical course of TURP-induced hyperammonemia?

The signs and symptoms of hyperammonemia usually appear within 1 hour of surgery. Typically, the patient becomes nauseated, vomits, and then becomes comatose. Blood ammonia level can rise to greater than 500 mM, with coma lasting 10 to 12 hours until ammonia blood level decreases to less than 150 mM. The hyperammonemia can linger postoperatively, probably because glycine absorption from the periprostatic space continues after surgery.

Malhotra V. Transurethral resection of prostate. *Anesthesiol Clin North Am*. 2000;18:883-897.

Roesch RP, Stoelting RK, Lingeman JE, et al. Ammonia toxicity resulting from glycine absorption during a transurethral resection of the prostate. *Anesthesiology*. 1983;58:577-579.

C.19. What are the clinical characteristics, causes, and prognosis of TURP-related blindness?

Transient blindness is one of the more alarming complications of TURP. The patient complains of blurred vision and of seeing halos around objects. This can occur either during surgery or later in the postanesthesia care unit (PACU). Although it is sometimes accompanied by other TURP-related complications, blindness can occur as an isolated complication. Examination of the eyes reveals dilated and unresponsive pupils. TURP-related blindness gradually recedes, and eyesight returns to normal 8 to 48 hours after surgery.

The cause of TURP-related blindness is unclear. The intraocular pressure and optic discs remain normal. In the past, edema of the cerebral optical cortex was suspected; however, the clinical signs of TURP-related blindness are consistent with retinal rather than cortical dysfunction. Unlike cortical blindness, TURP-related blindness allows perception of light, and the blink reflex is preserved. TURP-related blindness is most likely caused by a toxic effect of glycine on the retina. This is supported by the fact that glycine is an inhibitory neurotransmitter, and in animals, it has been shown to inhibit visual pathways.

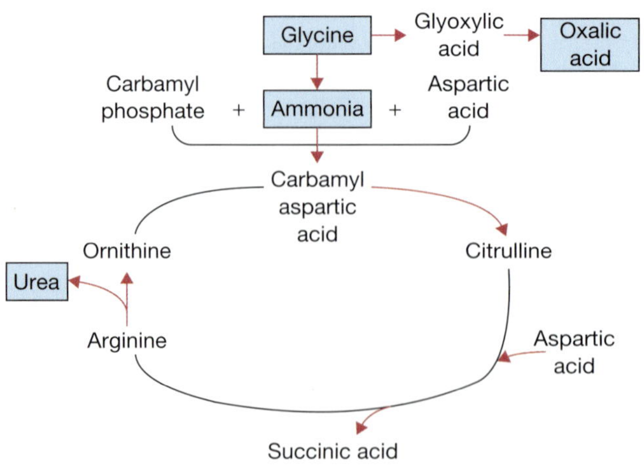

FIGURE 25.4. Metabolic pathways of glycine.

Also, the severity of TURP-related blindness is directly related to blood glycine level. Postoperatively, vision gradually improves as glycine level declines.

Gainsburg D, Pamnani A, Malhotra V. Anesthesia and the Renal and Genitourinary Systems. In: Gropper MA, Cohen NH, Eriksson LI, Fleisher LA, Johnson-Akeju S, Leslie K, eds. *Miller's Anesthesia.* 10th ed. Elsevier; 2025:1804-1832.

Gainsburg DM. Anesthesia for Urological Endoscopic Procedures. In: Gainsburg DM, Bryson EO, Frost EAM, eds. *Anesthesia for Urologic Surgery*. Springer; 2014:35-51.

C.20. What are the causes of excessive bleeding during TURP?

Patients undergoing TURP commonly bleed perioperatively, and 2.5% of patients undergoing M-TURP require transfusion. Possible causes include dilutional thrombocytopenia resulting from excessive absorption of irrigation solution and local release of fibrinolytic agents (plasminogen and urokinase) from the mucosa of the lower urinary tract. During and immediately after TURP, these factors cause local fibrinolysis and promote bleeding from the raw surfaces of the prostate. The existence of a local fibrinolytic mechanism is supported by the observation that prophylactic administration of ε-aminocaproic acid (an antifibrinolytic agent) reduces bleeding from the prostatic bed.

Systemic coagulopathy can also occur during TURP caused by disseminated intravascular coagulation (DIC) rather than by primary fibrinolysis. DIC is triggered during TURP by prostatic particles rich in thromboplastin that enter the bloodstream during resection. Characteristically, the platelet count and fibrinogen level are abnormally low. At autopsy, multiple widely distributed microthrombi are observed. The high level of fibrin-degradation products found in the blood of these patients is due to secondary fibrinolysis, which commonly accompanies DIC.

Gainsburg D, Pamnani A, Malhotra V. Anesthesia and the Renal and Genitourinary Systems. In: Gropper MA, Cohen NH, Eriksson LI, Fleisher LA, Johnson-Akeju S, Leslie K, eds. *Miller's Anesthesia*. 10th ed. Elsevier; 2025:1804-1832.

Gainsburg DM. Anesthesia for Urological Endoscopic Procedures. In: Gainsburg DM, Bryson EO, Frost EAM, eds. *Anesthesia for Urologic Surgery*. Springer; 2014:35-51.

SECTION 6

C.21. What are the causes, signs, symptoms, and treatment of bladder perforation during TURP?

The incidence of bladder perforation during TURP is approximately 1% as a result of trauma by surgical instrumentation, overdistension of the bladder, and, rarely, explosion of traces of hydrogen gas inside the bladder.

An early sign of bladder perforation is a sudden decrease in the return of irrigation solution from the bladder. This sign often goes unnoticed until a significant amount of irrigation solution accumulates in the abdomen, causing abdominal distress. Other clinical signs are hypotension, followed by hypertension and nausea. Reflex-type movements of the limbs have been observed under both general and regional anesthesia. When the perforation is intraperitoneal, symptoms develop faster and include severe shoulder pain caused by diaphragmatic irritation. Diagnosis of bladder perforation is confirmed by cystourethrography. Treatment is immediate suprapubic cystotomy.

Gainsburg D, Pamnani A, Malhotra V. Anesthesia and the Renal and Genitourinary Systems. In: Gropper MA, Cohen NH, Eriksson LI, Fleisher LA, Johnson-Akeju S, Leslie K, eds. *Miller's Anesthesia.* 10th ed. Elsevier; 2025:1804-1832.

C.22. What are the likely causes of hypotension during TURP?

The likely causes of hypotension during TURP are blood loss, circulatory overload with resulting CHF, myocardial ischemia or infarct, severe hyponatremia, and bacteremia or septicemia.

Gainsburg D, Pamnani A, Malhotra V. Anesthesia and the Renal and Genitourinary Systems. In: Gropper MA, Cohen NH, Eriksson LI, Fleisher LA, Johnson-Akeju S, Leslie K, eds. *Miller's Anesthesia*. 10th ed. Elsevier; 2025:1804-1832.

D. Postoperative Management

D.1. What is the source of postoperative bacteremia in patients who have undergone TURP? What factors increase the incidence of bacteremia?

The prostatic gland often harbors large amounts of bacteria. TURP facilitates the entry of bacteria into the bloodstream by opening venous sinuses, leading to postoperative bacteremia. About 30% of patients undergoing TURP have infected urine preoperatively, and half of them have transient bacteremia postoperatively, although most are asymptomatic; 6% to 7%, however, develop signs of sepsis. Also, a preoperative indwelling catheter promotes bacterial growth in the urethra. Surgical disruption of the prostatic venous sinuses and excessive hydrostatic pressure of the irrigation solution facilitate the entry of bacteria into the bloodstream.

Gainsburg D, Pamnani A, Malhotra V. Anesthesia and the Renal and Genitourinary Systems. In: Gropper MA, Cohen NH, Eriksson LI, Fleisher LA, Johnson-Akeju S, Leslie K, eds. *Miller's Anesthesia*. 10th ed. Elsevier; 2025:1804-1832.

D.2. What are the signs of post-TURP septicemia? What preventive measures are generally recommended?

The signs of septicemia usually appear postoperatively in the PACU. They include fever, chills, low blood pressure, and tachycardia. Symptoms can be due to bacterial endotoxins, in which case they are self-limited, or direct bloodstream seeding with bacteria.

Antibiotics administered prophylactically before TURP do not sterilize the urine because they do not easily penetrate the prostate gland. Nevertheless, preoperative administration of antibiotics is strongly recommended. If sepsis is suspected postoperatively in a patient who has undergone TURP, broad-spectrum antibiotics should be started immediately without waiting for blood culture results.

Gainsburg D, Pamnani A, Malhotra V. Anesthesia and the Renal and Genitourinary Systems. In: Gropper MA, Cohen NH, Eriksson LI, Fleisher LA, Johnson-Akeju S, Leslie K, eds. *Miller's Anesthesia*. 10th ed. Elsevier; 2025:1804-1832.

D.3. Is postoperative hypothermia a risk factor for myocardial ischemia?

Yes. Unexpected hypothermia and shivering are associated with a significantly higher incidence of postoperative myocardial ischemia due to increased oxygen demand. It is important to maintain normothermia during the perioperative period, particularly in older population at higher risk for hypothermia due to decreased subcutaneous fat. Also see Chapter 14: Ischemic Heart Disease and Noncardiac Surgery.

Frank SM, Beattie C, Christopherson R, et al. Unintentional hypothermia is associated with postoperative myocardial ischemia. The perioperative ischemia randomized anesthesia trial study group. *Anesthesiology*. 1993;78:468-476.

Frank SM, Fleisher LA, Olson KF et al. Consequences of hypothermia. *Curr Anaesth Crit Care*. 2001;12:79-86.

D.4. What is postoperative cognitive dysfunction (POCD)? How does this differ from delirium, and what is the time course to resolution?

POCD is a form of perioperative neurocognitive disorder defined by worsening cognitive performance postoperatively compared to preoperative baseline up to 12 months following the procedure. The deficit is present in multiple domains and presents days to weeks after surgery, highly correlated with age. POCD usually resolves within months; however, the time course varies, and sustained deficits have been reported.

Postoperative delirium, by contrast, manifests as acute fluctuation in orientation shortly following emergence, generally lasting 24 to 72 hours postoperatively.

For clinical purposes, a multispecialty working group recommends that "perioperative neurocognitive disorders" (PNDs) be used as an overarching term for cognitive impairment identified in the preoperative or postoperative period. This includes cognitive decline diagnosed before an operation (described as neurocognitive disorder), any form of acute event (postoperative delirium), and cognitive decline diagnosed up to 30 days after the procedure (delayed neurocognitive recovery) and up to 12 months after (postoperative neurocognitive disorder).

Evered LA, Silbert BS. Postoperative cognitive dysfunction and noncardiac surgery. *Anesth Analg*. 2018;127:496-505.

Evered L, Silbert B, Knopman DS, et al. Recommendations for the nomenclature of cognitive change associated with anaesthesia and surgery—2018. *Br J Anaesth*. 2018;121:1005-1012.

D.5. What are the mechanisms and risk factors for POCD? How would you mitigate the risk of POCD? Does the anesthetic technique influence the development of POCD?

The proposed mechanisms of POCD include preexisting neuroinflammation or neurodegeneration, which prime the brain to react more strongly to the systemic inflammatory response to the surgical procedure itself, resulting in accelerated progression of neuroinflammation and neurodegeneration with delayed neurocognitive recovery. Progression or eventual resolution of POCD can be impacted by several intraoperative and postoperative factors.

Preoperative risk factors include preexisting cognitive impairment, older age, and lower educational achievement. Intraoperative risk factors include major, prolonged, or emergency surgical procedures, as well as selection and dosing of certain anesthetic and adjunct agents, and possibly depth of general anesthesia.

Recommended strategies to mitigate the risk of POCD include:

- Minimize the use of benzodiazepines, opioids (particularly meperidine), anticholinergic drugs (particularly scopolamine), diphenhydramine, metoclopramide, and agents that can cause serotonin syndrome.

- Use raw or processed electroencephalography (EEG) or other neuromonitoring techniques, when available, as a supplemental guide to manage intraoperative dosing of anesthetic agents.
- Avoid hypotension and hypoxemia.
- Avoid hyperventilation because cerebral blood flow decreases by 2% to 4% for each mm Hg decrease in $Paco_2$. Prolonged $Paco_2$ below 30 mm Hg can result in cerebral ischemia and possibly POCD.
- Evidence suggests that postoperative administration of dexmedetomidine can reduce the incidence of delirium, although results are inconsistent for intraoperative administration, and there is scant evidence for other types of POCD.
- Inadequate postoperative pain control is associated with an increased incidence of delirium. A multimodal approach to analgesia can be employed to reduce the risk of opioid-related side effects.

Neuraxial or regional anesthesia with either light or deep sedation does not consistently decrease the incidence of postoperative neurocognitive disorders compared with general anesthesia. When general anesthesia is selected, the choice of either a total intravenous anesthesia (TIVA) technique or an inhalation-based anesthetic technique has been shown to affect the incidence of postoperative delirium in adult patients.

Small prospective studies have compared spinal anesthesia with intravenous sedation to general anesthesia in older patients undergoing TURP, with no difference in perioperative mental function between the groups at 30 days.

Berger M, Nadler JW, Browndyke J, et al. Postoperative cognitive dysfunction: minding the gaps in our knowledge of a common postoperative complication in the elderly. *Anesthesiol Clin*. 2015;33:517-550.

Berger M, Schenning KJ, Brown CH IV, et al. Best practices for postoperative brain health: recommendations from the Fifth International Perioperative Neurotoxicity Working Group. *Anesth Analg*. 2018;127:1406-1413.

Chung FF, Chung A, Meier RH, et al. Comparison of perioperative mental function after general anaesthesia and spinal anaesthesia with intravenous sedation. *Can J Anaesth*. 1989;36:382-387.

Cole DJ, Kharasch ED. Postoperative brain function: toward a better understanding and the American Society of Anesthesiologists perioperative brain health initiative. *Anesthesiology*. 2018;129:861-863.

Evered LA, Silbert BS. Postoperative cognitive dysfunction and noncardiac surgery. *Anesth Analg*. 2018;127:496-505.

Peden CJ, Miller TR, Deiner SG, et al; Members of the Perioperative Brain Health Expert Panel. Improving perioperative brain health: an expert consensus review of key actions for the perioperative care team. *Br J Anaesth*. 2021;126:423-432.

Silbert BS, Evered LA, Scott DA. Incidence of postoperative cognitive dysfunction after general or spinal anaesthesia for extracorporeal shock wave lithotripsy. *Br J Anaesth*. 2014;113:784-791.

E. Comparing M-TURP, B-TURP, and L-TURP

E.1. What differentiates M-TURP from B-TURP?

M-TURP uses high-energy cautery, which allows a fast-cutting technique of prostatic tissue with minimal coagulation in the process. The body is the conduit of the energy dispersed from the monopolar electrode to complete the electrical circuit to a large-surface skin grounding pad on the patient. It also requires the use of an electrolyte-free bladder-irrigating fluid. In B-TURP, the electrical circuit is completely contained within the resectoscope. This prevents energy from traveling through the body; the energy remains confined to the site of prostatic resection and is returned via the second limb of the bipolar resectoscope. With the bipolar electrode, less bleeding occurs and normal saline can be used as the bladder-irrigating fluid.

In a meta-analysis that compared the safety of M-TURP and B-TURP in a small number of patients undergoing TURP (1,802), a significant benefit was reported in the bipolar group in overall complication rate, need for transfusion, and the absence of TURP syndrome. Subsequent randomized controlled trials have confirmed this morbidity benefit.

Chen Q, Zhang L, Fan QL, et al. Bipolar transurethral resection in saline vs traditional monopolar resection of the prostate: results of a randomized trial with a 2-year follow-up. *BJU Int*. 2010;106:1339-1343.

Gainsburg D, Pamnani A, Malhotra V. Anesthesia and the Renal and Genitourinary Systems. In: Gropper MA, Cohen NH, Eriksson LI, Fleisher LA, Johnson-Akeju S, Leslie K, eds. *Miller's Anesthesia*. 10th ed. Elsevier; 2025:1804-1832.

Gainsburg DM. Anesthesia for Urological Endoscopic Procedures. In: Gainsburg DM, Bryson EO, Frost EAM, eds. *Anesthesia for Urologic Surgery*. Springer; 2014:35-51.

Issa MM. Technological advances in transurethral resection of the prostate: bipolar versus monopolar TURP. *J Endourol*. 2008;22:1587-1595.

Reich O, Gratzke C, Bachmann A, et al. Morbidity, mortality, and early outcome of transurethral resection of the prostate: a prospective multicenter evaluation of 10,654 patients. *J Urol*. 2008;180:246-249.

E.2. What differentiates the technologies for L-TURP?

L-TURP delivers light energy to coagulate or vaporize prostatic tissue. Holmium laser enucleation of the prostate (HoLEP), in particular, has been suggested as the new standard for surgical treatment of BPH. Prostatic tissue is vaporized, and the resulting heat dissipation coagulates small to medium blood vessels. HoLEP can be used safely on patients with larger prostatic glands, with similar outcomes as patients undergoing open prostatectomy or traditional M-TURP. HoLEP is associated with lower transfusion rates, shorter catheterization time, and shorter hospital stays. Photoselective vaporization and bipolar plasma vaporization have shown similar benefits.

There are five advantages of L-TURP: (1) use of normal saline as the bladder-irrigating solution, thus avoiding hyponatremia; (2) minimizes absorption of irrigating fluid; (3) minimizes or eliminates TURP syndrome; (4) produces significantly less bleeding, which allows the procedure to be performed on an anticoagulated patient if needed; and (5) de-emphasizes regional anesthesia as the preferred anesthetic technique.

Gainsburg D, Pamnani A, Malhotra V. Anesthesia and the Renal and Genitourinary Systems. In: Gropper MA, Cohen NH, Eriksson LI, Fleisher LA, Johnson-Akeju S, Leslie K, eds. *Miller's Anesthesia*. 10th ed. Elsevier; 2025:1804-1832.

Gainsburg DM. Anesthesia for Urological Endoscopic Procedures. In: Gainsburg DM, Bryson EO, Frost EAM, eds. *Anesthesia for Urologic Surgery*. Springer; 2014:35-51.

Geavlete B, Multescu R, Dragutescu M, et al. Transurethral resection (TUR) in saline plasma vaporization of the prostate vs standard TUR of the prostate: 'the better choice' in benign prostatic hyperplasia? *BJU Int*. 2010;106:1695-1699.

Michalak J, Tzou D, Funk J. HoLEP: the gold standard for the surgical management of BPH in the 21st century. *Am J Clin Exp Urol*. 2015;3:36-42.

E.3. Are there any alternatives to TURP for benign prostate hypertrophy (BPH)?

Although TURP is considered the standard surgical treatment of BPH, many advancements have been made with the goal of decreasing surgical morbidity and decreasing operative time while still achieving relief of lower urinary tract symptoms. Alternatives to conventional TURP and L-TURP include several novel BPH procedures, some of which can be done as outpatient or office-based procedures under local anesthesia. These relatively new procedures seek to ameliorate bladder outlet obstruction through multiple mechanisms, including displacement of prostate tissue through implant or mechanical dilation or through water-based ablation techniques. Many of these techniques, while currently in use, continue to be studied for the longevity of their outcomes and noninferiority to traditional TURP procedures.

Dornbier R, Pahouja G, Branch J, McVary KT. The New American Urological Association benign prostatic hyperplasia clinical guidelines: 2019 update. *Curr Urol Rep*. 2020;21:32.

Elterman D, Gao B, Lu S, Bhojani N, Zorn KC, Chughtai B. New technologies for treatment of benign prostatic hyperplasia. *Urol Clin North Am*. 2022;49:11-22.

Gainsburg D, Pamnani A, Malhotra V. Anesthesia and the Renal and Genitourinary Systems. In: Gropper MA, Cohen NH, Eriksson LI, Fleisher LA, Johnson-Akeju S, Leslie K, eds. *Miller's Anesthesia*. 10th ed. Elsevier; 2025:1804-1832.

26

Kidney Transplant

John E. Rubin and Christine M. Lennon

A 50-year-old male with rapid onset of end-stage renal disease (ESRD) prefers not to start hemodialysis. He would like to receive an organ transplant from a living related donor, but other options include a deceased-donor or a paired donor exchange program.

A. Medical Disease and Differential Diagnosis

1. What are the causes of chronic renal disease that can progress to renal failure?
2. How is chronic kidney disease (CKD) diagnosed?
3. What are the indications for hemodialysis?
4. What are the common clinical manifestations of ESRD?
5. What electrolyte imbalances occur in patients with impaired renal function, and how are they treated?
6. How is metabolic acidosis managed in chronic renal failure?
7. Are patients with renal disease at increased risk of cardiovascular disease?
8. When is the best time to receive a kidney transplant?
9. How are immunosuppressive drugs managed in kidney transplant recipients?
10. How are kidneys allocated to recipients on the waiting list in the United States?
11. What is donation after cardiac death (DCD)?
12. What is a living donor transplant program?
13. What is a paired donor exchange transplant program?
14. What are some barriers to receiving a kidney transplant?
15. What surgical techniques are available for donor nephrectomy?
16. How is a donor kidney preserved?
17. Describe the operative procedure of kidney transplantation.

B. Preoperative Evaluation and Preparation

1. What preoperative workup would you order for a recipient?
2. How does the presence of obesity affect the outcome of a transplanted kidney?
3. How are routine medications and immunosuppressive medications managed in the perioperative period?

C. Intraoperative Management

1. Are a central venous pressure (CVP) catheter, an arterial catheter, and a pulmonary artery catheter required for the transplant procedure?
2. What type of intravenous fluid should be used during surgery?
3. How would you conduct the induction of anesthesia?
4. Is succinylcholine contraindicated in patients with renal failure?
5. How are nondepolarizing neuromuscular blockers affected by renal failure?
6. How would you maintain anesthesia during the case?
7. What are the effects of inhalation anesthetics on renal blood flow (RBF), glomerular filtration (GFR), and urine output?
8. How does renal failure affect the pharmacology of opioids?
9. Can regional anesthesia be used to optimize postoperative analgesia?

D. Postoperative Management

1. How is the diagnosis of transplant rejection made?
2. What are immunosuppressive agents, and how do they affect anesthetic care?

A. Medical Disease and Differential Diagnosis

A.1. What are the causes of chronic renal disease that can progress to renal failure?

The most common etiologies of renal disease leading to kidney transplant are:

- Diabetes mellitus
- Hypertension
- Glomerular diseases
- Polycystic kidney disease
- Vascular diseases (eg, systemic lupus erythematosus)
- Congenital and metabolic diseases
- Tubular and interstitial diseases
- Neoplasms
- Retransplant and graft failure

Chronic kidney disease (CKD) has many potential causes that differ among the world's populations. In developed countries, age, hypertension, cardiovascular disease, diabetes mellitus, increased body mass index (BMI), and smoking are predominantly associated with CKD. In the developing world, unique causes of kidney failure include infections due to bacteria, viruses, and parasites.

The global increase in CKD parallels the obesity epidemic. Obesity has been associated with a secondary focal segmental glomerulosclerosis, which is referred to as obesity-related glomerulopathy (ORG). The accumulation of lipid in the cellular structure of the kidney is associated with structural and functional changes.

---

de Vries AP, Ruggenenti P, Ruan XZ, et al. Fatty kidney: emerging role of ectopic lipid in obesity-related renal disease. *Lancet Diabetes Endocrinol.* 2014;2:417-426.

Hart A, Smith JM, Skeans MA, et al. OPTN/SRTR 2017 annual data report: kidney. *Am J Transplant.* 2019;19:19-123.

A.2. How is chronic kidney disease (CKD) diagnosed?

CKD is defined as an abnormality of kidney structure or function that is present for more than 3 months, with implications for health. It is not dependent on the etiology leading to deteriorated kidney function.

The criteria for CKD include any of the following present for more than 3 months:

- Albuminuria
- Urine sediment abnormalities
- Electrolyte and other abnormalities due to tubular disorders
- Abnormalities detected by histology
- Structural abnormalities detected by imaging
- History of kidney transplantation
- GFR less than 60 mL/min/1.73 m^2

GFR and the progression of CKD can be estimated using several formulas, one of the most common being the Modification of Diet in Renal Disease (MDRD) formula. ESRD is established when GFR is <15 mL/min/1.73 m^2.

$$\text{GFR, in mL/min/1.73 m}^2 = 175 \times (\text{SCr})^{-1.154} \times (\text{age})^{-0.203} \times (0.742 \text{ if female}) \times (1.21 \text{ if black})$$

SCr is the serum creatinine (mg/dL). Among individuals with established CKD, progression is based on estimation of GFR and level of albuminuria.

Kidney Disease: Improving Global Outcomes. KDIGO 2012 clinical practice guideline for the evaluation and management of chronic kidney disease. *Kidney Int Suppl.* 2013;3:1-150.

National Kidney Foundation. KDOQI clinical practice guideline for hemodialysis adequacy: 2015 update. *Am J Kidney Dis.* 2015;66:884-930.

A.3. What are the indications for hemodialysis?

The decision about when to start hemodialysis is complex and patient specific, and generally depends on the estimated GFR, rate of decline in GFR, and presence of ESRD-related signs and symptoms. Recent data indicate that mortality may be higher when dialysis is initiated early, with no significant benefit in terms of quality of life. It is generally recommended that dialysis be initiated in patients with GFR between 5 and 15 mL/min/1.73 m^2 and concomitant signs and symptoms that could be due to ESRD, and in all patients with GFR less than 5 mL/min/1.73 m^2 regardless of the presence of additional signs or symptoms.

Patients with uremic symptoms (eg, encephalopathy, pericarditis, and pleuritis) should be started on hemodialysis even if GFR is not at critically low levels. Other indications for dialysis in CKD include refractory volume overload, refractory acidosis, hyperkalemia or hyperphosphatemia, declining nutritional status, fatigue and malaise, and mild cognitive impairment.

Cooper BA, Branley P, Bulfone L, et al. A randomized, controlled trial of early versus late initiation of dialysis. *N Engl J Med*. 2010;363:609-619.

Kalantar-Zadeh K, Jafar TH, Nitsch D, Neuen BL, Perkovic V. Chronic kidney disease. *Lancet*. 2021;398:786-802.

National Kidney Foundation. KDOQI clinical practice guideline for hemodialysis adequacy: 2015 update. *Am J Kidney Dis*. 2015;66:884-930.

A.4. What are the common clinical manifestations of ESRD?

The common problems related to ESRD are:

- Electrolytes: volume expansion, hyponatremia, hyperkalemia, metabolic acidosis, hyperuricemia, hyperphosphatemia, hypocalcemia
- Gastrointestinal: gastroparesis, nausea, vomiting, pancreatitis, anorexia, uremic gastroenteritis, peptic ulcer disease, gastrointestinal bleeding
- Cardiovascular: accelerated atherosclerosis, systemic hypertension, left ventricular hypertrophy, congestive heart failure, pulmonary edema, cardiomyopathy, pericarditis, hyperdynamic circulation
- Hematologic: anemia, B- and T-cell dysfunction, qualitative platelet dysfunction, bleeding diathesis
- Musculoskeletal: muscle weakness, uremic osteodystrophy (osteomalacia, osteosclerosis, osteitis fibrosa cystica)
- Neurologic: encephalopathy, loss of memory, seizures, peripheral neuropathy, autonomic dysfunction (postural hypotension), myoclonus, asterixis, dialysis disequilibrium (dehydration, weakness, nausea and vomiting, hypotension, and occasionally convulsion and coma)
- Endocrine: vitamin D deficiency, secondary hyperparathyroidism, carbohydrate intolerance, hypertriglyceridemia

Chronic pain is extremely common in ESRD and can result from renal and nonrenal etiologies. In a prospective study of 205 patients on hemodialysis, musculoskeletal pain was most common (63.1%), followed by dialysis-associated pain (13.6%), peripheral neuropathy (12.6%), and peripheral vascular disease/claudication pain (9.7%). Polycystic kidney disease can cause chronic abdominal pain. Analgesics should be initiated according to the World Health Organization (WHO) escalatory ladder guidelines. Ultimately, opioid pain medications are commonly prescribed for inadequate relief. Multiple factors contribute to altered opioid pharmacokinetics and pharmacodynamics in patients with chronic renal failure. Volume of distribution is altered, renal drug clearance is impaired, and hepatic drug metabolism is decreased. Fentanyl, methadone, and buprenorphine are considered the safest opioids for use in patients with ESRD, and other opioid pain medications should be used with caution with appropriate drug dosing reductions. Secondary hyperparathyroidism often results in bone pain.

O'Connor NR, Corcoran AM. End-stage renal disease: symptom management and advance care planning. *Am Fam Physician*. 2012;85:705-710.

Raina R, Krishnappa V, Gupta M. Management of pain in end-stage renal disease patients: short review. *Hemodial Int*. 2018;22:290-296.

Tobin DG, Lockwood MB, Kimmel PL, et al. Opioids for chronic pain management in patients with dialysis-dependent kidney failure. *Nat Rev Nephrol*. 2022;18:113-128.

A.5. What electrolyte imbalances occur in patients with impaired renal function, and how are they treated?

Chronic renal insufficiency and ESRD are associated with abnormalities in sodium, potassium, calcium, and magnesium balance, and metabolic acidosis.

Sodium and water (H_2O) balance are closely related. The kidney has its own inherent circadian rhythm involved in the transcription of genes for Na^+ excretion and blood pressure control. This function is impaired in renal disease. In patients with chronic renal failure, total body content of Na^+ and H_2O can be elevated. This can be due to glomerular disease promoting Na^+ retention or excessive ingestion of Na^+ leading to extracellular fluid (ECF) expansion. The ECF expansion and hyperosmolarity contribute to hypertension. Patients who are nonanuric can be treated with loop diuretics and salt restriction.

SECTION 6

TABLE 26.1 Treatment for Hyperkalemia

Drug	Dose
Calcium chloride	5 mL of 10% solution IV over 2 min (monitor for bradycardia)
Calcium gluconate	10 mL of 10% solution IV over 2 min (monitor for bradycardia)
Insulin	5-10 units regular insulin with 1-2 amps $D_{50}W$ IV bolus
Sodium bicarbonate	1 mEq/kg slow IV push or continuous drip; not to exceed 50-100 mEq
β-Agonists (albuterol)	2.5 mg mixed with 3 mL isotonic saline through nebulizer every 20 min as tolerated
Diuretic (furosemide)	20-40 mg IV push
Magnesium chloride	1-2 g IV over 30-60 s; repeat every 5-15 min as required or 3-10 mg/min IV infusion

$D_{50}W$, 50% dextrose in water; IV, intravenous.

The renal mechanisms for conserving Na^+ and H_2O are impaired in ESRD. Urine is isosthenuric in patients who are nonoliguric. This means the usual indices of detecting prerenal azotemia (high urine osmolality, low urine Na^+, and low fractional excretion of sodium [FE_{Na}]) are not applicable in such patients. If additional fluid loss (vomiting, fever) is imposed, patients can become severely hypovolemic, necessitating careful rehydration with normal saline.

Hyperkalemia rarely occurs in patients with a GFR >25 mL/min/1.73 m^2 in the absence of an endogenous or exogenous potassium load. Patients with GFR <25 mL/min/1.73 m^2 can be chronically hyperkalemic. Severe hyperkalemia increases cardiac and skeletal muscle excitability. The earliest changes begin with levels >6.5 mEq/L. The electrocardiogram (ECG) shows peaked T waves, flattened P waves, disappearance of P waves, increased PR interval, and a widened QRS complex that can progress to a "sine wave," ventricular asystole, or ventricular fibrillation. Muscle weakness can cause respiratory failure. Membrane excitability is more dependent on the rate of increase in K^+ than on K^+ concentration per se. Treatment of hyperkalemia includes a combination of insulin, glucose, loop diuretics (nonanuric), sodium bicarbonate, calcium, and magnesium (**Table 26.1**). The anesthetist might also institute hyperventilation in patients mechanically ventilated. Hemodialysis or peritoneal dialysis is the definitive treatment for severe hyperkalemia.

Magnesium imbalance can accompany chronic renal failure. High blood magnesium levels cause dose-dependent neuromuscular dysfunction and increased sensitivity to depolarizing and nondepolarizing neuromuscular blockers. Bradycardia, hypotension, and heart block are due to the calcium channel blocking effects of magnesium. The acute effects can be antagonized by intravenous infusion of calcium. Conversely, decreased dietary intake and impaired intestinal absorption can lead to hypomagnesemia. Magnesium deficiency has been related to progression of atherosclerosis and low parathyroid hormone (PTH) levels.

Phosphate retention occurs when GFR begins to decline. Retained phosphate promotes secondary hyperparathyroidism by lowering ionized plasma calcium levels, decreasing renal formation of calcitriol (1,25-dihydroxyvitamin D), and stimulating PTH gene expression.

Ionized and protein-bound calcium levels are lower in patients with uremia patients. This is the result of hyperphosphatemia and reduced gastrointestinal absorption secondary to the decreased production of vitamin D.

Kalantar-Zadeh K, Jafar TH, Nitsch D, Neuen BL, Perkovic V. Chronic kidney disease. *Lancet*. 2021;398:786-802.

Kanbay M, Goldsmith D, Uyar ME, et al. Magnesium in chronic kidney disease: challenges and opportunities. *Blood Purif*. 2010;29:280-292.

Malberti F. Hyperphosphataemia: treatment options. *Drugs*. 2013;73:673-688.

Nikolaeva S, Pradervand S, Centeno G, et al. The circadian clock modulates renal sodium handling. *J Am Soc Nephrol*. 2012;23:1019-1026.

Vervloet MG, Sezer S, Massy ZA, Johansson L, Cozzolino M, Fouque D. The role of phosphate in kidney disease. *Nat Rev Nephrol*. 2017;13:27-38.

A.6. How is metabolic acidosis managed in chronic renal failure?

A mild-to-moderate acidosis is commonly seen when GFR decreases to <20% to 25% of normal. The reduced renal mass results in decreased production and excretion of proton load. The plasma bicarbonate concentration ranges between 12 and 22 mEq/L, and blood pH remains >7.20. This does not routinely require correction. It may gradually evolve into a high anion gap acidosis when GFR is <20 mL/min/1.73 m^2. Some patients with ESRD maintain close to normal acid-base parameters even when renal function is severely compromised. However, when exposed to an increased dietary acid load, these patients can have decreased ability to increase bicarbonate generation. Correction of acidosis by oral sodium bicarbonate or a diet rich in fruits and vegetables can attenuate the rate of decline of renal function.

Goraya N, Wesson DE. Does correction of metabolic acidosis slow chronic kidney disease progression? *Curr Opin Nephrol Hypertens*. 2013;22:193-197.

Loniewski I. Combining a fruit and vegetable diet with sodium bicarbonate supplementation seems the best dietary option for chronic kidney disease patients. *Kidney Int*. 2012;82:937.

Zadeh KK, Fouque D. Nutritional management of chronic kidney disease. *N Engl J Med*. 2017;377:1765-1776.

A.7. Are patients with renal disease at increased risk of cardiovascular disease?

ESRD is associated with an increased incidence and prevalence of a wide range of cardiovascular morbidities including hypertension, coronary artery disease, stroke, congestive heart failure, atrial fibrillation, sudden cardiac death, pulmonary hypertension, and valvular heart disease.

Extensive vascular calcification contributes to early-onset cardiovascular disease and cardiovascular mortality. In addition to traditional cardiovascular risks, risk factors specific to CKD such as phosphate retention, hypercalcemia, history of dialysis, high-dose vitamin D therapy, and deficiency of calcification inhibitors promote arterial calcification. There is no specific therapy to reverse vascular calcification, but statin therapy is associated with decreased cardiovascular death. Additional measures such as reduction of calcium phosphate load, using non–calcium-containing phosphate binders, and moderate doses of active vitamin D can attenuate arterial hardening.

The rate of sudden cardiac death increases as the stage of CKD increases and could be responsible for 60% of cardiac deaths in patients undergoing dialysis. The uremic load results in cardiac fibrosis and left ventricular systolic and diastolic dysfunction. The occurrence of conduction abnormalities and arrhythmias is exacerbated by electrolyte shifts, diabetes mellitus, and autonomic neuropathy. Cardioverter-defibrillator implantation decreases the risk of sudden death in patients with CKD.

Hypertension has been reported to occur in 85% to 95% of patients with CKD (stages 3-5). Hypertension and CKD are interrelated: uncontrolled hypertension is a risk factor for developing CKD and leads to a more rapid progression of CKD, and CKD exacerbates uncontrolled hypertension due to volume expansion and increased systemic vascular resistance. An imbalanced autonomic system results in exaggerated sympathetic drive with loss of vagal tone. Autonomic neuropathy creates a setting for silent myocardial ischemia.

Correction of the uremic state and improved GFR after kidney transplantation can decrease the incidence and severity of cardiovascular complications.

Botdorf J, Chaudhary K, Whaley-Connell A. Hypertension in cardiovascular and kidney disease. *Cardiorenal Med*. 2011;1:183-192.

Disthabanchong S. Vascular calcification in chronic kidney disease: pathogenesis and clinical implication. *World J Nephrol*. 2012;1:43-53.

Glicklich D, Vohra P. Cardiovascular risk assessment before and after kidney transplantation. *Cardiol Rev*. 2014;22:153-162.

Matsushita L, Ballew SH, Wang AYM, Kalyesubula R, Schaeffner E, Agarwal R. Epidemiology and risk of cardiovascular disease in populations with chronic kidney disease. *Nat Rev Nephrol*. 2022;18:696-707.

Shamseddin MK, Parfrey PS. Sudden cardiac death in chronic kidney disease: epidemiology and prevention. *Nat Rev Nephrol*. 2011;7:145-154.

A.8. When is the best time to receive a kidney transplant?

In general, a patient is a candidate for kidney transplantation if their estimated GFR (eGFR) is 20 mL/min/1.73 m^2 or less, and renal function has irreversibly deteriorated to the point that a transplant or dialysis is inevitable. Survival of a transplanted kidney is incrementally worse if the recipient has been on long-term dialysis; the best outcomes in patients who are preemptively transplanted before dialysis is initiated. Therefore, if the patient will eventually require dialysis and a living donor is available, transplantation is practical and cost-effective option.

Candidates for transplantation with no known contraindications should be referred to a transplantation program early, when the eGFR is around 30 mL/min/1.73 m^2. Preparation for a transplant can take several months, involving thorough medical evaluation and optimization of cardiac and pulmonary status.

Lenihan CR, et al. Clinical management of the adult kidney transplant recipient. In: Yu A, ed. *Brenner and Rector's The Kidney*. 11th ed. Elsevier; 2019:2244-2287.

Link DK, Saxena R. The right patient, the right treatment, the right access and the right time. *Adv Chronic Kidney Dis*. 2014;21:360-364.

A.9. How are immunosuppressive drugs managed in kidney transplant recipients?

In order to decrease the incidence of graft rejection, several regimens of immunosuppressive agents have been devised. Centers throughout the world use various combinations of drugs, but the central purpose is to prevent acute and chronic T-cell alloimmune rejection. The regimens are separated into an induction phase and a long-term maintenance phase. Multiple classes of immunosuppressive medications are used: corticosteroids, calcineurin inhibitors (CNIs) (cyclosporine and tacrolimus), antimetabolites (mycophenolate mofetil, mycophenolate sodium, and azathioprine), target-of-rapamycin (TOR) inhibitor (sirolimus), and cell-depleting (eg, rabbit anti-thymocyte globulin [ATG]) and nondepleting antibodies (eg, basiliximab). Cell-depleting antibodies target receptors on T cells, B cells, or both, such as CD3, CD52, and CD20, while nondepleting antibodies target molecular targets like CD25 that react to robust inflammatory signals like interleukin-2. Conventional immunosuppressive treatment involves protein induction. The maintenance phase involves a combination of two or three nonprotein immunosuppressive medications, each from a separate class.

Immunosuppression therapy is started in the immediate preoperative period. In the intraoperative period, induction therapy is targeted to eliminate lymphoid cells that can cause acute rejection of the graft. An induction agent might be withheld if immediate graft function occurs from a living donor kidney. After surgery, maintenance therapy is initiated and continued for the lifetime of the recipient. Although lifelong immunosuppression helps prevent rejection of the allograft, it also increases the risk of malignancy and infectious diseases. The immunosuppressive regimens might not prevent the slow deterioration associated with chronic graft rejection.

In an effort to reduce the long-term toxicities of immunosuppressive drugs, corticosteroid- and CNI-sparing protocols have become popular in managing patients with kidney transplantation. Long-term use of corticosteroids contributes to cardiovascular disease and infectious disease complications. CNIs prevent acute rejection but are associated with reduced long-term allograft function. Protocols with agents such as mycophenolate mofetil, mycophenolate sodium, sirolimus, everolimus, and belatacept allow discontinuation of CNIs within 6 months or avoidance of the CNIs.

Halloran PF. Immunosuppressive drugs for kidney transplantation. *N Engl J Med*. 2004;351:2715-2729.

Helal I, Chan L. Steroid and calcineurin inhibitor-sparing protocols in kidney transplantation. *Transplant Proc*. 2011;43:472-477.

Tan HP, Smaldone MC, Shapiro R. Immunosuppression preconditioning or regimens: evidence to date. *Drugs*. 2006;66:1535-1545.

A.10. How are kidneys allocated to recipients on the waiting list in the United States?

A national allocation policy for deceased-donor kidneys was established in 1987 by the United Network for Organ Sharing (UNOS) and the Organ Procurement and Transplant Network (OPTN). In 2014, the kidney allocation system (KAS) was extensively revised in order to increase utilization of available kidneys, reduce regional variability in access to transplantation, and improve outcomes for individual kidneys that are transplanted. In 2019, UNOS and OPTN moved to a policy of prioritizing kidney offers for candidates listed within a 250 nautical-mile radius of the donor hospital in an effort to further reduce disparities and improve distribution.

Adult patients can be registered on the waiting list after the diagnosis of irreversible kidney disease is made and GFR less than or equal to 20 mL/min/1.73 m^2. The estimated post-transplant survival (EPTS) is a measure used to estimate the number of years of potential benefit from a kidney transplant, and is calculated for all candidates on the waiting list using candidate age, time on dialysis, presence or absence of diabetes mellitus, and prior history of solid organ transplant. A combination of EPTS score and time spent on the waiting list is used to determine ranked priority on the waiting list. Additional priority is given to candidates with rare blood types and high immune system sensitivity because these patients have fewer opportunities for a transplant.

The kidney donor risk index (KDRI) is a measure that provides information about the quality of a donor kidney graft based on how long it is estimated to function after transplant. The KDRI is calculated using donor age, ethnicity, creatinine, history of hypertension or diabetes mellitus, cause of death, height, weight, hepatitis C virus (HCV) status, and whether the kidney was donated after circulatory death. Kidneys with the highest KDRI score (ie, the shortest predicted lifespan) must be offered over a wider geographic area in order to increase the utilization of donated kidneys. Transplant programs must have informed consent from potential recipients to receive a kidney with a KDRI score more than 85%.

Hart A, Lentine KL, Smith JM, et al. OPTN/SRTR 2019 annual data report: kidney. *Am J Transplant.* 2021;21:21-137.

A.11. What is donation after cardiac death (DCD)?

DCD has opened new perspectives in the donor pool. It refers to kidney donation from patients with brain injuries who do not meet the criteria for brain death and who experience cardiopulmonary arrest after withdrawal of ventilatory support. This criterion increases the number of organs available, but DCD kidneys have a greater than 5-fold increase in incidence of delayed graft function and a higher primary nonfunction rate compared to donation after brain death. DCD kidneys also have a higher rate of discard and retrieval-associated injury. Long-term graft function is equivalent between brain death and cardiac death donors. Renal preservation fluid is delivered either with rapid laparotomy and direct aortic cannulation or using an intra-aortic catheter placed via the femoral artery. Rapid laparotomy is associated with lower kidney discard rate, shorter warm ischemia time, and higher graft survival rate. Newer preservation strategies using extracorporeal membrane oxygenation (ECMO) are under study to develop uniform guidelines for procurement.

Akoh JA. Kidney donation after cardiac death. *World J Nephrol.* 2012;1:79-91.

Morrissey PE, Monaco AP. Donation after circulatory death: current practices, ongoing challenges, and potential improvements. *Transplantation.* 2014;97:258-264.

Neyrinck A, Van Raemdonck D, Monbaliu D. Donation after circulatory death: current status. *Curr Opin Anaesthesiol.* 2013;26:382-390.

A.12. What is a living donor transplant program?

A living donor transplant program allows recipient and donor surgery to be scheduled simultaneously. It offers the advantage of minimal organ preservation time. The total ischemia time from removal of the kidney from the donor to restoration of blood flow in the recipient can be less than 1 hour. A short preservation time allows immediate graft function, high-volume urine output, and initiation of creatinine clearance.

A large number of recipients have preformed antibodies to potential living donors. These antibodies are the result of exposure to foreign antigens by blood transfusions, prior transplantation, or pregnancy. As a result, recipients have positive crossmatches against living donor tissue antigens. There are preoperative measures that can facilitate successful transplantation. One such regimen involves a combination of plasmapheresis and low-dose intravenous immunoglobulin with or without rituximab (a B-cell depleter) administered to a positive crossmatch and/or highly sensitized recipient. The living donor transplantation is conducted when the crossmatch converts to negative. The recipient usually has to undergo additional plasmapheresis treatments and immunoglobulin infusions postoperatively.

Husain SA, King KL, Sanichar N, Crew RJ, Schold JD, Mohan S. Association between donor-recipient biological relationship and allograft outcomes after living donor kidney transplant. *JAMA Netw Open.* 2021;4:e215718.

Jin MK, Cho JH, Kwon O, et al. Successful kidney transplantation after desensitization using plasmapheresis, low-dose intravenous immunoglobulin, and rituximab in highly sensitized patients: a single-center experience. *Transplant Proc.* 2012;44:200-203.

Tong A, Chapman JR, Wong G, et al. Living kidney donor assessment: challenges, uncertainties and controversies among transplant nephrologists and surgeons. *Am J Transplant.* 2013;13:2912-2923.

A.13. What is a paired donor exchange transplant program?

This program is sometimes referred to as a "kidney swap." For example, an incompatible donor-candidate pair is matched with another pair with a complementary incompatibility, such that the donor from one pair gives an organ to a compatible candidate in the other pair, and vice versa. Each kidney paired donation (KPD) has developed its own features to accommodate local needs. Reasons for participating in

KPD include blood group incompatibility, sensitization of the recipient against the donor, potential for improvement in transplant quality (eg, age difference or graft size), and tissue compatibility. Sophisticated algorithms allow simultaneous two-way, three-way, or four-way exchanges or nonsimultaneous chains of transplants over the course of months.

There are many benefits to a paired donor exchange program:

- It expands the pool of donors.
- With the use of ABO-compatible but nonidentical donors, transplants can be performed at individual centers without requiring large sharing networks.
- Type O recipients with incompatible donors are likely to be the primary beneficiary of exchange programs.
- These programs reflect a paradigm shift for live donation, converting a private resource (the donor) to a shared one.
- Both donors and recipients are more willing to participate if their intended recipient or donor is enthusiastic about participating.

Chkhotua A. Paired kidney donation: outcomes, limitations, and future perspectives. *Transplant Proc.* 2012;44: 1790-1792.

Mierzejewska B, Durlik M, Lisik W, et al. Current approaches in national kidney paired donation programs. *Ann Transplant.* 2013;18:112-124.

A.14. What are some barriers to receiving a kidney transplant?

Absolute contraindications to kidney transplantation include active infections, active malignancy, active substance misuse, reversible renal failure, uncontrolled psychiatric disease, documented active and ongoing treatment nonadherence, and a significantly shortened life expectancy. Recipient age alone is not a contraindication to transplant. However, recipients should have an estimated life expectancy longer than the anticipated waiting time for a kidney. A living donor transplant is often the best option for an older patient.

HIV infection is not a contraindication to acquiring a kidney. The US HIV Organ Policy Equity (HOPE) Act ended a federal ban on transplantation of organs from deceased HIV-infected donors to HIV-infected recipients. The new policy will expand the number of donor organs available for transplantation to patients who are HIV positive. The potential recipient should be clinically stable on highly active antiretroviral therapy (HAART), with an undetectable viral load and a CD4 count greater than or equal to 200 cells/μL.

Because the incidence of obesity has increased in the general population, more patients with higher weight are referred for kidney transplantation. Patients with higher weight have increased risk for delayed graft failure. Diet and/or bariatric surgery are beneficial for patients with a BMI of 40 kg/m^2 or more prior to transplantation. Improvements in postoperative management have resulted in similar graft survival and mortality in patients with higher weight compared to patients with normal weight.

Many patients on hemodialysis are infected with hepatitis B and/or hepatitis C. Currently, chronic hepatitis B is treated with interferon α-2a or interferon α-2b and lamivudine. Antiviral treatment with interferon is contraindicated after transplantation due to the risk of rejection, so treatment is recommended before transplant. Unlike interferon, lamivudine is a safe and effective antiviral treatment for hepatitis B virus (HBV) both before and after renal transplantation. New treatment strategies with oral nucleotide NS5B polymerase inhibitors (sofosbuvir) are revolutionizing therapy for HCV. A recipient infected with HCV can accept an organ from an HCV-positive donor. Established HBV or HCV with cirrhosis and active viral infection is a relative contraindication to renal transplantation.

Bahde R, Vowinkel T, Unser J, et al. Prognostic factors for kidney allograft survival in the Eurotransplant Senior Program. *Ann Transplant.* 2014;19:201-209.

Burra P, Rodríguez-Castro KI, Marchini F, et al. Hepatitis C virus infection in end-stage renal disease and kidney transplantation. *Transpl Int.* 2014;27:877-891.

Malani PN. New law allows organ transplants from deceased HIV-infected donors to HIV-infected recipients. *JAMA.* 2013;310:2492-2493.

Nicoletto BB, Fonseca NK, Manfro RC, et al. Effects of obesity on kidney transplantation outcomes: a systematic review and meta-analysis. *Transplantation.* 2014;98:167-176.

A.15. What surgical techniques are available for donor nephrectomy?

The standard techniques for donor nephrectomy are open, laparoscopic, and hand-assisted laparoscopic surgery. Laparoscopic living donor nephrectomy (LLDN) has increased in frequency. In some centers, it has replaced open donor nephrectomy as the standard technique. Laparoscopic donor nephrectomy results in less blood loss, reduced operative time, and shorter hospital stay than open donor nephrectomy. Hand-assisted laparoscopic donor nephrectomy has the potential to decrease warm ischemia time for renal allografts. Donors managed laparoscopically have fewer complications, significantly less wound-related morbidity, and less delayed graft function than patients who undergo open donor nephrectomy. Robotic nephrectomy offers several advantages compared to standard laparoscopic approaches. For example, a robotic system restores the three-dimensional vision lost in the laparoscopic approach and enhances the ability of the surgeon to perform complex tasks. Laparoendoscopic single-site surgery (LESS) uses one extraction site to place all ports to minimize the invasiveness of the planned procedure. A hybrid technique uses one periumbilical access and extraction site and an additional 2-mm needlescopic port. A robot can be used to aid in the surgery.

Caso JR. Minimally invasive donor nephrectomy: innovations. *Curr Urol Rep.*2014;15:378.

Giacomoni A, Di Sandro S, Lauterio A, et al. Evolution of robotic nephrectomy for living donation: from hand-assisted to totally robotic technique. *Int J Med Robot.* 2014;10:286-293.

A.16. How is a donor kidney preserved?

Currently, static cold storage and hypothermic pulsatile machine perfusion are the two methods most widely used to preserve donor kidneys. The benefit of one method over the other is debated. In static cold storage, the kidney is flushed, cooled with one of several cold preservation solutions, and transported on ice. In hypothermic machine perfusion, after an initial washout of blood, the kidney is connected to a perfusion device, and a solution is pumped continuously through the organ at temperatures between 1 °C and 10 °C until the moment of graft placement.

Preservation solutions are agents that do not readily permeate the cell membrane and have an electrolyte composition similar to the intracellular environment (low sodium, high potassium), thus preventing loss of cellular potassium. The organ-preserving cold storage interval is called cold ischemia time (CIT). It extends from the initiation of cold preservation of donor organs to restoration of warm circulation in the organ recipient. In general, kidneys with a CIT over 24 hours or more are susceptible to delayed graft function. Delayed graft function means a requirement for dialysis in the first week after transplantation.

As more suboptimal donor kidneys are used, machine perfusion has regained clinical interest. Hypothermic machine perfusion reduces delayed graft function compared with static cold. There is no difference in primary nonfunction, acute rejection, long-term renal function, or patient survival between the two methods.

As DCD donation becomes more widespread, newer strategies to minimize the ischemic injury to the donor organ are being developed, such as use of ECMO at body temperature to restore circulation with oxygenated blood to the abdominal organs in situ immediately following declaration of donor death; this is also referred to as normothermic regional perfusion.

Kidneys from living donors are easier to handle. The organ is flushed with preservation solution or iced Ringer's lactate solution containing heparin and mannitol. The ischemic time during implantation is usually 20 to 30 minutes because the transplant operation takes place immediately. Some practices place the living donor kidney in a pulsatile preservation machine that maintains organ viability for longer periods of time. Improved immunosuppression and lower CIT have contributed to improvements in graft function and survival.

Bathini V, McGregor T, McAlister VC, et al. Renal perfusion pump vs cold storage for donation after cardiac death kidneys: a systematic review. *J Urol.* 2013;189:2214-2220.

O'Callaghan JM, Morgan RD, Knight SR, et al. Systematic review and meta-analysis of hypothermic machine perfusion versus static cold storage of kidney allografts on transplant outcomes. *Br J Surg.* 2013;100:991-1001.

Padilla M, Coll E, Fernández-Pérez C, et al. Improved short-term outcomes of kidney transplants in controlled donation after the circulatory determination of death with the use of normothermic regional perfusion. *Am J Transplant.* 2021;21:3618-3628.

A.17. Describe the operative procedure of kidney transplantation.

Prior to the induction of anesthesia, a large-bore peripheral intravenous line (18- or 16-gauge) is required. If necessary for vascular access, following induction of anesthesia, a triple-lumen central line can be placed either via the internal jugular or subclavian vein. A urinary catheter is placed in the bladder, and the bladder is irrigated with an antibiotic solution. Fluids are infused liberally through the central

SECTION 6

line and intravenous line. An arterial catheter might also be placed depending on the patient's underlying clinical status.

A kidney is harvested from a living donor using a left-flank laparoscopic approach. Harvesting of the left kidney is favored because the left renal vein is longer. New surgical techniques allow preservation of longer arterial length on the harvested kidney. Longer vessel preservation facilitates right kidney donation.

The donor kidney is placed in either the right or left iliac fossa. The right kidney is usually placed in the left groin and vice versa. The renal artery of the donor kidney is connected to the external or internal iliac artery in the recipient. The renal vein of the donor kidney is connected to the external iliac vein in the recipient. Occasionally, a donor kidney has multiple renal arteries. This is addressed using primary or secondary anastomosis. A multiple-artery donor kidney has a longer operative and ischemic time than a kidney with a single artery. In the event that the recipient weighs less than 20 kg, the kidney is placed intra-abdominally posterior to the right colon. Urinary continuity is restored by placing the distal ureter into the bladder through a tunnel without opening the bladder.

In deceased-donor kidney transplant, prior to the release of the arterial clamp and following completion of the anastomosis, an intra-arterial injection of verapamil or papaverine can be given directly into the renal artery to prevent arterial vasospasm.

Chedid MF, Muthu C, Nyberg SL, et al. Living donor kidney transplantation using laparoscopically procured multiple renal artery kidneys and right kidneys. *J Am Coll Surg*. 2013;217:144-152.

B. Preoperative Evaluation and Preparation

B.1. What preoperative workup would you order for a recipient?

The transplant recipient should receive a thorough, multidisciplinary workup prior to being listed as a candidate on the waitlist. This workup should include routine tests such as ECG, chest radiography, complete blood count, serum electrolytes and glucose, blood urea nitrogen and creatinine concentration, coagulation tests, and liver function tests.

Because cardiac disease is prevalent in this population and cardiac events are the leading cause of posttransplant mortality, a thorough cardiac evaluation is recommended. In addition to adhering to the established 2024 American College of Cardiology/American Heart Association (ACC/AHA) guidelines on perioperative cardiovascular evaluation of patients undergoing noncardiac surgery, additional testing can be considered in pretransplant patients. Specifically, noninvasive stress testing can be considered in kidney transplantation candidates with no active cardiac conditions based on the presence of multiple coronary artery disease risk factors regardless of functional status. Relevant risk factors among transplantation candidates include diabetes mellitus, prior cardiovascular disease, more than 1 year on dialysis, left ventricular hypertrophy, age more than 60 years, smoking, hypertension, and dyslipidemia. Additionally, there is some recent evidence that the coronary artery calcium score (CACS), a noninvasive diagnostic test for advanced coronary artery disease performed by nonenhanced computed tomography with minimal radiation, can be useful as a primary risk stratification tool in this patient population. Medical treatment or intervention for coronary artery disease is recommended when indicated.

Routine hemodialysis should be avoided in the 24 hours prior to transplantation because it can increase the risk of delayed graft function. This recommendation is different for patients dependent on dialysis undergoing nontransplant surgery, for whom dialysis in the 24 hours prior to surgery is generally recommended. If hemodialysis needs to be done within 24 hours of the operation, it is best to avoid overzealous ultrafiltration as expanded filling pressures are desired, and intravascular volume depletion can result in severe hypotension during or after anesthetic induction.

Lentine KL, Costa SP, Weir MR, et al. Cardiac disease evaluation and management among kidney and liver transplantation candidates: a scientific statement from the American Heart Association and the American College of Cardiology Foundation. *J Am Coll Cardiol*. 2012;60:434-480.

Thompson A, et al. 2024 AHA/ACC/ACS/ASNC/HRS/SCA/SCCT/SCMR/SVM guideline for perioperative cardiovascular management for noncardiac surgery: a report of the American College of Cardiology/American Heart Association Joint Committee on Clinical Practice Guidelines. *Circulation*. 2024;150:e351-e442.

Winther S, Bøttcher M, Jørgensen HS, et al. Coronary calcium score may replace cardiovascular risk factors as primary risk stratification tool before kidney transplantation. *Transplantation*. 2016;100:2177-2187.

B.2. How does the presence of obesity affect the outcome of a transplanted kidney?

The benefit of renal transplantation in patients with higher weight is controversial, with many centers setting upper limits on BMI in consideration for listing patients for transplant. Historically, high BMI at transplant has been associated with increased risk of wound and surgical site infections, delayed graft function, acute rejection episodes, and graft loss. However, more recent evidence suggests that long-term overall outcomes are similar between patients with higher weight and normal weight. Prospective evaluations of the impact of targeted risk modification such as dietary changes and monitored exercise programs are being investigated at this time. Bariatric surgery is both safe and effective in patients with CKD and ESRD. A sleeve gastrectomy improves eligibility for transplant based on BMI and does not affect postoperative immunosuppressant dosing regimens. All patients presenting for kidney transplant should be considered to have a full stomach regardless of the period of preoperative fasting.

Lentine KL, Delos Santos R, Axelrod D, et al. Obesity and kidney transplant candidates: how big is too big for transplantation? *Am J Nephrol.* 2012;36:575-586.

Pham PT, Danovitch GM, Pham PC. Kidney transplantation in the obese transplant candidates: to transplant or not to transplant? *Semin Dial.* 2013;26:568-577.

Sureshkumar KK, Chopra B, Josephson MA, Shah PB, McGill RL. Recipient obesity and kidney transplant outcomes: a mate-kidney analysis. *Am J Kidney Dis.* 2021;78:501-510.

B.3. How are routine medications and immunosuppressive medications managed in the perioperative period?

Patients awaiting transplant often have comorbidities such as hypertension and diabetes mellitus. Antihypertensive drugs should be continued until the time of surgery. There are no rigorous studies in the transplant population regarding the protective value of β-blocker use. It is recommended that β-blockade be continued to reduce the risk of myocardial infarction. Medications such as angiotensin-converting enzyme inhibitors (ACE-I) and angiotensin II receptor blockers (ARB) should be omitted because of the risk of severe and refractory intraoperative hypotension. Despite careful antihypertensive therapy, patient hemodynamics can still be labile during induction, laryngoscopy, tracheal intubation, and extubation.

Oral hypoglycemic agents should be held on the morning of surgery. An insulin sliding scale can be used to manage patients on insulin. The sliding scale may be used intraoperatively if high blood glucose levels are measured. Antibiotic prophylaxis for infectious complications includes a first-generation cephalosporin (cefazolin 2 g IV), or an alternative such as vancomycin (1 g IV).

Anxiolytics should be titrated carefully because these patients can have increased sensitivity to premedication. For example, diazepam is highly bound to albumin, but with decreased albumin levels, the effect of the drug is increased. Midazolam is water soluble and so less affected by albumin levels, and can be useful prior to induction.

Prior to entering the operating room, patients are given intravenous corticosteroids and an immunosuppressive agent. Diphenhydramine and acetaminophen should be given before rabbit antithymocyte globulin (Thymoglobulin) is infused intraoperatively. Under specific circumstances, basiliximab (Simulect) is substituted for Thymoglobulin. This is typically done if the patient has history of reaction to Thymoglobulin, has significantly decreased cardiac function, or is not a perfect match to the donor kidney. Both Thymoglobulin and basiliximab can be administered either peripherally or centrally. No prophylactic premedication is required with basiliximab. Rituximab and plasmapheresis followed by intravenous immunoglobulin are incorporated into the regimens of those patients with a positive crossmatch. A steroid-sparing regimen includes intraoperative methylprednisolone, which is tapered over 4 days. Patients go home taking only tacrolimus (Prograf) and mycophenolate mofetil (CellCept). In the steroid protocol, patients are continued on prednisone.

Spiro MD, Eilers H. Intraoperative care of the transplant patient. *Anesthesiol Clin.* 2013;31:705-721.

C. Intraoperative Management

C.1. Are a central venous pressure (CVP) catheter, an arterial catheter, and a pulmonary artery catheter required for the transplant procedure?

Measuring the CVP is not an absolute requirement; however, ensuring adequate hydration is an important part of the anesthetic management in renal transplantation. Most patients will have undergone

SECTION 6

hemodialysis within 48 hours of surgery and can thus be hypovolemic. To decrease the incidence of postoperative acute tubular necrosis (ATN), a liberal hydration policy is employed intraoperatively. However, current guidelines from the Transplant Anesthesia Committee of the American Society of Anesthesiologists state that CVP is a poor indicator for intraoperative volume status, and static CVP measurements should not be used to guide volume resuscitation. Alternate dynamic measurements, such as pulse-pressure variation, are better for assessing volume responsiveness.

An arterial line is not absolutely required for the transplant procedure. It should be placed if a patient has an advanced comorbid condition that requires close monitoring of blood pressure or acid-base status. Placement of an intra-arterial line can be difficult because many recipients have poor arterial access secondary to diabetes mellitus, peripheral vascular disease, arteriovenous fistulas, and shunts. Major changes in blood pressure can occur, with hypotension (49.6%) being more likely than hypertension (26.8%). Induction drugs and maintenance agents should be titrated carefully. The main utility of instantaneous blood pressure reading is toward the end of the procedure. Hypotension can occur after unclamping of the iliac vessels and/or from partial systemic absorption of the vasodilator (verapamil or papaverine) injected by the surgeon into the graft vessels. Hypotension must be avoided during this period because it can lead to delayed graft function and/or renal vein thrombosis. For example, evidence suggests that mean arterial pressure (MAP) less than 70 mm Hg is associated with delayed graft function.

A pulmonary artery catheter is not routinely placed for kidney transplantation. Patients with severe comorbid conditions, such as symptomatic coronary artery disease, left ventricular dysfunction, congestive heart failure, valvular heart disease, or severe chronic obstructive pulmonary disease, can be monitored precisely with a pulmonary artery catheter. Transesophageal echocardiography can help determine if hypotension is caused by hypovolemia or myocardial dysfunction.

Kannan G, Loganathan S, Kajal K, et al. The effect of pulse pressure variation compared with central venous pressure on intraoperative fluid management during kidney transplant surgery: a randomized controlled trial. *Can J Anaesth.* 2022;69:62-71.

Othman MM, Ismael AZ, Hammouda GE. The impact of timing of maximal crystalloid hydration on early graft function during kidney transplantation. *Anesth Analg.* 2010;110:1440-1446.

Wagener G, Bezinover D, Wang C, et al. Fluid management during kidney transplantation: a consensus statement of the committee on transplant anesthesia of the American Society of Anesthesiologists. *Transplantation.* 2021;105:1677-1684.

C.2. What type of intravenous fluid should be used during surgery?

Administration of normal saline and normal saline-based fluids (5% albumin) has been the standard of care for fluid management in patients undergoing renal transplant surgery. This practice is primarily based on avoidance of potassium-containing fluids, which could contribute to intraoperative hyperkalemia. However, several recent studies suggest a higher risk of acidosis and hyperkalemia when using normal saline solutions versus balanced saline solutions such as Ringer's lactate or Plasma-Lyte, and no difference in clinical outcomes. Therefore, many transplant centers have made the switch to administering balanced, potassium-containing solutions. The typical fluid requirement for a 70-kg adult is about 3,000 to 4,000 mL. Often, 500 mL of 5% albumin is given as a colloid.

Recipients typically undergo blood type testing and screening, but because blood loss is minimal, transfusion is unlikely. Administration of adequate volumes of fluid is associated with earlier onset of graft function, lower postoperative serum creatinine, higher postoperative creatinine clearance, reduced incidence of delayed graft function, and improved graft survival.

Nesseler N, Rached A, Ross JT, et al. Association between perioperative normal saline and delayed graft function in deceased-donor kidney transplantation: a retrospective observational study. *Can J Anaesth.* 2020;67:421-429.

Wagener G, Bezinover D, Wang C, et al. Fluid management during kidney transplantation: a consensus statement of the committee on transplant anesthesia of the American Society of Anesthesiologists. *Transplantation.* 2021;105:1677-1684.

Wan S, Roberts MA, Mount P. Normal saline versus lower-chloride solutions for kidney transplantation. *Cochrane Database Syst Rev.* 2016;2016:CD010741.

Weinberg L, Harris L, Bellomo R, et al. Effects of intraoperative and early postoperative normal saline or Plasma-Lyte 148® on hyperkalaemia in deceased donor renal transplantation: a double-blind randomized trial. *Br J Anaesth.* 2017;119:606-615.

C.3. How would you conduct the induction of anesthesia?

Renal transplantation can be a scheduled or emergent procedure. Living donor transplants are scheduled. Patients receiving cadaver kidneys might learn of the surgical procedure on short notice. Standard anesthesia monitors are required prior to induction. If needed, a central venous line and/or arterial line are usually placed after induction of anesthesia unless indicated for induction itself.

The induction of general anesthesia and tracheal intubation can be safely accomplished with commonly used drugs. The induction drugs should be given slowly to minimize the chance of drug-induced hypotension. Regardless of blood volume status, these patients often respond to induction of anesthesia as if they were hypovolemic. The sympathetic nervous system response can be attenuated by antihypertensive therapy or diabetic autonomic neuropathy. A blunted sympathetic response impairs compensatory peripheral vasoconstriction. In addition, the central nervous system (CNS) can exhibit increased sensitivity to the induction drugs. Low serum protein and albumin levels can increase the level of unbound drug crossing the blood-brain barrier into CNS receptors. Uremia can also disrupt the blood-brain barrier. The dose of induction agent might need to be adjusted based on volume status, acidic pH, and comorbidities. Propofol or etomidate can be used in routine circumstances. A reduced induction dose of propofol might be considered because lower plasma protein levels and post-hemodialysis hypovolemia can exaggerate its cardiac depressant effects. Ketamine pharmacokinetics are not significantly altered by renal disease, but its hypertensive effects make it undesirable in patients with underlying hypertension. Etomidate is well tolerated and preserves hemodynamic stability.

Large fluctuations in blood pressure and heart rate can occur in patients with preexisting hypertension during intubation. Underlying coronary artery disease should be carefully managed. Opioids can blunt the response to laryngoscopy. Fentanyl can be used in moderate doses, but there is a risk of hypotension after induction with lack of stimulation. Remifentanil is also effective for heart rate control. A short-acting β-blocker such as esmolol (0.5-1.0 mg/kg) can blunt the response to tracheal intubation.

A number of neuromuscular blocking agents can be used to facilitate tracheal intubation. A rapid sequence induction with cricoid pressure using either succinylcholine or rocuronium can be used to prevent reflux and aspiration. Succinylcholine can be used safely because potassium release is not exaggerated in patients with chronic renal failure. If the preoperative potassium is in the high normal range or if there is underlying metabolic acidosis, an additional increase of 0.5 to 1.0 mEq/L should be considered. A nondepolarizing neuromuscular blocking agent is used for the maintenance phase of anesthesia.

Schmid S, Jungwirth B. Anaesthesia for renal transplant surgery: an update. *Eur J Anaesthesiol.* 2012;29:552-558.

SECTION 6

C.4. Is succinylcholine contraindicated in patients with renal failure?

Normally, succinylcholine causes an increase in serum potassium of 0.5 to 1.0 mEq/L within 3 to 5 minutes after intravenous administration, which lasts for less than 10 to 15 minutes. Succinylcholine can be used safely in patients with chronic renal failure if the potassium concentration is less than 5.5 mEq/L and repeated doses are avoided. Potassium flux after administration of succinylcholine in patients with renal failure does not differ from normal patients. Plasma cholinesterase activity can be below normal in more than 20% of patients with ESRD whether they are receiving any form of hemodialysis. Values are rarely so low that they cause a prolonged block.

Brull SJ, et al. Pharmacology of neuromuscular blocking drugs and antagonists (reversal agents). In: Gropper M, ed. *Miller's Anesthesia*. 10th ed. Elsevier; 2025:674-741.

C.5. How are nondepolarizing neuromuscular blockers affected by renal failure?

Table 26.2 notes the commonly used nondepolarizing neuromuscular blocking agents and how they are affected by renal failure. The prolonged duration of action to nondepolarizing agents is primarily due to

TABLE 26.2 Pharmacokinetics of Neuromuscular Blocking Agents in Normal Patients Versus Patients in Anephric State

Drug	Renal Excretion (%)	Normal $T_{1/2}$ (min)	Anephric $T_{1/2}$ (min)
Pancuronium	85	132	258
Rocuronium	10	42	58
Vecuronium	40-50	54	84
Atracurium	10-40	18	24
Cisatracurium	16	34	No effect
Mivacurium	<5	1.8	3.6
Succinylcholine	<25	1	1

$T_{1/2}$, half-life.

slow renal clearance. Cisatracurium mainly undergo Hofmann elimination that is not altered in patients with CKD. Renal failure can delay clearance of laudanosine, the principal metabolite of cisatracurium. Laudanosine does not have effect at the neuromuscular junction, but at high plasma levels, it can act as a CNS stimulant. The long-acting neuromuscular blocking agent pancuronium is not suitable for use because the kidneys excrete most of the drug and its metabolite. The prolonged effect of a nondepolarizing agent is not usually apparent after a single small dose. After a small dose, the termination of action is by redistribution rather than elimination. It is only after a single large dose, repeated dosing, or prolonged infusion that the increased elimination half-life becomes clinically apparent. It has also been shown that there are large differences in pharmacokinetics in patients with renal failure receiving rocuronium. Maintenance doses for patients with decreased renal function should be smaller, and the interval between doses should be increased. Monitoring of neuromuscular blockade with a nerve stimulator is recommended.

If steroidal nondepolarizing neuromuscular blocking agents were used during induction and maintenance of anesthesia, novel aminosteroid reversal agents such as sugammadex can be safely used in patients with ESRD. Observational studies demonstrate that sugammadex results in full reversal of neuromuscular blockade without adverse postoperative outcomes during the first 48 hours. Long-term safety of rocuronium-sugammadex complexes is still unknown, but no evidence to date suggests significant adverse safety profiles.

Adams DR, Tollinche LE, Yeoh CB, et al. Short-term safety and effectiveness of sugammadex for surgical patients with end-stage renal disease: a two-centre retrospective study. Anaesthesia. 2020;75:348-352.

Brull SJ, et al. Pharmacology of neuromuscular blocking drugs and antagonists (reversal agents). In: Gropper M, ed. *Miller's Anesthesia*. 10th ed. Elsevier; 2025:674-741.

Staals LM, de Boer HD, van Egmond J, et al. Reversal of rocuronium-induced neuromuscular block by sugammadex is independent of renal perfusion in anesthetized cats. *J Anesth*. 2011;25:241-246.

Staals LM, Snoeck MM, Driessen JJ, et al. Reduced clearance of rocuronium and sugammadex in patients with severe to end-stage renal failure: a pharmacokinetic study. *Br J Anaesth*. 2010;104:31-39.

C.6. How would you maintain anesthesia during the case?

General anesthesia is the preferred technique for kidney transplantation. Volatile agents, opioids, and a neuromuscular blocking agent are required to provide optimal operating conditions.

The choice of inhaled anesthetic includes sevoflurane or isoflurane. While desflurane is also an option, it has fallen out of favor as an inhalational anesthetic due to its contributions to greenhouse gas emissions. Neither desflurane nor isoflurane have nephrotoxic potential secondary to fluoride accumulation. There was concern that sevoflurane might contribute to renal toxicity due to the accumulation of Compound A as a metabolite. While Compound A does accumulate and cause renal toxicity in rats, there is no evidence that it has any clinical effects in humans. Furthermore, newer carbon dioxide absorbents made from calcium chloride and calcium hydroxide produce negligible amounts of Compound A.

Opioids such as fentanyl, sufentanil, and remifentanil can be used during the procedure. Morphine and meperidine have active metabolites that depend on renal clearance and can accumulate and should be avoided if possible.

Hypotension can occur after unclamping the iliac vessels and reperfusion of the graft. It is important to maintain the blood pressure because renal function is critically dependent on adequate perfusion. It is crucial that the patient is adequately hydrated throughout surgery in preparation for reperfusion of the graft. Close monitoring of volume status and reducing the level of anesthesia during hemodynamic instability can prevent hypotension. Vasopressors with α-agonist action should be avoided because they can compromise blood flow to the transplanted kidney. Additional fluid may be required to maintain blood pressure and replace urine output. Furosemide or mannitol can enhance urine output. Loop diuretics block the Na/K transporters in the thin ascending loop of Henle. This prevents reabsorption of electrolytes in this part of the nephron. The high-osmolar fluid then prevents reabsorption of water in the distal tubule. A large volume of fluid with high electrolyte content is excreted. Mannitol is freely filtered in the glomerulus but not reabsorbed. It causes osmotic expansion of urine volume.

Estimated blood loss is usually between 200 and 500 mL. In some cases, greater blood loss requires transfusion of packed red blood cells. Packed red blood cells should be cytomegalovirus negative. At the end of surgery, patients can be given reversal agents and extubated promptly. Patients are then transferred to the postanesthesia care unit (PACU) for continued monitoring of urine output and electrolytes.

Devlin-Hegedus JA, McGain F, Harris RD, Sherman JD. Action guidance for addressing pollution from inhalational anaesthetics. *Anaesthesia*. 2022;77:1023-1029.

Morris P, Knechtle SJ. *Kidney Transplantation: Principles and Practice*. 7th ed. Saunders Elsevier; 2014.

Park M, Jung K, Cho HS, Min JJ. Renal injury from sevoflurane in noncardiac surgery: a retrospective cohort study. *Br J Anaesth.* 2022;129:182-190.

Spiro MD, Eilers H. Intraoperative care of the transplant patient. *Anesthesiol Clin.* 2013;31:705-721.

Yamakage M, Takahashi K, Takahashi M, Satoh JI, Namiki A. Performance of four carbon dioxide absorbents in experimental and clinical settings. *Anaesthesia.* 2009;64:287-292.

C.7. What are the effects of inhalation anesthetics on renal blood flow (RBF), glomerular filtration (GFR), and urine output?

All volatile anesthetics produce a dose-related transient and reversible decrease in RBF, GFR, urine output, and the urinary excretion of sodium. This is primarily in response to a decline in systemic blood pressure and cardiac output. Reduced RBF, loss of renal autoregulation, and neurohumoral and neuroendocrine factors also contribute. Specific differences between agents on renal function are to be noted. Desflurane and sevoflurane are two most frequently used inhalational anesthetics. Use of desflurane has demonstrated better hepatic and renal function tests after surgery compared to sevoflurane.

Brull SJ, et al. Pharmacology of neuromuscular blocking drugs and antagonists (reversal agents). In: Gropper M, ed. *Miller's Anesthesia.* 10th ed. Elsevier; 2025:674-741.

Ko JS, Gwak MS, Choi SJ, et al. The effects of desflurane and sevoflurane on hepatic and renal functions after right hepatectomy in living donors. *Transpl Int.* 2010;23:736-744.

C.8. How does renal failure affect the pharmacology of opioids?

The effect of renal failure on individual opioids varies, so one must consider the effect of renal failure on drug metabolites as well as the parent compound.

Morphine is metabolized in the liver to morphine-6-glucuronide (M6G) (10%), morphine-3-glucuronide (M3G) (55%), and normorphine (4%), all of which are excreted by the kidneys, along with about 10% of the parent compound, in subjects with normal renal function. M6G can produce CNS and respiratory depression when it accumulates in renal failure.

Meperidine is metabolized in the liver to normeperidine, which is also excreted by the kidneys. Accumulation of this metabolite can lead to excitatory CNS effects including convulsions.

Fentanyl is metabolized by the liver, with only 7% excreted unchanged in the urine. Fentanyl is suitable for use during surgery and is safe in the short term. There are reports of the parent compound accumulating during renal failure, but clinical experience is that there are no adverse effects. However, if being used long term in patients with renal failure, the pharmacodynamic effects should be monitored carefully.

Alfentanil metabolism occurs by inducible cytochrome C enzymes in the liver, making it suitable for patients with renal failure. The clearance and half-life of sufentanil and alfentanil are not significantly different in patients with reduced renal function.

Remifentanil is metabolized by blood and tissue esterases. The principle metabolite of remifentanil (GR90291) is eliminated by the kidney. The reduced renal elimination of this metabolite is not of clinical significance because the potency is 4,000-fold less that of the parent compound.

Nayak-Rao S. Achieving effective pain relief in patients with chronic kidney disease: a review of analgesics in renal failure. *J Nephrol.* 2011;24:35-40.

Niscola P, Scaramucci L, Vischini G, et al. The use of major analgesics in patients with renal dysfunction. *Curr Drug Targets.* 2010;11:752-758.

C.9. Can regional anesthesia be used to optimize postoperative analgesia?

Because systemic opioids have altered pharmacokinetics and pharmacodynamics in the setting of renal failure, postoperative opioids can have deleterious effects on patients who have undergone a kidney transplant. A multimodal approach to analgesia is optimal, and regional anesthesia can help to reduce postoperative opioid consumption.

The gold standard for open intra-abdominal surgeries is analgesia using a thoracic epidural. A standard postoperative infusion would involve an opioid and local anesthetic solution. However, due to the risk of postoperative hypotension in patients with kidney transplant, epidural analgesia might not be optimal due to the risk of further potentiating hypotension from the partial sympathectomy induced by the analgesic infusion.

Given that the surgical incision is in the right or left flank of the anterior abdominal wall, the anatomy of the procedure lends itself well to the use of regional anesthesia. Specifically, truncal blocks, such as a transversus abdominis plane (TAP) block, can be used to anesthetize the abdominal wall to treat somatic incisional pain. Patients undergoing kidney transplant can have multiple risk factors for developing local anesthetic systemic toxicity (LAST) including cardiac disease, renal disease, and variable volume of distribution, so care must be taken to use an appropriate amount of local anesthetic during block placement. The addition of epinephrine to the peripheral nerve block should aid in reducing the risk of LAST while having no effect hemodynamic status.

Hanson NA, Strunk J, Saunders G, et al. Comparison of continuous intravenous lidocaine versus transversus abdominis plane block for kidney transplant surgery: a randomized, non-inferiority trial. *Reg Anesth Pain Med.* 2021;46:955-959.

Johnson MD, Mickler T, Arthur GR, Rosenburg S, Wilson R. Bupivacaine with and without epinephrine for intercostal nerve block. *J Cardiothorac Anesth.* 1990;4:200-203.

Neal JM, Barrington MJ, Fettiplace MR, et al. The Third American Society of Regional Anesthesia and Pain Medicine Practice Advisory on local anesthetic systemic toxicity: executive summary 2017. *Reg Anesth Pain Med.* 2018;43:113-123.

D. Postoperative Management

D.1. How is the diagnosis of transplant rejection made?

There are various forms of rejection such as hyperacute, accelerated acute, acute, and chronic. Acute rejection is the most common, but less common with immunosuppressive agents. It is usually seen within days to a few months posttransplant. The diagnosis is made with a renal biopsy. In patients with prolonged delayed graft function, surveillance biopsies can detect or exclude acute rejection episodes. The process is associated with systemic symptoms such as fever, chills, malaise, and arthralgias. However, with current immunosuppressive drugs, most acute rejection episodes are asymptomatic. A rapid increase in creatinine of 10% to 25% over baseline with or without a decrease in urine output can occur with rejection.

Nankivell BJ, Alexander SI. Rejection of the kidney allograft. *N Engl J Med.* 2010;363:1451-1462.

D.2. What are immunosuppressive agents, and how do they affect anesthetic care?

Induction antirejection drugs are used at the time of transplantation. The patient is then placed on long-term maintenance drugs. There are generally four classes of maintenance drugs:

- CNIs: tacrolimus, belatacept, cyclosporine
- Antiproliferative agents: mycophenolate mofetil, mycophenolate sodium, azathioprine
- TOR inhibitors: sirolimus, everolimus
- Steroids: prednisone

Some of the side effects of immunosuppressive agents can be encountered if a posttransplant patient presents for other surgeries and are pertinent to anesthetic care:

- Calcineurin inhibitors: nephrotoxicity, hypertension, hyperchloremic acidosis, hyperkalemia, hypomagnesemia, hypocalcemia, glucose intolerance, coarse tremor, dysesthesia, headache, seizure, prolonged QT interval, hypercoagulability, acute microvascular disease (similar to thrombotic thrombocytopenic purpura)
- Mycophenolate mofetil: nausea, vomiting, cytopenia (leukopenia, anemia, thrombocytopenia), leukocytosis
- TOR inhibitors: mucocutaneous ulceration, hypokalemia, hypomagnesemia, impaired wound healing, interstitial pneumonia, cytopenia
- Azathioprine: cytopenia, hepatitis

Halleck F, Friedersdorff F, Fuller TF, et al. New perspectives of immunosuppression. *Transplant Proc.* 2013;45:1224-1231.

Laftavi MR, Sharma R, Feng L, et al. Induction therapy in renal transplant recipients: a review. *Immunol Invest.* 2014;43:790-806.

Acknowledgment

We gratefully acknowledge the contributions of previous editions author, Fun-Sun F. Yao, as portions of those chapters have been retained in this revision.

SECTION 7 The Reproductive System

27 Placenta Previa/Placenta Accreta Spectrum

Danielle McCullough and Joe E.L. Bryant-Huppert

A 40-year-old female, gravida 6 para 5, is electively scheduled for her fourth cesarean section at 36 weeks of gestation. She has placenta previa that was diagnosed by sonography after a single episode of painless vaginal bleeding at 27 weeks of gestation, which resolved spontaneously. Her vital signs are as follows: blood pressure, 110/56 mm Hg; heart rate, 85 beats per minute; respiratory rate, 18 breaths per minute; and oxygen saturation (Spo_2), 98% on room air. Her hematocrit (Hct) is 35%.

A. Medical Disease and Differential Diagnosis

1. What are the leading causes of maternal mortality, and what role does anesthesia play in this mortality?
2. What is your differential diagnosis for this patient's antepartum hemorrhage?
3. How would you quickly differentiate and diagnose the most urgent, concerning, and likely etiologies of this patient's antepartum bleeding?
4. As your obstetric colleagues work to determine the etiology of bleeding, what is your initial management for maternal antepartum hemorrhage?
5. What is the incidence of placenta previa, and what are the associated conditions?
6. What is the usual obstetric management for placenta previa?
7. What is vasa previa and how is it managed?
8. What are the risk factors of this patient for the development of placental abruption?
9. How is placental abruption managed, and what complications can be associated with placental abruption?
10. Does this patient have any risk factors for uterine rupture?
11. What is the treatment for uterine rupture?
12. Is this patient at risk for postpartum bleeding?
13. What is placenta accreta spectrum (PAS)?
14. How is PAS diagnosed?
15. How is PAS managed obstetrically?
16. What tests and/or interventions can improve neonatal outcome of a preterm birth?

B. Preoperative Evaluation and Preparation

1. How does pregnancy change respiratory function, and what impact does this have on anesthetic care?
2. What are the maternal cardiovascular changes of pregnancy?
3. What are the maternal gastrointestinal changes of pregnancy?
4. What hematologic changes occur during pregnancy?
5. What laboratory data do you need before taking this patient to the operating room?
6. What preoperative medications would you administer to this patient?

C. Intraoperative Management

1. What monitors would you use for this patient?
2. What anesthetic approaches could be used in this patient?
3. What are the absolute and relative contraindications for neuraxial anesthesia?
4. How is postpartum hemorrhage (PPH) defined, and what are the etiologies of this bleeding?
5. After delivery of the fetus, the placenta is removed with some difficulty in one small area, and generalized oozing from the placental implantation site is noted. What is the most likely cause of this patient's bleeding?
6. After delivery of the placenta in a cesarean delivery, what maneuvers and drugs can enhance myometrial contractility and therefore decrease blood loss?
7. When should this patient receive tranexamic acid (TXA)?
8. If this patient had ongoing bleeding intraoperatively, what guidelines help determine when red blood cell (RBC) transfusions should be given?
9. What laboratory tests should be ordered during the resuscitation of this patient?
10. If this patient had a massive blood loss, what blood replacement therapy would be indicated?
11. What is the role of recombinant activated factor VII (rFVIIa) in the hemorrhaging obstetric patient?
12. What is the role of type O Rh-negative (universal donor) uncrossmatched blood in emergency transfusions, and how does this change your future management?
13. What complications can occur from transfusion of blood products?
14. What is the role of autologous transfusion in obstetric patients?
15. Significant intraoperative blood loss required the transfusion of 8 units of type-specific, crossmatched packed RBCs (pRBCs). This patient had generalized oozing in the surgical site and hematuria. What is your differential diagnosis?
16. What is disseminated intravascular coagulation (DIC)?
17. Define amniotic fluid embolism (AFE) syndrome and discuss treatment.

D. Postoperative Management

1. If the patient received epidural anesthesia and subsequently developed DIC, when should the epidural catheter be removed?
2. You have successfully treated the patient's massive hemorrhage. The laboratory values have returned to normal. The patient, however, is still hypotensive despite appropriate intravascular volume replacement and support with vasopressors. What is your concern in this case?

A. Medical Disease and Differential Diagnosis

A.1. What are the leading causes of maternal mortality, and what role does anesthesia play in this mortality?

According to 2018 World Health Organization (WHO) reporting, 99% of maternal deaths occur in developing countries. The WHO defines the maternal mortality ratio (MMR) as the number of direct and indirect maternal deaths per 100,000 live births; it does not include late maternal deaths occurring more than 42 days but less than 1 year after pregnancy termination. In the United States, based on data from the Pregnancy Mortality Surveillance System of the Centers for Disease Control and Prevention, the pregnancy-related mortality ratio (PRMR) fell significantly during the 20th century. However, more recently there has been a significant increase in documented cases of maternal mortality, from 7.2 deaths per 100,000 live births in 1987 to more than 17 deaths per 100,000 live births from 2017 onwards. This increase may be partly secondary to an artifact of changes in surveillance and increased identification of maternal deaths rather than a true increase in incidence. Nevertheless, these rates are dramatically higher for the United States compared with most other high-income countries, despite having higher overall medical spending.

The leading causes of pregnancy-related deaths in the United States in recent years are cardiovascular conditions (16.2%), sepsis (13.9%), cardiomyopathy (12.5%), and hemorrhage (11.0%). Other significant, yet less common, causes include embolism, cerebrovascular accidents, hypertensive disorders of pregnancy, amniotic fluid embolism (AFE), and complications of anesthesia. Of note, the incidence of mortality due to anesthetic complications, hemorrhage, and hypertensive disorders of pregnancy are trending down in the most recent decade. In the United States, the risk of maternal death is increased in non-Hispanic Black females compared to non-Hispanic White females and in females of advanced maternal age.

In the 21st century, MMR (the number of maternal deaths divided by the total number of live births) dropped by about 34% worldwide, with nearly 95% of deaths occurring in low- and lower middle-income countries. In these instances, nearly 75% of all maternal deaths are due to severe bleeding, infections, hypertensive disorders of pregnancy, delivery complications, and unsafe abortions. Most maternal deaths are considered preventable, as the medical management and prevention of the most common complications are well known yet not universally accessible, notably for hemorrhage, infection and sepsis, and hypertensive disorders of pregnancy. Additionally, complications in pregnancy and childbirth are a leading cause of death among adolescent girls in developing countries.

In developed regions, the estimated anesthesia-related MMR ranges between 1 and 3 deaths per 1,000,000 live births. If a maternal death can be attributed to an anesthetic complication and if an ideal anesthetic would have likely avoided this death, the death is considered anesthetic related. The most common serious anesthesia-related complications include high neuraxial block, respiratory arrest in the labor suite, and unrecognized spinal catheters. The role of anesthesiologists working as part of a skilled multidisciplinary health care team has helped to make labor and delivery not only a more pleasant experience for parturients, but they also play an essential role in ensuring the safety throughout the peripartum period for both mother and fetus.

Centers for Disease Control and Prevention. Pregnancy mortality surveillance system. Accessed July 25, 2023. https://www.cdc.gov/maternal-mortality/php/pregnancy-mortality-surveillance/index.html

Creanga AA, Syverson C, Seed K, et al. Pregnancy-related mortality in the United States, 2011–2013. *Obstet Gynecol.* 2017;130:366-373.

MacDorman MF, Declercq E, Thoma ME. Trends in maternal mortality by sociodemographic characteristics and cause of death in 27 states and the District of Columbia. *Obstet Gynecol.* 2017;129:811-818.

Say L, Chou D, Gemmill A, et al. Global causes of maternal death: a WHO systematic analysis. *Lancet Glob Health.* 2014;6:323-333.

Sobhy S, Zamora J, Dharmarajah K, et al. Anesthesia-related maternal mortality in low-income and middle-income countries: a systemic review and meta-analysis. *Lancet Glob Health.* 2016;4:e320-e327.

A.2. What is your differential diagnosis for this patient's antepartum hemorrhage?

Up to one-fourth of pregnant females may have antepartum vaginal bleeding, but only a small fraction experiences an antepartum hemorrhage. Most of this bleeding occurs in the first trimester, and bleeding in the first 20 weeks is presumed to be a threatened abortion or an ectopic pregnancy. Even if pregnancy loss does not occur, the risk for adverse outcomes later in pregnancy is increased.

For this patient, and all pregnancies with a viable living fetus, antepartum bleeding generally poses a greater threat to the fetus than the mother. The most concerning causes of antepartum hemorrhage are placenta previa, vasa previa, placental abruption, and uterine rupture. Other lesser emergent and concerning differentials include bloody show and lesions of the urogenital tract such as trauma, cervicitis, infection, erosion, tumors, or vulvovaginal varicosities.

In some cases, it is not always possible to identify the source of antepartum bleeding. Usually, this type of bleeding begins with minimal symptoms, if any, and stops; no anatomic cause is identified at delivery, and it is likely attributable to marginal placenta separation. However, these pregnancies have a higher risk of poor neonatal outcome and preterm delivery.

Battula SP, Mohammed NH, Datta S. Antepartum haemorrhage. *Obstet Gynaecol Reprod Med.* 2021;31:117-123.

Cunningham FG, Leveno KJ, Bloom SL, et al., eds. Causes of Obstetrical Hemorrhage. In: *Williams Obstetrics.* 26th ed. McGraw-Hill Education; 2022:731-748.

Gyamfi-Bannerman C. Society for maternal-fetal medicine (SMFM) consult series #44: management of bleeding in the late preterm period. *Am J Obstet Gynecol.* 2018;218:B2-B8.

McCormack RA, Doherty DA, Magann EF, et al. Antepartum bleeding of unknown origin in the second half of pregnancy and pregnancy outcomes. *BJOG.* 2008;115:1451-1457.

A.3. How would you quickly differentiate and diagnose the most urgent, concerning, and likely etiologies of this patient's antepartum bleeding?

With antepartum uterine bleeding after midpregnancy, placenta previa, placenta abruption, vasa previa, and uterine rupture should be at the top of your differential, as they pose the most imminent threat to the mother and fetus.

Classically, painless uterine bleeding is indicative of placenta previa, or possibly vasa previa after rupture of membranes with concordant fetal distress, whereas painful uterine bleeding signifies placental abruption, or uterine rupture when there is concordant loss of fetal station and fetal distress. The differential diagnosis, however, is not actually straightforward; for instance, labor or placental separation accompanying placenta previa can cause pain, whereas pain from placental abruption can mimic normal labor. Digital examination of the cervix *should be avoided* until the diagnosis of placenta previa has been excluded because it can cause immediate, severe hemorrhage.

Transabdominal sonography is a simple and safe method of locating the placenta in suspected placenta previa. Transvaginal sonography has been shown to be superior to transabdominal sonography and is currently the imaging modality of choice. On the other hand, sonography infrequently aids in the diagnosis of acute placental abruption because fresh clot and placenta appear sonographically similar. Negative findings on sonographic examination do not rule out placental abruption. Magnetic resonance imaging (MRI) has been used by numerous investigators to visualize placental abnormalities, including placenta previa and placental abruption, and it should be considered if time allows and if the diagnostic information would change patient management.

Vaginal bleeding with fetal distress or death when the membranes rupture is seen in an undiagnosed vasa previa and necessitate an emergency cesarean section based on fetal distress. If vaginal blood is present, the presence of fetal blood (RBCs) can be determined using a Kleihauer-Betke test or flow cytometry, although there is rarely time in emergent situations with fetal distress.

Uterine rupture can be difficult to diagnose because of the varied symptoms and physical findings that can occur. The most consistent sign of uterine rupture is a nonreassuring fetal heart rate pattern. In some patients, the symptoms of uterine rupture will be indistinguishable from those of placental abruption. Other signs that may be present include maternal hypotension, tachycardia, vaginal bleeding, abdominal pain, change in the uterine contour, changes in the uterine contraction pattern, and cessation of labor. There may be little pain, and because most of these ruptures occur during labor, any pain may be masked by the analgesics given to treat the discomfort of labor.

Al-Zirqi L, Stray-Pedersen B, Forsén L, et al. Uterine rupture: trends over 40 years. *BJOG*. 2016;123:780-787.

Gyamfi-Bannerman C. Society for maternal-fetal medicine (SMFM) consult series #44: management of bleeding in the late preterm period. *Am J Obstet Gynecol*. 2018;218:B2-B8.

Kulkarni A, Powel J, Aziz M, et al. Vasa previa: prenatal diagnosis and outcomes: thirty-five cases from a single maternal-fetal medicine practice. *J Ultrasound Med*. 2018;37:1017-1024.

Masselli G, Brunelli R, Di Tola M, et al. MR imaging in the evaluation of placental abruption: correlation with sonographic findings. *Radiology*. 2011;259:222-230.

Quant HS, Friedman AM, Wang E, et al. Transabdominal ultrasonography as a screening test for second-trimester placenta previa. *Obstet Gynecol*. 2014;123:628-633.

A.4. As your obstetric colleagues work to determine the etiology of bleeding, what is your initial management for maternal antepartum hemorrhage?

Initial management of the parturient should include a thorough history and physical, and evaluation of signs of hemorrhagic shock. Monitoring should include continuous pulse oximetry as well as frequent blood pressure monitoring to rule out potential hemodynamic compromise; invasive arterial monitoring may be indicated. As needed, adequate intravenous access and laboratory studies, including a complete blood count (CBC), coagulation profile, and a type and screen/crossmatch, should be obtained.

In the United States, Rh (anti-D) immunoglobulin (Ig) is offered to unsensitized Rh-negative females at 28 weeks of gestation when the fetal blood type is unknown or known to be Rh-positive and again after delivery if the neonate is Rh-positive. Anti-D Ig should be administered to Rh-negative females who have an antenatal hemorrhage after 20 weeks. Management of the patient who has intermittent antenatal bleeding is complex. With an acute bleeding episode in an Rh-negative parturient, the most conservative approach is to do a quantitative Kleihauer-Betke test to determine if a fetal-maternal transfusion has occurred and if additional Ig is required. It has been proposed that cell-free DNA testing to determine the fetal Rh D status be done to avoid repeated administration of anti-D Ig if the fetus is Rh-D negative.

American College of Obstetricians and Gynecologists Committee on Practice Bulletins—Obstetrics. Practice bulletin no. 181: prevention of Rh D alloimmunization. *Obstet Gynecol*. 2017;130:e57-e70.

Battula SP, Mohammed NH, Datta S. Antepartum haemorrhage. *Obstet Gynaecol Reprod Med*. 2021;31:117-123.

A.5. What is the incidence of placenta previa, and what are the associated conditions?

The incidence of placenta previa in the United States is about 1 in 300 to 400 deliveries. The risk of placenta previa increases with advancing maternal age, multiparity, multifetal gestations, previous cesarean delivery, prior uterine surgery, cigarette smoking, cocaine use, infertility treatments, and unexplained increases in maternal serum α-fetoprotein levels. In approximately 90% of the patients with sonographic evidence of placenta previa at 20 weeks, the placenta moved away from the cervix and out of the lower uterine segment by term.

Placenta previa is associated with an increased risk of antepartum bleeding, intrapartum and PPH, abnormalities of placental adherence, peripartum hysterectomy, blood transfusions, preterm birth with perinatal morbidity and mortality, congenital malformations, and septicemia. In the presence of a prior cesarean section, the patient with placenta previa is at greater risk for having PAS; this risk increased as the number of cesarean deliveries increased. In patients with placenta previa, the risk of placenta accreta was 3%, 11%, 40%, 61%, and 67% for the first, second, third, fourth, and fifth or greater repeat cesarean deliveries, respectively.

Cunningham FG, Leveno KJ, Bloom SL, et al., eds. Hemorrhagic Placental Disorders. In: Cunningham FG, Leveno KJ, Dashe JS, Hoffman BL, Spong CY, Casey BM, eds. *Williams Obstetrics*. 26th ed. McGraw-Hill Education; 2022:749-769.

Gibbins KJ, Einerson BD, Varner MW, et al. Placenta previa and maternal hemorrhagic morbidity. *J Matern Fetal Neonatal Med*. 2018;31:494-499.

Oyelese Y, Smulian JC. Placenta previa, placenta accreta, and vasa previa. *Obstet Gynecol*. 2006;107:927-941.

Silver RM, Landon MB, Rouse DJ, et al. Maternal morbidity associated with multiple repeat cesarean deliveries. *Obstet Gynecol*. 2006;107:1226-1232.

A.6. What is the usual obstetric management for placenta previa?

Obstetric management for patients with placenta previa depends on three things: fetal age and maturity, presence or absence of labor, and severity of bleeding. The goal of management is to maximize fetal growth and minimize the possibility of antepartum hemorrhage. With many patients, the first episode of bleeding begins without warning or pain, stops spontaneously, and rarely causes maternal or fetal compromise, but bleeding often recurs. A mature fetus with or without labor should be delivered; if bleeding occur at or beyond 36 weeks, immediate delivery is indicated. If hemorrhaging is severe or there is concern about the fetal condition, delivery should take place regardless of gestational age. Otherwise, conservative management can safely prolong the pregnancy by an average of 4 weeks after the initial bleed. Between 24 and 34 weeks of gestation, betamethasone, a corticosteroid, often is given to the patient with placenta previa to accelerate fetal lung maturity (FLM), and the Society for Maternal-Fetal Medicine (SMFM) recommends that antenatal steroids be given to patients being managed expectantly if delivery is likely within 7 days, the gestational age is between 34 0/7 and 36 6/7 weeks of gestation, and antenatal corticosteroids have not been given previously.

With a preterm fetus and no persistent active uterine bleeding, management consists of close observation for bleeding and activity restriction in an inpatient setting or, in certain selected patients, an outpatient setting. For stable patients with no bleeding in the previous 48 hours and who have ready access to hospital care, maternal and fetal outcome did not differ between outpatient and inpatient management. Maternal vital signs and hemoglobin (Hgb) are checked at regular intervals depending on when the bleeding, if it exists, subsides. The American Association of Blood Banks recommends that a blood type and screen be done every 3 days in actively bleeding pregnant females because of the risk for developing new alloantibodies. Fetal well-being also is assessed regularly. The use of tocolytic therapy in patients with placenta previa with preterm labor and bleeding is controversial; it has been used to prolong gestation if both the mother and fetus are stable, however, has not shown to decrease the incidence of hemorrhage or blood loss.

The SMFM recommends that delivery for stable females with placenta previa without bleeding should take place at 36 to 37 6/7 weeks, and if a placenta accreta is suspected, it has been recommended that delivery take place between 34 and 37 weeks. As gestational age increases, there is an increased risk of significant bleeding that would necessitate delivery: 4.7% rebleed at 35 weeks, 15% at 36 weeks, 30% at 37 weeks, and 59% at 38 weeks. If an indication for delivery is present, FLM testing does not aid in guiding management in the late preterm period when an indication for delivery is present.

Patients with placenta previa almost always are delivered by cesarean delivery. The optimal route of delivery for patients whose placenta lies within 2 cm of the cervical os is contentious as there is increased risk of hemorrhage and conversion to cesarean delivery. Therefore, shared decision-making should be undertaken between the obstetrician and patient for an attempted trial of labor, and these patients should be managed in a setting that has capability to manage appropriately.

Normally, with placenta removal, the myometrium of the uterus contracts and reestablishes vascular integrity by constricting the open vessels in the placental bed. In patients with placenta previa, bleeding after placenta removal can be brisk because the lower uterine segment contracts poorly and therefore does not constrict the avulsed vessels. There is a known association between placenta previa and placenta accreta syndrome that can further exacerbate uterine bleeding and require additional surgical and/or radiologic interventions to staunch the bleeding.

Cunningham FG, Leveno KJ, Bloom SL, et al., eds. Hemorrhagic Placental Disorders. In: Cunningham FG, Leveno KJ, Dashe JS, Hoffman BL, Spong CY, Casey BM, eds. *Williams Obstetrics*. 26th ed. McGraw-Hill Education; 2022:749-769.

Gyamfi-Bannerman C; Society for Maternal-Fetal Medicine. Society for maternal-fetal medicine (SMFM) consult series #44: management of bleeding in the late preterm period. *Am J Obstet Gynecol*. 2018;218:B2-B8.

Jansen CH, de Mooij YM, Blomaard CM, et al. Vaginal delivery in women with a low-lying placenta: a systematic review and meta-analysis. *BJOG*. 2019;126:1118-1126.

Spong CY, Mercer BM, D'alton M, et al. Timing of indicated late-preterm and early-term birth. *Obstet Gynecol*. 2011;118:323-333.

A.7. What is vasa previa and how is it managed?

Vasa previa refers to intramembranous fetal vessels, unprotected by placenta or umbilical cord, coursing through the membranes over the cervical os and under the fetal presenting part. The incidence is approximately 1 in 2,500 deliveries and associated risk factors include a second-trimester low-lying placenta/placenta previa, a placenta with accessory lobes, velamentous umbilical cord insertions, multiple pregnancies, and pregnancies from in vitro fertilization. Undiagnosed vasa previa is associated with a high fetal mortality (~60%). Because fetal blood volume is small, any detectable bleeding puts the fetus in jeopardy. When membranes rupture, either spontaneously or artificially, the fetal vessels running through these membranes often rupture. Fortunately, the majority of cases of vasa previa can be diagnosed prenatally by routinely evaluating placental cord insertion by ultrasound examination and transvaginal sonographic color Doppler if the insertion site cannot be delineated clearly. Good outcomes in patients with vasa previa require a prenatal diagnosis and delivery by cesarean delivery before the membranes rupture. If stable, the SMFM recommends that patients with vasa previa be delivered between 34 and 37 weeks of gestation.

Bronsteen R, Whitten A, Balasubramanian M, et al. Vasa previa: clinical presentations, outcomes, and implications for management. *Obstet Gynecol*. 2013;122:352-357.

Gyamfi-Bannerman C; Society for Maternal-Fetal Medicine. Society for maternal-fetal medicine (SMFM) consult series #44: management of bleeding in the late preterm period. *Am J Obstet Gynecol*. 2018;218:B2-B8.

Kulkarni A, Powel J, Aziz M, et al. Vasa previa: prenatal diagnosis and outcomes: thirty-five cases from a single maternal-fetal medicine practice. *J Ultrasound Med*. 2018;37:1017-1024.

Oyelese Y, Smulian JC. Placenta previa, placenta accreta, and vasa previa. *Obstet Gynecol*. 2006;107:927-941.

A.8. What are the risk factors of this patient for the development of placental abruption?

The frequency of placental abruption is about 1 in 200 deliveries. Premature separation of the normally implanted placenta can be total or partial and can lead to external or concealed bleeding. Concealed hemorrhage is associated with greater maternal and fetal risks. The most common condition associated with placental abruption is some type of hypertension, either gestational hypertension, preeclampsia, chronic hypertension, or some combination thereof. The incidence of placental abruption is increased with increased maternal age, body mass index, use of assisted fertility methods, Black or Caucasian race, prematurely ruptured membranes, a history of previous abruption, cigarette smoking, cocaine use, leiomyoma, an isolated uterine artery, and external trauma. Bleeding in nontraumatic placental abruption almost always is maternal because the placental separation is within the maternal decidua.

Cunningham FG, Leveno KJ, Bloom SL, et al., eds. Hemorrhagic Placental Disorders. In: Cunningham FG, Leveno KJ, Dashe JS, Hoffman BL, Spong CY, Casey BM, eds. *Williams Obstetrics*. 26th ed. McGraw-Hill Education; 2022:749-769.

Downes KL, Grantz KL, Shenassa ED. Maternal, labor, delivery, and perinatal outcomes associated with placental abruption: a systematic review. *Am J Perinatol*. 2017;34:935-957.

A.9. How is placental abruption managed, and what complications can be associated with placental abruption?

Maternal complications with severe abruption can include PPH, hemorrhagic shock, consumptive coagulopathy, acute renal injury, and Sheehan syndrome (pituitary failure).

Management and treatment of placental abruptions for the fetus depend on fetal gestational age and fetal and maternal condition. If the diagnosis is uncertain and the fetus is uncompromised, inpatient expectant management with close observation can be practiced. However, further placental separation can occur any time and lead to serious fetal compromise or death. Use of tocolytics to prolong pregnancy is controversial. Rapid delivery of the compromised, but alive, fetus is by cesarean delivery.

If placental separation has led to fetal death, vaginal delivery usually is preferred; there are two exceptions: massive hemorrhage that cannot be managed with vigorous blood replacement, and obstetric complications that prevent vaginal delivery will necessitate an operative delivery.

Battula SP, Mohammed NH, Datta S. Antepartum haemorrhage. *Obstet, Gynaeco and Reprod Med.* 2021;31: 117-123.

Cunningham FG, Leveno KJ, Bloom SL, et al., eds. Hemorrhagic Placental Disorders. In: Cunningham FG, Leveno KJ, Dashe JS, Hoffman BL, Spong CY, Casey BM, eds. *Williams Obstetrics.* 26th ed. McGraw-Hill Education; 2022:749-769.

Kayani SI, Walkinshaw SA, Preston C. Pregnancy outcome in severe placental abruption. *BJOG.* 2003;110:679-683.

A.10. Does this patient have any risk factors for uterine rupture?

This patient's risk factors for uterine rupture include grand multiparity (more than five births) and prior cesarean delivery.

Patients who have had a uterine rupture in a prior pregnancy have a higher risk of having another one. Prior cesarean delivery increases the risk of uterine rupture with a classical, T-shaped, or low vertical uterine incision increasing the incidence when compared to a low transverse incision. Other risk factors associated with uterine rupture include previous uterine surgery involving the myometrium, a tumultuous labor difficult forceps delivery, uterine trauma, breech extraction, external and internal version, labor stimulation with oxytocin or prostaglandins, inappropriate uterotonic medication use, uterine anomalies; placenta increta/percreta, connective tissue defects such as Marfan or Ehlers-Danlos syndrome, and uterine overdistention by fetal macrosomia, hydramnios, or multifetal pregnancy.

Primary uterine rupture is defined as a rupture occurring in a previously intact unscarred uterus, whereas a secondary rupture is associated with a preexisting myometrial incision, injury, or anomaly. Uterine rupture is typically classified as either complete, with all of the uterine wall layers separated, or incomplete (uterine dehiscence), with the uterine muscle separated but the visceral peritoneum intact. Uterine dehiscence is more common; it is less likely to cause adverse maternal and fetal derangements or necessitate cesarean delivery. The morbidity and mortality rates are higher when the rupture is complete. Fortunately, uterine ruptures are rare. In developed countries, uterine rupture incidence is approximated at 1 in 4,800, whereas in developing countries, the incidence is higher. The frequency of primary rupture is about 1 in 10,000 to 15,000 births, whereas the incidence in females attempting a trail of labor after previous cesarean delivery varies between about 0.5% and 4%.

American College of Obstetricians and Gynecologists Committee on Practice Bulletins—Obstetrics. Practice bulletin no. 205: vaginal birth after cesarean delivery. *Obstet Gynecol.* 2019;133:e110-e127.

Cunningham FG, Leveno KJ, Bloom SL, et al., eds. Causes of Obstetrical Hemorrhage. In: Cunningham FG, Leveno KJ, Dashe JS, Hoffman BL, Spong CY, Casey BM, eds. *Williams Obstetrics.* 26th ed. McGraw-Hill Education; 2022:742-743.

Gibbins KJ, Weber T, Holmgren CM, et al. Maternal and fetal morbidity associated with uterine rupture of the unscarred uterus. *Am J Obstet Gynecol.* 2015;213:382.e1-382.e6.

Porreco RP, Clark SL, Belfort MA, et al. The changing specter of uterine rupture. *Am J Obstet Gynecol.* 2009;200: 269.e1-269.e4.

A.11. What is the treatment for uterine rupture?

With a complete uterine rupture, fetal distress and maternal bleeding occur. Emergent cesarean delivery is imperative to deliver the fetus and stabilize the mother. After delivery of the fetus, the uterus can be repaired, the uterine arteries can be ligated, or a hysterectomy can be performed, depending on the size of the rupture and the patient's condition. Fetal distress and/or death are common, whereas maternal death in the developed world is not.

Cunningham FG, Leveno KJ, Bloom SL, et al., eds. Causes of Obstetrical Hemorrhage. In: Cunningham FG, Leveno KJ, Dashe JS, Hoffman BL, Spong CY, Casey BM, eds. *Williams Obstetrics.* 26th ed. McGraw-Hill Education; 2022:731-748.

A.12. Is this patient at risk for postpartum bleeding?

Yes, this patient has a higher chance of postpartum bleeding because of her known placenta previa and the increased risk of having an associated PAS. There is a strong association between placenta previa, prior cesarean delivery, prior uterine surgery, and PAS.

The risk of PAS greatly increases for patients with known placenta previa for each successive cesarean delivery. This risk is 3% for the primary cesarean delivery and increases to 11% after for the second cesarean delivery, up to 67% for the fifth or greater cesarean delivery. In patients without placenta previa, the risk still increases with each successive cesarean delivery, but at a much lower incidence, from 0.03% for the first cesarean delivery up to 4.7% for the sixth or greater cesarean delivery.

Baldwin HJ, Patterson JA, Nippita TA, et al. Antecedents of abnormally invasive placenta in primiparous women: risk associated with gynecologic procedures. *Obstet Gynecol.* 2018;131:227.

Silver RM. Abnormal placentation: placenta previa, vasa previa, and placenta accreta. *Obstet Gynecol.* 2015;126:654-668.

A.13. What is placenta accreta spectrum(PAS)?

Placenta acreta spectrum (PAS), which includes placenta accreta, increta, and percreta, refers to a placenta that adheres abnormally to the myometrium of the uterus due to a partial or total absence of the decidua basalis and an incomplete development of the fibrinoid layer. It was formerly referred to as morbidly adherent placenta. The normal placenta has three general layers: the decidua, which is maternal in origin and adherent to the uterus; the chorion, including the chorionic villi; and the amnion. Both the chorion and amnion are of fetal origin. Normally, in the first few minutes after delivery of the neonate, the placenta separates from its implantation site at a physiologic cleavage line through the spongy layer of the decidua basalis. In PAS, evidence suggests that not only is the decidua basalis scant or absent, but also that the cytotrophoblasts may exert some control of over decidua invasion via angiogenesis and growth expression allowing chorionic villi to attach to and invade uterine myometrium. Placenta accreta occurs when the placental chorionic villi are attached directly to the uterine myometrium without a decidua layer. With placenta increta, the villi invade into the myometrium, and with placenta percreta, the villi penetrate through the myometrium and serosa of the uterus and, sometimes, into adjacent organs. The abnormal adherence may involve the entire placenta (total placenta accreta), several placental lobules (partial accreta), or part or all of a single lobule (focal placenta accreta).

The incidence was approximately 1 in 2,510 deliveries in the 1980s versus 1 in 533 deliveries for the period from 1982 to 2002, and most recently 1 in 272 deliveries in 2016. Among patients with PAS, approximately 63% are placenta accreta, 15% are placenta increta, and 22% are placenta percreta. Increasing cesarean delivery rates and placenta previa are by far the two most important risk factors. Decidua formation is commonly defective over a previous cesarean section scar, in the lower uterine segment, and/or after uterine surgery. Maternal age of more than 35 years, multiparity, Asherman syndrome, and otherwise unexplained elevations in maternal serum α-fetoprotein concentration and β-human chorionic gonadotropin (β-hCG) are other risk factors associated with placenta accreta.

Cahill AG, Beigi R, Heine RP, et al; for Society of Gynecologic Oncology, American. American College of Obstetricians and Gynecologists Committee on Obstetric Practice. Committee opinion no. 529: placenta accreta. *Obstet Gynecol.* 2018;132:E259-E275.

Cunningham FG, Leveno KJ, Bloom SL, et al., eds. Hemorrhagic Placental Disorders. In: Cunningham FG, Leveno KJ, Dashe JS, Hoffman BL, Spong CY, Casey BM, eds. *Williams Obstetrics.* 26th ed. McGraw-Hill Education; 2022:749-761.

Jauniaux ER, Alfirevic Z, Bhide AG, et al; on behalf of the Royal College of Obstetricians and Gynaecologists. Placenta praevia and placenta accreta: diagnosis and management: green-top guideline no. 27a. *BJOG.* 2019;126:E1-E48.

Jauniaux E, Bunce C, Grønbeck L, et al. Prevalence and main outcomes of placenta accreta spectrum: a systematic review and meta-analysis. *Am J Obstet Gynecol.* 2019;221:208-218.

Silver RM. Abnormal placentation: placenta previa, vasa previa, and placenta accreta. *Obstet Gynecol.* 2015;126:654-668.

A.14. How is placenta accreta spectrum diagnosed?

In patients with conditions such as placenta previa and previous uterine surgery that are highly associated with PAS, it is important to have a high index of suspicion and to look carefully for signs of PAS. Transabdominal and transvaginal ultrasonography are useful for evaluating placental position and implantation; perhaps the most important ultrasonographic association in the second and third trimesters is the presence of placenta previa, which is present in more than 80% of accreta in most large series. Intraplacental vascular lacunae, the loss of the hypoechoic (ie, clear space) boundary between the placenta and myometrium and/or bladder, decreased retroplacental myometrial thickness, and increased vascularity of the uterine serosa-bladder interface are strongly suggestive of PAS. Although ultrasound evaluation is important, the lack of ultrasound findings does not rule out a diagnosis of PAS. Clinical factors remain equally important predictors of PAS; there is no single diagnostic modality that determines the diagnosis of PAS with absolute accuracy. Color flow Doppler and MRI can be used as adjunctive diagnostic tools. Placental biomarkers, such as α-fetoprotein, are too nonspecific for clinical use.

Cahill AG, Beigi R, Heine RP, et al; for Society of Gynecologic Oncology, American. American College of Obstetricians and Gynecologists Committee on Obstetric Practice. Committee opinion no. 529: placenta accreta. *Obstet Gynecol.* 2018;132:E259-E275.

Jauniaux ER, Alfirevic Z, Bhide AG, et al; on behalf of the Royal College of Obstetricians and Gynaecologists. Placenta praevia and placenta accreta: diagnosis and management: green-top guideline no. 27a. *BJOG.* 2019;126:E1-E48.

Jauniaux E, Collins S, Burton GJ. Placenta accreta spectrum: pathophysiology and evidence-based anatomy for prenatal ultrasound imaging. *Am J Obstet Gynecol.* 2018;218:75-87.

A.15. How is placenta acreta spectrum managed obstetrically?

Optimal management of PAS has yet to be defined. Care should be individualized for each patient, and a multidisciplinary approach to delivery planning should be taken. Prenatal diagnosis and management are important and provide the opportunity to optimize outcome. The problems associated with PAS depend on the site of implantation, depth of myometrial penetration, and the number of placental lobules involved. Only a focal placenta accreta may not require aggressive surgical intervention. Otherwise, surgical management can be difficult and requires a multidisciplinary approach in order to minimize maternal complications. If PAS is known to exist antenatally, it is usually treated with elective cesarean delivery and hysterectomy; the placenta should be left in place during surgery. The optimal timing for the delivery of the patient with PAS remains controversial; however, planned en bloc hysterectomy without removal of the placenta at 34 to 35 weeks of gestation after betamethasone administration has been shown to decrease maternal hemorrhagic morbidity without a significant increase in neonatal morbidity.

Preoperative placement of balloon catheters into the internal iliac arteries has been used in attempts to decrease blood loss and provide optimum exposure of the operative field, and can also be used for intraoperative or postoperative embolization with persistent bleeding. However, the placement of these catheters is not risk free as thrombosis and thromboemboli have been reported; thus, the efficacy of this intervention is unclear. Some suggest that placement of preoperative ureteral stents reduces morbidity in cesarean hysterectomies; others use stents intraoperatively as needed.

Because a hysterectomy renders the patient infertile, there has been some interest in attempting to leave the uterus intact in those patients with a strong desire to maintain fertility. The success of "conservative" expectant management, which is defined as leaving all or part of the placenta in situ without removing the uterus, seems to correlate to the degree of the placental attachment abnormality. Overall, 15% to 22% of conservatively management patients had eventual hysterectomy due to hemorrhage or infection, whereas approximately 13% of conservatively managed patients had subsequent pregnancies. Only in highly select cases when blood loss is minimal and maintenance of fertility is desired should conservative management be considered.

Cahill AG, Beigi R, Heine RP, et al; for Society of Gynecologic Oncology, American. American College of Obstetricians and Gynecologists Committee on Obstetric Practice. Committee opinion no. 529: placenta accreta. *Obstet Gynecol.* 2018;132:E259-E275.

Fox KA, Shamshirsaz AA, Carusi D, et al. Conservative management of morbidly adherent placenta: expert review. *Am J Obstet Gynecol.* 2015;213:755-760.

Jauniaux ER, Alfirevic Z, Bhide AG, et al; on behalf of the Royal College of Obstetricians and Gynaecologists. Placenta praevia and placenta accreta: diagnosis and management: green-top guideline no. 27a. *BJOG.* 2019;126:E1-E48.

Sentilhes L, Ambroselli C, Kayem G, et al. Maternal outcome after conservative treatment of placenta accreta. *Obstet Gynecol.* 2010;115:526-534.

A.16. What tests and/or interventions can improve neonatal outcome of a preterm birth?

Because significant neonatal morbidity has been reported with elective delivery before 39 weeks of gestation, planned repeat cesarean deliveries should be performed after 39 weeks of gestation. Neonatal survival increases as birth weight and/or gestational age increases. The pivotal complication of preterm delivery is respiratory distress syndrome (RDS). The American College of Obstetricians and Gynecologists (ACOG) considers first-trimester ultrasonography the most accurate method for establishing or confirming gestational age. Pregnancies without an ultrasound confirming or revising the estimated due date before 22 weeks of gestation should be considered suboptimally dated. If an indication for delivery is present, use of amniocentesis to assess FLM does not aid in guiding management. In our case of preterm vaginal bleeding from sonographically documented placenta previa, the patient should be electively delivered before 39 weeks because the risk of bleeding increases as gestation progresses. If there is maternal hemorrhage, fetal maturity would not impact the decision to perform an immediate cesarean delivery.

Respiratory distress syndrome is the leading cause of morbidity and mortality in preterm infants. Sixty percent of infants born below 28 weeks of gestation will develop RDS, whereas the incidence of RDS is 30% and less than 5% in infants born between 28 and 34 weeks and after 34 weeks, respectively. Use of maternal antenatal corticosteroids, neonatal nasal continuous positive airway pressure (nCPAP), and neonatal exogenous surfactant, if needed, can help decrease neonatal morbidity and mortality.

Antenatal corticosteroids should be administered when a female is at risk of preterm delivery within 7 days to decrease the rate of neonatal respiratory complications. Between 24 and 34 weeks of gestation, a single-dose course of a corticosteroid, such as betamethasone (two doses of 12 mg intramuscularly, 24 hours apart) or dexamethasone (four doses of 6 mg intramuscularly, 12 hours apart), should be given to accelerate FLM in a parturient who is at risk for imminent preterm delivery. A single repeat course of antenatal steroids should be considered if the first course was greater than 14 days, the fetus is less than 34 0/7 weeks of gestation, and the delivery is likely within the next 7 days. At 23 0/7 weeks of gestation, corticosteroids can be considered based on a family's decision about resuscitation, irrespective of membrane rupture status and fetal number. A single course of betamethasone is recommended for pregnant patients at risk for late preterm delivery, 34 0/7 to 36 6/7 weeks of gestation, who have not had a previous course of antenatal corticosteroids.

Early CPAP with subsequent selective surfactant administration in extremely preterm infants, defined as less than 32 weeks of gestation or weighing less than 1,500 g, results in lower rates of mechanical ventilation, surfactant administration, and bronchopulmonary dysplasia (BPD)/death when compared to treatment with prophylactic or early surfactant treatment. In neonates who receive a combination of maternal antenatal steroids and early nCPAP in the delivery room, prophylactic surfactant therapy is no longer recommended. Infants with RDS on CPAP who fail to maintain Spo_2 more than 90% on a fraction of inspired oxygen (Fio_2) of 0.40 or higher have respiratory acidosis (arterial pH <7.2 and partial pressure of arterial carbon dioxide [$Paco_2$] >60-65 mm Hg), or are apneic, or require tracheal intubation and surfactant administration. Surfactant is most effective when given within the first 30 to 60 minutes of life.

Use of magnesium sulfate for fetal neuroprotection in threatened preterm delivery is recommended; recommendations about dose, duration, upper gestational age, and repeating treatment vary and differ. ACOG recommends that females at risk for imminent delivery before 32 0/7 weeks of gestation be considered candidates for fetal neuroprotection treatment with magnesium sulfate.

Use of amniocentesis for FLM tests is rarely done in the United States. ACOG does not recommend it for assessment to guide the timing of delivery. Some still use it in patients with poorly dated gestations when FLM can influence plans for delivery (eg, repeat cesarean delivery in a female with a prior classical cesarean delivery and unconfirmed gestational age). FLM is not generally assessed before 32 weeks of gestation because pulmonary maturity is unlikely before this time and is not assessed after 39 weeks.

Borders A, Birsner M, Gyamfi-Bannerman C, et al. American College of Obstetricians and Gynecologists. Committee opinion no. 761: nonmedically indicated early-term deliveries. *Obstet Gynecol.* 2019;133:E156-E162.

Cunningham FG, Leveno KJ, Bloom SL, et al., eds. Hemorrhagic Placental Disorders. In: Cunningham FG, Leveno KJ, Dashe JS, Hoffman BL, Spong CY, Casey BM, eds. *Williams Obstetrics.* 26th ed. McGraw-Hill Education; 2022:761-762.

El-Sayed Y, Borders A, Gyamfi-Bannerman C, et al. American College of Obstetricians and Gynecologists. Committee opinion no. 713: antenatal corticosteroid therapy for fetal maturation. *Obstet Gynecol.* 2017;130:e102-e109.

Jayaram PM, Mohan MK, Farid I, et al. Antenatal magnesium sulfate for fetal neuroprotection: a critical appraisal and systematic review of clinical practice guidelines. *J Perinat Med.* 2019;47:262-269.

Miller RS, Heine RP. American College of Obstetricians and Gynecologists. Committee opinion no. 688 management of suboptimally dated pregnancies. *Obstet Gynecol.* 2017 (Reaffirmed 2021);129:591-592.

Papile L, Baley J, Benitz W, et al; American Academy of Pediatrics Committee on Fetus and Newborn. Respiratory support in preterm infants at birth. *Pediatrics.* 2014;133:171-174.

B. Preoperative Evaluation and Preparation

B.1. How does pregnancy change respiratory function, and what impact does this have on anesthetic care?

A number of respiratory changes are seen in pregnancy:

- Capillary engorgement of the mucosa is found throughout the respiratory tract, causing swelling of the nasal and oral pharynx, larynx, and trachea; this begins in the first trimester and increases progressively throughout pregnancy, putting the patient at risk for epistaxis and serving as a relative contraindication to nasal intubation in pregnancy. Tracheal intubation of the edematous and possibly friable airway requires careful selection of a smaller diameter endotracheal tube. These anatomic changes also put the patient at risk for a more difficult intubation, although the advent of videolaryngoscopy might lessen this risk. Mallampati class can worsen during pregnancy and labor irrespective of other patient characteristics such as obesity; thorough and serial airway examinations are important in this population.

- At term, there are increases in minute ventilation (45%), tidal volume (45%), and oxygen consumption (30%-40%); respiratory rate does not change. These changes do not return to their prepregnancy state for at least 6 to 8 weeks after delivery.
- Arterial $Paco_2$ decreases to about 30 mm Hg by 12 weeks of gestation and remains there until it slowly increases after delivery over about 6 to 8 weeks postpartum.
- Arterial pH increases to about 7.44, and there is a partial metabolic compensation for the respiratory alkalosis (20 mEq/L).
- Functional residual capacity (FRC) begins to decrease by the fifth month and by term is 20% below prepregnancy values. After delivery, FRC increases and by 1 to 2 weeks postpartum returns to its prepregnant level. Additionally, the supine position will further decrease the FRC to approximately 70% of prepregnancy volume. The combination of decreased FRC and increased oxygen consumption makes the pregnant patient more susceptible to the rapid onset of hypoxemia in the apneic state. Therefore, before induction of general anesthesia, the parturient should be "preoxygenated" with 100% oxygen for 3 to 5 minutes while taking normal tidal breaths or, if time is limited, for four vital capacity breaths. The reduced FRC combined with the increased minute ventilation increase the rapidity of changes in the depth of anesthesia while employing an inhaled anesthetic technique.
- Minimum alveolar concentration (MAC) of inhaled anesthetic agents is decreased by approximately 40% in pregnancy.

Bobrowski RA. Pulmonary physiology in pregnancy. *Clin Obstet Gynecol.* 2010;53:285-300.

Boutonnet M, Faitot V, Katz A, et al. Mallampati class changes during pregnancy, labour, and after delivery: can these be predicted? *Br J Anaesth.* 2010;104:67-70.

Cunningham F, Leveno KJ, Dashe JS, Hoffman BL, Spong CY, Casey BM, eds. Hemorrhagic Placental Disorders. *Williams Obstetrics.* 26th ed. McGraw-Hill; 2022:762-765.

Pilkington S, Carli F, Dakin MJ, et al. Increase in Mallampati score during pregnancy. *Br J Anaesth.* 1995;74:638-642.

Scott-Brown S, Russel R. Video laryngoscopes and the obstetric airway. *Int J Obstet Anesth.* 2015;24:137-146.

Ueyama H, Hagihira S, Takashina M, et al. Pregnancy does not enhance volatile anesthetic sensitivity on the brain: an electroencephalographic analysis study. *Anesthesiology.* 2010;113:577-584.

SECTION 7

B.2. What are the maternal cardiovascular changes of pregnancy?

Most cardiovascular changes of pregnancy begin early in the first trimester and peak by 30 to 34 weeks of gestation. At term, cardiovascular changes include:

- Cardiac output increases 40% to 50%. During the first trimester of pregnancy, cardiac output increases to 40% or 50% above normal and plateaus by approximately 28 weeks of gestation. It remains fairly stable until the stresses imposed by labor increase it further. During labor, cardiac output increases approximately 15% with uterine contractions during the latent phase, 30% in the active phase, and 45% in the expulsive phase when compared to prelabor values. The greatest increase in cardiac output occurs immediately postpartum when it increases on an average by 80% above prelabor values. Cardiac output and heart rate decline to prelabor values within 1 hour of delivery. Postpartum, over the next 2 to 4 weeks, cardiac hemodynamic parameters return toward pregravid levels. It can take a year, however, for the residual effects of cardiovascular remodeling to subside.
- Stroke volume increases approximately 30%.
- Heart rate increases approximately 15%.
- Systolic blood pressure is minimally affected by pregnancy.
- Diastolic blood pressure decreases up to 20% by midpregnancy but returns to prepregnancy level at term.
- Systemic vascular resistance decreases 20%.
- Central venous pressure (CVP) remains unchanged.
- Aortocaval compression refers to the gravid uterus compressing the inferior vena cava (IVC) and/or the abdominal aorta. The extent of the compression depends on patient position and weeks of gestation. In the supine position, compression of the IVC begins by 20 weeks of gestation. At term in the supine position, the IVC is occluded almost completely, with venous return from the lower extremities occurring

through the dilated azygos system of veins as the dominant pathway of collateral circulation. Despite this impaired blood flow and concomitant decrease in cardiac output, the majority of supine females are not hypotensive or symptomatic because of the compensatory rise in systemic vascular resistance and venous return via collateral circulation. However, up to 11% of supine females at term develop supine hypotension syndrome with hypotension, bradycardia, and symptoms of dizziness, light-headedness, nausea, and even syncope. It is standard practice for patients after 20 weeks of gestation to be positioned with left lateral uterine displacement. Recently, however, this practice has been questioned, with some suggesting that neonatal and maternal outcomes are preserved without tilt as long as hemodynamic support with phenylephrine and fluid co-loading during spinal anesthesia are given.

Armstrong S, Fernando R, Columb M, et al. Cardiac index in term pregnant women in the sitting, lateral, and supine positions: an observational, crossover study. *Anesth Analg*. 2011;113:318-322.

Chestnut DH. The aortocaval compression conundrum. *Anesth Analg*. 2017;125:1838-1839.

Kacmar R, Gaiser R. Chapter 2: Physiologic changes of pregnancy. In: Chestnut DH, Wong CA, Tsen LC, et al, eds. *Chestnut's Obstetric Anesthesia: Principles and Practice*. 6th ed. Elsevier; 2019:13-17.

Higuchi H, Takagi S, Zhang K, et al. Effect of lateral tilt angle on the volume of the abdominal aorta and inferior vena cava in pregnant and nonpregnant women determined by magnetic resonance imaging. *Anesthesiology*. 2015;122:286-293.

Humphries A, Mirjalili SA, Tarr GP, et al. The effect of supine positioning on maternal hemodynamics during late pregnancy. *J Matern Fetal Neonatal Med*. 2019;32:3923-3930.

Lee AJ, Landau R. Aortocaval compression syndrome: time to revisit certain dogmas. *Anesth Analg*. 2017;125: 1975-1985.

Lee AJ, Landau R, Mattingly JL, et al. Left lateral table tilt for elective cesarean delivery under spinal anesthesia has no effect on neonatal acid-base status: a randomized controlled trial. *Anesthesiology*. 2017;127:241-249.

Practice guidelines for obstetric anesthesia: an updated report by the American Society of Anesthesiologists Task Force on Obstetric Anesthesia and the Society for Obstetric Anesthesia and Perinatology. *Anesthesiology*. 2016;124:270-300.

B.3. What are the maternal gastrointestinal changes of pregnancy?

Parturients are considered to be at increased risk for aspiration of gastric contents. Pregnancy itself does not alter gastric emptying of liquid or solid materials, but during labor, gastric motility decreases. Gastric acid secretion appears to be unchanged. Because of the upward displacement of the stomach by the gravid uterus, tone in lower esophageal high-pressure zone, however, is decreased. This zone normally prevents the reflux of gastric contents. In the first trimester, the tone in this zone can be unchanged, but in the second and third trimesters, the tone in lower esophageal high-pressure zone falls gradually to about 50% of its preconceptual level. By 36 weeks of gestation, it reaches its lowest point and does not return to prepregnancy levels until 1 to 4 weeks postpartum. As a result, 30% to 50% of females experience heartburn during pregnancy. The increased aspiration risk is thought to be due to decreased lower esophageal high-pressure zone tone. The increased risk of difficult intubation adds to concern for aspiration in this population. NPO (nothing by mouth) guidelines should be strictly observed, although balanced with the urgency of active labor requiring surgical interventions.

Farber MK. Aspiration: Risk, Prophylaxis, and Treatment. In: Chestnut DH, Wong CA, Tsen LC, et al., eds. *Chestnut's Obstetric Anesthesia: Principles and Practice*. 6th ed. Elsevier; 2019:671-675.

Ramu B, Mohan P, Rajasekaran MS, et al. Prevalence and risk factors for gastroesophageal reflux in pregnancy. *Indian J Gastroenterol*. 2011;30:144-147.

B.4. What hematologic changes occur during pregnancy?

The hematologic changes seen by term are as follows:

- Intravascular fluid volume increases 45%.
- Plasma volume increases 55%.
- RBC volume increases 30%.

The disproportionate increase in plasma volume compared to RBC volume results in the relative, or physiologic, anemia of pregnancy. By midgestation, hematocrit has typically fallen approximately 15% below prepregnant levels. In late gestation, RBC volume increases. This decreased viscosity can aid in maintaining the patency of the uteroplacental vascular bed.

In addition, the following coagulation factors are increased at term: factors I (fibrinogen), VII, VIII, IX, X, and XII. Plasminogen, fibrin degradation products, and fibrinopeptide A are also increased. Factors

II and V are unchanged. Factors XI and XIII are decreased as is antithrombin III. Overall, pregnancy is associated with an accelerated, but compensated, rate of intravascular coagulation. Both, prothrombin time (PT) and activated partial thromboplastin time (aPTT) are shortened 20%, and thromboelastography (TEG) suggests a hypercoagulable state. Platelet count is typically unchanged at term. Gestational thrombocytopenia is common (7%-12% of term pregnancies) and refers to maternal platelet counts less than 150,000/μL in otherwise normal females.

Boehlen F, Hohlfeld P, Extermann P, Perneger TV, de Moerloose P. Platelet count at term pregnancy: a reappraisal of the threshold. *Obstet Gynecol.* 2000;95:29-33.

Kacmar R, Gaiser R. Physiologic Changes of Pregnancy. In: Chestnut DH, Wong CA, Tsen LC, et al., eds. *Chestnut's Obstetric Anesthesia: Principles and Practice.* 6th ed. Elsevier; 2019:22-25.

B.5. What laboratory data do you need before taking this patient to the operating room?

The laboratory values needed in this healthy parturient having an elective scheduled cesarean delivery are minimal. A type and crossmatch should be sent because this patient is at an increased risk for bleeding due to placenta previa and the increased likelihood of an associated placenta accreta in the setting of a third cesarean delivery. A CBC should be sent for baseline reference. If the patient in labor, there is no need to delay neuraxial anesthesia for the CBC results in the absence of risk factors for thrombocytopenia with platelets less than 70,000/μL (eg, preeclampsia, hypertensive spectrum disorders, or history of low platelet count). Unless the patient has a coagulation disorder or is actively bleeding, PT, aPTT, and fibrinogen levels are not needed because the values should be within normal limits.

Banayan J, Hofer J, Scavone B. Antepartum and Postpartum Hemorrhage. In: Chestnut DH, Wong CA, Tsen LC, et al, eds. *Chestnut's Obstetric Anesthesia: Principles and Practice.* 6th ed. Elsevier; 2019:917-918.

Tsen L, Bateman B. Anesthesia for Cesarean Delivery. In: Chestnut DH, Wong CA, Tsen LC, et al, eds. *Chestnut's Obstetric Anesthesia: Principles and Practice.* 6th ed. Elsevier; 2019:571-572.

B.6. What preoperative medications would you administer to this patient?

Although not required, patients at increased risk for aspiration may receive a nonparticulate oral antacid such as sodium citrate 30 minutes prior to the induction of anesthesia. Intravenous H_2-receptor antagonists, such as ranitidine and/or metoclopramide, can also be given preoperatively for aspiration prophylaxis. This patient is having an elective cesarean delivery; standard NPO guidelines must be observed.

This patient should receive antimicrobial prophylaxis within the 60-minute period before skin incision for the cesarean delivery. As per the 2018 ACOG guidelines, a single dose of the first-generation cephalosporin, cefazolin is the first-line antibiotic of choice unless a patient is allergic to this medication. If an allergy exists, a single intravenous dose of clindamycin (900 mg) and an aminoglycoside (eg, gentamicin 5 mg/kg infused over 30-120 minutes) should be given. In addition, azithromycin 500 mg infused over 1 hour can be added to the standard antibiotic regimen if a patient is undergoing a nonelective cesarean delivery.

American College of Obstetricians and Gynecologists Committee on Practice Bulletins—Obstetrics. ACOG practice bulletin no. 199: use of prophylactic antibiotics in labor and delivery. *Obstet Gynecol.* 2018;132:e103-e119.

Practice guidelines for obstetric anesthesia: an updated report by the American Society of Anesthesiologists Task Force on Obstetric Anesthesia and the Society for Obstetric Anesthesia and Perinatology. *Anesthesiology.* 2016;124:270-300.

SECTION 7

C. Intraoperative Management

C.1. What monitors would you use for this patient?

Standard monitors should be used and include the following: electrocardiogram (ECG), blood pressure, pulse oximetry, end-tidal carbon dioxide, temperature when feasible, and Foley catheter. In addition, two large-bore intravenous lines, a forced air body warming blanket, intravenous fluid warmers, and intermittent pneumatic compression stockings should be used. A radial arterial line should also be considered if multiple blood samples are needed and/or hemodynamic instability is anticipated or occurs. Central venous access, placed above the diaphragm, should be considered if vasoactive drugs and additional volume are required for hemodynamic resuscitation. Equipment for rapid infusion of intravenous fluids and blood products should be readily available.

Kolettis D, Craigo S. Thromboprophylaxis in pregnancy. *Obstet Gynecol Clin North Am*. 2018;45:389-402.

Lier H, von Heymann C, Korte W, et al. Peripartum haemorrhage: haemostatic aspects of the new German PPH guideline. *Transfus Med Hemother*. 2018;45:127-135.

Tsen LC, Bateman B. Anesthesia for Cesarean Delivery. In: Chestnut DH, Wong CA, Tsen LC, et al., eds. *Chestnut's Obstetric Anesthesia: Principles and Practice*. 6th ed. Elsevier; 2019:572-574.

C.2. What anesthetic approaches could be used in this patient?

In the patient with placenta previa, a regional or general anesthetic technique could be used. A continuous neuraxial anesthetic is reasonable for this patient when a prolonged or technically difficult procedure is anticipated. The choice of anesthetic depends on the cesarean delivery indication, urgency, and maternal comorbidities. All patients with placenta previa are at risk for increased intraoperative blood loss due to poor contractility of the lower uterine segment, increased risk of associated placenta accreta, and the possibility of an anterior placenta being cut during uterine incision. Of patients having nonemergent cesarean deliveries for placenta previa with suspected PAS, 95% had some form of neuraxial anesthesia as their primary anesthetic, and 21% neuraxial anesthesia who needed a hysterectomy had their anesthetic converted to general anesthesia intraoperatively.

Options for neuraxial anesthesia include continuous spinal, combined spinal and epidural, and continuous epidural anesthesia. Single-injection spinal anesthesia can be used, but the unpredictable length of surgery makes this a poor choice. All patients having neuraxial anesthesia should be informed that if the need arises, general anesthesia might be induced. If the patient has suspected placenta percreta, general anesthesia is the usual choice for cesarean delivery and hysterectomy because of the extensive surgery that can be required. Cesarean delivery can still take place under continuous neuraxial anesthesia in specific patients, and discussion between the patient, anesthesiologist, and surgical team should aim to determine whether patients are suitable candidates.

If postpartum hemorrhage occurs, a coordinated multidisciplinary team approach aimed at early recognition and treatment is essential.

American College of Obstetricians and Gynecologists Committee on Practice Bulletins—Obstetrics. Practice bulletin no. 183: postpartum hemorrhage. *Obstet Gynecol*. 2017;130:e168-e186.

Markley JC, Farber MK, Perlman NC, et al. Neuraxial anesthesia during cesarean delivery for placenta previa with suspected morbidly adherent placenta: a retrospective analysis. *Anesth Analg*. 2018;127:930-938.

C.3. What are the absolute and relative contraindications for neuraxial anesthesia?

Absolute contraindications:

- Patient inability to tolerate or patient refusal
- Uncorrected maternal hypovolemia or hypovolemic shock
- Infection at the site of needle insertion
- Frank coagulopathies
- Recent pharmacologic anticoagulation
- Mass lesions causing increased intracranial pressure
- Lack of appropriate monitoring and/or resuscitative equipment

Relative contraindications include maternal systemic infection, neurologic disease, severe stenotic cardiac valve lesions, and some isolated blood coagulation test abnormalities. Each patient should be treated individually with careful consideration of the benefits and risks of neuraxial anesthesia.

Wong CA. Epidural and Spinal Analgesia: Anesthesia for Labor and Vaginal Delivery. In: Chestnut DH, Wong CA, Tsen LC, et al., eds. *Chestnut's Obstetric Anesthesia: Principles and Practice*. 6th ed. Elsevier; 2019:475-478.

C.4. How is postpartum hemorrhage (PPH) defined, and what are the etiologies of this bleeding?

The ACOG reVITALize program currently defines PPH as cumulative blood loss equal to or more than 1 L or blood loss accompanied by signs and symptoms of hypovolemia within 24 hours of delivery regardless of the delivery route. This differs from the more traditionally accepted definition, which states that estimated blood loss more than 500 mL for vaginal deliveries and 1 L for cesarean delivery constitutes PPH. Despite this new definition, ACOG suggests that a blood loss more than 500 mL after a vaginal delivery should be considered abnormal and be investigated.

Depending on nonpregnant blood volume and the corresponding magnitude of pregnancy-induced hypervolemia, a dangerous feature of postpartum bleeding is the failure of pulse and blood pressure to undergo more than moderate alterations until large amounts of blood are lost. This is seen typically after loss of nearly 25% of the blood volume, which is approximately more than or equal to 1.5 L. Recognition of PPH before vital sign deterioration can improve outcomes. Risk assessment tools are available to help. About 60% to 85% of patients who will experience a significant obstetrical bleed can be identified, but diligent surveillance of all patients is prudent.

Visual estimations of blood loss are inaccurate and usually underestimate true blood loss. Quantification of blood loss by measuring the amount of blood in the suction canister, drapes, and weighing surgical lap pads is significantly more accurate than estimated blood loss.

The causes of PPH generally can be categorized as those occurring early within 24 hours of delivery and those occurring late, 24 hours after delivery. Because the obstetrician typically is faced with early PPH, the remainder of this discussion focuses on its causes. The two broad etiologies of early PPH are based on bleeding from the placental implantation site and genital tract trauma. Placental site bleeding is usually due to either myometrial hypotonia, as seen with uterine atony and placenta previa, or retained placental tissue as can be seen with invasive placentation, such as PAS and uterine inversion. Genital tract trauma that leads to postpartum bleeding includes genital tract lacerations and uterine rupture. Coagulation defects intensify the bleeding that occurs with any of the earlier abnormalities.

American College of Obstetricians and Gynecologists Committee on Practice Bulletins—Obstetrics. Practice bulletin no. 183: postpartum hemorrhage. *Obstet Gynecol.* 2017;130:e168-e186.

Association of Women's Health, Obstetric and Neonatal Nurses. Quantification of blood loss: AWHONN practice brief number 1. *J Obstet Gynecol Neonatal Nurs.* 2015;44:158-160.

Cunningham FG, Leveno KJ, Bloom SL, et al., eds. Causes of Obstetrical Hemorrhage. In: Cunningham FG, Leveno KJ, Dashe JS, Hoffman BL, Spong CY, Casey BM, eds. *Williams Obstetrics.* 26th ed. McGraw-Hill Education; 2022:731-748.

Hamm RF, Wang EY, Bastek JA, et al. Assessing reVITALize: should the definition of postpartum hemorrhage differ by mode of delivery? *Am J Perinatol.* 2017;34:503-507.

Sentilhes L, Goffinet F, Vayssière C, et al. Comparison of postpartum haemorrhage guidelines: discrepancies underline our lack of knowledge. *BJOG.* 2017;124:718-722.

Sentilhes L, Vayssière C, Deneux-Tharaux C, et al. Postpartum hemorrhage: guidelines for clinical practice from the French College of Gynaecologists and Obstetricians (CNGOF): in collaboration with the French Society of Anesthesiology and Intensive Care (SFAR). *Eur J Obstet Gynecol Reprod Biol.* 2016;198:12-21.

C.5. After delivery of the fetus, the placenta is removed with some difficulty in one small area, and generalized oozing from the placental implantation site is noted. What is the most likely cause of this patient's bleeding?

The most likely causes of bleeding in this patient are focal placenta accreta and myometrial hypotonia due to poor contraction of the lower uterine segment. Near term, at least 600 mL/min of blood flows through the intervillous space carried by about 120 spiral arteries and their accompanying veins. Due to endotrophoblastic remodeling to create a low-pressure system, these arteries have no muscular layer. With placental separation, these vessels are avulsed; hemostasis at the placental implantation site is first achieved by contraction of the myometrium that compresses these relatively large vessels and reestablishes vascular integrity. Subsequently, clotting occurs, and vessel lumens are obliterated. Ineffective myometrial contractions, such as those occurring with retained placenta or massive blood clots, can impair hemostasis at the implantation site. In this patient, the lower uterine segment contracts poorly as it contains less myometrial tissue, and hemorrhage can result despite normal coagulation. Bleeding that occurs after placenta delivery is usually a steady insidious hemorrhage that can lead to enormous blood loss. Severe PPH, therefore, can result from uterine atony despite normal coagulation. During rapid bleeding, hematocrit might not accurately reflect the amount of blood lost due to the lack of equilibration with other fluid compartments.

Cunningham FG, Leveno KJ, Bloom SL, et al., eds. Causes of Obstetrical Hemorrhage. In: Cunningham FG, Leveno KJ, Dashe JS, Hoffman BL, Spong CY, Casey BM, eds. *Williams Obstetrics.* 26th ed. McGraw-Hill Education; 2022:731-748.

Silver RM. Abnormal placentation: placenta previa, vasa previa, and placenta accreta. *Obstet Gynecol.* 2015;126:654-668.

C.6. After delivery of the placenta in a cesarean delivery, what maneuvers and drugs can enhance myometrial contractility and therefore decrease blood loss?

Uterotonic medications cause myometrial contractions and decrease postpartum bleeding. They should be the first-line treatment for PPH caused by uterine atony, which accounts for 70% to 80% of PPH cases. Given prophylactically, uterotonics prevent most cases of uterine atony.

Synthetic oxytocin (Pitocin, Syntocinon) is usually recommended as the drug of choice and is given once the fetus is delivered. Oxytocin increases the frequency and duration of uterine contraction; these contractions are mediated through an increase in intracellular calcium levels. The number of oxytocin receptors in the uterus increases from about 20 weeks of gestation to 34 weeks of gestation, and receptor sensitivity increases during labor. Although oxytocin is routinely given, there is no standard prophylactic dose for either vaginal or cesarean delivery. Intravenous therapy is often the preferred route of administration, but intramuscular (IM) dosing is possible. Intravenous oxytocin has a rapid onset of about 1 minute and a fast mean elimination half-life of 3 to 5 minutes. A commonly used dose is 10 to 40 international units (IU) of oxytocin in 500 to 1,000 mL of normal saline, with the rate of infusion adjusted according to uterine tone. When uterine tone is maintained and bleeding is not excessive, this rate is generally decreased. Many protocols have been developed, most of which have an initial bolus over 1 hour of 10 to 30 IUs, followed by 1 to 4 hours of an additional 10 to 40 IUs of oxytocin. Administration in a standardized concentration under site-specific protocol can reduce risk of medication errors.

Studies show that females having cesarean delivery after exposure to exogenous oxytocin during labor required higher infusion rates of oxytocin to prevent uterine atony than females without prior exposure. The posterior pituitary produces the polypeptide hormones, oxytocin, and antidiuretic hormone. Because they differ from one another by only two amino acids, oxytocin exhibits a small antidiuretic effect that is clinically insignificant unless very large doses are given; in this situation, water intoxication can occur. A bolus of oxytocin can decrease peripheral vascular resistance due to a direct relaxing effect on vascular smooth muscle leading to hypotension that on occasion requires treatment with vasopressors. Patients can also exhibit tachycardia and arrhythmias. When oxytocin fails to produce adequate uterine tone and uterine atony is present, other uterotonic medications are often used in prompt succession.

Second-line uterotonic agents depend on side effect profiles and contraindications. Ergot alkaloids, methylergonovine (Methergine), and ergonovine (ergometrine) are effective uterotonic agents; they are usually given intramuscularly and produce tetanic contractions of the uterus that may be mediated through α-adrenergic receptors. Their usefulness is limited because vasoconstriction-induced hypertension can be prominent. These agents should be avoided in patients with preexisting hypertensive disease. Other deleterious effects include coronary artery spasm leading to myocardial infarction or arrhythmia, and possible cerebrovascular accidents. Pulmonary complications have been reported including pulmonary artery vasoconstriction and pulmonary hypertension. Associated side effects include headache, dizziness, nausea, and vomiting.

Prostaglandins are uterotonic agents that cause an increase in myometrial intracellular calcium levels leading to an increase in myosin light-chain kinase activity and uterine contraction. IM and intrauterine administration of 15-methyl prostaglandin $F_{2\alpha}$ (carboprost tromethamine [Hemabate]) can be used to control uterine atony. Due to its bronchoconstrictive properties, its use is strongly contraindicated in asthmatic patients. Rectally administered prostaglandin E_2 (Prostin E_2) is a naturally occurring uterotonic agent that has not been tested in clinical trials for postpartum bleeding, and its unfavorable side effects include fever, chills, nausea, vomiting, diarrhea, and headaches.

Misoprostol (Cytotec), a synthetic prostaglandin E1 analogue, causes uterine contractions and can be administered orally, sublingually, buccally, or per rectum. Common side effects include shivering and fever. Misoprostol has been found to have no added benefit when compared to standard therapy with oxytocin and ergometrine (ergonovine) in primary PPH.

Manual uterine massage is often done and is thought to stimulate the myometrium to contract. The evidence for this common practice, however, is not strong, and research has shown it is ineffective at reducing the incidence of PPH in patients receiving other uterotonic medications.

If pharmacologic methods fail to control atony-related hemorrhage, prompt alternative measures, including uterine tamponade, selective arterial embolization, and surgical intervention must be undertaken.

Lavoie A, McCarthy RJ, Wong CA. The ED90 of prophylactic oxytocin infusion after delivery of the placenta during cesarean delivery in laboring compared with nonlaboring women: an up-down sequential allocation dose-response study. *Anesth Analg*. 2015;121:159-164.

Schmitz T, Tararbit K, Dupont C, et al. Prostaglandin E2 analogue sulprostone for treatment of atonic postpartum hemorrhage. *Obstet Gynecol*. 2011;118:257-265.

Sentilhes L, Goffinet F, Vayssière C, et al. Comparison of postpartum haemorrhage guidelines: discrepancies underline our lack of knowledge. *BJOG*. 2017;124:718-722.

Sentilhes L, Vayssière C, Deneux-Tharaux C, et al. Postpartum hemorrhage: guidelines for clinical practice from the French College of Gynaecologists and Obstetricians (CNGOF): in collaboration with the French Society of Anesthesiology and Intensive Care (SFAR). *Eur J Obstet Gynecol Reprod Biol*. 2016;198:12-21.

Vallera C, Choi LO, Cha CM, et al. Uterotonic medications: oxytocin, methylergonovine, carboprost, misoprostol. *Anesthesiol Clin*. 2017;35:207-219.

C.7. When should this patient receive tranexamic acid (TXA)?

Once this patient has an estimated blood loss of more than 1,000 mL after cesarean delivery or any blood loss sufficient to compromise hemodynamic stability, the patient should receive intravenous TXA. TXA should be given in all cases of PPH, regardless of whether the bleeding is due to genital tract trauma or other causes, unless there is a clear contraindication to antifibrinolytic therapy. Administration should start as soon as possible after the onset of bleeding and within 3 hours of birth. TXA is a competitive inhibitor of plasminogen activation and can reduce bleeding by inhibiting fibrinolysis. TXA should be administered intravenously over 10 minutes in a fixed dose of 1 g in 10 mL; if bleeding continues after 30 minutes or restarts within 24 hours of completing the first dose, a second dose of 1 g should be given. Studies show that TXA administration reduced death caused by bleeding in females with PPH with no adverse effects.

Gayet-Ageron A, Prieto-Merino D, Ker K, et al. Effect of treatment delay on the effectiveness and safety of antifibrinolytics in acute severe haemorrhage: a meta-analysis of individual patient-level data from 40 138 bleeding patients. *Lancet*. 2018;391:125-132.

Shakur H, Beaumont D, Pavord S, et al. Antifibrinolytic drugs for treating primary postpartum haemorrhage. *Cochrane Database Syst Rev*. 2018;2:CD012964.

WOMAN Trial Collaborators. Effect of early tranexamic acid administration on mortality, hysterectomy, and other morbidities in women with post-partum haemorrhage (WOMAN): an international, randomised, double-blind, placebo-controlled trial. *Lancet*. 2017;389:2105-2116.

World Health Organization. *Updated WHO Recommendation on Tranexamic Acid for the Treatment of Postpartum Haemorrhage*. World Health Organization; 2017.

C.8. If this patient had ongoing bleeding intraoperatively, what guidelines help determine when red blood cell (RBC) transfusions should be given?

Treatment of serious bleeding demands prompt and adequate refilling of the intravascular compartment. Normovolemia should be maintained, and crystalloid solutions are used for initial volume resuscitation. Optimal crystalloid type and volume resuscitation have not been identified for the obstetric patient, yet the transition from crystalloid to blood should occur as early as possible, as excessive infusion of crystalloid solution has been associated with worse outcomes in patients with severe hemorrhage. Colloid solutions can also be used to maintain normovolemia but confer no greater benefit than crystalloid solutions

After the hypervolemia of pregnancy is lost at delivery, blood loss can be estimated by every 3 vol% drop in hematocrit representing a 500-mL loss of blood. With acute blood loss, real-time hematocrit measured in the delivery or operating room is often at a maximum. In PPH, the reason for hypoperfusion is blood loss. If the patient is not receiving diuretics, urine output reflects renal perfusion, which in turn reflects perfusion of other vital organs, and should be maintained at greater than or equal to 0.3 mL/kg/h or at least 30 mL/h but preferably greater than 50 mL/h. Although physiologic parameters, such as blood pressure, heart rate, urine output, and perhaps CVP, are monitored during surgery, use of these static parameters to guide fluid therapy can result in either hypovolemia or hypervolemia and might not recognize significant intraoperative reductions in tissue perfusion. Dynamic hemodynamic parameters, such as pulse pressure variation, however, are often not practical in the hemorrhaging obstetrical patient if they are awake and breathing spontaneously with neuraxial anesthesia.

Defining a universal Hct or Hgb value below or above which transfusion is either mandatory or contraindicated is difficult. RBCs carry oxygen to the tissues, and the goal of RBC transfusion is to maintain adequate tissue oxygenation. The 2015 American Society of Anesthesiologists Practice Guidelines state that determining whether patients with Hgb concentrations of 6 to 10 g/dL require RBC transfusion should be based on potential or actual ongoing bleeding, intravascular volume status, signs of organ ischemia, and adequacy of cardiorespiratory reserve. RBC transfusions should be considered in all patients with clinical evidence of inadequate oxygen carrying capacity. In most bleeding obstetric patients, maintaining an Hgb level above 7 g/dL is suggested unless evidence of impaired pulmonary or cardiac function indicates a need for a higher Hgb level.

American Society of Anesthesiologists Task Force on Perioperative Blood Management. Practice guidelines for perioperative blood management: an updated report by the American Society of Anesthesiologists Task Force on Perioperative Blood Management. *Anesthesiology*. 2015;122:241-275.

Bienstock JL, Ahizechukwu CE, Longo NA, et al. Postpartum hemorrhage. *N Engl Med J*. 2021;384:1635-1645.

California Maternal Quality Care Collaborative. Obstetric Hemorrhage Toolkit 2.0, OB Hemorrhage Toolkit V3.0. California Maternal Quality Care Collaborative. 2015. Accessed March 31, 2023. cmqcc.org

Cunningham FG, Leveno KJ, Bloom SL, et al., eds. Management of Obstetrical Hemorrhage. In: Cunningham FG, Leveno KJ, Dashe JS, Hoffman BL, Spong CY, Casey BM, eds. *Williams Obstetrics*. 26th ed. McGraw-Hill Education; 2022:770-775.

Kunst G, Ostermann M. Intraoperative permissive oliguria—how much is too much? *Br J Anaesth*. 2017;119:1075-1077.

C.9. What laboratory tests should be ordered during the resuscitation of this patient?

Once the patient loses 1 L of blood with ongoing bleeding occurring, blood specimens for Hct, Hgb level, platelet count, and coagulation tests (aPTT, PT, and fibrinogen levels) should be sent. Arterial blood gas analysis and lactate level can be done to establish an early baseline. *Blood products should be administered without waiting for results if needed based on clinical assessment.* During resuscitation, the aforementioned tests should be sent periodically to help guide treatment including blood component therapy. Point-of-care bedside testing of blood gases, electrolytes, lactate, Hct, Hgb, and viscoelastic assays of coagulation, such as TEG or rotational thromboelastometry (ROTEM), should be used if available (see Chapter 12: Cardiac Tamponade, Sections B.8, B.9, and B.10; Chapter 31: Coagulopathy, Section A.1; and Chapter 57: Trauma, Section C.25). These results will be more immediate and reflective of the ongoing resuscitation.

If the volume of blood lost requires treatment with a massive transfusion, then electrolyte levels, including potassium and calcium, should be followed. Patients can develop hyperkalemia due to the elevated potassium levels in transfused blood and the cellular shifts caused by acidosis. Patients can develop hypocalcemia from citrate toxicity; citrate is the anticoagulant found in transfused pRBCs. Arterial blood gases and serum lactate levels also should be monitored to evaluate the acidosis that can develop due to poor tissue perfusion and development of shock. Changes in lactate levels have been used to follow the response to treatment. If DIC is a concern, the level of fibrin degradation products should be checked.

American College of Obstetricians and Gynecologists Committee on Practice Bulletins—Obstetrics. Practice bulletin no. 183: postpartum hemorrhage. *Obstet Gynecol.* 2017;130:e168-e186.

Cunningham FG, Leveno KJ, Bloom SL, et al., eds. Causes of Obstetrical Hemorrhage. In: Cunningham FG, Leveno KJ, Dashe JS, Hoffman BL, Spong CY, Casey BM, eds. *Williams Obstetrics.* 26th ed. McGraw-Hill Education; 2022:770-777.

Kraut JA, Madias NE. Lactic acidosis. *N Engl J Med.* 2014;371:2309-2319.

Lier H, von Heymann C, Korte W, et al. Peripartum haemorrhage: haemostatic aspects of the new German PPH guideline. *Transfus Med Hemother.* 2018;45:127-135.

C.10. If this patient had a massive blood loss, what blood replacement therapy would be indicated?

When blood replacement therapy is indicated, compatible whole blood is ideal for maintaining intravascular volume in the treatment of hypovolemia from catastrophic acute hemorrhage. One unit of whole blood raises Hct by 3 vol% to 4 vol% and replaces many coagulation factors, especially fibrinogen. Importantly, using whole blood versus pRBCs and components decreases the exposure of females with severe hemorrhage to blood donors. However, availability of whole blood is limited. Few units of whole blood are kept in the modern blood bank because over 85% of globally collected donor blood is fractionated into blood components. In high-income countries compared to low-income countries, 97% versus 50% of whole blood is fractionated into components. For females who do not have massive blood loss, pRBC transfusions are suitable, and component therapy provides better treatment because only the specific component needed is given.

Products available for component-targeted therapy include pRBCs, fresh frozen plasma (FFP), cryoprecipitate, platelets, and fibrinogen concentrate. A unit of pRBCs increases the patient's Hct approximately by 3 vol% and Hgb by about 1 g/dL. Crystalloid infusion and pRBC transfusion are the mainstays of therapy in the bleeding obstetric patient.

FFP contains all the necessary coagulation factors including 660 to 700 mg of fibrinogen per unit; each unit has a volume of approximately 250 mL and takes about 30 minutes to thaw. Fibrinogen falls earlier than other coagulation factors during postpartum hemorrhaging and can be low despite a normal PT and aPTT. Thromboelast-ography/-ometry (eg, TEG and ROTEM) can identify in real time which components are needed, including fibrinogen. When replacement of coagulation factors is needed for hemostasis during massive transfusion, FFP transfusion is indicated. Cryoprecipitate and fibrinogen concentrate are appropriate choices for fibrinogen replacement. Ten pooled bags (10-15 mL/bag) of cryoprecipitate will increase fibrinogen level by 65 to 70 mg/dL. A critically low fibrinogen level should be anticipated in PPH due to placental abruption or AFE, and early use of cryoprecipitate is commonly used as part of the resuscitation. Fibrinogen concentrate, if it is readily available on the unit, can be more quickly administered than cryoprecipitate, as it does not need thawing. Further, it provides a known and standardized dose.

With obstetric hemorrhage, platelet count should be maintained greater than 50,000/μL with infusion of platelet concentrates. One unit of platelets increases the platelet count from 5,000 to 10,000/μL in an adult. Platelets are difficult to store and have a short shelf life (5 days). Typically, the blood bank provides platelets from ABO- and Rh-compatible donors. Platelet unit donor plasma must be compatible with, not identical to, recipient erythrocytes, but only units from D-negative donors should go to D-negative recipients.

Massive transfusion protocols (MTP) function to speed blood product delivery to the operating room and permit product infusion early in the resuscitation process to prevent the adverse effects of aggressive resuscitation with only crystalloid and pRBC transfusions. Massive transfusion is often defined as transfusing 10 or more RBC units in a 24-hour period, 4 units of RBCs within 1 hour with an anticipated ongoing need for more blood, or replacement of a complete blood volume.

Recommendations for the rapid transfusion protocols have been adapted from trauma literature and a few clinical reports. Although replacement therapy with plasma, platelets, and RBCs generally should not be based on any set formula, the results from these studies suggest that patients with severe trauma, massive blood replacement, and coagulopathy have improved survival when the ratio of transfused RBCs (units) to FFP (units) to platelet (units) approaches 1:1:1.

Data concerning the use of prothrombin concentrates (PCCs) are limited. The ACOG recommends that their use should only be considered after multiple rounds of standard massive transfusion agents and in consultation with an expert in massive transfusion. Different preparations of PCCs, the human plasma–derived concentrates of vitamin K–dependent clotting factors, are available containing either three factors (factors II, IX, and X) or four factors (factors II, VII, IX, and X). Each gram of fibrinogen concentrate increases the fibrinogen level approximately 40 mg/dL.

Alexander JM, Sarode R, McIntire DD, et al. Whole blood in the management of hypovolemia due to obstetric hemorrhage. *Obstet Gynecol.* 2009;113:1320-1326.

American College of Obstetricians and Gynecologists Committee on Practice Bulletins—Obstetrics. Practice bulletin no. 183: postpartum hemorrhage. *Obstet Gynecol.* 2017;130:e168-e186.

Charbit B, Mandelbrot L, Samain E, et al. The decrease of fibrinogen is an early predictor of the severity of postpartum hemorrhage. *J Thromb Haemost.* 2007;5:266-273.

Collins P, Abdul-Kadir R, Thachil J, et al. Management of coagulopathy associated with postpartum hemorrhage: guidance from the SSC of the ISTH. *J Thromb Haemost.* 2016;14:205-210.

Cunningham FG, Leveno KJ, Bloom SL, et al., eds. Causes of Obstetrical Hemorrhage. In: Cunningham FG, Leveno KJ, Dashe JS, Hoffman BL, Spong CY, Casey BM, eds. *Williams Obstetrics.* 26th ed. McGraw-Hill Education; 2022:770-777.

FIBRYGA. Package insert. Octapharma; 2017. Accessed March 29, 2023. Available from: www.fda.gov/media/105864/download

Lier H, von Heymann C, Korte W, et al. Peripartum haemorrhage: haemostatic aspects of the new German PPH guideline. *Transfus Med Hemother.* 2018;45:127-135.

Pasquier P, Gayat E, Rackelboom T, et al. An observational study of the fresh frozen plasma: red blood cell ratio in postpartum hemorrhage. *Anesth Analg.* 2013;116:155-161.

Shields LE, Wiesner S, Fulton J, et al. Comprehensive maternal hemorrhage protocols reduce use of blood products and improve patient safety. *Am J Obstet Gynecol.* 2015;212:272-280.

Treml AB, Gorlin JB, Dutton RP, et al. Massive transfusion protocols: a survey of academic medical centers in the United States. *Anesth Analg.* 2017;124:277-281.

World Health Organization. *Global Status Report on Blood Safety and Availability 2016.* World Health Organization; 2017.

C.11. What is the role of recombinant activated factor VII (rFVIIa) in the hemorrhaging obstetric patient?

Recombinant activated factor VII (rFVIIa) (NovoSeven), a synthetic vitamin K–dependent glycoprotein, has been used to facilitate hemostasis in patients bleeding from coagulopathies, surgery, trauma, and severe obstetric hemorrhage. Use of rFVIIa in obstetrics has been reported in case series and international registries; no randomized controlled trials have been published. The ACOG recommends that its use be reserved for extenuating circumstances after multiple rounds of standard transfusion agents and in consultation with an expert in massive hemorrhage.

At pharmacologic doses, rFVIIa promotes hemostasis by activating the extrinsic pathway of the coagulation cascade; it replaces deficient activated factor VII. It complexes with tissue factor and may activate the conversion of factor X to Xa and factor IX to IXa; when complexed with other factors, factor Xa converts prothrombin to thrombin, which is a key step in the formation of a fibrin-platelet plug that may control bleeding. A median dose of 81.5 μg/kg of rFVIIa has been found to be effective in stopping or decreasing bleeding in 85% of obstetric cases where it has been utilized. rFVIIa should be considered only after the failure of medical treatment, blood component therapy, and conservative surgical/

invasive treatment. Before administering rFVIIa, acidosis, thrombocytopenia, hypofibrinogenemia, hypocalcemia, and hypothermia should be corrected. Although the optimal dose of rFVIIa for PPH has not been determined, 90 μg/kg can be given intravenously over 3 to 5 minutes. If no response has occurred 20 minutes later, a second dose of 90 μg/kg may be given. Because to date all the information about rFVIIa in obstetrics is anecdotal, use of rFVIIa should be determined on an individual case basis. There are unanswered concerns about the increased likelihood of thrombotic events, and the role of rFVIIa remains undefined. In any uncontrolled obstetrical hemorrhage, hysterectomy should be considered after all hemostasis options have been exhausted. In recent years, pelvic vessel embolization by interventional radiologists has played an increasingly important role in control of obstetrical hemorrhage, allowing preservation of fertility in appropriate cases.

American College of Obstetricians and Gynecologists Committee on Practice Bulletins—Obstetrics. Practice bulletin no. 183: postpartum hemorrhage. *Obstet Gynecol.* 2017;130:e168-e186.

Collins P, Abdul-Kadir R, Thachil J, et al. Management of coagulopathy associated with postpartum hemorrhage: guidance from the SSC of the ISTH. *J Thromb Haemost.* 2016;14:205-210.

Franchini M, Franchi M, Bergamini V, et al. The use of recombinant activated FVII in postpartum hemorrhage. *Clin Obstet Gynecol.* 2010;53:219-227.

Gonsalves M, Belli A. The role of interventional radiology in obstetric hemorrhage. *Cardiovasc Interv Radiol.* 2010;33:887-895.

Lier H, von Heymann C, Korte W, et al. Peripartum haemorrhage: haemostatic aspects of the new German PPH guideline. *Transfus Med Hemother.* 2018;45:127-135.

C.12. What is the role of type O Rh-negative (universal donor) uncrossmatched blood in emergency transfusions, and how does this change your future management?

When typed and screened/crossed blood is unavailable and crystalloid/vasopressor support have been initiated, uncrossmatched type O Rh-negative blood can and should be given in the hemodynamically unstable, hemorrhaging obstetric patient. People with type O blood are considered universal donors because they lack A and B antigens; therefore, their erythrocytes will not be hemolyzed by a recipient's anti-A or anti-B antibodies if present. Some type O donors, however, produce high titers of hemolytic anti-A and anti-B antibodies. RBCs, therefore, are preferable to whole blood because pRBCs have a smaller volume of plasma and therefore a minimal amount of anti-A and anti-B antibodies if present. If whole blood is to be used, the blood bank should supply type O blood that is free of anti-A and anti-B antibodies.

Some confusion exists as to when it is safe to switch back to the patient's native blood type. After a patient has received 2 units of type O Rh-negative uncrossmatched whole blood, the patient should not be switched to their type-specific (A, B, AB) blood; additional transfusions should be continued with type O blood. The patient must not receive a transfusion of their correct blood type until the blood bank determines that switching back to the patient's native blood type is safe. Patients who have received uncrossmatched type O Rh-negative pRBCs can receive many more units without concern for antibody reactions. Individual centers have different policies governing the maximum number of uncrossmatched type O Rh-negative blood units that can be given before switching back to the patient's specific blood type. Most centers do recommend switching to the patient's native blood type as soon as safely possible in order to conserve the emergency supply of type O Rh-negative blood. Recommendations should be obtained from your local blood bank.

Martinez R, Dudley M. Patient Blood Management: Transfusion Therapy. In: Gropper MA, ed. *Miller's Anesthesia.* 10th ed. Elsevier; 2025:1416-1419.

C.13. What complications can occur from transfusion of blood products?

Allogenic blood transfusion safety has improved over the past several decades. Deaths from allogenic transfusions are rare. When they occur, they are primarily due to transfusion-related acute lung injury (TRALI), ABO- and non-ABO hemolytic transfusion reactions (HTRs), and transfusion-related sepsis. Other transfusion-related adverse reactions include transfusion-associated circulatory overload, delayed HTRs, febrile and allergic non-HTRs, infection due to bacterial and/or viral contamination of blood products, transfusion-associated graft-versus-host disease, transfusion-related immunomodulation, and posttransfusion purpura.

TRALI is the most common cause of transfusion-related mortality. TRALI is a noncardiogenic pulmonary edema that occurs within 6 hours after transfusion; this life-threatening complication is characterized by severe dyspnea and hypoxia. A delayed form of TRALI has been reported to occur 6 to 72 hours after transfusion. All blood products can cause TRALI, but plasma-containing products account for 50% to

63% of the fatalities. Its pathogenesis is incompletely understood, but the lung injury appears to involve the activation of recipient white blood cells by human leukocyte antigen antibodies and/or human neutrophil antigen antibodies in the donor plasma. Because the risk of multiparous female donors having these offending antibodies is increased, male-only plasma donation policies have decreased the TRALI rate. Currently, the American Red Cross plasma distribution from male donors exceed 99% for blood groups A, B, and O but is only 60% for group AB. The risk of TRALI after plasma transfusion has been markedly reduced for groups A, B, and O (1.8 per million distributed products) but not for AB (26.3 per million distributed products) due to the continuing use of AB plasma from female donors to meet demand.

HTRs can be acute or delayed. Fatalities from HTRs are rare but do continue to occur in 1 in 1.5 million to 1.8 million transfusions. The severity of an HTR depends on the incompatible recipient antibody, which is most severe in an ABO mismatch, and the volume of blood transfused, with more than 200 mL transfused usually needed to cause a fatality. Accidental transfusion of ABO-incompatible blood can result in acute intravascular hemolysis. This is typically characterized by the symptoms of fever, chills, nausea, flushing, chest and flank pain, tachycardia, hypotension, DIC, hemoglobinuria, acute renal failure, and potentially death. Immediate supportive care includes the discontinuation of the transfusion, treatment of the hypotension and hyperkalemia, administration of a diuretic, and urine alkalinization. The unused blood product should be sent back to the blood bank along with a new patient specimen for a second crossmatch. Assays for urine and plasma Hgb concentration and a direct antiglobulin antibody screen confirm the diagnosis. Reported fatalities due to acute HTRs secondary to non-ABO antibody incompatibilities have increased in the United States and were implicated in 69.2% of all fatal HTRs. Although acute HTRs occur within 24 hours of the transfusion, delayed reactions occur approximately 7 to 10 days after the transfusion of seemingly compatible blood. Death from delayed HTRs occurs much more infrequently than those from an acute reaction.

Because they are stored at room temperature, platelets present the greatest risk of bacterial contamination that can lead to transfusion-related sepsis. The introduction of culture-negative platelets has decreased the risk of receiving an infected platelet transfusion.

The risk of viral infection transmission is low. The risk of contracting human immunodeficiency virus (HIV) or hepatitis C is approximately 1 in 2 million units transfused. The risk of *hepatitis B* transmission is estimated to be less than 1 per 200,000 to 500,000 units transfused. The risk of transfusion-transmitted cytomegalovirus (CMV) can lead to serious morbidity in the immunocompromised patient and/or the fetus or neonate; therefore, pregnant patients should receive blood that is seronegative and leukocyte-depleted to decrease the risk of CMV infection. There have been rare reports of West Nile virus infection, variant Creutzfeldt-Jakob disease, human T-lymphocyte virus type 1, toxoplasmosis, and parvovirus B19 acquired via transfusion. In the United States, blood products are screened for the following infectious agents: HIV-1, HIV-2, human T-lymphocyte virus type I and II, Hepatitis B and C, West Nile virus, Zika virus, *Treponema pallidum* (syphilis), *Trypanosoma cruzi*, CMV (only on enough units to have a sufficient inventory for at-risk recipients), and *Babesia microti* (in high-risk regions only).

The biochemical changes that occur with the storage of blood can lead to problems in the recipient especially when large amounts are rapidly infused. Hypocalcemia, hyperkalemia, and hypothermia can occur and should be promptly corrected.

Cunningham FG, Leveno KJ, Bloom SL, et al., eds. Causes of Obstetrical Hemorrhage. In: Cunningham FG, Leveno KJ, Dashe JS, Hoffman BL, Spong CY, Casey BM, eds. *Williams Obstetrics*. 26th ed. McGraw-Hill Education; 2022:774-775.

Eder AF, Dy BA, Perez JM, et al. The residual risk of transfusion-related acute lung injury at the American Red Cross (2008-2011): limitations of a predominantly male-donor plasma mitigation strategy. *Transfusion*. 2013;53:1442-1449.

Müller MC, van Stein D, Binnekade JM, et al. Low-risk transfusion-related acute lung injury donor strategies and the impact on the onset of transfusion-related acute lung injury: a meta-analysis. *Transfusion*. 2015;55:164-175.

Osterman JL, Arora S. Blood product transfusions and reactions. *Hematol Oncol Clin North Am*. 2017;31:1159-1170.

Vamvakas EC, Blajchman MA. Transfusion-related mortality: the ongoing risks of allogeneic blood transfusion and the available strategies for their prevention. *Blood*. 2009;113:3406-3417.

C.14. What is the role of autologous transfusion in obstetric patients?

Autologous blood transfusion may avoid the risks of alloimmunization, hemolytic reactions, and viral infections; potentially decrease the demands on the allogenic blood supply; and provide a psychological benefit to the patient. There are three methods of autologous transfusion: preoperative (antepartum) donation, normovolemic hemodilution, and intraoperative blood salvage.

SECTION 7

Due to the inability to correctly anticipate which patients will require transfusions and the limited amount of transfusable blood obtained, preoperative donation and normovolemic hemodilution are ineffective strategies for avoiding allogenic transfusions in the obstetric patient. Females with rare blood types or unusual antibodies, however, may benefit from preoperative donation, as well as females with scheduled cesarean deliveries and risk factors for postpartum hemorrhage, or those who are unwilling to accept allogenic blood.

Intraoperative blood salvage has been used in obstetric patients and is considered safe. The limitations are primarily due to the availability of equipment and the appropriate staff, and it only provides RBCs (thus diluting clotting factors). During cesarean delivery after placenta removal, blood is suctioned from the surgical site, collected, and processed through a cell salvage machine that yields a washed, pRBC product for transfusion. Earlier concerns about the safety of blood salvage during cesarean section related to contamination with amniotic fluid have been dispelled with higher quality filtering. Leukocyte depletion filters may improve the margin of safety of the salvaged pRBC product. Because washed pRBCs may contain fetal RBCs, isoimmunization of the mother is possible; anti-D Ig should be given when appropriate.

Patients who are Jehovah's Witnesses have an increased risk of maternal death due to maternal hemorrhage because their religious beliefs prevent them from receiving blood transfusions. The use of intraoperative blood salvage during surgery sometimes is accepted by the patient, because continuity of the salvaged blood with the patient's circulatory system can be maintained. The possibilities for acceptable treatment options should be discussed with each individual patient early in pregnancy, ensuring that they truly have an informed consent regarding each resuscitation product in order to preserve autonomy.

American College of Obstetricians and Gynecologists Committee on Practice Bulletins—Obstetrics. Practice bulletin no. 183: postpartum hemorrhage. *Obstet Gynecol.* 2017;130:e168-e186.

Goucher H, Wong C, Patel SK, et al. Cell salvage in obstetrics. *Anesth Analg.* 2015;121:465-468.

Lier H, von Heymann C, Korte W, et al. Peripartum haemorrhage: haemostatic aspects of the new German PPH guideline. *Transfus Med Hemother.* 2018;45:127-135.

Van Wolfswinkel ME, Zwart JJ, Schutte JM, et al. Maternal mortality and serious maternal morbidity in Jehovah's Witnesses in the Netherlands. *BJOG.* 2009;116:1103-1110.

C.15. Significant intraoperative blood loss required the transfusion of 8 units of type-specific, crossmatched packed RBCs (pRBCs). This patient had generalized oozing in the surgical site and hematuria. What is your differential diagnosis?

The obstetric patient can rapidly develop coagulopathy. It can be dilutional coagulopathy or DIC. Dilutional coagulopathy occurs when massive blood loss is replaced with only crystalloid solutions and pRBCs, leading to a relative depletion of platelets and soluble clotting factors. Thrombocytopenia, hypofibrinogenemia, and factor depletion occur. Pregnancy-related causes of DIC include hemorrhagic shock, AFE, placental abruption, intrauterine fetal demise, preeclampsia/hemolysis, elevated liver enzymes, low platelet count (HELLP) syndrome, sepsis, and acute fatty liver of pregnancy. Additionally, HTRs can cause DIC. Acidosis and hypothermia both interfere with the normal functioning of the coagulation system and worsen coagulopathy.

Cunningham FG, Leveno KJ, Bloom SL, et al., eds. Causes of Obstetrical Hemorrhage. In: Cunningham FG, Leveno KJ, Dashe JS, Hoffman BL, Spong CY, Casey BM, eds. *Williams Obstetrics.* 26th ed. McGraw-Hill Education; 2022:770-777.

Erez O. Disseminated intravascular coagulation in pregnancy—clinical phenotypes and diagnostic scores. *Thromb Res.* 2017;151:S56-S60.

C.16. What is disseminated intravascular coagulation (DIC)?

DIC, a consumptive coagulopathy, is a pathologic activation of the coagulation system that occurs in response to a variety of diseases. The domino effect of widespread intravascular clotting causes uncontrolled bleeding due to the depletion of factors and platelets. Dysregulated clotting deposits thrombi in the microcirculation, diminishing blood flow to the organs and eventually leading to multisystem organ failure. Simultaneously, increased fibrinolysis occurs with the formation of fibrin degradation products. Once DIC begins, the pathophysiology is the same regardless of the inciting cause. Supportive treatment is aimed at replacing the consumed blood products, which "feeds the fire" of inappropriate consumption. Resolution of DIC requires treatment of the underlying cause, allowing reestablishment of homeostasis of clot formation and breakdown. Laboratory values (eg, thromboelastography, traditional coagulation tests) can help guide management by indicating where in the balance of clot formation and breakdown the patient is at any given moment in the resuscitation. Thrombocytopenia, decreased levels of fibrinogen and coagulation factors, increased levels of fibrin degradation products (D-dimers), increased PT, and increased aPTT are seen.

Cunningham FG, Leveno KJ, Bloom SL, et al., eds. Causes of Obstetrical Hemorrhage. In: Cunningham FG, Leveno KJ, Dashe JS, Hoffman BL, Spong CY, Casey BM, eds. *Williams Obstetrics*. 26th ed. McGraw-Hill Education; 2022:775-777.

Erez O. Disseminated intravascular coagulation in pregnancy—clinical phenotypes and diagnostic scores. *Thromb Res*. 2017;151:S56-S60.

C.17. Define amniotic fluid embolism (AFE) syndrome and discuss treatment.

The typical presentation of AFE includes a triad of sudden cardiac and respiratory compromise with DIC occurring in relation to labor and delivery. Classically, it is characterized by the abrupt onset of maternal hypotension, dyspnea, hypoxemia, cyanosis, loss of consciousness, seizures, cardiopulmonary arrest, and hemorrhage due to DIC. AFE is a complex disorder that is poorly understood.

The cause of AFE syndrome is unknown. The diagnosis of AFE is a clinical one of exclusion; no diagnostic tests exist. The pathophysiology seems to involve an abnormal activation of maternal pro-inflammatory mediators in response to fetal tissue exposure during breaks in the maternal-fetal barrier during parturition. Multiple possible mechanisms have been proposed, but none adequately explains this complex syndrome. The abnormal endogenous mediator release has clinical similarities to the systemic inflammatory response syndrome (SIRS) seen with severe sepsis and anaphylaxis. Laboratory findings are nonspecific. The detection of squamous cells, trophoblasts, and other debris of fetal origin is neither sensitive nor specific for AFE.

The estimated AFE incidence is 1 in 40,000 deliveries. Cesarean delivery or instrumented vaginal delivery, precipitous labor, advanced maternal age, placental abruption, placenta previa, PAS, grand multiparity, cervical lacerations, uterine rupture, uterine or pelvic vein tears, eclampsia, pharmacologic labor induction, and polyhydramnios are risk factors.

The overall maternal mortality was reported as 11% to 90% in the past but is currently reported as 20% to 60%. The reported incidence and outcome vary in part because AFE is a diagnosis of exclusion, and perhaps the changing mortality rates reflect improved intensive care. In survivors, the neurologic outcome is often poor, with as many as 85% suffering significant neurologic dysfunction. The neonatal mortality rate is estimated to be between 20% and 60%, and up to 50% of the survivors are neurologically intact. Overall, neonatal outcomes have improved with prompt delivery.

Maternal treatment is primarily prompt supportive resuscitation. The need for delivery is made on a case-by-case basis, but prompt delivery of the fetus in the mother who has sustained a cardiopulmonary arrest is critical. There are no data that any type of intervention improves maternal prognosis with AFE, although case reports using hemofiltration, exchange transfusion, cardiopulmonary bypass, or extracorporeal membrane oxygenation exist.

Clark SL. Amniotic fluid embolism. *Obstet Gynecol*. 2014;123:337-348.

Clark SL, Romero R, Dildy GA, et al. Proposed diagnostic criteria for the case definition of amniotic fluid embolism in research studies. *Am J Obstet Gynecol*. 2016;215:408-412.

Fitzpatrick KE, Tuffnell D, Kurinczuk JJ, et al. Incidence, risk factors, management and outcomes of amniotic-fluid embolism: a population-based cohort and nested case-control study. *BJOG*. 2016;123:100-109.

Pacheco LD, Saade G, Hankins GD, et al; for Society for Maternal-Fetal Medicine. Amniotic fluid embolism: diagnosis and management. *Am J Obstet Gynecol*. 2016 (Reaffirmed 2022);215:B16-B24.

D. Postoperative Management

D.1. If the patient received epidural anesthesia and subsequently developed DIC, when should the epidural catheter be removed?

There is little information available concerning this topic. Neurologic status should be evaluated frequently, and the coagulopathy treated; if there is no indication of intraspinal bleeding, the catheter should be removed as early as possible. If, however, bleeding is present around the catheter insertion site, the catheter can be left in place for tamponade. Any neurologic deficits should be evaluated immediately; prompt surgical decompression may be necessary. However, if neurologic status cannot be evaluated (eg, postoperative intubation and sedation), an argument can be made for removal of an indwelling catheter as soon as possible after replacement of coagulation factors has created a state of normal coagulation (even if this status is presumed temporary).

Horlocker TT, Vandermeuelen E, Kopp SL, et al. Regional anesthesia in the patient receiving antithrombotic or thrombolytic therapy: American Society of Regional Anesthesia and Pain Medicine evidence-based guidelines (fourth edition). *Reg Anesth Pain Med.* 2018;43:263-309.

Sprung J, Cheng EY, Patel S. When to remove an epidural catheter in a parturient with disseminated intravascular coagulation? *Reg Anesth.* 1992;17:351-354.

D.2. You have successfully treated the patient's massive hemorrhage. The laboratory values have returned to normal. The patient, however, is still hypotensive despite appropriate intravascular volume replacement and support with vasopressors. What is your concern in this case?

The patient could have developed Sheehan syndrome. Sheehan syndrome refers to the development of a postpartum pituitary infarction with necrosis, typically precipitated by an obstetric hemorrhage with severe hypotension. Sheehan syndrome is a rare complication. The damage to the pituitary may affect the secretion of one or several hormones. Any of the manifestations of hypopituitarism (eg, failure of lactation, amenorrhea/oligomenorrhea, hypotension, hyponatremia, hypothyroidism) can occur at any time from the immediate postpartum period to years after delivery. If the patient remains hypotensive after control of hemorrhage and adequate volume replacement, the patient should be evaluated and treated for adrenal insufficiency immediately; treatment of possible adrenal crisis should not be delayed while diagnostic tests are performed. Glucocorticoids have a role in maintaining peripheral vascular adrenergic tone, and the sudden loss of corticotropin (adrenocorticotropic hormone) secretion, particularly in conjunction with other serious physical stress, can lead to hypotension and shock. Prompt treatment with stress doses of glucocorticoids may be necessary. The workup includes measuring adrenocorticotropic hormone, cortisol, thyroxine, prolactin, and growth hormone levels. The evaluation of other hormonal deficiencies is not urgent and can be deferred until 4 to 6 weeks postpartum.

Diri H, Karaca Z, Tanriverdi F, et al. Sheehan's syndrome: new insights into an old disease. *Endocrine.* 2016;51:22-31.

Matsuzaki S, Endo M, Ueda Y, et al. A case of acute Sheehan's syndrome and literature review: a rare but life-threatening complication of postpartum hemorrhage. *BMC Pregnancy Childbirth.* 2017;17:188.

Acknowledgment

We gratefully acknowledge the contributions of previous edition author Jill Fong, as portions of those chapters have been retained in this revision.

28 Hypertensive Disorders of Pregnancy

Sharon E. Abramovitz, Joe E.L. Bryant-Huppert, and Jennifer Landon Wagner

A 39-year-old female gravida 1 para 0 at 29 weeks gestation was admitted to the hospital because of an elevated blood pressure (182/111 mm Hg) and headache.

A. Medical Disease and Differential Diagnosis

1. What is the classification of hypertension disorders in pregnancy as defined by the American College of Obstetricians and Gynecologists?
2. What is preeclampsia?
3. What is preeclampsia with severe features?
4. What is eclampsia?
5. What is HELLP syndrome?
6. What are the risk factors for developing preeclampsia?
7. What is the mortality associated with preeclampsia?
8. Discuss the pathogenesis of preeclampsia.
9. Discuss the pathologic alterations of preeclampsia.
10. What are some of the complications associated with preeclampsia?

B. Preoperative Evaluation and Preparation

1. What initial laboratory studies are recommended for patients with preeclampsia?
2. Discuss bleeding time and platelet count evaluation during preoperative assessment of a patient with preeclampsia requesting epidural analgesia/anesthesia for labor and delivery.
3. What types of monitoring are important for patients with preeclampsia with severe features? When is a central venous pressure (CVP) monitor indicated?
4. Discuss the obstetric management of preeclampsia with severe features.
5. What are the goals and agents of choice for severe hypertension seen with preeclampsia?
6. What drug therapy is the treatment of choice for seizure prophylaxis?
7. Discuss the mechanism of action of magnesium sulfate therapy.
8. What are the fetal effects of magnesium sulfate therapy?
9. Discuss the treatment of magnesium sulfate toxicity.
10. What conditions mandate immediate delivery, regardless of gestational age?
11. Discuss the management of eclampsia.

C. Intraoperative Management

1. What is your choice of labor analgesia for patients with preeclampsia?
2. Discuss prehydration prior to initiation of neuraxial analgesia.
3. What sensory level of analgesia is required for labor and delivery?
4. Discuss the commonly used local anesthetics for labor analgesia.
5. Is the addition of epinephrine to local anesthetics advisable in patients with preeclampsia?
6. What is the treatment for abnormal fetal heart rate pattern seen with maternal hypotension after neuraxial analgesia is instituted?
7. What would you do after accidental dural puncture? How do you treat postdural puncture headache (PDPH)?
8. How would you manage total spinal anesthesia?
9. Should methylergonovine be given to patients with preeclampsia?
10. When and how would you administer spinal anesthesia?

11. Discuss a general anesthesia technique for the patient with preeclampsia presenting for cesarean delivery.
12. What agents can you use to prevent hypertension during induction of general anesthesia for cesarean delivery?

D. Postoperative Management

1. Discuss the postpartum management of patients with preeclampsia.
2. Can nonsteroidal anti-inflammatory drugs (NSAIDs) be used to treat postpartum pain in patients with preeclampsia?

A. Medical Disease and Differential Diagnosis

A.1. What is the classification of hypertension disorders in pregnancy as defined by the American College of Obstetricians and Gynecologists?

Hypertensive disorders of pregnancy are classified as follows:

- Gestational hypertension
- Preeclampsia (and related disorders)
  - Preeclampsia
  - Preeclampsia with severe features
  - HEELP (hemolysis, elevated liver enzymes, and low platelet count) syndrome
  - Eclampsia
- Chronic hypertension preceding pregnancy
- Chronic hypertension with superimposed preeclampsia

Gestational hypertension and preeclampsia: ACOG practice bulletin, number 222. *Obstet Gynecol.* 2020;135:e237-e260.

A.2. What is preeclampsia?

Preeclampsia is a multiorgan disease characterized by development of hypertension, along with proteinuria or end-organ dysfunction, after the 20th week of gestation. It is a disorder affecting 2% to 8% of all pregnancies worldwide, with most cases occurring during the first pregnancy, and is unique to humans. Preeclampsia is a leading cause of maternal and perinatal morbidity and mortality worldwide, particularly in developing countries. Hypertension is defined as a systolic blood pressure (BP) of at least 140 mm Hg or a diastolic BP of at least 90 mm Hg on two occasions at least 4 hours apart in a previously normotensive patient. A single reading of a systolic BP of 160 mm Hg or more or diastolic BP of 110 mg Hg or more also defines hypertension. Proteinuria is defined as 300 mg or more of protein in a 24-hour urine collection, a protein-creatinine ratio of 0.3 or greater, or 2+ protein on a urine dipstick. (Dipstick results can be variable and should only be used if other tests are not readily available.) Signs of end-organ dysfunction include thrombocytopenia (platelet count <100,000 per μL), elevated liver transaminases (twice normal concentration), elevated serum creatinine (>1.1 mg/dL or a doubling of serum creatinine in the absence of other renal disease), pulmonary edema, or new-onset cerebral or visual disturbances. Peripheral edema is no longer part of the diagnostic criteria because it lacks specificity and is found in many healthy pregnant females.

Dyer RA, Swanevelder JL, Bateman BT. Hypertensive Disorders. In: Chestnut DH, Wong CA, Tsen LC, et al., eds. *Chestnut's Obstetric Anesthesia: Principles and Practice.* 6th ed. Elsevier; 2019:35, 840-878.

Gestational hypertension and preeclampsia: ACOG practice bulletin, number 222. *Obstet Gynecol.* 2020;135: e237-e260.

Hypertension in pregnancy. Report of the American College of Obstetricians and Gynecologists' Task Force on hypertension in pregnancy. *Obstet Gynecol.* 2013;122:1122-1131.

A.3. What is preeclampsia with severe features?

Preeclampsia with severe features includes at least one of the following features:

- BP: systolic BP greater than or equal to 160 mm Hg or diastolic BP greater than or equal to 110 mm Hg on two occasions at least 4 hours apart while the patient is on bedrest
- Thrombocytopenia (platelet count less than 100,000 per μL)
- Serum creatinine concentration greater than 1.1 mg/dL or greater than 2 times the baseline serum creatinine concentration

- Pulmonary edema
- New-onset cerebral or visual disturbances (headache, scotoma, photopsia)
- Impaired liver function, indicated by elevated blood concentrations of liver enzymes (twice baseline values) or severe, persistent right upper quadrant or epigastric pain
- Fetal growth restriction and severe proteinuria (>5 g in 24 hours) are *no* longer considered features of preeclampsia with severe features

Dyer RA, Swanevelder JL, Bateman BT. Hypertensive Disorders. In: Chestnut DH, Wong CA, Tsen LC, et al., eds. *Chestnut's Obstetric Anesthesia: Principles and Practice*. 6th ed. Elsevier; 2019:35, 840-878.

Gestational hypertension and preeclampsia: ACOG practice bulletin, number 222. *Obstet Gynecol.* 2020;135: e237-e260.

A.4. What is eclampsia?

Eclampsia is defined as convulsions and/or coma not caused by coexisting neurologic disease (eg, epilepsy), which occurs during pregnancy or the puerperium in a female whose condition also meets the criteria for preeclampsia.

Dyer RA, Swanevelder JL, Bateman BT. Hypertensive Disorders. In: Chestnut DH, Wong CA, Tsen LC, et al., eds. *Chestnut's Obstetric Anesthesia: Principles and Practice*. 6th ed. Elsevier; 2019:35, 840-878.

Gestational hypertension and preeclampsia: ACOG practice bulletin, number 222. *Obstet Gynecol.* 2020;135: e237-e260.

A.5. What is HELLP syndrome?

HELLP syndrome is a severe form of preeclampsia characterized by hemolysis (*H*), elevated liver enzymes (*EL*), and low platelets (*LP*). It can occur antepartum or postpartum and complicates 0.2 to 7.6 per 1,000 pregnancies. Delivery represents the only definitive treatment of HELLP syndrome. HELLP syndrome is associated with maternal and neonatal morbidity and mortality and has a high incidence of serious maternal complications including disseminated intravascular coagulation, placental abruption, need for blood transfusion, pleural effusion, acute renal failure, and wound infection. Hemolysis is defined by at least two of the following criteria: abnormal peripheral blood smear, increased bilirubin level (1.2 mg/dL or greater), low haptoglobin or lactate dehydrogenase more than twice the upper limit of normal, or anemia unrelated to blood loss. Elevated liver enzymes are defined as an increased aspartate aminotransferase (AST) or alanine aminotransferase (ALT) twice the upper limit of normal. A low platelet count is defined as a count of less than 100,000 per µL.

Gestational hypertension and preeclampsia: ACOG practice bulletin, number 222. *Obstet Gynecol.* 2020;135: e237-e260.

Lisonkova S, Razaz N, Sabr Y, et al. Maternal risk factors and adverse birth outcomes associated with HELLP syndrome: a population-based study. *BJOG.* 2020;127:1189-1198.

Pauli JM, Repke JT. Preeclampsia: short-term and long-term implications. *Obstet Gynecol Clin North Am.* 2015;42: 299-313.

A.6. What are the risk factors for developing preeclampsia?

The risk factors for developing preeclampsia are:

Hypertensive disease

- Preeclampsia in prior pregnancy
- History of chronic hypertension
- Family history of hypertensive disorder during pregnancy
- Systolic hypertension during early pregnancy

Coexisting vascular and endothelial disease

- Diabetes mellitus (pregestational or gestational)
- Chronic renal disease
- Systemic lupus erythematosus
- Protein S deficiency
- Activated protein C resistance
- Antiphospholipid antibody syndrome
- Angiotensinogen gene *T235*
- Thrombophilia

Obstetric factors
- Nulliparity
- Increased trophoblastic mass (eg, multiple gestation, molar pregnancy)
- Large-for-gestational-age fetus
- Polyhydramnios, particularly in young primigravidas
- Use of assisted reproductive technology
- Erythroblastosis fetalis

Other
- African American race
- Obesity
- Obstructive sleep apnea
- Advanced maternal age (>35 years)

Bartsch E, Medcalf KE, Park AL, Ray JG; High Risk of Pre-eclampsia Identification Group. Clinical risk factors for pre-eclampsia determined in early pregnancy: systematic review and meta-analysis of large cohort studies. *BMJ.* 2016;353:i1753.

Dyer RA, Swanevelder JL, Bateman BT. Hypertensive Disorders. In: Chestnut DH, Wong CA, Tsen LC, et al., eds. *Chestnut's Obstetric Anesthesia: Principles and Practice.* 6th ed. Chestnut DH, ed. Elsevier; 2019:35, 840-878.

Gestational hypertension and preeclampsia: ACOG practice bulletin, number 222. *Obstet Gynecol.* 2020;135: e237-e260.

A.7. What is the mortality associated with preeclampsia?

In 2023, hypertensive disorders of pregnancy accounted for 6.4% of pregnancy-related deaths in the United States. Worldwide this incidence is much higher, with 10% to 15% of maternal mortality being attributed to preeclampsia and its associated complications.

Centers for Disease Control and Prevention. Pregnancy mortality surveillance system. Accessed May 28, 2025. https://www.cdc.gov/maternal-mortality/php/pregnancy-mortality-surveillance-data/index.html?cove-tab=2

Duley L. The global impact of pre-eclampsia and eclampsia. *Semin Perinatol.* 2009;33:130-137.

Khan KS, Wojdyla D, Say L, Gülmezoglu AM, Van Look PF. WHO analysis of causes of maternal death: a systematic review. *Lancet.* 2006;367:1066-1074.

A.8. Discuss the pathogenesis of preeclampsia.

Preeclampsia is a disease of heterogeneous causes of both maternal and placental origin that are not yet fully understood. In the current understanding, preeclampsia is seen as a two-stage disorder, with the first stage owing to abnormal vascularization of the placenta, and the second due to the release of antiangiogenic factors into maternal circulation from this abnormal placentation.

Abnormal Placentation

In normal pregnancy, the spiral arteries of the decidual and myometrial segments undergo vascular remodeling allowing them to increase in diameter to create a low-resistance pathway to facilitate profusion of the placenta. This remodeled vasculature is resistant to vasoactive mediators to ensure maximal blood flow. In patients with abnormal placentation and preeclampsia, spiral arteries are largely not remodeled the same way and remain small and susceptible to maternal vasoactive constriction. This process leads to placentation that is more superficial, with increased incidence of placental infarcts and decreased profusion. Defective trophoblast differentiation has also been implicated in the abnormal invasion of trophoblasts into the spiral arteries seen in preeclampsia. These processes are thought to be multifactorial due to inflammatory, immunologic, genetic, hemostatic, environmental, and vascular factors, as well as oxidative stress.

Endothelial and Inflammatory Factors

Vascular endothelial damage, inflammation, and dysfunction are the common pathologic features of preeclampsia and occur in the placental decidual vessels. Normal placentation and invasion of the trophoblasts into the decidua involves several inflammatory modulators, as well as macrophages, natural killer cells, dendritic cells, and T cells. Endothelial cell dysfunction in response to imbalance of these factors has been noted in many patients who develop preeclampsia and remains a focus of ongoing research.

Immunologic Factors

Immunologic disorders can arise from an abnormal maternal-fetal antigen-antibody response or from the contents of seminal fluids; spermatozoa can cause antibody formation, and prostaglandins can initiate uterine vasoconstriction. The fetus acquires 50% of its genes from the father, which represents in part a paternal allograft that interacts with maternal tissue as the fetal trophoblast migrates into the maternal decidua after implantation. Those patients who have less exposure to paternal antigens, such as those who are nulliparous or use barrier protection, have higher incidence of developing preeclampsia. Additionally, preeclampsia is more prevalent among patients who conceive with reproductive assistive techniques, particularly with oocyte donation, implying such an immunologic difference might play a role in this pathogenesis.

Genetic Factors

A familial tendency toward preeclampsia exists in some populations, and genome-wide association studies are attempting to identify potentially significant genetic loci associated with development of the disorder.

Platelet and Coagulation Factors

In mild preeclampsia, serotonin (5-HT) released from aggregating platelets interacts with endothelial 5-HT_1 receptors, resulting in release of prostacyclin and nitric oxide (NO; *endothelium-derived relaxing factor*. Prostacyclin induces angiotensin II release, improving uteroplacental perfusion. In early-onset severe preeclampsia, damaged uteroplacental vessels cannot respond to 5-HT_1 effects. Instead, serotonin interacts with 5-HT_2 receptors on vascular smooth muscle, inducing vasoconstriction. Platelet-derived serotonin also activates 5-HT_2 platelet receptors, establishing a positive feedback loop and intensifying platelet aggregation. The loss of 5-HT_1 receptors prevents stimulation of angiotensin II release.

Patients with preeclampsia also have an increased tendency toward thromboembolism, which results in part from an alteration in the ratio between plasma von Willebrand factor and factor VIII coagulant activity.

Calcium

In normal pregnancy, intracellular free calcium concentration increases slowly, but this increase is greater in the third trimester in females with preeclampsia. The increase in cytoplasmic calcium levels is enhanced by angiotensin II, and the enhancement is greater in females with preeclampsia compared with normotensive females. Calcium supplementation can reduce the risk of preeclampsia, especially in patients with low baseline calcium.

Vascular Factors

Patients with preeclampsia have elevated plasma levels of endoglin and soluble FLT-1, the receptor for vascular endothelial growth factor, throughout gestation. Nitric oxide also plays a vital role in regulating vascular blood flow, arterial pressure, and maternal and placental perfusion. Recent research suggests that these molecules are not just disease markers but are involved in the pathogenesis of preeclampsia.

Oxidative Stress

Imbalance between oxidants and antioxidants, or oxidative stress, can lead to abnormal cell signaling and molecular damage, and has also been implicated in the pathogenesis of preeclampsia. In the first trimester, the placenta has a relatively hypoxic environment; with increasing perfusion, reactive oxygen species such as free radicals and toxic lipid peroxides are generated. The normal placental response is an increase in antioxidants to protect from oxidative stress, whereas in preeclampsia there might be a reduction of such protective antioxidants.

Ditisheim A, Sibai B, Tatevian N. Placental findings in postpartum preeclampsia: a comparative retrospective study. *Am J Perinatol.* 2020;37:1217-1222.

Dyer RA, Swanevelder JL, Bateman BT. Hypertensive Disorders. In: Chestnut DH, Wong CA, Tsen LC, et al., eds. *Chestnut's Obstetric Anesthesia: Principles and Practice.* 6th ed. Chestnut DH, ed. Elsevier; 2019:35, 840-878.

Lian R, Zhu BS, Zeng X. An update review of the pathogenesis hypothesis in preeclampsia. *Clin Exp Obstet Gynecol.* 2022;49:170.

Woo Kinshella ML, Sarr C, Sandhu A, et al; PRECISE Network. Calcium for pre-eclampsia prevention: a systematic review and network meta-analysis to guide personalised antenatal care. *BJOG.* 2022;129:1833-1843.

A.9. Discuss the pathologic alterations of preeclampsia.

Cardiovascular Changes

- *Blood pressure.* Blood pressure is increased due to an increase in peripheral vascular resistance secondary to a state of sympathetic overactivity.
- *Blood volume.* Intravascular volume is decreased due to vasoconstriction, leading to hemoconcentration.

Hemodynamic Changes

Three hemodynamic subsets of preeclampsia exist:

- Normal or slightly increased systemic vascular resistance (SVR), normal or slightly decreased blood volume and filling pressures and hyperdynamic with increased cardiac output

SECTION 7

- High SVR and lower filling pressures with normal cardiac output
- Markedly increased SVR and decreased blood volume with depressed left ventricular function and cardiac output

  There is poor correlation between CVP and pulmonary artery (PA) occlusion pressure.
- Decreased colloid oncotic pressure occurs in pregnancy with further reduction in preeclampsia. The low colloid oncotic pressure, coupled with increased vascular permeability and loss of intravascular fluid and protein into interstitial tissues, increases the risk of pulmonary edema.

Hematologic Changes

- *Platelet activation*: Thrombocytopenia occurs in 15% to 30% of females with preeclampsia or eclampsia. Preeclampsia can be associated with a defect in *both* platelet function and platelet number. Thrombocytopenia with evidence of hemolysis and increased liver enzymes characterizes HELLP syndrome.
- *Disseminated Intravascular Coagulation (DIC)*: DIC can be present in the patient with preeclampsia; this is generally seen in patients with liver involvement, intrauterine fetal demise, placental abruption, or postpartum hemorrhage.

Renal Changes

- Glomerular enlargement results in ischemia, leading to decreased glomerular filtration rate. This can be seen by measured decreases in markers of renal clearance, such as creatinine and blood urea nitrogen (BUN).
- Proteinuria occurs as a result of an increased permeability to most large-molecular weight proteins.
- Urate clearance decreases and serum uric acid concentration increases. Hyperuricemia might provide an early indication of preeclampsia.
- Oliguria parallels the severity of preeclampsia.

Respiratory Changes

- Pharyngeal and laryngeal edema can make airway management difficult, necessitating use of smaller endotracheal tubes.
- Pulmonary edema occurs in 3% of cases, with some cases occurring postpartum. The etiology can be multifactorial, due to decreased colloid osmotic pressure, increased vascular permeability, increased intravascular pressure due to fluid overload, or ventricular dysfunction.

Hepatic Changes

- Serum transaminase levels frequently increase in patients with preeclampsia.
- Epigastric or subcostal pain is an ominous symptom that is typically caused by distension of the liver capsule by edema or subcapsular or parenchymal bleeding. Hepatic swelling produces epigastric pain.
- Liver rupture is a rare complication but is associated with a 32% mortality rate.

Neurologic Changes

- The classic manifestations of preeclampsia include severe headache, visual disturbances, central nervous system hyperexcitability, and hyperreflexia.
- The occurrence of seizures indicates eclampsia until proven otherwise. Etiologies of seizures include hypertonic encephalopathy, vasospasm, microinfarctions and punctate hemorrhages, thrombosis, and cerebral edema.
- Postpartum eclampsia can occur up to 4 weeks after delivery.
- Reversible posterior leukoencephalopathy syndrome (RPLS) is a neurologic syndrome associated with headache, confusion, visual symptoms, and seizures defined by clinical and radiologic features. MRI findings are consistent with vasogenic edema and need to be closely evaluated to differentiate from stroke. Most patients recover within weeks; however, some have residual neurologic deficits resulting from cortical infarction or hemorrhage.

Uteroplacental Perfusion

- Uteroplacental perfusion is decreased in preeclampsia with the potential for intrauterine growth retardation, oligohydramnios, and stillbirth. Placental abruption is more likely in patients with preeclampsia.

Dyer RA, Swanevelder JL, Bateman BT. Hypertensive Disorders. In: Chestnut DH, Wong CA, Tsen LC, et al., eds. *Chestnut's Obstetric Anesthesia: Principles and Practice*. 6th ed. Chestnut DH, ed. Elsevier; 2019:35, 840-878.

Gestational hypertension and preeclampsia: ACOG practice bulletin, number 222. *Obstet Gynecol.* 2020;135:e237-e260.

Mayama M, Uno K, Tano S, et al. Incidence of posterior reversible encephalopathy syndrome in eclamptic and patients with preeclampsia with neurologic symptoms. *Am J Obstet Gynecol.* 2016;215:239.e1-239.e5.

Melchiorre K, Sharma R, Thilaganathan B. Cardiovascular implications in preeclampsia: an overview. *Circulation.* 2014;130:703-714.

Yancey LM, Withers E, Bakes K, Abbott J. Postpartum preeclampsia: emergency department presentation and management. *J Emerg Med.* 2011;40:380-384.

A.10. What are some of the complications associated with preeclampsia?

Maternal complications include seizure, stroke, cardiomyopathy, pulmonary edema, disseminated intravascular coagulation, postpartum hemorrhage, acute kidney injury, and rupture or failure of the liver. The leading cause of maternal death is intracranial hemorrhage. Patients with preeclampsia are at risk for recurrence in subsequent pregnancies, as well as at increased risk of cardiovascular disease later in life.

Fetal complications include either intrauterine growth retardation, oligohydramnios, intracranial hemorrhage, increased risk of prematurity, and meconium aspiration syndrome. The leading cause of intrauterine morbidity and mortality is uteroplacental insufficiency caused by placental infarcts, followed by placental abruption, and chorioamnionitis.

Bramham K, Briley AL, Seed P, Poston L, Shennan AH, Chappell LC. Adverse maternal and perinatal outcomes in women with previous preeclampsia: a prospective study. *Am J Obstet Gynecol.* 2011;204:512.e1-512.e9.

Gatt SP, Elliott D. Preeclampsia and Eclampsia. In: Datta S, ed. *Anesthetic and Obstetric Management of High-Risk Pregnancy.* 3rd ed. Springer; 2004:279-289.

Ghulmiyyah L, Sibai B. Maternal mortality from preeclampsia/eclampsia. *Semin Perinatol.* 2012;36:56-59.

Magee LA, Nicolaides KH, von Dadelszen P. Preeclampsia. *N Engl J Med.* 2022;386:1817-1832.

B. Preoperative Evaluation and Preparation

B.1. What initial laboratory studies are recommended for patients with preeclampsia?

- Hemoglobin and hematocrit
- Platelet count: If less than 100,000 mm^{-3}, further coagulation studies (activated partial thromboplastin time, prothrombin time, fibrinogen) can be useful
- Serum electrolytes
- Serum creatinine and uric acid concentrations
- Liver function tests
- Serum lactate dehydrogenase (LDH)
- Urine protein-creatinine ratio or 24-hour urine protein excretion
- Type and screen (crossmatch if antibodies present)

SECTION 7

Dyer RA, Swanevelder JL, Bateman BT. Hypertensive Disorders. In: Chestnut DH, Wong CA, Tsen LC, et al., eds. *Chestnut's Obstetric Anesthesia: Principles and Practice.* 6th ed. Chestnut DH, ed. Elsevier; 2019:35, 840-878.

Publications Committee, Society for Maternal-Fetal Medicine; Sibai BM. Evaluation and management of severe preeclampsia before 34 weeks' gestation. *Am J Obstet Gynecol.* 2011;205:191-198.

B.2. Discuss bleeding time and platelet count evaluation during preoperative assessment of a patient with preeclampsia requesting epidural analgesia/anesthesia for labor and delivery.

The bleeding time does not specifically measure platelet function, and it can be abnormal in a number of coagulation disorders, including factor deficiencies. No evidence suggests that the skin bleeding time predicts the potential for bleeding from a traumatized epidural vein in a female with preeclampsia. Therefore, the bleeding time should not be used to measure platelet function. The *trend* in platelet count is important because preeclampsia is a dynamic disorder, and a rapid decrease in platelet count in a short interval warrants concern.

Many anesthesiologists will place an epidural catheter with a platelet count of more than 70,000 per μL and some at lower platelet counts, especially in otherwise healthy parturients. The patient with preeclampsia must be individualized and a thorough bleeding history, along with the trend in platelet count, should be considered. If the platelet count is less than 100,000 per μL, serial platelet counts as well as prothrombin time, partial thromboplastin time, and fibrinogen levels should be measured. If concomitant signs of HELLP are present, a platelet count within 6 hours is recommended due to the potential for rapid depletion of platelets.

Abramovitz S, Beilin Y. Thrombocytopenia, low molecular weight heparin, and obstetric anesthesia. *Anesthesiol Clin North Am.* 2003;21:99-109.

Bauer ME, Arendt K, Beilin Y, et al. The society for obstetric anesthesia and perinatology interdisciplinary consensus statement on neuraxial procedures in obstetric patients with thrombocytopenia. *Anesth Analg.* 2021;132:1531-1544.

Laskin S, Payne B, Hutcheon JA, et al. The role of platelet counts in the assessment of inpatient women with preeclampsia. *J Obstet Gynaecol Can*. 2011;33:900-908.

Lee LO, Bateman BT, Kheterpal S, et al; Multicenter Perioperative Outcomes Group Investigators. Risk of epidural hematoma after neuraxial techniques in thrombocytopenic parturients: a report from the multicenter perioperative outcomes group. *Anesthesiology*. 2017;126:1053-1063.

B.3. What types of monitoring are important for patients with preeclampsia with severe features? When is a central venous pressure (CVP) monitor indicated?

- Noninvasive BP monitoring
- Maternal respiratory function assessment by pulse oximetry
- Urine output monitoring
- Monitoring of deep tendon reflexes and serial magnesium levels
- Tocodynamometer and continuous fetal heart rate monitoring
- Ongoing maternal physical assessment and report for development of symptoms
- Consider invasive BP monitoring with an arterial line when severe refractory hypertension is present, or when noninvasive BP measurement proves difficult (eg, obesity).
- A CVP monitor or PA catheter were commonly used in the past to inform fluid management; however, they are now reserved for cases of severe organ failure, valvular or congenital heart disease, and critically unstable patients requiring vasoactive medications.

Pulmonary edema can be due to an increase in capillary permeability as well as from diastolic dysfunction, complicating assessment of cardiac function and volume status. Furthermore, there can be technical difficulties with placing the PA catheter that are both patient related (awake, anxious, short neck with poorly visible landmarks, coagulopathy) and physician related (inexperience with central venous catheterization), which alters the balance between benefit and risk of invasive monitoring. Whenever possible, a bedside transthoracic echocardiogram can be obtained; however, there can be limited windows for imaging due to the gravid uterus causing distention of the abdomen.

Dyer RA, Swanevelder JL, Bateman BT. Hypertensive Disorders. In: Chestnut DH, Wong CA, Tsen LC, et al., eds. *Chestnut's Obstetric Anesthesia: Principles and Practice*. 6th ed. Chestnut DH, ed. Elsevier; 2019:35, 840-878.

Li YH, Novikova N. Pulmonary artery flow catheters for directing management in pre-eclampsia. *Cochrane Database Syst Rev*. 2012:CD008882.

B.4. Discuss the obstetric management of preeclampsia with severe features.

Multidisciplinary planning can be of benefit with input from obstetric, nursing, and anesthesia staff. Overall obstetric management aims to stabilize the mother and safely deliver the fetus.

- Administer antihypertensive agents to prevent stroke, myocardial ischemia, or heart failure.
- Administer seizure prophylaxis.
- Determine timing of delivery.

B.5. What are the goals and agents of choice for severe hypertension seen with preeclampsia?

Severe hypertension, defined as greater than 160 mm Hg systolic or greater than 110 mm Hg diastolic, confirmed by a repeat measurement within 15 minutes, mandates prompt treatment. If left untreated, there are increased maternal complications such as stroke and heart failure; however, this must be weighed against the concerns of lowering maternal BP excessively as this can lead to decreased uteroplacental perfusion. Most guidelines recommend intravenous labetalol, intravenous hydralazine, or oral nifedipine as first-line agents. There is insufficient evidence regarding superiority among these three agents.

Labetalol, a combined nonselective β- and α_1-receptor blocker, decreases maternal SVR without increasing maternal heart rate or decreasing cardiac index, uterine blood flow, or fetal heart rate when it is given in a total dose of less than 1 mg/kg. When given in an initial bolus dose of 10 to 20 mg, it has a faster onset of action than hydralazine, and, if necessary, the dose can be doubled every 10 minutes. If a second antihypertensive agent is needed (eg, hydralazine or nicardipine), labetalol helps to prevent reflex tachycardia. Labetalol should be used cautiously in females with asthma due to risk of bronchospasm.

Hydralazine is used as antihypertensive agent because of its direct vasodilating effect. The full extent of its effect is evident in 20 minutes; therefore, if sufficient time is not allowed between doses, severe hypotension can be seen. It is used in 5 to 10-mg increments intravenously every 20 to 30 minutes until the BP is below threshold, with a cumulative dose of 20 mg. Hydralazine directly decreases SVR. Reflex sympathetic activity can result in tachycardia and increased stroke volume and cardiac output. Tachycardia can be treated with labetalol, 10 to 20 mg intravenously.

Nifedipine is a calcium channel blocker that affects predominantly arterial and arteriolar smooth muscle. Common maternal side effects include facial flushing, headache, and tachycardia. Nifedipine rapidly lowers BP after oral or sublingual administration. After an initial dose of 10 mg orally, a dose of 20 mg can be repeated in 20 minutes and subsequently given in a maintenance dose of 10 to 20 mg every 3 to 6 hours. Caution must be exercised in patients receiving both magnesium sulfate and calcium channel blockers because of potential myocardial depression and resultant pulmonary edema.

Nitroglycerin (NTG) causes vascular smooth muscle relaxation by means of its intracellular generation of NO. The primary effect of NTG is venodilation, but it is less effective in prehydrated patients. NTG readily crosses the placenta. It is most useful for short-term treatment (eg, to control the response to tracheal intubation). Small doses (50-100 μg) can be given intravenously or sublingually in a 400-μg metered spray.

Sodium nitroprusside (SNP) relaxes arterial vessels, thereby reducing afterload, and also reduces venous return. It was previously used for short-term treatment, similar to NTG, but cyanide toxicity is problematic with prolonged infusions that exceed 4 μg/kg/min over several hours to days. Given the availability of better alternatives, it is now rarely used. Coadministration of sodium thiosulfate can help prevent fetal and maternal cyanide toxicity in animal models. It is not known whether these findings are transferable to humans, raising major concern over ongoing clinical use of nitroprusside in obstetrics when safer drugs such as nicardipine and labetalol are available.

Alavifard S, Chase R, Janoudi G, et al. First-line antihypertensive treatment for severe hypertension in pregnancy: a systematic review and network meta-analysis. *Pregnancy Hypertens.* 2019;18:179-187.

Curry SC, Carlton MW, Raschke RA. Prevention of fetal and maternal cyanide toxicity from nitroprusside with coinfusion of sodium thiosulfate in gravid ewes. *Anesth Analg.* 1997;84:1121-1126.

Duley L, Meher S, Jones L. Drugs for treatment of very high blood pressure during pregnancy. *Cochrane Database Syst Rev.* 2013;2013:CD001449.

Dyer RA, Swanevelder JL, Bateman BT. Hypertensive Disorders. In: Chestnut DH, Wong CA, Tsen LC, et al., eds. *Chestnut's Obstetric Anesthesia: Principles and Practice.* 6th ed. Chestnut DH, ed. Elsevier; 2019:35, 840-878.

Magee LA, Nicolaides KH, von Dadelszen P. Preeclampsia. *N Engl J Med.* 2022;386:1817-1832.

Gestational hypertension and preeclampsia: ACOG practice bulletin, number 222. *Obstet Gynecol.* 2020;135: e237-e260.

Publications Committee, Society for Maternal-Fetal Medicine; Sibai BM. Evaluation and management of severe preeclampsia before 34 weeks' gestation. *Am J Obstet Gynecol.* 2011;205:191-198.

B.6. What drug therapy is the treatment of choice for seizure prophylaxis?

Magnesium sulfate is the initial therapy for seizure prophylaxis in females with preeclampsia with severe features. The Eclampsia Trial Collaborative Group compared magnesium sulfate, phenytoin, and diazepam administration for prevention of recurrent seizures in females with preeclampsia. Magnesium sulfate was more effective in preventing seizures than either phenytoin or diazepam. Current research supports continuing magnesium sulfate therapy for 24 hours after delivery for seizure prophylaxis.

An initial bolus of 4 to 6 g of magnesium sulfate is administered over 20 to 30 minutes and followed with an intravenous infusion of 1 to 2 g/h. Urine output, respiratory rate, and patellar reflexes are monitored, and serum magnesium sulfate concentration should be measured at least 4 hours after initiation of therapy. The therapeutic range for serum magnesium sulfate is 4 to 7 mEq/L. Loss of deep tendon reflexes occurs at 7 mEq/L with evidence of prolonged PQ intervals and widening QRS complexes. Respiratory depression occurs at 10 mEq/L, and asystole or cardiac arrest occurs at 25 mEq/L.

Gestational hypertension and preeclampsia: ACOG practice bulletin, number 222. *Obstet Gynecol.* 2020;135: e237-e260.

Pauli JM, Repke JT. Preeclampsia: short-term and long-term implications. *Obstet Gynecol Clin North Am.* 2015; 42:299-313.

Sullivan M, Cunningham K, Angras K, Mackeen AD. Duration of postpartum magnesium sulfate for seizure prophylaxis in women with preeclampsia: a systematic review and meta-analysis. *J Matern Fetal Neonatal Med.* 2022;35:7188-7193.

The Eclampsia Trial Collaborative Group. Which anticonvulsant for women with eclampsia? Evidence from the collaborative eclampsia trial. *Lancet.* 1995;345:1455-1463.

B.7. Discuss the mechanism of action of magnesium sulfate therapy.

The mechanism of action of magnesium sulfate for prevention of seizures is not entirely understood, however, the following effects are considered possible:

- It acts as a central nervous system depressant and anticonvulsant.
- It can protect the blood-brain barrier, decrease cerebral edema, or act centrally at *N*-methyl-D-aspartate receptors to raise the seizure threshold.

- It inhibits the release of acetylcholine at the neuromuscular junction, decreases the sensitivity of the motor end plate to acetylcholine, and decreases muscle membrane excitability, thereby potentiating the effects of nondepolarizing and depolarizing neuromuscular blockers.
- It decreases uterine hyperactivity by a mild relaxant effect on vascular and uterine smooth muscle; it might improve uterine blood flow. Postpartum, it can lead to uterine atony and increased hemorrhage risk.
- It is a mild vasodilator in vascular beds (including small-diameter cerebral vessels) by a direct or indirect (calcium-competing) effect, and it has a mild antihypertensive effect.

Dyer RA, Swanevelder JL, Bateman BT. Hypertensive Disorders. In: Chestnut DH, Wong CA, Tsen LC, et al., eds. *Chestnut's Obstetric Anesthesia: Principles and Practice*. 6th ed. Chestnut DH, ed. Elsevier; 2019:35, 840-878.

Imaralu JO. Evolution of magnesium sulphate for eclampsia. *Obstet Gynecol Int J*. 2018;9:483-486.

B.8. What are the fetal effects of magnesium sulfate therapy?

Magnesium sulfate crosses the placenta. There can be decreased beat-to-beat variability in fetal heart rate. Neonatal depression (eg, respiratory depression and hyporeflexia) can also occur.

Pauli JM, Repke JT. Preeclampsia: short-term and long-term implications. *Obstet Gynecol Clin North Am*. 2015;42:299-313.

B.9. Discuss the treatment of magnesium sulfate toxicity.

Magnesium sulfate is excreted by the kidneys. Therefore, urine output must be followed closely, and serial serum concentrations of magnesium sulfate must be checked, especially in females with renal dysfunction. If magnesium sulfate toxicity is suspected, the magnesium sulfate infusion should be immediately discontinued. Intravenous calcium gluconate, 1 g, or calcium chloride, 300 mg, should be administered if needed to antagonize the effects of magnesium sulfate along with intravenous furosemide to accelerate urinary excretion. If respiratory distress occurs, the patient might require tracheal intubation and mechanical ventilation.

Dyer RA, Swanevelder JL, Bateman BT. Hypertensive Disorders. In: Chestnut DH, Wong CA, Tsen LC, et al., eds. *Chestnut's Obstetric Anesthesia: Principles and Practice*. 6th ed. Chestnut DH, ed. Elsevier; 2019:35, 840-878.

Gestational hypertension and preeclampsia: ACOG practice bulletin, number 222. *Obstet Gynecol*. 2020;135:e237-e260.

Imaralu JO. Evolution of magnesium sulphate for eclampsia. *Obstet Gynecol Int J*. 2018;9:483-486.

B.10. What conditions mandate immediate delivery, regardless of gestational age?

- Severe hypertension that is unresponsive to antihypertensive medications
- HELLP syndrome
- Epigastric or right upper quadrant (RUQ) pain that is unresponsive to analgesics
- Persistent headache or other neurologic sequela of preeclampsia (including seizure or stroke)
- New or worsening renal dysfunction (including severe oliguria)
- Pulmonary edema
- Evidence of deteriorating fetal status

Gatt SP, Elliott D. Preeclampsia and Eclampsia. In: Datta S, ed. *Anesthetic and Obstetric Management of High-Risk Pregnancy*. 3rd ed. Springer; 2004:279-289.

Gestational Hypertension and Preeclampsia: ACOG Practice Bulletin, Number 222. *Obstet Gynecol*. 2020;135:e237-e260.

Publications Committee, Society for Maternal-Fetal Medicine; Sibai BM. Evaluation and management of severe preeclampsia before 34 weeks' gestation. *Am J Obstet Gynecol*. 2011;205:191-198.

B.11. Discuss the management of eclampsia.

- Turn patient to the left side; apply jaw thrust.
- Administer oxygen.
- Apply pulse oximeter and monitor.
- Secure intravenous access.
- Check BP at frequent intervals.
- Monitor electrocardiogram (ECG) recordings.
- If recurrent seizures, secure airway with aspiration precautions and administer anticonvulsants (lorazepam 2-4 mg IV or diazepam 5-10 mg IV).
- Administer magnesium sulfate to prevent recurrent seizures.
- Develop delivery plan.

Dyer RA, Swanevelder JL, Bateman BT. Hypertensive Disorders. In: Chestnut DH, Wong CA, Tsen LC, et al., eds. *Chestnut's Obstetric Anesthesia: Principles and Practice*. 6th ed. Chestnut DH, ed. Elsevier; 2019:35, 840-878.

Gestational hypertension and preeclampsia: ACOG practice bulletin, number 222. *Obstet Gynecol*. 2020 Jun;135: e237-e260.

C. Intraoperative Management

C.1. What is your choice of labor analgesia for patients with preeclampsia?

Continuous epidural and combined-spinal epidural (CSE) analgesia are safe and preferred methods of pain relief for labor and delivery in females with preeclampsia. Epidural and CSE analgesia provide the following advantages:

- Pain relief that is superior to other analgesic methods
- Attenuation of the exaggerated hypertensive response to pain
- Decrease in circulating levels of catecholamines and stress-related hormones, which facilitates BP control
- Improvement of intervillous blood flow
- Stable cardiac output
- Females with preeclampsia are at increased risk for cesarean delivery compared to other parturients, and early administration of epidural analgesia for labor facilitates subsequent administration of epidural anesthesia for emergent cesarean delivery while avoiding the risks of general anesthesia.

Dyer RA, Swanevelder JL, Bateman BT. Hypertensive Disorders. In: Chestnut DH, Wong CA, Tsen LC, et al., eds. *Chestnut's Obstetric Anesthesia: Principles and Practice*. 6th ed. Chestnut DH, ed. Elsevier; 2019:35, 840-878.

Pauli JM, Repke JT. Preeclampsia: short-term and long-term implications. *Obstet Gynecol Clin North Am*. 2015;42:299-313.

C.2. Discuss prehydration prior to initiation of neuraxial analgesia.

Prehydration with intravenous crystalloid solution has been used to reduce the incidence and severity of hypotension after initiation of neuraxial analgesia. However, in current practice, lower concentrations of local anesthetics combined with an opioid are used for labor analgesia, and fluid preloading is of less clinical relevance, and several randomized controlled trials show no benefit in hypotension reduction or severity with prehydration. For spinal anesthesia for cesarean delivery, co-loading of IV fluids at the time of spinal anesthesia has been shown to be equally as effective as prehydration. One must be vigilant regarding the risk of pulmonary edema in patient with preeclampsia with severe features because the incidence of global diastolic dysfunction is about 40% although it is usually mild.

Melchiorre K, Sutherland GR, Baltabaeva A, Liberati M, Thilaganathan B. Maternal cardiac dysfunction and remodeling in women with preeclampsia at term. *Hypertension*. 2011;57:85-93.

Wong CA. Epidural and Spinal Analgesia: Anesthesia for Labor and Vaginal Delivery. In: Chestnut DH, Wong CA, Tsen LC, et al., eds. *Chestnut's Obstetric Anesthesia: Principles and Practice*. 6th ed. Chestnut DH, ed. Elsevier; 2019:23, 474-539.

C.3. What sensory level of analgesia is required for labor and delivery?

- First stage of labor: T10-L1
- Second stage of labor: S2-S4

Wong CA. Epidural and Spinal Analgesia: Anesthesia for Labor and Vaginal Delivery. In: Chestnut DH, Wong CA, Tsen LC, et al., eds. *Chestnut's Obstetric Anesthesia: Principles and Practice*. 6th ed. Elsevier; 2019:474-539.

C.4. Discuss the commonly used local anesthetics for labor analgesia.

Bupivacaine, ropivacaine, and levobupivacaine (all amide local anesthetics) are commonly used because they provide potent analgesia, a longer duration, and less motor block compared to lidocaine. Labor analgesia using local anesthetic agents at low concentrations is favored as opposed to local anesthetics at higher concentrations as it is not associated with a prolonged duration of the second stage of labor or increased instrumental birth rate.

Bupivacaine is 4 times more potent than lidocaine. However, it is also more cardiotoxic due to its action on cardiac sodium channels. Bupivacaine is a "fast-on, slow-off" agent. While bupivacaine and lidocaine both rapidly block sodium channels on nerves and heart, bupivacaine is 5 times slower; this delayed recovery can precipitate arrhythmias.

Ropivacaine is a homolog of mepivacaine and bupivacaine, but is formulated as a single levorotatory racemate rather than as a racemic mixture. It appears to be less cardiotoxic than bupivacaine.

Levobupivacaine is also a single levorotatory racemate formulation of a local anesthetic, and appears to be less cardiotoxic than bupivacaine.

Wang TT, Sun S, Huang SQ. Effects of epidural labor analgesia with low concentrations of local anesthetics on obstetric outcomes: a systematic review and meta-analysis of randomized controlled trials. *Anesth Analg*. 2017;124: 1571-1580.

Wong CA. Epidural and Spinal Analgesia: Anesthesia for Labor and Vaginal Delivery. In: Chestnut DH, Wong CA, Tsen LC, et al., eds. *Chestnut's Obstetric Anesthesia: Principles and Practice.* 6th ed. Elsevier; 2019:474-539.

C.5. Is the addition of epinephrine to local anesthetics advisable in patients with preeclampsia?

Clinical evidence supports the safety of epidural administration of epinephrine-containing local anesthetic in females with preeclampsia. However, care must be taken when using epinephrine-containing local anesthetic solutions in females with preeclampsia with severe features because inadvertent intravascular injection can result in severe acute hypertension. Epinephrine in epidural test doses might not be diagnostic in patients with preeclampsia who have received β-adrenergic receptor antagonists as they might not produce the typical tachycardia after intravascular injection of epinephrine.

Dror A, Abboud TK, Moore J, et al. Maternal hemodynamic responses to epinephrine-containing local anesthetics in mild pre-eclampsia. *Reg Anesth*. 1988;13:107-111.

Dyer RA, Swanevelder JL, Bateman BT. Hypertensive Disorders. In: Chestnut DH, Wong CA, Tsen LC, et al., eds. *Chestnut's Obstetric Anesthesia: Principles and Practice*. 6th ed. Chestnut DH, ed. Elsevier; 2019:35, 840-878.

Heller PJ, Goodman C. Use of local anesthetics with epinephrine for epidural anesthesia in preeclampsia. *Anesthesiology*. 1986;65:224-226.

C.6. What is the treatment for abnormal fetal heart rate pattern seen with maternal hypotension after neuraxial analgesia is instituted?

- Left uterine displacement
- Administration of intravenous fluids
- Elevation of lower extremities to facilitate venous return
- Administration of small increments of phenylephrine (40-100 μg) or ephedrine (5-10 mg) intravenously if BP is less than 20% of baseline

Tsen LC, Bateman BT. Anesthesia for cesarean delivery. In: *Chestnut DH, ed. Chestnut's Obstetric Anesthesia: Principles and Practice*. 6th ed. Elsevier; 2019;23: 474-539.

Vercauteren M. Obstetric spinal analgesia and anesthesia. *Curr Opin Anaesthesiol*. 2003;16:503-507.

C.7. What would you do after accidental dural puncture? How do you treat postdural puncture headache (PDPH)?

Accidental dural puncture can be managed with one of two major options. First, the epidural needle can be removed, and the placement of epidural catheter can be reattempted in another interspace. Local anesthetic must be administered cautiously, as direct communication with the intrathecal space through the dural hole could lead to a more profound block. Alternatively, a catheter can be threaded into the intrathecal space and maintained for continuous spinal labor analgesia. This approach is prudent when the initial placement of the epidural catheter was difficult, allowing for faster pain relief and eliminating the risk of a second dural puncture. Great caution should be exercised in maintaining an intrathecal catheter, and all staff should be informed of the status of the catheter, with judicious monitoring and consideration of any bolus medications.

The incidence of a postdural puncture headache (PDPH) after accidental wet tap with an epidural needle is more than 50%. The headache occurs within 5 days of dural puncture and symptoms include nausea and vomiting, tinnitus, blurry vision, and neck pain. Prior treatment strategies endorsed bedrest, increased hydration, caffeine intake, sphenopalatine ganglion block, and neuraxial opioids as potential therapeutic options, however, their efficacy has not been proven. Epidural blood patch is the gold standard for treatment of PDPH. Immediate relief occurs in almost 80% of patients on the first attempt, and a blood patch can be repeated if the initial procedure does not help with symptomatic relief, usually with good efficacy. Transient side effects include backache and neck pain.

Gaiser RR. Postdural puncture headache: an evidence-based approach. *Anesthesiol Clin*. 2017;35:157-167.

Peralta F, Macarthur A. Postpartum Headache. In: Chestnut DH, Wong CA, Tsen LC, et al., eds. *Chestnut's Obstetric Anesthesia: Principles and Practice*. 6th ed. Chestnut DH, ed. Elsevier; 2019:724-761.

C.8. How would you manage total spinal anesthesia?

- High spinal anesthesia can occur several minutes after an inadvertent injection of local anesthetic into the subarachnoid or subdural space. It is vitally important to communicate with the patient. Agitation, dyspnea, and difficulty speaking can indicate onset of total spinal anesthesia.
- Avoid aortocaval compression.
- Administer 100% oxygen.
- Provide positive pressure ventilation if necessary, preferably through an endotracheal tube.
- Monitor maternal BP, ECG, and fetal heart rate.
- Support maternal circulation with intravenous fluids and vasopressors as needed. Give epinephrine if needed.

Tsen LC, Bateman BT. Anesthesia for cesarean delivery. In: Chestnut DH, ed. *Chestnut's Obstetric Anesthesia: Principles and Practice*. 6th ed. Elsevier; 2019;23: 474-539.

C.9. Should methylergonovine be given to patients with preeclampsia?

Preeclampsia is a relative contraindication to the use of ergot alkaloids because of the risk of inducing a hypertensive crisis. In patients with preeclampsia, uterine atony unresponsive to oxytocin can be treated with 15-methylprostaglandin $F_{2\alpha}$.

Balki M, Wong CA. Refractory uterine atony: still a problem after all these years. *Int J Obstet Anesth*. 2021;48: 103207.

Dyer RA, Swanevelder JL, Bateman BT. Hypertensive Disorders. In: Chestnut DH, Wong CA, Tsen LC, et al., eds. *Chestnut's Obstetric Anesthesia: Principles and Practice*. 6th ed. Chestnut DH, ed. Elsevier; 2019:35, 840-878.

C.10. When and how would you administer spinal anesthesia?

Spinal anesthesia can be used for cesarean delivery in patients with preeclampsia. Hyperbaric bupivacaine 0.75% at a dose of 11.25 to 12 mg with or without fentanyl, 15 to 20 μg, and morphine, 100 to 200 μg, can be given.

Advantages of spinal anesthesia in patients with preeclampsia with severe features include:

- Avoidance of general anesthesia and risks of the difficulty with an edematous airway
- Avoidance of severe hypertensive response to laryngoscopy and tracheal intubation, which can result in intracranial hemorrhage
- More reliable anesthesia than with an epidural anesthetic technique
- Better postoperative analgesia with administration of intrathecal long-lasting opioids such as morphine
- Smaller needle size than an epidural needle and therefore possibly less risk of trauma to epidural veins

Hypotension is almost 6 times less likely in patients with preeclampsia with severe features than in healthy pregnant females receiving spinal anesthesia for elective cesarean delivery. Despite this, spinal anesthesia can still cause a higher incidence of hypotension compared to epidural anesthesia. However, this is typically easily treatable and short-lived and has not been linked to clinically significant differences in maternal or neonatal outcomes.

Aya AGM, Mangin R, Vialles N, et al. Patients with severe preeclampsia experience less hypotension during spinal anesthesia for elective cesarean delivery than healthy parturients: a prospective cohort comparison. *Anesth Analg*. 2003;97:867-872.

Henke VG, Bateman BT, Leffert LR. Focused review: spinal anesthesia in severe preeclampsia [published correction appears in *Anesth Analg*. 2013;117:1263]. *Anesth Analg*. 2013;117:686-693.

Russell R. Preeclampsia and the anaesthesiologist: current management. *Curr Opin Anaesthesiol*. 2020;33:305-310.

C.11. Discuss a general anesthesia technique for the patient with preeclampsia presenting for cesarean delivery.

- Aspiration prophylaxis. Acceptable methods include 30 mL of an oral nonparticulate antacid, and/or an H_2-blocker IV, and possibly metoclopramide, 10 mg IV.
- Consider arterial line placement before induction of anesthesia in patients with preeclampsia with severe features for continuous BP measurement. The transient but severe hypertension that accompanies tracheal intubation in females with preeclampsia can increase maternal intracranial pressure, with the attendant risks of intracerebral hemorrhage. Prepare for possible difficult airway, with available equipment such as a videolaryngoscope.
- Preoxygenation and denitrogenation with 100% oxygen by face mask

- Induction of anesthesia with rapid sequence induction with either propofol or etomidate and succinylcholine
- Use a smaller endotracheal tube (6.0 or 6.5 mm internal diameter) because of airway edema.
- Continue magnesium sulfate administration during the intraoperative and postoperative periods; magnesium sulfate potentiates the effects of both depolarizing and nondepolarizing neuromuscular blockers.
- Administer volatile anesthetics until delivery to prevent awareness under anesthesia.
- Consider adding nitrous oxide (N_2O) and reducing volatile anesthetic to 0.5 to 0.75 minimum alveolar concentration (MAC) after delivery to minimize uterine atony and bleeding, or transition to a total intravenous anesthetic approach with propofol infusion.

Dyer RA, Swanevelder JL, Bateman BT. Hypertensive Disorders. In: Chestnut DH, Wong CA, Tsen LC, et al., eds. *Chestnut's Obstetric Anesthesia: Principles and Practice*. 6th ed. Chestnut DH, ed. Elsevier; 2019:35, 840-878.

Russell R. Preeclampsia and the anaesthesiologist: current management. *Curr Opin Anaesthesiol*. 2020;33:305-310.

C.12. What agents can you use to prevent hypertension during induction of general anesthesia for cesarean delivery?

Before induction, labetalol in 5 to 10 mg increments or NTG in 50 to 100 μg increments can be used to attenuate the pressor response to laryngoscopy and intubation. The short-acting opioid remifentanil or lidocaine 1.5 mg/kg can also be used.

Dyer RA, Swanevelder JL, Bateman BT. Hypertensive Disorders. In: Chestnut DH, Wong CA, Tsen LC, et al., eds. *Chestnut's Obstetric Anesthesia: Principles and Practice*. 6th ed. Chestnut DH, ed. Elsevier; 2019:35, 840-878.

Pant M, Fong R, Scavone B. Prevention of peri-induction hypertension in preeclamptic patients: a focused review. *Anesth Analg*. 2014;119:1350-1356.

D. Postoperative Management

D.1. Discuss the postpartum management of patients with preeclampsia.

- Provide adequate analgesia.
- Continue magnesium sulfate for at least 24 hours after delivery, regardless of mode of delivery.
- Maintain strict fluid intake/output during magnesium infusion.
- Maintain hemodynamic control with antihypertensives if necessary.
- Continue to monitor for symptoms of eclampsia, stroke, and pulmonary edema in the postpartum period.

Dyer RA, Swanevelder JL, Bateman BT. Hypertensive Disorders. In: Chestnut DH, Wong CA, Tsen LC, et al., eds. *Chestnut's Obstetric Anesthesia: Principles and Practice*. 6th ed. Chestnut DH, ed. Elsevier; 2019:35, 840-878.

Gestational hypertension and preeclampsia: ACOG practice bulletin, number 222. *Obstet Gynecol*. 2020;135: e237-e260.

D.2. Can nonsteroidal anti-inflammatory drugs (NSAIDs) be used to treat postpartum pain in patients with preeclampsia?

Increasing concerns surrounding the opioid epidemic as well as opioid use in breastfeeding females have led to a preference for administration of NSAIDs over opioids for postpartum pain. NSAIDs do not cause a significant elevation of BP in nonpregnant, normotensive individuals but can lead to increased BP in patients with chronic hypertension. However, data suggest NSAID use in hypertensive postpartum patients is safe and not associated with persistent postpartum hypertension or adverse outcomes. Administration of ibuprofen, compared to acetaminophen, does not prolong the duration of severe BP elevations in patients with preeclampsia. The American College of Obstetricians and Gynecologists recommends use of NSAIDs over opioid analgesics in this patient population.

Blue NR, Murray-Krezan C, Drake-Lavelle S, et al. Effect of ibuprofen vs acetaminophen on postpartum hypertension in preeclampsia with severe features: a double-masked, randomized controlled trial. *Am J Obstet Gynecol*. 2018;218:616.e1-616.e8.

Gestational hypertension and preeclampsia: ACOG practice bulletin, number 222. *Obstet Gynecol*. 2020;135: e237-e260.

Viteri OA, England JA, Alrais MA, et al. Association of nonsteroidal antiinflammatory drugs and postpartum hypertension in women with preeclampsia with severe features. *Obstet Gynecol*. 2017;130:830-835.

Wasden SW, Ragsdale ES, Chasen ST, Skupski DW. Impact of non-steroidal anti-inflammatory drugs on hypertensive disorders of pregnancy. *Pregnancy Hypertens*. 2014;4:259-263.

29

Breech Presentation, Fetal Distress, and Mitral Stenosis

Jill Fong, Jaime Aaronson, and Jason J. White

A 24-year-old primigravida at 37 weeks of gestation with fetal breech position presents to the labor and delivery unit for an external cephalic version (ECV). The patient has a history of rheumatic fever with no subsequent medical follow-up. On physical examination, she has an opening snap and a diastolic murmur. She reports having shortness of breath when climbing two flights of stairs. Prior to attempting ECV, an epidural catheter is placed without event. After adequate analgesia is achieved, the obstetrician begins to rotate the fetus. Several minutes into the attempted ECV, the fetal heart rate (FHR) decreases to 60 beats per minute. Despite intrauterine resuscitative efforts, the FHR remains at 60 beats per minute. The patient is rushed to the operating room for an emergency cesarean delivery. Her blood pressure is 100/60 mm Hg; pulse rate, 100 beats per minute; and respiratory rate, 18 breaths per minute.

A. Medical Disease and Differential Diagnosis

1. How are fetal lie, presentation, and position defined and determined?
2. What is the approximate frequency of the various lies and presentations at or near term?
3. What are the different types of breech presentation, and what is their incidence?
4. What is the cause of breech presentation?
5. What are the delivery problems associated with breech presentation?
6. What is the usual obstetrical management for patients with breech presentation?
7. What is the incidence of heart disease in pregnancy and the mortality rate associated with maternal cardiac disease?
8. How is peripartum cardiomyopathy defined?
9. What classifications help predict an individual pregnant person's cardiac risk?
10. What are the cardiovascular changes of pregnancy?
11. What changes normally occur in heart sounds during pregnancy?
12. What are the normal electrocardiographic and echocardiographic changes seen during pregnancy?
13. What causes rheumatic heart disease?
14. What are the physiologic consequences of mitral stenosis?
15. What are the auscultatory findings associated with mitral stenosis?
16. What changes in the electrocardiogram (ECG) can be seen in patients with mitral stenosis?
17. What are the echocardiographic findings in patients with mitral stenosis?
18. What is the effect of the physiologic changes of pregnancy on patients with mitral stenosis?
19. If mitral stenosis is first recognized during pregnancy and symptoms develop, how would you treat the patient?
20. What are the determinants of fetal oxygenation?
21. What are the determinants of uterine blood flow?

B. Preoperative Evaluation and Preparation

1. How is fetal well-being assessed during labor?
2. How are FHR and maternal contractions monitored?
3. What is the normal FHR with beat-to-beat variability?
4. What are FHR decelerations?

5. How accurate is FHR monitoring in predicting fetal well-being?
6. In a fetus with minimal FHR variability, what other modalities can be used to assess fetal well-being?
7. What is the significance of meconium-stained amniotic fluid?
8. What is meconium aspiration syndrome?
9. What are the usual noninvasive tests used to evaluate the pregnant cardiac patient?
10. What preoperative medications, if any, would you give this patient?

C. Intraoperative Management

1. What monitors would you use in this functional New York Heart Association (NYHA) class II patient during cesarean delivery?
2. When would you use invasive monitoring in a pregnant patient with cardiac disease?
3. What are the hemodynamic goals of intraoperative management of the pregnant patient with mitral stenosis?
4. What anesthetic technique would you use for this emergency cesarean delivery?
5. How would you manage local anesthetic systemic toxicity (LAST) in this patient?
6. If cardiac arrest were to occur prior to delivery, how would you proceed?
7. What technique could you use for general anesthesia in this patient?
8. If you are unexpectedly unable to intubate the trachea of this patient, how would you manage the airway?
9. Would this patient benefit from the use of β-blockers?
10. What is the effect of the inhalation agents on uterine contractility?
11. What is the Apgar scoring system?
12. What is the significance of the Apgar score?
13. At birth, what should be done to minimize an infant's risk of meconium aspiration syndrome?
14. If the Apgar score of the newborn is 3 at 1 minute, how would you treat the newborn?
15. Blood gas analysis is sent immediately after delivery. What are the normal values for umbilical vein and artery blood gases?

D. Postoperative Management

1. Immediately after the baby is delivered, the mother's oxygen saturation decreases. What is the differential diagnosis?
2. Additional bleeding occurs in the postanesthesia care unit, and the obstetrician diagnoses retained placenta. What, if any, antibiotics are indicated to prevent endometritis after manual extraction of retained placenta?

A. Medical Disease and Differential Diagnosis

A.1. How are fetal lie, presentation, and position defined and determined?

- Fetal lie can be longitudinal, transverse, or oblique; this describes the position of the long axis of the fetus relative to the long axis of the mother. Longitudinal lies are either cephalic or pelvic (breech), depending on which fetal structure enters the maternal pelvis. Transverse lies are either back up or back down with the long axis of the fetus perpendicular to the mother's long axis. An oblique lie results when the long axis of the fetus is at an acute angle to that of the mother; it is usually transitory and converts to transverse or longitudinal when labor begins.
- Presentation describes the part of the fetus that is lowermost in the pelvis: cephalic or breech if the lie is longitudinal, or shoulder if the lie is transverse. Cephalic presentations are further subdivided into vertex, sinciput (anterior fontanel), brow, and face.
- Position describes the relationship of the presenting part to either side (right or left) of the birth canal. For vertex, face, and breech presentations, the determining points are the fetal occiput, chin (mentum), and sacrum, respectively.
- Fetal lie, presentation, and position are determined by manual pelvic and abdominal examination. Ultrasonography is also useful, particularly when palpation is inconclusive, as can occur with maternal obesity, multiple gestations, placenta previa, and/or polyhydramnios.

Cunningham FG, Leveno KJ, Dashe JS, et al. Normal labor. In: *Williams Obstetrics*. 26th ed. McGraw-Hill; 2022:417-432.

A.2. What is the approximate frequency of the various lies and presentations at or near term?

Longitudinal lie, greater than 99%, which includes cephalic (97%) and breech (3%-4%); transverse lie, 0.3%. Frequencies of the various presentations are as follows: compound (an extremity prolapses alongside the presenting part), 0.1%; face, 0.05%; and brow, 0.01%.

Cunningham FG, Leveno KJ, Dashe JS, et al, eds. Normal labor. In: *Williams Obstetrics*. 26th ed. McGraw-Hill; 2022:417-432.

Cunningham FG, Leveno KJ, Dashe JS, et al, eds. Abnormal labor. In: *Williams Obstetrics*. 26th ed. McGraw-Hill; 2022:433-445.

A.3. What are the different types of breech presentation, and what is their incidence?

- *Frank breech*: Both fetal lower extremities are flexed at the hips and extended at the knees; the incidence is approximately 60% (48%-73%).
- *Complete breech*: One or both knees are flexed; the incidence is approximately 10% (4.6%-11.5%).
- *Incomplete or footling breech*: One or both hips are extended, and one or both feet or knees hang below the breech; the incidence is approximately 30% (12%-38%).

Cunningham FG, Leveno KJ, Dashe JS, et al. Singleton breech delivery. In: *Williams Obstetrics*. 26th ed. McGraw-Hill; 2022:518-532.

A.4. What is the cause of breech presentation?

Although the etiology of breech presentation is unknown, certain factors are associated with it; these include prematurity, polyhydramnios, uterine relaxation secondary to high parity, multiple fetuses, oligohydramnios, hydrocephaly, anencephaly, uterine anomalies (eg, a uterine septum), pelvic tumors, placenta previa, cornual-fundal placenta implantation, and previous breech delivery. Ford et al found the rate of breech recurrence after a previous breech pregnancy to be 9.9% and after two prior breech pregnancies to be 27.5%. After a prior cesarean delivery, a 2-fold increase in the incidence of breech presentation has been reported.

Cunningham FG, Leveno KJ, Dashe JS, et al. Singleton breech delivery. In: *Williams Obstetrics*. 26th ed. McGraw-Hill; 2022:518-532.

Ford JB, Roberts CL, Nassar N, et al. Recurrence of breech presentation in consecutive pregnancies. *BJOG*. 2010;117:830-836.

A.5. What are the delivery problems associated with breech presentation?

There is an increased incidence of both maternal and fetal morbidity with breech presentation. For the mother, the mode of delivery (vaginal versus cesarean) correlates with the nature of the morbidity. With a vaginal delivery, for example, genital tract laceration is a concern, whereas with cesarean delivery, extraction of the head may require an extension of the hysterotomy. Fetal morbidity occurs in the way of birth trauma, prolapsed umbilical cord, preterm delivery, and fetal anomalies.

Cunningham FG, Leveno KJ, Dashe JS, et al. Singleton breech delivery. In: *Williams Obstetrics*. 26th ed. McGraw-Hill; 2022:518-532.

A.6. What is the usual obstetrical management for patients with breech presentation?

ECV is a procedure whereby a breech fetus is rotated to the vertex position before the onset of labor. The American College of Obstetricians and Gynecologists (ACOG) recommends that ECV be offered to patients with a term singleton breech fetus who desire a planned vaginal delivery (of a vertex-presenting fetus) and have no contraindications. The reported success rate of ECV is from 35% to 86% and is associated with multiparity, abundant amniotic fluid, a nonengaged presenting part, fetal size ranging from 2,500 to 3,000 g, a posterior placenta, and nonobesity. Tocolysis is variably effective in improving ECV success rates, and there is more evidence to support betamimetic tocolysis than, for example, oral nifedipine (10-20 mg) or IV nitroglycerin (50-100 μg). The use of neuraxial techniques increases the success rate of ECV and reduces cesarean delivery rates for fetal malpresentation. There is no consensus, however, regarding the optimal dose of local anesthetic to facilitate ECV. According to available data, anesthetic doses of neuraxial blockade are better than analgesic doses.

According to ACOG, the decision regarding the mode of delivery depends on the experience of the health care provider and should consider the patient's wishes. To this end, planned vaginal delivery of a term singleton breech fetus can be reasonable under hospital-specific protocol guidelines with detailed informed consent, including perinatal/neonatal morbidity and mortality. Cesarean delivery is commonly performed in the following circumstances: lack of operator experience, incomplete or footling breech, hyperextended fetal head, fetal macrosomia, unfavorable pelvic shape, severe fetal growth restriction, fetal anomaly incompatible with vaginal delivery, a healthy preterm fetus with maternal labor or indicated delivery, previous perinatal death/trauma, maternal request, and possibly previous cesarean delivery. The availability of skilled operators to perform safe vaginal delivery of breech fetuses seems to be declining. This trend is likely related to the publication of the Term Breech Trial in 2000, a large, international, multicenter, randomized trial that compared planned, breech vaginal delivery to planned cesarean delivery. The trial found perinatal mortality, neonatal mortality, and serious neonatal morbidity to be significantly lower in the planned cesarean group. The same authors published additional follow-up studies 2 years postpartum, demonstrating no difference in maternal parameters or risk of neonatal death based on the method of delivery.

American College of Obstetricians and Gynecologists. ACOG committee opinion no. 745: mode of term singleton breech delivery. *Obstet Gynecol.* 2018;132:e60-e63.

American College of Obstetricians and Gynecologists, Society for Maternal-Fetal Medicine. Obstetric care consensus no. 1: safe prevention of the primary cesarean delivery. *Obstet Gynecol.* 2014 (reaffirmed 2023);123:693-711.

Chalifoux LA, Bauchat JR, Higgins N, et al. Effect of intrathecal bupivacaine dose on the success of external cephalic version for breech presentation: a prospective, randomized, blinded clinical trial. *Anesthesiology.* 2017;127:625-632.

Goetzinger KR, Harper LM, Tuuli MG, et al. Effect of regional anesthesia on the success rate of external cephalic version: a systematic review and meta-analysis. *Obstet Gynecol.* 2011;118:1137-1144.

Hannah ME, Hannah WJ, Hewson SA, et al. Planned caesarean section versus planned vaginal birth for breech presentation at term: a randomised, multicentre trial. Term breech trial collaborative group. *Lancet.* 2000;356:1375-1383.

Hannah ME, Whyte H, Hannah WJ. Maternal outcomes at two years after a planned cesarean section versus planned vaginal birth for breech presentation at term: the international randomized breech trial. *Am J Obstet Gynecol.* 2004;191:917-927.

Weiniger, CF. Analgesia/anesthesia for external cephalic version. *Curr Opin Anaesthesiol.* 2013;26:278-287.

A.7. What is the incidence of heart disease in pregnancy and the mortality rate associated with maternal cardiac disease?

Cardiac disease occurs in 1% to 4% of pregnancies and is the leading cause of indirect (ie, nonobstetric) maternal deaths. In developing nations, rheumatic fever remains the main cause of valvular disease in pregnancy, and it also continues to be a problem in immigrants to developed countries. In developed countries, congenital, not rheumatic, heart disease is the major cause of heart disease in pregnancy. Cardiovascular disease is currently responsible for approximately 13% of maternal deaths in the United States. Other cardiac conditions encountered in pregnancy include cardiomyopathy (peripartum and nonperipartum), pulmonary hypertension, and ischemic heart disease.

Centers for Disease Control and Prevention. Pregnancy mortality surveillance system. Accessed February 7, 2019. https://www.cdc.gov/maternal-mortality/php/pregnancy-mortality-surveillance/index.html

Elkayam U, Goland S, Pieper PG, et al. High-risk cardiac disease in pregnancy: part I. *J Am Coll Cardiol.* 2016;68:396-410.

Meng ML, Arendt KW. Obstetric anesthesia and heart disease: practical clinical considerations. *Anesthesiology.* 2021;135:164-183.

Simpson LL. Maternal cardiac disease: update for the clinician. *Obstet Gynecol.* 2012;119:345-359.

Small MJ, James AH, Kershaw T, et al. Near-miss maternal mortality: cardiac dysfunction as the principal cause of obstetric intensive care unit admission. *Obstet Gynecol.* 2012;119:250-255.

A.8. How is peripartum cardiomyopathy defined?

Peripartum cardiomyopathy is an idiopathic cardiomyopathy that presents toward the end of pregnancy or in the months following delivery with heart failure due to left ventricular systolic dysfunction. Unlike valvular heart disease in pregnancy, peripartum cardiomyopathy is a diagnosis of exclusion, and although the left ventricle might not be dilated, the ejection fraction is almost always less than 45%. Because early symptoms may mimic those of normal pregnancy, the index of suspicion for peripartum cardiomyopathy must be high. The incidence worldwide is about 1 per 1,000 pregnancies.

Cunningham FG, Byrne JJ, Nelson DB. Peripartum cardiomyopathy. *Obstet Gynecol.* 2019;133:167-179.

Sliwa K, Hilfiker-Kleiner D, Petrie MC, et al; for Heart Failure Association of the European Society of Cardiology Working Group on Peripartum Cardiomyopathy. Current state of knowledge on aetiology, diagnosis, management, and therapy of peripartum cardiomyopathy: a position statement from the Heart Failure Association of the European Society of Cardiology Working Group on peripartum cardiomyopathy. *Eur J Heart Fail.* 2010;12:767-778.

A.9. What classifications help predict an individual pregnant person's cardiac risk?

There are three models for maternal cardiac risk stratification: Cardiac Disease in Pregnancy (CARPREG), Zwangerschap bij Aangeboren Hartafwijkingen I (ZAHARA), and World Health Organization (WHO) (**Table 29.1**). The NYHA classification, although not widely used to determine overall risk, is included in each of the models:

- *Class I*: no limitation of physical activity
- *Class II*: slight limitation of physical activity; symptoms with ordinary activity
- *Class III*: marked limitation of physical activity; symptoms with less than ordinary activity
- *Class IV*: unable to carry out any physical activity without discomfort; symptoms can be present at rest

According to the American College of Cardiology, the WHO model best predicts cardiovascular risk in pregnant patients with congenital heart disease. The Task Force for the Management of Cardiovascular Diseases during Pregnancy of the European Society of Cardiology recommends that disease-specific risk be assessed using the modified WHO classification and that risk estimation should be further refined by CARPREG, ZAHARA, and the European Society of Cardiologist's Registry of Pregnancy and Cardiac Disease (ROPAC).

Neonatal and maternal adverse events are highly correlated; specifically, maternal cardiac disease is associated with neonatal complications, which include small for gestational age, prematurity, and death. In females with cardiac disease, maternal predictors of increased neonatal adverse events include baseline

TABLE 29.1 World Health Organization (WHO) Risk Classification for Cardiovascular Disease in Pregnancy

WHO class I: no increase mortality risk; no/mild increase morbidity	• Uncomplicated, small or mild
	  • Pulmonary stenosis
	  • Patent ductus arteriosus
	  • Mitral valve prolapse
	• Successfully repaired simple lesions (atrial or ventricular septal defect, patent ductus arteriosus, anomalous pulmonary venous drainage)
	• Atrial or ventricular ectopic beats, isolated

WHO class II: small increase mortality risk; moderate increase morbidity	• Unoperated atrial or ventricular septal defect • Repaired tetralogy of Fallot • Most arrhythmias
WHO classes II to III (depends on the individual)	• Mild left ventricular impairment • Hypertrophic cardiomyopathy • Native or tissue valvular heart disease not considered WHO class I or IV • Marfan syndrome without aortic dilation • Aorta <45 mm in aortic disease associated with bicuspid aortic valve • Repaired coarctation
WHO class III: significant increase mortality risk; severe increase morbidity	• Mechanical valve • Systemic right ventricle • Fontan circulation • Cyanotic heart disease (unrepaired) • Other complex congenital heart disease • Aortic dilation 40-45 mm in Marfan syndrome • Aortic dilation 45-50 mm in aortic disease associated with bicuspid aortic valve
WHO class IV: extremely high-risk mortality/morbidity; pregnancy contraindicated; discuss termination	• Pulmonary arterial hypertension of any cause • Severe systemic ventricular dysfunction (LVEF <30%, NYHA III-IV) • Severe mitral stenosis, severe symptomatic aortic stenosis • Marfan syndrome with aorta dilated >45 mm • Aortic dilation >50 mm in aortic disease associated with bicuspid aortic valve • Native severe coarctation

LVEF, left ventricular ejection fraction; NYHA, New York Heart Association.
Modified from Thorne S, MacGregor A, Nelson-Piercy C. Risks of contraception and pregnancy in heart disease. *Heart.* 2006;92:1520-1525; with permission from BMJ Publishing Group Ltd.; Regitz-Zagrosek V, Blomstrom Lundqvist C, Borghi C, et al. ESC guidelines on the management of cardiovascular diseases during pregnancy: the task force on the management of cardiovascular diseases during pregnancy of the European Society of Cardiology (ESC). *Eur Heart J.* 2011;32:3147-3197.

SECTION 7

NYHA class more than II, cyanosis, smoking during pregnancy, left-sided heart obstruction, multiple gestations, oral anticoagulation during pregnancy, and the presence of a mechanical valve prosthesis.

Drenthen W, Boersma E, Balci A, et al. Predictors of pregnancy complications in women with congenital heart disease. *Eur Heart J*. 2010;31:2124-2132.

Furenäs E, Eriksson P, Wennerholm UB, et al. Effects of maternal age and cardiac disease severity on outcome of pregnancy in women with congenital heart disease. *Int J Cardiol*. 2017;243:197-203.

Owens A, Yang J, Nie L, et al. Neonatal and maternal outcomes in pregnant women with cardiac disease. *J Am Heart Assoc*. 2018;7:e009395.

Retitz-Zagrosek V, Roos-Hesselink JW, Bauersachs J, et al. 2018 ESC Guidelines for the management of cardiovascular diseases during pregnancy. *Eur Heart J*. 2018;39:3165-3241.

Siu SC, Sermer M, Colman JM, et al. Prospective multicenter study of pregnancy outcomes in women with heart disease. *Circulation*. 2001;104:515-521.

Stangl V, Schad J, Gossing G, et al. Maternal heart disease and pregnancy outcome: a single-centre experience. *Eur J Heart Fail*. 2008;10:855-860.

A.10. What are the cardiovascular changes of pregnancy?

During the first trimester of pregnancy, cardiac output increases 40% to 50% above the normal nonpregnant level and plateaus at about 28 weeks of gestation. It remains fairly stable until the stresses imposed by labor increase it further. The increase in cardiac output is due to a 25% increase in stroke volume and a 10% increase in heart rate. Blood pressure, however, is not elevated because peripheral vascular resistance decreases. Central venous pressure, pulmonary capillary wedge pressure, pulmonary artery diastolic pressure, and left ventricular stroke work index are unchanged compared to nonpregnant values.

During labor, cardiac output increases approximately 10%, with uterine contractions during the latent phase, 25% in the active phase, and 40% in the expulsive phase compared to prelabor values. The greatest increase in cardiac output occurs immediately postpartum when it increases about 80% above prelabor values. Cardiac output and heart rate decline to prelabor values within 1 hour of delivery, and by approximately 24 hours, mean blood pressure and stroke volume return to prelabor baseline. The cardiovascular changes of pregnancy resolve in the first 3 to 6 months after delivery. It can take up to a year, however, for the residual effects of cardiovascular remodeling to subside.

Kacmar R, Gaiser R. Physiologic changes of pregnancy. In: Chestnut DH, Wong CA, Tsen LC, et al, eds. *Chestnut's Obstetric Anesthesia: Principles and Practice*. 6th ed. Elsevier; 2019:12-37.

A.11. What changes normally occur in heart sounds during pregnancy?

It is normal for changes in heart sounds to occur in pregnancy, for example, an exaggerated splitting of the first heart sound and increased loudness of both components. There can also be a loud third heart sound. Soft diastolic murmurs occur, as do continuous murmurs arising from the breast vasculature.

Cunningham FG, Leveno KJ, Dashe JS, et al. Maternal Physiology. In: *Williams Obstetrics*. 26th ed. McGraw-Hill; 2022:51-79.

A.12. What are the normal electrocardiographic and echocardiographic changes seen during pregnancy?

Normal changes in the ECG in pregnancy commonly seen include slight left axis deviation as well as Q waves in leads II, III, and avF. Flat or inverted T waves can also occur. ST elevations, however, do not occur normally and should be considered pathologic. Normal echocardiographic findings include an increase in both left ventricular wall mass and atrial diameters bilaterally, whereas left ventricular function can be unchanged or slightly improved. The annuli of the pulmonary, tricuspid, and mitral valves dilate progressively, and term pregnant patients can have mild tricuspid, pulmonic, and/or (but much more infrequently) mitral regurgitation. A small pericardial effusion can develop as well.

Cunningham FG, Leveno KJ, Dashe JS, et al, eds. Maternal physiology. In: *Williams Obstetrics*. 26th ed. McGraw-Hill; 2022:63.

Kacmar R, Gaiser R. Physiologic changes of pregnancy. In: Chestnut DH, Wong CA, Tsen LC, et al, eds. *Chestnut's Obstetric Anesthesia: Principles and Practice*. 6th ed. Elsevier; 2019:12-37.

A.13. What causes rheumatic heart disease?

Rheumatic heart disease occurs in patients who have had acute rheumatic fever (ARF), an immune-mediated illness that develops after an untreated group A streptococcal infection. It predominantly affects the heart and joints and can lead to chronic rheumatic heart disease. ARF occurs most commonly in the winter and spring in children between 5 and 15 years old. In developed countries, ARF is much less common than it was decades ago.

The pathogenetic mechanism of ARF is unknown. The manifestations are extremely variable, and specific laboratory tests to confirm the diagnosis do not exist. The diagnosis is clinical and made using the Jones Criteria, revised by the American Heart Association in 1992 and again in 2000. Diagnosis of ARF requires evidence of a preceding group A streptococcal infection in conjunction with two major or one major plus two minor manifestations (**Table 29.2**).

Of note, rheumatic heart disease is the only long-term sequelae of ARF. With an improved ability to prevent recurrent attacks, prognosis has improved and is related directly to the severity of cardiac involvement during the acute phase. More widespread use of echocardiography has revealed the prevalence of rheumatic heart disease in developing countries to be about 10-fold greater than that recognized by conventional screening.

In almost all adults, mitral stenosis is caused by previous rheumatic carditis, although approximately 60% of patients with rheumatic mitral valve disease do not report a history of rheumatic fever or chorea. In about 40% of all patients with rheumatic heart disease, isolated mitral stenosis occurs. Mitral valve insufficiency and aortic valve stenosis and insufficiency can also occur in these patients.

Gewitz MH, Baltimore RS, Tani LY, et al. Revision of the Jones Criteria for the diagnosis of acute rheumatic fever in the era of Doppler echocardiography: a scientific statement from the American Heart Association. *Circulation*. 2015;131:1806-1818.

Karthikeyan G, Guilherme L. Acute rheumatic fever. *Lancet*. 2018;392:161-174.

Otto CM, Nishimura RA, Bonow RO, et al. 2020 ACC/AHA guideline for the management of patients with valvular heart disease: executive summary: a report of the American College of Cardiology/American Heart Association Joint Committee on clinical practice guidelines. *Circulation*. 2021;143:e35-e71.

A.14. What are the physiologic consequences of mitral stenosis?

The normal mitral valve orifice area is 4 to 6 cm^2, but with mitral stenosis, the valve area is reduced to varying degrees. When it reaches 2 cm^2, cardiovascular hemodynamics are impaired. A valve area of less than or equal to 1.5 cm^2 is considered moderate mitral stenosis, and as the cross-sectional area decreases to 1 cm^2 and mean left atrial pressure increases to at least 25 mm Hg to maintain an adequate cardiac output, it is considered severe. The pathophysiology of mitral stenosis results from obstruction of blood flow from the left atrium into the left ventricle.

SECTION 7

TABLE 29.2 Revised Jones Criteria

For all patients with a preceding group A streptococcus infection • Diagnosis: initial ARF • Diagnosis: recurrent ARF	Two major or one major plus two minor manifestations Two major or one major and two or three minor manifestations
Major criteria—low-risk populations • Carditis (clinical and/or subclinical) • Arthritis (polyarthritis only) • Chorea • Erythema marginatum • Subcutaneous nodules	Major criteria—moderate-/high-risk populations • Carditis (clinical and/or subclinical) • Arthritis (mono- or polyarthritis; polyarthralgia) • Chorea • Erythema marginatum • Subcutaneous nodules
Minor criteria—Low-risk populations • Polyarthralgia • Fever (≥38.5 °C) • ESR ≥60 mm in the first hour and/or CRP ≥3.0 mg/dL (or upper limit of normal for laboratory; use peak value) • Prolonged PR interval, after accounting for age (unless carditis is a major criterion)	Minor criteria—moderate-/high-risk populations • Monoarthralgia • Fever (≥38 °C) • ESR ≥30 mm/h and/or CRP ≥3.0 mg/dL (or upper limit of normal for laboratory; use peak value) • Prolonged PR interval, after accounting for age (unless carditis is a major criterion)

ARF, acute rheumatic fever; CRP, C-reactive protein; ESR, erythrocyte sedimentation rate.
Reprinted with permission from Gewitz MH, Baltimore RS, Tani LY, et al. Revision of the Jones Criteria for the diagnosis of acute rheumatic fever in the era of Doppler echocardiography: a scientific statement from the American Heart Association. *Circulation*. 2015;131:1806-1818.

The increase in heart rate, cardiac output, red blood cell mass, and plasma volume that occurs with pregnancy can lead to increased atrial pressure and cardiac decompensation in patients with mitral stenosis. Consequences include a decline in functional capacity, atrial arrhythmias, and pulmonary edema. Pulmonary hypertension can also result due to elevated left atrial pressure and pulmonary arteriolar constriction. If severe pulmonary hypertension develops, right-sided heart failure can ensue.

Elkayam U, Goland S, Pieper PG, et al. High-risk cardiac disease in pregnancy: part I. *J Am Coll Cardiol.* 2016;68:396-410.

Otto CM, Nishimura RA, Bonow RO, et al. 2020 ACC/AHA guideline for the management of patients with valvular heart disease: executive summary: a report of the American College of Cardiology/American Heart Association Joint Committee on clinical practice guidelines. *Circulation.* 2021;143:e35-e71.

A.15. What are the auscultatory findings associated with mitral stenosis?

The first heart sound is accentuated, whereas the second heart sound is normal or accentuated. There can be an opening snap, which is usually loudest at the apex. A diastolic rumbling murmur is best heard at the apex with the patient in the left lateral decubitus position and usually starts with or shortly after the opening snap and can continue through the entire diastolic phase. The presence of pulmonary hypertension can alter the auscultatory findings associated with mitral stenosis such that the first heart sound is normal or only slightly accentuated, and the opening snap and diastolic murmur are absent.

Dack S, Bleifer S, Grishman A, et al. Mitral stenosis: auscultatory and phonocardiographic findings. *Am J Cardiol.* 1960;5:815-835.

A.16. What changes in the electrocardiogram (ECG) can be seen in patients with mitral stenosis?

Broad diphasic P waves with tall R waves may be present in the right precordial leads.

Bahl VK, Math RS. Mitral stenosis. In: Fuster V, Narula JVaishnava P, et al, eds. *Fuster and Hurst's The Heart.* 15th ed. McGraw-Hill; 2022:981.

A.17. What are the echocardiographic findings in patients with mitral stenosis?

Mitral stenosis is characterized by both thickening and shortening of the leaflets and chordae and fusion of the commissures, which results in the doming of the leaflets in diastole. Together, these changes restrict valve opening, leading to varying degrees of mitral stenosis. On echocardiography, the anterior leaflet is commonly described as having a "hockey stick" appearance (**Figure 29.1**).

With mitral stenosis, diastolic filling of the left ventricle is compromised, and in turn, left atrial pressure increases and the left atrium can become dilated. Long-standing mitral stenosis leads to pulmonary hypertension by way of increased pulmonary vascular resistance. Two-dimensional echocardiography is used to evaluate mitral valve area and morphology. Three-dimensional echocardiography enhances the

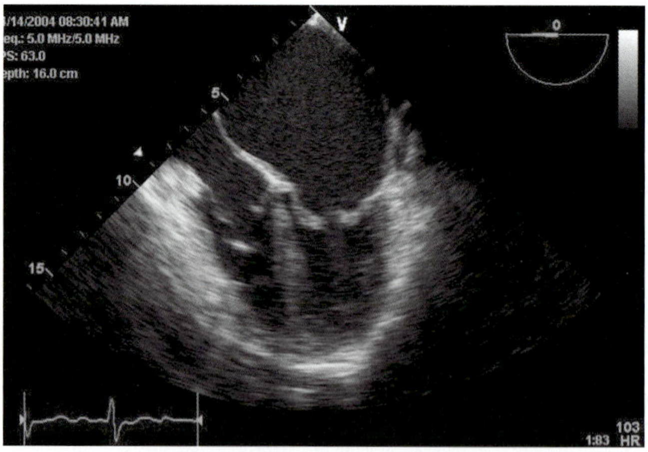

FIGURE 29.1. Two-dimensional echocardiography of the mitral valve showing severe mitral stenosis with a typical "hockey stick" appearance.

ability to examine mitral valve morphology and allows for complete assessment in a single-imaging plane. Continuous Doppler across the mitral valve best measures the severity of the lesion.

Wunderlich NC, Beigel R, Siegel RJ. Management of mitral stenosis using 2D and 3D echo-Doppler imaging. *JACC Cardiovasc Imaging*. 2013;6:1191-1205.

A.18. What is the effect of the physiologic changes of pregnancy on patients with mitral stenosis?

The increased cardiovascular load of pregnancy can cause patients to deteriorate and even advance from one NYHA classification to another. Increased cardiac output, tachycardia, and fluid retention increase the pressure gradient across the stenotic valve, which explains why more than half of NYHA class I and II patients with mitral stenosis have worsening clinical symptoms during pregnancy. A decline in functional capacity, atrial fibrillation, and pulmonary edema can occur. Decreased oncotic pressure increases the risk of pulmonary edema. The incidence of maternal and fetal complications is related to the severity of stenosis, and maternal and perinatal outcomes depend largely on maternal functional status during pregnancy. Maternal mortality and morbidity are increased in parturients with NYHA III and IV disease.

Hameed A, Karaalp IS, Tummala PP, et al. The effect of valvular heart disease on maternal and fetal outcome of pregnancy. *J Am Coll Cardiol*. 2001;37:893-899.

Nanna M, Stergiopoulos K. Pregnancy complicated by valvular heart disease: an update. *J Am Heart Assoc*. 2014;3:e000712.

Silversides CK, Colman JM, Sermer M, et al. Cardiac risk in pregnant women with rheumatic mitral stenosis. *Am J Cardiol*. 2003;91:1382-1385.

A.19. If mitral stenosis is first recognized during pregnancy and symptoms develop, how would you treat the patient?

Heart rate reduction and decreased left atrial pressure are the standard therapeutic goals for females with moderate to severe mitral stenosis. Therefore, β-adrenergic receptor blockade is the cornerstone of medical therapy in the symptomatic patient and should be continued through labor and delivery. It is useful in preventing tachycardia and prolonging diastolic filling time, which can markedly improve symptoms.

Atrial fibrillation or flutter should be treated aggressively; a rapid ventricular response compromises diastolic flow time and can lead to pulmonary edema. For rate control, digoxin or a β-adrenergic receptor blocker should be given. Calcium channel blockers are also thought to be safe in pregnancy, although there are fewer data to support their use. If the patient is unstable, synchronized cardioversion should be performed. Atrial fibrillation increases not only the risk of pulmonary edema but also the likelihood of a thromboembolic event, which is why patients with persistent atrial fibrillation should be anticoagulated. There are some data to suggest that patients with severe mitral stenosis should receive antithrombotic therapy even if they are in sinus rhythm because of the potential for thrombotic events.

If symptoms of pulmonary congestion develop, salt restriction and cautious use of diuretics decrease left atrial pressure by decreasing blood volume. Avoidance of both hypovolemia and decreased uteroplacental perfusion is essential. If symptoms are uncontrolled by medical therapy, the mitral valve should be repaired or replaced. Percutaneous balloon valvuloplasty can be done using echocardiographic or radiographic imaging, with appropriate shielding of the fetus, which has a low morbidity rate for both the mother and fetus and favorable long-term results when performed in NYHA functional class III and IV patients. If a contraindication to balloon valvuloplasty exists, surgical commissurotomy or valve replacement should be done; although it is usually well tolerated by the mother (ie, comparable to nonpregnant females), fetal loss of over 20% has been reported.

Esteves CA, Munoz JS, Braga S, et al. Immediate and long-term follow-up of percutaneous balloon mitral valvuloplasty in pregnant patients with mitral stenosis. *Am J Cardiol*. 2006;98:812-816.

Hameed A, Akhter M, Bitar F, et al. Left atrial thrombosis in pregnant women with mitral stenosis and sinus rhythm. *Am J Obstet Gynecol*. 2005;193:501-504.

Katsi V, Georgiopoulos G, Marketou M, et al. Atrial fibrillation in pregnancy: a growing challenge. *Curr Med Res Opin*. 2017;33:1497-1504.

Otto CM, Nishimura RA, Bonow RO, et al. 2020 ACC/AHA guideline for the management of patients with valvular heart disease: executive summary: a report of the American College of Cardiology/American Heart Association Joint Committee on clinical practice guidelines. *Circulation*. 2021;143:e35-e71.

Sutton SW, Duncan MA, Chase VA, et al. Cardiopulmonary bypass and mitral valve replacement during pregnancy. *Perfusion*. 2005;20:359-368.

A.20. What are the determinants of fetal oxygenation?

Oxygen delivery to the fetal circulation occurs via the placenta. Factors that affect oxygen exchange across the placenta include blood flow (maternal placental and fetal placental), maternal blood oxygen capacity, maternal and fetal hemoglobin oxygen affinity, placental oxygen diffusion capacity, and oxygen consumption.

Carter AM. Evolution of factors affecting placental oxygen transfer. *Placenta*. 2009;30:S19-S25.

A.21. What are the determinants of uterine blood flow?

Uterine blood flow is described by the following equation:

$$\text{Uterine blood flow} = \frac{\text{uterine artery pressure} - \text{uterine venous pressure}}{\text{uterine artery resistance}}$$

At term, uterine blood flow is 17% of cardiac output (450-650 mL/min). Uterine blood flow is directly related to maternal blood pressure because the uterine vessels do not autoregulate.

Segal S, Kodali BS. Uteroplacental Blood Flow. In: Datta S, Kodali BS, Segal S, eds. *Obstetric Anesthesia Handbook*. 6th ed. Springer; 2023:71-88.

Antony KM, Racusin DA, Aagaard K. Maternal physiology. In: Landon MB, Galan HL, Jauniaux ERM, et al, eds. *Gabbe's Obsterics: Normal and Problem Pregnancies*. 9th ed. 2025:42-65.

B. Preoperative Evaluation and Preparation

B.1. How is fetal well-being assessed during labor?

Fetal well-being depends on an intact uteroplacental unit. Simultaneous monitoring of FHR and uterine contractions aids in the detection of fetal distress.

American College of Obstetricians and Gynecologists. Practice bulletin no. 106: intrapartum fetal heart rate monitoring: nomenclature, interpretation, and general management principles. *Obstet Gynecol*. 2009;114:192-202.

B.2. How are FHR and maternal contractions monitored?

FHR can be monitored noninvasively using Doppler ultrasonography or invasively using a fetal scalp electrode. Uterine contractions can be monitored noninvasively by a tocodynamometer, which measures the tightening of maternal abdominal muscles, or invasively by a transcervical pressure catheter connected to a strain gauge.

American College of Obstetricians and Gynecologists. Practice bulletin no. 106: intrapartum fetal heart rate monitoring: nomenclature, interpretation, and general management principles. *Obstet Gynecol*. 2009;114:192-202.

Bakker JJ, Janssen PF, van Halem K, et al. Internal versus external tocodynamometry during induced or augmented labor. *Cochrane Database Syst Rev*. 2013;2013:CD006947.

B.3. What is the normal FHR with beat-to-beat variability?

In the third trimester, the normal baseline FHR is 110 to 160 beats per minute with beat-to-beat variability (6-25 beats per minute). Baseline FHR less than 110 beats per minute is *bradycardia* and greater than 160 beats per minute is *tachycardia*.

American College of Obstetricians and Gynecologists. Practice bulletin no. 116: management of intrapartum fetal heart rate tracings. *Obstet Gynecol*. 2010;116:1232-1240.

B.4. What are FHR decelerations?

A deceleration is a decrease in FHR from baseline. Decelerations fall into three categories, early, late, or variable, depending on their shape and timing with respect to maternal contractions (**Figure 29.2**).

- Early deceleration—symmetrical, gradual decrease and return of FHR that coincides with the onset, peak, and end of a uterine contraction. They are thought to be a vagal response caused by fetal head compression and are not associated with fetal hypoxia, acidemia, or low Apgar scores.
- Late deceleration—symmetrical, gradual decrease and return of FHR that begins after the onset of a contraction and lasts beyond the end. They indicate uteroplacental insufficiency and require prompt evaluation and treatment.

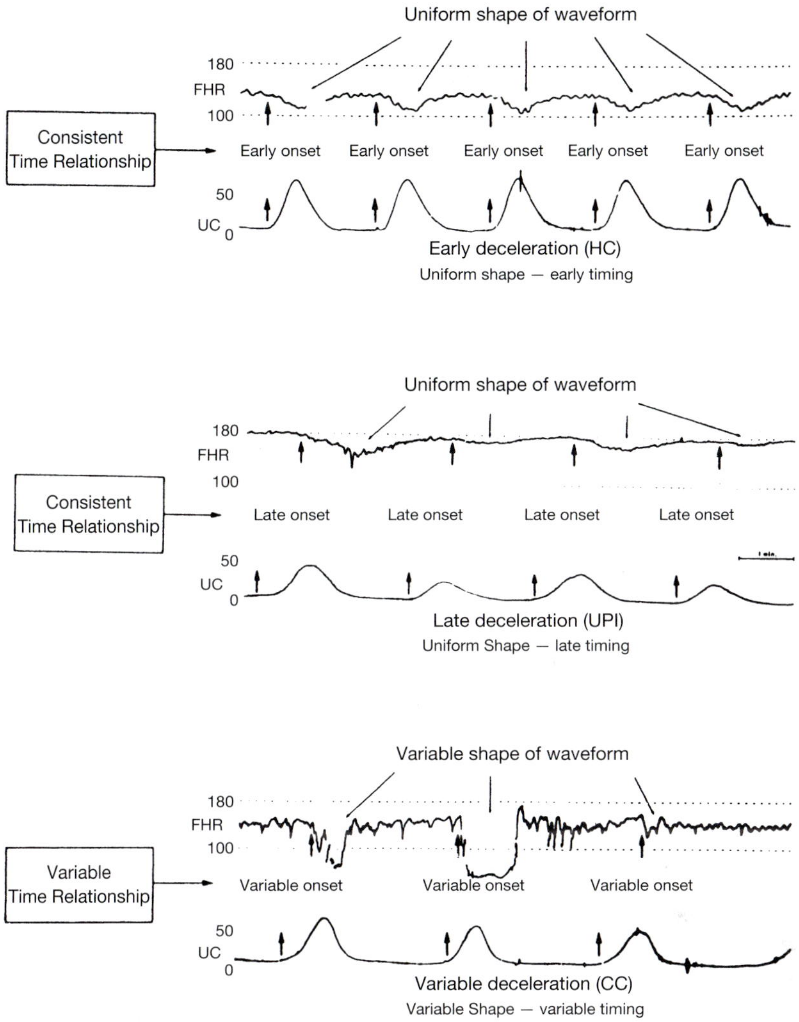

FIGURE 29.2. Fetal heart rate (FHR) decelerations in relation to the time of onset of uterine contractions (UCs). CC, cord compression; HC, head compression; UPI, uteroplacental insufficiency. (Based on Hon EH. *An Atlas of Fetal Heart Rate Patterns.* Harty Press; 1968.)

- Variable deceleration—abrupt decrease in FHR with an onset, depth, and duration that varies with successive uterine contractions. The decrease in FHR is 15 beats per minute or greater and lasts from 15 seconds to 2 minutes. They are FHR reflexes that reflect fetal blood pressure changes due to umbilical cord compression or changes in fetal oxygenation.

A prolonged deceleration is a decrease from baseline that is 15 beats per minute or more and lasts 2 or more minutes but less than 10 minutes.

American College of Obstetricians and Gynecologists. Practice bulletin no. 116: management of intrapartum fetal heart rate tracings. *Obstet Gynecol.* 2010;116:1232-1240.

B.5. How accurate is FHR monitoring in predicting fetal well-being?

FHR monitoring is used to determine fetal oxygenation (ie, fetal well-being). This is because the fetal brain, via a combination of sympathetic and parasympathetic pathways, modulates the FHR. The accuracy of FHR monitoring is thought to be limited, however, by various factors, which include questions about its overall efficacy as well as clinician reliability.

A three-tiered system is currently used to evaluate and manage intrapartum electronic FHR patterns. Category I FHR tracings are normal and include a baseline heart rate of 110 to 160 beats per minute, moderate beat-to-beat variability, and no late or variable decelerations; early decelerations and accelerations may or may not be present. Category I tracings are not associated with fetal acidemia. Category III FHR tracings are abnormal and are characterized by the absence of variability and recurrent late decelerations, recurrent variable decelerations, bradycardia, or a sinusoidal pattern. Unlike category I FHR tracings, category III tracings are associated with an increased risk for fetal acidemia (at the time of interpretation). Category II FHR tracings are considered to be indeterminate and include all those not categorized as either category I or III. They are not predictive of abnormal fetal acid-base status but require evaluation, intervention when applicable, and continuous surveillance. Cahill et al conducted a retrospective cohort study of more than 5,000 term births and found that none of the three categories had a significant association with neonatal blood acidemia (pH $\leq$ 7.10) when considered in the last 10 or 30 minutes prior to delivery. *Minimal variability without an identifiable cause or that does not resolve with appropriate resuscitative measures can indicate fetal acidemia.*

American College of Obstetricians and Gynecologists. Practice Bulletin No. 106: intrapartum fetal heart rate monitoring: nomenclature, interpretation, and general management principles. *Obstet Gynecol.* 2009;114:192-202.

American College of Obstetricians and Gynecologists. Practice Bulletin No. 116: management of intrapartum fetal heart rate tracings. *Obstet Gynecol.* 2010;116:1232-1240.

Cahill AG, Roehl KA, Odibo AO, et al. Association and prediction of neonatal acidemia. *Am J Obstet Gynecol.* 2012;207:206.e1-206.e8.

Macones GA, Hankins GD, Spong CY, et al. The 2008 National Institute of Child Health and Human Development workshop report on electronic fetal monitoring: update on definitions, interpretations, and research guidelines. *Obstet Gynecol.* 2008;112:661-666.

B.6. In a fetus with minimal FHR variability, what other modalities can be used to assess fetal well-being?

Four techniques can be used to elicit or improve FHR variability—fetal scalp sampling, Allis clamp scalp stimulation, vibroacoustic stimulation, and digital scalp stimulation. The latter two options are preferred, given the invasiveness of the former. In a parturient with a breech fetus, any technique that requires access to the fetal head is not applicable.

American College of Obstetricians and Gynecologists. Practice bulletin no. 106: intrapartum fetal heart rate monitoring: nomenclature, interpretation, and general management principles. *Obstet Gynecol.* 2009;114:192-202.

Skupski DW, Rosenberg CR, Eglinton GS. Intrapartum fetal stimulation tests: a meta-analysis. *Obstet Gynecol.* 2002;99:129-134.

B.7. What is the significance of meconium-stained amniotic fluid?

Meconium-stained amniotic fluid occurs in 4% to 22% of births. In and of itself, it does not indicate an adverse outcome. It has been suggested that meconium is released with fetal acidemia occurring rather than meconium release being a marker of preexisting fetal compromise.

Blackwell SC, Moldenhauer J, Hassan SS, et al. Meconium aspiration syndrome in term neonates with normal acid-base status at delivery: is it different? *Am J Obstet Gynecol.* 2001;184:1422-1426.

Greenwood C, Lalchandani S, MacQuillan K, et al. Meconium passed in labor: how reassuring is clear amniotic fluid? *Obstet Gynecol.* 2003;102:89-93.

Ramin KD, Leveno KJ, Kelly MA, et al. Amniotic fluid meconium: a fetal environmental hazard. *Obstet Gynecol.* 1996;87:181-184.

B.8. What is meconium aspiration syndrome?

Meconium aspiration syndrome is a respiratory condition that occurs in neonates born through meconium-stained amniotic fluid. The degree of respiratory distress is variable, but severe cases are associated with perinatal mortality. The pathophysiology of meconium aspiration is incompletely understood and complex, with a number of contributing factors: airway obstruction, surfactant dysfunction, chemical pneumonitis, and persistent pulmonary hypertension of the newborn. Treatment is mainly supportive, although infants who fail conventional ventilation strategies can benefit from extracorporeal membrane oxygenation (ECMO).

Chettri S, Bhat BV, Adhisivam B. Current concepts in the management of meconium aspiration syndrome. *Indian J Pediatr.* 2016;83:1125-1130.

Swarnam K, Soraisham AS, Sivanandan S. Advances in the management of meconium aspiration syndrome. *Int J Pediatr.* 2012;2012:359571.

Vain NE, Batton DG. Meconium "aspiration" (or respiratory distress associated with meconium-stained amniotic fluid?). *Semin Fetal Neonatal Med.* 2017;22:214-219.

B.9. What are the usual noninvasive tests used to evaluate the pregnant cardiac patient?

Physical examination, exercise tolerance, ECG, pulse oximetry, Holter monitoring, and echocardiography with Doppler flow studies are all useful to evaluate these patients. Cardiac magnetic resonance imaging is safe in pregnant females, but the use of contrast dye should be limited to situations in which its use will improve diagnostic performance. Tests using radiation should be avoided unless absolutely necessary; it is best to delay radiologic exams until as late as possible in the pregnancy and to use protective fetal radiation shielding. The risk of fetal anomalies is low with less than 50 mGy of radiation exposure. Radiation exposure with a chest radiograph is less than 0.1 mGy, whereas fetal exposure is 0.0005 to 0.01 mGy.

Brent RL. Saving lives and changing family histories: appropriate counseling of pregnant women and men and women of reproductive age, concerning the risk of diagnostic radiation exposures during and before pregnancy. *Am J Obstet Gynecol.* 2009;200:4-24.

Jain C. ACOG committee opinion no. 723: guidelines for diagnostic imaging during pregnancy and lactation. *Obstet Gynecol.* 2019;133:186.

B.10. What preoperative medications, if any, would you give this patient?

Prophylactic antibiotics to prevent endocarditis are not recommended for females with acquired (or congenital) heart disease for either vaginal or cesarean delivery in the absence of infection. According to the American Heart Association, it is reasonable to consider antibiotic prophylaxis only for those females at highest risk of an adverse outcome from infective endocarditis (eg, prosthetic cardiac valve or material, previous endocarditis, unrepaired cyanotic heart disease, during the first 6 months after complete repair of congenital heart disease, presence of residual defects after repair of congenital heart disease, and valvulopathy after heart transplant). When prophylactic antibiotics are indicated, the regimens are as follows: amoxicillin (2 g orally), or in patients unable to take anything by mouth, ampicillin (2 g intravenous [IV]), cefazolin (1 g IV), or ceftriaxone (1 g IV) should be given 30 to 60 minutes before the procedure. If the patient is allergic to ampicillin or penicillin, cefazolin (1 g IV), ceftriaxone (1 g IV), or clindamycin (600 mg IV) should be given.

Prophylactic antibiotics are indicated for patients undergoing cesarean delivery to prevent endometritis, febrile morbidity, and wound infections. ACOG recommends a first-generation cephalosporin (ie, cefazolin; if $<$80 kg, 1 g; if $>$80 kg, 2 g; if $>$120 kg, 3 g) be given within 1 hour of surgical incision to reduce maternal infections without adverse neonatal effects.

Pregnant patients are considered at increased risk for aspiration of gastric contents. Gastric fluid volume, though, is not different in pregnant patients compared with their nonpregnant counterparts, and pregnancy itself does not decrease gastric emptying (except during labor). The increased risk for aspiration is thought to be due to a decrease in lower esophageal sphincter tone as well as an increased risk of difficult intubation. Although the exact time at which the risk increases is unclear, it is prudent to consider pregnant patients to be at increased risk for aspiration of gastric contents after 16 to 20 weeks of gestation.

In this patient for emergency cesarean delivery, an oral nonparticulate antacid, such as 15 to 30 mL of 0.3 M sodium citrate, given immediately before induction of anesthesia, reduces the risk of developing aspiration pneumonitis. H_2-receptor antagonists (ranitidine and famotidine), as well as metoclopramide can also decrease the risk, but require at least 30 to 40 minutes to be effective. These drugs can be given after induction of anesthesia if time does not allow for dosing before. Avoiding general anesthesia is the most effective way to reduce the risk of aspiration.

American College of Obstetricians and Gynecologists Committee on Practice Bulletins-Obstetrics. ACOG practice bulletin No. 199: use of prophylactic antibiotics in labor and delivery. *Obstet Gynecol.* 2018;132:e103-e119.

Apfelbaum J, Hawkins J, Madhulika A, et al. Practice guidelines for obstetric anesthesia: an updated report by the American Society of Anesthesiologists Task Force on obstetric anesthesia and the society for obstetric anesthesia and perinatology. *Anesthesiology.* 2016;124:270-300.

Bedson R. Physiology of pregnancy: clinical anesthetic implications. *Contin Educ Anaesth Critic Care Pain.* 2013;14:69-72.

Tita AT, Rouse DJ, Blackwell S, et al. Emerging concepts in antibiotic prophylaxis for cesarean delivery: a systematic review. *Obstet Gynecol.* 2009;113:675-682.

Van de Putte P, Vernieuwe L, Perlas A. Term pregnant patients have a similar gastric volume to non-pregnant females: a single-centre cohort study. *Br J Anaesth.* 2019;122:79-85.

Wilson W, Taubert KA, Gewitz M, et al. Prevention of infective endocarditis: guidelines from the American Heart Association: a guideline from the rheumatic fever, endocarditis, and Kawasaki disease committee, council on cardiovascular disease in the young, and the council on clinical cardiology, council on cardiovascular surgery and anesthesia, and the quality of care and outcomes research interdisciplinary working group. *Circulation.* 2007;116:887-896.

C. Intraoperative Management

C.1. What monitors would you use in this functional New York Heart Association (NYHA) class II patient during cesarean delivery?

Heart rate (via ECG), blood pressure, oxygen saturation, and temperature need to be monitored throughout the procedure. A urinary catheter should also be used to monitor urine output and decompress the bladder. For patients undergoing general anesthesia, continuous end-tidal carbon dioxide monitoring is needed. Assessment of neuromuscular function using a peripheral nerve stimulator is critical. In addition, processed electroencephalogram monitors can be used, although they probably do not reduce the incidence of intraoperative awareness during general anesthesia when end-tidal gas monitoring is used.

Standards for Basic Anesthetic Monitoring. Committee of origin: standards and practice parameters (approved by the ASA House of Delegates on October 21, 1986, last amended on October 20, 2010, and last affirmed on October 28, 2016). Accessed May 30, 2025. https://www.asahq.org/standards-and-practice-parameters/standards-for-basic-anesthetic-monitoring

C.2. When would you use invasive monitoring in a pregnant patient with cardiac disease?

NYHA class I and II patients do not routinely require invasive hemodynamic monitoring. In the past, parturients in class III or IV were often monitored with a pulmonary artery catheter; routine use has fallen out of favor, given its invasiveness. Transthoracic echocardiography is far less invasive, yet both safe and effective, a combination that has led to its increasing popularity in the perioperative period. An arterial line is warranted if serial blood gas determinations or continuous blood pressure monitoring is needed. Intra-arterial blood pressure monitoring during labor and delivery is especially helpful with severe mitral stenosis. Central venous pressure monitoring has low utility in labor, but should be placed if vasoactive medications or inotropes are required or as a conduit for a pulmonary artery catheter. Hemodynamic monitoring should be continued for at least 24 hours postdelivery because the sudden increase in preload can precipitate pulmonary edema.

Canobbio MM, Warnes CA, Aboulhosn J, et al. Management of pregnancy in patients with complex congenital heart disease: a scientific statement for healthcare professionals from the American Heart Association. *Circulation.* 2017;135:e50-e87.

Meng ML, Arendt KW. Obstetric Anesthesia and heart disease: practical clinical considerations. *Anesthesiology.* 2021;135:164-183.

Meng ML, Arendt KW, Banayan JM, et al. Anesthetic care of the pregnant patient with cardiovascular disease: a scientific statement from the American Heart Association. *Circulation.* 2023;147:e657-e673.

C.3. What are the hemodynamic goals of intraoperative management of the pregnant patient with mitral stenosis?

- Avoid tachycardia.
- Maintain sinus rhythm.
- Avoid marked decreases in systemic vascular resistance.
- Avoid marked increases in blood volume.
- Avoid increases in pulmonary vascular resistance.

Increased heart rate should be avoided because decreasing the amount of diastolic time for blood to flow across the stenotic mitral valve can lead to pulmonary edema and decreased cardiac output. Atrial fibrillation with a rapid ventricular response, similarly, can result in cardiac decompensation, and the loss of atrial contraction is detrimental. Marked decreases in systemic vascular resistance should be avoided because a compensatory increase in heart rate can result. Elevation of pulmonary vascular resistance, which can occur with hypercarbia, hypoxia, and acidosis, is poorly tolerated by these patients.

Kannan M, Vijayanand G. Mitral stenosis and pregnancy: current concepts in anaesthetic practice. *Indian J Anaesth.* 2010;54:439-444.

C.4. What anesthetic technique would you use for this emergency cesarean delivery?

The choices of anesthetic techniques are neuraxial (spinal, epidural, and combined spinal-epidural) or general anesthesia. In this case, the patient's epidural catheter should be dosed with additional local anesthetic to provide surgical anesthesia to a T4 level. If an adequate level of anesthesia cannot be achieved via an existing epidural catheter, conversion to general anesthesia is needed, specifically in the setting of abnormal FHR tracing. It is advisable to replace a nonfunctioning epidural catheter (before converting to general anesthesia) if the FHR tracing permits.

In the nonemergent setting, patients with mitral stenosis are good candidates for epidural anesthesia for cesarean (or vaginal) delivery. Combined spinal-epidural analgesia, particularly when an opioid-only spinal dose is used, is also a reasonable option. Spinal anesthesia with local anesthetic, on the other hand, can lead to a sudden and profound decrease in systemic vascular resistance with hypotension and reflex tachycardia, which can exacerbate fetal distress and lead to maternal decompensation in patients with mitral stenosis.

Cohen K, Minehart R, Leffert L. Anesthetic treatment of cardiac disease during pregnancy. *Curr Treat Options Cardiovasc Med.* 2018;20:66.

C.5. How would you manage local anesthetic systemic toxicity (LAST) in this patient?

LAST is a serious and potentially fatal complication of regional/neuraxial anesthesia. It is caused by a high plasma concentration of local anesthetic, either as a result of direct IV injection or from delayed absorption at the injection site. Pregnant patients appear to be at higher risk of refractory cardiac arrest in the setting of local anesthetic overdose, and it appears that epidural conversion from labor analgesia to surgical anesthesia puts patients at particular risk. Management of LAST includes the use of lipid emulsion according to the most current practice advisory by the American Society of Regional Anesthesia and Pain Medicine in conjunction with advanced cardiovascular life support (ACLS) guidelines, although there have been no trials to determine differences in either timing or dosing in pregnancy (**Figure 29.3**).

Bern S, Weinberg G. Local anesthetic toxicity and lipid resuscitation in pregnancy. *Curr Opin Anaesthesiol.* 2011;24:262-267.

Bucklin B, Santos A. Local Anesthetics and Opioids. In: Chestnut DH, Wong CA, Tsen LC, et al., eds. *Chestnut's Obstetric Anesthesia: Principles and Practice.* 6th ed. Elsevier; 2019:271-311.

Neal JM, Bernards CM, Butterworth JF IV, et al. ASRA practice advisory on local anesthetic systemic toxicity. *Reg Anesth Pain Med.* 2010;35:152-161.

C.6. If cardiac arrest were to occur prior to delivery, how would you proceed?

High-quality chest compressions and oxygenation must be performed along with manual left lateral uterine displacement; this is true for all pregnant patients when the uterine size is greater than or equal to 20 weeks. When the rhythm is shockable, defibrillation is appropriate (without risk to the fetus) in pregnancy. If the return of spontaneous circulation fails to occur within 4 minutes of resuscitation efforts, perimortem cesarean delivery is advised. Of note, IV access should be obtained above the diaphragm because compression of the inferior vena cava by the gravid uterus can prevent both fluids and medications from reaching the heart.

Jeejeebhoy FM, Zelop CM, Lipman S, et al. Cardiac arrest in pregnancy: a scientific statement from the American Heart Association. *Circulation.* 2015;132:1747-1773.

Zelop CM, Einav S, Mhyre JM, et al. Cardiac arrest during pregnancy: ongoing clinical conundrum. *Am J Obstet Gynecol.* 2018;219:52-61.

C.7. What technique could you use for general anesthesia in this patient?

- Induction
  - Crystalloid hydration through a large-bore, peripheral cannula
  - Supine position with a left lateral tilt to avoid aortocaval compression

SECTION 7

AMERICAN SOCIETY OF REGIONAL ANESTHESIA AND PAIN MEDICINE

CHECKLIST FOR TREATMENT OF LOCAL ANESTHETIC SYSTEMIC TOXICITY (LAST)

The Pharmacologic Treatment of LAST is Different from Other Cardiac Arrest Scenarios

- ¤ **Reduce** individual **epinephrine** boluses to ≤ 1 mcg/kg
- ¤ **Avoid** vasopressin, calcium channel blockers, beta blockers, or other local anesthetics

- Stop injecting local anesthetic
- Get help
  - Consider lipid emulsion therapy at the first sign of a serious LAST event
  - Call for the LAST Rescue Kit
  - Alert the nearest cardiopulmonary bypass team – resuscitation may be prolonged
- Airway management
  - Ventilate with 100% oxygen / avoid hyperventilation / advanced airway device if necessary
- Control seizures
  - Benzodiazepines preferred
  - **Avoid** large doses of **propofol**, especially in hemodynamically unstable patients
- Treat hypotension and bradycardia – **If pulseless, start CPR**

Lipid Emulsion 20% (Precise volume and flow rate are not crucial)	
Greater than 70 kg patient	Less than 70 kg patient
Bolus 100 mL Lipid Emulsion 20% Rapidly over 2–3 minutes • Lipid emulsion infusion 200–250 mL over 15–20 minutes	**Bolus 1.5 mL/kg Lipid Emulsion 20%** Rapidly over 2–3 minutes • Lipid emulsion infusion ~0.25 mL/kg/min (ideal body weight)
If patient remains unstable: • Re-bolus once or twice at the same dose and double infusion rate; be aware of dosing limit (12 mL/kg) • Total volume of lipid emulsion can approach 1 L in a prolonged resuscitation (e.g., > 30 minutes)	

- Continue monitoring
  - At least 4–6 hours after a cardiovascular event
  - Or, at least 2 hours after a limited CNS event
- Do not exceed 12 mL/kg lipid emulsion (particularly important in the small adult or child)
  - Much smaller doses are typically needed for LAST treatment
- See reverse side of this checklist for further details

ASRA

FIGURE 29.3. Checklist for treatment of LAST. (Reprinted from Neal JM, Barrington MJ, Fettiplace MR, et al. The Third American Society of Regional Anesthesia and Pain Medicine Practice Advisory on local anesthetic systemic toxicity: executive summary 2017. *Reg Anesth Pain Med.* 2018;43:113-123; with permission from BMJ Publishing Group Ltd.)

Risk Reduction (Be sensible)

- Use the least dose of local anesthetic necessary to achieve the desired extent and duration of block.
- Local anesthetic blood levels are influenced by site of injection and dose. It is important to identify patients at increased risk of LAST prior to using local anesthetics, eg, infants <6 months old, small patient size, advanced age and frailty, heart failure, ischemic heart disease, conduction abnormalities, or rhythm disorders, metabolic (eg, mitochondrial) disease, liver disease, low plasma protein concentration, acidosis, and medications that inhibit sodium channels. Patients with very low ejection fraction are more sensitive to LAST and may be especially prone to elevated local anesthetic levels associated with "stacked" injections.
- Consider using a pharmacologic marker and/or test dose, eg, epinephrine 2.5 to 5 mcg/mL (total 10–15 mcg). Know the expected response, onset, duration, and limitations of a "test dose" in identifying intravascular injection.
- Aspirate the syringe prior to each injection while observing for blood in the syringe or tubing
- Inject incrementally, while observing for signs and inquiring for symptoms of toxicity between each injection.
- Consider discussing local anesthetic dose as part of the pre-procedural or pre-surgical pause ("time out").

Detection (Be vigilant)

- Monitor the patient during and after completing injection. Clinical toxicity can be delayed 30 minutes or longer.
- Use standard American Society of Anesthesiologists (ASA) monitors.
- Communicate frequently with the patient to query for symptoms of toxicity.
- Consider LAST in any patient with altered mental status, neurological symptoms or signs of cardiovascular instability after a regional anesthetic (eg, change in HR, BP, ECG). Consider LAST even when the local anesthetic doses is 1) small (susceptible patient), 2) atypically administered (subcutaneous, mucosal, topical), 3) administered by the surgeon, or 4) after recent tourniquet deflation.
- Central nervous system signs (may be subtle, atypical, or absent)
  - Excitation (agitation, confusion, vocalization, muscle twitching, seizure)
  - Depression (drowsiness, obtundation, coma, or apnea)
  - Non-specific (metallic taste, circumoral numbness, diplopia, tinnitus, dizziness)
- Cardiovascular signs (occasionally the only manifestation of severe LAST)
  - Initially may be hyperdynamic (hypertension, tachycardia, ventricular arrhythmias), then
    - Progressive hypotension
    - Conduction block, bradycardia or asystole
    - Ventricular arrhythmia (ventricular tachycardia, Torsades de Pointes, ventricular fibrillation or asystole)
- Sedation may abolish the patient's ability to recognize or report LAST-related symptoms.

Treatment

Suggested components of a "LAST Rescue Kit"
• 1 L (total) lipid emulsion 20%
• Several large syringes and needles for administration
• Standard IV tubing
• ASRA Last Checklist

- Administer lipid emulsion at the first sign of a serious LAST event.
- Lipid emulsion can be used to treat LAST caused by any local anesthetic.
- Standard dose epinephrine (1 mg) can impair resuscitation from LAST and reduce the efficacy of lipid rescue. Use smaller doses than typical for ACLS, eg, ≤1 mcg/kg boluses, or for treating hypotension.
- Propofol should not be used when there are signs of cardiovascular instability.
- Prolonged monitoring (2–6 hours) is recommended after any signs of LAST, since cardiovascular depression due to local anesthetics can persist or recur after treatment.
  - If LAST event is short-lived and without signs of cardiovascular instability, one may consider proceeding with surgery after an uneventful ~30 minute interval of monitoring.

Please report LAST events to www.lipidrescue.org

The Third American Society of Regional Anesthesia and Pain Medicine Practice Advisory on Local Anesthetic Systemic Toxicity. Executive Summary 2017. Reg Anesth Pain Med 2018;43:113–123

The ASRA LAST™ smart phone app can be purchased from The Apple App Store or Google Play

ASRA LAST

FIGURE 29.3. Checklist for treatment of LAST. *(continued)*

- Preoxygenation with 100% inspired oxygen (FIO_2 = 1.0) by face mask for 3 to 5 minutes if time permits or four maximally deep inspirations (vital capacity breaths) if time is limited
- Rapid sequence induction (after a team "time-out" and abdominal preparation and draping) with thiopental (4 mg/kg; not available in the United States) or etomidate (0.2-0.3 mg/kg) and succinylcholine (1 mg/kg)
  - Although propofol (2 mg/kg) is otherwise most often used for induction of general anesthesia for cesarean delivery, it can cause hypotension.
  - Ketamine should also be avoided because it increases heart rate.
  - Because pregnant patients tend not to experience severe fasciculations, a defasciculating dose of a nondepolarizing muscle-blocking drug is not recommended.
  - Depending on the severity of the lesion, patients with mitral stenosis benefit from the use of a β-adrenergic receptor antagonist, such as esmolol, or a modest dose of opioid (eg, remifentanil) during induction of general anesthesia.
  - If hypotension occurs, phenylephrine, not ephedrine, is the vasopressor of choice because it does not cause tachycardia in the mother (and is less likely than ephedrine to cross the placenta and increase concentrations of lactate, glucose, and catecholamines in the fetal circulation).
- It is important to inform the neonatologist in the delivery room about medications given to the mother.
- Mucosal swelling and capillary engorgement in pregnancy can make tracheal intubation more difficult. Using a smaller endotracheal tube, such as a 7-mm internal diameter, can increase the likelihood of successful tracheal intubation on the first attempt. The value of cricoid pressure, traditionally maintained until the endotracheal tube cuff is inflated and the position of the tube verified, is unknown. In human cadavers, it seems to effectively prevent regurgitation with gastric pressures as high as 50 to 94 cm H_2O. Rice et al showed that cricoid pressure compresses the hypopharynx, leading to effective compression of the conduit between the stomach and the pharynx. Smith et al found, however, that cricoid pressure in awake volunteers leads to airway displacement and does not reliably produce midline esophageal compression. In practice, its protective effect against passive reflux appears limited and can even make intubation more difficult.

- Maintenance—prior to delivery of the neonate
  - 50% oxygen and volatile anesthetic (eg, 1% sevoflurane)
    - If pulmonary hypertension is present, N_2O should be avoided because it increases pulmonary vascular resistance.
    - No more than 0.5 minimum alveolar concentration (MAC) should be used because halogenated anesthetic agents promote uterine atony. In this patient, both isoflurane and desflurane are best avoided because they can cause tachycardia.
  - Neuromuscular blocking drug (vecuronium, cisatracurium, or rocuronium), as needed
  - Maintenance of eucapnia
  - As always, the anesthetic technique should be tailored to the severity of the patient's underlying condition.
- Maintenance—after delivery of the neonate
  - Use of midazolam, fentanyl (or other opioid), neuromuscular blocking drug, and oxygen
  - The MAC of volatile agents is decreased by up to 40% in pregnant patients. MAC is a spinal nociceptive reflex involving both sensory and motor components; the decrease in MAC has been interpreted to mean that pregnant patients have a decreased inhalational anesthetic requirement. In a small study of 30 patients, however, there was no difference in bispectral index (BIS) values between cesarean delivery patients and nonpregnant gynecologic patients undergoing general anesthesia with sevoflurane. According to Zand et al, BIS is not reliable for monitoring the depth of anesthesia during cesarean delivery. Regardless of the anesthetic agents chosen, the aim is to achieve a satisfactory balance between hemodynamic stability, maternal amnesia, adequate uterine tone, and minimal neonatal depression.
- IV oxytocin infusion—begin immediately after delivery of the neonate.
  - Bolus administration of oxytocin, methylergonovine, or 15-methyl prostaglandin $F_2\alpha$ should be avoided.
- Tracheal extubation—after protective laryngeal reflexes have returned and the patient has regained consciousness

de Souza DG, Doar LH, Mehta SH, et al. Aspiration prophylaxis and rapid sequence induction for elective cesarean delivery: time to reassess old dogma? *Anesth Analg*. 2010;110:1503-1505.

Norris MC, Dewan DM. Preoxygenation for cesarean section: a comparison of two techniques. *Anesthesiology*. 1985;62:827-829.

Rice MJ, Mancuso AA, Gibbs C, et al. Cricoid pressure results in compression of the postcricoid hypopharynx: the esophageal position is irrelevant. *Anesth Analg*. 2009;109:1546-1552.

Schulte-Sasse U, Hess W, Tarnow J. Pulmonary vascular response to nitrous oxide in patients with normal and high pulmonary vascular resistance. *Anesthesiology*. 1982;57:9-13.

Smith KJ, Dobranowski J, Yip G, et al. Cricoid pressure displaces the esophagus: an observational study using magnetic resonance imaging. *Anesthesiology*. 2003;99:60-64.

Ueyama H, Hagihira S, Takashina M, et al. Pregnancy does not enhance volatile anesthetic sensitivity on the brain: an electroencephalographic analysis study. *Anesthesiology*. 2010;113:577-584.

Zand F, Hadavi SM, Chohedri A, et al. Survey on the adequacy of depth of anaesthesia with bispectral index and isolated forearm technique in elective caesarean section under general anaesthesia with sevoflurane. *Br J Anaesth*. 2014;112:871-878.

C.8. If you are unexpectedly unable to intubate the trachea of this patient, how would you manage the airway?

Figure 29.4 illustrates the management of failed intubation in an obstetric patient with an unrecognized difficult airway. In the case of failed intubation when delivery of the neonate must occur, it is of utmost importance to maintain maternal oxygenation either via a facemask or supraglottic airway device. The mother's life should not be endangered to deliver a distressed fetus. Calling for help promptly when difficulties arise is essential.

American Society of Anesthesiologists Task Force on Obstetric Anesthesia. Practice guidelines for obstetric anesthesia: an updated report by the American Society of Anesthesiologists Task Force on obstetric anesthesia. *Anesthesiology*. 2007;106:843-863.

Apfelbaum JL, Hagberg CA, Caplan RA, et al; for American Society of Anesthesiologists Task Force on Management of the Difficult Airway. Practice guidelines for the management of the difficult airway: an updated report by the American Society of Anesthesiologists Task Force on management of the difficult airway. *Anesthesiology*. 2013;118:251-270.

Frerk C, Mitchell VS, McNarry AF, et al; Difficult Airway Society Intubation Guidelines Working Group. Difficult airway society 2015 guidelines for management of unanticipated difficult intubation in adults. *Br J Anaesth*. 2015;115:827-848.

Mushambi MC, Kinsella SM, Popat M, et al. Obstetric anaesthetists' association and difficult airway society guidelines for the management of difficult and failed tracheal intubation in obstetrics. *Anaesthesia*. 2015;70:1286-1306.

C.9. Would this patient benefit from the use of β-blockers?

Because this patient is asymptomatic, β-blockade is unnecessary. Should tachycardia occur, β-blockade with drugs such as propranolol, atenolol, or esmolol can be useful, as can digoxin or cardioversion, depending on the dysrhythmia. It has been shown that pregnant patients with symptomatic mitral stenosis who receive β-blockade with propranolol or atenolol to attenuate tachycardia have a significant decrease in the incidence of pulmonary edema with no adverse neonatal side effects.

al Kasab SM, Sabag T, al Zaibag M, et al. Beta-adrenergic receptor blockage in the management of pregnant women with mitral stenosis. *Am J Obstet Gynecol*. 1990;163:37-40.

C.10. What is the effect of the inhalation agents on uterine contractility?

At less than 1 MAC, there is no decrease in uterine contractility (or increase in blood loss) because the uterus still responds to oxytocin. At higher concentrations, uterine contractility is decreased, and as a result, blood loss is increased.

Tjeuw MT, Yao FS, van Poznak A. Depressant effects of anesthetics on isolated human gravid and non-gravid uterine muscle. *Chinese Med J (Engl)*. 1986;99:235-242.

Warren TM, Datta S, Ostheimer GW, et al. Comparison of the maternal and neonatal effects of halothane, enflurane, and isoflurane for cesarean delivery. *Anesth Analg*. 1983;62:516-520.

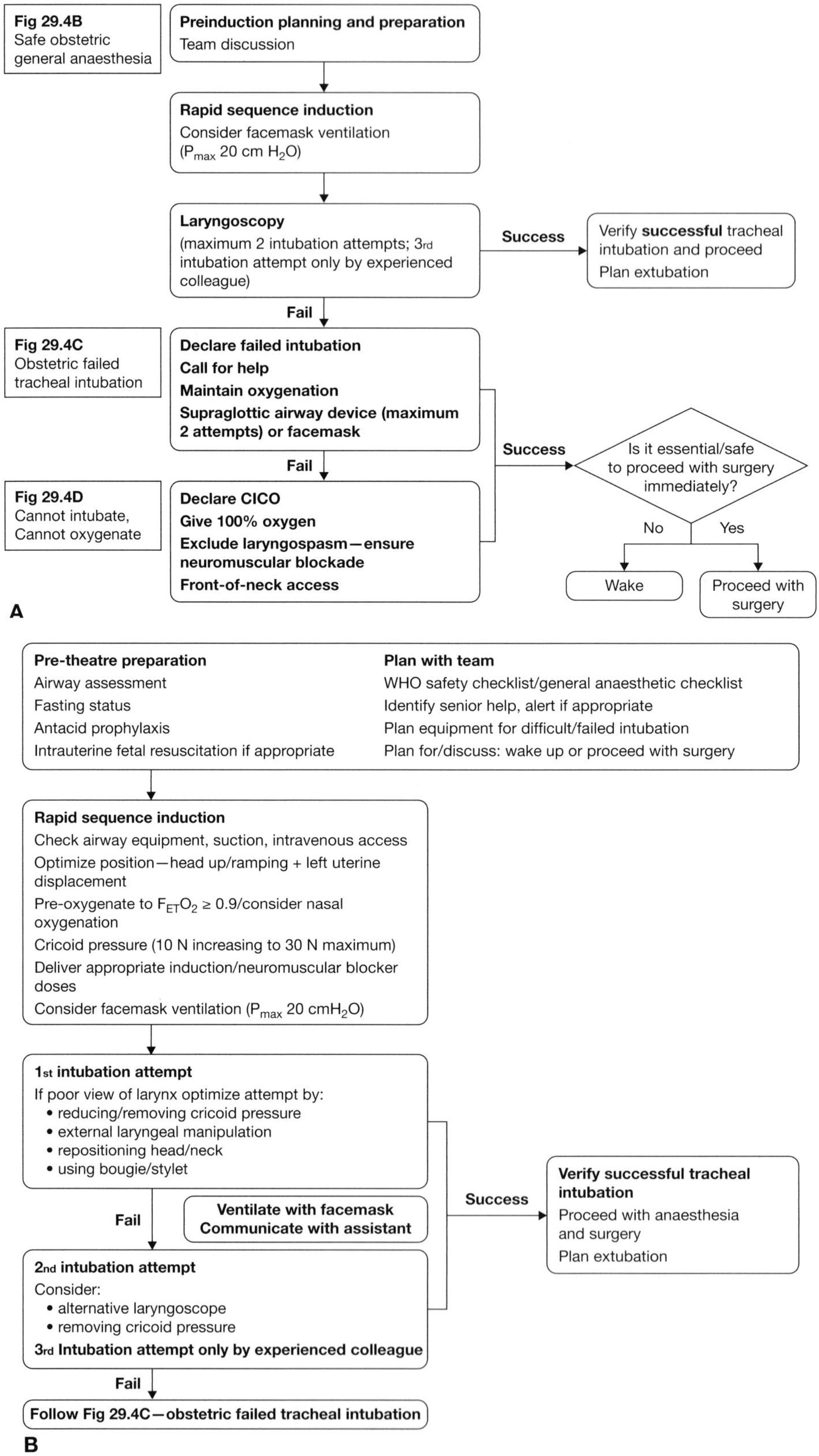

FIGURE 29.4. Algorithms for management of failed tracheal intubation in obstetric patients. A. Master algorithm. **B.** Safe obstetric general anesthesia.

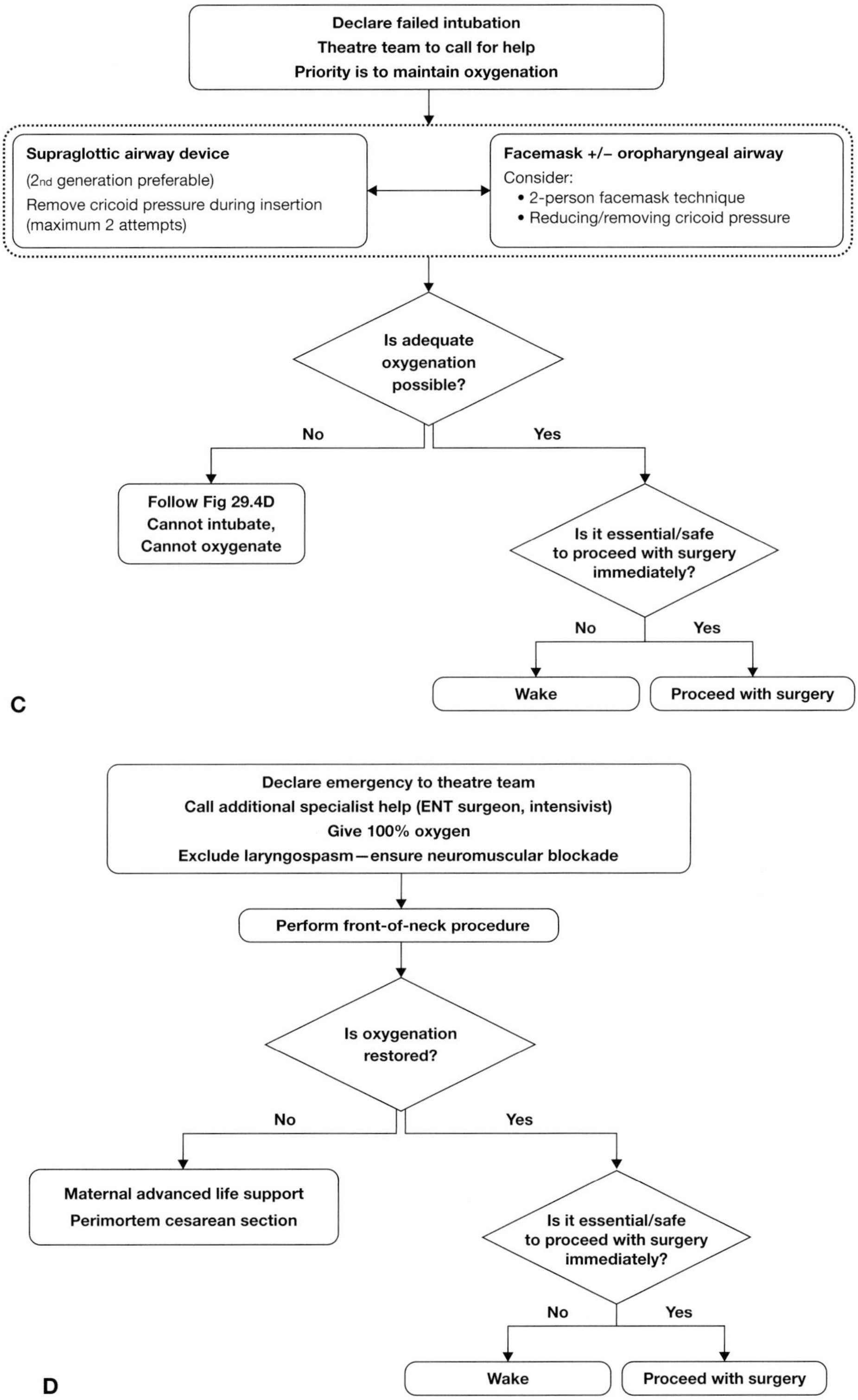

FIGURE 29.4. (*continued*) **C.** Obstetric failed tracheal intubation. **D.** Cannot intubate, cannot oxygenate (CICO). ENT, ear, nose, and throat. (Reproduced from Mushambi MC, Kinsella SM, Popat M, et al. Obstetric Anaesthetists' Association and difficult airway society guidelines for the management of difficult and failed tracheal intubation in obstetrics. *Anaesthesia.* 2015;70:1286-1306, with permission from Obstetric Anaesthetists' Association/Difficult Airway Society.)

TABLE 29.3 Apgar Scoring System

		Score		
Mnemonic	**Sign**	**0**	**1**	**2**
A	Appearance (color)	Blue, pale	Body pink, extremities blue	Pink
P	Pulse	Absent	<100/min	>100/min
G	Grimace (reflex irritability; response to catheter in the nose)	Absent	Grimace	Cough, sneeze
A	Activity (muscle tone)	Limp	Some extremity flexion	Active motion
R	Respiratory effect	Absent	Slow, irregular	Good cry

C.11. What is the Apgar scoring system?

The Apgar scoring system is used to assess the neonate's condition at 1 and 5 minutes of life. Each of the five categories is given a rating of 0 to 2, and the final score at each time is the sum of the individual category scores. Ten points is the best possible score (**Table 29.3**).

Apgar V. A proposal for a new method of evaluation of the newborn infant. *Curr Res Anesth Analg*. 1953;32:260-267.

C.12. What is the significance of the Apgar score?

The Apgar score is a standardized assessment of neonates at the time of delivery. It is measured at 1 and 5 minutes of life for all infants and then every 5 minutes up to 20 minutes for those with a score less than 7. The Apgar score provides information about the response to resuscitation but does not predict mortality or neurologic outcome.

American Academy of Pediatrics Committee on Fetus and Newborn, American College of Obstetricians and Gynecologists Committee on Obstetric Practice. The Apgar score. *Pediatrics*. 2015;136:819-822.

Casey BM, McIntire DD, Leveno KJ. The continuing value of the Apgar score for the assessment of newborn infants. *N Engl J Med*. 2001;344:467-471.

Silverman F, Suidan J, Wasserman J, et al. The Apgar score: is it enough? *Obstet Gynecol*. 1985;66:331-336.

C.13. At birth, what should be done to minimize an infant's risk of meconium aspiration syndrome?

For many years, obstetricians suctioned the mouth and nose of the newborn before its first breath and delivery of the shoulders. Now, neither routine suctioning (oropharyngeal/nasopharyngeal) nor tracheal intubation, even in the presence of meconium-stained fluid, is recommended. In the case of neonatal depression, it is recommended that emphasis be placed on initiating positive pressure ventilation; routine intubation, even in this situation, is not supported.

American College of Obstetricians and Gynecologists Committee on Obstetric Practice. ACOG committee opinion no. 689: delivery of a newborn with meconium-stained amniotic fluid. *Obstet Gynecol*. 2017;129:e33-e34.

American Heart Association, American Academy of Pediatrics. 2005 American Heart Association (AHA) guidelines for cardiopulmonary resuscitation (CPR) and emergency cardiovascular care (ECC) of pediatric and neonatal patients: neonatal resuscitation guidelines. *Pediatrics*. 2006;117:e1029-e1038.

Polin RA, Carlo WA. Surfactant replacement therapy for preterm and term neonates with respiratory distress. *Pediatrics*. 2014;133:156-163.

Vain NE, Szyld EG, Prudent LM, et al. Oropharyngeal and nasopharyngeal suctioning of meconium-stained neonates before delivery of their shoulders: multicentre, randomised controlled trial. *Lancet*. 2004;364:597-602.

Wyckoff MH, Aziz K, Escobedo MB, et al. Part 13: neonatal resuscitation: 2015 American Heart Association guidelines update for cardiopulmonary resuscitation and emergency cardiovascular care. *Circulation*. 2015;132:S543-S560.

C.14. If the Apgar score of the newborn is 3 at 1 minute, how would you treat the newborn?

Positive pressure ventilation and preductal pulse oximetry (right upper extremity) should be initiated at 1 minute of life when the heart rate is less than 100 beats per minute or the infant is gasping or apneic.

If the heart rate remains less than 100 beats per minute, an attempt to correct ventilation should occur; but if it is less than 60, chest compressions are indicated. The FIO_2 used during the initial resuscitation should be low (21% in term infants and 21%-30% in infants ≤35 weeks) because hyperoxia can lead to tissue and organ injury. If chest compressions are needed, FIO_2 can be increased. For term infants born at sea level, target preductal SpO_2 levels based on the time after delivery are as follows:

- 1 minute, 60% to 65%
- 2 minutes, 65% to 70%
- 3 minutes, 70% to 75%
- 4 minutes, 75% to 80%
- 5 minutes, 80% to 85%
- 10 minutes, 85% to 95%

Target data on SpO_2 levels do not exist for preterm or term infants born at different altitudes, but the above levels are thought to be reasonably usable in both of these patient populations.

Medications are rarely needed during neonatal resuscitation. However, if the heart rate remains less than 60 beats per minute despite adequate ventilation and chest compressions, IV epinephrine (0.01-0.03 mg/kg) should be given. Umbilical vein catheterization is the quickest way to gain IV access.

Dawson JA, Vento M, Finer NN, et al. Managing oxygen therapy during delivery room stabilization of preterm infants. *J Pediatr.* 2012;160:158-161.

Perlman JM, Wyllie J, Kattwinkel J, et al. Part 7: neonatal resuscitation: 2015 International Consensus on Cardiopulmonary Resuscitation and Emergency Cardiovascular Care Science with Treatment Recommendations. *Circulation.* 2015;132:S204-S241.

Rook D, Schierbeek H, Vento M, et al. Resuscitation of preterm infants with different inspired oxygen fractions. *J Pediatr.* 2014;164:1322.e3-1326.e3.

C.15. Blood gas analysis is sent immediately after delivery. What are the normal values for umbilical vein and artery blood gases?

In term infants, normal blood gases are as follows:

Umbilical artery

- pH, 7.27 ± 0.069
- PCO_2, 50.3 ± 11.1 mm Hg
- PO_2, 22.0 ± 3.6 mm Hg
- Bicarbonate, 22.3 ± 2.5 mEq/L

Umbilical vein

- pH, 7.35 ± 0.05
- PCO_2, 38.2 ± 5.6 mm Hg
- PO_2, 29.2 ± 5.9 mm Hg
- Bicarbonate, 20.4 ± 2.1 mEq/L

Umbilical artery blood gas values reflect fetal conditions, whereas umbilical vein blood gas values represent those of the uteroplacental unit and mother. ACOG recommends that cord blood gas measurements be obtained in the following circumstances: cesarean delivery for fetal compromise, low 5-minute Apgar score, severe fetal growth restriction, abnormalities in the FHR tracing, maternal thyroid disease, intrapartum maternal fever, or multiple gestation. In 2003, the American Academy of Pediatrics and ACOG defined metabolic acidosis as umbilical arterial pH less than 7.0 and a base deficit of at least 12 mmol/L. Umbilical cord blood gas and pH measurements alone, however, are poorly predictive of immediate- or long-term adverse neurologic outcome, but they do provide objective evidence of the fetal metabolic state at birth.

American College of Obstetricians and Gynecologists Committee on Obstetric Practice. ACOG committee opinion no. 348, November 2006: umbilical cord blood gas and acid-base analysis. *Obstet Gynecol.* 2006;108:1319-1322.

American College of Obstetricians and Gynecologists' Task Force on Neonatal Encephalopathy. Executive summary: neonatal encephalopathy and neurologic outcome, second edition. Report of the American College of Obstetricians and Gynecologists' Task Force on neonatal encephalopathy. *Obstet Gynecol.* 2014;123:896-901.

Cunningham FG, Leveno KJ, Dashe JS, et al., eds. The Newborn. In: *Williams Obstetrics.* 26th ed. McGraw-Hill; 2022:586-598.

Phelan JP, Korst LM, Martin GI. Application of criteria developed by the task force on neonatal encephalopathy and cerebral palsy to acutely asphyxiated neonates. *Obstet Gynecol.* 2011;118:824-830.

D. Postoperative Management

D.1. Immediately after the baby is delivered, the mother's oxygen saturation decreases. What is the differential diagnosis?

The following are possible causes of hypoxemia in the mother:

- Mechanical problems with the endotracheal tube (eg, kinking)
- Cardiac decompensation with pulmonary edema
- Pulmonary venous embolism: air, amniotic, or thrombotic

Fong J, Gadalla F, Pierri MK, et al. Are Doppler-detected venous emboli during cesarean section air emboli? *Anesth Analg*. 1990;71:254-257.

Toledo P. Embolic Disorders. In: Chestnut DH, Wong CA, Tsen LC, et al., eds. *Chestnut's Obstetric Anesthesia: Principles and Practice*. 6th ed. Elsevier; 2019:937-955.

D.2. Additional bleeding occurs in the postanesthesia care unit, and the obstetrician diagnoses retained placenta. What, if any, antibiotics are indicated to prevent endometritis after manual extraction of retained placenta?

Manual extraction of the placenta is indicated when excessive bleeding occurs and/or when part of the placenta is retained after delivery. There are conflicting data regarding the risk for endometritis after manual extraction of the placenta, and the need for antibiotic prophylaxis, therefore, remains in question. Despite a lack of consensus regarding the need for routine antibiotics, the WHO recommends one dose of ampicillin IV or a first-generation cephalosporin. In a retrospective cohort study of more than 400 females who delivered vaginally, there was no statistically significant difference in the rate of postpartum endometritis after manual extraction of the placenta with or without prophylactic antibiotics.

Safrai M, Kabiri D, Haj-Yahya R, et al. The effect of prophylactic antibiotic treatment for manual removal of the placenta on frequency of postpartum endometritis. *Int J Gynaecol Obstet*. 2017;139:45-49.

World Health Organization. *WHO Recommendations for the Prevention and Treatment of Postpartum Haemorrhage*. World Health Organization. Accessed February 7, 2019. https://www.who.int/reproductivehealth/publications/maternal_perinatal_health/9789241548502/en/

30 Appendectomy for a Pregnant Patient

Robert S. White and Farida Gadalla

A 25-year-old female at 32 weeks of gestation presented to the emergency room with vague right-sided abdominal pain. She had lost her appetite and experienced two episodes of emesis. Her temperature was 37.5 °C (99.5 °F); pulse rate, 100 beats per minute; hematocrit, 34%; and white blood cell (WBC) count, 15,000 per μL.

A. Medical Disease and Differential Diagnosis

1. What is the differential diagnosis for acute abdomen in a pregnant patient?
2. How would you make the clinical diagnosis of acute appendicitis?
3. What is the incidence of emergency surgery during pregnancy? What is the incidence of appendicitis during pregnancy?
4. What is the incidence of gangrenous appendicitis/peritonitis during pregnancy? Is this incidence higher in pregnant than in nonpregnant females?
5. What are the main concerns associated with nonobstetric surgery in the pregnant patient?
6. What are the factors influencing the teratogenicity of anesthetic agents in humans?
7. Are there any specific concerns regarding neurotoxicity and cognitive development in the developing fetus?
8. What factors influence fetal oxygenation, and how would you prevent intrauterine fetal asphyxia?
9. What is the incidence of trauma during pregnancy, and what are the risks to the mother and the fetus secondary to trauma?
10. What are other common surgeries performed during pregnancy?

B. Preoperative Evaluation and Preparation

1. What would you discuss with this patient preoperatively? Are any additional medical consultations warranted?
2. Is there a difference in the goal of anesthesia for delivery and for nonobstetric surgery in a pregnant patient?
3. How would you premedicate this patient?

C. Intraoperative Management

1. What factors would alter your anesthetic technique from that used for a nonpregnant patient?
2. If you choose epidural anesthesia, describe your technique and dosage.
3. If the patient needs supplemental analgesia, what would be your choice?
4. What vasopressor would you choose to improve uteroplacental perfusion?
5. When this patient arrived in the operating room, she desired a general anesthetic. Describe your technique.
6. Does any controversy exist surrounding the use of nitrous oxide?
7. Does any controversy exist surrounding operating room personnel, anesthetic exposure, and pregnancy outcomes?
8. What is the impact of nonobstetric surgery on maternal mortality, birth defects, and fetal loss? What factors influence it?
9. Should intraoperative fetal heart rate (FHR) monitoring be used? What would you expect to see on the electronic fetal monitor during anesthesia?
10. How would your anesthetic management differ if the patient were having upper extremity surgery?
11. The surgeon schedules the procedure to be performed laparoscopically. Does this pose any additional problems?

D. Postoperative Management

1. When would you extubate the trachea for this patient?
2. Postoperatively, what monitors would you use?
3. What other postoperative precautions would you take? What is the incidence of preterm delivery following nonobstetric surgery during pregnancy?
4. The next day, the patient went into premature labor and now needs a cesarean section for prematurity and breech presentation. She requires another general anesthetic. In what way would your technique differ from your previous anesthetic technique?

A. Medical Disease and Differential Diagnosis

A.1. What is the differential diagnosis for acute abdomen in a pregnant patient?

The differential diagnosis for acute abdomen in a pregnant patient includes appendicitis, cholecystitis, and intestinal obstruction as the most common nonobstetric surgical emergencies.

Medical Conditions

- Sickle cell disease
- Porphyria
- Glomerulonephritis
- Inflammatory bowel disease
- Pyelonephritis
- Pneumonia
- Splenic disorders
- Withdrawal from drug addiction

Obstetric Conditions

- Ectopic pregnancy
- Hemolysis, elevated liver enzymes, low platelet count (HELLP) syndrome
- Labor
- Abruptio placentae
- Chorioamnionitis

Gynecologic Conditions

- Fibroid degeneration
- Salpingitis
- Degenerating myoma
- Ovarian cyst or tumor, either torted or ruptured
- Tubo-ovarian abscess

Surgical Conditions

- Appendicitis
- Cholecystitis
- Pancreatitis
- Mesenteric adenitis
- Intestinal obstruction
- Maternal trauma

Bauchat JR, Van de Velde M. Nonobstetric Surgery during Pregnancy. In: Chestnut DH, Wong CA, Tsen LC, et al., eds. *Chestnut's Obstetric Anesthesia: Principles and Practice*. 6th ed. Elsevier; 2020:368-391.

Tase A, Kamarizan MF, Swarnkar K. Appendicitis in pregnancy: difficulties in diagnosis and management. Guidance for the emergency general surgeon: a systematic review. *Int J Surg Open*. 2017;6:5-11.

A.2. How would you make the clinical diagnosis of acute appendicitis?

The diagnosis is based on a detailed history, physical exam, imaging, and the following symptoms:

- Vague abdominal pain (right flank or upper quadrant): The position is variable because of the cephalad displacement of appendix due to the growing uterus, but the most common presenting symptom is right lower quadrant pain.

- Gastrointestinal distress: anorexia, nausea, vomiting
- Abdominal tenderness, guarding, rebound pain, rectal tenderness
- Mildly elevated temperature, 37 °C to 38 °C (98.6 °F-100.4 °F)
- Mildly elevated pulse rate
- An increase in WBC count: Because pregnant patients normally have a higher WBC count, a physiologic leukocytosis, than nonpregnant patients, an increased WBC count might not be a reliable marker.

Ultrasonography is the most frequently used imaging technique, is not associated with risk, and allows for exclusion of other causes of acute abdominal pain and for assessment of fetal condition. The use is operator dependent, and acute appendicitis can have normal abdominal findings. When the ultrasound is equivocal, magnetic resonance imaging (MRI) has lower rates of nonvisualization. Gadolinium-based contrast during pregnancy is controversial with restricted use. Computed tomography (CT) scan has a limited role in pregnancy because of radiation and contrast risks; however, radiation exposure is at a much lower dose than the exposure associated with fetal harm, and clinically necessary imaging should not be withheld.

Bauchat JR, Van de Velde M. Nonobstetric Surgery during Pregnancy. In: Chestnut DH, Wong CA, Tsen LC, et al., eds. *Chestnut's Obstetric Anesthesia: Principles and Practice*. 6th ed. Elsevier; 2020:368-391.

Committee on Obstetric Practice. Committee opinion no. 723: guidelines for diagnostic imaging during pregnancy and lactation. *Obstet Gynecol*. 2017;130:e210-e216.

Walker HG, Al Samaraee A, Mills SJ, et al. Laparoscopic appendicectomy in pregnancy: a systematic review of the published evidence. *Int J Surg*. 2014;12:1235-1241.

A.3. What is the incidence of emergency surgery during pregnancy? What is the incidence of appendicitis during pregnancy?

Between 0.75% and 2% or approximately 75,000 pregnant patients require emergency nonobstetric surgery yearly, mostly for acute appendicitis, cholecystitis (6:1,000 pregnancies), maternal trauma, and cancer. Gastrointestinal surgery accounts for 45% of nonobstetric surgeries in the pregnant patients, and orthopedic procedures account for 24%. Appendicitis is the most common surgical emergency with varying incidence between 1:500 and 1:635 and has been reported as low as 1:2,000. It occurs more frequently in the second (45%) than in the first (30%) or third trimesters (25%). In epidemiologic studies, the reduced incidence of appendicitis in pregnant patients compared to matched controls suggests a protective effect of pregnancy.

Lee SH, Lee JY, Choi YY, et al. Laparoscopic appendectomy versus open appendectomy for suspected appendicitis during pregnancy: a systematic review and updated meta-analysis. *BMC Surg*. 2019;19:41.

Tolcher MC, Fisher WE, Clark SL. Nonobstetric surgery during pregnancy. *Obstet Gynecol*. 2018;132:395-403.

Walker HG, Al Samaraee A, Mills SJ, et al. Laparoscopic appendicectomy in pregnancy: a systematic review of the published evidence. *Int J Surg*. 2014;12:1235-1241.

A.4. What is the incidence of gangrenous appendicitis/peritonitis during pregnancy? Is this incidence higher in pregnant than in nonpregnant females?

During pregnancy, the gravid uterus pushes the appendix cephalad away from the omentum (**Figure 30.1**), thereby causing the diseased appendix to produce little pain typically in the right lower quadrant and obfuscating the classic symptoms with flank pain. Imaging studies have confirmed that the appendix is displaced upward to a mean distance of 45 mm above the iliac crest at term. This delays diagnosis and surgical intervention, allowing the appendix to progress to gangrenous without detection. Also, contributing to diagnostic delay is postponement in diagnostic procedures such as radiography and laparoscopy for fetal concerns. A 24-hour surgical delay can cause a 66% increase in perforation rate. The incidence of perforation of the appendix is approximately 15%. The perforation rates for first, second, and third trimesters are about 8.7%, 12.1%, and 26.1%, respectively.

Andersson RE, Lambe M. Incidence of appendicitis during pregnancy. *Int J Epidemiol*. 2001;30:1281-1285.

Kumamoto K, Imaizumi H, Hokama N, et al. Recent trend of acute appendicitis during pregnancy. *Surg Today*. 2015;45:1521-1526.

Tase A, Kamarizan MF, Swarnkar K. Appendicitis in pregnancy: difficulties in diagnosis and management. Guidance for the emergency general surgeon: a systematic review. *Int J Surg Open*. 2017;6:5-11.

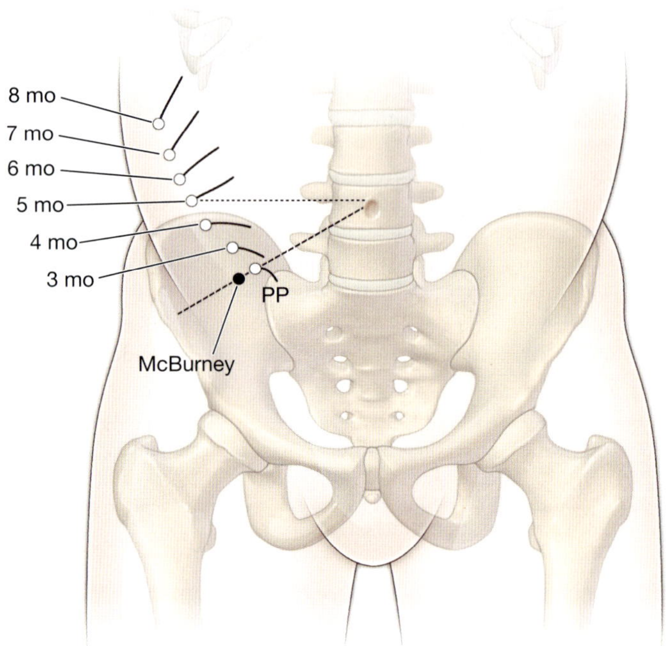

FIGURE 30.1. Changes in position and direction of the appendix during pregnancy. McBurney, McBurney's point; PP, prepregnancy. (Adapted from Baer JL, Reis RA, Arens RA. Appendicitis in pregnancy with changes in position and axis of the normal appendix in pregnancy. *JAMA.* 1932;98:1359.)

A.5. What are the main concerns associated with nonobstetric surgery in the pregnant patient?

Abdominal surgeries during pregnancy have an increased risk of poor pregnancy outcomes, including premature delivery, spontaneous abortion, premature labor, and perinatal morbidity and mortality. Maternal mortality rate is very low, and to ensure maternal safety, awareness of the physiologic changes of the parturient is of great importance. Special care should be taken to prevent aspiration pneumonitis especially after midgestation. The risk of failed tracheal intubation is increased. Faster uptake of anesthetics and a decrease in minimum alveolar concentration (MAC) for volatile anesthetics rapidly render patients unconscious at lower doses.

As early as 8 weeks of gestation, most of the increases in cardiac output and stroke volume and decreases in vascular resistance are apparent. There is the risk of supine hypotensive syndrome (aortocaval compression). For fetal safety, it is essential to avoid teratogenic anesthetic agents and intrauterine fetal asphyxia. Maintenance of adequate maternal oxygenation, blood oxygen-carrying capacity, and uteroplacental perfusion are critical to fetal well-being.

The American College of Obstetricians and Gynecologists (ACOG) and the American Society of Anesthesiologists (ASA) have recommended that medically necessary surgery should never be denied to a pregnant patient, regardless of trimester, because delaying surgery can adversely affect both the pregnant patient and her fetus. However, elective surgery should be postponed until after delivery. Additional concerns exist for preterm delivery potential, and consideration should be given to corticosteroid administration for benefit of fetuses at viable premature gestational ages. During the perioperative period, patients should be monitored for signs and symptoms of preterm labor and screened for venous thromboembolism risk with appropriate perioperative prophylaxis administration.

Bauchat JR, Van de Velde M. Nonobstetric Surgery during Pregnancy. In: Chestnut DH, Wong CA, Tsen LC, et al., eds. *Chestnut's Obstetric Anesthesia: Principles and Practice*. 6th ed. Elsevier; 2020:368-391.

Committee on Obstetric Practice, American Society of Anesthesiologists. Committee opinion no. 775: nonobstetric surgery during pregnancy. *Obstet Gynecol.* 2019;129:777-778.

Haggerty E, Daly J. Anaesthesia and non-obstetric surgery in pregnancy. *BJA Educ.* 2021;21:42-43.

A.6. What are the factors influencing the teratogenicity of anesthetic agents in humans?

The ACOG/ASA committee opinion states: "No currently used anesthetic agents have been shown to have any teratogenic effects in humans when using standard concentrations at any gestational age." Nevertheless, most anesthesiologists adhere to the use of only time-tested anesthetics with the goal of minimizing anesthetic exposures and exposure time. The factors influencing teratogenicity are genetic predisposition, inherent toxicity of the administered drug, drug dosage and duration, placental transfer to the fetus, and fetal developmental stage at the time of exposure.

Almost all anesthetics are teratogenic in some animals, but no animal model is perfectly applicable to humans. There are no documented reports of teratogenicity, congenital anomalies, or increase in birth defects in humans ascribed to any anesthetic agent used during pregnancy. The most susceptible time for human teratogenicity is during organogenesis between days 31 and 71 after the last menstrual period. Before implantation of the ovum, teratogenicity leads to abortion. Later, malformation, functional deficiencies, and even death can occur. Associations between the use of benzodiazepines and cleft palate and cardiac anomalies have been refuted; no evidence exists that a single dose of a benzodiazepine is harmful.

Bauchat JR, Van de Velde M. Nonobstetric Surgery during Pregnancy. In: Chestnut DH, Wong CA, Tsen LC, et al., eds. *Chestnut's Obstetric Anesthesia: Principles and Practice*. 6th ed. Elsevier; 2020:368-391.

Committee on Obstetric Practice, American Society of Anesthesiologists. Committee opinion no. 775: nonobstetric surgery during pregnancy. *Obstet Gynecol*. 2019;129:777-778.

Vasco Ramirez M, Valencia GCM. Anesthesia for nonobstetric surgery in pregnancy. *Clin Obstet Gynecol*. 2020;63:351-363.

A.7. Are there any specific concerns regarding neurotoxicity and cognitive development in the developing fetus?

Concern exists regarding exposure to anesthesia and potential neurotoxicity impacting neurodevelopment. A single and relatively brief exposure to general anesthesia is not associated with detectable deficits in most cognitive domains or academic achievement. The ACOG/ASA committee opinion states: "There is no evidence that in utero human exposure to anesthetic or sedative drugs has any effect on the developing fetal brain; and there are no animal data to support an effect with limited exposures less than 3 hours in duration."

In December 2016, the US Food and Drug Administration (FDA) released a Drug Safety Communications warning and medication labeling changes that stated: "repeated or lengthy use of general anesthetic and sedation drugs during surgeries or procedures in children younger than 3 years or in pregnant women during their third trimester may affect the development of children's brains." The response to this FDA rule change from concerned medical societies has been critical for the poor quality of scientific evidence used, lack of involvement of stakeholder medical societies, and its untoward impact on appropriate medical care with possible patient reluctance to undergo medically necessary procedures.

Committee on Obstetric Practice, American Society of Anesthesiologists. Committee opinion no. 775: nonobstetric surgery during pregnancy. *Obstet Gynecol*. 2019;129:777-778.

O'Leary JD, Warner DO. What do recent human studies tell us about the association between anaesthesia in young children and neurodevelopmental outcomes? *Br J Anaesth*. 2017;119:458-464.

U.S. Food and Drug Administration. FDA drug safety communication: FDA review results in new warnings about using general anesthetics and sedation drugs in young children and pregnant women. Accessed December 2, 2018. https://www.fda.gov/drugs/drug-safety-and-availability/fda-drug-safety-communication-fda-review-results-new-warnings-about-using-general-anesthetics-and

A.8. What factors influence fetal oxygenation, and how would you prevent intrauterine fetal asphyxia?

Maintaining maternal homeostasis (ie, prevention of hypoxemia, hypotension, acidosis, and hyperventilation) is essential to fetal well-being. Fetal oxygenation is directly dependent on maternal oxygen tension, oxygen saturation, hemoglobin content, oxygen affinity, and uteroplacental perfusion. Maternal hypoxia will result in fetal hypoxia; if uncorrected, fetal abnormalities or death can occur. Uterine blood flow is determined by uterine vascular resistance and uterine perfusion pressure (relative passive perfusion);

factors that decrease uterine blood flow must be avoided. Uterine blood flow can be decreased by the following: maternal hypotension; stress, pain, or anxiety (due to the release of maternal catecholamines); hypoxia; hypercarbia, which also directly results in fetal respiratory acidosis; hyperventilation (hypocapnia); positive pressure ventilation; and vasopressor agents. Overall, one should place greater importance on anesthetic management than on the agents used, and fluid administration should be appropriate for estimated or anticipated blood loss.

Bauchat JR, Van de Velde M. Nonobstetric Surgery during Pregnancy. In: Chestnut DH, Wong CA, Tsen LC, et al., eds. *Chestnut's Obstetric Anesthesia: Principles and Practice*. 6th ed. Elsevier; 2020:368-391.

Haggerty E, Daly J. Anaesthesia and non-obstetric surgery in pregnancy. *BJA Educ*. 2021;21:42-43.

Vasco Ramirez M, Valencia GCM. Anesthesia for nonobstetric surgery in pregnancy. *Clin Obstet Gynecol*. 2020;63:351-363.

A.9. What is the incidence of trauma during pregnancy, and what are the risks to the mother and the fetus secondary to trauma?

Trauma occurs in 6% to 8% of all pregnancies and is the leading cause of nonobstetric maternal mortality. To optimize outcomes, urgent multidisciplinary care is required. Most common causes of trauma during pregnancy are motor vehicle accidents (207:100,000 live births), falls and slips (48.9:100,000), and domestic violence (8,307:100,000). Maternal mortality and fetal mortality due to trauma are 1.4/100,000 and 3.7/100,000 pregnancies, respectively. Death rates and complications are higher in mothers at term compared to nonpregnant females. Maternal complications are due to uterine rupture, placental abruption, and premature rupture of membranes. Fetal complications are due to these factors as well as to prematurity and stillbirths.

The primary goal of initial management is maternal assessment and stabilizing the mother with aggressive resuscitation. Uterine displacement is used, and initial evaluation should be based on standard trauma guidelines. Maternal stability might not be accomplishable without obstetric intervention, and emergent delivery might be necessary. Radiographic studies, if indicated, should be done. CT imaging produces a radiation exposure dose lower than that associated with fetal harm.

Committee on Obstetric Practice. Committee opinion no. 723: guidelines for diagnostic imaging during pregnancy and lactation. *Obstet Gynecol*. 2017;130:e210-e216.

Irving T, Menon R, Ciantar E. Trauma during pregnancy. *BJA Educ*. 2021;21:10-19.

Mendez-Figueroa H, Dahlke JD, Vrees RA, et al. Trauma in pregnancy: an updated systematic review. *Am J Obstet Gynecol*. 2013;209:1-10.

A.10. What are other common surgeries performed during pregnancy?

Cardiac surgery: The physiologic changes of pregnancy (ie, increases in blood volume, cardiac output, and decrease in systemic vascular resistance) can exacerbate preexisting heart disease, leading to congestive heart failure, particularly in patients with stenotic mitral or aortic valvular disease and pulmonary hypertension. Two periods are especially associated with cardiac decompensation: at 24 to 28 weeks when cardiac output reaches a maximum and immediately after delivery when uterine autotransfusion increases venous return causing volume overload. Procedures consist of surgical repair and percutaneous balloon valvuloplasty.

Neurosurgical procedures: The physiologic changes of pregnancy resulting in cardiac and hormonal (ie, softening of vascular connective tissue) system changes can increase the risk of hemorrhage from intracranial saccular aneurysms or arteriovenous malformations. Other common conditions encountered include brain tumors, traumatic brain injury, and spinal surgery. Specific considerations include use of "controlled hypotension," prone positioning, and intraoperative maternal hypothermia.

In these unique surgical situations, a multidisciplinary approach involving anesthesia, obstetric, and surgical services is critical.

Reitman E, Flood P. Anaesthetic considerations for non-obstetric surgery during pregnancy. *Br J Anaesth*. 2011;107:i72-i78.

Tolcher MC, Fisher WE, Clark SL. Nonobstetric surgery during pregnancy. *Obstet Gynecol*. 2018;132:395-403.

Vasco Ramirez M, Valencia GCM. Anesthesia for nonobstetric surgery in pregnancy. *Clin Obstet Gynecol*. 2020;63:351-363.

B. Preoperative Evaluation and Preparation

B.1. What would you discuss with this patient preoperatively? Are any additional medical consultations warranted?

The pregnant patient undergoing nonobstetric surgery requires a standard anesthesia preoperative assessment and reevaluation with discussion regarding anesthetic and surgical risks to the pregnancy and fetus. Obstetric consultation before surgery is essential as is utilization of a multidisciplinary team approach to provide for optimal safety of the patient and the fetus. The primary obstetric care provider should be notified and an obstetrician with hospital privileges at the institution where surgery is to be performed should be involved. Use of fetal monitoring should also be discussed, again emphasizing communication, coordination, and planning between the different physician services. Fetal heart rate (FHR) monitoring can assist in maternal positioning during the procedure and maternal cardiorespiratory management; FHR monitoring can also influence a decision for fetal delivery. If fetal monitoring is used, the surgery should be done at an institution with neonatal and pediatric services; an obstetric care provider with privileges for cesarean delivery should be readily available; and a qualified individual who can interpret FHR patterns should be readily available. When possible, informed consent should be obtained that allows for emergency cesarean delivery. Decisions regarding preterm labor and tocolysis should be delineated.

It is important to discuss the patient's options concerning regional versus general anesthesia, emphasizing that the fetal outcome is statistically similar, but regional anesthesia is the technique of choice for the mother whenever possible (avoids fetal exposure to drugs and need for airway protection). In this case, if the appendectomy is planned laparoscopically, general anesthesia with airway control is preferred. Outcome studies show that patients who undergo surgery during pregnancy deliver earlier and have smaller babies than those who do not. Any increase in miscarriage or preterm birth is mostly attributable to surgical concerns.

Cheek TG, Baird E. Anesthesia for nonobstetric surgery: maternal and fetal considerations. *Clin Obstet Gynecol.* 2009;52:535-545.

Committee on Obstetric Practice, American Society of Anesthesiologists. Committee opinion no. 775: nonobstetric surgery during pregnancy. *Obstet Gynecol.* 2019;129:777-778.

Reitman E, Flood P. Anaesthetic considerations for non-obstetric surgery during pregnancy. *Br J Anaesth.* 2011;107:i72-i78.

SECTION 7

B.2. Is there a difference in the goal of anesthesia for delivery and for nonobstetric surgery in a pregnant patient?

The aim of obstetric anesthesia is to permit pain-free labor and delivery without interfering with the progress of childbirth. Obstetric anesthesia should provide maternal analgesia without fetal or newborn neurologic or respiratory depression. Conversely, the aim of surgical anesthesia is to provide maternal anesthesia without stimulating uterine activity and precipitating premature labor. Surgical anesthesia is designed to maintain uteroplacental perfusion.

Bauchat JR, Van de Velde M. Nonobstetric Surgery during Pregnancy. In: Chestnut DH, Wong CA, Tsen LC, et al., eds. *Chestnut's Obstetric Anesthesia: Principles and Practice.* 6th ed. Elsevier; 2020:368-391.

Tsen LC, Bateman BT. Anesthesia for Cesarean Delivery. In: Chestnut DH, Wong CA, Tsen LC, et al., eds. *Chestnut's Obstetric Anesthesia: Principles and Practice.* 6th ed. Elsevier; 2020:568-626.

B.3. How would you premedicate this patient?

Premedication is usually avoided in favor of verbal anxiolysis, reassurance, and support. If necessary, benzodiazepines can be given to relieve maternal anxiety and to avoid increased maternal catecholamine levels. Glycopyrrolate, which does not cross the placental barrier, can be used as a vagolytic and antisialagogue. For general anesthesia, a nonparticulate antacid, such as 30 mL of 0.3 M sodium citrate, is given about 30 minutes before surgery to reduce aspiration pneumonitis; an H_2-receptor antagonist (ranitidine) or metoclopramide can also be given. Standard adult fasting guidelines should be followed for elective procedures.

Bauchat JR, Van de Velde M. Nonobstetric Surgery during Pregnancy. In: Chestnut DH, Wong CA, Tsen LC, et al., eds. *Chestnut's Obstetric Anesthesia: Principles and Practice.* 6th ed. Elsevier; 2020:368-391.

Tsen LC, Bateman BT. Anesthesia for Cesarean Delivery. In: Chestnut DH, Wong CA, Tsen LC, et al., eds. *Chestnut's Obstetric Anesthesia: Principles and Practice.* 6th ed. Elsevier; 2020:568-626.

Cheek TG, Baird E. Anesthesia for nonobstetric surgery: maternal and fetal considerations. *Clin Obstet Gynecol.* 2009;52:535-545.

Vasco Ramirez M, Valencia GCM. Anesthesia for nonobstetric surgery in pregnancy. *Clin Obstet Gynecol.* 2020;63:351-363.

C. Intraoperative Management

C.1. What factors would alter your anesthetic technique from that used for a nonpregnant patient?

The maternal anatomic and physiologic changes of pregnancy have anesthetic implications.

Cardiovascular System

- A 40% to 50% increase in blood volume (20% reduction in hematocrit due to physiologic anemia of pregnancy with a greater increase in plasma volume than in red blood cell volume)
- A 40% to 50% increase in cardiac output (stroke volume and heart rate)
- Decreased peripheral vascular resistance
- Decreased mean arterial blood pressure
- Aortocaval compression in the supine position secondary to growing uterus (**Figure 30.2**). This can reduce venous return and cardiac output by 30%. Left uterine displacement (supine patient tilted by a wedge under the right hip) should be used.
- Lower extremity venous stasis can lead to pedal edema and deep venous thrombosis (also affected by hypercoagulable state of pregnancy).

Respiratory System

- Increased minute ventilation (hyperventilation from progesterone shifting $Paco_2$ curve); chronic respiratory alkalosis with subsequent decrease in bicarbonate buffering capacity
- Increased oxygen consumption by 20%
- Decreased functional residual capacity (FRC) by 20% (**Figure 30.3**)
- Both factors contribute to a rapid decrease in Pao_2 during apneic periods.

Gastrointestinal System

- Decreased esophageal and intestinal motility
- Gastric emptying time is normal except for laboring patient.
- Decreased volume of gastrointestinal secretions
- Distortion of gastric anatomy secondary to growing uterus
- Increased gastric acidity
- Decreased lower esophageal (gastroesophageal) sphincter tone secondary to increased progesterone level. Increased incidence of heartburn/reflux. A pregnant patient after 18 weeks should always be considered as having a full stomach and must be considered at risk for regurgitation and aspiration (cautious use of mask ventilation or laryngeal mask airway [LMA]).

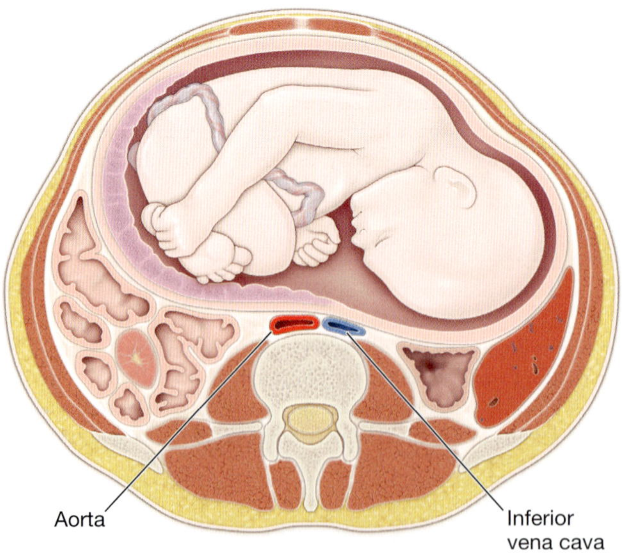

FIGURE 30.2. The pregnant uterus compressing the aorta and the inferior vena cava (aortocaval compression) in the supine position. (Redrawn from Ostheimer GW. *Regional Anesthesia Techniques in Obstetrics*. Breon Laboratories; 1980.)

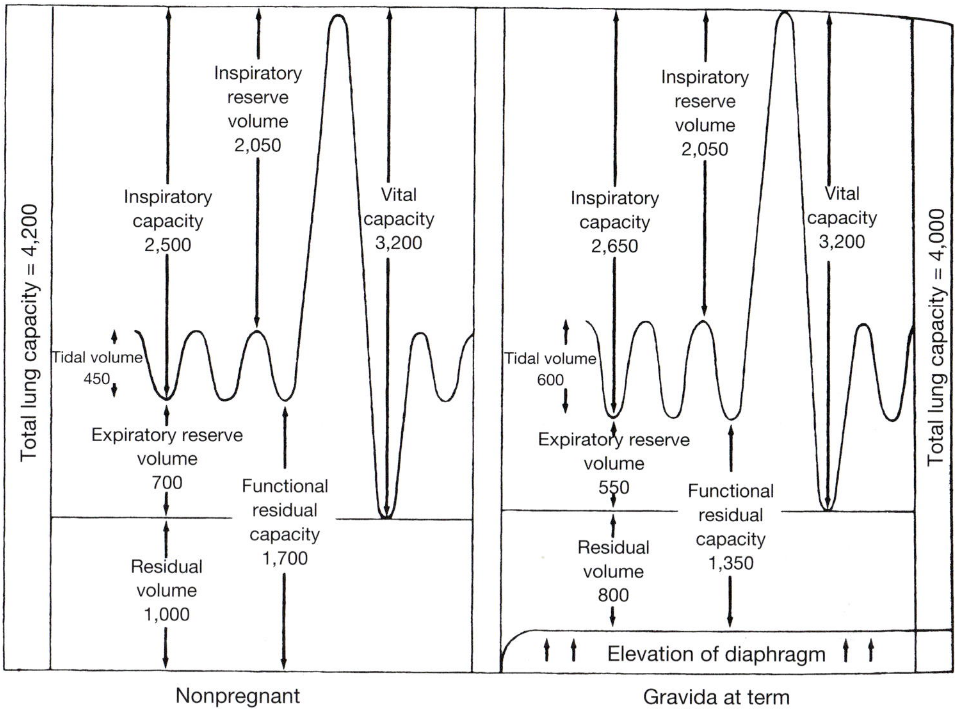

FIGURE 30.3. Pulmonary volumes and capacities during pregnancy. (From Bonica JJ, McDonald JS. Maternal anatomic and physiologic alterations during pregnancy and parturition. In: Bonica JJ, McDonald JS, eds. *Principles and Practice of Obstetric Analgesia and Anesthesia.* 2nd ed. Baltimore, MD: Williams & Wilkins; 1995:49. Figures 2-4.)

Central Nervous System

- A 30% to 40% decrease in MAC for inhaled anesthetics
- Increased sensitivity to local anesthetics
- Decreased volume of epidural anesthetic required because of engorgement of epidural veins and consequent decrease in size of epidural space; also increases risk of intravascular injection

Airway, Skin, and Mucous Membranes

- Swelling of oropharyngeal tissues with decreased caliber of glottic opening (difficulty performing mask ventilation and intubation; increased risk of failed intubation)
- More friable mucous membranes and engorged mucosal capillaries. Avoid nasal manipulation such as insertion of nasal airway, nasotracheal tube, and nasogastric tube.
- Mallampati classification may be more predictive of difficult intubation.

Haggerty E, Daly J. Anaesthesia and non-obstetric surgery in pregnancy. *BJA Educ.* 2021;21:42-43.

Kacmar RM, Gaiser R. Physiologic Changes of Pregnancy. In: Chestnut DH, Wong CA, Tsen LC, et al., eds. Chestnut's Obstetric Anesthesia: Principles and Practice. 6th ed. Elsevier; 2020:13-37.

Vasco Ramirez M, Valencia GCM. Anesthesia for nonobstetric surgery in pregnancy. *Clin Obstet Gynecol.* 2020;63:351-363.

C.2. If you choose epidural anesthesia, describe your technique and dosage.

The patient is placed either in the sitting position or on their side for epidural placement at L2-L3 or L3-L4. Adequate hydration is achieved with intravenous fluids. After testing for inadvertent spinal or intravascular placement, the local anesthetic solution is given in divided doses to attain a T4 sensory level. Inadvertent spinal injection is detected by rapid onset of a solid motor block; intravascular injection is evidenced by signs of systemic toxicity (dizziness, tinnitus, circumoral numbness, metallic taste). Local anesthetics used are 2% lidocaine, 0.5% bupivacaine, or 0.5% or 0.75% ropivacaine. These agents provide good analgesia with a degree of motor blockade for muscular relaxation. Epidural fentanyl promotes quicker onset and more solid block. The patient is again positioned with a left uterine wedge, oxygen is delivered by nasal cannula, and blood pressure is monitored closely. Consideration should be given to thromboprophylaxis in a pregnant patient (especially those with increased risk factors for thromboembolic events). Interruption of pharmacologic thromboprophylaxis is safe for use of neuraxial techniques with consideration of medication specific timing of last anticoagulant use.

Horlocker TT, Vandermeulen E, Kopp SL, et al. Regional anesthesia in the patient receiving antithrombotic or thrombolytic therapy: American Society of Regional Anesthesia and Pain Medicine Evidence-Based Guidelines (Fourth Edition). *Reg Anesth Pain Med.* 2018;43:263-309.

Leffert L, Butwick A, Carvalho B, et al; members of the SOAP VTE Taskforce. The Society for Obstetric Anesthesia and Perinatology consensus statement on the anesthetic management of pregnant and postpartum women receiving thromboprophylaxis or higher dose anticoagulants. *Anesth Analg.* 2018;126:928-944.

Nathan N, Wong CA. Spinal, Epidural, and Caudal Anesthesia: Anatomy, Physiology, and Technique. In: Chestnut DH, Wong CA, Tsen LC, et al., eds. *Chestnut's Obstetric Anesthesia: Principles and Practice.* 6th ed. Elsevier; 2020:238-270.

C.3. If the patient needs supplemental analgesia, what would be your choice?

Morphine and fentanyl are opioids that have been time tested. Small doses of ketamine (0.25 mg/kg intravenously) can also be given.

Bauchat JR, Van de Velde M. Nonobstetric Surgery during Pregnancy. In: Chestnut DH, Wong CA, Tsen LC, et al., eds. *Chestnut's Obstetric Anesthesia: Principles and Practice.* 6th ed. Elsevier; 2020:368-391.

Sharpe EE, Arendt KW. Anesthesia for Obstetrics. In: Gropper MA, Cohen NH, Eriksson LI, et al., eds. *Miller's Anesthesia.* 9th ed. Elsevier; 2020:2006-2041.

Zakowski MI, Geller A. The placenta: anatomy, physiology, and transfer of drugs. In: Chestnut DH, Wong CA, Tsen LC, et al, eds. *Chestnut's Obstetric Anesthesia: Principles and Practice.* 6th ed. Elsevier; 2020:56-76.

C.4. What vasopressor would you choose to improve uteroplacental perfusion?

The ASA practice guidelines state that "either IV ephedrine or phenylephrine may be used for treating hypotension during neuraxial anesthesia" and that "in the absence of maternal bradycardia, consider selecting phenylephrine because of improved fetal acid-base status in uncomplicated pregnancies." Ephedrine was previously considered the safest vasopressor because its β-adrenergic effects increase cardiac output, mean arterial pressure, and uterine artery blood flow without a concomitant decrease in uteroplacental perfusion. However, the use of ephedrine has been associated with adverse effects on fetal acid-base status (lower neonatal pH and fetal acidosis). Phenylephrine (a pure α-agonist) use is now preferred because phenylephrine does not adversely affect neonatal outcome and decreases the incidence of fetal acidosis. This evidence is based on studies conducted in elective cesarean section, and there is a paucity of evidence on the vasopressor of choice for nonelective cesarean deliveries or other surgical procedures.

Habib AS. A review of the impact of phenylephrine administration on maternal hemodynamics and maternal and neonatal outcomes in women undergoing cesarean delivery under spinal anesthesia. *Anesth Analg.* 2012;114:377-390.

Ngan Kee WD, Khaw KS, Tan PE, et al. Placental transfer and fetal metabolic effects of phenylephrine and ephedrine during spinal anesthesia for cesarean delivery. *Anesthesiology.* 2009;111:506-512.

Practice guidelines for obstetric anesthesia: an updated report by the American Society of Anesthesiologists Task Force on Obstetric Anesthesia and the Society for Obstetric Anesthesia and Perinatology. *Anesthesiology.* 2016;124:270-300.

C.5. When this patient arrived in the operating room, she desired a general anesthetic. Describe your technique.

- Apply standard ASA monitors, ensure a free-flowing intravenous catheter, use left uterine displacement, and consider blood glucose monitoring for long procedures.
- Preoxygenate for at least 3 minutes to ensure denitrogenation.
- Induction by rapid sequence induction and intubation (intubation using a cuffed endotracheal tube with a 7-mm internal diameter or less)
- Anesthesia maintenance using time-tested agents: morphine, fentanyl, a nondepolarizing neuromuscular blocker, and sevoflurane or desflurane. Inhalation anesthetics relax the uterus and can aid in preventing premature labor.
- Maintain appropriate maternal oxygenation and blood pressure to ensure uteroplacental perfusion, and avoid hyperventilation and hypoventilation.

- Neuromuscular block reversal should be monitored with a nerve stimulator to ensure adequate muscle reversal before tracheal extubation. Neuromuscular block reversal should be done using neostigmine and atropine. The Society for Obstetric Anesthesia and Perinatology (SOAP) released a statement on sugammadex use during pregnancy and lactation (April 2019) because of concerns about sugammadex binding maternal plasma progesterone: "The literature is insufficient to evaluate the safety of sugammadex with regards to effects on plasma hormone levels and teratogenicity. Therefore, the SOAP task force recommends traditional neuromuscular blockade reversal during pregnancy."
- Extubate the trachea when the patient is fully awake and following commands and has regained laryngeal reflexes. Stricter extubation criteria help to prevent postextubation aspiration and hypoxemia.

Bauchat JR, Van de Velde M. Nonobstetric Surgery during Pregnancy. In: Chestnut DH, Wong CA, Tsen LC, et al., eds. *Chestnut's Obstetric Anesthesia: Principles and Practice*. 6th ed. Elsevier; 2020:368-391.

Society for Obstetric Anesthesia and Perinatology. Statement on sugammadex during pregnancy and lactation. Published 2019. Accessed June 20, 2023. https://www.soap.org/assets/docs/SOAP_Statement_Sugammadex_During_Pregnancy_Lactation_APPROVED.pdf

Vasco Ramirez M, Valencia GCM. Anesthesia for nonobstetric surgery in pregnancy. *Clin Obstet Gynecol.* 2020;63:351-363.

Zakowski MI, Geller A. The Placenta: Anatomy, Physiology, and Transfer of Drugs. In: Chestnut DH, Wong CA, Tsen LC, et al., eds. *Chestnut's Obstetric Anesthesia: Principles and Practice*. 6th ed. Elsevier; 2020:56-76.

C.6. Does any controversy exist surrounding the use of nitrous oxide?

Nitrous oxide inhibits methionine synthase, potentially affecting DNA synthesis and myelin deposition, and has been shown to be teratogenic in rats and mice. Increased neuronal apoptosis and learning impairment observed in animals after prolonged exposure to high concentrations of nitrous oxide remains to be determined in humans, and is unlikely to be encountered in humans during clinical anesthesia. At this time, no detrimental effects of nitrous oxide on the development of the human fetus have been demonstrated. Nitrous oxide also increases adrenergic tone and decreases uterine blood flow. This can be prevented by the addition of a volatile agent. Nitrous oxide can be used as a component of the inhalational anesthetic.

Bauchat JR, Van de Velde M. Nonobstetric Surgery during Pregnancy. In: Chestnut DH, Wong CA, Tsen LC, et al., eds. *Chestnut's Obstetric Anesthesia: Principles and Practice*. 6th ed. Elsevier; 2020:368-391.

Tolcher MC, Fisher WE, Clark SL. Nonobstetric surgery during pregnancy. *Obstet Gynecol.* 2018;132:395-403.

Vasco Ramirez M, Valencia GCM. Anesthesia for nonobstetric surgery in pregnancy. *Clin Obstet Gynecol.* 2020;63:351-363.

SECTION 7

C.7. Does any controversy exist surrounding operating room personnel, anesthetic exposure, and pregnancy outcomes?

Case reports and epidemiologic studies from the 1960s and 1970s showed associations between anesthetic exposure and increased spontaneous abortions (increased miscarriage rates) in operating room and dental surgical personnel. Subsequent independent analysis of this work identified methodologic flaws and bias in data collection, causing spurious findings. Prospective studies have found no causal relationships. Additionally, modern volatile anesthetic exposure can be reduced by more than 90% with the use of modern scavenging systems.

Bauchat JR, Van de Velde M. Nonobstetric Surgery during Pregnancy. In: Chestnut DH, Wong CA, Tsen LC, et al., eds. *Chestnut's Obstetric Anesthesia: Principles and Practice*. 6th ed. Elsevier; 2020:368-391.

Cheek TG, Baird E. Anesthesia for nonobstetric surgery: maternal and fetal considerations. *Clin Obstet Gynecol.* 2009;52:535-545.

Vasco Ramirez M, Valencia GCM. Anesthesia for nonobstetric surgery in pregnancy. *Clin Obstet Gynecol.* 2020;63:351-363.

C.8. What is the impact of nonobstetric surgery on maternal mortality, birth defects, and fetal loss? What factors influence it?

A meta-analysis including 12,452 pregnant patients having surgery estimated maternal mortality at 0.006% (<1/10,000). Surgery and anesthesia did not increase the risk of major birth defects and were not major risk factors for spontaneous abortion. However, acute appendicitis with peritonitis poses a significant risk for fetal loss. Fetal loss was estimated at less than 5% in cases of uncomplicated acute appendicitis; the rate of fetal loss increased to 20% with perforated appendicitis and 35.7% with generalized peritonitis. Miscarriage and preterm birth slightly increased after surgery with the severity of the disease process requiring surgery or the site of surgery having the strongest influence.

Bauchat JR, Van de Velde M. Nonobstetric Surgery during Pregnancy. In: Chestnut DH, Wong CA, Tsen LC, et al., eds. Chestnut's Obstetric Anesthesia: Principles and Practice. 6th ed. Elsevier; 2020:368-391.

Cheek TG, Baird E. Anesthesia for nonobstetric surgery: maternal and fetal considerations. *Clin Obstet Gynecol.* 2009;52:535-545.

Vasco Ramirez M, Valencia GCM. Anesthesia for nonobstetric surgery in pregnancy. *Clin Obstet Gynecol.* 2020;63:351-363.

C.9. Should intraoperative fetal heart rate (FHR) monitoring be used? What would you expect to see on the electronic fetal monitor during anesthesia?

Use of intraoperative FHR monitoring is recommended only if it will alter case management. This decision is individualized and dependent on gestational age, type of surgery, and facilities available. FHR monitoring is practical from 18 to 22 weeks, and heart rate variability can be observed from 25 weeks on. The ACOG/ASA guidelines for fetal monitoring state that for a previable fetus, it is generally sufficient to ascertain FHR by Doppler before and after the procedure. For a viable fetus, a minimum simultaneous electronic FHR and contraction monitoring should be performed before and after the procedure to assess fetal well-being and the absence of contractions. Intraoperative electronic fetal monitoring might be appropriate when the following conditions are present: the fetus is viable; it is physically possible to perform intraoperative electronic fetal monitoring; a health care provider with obstetric surgery privileges is available; consideration for provision of informed consent that allows for emergency cesarean delivery for fetal indications; and the nature of planned surgery allows for safe interruption or alteration of the procedure to allow for emergency delivery.

One would expect to see a decrease in beat-to-beat FHR variability during general anesthesia using inhalational agents. FHR slowing (bradycardia) can also be observed, but this could also be secondary to nonbenign situations such as fetal hypoxemia and acidosis. FHR variability is also decreased by the use of opioids and induction agents.

Committee on Obstetric Practice, American Society of Anesthesiologists. Committee opinion no. 775: nonobstetric surgery during pregnancy. *Obstet Gynecol.* 2019;129:777-778.

Reitman E, Flood P. Anaesthetic considerations for non-obstetric surgery during pregnancy. *Br J Anaesth.* 2011;107:i72-i78.

Vasco Ramirez M, Valencia GCM. Anesthesia for nonobstetric surgery in pregnancy. *Clin Obstet Gynecol.* 2020;63:351-363.

C.10. How would your anesthetic management differ if the patient were having upper extremity surgery?

A brachial plexus block regional anesthetic technique could be used. It would be possible to monitor FHR during surgery and to monitor uterine contractions using a tocodynamometer.

Bauchat JR, Van de Velde M. Nonobstetric Surgery during Pregnancy. In: Chestnut DH, Wong CA, Tsen LC, et al., eds. *Chestnut's Obstetric Anesthesia: Principles and Practice.* 6th ed. Elsevier; 2020:368-391.

Committee on Obstetric Practice, American Society of Anesthesiologists. Committee opinion no. 775: nonobstetric surgery during pregnancy. *Obstet Gynecol.* 2019;129:777-778.

C.11. The surgeon schedules the procedure to be performed laparoscopically. Does this pose any additional problems?

Laparoscopy has been performed during pregnancy both for diagnostic and procedural surgery. Benefits appear similar to those in nonpregnant patients: reduced postoperative pain, postoperative ileus, and other complications, and decreased length of hospital stay with faster recovery. There has been a concern for direct fetal and uterine trauma and increased intra-abdominal pressure, causing a decrease in maternal cardiac output and uteroplacental perfusion. Carbon dioxide (CO_2) pneumoperitoneum can cause fetal respiratory acidosis. General guidelines are to maintain low intra-abdominal insufflation pressure of 10 to 15 mm Hg, limiting extremes in positioning (Trendelenburg or reverse Trendelenburg), and limiting surgery duration. Intraoperative CO_2 monitoring via capnography is adequate to guide ventilation, and end-tidal CO_2 should be maintained at approximately 32 mm Hg.

Laparoscopic appendectomy is associated with a low rate of intraoperative complications in all three trimesters. Results of multiple meta-analyses, however, have found that fetal loss was significantly more likely with laparoscopic compared to open appendectomy. These findings concerning fetal loss were largely dominated by one large study, and with exclusion of that study from pooled meta-analysis, there was no effect of laparoscopy on fetal loss. In summary, the current literature is inconclusive, and further larger studies are needed to better elucidate the association between fetal loss and laparoscopic appendectomy. The Society of American Gastrointestinal and Endoscopic Surgeons states that "laparoscopic appendectomy is the treatment of choice for pregnant patients with acute appendicitis." Furthermore, "Laparoscopy can be safely performed during any trimester of pregnancy when operation is indicated" and "postponing necessary operations until after parturition has been shown in some cases to increase the rates of complications for both mother and fetus."

Lee SH, Lee JY, Choi YY, Lee JG. Laparoscopic appendectomy versus open appendectomy for suspected appendicitis during pregnancy: a systematic review and updated meta-analysis. *BMC Surg.* 2019;19:41.

Pearl JP, Price RR, Tonkin AE, et al. SAGES guidelines for the use of laparoscopy during pregnancy. *Surg Endosc.* 2017;31:3767-3782.

Prodromidou A, Machairas N, Kostakis ID, et al. Outcomes after open and laparoscopic appendectomy during pregnancy: a meta-analysis. *Eur J Obstet Gynecol Reprod Biol.* 2018;225:40-50.

D. Postoperative Management

D.1. When would you extubate the trachea for this patient?

The patient can be extubated when she is fully awake, in control of her airway reflexes, and able to avoid pulmonary aspiration. Neuromuscular block reversal should be monitored with a nerve stimulator to ensure adequate neuromuscular reversal before extubating. Neuromuscular block reversal should be performed using neostigmine and atropine. The Society for Obstetric Anesthesia and Perinatology (SOAP) released a statement on the use of sugammadex during pregnancy and lactation (April 2019) because of concerns about sugammadex binding to maternal progesterone: "The literature is insufficient to evaluate the safety of sugammadex with regards to effects on plasma hormone levels and teratogenicity. Therefore, the SOAP task force recommends traditional neuromuscular blockade reversal during pregnancy."

Bauchat JR, Van de Velde M. Nonobstetric Surgery during Pregnancy. In: Chestnut DH, Wong CA, Tsen LC, et al., eds. Chestnut's Obstetric Anesthesia: Principles and Practice. 6th ed. Elsevier; 2020:368-391.

Society for Obstetric Anesthesia and Perinatology. Statement on sugammadex during pregnancy and lactation. Published 2019. Accessed June 20, 2023. https://www.soap.org/assets/docs/SOAP_Statement_Sugammadex_During_Pregnancy_Lactation_APPROVED.pdf

Vasco Ramirez M, Valencia GCM. Anesthesia for nonobstetric surgery in pregnancy. *Clin Obstet Gynecol.* 2020;63:351-363.

D.2. Postoperatively, what monitors would you use?

Postoperative monitors should include electrocardiography, pulse oximetry, intermittent blood pressure and temperature monitoring, urinary catheter (to be discontinued within 24 hours, unless specifically indicated), FHR monitor to ensure fetal well-being, and tocodynamometer to detect premature labor.

Bauchat JR, Van de Velde M. Nonobstetric Surgery during Pregnancy. In: Chestnut DH, Wong CA, Tsen LC, et al., eds. *Chestnut's Obstetric Anesthesia: Principles and Practice*. 6th ed. Elsevier; 2020:368-391.

Sharpe EE, Arendt KW. Anesthesia for Obstetrics. In: Gropper MA, Cohen NH, Eriksson LI, et al., eds. *Miller's Anesthesia*. 9th ed. Elsevier; 2020:2006-2041.

D.3. What other postoperative precautions would you take? What is the incidence of preterm delivery following nonobstetric surgery during pregnancy?

Postoperative precautions include adequate hydration, supplemental oxygen as needed, continued left uterine displacement, early mobilization, and use of antiembolic massage devices and/or anticoagulation to prevent deep venous thrombosis.

Many obstetricians use intravenous fluids and β-agonist drugs to prevent premature labor. It is recommended that pregnant patients be observed postoperatively on the obstetric floor for a minimum of 12 hours. Magnesium sulfate is given intravenously if preterm labor occurs.

In a study of 778 females who underwent appendectomy while pregnant, 22% delivered within the following week if surgery occurred between 24 and 36 weeks of gestation. There is an increased risk of low-birth weight infants (<2,500 g) and premature labor before 37 weeks.

Augustin G. *Acute Abdomen during Pregnancy*. 3rd ed. Springer; 2014:371-419.

Bauchat JR, Van de Velde M. Nonobstetric Surgery during Pregnancy. In: Chestnut DH, Wong CA, Tsen LC, et al., eds. *Chestnut's Obstetric Anesthesia: Principles and Practice*. 6th ed. Elsevier; 2020:368-391..

Cheek TG, Baird E. Anesthesia for nonobstetric surgery: maternal and fetal considerations. *Clin Obstet Gynecol.* 2009;52:535-545.

D.4. The next day, the patient went into premature labor and now needs a cesarean section for prematurity and breech presentation. She requires another general anesthetic. In what way would your technique differ from your previous anesthetic technique?

Magnesium sulfate will both prevent the muscle fasciculations that normally occur following the administration of succinylcholine and will potentiate the effects of nondepolarizing neuromuscular blockers (necessitating smaller doses). Avoid the use of opioids until after delivery, and after delivery discontinue the volatile agent and initiate an intravenous technique.

Bauchat JR, Van de Velde M. Nonobstetric Surgery during Pregnancy. In: Chestnut DH, Wong CA, Tsen LC, et al., eds. *Chestnut's Obstetric Anesthesia: Principles and Practice*. 6th ed. Elsevier; 2020:368-391.

Sharpe EE, Arendt KW. Anesthesia for Obstetrics. In: Gropper MA, Cohen NH, Eriksson LI, et al., eds. *Miller's Anesthesia*. 9th ed. Elsevier; 2020:2036-2041.

Tsen LC, Bateman BT. Anesthesia for Cesarean Delivery. In: Chestnut DH, Wong CA, Tsen LC, et al., eds. *Chestnut's Obstetric Anesthesia: Principles and Practice*. 6th ed. Elsevier; 2020:568-626.

31 Coagulopathy

Meghann M. Fitzgerald and Thorsten Haas

A 26-year-old male with a history of scoliosis and seizure disorder presents for a multilevel interbody fusion (T3-S1) in the prone position. His medications include valproic acid for seizure control. His weight is 52 kg and laboratory studies indicate a hemoglobin of 11.2 g/dL, hematocrit 32%, platelet count 173,000 per μL.

A. Medical Disease and Differential Diagnosis

1. What are the normal hemoglobin values for healthy males and females?
2. What are the common etiologies of anemia?
3. What underlying medical conditions can contribute to anemia?
4. What are the perioperative outcomes associated with preoperative anemia?
5. Describe the hematologic side effects of chronic valproic acid therapy.

B. Preoperative Evaluation and Preparation

1. What preoperative evaluation and testing would you recommend for this patient prior to anesthesia?
2. Describe the efficacy of oral versus intravenous iron supplementation. What additional therapies can be used to increase red blood cell mass?
3. Describe the advantages and limitations of preoperative autologous blood donation.
4. Discuss the clinical value of assessing standard plasma coagulation testing to predict perioperative bleeding.

C. Intraoperative Management

1. Discuss the anesthetic plan for this patient.
2. Discuss the indications and use of available antifibrinolytic drugs. What dose should be given? Describe the side effects of antifibrinolytic therapy.
3. After 3 hours of surgery, the surgeon noticed increased bleeding with oozing from all surgical sites. Blood gas analysis revealed a hemoglobin of 7 g/dL. Describe the pathophysiology of acquired coagulopathy. What are the factors that lead to acquired coagulopathy?
4. What are the laboratory methods to confirm acquired coagulopathy?
5. Describe the clinical use of viscoelastic testing for timely detection of acquired coagulopathy.
6. What are the options to treat acquired hypofibrinogenemia?
7. Discuss the use of plasma to maintain perioperative hemostasis.

D. Postoperative Management

1. Discuss the postoperative management of this patient. What laboratory testing should be used to detect further deterioration of hemostasis?
2. What is the target hemoglobin level during the postoperative period? What are the advantages and disadvantages of common transfusion triggers?

3. Describe the pathophysiology of potential complications following massive transfusion and hematologic resuscitation. What are the risks of thromboembolic complications after intraoperative administration of procoagulants?
4. At what point can antithrombotic therapy be initiated after surgery in the presence of acquired coagulopathy?

A. Medical Disease and Differential Diagnosis

A.1. What are the normal hemoglobin values for healthy males and females?

Anemia is defined as hemoglobin (Hb) concentration less than or equal to 12.0 g/dL in females and less than or equal to 13.0 g/dL in males, according to a 1968 World Health Organization report. Data for the US population collected from 1988 through 1994 in the third National Health and Nutrition Examination Survey (NHANES III) delineates the variation of normal hemoglobin values based on ethnicity, sex, and age.

Blanc B, Finch CA, Hallberg L, Herbert V, Lawkowicz W, Layrisse M. Nutritional anaemias. Report of a WHO scientific group. *World Health Organ Tech Rep Ser*. 1968;405:5-37.

Hollowell JG, van Assendelft OW, Gunter EW, et al. Hematological and iron-related analytes—reference data for persons aged 1 year and over: United States, 1988-1994. *Vital Health Stat*. 2005;11:1-156.

A.2. What are the common etiologies of anemia?

The causes of anemia can be grossly divided into three major categories: red blood cell loss, decreased red blood cell production, and increased red blood cell destruction. Basic hematologic laboratory tests, the clinical history, and physical exam findings are useful in determining the etiology. Low transferrin saturation, ferritin, and reticulocyte hemoglobin content in conjunction with a low mean corpuscular volume indicate iron deficiency. A high reticulocyte count reflects appropriate bone marrow response to red blood cell loss or hemolysis, which can be differentiated with hemolysis markers: lactate dehydrogenase, haptoglobin, and bilirubin levels. A low reticulocyte count reflects inadequate red blood cell production and suggests anemia of chronic inflammation or chronic kidney disease.

Warner MA, Shore-Lesserson L, Shander A, Patel SY, Perelman SI, Guinn NR. Perioperative anemia: prevention, diagnosis, and management throughout the spectrum of perioperative care. *Anesth Analg*. 2020;130:1364-1380.

A.3. What underlying medical conditions can contribute to anemia?

After excluding acute red blood cell loss and hemolysis-related red blood cell destruction, hypoproliferative anemia can be narrowed down to three etiologies: nutritional deficiencies, chronic disease, and myelosuppressive drugs and toxins. The most common cause of hypoproliferative anemia globally is iron deficiency. Chronic hematologic diseases causing hypoproliferative anemia include thalassemias, hemoglobinopathies, myelodysplastic syndromes, sideroblastic anemia, and other less common disorders of bone marrow causing decreased red cell production. Many chronic systemic diseases cause anemia through iron sequestration and elevated hepcidin levels. Hepcidin is a protein secreted by hepatocytes during exposure to high levels of iron that blocks further absorption of iron from the small bowel. Anemia related to renal dysfunction attributed to decreased erythropoietin production in response to hypoxemia, as well as a general decreased capacity for erythropoietin production. Anemia in patients with chronic kidney disease is also compounded by increased hepcidin levels

Ginzburg YZ. Anemia of chronic inflammation. In: Hoffman R, ed. *Hematology, Basic Principles and Practice*. 8th ed. Elsevier; 2023:498-506.

Laureano M, Hillis C. Hematologic manifestations of end-organ failure download. In: Hoffman R, ed. *Hematology, Basic Principles and Practice*. 8th ed. Elsevier; 2023:2305-2311.

Lin JC, Benz EJ. Approach to anemia in the adult and child. In: Hoffman R, ed. *Hematology, Basic Principles and Practice*. 8th ed. Elsevier; 2023:463-472.

A.4. What are the perioperative outcomes associated with preoperative anemia?

Mild, moderate, and severe degrees of anemia have been associated with increased risk of 30-day morbidity and mortality in patients undergoing major noncardiac surgery. Thirty-day morbidities include cardiac, respiratory, urinary tract, and wound complications, sepsis, and venous thromboembolism. In the cardiac surgery population, anemia is also associated with stroke. The impact of anemia on morbidity and mortality occurs across multiple surgical specialties, including general, orthopedic, cardiac, hepatic, and neonatal surgeries.

Fowler AJ, Ahmad T, Phull MK, Allard S, Gillies MA, Pearse RM. Meta-analysis of the association between preoperative anaemia and mortality after surgery. *Br J Surg*. 2015;102:1314-1324.

Goobie SM, Faraoni D, Zurakowski D, DiNardo JA. Association of preoperative anemia with postoperative mortality in neonates. *JAMA Pediatr*. 2016;170:855-862.

Lu M, Sing DC, Kuo AC, Hansen EN. Preoperative anemia independently predicts 30-day complications after aseptic and septic revision total joint arthroplasty. *J Arthroplasty*. 2017;32:S197-S201.

Musallam KM, Tamim HM, Richards T, et al. Preoperative anaemia and postoperative outcomes in non-cardiac surgery: a retrospective cohort study. *Lancet*. 2011;378:1396-1407.

Oprea AD, Del Rio JM, Cooter M, et al. Pre- and postoperative anemia, acute kidney injury, and mortality after coronary artery bypass grafting surgery: a retrospective observational study. *Can J Anaesth*. 2018;65:46-59.

Spiegelstein D, Holmes SD, Pritchard G, Halpin L, Ad N. Preoperative hematocrit as a predictor of perioperative morbidities following nonemergent coronary artery bypass surgery. *J Card Surg*. 2015;30:20-26.

A.5. Describe the hematologic side effects of chronic valproic acid therapy.

A variety of coagulation disorders have been linked to valproic acid use, including thrombocytopenia, platelet dysfunction, hypofibrogenemia, factor XIII deficiency, and acquired von Willebrand disease. The most consistently reported associated coagulopathy is thrombocytopenia and platelet dysfunction. There is an increased risk of perioperative hemorrhage in pediatric surgical patients taking valproic acid, but this association has not been demonstrated in the adult surgical population.

Abdallah C. Considerations in perioperative assessment of valproic acid coagulopathy. *J Anaesthesiol Clin Pharmacol*. 2014;30:7-9.

Kumar R, Vidaurre J, Gedela S. Valproic acid-induced coagulopathy. *Pediatr Neurol*. 2019; 98:25-30.

B. Preoperative Evaluation and Preparation

B.1. What preoperative evaluation and testing would you recommend for this patient prior to anesthesia?

Preoperative assessment should include a comprehensive medical, surgical, and anesthetic history. In addition to a focused physical exam, an airway examination should be performed with attention to neck mobility. A complete blood count with differential is indicated in this patient due to valproic acid use and anticipated blood loss associated with the proposed surgery. Once anemia has been identified, additional studies to determine the etiology include transferrin saturation, ferritin levels, reticulocyte hemoglobin content, Vitamin B_{12}, and folate levels. A basic metabolic panel could reveal or exclude previously undiagnosed renal dysfunction.

SECTION 8

Warner MA, Shore-Lesserson L, Shander A, Patel SY, Perelman SI, Guinn NR. Perioperative anemia: prevention, diagnosis, and management throughout the spectrum of perioperative care. *Anesth Analg*. 2020;130:1364-1380.

B.2. Describe the efficacy of oral versus intravenous iron supplementation. What additional therapies can be used to increase red blood cell mass?

Treatment of iron-deficiency anemia is usually based on the rapidity with which red blood cell mass must be normalized. Diet modification to include foods high in iron content has limited efficacy due to the low absorption of dietary iron, and is usually insufficient. Oral supplementation can include common over-the-counter-preparations such as ferrous sulfate, but low rates of absorption and high incidence of side effects including constipation and nausea limit its efficacy and compliance with treatment. Even with consistent use, oral iron replacement requires 3 to 6 months to substantially improve red cell mass.

Administration of parenteral iron can rapidly increase red cell mass, but its application is most often limited due to high cost and logistical barriers. Older formulations had high rates of severe hypersensitivity reactions requiring slower infusion rates under observation and led to hesitancy about intravenous administration. A mounting body of evidence suggests that there are both morbidity reduction and economic benefits to detecting and treating iron-deficiency anemia with intravenous iron supplementation before elective surgery. The optimal window for intravenous iron supplementation to restore red cell mass is 3 to 4 weeks, but benefits have been demonstrated in cardiac surgery when given as little as 1 day preoperatively.

There are additional methods to increase physiological oxygen-carrying capacity. Exercise or other conditions of chronic hypoxemia can increase total hemoglobin and red cell mass. Preoperative allogenic red blood cell transfusion in asymptomatic patients should be avoided as benefits do not outweigh associated disadvantages.

Camaschella C. Disorders of iron homeostasis: iron deficiency and overload. In: Hoffman R, ed. *Hematology, Basic Principles and Practice*. 8th ed. Elsevier; 2023:483-497.

Meyer J, Cirocchi R, Di Saverio S, Ris F, Wheeler J, Davies RJ. Pre-operative iron increases haemoglobin concentration before abdominal surgery: a systematic review and meta-analysis of randomized controlled trials. *Sci Rep*. 2022;12:2158. Published correction appears in *Sci Rep*. 2022;12:6084.

Spahn DR, Schoenrath F, Spahn GH, et al. Effect of ultra-short-term treatment of patients with iron deficiency or anaemia undergoing cardiac surgery: a prospective randomised trial. *Lancet*. 2019;393:2201-2212.

Warner MA, Shore-Lesserson L, Shander A, Patel SY, Perelman SI, Guinn NR. Perioperative anemia: prevention, diagnosis, and management throughout the spectrum of perioperative care. *Anesth Analg*. 2020; 130:1364-1380.

B.3. Describe the advantages and limitations of preoperative autologous blood donation.

Preoperative autologous blood donation has been shown to reduce the incidence and volume of allogeneic transfusions in certain noncardiac surgeries. Limitations to autologous blood donation are numerous. Urgent and emergent surgeries will not allow for adequate time to restore red cell mass following autologous donation. For elective surgeries, specific patient populations and surgery types have not been identified as benefiting from autologous donation, making it difficult to justify the procedure in patients who are unlikely to require transfusion anyway. Many centers lack resources to support programs for which compelling economic benefit is difficult to demonstrate.

ASA Task Force on Perioperative Blood Management. Practice guidelines for perioperative blood management—an updated report by the ASA task force on perioperative blood management. *Anesthesiology*. 2015;122:241-275.

B.4. Discuss the clinical value of assessing standard plasma coagulation testing to predict perioperative bleeding.

Standard laboratory testing (SLT) of coagulation encompasses measurement of prothrombin time (PT), international normalized ratio (INR), and activated partial thromboplastin time (aPTT). Although SLT shows good reproducibility and is the gold standard to guide oral anticoagulation therapy and for monitoring heparin effect, there is poor correlation with intraoperative bleeding risk. In addition, SLT poorly reflects compromised thrombin generation in the perioperative setting. Sound evidence from well-controlled studies is lacking to give clear thresholds to guide hemostatic therapy.

Dzik WH. Predicting hemorrhage using preoperative coagulation screening assays. *Curr Hematol Rep*. 2004;3:324-330.

Haas T, Fries D, Tanaka KA, et al. Usefulness of standard plasma coagulation tests in the management of perioperative coagulopathic bleeding: is there any evidence? *Br J Anaesth*. 2015;114:217-224.

C. Intraoperative Management

C.1. Discuss the anesthetic plan for this patient.

General anesthesia is the only established anesthetic technique for multilevel spinal fusion surgery. Airway management including advanced techniques of tracheal intubation should be planned according to preoperative evaluation. The selection of anesthetic agents depends on the performance of neuromonitoring. One of the main advantages of neuromonitoring is that intraoperative wake-up testing can be omitted. However, important anesthetic drug-related interactions need to be considered. First, electromyography and motor evoked potentials cannot be performed with complete paralysis. A bite block should be taped in place to prevent injuries of the tongue and lips if neuromonitoring with evoked potentials will be used. Second, most anesthetic drugs interfere with electroencephalogram (EEG), with volatile inhalation agents including nitrous oxide showing the most pronounced decrease in EEG, depending on their concentration. Most intravenous anesthetic agents including opioids and ketamine have fewer effects on

EEG. Total intravenous anesthesia (TIVA) or balanced anesthesia including low levels (<0.5 MAC) of volatile agents allows neuromonitoring. A constant depth of anesthesia should be maintained to avoid confounding interpretation of neuromonitoring.

As major spine surgery can result in significant blood loss, at least two large-bore intravenous catheters (14 or 16 gauge) should be placed. An arterial catheter should be established, as repeated blood samplings are expected, and it allows for continuous monitoring of arterial pressure. Intraoperative infusion of vasopressors such as norepinephrine or phenylephrine might be needed to maintain mean arterial blood pressure in the range of the targeted perioperative pressure. Hypotension should be avoided to ensure adequate perfusion of the spinal cord, optic nerve, and other organs. Long procedures in prone position call for bladder catheterization and placement of an orogastric tube.

Enhanced recovery after surgery (ERAS) protocols for scoliosis surgery have been successfully established in adults and adolescent patients, including a standardized approach to improve preoperative conditions such as anemia treatment, intraoperative management, and postoperative rehabilitation.

Glover CD, Carling NP. Neuromonitoring for scoliosis surgery. *Anesthesiology Clin*. 2014;32:101-114.

Khanna P, Sarkar S, Garg B. Anesthetic considerations in spine surgery: what orthopaedic surgeons should know! *J Clin Orthop Trauma*. 2020;11:742-748.

Soldozy S, Patel P, Elsarrag M, et al. The implementation of enhanced recovery after surgery (ERAS) in complex spinal surgery. *J Spine Surg*. 2019;5:116-123.

C.2. Discuss the indications and use of available antifibrinolytic drugs. What dose should be given? Describe the side effects of antifibrinolytic therapy.

Perioperative administration of antifibrinolytics can reduce perioperative blood loss and to reduce allogeneic blood transfusion in a variety clinical of settings including major spinal surgery, and is an integral part of current perioperative bleeding management guidelines and recommendations. The mechanism of action of the available lysine analogs tranexamic acid (TXA) and epsilon aminocaproic acid (EACA) is the prevention of clot breakdown by plasmin by competitive and reversible binding of the antifibrinolytic agent to plasminogen, thus preserving clot strength. For orthopedic surgery, antifibrinolytic drugs can be administered either as single bolus (TXA 10-20 mg/kg; EACA 100 mg/kg) or single bolus followed by continuous infusion (TXA 2-5 mg/kg/h; EACA 10-15 mg/kg/h). A target plasma concentration of greater than or equal to 10 μg/mL for TXA should be achieved. A systematic review in 1,158 patients who underwent scoliosis surgery demonstrated that use of TXA or EACA versus placebo led to a significant decrease in blood loss, and the rate of transfusion decreased from 68.3% in the placebo group to 44.6% in the antifibrinolytic group. In this study, antifibrinolytics did not increase adverse events including thromboembolism. TXA also appeared more effective than EACA in reducing total blood and transfusion requirements in a meta-analysis in 1,191 patients who underwent spine surgery. There are far more published studies investigating the overall clinical efficacy of TXA as compared to EACA, although the latter is more extensively used in the United States. Despite the clinical concern of increased risk of venous thromboembolism by using antifibrinolytics, data from meta-analyses in orthopedic surgery and spinal surgery did not show a higher incidence of thromboembolic events. The occurrence of convulsive seizures has only been observed using high-doses of TXA following cardiac surgery.

Levy JH, Koster A, Quinones QJ, et al. Antifibrinolytic therapy and perioperative considerations. *Anesthesiology*. 2018;128:657-670.

Li G, Sun TW, Luo G. et al. Efficacy of antifibrinolytic agents on surgical bleeding and transfusion requirements in spine surgery: a meta-analysis. *Eur Spine J*. 2017;26:140-154.

Patel PA, Wyrobek JA, Butwick AJ, et al. Update on applications and limitations of perioperative tranexamic acid. *Anesth Analg*. 2022;135:460-473.

Soroceanu A, Oren JH, Smith JS, et al. Effect of antifibrinolytic therapy on complications, thromboembolic events, blood product utilization, and fusion in adult spinal deformity surgery. *Spine*. 2016;41:E879-E886.

C.3. After 3 hours of surgery, the surgeon noticed increased bleeding with oozing from all surgical sites. Blood gas analysis revealed a hemoglobin of 7 g/dL. Describe the pathophysiology of acquired coagulopathy. What are the factors that lead to acquired coagulopathy?

Acquired coagulopathy occurs due to a combination of significant surgical bleeding and resuscitation with fluids without hemostatic activity. This dilutional coagulopathy results in impaired hemostasis and reduced clot activity. The first coagulation factor that becomes critically low is fibrinogen which plays an essential role in hemostasis as the foundation of fibrin clot formation at the site of vessel injury. The greater the tissue injury, the more fibrinogen is consumed. Hypofibrinogenemia combined with hemodilution results in an inability to establish a tight fibrinogen-fibrin network, impaired clot stability, and increased bleeding tendency. Fibrin polymerization can be further impaired with colloid administration, particularly high-molecular weight starch solutions.

Following initial clot destabilization, coagulopathy is compounded by impaired thrombin generation, primary hemostasis, and clot resistance to fibrinolysis. Dilutional coagulopathy is further exacerbated by mild-to-moderate von Willebrand factor deficiency, preexisting coagulopathy and platelet disorders, anticoagulant medications, hypothermia, acidosis, and hypocalcemia. A reduction in factor XIII, which is necessary to cross-link the fibrin mesh, might also contribute to development of perioperative coagulopathy.

Besser MW, MacDonald SG. Acquired hypofibrinogenemia: current perspectives. *J Blood Med.* 2016;7:217-225.

Innerhofer P, Kienast J. Principles of perioperative coagulopathy. *Best Pract Res Clin Anaesthesiol.* 2010;24:1-14.

Korte WF. XIII in perioperative coagulation management. *Best Pract Res Clin Anaesthesiol.* 2010;24:85-93.

C.4. What are the laboratory methods to confirm acquired coagulopathy?

The turnaround time for SLTs hampers their use for quick decision-making in scenarios of critical bleeding and leave most clinicians to make bleeding management decisions based on the clinical situation rather than laboratory thresholds. The first sign of dilutional coagulopathy is weakening of the fibrin network. The Clauss method is the most frequently used assay for measuring plasma fibrinogen concentration. In the presence of increased bleeding tendency, treatment of hypofibrinogenemia is recommended if the Clauss fibrinogen level is less than 150 to 200 mg/dL. The contribution of low platelets to clot firmness is usually a late finding in dilutional coagulopathy because reserve platelets are released from the bone marrow or spleen during bleeding. There is limited data to suggest that a platelet count of less than 50,000 per μL during perioperative bleeding is a reasonable transfusion threshold.

American Society of Anesthesiologists Task Force on Perioperative Blood Management. Practice guidelines for perioperative blood management: an updated report by the American Society of Anesthesiologists Task Force on Perioperative Blood Management. *Anesthesiology.*2015;122:241-275.

Haas T, Fries D, Tanaka KA, et al. Usefulness of standard plasma coagulation tests in the management of perioperative coagulopathic bleeding: is there any evidence? *Br J Anaesth.* 2015;114:217-224.

Innerhofer P, Kienast J. Principles of perioperative coagulopathy. *Best Pract Res Clin Anaesthesiol.* 2010;24:1-14.

Kietaibl S, Ahmed A, Afshari A, et al. Management of severe peri-operative bleeding: guidelines from the European Society of Anaesthesiology and Intensive Care: Second update 2022. *Eur J Anaesthesiol.* 2023;40:226-304.

C.5. Describe the clinical use of viscoelastic testing for timely detection of acquired coagulopathy.

There have been many studies over the past decade addressing goal-directed bleeding management favoring the use of viscoelastic testing (VET) with a tailored bleeding management algorithm in various clinical settings. There are several VET devices available to demonstrate whole blood hemostasis from clot initiation to clot lysis by analyzing the changes in clot characteristics from viscous to elastic over time by inducing a shear stress. There are several advantages of VET over SLT. First, it can be used as true point-of-care testing (POCT), thus allowing for immediate performance. Second, there is an array of VET assays available, using different steps of activating the whole blood sample, reflecting the extrinsic and intrinsic pathways of hemostasis. In addition, the platelet contribution to clot firmness can be pharmacologically blocked to assess the contribution of fibrinogen/fibrin polymerization. Finally, VET offers the only timely laboratory method to investigate lysis of the clot, including detection of hyperfibrinolysis (**Table 31.1**).

In a systematic review and meta-analysis of 17 trials including 1,493 patients, use of VET to guide bleeding management significantly decreased the proportion of patients transfused with red blood cells, plasma, or platelets, and demonstrated reduced overall mortality versus any comparator (3.9% vs 7.4%). It should be noted that this review study included mostly patients undergoing cardiac surgery. However, decreased blood loss and transfusion requirements following VET-guided bleeding management have also been described in pediatric, adolescent, and adult scoliosis surgery.

American Society of Anesthesiologists Task Force on Perioperative Blood Management. Practice guidelines for perioperative blood management: an updated report by the American Society of Anesthesiologists Task Force on Perioperative Blood Management. *Anesthesiology.* 2015;122:241-275.

TABLE 31.1 Description of Coagulation Measurement Capabilities in Currently Available Viscoelastic Testing Devices

	Clot Initiation (Assay/Unit)	Clot Firmness (Assay/Unit)	Clot Lysis (Assay/Unit)	Fibrinogen Activity (Assay/Unit)
ROTEM	INTEM (kaolin) EXTEM (tissue factor) Clot time (CT in secs)	INTEM/EXTEM Maximum clot firmness (MCF in mm) Clot amplitude after 5/10/20 min after CT (A5/A10/A20 in mm)	EXTEM/INTEM/FIBTEM Clot Lysis Index 30/60 mins after MCF (CLI30/CLI60 in %) Maximum lysis (ML in %)	FIBTEM (EXTEM test plus Cytochalasin) Maximum clot firmness (MCF in mm) Clot amplitude after 5/10/20 min after CT (A5/A10/A20 in mm)
TEG	Kaolin TEG (Kaolin) Rapid TEG (Kaolin and tissue factor) Reaction time (R time in mins)	Kaolin TEG Rapid TEG Maximum amplitude (MA in mm)	Kaolin TEG Rapid TEG Functional fibrinogen Lysis Index 30 min after MA (LY30 in %)	Functional Fibrinogen (Abciximab) Maximum amplitude (MA in mm)
Quantra	Quantra QPlus Cartridge (Kaolin) Quantra QStat Cartridge Clot time (CT in seconds)	Quantra QPlus Quantra QStat Clot stiffness (CS in hPa)	Quantra QStat Clot stability to lysis (CSL in %)	Quantra QPlus (Thromboplastin plus abciximab) Fibrinogen contribution to clot stiffness (FCS in hPa)

ROTEM, Werfen, USA; TEG, Haemonetics, USA; Quantra, Hemosonics, USA.
ROTEM, rotational thromboelastometry; TEG, thromboelastography.

Hartman J, Murphy M, Dias JD. Viscoelastic hemostatic assays: moving from the laboratory to the site of care—a review of established and emerging technologies. *Diagnostics*. 2020;10;1-14.

Jonas J, Durila M, Malosek M, et al. Usefulness of perioperative rotational thrombelastometry during scoliosis surgery in children. *J Neurosurg Spine*. 2020;32:865-870.

Kietaibl S, Ahmed A, Afshari A, et al. Management of severe peri-operative bleeding: guidelines from the European Society of Anaesthesiology and Intensive Care: second update 2022. *Eur J Anaesthesiol*. 2023;40:226-304.

Wikkelsø A, Wetterslev J, Møller AM, Afshari A. Thromboelastography (TEG) or rotational thromboelastometry (ROTEM) to monitor haemostatic treatment in bleeding patients: a systematic review with meta-analysis and trial sequential analysis. *Anaesthesia*. 2017;72:519-531.

SECTION 8

C.6. What are the options to treat acquired hypofibrinogenemia?

Acquired hypofibrinogenemia is most frequently caused by hemodilution and/or consumption of coagulation factors. There are several strategies to replenish plasma fibrinogen concentrations. Fibrinogen content in various blood products varies by product:

- Cryoprecipitate: 5-unit pool contains at least 750 mg fibrinogen in about 100 mL
- Fibrinogen concentrate: 1,000 mg vial (50 mL)
- Plasma: approximately 400 mg 200 to 250 mL

Fibrinogen concentrate can be stored at room temperature, and reconstitution of the powder takes several minutes. By contrast, cryoprecipitate or plasma require thawing which is time consuming and can delay therapy. In addition to the logistical disadvantages of cryoprecipitate, it contains other factors such as factor VIII (FVIII) and von Willebrand factor (vWF). These factors might not become depleted early during dilutional coagulopathy, such that cryoprecipitate transfusion could result in elevated levels of FVIII and vWF.

A recently published guideline for perioperative bleeding management is recommending the use of cryoprecipitate or fibrinogen concentrate if viscoelastic signs of hypofibrinogenemia are present, such as FIBTEM A10 less than 10 mm using the ROTEM device, or if plasma Clauss testing fibrinogen level is less than or equal to 150 mg/dL. Regardless of which product (cryoprecipitate or fibrinogen concentrate) used, the importance of a targeted treatment of acquired hypofibrinogenemia cannot be underestimated.

Besser MW, MacDonald SG. Acquired hypofibrinogenemia: current perspectives. *J Blood Med*. 2016;7:217-225.

Collins PW, Solomon C, Sutor K, et al. Theoretical modelling of fibrinogen supplementation with therapeutic plasma, cryoprecipitate, or fibrinogen concentrate. *Br J Anaesth*. 2014;113:585-595.

Cushing MM, Haas T, Karkouti K, Callum J. Which is the preferred blood product for fibrinogen replacement in the bleeding patient with acquired hypofibrinogenemia-cryoprecipitate or fibrinogen concentrate? *Transfusion.* 2020;60:S17-S23.

Hofer S, Schlimp CJ, Casu S, et al. Management of coagulopathy in bleeding patients. *J Clin Med.* 2022;11:1-14.

Kietaibl S, Ahmed A, Afshari A, et al. Management of severe peri-operative bleeding: guidelines from the European Society of Anaesthesiology and Intensive Care: second update 2022. *Eur J Anaesthesiol.* 2023;40:226-304.

C.7. Discuss the use of plasma to maintain perioperative hemostasis.

Although plasma transfusions are frequently used to prevent or treat bleeding, there is ample evidence for both inadequate dosing and the use for indications outside of recent, published guidelines. Recommendations and limitations described in current guidelines include:

- Plasma transfusion is recommended in the setting of massive transfusion.
- Plasma should not be used for volume replacement in the absence of massive bleeding and coagulation deficiencies.
- There is limited potential to correct a mild-to-moderately prolonged PT ratio or INR more than 1.5 with plasma transfusion.
- There is no evidence to support the prophylactic use of plasma in nonbleeding patients with abnormal routine coagulation tests.
- Plasma contains insufficient amounts of fibrinogen to treat acquired hypofibrinogenemia.

Adam EH, Fischer D. Plasma transfusion practice in adult surgical patients: systematic review of the literature. *Transfus Med Hemother.* 2020;47:347-359.

Stanworth SJ, Brunskill SJ, Hyde CJ, et al. Is fresh frozen plasma clinically effective? A systematic review of randomized controlled trials. *Br J Haematol.* 2004;126:139-152.

D. Postoperative Management

D.1. Discuss the postoperative management of this patient. What laboratory testing should be used to detect further deterioration of hemostasis?

Postoperative management of patients undergoing complex spine surgery often includes admission to the intensive care unit for appropriate hemodynamic and neurologic monitoring as well as continued hematologic resuscitation. A similar rationale for viscoelastic testing in the intraoperative period is applied in the setting of postoperative hemorrhage. The majority of evidence in support of viscoelastic testing for postoperative hemorrhage exists in the cardiac surgery population. In a Cochrane analysis including both cardiac and noncardiac surgery, with 96% of the patients having cardiac surgery, viscoelastic testing was associated with a decrease in both overall mortality and all types of allogeneic transfusions.

Shen L, Tabaie S, Ivascu N. Viscoelastic testing inside and beyond the operating room. *J Thorac Dis.* 2017;9: S299-S308.

Wikkelsø A, Wetterslev J, Møller AM, Afshari A. Thromboelastography (TEG) or thromboelastometry (ROTEM) to monitor haemostatic treatment versus usual care in adults or children with bleeding. *Cochrane Database Syst Rev.* 2016;2016:CD007871.

D.2. What is the target hemoglobin level during the postoperative period? What are the advantages and disadvantages of common transfusion triggers?

While there have been many attempts to define an absolute threshold hemoglobin level for transfusion, the heterogeneity of settings, patient populations, and comorbidities make it nearly impossible to apply one universal value. The most widely accepted lower limit hemoglobin level is 7 to 8 g/dL in most patient populations, with multiple well-designed studies demonstrating at least noninferiority of a restrictive (lower target Hb) versus liberal (higher target Hb) approach to transfusion.

Using the hemoglobin level as an indication for transfusion is easy and convenient, but might not be the best method of determining appropriateness of a specific transfusion. Studies assessing transfusion thresholds report differences in mortality or surrogate outcomes like hospital length of stay, without comparing intangible outcomes such as ability to participate in rehabilitation or quality of life following discharge. Physiologic transfusion triggers based on mixed venous oxygen content, global oxygen delivery, or surrogates of end-organ perfusion are neither clinically applicable for a general population nor proven to be clinically superior to hemoglobin levels.

Shander A, Kim TY, Goodnough LT. Thresholds, triggers or requirements-time to look beyond the transfusion trials. *J Thorac Dis*. 2018;10:1152-1157.

Trentino KM, Farmer SL, Leahy MF, et al. Systematic reviews and meta-analyses comparing mortality in restrictive and liberal haemoglobin thresholds for red cell transfusion: an overview of systematic reviews. *BMC Med*. 2020;18:154.

D.3. Describe the pathophysiology of potential complications following massive transfusion and hematologic resuscitation. What are the risks of thromboembolic complications after intraoperative administration of procoagulants?

Massive transfusion and hematologic resuscitation are a balance between promoting clot formation and avoiding hypercoagulability. Dilutional coagulopathy is a multifactorial result of fibrinogen depletion by clot formation and subsequent hemodilution during resuscitation, altered activity of coagulation factors, impaired thrombin generation, and inappropriate fibrinolysis (Section C.3). Two major phenotypes have been described following minor to massive trauma: a bleeding phenotype in the presence of shock accompanied by sympathetic hyperstimulation, and a thrombotic phenotype without shock or pronounced sympathetic activation. In the shock state, hypocoagulation is the result of activation of protein C, release of tissue plasminogen activator (tPA), and hyperfibrinolysis. The proposed mechanism for the thrombotic phenotype is increases in procoagulation factors and impaired endogenous anticoagulant activity in the setting of massive injury and tissue factor exposure.

In the controlled environment of the operating room, goal-directed resuscitation with POCT can be applied to target transfusion of specific factors, potentially avoid unnecessary blood product transfusion, and ultimately avoid the hypercoagulable complications of hematologic resuscitation. Putting cost aside, one of the greatest deterrents to administration of factor concentrates is the associated potential thrombotic complications and lack of experience or regulatory approval for many of these products in certain patient populations. Factor or fibrinogen concentrates should be used with caution in patients with previous thrombotic events and potentially avoided in patients with recent coronary artery bypass grafting. Additional investigation is necessary to identify the patients in whom the benefit of these formulations outweighs their risk profile.

Duque P, Mora L, Levy JH, et al. Response to trauma-induced coagulopathy: a comprehensive review. *Anesth Analg*. 2020;130:654-664.

Napolitano LM. Hemostatic defects in massive transfusion: an update and treatment recommendations. *Expert Rev Hematol*. 2021;14:219-239.

D.4. At what point can antithrombotic therapy be initiated after surgery in the presence of acquired coagulopathy?

The risk of postoperative venous thromboembolism varies in different surgical populations, with the highest rates in patients undergoing hip and knee arthroplasty, neurologic surgery, and vascular surgery. Following surgery with acquired coagulopathy and massive hemorrhagic resuscitation, initiation of prophylactic or therapeutic antithrombotic therapy must be weighed against thrombotic risk to the patient. Arbitrary time points of 12 to 24 hours postoperatively can be used or alternatively, other indicators of lowered bleeding risk such as drain or chest tube output can be used to assess appropriateness of pharmacologic thromboembolic prophylaxis.

Anderson DR, Morgano GP, Bennett C, et al. American Society of Hematology 2019 guidelines for management of venous thromboembolism: prevention of venous thromboembolism in surgical hospitalized patients. *Blood Adv*. 2019;3:3898-3944.

32 Sickle Cell Disease

Chris R. Edmonds and Vinod Malhotra

A 30-year-old AfricanAmerican female with avascular necrosis of her right hip was admitted for a total hip arthroplasty. Her hematocrit was 22%, blood pressure was 130/90 mm Hg, and pulse was 107 beats per minute. Her medications included hydroxyurea and oxycodone. She has a past medical history of recurrent joint pain, bone pain, acute chest syndrome, dyspnea, multiple transfusions, jaundice, and abdominal pain requiring multiple hospitalizations for analgesia. Her past surgical history was remarkable for cholecystectomy, and her postoperative course was remarkable for a prolonged hospitalization for respiratory complications.

A. Medical Disease and Differential Diagnosis

1. What was the most likely underlying medical condition in this patient? How would you confirm the diagnosis of sickle cell anemia?
2. What is sickle cell disease?
3. What is sickle cell trait?
4. What are some other common hemoglobinopathies and what are their clinical features?
5. What are the clinical features of sickle cell disease?
6. Describe the different types of sickle cell crisis.
7. Discuss the pathophysiologic effects of sickle cell disease.
8. What is acute chest syndrome?

B. Preoperative Evaluation and Preparation

1. What preoperative evaluation and testing would you perform on this patient prior to anesthesia? Would you request a hematology consult, and what question(s) would you ask?
2. What preoperative instructions would you give this patient prior to being admitted to the hospital? How would you prepare this patient for general anesthesia and regional anesthesia?
3. Discuss the indications for perioperative exchange transfusion in this patient.
4. What are the indications for blood transfusion in sickle cell disease?

C. Intraoperative Management

1. Discuss the anesthetic management for this patient. Discuss both regional and/or general anesthesia considerations.
2. Discuss how the comorbidities associated with sickle cell disease can affect your anesthetic management.
3. What precautions should one take to prevent sickling in this patient?
4. Discuss what issues or concerns should be brought up by the team during the debrief at the conclusion of the case. How would you sign out to the postanesthesia care unit (PACU) staff?

D. Postoperative Management

1. Discuss the postoperative management of this patient. What opioid-sparing techniques can you use and discuss a multimodal analgesic plan?
2. What complications might occur in this patient in the immediate postoperative period?
3. What is the treatment of vaso-occlusive sickle cell crisis?
4. What is the role of hyperbaric oxygen therapy in the treatment of acute vaso-occlusive sickle cell crisis?

A. Medical Disease and Differential Diagnosis

A.1. What was the most likely underlying medical condition in this patient? How would you confirm the diagnosis of sickle cell anemia?

For a young AfricanAmerican patient presenting with a history of joint pain, bone pain, abdominal pain, and anemia, the most likely diagnosis is sickle cell disease (SCD). Other diagnoses to consider include other hemoglobinopathies, dermatomyositis, glucose-6-phosphate dehydrogenase (G6PD) deficiency, and porphyria. Nevertheless, given the constellation of symptoms and the laboratory findings, SCD is the most likely diagnosis. Hemoglobin (Hgb) electrophoresis will confirm the diagnosis and provide the percentage of abnormal hemoglobin S (HgbS) relative to the percentage of normal hemoglobin (HbAA).

Adjepong KO, Otegbeye F, Adjepong YA. Perioperative management of sickle cell disease. *Mediterr J Hematol Infect Dis*. 2018;10:e2018032.

Firth PG. Anaesthesia for peculiar cells–a century of sickle cell disease. *Br J Anaesth*. 2005;95:287-299.

Firth PG. Anesthesia and hemoglobinopathies. *Anesthesiol Clin*. 2009;27:321-336.

Firth PG, Head A. Sickle cell disease and anesthesia. *Anesthesiology*. 2004;101:766-785.

Khurmi N, Gorlin A, Misra L. Perioperative considerations for patients with sickle cell disease: a narrative review. *Can J Anaesth*. 2017;64:860-869.

Stasic AF, Heine CL, Fisher G, Choi SW, Smith J. Rare coexisting diseases. In: Cullen BF, Stock MC, Ortega R, et al, eds. *Barash, Cullen, and Stoelting's Clinical Anesthesia*. 9th ed. Wolters Kluwer; 2024:577-610.

A.2. What is sickle cell disease?

SCD is a hereditary hemoglobinopathy resulting from inheritance of a β-*globin* gene mutation located on chromosome 11. This single-point mutation involves an adenine substitution with thymine. The mutant β-allele codes for production and assembly of a variant Hgb (β-S). The molecular basis of SCD is the substitution of valine for glutamic acid in the sixth position from the *N*-terminus of the Hgb β-chains. This substitution replaces a hydrophilic negative-charged amino acid (glutamic acid) with a hydrophobic nonpolar amino acid (valine) which greatly destabilizes the structure of Hgb and exposes highly reactive hydroxyl groups on the protein surface. The mutation in β-S Hgb accelerates denaturation of the Hgb protein and significantly decreases its solubility. Decreased oxygen tension causes conformational changes in Hgb, allowing hydrophobic bonds to form between valine-6 of one chain and phenylalanine-85 and leucine-88 of a second chain. This forms insoluble tetramers that interact with other tetramers to form long helical strands that subsequently polymerize, causing deformation of the red blood cell membrane into a sickle shape. The result is a red blood cell that is less able to transverse capillaries of the microcirculation, disposing end organs to hypoxia and ischemic damage when sickle cells are present in sufficient quantity. In the United States, the estimated prevalence of Hgb SS disease is 1:625 (0.2%) in people of African descent. Patients with sickle cell anemia (SCA) have early mortality, with a median age at death in the late 40s to early 50s. They have a "300-fold" higher risk of stroke by 45 years of age.

Bunn HF. Pathogenesis and treatment of sickle cell disease. *N Engl J Med*. 1997;337:762-769.

Firth PG. Anaesthesia for peculiar cells—a century of sickle cell disease. *Br J Anaesth*. 2005;95:287-299.

Firth PG. Anesthesia and hemoglobinopathies. *Anesthesiol Clin*. 2009;27:321-336.

Firth PG, Head A. Sickle cell disease and anesthesia. *Anesthesiology*. 2004;101:766-785.

Stasic AF, Heine CL, Fisher G, Choi SW, Smith J. Rare coexisting diseases. In: Cullen BF, Stock MC, Ortega R, et al, eds. *Barash, Cullen, and Stoelting's Clinical Anesthesia*. 9th ed. Wolters Kluwer; 2024:577-610.

Steinberg MH. Management of sickle cell disease. *N Engl J Med*. 1999;340:1021-1030.

A.3. What is sickle cell trait?

Sickle cell trait (SCT) is the heterozygous or carrier state of SCD. Large-scale screening for SCD in American military recruits revealed an incidence of SCT (HbAS) of 8% to 10% in African Americans and 0.05% to 0.08% in other ethnic groups. HbAS cells begin to sickle only when Hgb oxygen saturation is less than 20%. No difference in survival rates or incidence of severe disease has been found between those with and without SCT with one exception: patients with HbAS have a 50% increased risk for pulmonary infarction. Studies suggest that SCT provides a survival advantage over HbAA individuals when infected by the malarial parasite *Plasmodium falciparum*.

Firth PG. Anaesthesia for peculiar cells—a century of sickle cell disease. *Br J Anaesth*. 2005;95:287-299.

Firth PG. Anesthesia and hemoglobinopathies. *Anesthesiol Clin*. 2009;27:321-336.

Firth PG, Head A. Sickle cell disease and anesthesia. *Anesthesiology*. 2004;101:766-785.

Gong L, Parikh S, Rosenthal PJ, et al. Biochemical and immunological mechanisms by which sickle cell trait protects against malaria. *Malar J*. 2013;12:317.

Stasic AF, Heine CL, Fisher G, Choi SW, Smith J. Rare coexisting diseases. In: Cullen BF, Stock MC, Ortega R, et al, eds. *Barash, Cullen, and Stoelting's Clinical Anesthesia*. 9th ed. Wolters Kluwer; 2024:577-610.

A.4. What are some other common hemoglobinopathies and what are their clinical features?

Other common hemoglobinopathies include the thalassemias and Hgb C disease. Thalassemia arises from alterations in one or more of the four genes that code for the α-chain. The mildest form of thalassemia (loss of one α-gene) presents as a mild form of anemia, whereas the most severe form (loss of all four genes) is incompatible with life. Hgb C results from a mutation in the β-*globin* gene. Hgb C disease is a relatively benign disease producing a mild hemolytic anemia and splenomegaly. However, when it is paired with a β-S mutation, the disease is more severe. Other rare hemoglobinopathies will not be discussed further.

Each Hgb gene mutation of the heterozygous form causes little or no clinical consequence, but when both genes of a heterozygote are abnormal, a disease state is evident. Heterozygous combinations such as HbS and HbC (HbSC disease), and β-thalassemia mutation (HbS-β-thalassemia) usually cause a milder clinical course than that of SCD.

Firth PG. Anesthesia and hemoglobinopathies. *Anesthesiol Clin*. 2009;27:321-336.

Park KW. Sickle cell disease and other hemoglobinopathies. *Int Anesthesiol Clin*. 2004;42:77-93.

Stasic AF, Heine CL, Fisher G, Choi SW, Smith J. Rare coexisting diseases. In: Cullen BF, Stock MC, Ortega R, et al, eds. *Barash, Cullen, and Stoelting's Clinical Anesthesia*. 9th ed. Wolters Kluwer; 2024:577-610.

A.5. What are the clinical features of sickle cell disease?

The clinical features of SCD include indolent end-organ damage with intermittent acute episodes of severe pain and pulmonary complications. Although SCD is a disease of Hgb, it ultimately affects all organ systems. It is usually the acute problems that bring these individuals to the attention of a physician. The clinical manifestations by organ systems are presented in **Table 32.1**.

The progression and severity of SCD is variable. Many patients have an indolent course, whereas a smaller subset suffers from an early end-organ failure and early death. The leading causes of morbidity and mortality are pulmonary, neurologic, and renal disease. Hydroxyurea is a drug that increases the percentage of fetal Hgb, thereby decreasing the severity of the disease. However, it does not seem to decrease the perioperative complications of the disease.

Adjepong KO, Otegbeye F, Adjepong YA. Perioperative management of sickle cell disease. *Mediterr J Hematol Infect Dis*. 2018;10:e2018032.

Ataga KI, Derebail VK, Archer DR. The glomerulopathy of sickle cell disease. *Am J Hematol*. 2014;89:907-914.

Firth PG. Anesthesia and hemoglobinopathies. *Anesthesiology Clin*. 2009;27:321-336.

Stasic AF, Heine CL, Fisher G, Choi SW, Smith J. Rare coexisting diseases. In: Cullen BF, Stock MC, Ortega R, et al, eds. *Barash, Cullen, and Stoelting's Clinical Anesthesia*. 9th ed. Wolters Kluwer; 2024:577-610.

A.6. Describe the different types of sickle cell crisis.

Sickle cell crisis refers to the acute clinical picture generally caused by sickling of red blood cells in the *microcirculation*. Four main clinical types of crisis have been described as shown in **Table 32.2**.

The most common crisis in SCD is the vaso-occlusive crisis, characterized by intermittent, recurrent acute episodes of severe pain. The central cause of pain is thought to be ongoing acute ischemia, vaso-occlusion, and infarction. The detailed pathophysiology and nociceptive pathways have not been elucidated. Patients in vaso-occlusive crisis present with fever, anemia, spine pain, limb pain, and abdominal pain. They are tachypneic and can have hepatomegaly and splenomegaly in addition to abdominal tenderness. A study reported that in 118 patients having 183 painful crises, the pain was in the lumbar spine (49%), abdomen (32%), femoral shaft (30%), and the knee (21%). Often, no trigger is identified for most vaso-occlusive crisis. The average rate of painful crises per patient year is 0.8%. A subset of patients

(5.2%) experience an average of 8 to 10 crises each year, which accounts for 33% of all hospitalizations. Mortality positively correlates with increased pain rate in adults.

Brandow AM, Carroll CP, Creary S, et al. American Society of Hemotology 2020 guidelines for sickle cell disease: management of acute and chronic pain. *Blood Adv.* 2020;4:2656-2701.

Firth PG. Anesthesia and hemoglobinopathies. *Anesthesiol Clin.* 2009;27:321-336.

Serjeant GR, Ceulaer CD, Lethbridge R, et al. The painful crisis of homozygous sickle cell disease: clinical features. *Br J Haematol.* 1994;87:586-591.

Vijay V, Cavenagh JD, Yate P. The anaesthetist's role in acute sickle cell crisis. *Br J Anaesth.* 1998;80:820-828.

TABLE 32.1 Clinical Manifestations of Sickle Cell Disease

System	Symptoms
Central nervous system/Neurologic	• Stroke (cerebrovascular accident) in children as well as adults (50%-70% recurrence within 3 y) • Proliferative retinopathy/blindness • Painful crisis (>70%) • Chronic pain (not common) • Peripheral neuropathy (not common) • Poor school performance
Cardiovascular	• Conduction abnormalities secondary to iron overload • Hypertension • Cor pulmonale • Left and right ventricular dysfunction • Chronic ulcers
Pulmonary	• Infarction, pulmonary fibrosis • Infection • Restrictive/obstructive lung disease (10%-15%) • Acute chest syndrome (40%) • Pulmonary hypertension (30%-40%) • Airway hyperactivity
Genitourinary	• Hyposthenuria, hematuria, proteinuria • Chronic renal insufficiency (5%-20%) • Renal failure • Priapism (10%-40% of males) • Urinary tract infection
Gastrointestinal	• Cholelithiasis (70%) • Acute hepatic syndrome • Elevated liver function tests, hyperbilirubinemia • Hepatopathy • Cirrhosis (16%-29%) • Dyspepsia secondary to mucosal ischemia • Sickle girdle syndrome (mesenteric ischemia)
Musculoskeletal	• Osteomyelitis (*Staphylococcus*/*Salmonella*) • Dactylitis • Avascular necrosis (50%) • Infarction
Hematologic/Immunologic	• Chronic anemia • Autosplenectomy/hyposplenism • Susceptibility to infections with encapsulated organisms • Erythrocyte alloimmunization from blood transfusions • Sequestration crisis • Hemolytic crisis • Aplastic crisis • Immune dysfunction/neutrophil dysfunction • Opsonization dysfunction • Hypercoagulability • Chronic inflammation

TABLE 32.2 Types of Sickle Cell Crises

Type	Pathophysiology	Treatment
Vaso-occlusive	Pain secondary to obstruction of flow in the microvascular beds leading to localized ischemia	• Hydration • Analgesia • Incentive spirometry
Splenic sequestration	Acute painful enlargement of the spleen Acute hypovolemia	• Restore circulatory volume, possible splenectomy
Aplastic	Sudden cessation of bone marrow activity Acute worsening of anemia usually associated with viral infection (parvovirus B19) Recovery in 7-10 d	• Supportive therapy • Blood transfusion
Hemolytic crisis	Acute accentuated decrease in hemoglobin level Secondary to red cell destruction Usually associated with coexisting G6PD deficiency	• Supportive therapy • Blood transfusion

G6PD, glucose-6-phosphate dehydrogenase.

A.7. Discuss the pathophysiologic effects of sickle cell disease.

The pathophysiologic effects of SCD are not limited to the structure or deformation of the erythrocyte. The interaction and balance between the Hgb molecule, cytoplasm, cell membrane and vascular endothelium is drastically altered to create chronic systemic biochemical alterations that produce the clinical features of SCD. A triggering insult, such as infection, surgical stress, or ischemia-reperfusion injury, catalyzes a complex interaction among sickled cells, endothelial regulation of flow, inflammatory cytokines, platelet aggregation factors, and vasoconstriction leading eventually to ischemia, infarction, and cell death. This cascade promotes a vicious cycle that eventually causes end-organ damage and dysfunction.

End-organ damage that occurs in sickle cell states is attributable to three pathways. In the erythrocyte cytoplasm, the loss of Hgb structural stability leads to increased heme oxidation with subsequent denaturation, deterioration, and polymerization. Iron oxidation produces superoxide (O_2^-) and hydrogen peroxide ($H_2O_2^-$), which increases formation of highly reactive hydroxyl radicals (−OH). In the cell membrane, free iron and iron-containing compounds accumulate, leading to clustering of membrane surface proteins, abnormal cation permeability, and cellular dehydration. These events within the erythrocyte increase adherence to the vascular endothelium, exposing it to shear and oxidative stress. The interaction between the abnormal erythrocytes and the vascular endothelium produces chronic inflammation, upregulation of endothelial cell adhesion molecules, and altered expression of endothelial nitric oxide synthetase. Systemically, there is an increase in leukocyte counts, activation of coagulation pathways, increase in inflammatory compounds, and increase in circulating endothelial cells in the plasma. This complex pathologic interaction between sickling cells in blood vessels and the vascular endothelium leads to infarcts, tissue destruction, and end-organ failure. The pathogenesis of sickle cell disease is depicted in **Figure 32.1**.

Adjepong KO, Otegbeye F, Adjepong YA. Perioperative management of sickle cell disease. *Mediterr J Hematol Infect Dis*. 2018;10:e2018032.

Conran N, Franco-Penteado CF, Costa FF. Newer aspects of the pathophysiology of sickle cell disease vaso-occlusion. *Hemoglobin*. 2009;33:1-16.

Firth PG. Anesthesia and hemoglobinopathies. *Anesthesiology Clin*. 2009; 27:321-336.

Strijbos MH, Landburg PP, Nur E, et al. Circulating endothelial cells: a potential parameter of organ damage in sickle cell anemia? *Blood Cells Mol Dis*. 2009;43:63-67.

A.8. What is acute chest syndrome?

Acute chest syndrome is a term used to describe an acute pulmonary complication of SCD. It is defined by the finding of a new pulmonary infiltrate involving at least one complete lung segment on chest radiograph that is not due to atelectasis. It presents with a constellation of pulmonary symptoms and

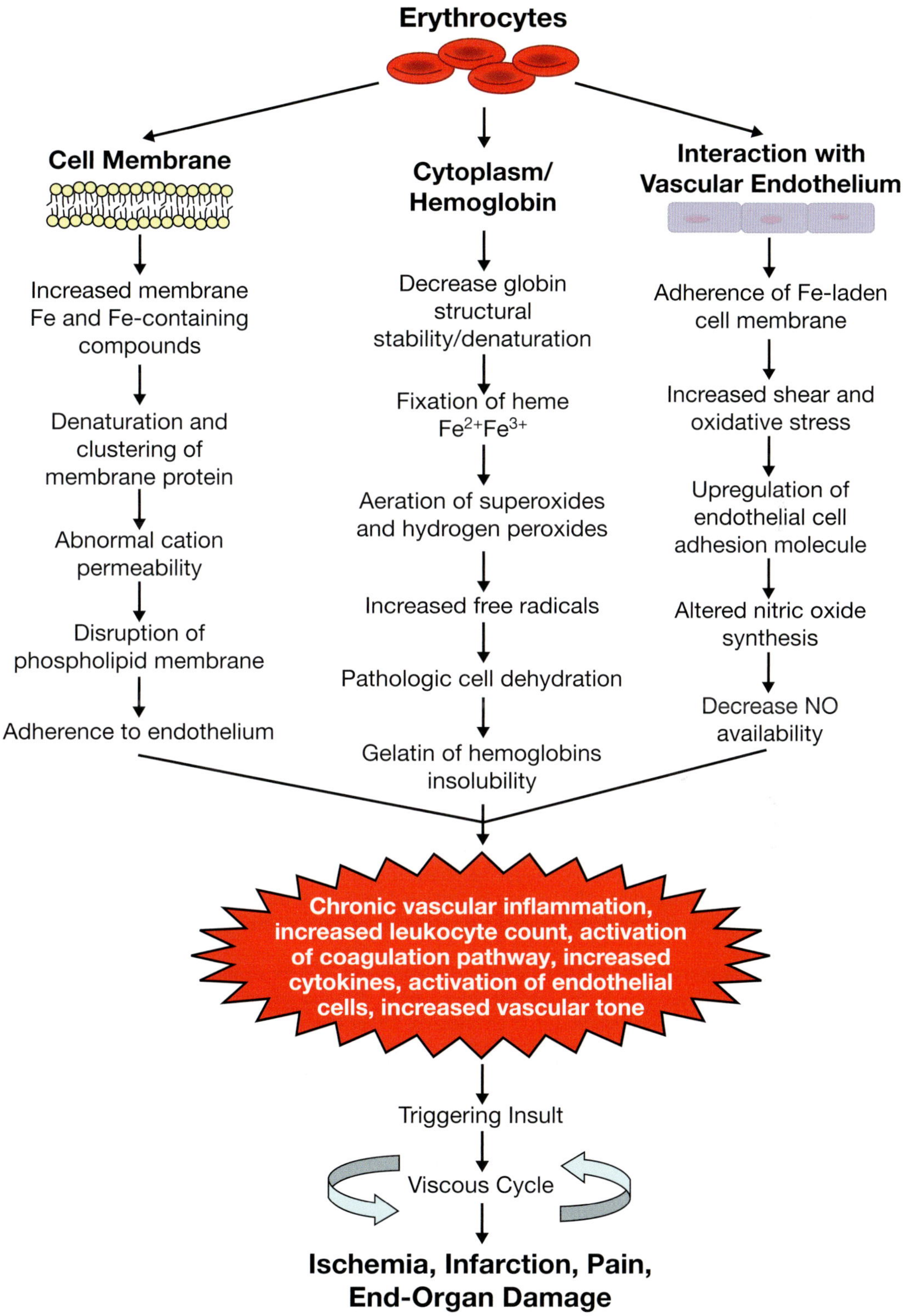

FIGURE 32.1. Pathogenesis of sickle cell damage. Fe, iron; NO, nitric oxide.

signs in a patient with SCD. These include fever (temperature 38.5 °C [101.3 °F]), wheezing, coughing, tachypnea, chest pain, and hypoxemia (<92% Spo_2 on room air). Pleural effusions are commonly (55%) seen on chest radiography. Acute chest syndrome frequently follows vaso-occlusive crisis, and vaso-occlusive pulmonary infarction might be the precipitating factor. Other causes include infection (viral, *Chlamydia*, *Mycoplasma*, and bacterial) and pulmonary fat embolism resulting from bone marrow necrosis.

Acute chest syndrome is a common postoperative complication in patients with SCD who have a history of pulmonary disease following general anesthesia. It is one of the most common causes of death in adults with SCD. Acute chest syndrome can be prevented by judicious hydration, incentive spirometry, effective analgesia, and avoidance of even mild hypothermia during the crises. Acute chest syndrome should be treated with bronchodilators, antibiotics, and exchange transfusion, when necessary. An exchange transfusion is recommended if the patient is clinically deteriorating.

Adjepong KO, Otegbeye F, Adjepong YA. Perioperative management of sickle cell disease. *Mediterr J Hematol Infect Dis*. 2018;10:e2018032.

Brandow AM, Carroll CP, Creary S, et al. American Society of Hemotology 2020 guidelines for sickle cell disease: management of acute and chronic pain. *Blood Adv*. 2020;4:2656-2701.

Chou ST, Alsawas M, Fasano RM, et al. American Society of Hemotology 2020 guidelines for sickle cell disease: transfusion support. *Blood Adv*. 2020;4:327-355.

Emre U, Miller ST, Gutierez M, et al. Effect of transfusion in acute chest syndrome of sickle cell disease. *J Pediatr*. 1995;127:901-904.

Stuart MJ, Yamaja S. Sickle cell acute chest syndrome: pathogenesis and rationale for treatment. *Blood*. 1999;94:1555-1560.

Vichinsky EP, Haberkern CM, Neumayr L, et al. A comparison of conservative and aggressive transfusion regimens in the perioperative management of sickle cell disease. The preoperative transfusion in sickle cell disease study group. *N Engl J Med*. 1995;333:206-213.

Vichinsky EP, Neumayr LD, Earles AN, et al. Causes and outcomes of the acute chest syndrome in sickle cell disease. National acute chest syndrome study group. *N Engl J Med*. 2010;342:1855-1865.

B. Preoperative Evaluation and Preparation

B.1. What preoperative evaluation and testing would you perform on this patient prior to anesthesia? Would you request a hematology consult, and what question(s) would you ask?

The aim of preoperative assessment in a patient with SCD is to determine preoperative risks of this multi-systemic disease and how potential end-organ damage will affect the anesthetic management (**Table 32.1**). A careful history should be obtained with a complete physical examination. Cardiopulmonary status should be thoroughly investigated in view of the increased incidence of cardiac and pulmonary morbidity in these patients, especially those with a history of acute chest syndrome and dyspnea.

A history of frequent hospitalizations in the year before surgery significantly increases the likelihood of a vaso-occlusive crisis in the perioperative period. Vaccination status for pneumococcal and *Haemophilus influenzae* pneumonia should be checked. Other characteristics that increase the perioperative risk are age, pregnancy, smoking, and infection. Cessation of smoking prior to elective surgery should be strongly encouraged because smoking increases the risk of acute chest syndrome and pain in the preoperative period. One should correct hypovolemia and treat infection appropriately preoperatively. Laboratory investigation should include complete blood count, blood urea nitrogen, serum creatinine, urinalysis, electrocardiogram, chest radiograph, pulse oximetry, and liver function tests. In addition, the following tests might be indicated:

- Arterial blood gas analysis
- Sickle cell preparation (if diagnosis is unclear)
- Hgb electrophoresis to determine HbS quantitatively
- Reticulocyte count
- Type and crossmatching of blood (alloimmunization can make this difficult)
- Pulmonary function testing (if severe pathology, paroxysmal dyspnea, or history of acute chest syndrome)
- Echocardiogram in patients with history of pulmonary hypertension or cardiomegaly
- Neurologic imaging (if there are neurological, psychological, or behavioral changes)

A hematology consult should be requested if the diagnosis of SCD is unclear or to obtain Hgb electrophoresis to determine the percentage of HgbS. A hematologist can also help patients with difficulty in blood crossmatching.

Adjepong KO, Otegbeye F, Adjepong YA. Perioperative management of sickle cell disease. *Mediterr J Hematol Infect Dis*. 2018;10:e2018032.

Cohen RT, DeBaun MR, Blinder MA, et al. Smoking is associated with an increased risk of acute syndrome and pain among adults with sickle cell disease. *Blood*. 2010;115:3852-3854.

Firth PG. Anesthesia and hemoglobinopathies. *Anesthesiol Clin*. 2009;27:321-336.

Firth PG, Head A. Sickle cell disease and anesthesia. *Anesthesiology*. 2004;101:766-785.

Knight-Madden JM, Barton-Gooden A, Weaver SR, et al. Mortality, asthma, smoking and acute chest syndrome in young adults with sickle cell disease. *Lung*. 2013;191:95-100.

Stasic AF, Heine CL, Fisher G, Choi SW, Smith J. Rare coexisting diseases. In: Cullen BF, Stock MC, Ortega R, et al, eds. *Barash, Cullen, and Stoelting's Clinical Anesthesia*. 9th ed. Wolters Kluwer; 2024:577-610.

B.2. What preoperative instructions would you give this patient prior to being admitted to the hospital? How would you prepare this patient for general anesthesia and regional anesthesia?

Prior to being admitted to the hospital for elective surgery, this patient should be given fasting instructions, to include clear fluids up to 2 hours prior to surgery and carbohydrate loading to maintain baseline metabolic state.

- Informed consent should be obtained to explain the options, risks, and benefits of different types of anesthesia used.
- Preoperative hydration should be initiated to treat baseline volume deficit.
- Euvolemia should be maintained preoperatively remembering that the patient is fasting and could also have a urine concentration defect requiring volume replacement.
- Any infections should be treated preoperatively, if possible.
- End-organ dysfunction should be identified and treated appropriately.
- Type and crossmatching can be difficult in these patients because of alloimmunization.

Consider transfusion of red blood cells to maintain oxygen-carrying capacity. Transfusion guidelines should be based on comorbidities, surgical risk, and degree of anemia. Transfusion should be individualized and based on the patient's individual risks and benefits. Efforts should be made for leukocyte reduction techniques, as with buffy coat–poor red cells, to reduce the incidence of leukocyte antigen alloimmunization. The goals of transfusion are to achieve an Hgb concentration of more than 8 g/dL and to ensure that Hgb A represents more than 40% of total Hgb. Past practices of reducing HgbS levels to less than 30% do not appear to improve outcomes but increase transfusion-related complications.

Chou ST, Alsawas M, Fasano RM, et al. American Society of Hemotology 2020 guidelines for sickle cell disease: transfusion support. *Blood Adv*. 2020;4:327-355.

Fawcett WJ, Thomas M. Preoperative fasting in adults and children: clinical practice and guidelines. *Anaesthesia*. 2019;74:83-88.

Firth PG. Anesthesia and hemoglobinopathies. *Anesthesiol Clin*. 2009;27:321-336.

Khurmi N, Gorlin A, Misra L. Perioperative considerations for patients with sickle cell disease: a narrative review. *Can J Anaesth*. 2017;64:860-869.

Soffin EM, Gibbons MM, Ko CY, et al. Evidence review conducted for the Agency for Healthcare Research and Quality safety program for improving surgical care and recovery: focus on anesthesiology for total hip arthroplasty. *Anesth Analg*. 2019;128:454-465.

Stasic AF, Heine CL, Fisher G, Choi SW, Smith J. Rare coexisting diseases. In: Cullen BF, Stock MC, Ortega R, et al, eds. *Barash, Cullen, and Stoelting's Clinical Anesthesia*. 9th ed. Wolters Kluwer; 2024:577-610.

B.3. Discuss the indications for perioperative exchange transfusion in this patient.

Controversy exists as to whether these patients benefit from preoperative exchange transfusion. For high-risk surgical procedures such as cardiopulmonary bypass, an exchange transfusion could be appropriate. Nevertheless, there are reports of cardiopulmonary bypass cases in which exchange transfusions were not performed or only a partial exchange was performed with good outcomes. If an exchange transfusion is required, it should be performed with buffy coat–free packed red blood cells to reduce the HbS fraction to less than 40%. Nevertheless, growing evidence indicates that most surgical procedures can be safely performed in patients with SCD without aggressive transfusion. For example, for certain surgical procedures, a packed red blood cell transfusion done simply to increase the Hgb level to 10 g/dL is as effective in decreasing perioperative morbidity as an exchange transfusion aimed at lowering HbS(S) levels to less than 40%. Exchange transfusion is a therapy often used in patients with SCD complicated by acute chest syndrome. It is beneficial to keep the hematocrit less than 35% with an exchange transfusion, because increased hematocrit increases blood viscosity and stasis in the circulation.

Adhikari RK, Maddali MM, Zacharias S. Preoperative exchange transfusion for sickle cell disease patients undergoing open-heart surgery: exception to the rule. *J Card Surg*. 2010;25:691-693.

Adjepong KO, Otegbeye F, Adjepong YA. Perioperative management of sickle cell disease. *Mediterr J Hematol Infect Dis*. 2018;10:e2018032.

Chou ST, Alsawas M, Fasano RM, et al. American Society of Hemotology 2020 guidelines for sickle cell disease: transfusion support. *Blood Adv*. 2020;4:327-355.

Stasic AF, Heine CL, Fisher G, Choi SW, Smith J. Rare coexisting diseases. In: Cullen BF, Stock MC, Ortega R, et al, eds. *Barash, Cullen, and Stoelting's Clinical Anesthesia*. 9th ed. Wolters Kluwer; 2024:577-610.

Vichinsky EP, Haberkern CM, Neumayr L, et al. A comparison of conservative and aggressive transfusion regimens in the perioperative management of sickle cell disease. The preoperative transfusion in sickle cell disease study group. *N Engl J Med*. 1995;333:206-213.

B.4. What are the indications for blood transfusion in sickle cell disease?

Blood transfusions should be guided by the clinical picture and the potential for blood loss. Prophylactic transfusion remains controversial and is of questionable benefit in mild-to-moderate risk cases. Some of the clinical indications for blood transfusion in SCD include:

Acute Conditions

- Vaso-occlusive crisis with organ infarction and dysfunction
- Sequestration syndrome
- Acute hemolysis with exacerbation of anemia
- Aplastic crisis
- Acute chest syndrome
- Acute multiorgan failure
- Severe unresponsive priapism
- Protracted painful crisis
- High-risk surgery (eg, cardiovascular, thoracic)

Chronic Conditions

- Intractable leg ulcers
- Complicated pregnancy
- Stroke
- Recurrent SCD pain syndrome
- Recurrent acute chest syndrome

Chou ST, Alsawas M, Fasano RM, et al. American Society of Hemotology 2020 guidelines for sickle cell disease: transfusion support. *Blood Adv*. 2020;4:327-355.

Howard J, Malfroy M, Llewelyn C, et al. The transfusion alternatives preoperatively in sickle cell disease (TAPS) study: a randomized, controlled, multicentre clinical trial. *Lancet*. 2013;381:930-938.

Wun T, Hassell K. Best practices for transfusion for patients with sickle cell disease. *Hematol Rev*. 2009;1:e22.

C. Intraoperative Management

C.1. Discuss the anesthetic management for this patient. Discuss both regional and/or general anesthesia considerations.

The definitive anesthetic technique has not been established secondary to the wide clinical spectrum of SCD and the different severities in the surgical procedures. A retrospective study reviewed 1,079 anesthetic procedures and noted an apparent association between postoperative complications and use of regional anesthesia. Nevertheless, this study did not control obstetric procedures and the tendency that clinicians often use regional anesthesia for sicker patients. Other studies did not find an adverse effect of regional anesthesia. Regional anesthesia, especially when used with epinephrine, could produce compensatory vasoconstriction in the nonblocked area, but this has not been supported in the literature. An additional study found that epidural analgesia markedly improved oxygenation in children in vaso-occlusive crisis, either through superior pain control or opioid-sparing effects. Therefore, almost any anesthetic technique can be used, provided the following principles are considered:

- Good intravenous access for maintenance of intravascular volume
- Adequate oxygenation
- Denitrogenating before induction of general anesthesia
- Tracheal intubation for general anesthesia to ensure a controlled airway and adequate ventilation
- Maintenance of adequate oxygen-carrying capacity through judicious use of red blood cell transfusions
- Maintenance of normothermia
- Careful use of opioids for perioperative and postoperative analgesia to avoid oversedation and respiratory depression
- Avoidance of tourniquet use
- Use of regional analgesia both intraoperatively and postoperatively
- Avoidance of hypotension and venous stasis to prevent sickling of red blood cells
- Use of invasive monitoring (arterial catheter, central venous pressure catheter) for continuous blood pressure monitoring, volume monitoring, and frequent laboratory tests
- Avoidance of hypoventilation to prevent acidosis
- Use of increased inspired oxygen concentration to ensure maintenance of normal to increased Pao_2

Adjepong KO, Otegbeye F, Adjepong YA. Perioperative management of sickle cell disease. *Mediterr J Hematol Infect Dis*. 2018;10:e2018032.

Brandow AM, Carroll CP, Creary S, et al. American Society of Hemotology 2020 guidelines for sickle cell disease: management of acute and chronic pain. *Blood Adv*. 2020;4:2656-2701.

Chou ST, Alsawas M, Fasano RM, et al. American Society of Hemotology 2020 guidelines for sickle cell disease: transfusion support. *Blood Adv*. 2020;4:327-355.

Firth PG. Anesthesia and hemoglobinopathies. *Anesthesiol Clin*. 2009;27:321-336.

Khurmi N, Gorlin A, Misra L. Perioperative considerations for patients with sickle cell disease: a narrative review. *Can J Anaesth*. 2017;64:860-869.

Koshy M, Weiner SJ, Miller ST, et al. Surgery and anesthesia in sickle cell disease. Cooperative study of sickle cell diseases. *Blood*. 1995;86:3676-3684.

Stasic AF, Heine CL, Fisher G, Choi SW, Smith J. Rare coexisting diseases. In: Cullen BF, Stock MC, Ortega R, et al, eds. *Barash, Cullen, and Stoelting's Clinical Anesthesia*. 9th ed. Wolters Kluwer; 2024:577-610.

Yaster M, Tobin JR, Billet C, et al. Epidural analgesia in the management of severe vaso-occlusive sickle cell crises. *Pediatrics*. 1994;93:310-315.

C.2. Discuss how the comorbidities associated with sickle cell disease can affect your anesthetic management.

SCD can affect every organ. Therefore, evaluating the patient for end-organ dysfunction is paramount. This patient is anemic, tachycardic, and hypertensive. She could have dyspepsia, hyperreactive airways, chronic renal insufficiency, and liver disease, and might be debilitated with cardiopulmonary complications. Patients with SCD often present with cardiomegaly, pulmonary hypertension, and heart failure. For this surgery, the patient will probably require transfusion, and it might be difficult to crossmatch.

In the postoperative period, pulmonary infarcts and infections are common, which can lead to acute chest syndrome. These problems, in addition to the potential for a sickling crisis or sequestration syndrome, pose a greater risk than normal for perioperative morbidity and mortality. Patients at greater risk include those with a homozygous state SCD, Hgb C disease (HbSC), and HgbS thalassemia. In contrast, patients with SCT do not present an increased risk for intraoperative morbidity. As a perioperative specialist, one can have a profound effect on the outcome in these patients by attention to detail, with a multisystem approach to address all end-organ dysfunction to reduce morbidity by maintaining oxygen delivery and preventing ongoing sickling.

Firth PG. Anesthesia and hemoglobinopathies. *Anesthesiol Clin*. 2009;27:321-336.

Khurmi N, Gorlin A, Misra L. Perioperative considerations for patients with sickle cell disease: a narrative review. *Can J Anaesth*. 2017;64:860-869.

C.3. What precautions should one take to prevent sickling in this patient?

Sickling of red blood cells is triggered by a variety of factors. One should avoid or correct factors that can precipitate sickling. Special precautions include the following:

- Avoid hypoxemia by preoxygenation and employing higher than usual concentrations of inspired oxygen.
- Prevent acidosis by maintaining adequate oxygenation, normovolemia, and cardiac output.
- Prevent respiratory acidosis by avoiding hypoventilation.
- Prevent stasis. This requires proper hydration and good regional blood flow. Blood viscosity should be maintained at a low level by limiting a rise in hematocrit to 35% and avoiding over transfusion.
- Avoid hypovolemia.
- Avoid hypothermia by using body-warming and intravenous fluid–warming devices perioperatively.
- Replace blood loss to prevent anemia.
- The use of tourniquets is controversial. Some advice against the use of tourniquets although they have been used without ill effects by others. If a tourniquet is to be used, it should only be used when absolutely necessary and for as short a period as possible. Special attention should be paid to maintain adequate oxygenation and to prevent respiratory or metabolic acidosis at the time of tourniquet release.
- Thromboembolic prophylaxis such as mechanical compresion, oral anticoagulants, heparin or heparin analogues have been used to reduce the incidence of thromboembolic events, and the results are promising. However, more studies are needed to determine the best preventative treatment

Chou ST, Alsawas M, Fasano RM, et al. American Society of Hemotology 2020 guidelines for sickle cell disease: transfusion support. *Blood Adv*. 2020;4:327-355.

Davila J, Stanek J, O'Brien S. Venous thromboembolism prophylaxis in sickle cell disease: a multicenter cohort study of adolescent inpatients. *Blood Adv*. 2023;9:1792-1768.

Firth PG. Anesthesia and hemoglobinopathies. *Anesthesiol Clin*. 2009;27:321-336.

Khurmi N, Gorlin A, Misra L. Perioperative considerations for patients with sickle cell disease: a narrative review. *Can J Anaesth*. 2017;64:860-869.

Stasic AF, Heine CL, Fisher G, Choi SW, Smith J. Rare coexisting diseases. In: Cullen BF, Stock MC, Ortega R, et al, eds. *Barash, Cullen, and Stoelting's Clinical Anesthesia*. 9th ed. Wolters Kluwer; 2024:577-610.

C.4. Discuss what issues or concerns should be brought up by the team during the debrief at the conclusion of the case. How would you sign out to the postanesthesia care unit (PACU) staff?

Checklists, surgical time-outs, and a postoperative debrief can improve patient safety by creating an environment where there is team involvement and communication is enhanced. They promote collaborative information sharing by pausing to allow the team as a whole to address positive aspects of the case as well as giving opportunity to address deficiencies and areas for improvement in a nonpunitive way with the goal of improving operating room efficiency, patient safety, and to learn from each case. For a patient with SCD who underwent total hip arthroplasty (THA), postoperative concerns include pain control, adequate hydration, cardiopulmonary monitoring, and hematologic monitoring. Early ambulation, incentive spirometry, supplemental oxygen, multimodal analgesia, and laboratory evaluation of hematocrit and renal function are paramount until the patient is stable. The sign out to the PACU team should include all these concerns and any issues that occurred preoperatively, intraoperatively, or might occur postoperatively.

Brandow AM, Carroll CP, Creary S, et al. American Society of Hemotology 2020 guidelines for sickle cell disease: management of acute and chronic pain. *Blood Adv*. 2020;4:2656-2701.

Chou ST, Alsawas M, Fasano RM, et al. American Society of Hemotology 2020 guidelines for sickle cell disease: transfusion support. *Blood Adv*. 2020;4:327-355.

Magill ST, Wang DD, Rutledge WC, et al. Changing operating room culture: implementation of a postoperative debrief and improved safety culture. *World Neurosurg*. 2017;107:597-603.

Rose MR, Rose KM. Use of a surgical debriefing checklist to achieve higher value health care. *AM J Med Qual*. 2018;33:514-522.

Sew Lan Leong KBM, Hanskamp-Sebregts M, van der Wal RA, et al. Effects of perioperative briefing and debriefing on patient safety: a prospective intervention study. *BMJ Open*. 2017;7:e018367.

D. Postoperative Management

D.1. Discuss the postoperative management of this patient. What opioid-sparing techniques can you use and discuss a multimodal analgesic plan?

The postoperative period is a crucial time for patients with SCD. Surgical pain, hypoventilation, a high incidence of pulmonary infarction, and an expected decrease in Pao_2 predisposes these patients to formation of sickle cells, leading to the possibility of developing vaso-occlusive crisis or acute chest syndrome. The mainstay of postoperative management is supportive and preventive care. Supplemental oxygen, maintenance of intravascular fluid volume, maintenance of normothermia, glycemic control, blood transfusion management, and adequate analgesia are important considerations.

There is evidence suggesting that patients with SCD have an altered pain response but both intravenous patient-controlled analgesia and epidural patient-controlled analgesia can improve postoperative pain control. Regional analgesia has been shown to decrease pain scores while improving oxygenation. A multimodal analgesia approach to pain control is paramount, which improves patient recovery and reduces reliance on opioids, including gabapentinoids, acetaminophen, and NSAIDs.

Supportive and preventive care should be continued in the extended postoperative period. The basic outline of routine postoperative care includes:

- Early mobilization
- Maintenance of normothermia
- Supplemental oxygen
- Early effective multimodal analgesia or adjunctive analgesic extending into the postoperative period
- Maintenance of euvolemia and adequate circulation
- Conservative transfusion therapy and Hgb management
- Incentive spirometry
- Pulse oximetry
- Pulmonary monitoring
- Psychological support
- Consider extended postoperative cardiovascular monitoring
- Consider regional analgesia for postoperative pain management

Brandow AM, Carroll CP, Creary S, et al. American Society of Hemotology 2020 guidelines for sickle cell disease: management of acute and chronic pain. *Blood Adv*. 2020;4:2656-2701.

Khurmi N, Gorlin A, Misra L. Perioperative considerations for patients with sickle cell disease: a narrative review. *Can J Anaesth*. 2017;64:860-869.

Soffin EM, Gibbons MM, Ko CY, et al. Evidence review conducted for the agency for healthcare research and quality safety program for improving surgical care and recovery: focus on anesthesiology for total hip arthroplasty. *Anesth Analg*. 2019;128:454-465.

Stasic AF, Heine CL, Fisher G, Choi SW, Smith J. Rare coexisting diseases. In: Cullen BF, Stock MC, Ortega R, et al, eds. *Barash, Cullen, and Stoelting's Clinical Anesthesia*. 9th ed. Wolters Kluwer; 2024:577-610.

D.2. What complications might occur in this patient in the immediate postoperative period?

Postoperative complications most likely to occur in this patient with SCD include deep vein thrombosis, vaso-occlusive crisis, pulmonary infarction, acute chest syndrome, and infection. Hypoxemic episodes are always a threat in the postoperative period secondary to pain, splinting, or oversedation and can precipitate a sickling crisis. The incidence of postoperative respiratory infection is high and is a leading cause of morbidity and mortality. Acute chest syndrome is one of the most common causes of death in adult patients and is a potentially lethal postoperative complication in patients with SCD who undergo major or high-risk surgery. Sequestration syndrome with shock is another potentially lethal complication, especially in obstetric patients immediately postpartum. Patients with cardiomegaly and pulmonary hypertension are susceptible to heart failure. Renal and hepatic dysfunction can result in prolongation of the effects of certain medications. Orthopedic patients with SCD are at risk for deep vein thrombosis, acute thrombosis, and pulmonary embolism. Antithrombotic therapy should be tailored to reduce this common complication.

Adjepong KO, Otegbeye F, Adjepong YA. Perioperative management of sickle cell disease. *Mediterr J Hematol Infect Dis*. 2018;10:e2018032.

Brandow AM, Carroll CP, Creary S, et al. American Society of Hemotology 2020 guidelines for sickle cell disease: management of acute and chronic pain. *Blood Adv*. 2020;4:2656-2701.

Chou ST, Alsawas M, Fasano RM, et al. American Society of Hemotology 2020 guidelines for sickle cell disease: transfusion support. *Blood Adv*. 2020;4:327-355.

Khurmi N, Gorlin A, Misra L. Perioperative considerations for patients with sickle cell disease: a narrative review. *Can J Anaesth*. 2017;64:860-869.

Stasic AF, Heine CL, Fisher G, Choi SW, Smith J. Rare coexisting diseases. In: Cullen BF, Stock MC, Ortega R, et al, eds. *Barash, Cullen, and Stoelting's Clinical Anesthesia*. 9th ed. Wolters Kluwer; 2024:577-610.

D.3. What is the treatment of vaso-occlusive sickle cell crisis?

The treatment of vaso-occlusive sickle cell crisis is to break the vicious cycle of sickling, ischemia, infarction, pain, and end-organ failure. Aggressive multimodal therapy can reduce clinical symptoms of the crises. The principles of treatment for painful sickle cell crisis include:

- Rest
- Hydration
- Oxygen therapy
- Treatment of infection
- Analgesics (consider patient-controlled analgesia)
- Consider regional analgesia
- Transfusion to reduce Hgb SS concentration
- Incentive spirometry
- Maintenance of normothermia

Adjepong KO, Otegbeye F, Adjepong YA. Perioperative management of sickle cell disease. *Mediterr J Hematol Infect Dis*. 2018;10:e2018032.

Brandow AM, Carroll CP, Creary S, et al. American Society of Hemotology 2020 guidelines for sickle cell disease: management of acute and chronic pain. *Blood Adv*. 2020;4:2656-2701.

Chou ST, Alsawas M, Fasano RM, et al. American Society of Hemotology 2020 guidelines for sickle cell disease: transfusion support. *Blood Adv*. 2020;4:327-355.

Khurmi N, Gorlin A, Misra L. Perioperative considerations for patients with sickle cell disease: a narrative review. *Can J Anaesth*. 2017;64:860-869.

Stasic AF, Heine CL, Fisher G, Choi SW, Smith J. Rare coexisting diseases. In: Cullen BF, Stock MC, Ortega R, et al, eds. *Barash, Cullen, and Stoelting's Clinical Anesthesia*. 9th ed. Wolters Kluwer; 2024:577-610.

D.4. What is the role of hyperbaric oxygen therapy in the treatment of acute vaso-occlusive sickle cell crisis?

Hyperbaric oxygen has been used empirically in some institutions for treatment of acute sickle cell crisis. However, it is not widely available. Although some reports claim instant improvement of symptoms, others have failed to show beneficial effects. There is better evidence that therapy is useful in management of ischemic disorders of the anterior segment of the eye or in chronic leg ulcers. Studies have shown no apparent effects of hyperbaric oxygen on sickle cell morphology in vitro. Thus, reported benefits in vivo might be due to a decrease in the rate of sickling or improved tissue oxygenation by direct diffusion. Despite some case series supporting its use, there is not enough evidence to recommend routine use over conventional therapy.

Butler FK Jr, Hagan C, Murphy-Lavoie H. Hyperbaric oxygen therapy and the eye. *Undersea Hyperb Med*. 2008;35:333-387.

Mychaskiw G II, Woodyard SA, Brunson CD, et al. In vitro effects of hyperbaric oxygen on sickle cell morphology. *J Clin Anesth*. 2001;13:255-258.

Reynolds JD. Painful sickle cell crisis. Successful treatment with hyperbaric oxygen therapy. *JAMA*. 1971;216:1977-1978.

Stirnemann J, Letellier E, Aras N, et al. Hyperbaric oxygen therapy for vaso-occlusive crises in nine patients with sickle-cell disease. *Diving Hyperb Med*. 2012;42:82-84.

Wallyn CR, Jampol LM, Goldberg MF, et al. The use of hyperbaric oxygen in treatment of sickle cell hyphema. *Invest Ophthalmol Vis Sci*. 1985;26:1155-1158.

SECTION 9 Eye, Ear, Nose, and Throat

33 Airway Trauma

Rohan K. Panchamia, Jonathan St. George, and
Jon D. Samuels

A 46-year-old male was thrown from his motorcycle at a high speed and impaled in the base of the neck by a tree branch. Upon presentation to the trauma center, he is awake and alert with a heart rate (HR) of 122 beats per minute, blood pressure of 143/85 mm Hg, respiratory rate of 20 breaths per minute, and oxygen saturation of 98% on 100% nonrebreathing mask. There is a 5-cm-wide piece of wood protruding from his anterior lower neck at the sternal notch, without visible bleeding. The patient is neurologically intact but admits to consuming six beers in the hours before injury. His medical history is unremarkable.

A. Medical Disease and Differential Diagnosis

1. What variables mitigate injury from motorcycle collisions?
2. What other significant traumas can be present?
3. How is the initial assessment of a patient with trauma organized?
4. How would you evaluate airway and breathing?
5. How would you classify traumatic neck injuries?
6. What signs and symptoms are concerning for direct airway trauma?
7. How would you evaluate the circulation?
8. How would you evaluate mental status and neurologic condition?
9. What are the zones of the neck, and what is their clinical significance?
10. What diagnostic tests are indicated for this patient based on the mechanism of injury?
11. What immediate treatment is necessary before diagnostic studies?
12. When and where should the impaling piece of wood be removed?

B. Preoperative Evaluation and Preparation

1. What laboratory tests would you want?
2. What radiographic studies are most important to the anesthesiologist?
3. Should this patient's trachea be intubated before going for computed tomography (CT) scanning?
4. Are any prophylactic medications indicated?

C. Intraoperative Management

1. What monitors would you use? Is invasive monitoring necessary before definitive airway control?
2. What is the surgical approach to a zone I neck injury?
3. Is the patient likely to require tube thoracostomy? Should this be placed before managing the airway?
4. What are the options for managing this patient's airway?
5. What are the risks of rapid sequence induction of anesthesia in this patient?
6. What anesthetic agents would you use for a rapid sequence induction?
7. How can you minimize the risk of exacerbating cervical spine trauma?
8. How can you minimize the risks of aspiration?

9. How would you anesthetize the airway for awake tracheal intubation?
10. What are the risks of awake fiberoptic tracheal intubation?
11. If the patient cannot be ventilated, what options are available?
12. Would a supraglottic airway (SGA) or other pharyngeal airway device be of assistance?
13. What surgical airway options are available in this case?
14. What maintenance anesthetics are indicated or contraindicated in this patient?
15. What complications will the surgical plan introduce?

D. Postoperative Management

1. What are the criteria for tracheal extubation?
2. What techniques may be used during extubation?
3. How does alcohol misuse affect postoperative management?
4. What pain medications should be used for analgesia?

A. Medical Disease and Differential Diagnosis

A.1. What variables mitigate injury from motorcycle collisions?

Trauma involving motorcycles accounts for only 2% to 5% of all motor vehicle traumas, but there is a higher proportion of death and serious injury because of the relative exposure of the motorcycle rider to the environment. Factors such as youth, high speed, and impairment contribute to motorcycle collisions just as they do for automobiles. Motorcycle riders also are much more susceptible to factors beyond their own control, such as lack of vigilance on the part of automobile and truck drivers, road conditions (oil or debris) and design, and the weather.

Factors that can reduce the seriousness of motorcycle collisions when they do occur include helmets and protective clothing. Helmets have been shown to be one of the most effective measures for preventing head injuries in motorcycle collisions, reducing the risk of head injury by 69%, and the risk of death by 37% in motorcycle crashes. Full leather or synthetic "armor" reduces the risk of massive skin and soft-tissue injuries in the event of a high-speed collision.

Liu BC, Ivers R, Norton R, et al. Helmets for preventing injury in motorcycle riders. *Cochrane Database Syst Rev.* 2008:CD004333.

Meredith L, Brown J, Ivers R, et al. Distribution and type of crash damage to motorcyclists' clothing: validation of the zone approach in the European Standard for motorcycle protective clothing, EN13595. *Traffic Inj Prev.* 2014;15:501-507.

National Highway Traffic Safety Administration. *Motorcycles* (Traffic Safety Facts. Report no. DOT HS 813 112). U.S. Department of Transportation; 2021. Accessed April 7, 2025. https://crashstats.nhtsa.dot.gov/Api/Public/ViewPublication/813112external icon

A.2. What other significant traumas can be present?

Motorcycle collisions are high-energy trauma that can result in injury to any organ system or region of the body. This patient will need a complete head-to-toe assessment and a number of diagnostic studies to establish the full extent of injury. Common injuries in motorcyclists include brain trauma from direct impact with the road and with other vehicles, pelvic fractures from impact with the frame of the motorcycle, abdominal trauma from impact with the handlebars, and lower extremity orthopedic and soft-tissue trauma from impact with the road.

A.3. How is the initial assessment of a patient with trauma organized?

The initial management of patients with trauma is best described by the tenets of the Advanced Trauma Life Support (ATLS) course, published by the American College of Surgeons Committee on Trauma. Assessment of the seriously injured patient begins with the ABCs: *A*irway, *B*reathing, and *C*irculation; followed by a brief neurologic examination and a catalog of visible injuries. This "primary survey" is followed by diagnostic testing and a more detailed secondary survey to discover all of the patient's injuries. Despite revision of this assessment in the combat and disaster setting to follow a CCAB approach (catastrophic hemorrhage, circulation restoration, airway management, breathing/respiratory support), ATLS continues to support prioritizing rapid assessment and treatment of life-threatening airway and breathing problems ahead of circulation problems. No evidence-based data were identified that justified a modification to this approach in the care of civilian patients. One important principle of ATLS is interruption of the diagnostic sequence as necessary to provide lifesaving resuscitative care, up to and including surgery for airway compromise or hemorrhage control prior to completion of diagnostic studies.

American College of Surgeons. Initial assessment and management. In: *Advanced Trauma Life Support (ATLS) Student Course Manual.* 11th ed. American College of Surgeons; 2023:1–28.

Breeding T, Martinez B, Katz J, et al. CAB versus ABC approach for resuscitation of patients following traumatic injury: toward improving patient safety and survival. *Am J Emerg Med.* 2023;68:28-32.

A.4. How would you evaluate airway and breathing?

On first contact with the patient, the provider should attempt verbal communication: "How are you?" A patient who answers coherently in a normal voice has no immediate airway issue, adequate circulatory function, and minimal traumatic brain injury. In an unconscious patient, initial assessment is made by looking, listening, and feeling for airflow. If airflow is absent, the airway should be opened by jaw thrust (*not* head tilt because this may exacerbate a cervical spinal column injury), cleared of any visible foreign bodies or secretions, and an oral or nasopharyngeal airway should be placed.

Breathing is assessed by observation of the chest wall and diaphragm once the airway is open and by immediate placement of a pulse oximeter probe. Patients who are not breathing adequately and/or are failing to maintain and protect their airway should be assisted with bag-valve-mask ventilation while preparations are made for securing a definitive airway and instituting mechanical ventilation.

A.5. How would you classify traumatic neck injuries?

Traumatic neck injuries can be broadly categorized into two groups: blunt trauma and penetrating trauma. Although a rare occurrence, due to the protection provided by the mandible, traumatic neck injuries carry a high rate of morbidity and mortality, with blunt trauma more so than penetrating trauma. The most common cause of blunt neck trauma is motor vehicle crashes, whereas gunshot and stab wounds account for most penetrating neck trauma incidents.

A.6. What signs and symptoms are concerning for direct airway trauma?

In addition to the mechanism of injury, various clinical signs and symptoms can increase suspicion for direct airway trauma. Red flag symptoms of airway trauma include neck and laryngeal pain, dysphonia, dysphagia, dyspnea, and odynophagia. Pain out of proportion with physical exam findings warrants further investigation, such as performing a nasopharyngoscopy. Direct and indirect exam findings of a compromised airway include stridor, ecchymosis, tracheal deviation, crepitus, subcutaneous emphysema, and an expanding neck hematoma.

American College of Surgeons. Initial assessment and management. In: *Advanced Trauma Life Support (ATLS) Student Course Manual.* 11th ed. American College of Surgeons; 2023:1–28.

DePorre AR, Schechtman SA, Hogikyan ND, et al. Airway management and clinical outcomes in external laryngeal trauma: a case series. *Anesth Analg.* 2019;129:e52-e54.

Shilston J, Evans DL, Simons A, et al. Initial management of blunt and penetrating neck trauma. *BJA Educ.* 2021;21:329-335.

A.7. How would you evaluate the circulation?

Penetrating neck trauma can be associated with major hemorrhage due to the proximity of major vessels, with a mortality rate as high as 50%; therefore, achieving hemorrhage control (following the CCAB approach) might be necessary to immediately address life-threatening bleeding prior to securing the airway. Initial assessment for shock is by vital signs (HR, blood pressure, pulse oximetry) and physical examination (pallor, diaphoresis, delayed capillary refill). In the setting of traumatic neck injury, visible hemorrhage, a rapidly expanding neck hematoma, and/or shock physiology that does not respond appropriately to resuscitation suggest uncontrolled vascular injury. Additional data points useful in diagnosing shock include an elevated blood lactate and base deficit. Mental status is also a useful sign; the patient in hemorrhagic shock will be first agitated and then lethargic. It is important to recognize that young patients have significant compensatory reserves and maintain a normal systolic blood pressure even in the face of hemorrhage as great as 40% of their blood volume. Shock in this patient could be the result of hemorrhage or a tension pneumothorax.

A.8. How would you evaluate mental status and neurologic condition?

The quick neurologic examination consists of questions to determine the level of consciousness and the presence of focal neurologic deficits. In the less responsive patient, the Glasgow Coma Score (GCS) (**Table 33.1**) is used to stratify the degree of impairment: GCS 3 to 8 is a severe injury, GCS 9 to 13 is

TABLE 33.1 Glasgow Coma Scale

Eye-Opening Response	Verbal Response	Motor Response
4 = Spontaneous	5 = Oriented to name	6 = Follows commands
3 = To speech	4 = Confused	5 = Localizes to painful stimuli
2 = To pain	3 = Inappropriate speech	4 = Withdraws from painful stimuli
1 = None	2 = Incomprehensible sounds	3 = Abnormal flexion (decorticate posturing)
	1 = None	2 = Abnormal extension (decerebrate posturing)
		1 = None

The Glasgow Coma Score is the sum of the best scores in each of three categories.

moderate traumatic brain injury, and GCS 14 to 15 is mild injury. Cranial nerves, spinal cord, and peripheral nervous system function are assessed by specific motor and sensory testing; zone III injuries carry the highest risk of damage to these neurologic structures.

American College of Surgeons. Initial assessment and management. In: *Advanced Trauma Life Support (ATLS) Student Course Manual.* 11th ed. American College of Surgeons; 2023:1–28.

Bouglé A, Harrois A, Duranteau J. Resuscitative strategies in traumatic hemorrhagic shock. *Ann Intensive Care.* 2013;3:1.

Duggan LV, Doyle LN, Zunder JS, et al. Blunt and penetrating airway trauma. *Emerg Med Clin North Am.* 2023; 41:e1-e15.

Dutton RP. Initial resuscitation of the hemorrhaging patient. In: Spiess B, Spence R, Shander A, eds. *Perioperative Transfusion Medicine.* 2nd ed. Lippincott Williams & Wilkins; 2006:289-300.

Nowicki JL, Stew B, Ooi E. Penetrating neck injuries: a guide to evaluation and management. *Ann R Coll Surg Engl.* 2018;100:6-11.

Teasdale G, Jennett B. Assessment of coma and impaired consciousness. A practical scale. *Lancet.* 1974;2:81-84.

A.9. What are the zones of the neck, and what is their clinical significance?

Historically, the clinical management of penetrating neck injuries has been based on the anatomic location or "zone" of injury.

Zone I of the neck includes the area from the inferior aspect of the cricoid cartilage down to the thoracic outlet; structures of interest include the trachea and esophagus. Zone I injuries could require a surgical approach that allows access to both the neck and chest. Zone II of the neck includes the area from the angle of the mandible down to the cricoid cartilage, encompassing the laryngotracheal complex, carotid and vertebral arteries, jugular veins, and vagus and phrenic nerves. Injuries in zone II may need to be addressed through a lateral or transverse cervical incision, with the surgeon being able to achieve both proximal and distal control of the carotid or jugular vessels before exploring the wound itself. Zone III of the neck includes the area from the angle of the mandible upward to the base of the skull. Sympathetic chain, pharynx, and cranial nerves can be found in this zone. Zone III vascular injuries pose a significant operative risk because distal control of an injured vessel cannot be achieved; they are therefore approached angiographically.

In recent decades, surgical management of penetrating neck trauma has evolved, moving away from the rigid framework of the zone approach, which required neck exploration for zone II injuries or mandatory endoscopy and angiography for zone I and III injuries. Current management follows a "no zone" approach, relying on the physical exam and computed tomography angiography (CTA) findings in triage and workup for vascular and aerodigestive damage after penetrating neck trauma. Patients with airway compromise or hemodynamic instability should be brought to the operating room without delay for surgical exploration.

Shilston J, Evans DL, Simons A, et al. Initial management of blunt and penetrating neck trauma. *BJA Educ.* 2021;21:329-335.

Shiroff AM, Gale SC, Martin ND, et al. Penetrating neck trauma: a review of management strategies and discussion of the 'No Zone' approach. *Am Surg.* 2013;79:23-29.

Sperry JL, Moore EE, Coimbra R, et al. Western Trauma Association critical decisions in trauma: penetrating neck trauma. *J Trauma Acute Care Surg.* 2013;75:936-940.

A.10. What diagnostic tests are indicated for this patient based on the mechanism of injury?

Because of high-energy mechanism of injury, this patient must be assessed from head to toe. Focused ultrasonography examination of the abdomen and thorax is used to diagnose free peritoneal fluid, pneumothorax, and pericardial effusion. Chest and pelvis plain-film radiography will reveal fractures, pneumothorax, and hemothorax. CT scanning should include the head, neck, chest, abdomen, and pelvis; newer technology will allow for three-dimensional (3D) reconstructions of organs and vasculature with sensitivity and specificity equivalent to more traditional angiographic imaging.

This patient's injury to zone I of the neck will necessitate a focused assessment of the trachea, great vessels, esophagus, and bilateral pleural cavities. Traditionally, this has been accomplished by a combination of plain-film radiography, angiography, bronchoscopy, and esophagoscopy. Increasing CT speed and resolution as well as point-of-care ultrasonography is leading to the increased use of these tests at centers with experienced radiographers and traumatologists. The sequencing of diagnostic studies will depend on the patient's stability. In this case, the patient is likely to require intubation and perhaps exploratory surgery first. A CTA may help guide the surgical approach to removal of the impaling object if the patient is calm, able to lay flat, and stable enough to tolerate the test. An underutilized tool in evaluating penetrating neck trauma is nasopharyngoscopy, which allows a real-time view of the glottis and surrounding anatomy throughout respiration.

Duggan LV, Doyle LN, Zunder JS, et al. Blunt and penetrating airway trauma. *Emerg Med Clin North Am*. 2023;41:e1-e15.

Fox AD, Livingston DH. Initial assessment. In: Feliciano DV, Mattox KL, Moore EE, eds. *Trauma*. 9th ed. McGraw Hill; 2020. Accessed May 1, 2025. https://accesssurgery-mhmedical-com.ezproxy.med.cornell.edu/content.aspx?bookid=2952&sectionid=249117545

A.11. What immediate treatment is necessary before diagnostic studies?

The key to this case will be control of the patient's airway. Once hemodynamic stability is confirmed, the timing and sequence of diagnostic studies will be determined by the patient's degree of cooperation and ability to spontaneously ventilate. Although a CT scan before a controlled intubation in the operating room (OR) would be ideal, it is possible that the patient will decompensate before this can be accomplished. Preemptive airway control will allow for a more secure and safer diagnostic workup before the operation.

A.12. When and where should the impaling piece of wood be removed?

The impaling piece of wood is best removed in the OR under anesthesia to reduce the possibility of uncontrolled hemorrhage. All the personnel and equipment should be present to perform an emergent median sternotomy and major vascular and/or tracheal surgery if necessary.

B. Preoperative Evaluation and Preparation

B.1. What laboratory tests would you want?

The patient should have a full set of laboratory studies, both to identify abnormalities and to establish a baseline for future changes. Hemoglobin and hematocrit might not indicate hemorrhage initially since the bleeding patient with trauma is losing whole blood but will likely drop with subsequent fluid resuscitation. Lactate and standard base excess measurements seen on blood gas analysis will be the most sensitive indicators of hypoperfusion and shock. Serum electrolytes will reveal baseline abnormalities, if any, and the effects of alcohol consumption and dehydration. Clotting studies are important to rule out congenital abnormalities or the effects of liver disease before what could be a major surgical procedure; coagulopathy at the time of admission is an indicator of substantial blood loss and severe hemorrhagic shock. Toxicology screening is indicated in every patient with trauma and is important to rule out the use of drugs, such as heroin or cocaine, which have implications for the anesthesiologist.

Initial laboratory studies also should include a sample for the blood bank with the request for an urgent crossmatch of red blood cells and plasma. If there has been a major vascular injury, substantial blood loss is a possibility and should be treated with immediate transfusion therapy.

American College of Surgeons. Initial assessment and management. In: *Advanced Trauma Life Support (ATLS) Student Course Manual*. 11th ed. American College of Surgeons; 2023:1–28.

Hess JR, Lindell AL, Stansbury LG, et al. The prevalence of abnormal results of conventional coagulation tests on admission to a trauma center. *Transfusion*. 2009;49:34-39.

B.2. What radiographic studies are most important to the anesthesiologist?

Although all of the studies described in the preceding text will have some relevance, there are a few that have particular implications for anesthesiologist. The CT scan helps to evaluate tracheal involvement by the impaling object, evidence of major vascular injury, and presence of pneumothorax. Furthermore, CT scan of the cervical spine can assess for bony or ligamentous injury that might be exacerbated by manipulation of the neck during airway management.

B.3. Should this patient's trachea be intubated before going for computed tomography (CT) scanning?

The answer requires an assessment of risks and benefits. If the patient is cooperative, able to lay flat, vital signs are stable, a CT scanner is close at hand, and anesthesia personnel are available to accompany the patient, then an immediate CT scan would be indicated. If the patient is deteriorating, his degree of cooperation is in doubt, or a CT scan would place the patient far from expert resources for an extended period, then it would be wise to secure the airway first. In this case, there is a possibility that airway management could precipitate patient deterioration (eg, hemorrhage, conversion from simple to tension pneumothorax), which suggests that if airway management is attempted before CT, it should probably be done in the OR with the surgical team on hand; instruments should be available for videolaryngoscopy and bronchoscopy, emergent tracheostomy, control of large vessel bleeding, and median sternotomy.

One approach to this kind of complex decision is to define an ideal course of care that provides the best information for each of the team of experts involved while minimizing risk to the patient and maximizing flexibility in dealing with changing circumstances. In this case, the surgeon and anesthesiologist might define a plan that includes transport to the OR; induction, tracheal intubation, and mechanical ventilation in the OR (safest possible environment); transport to CT or angiography with the anesthesiologist in attendance for diagnostic studies; and return to the OR for definitive surgery.

B.4. Are any prophylactic medications indicated?

Tetanus toxoid treatment is indicated for any patient with trauma with an open wound who has not received a booster in the past 5 years. Any patient with a significant open wound should receive prophylactic antibiotic therapy that covers Gram-positive organisms for at least the first 24 hours following injury.

Prophylactic treatment to reduce the consequences of aspiration would be considered but probably rejected in this case. Promotility agents such as metoclopramide and histamine H_2-receptor antagonists such as ranitidine will not have time to work before definitive airway control is achieved and the more immediate approach of administering oral sodium citrate/citric acid (eg, Bicitra) would be contraindicated because of the possibility of esophageal injury.

Because of the patient's history of intoxication, prophylactic intravenous administration of vitamins and thiamine is indicated. Prophylaxis against alcohol withdrawal and deep venous thrombosis are indicated in the immediate postoperative period.

C. Intraoperative Management

C.1. What monitors would you use? Is invasive monitoring necessary before definitive airway control?

Blood pressure, electrocardiography, capnography, and pulse oximetry should be employed as with any patient. A urinary catheter should be inserted once the patient is anesthetized, although urine output is not an accurate measure of intravascular volume status in a recently intoxicated patient. An arterial line is useful for continuous measurement of blood pressure and for easy access to blood for laboratory assay including arterial blood gases. A central venous catheter should be placed if there is a need for rapid intravascular expansion and administration of vasoactive medications. Because of the potential for great vessel injury in this case, initial central access should be through the femoral vein. A pulmonary artery catheter is rarely indicated and used acutely for resuscitation, although it can be helpful in selected patients presenting in undifferentiated shock, decompensated heart failure, or pulmonary hypertensive crisis.

Invasive monitoring lines are usually placed after induction and intubation, when the patient is anesthetized. Surgical hemostasis should not be delayed unnecessarily in an unstable patient. In this case, it would be appropriate to place an arterial line in the OR before airway management, as long as the patient remains cooperative and stable, and to place a femoral venous line thereafter. Placing the arterial line on the right side will allow assessment of blood flow in the innominate artery during surgical exploration.

Steurer MP, Sikorski RA, Richards JE, Galvagno SM. Anesthesia for trauma. In: Gropper MA, Eriksson LI, Fleisher LA, Cohen NH, Leslie K, Johnson-Akeju O, eds. *Miller's Anesthesia*. 10th ed. Vol 2. Elsevier; 2025:2000-2043.

C.2. What is the surgical approach to a zone I neck injury?

The surgery is likely to start with a collar incision through the impalement wound to allow for better visualization of the path of injury. If an injury to the trachea or a great vessel is discovered, a partial or complete median sternotomy would be the next step. The uncertain nature of this patient's injuries makes preoperative diagnostic information so critical that the requirement of a CT scan before definitive surgery after airway management is a strong consideration.

C.3. Is the patient likely to require tube thoracostomy? Should this be placed before managing the airway?

Pneumothorax and hemothorax are common in patients with trauma and should be suspected and definitively ruled out following any high-energy blunt trauma (eg, motor vehicle accident, pedestrian struck, fall from a height) or any penetrating trauma to the neck, thorax, or upper abdomen. Immediate needle decompression and/or tube thoracostomy are indicated in any hemodynamically unstable patient with a suspicious injury, even before imaging studies are performed. Tracheal intubation and positive pressure ventilation can precipitate hemodynamic decompensation in a patient with a chest injury due to decreased preload in the setting of hemorrhage or increased intrathoracic pressure caused by conversion from a simple to a tension pneumothorax.

In this case, there is a possibility of unilateral or bilateral thoracic injury with hemithorax. A portable anterior-posterior chest radiograph should be obtained as early as possible, followed by a CT of the chest. If a simple pneumothorax is present, prepare for chest tube placement (personnel, equipment) before airway management but wait until the airway is secure before actually placing the chest tube. If a large air leak is present after chest tube placement, injuries to the airway must be assessed and ruled out.

C.4. What are the options for managing this patient's airway?

Choices for induction of anesthesia should be considered in concert with choices for securing the airway and transitioning to positive pressure ventilation. In a cooperative patient, awake fiberoptic intubation with topicalization of the airway is the preferred technique, as it maintains spontaneous ventilation, allows direct visualization, and facilitates tracheal access and inspection of the airway distal to the entry wound. Awake surgical tracheostomy is another option, although in this case it would be challenging to perform given that the site of injury is at the level of the sternal notch. A rapid sequence intubation (RSI) with videolaryngoscopy (VL) is expedient but does not have the benefit of spontaneous ventilation and creates the potential of further airway injury.

Duggan LV, Doyle LN, Zunder JS, et al. Blunt and penetrating airway trauma. *Emerg Med Clin North Am.* 2023; 41:e1-e15.

Shilston J, Evans DL, Simons A, et al. Initial management of blunt and penetrating neck trauma. *BJA Educ.* 2021; 21:329-335.

C.5. What are the risks of rapid sequence induction of anesthesia in this patient?

The primary risk of rapid sequence induction and intubation is creation of a "cannot intubate, cannot oxygenate" (CICO) situation in a patient who was previously oxygenating adequately, even though placement of a secure airway is clearly indicated.

For all patients with trauma, the risks of RSI must always be balanced with the patient's current airway status and predicted ability to deliver oxygen to the alveoli, and the competing necessities of lifesaving time-dependent interventions. In most trauma cases, RSI is the fastest way to establish optimal intubating conditions and secure the airway.

In this case, however, with an awake and alert patient, if time and conditions allow, intubation by means other than RSI can be advantageous. Physical trauma to the airway by a penetrating foreign body can create difficulties that prevent the passage of an endotracheal tube. Blood, secretions, anatomic distortion, false passages, and physical obstruction can precipitate a CICO situation that might be avoided with an awake approach to tracheal access. This is a context-specific clinical decision that requires weighing the risks of RSI and evaluating the clinical conditions to assess if they are suitable for a non-RSI approach.

Stephens CT, Kahntroff S, Dutton RP. The success of emergency endotracheal intubation in trauma patients: a 10-year experience at a major adult trauma referral center. *Anesth Analg.* 2009;109:866-872.

C.6. What anesthetic agents would you use for a rapid sequence induction?

For patients in shock, administering a low dose of an induction agent and a high dose of neuromuscular blocking agent (NMBA) is the best approach. Patients in shock, particularly those with hypotension and altered mental status, require reduced doses of anesthetic agents that act centrally, such as etomidate or ketamine, but higher doses of NMBAs that act peripherally due to reduced cardiac output and shock physiology.

Rocuronium is currently the NMBA of choice for RSI due to its safety profile over succinylcholine, but both agents are effective, and they are the key components required to create optimal intubating conditions if RSI is to be effective. Dosing for either of these agents should be in the higher range. The onset of action of rocuronium is longer than that of succinylcholine and is dose dependent. For patients in shock, a minimum of 1.2 mg/kg rocuronium is recommended, and higher doses up to 2 mg/kg have been used safely. For succinylcholine, 1.5 mg/kg should be used. It has a faster onset of action, but should be avoided in patients with suspected crush injuries or with chronic conditions such as renal failure or prior stroke that put them at a higher risk of hyperkalemia induced by its depolarizing effects. The medical history of patients with trauma is often uncertain, which is one reason why rocuronium is often the preferred agent.

Guihard B, Chollet-Xémard C, Lakhnati P, et al. Effect of rocuronium vs succinylcholine on endotracheal intubation success rate among patients undergoing out-of-hospital rapid sequence intubation: a randomized clinical trial. *JAMA*. 2019;322:2303-2312.

Steurer MP, Sikorski RA, Richards JE, Galvagno SM. Anesthesia for trauma. In: Gropper MA, Eriksson LI, Fleisher LA, Cohen NH, Leslie K, Johnson-Akeju O, eds. *Miller's Anesthesia*. 10th ed. Vol 2. Elsevier; 2025:2000-2043.

C.7. How can you minimize the risk of exacerbating cervical spine trauma?

All patients with trauma undergoing tracheal intubation must be considered to have a potential cervical spine injury and should be placed in a cervical collar until cervical injury is excluded. This requires imaging, a physical exam done by an experienced clinician, and a cooperative patient without distracting injuries.

During intubation, cervical collars restrict mouth opening and the ability to place the patient in an ideal ear-to-sternal notch, or "sniffing" position. In addition, the forces used during laryngoscopy to displace tissue and access the trachea can potentially cause injury. Several steps can be taken to minimize the risk of further injury to a patient with trauma with a suspected cervical spine injury and improve first-pass intubation success. Maintenance of manual inline stabilization by an assistant during intubation allows temporary removal of the cervical collar and is considered safe. This allows jaw mobility and creates more space for the laryngoscope and endotracheal tube. Some collars, such as the Aspen collar, which can be adjusted, can be left in place to provide stabilization, and allow mouth opening. The collar can then be adjusted after intubation for a snugger fit.

Use of a videolaryngoscope is recommended in preference to a direct laryngoscope. A hyperangulated videolaryngoscope blade (HAVL) allows visualization around the base of the tongue and insertion of the endotracheal tube with minimal displacement of tissue, thus reducing the force required during intubation. Although the risk of injury is low, particularly with HAVL, awake intubation with a fiberoptic bronchoscope transfers the least amount of force to a potentially unstable cervical spine injury.

Cranshaw J, Nolan J. Airway management after major trauma. *Contin Educ Anaesth Crit Care Pain*. 2006;6:124-127.

Steurer MP, Sikorski RA, Richards JE, Galvagno SM. Anesthesia for trauma. In: Gropper MA, Eriksson LI, Fleisher LA, Cohen NH, Leslie K, Johnson-Akeju O, eds. *Miller's Anesthesia*. 10th ed. Vol 2. Elsevier; 2025:2000-2043.

Pierre EJ, McNeer RR, Shamir MY. Early management of the traumatized airway. *Anesthesiol Clin*. 2007;25:1-11.

C.8. How can you minimize the risks of aspiration?

Because significant injury is associated with decreased gastrointestinal motility, all patients with trauma are considered to have full stomachs and thus at risk of regurgitation of gastric contents and pulmonary aspiration. The risk of aspiration is further increased by intoxication with drugs including alcohol; obesity; opioid analgesics; and injuries to the face, neck, or abdomen that lead to bleeding within the gastrointestinal tract.

Minimizing the time to intubation decreases the risk of aspiration in an unsecured airway. The use of RSI and intubation minimizes the time during which the airway is at risk while optimizing intubating conditions. RSI also reduces iatrogenic aspiration caused by stimulation of the trachea and pharynx during intubation that can trigger retching or vomiting.

While patients with trauma should have their cervical spine in a neutral position, they do not need to be lying flat. Elevating the head of the bed to 30° can improve intubating conditions and reduce passive flow of gastric contents into the oropharynx.

Use of cricoid pressure (Sellick maneuver) to obstruct the upper esophagus against passive reflux has been questioned. Most studies find that not only is cricoid pressure ineffective in occluding the esophagus and preventing aspiration, but it can also worsen views during laryngoscopy, prolong laryngoscopy time, and impair bag-valve-mask ventilation. In this patient, there would be a risk of dislodging the impaling object rendering cricoid pressure inappropriate. Cricoid pressure also applies undue force to the cervical spine and is impractical when intubating with the cervical collar in place.

Birenbaum A, Hajage D, Roche S et al. Effect of cricoid pressure compared with a sham procedure in the rapid sequence induction of anesthesia. The IRIS randomized clinical trial. *JAMA Surg*. 2019;154:9-17.

Smith KJ, Dobranowski J, Yip G, et al. Cricoid pressure displaces the esophagus: an observational study using magnetic resonance imaging. *Anesthesiology*. 2003;99:60-64.

Stewart JC, Bhananker S, Ramaiah R. Rapid-sequence intubation and cricoid pressure. *Int J Crit Illn Inj Sci*. 2014;4:42-49.

C.9. How would you anesthetize the airway for awake tracheal intubation?

Innervation of the airway includes three neural pathways: cranial nerves V, IX, and X. The nasal airway is innervated by the maxillary branch of the *trigeminal nerve* (V), from the nares to the base of the uvula. The *facial nerve* (VII) supplies motor distribution to the facial muscles, parasympathetic supply to the oral cavity and lacrimal gland, and sensory distribution to the anterior two-thirds of the tongue. The *glossopharyngeal nerve* (IX) includes the pharyngeal branch innervating the walls of the pharynx, the posterior third of the tongue, and the vallecula, the lingual branch innervating the anterior surface of the epiglottis, and the tonsillar branch innervating the tonsils are respectively innervated by. Branches of the *vagus nerve* (X) innervate the posterior surface of the epiglottis, the larynx, and the lower airway. The *hypoglossal nerve* (XII) innervates the tongue musculature, acting as the physiologic obturator and opening the hypopharynx. Sensory innervation of the anterior two-thirds of the tongue is provided by the lingual branch of the trigeminal nerve (V), including taste; it is not essential to airway anesthesia.

Anesthetizing the airway is best understood by anatomic territory and technique, whether performed awake or sedated. Awake, the nasal cavity should be thoroughly prepared in order to minimize the risk of bleeding. Nasal techniques should always be performed bilaterally and begin with oxymetazoline 0.05% spray in single-use metered dispensers, plus glycopyrrolate 0.2 mg IV to provide a dry, insensate naris. *When awake*, dense anesthesia is provided by topical 4% cocaine or 2% lidocaine mixed with phenylephrine (10 mg) administered using soaked pledgets. It is important to thoroughly apply the anesthetizing mixture, as well as give an adequate soak time of approximately 10 minutes for a satisfactory block and to allow for vasoconstriction. The nervous structures are the ethmoid nerve and the sphenopalatine ganglion. *Following sedation*, the nares are lubricated with 6 mL mixture of 5% lidocaine jelly and 1% lidocaine in each naris. Sequential insertion of lubricated nasopharyngeal airways, typically starting at 28F and up to 36F, is a common practice during nasal intubation, but it is possible that there is little to no benefit in further dilating the nostril, and the maneuver could increase bleeding. An alternative approach is inserting an appropriately sized nasopharyngeal airway and keeping it in place for at least 1 minute to facilitate anesthesia and vasoconstriction.

Oral techniques in the awake patient include topical or nebulized lidocaine, followed by oral airway blocks. Superior laryngeal nerve blocks are performed bilaterally near the greater cornu of the hyoid bone with 2% lidocaine injections of 3 mL each. Glossopharyngeal nerve blocks are performed bilaterally in the palatoglossal arch, and 5% lidocaine is placed on an oral airway that is gradually advanced into the oral cavity until fully seated, when it is then replaced by a flexible fiberoptic bronchoscope with a lubricated and sheathed endotracheal tube. With manual jaw thrust by an assistant, judicious advancement of the bronchoscope is generally well tolerated. If stability of the cervical spine is in doubt, inline stabilization should be held while the blocks are performed and coughing occurs. In the present case, both superior laryngeal and transtracheal blocks would be difficult to perform, and induced coughing might exacerbate the injury. Administration of nebulized lidocaine might be a safer choice.

Gotta AW, Sullivan CA. Anaesthesia of the upper airway using topical anaesthetic and superior laryngeal nerve block. *Br J Anaesth*. 1981;53:1055-1058.

Hawke A, Stamper S. Cervical plexus block. In: Farag E, Mounir-Soliman L, eds. *Brown's Atlas of Regional Anesthesia*. 7th ed. Elsevier; 2024: 215-217.

Iowa head and neck protocols: glossopharyngeal nerve block (gag reflex, transoral vocal cord surgery). n.d. Accessed October 31, 2024. https://medicine.uiowa.edu/iowaprotocols/glossopharyngeal-nerve-block-gag-reflex-transoral-vocal-cord-surgery

NYSORA—World Leader in Anesthesiology Education. Published April 21, 2023. Accessed October 31, 2024. https://www.nysora.com/

C.10. What are the risks of awake fiberoptic tracheal intubation?

Successful execution of this technique requires an experienced practitioner, a cooperative, lightly or non-sedated patient, and an adequate soak time for local anesthetic topicalization. This technique is not to be rushed and requires several minutes to prevent the airway from becoming bloody and ruin fiberoptic visualization. Trauma patients with hypoxemia should be managed with other techniques. Backup techniques, including orotracheal intubation following induction of general anesthesia and surgical airway management, should be readily available. The greatest risk of awake fiberoptic intubation is deterioration of the patient's airway or mental status during the procedure. Increased intravenous sedation is not a substitute for inadequate topical anesthesia. Uncommon complications include injury to nerves or vessels during nerve blocks, toxicity from local anesthetics, and direct injury to the pharyngeal or laryngeal mucosa.

In this case, the possibility of dislodgment of the impaling tree branch during sedation and nerve blocks or during tracheal intubation is an additional risk. Bleeding from a loss of tamponade, both external and concealed, or disruption could necessitate a sudden change in the anesthetic or surgical plans. Although awake fiberoptic intubation in the OR is a reasonable starting point, the team must be prepared to escalate care to RSI or emergent surgical airway access. The OR is the best place for management of this patient, provided the patient is stable for transport.

Joseph TT, Gal JS, DeMaria S, et al. A retrospective study of success, failure, and time needed to perform awake intubation. *Anesthesiology*. 2016;125:105-114.

C.11. If the patient cannot be ventilated, what options are available?

Failure of awake fiberoptic intubation should be followed by an immediate attempt at RSI. If RSI is not possible and the patient cannot be ventilated by mask or supraglottic airway (SGA), a surgical airway must be established. The anesthesiologist should attempt to awaken the patient. Use of transnasal humidified rapid-insufflation ventilatory exchange (THRIVE) can provide a bridge until a surgical airway is established, but it requires a patent airway in order to work. If intubation is not feasible because of blockage of the upper airway, the team should proceed promptly with emergency front-of-neck access (eFONA). This equipment should be available at all airway management sites. Early invasive airway access, when appropriate, is associated with improved outcome. The airway practitioner should be trained in this technique and have periodic retraining.

Cook TM, Woodall N, Frerk C; Fourth National Audit Project. Major complications of airway management in the UK: results of the Fourth National Audit Project of the Royal College of Anaesthetists and the Difficult Airway Society. Part 1: anaesthesia. *Br J Anaesth*. 2011;106:617-631.

Sud A, Patel A. THRIVE: five years on and into the COVID-19 era. *Br J Anaesth*. 2021;126:768-773.

C.12. Would a supraglottic airway (SGA) or other pharyngeal airway device be of assistance?

Although a supraglottic airway (SGA) is an integral part of the American Society of Anesthesiologists Difficult Airway Algorithm and the Difficult Airway Society 2015 Guidelines for management of the unanticipated difficult intubation in adults, this case could represent an exception. Establishing an effective airway by mask or SGA is beneficial when the etiology is neurologic (diminished respiratory drive due to sedatives) or related to changes in pharyngeal anatomy (obstruction following administration of a NMBA). The SGA is not helpful with distal airway obstruction, such as bronchospasm, tracheal disruption, massive aspiration, or penetrating foreign airway in or near the airway.

Apfelbaum JL, Hagberg CA, Connis RT, et al. 2022 American Society of Anesthesiologists practice guidelines for management of the difficult airway. *Anesthesiology*. 2022;136:31-81.

Frerk C, Mitchell VD, McNarry AF, et al. Difficult Airway Society intubation guidelines working group. Difficult Airway Society 2015 guidelines for management of unanticipated difficult intubation in adults. *Br J Anaesth*. 2015; 115:827-848.

C.13. What surgical airway options are available in this case?

Surgical airway access is beneficial when the cause of airway obstruction is proximal to the site of surgical access. eFONA access, for example cricothyroidotomy, is the fastest and most readily available surgical airway procedure. It is of benefit in CICO situations where the airway obstruction is in the pharynx, hypopharynx, or larynx. Current recommendations are to perform eFONA using a scalpel and bougie with a 6.0-cuffed endotracheal tube. eFONA is faster than conventional tracheostomy and can be performed by trained nonsurgical clinicians. It is, however, more traumatic and less stable. The eFONA airway should be either surgically closed or revised to a conventional tracheostomy in the OR.

Emergent surgical tracheostomy is performed lower in the airway, usually between the first and second tracheal rings. It requires more time for airway access due to the need for tissue dissection and the greater risk of hemorrhage. In this case, surgical access to the lower trachea might be required if the impaling object has disrupted or transected the upper trachea, which would require the full resources of the OR including a rigid bronchoscopy with jet ventilation and a full or partial median sternotomy. Disruption of the major vessels at the base of the neck and mediastinum could require massive transfusion. Extracorporeal membrane oxygenation (ECMO) might be necessary for tracheal repair.

DeVore EK, Redmann A, Howell R, et al. Best practices for emergency surgical airway: a systematic review. *Laryngoscope Investig Otolaryngol*. 2019;4:602-608.

Kempema JM, D. Trust M, Brown CR. Management of the airway. In: Feliciano DV, Mattox KL, Moore EE. eds. *Trauma*. 9th ed. McGraw Hill; 2020. Accessed April 17, 2025. https://accesssurgery-mhmedical-com.ezproxy.med.cornell.edu/content.aspx?bookid=2952&sectionid=249117625

C.14. What maintenance anesthetics are indicated or contraindicated in this patient?

If initial awake fiberoptic examination of the larynx and trachea at the time of intubation rules out airway injury, then the use of NMBAs to facilitate surgical exposure is appropriate for the duration of the case. If, however, there is an airway injury, volatile anesthetics alone, with continued spontaneous ventilation, offer additional security in the event of airway discontinuity during the surgical repair. Sevoflurane, because of its greater palatability, is the least irritating volatile anesthetic. Care must be taken to ensure adequate fluid volume replacement during a pure inhalational anesthetic to avoid hemodynamic instability. Nitrous oxide is contraindicated when the potential for pneumothorax exists or when airway continuity is in doubt.

Opioids are frequently required for postoperative analgesia and offer some intraoperative advantages. Once airway patency is confirmed, an opioid-based anesthetic technique lowers the level of circulating catecholamines, simplifying physiologic assessment and management of fluid resuscitation. The usual concern with delayed emergence in a patient receiving a larger dose of opioids is not relevant here because the patient will most likely require postoperative mechanical ventilation. The only caveat to an opioid-based technique here is the potential need to sustain spontaneous ventilation postoperatively while the airway is assessed; one should therefore implement this technique after patient disposition, surgical and anesthetic plans are jointly decided.

Lodhia VJ, Eyre L, Smith M, et al. Management of thoracic trauma. *Anaesthesia*. 2022;78:225-235.

C.15. What complications will the surgical plan introduce?

Maintenance of homeostasis in the face of surgical intervention is a common concern. At some point, ideally after anesthetic induction, successful airway management, and placement of lines and monitors, the impaling object will be removed from the patient's neck. Blunt object impalements in patients seen alive in the trauma center produce less organ-specific damage than predicted from the location and course of the injury due to the ability of mobile anatomic structures to deform away from low-speed penetrations. Even so, it is possible that this object injured one of the great vessels or the trachea and that removing it might lead to heavy bleeding or disruption of the airway. The anesthesia team must be prepared to change course rapidly from a spontaneous breathing inhalational approach (assuming that airway continuity is the initial concern) to an opioid-based approach if blood loss and hemorrhagic shock become the major issue. An open team discussion of both surgical and anesthetic plans, including likely contingencies, is essential before beginning definitive treatment.

Dutton RP. Shock management. In: Smith CE, ed. *Trauma Anesthesia*. 2nd ed. Cambridge University Press; 2015:65-78.

D. Postoperative Management

D.1. What are the criteria for tracheal extubation?

Assuming that the case goes well, and the patient's anatomic injuries are successfully repaired, it is appropriate to consider emergence and tracheal extubation when the following criteria are satisfied:

- Hemodynamic stability with complete cessation of bleeding and normal coagulation
- Adequate respiratory drive and reserve, including complete return of neuromuscular function and minimal requirement for ventilator support
- Acceptable mental status; the patient should be calm, cooperative, comfortable, not overly sedated, and recovered from acute intoxication.

- Evidence of airway patency. Edema at the site of injury will not be an issue with a tracheal tube in place but might obstruct the airway quickly following extubation. Although not 100% predictive, the presence of an air leak around the tracheal tube when the cuff is deflated is reassuring.
- Completion of the diagnostic workup for high-energy trauma, including indicated CT scans, laboratory studies, and completion of all procedures that are likely to require general anesthesia. Extubation should be deferred if there is a likelihood for other urgently planned surgery such as orthopedic procedures.

Steurer MP, Sikorski RA, Richards JE, Galvagno SM. Anesthesia for trauma. In: Gropper MA, Eriksson LI, Fleisher LA, Cohen NH, Leslie K, Johnson-Akeju O, eds. *Miller's Anesthesia*. 10th ed. Vol 2. Elsevier; 2025:2000-2043.

D.2. What techniques may be used during extubation?

The best results from extubation will be achieved when the patient is calm and comfortable and when the extubation itself is as nonstimulating as possible. The appropriate level of sedation and analgesia is complex, controversial, and important. Sedatives and hypnotics, such as benzodiazepines and propofol, diminish respiratory drive, cooperation, and ability to protect the airway, and should be minimized. An appropriate dose of opioids can allow for a comfortable patient with diminished airway reactivity who can open their eyes and follow commands but is not otherwise distressed by tubes or the ventilator. The tracheal tube should be suctioned ahead of time, and extubation should be delayed if copious secretions are present. The posterior pharynx is suctioned, the patient is asked to inhale deeply, the tracheal cuff is deflated, and the tracheal tube is removed as the patient exhales.

The airway is in jeopardy immediately after extubation by edema and secretions. Continuous pulse oximetry in a monitored setting is required, and humidified oxygen should be administered for 24 hours following extubation.

D.3. How does alcohol misuse affect postoperative management?

Symptomatic withdrawal from alcohol usually occurs within 24 hours and manifests as agitation, tachycardia, and hypertension. Delirium tremens can occur thereafter if prophylactic therapy is not initiated. Prophylaxis should consist of a small basal dose of a benzodiazepine or a low-dose intravenous alcohol infusion, with frequent assessment of mental status and supplemental short-acting benzodiazepines if symptoms develop. The plan for delirium tremens prophylaxis should be coordinated with the pain management plan, ideally under the direction of a single individual, to assure overall consistency while avoiding oversedation and respiratory arrest secondary to the synergistic central respiratory depressant effects of multiple drugs.

D.4. What pain medications should be used for analgesia?

Postoperative analgesia in this case will depend on the extent of the surgical procedure and on the individual tolerance of the patient. Soft-tissue exploration of the neck, including surgery on the trachea or major vessels, requires relatively little postoperative analgesia. Titrated intravenous opioids can be used in the first 24 hours, with a rapid transition to an oral opioid/acetaminophen preparation thereafter. Median sternotomy or other significant extension of the surgery into the chest will necessitate more intensive postoperative analgesia, including a continuous opioid infusion while the patient remains intubated, followed by intravenous patient-controlled analgesia after emergence and extubation. Nonsteroidal anti-inflammatory drugs are an appropriate adjuvant therapy once the risk of traumatic hemorrhage is past.

34 Open-Eye Injury and Cataract Surgery

Alaeldin A. Darwich and Joe E.L. Bryant-Huppert

CASE 1

A 28-year-old, otherwise healthy male presented to the emergency room with a fishhook embedded in his eye. He had eaten a full meal just before the fishing accident.

A. Medical Disease and Differential Diagnosis

1. Why is this patient a particular challenge to the anesthesiologist?
2. What are the determinants of intraocular pressure (IOP) under normal circumstances? What is the normal range? What was the expected IOP in this patient's injured eye?
3. How is aqueous humor formed and eliminated?
4. How is IOP affected by arterial Pco_2, systemic arterial pressure, coughing and vomiting, deep inspiration, and hypoxemia?
5. What is the impact of central nervous system (CNS) on IOP?
6. What is glaucoma?
7. Is atropine contraindicated in patients with glaucoma?
8. How do carbonic anhydrase inhibitors decrease IOP? By what mechanism can osmotic agents decrease IOP?
9. Are carbonic anhydrase inhibitors or osmotic diuretics indicated in open-globe eye injuries?
10. Are topically applied ophthalmic medications absorbed systemically? How can this absorption be reduced? Which eye drops can have effects that are of concern to the anesthesiologist?

B. Preoperative Evaluation and Preparation

1. Is an open-globe eye injury always a surgical emergency?
2. What preoperative evaluation would you require?
3. The patient ate shortly before the accident. Would you attempt to pass a nasogastric tube or administer emetics to empty the stomach?
4. Could this case be done with topical anesthesia or a retrobulbar block?
5. How would you premedicate this patient?

C. Intraoperative Management

1. What factors can increase the risk of vitreous herniation during induction and maintenance of anesthesia?
2. Will you intubate the trachea of this patient? Would you consider a laryngeal mask airway? How does tracheal intubation affect IOP? How can this effect be minimized?
3. Would you consider awake tracheal intubation?
4. Is succinylcholine contraindicated in open-globe eye injuries? How does succinylcholine affect IOP?
5. Does pretreatment with nondepolarizing neuromuscular blocking agents prevent succinylcholine-induced elevation in IOP?
6. How do nondepolarizing neuromuscular blocking agents affect IOP?
7. How will you perform a rapid sequence induction of anesthesia and tracheal intubation without using succinylcholine?
8. What are the effects of ketamine on the eye?
9. Would you consider the use of etomidate as an induction agent or prefer the use of propofol?
10. How do inhalation agents affect IOP and by what mechanism?

11. During the procedure, the patient's pulse rate suddenly decreased to 40 beats per minute. What do you think was happening? What is oculocardiac reflex (OCR)?
12. What are afferent and efferent pathways of OCR?
13. What factors increase the incidence of OCR?
14. How do you diagnose and treat OCR?
15. Is atropine or glycopyrrolate useful for treating OCR?
16. Can a retrobulbar block prevent OCR? Is it appropriate for this patient?

D. Postoperative Management

1. Would you reverse the neuromuscular blockade in this patient?
2. Do reversal doses of atropine affect IOP?
3. What would you do before tracheal extubation of this patient?
4. What can you do to reduce coughing during emergence?
5. When would you extubate this patient?
6. The patient awoke in the recovery room and complained of pain and tearing in the opposite eye. The conjunctiva was inflamed. What was the probable cause?
7. Will taping the eyes shut or applying ointment prevent corneal abrasions? Are there any contributing factors?
8. What should you do when you suspect a corneal abrasion?
9. A month after surgical repair, the patient complained of impaired vision in the operative eye. He was examined and found to have a detached retina. As part of the surgical treatment, the ophthalmologist injected a gas bubble into the patient's posterior chamber. Why is this important to an anesthesiologist?

CASE 2

A 77-year-old male is scheduled for cataract surgery. His medical history is significant for hypertension, diabetes mellitus type 2, chronic atrial fibrillation, coronary artery disease, and three coronary drug-eluding stents placed 5 years ago. He is on multiple medications related to his condition.

E. Anesthesia for Cataract Surgery

1. What is a cataract?
2. What are the causes and risk factors of cataract formation?
3. How would you conduct the preoperative medical evaluation for a patient having cataract surgery?
4. What is the cardiac risk for this patient? If this patient is on anticoagulant and/or antiplatelet medications, should the patient stop or continue these medications?
5. What are the anesthetic options for cataract surgery?
6. What is the postoperative course after cataract surgery?

CASE 1

A. Medical Disease and Differential Diagnosis

A.1. Why is this patient a particular challenge to the anesthesiologist?

The combination of a full stomach and an open-globe eye injury presents a unique challenge to the anesthesiologist. In addition to the increased risk of aspiration of gastric contents, any drug or maneuver that raises intraocular pressure (IOP) in the injured, open eye can cause extrusion of the vitreous humor and loss of vision when the globe is opened.

Kelly DJ, Farrell SM. Physiology and role of intraocular pressure in contemporary anesthesia. *Anesth Analg*. 2018; 126:1551-1562.

Pucchio A, Pur DR, Dhawan A, Sodhi SK, Pereira A, Choudhry N. Anesthesia for ophthalmic surgery: an educational review. *Int Ophthalmol*. 2023;43:1761-1769.

A.2. What are the determinants of intraocular pressure (IOP) under normal circumstances? What is the normal range? What was the expected IOP in this patient's injured eye?

IOP is determined by the balance between production and drainage of aqueous humor, by changes in choroidal blood volume, and by vitreous volume and extraocular muscle tone. Resistance to outflow of aqueous humor in the trabecular tissue is the factor that maintains IOP within physiologic range, but the mechanism of homeostasis is unknown.

Normal IOP is 12 to 16 mm Hg in the upright posture and increases by 2 to 4 mm Hg in the supine position. IOP has been observed to nearly double in steep head-down Trendelenburg position (SHDT) within 60 minutes in the operating room and it continues to increase over time.

When the globe is open, IOP is lowered and can be as low as ambient pressure. The concern in this case is for the relative volume of choroid and vitreous humor within the eye. If this volume increases while the eye is open, the vitreous humor can be lost. Any eye deformation by external pressure in the globe can increase IOP.

Jay JL. Functional organization of the human eye. *Br J Anaesth*. 1980;52:649-654.

Kohli R, Ramsingh H, Makkad B. The anesthetic management of ocular trauma. *Int Anesthesiol Clin*. 2007;45:83-98.

Ripa M, Shipa C, Kopsacheilis N, et al. The impact of steep Trendelenburg position on intraocular pressure. *J Clin Med*. 2022; 11:2844.

A.3. How is aqueous humor formed and eliminated?

Aqueous humor is a clear fluid that occupies the anterior and posterior chambers of the eye; its total volume is 0.3 mL. Aqueous humor is produced primarily by an active secretory process from the ciliary body in the posterior chambers at an equilibrium rate of 2 μL/min. The aqueous humor then circulates through the pupil to the anterior chamber, passes through the trabeculated Fontana spaces, and enters the canal of Schlemm. From there, fluid drains into the episcleral veins and finally into the cavernous sinus or jugular venous systems (**Figure 34.1**).

Kelly DJ, Farrell SM. Physiology and role of intraocular pressure in contemporary anesthesia. *Anesth Analg*. 2018;126:1551-1562.

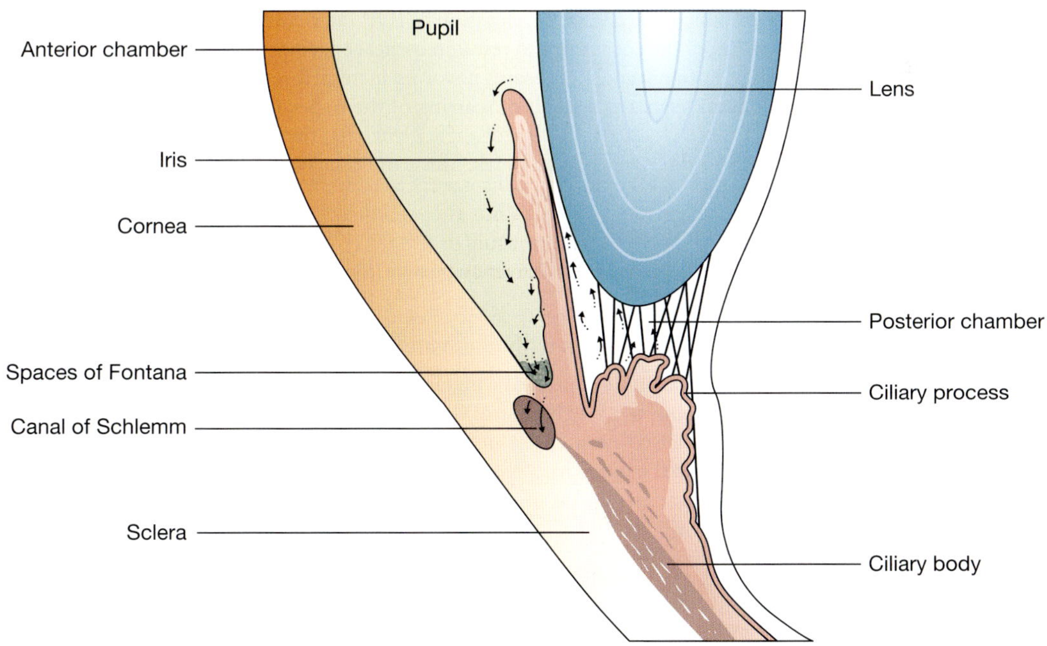

FIGURE 34.1. Sites of formation, circulation, and drainage of aqueous humor. (Modified by permission from Springer: Cunningham AJ, Barry P. Intraocular pressure—physiology and implications for anaesthetic management. *Can Anaesth Soc J*. 1986;33:195-208. Copyright © 1986 Canadian Anesthesiologists.)

SECTION 9

A.4. How is IOP affected by arterial P_{CO_2}, systemic arterial pressure, coughing and vomiting, deep inspiration, and hypoxemia?

The choroidal arterioles vasodilate in response to hypercapnia and constrict during hypocapnia, thereby changing intraocular volume and pressure. However, the effect is minimal within the normal physiologic range of P_{CO_2}.

Minor fluctuations in the arterial blood pressure also have minimal effects on IOP, although IOP can increase when hypertension is sustained and can fall with induced hypotension. Changes in venous pressure, on the other hand, greatly impact IOP. Vomiting, coughing, and bucking on an endotracheal tube cause a large increase in IOP of 30 to 40 mm Hg. These actions and the Valsalva maneuver cause congestion in the venous system, which impedes outflow of aqueous humor and increases the volume of choroidal blood. Deep inspiration can reduce IOP by 5 mm Hg. Hypoxemia can increase IOP through choroidal vasodilation.

Beulen P, Rotteveel J, de Haan A, et al. Ultrasonographic assessment of congestion of the choroid plexus in relation to carbon dioxide pressure. *Eur J Ultrasound*. 2000;11:25-29.

Calobrisi BL, Lebowitz P. Muscle relaxants and the open globe. *Int Anesthesiol Clin*. 1990;28:83-88.

Gayer S, Palte HD. Ophthalmology and otolaryngology. In: Pardo MC, ed. *Miller's Basics of Anesthesia*. 8th ed. Elsevier, 2023;31:546-558.

Kelly DJ, Farrell SM. Physiology and role of intraocular pressure in contemporary anesthesia. *Anesth Analg*. 2018;126:1551-1562.

A.5. What is the impact of central nervous system (CNS) on IOP?

The CNS influences IOP through alterations in extraocular muscle tone or, indirectly, by hormonal or hemodynamic changes.

Cunningham AJ, Barry P. Intraocular pressure—physiology and implications for anaesthetic management. *Can Anaesth Soc J*. 1986;33:195-208.

Kelly DJ, Farrell SM. Physiology and role of intraocular pressure in contemporary anesthesia. *Anesth Analg*. 2018;126:1551-1562.

A.6. What is glaucoma?

Glaucoma is a pathologic elevation of IOP caused by increased resistance to outflow of aqueous humor from the anterior chamber of the eye. It is classified as either open-angle or closed-angle glaucoma, depending on the anatomy and pathophysiology. Chronic elevation of IOP interferes with the intraocular blood supply and normal metabolism of the cornea. It can result in corneal opacities or decreased retinal blood flow.

The pathophysiology in open-angle glaucoma involves increased resistance to the flow of aqueous humor through the Fontana spaces as a result of scarring of the trabecular network or thickening of the endothelial covering of these channels. In closed-angle glaucoma, the iris bulges forward blocking the access of aqueous humor to the trabecular network. This can occur with pupillary dilation or an acutely swollen lens.

Johnson DH, Brubaker RF. Glaucoma: an overview. *Mayo Clin Proc*. 1986;61:59-67.

Kelly DJ, Farrell SM. Physiology and role of intraocular pressure in contemporary anesthesia. *Anesth Analg*. 2018;126:1551-1562.

A.7. Is atropine contraindicated in patients with glaucoma?

Topical atropine in the eye is generally contraindicated in patients with glaucoma, especially in those with closed-angle glaucoma. Atropine, in a single dose of 0.01 mg/kg intramuscularly (IM) or orally as 0.6 mg in two doses 4 hours apart, caused no increase in IOP in either open-angle or closed-angle glaucoma since only ~0.0001 mg reaches the eye, which is far less than a topical dose. Intravenous (IV) atropine is minimally associated with mydriasis and is minimally absorbed by the eye, and can be used when indicated during anesthesia. Preemptive topical use of pupillary constrictors such as pilocarpine and Timolol can help prevent this problem.

Gayer S, Palte HD. Ophthalmology and otolaryngology. In: Pardo MC, ed. *Miller's Basics of Anesthesia*. 8th ed. Elsevier, 2023;31:546-558

Greenstein SH, Abramson DH, Pitts WR III. Systemic atropine and glaucoma. *Bull N Y Acad Med*. 1984;60:961-968.

Kelly DJ, Farrell SM. Physiology and role of intraocular pressure in contemporary anesthesia. *Anesth Analg*. 2018;126:1551-1562.

A.8. How do carbonic anhydrase inhibitors decrease IOP? By what mechanism can osmotic agents decrease IOP?

Carbonic anhydrase inhibitors, such as acetazolamide, reduce secretion of aqueous humor. An IV dose acts in 5 minutes, with maximal effect in 20 to 30 minutes. Chronic acetazolamide therapy can result in potassium depletion.

Osmotic agents, such as mannitol, increase plasma oncotic pressure relative to that of aqueous humor and produce an acute, transient drop in IOP. The maximum reduction in IOP occurs after 30 to 45 minutes, and the effect lasts 5 to 6 hours.

Kelly DJ, Farrell SM. Physiology and role of intraocular pressure in contemporary anesthesia. *Anesth Analg.* 2018;126:1551-1562.

McGoldrick KE. Ocular drugs and anesthesia. *Int Anesthesiol Clin.* 1990;28:72-77.

Pritchard NC. General anaesthesia for ophthalmic surgery. *Anaesth Intensive Care Med.* 2017;18:33-36.

A.9. Are carbonic anhydrase inhibitors or osmotic diuretics indicated in open-globe eye injuries?

No. If the globe is open, the IOP is low, and these agents are not useful. In addition, they can cause transient choroidal congestion, which could lead to loss of ocular contents.

Smith GB. *Ophthalmic Anaesthesia.* University Park Press; 1983.

A.10. Are topically applied ophthalmic medications absorbed systemically? How can this absorption be reduced? Which eye drops can have effects that are of concern to the anesthesiologist?

Topical ophthalmic drugs can be absorbed through the conjunctiva or drain through the nasolacrimal duct and be absorbed through the nasal mucosa. Absorption is increased when the eye is instrumented, diseased, or traumatized. Finger pressure on the inner canthus for a few minutes after instillation of eye drops can impede absorption by occluding the nasolacrimal duct. The following topical medications have implications for the anesthesiologist:

Atropine

Atropine is used to produce mydriasis and cycloplegia. The 1% solution contains 0.2 to 0.5 mg of atropine per drop (there are 20 drops per milliliter). Systemic antimuscarinic effects, seen primarily in children and older adults, include tachycardia, flushing, thirst, dry skin, and agitation. Atropine is contraindicated in closed-angle glaucoma.

Scopolamine

One drop of 0.5% solution has 0.2 mg of scopolamine. CNS excitement can be treated with physostigmine, 0.015 mg/kg IV, repeated 1 or 2 times in a 15-minute period. Scopolamine is contraindicated in closed-angle glaucoma.

Cyclopentolate (Cyclogyl)

Cyclopentolate, a short-acting mydriatic and cycloplegic, can cause transient neurotoxic effects such as incoherence, visual hallucinations, slurred speech, ataxia, and seizures. It is contraindicated in closed-angle glaucoma.

Tropicamide (Mydriacyl)

Tropicamide is used to produce mydriasis for refraction or funduscopic examination. It can have CNS effects and can elevate IOP in closed-angle glaucoma.

Phenylephrine Hydrochloride (Neo-Synephrine)

Phenylephrine hydrochloride is used to produce capillary decongestion and pupillary dilatation. Applied to the cornea, phenylephrine hydrochloride can cause palpitations, nervousness, tachycardia, headache, nausea and vomiting, severe hypertension, reflex bradycardia, and subarachnoid hemorrhage. The dose is one drop per eye per hour of the 2.5% solution (children) or the 5% solution (adults).

Epinephrine

Topical 2% epinephrine will decrease aqueous secretion, improve outflow, and lower IOP. Side effects include hypertension, palpitations, fainting, pallor, and tachycardia. The effects last approximately 15 minutes. One drop of 2% solution contains 0.5 to 1 mg of epinephrine. Epinephrine 1:200,000 in a balanced salt solution is sometimes continuously infused into the anterior chamber during cataract surgery.

Timolol Maleate (Timoptic)

Timolol maleate is a β-blocker used in the treatment of chronic glaucoma as it lowers IOP. Side effects include light-headedness, fatigue, disorientation, depressed CNS function, and exacerbation of asthma. Bradycardia and bronchospasm can occur as well as potentiation of systemic β-blockers.

Betaxolol Hydrochloride (Betoptic)

Betaxolol HCl is a cardioselective (β_1) blocking agent used to treat glaucoma, similarly through lowering IOP. It has a lesser systemic effect but should be used with caution in patients with sinus bradycardia, heart block, or heart failure.

Acetylcholine

Acetylcholine can be injected intraoperatively into the anterior chamber to produce miosis. Side effects are due to its parasympathetic action and include hypotension, bradycardia, and bronchospasm. IV atropine is an effective treatment.

Echothiophate Iodide (Phospholine Iodide)

Echothiophate iodide, a cholinesterase inhibitor, is used as a miotic agent. It can prolong the effect of both succinylcholine and ester-type local anesthetics. Levels of pseudocholinesterase decrease by 80% after 2 weeks on the drug. It takes 3 to 6 weeks to return to normal pseudocholinesterase activity after stopping the drug (4 weeks for return to 75% activity). Succinylcholine and ester-type local anesthetics should be avoided.

Cocaine

Cocaine is used to produce vasoconstriction and to shrink mucous membranes during dacryocystorhinostomy. One drop of 4% solution contains approximately 1.5 mg of cocaine, and the maximum dose is 3 mg/kg. Systemic effects can be seen with a dose as low as 20 mg, and involve the CNS, respiratory system, and cardiovascular system.

Fong ZT, Liew EC, Keyes MA. Anesthesia for opthalmic surgery. In: Gropper MA, Cohen NH, Eriksson LI , et al, eds. *Miller's Anesthesia*. 10th ed. Elsevier; 2025;65:2085-2102.

Gayer S, Palte HD. Ophthalmology and otolaryngology. In: Pardo MC, ed. *Miller's Basics of Anesthesia*. 8th ed. Elsevier; 2023;31: 546-558.

Gayer SI, Stein ALS. Anesthesia for ophthalmologic surgery. In: Cullen BF, Stock MC, Ortega R, et al, eds. *Barash, Cullen, and Stoelting's Clinical Anesthesia*. 9th ed. Wolters Kluwer; 2024:1321-1348.

Kelly DJ, Farrell SM. Physiology and role of intraocular pressure in contemporary anesthesia. *Anesth Analg*. 2018;126:1551-1562.

McGoldrick KE. Ocular drugs and anesthesia. *Int Anesthesiol Clin*. 1990;28:72-77.

B. Preoperative Evaluation and Preparation

B.1. Is an open-globe eye injury always a surgical emergency?

No. In most cases, surgery is not required immediately, and some time can be taken to adequately prepare the patient for anesthesia and surgery. However, surgery should be performed within 12 to 24 hours to minimize infection and other complications. Delaying surgery for gastric emptying to occur is not reliable because gastric emptying can be prolonged by this stressful situation.

Blanch RJ, Bishop J, Javidi H, et al. Effect of time to primary repair on final visual outcome after open globe injury. *Br J Ophthalmol*. 2019;10:1491-1494.

Lewis H, James I. Update on anaesthesia for paediatric ophthalmic surgery. *BJA Educ*. 2021;21:32-38.

B.2. What preoperative evaluation would you require?

An accurate, thorough history and physical examination are the best means of evaluating this patient preoperatively, and should reveal any existing medical problems that will guide selection of preoperative laboratory tests. In this otherwise healthy young patient, no routine laboratory tests are indicated for this surgery. In cases where more extensive trauma is suspected, other injuries must also be addressed such as fractures to the skull and orbit, intracranial hemorrhage, and any other injuries suggested by history and physical examination.

Fong ZT, Liew EC, Keyes MA. Anesthesia for opthalmic surgery. In: Gropper MA, Cohen NH, Eriksson LI , et al, eds. *Miller's Anesthesia*. 10th ed. Elsevier; 2025;65:2085-2102.

Gayer SI, Stein ALS. Anesthesia for ophthalmologic surgery. In: Cullen BF, Stock MC, Ortega R, et al, eds. *Barash, Cullen, and Stoelting's Clinical Anesthesia*. 9th ed. Wolters Kluwer; 2024:1321-1348.

Pucchio A, Pur DR, Dhawan A, Sodhi SK, Pereira A, Choudhry N. Anesthesia for ophthalmic surgery: an educational review. *Int Ophthalmol*. 2023;43:1761-1769.

B.3. The patient ate shortly before the accident. Would you attempt to pass a nasogastric tube or administer emetics to empty the stomach?

No. This is contraindicated when there has been a perforation of the eye since gagging, vomiting, and straining could cause a potentially disastrous increase in IOP and extrusion of intraocular contents. A cough can increase central venous pressure and choroidal blood volume and raise IOP by 34 to 40 mm Hg.

Kelly DJ, Farrell SM. Physiology and role of intraocular pressure in contemporary anesthesia. *Anesth Analg.* 2018;126:1551-1562.

Zhou Y, DiSclafani M, Jeang L, et al. Open globe injuries: review of evaluation, management, and surgical pearls. *Clin Ophthalmol.* 2022;16:2545-2559.

B.4. Could this case be done with topical anesthesia or a retrobulbar block?

General anesthesia has been the preferred technique for open-globe eye injuries. It can provide akinesia and allow for unpredictable surgical time. In this case, because the patient is not fasting, an endotracheal tube has an additional advantage as protection against aspiration, but comes with the risk of increased IOP during laryngoscopy and mask ventilation.

A retrobulbar or peribulbar injection can increase IOP because of the volume of local anesthetic used and the likelihood of the patient squeezing his eyes during injection. However, it provides akinesia and anesthesia for procedures of predicable length and complexity. Topical anesthesia with IV sedation also has been used to repair the globe in select patients with limited injury. In general, topical or regional anesthesia has been limited to smaller and/or anterior injuries than those with more complex and deeper trauma.

Of all forms of anesthesia, each has been proven to have comparable time-to-surgery and visual outcomes. Conversation around the risks (ie, aspiration, increased IOP, unpredictable duration of surgery), surgical preferences and considerations, and patient comorbidities, needs, and preferences should be navigated by the anesthesia provider.

Gayer S. Rethinking anaesthesia strategies for patients with traumatic eye injuries: Alternatives to general anaesthesia. *Curr Anaesth Crit Care.* 2006;17:191-196.

Gayer S, Palte HD. Ophthalmology and otolaryngology. In: Pardo MC, ed. *Miller's Basics of Anesthesia.* 8th ed. Elsevier; 2023:31, 546-558.

McClellan AJ, Daubert JJ, Relhan N, et al. Comparison of regional vs general anesthesia for surgical repair of open-globe injuries at a university referral center. *Ophthalmol Retina.* 2017;3:188-191.

Young S, Basavaraju A. General anaesthesia for ophthalmic surgery. *Anaesth Intensive Care Med.* 2019;20:716-720.

B.5. How would you premedicate this patient?

Sedatives and anxiolytics can be given, as necessary. Metoclopramide (0.15 mg/kg IM or IV) can be used to facilitate gastric emptying and to increase lower esophageal sphincter tone. Opioids should be used cautiously since they can cause nausea and vomiting. Nonparticulate antacids and H_2 receptor antagonists can be considered to reduce the risk of aspiration pneumonitis. IV ondansetron (0.15 mg/kg) can be given for antiemesis. Atropine or glycopyrrolate can be useful to reduce secretions, gastric acidity, and the likelihood of bradycardia due to OCR.

Gayer SI, Stein ALS. Anesthesia for ophthalmologic surgery. In: Cullen BF, Stock MC, Ortega R, et al, eds. *Barash, Cullen, and Stoelting's Clinical Anesthesia.* 9th ed. Wolters Kluwer; 2024:1321-1348.

Zhou Y, DiSclafani M, Jeang L, et al. Open globe injuries: review of evaluation, management, and surgical pearls. *Clin Ophthalmol.* 2022;16:2545-2559.

C. Intraoperative Management

C.1. What factors can increase the risk of vitreous herniation during induction and maintenance of anesthesia?

Factors that can increase the risk of vitreous herniation during induction and maintenance of anesthesia include the following:

- Face mask pressing on the eye
- Increased pressure from coughing, straining, bucking, and head-down position
- Extraocular muscle spasm induced by depolarizing neuromuscular blockers or surgical stimulation during light anesthesia

- Poorly applied cricoid pressure that blocks venous drainage from the eye
- Choroidal congestion from hypercarbia, hypoxia, osmotic diuretics, intubation, or increases in blood pressure

Gayer SI, Stein ALS. Anesthesia for ophthalmologic surgery. In: Cullen BF, Stock MC, Ortega R, et al, eds. *Barash, Cullen, and Stoelting's Clinical Anesthesia*. 9th ed. Wolters Kluwer; 2024:1321-1348.

Kelly DJ, Farrell SM. Physiology and role of intraocular pressure in contemporary anesthesia. *Anesth Analg*. 2018;126:1551-1562.

Kohli R, Ramsingh H, Makkad B. The anesthetic management of ocular trauma. *Int Anesthesiol Clin*. 2007;45:83-98.

C.2. Will you intubate the trachea of this patient? Would you consider a laryngeal mask airway? How does tracheal intubation affect IOP? How can this effect be minimized?

If electing general anesthesia, the trachea should be intubated not only to maintain the airway, which is close to the surgical field, but also to avoid pressure by a face mask on the eye and to minimize the risk of aspiration. Although a laryngeal mask airway can be successful in ophthalmologic anesthesia, it is not appropriate with a full stomach since it does not protect the airway from aspiration as well as a tracheal tube. Many studies have demonstrated a significant increase in IOP caused by laryngoscopy and intubation under varying states of anesthetic depth and neuromuscular blockade. IOP can be increased even when there is no major reaction to intubation. This increase in IOP can be attenuated by topical laryngeal anesthesia and by increased depth of anesthesia to reduce coughing, straining, and increases in blood pressure. The cardiovascular response to intubation can also be reduced by IV lidocaine (1.5 mg/kg), β-blockers, α_2-adrenergic receptor agonists, or calcium channel blockers. Topical anesthesia of the larynx is not recommended in a full-stomach situation because of the increased risk of aspiration.

Akhtar TM, McMurray P, Kerr WJ, et al. A comparison of laryngeal mask airway with tracheal tube for intra-ocular ophthalmic surgery. *Anaesthesia*. 1992;47:668-671.

Gayer SI, Stein ALS. Anesthesia for ophthalmologic surgery. In: Cullen BF, Stock MC, Ortega R, et al, eds. *Barash, Cullen, and Stoelting's Clinical Anesthesia*. 9th ed. Wolters Kluwer; 2024:1321-1348.

Kelly DJ, Farrell SM. Physiology and role of intraocular pressure in contemporary anesthesia. *Anesth Analg*. 2018;126:1551-1562.

C.3. Would you consider awake tracheal intubation?

Awake tracheal intubation is frequently accompanied by coughing and bucking and is risky in an open-globe eye injury when other safe methods of intubation are available. However, when dealing with a possible compromised airway or difficult intubation, awake flexible fiberoptic intubation expertly done under careful sedation might be indicated to safely secure the airway.

Gayer SI, Stein ALS. Anesthesia for ophthalmologic surgery. In: Cullen BF, Stock MC, Ortega R, et al, eds. *Barash, Cullen, and Stoelting's Clinical Anesthesia*. 9th ed. Wolters Kluwer; 2024:1321-1348.

Kelly DJ, Farrell SM. Physiology and role of intraocular pressure in contemporary anesthesia. *Anesth Analg*. 2018;126:1551-1562.

Kohli R, Ramsingh H, Makkad B. The anesthetic management of ocular trauma. *Int Anesthesiol Clin*. 2007;45:83-98.

C.4. Is succinylcholine contraindicated in open-globe eye injuries? How does succinylcholine affect IOP?

Use of succinylcholine in open-globe eye injuries is controversial. In the intact eye, following thiopental induction, succinylcholine can increase IOP by 6 to 8 mm Hg between 1 and 4 minutes after administration. Tracheal intubation further increases IOP, which returns to baseline in 5 to 7 minutes. In open-globe injuries, succinylcholine use has been associated with a theoretical loss of ocular contents. The increase in IOP can be mediated by prolonged tonic contraction of the extraocular muscles, although IOP can rise after succinylcholine even when the extraocular muscles have been severed. Other factors that can contribute include choroidal blood flow, increased central venous pressure, and increased resistance to outflow of aqueous humor resulting from the cycloplegic effects of succinylcholine. Traditionally, succinylcholine use has been avoided due to these reasons, however, it is not contraindicated based on current evidence.

The hemodynamic response to laryngoscopy or tracheal intubation can have a much more significant effect on IOP than succinylcholine alone. Simply blinking will increase IOP in a normal eye by 10 to 15 mm Hg, similar to the effect of succinylcholine. Pretreatment with nifedipine or lidocaine can attenuate the increase in IOP following succinylcholine and intubation.

Fong ZT, Liew EC, Keyes MA. Anesthesia for opthalmic surgery. In: Gropper MA, Cohen NH, Eriksson LI , et al, eds. *Miller's Anesthesia*. 10th ed. Elsevier; 2025;65:2085-2102.

Kelly DJ, Farrell SM. Physiology and role of intraocular pressure in contemporary anesthesia. *Anesth Analg*. 2018;126:1551-1562.

Kelly RE, Dinner M, Turner LS, et al. Succinylcholine increases intraocular pressure in the human eye with the extraocular muscles detached. *Anesthesiology*. 1993;79:948-952.

C.5. Does pretreatment with nondepolarizing neuromuscular blocking agents prevent succinylcholine-induced elevation in IOP?

Available data are contradictory, reflecting the different methods of IOP measurement under varying depths of anesthesia with a variety of anesthetic adjuvant agents. Many techniques have been tried to prevent succinylcholine-induced elevation of IOP, and none has been consistently effective. However, there are no published reports of loss of ocular contents when succinylcholine use has been preceded by pretreatment with a nondepolarizing neuromuscular blocking agent for induction.

Gayer SI, Stein ALS. Anesthesia for ophthalmologic surgery. In: Cullen BF, Stock MC, Ortega R, et al, eds. *Barash, Cullen, and Stoelting's Clinical Anesthesia*. 9th ed. Wolters Kluwer; 2024:1321-1348.

Kelly DJ, Farrell SM. Physiology and role of intraocular pressure in contemporary anesthesia. *Anesth Analg*. 2018; 126:1551-1562.

C.6. How do nondepolarizing neuromuscular blocking agents affect IOP?

Nondepolarizing neuromuscular blocking agents either decrease or have no effect on IOP.

Calobrisi BL, Lebowitz P. Muscle relaxants and the open globe. *Int Anesthesiol Clin*. 1990;28:83-88.

Kelly DJ, Farrell SM. Physiology and role of intraocular pressure in contemporary anesthesia. *Anesth Analg*. 2018; 126:1551-1562.

C.7. How will you perform a rapid sequence induction of anesthesia and tracheal intubation without using succinylcholine?

Safety of the patient must always be the primary concern; preservation of the injured eye is secondary. Measures must be taken to guarantee adequate anesthetic depth and to blunt the hemodynamic responses to laryngoscopy and tracheal intubation. Pretreatment measures such as opioids, β-blockers, calcium channel blockers, lidocaine, or midazolam should be considered. Before induction, the patient should breathe 100% oxygen for several minutes via a gently applied face mask. Anesthesia can then be induced with IV propofol (2-3 mg/kg) and one of several alternatives to succinylcholine to achieve optimal intubating conditions:

- Atracurium (0.5 mg/kg) will allow safe intubation in 3 minutes. A larger bolus (1.5 mg/kg) will allow intubation in 60 to 90 seconds but can cause hypotension, tachycardia, and histamine release.
- Cisatracurium (0.10-0.15 mg/kg), because of its intermediate onset of action, is not recommended for rapid sequence tracheal intubations. Cisatracurium (0.4 mg/kg) 8 × effective dose (ED_{95}) will allow intubation in 90 seconds without histamine release, but duration of action can exceed for 60 minutes.
- Rocuronium in a large dose (1.2 mg/kg) can create adequate intubating conditions in 60 seconds. Sugammadex, in appropriate doses, can be used to reverse the profound rocuronium blockade quickly and effectively in case of difficult airway or short surgical time.
- Vecuronium (0.2 mg/kg) should provide adequate intubating conditions after 90 seconds.
- An alternative is to pretreat the patient with a small dose of nondepolarizing neuromuscular blocking agent several minutes before induction, which can shorten the onset of action and lessen the dose required of subsequently administered drug. This has been referred to as a priming dose, which is controversial in that it can lead to diplopia, muscle weakness, respiratory distress, and aspiration while

offering no definite advantage over the use of larger initial doses of nondepolarizing neuromuscular blocking agents.

- Disadvantages of use of nondepolarizing neuromuscular blocking agents include risk of pulmonary aspiration of gastric contents during the longer period (compared to succinylcholine) when the airway is unprotected. Attempts to perform laryngoscopy and intubation prematurely, before full onset of neuromuscular blockade, can result in coughing and straining with a major increase in IOP. For this reason, a peripheral neuromuscular function monitor should be used to confirm paralysis prior to laryngoscopy and tracheal intubation.

Remifentanil is another option when use of succinylcholine or prolonged duration of neuromuscular blockade are unwanted. Remifentanil bolus (3-5 μg/kg IV) provides desirable intubating conditions within 1 to 2.5 minutes. Bradycardia and hypotension from remifentanil can be attenuated with ephedrine administration upon induction.

Gayer SI, Stein ALS. Anesthesia for ophthalmologic surgery. In: Cullen BF, Stock MC, Ortega R, et al, eds. *Barash, Cullen, and Stoelting's Clinical Anesthesia*. 9th ed. Wolters Kluwer; 2024:1321-1348.

Kelly DJ, Farrell SM. Physiology and role of intraocular pressure in contemporary anesthesia. *Anesth Analg*. 2018; 126:1551-1562.

Mehta MP, Choi WW, Gergis SD, et al. Facilitation of rapid endotracheal intubations with divided doses of nondepolarizing neuromuscular blocking drugs. *Anesthesiology*. 1985;62:392-395.

C.8. What are the effects of ketamine on the eye?

Ketamine can cause nystagmus and blepharospasm and is therefore not suitable for ophthalmic surgery. Studies with respect to the effect of ketamine on IOP have shown both increased and decreased IOP in children and no change in IOP in adults premedicated with diazepam and meperidine. This may depend on the dose and whether ketamine is administered through the IM or IV route.

Antal M, Mucsi G, Faludi A. Ketamine anesthesia and intraocular pressure. *Ann Ophthalmol*. 1978;10:1281-1289.

Drayna PC, Estrada C, Wang W, et al. Ketamine sedation is not associated with clinically meaningful elevation of intraocular pressure. *Am J Emerg Med*. 2012;30:1215-1218.

Kelly DJ, Farrell SM. Physiology and role of intraocular pressure in contemporary anesthesia. *Anesth Analg*. 2018; 126:1551-1562.

Nagdeve NG, Yaddanapudi S, Pandav SS. The effect of different doses of ketamine on intraocular pressure in anesthetized children. *J Peditr Ophtalmol Strabismus*. 2006;43:219-223.

C.9. Would you consider the use of etomidate as an induction agent or prefer the use of propofol?

Although etomidate has been associated with a decrease in IOP when used as an induction agent, the unpredictable incidence of generalized myoclonus seen with etomidate use and the resultant elevation of IOP can preclude use in open-globe eye injuries, unless rapid and complete prior neuromuscular block can be guaranteed. Propofol can decrease IOP, and would be an excellent choice for induction.

Berry JM, Merin RG. Etomidate myoclonus and the open globe. *Anesth Analg*. 1989;69:256-259.

Calla S, Gupta A, Sen N, et al. Comparison of the effects of etomidate and thiopentone on intraocular pressure. *Br J Anaesth*. 1987;59:437-439.

Ferrari LR, Donlon JV. A comparison of propofol, midazolam, and methohexital for sedation during retrobulbar and peribulbar block. *J Clin Anesth*. 1992;4:93-96.

Kelly DJ, Farrell SM. Physiology and role of intraocular pressure in contemporary anesthesia. *Anesth Analg*. 2018; 126:1551-1562.

Kohli R, Ramsingh H, Makkad B. The anesthetic management of ocular trauma. *Int Anesthesiol Clin*. 2007;45:83-98.

C.10. How do inhalation agents affect IOP and by what mechanism?

Nitrous oxide has no effect in IOP, while all volatile inhalation agents cause dose-related decreases in IOP as a consequence of:

- Reduced aqueous humor production
- Depression of the CNS control center
- Facilitation of aqueous humor outflow
- Decreased extraocular muscle tension
- Lowered arterial blood pressure

The degree of IOP reduction is proportional to the depth of anesthesia.

Fong ZT, Liew EC, Keyes MA. Anesthesia for opthalmic surgery. In: Gropper MA, Cohen NH, Eriksson LI , et al, eds. *Miller's Anesthesia*. 10th ed. Elsevier; 2025;65:2085-2102.

Kelly DJ, Farrell SM. Physiology and role of intraocular pressure in contemporary anesthesia. *Anesth Analg*. 2018; 126:1551-1562.

C.11. During the procedure, the patient's pulse rate suddenly decreased to 40 beats per minute. What do you think was happening? What is oculocardiac reflex (OCR)?

The OCR is manifested by bradycardia, bigeminy, ectopy, nodal rhythms, atrioventricular block, and cardiac arrest. It is caused by traction on the extraocular muscles (especially medial rectus), ocular manipulation, or manual pressure on the globe. The OCR is commonly seen during eye muscle surgery, detached retina repair, enucleation, or whenever there is extensive traction or rotation of the globe.

Fong ZT, Liew EC, Keyes MA. Anesthesia for opthalmic surgery. In: Gropper MA, Cohen NH, Eriksson LI , et al, eds. *Miller's Anesthesia*. 10th ed. Elsevier; 2025;65:2085-2102.

Gayer SI, Stein ALS. Anesthesia for ophthalmologic surgery. In: Cullen BF, Stock MC, Ortega R, et al, eds. *Barash, Cullen, and Stoelting's Clinical Anesthesia*. 9th ed. Wolters Kluwer; 2024:1321-1348.

C.12. What are afferent and efferent pathways of OCR?

The OCR is a trigeminovagal reflex. The afferent pathway is by way of the ciliary ganglion to the ophthalmic division of the trigeminal nerve and through the Gasserian ganglion to the main sensory nucleus in the fourth ventricle. The efferent pathway is the vagus nerve.

Fong ZT, Liew EC, Keyes MA. Anesthesia for opthalmic surgery. In: Gropper MA, Cohen NH, Eriksson LI , et al, eds. *Miller's Anesthesia*. 10th ed. Elsevier; 2025;65:2085-2102.

Gayer SI, Stein ALS. Anesthesia for ophthalmologic surgery. In: Cullen BF, Stock MC, Ortega R, et al, eds. *Barash, Cullen, and Stoelting's Clinical Anesthesia*. 9th ed. Wolters Kluwer; 2024:1321-1348.

C.13. What factors increase the incidence of OCR?

Preoperative anxiety, light general anesthesia, hypoxemia, hypercarbia, and increased vagal tone because of age or drugs are associated with an increased incidence of the OCR. The reported incidence of cardiac rhythm changes during eye muscle surgery is 32% to 82%, and is higher in children.

Fong ZT, Liew EC, Keyes MA. Anesthesia for opthalmic surgery. In: Gropper MA, Cohen NH, Eriksson LI , et al, eds. *Miller's Anesthesia*. 10th ed. Elsevier; 2025;65:2085-2102.

C.14. How do you diagnose and treat OCR?

- Monitor the electrocardiogram intraoperatively and during any eye manipulation.
- Stop the surgical stimulus immediately.
- Ensure that ventilation and oxygenation is adequate.
- Ensure sufficient anesthetic depth.

The OCR can fatigue with repeated stimulation.

Fang ZT, Liew EC, Keyes MA. Anesthesia for ophthalmic surgery. In: Gropper A, ed. *Miller's Anesthesia*. 9th ed. Elsevier; 2020:69, 2194-2209.

C.15. Is atropine or glycopyrrolate useful for treating OCR?

Although anticholinergics do not preclude occurrence of bradycardia, they decrease the incidence and severity. Atropine 0.02 mg/kg or glycopyrrolate 0.01 mg/kg IV are effective for up to 30 minutes in preventing bradycardia associated with OCR. Additional doses can be given should bradycardia recur. Doses greater than 0.5 mg IV can cause tachycardia that can be detrimental in certain patients with heart disease. At least 2 to 3 mg is required to ensure a complete vagal block. IV epinephrine is rarely necessary but should always be available.

Fong ZT, Liew EC, Keyes MA. Anesthesia for opthalmic surgery. In: Gropper MA, Cohen NH, Eriksson LI , et al, eds. *Miller's Anesthesia*. 10th ed. Elsevier; 2025;65:2085-2102.

C.16. Can a retrobulbar block prevent OCR? Is it appropriate for this patient?

Retrobulbar block injection is not only unreliable in preventing OCR but can also, during the injection, cause OCR, cardiac arrest, or retrobulbar hemorrhage.

Local infiltration of the rectus muscles and a delicate operating technique can decrease the incidence of OCR. In this patient, retrobulbar block is relatively contraindicated because it can increase IOP.

Fong ZT, Liew EC, Keyes MA. Anesthesia for opthalmic surgery. In: Gropper MA, Cohen NH, Eriksson LI , et al, eds. *Miller's Anesthesia*. 10th ed. Elsevier; 2025;65:2085-2102.

McGoldrick KE. Complications of regional anesthesia for ophthalmic surgery. *Yale J Biol Med*. 1993;66:443-445.

Singh RB, Khera T, Ly V, et al. Ocular complications of perioperative anesthesia: a review. *Graefes Arch Clin Exp Ophthalmol*. 2021;259:2069-2083.

D. Postoperative Management

D.1. Would you reverse the neuromuscular blockade in this patient?

There is no contraindication to reversal provided that efforts are made to minimize coughing or bucking on the endotracheal tube.

D.2. Do reversal doses of atropine affect IOP?

Reversal doses of atropine, when given with neostigmine, do not significantly alter IOP. This combination can be used safely even in patients with glaucoma.

Gayer SI, Stein ALS. Anesthesia for ophthalmologic surgery. In: Cullen BF, Stock MC, Ortega R, et al, eds. *Barash, Cullen, and Stoelting's Clinical Anesthesia*. 9th ed. Wolters Kluwer; 2024:1321-1348.

D.3. What would you do before tracheal extubation of this patient?

- Empty the stomach with an orogastric tube while the patient is still paralyzed.
- Suction the pharynx with the patient still paralyzed or deeply anesthetized.
- Give IV antiemetics, based on the current postoperative nausea and vomiting (PONV) guidelines before the end of surgery.

Gan TJ, Belani KG, BergeseS, et al. Fourth consensus guidelines for the management of postoperative nausea and vomiting. *Anesth Analg*. 2020;131:411-448.

Zhou Y, DiSclafani M, Jeang L, et al. Open globe injuries: review of evaluation, management, and surgical pearls. *Clin Ophthalmol*. 2022;16:2545-2559.

D.4. What can you do to reduce coughing during emergence?

There are several pharmacologic options to help reduce the incidence of coughing and bucking on the endotracheal tube prior to emergence, and can help facilitate a smooth extubation:

- Lidocaine 1 to 2 mg/kg IV bolus extubation or 2% instilled into the endotracheal tube cuff or administered topically to the vocal cords or transtracheally prior to extubation
- Remifentanil 0.5 to 0.8 μg/kg IV bolus extubation or 0.1 to 0.3 ng/kg/min infusion during emergence
- Dexmedetomidine 0.25 to 1 μg/kg IV slow bolus prior to emergence

Alan T, Fergusson NA, Ng N, et al. Medications to reduce emergence coughing after general anaesthesia with tracheal intubation: a systematic review and network meta-analysis. *Br J Anaesth*. 2020;124:480-495.

Aouad MT, Al-Alami AA, Nasr VG, Souki FG, Zbeidy RA, Siddik-Sayyid SM. The effect of low-dose remifentanil on responses to the endotracheal tube during emergence from general anesthesia. *Anesth Analg*. 2009;108:1157-1160.

Gefke K, Andersen LW, Friesel E. Lidocaine given intravenously as a suppressant of cough and laryngospasm in connection with extubation after tonsillectomy. *Acta Anaesthesiol Scand*. 1983;27:111-112.

Gonzalez RM, Bjerke RJ, Drobycki T, et al. Prevention of endo-tracheal tube-induced coughing during emergence from general anesthesia. *Anesth Analg*. 1994;79:792-795.

D.5. When would you extubate this patient?

There may be a conflict between the desire to extubate awake because of the full stomach and the desire to extubate deep to prevent coughing and bucking. Because modern techniques of eye repair involve minimal risk of suture disruption with coughing, one can extubate the trachea awake, thereby protecting the airway.

Gayer S, Palte HD. Ophthalmology and otolaryngology. In: Pardo MC, ed. *Miller's Basics of Anesthesia*. 8th ed. Elsevier; 2023:31, 546-558.

D.6. The patient awoke in the recovery room and complained of pain and tearing in the opposite eye. The conjunctiva was inflamed. What was the probable cause?

General anesthesia decreases tear production and reduces normal mechanical eyelid closure. Corneal abrasions are the most common perioperative ocular injury, and this patient's complaints are consistent with that diagnosis.

Gayer SI, Stein ALS. Anesthesia for ophthalmologic surgery. In: Cullen BF, Stock MC, Ortega R, et al, eds. *Barash, Cullen, and Stoelting's Clinical Anesthesia*. 9th ed. Wolters Kluwer; 2024:1321-1348.

Grixti A, Sadri M, Watts MT. Corneal protection during general anesthesia for nonocular surgery. *Ocul Surf.* 2013; 11:109-118.

D.7. Will taping the eyes shut or applying ointment prevent corneal abrasions? Are there any contributing factors?

Even an eye that has been taped shut or lubricated can sustain a corneal abrasion. Most anesthesiologists protect the eyes in some way; abrasions, however, still occur. Corneal abrasions represent the most common ophthalmic complication associated with general anesthesia. The incidence can be as high as 44% when no preventive measures have been taken and the cornea is exposed. The mechanism is thought to be drying of or direct trauma to exposed cornea. Possible contributing factors include mask anesthesia; the prone, lateral, or Trendelenburg position; or having the patient's face in the surgical field.

Gayer SI, Stein ALS. Anesthesia for ophthalmologic surgery. In: Cullen BF, Stock MC, Ortega R, et al, eds. *Barash, Cullen, and Stoelting's Clinical Anesthesia*. 9th ed. Wolters Kluwer; 2024:1321-1348.

McKevitt I, Ward C, Robertson E. Care of the eye during anaesthesia and intensive care. *Anaesth & Intens Care Med.* 2022;23:718-722.

D.8. What should you do when you suspect a corneal abrasion?

Prompt consultation with an ophthalmologist should be solicited for precise diagnosis and treatment. The patient should be reassured that corneal abrasions heal and that relief of pain occurs within 24 to 48 hours. Possible treatments include eye patching and topical administration of antibiotics, short-acting cycloplegics, or anti-inflammatory agents. Use of eye patches is controversial. A topical anesthetic for the cornea should not be given to a patient for self-administration; misuse can cause delayed wound healing and keratopathy.

McKevitt I, Ward C, Robertson E. Care of the eye during anaesthesia and intensive care. *Anaesth Intensive Care Med.* 2022;23:718-722.

Turner A, Rabiu M. Patching for corneal abrasion. *Cochrane Database Syst Rev.* 2006;CD004764. Published April 19, 2006. doi:10.1002/14651858.CD004764.pub2

D.9. A month after surgical repair, the patient complained of impaired vision in the operative eye. He was examined and found to have a detached retina. As part of the surgical treatment, the ophthalmologist injected a gas bubble into the patient's posterior chamber. Why is this important to an anesthesiologist?

If a patient with intraocular gas needs to undergo general anesthesia before the gas bubble resorbs, nitrous oxide must be avoided because the gas will expand thereby increasing IOP. The effects on the eye can be disastrous. Various types of gases can be injected, with different durations. Patients are usually given bracelets to inform anesthesiologists that they have gas in their eye and nitrous oxide must be avoided.

Fu AD, McDonald HR, Eliott D, et al. Complications of general anesthesia using nitrous oxide in eyes with preexisting gas bubbles. *Retina.* 2002;22:569-574.

Hart RH, Vote BJ, Borthwick JH, et al. Loss of vision caused by expansion of intraocular perfluoropropane (C_3F_8) gas during nitrous oxide anesthesia. *Am J Ophthalmol.* 2002;134:761-763.

CASE 2

E. Anesthesia for Cataract Surgery

E.1. What is a cataract?

A cataract is an opacity of the lens of the eye, which interferes with clear vision.

E.2. What are the causes and risk factors of cataract formation?

Aging is the most common cause of cataracts, and exposure to oxidative stress is the second most common cause. Other risk factors linked to cataract development are diabetes mellitus, hypertension, long-term corticosteroid use (topical, systemic, oral, or inhaled), obesity, and intraocular surgeries. Modifiable risk factors include smoking, exposure to ionizing radiation, and ultraviolet light.

Cicinelli MV, Buchan JC, Nicholson M, et al. Cataracts. *Lancet.* 2023;401:377-389.

E.3. How would you conduct the preoperative medical evaluation for a patient having cataract surgery?

The majority of patients with cataracts are older adults with chronic multiple coexisting diseases. They can proceed with cataract surgery if their comorbidities are controlled. Routine preoperative testing before cataract surgery does not improve outcomes (and can even worsen outcomes due to delay in vision improvement) or patient safety and is not indicated. Medical history and physical examination should direct the need to order any test.

The evaluation should be focused on the patient's ability to understand and communicate since cataract surgery is done mostly under topical or regional anesthesia, and the patient needs to be still and cooperative. Any condition that interferes with maintaining a supine position should be evaluated, for example, chronic obstructive pulmonary disease, congestive heart failure, or claustrophobia.

Lee RM, Eke T. Choice of anaesthesia. In: Liu C, Shalaby Bardan A. *Cataract Surgery.* 1st ed. Springer; 2021:4, 29-43.

Mafi JN, Godoy-Travieso P, Wei E, et al. Evaluation of an intervention to reduce low-value preoperative care for patients undergoing cataract surgery at a safety-net health system. *JAMA Intern Med.* 2019;179:648-657.

E.4. What is the cardiac risk for this patient? If this patient is on anticoagulant and/or antiplatelet medications, should the patient stop or continue these medications?

Cataract surgery is a low-risk procedure. The risk of major adverse cardiac events or death is less than 1%. Cataract surgery has a low risk of bleeding. Anticoagulants or aspirin can be continued in the perioperative period as their benefits outweigh the bleeding risks in most cases.

Chen CL, Lin GA, Bardach NS, et al. Preoperative medical testing in medicare patients undergoing cataract surgery. *N Engl J Med.* 2015;372:1530-1538.

Cheung JJC, Liu S, Li KKW. Phacoemulsification cataract surgery in patients receiving novel oral anticoagulant medications. *Int Ophthalmol.* 2019;39:623-630.

Kumar CM, Seet E. Stopping antithrombotics during regional anaesthesia and eye surgery: crying wolf? *Br J Anaesth.* 2017;118:154-158.

E.5. What are the anesthetic options for cataract surgery?

The majority of cataract surgery is performed with local anesthesia or topical anesthetics with or without sedation. Some patients require general anesthesia if they cannot maintain a supine position or remain still and cooperative during surgery (eg, children, patients with severe dementia or neurocognitive impairment).

Topical anesthesia is the most common technique used in the United States followed by peribulbar and retrobulbar blocks. The goal of sedation is to minimize anxiety and maintain a cooperative patient during the procedure. Short-acting agents are used, for example, midazolam, remifentanil, or small doses of propofol.

To prevent rebreathing of CO_2, medical air can be flushed under the surgical drapes as administration of exogenous oxygen is a risk factor for surgical fire if electrocautery is used.

Gayer SI, Stein ALS. Anesthesia for Ophthalmologic Surgery. In: Cullen BF, Stock MC, Ortega R, et al, eds. *Barash, Cullen, and Stoelting's Clinical Anesthesia.* 9th ed. Wolters Kluwer; 2024:1321-1348.

Lee RM, Eke T. Choice of anaesthesia. In: Liu C, Shalaby Bardan A. *Cataract Surgery.* 1st ed. Springer; 2021;4:29-43.

E.6. What is the postoperative course after cataract surgery?

Hospitalization on the same day after cataract surgery is exceedingly rare (0.3%). The majority of patients are discharged from the recovery room once the discharge criteria are met. Complications that can require admission include uncontrolled elevation in the intraocular pressure, retrobulbar hemorrhage, and suprachoroidal hemorrhage. Other indications for admission are related to patient's coexisting diseases (e.g., uncontrolled hypertension, diabetes mellitus, unstable respiratory or cardiovascular conditions).

Gayer SI, Stein ALS. Anesthesia for ophthalmologic surgery. In: Cullen BF, Stock MC, Ortega R, et al, eds. *Barash, Cullen, and Stoelting's Clinical Anesthesia.* 9th ed. Wolters Kluwer; 2024:1321-1348.

Shoss BL, Tsai LM. Postoperative care in cataract surgery. *Curr Opin Ophthalmol.* 2013;24:66-73.

35 Laser Treatment for Laryngeal Lesions

Jennifer K. Lee and Yang Long

A 7-year-old girl with a history of recurrent respiratory papillomatosis (RRP) is scheduled for direct laryngoscopy and possible re-excision. The patient has had 10 papilloma excisions in the past 2 years. Currently, she is undergoing adjuvant treatment with α-interferon (IFN) but now presents with slowly progressive hoarseness.

A. Pathophysiology and Differential Diagnosis

1. What is the differential diagnosis of hoarseness in this child?
2. What causes RRP?
3. What is the typical presentation of RRP?
4. How is RRP diagnosed?
5. What treatment options are available?
6. What are the common adverse effects of α-interferon (IFN) therapy?

B. Preoperative Evaluation and Preparation

1. What are the key points in the preoperative evaluation of this patient?
2. Are any preoperative laboratory tests necessary?
3. Is it safe to premedicate this child?
4. What are the special anesthetic considerations prior to bringing the child to the operating room?

C. Intraoperative Management

1. How would you induce anesthesia in a patient with RRP?
2. Discuss airway management options during laryngeal papilloma resection.
3. What is a laser and how does it work?
4. What are the characteristics of laser radiation?
5. What are some advantages of using lasers for laryngeal surgery?
6. What are some disadvantages of lasers compared to microdebriders?
7. What special endotracheal tubes (ETTs) are available for laser surgery?
8. How would you protect the external surface of a conventional ETT for use during laser microlaryngoscopy?
9. How would you manage an airway fire?
10. What is the Venturi effect?
11. What is Venturi jet ventilation?
12. How would you institute and maintain jet ventilation?
13. How is anesthesia maintained during jet ventilation?
14. What are the complications of jet ventilation?
15. Are there contraindications to the use of jet ventilation?
16. How will you monitor this patient?

D. Postoperative Anesthetic Management

1. What are the common postoperative complications?

A. Differential Diagnosis and Medical Disease

A.1. What is the differential diagnosis of hoarseness in this child?

Given the patient's history, recurrence of laryngeal papilloma or postoperative scarring of laryngeal structures is most likely. A broader differential diagnosis for hoarseness in children includes:

Anatomic and congenital causes
- Cystic lesions (laryngocele, thyroglossal cyst)
- Vocal fold nodule, cyst, or polyp
- Glottic webs

Neoplasms
- Squamous cell carcinoma

Neurologic causes
- Vocal fold paralysis
- Spasmodic dysphonia

Inflammatory causes
- Gastroesophageal reflux
- Eosinophilic esophagitis
- Rheumatoid arthritis
- Angioneurotic edema

Infectious causes
- Croup
- Laryngotracheobronchitis
- Epiglottitis

McMurray JS. Disorders of phonation in children. *Pediatr Clin North Am*. 2003;50:363-380.

Stachler RJ, Francis DO, Schwartz SR, et al. Clinical practice guideline: hoarseness (dysphonia)(update). *Otolaryngol Head Neck Surg*. 2018;158:S1-S42.

A.2. What causes RRP?

RRP is characterized by recurring benign papillomatous lesions in the respiratory tract, particularly the larynx, caused by human papilloma virus (HPV), most commonly HPV 6 and 11. Lesions undergo malignant transformation at a rate of 2% to 4%.

Derkay CS, Campisi P. Recurrent respiratory papillomatosis. In: Flint PW, Haughey BH, Lund VJ, et al, eds. *Cummings Otolaryngology: Head and Neck Surgery*. 7th ed. Elsevier; 2020:3076-3091.

Welschmeyer A, Berke GS. An updated review of the epidemiological factors associated with recurrent respiratory papillomatosis. *Laryngoscope Investig Otolaryngol*. 2021;6:226-233.

A.3. What is the typical presentation of RRP?

RRP most commonly presents with hoarseness. Other symptoms can include dysphonia (more commonly in adults), stridor, dyspnea, chronic cough, recurrent upper respiratory infections, and dysphagia. The average age of diagnosis in children is 5 years, and in adults, the third decade of life, with a second peak in the sixth decade of life.

Moreddu E, Lambert E, Kacmarynski D, et al. Risk factors for severity of juvenile-onset recurrent respiratory papillomatosis at first endoscopy. *Eur Ann Otorhinolaryngol Head Neck Dis*. 2019;136:25-28.

Welschmeyer A, Berke GS. An updated review of the epidemiological factors associated with recurrent respiratory papillomatosis. *Laryngoscope Investig Otolaryngol*. 2021;6:226-233.

A.4. How is RRP diagnosed?

A pediatric patient presenting with a persistent change in voice quality should undergo a diagnostic flexible fiberoptic laryngoscopy by an otolaryngologist. Typical findings include multiple fragile grapelike clusters (**Figure 35.1**). Definitive diagnosis requires direct laryngoscopy with biopsy for tissue diagnosis and viral typing. HPV 11 is the more aggressive strain presenting at younger age and associated with a worse prognosis.

Derkay CS, Bluher AE. Update on recurrent respiratory papillomatosis. *Otolaryngol Clin North Am*. 2019;52:669-679.

Welschmeyer A, Berke GS. An updated review of the epidemiological factors associated with recurrent respiratory papillomatosis. *Laryngoscope Investig Otolaryngol*. 2021;6:226-233.

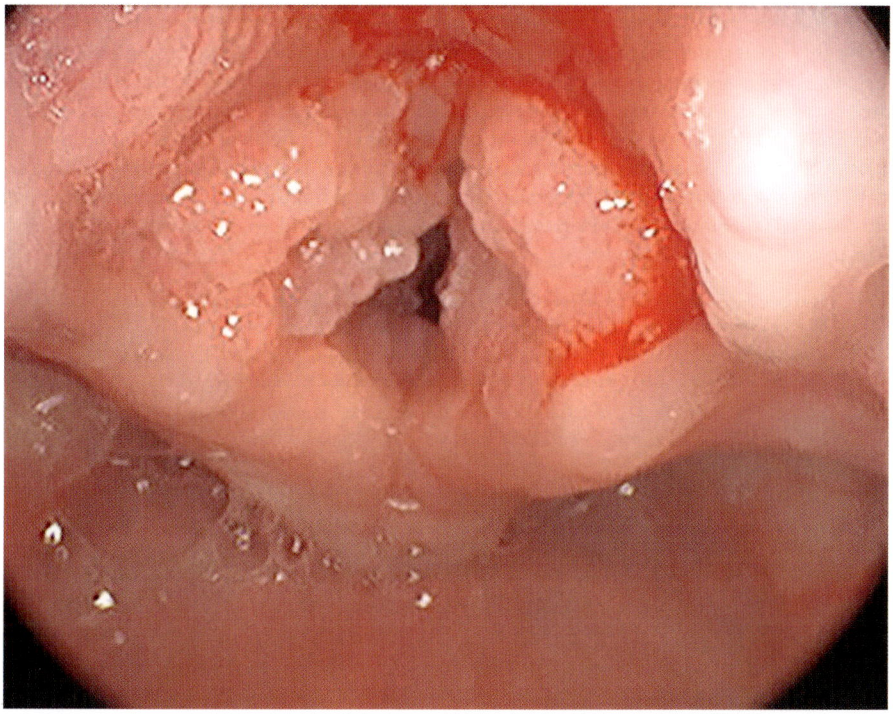

FIGURE 35.1. Laryngoscopic view of pediatric larynx with multiple papillomata. (From Derkay CS, Bluher AE. Update on recurrent respiratory papillomatosis. *Otolaryngol Clin North Am*. 2019;52:669-679.)

A.5. What treatment options are available?

Though there is no cure for RRP, standard management includes both surgical excision and adjuvant therapy. On average, patients with RRP undergo four surgeries per year. Surgical excision of lesions is typically performed using carbon dioxide (CO_2) laser and/or a microdebrider under direct laryngoscopy. Other options include "coblation" (controlled ablation) or sharp dissection. The goal of treatment is to improve airway patency while preserving voice quality. Subtotal excision might be necessary to preserve normal structures and prevent later stenosis. Even with removal of all clinically evident papilloma, latent virus remains.

Microdebriders allow precise resection without the risk of thermal damage but can lead to scarring. Certain lesions, such as sessile lesions, those with ventricular involvement, or in areas of significant scarring, are best treated using laser. An N95 mask respirator should be worn by health care workers in the operating room when a laser is used to treat RRP.

Adjuvant therapies include IFN-α, antiviral agents (most commonly intralesional cidofovir), bevacizumab (a vascular endothelial growth factor [VEGF] monoclonal antibody), indole-3-carbinol (found in cruciferous vegetables), and vaccines (9-valent and quadrivalent HPV vaccines).

Derkay CS, Bluher AE. Update on recurrent respiratory papillomatosis. *Otolaryngol Clin North Am*. 2019;52:669-679.

Derkay CS, Campisi P. Recurrent respiratory papillomatosis. In: Flint PW, Haughey BH, Lund VJ, et al, eds. *Cummings Otolaryngology: Head and Neck Surgery*. 7th ed. Elsevier; 2020:3076-3091.

Manley C, Hutchinson C, Mahajan A, et al. Treatment of recurrent respiratory papillomatosis: case series and review of technique. *Surg Technol Int*. 2021;38:139-143.

Rasmussen ER, Schnack DT, Jorkov AS, et al. Long-term follow-up and outcome in patients with recurrent respiratory laryngeal papillomatosis. *Dan Med J*. 2017;64:A5424.

Welschmeyer A, Berke GS. An updated review of the epidemiological factors associated with recurrent respiratory papillomatosis. *Laryngoscope Investig Otolaryngol*. 2021;6:226-233.

A.6. What are the common adverse effects of α-interferon (IFN) therapy?

IFNs are potent cytokines that possess antiviral, immunomodulating, and antiproliferative activities. Only IFN-α is clinically used in RRP. Adverse effects associated with systemic use (subcutaneous injections) are an influenza-like syndrome, characterized by fever, chills, headache, myalgias, arthralgias, nausea, vomiting, and diarrhea as well as more serious dose-limiting effects like myelosuppression and neurotoxicity. Neurotoxicity can manifest as somnolence, confusion, behavioral disturbances, and rarely, seizures, debilitating neurasthenia, and depression (up to and including suicidal ideation). Alopecia and personality changes are common in IFN-treated children. Cardiovascular toxicity (hypotension and tachycardia) and hepatotoxicity are rare.

Acosta EP. Antiviral Agents (Nonretroviral). In: Brunton LL, Knollmann BC. eds. *Goodman & Gilman's: The Pharmacological Basis of Therapeutics,* 14th Edition. McGraw-Hill Education; 2023. Accessed May 20, 2025.

Derkay CS, Campisi P. Recurrent respiratory papillomatosis. In: Flint PW, Haughey BH, Lund VJ, et al, eds. *Cummings Otolaryngology: Head and Neck Surgery*. 7th ed. Elsevier; 2020:3076-3091.

Ghazal EA, Carter H, Mason LJ, et al. Preoperative evaluation, premedication, and induction of anesthesia. In: Cote CJ, Lerman J, Anderson B, eds. *A Practice of Anesthesia for Infants and Children*. 7th ed. Elsevier; 2024: 22-64.

B. Preoperative Evaluation and Preparation

B.1. What are the key points in the preoperative evaluation of this patient?

It is important to quickly detect and address respiratory compromise. The team should observe the child for tachypnea, flaring of the nares, or use of accessory neck and chest muscles. In the absence of severe respiratory distress, a detailed history and physical should be obtained. Were there any problems with previous anesthetics particularly related to airway management? Are there signs of airway obstruction (eg, stridor, snoring)? What position does the child sleep in? Has there been a recent respiratory infection? Has the child had difficulty swallowing? If the patient has received IFN therapy, any adverse side effects should be discussed.

A detailed inquiry regarding voice changes can provide insight to where the papillomatous lesions are located if recent flexible fiberoptic laryngoscopy has not been performed. A low-pitched, coarse, fluttering voice suggests a subglottic lesion, whereas a high-pitched, cracking voice, aphonia, or breathy voice suggests a glottic lesion. High-pitched stridor suggests a glottic or subglottic lesion. On exam, stridor due to laryngeal obstruction is often musical and can begin as inspiratory but will progress to biphasic with increased airway narrowing.

The goal is to recognize a lesion that might result in partial or complete airway obstruction during induction of anesthesia. A preoperative flexible nasopharyngoscopic examination is routinely performed mostly in ear, nose, and throat offices. If this has not been done, an immediate preoperative flexible nasopharyngoscopic examination should be considered.

Derkay CS. Recurrent respiratory papillomatosis. *Laryngoscope*. 2001;111:57-69.

B.2. Are any preoperative laboratory tests necessary?

For a surgical procedure that is not expected to have significant intraoperative blood loss in a child without risk factors for severe anemia, preoperative laboratory tests are not required. However, if the patient has been receiving IFN-α, myelosuppression is a possible side effect with resultant anemia. In this case, a preoperative complete cell blood count might be helpful.

Ghazal EA, Vadi MG, Mason LJ, et al. Preoperative evaluation, premedication, and induction of anesthesia. In: Coté CJ, Lerman J, Anderson MB, eds. *A Practice of Anesthesia for Infants and Children*. 6th ed. Elsevier; 2019:35-68.

B.3. Is it safe to premedicate this child?

Given the need for repeat surgical excision, children with RRP can be quite anxious in the hospital setting. Reassurance by the anesthesiologist and the child life staff, who can employ distraction techniques during induction, can be helpful. Sedative premedication should only be considered in children without signs of suspected potential of airway obstruction.

Dexmedetomidine, an α_2-adrenergic receptor agonist, given intranasally, has minimal effect on respiration and would be preferred over oral midazolam. If proceeding with premedication, the child should be placed on continuous pulse oximetry monitoring with immediate availability of supplemental oxygen, suction, and positive pressure ventilation. Anticholinergic premedication can also be given to reduce oral secretions.

Ghazal EA, Vadi MG, Mason LJ, et al. Preoperative evaluation, premedication, and induction of anesthesia. In: Coté CJ, Lerman J, Anderson MB, eds. *A Practice of Anesthesia for Infants and Children*. 6th ed. Elsevier; 2019:35-68.

B.4. What are the special anesthetic considerations prior to bringing the child to the operating room?

The anesthesiologist should discuss the surgical and airway management plan with the surgeon. Close communication will be important throughout the procedure to ensure adequate oxygenation and ventilation while allowing adequate surgical exposure and reducing the risk of airway fire. Special equipment (eg, laser, jet ventilator, bronchoscope, laser-resistant endotracheal tube) must be physically present in the operating room and checked to be properly functioning. Equipment for a potentially difficult pediatric airway should be present in the operating room, including a tracheostomy-cricothyrotomy kit. Laser safety eyewear must be available for all operating room personnel.

Derkay CS. Recurrent respiratory papillomatosis. *Laryngoscope*. 2001;111:57-69.

C. Intraoperative Management

C.1. How would you induce anesthesia in a patient with RRP?

The mode of induction will depend on the presence of signs and symptoms of airway compromise which can be exacerbated with induction and relaxation of upper airway and pharyngeal muscles. In an adult patient with potential for airway obstruction, awake fiberoptic intubation can be performed. In children and uncooperative adults, inhalational induction with sevoflurane can be performed while maintaining spontaneous respiration. Neuromuscular blockers should not be administered until it is clear that the patient can be ventilated and/or the trachea intubated.

If the patient has had a very recent flexible nasopharyngoscopic examination that is reassuring and there is no concern for airway compromise, intravenous induction can be used. However, papillomata are dynamic lesions that can grow very rapidly. The lack of preoperative signs and symptoms of airway obstruction does not guarantee a patent airway following induction of anesthesia. Thus, it is better to err on the side of caution when managing these patients. An experienced otolaryngologist should be present in the operating room for induction.

Gerstein NS, Spafford MF. Obstructing respiratory papillomatosis. *Anesthesiology*. 2018;128:1239.

Patel A. Anesthesia for otolaryngologic and head-neck surgery. In: Gropper MA, Cohen NH, Eriksson LI, et al, eds. *Miller's Anesthesia*. 9th ed. Elsevier, 2020:2210-2235.

C.2. Discuss airway management options during laryngeal papilloma resection.

In addition to maintaining spontaneous ventilation with total intravenous anesthesia, other options include manual Venturi jet ventilation, controlled mechanical ventilation through a smaller ETT, or apnea with intermittent ventilation. With jet ventilation, there is an increased risk of barotrauma, and appropriate exhalation needs to be assured. The downsides of using an ETT during airway laser surgery is the risk of airway fire as well as suboptimal surgical exposure of the larynx. In the pediatric population, maintenance of spontaneous ventilation without an airway device using total intravenous anesthesia is the preferred technique.

With an intermittent apnea technique, the patient is hyperventilated either via ETT or mask, followed by a period of apnea during which the surgeon operates. If an ETT is used, it is removed periodically to allow for surgical exposure as well as to diminish airway fire risk. The cycle is repeated until resection of the lesion is complete. It is best to use neuromuscular blockers with this technique to prevent inadvertent movement.

The inspired oxygen concentration should be minimized to avoid hypoxia, and nitrous oxide should be avoided as it also supports combustion. Reducing the inspired oxygen concentration to below 30% seems to prevent combustion.

Derkay CS, Campisi P. Recurrent respiratory papillomatosis. In: Flint PW, Haughey BH, Lund VJ, et al, eds. *Cummings Otolaryngology: Head and Neck Surgery*. 7th ed. Elsevier; 2020:3076-3091.

Gerstein NS, Spafford MF. Obstructing respiratory papillomatosis. *Anesthesiology*. 2018;128:1239.

Roy S, Smith LP. Surgical fires in laser laryngeal surgery: are we safe enough? *Otolaryngol Head Neck Surg*. 2015;152:67-72.

C.3. What is a laser and how does it work?

Laser is an acronym for light amplification by stimulated emission of radiation. The necessary components of a laser system consist of a laser medium (gas, liquid, or solid) containing the atoms whose electrons create the laser light, resonating mirrors to enhance laser efficiency, and an energy source to excite the atoms of the laser medium into generating laser light.

The laser produces high energy, focused electromagnetic radiation that can cut or coagulate tissue. Named for the active medium between the mirrors, lasers commonly used in ear, nose, throat (ENT) surgery include CO_2, potassium titanyl phosphate (KTP), neodymium:yttrium-aluminum-garnet (Nd:YAG), and pulse dye lasers (PDL).

O'Connell Ferster AP. Lasers in laryngeal surgery. *Oper Tech Otolayngol Head Neck Surg*. 2019;30:279-283.

Patel A. Anesthesia for otolaryngologic and head-neck surgery. In: Gropper MA, Cohen NH, Eriksson LI, et al, eds. *Miller's Anesthesia*. 9th ed. Elsevier; 2020:2210-2235.

C.4. What are the characteristics of laser radiation?

The high energy density of a laser is the result of three characteristics:

- Monochromaticity: All photons in a laser beam have the same wavelength.
- Coherence: Electromagnetic fields of all photons in a laser beam oscillate in identical phase, unlike in ordinary light where the electromagnetic fields are randomly phased.
- Directionality: Laser light remains in a narrow collimated beam with the elements of the laser beam parallel, unlike ordinary light beams that spread out in many directions from a point source.

These properties permit lasers to deliver intense energy via powerful light beams efficiently and accurately through lenses to small targets. They also allow the surgeon to control several parameters and alter laser interaction with the target tissue:

- Power: rate at which energy is transmitted by laser beam
- Spot size: radius of laser beam. A larger spot size results in an overall lower power density.
- Exposure time: time that laser energy is delivered to tissues. Pulse modes result in less tissue damage by allowing heated tissues time to cool in between laser applications compared to continuous modes.

O'Connell Ferster AP. Lasers in laryngeal surgery. *Oper Tech Otolayngol Head Neck Surg*. 2019;30:279-283.

Patel A. Anesthesia for otolaryngologic and head-neck surgery. In: Gropper MA, Cohen NH, Eriksson LI, et al, eds. *Miller's Anesthesia*. 9th ed. Elsevier; 2020:2210-2235.

Yan Y, Olszewski AE, Hoffman MR, et al. Use of lasers in laryngeal surgery. *J Voice*. 2010;24:102-109.

C.5. What are some advantages of using lasers for laryngeal surgery?

Lasers are precise, minimize damage to surrounding tissues, improve intraoperative hemostasis, and decrease postoperative bleeding. They also allow the surgeon a longer working distance with minimal tissue manipulation in an unobstructed operating field.

The CO_2 laser is one of the first lasers developed and most widely used for treating laryngeal lesions such as RRP. Its wavelength is in the infrared spectrum (10,600 nm), which is absorbed by water in the first few layers of cells. The thermal effect is therefore largely limited to the point of entry into the target tissue with little damage to surrounding laryngeal structures.

PDL (585 nm) and KTP (532 nm) lasers, both in the visible light spectrum, target hemoglobin in the microvascular supply of the lesion. In highly vascularized papillomatous tissue, they are thought to have better hemostatic effects and preservation of surrounding normal tissue than the CO_2 laser. An added benefit, at least in the adult population, is that the PDL and KTP lasers can be used safely and effectively in the office with topical anesthesia, thereby avoiding general anesthesia risks, decreasing procedural times, and reducing health care costs.

Ivancic R, Iqbal H, deSilva B, et al. Current and future management of recurrent respiratory papillomatosis. *Laryngoscope Investig Otolaryngol*. 2018;3:22-34.

O'Connell Ferster AP. Lasers in laryngeal surgery. *Oper Tech Otolayngol Head Neck Surg*. 2019;30:279-283.

Patel A. Anesthesia for otolaryngologic and head-neck surgery. In: Gropper MA, Cohen NH, Eriksson LI, et al, eds. *Miller's Anesthesia*. 9th ed. Elsevier; 2020:2210-2235.

C.6. What are some disadvantages of lasers compared to microdebriders?

Although laser surgery has benefits as noted in the previous section, there are significant risks associated with their use for laryngeal surgery. All operating room personnel should be appropriately trained for the safe operation of laser equipment. Special eye protection for both patient and staff is required because the laser beam can cause serious retinal injury. Other body parts might need to be carefully protected from inadvertent laser exposure in order to prevent tissue injury (burns).

The biggest concern with laser use, however, is the risk of an airway fire through ignition of the ETT by inadvertent laser strike. This is a potentially fatal complication if not managed quickly. Precautions to minimize the risk of an airway fire include using a laser-resistant ETT, lowering inspired oxygen concentration, avoiding nitrous oxide, and protecting surrounding tissue in the surgical field with moist packing.

Inappropriate and aggressive use of the laser can injure mucosa unaffected by disease and create an environment suitable for implantation of viral particles which can actually promote spread of the disease. Although the thermal effect is largely limited to the point of entry into the target tissue, if not used judiciously especially near delicate structures such as the anterior or posterior laryngeal commissure, the laser can cause unacceptable scarring and subsequent abnormal vocal fold function.

Laser smoke contains water vapor and vaporized tissue. It has been found to contain active viral DNA, a potential source of infection for operating room personnel as these small particles can be inhaled. Smoke can also obstruct the surgeon's view during the resection. An efficient smoke evacuator and N95 face masks are necessary.

When comparing the microdebrider to the CO_2 laser, removing papillomata using the microdebrider is associated with better short-term improvement in voice quality and a shorter procedure time, which can ultimately translate to reduced operative cost. Furthermore, heat-induced scarring of nearby tissues is not a concern, there is no need for protection from an inadvertent laser strike, and the risk for an airway fire is no higher than in a standard case. In fact, microdebriders are often used in conjunction with lasers by first removing the bulk of the papilloma and then lasers used to provide hemostasis and more targeted treatment.

Derkay CS, Campisi P. Recurrent respiratory papillomatosis. In: Flint PW, Haughey BH, Lund VJ, et al, eds. *Cummings Otolaryngology: Head and Neck Surgery*. 7th ed. Elsevier; 2020:3076-3091.

Ivancic R, Iqbal H, deSilva B, et al. Current and future management of recurrent respiratory papillomatosis. *Laryngoscope Investig Otolaryngol*. 2018;3:22-34.

Liu S, Wang J, Shao J. Safety of different surgical modalities for recurrent respiratory papillomatosis resection: a systematic review and meta-analysis. *Clin Otolaryngol*. 2023;48:403-413.

Patel A. Anesthesia for otolaryngologic and head-neck surgery. In: Gropper MA, Cohen NH, Eriksson LI, et al, eds. *Miller's Anesthesia*. 9th ed. Elsevier; 2020:2210-2235.

C.7. What special endotracheal tubes (ETTs) are available for laser surgery?

Because of their proximity to the operative field, ETTs pose a serious fire hazard during laser use, especially in the oxygen-enriched environment. The US Food and Drug Administration (FDA)-approved specialized tubes for laser surgery are commercially available. Although these laser-resistant ETTs can withstand laser strikes longer than conventional tubes, they will ignite with prolonged exposure. Laser-resistant tubes are made of metal or have a metallic overlay on a nonmetal core **(Figure 35.2)**. The most commonly used laser-resistant ETTs are the Mallinckrodt Laser-Flex (Covidien) and Rusch LaserTubus (Teleflex).

The Rusch LaserTubus has a rubber latex core with a copper foil overlay covered by latex coating; it has dual inner and outer cuffs made of latex. It cannot be used in patients with latex allergy and tends to kink easily when bent at acute angles. The Mallinckrodt Laser-Flex is a stainless steel spiral ETT; it has dual cuffs in series made of polyvinyl chloride (PVC). Its rigidity makes it an unpopular choice in pediatric patients. For both tubes, if one cuff ruptures, the second cuff will still limit egress of oxygen-rich gas. The American Society of Anesthesiologists (ASA) guidelines recommend the cuffs be filled with saline as this will allow additional protection in case of rupture. Methylene blue can be added to help aid detection of cuff rupture. The cuffs take longer to deflate when filled with saline compared to air.

SECTION 9

Apfelbaum JL, Caplan RA, Barker SJ, et al; American Society of Anesthesiologists Task Force on Operating Room Fires. Practice advisory for the prevention and management of operating room fires: an updated report by the American Society of Anesthesiologists Task Force on Operating Room Fires. *Anesthesiology*. 2013;118:271-290.

Burns JA, Adlard SD, Kobler JB, et al. A comparison of laser-protected endotracheal tubes. *Otolaryngol Head Neck Surg*. 2018;159:871-878.

Patel A. Anesthesia for otolaryngologic and head-neck surgery. In: Gropper MA, Cohen NH, Eriksson LI, et al, eds. *Miller's Anesthesia*. 9th ed. Elsevier; 2020:2210-2235.

C.8. How would you protect the external surface of a conventional ETT for use during laser microlaryngoscopy?

The most recent practice advisory published by the ASA for the prevention and management of operating room fires recommends using laser-resistant ETTs for laser surgery. If none are available, conventional polyvinylchloride (PVC) tubes can be wrapped with reflective tape to make them safer. PVC tubes are more flammable than older red rubber tubes, which also produce less toxic combustion products once ignited. Aluminum or copper tape is an inexpensive (though not FDA-approved) way to provide protection against a brief laser strike. FDA-approved tape is also available (Merocel Laser-Guard).

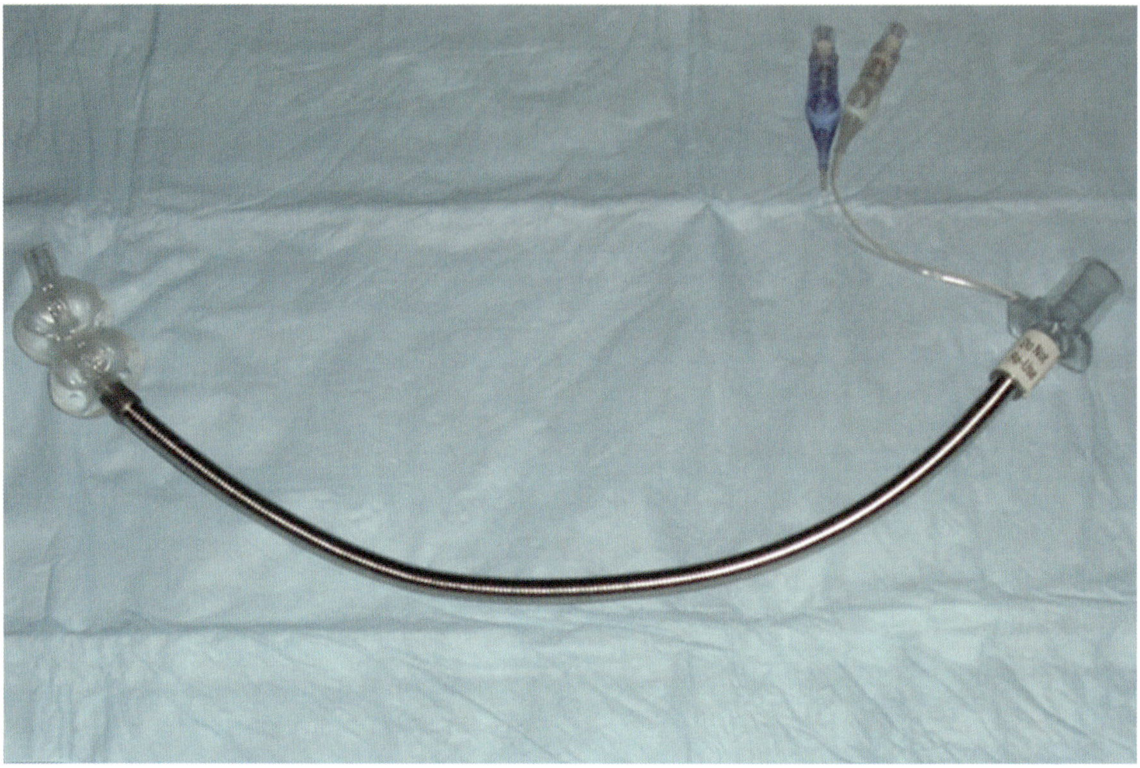

FIGURE 35.2. Example of laser-resistant endotracheal tubes. (From Botney R. Fire safety. In: Woodworth G, Kirsch JR, Sayers-Rana S, eds. *Anesthesia Technician and Technologist's Manual.* Wolters Kluwer; 2012:506.)

Apfelbaum JL, Caplan RA, Barker SJ, et al; American Society of Anesthesiologists Task Force on Operating Room Fires. Practice advisory for the prevention and management of operating room fires: an updated report by the American Society of Anesthesiologists Task Force on Operating Room Fires. *Anesthesiology*. 2013;118:271-290.

Patel A. Anesthesia for otolaryngologic and head-neck surgery. In: Gropper MA, Cohen NH, Eriksson LI, et al, eds. *Miller's Anesthesia*. 9th ed. Elsevier; 2020:2210-2235.

Wöllmer W, Schade G, Kessler G. Endotracheal tube fires still happen–A short overview. *Med Laser Appl*. 2010;25:118-125.

C.9. How would you manage an airway fire?

An airway fire can occur with the close proximity of three components ("fire triad"): an ignition source (laser strike), a fuel (ETT), and an oxidizing agent (oxygen). In the event of an airway fire, immediate and effective action is needed. The "4 *Es*" mnemonic provides focus in this crisis situation: *E*xtract, *E*liminate, *E*xtinguish, *E*valuate.

All combustible material (ETTs, pledgets) must be *E*xtracted from the airway at once. Oxygen supply through the tube must be quickly *E*liminated by disconnecting the circuit. Continued oxygen flow through a burning ETT can lead to a blowtorch effect. Residual fire needs to be *E*xtinguished with normal saline. Ventilation with 100% oxygen should then be provided by mask. *E*valuation of the injury should follow via direct laryngoscopy and rigid bronchoscopy to assess the upper and lower airway. Any airway damage makes reintubation the most prudent approach. For severe injury, a low tracheotomy might be indicated.

According to the most recent practice advisory from the ASA for the prevention and management of operating room fires, when a suspected airway fire has occurred and has not been extinguished with the use of saline, a CO_2 fire extinguisher should be used. The ETT should also be examined and assessed to exclude any fragments left behind in the airway.

Apfelbaum JL, Caplan RA, Barker SJ, et al; American Society of Anesthesiologists Task Force on Operating Room Fires. Practice advisory for the prevention and management of operating room fires: an updated report by the American Society of Anesthesiologists Task Force on Operating Room Fires. *Anesthesiology*. 2013;118:271-290.

Patel A. Anesthesia for otolaryngologic and head-neck surgery. In: Gropper MA, Cohen NH, Eriksson LI, et al, eds. *Miller's Anesthesia*. 9th ed. Elsevier; 2020:2210-2235.

Roy S, Smith LP. Preventing and managing operating room fires in otolaryngology-head and neck surgery. *Otolaryngol Clin North Am*. 2019;52:163-171.

C.10. What is the Venturi effect?

The Venturi effect originally described the impact of constricted channels on fluid flow. As fluid passes through the constriction of a Venturi tube (a tube with a narrowing), it must speed up through the constriction, and its hydrostatic pressure drops. The pressure drop is proportional to the flow and can be used to measure the flow rate in pipes without interfering with the flow. The Venturi effect has many applications as different gases and liquids can be mixed; the pressure drop allows a second gas or liquid to be drawn into the primary stream.

Ihra G, Aloy A. On the use of Venturi's principle to describe entrainment during jet ventilation. *J Clin Anesth*. 2000;12:417-419.

C.11. What is Venturi jet ventilation?

The jet injector technique of ventilation for upper airway surgery involves a high-pressure gas source connected to a stiff, narrow cannula positioned at the inlet of the laryngoscope. With a manual switch, intermittent gas boluses are delivered. In the lumen of the laryngoscope, the high-velocity stream of gas encounters stationary gas, which it draws forward. Each jet bolus entrains ambient air through the open laryngoscope entrance, substantially augmenting the volume of the gas bolus and diluting the oxygen fraction of the jet. Whether or not it is truly based on the phenomenon known as the Venturi effect, the jet injector provides a simple approach to delivering physiologic tidal volumes in an "open" delivery system. Venturi ventilation has become synonymous with jet ventilation.

Ihra G, Aloy A. On the use of Venturi's principle to describe entrainment during jet ventilation. *J Clin Anesth*. 2000;12:417-419.

Sikora M, Sonal P, Maurtua M. Jet ventilation a review. *Adv Case Stud*. 2019;2:1-5.

C.12. How would you institute and maintain jet ventilation?

Before effective jet ventilation can begin, the operating laryngoscope must be inserted, the larynx adequately exposed and evaluated for jet ventilation, the suspension system installed, and the jet injector needle attached to the laryngoscope in alignment with the axis of the trachea. This takes time in an anesthetized patient with apnea. One option is to begin with laryngoscopy and intubation using a standard ETT if the airway appears appropriate for jet ventilation. Uninterrupted ventilation can then be performed while the operating laryngoscope and jet injector are positioned. When ready, the ETT is removed, and jet ventilation begins. Alternatively, following induction of anesthesia and adequate mask airway ventilation, the patient is paralyzed and the operating laryngoscope and jet injector are inserted and positioned while the patient is apneic.

Ventilation begins with a jet pressure of 5 to 10 psi in infants and children and 15 to 20 psi in adults. The jet pressure is gradually increased until adequate chest excursions are evident. Jet ventilation should produce good clinical expansion of the chest at a rate appropriate for patient age. The inspiratory-to-expiratory (I:E) ratio should allow for complete passive exhalation between jet applications. Monitoring of peripheral arterial saturation is mandatory as is monitoring ventilation both by auscultation and palpation.

Derkay CS, Campisi P. Recurrent respiratory papillomatosis. In: Flint PW, Haughey BH, Lund VJ, et al, eds. *Cummings Otolaryngology: Head and Neck Surgery*. 7th ed. Elsevier; 2020:3076-3091.

Patel A. Anesthesia for otolaryngologic and head-neck surgery. In: Gropper MA, Cohen NH, Eriksson LI, et al, eds. *Miller's Anesthesia*. 9th ed. Elsevier; 2020:2210-2235.

C.13. How is anesthesia maintained during jet ventilation?

Total intravenous anesthesia is preferred technique with jet ventilation. By combining a hypnotic agent such as propofol with a short-acting opioid such as remifentanil, hypnosis, amnesia, and analgesia can all be achieved, while allowing for a relatively quick recovery at the end of the procedure. Temporary neuromuscular blockers can be achieved with either a short-acting or an intermediate-duration neuromuscular blocker.

Patel A. Anesthesia for otolaryngologic and head-neck surgery. In: Gropper MA, Cohen NH, Eriksson LI, et al, eds. *Miller's Anesthesia*. 9th ed. Elsevier; 2020:2210-2235.

C.14. What are the complications of jet ventilation?

Complications associated with jet ventilation include drying of the mucosa and subsequent mucosal damage, inadequate oxygenation and ventilation, gastric distention (due to inadvertent gas delivery to the gastrointestinal tract, which may lead to aspiration, perforation, or bleeding), and barotrauma. Subcutaneous emphysema, pneumomediastinum, and pneumothorax have been reported, and seem to occur most frequently with subglottic (as opposed to supraglottic) jet ventilation and in patients with a (partially) obstructed airway. Laryngospasm causing an obstructed airway is best avoided by using adequate local anesthesia and neuromuscular block during jet ventilation. In addition, particulate matter and virus particles can be spread down the distal airway.

Derkay CS, Campisi P. Recurrent respiratory papillomatosis. In: Flint PW, Haughey BH, Lund VJ, et al, eds. *Cummings Otolaryngology: Head and Neck Surgery*. 7th ed. Elsevier; 2020:3076-3091.

Jaquet Y, Monnier P, Van Melle G, et al. Complications of different ventilation strategies in endoscopic laryngeal surgery: a 10-year review. *Anesthesiology*. 2006;104:52-59.

Schiff J, Walther A, Krier C, et al. Complications of managing the airway. In: Hagberg CA, Artime CA, Aziz MF, eds. *Benumof and Hagberg's Airway Management*. 5th ed. Elsevier; 2023:876-895.

C.15. Are there contraindications to the use of jet ventilation?

Jet ventilation is most suited for patients with normal, unobstructed airways and normal lung and chest wall compliance. The ability to fully exhale between jet applications is crucial. If this is not possible (glottic lesion, significant interarytenoid scarring, laryngospasm), jet ventilation might not be appropriate. Decreased chest wall compliance, such as in patients with higher weight, can lead to inadvertent gastric distension, further worsening respiratory compliance. Advanced chronic obstructive pulmonary disease with its inherent prolonged exhalation phase can make jet ventilation impractical and, in the presence of pulmonary bullae, even hazardous.

Helmstaedter V, Tellkamp R, Majdani O, et al. High-frequency jet ventilation for endolaryngotracheal surgery–chart review and procedure analysis from the surgeon's and the anaesthesiologist's point of view. *Clin Otolaryngol*. 2015;40:341-348.

Jaquet Y, Monnier P, Van Melle G, et al. Complications of different ventilation strategies in endoscopic laryngeal surgery: a 10-year review. *Anesthesiology*. 2006;104:52-59.

C.16. How will you monitor this patient?

Routine monitors include pulse oximetry, noninvasive blood pressure measurements, electrocardiography, precordial stethoscope, temperature probe, end-tidal CO_2 detector, oxygen analyzer, and neuromuscular function monitor, if relevant. If maintaining spontaneous ventilation, exposing the patient's chest is helpful for assessing adequate chest rise.

American Society of Anesthesiologists. Standards for basic anesthetic monitoring. Reaffirmed December 13, 2020. Accessed November 30, 2022. https://www.asahq.org/standards-and-guidelines/standards-for-basic-anesthetic-monitoring

D. Postoperative Anesthetic Management

D.1. What are the common postoperative complications?

Laryngeal edema can occur early in the postoperative period, and usually manifests with chest retractions and inspiratory stridor. After microlaryngeal surgery, patients benefit from humidified oxygen, intravenous steroids (eg, dexamethasone, if not already administered intraoperatively), and inhaled racemic epinephrine. Laryngospasm can develop because of laryngeal hyperactivity. To reduce the incidence of laryngospasm, lidocaine can be sprayed on the vocal cords in the operating room. If laryngospasm develops postoperatively, it is treated with standard maneuvers, including a jaw thrust and positive pressure ventilation. More severe laryngospasm can require use of succinylcholine (1-2 mg/kg intravenously). Pulmonary complications can result from retained secretions, atelectasis, or barotrauma (if jet ventilation was used).

Altun D, Camci E, Orhan-Sungur, et al. High frequency jet ventilation during endolaryngeal surgery: risk factors for complications. *Auris Nasus Larynx*. 2018;45:1047-1052.

Jaquet Y, Monnier P, Van Melle G, et al. Complications of different ventilation strategies in endoscopic laryngeal surgery: a 10-year review. *Anesthesiology*. 2006;104:52-59.

Patel A. Anesthesia for otolaryngologic and head-neck surgery. In: Gropper MA, Cohen NH, Eriksson LI, et al, eds. *Miller's Anesthesia*. 9th ed. Elsevier; 2020:2210-2235.

36

Tracheoesophageal Fistula

Jacques H. Scharoun

A 12-hour-old full-term infant weighing 2.5 kg presents with choking and cyanosis upon his first feed. Neonatal intensive care unit (NICU) staff are unable to pass a feeding tube into the stomach. The baby also has copious oral secretions. Before birth, polyhydramnios was detected.

A. Pathophysiology and Differential Diagnosis

1. What is the diagnosis? What are the clinical features of this disease?
2. What is the pathophysiology of this disease?
3. Describe the normal development of the trachea and esophagus.
4. Are tracheoesophageal fistula (TEF) and esophageal atresia (EA) inherited?
5. How are the different types of TEF and EA classified?
6. What other anomalies might this child have, and when should these be investigated?
7. What should the parents be told regarding perioperative risk?

B. Preoperative Evaluation and Preparation

1. What laboratory workup should be obtained before surgery?
2. Describe management in the NICU before surgery.
3. How is severe lung disease managed before the repair of TEF?
4. Should this patient be intubated preoperatively for airway protection?
5. Discuss optimal timing for surgical repair.

C. Intraoperative Management

1. What invasive lines and monitoring are appropriate before induction of anesthesia? After induction?
2. Discuss fluid and temperature management for this neonate.
3. What are the options regarding induction of anesthesia and tracheal intubation?
4. What is the role of rigid and fiberoptic bronchoscopy in this patient prior to incision?
5. Describe the steps of an open repair of TEF and EA.
6. What are common intraoperative problems, and how can they be managed?
7. If the surgeon decides to proceed thoracoscopically, how will you perform your anesthetic? Is one-lung ventilation required? What are some complications unique to thoracoscopy in the newborn?

D. Postoperative Management

1. When should the trachea be extubated?
2. What options are available for postoperative analgesia?
3. What are the early and late complications of TEF repair?

A. Pathophysiology and Differential Diagnosis

A.1. What is the diagnosis? What are the clinical features of this disease?

This infant has EA with a TEF. This occurs in approximately 1 per 3,000 live births. The diagnosis is suspected prenatally by the presence of polyhydramnios, which is caused by the failure of the fetus to swallow amniotic fluid (secondary to EA). Polyhydramnios is a nonspecific prenatal finding; the combination of polyhydramnios and absent stomach bubble on prenatal ultrasound gives a 44% to 56% likelihood of EA/TEF. Only 20% to 30% of cases are diagnosed prenatally. After birth, the neonate will have copious drooling from an inability to swallow secretions, and attempts to feed result in coughing and cyanosis. An orogastric tube (OGT) will coil in the upper esophageal pouch rather than pass into the stomach.

Hunt RW, Perkins EJ, King S. Peri-operative management of neonates with oesophageal atresia and tracheo-oesophageal fistula. *Paediatr Respir Rev*. 2016;19:3-9.

Parolini F, Bulotta AL, Battaglia S, Alberti D. Preoperative management of children with esophageal atresia: current perspectives. *Ped Health Med Ther*. 2017;8:1-7.

Walk RM. Esophageal atresia and tracheoesophageal fistula: overview and considerations for the general surgeon. *Surg Clin North Am*. 2022;102:759-778.

A.2. What is the pathophysiology of this disease?

This infant has two distinct issues related to TEF and EA. In TEF, the trachea is connected to the esophagus through a fistula, which causes two problems. First, inhaled air can bypass the lungs through the fistula and enter the stomach. This is typically not a problem while the infant is breathing spontaneously. However, if the lungs are noncompliant due to prematurity or pneumonia or if the fistula is large, positive pressure ventilation (PPV) can result in poor gas exchange and gastric distension. This increased abdominal pressure can further compromise ventilation by requiring higher inspiratory pressure, which further increases the gas leak into the fistula. Second, there is the continual risk of acidic stomach contents refluxing via the fistula into the trachea, causing aspiration pneumonitis. Spontaneous ventilation, with cyclical negative intrathoracic pressure, can contribute to suctioning of gastric contents into the lung.

With EA, the esophagus is divided into a proximal and distal portion. The proximal portion ends in a blind pouch. Secretions from the hypopharynx pool here and cause drooling, coughing, and choking with feeds such that children are unable to feed orally.

Hunt RW, Perkins EJ, King S. Peri-operative management of neonates with oesophageal atresia and tracheo-oesophageal fistula. *Paediatr Respir Rev*. 2016;19:3-9.

Morini F, Conforti A, Bagolan P. Perioperative complications of esophageal atresia. *Eur J Pediatr Surg*. 2018;28:133-140.

Parolini F, Bulotta AL, Battaglia S, Alberti D. Preoperative management of children with esophageal atresia: current perspectives. *Ped Health Med Ther*. 2017;8:1-7.

Walk RM. Esophageal atresia and tracheoesophageal fistula: overview and considerations for the general surgeon. *Surg Clin North Am*. 2022;102:759-778.

A.3. Describe the normal development of the trachea and esophagus.

The foregut arises first from primitive endoderm, which will eventually differentiate into trachea and esophagus. Lung buds form anteriorly at the pharyngeal arch 6. Differential expression of various growth factors results in the anterior foregut developing into trachea and lung tissue, whereas the posterior portion develops into the esophagus. The septation process is believed to arise at the level of the lung bud and proceed toward the pharynx. This process requires *multiple* gene signals, including Sonic hedgehog, Sox2, and NKX2.1. Errors in this process of separation of the trachea from the foregut result in a residual fistula between the esophagus and the trachea.

Brosens E, Brouwer RWW, Douben H, et al. Heritability and de novo mutations in oesophageal atresia and tracheo-esophageal fistula aetiology. *Genes (Basel)*. 2021;12:1595.

Brosens E, Ploeg M, van Bever Y, et al. Clinical and etiological heterogeneity in patients with tracheo-esophageal malformations and associated anomalies. *Eur J Med Genet*. 2014;57:440-452.

Raad S, David A, Que J, Faure C. Genetic mouse models and induced pluripotent stem cells for studying tracheal-esophageal separation and esophageal development. *Stem Cells Dev*. 2020;29:953-966.

A.4. Are tracheoesophageal fistula (TEF) and esophageal atresia (EA) inherited?

TEF with EA usually occurs de novo and is multifactorial in etiology. Rarely, it is associated with a specific genetic mutation or syndrome, which includes trisomy 18, Hall-Hittner syndrome, anophthalmia-esophageal-genital (AEG) syndrome, Feingold syndrome, and 16q24.1 deletion syndrome. Most of the cases, however, are nonfamilial. There is a 1% to 3% chance of recurrence in each sibling of someone with EA.

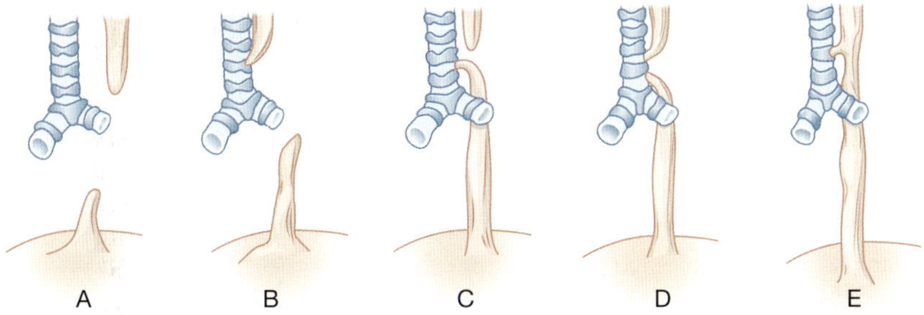

FIGURE 36.1. Gross classification of tracheoesophageal fistula and esophageal atresia. Type A: isolated esophageal atresia; Type B: esophageal atresia, proximal esophageal pouch attached to trachea; Type C: esophageal atresia, distal esophagus attached to trachea; Type D: esophageal atresia, both proximal and distal esophagus attached to trachea via 2 fistula; Type E: no esophageal atresia, a fistula connects intact esophagus to intact trachea. (Modified from Gregory GA, ed. *Pediatric Anesthesia.* 2nd ed. Churchill Livingstone; 1989:921, with permission.)

Brosens E, Brouwer RWW, Douben H, et al. Heritability and de novo mutations in oesophageal atresia and tracheoesophageal fistula aetiology. *Genes (Basel).* 2021;12:1595.

Brosens E, Ploeg M, van Bever Y, et al. Clinical and etiological heterogeneity in patients with tracheo-esophageal malformations and associated anomalies. *Eur J Med Genet.* 2014;57:440-452.

A.5. How are the different types of TEF and EA classified?

There are five types of TEF according to the classic Gross classification (**Figure 36.1**). Type A is pure EA with no involvement of the respiratory tree; this occurs in 8% of cases. This type is most frequently detected prenatally. Gross type B has EA and a fistula connecting the proximal esophageal pouch to the trachea; this occurs in less than 1% of cases. The most common is type C, with EA and a fistula linking the distal esophagus to the trachea; this occurs in 75% to 80% of cases. Rarely, type D occurs with two fistulae connecting both proximal and distal esophagus to the trachea (2%). Type E, known as an H-type fistula, has no atresia. Instead, an intact esophagus has a linkage with the trachea through a fistula, which occurs in 4% of cases.

Lal DR, Gadepalli SK, Downard CD, et al. Perioperative management and outcomes of esophageal atresia and tracheoesophageal fistula. *J Pediatr Surg.* 2017;52:1245-1251.

Parolini F, Bulotta AL, Battaglia S, Alberti D. Preoperative management of children with esophageal atresia: current perspectives. *Ped Health Med Ther.* 2017;8:1-7.

Walk RM. Esophageal atresia and tracheoesophageal fistula: overview and considerations for the general surgeon. *Surg Clin North Am.* 2022;102:759-778.

A.6. What other anomalies might this child have, and when should these be investigated?

Fifty percent of children with EA/TEF have additional anomalies. Most often, they occur in the spectrum known as the *VACTERL* association.

V = vertebral anomalies (10%)
A = anal canal defect (14%)
C = cardiac malformations (29%), including septal defects, tetralogy of Fallot, right-sided aortic arch, patent ductus arteriosus
TE = tracheoesophageal fistula
R = renal dysplasia
L = limb defect (radial aplasia)

A patient is considered to have the VACTERL association with the presence of three or more of these lesions. Nearly one-third of TEF patients have an additional VACTERL lesion, and an additional one-fifth have two. Other possible gastrointestinal problems include malrotation of the midgut and duodenal atresia. Renal problems include malposition, hydronephrosis, and ureteral abnormalities. Most of these issues are not emergent, and evaluation can proceed after the repair of the TEF.

However, the cardiac anatomy must be assessed by echocardiography prior to surgery for two reasons. First, the presence of major congenital heart disease can alter the anesthetic management, including the choice of monitors and ventilation strategy. Second, the presence of a right-sided aortic arch, if known in advance, might lead the surgeon to approach the fistula by a left thoracotomy instead of the conventional right thoracotomy.

Dingemann C, Eaton S, Aksnes G, et al. ERNICA consensus conference on the management of patients with esophageal atresia and tracheoesophageal fistula: diagnostics, preoperative, operative, and postoperative management. *Eur J Pediatr Surg.* 2020;30:326-336.

Hunt RW, Perkins EJ, King S. Peri-operative management of neonates with oesophageal atresia and tracheo-oesophageal fistula. *Paediatr Respir Rev.* 2016;19:3-9.

Husain M, Dutra-Clarke M, Lemieux B, et al. Phenotypic diversity of patients diagnosed with VACTERL association. *Am J Med Genetics.* 2018;176:1830-1837.

Lal DR, Gadepalli SK, Downard CD, et al. Perioperative management and outcomes of esophageal atresia and tracheoesophageal fistula. *J Pediatr Surg.* 2017;52:1245-1251.

A.7. What should the parents be told regarding perioperative risk?

The survival of TEF babies has improved over the years because of improvements in intensive care unit care, anesthesia, and surgical technique. The risk of perioperative mortality remains well stratified by the Spitz Classification of a recent series of 248 neonates over a 20-year period. In the modern era, the presence of major cardiac disease remains the primary risk factor for mortality.

- Spitz group I: birth weight greater than 1.5 kg, no major cardiac disease, survival 96%
- Spitz group II: birth weight less than 1.5 kg, or major cardiac disease, survival 79%
- Spitz group III: birth weight less than 1.5 kg and major cardiac disease, survival 38%

Lal DR, Gadepalli SK, Downard CD, et al. Perioperative management and outcomes of esophageal atresia and tracheoesophageal fistula. *J Pediatr Surg.* 2017;52:1245-1251.

Lazow SP, Ben-Ishay O, Aribindi VK, et al. Predictors of index admission mortality and morbidity in contemporary esophageal atresia patients. *J Pediatr Surg.* 2020;55:2322-2328.

Peters RT, Ragab H, Columb MO, et al. Mortality and morbidity in oesophageal atresia. *Pediatr Surg Int.* 2017;33:989-994.

B. Preoperative Evaluation and Preparation

B.1. What laboratory workup should be obtained before surgery?

First, a plain chest x-ray is used to assess the presence and severity of pulmonary disease, especially aspiration pneumonia and bronchopulmonary dysplasia. It can also show the presence of congestive heart failure in the setting of associated cardiac disease, which can be optimized by administering a diuretic. A radiopaque OGT can be seen coiled in the proximal esophageal pouch, whereas an abdominal x-ray can show air in the bowels entering through the fistula. Because of the risk of aspiration, contrast dye to delineate the fistula should be used only when there is diagnostic uncertainty. An OGT that appears to enter the stomach can in fact have passed through an esophageal perforation caused by repeated traumatic insertion attempts.

Second, an echocardiogram is *mandatory* because major cardiac defects strongly influence survival and have an impact on anesthetic management. If the child has severe tetralogy of Fallot, they might require placement of a temporary shunt between the systemic arterial and pulmonary circulation prior to repair of the TEF. The presence of a right-sided aortic arch will require positioning the infant in the right lateral decubitus position instead of the usual left side down.

Spinal plain films and/or ultrasound should be done to exclude vertebral anomalies if epidural pain management is being considered.

Complete blood count (CBC), arterial blood gas, and electrolytes should be drawn, and at least 1 unit of packed red blood cells should be typed and crossed.

Dingemann C, Eaton S, Aksnes G, et al. ERNICA consensus conference on the management of patients with esophageal atresia and tracheoesophageal fistula: diagnostics, preoperative, operative, and postoperative management. *Eur J Pediatr Surg.* 2020;30:326-336.

Hunt RW, Perkins EJ, King S. Peri-operative management of neonates with oesophageal atresia and tracheo-oesophageal fistula. *Paediatr Respir Rev.* 2016;19:3-9.

Parolini F, Bulotta AL, Battaglia S, Alberti D. Preoperative management of children with esophageal atresia: current perspectives. *Ped Health Med Ther.* 2017;8:1-7.

B.2. Describe management in the NICU before surgery.

After the diagnosis of TEF is established, the baby should not be fed orally, and intravenous (IV) replacement of fluid and glucose is provided. A drainage tube should be placed in the proximal esophageal pouch and kept on intermittent suction to minimize aspiration of oral secretions. Patients should be positioned either prone or supine with the head up 30° to minimize reflux of gastric fluids into the lungs via the fistula. Antibiotics should be given if pneumonia is present but are not administered prophylactically.

Ensure that blood is available from the blood bank. Because the patient will require a thoracotomy with lung retraction and intermittent compression of the trachea and great vessels, an arterial catheter is mandatory. An umbilical artery catheter can be conveniently placed by a neonatologist in the NICU. Two additional IV catheters should also be placed. A central venous catheter is not necessary. Avoid placing IV catheters in the right arm since this arm will most likely be elevated during right thoracotomy, and access to it might be limited.

Dingemann C, Eaton S, Aksnes G, et al. ERNICA consensus conference on the management of patients with esophageal atresia and tracheoesophageal fistula: diagnostics, preoperative, operative, and postoperative management. *Eur J Pediatr Surg*. 2020;30:326-336.

Hunt RW, Perkins EJ, King S. Peri-operative management of neonates with oesophageal atresia and tracheo-oesophageal fistula. *Paediatr Respir Rev*. 2016;19:3-9.

Walk RM. Esophageal atresia and tracheoesophageal fistula: overview and considerations for the general surgeon. *Surg Clin North Am*. 2022;102:759-778.

B.3. How is severe lung disease managed before the repair of TEF?

Very early primary repair is the standard of care. However, there remains a subset of neonates with either severe pneumonia or respiratory distress syndrome (from prematurity), who are at poor risk for anesthesia and surgery, and who need to be intubated because of respiratory disease. The baby can be intubated conventionally while a simple gastrostomy is simultaneously placed to relieve gastric distension that can occur with PPV in the setting of a type C TEF. This can be performed under local anesthesia. The problem with this approach is that by decompressing the stomach, gas from the trachea can now bypass the lungs and exit through the stomach. This is especially a concern if the lungs are noncompliant, which can make it difficult or impossible to ventilate adequately. Alternately, the baby can be ventilated using a high-frequency oscillator, which has the advantage of providing oxygenation and carbon dioxide (CO_2) removal while minimizing the peak inspiratory pressure and therefore gastric distension.

Ho AM, Dion JM, Wong JC. Airway and ventilatory management options in congenital tracheoesophageal fistula repair. *J Cardiothorac Vasc Anesth*. 2016;30:515-520.

Holcomb GW III. Thoracoscopic surgery for esophageal atresia. *Pediatr Surg Int*. 2017;33:475-481.

Hunt RW, Perkins EJ, King S. Peri-operative management of neonates with oesophageal atresia and tracheo-oesophageal fistula. *Paediatr Respir Rev*. 2016;19:3-9.

B.4. Should this patient be intubated preoperatively for airway protection?

Unless mandated by severe pulmonary disease, the child is not intubated preoperatively to minimize the possibility of gastric distension from PPV through the fistula. Intubation does not protect the child from aspiration of gastric contents through the fistula.

Dingemann C, Eaton S, Aksnes G, et al. ERNICA consensus conference on the management of patients with esophageal atresia and tracheoesophageal fistula: diagnostics, preoperative, operative, and postoperative management. *Eur J Pediatr Surg*. 2020;30:326-336.

Hunt RW, Perkins EJ, King S. Peri-operative management of neonates with oesophageal atresia and tracheo-oesophageal fistula. *Paediatr Respir Rev*. 2016;19:3-9.

Morini F, Conforti A, Bagolan P. Perioperative complications of esophageal atresia. *Eur J Pediatr Surg*. 2018;28:133-140.

B.5. Discuss optimal timing for surgical repair.

Tracheoesophageal repair is urgent, but not an emergency. For a stable infant without pulmonary compromise, there is no reason to operate on the child outside of normal hours. Late-night surgery adds operator fatigue to the complexity of a potentially chaotic pre-ligation course and esophageal anastomosis. A series of 28 cases showed a substantial increase in the rate of postoperative esophageal anastomosis leak for patients who underwent surgery late at night.

However, delaying surgery allows more opportunity for gastric regurgitation via the fistula into the lungs, especially if the fistula is large. The resulting pneumonia leads to two problems. First, it will cause decreased pulmonary compliance, with resulting higher airway pressure and gastric distension when positive pressure is initiated during surgery. Second, the infant will be less able to tolerate lung retraction without significant desaturation. Therefore, TEF/EA repair should be done at the earliest daytime opportunity, after all mandatory workup is completed, typically on or before the third day of life.

Infants who develop severe gastric distension or rupture can need immediate laparotomy for gastric decompression. During this procedure, the surgeon can occlude the esophagus with a balloon to stabilize ventilation. A special case is infants who have associated anal canal defects. In these patients, lack of egress for air that passes through the fistula can lead to rapid distension of the entire gut. These infants should undergo surgery within 24 hours of birth.

Dingemann C, Eaton S, Aksnes G, et al. ERNICA consensus conference on the management of patients with esophageal atresia and tracheoesophageal fistula: diagnostics, preoperative, operative, and postoperative management. *Eur J Pediatr Surg*. 2020;30:326-336.

Morini F, Conforti A, Bagolan P. Perioperative complications of esophageal atresia. *Eur J Pediatr Surg*. 2018;28:133-140.

Walk RM. Esophageal atresia and tracheoesophageal fistula: overview and considerations for the general surgeon. *Surg Clin North Am*. 2022;102:759-778.

Yeung A, Butterworth SA. A comparison of surgical outcomes between in-hours and after-hours tracheoesophageal fistula repairs. *J Pediatr Surg*. 2015;50:805-808.

C. Intraoperative Management

C.1. What invasive lines and monitoring are appropriate before induction of anesthesia? After induction?

At least one peripheral IV catheter should be in place before induction of anesthesia. A second catheter can be placed after the patient is anesthetized. An arterial catheter for blood gas and hemodynamic monitoring should be in place before incision. It is especially useful if thoracoscopy is planned. If a peripheral arterial catheter is not feasible, an umbilical arterial line can be placed by a skilled NICU practitioner.

Electrocardiogram, oxygen saturation, end-tidal CO_2, and rectal temperature should be monitored. A precordial stethoscope should be placed over the left axilla to assess breath sounds in case of inadvertent movement of the endotracheal tube (ETT) during surgical retraction or positioning.

Pre- and postductal oxygen saturation should be continuously measured by placing one probe on the right hand and the other probe on either foot. A sudden relative decrease in postductal saturation with a normal preductal saturation is an early indication of elevated pulmonary vascular resistance, which should be treated. Pre- and post-ductal oxygen monitoring is particularly helpful in managing newborns with many types of congenital cardiac disease.

Dingemann C, Eaton S, Aksnes G, et al. ERNICA consensus conference on the management of patients with esophageal atresia and tracheoesophageal fistula: diagnostics, preoperative, operative, and postoperative management. *Eur J Pediatr Surg*. 2020;30:326-336.

Ho AM-H, Dion JM, Wong JCP. Airway and ventilatory management options in congenital tracheoesophageal fistula repair. *J Cardiothorac Vasc Anesth*. 2016;30:515-520.

C.2. Discuss fluid and temperature management for this neonate.

As with all neonates undergoing surgery, meticulous attention to fluid management and temperature is essential. Limited subcutaneous fat renders neonates prone to hypothermia. Hypothermia is dangerous because it will increase pulmonary vascular resistance and can result in a reversion to transitional circulation, greatly complicating intraoperative care. The child should be transported to the operating room (OR) in a warmed isolette, with a stocking cap to minimize heat loss. The OR should be prewarmed to at least 30 °C. Surgical irrigation and red blood cells (RBCs) should be warmed. Using a forced-air convective warming system is strongly recommended.

The baby will require intraoperative glucose infusion. Once infused, glucose is rapidly metabolized, leaving a potentially hypotonic solution. In the past, free water was routinely infused in the form of a hypotonic glucose solution such as D10/0.2 normal saline (NS) administered at 4 mL/kg/h, which is sufficient to prevent hypoglycemia. Recent studies have focused on the role of increased antidiuretic hormone (ADH) secretion, which occurs during surgery. This ADH secretion renders the infant at a 5-fold increased risk of severe hyponatremia when given free water. Current recommendations include infusing an *isotonic* glucose solution for maintenance. Insensible losses should be estimated at 3 to 4 mL/kg/h and replaced with an isotonic (non-glucose-containing) solution. Urine output (ideally 1 mL/kg/h) can be difficult to assess accurately in a low-birth-weight baby.

Engorn BM, Kahntroff SL, Frank KM, et al. Perioperative hypothermia in neonatal intensive care unit patients: effectiveness of a thermoregulation intervention and associated risk factors. *Paediatr Anaesth*. 2017;27:196-204.

Kuan CC, Shaw SJ. Anesthesia for major surgery in the neonate. *Anesthesiol Clin*. 2020;38:1-18.

Nkilly GE, Michelet D, Hilly J, et al. Postoperative decrease in plasma sodium concentration after infusion of hypotonic intravenous solutions in neonatal surgery. *Br J Anaesth.* 2014;112:540-545.

Wang J, Xu E, Xiao Y. Isotonic versus hypotonic maintenance IV fluids in hospitalized children: a meta-analysis. *Pediatrics.* 2014;133:105-113.

C.3. What are the options regarding induction of anesthesia and tracheal intubation?

The goal is to intubate the baby to allow adequate gas exchange with the lowest possible inspiratory pressure needed to inflate the lungs, avoid atelectasis, and minimize gas flow through the fistula. One-lung ventilation is generally not required. The most important aspect of the intubation is the correct positioning of the ETT. The goal is to have the tip of the ETT distal to the fistula yet proximal to the carina. If the tube is deliberately placed deep (into the right mainstem) with the bevel facing forward and then slowly pulled back just until breath sounds occur on the left equal to the right, the tube is likely to be in a good position. Consider the following options:

1. Avoidance of PPV until the fistula is ligated decreases the risk of gastric distension. One can intubate awake in the smallest neonates (which can be difficult) or after inhalation induction while maintaining spontaneous ventilation in the term infant of normal size. If one chooses to intubate after induction, the airway should be topicalized with a weight-based dose of atomized lidocaine. The lowest inspiratory pressure assistance is used to prevent atelectasis while minimizing distension of the stomach. If the lungs are suspected of being poorly compliant due to pneumonia or prematurity, then mask ventilation should be avoided. Good intubating conditions can be achieved with a volatile agent; however, maintaining adequate ventilation and surgical conditions during a thoracotomy without neuromuscular block can be challenging.
2. Rapid-sequence induction and placement of the ETT above the carina but below the fistula is another option. If the ETT is in a good position, then neuromuscular blocking agents can be given, and normal PPV can be maintained. A cuffed ETT will more effectively occlude the fistula. A microcuffed ETT is preferred because it lacks a Murphy eye, which may allow air to pass into the fistula. The bevel of the ETT should be positioned anteriorly, if possible. The difficulty lies in maintaining a good position of the ETT during surgical manipulation and turning the patient laterally. It is possible for the tip of the tube to migrate directly into the fistula, with resultant high airway pressure, loss of end-tidal CO_2, and desaturation.
3. Another option to avoid the risk of ETT malposition is to deliberately keep the tip of the tube *above* the fistula (if it is shown by bronchoscopy to be small) and keep ventilation pressures low until the fistula is ligated. This comes with a higher risk of gastric distension.
4. In cases where the fistula is very close to or at the carina, one can consider deliberately intubating the left mainstem bronchus. One-lung ventilation can be poorly tolerated in the neonate, however, especially if there is a preexisting lung disease.
5. In cases where the lung compliance is poor, or the fistula is located near the carina, high-frequency oscillating ventilation (HFOV) can be used because it provides gas exchange with a much lower inspiratory pressure. This technique is technically cumbersome and requires the use of total IV anesthesia. It is also difficult to measure end-tidal CO_2 with this technique.

Ahmad NS, Dobby N, Walker E, et al. A multicenter audit of the use of bronchoscopy during open and thoracoscopic repair of esophageal atresia with tracheoesophageal fistula. *Paediatr Anaesth.* 2019;29:640-647.

Ho AM, Dion JM, Wong JC. Airway and ventilatory management options in congenital tracheoesophageal fistula repair. *J Cardiothorac Vasc Anesth.* 2016;30:515-520.

Mathew PJ, Ashok V, Malik MA. Ventilation failure due to endotracheal tube migration into a tracheal pouch in a toddler with a repaired tracheoesophageal fistula: a case report. *Anes Analg Pract.* 2020;14:48-50.

Morini F, Conforti A, Bagolan P. Perioperative complications of esophageal atresia. *Eur J Pediatr Surg.* 2018;28:133-140.

C.4. What is the role of rigid and fiberoptic bronchoscopy in this patient prior to incision?

Perioperative bronchoscopy before commencing TEF repair allows assessment of the size and location of the fistula. A cervical-level fistula does not require a thoracotomy to repair. A low-lying or subcarinal fistula predicts difficulty in placing an ETT that does not ventilate the fistula. The presence of a second fistula can be ruled out. If deemed appropriate, the fistula can be occluded using a 3F Fogarty occlusion catheter, thereby allowing normal PPV without distending the abdomen. Following placement of the balloon, the rigid bronchoscope is removed and the child is intubated with a microcuff ETT *alongside* the catheter. During positioning or surgical manipulation, the Fogarty balloon can slide back into the trachea. This could precipitate immediate, complete airway obstruction if not promptly recognized and treated by deflating the cuff.

Ahmad NS, Dobby N, Walker E, et al. A multicenter audit of the use of bronchoscopy during open and thoracoscopic repair of esophageal atresia with tracheoesophageal fistula. *Paediatr Anaesth.* 2019;29:640-647.

Ho AM, Dion JM, Wong JC. Airway and ventilatory management options in congenital tracheoesophageal fistula repair. *J Cardiothorac Vasc Anesth.* 2016;30:515-520.

Hunt RW, Perkins EJ, King S. Peri-operative management of neonates with oesophageal atresia and tracheo-oesophageal fistula. *Paediatr Respir Rev.* 2016;19:3-9.

Pepper VK, Boomer LA, Thung AK, et al. Routine bronchoscopy and Fogarty catheter occlusion of tracheoesophageal fistulas. *J Laparoendosc Adv Surg Tech A.* 2017;27:97-100.

Rinkel R, Van Poll D, Sibarani-Ponsen R, et al. Bronchoscopy and Fogarty balloon insertion of distal tracheo-oesophageal fistula for oesophageal atresia repair with video illustration. *Ann Otol Rhinol Laryngol.* 2017;126:6-8.

C.5. Describe the steps of an open repair of TEF and EA.

Usually, the patient is positioned in the lateral position, left side down. If the patient has a right-sided aortic arch (rare), the surgeon might position the patient with the right side down. A retropleural approach is used, which decreases the consequence of any postoperative esophageal anastomosis leak. The azygos vein is often ligated to better visualize the fistula. The right lung is retracted to expose and identify the fistula. The fistula is then ligated, leaving a stump; this usually occurs within 45 minutes. If the patient is stable, normal PPV can commence while the repair of the esophagus begins. The upper esophagus is mobilized, followed by the distal esophagus, and the esophagus is joined together. If there is a long gap between the proximal and distal portions, the esophageal repair can follow in a staged procedure. Following this, a feeding tube is placed across the anastomosis to allow feeding (if the patient does not have a gastrostomy). The lung should be carefully reexpanded to eliminate atelectasis before closure. Chest tubes are not routinely placed following repair.

Dingemann C, Eaton S, Aksnes G, et al. ERNICA consensus conference on the management of patients with esophageal atresia and tracheoesophageal fistula: diagnostics, preoperative, operative, and postoperative management. *Eur J Pediatr Surg.* 2020;30:326-336.

Slater BJ, Rothenberg SS. Tracheoesophageal fistula. *Semin Pediatr Surg.* 2016;25:176-178.

Walk RM. Esophageal atresia and tracheoesophageal fistula: overview and considerations for the general surgeon. *Surg Clin North Am.* 2022;102:759-778.

C.6. What are common intraoperative problems, and how can they be managed?

1. Lung retraction leads to atelectasis (with desaturation) and hypercapnia. If desaturation persists, the surgeon might need to temporarily release traction to allow the right lung to reexpand. Hypercapnia (Pco_2 > 70 mm Hg) can occur.
2. Surgical manipulation can kink the trachea or displace the ETT into the fistula or above the fistula. The patient can be accidentally extubated during positioning.
3. A balloon placed into the fistula can dislodge and occlude the trachea.
4. Blood and secretions can obstruct the ETT, especially if using a microcuffed ETT without a Murphy eye. The ETT can require frequent suctioning.
5. Frequent compression of vital structures in the mediastinum can lead to profound hemodynamic compromise. In this event, the surgeon might have to release pressure on involved structures temporarily. Close communication with the surgeon is essential.
6. Severe gastric distension before ligation of the TEF can require emergent gastric needle decompression.
7. Major blood loss is uncommon.

Ahmad NS, Dobby N, Walker E, et al. A multicenter audit of the use of bronchoscopy during open and thoracoscopic repair of esophageal atresia with tracheoesophageal fistula. *Paediatr Anaesth.* 2019;29:640-647.

Ho AM, Dion JM, Wong JC. Airway and ventilatory management options in congenital tracheoesophageal fistula repair. *J Cardiothorac Vasc Anesth.* 2016;30:515-520.

Walk RM. Esophageal atresia and tracheoesophageal fistula: overview and considerations for the general surgeon. *Surg Clin North Am.* 2022;102:759-778.

C.7. If the surgeon decides to proceed thoracoscopically, how will you perform your anesthetic? Is one-lung ventilation required? What are some complications unique to thoracoscopy in the newborn?

Thoracoscopy to repair TEF/EA has gained popularity recently. Major advantages are (1) the approach provides excellent visualization of the fistula, which allows rapid ligation and stabilization of ventilation;

(2) avoidance of thoracotomy results in less postoperative pain; and (3) avoiding posterolateral thoracotomy results in better chest wall symmetry and less long-term scoliosis. The anastomosis leak rate is not increased by thoracoscopic repair.

For anesthesia, an arterial line is mandatory due to the significant gradient between end-tidal and arterial CO_2. Concerns regarding tracheal intubation, PPV, paralysis, fluid, and temperature management are identical to those for an open repair. Opioid requirements can be reduced. Isolating the right lung is *not* required for successful thoracoscopy. One-lung ventilation is helpful but not necessary and might not be tolerated in a neonate. Deliberate left mainstem ETT intubation to collapse the right lung can result in prolonged left upper lobe lung collapse. Exposure of the fistula is attained by insufflation of the right chest cavity with CO_2 to a pressure of 5 mm Hg. Higher inflation pressure is unnecessary and leads to increased complications. Hypercapnia and acidosis are expected with both open repair and thoracoscopic repair, but the degree of hypercapnia and acidosis is worse with thoracoscopy. The impact of the increased intrathoracic pressure and hypercapnia associated with thoracoscopy on neonatal brain oxygenation has been explored. A single-center study found no significant effect on brain cerebral oximetry measurement in infants having repair thoracoscopically compared to open repair, provided mean arterial pressure was maintained with a combination of fluid and inotropic support.

Stolwijk LJ, Tytgat SH, Keunen K, et al. The effects of CO_2-insufflation with 5 and 10 mmHg during thoracoscopy on cerebral oxygenation and hemodynamics in piglets: an animal experimental study. *Surg Endosc*. 2015;29: 2781-2788.

Tytgat SH, van Herwaarden MY, Stolwijk LJ, et al. Neonatal brain oxygenation during thoracoscopic correction of esophageal atresia. *Surg Endosc*. 2016;30:2811-2817.

van Hoorn CE, Costerus SA, Lau J, et al. Perioperative management of esophageal atresia/tracheo-esophageal fistula: an analysis of data of 101 consecutive patients. *Paediatr Anaesth*. 2019;29:1024-1032.

Way C, Wayne C, Grandpierre V, et al. Thoracoscopy vs. thoracotomy for the repair of esophageal atresia and tracheoesophageal fistula: a systematic review and meta-analysis. *Pediatr Surg Int*. 2019;35:1167-1184.

Zani A, Lamas-Pinheiro R, Paraboschi I, et al. Intraoperative acidosis and hypercapnia during thoracoscopic repair of congenital diaphragmatic hernia and esophageal atresia/tracheoesophageal fistula. *Paediatr Anesth*. 2017;27: 841-848.

D. Postoperative Management

D.1. When should the trachea be extubated?

Although some surgeons prefer to extubate immediately in the OR to minimize tension on the tracheal suture line, this can be risky. Many infants with TEF have a deficiency of tracheal cartilage at the level of the fistula predisposing to tracheomalacia. This can result in airway obstruction requiring immediate reintubation. Many children have significant lung disease from prematurity or aspiration pneumonia; they should remain intubated. For patients with long-gap EA, it might be safer to leave the infant intubated and paralyzed in a flexed position for several days. If the child is to remain intubated, care should be taken to limit inspiratory pressure to protect the repair from disruption. If opioid-based postoperative analgesia is planned, mechanical ventilation is preferred due to the risk of hypoventilation. If the trachea is extubated to noninvasive PPV, there is an increased risk of anastomotic leak and mediastinitis.

De Rose DU, Landolfo F, Giliberti P, et al. Post-operative ventilation strategies after surgical repair in neonates with esophageal atresia: A retrospective cohort study. *J Pediatr Surg*. 2022;57:801-805.

Ferrand A, Roy SK, Faure C, et al. Postoperative noninvasive ventilation and complications in esophageal atresia-tracheoesophageal fistula. *J Pediatr Surg*. 2019;54:945-948.

Morini F, Conforti A, Bagolan P. Perioperative complications of esophageal atresia. *Eur J Pediatr Surg*. 2018;28: 133-140.

Walk RM. Esophageal atresia and tracheoesophageal fistula: overview and considerations for the general surgeon. *Surg Clin North Am*. 2022;102:759-778.

SECTION 10

D.2. What options are available for postoperative analgesia?

For patients who are to remain intubated postoperatively, a fentanyl infusion (1 μg/kg/h) can give effective postoperative analgesia and facilitate tolerance of the ETT. An epidural catheter inserted through the caudal space can be easily threaded up to the thoracic epidural space. The position of the catheter placed in this way should be confirmed with fluoroscopy or ultrasound prior to use. There is increasing interest in performing right-sided ultrasound-guided erector spinae block for postoperative analgesia.

Altıparmak B, Toker MK, Uysal Aİ, Özcan M, Demirbilek SG. Erector spinae plane block for pain management of esophageal atresia in a preterm neonate. *J Clin Anesth.* 2019;56:115-116.

Nagappa S, Kalappa S, Vijayakumar HN, et al. Comparison of the effectiveness of intravenous fentanyl versus caudal epidural in neonates undergoing tracheoesophageal fistula surgeries. *Saudi J Anaesth.* 2022;16:182-187.

Oliveira I, Marinho S, Gonçalves M. Erector spinae plane block for surgery of esophageal atresia in a preterm neonate. *Rev Esp Anestesiol Reanim.* 2022;69:680-682.

D.3. What are the early and late complications of TEF repair?

Early anastomosis leakage occurs in up to 15% of patients. This can require immediate exploration or can be managed expectantly. Esophageal dysmotility and gastroesophageal reflux disease (GERD) are common. The dysmotility can be from abnormal innervation of the distal esophagus or be related to vagal nerve injury during the repair. Stricture of the esophageal anastomosis can require repeated dilatations. Tracheomalacia can be evident postoperatively, and vocal cord paresis has been reported in 5% of Type C repairs.

A fistula stump remains after repair, at least initially. When the patient is intubated in future operations, the ETT might be observed to pass through the vocal cords, but the tip might be in the stump, precluding effective ventilation. An anterior-posterior chest radiograph will not show this, but a lateral film will. This possibility should always be entertained if unable to ventilate despite apparent successful intubation.

Ferrand A, Roy SK, Faure C, et al. Postoperative noninvasive ventilation and complications in esophageal atresia-tracheoesophageal fistula. *J Pediatr Surg.* 2019;54:945-948.

Friedmacher F, Kroneis B, Huber-Zeyringer A, et al. Postoperative complications and functional outcome after esophageal atresia repair: results from longitudinal single-center follow-up. *J Gastrointest Surg.* 2017;21:927-935.

Lal DR, Gadepalli SK, Downard CD, et al. Perioperative management and outcomes of esophageal atresia and tracheoesophageal fistula. *J Pediatr Surg.* 2017;52:1245-1251.

Mathew PJ, Ashok V, Malik MA. Ventilation failure due to endotracheal tube migration into a tracheal pouch in a toddler with a repaired tracheoesophageal fistula: a case report. *Anes Analg Pract.* 2020;14:48-50.

Wu Y, Kuang H, Ly T, et al. Comparison of clinical outcomes between open and thoracoscopic repair for esophageal atresia with tracheoesophageal fistula: a systematic review and meta-analysis. *Pediatr Surg Int.* 2017;33:1147-1157.

37

Congenital Diaphragmatic Hernia

Dana L. Gurvitch and Michael D. Green

A full-term male infant was born with respiratory distress and cyanosis. Physical examination showed a barrel chest and a scaphoid abdomen. Breath sounds were absent on the left side of the chest; heart sounds were best heard on the right side of the chest. Labored respiration, nasal flaring, and sternal retraction were present. The newborn weighed 2,800 g. Blood pressure was 60/30 mm Hg; heart rate, 160 beats per minute; respiration, 70 breaths per minute; and temperature, 36 °C (96.8 °F). Arterial blood gas analysis on room air showed: pH, 7.20; $Paco_2$, 55 mm Hg; Pao_2, 35 mm Hg; and CO_2 content, 19 mEq/L.

A. Medical Disease and Differential Diagnosis

1. What differential diagnoses are compatible with the signs and symptoms?
2. Describe the incidence and classification of congenital diaphragmatic hernia (CDH).
3. What are the causes of hypoxemia in patients with CDH?
4. How do you assess the severity of pulmonary hypoplasia?
5. How do you make a diagnosis of right-to-left shunting through a patent ductus arteriosus?
6. What other congenital anomalies are usually associated with CDH?

B. Preoperative Evaluation and Preparation

1. How would you interpret the following arterial blood gas analysis: pH, 7.20; $Paco_2$, 55 mm Hg; Pao_2, 35 mm Hg; and CO_2 content, 19 mEq/L? How would you correct this?
2. What immediate treatment should be given to improve respiratory status preoperatively?
3. Should CDH be repaired urgently once the diagnosis is made and confirmed?
4. What are the effects of inhaled nitric oxide (NO) on the pulmonary and systemic circulations?
5. What is the current role of extracorporeal membrane oxygenation (ECMO) in the management of CDH?

C. Intraoperative Management

1. What monitors would you use for this neonate during surgery?
2. How would you induce and maintain anesthesia?
3. Would you use nitrous oxide for anesthesia? Why?
4. How would you ventilate the patient?
5. Is the infant with CDH at greater risk for hypothermia?
6. The surgeon returned the intrathoracic stomach and intestine to the peritoneal cavity, and the ipsilateral lung was found to be hypoplastic and collapsed. Attempts were made to manually expand the collapsed lung with positive airway pressure. Five minutes after the abdomen was closed, the blood pressure suddenly decreased from 70/40 mm Hg to 30/20 mm Hg, the heart rate decreased from 150 to 80 beats per minute, and the Spo_2 decreased from 95% to 60%. What would you immediately do?
7. Discuss fluid therapy in this patient.
8. At the conclusion of surgery, would you extubate the patient in the operating room?

D. Postoperative Management

1. What is the mortality rate in patients with CDH? What postoperative problems would you expect in this patient?

A. Medical Disease and Differential Diagnosis

A.1. What differential diagnoses are compatible with the signs and symptoms?

The differential diagnosis of cyanosis and respiratory distress in the newborn is broad and includes respiratory distress syndrome, meconium aspiration, diaphragmatic hernia, persistent pulmonary hypertension (PPH) of the newborn, cyanotic congenital heart disease, choanal atresia, airway abnormalities, and bronchopulmonary sequestration. However, congenital diaphragmatic hernia (CDH) should be suspected in any infant with respiratory distress, shift of cardiac sounds to the right, decreased breath sounds ipsilateral to the side of the hernia, bowel sounds heard in the chest and a concave/scaphoid abdomen. Confirmation of diagnosis includes chest radiography demonstrating herniation of abdominal contents into the hemithorax, little or no visible aerated lung on the affected side and mediastinal shift (**Figure 37.1**). If in

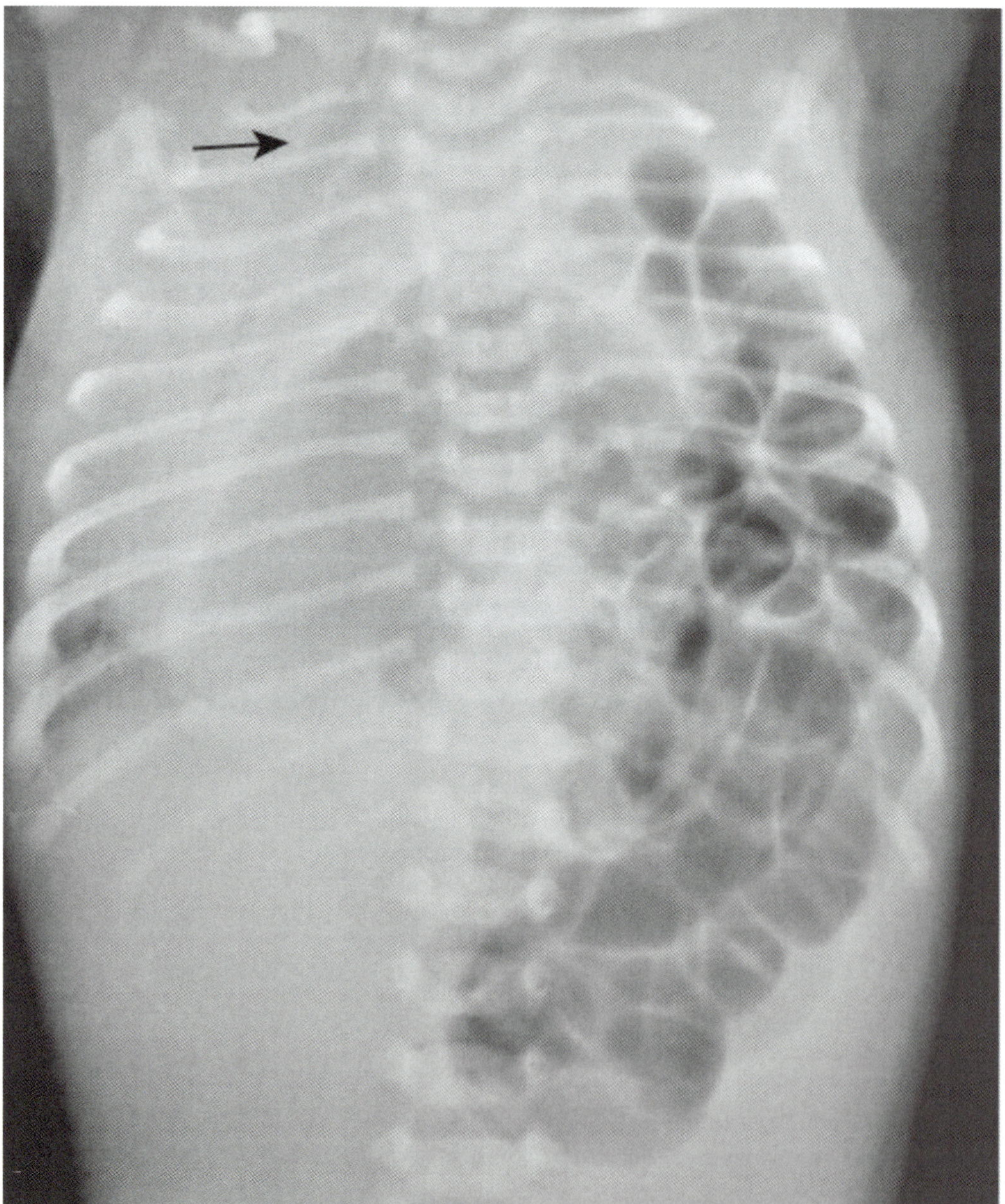

FIGURE 37.1. Chest radiograph of a neonate with a left diaphragmatic hernia. Note shifting of the trachea and bronchi into the right chest (*arrow*). (Reprinted from Spaeth JP, Lam JE. The extremely premature infant [micropremie] and common neonatal emergencies. In: Coté CJ, Lerman J, Anderson BJ, eds. *Coté and Lerman's A Practice of Anesthesia for Infants and Children.* 7th ed. Saunders/Elsevier; 2025:953-981. Copyright © 2018 Elsevier. With permission.)

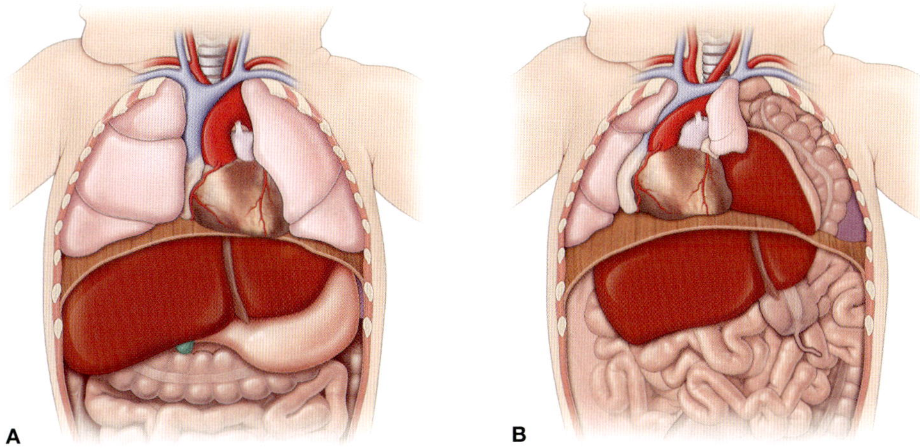

FIGURE 37.2. Congenital diaphragmatic hernia (CDH) internal abdominal view. The diaphragm (**A**, *left*) is a sheet of flat muscle that separates the heart and lungs from the abdominal cavity. In CDH, a hole in the diaphragm (**B**, *right*) allows abdominal organs to move into the chest and restrict lung development.

doubt, a radiopaque dye can be injected through a nasogastric tube to delineate the stomach and intestine in the chest cavity. If the CDH is right sided, the liver might be the only herniated organ and appear as a thoracic soft tissue mass. The internal abdominal view of CDH is shown in Figure 37.2.

Diu M, Walker K. Pediatric diseases. In: Hines RL, Maschall KE. *Stoelting's Anesthesia and Co-existing Disease.* 8th ed. Elsevier; 2021:663-696.

Steinhorn RH, Abman SH, Lakshminrusimha S. Vascular development and pulmonary hypertension. In: Kliegman RM, Stanton BF, St Geme JW, et al, eds. *Nelson Textbook of Pediatrics.* 22nd ed. Elsevier; 2025:1094-1096.

A.2. Describe the incidence and classification of congenital diaphragmatic hernia (CDH).

The incidence of CDH is between 1 per 2,000 and 1 per 3,000 births. Eighty-five percent of defects are left sided and less than 5% are bilateral, and 90% are posterolateral (Bochdalek hernia). Anteromedial and paraesophageal hernias and eventrations make up the remainder (Figure 37.3). There is no difference in mortality between left- and right-sided herniation, although right-sided CDH can have a higher incidence of pulmonary complications. Associated anomalies include central nervous system (CNS) lesions, esophageal atresia, omphalocele, and cardiovascular lesions. Trisomy 21, trisomy 13, trisomy 18, and tetrasomy 12p are examples of syndromes associated with CDH.

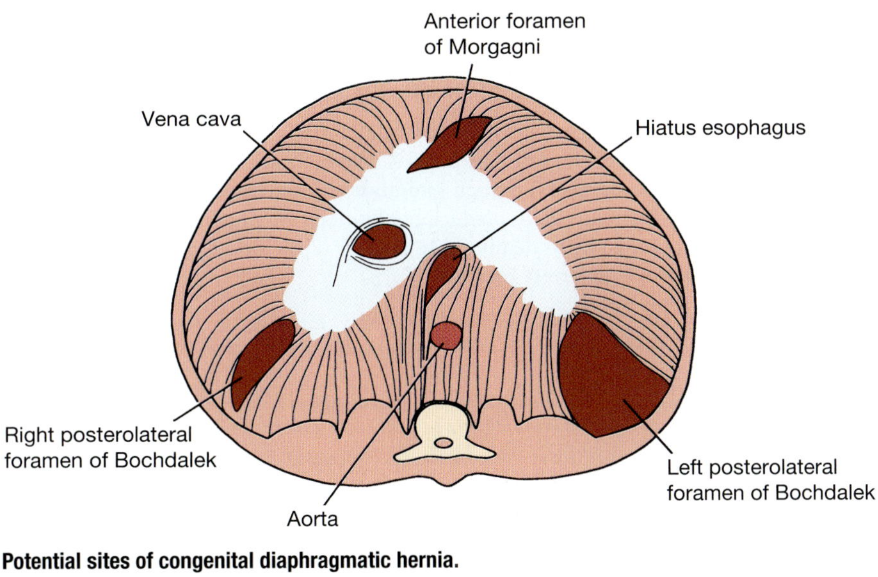

FIGURE 37.3. Potential sites of congenital diaphragmatic hernia.

Barnes SS, Davis PJ, Brett C. Anesthesia for general surgery in neonates. In: Davis PJ, Cladis FP, eds. *Smith's Anesthesia for Infants and Children*. 10th ed. Elsevier; 2022:669-708.

Spaeth JP, Lam JE. The extremely premature infant (micropremie) and common neonatal emergencies. In: Coté CJ, Lerman J, Anderson BJ, eds. *Coté and Lerman's A Practice of Anesthesia for Infants and Children*. 7th ed. Saunders/Elsevier; 2025:953-981.

Partidge EA, Peranteau WH, Herkert L, et al. Right- versus left-sided congenital diaphragmatic hernia: a comparative outcomes analysis. *J Pediatr Surg*. 2016;51:900-902.

A.3. What are the causes of hypoxemia in patients with CDH?

Infants with CDH have deficient bilateral major airway and vessel branching, which cannot be explained by simple compression of the ipsilateral and contralateral lungs. The severity of pulmonary vascular hypoplasia correlates with mortality in CDH. Airway maldevelopment leads to reduced total number of bronchi and alveoli at birth with resulting decreased lung compliance and decreases in both ventilation and surface area for gas exchange, with impaired oxygenation. Pulmonary vascular hypoplasia results in pulmonary hypertension, causing right-to-left shunting through the patent ductus arteriosus, with resultant hypoxemia.

Ruano R, Okpaise OO. Fetal intervention in congenital malformations of the respiratory system. In: Bancalari E, Keszler M, Davis P, Polin R, ed. *The Newborn Lung: Neonatology Questions and Controversies*. 4th ed. Elsevier; 2023:349-358.

A.4. How do you assess the severity of pulmonary hypoplasia?

Most infants with CDH are diagnosed prenatally by ultrasonography, which demonstrates herniated viscera with or without liver in the fetal thorax. The degree of pulmonary hypoplasia is estimated by calculating the lung-to-head ratio where a high ratio (>1.4) indicates good lung size and predicts a good outcome compared to a low ratio (<1.0). In addition, color-flow Doppler ultrasound can be used to assess positioning of the umbilical and portal veins, which are indicative of liver herniation. Fetal magnetic resonance imaging (MRI) is increasingly used for confirmation of CDH and for anatomy delineation, with fast spin echo MRI for lung volume calculation and further assessment of pulmonary hypoplasia.

Postnatally, the degree of pulmonary hypoplasia can be assessed by the degree of respiratory distress, hypoxemia, acidosis, and ensuing PPH in the newborn. Severe hypoplasia necessitates immediate tracheal intubation and mechanical ventilation and ECMO for neonates with critical cardiopulmonary deterioration. Inability to resuscitate in the delivery room is a marker of lethal lung hypoplasia, and most centers will not attempt emergency ECMO in this situation.

Ferschl MB, Rollins MD. Fetal intervention and the EXIT procedure. In: Coté CJ, Lerman J, Anderson BJ, eds. *Coté and Lerman's A Practice of Anesthesia for Infants and Children*. 7th ed. Saunders/Elsevier; 2025:982-999.

Gorincour G, Bouvenot J, Mourot MG, et al. Prenatal prognosis of congenital diaphragmatic hernia using magnetic resonance imaging measurement of fetal lung volume. *Ultrasound Obstet Gynecol*. 2005;26:738-744.

Hedrick HL, Crombleholme TM, Flake AW, et al. Right congenital diaphragmatic hernia: prenatal assessment and outcome. *J Pediatr Surg*. 2004;39:319-323.

Ruano R, Okpaise OO. Fetal intervention in congenital malformations of the respiratory system. In: Bancalari E, Keszler M, Davis P, Polin R, ed. *The Newborn Lung: Neonatology Questions and Controversies*. 4th ed. Elsevier; 2023:349-358.

A.5. How do you make a diagnosis of right-to-left shunting through a patent ductus arteriosus?

Clinical signs of ductal patency include murmur, tachycardia, bounding peripheral pulses with wide pulse pressure, congestive heart failure, and unexplained metabolic acidosis. Preductal (upper extremity) and postductal (lower/umbilical arteries) oxygen saturation measurements by pulse oximetry demonstrate a 10% or more gradient difference (with preductal saturation being higher). The gold standard for diagnosis is Doppler echocardiography to demonstrate the size of the ductal opening and the shunt and allow estimation of mean pulmonary artery pressure.

Holinski P, Turi J, Allareddy V, Ben Sivarajan V, Rotta AT. Critical care after surgery for congenital cardiac disease. In: Zimmerman JJ, Clark SB, *Furhrman BP, et al, eds. Fuhrman & Zimmerman's Pediatric Critical Care*. 6th ed. Elsevier; 2022:380-410.

Kussman BD, McGowan FX, Powell AJ, DiNardo JA. Anesthesia for congenital heart disease. In: Davis PJ, Cladis FP, eds. *Smith's Anesthesia for Infants and Children*. 10th ed. Elsevier; 2024:732-831.

Mariani G, Dik PB, Ezquer A, et al. Pre-ductal and post-ductal O_2 saturation in healthy term neonates after birth. *J Pediatr*. 2007;150:418-421.

A.6. What other congenital anomalies are usually associated with CDH?

About one-third of patients born with CDH have major congenital abnormalities.

- 10% have chromosome abnormality, most commonly trisomy 18 and isochromosome 12p
- 25% have cardiovascular malformations including ventricular septal defect (VSD), atrial septal defect (ASD), tetralogy of Fallot (TOF), and hypoplastic left heart syndrome
- 28% have CNS abnormalities including neural tube defects, hydrocephalus, agenesis of corpus callous, and sensorineural hearing loss
- 15% have genitourinary abnormalities including undescended testis and hypospadias
- 20% have gastrointestinal malformations including malrotation, atresia, omphalocele, and gastroesophageal reflux

B. Preoperative Evaluation and Preparation

B.1. How would you interpret the following arterial blood gas analysis: pH, 7.20; $Pa{CO_2}$, 55 mm Hg; $Pa{O_2}$, 35 mm Hg; and CO_2 content, 19 mEq/L? How would you correct this?

The blood gas analysis demonstrates an acute mixed respiratory and metabolic acidosis with severe hypoxemia. The typical compensatory relationship between HCO_3^- and $Pa{CO_2}$ is represented by the equation: $Pa{CO_2}$ (expected) = $(1.5 \times HCO_3^-) + 8 \pm 2$. A $Pa{CO_2}$ of 55 mm Hg suggests a concomitant respiratory acidosis. The severe hypoxemia is due to pulmonary hypoplasia and PPH. As alveolar $P{O_2}$ decreases below a threshold of 50 mm Hg at normal $Pa{CO_2}$, ventilation initially increases leading to respiratory alkalosis. However, if hypoxemia is not corrected, patient fatigue will result in CO_2 retention and respiratory acidosis. In addition, the hypoxemia results in anaerobic metabolism and lactic (metabolic) acidosis.

Treatment includes immediate tracheal intubation with gentle, conventional mechanical ventilation, $F{IO_2}$ less than 100%, avoiding any manual ventilation with a bag-valve mask. $F{IO_2}$ can be adjusted to achieve preductal O_2 saturation of 80% to 95%, or postductal O_2 saturation greater than 70%. Permissive hypercapnia to $Pa{CO_2}$ of 60 mm Hg or less can be employed to reduce ventilator-induced lung injury by keeping peak inspiratory pressures (PIPs) less than 25 cm H_20. For frequent blood gas monitoring, an intra-arterial catheter should be placed in a preductal location like the right radial artery, or a postductal location like the umbilical artery. Perfusion can be augmented using fluid therapy as a 10 mL/kg bolus of crystalloid to further normalize pH, oxygen content, and tissue perfusion. If pH is not within normal limits after 20 mL/kg of crystalloid, a vasopressor can be started. Inhaled NO can be utilized if there is difficulty achieving oxygenation and ventilation goals. If peak airway pressures continue to rise above 25 cm H_2O, one can consider changing ventilation strategies to high-flow oscillatory ventilation or ECMO. The risks of sodium bicarbonate administration preclude its utility at this pH.

Greenbaum LA. Electrolyte and acid-base disorders. In: Kliegman RM, Stanton BF, St Geme JW, et al, eds. *Nelson Textbook of Pediatrics*. 22nd ed. Elsevier; 2025:485-525.

Pittman RN. Oxygen transport in normal and pathological situations: defects and compensations. Pittman RN, ed. *Regulation of Tissue Oxygenation*. Morgan & Claypool Life Sciences; 2011:33-35.

Yamada NK, Szyld E, Strand ML, et al; American Heart Association and American Academy of Pediatrics. 2023 American Heart Association and American Academy of Pediatrics Focused Update on Neonatal Resuscitation: an update to the American Heart Association Guidelines for Cardiopulmonary Resuscitation and Emergency Cardiovascular Care. *Pediatrics*. 2024;153:e2023065030.

Zaki SA, Shanbag P. Metabolic acidosis in children: a literature review. *EMJ*. 2023:47-58.

B.2. What immediate treatment should be given to improve respiratory status preoperatively?

Immediate treatment should include tracheal intubation with mechanical ventilation (most of these patients are intubated immediately after delivery). The carina is elevated so there is increased potential to intubate the right mainstem bronchus. The intrathoracic bowel should be decompressed with a nasogastric tube. PIPs should be maintained at less than 25 cm H_2O, which often requires employing permissive hypercarbia to avoid barotrauma, reduce risk of pneumothorax, and further pulmonary damage. The $F{IO_2}$ should be adjusted to maintain preductal arterial saturation 85% or more (or >70% postductal). Spontaneous ventilatory mode is initially preferred over paralysis with neuromuscular blockade to reduce intrathoracic pressure, increase preload, and allow the patient to participate in ventilation to assess clinical status. Paralytics can be utilized if the patient remains difficult to ventilate at acceptable pressures or has significant risk factors (ie, liver herniating into right thorax, observed-to-expected lung-to-head ratio of <50%). Use of high-frequency oscillatory ventilation (HFOV) can be attempted if PIPs climb to 28 cm H_2O or oxygenation does not improve. Echocardiography should be performed to inform treatment decisions regarding pulmonary hypertension, evaluating shunt direction and patency of ductus arteriosus (PDA) as maintaining a PDA with prostaglandin can improve systemic perfusion. For patients weighing more than 2 kg who cannot be ventilated adequately with mean airway pressure less than 16 cm H_2O on HFOV, and who have been refractory to interventions for PPH (sildenafil, iNO, milrinone, bosentan, PGE1), can be considered for extracorporeal membrane oxygenation (ECMO).

Chatterjee D, Ing RJ, Gien J. Update on congenital diaphragmatic hernia. *Anesth Analg*. 2020;131:808-821.

Duncan KV, Polites S, Krishnaswami S, Scottoline BP. Congenital diaphragmatic hernia management: a systematic review and care pathway description including volume-targeted ventilation. *Adv Neonatal Care*. 2021;21:E138-E143.

King H, Booker PD. Congenital diaphragmatic hernia in the neonate. *Contin Educ Anaesth Crit Care Pain*. 2005; 5:171-174.

Lefebvre C, Rakza T, Weslinck N, et al; French CDH Study Group. Feasibility and safety of intact cord resuscitation in newborn infants with congenital diaphragmatic hernia (CDH). *Resuscitation*. 2017;120:20-25.

Noori S, Fisher ER, Kluckow M. Pulmonary and cardiovascular interaction. In: Bancalari E, Polin RA, Keszler M, Davis PG, eds. *The Newborn Lung: Neonatology Questions and Controversies*. 4th ed. Elsevier; 2025:165-188.

Quinney M, Wellesley H. Anaesthetic management of patients with a congenital diaphragmatic hernia. *BJA Educ*. 2018;18:95-101.

Snoek KG, Reiss IK, Greenough A, et al. Standardized postnatal management of infants with congenital diaphragmatic hernia in Europe: the CDH EURO Consortium Consensus-2015 update. *Neonatology*. 2016;110:66-74.

Spaeth JP, Lam JE. The extremely premature infant (micropremie) and common neonatal emergencies. In: Coté CJ, Lerman J, Anderson BJ, eds. *Coté and Lerman's A Practice of Anesthesia for Infants and Children*. 7th ed. Saunders/ Elsevier; 2025:953-981.

B.3. Should CDH be repaired urgently once the diagnosis is made and confirmed?

Surgical repair of CDH was once treated as a surgical emergency. However, improvements in gas exchange, thoracic compliance, $Paco_2$, or mortality were not immediately improved with this approach. Delaying surgery for clinical stabilization of respiratory and cardiovascular status by ensuring adequate end-organ perfusion, as evidenced by improved oxygenation, decreasing pulmonary vascular hypertension, and correction of metabolic acidosis, has become standard. The duration of delay is still a matter of controversy and often depends on severity by looking at risk factors including side, liver involvement, observed-to-expected lung-to-head ratio less than 50%, presence of a hernia sac, and cardiovascular status. Regarding severity of pulmonary hypertension, waiting for left-to-right shunting across the PDA before repair appears to be safe, even if there is some residual pulmonary hypertension.

Boloker J, Bateman DA, Wung JT, et al. Congenital diaphragmatic hernia in 120 infants treated consecutively with permissive hypercapnia/spontaneous respiration/elective repair. *J Pediatr Surg*. 2002;37:357-366.

Chatterjee D, Ing RJ, Gien J. Update on congenital diaphragmatic hernia. *Anesth Analg*. 2020;131:808-821.

Levesque M, Derraugh G, Schantz D, et al. The presence of a hernia sac in isolated congenital diaphragmatic hernia is associated with less disease severity: a retrospective cohort study. *J Pediatr Surg*. 2019;54:899-902.

Mohseni-Bod H, Bohn D. Pulmonary hypertension in congenital diaphragmatic hernia. *Semin Pediatr Surg*. 2007;16:126-133.

Noori S, Fisher ER, Kluckow M. Pulmonary and cardiovascular interaction. In: Bancalari E, Polin RA, Keszler M, Davis PG, eds. *The Newborn Lung: Neonatology Questions and Controversies*. 4th ed. Elsevier; 2025:165-188.

Quinney M, Wellesley H. Anaesthetic management of patients with a congenital diaphragmatic hernia. *BJA Educ*. 2018;18:95-101.

Snoek KG, Derraugh G, Schantz D, et al. Standardized postnatal management of infants with congenital diaphragmatic hernia in Europe: the CDH EURO Consortium Consensus-2015 update. *Neonatology*. 2016;110:66-74.

Spaeth JP, Lam JE. The extremely premature infant (micropremie) and common neonatal emergencies. In: Coté CJ, Lerman J, Anderson BJ, eds. *Coté and Lerman's A Practice of Anesthesia for Infants and Children*. 7th ed. Saunders/ Elsevier; 2025:953-981.

Wung JT, Sahni R, Moffitt ST, et al. Congenital diaphragmatic hernia: survival treated with very delayed surgery, spontaneous respiration, and no chest tube. *J Pediatr Surg*. 1995;30:406-409.

B.4. What are the effects of inhaled nitric oxide (NO) on the pulmonary and systemic circulations?

NO is endothelium-derived relaxing factor, which causes smooth muscle relaxation and vasodilation. Inhaled NO (iNO) is unique as a selective pulmonary vasodilator with no effect on systemic circulation. In low concentrations, iNO diffuses into pulmonary smooth muscle, increases the concentration of cyclic guanosine monophosphate (cGMP), which induces selective vasodilation and decreased vascular tone.

Unfortunately, most neonates with CDH with pulmonary hypertension plus lung hypoplasia do not have a dramatic response to iNO. A Cochrane review concluded that iNO does not improve outcomes in neonates with CDH and can even worsen outcomes. However, it has been shown to decrease duration of mechanical ventilation, need for ECMO, and severity of pulmonary hypertension, and therefore, continues to have a place in many protocols internationally. It must be discontinued if no improvement is demonstrated, as there are other options like milrinone available. Hyperoxygenation has also been reported to affect the efficacy of some pulmonary vasodilators, underscoring the importance of maintaining preductal saturations of 80% to 95%.

Barnes SS, Davis PJ, Brett C. Anesthesia for general surgery in neonates. In: Davis PJ, Cladis FP, eds. *Smith's Anesthesia for Infants and Children*. 10th ed. Elsevier; 2022:669-708.

Barrington KJ, Finer N, Pennaforte T, Altit G. Nitric oxide for respiratory failure in infants born at or near term. *Cochrane Database Syst Rev*. 2017;1:CD000399.

Campbell BT, Herbst KW, Briden KE, et al. Inhaled nitric oxide use in neonates with congenital diaphragmatic hernia. *Pediatrics*. 2014;134:e420-e426.

Kumar VHS, Dadiz R, Koumoundouros J, Guilford S, Lakshminrusimha S. Response to pulmonary vasodilators in infants with congenital diaphragmatic hernia. *Pediatr Surg Int*. 2018;34:735-742.

B.5. What is the current role of extracorporeal membrane oxygenation (ECMO) in the management of CDH?

While CDH is the most common indication for ECMO in neonates with respiratory distress, survival of patients with CDH treated with ECMO remains unchanged at 50%. Utilization has decreased precipitously over time, largely due to the employment of gentle mechanical ventilation with permissive hypercapnia, delayed surgical timing, and pulmonary vasodilators. There is great variation in utilization of ECMO across the United States with southern regions employing it more frequently than other regions. A recent UK study showed that infants who received ECMO for CDH had significant mortality in the first year of life with long-term physical and neurodevelopmental morbidity in the majority of survivors. Consensus on significant risks associated with ECMO, such as bleeding, intracranial hemorrhage, and sepsis, has shifted the implementation of ECMO, as a rescue therapy for infants with persistent preductal hypoxemia and acidosis despite inotropic and ventilator support. Some indications for ECMO in infants with CDH include refractory hypotension secondary to left ventricular (LV) systolic dysfunction, preductal saturation less than 80% refractory to ventilator manipulation and medical therapy, oxygenation index greater than 40, severe air leak, and mixed acidosis (pH <7.2). Some risk factors have been correlated with increased use as well. Newborns with a percent predicted lung volume (PPLV) of less than 15% and those with liver herniation and LV failure after initiation of milrinone and vasopressin had significantly higher ECMO use and poor outcomes. For patients placed on ECMO, there is some evidence supporting surgery within 48 to 72 hours, but patients must be optimized as far as ventilation and pulmonary hypertension.

Barnes SS, Davis PJ, Brett C. Anesthesia for general surgery in neonates. In: Davis PJ, Cladis FP, eds. *Smith's Anesthesia for Infants and Children*. 10th ed. Elsevier; 2022:669-708.

Davis PJ, Firmin RK, Manktelow B, et al. Long-term outcome following extracorporeal membrane oxygenation for congenital diaphragmatic hernia: the UK experience. *J Pediatr*. 2004;144:309-315.

Kays DW. ECMO in CDH: is there a role? *Semin Pediatr Surg*. 2017;26:166-170.

Kokhanov A, Lau C, Garg M, Jen H, Chu A. ECMO utilization in infants with congenital diaphragmatic hernia in the USA. *World J Pediatr Surg*. 2022;5:e000393.

Smithers CJ, Zalieckas JM, Rice-Townsend SE, Kamran A, Zurakowski D, Buchmiller TL. The timing of congenital diaphragmatic hernia repair on extracorporeal membrane oxygenation impacts surgical bleeding risk. *J Pediatr Surg*. 2023;58:1656-1662.

C. Intraoperative Management

C.1. What monitors would you use for this neonate during surgery?

Respiratory Monitors

- Two pulse oximeters, for preductal and postductal oxygen saturation
- Capnometry
- Inspiratory pressure measurement
- Inspiratory oxygen concentration
- Intraoperative arterial blood gas analysis

Cardiovascular Monitors

- Five-lead electrocardiogram
- Blood pressure cuff
- Arterial catheter in right radial artery for preductal Pao_2
- Central venous pressure (CVP) catheter for evaluating intravascular volume and right ventricular performance

Thermoregulatory Monitor

- Esophageal or rectal temperature probe

C.2. How would you induce and maintain anesthesia?

In general, the preoperative care of the neonate is continued into the operating room with the addition of high-dose opioids (fentanyl 10-30 µg/kg) and a nondepolarizing neuromuscular blocking agent. Ventilation strategies focus on permissive hypercarbia (50-70 mm Hg), preductal oxygen saturation of 80% to 95%, and peak pressures less than 25 cm H_2O. Volatile anesthetics should be administered with caution because systemic vascular resistance can decrease more than pulmonary vascular resistance (PVR) thus increasing the right-to-left shunt. Frequent blood gas sampling guides changes in respiratory management and assessment of acid-base status. Goals include normal mean arterial blood pressure guided by preductal oxygen saturations of 85% to 95%, lactate level less than 3 mM, and urine output more than 1 mL/kg/h. Availability of drugs to maintain blood pressure support should be readily available and include isotonic fluids and inotropes such as milrinone, vasopressin, dopamine and/or dobutamine, and hydrocortisone. Meticulous attention to temperature is essential because hypothermia can increase PVR and thus increase right-to-left shunting. Regional analgesia has been safely incorporated into the postoperative pain plan for select cases in this population with use of a caudal epidural catheters and erector spinae blocks.

Aggarwal A, Lohani R, Suresh V. Case series on anesthesia for video-assisted thoracoscopic surgery for congenital diaphragmatic hernia in children. *Anesth Essays Res*. 2016;10:128-131.

Barnes SS, Davis PJ, Brett C. Anesthesia for general surgery in neonates. In: Davis PJ, Cladis FP, eds. *Smith's Anesthesia for Infants and Children*. 10th ed. Elsevier; 2022:669-708.

Bosenberg AT. Epidural analgesia for major neonatal surgery. *Paediat Anaesth*. 1998;8:479-483.

Kulkarni K, Patil S, Mubarizuddin A, Malager A. Management of congenital diaphragmatic hernia with epidural and general anaesthesia. *J Anesth Clin Care*. 2018;5:30.

Kumar VHS, Dadiz R, Koumoundouros J, Guilford S, Lakshminrusimha S. Response to pulmonary vasodilators in infants with congenital diaphragmatic hernia. *Pediatr Surg Int*. 2018;34:735-742.

Spaeth JP, Lam JE. The extremely premature infant (micropremie) and common neonatal emergencies. In: Coté CJ, Lerman J, Anderson BJ, eds. *Coté and Lerman's A Practice of Anesthesia for Infants and Children*. 7th ed. Saunders/ Elsevier; 2025:953-981.

Wiegele M, Marhofer P, Lönnqvist PA. Caudal epidural blocks in paediatric patients: a review and practical considerations. *Br J Anaesth*. 2019;122:509-517.

Yadav RK, Acharya U, Malla SS. Ultrasound guided erector spinae and celiac plexus block for postoperative analgesia following surgical repair of congenital diaphragmatic hernia. *Bali J Anaesthesiol*. 2021;5:198-200.

C.3. Would you use nitrous oxide for anesthesia? Why?

Nitrous oxide is avoided because it can expand air-filled cavities (such as bowel) and potentially compress functioning lung tissue further, and because it limits the inspired oxygen concentration that can be provided to a compromised neonate.

Spaeth JP, Lam JE. The extremely premature infant (micropremie) and common neonatal emergencies. In: Coté CJ, Lerman J, Anderson BJ, eds. *Coté and Lerman's A Practice of Anesthesia for Infants and Children*. 7th ed. Saunders/ Elsevier; 2025:953-981.

C.4. How would you ventilate the patient?

The goals of ventilation and oxygenation in the operating room are the same as preoperatively: Avoid volutrauma by using small tidal volumes (3-6 mL/kg) and low-peak inspiratory pressures (<25 cm H_2O), adequate oxygenation to preductal O_2 saturations of 80% to 95%, and permissive hypercapnia with maintenance of pH more than 7.20 at respiratory rates of 40 to 60 breaths per minute with positive end-expiratory pressure (PEEP) of 3 to 5 cm H_2O. Neuromuscular blocking agents should be used intraoperatively to facilitate reduction of bowel contents and closure.

Chatterjee D, Ing RJ, Gien J. Update on congenital diaphragmatic hernia. *Anesth Analg*. 2020;131:808-821.

Spaeth JP, Lam JE. The extremely premature infant (micropremie) and common neonatal emergencies. In: Coté CJ, Lerman J, Anderson BJ, eds. *Coté and Lerman's A Practice of Anesthesia for Infants and Children*. 7th ed. Saunders/Elsevier; 2025:953-981.

Barnes SS, Davis PJ, Brett C. Anesthesia for general surgery in neonates. In: Davis PJ, Cladis FP, eds. *Smith's Anesthesia for Infants and Children*. 10th ed. Elsevier; 2022:669-708.

Snoek KG, Capolupo I, van Rosmalen J, et al; CDH EURO Consortium. Conventional mechanical ventilation versus high-frequency oscillatory ventilation for congenital diaphragmatic hernia: a randomized clinical trial (the VICI-trial). *Ann Surg*. 2016;263:867-874.

C.5. Is the infant with CDH at greater risk for hypothermia?

All neonates are susceptible to heat loss because of a high ratio of surface area to body weight, reduced subcutaneous fat, and an underdeveloped ability to shiver (thermogenesis) in response to cold. However, infants with CDH have increased morbidity and mortality secondary to hypothermia because the resulting increased PVR can cause decreased oxygen delivery, worsening acidosis, shunting, and continued increases in PVR. Concerted efforts to maintain normothermia are mandatory and include maintaining ambient operating room temperature more than 23 °C, use of warmed intravenous fluids, passive insulation with drapes and blankets, forced air warming, and passive humidification of inspired anesthetic gases.

Bajwa SJ, Jindal S. Perioperative hypothermia in pediatric patients: diagnosis, prevention and management. *Anaesth Pain Intensive Care*. 2014;18:97-100.

Engorn B, Harvey H, Davis PJ, Lunginbuehl I, Bissonnette B. Thermoregulation. In: Davis PJ, Cladis FP, eds. *Smith's Anesthesia for Infants and Children*. 10th ed. Elsevier; 2022:158-177.

C.6. The surgeon returned the intrathoracic stomach and intestine to the peritoneal cavity, and the ipsilateral lung was found to be hypoplastic and collapsed. Attempts were made to manually expand the collapsed lung with positive airway pressure. Five minutes after the abdomen was closed, the blood pressure suddenly decreased from 70/40 mm Hg to 30/20 mm Hg, the heart rate decreased from 150 to 80 beats per minute, and the Spo_2 decreased from 95% to 60%. What would you immediately do?

Sudden deterioration in blood pressure, heart rate, oxygen saturation, or pulmonary compliance is suggestive of tension pneumothorax. Auscultation of the chest, particularly the contralateral side, should be performed immediately. If absent or diminished breath sounds confirm the diagnosis, a chest tube should be inserted immediately. A large-bore intravenous catheter with needle can be inserted to release the tension pneumothorax if a chest tube is not immediately available. Importantly, the thoracostomy tube should be placed to a water seal and not suction, as excessive suction could pull the entire mediastinum over creating a tension effect.

The tension pneumothorax is usually on the contralateral side because the high airway pressure required to inflate the hypoplastic lung can rupture normal alveoli on the contralateral side, resulting in pneumothorax. Moreover, the ipsilateral chest usually already has a chest tube after surgery. If there is any question, lung point-of-care ultrasound (POCUS) can be employed to look for lung sliding.

If there is no pneumothorax, or if deterioration is not improved after insertion of a chest tube, inferior vena cava compression resulting in decreased venous return and decreased cardiac output should be considered. The abdominal cavity is often underdeveloped and unable to fully accommodate the returned abdominal organs, which increases intra-abdominal pressure, displaces the diaphragm cephalad, and ultimately decreases pulmonary compliance in the healthy lung. The result is arterial desaturation, hypercarbia, and overall instability. In this circumstance, the abdominal wound should be reopened to relieve compression on the great vessels and displacement of the diaphragm. A patch closure of the abdomen can be attempted, or a silo pouch can be placed until growth allows safe return of organs to the abdominal cavity.

Barnes SS, Davis PJ, Brett C. Anesthesia for general surgery in neonates. In: Davis PJ, Cladis FP, eds. *Smith's Anesthesia for Infants and Children*. 10th ed. Elsevier; 2022:669-708.

Chatterjee D, Ing RJ, Gien J. Update on congenital diaphragmatic hernia. *Anesth Analg*. 2020;131:808-821.

Spaeth JP, Lam JE. The extremely premature infant (micropremie) and common neonatal emergencies. In: Coté CJ, Lerman J, Anderson BJ, eds. *Coté and Lerman's A Practice of Anesthesia for Infants and Children*. 7th ed. Saunders/Elsevier; 2025:953-981.

Stewart DL, Elsayed Y, Fraga MV, et al. Use of point-of-care ultrasonography in the NICU for diagnostic and procedural purposes. *Pediatrics*. 2022;150:e2022060053.

C.7. Discuss fluid therapy in this patient.

Fluid and electrolyte management in newborns should be focused on maintaining homeostasis while recognizing the impact of gestational age, physiologic changes in renal function, redistribution of total body water, water loss secondary to environmental factors, underlying medical condition of neonate, and surgical stress on fluid requirements. Neonates are obligate sodium losers, and therefore, exogenous sodium should be supplied. In addition, urine concentrating ability is limited in the newborn and as a result, the risk of volume depletion is increased due to the inability to maximally concentrate urine, decreased response to antidiuretic hormone (ADH), limited sodium reabsorption due to tubular immaturity, and reduced responsiveness to aldosterone.

The preoperative fluid deficit can be evaluated by careful history taking, signs and symptoms of dehydration, urine output, and bedside ultrasonography. Maintenance fluids consisting of 5% dextrose in 0.25 or 0.5 normal saline are given at 4 mL/kg/h. Intraoperative evaporative and third-space losses are replaced with lactated Ringer's, Plasma-Lyte, or saline at 6 to 8 mL/kg/h. Each milliliter of blood loss is replaced with 3 mL of lactated Ringer's or 1 mL of 5% albumin. Blood pressure, heart rate, urine output, CVP, hematocrit, and electrolytes should guide fluid therapy. POCUS has been shown to be useful in this population for determining fluid status.

Feld LG, Neuspiel DR, Foster BA, et al. Clinical practice guideline: maintenance intravenous fluids in children. *Pediatrics*. 2018;142:e20183083.

Greenbaum LA. Electrolyte and acid-base disorders. In: Kliegman RM, Stanton BF, St Geme JW, et al, eds. *Nelson Textbook of Pediatrics*. 22nd ed. Elsevier; 2025:485-525.

Stewart DL, Elsayed Y, Fraga MV, et al. Use of point-of-care ultrasonography in the NICU for diagnostic and procedural purposes. *Pediatrics*. 2022;150:e2022060053.

C.8. At the conclusion of surgery, would you extubate the patient in the operating room?

No, the patient should remain intubated at the conclusion of surgery. Varying degrees of pulmonary dysfunction, fluid shifts, and changes in abdominal compliance must be anticipated, including the need for postoperative mechanical ventilation and stabilization.

D. Postoperative Management

D.1. What is the mortality rate in patients with CDH? What postoperative problems would you expect in this patient?

Despite advances in medical and surgical treatment, the mortality rate in patients with CDH has remained at 20% to 30% over the past two decades. Pulmonary hypoplasia and PPH are the two main risk factors although these have expanded to include associated cardiac or chromosomal anomalies, liver herniation, observed-to-expected lung-to-head ratio less than 25%, predicted lung volume less than 15%, total lung volume less than 20 mL, left ventricular hypoplasia, right-sided diaphragmatic hernia and hernia sac involvement. Survival is complicated by both restrictive and obstructive lung disease patterns and bronchopulmonary dysplasia (BPD) is often documented radiographically. By childhood or adolescence, survivors of CDH often recover and remodel achieving near-normal lung volumes and mechanics. Gastroesophageal reflux disease, intestinal obstruction, delayed growth, neurocognitive defects, sensorineural hearing loss, and musculoskeletal abnormalities (mainly scoliosis and pectus excavatum) also complicate long-term survival. There is evidence that neonates treated with high-dose opioids can have decreased neurocognitive and social development in early childhood; techniques that decrease opioid use in these patients could help improve their long-term well-being.

Barnes SS, Davis PJ, Brett C. Anesthesia for general surgery in neonates. In: Davis PJ, Cladis FP, eds. *Smith's Anesthesia for Infants and Children*. 10th ed. Elsevier; 2022:669-708.

Chatterjee D, Ing RJ, Gien J. Update on congenital diaphragmatic hernia. *Anesth Analg*. 2020;131:808-821.

Grabski DF, Vavolizza RD, Roecker Z, et al. Reduction of post-operative opioid use in neonates following open congenital diaphragmatic hernia repairs: a quality improvement initiative. *J Pediatr Surg*. 2022;57:45-51.

Rintoul NE, Partridge EA, Hedrick HL. Fetal intervention and surgery. In: Kliegman RM, Stanton BF, St Geme JW, et al, eds. *Nelson Textbook of Pediatrics*. 22nd ed. Elsevier; 2025:1028-1037.

38

Tetralogy of Fallot

David Whiting and James A. DiNardo

A 5-month-old infant is being evaluated for stable persistent cyanosis with arterial oxygen saturation (Sa_{O_2}) of 70% to 80% since birth. She eats well and is in the 70th percentile for weight (6.5 kg). A transthoracic echocardiogram done before her arrival at your institution suggests that she has tetralogy of Fallot (TOF). Although she has never been noted to have a "Tet spell," her Sa_{O_2} was noted to decrease to 60% during a recent febrile illness. A repeat echocardiogram reveals TOF with severe valvular pulmonary stenosis (PS) and mild subvalvular PS secondary to anterior deviation of the conal septum into the right ventricle outflow tract (RVOT). There is a peak instantaneous pressure gradient of 70 mm Hg across the RVOT as determined by continuous wave Doppler.

A. Medical Disease and Differential Diagnosis

1. What is TOF?
2. What is the pathophysiology of TOF/PS?
3. What is shunting, and how is $Q_P:Q_S$ calculated?
4. What is the pathophysiology of TOF with pulmonary atresia?
5. How is Sa_{O_2} determined in single ventricle physiology?
6. What is a "pink Tet"?
7. What are hypercyanotic spells? How are they treated?
8. What palliative surgical procedures are available for treating patients with TOF/PS?
9. What palliative catheter-based procedures are available for patients with TOF?
10. What definitive surgical procedures are available for treating patients with TOF/PS?
11. What palliative and definitive surgical procedures are available for patients with TOF with pulmonary atresia?
12. What are the long-term outcomes of patients with TOF/PS?

B. Preoperative Evaluation and Preparation

1. What preoperative history and physical examination information do you need for this patient?
2. Which other abnormalities need to be considered in this patient?
3. What premedication will you give to a child with congenital heart disease?

C. Intraoperative Management

1. How will you induce anesthesia in this patient if intravenous access cannot be obtained?
2. Why would end-tidal carbon dioxide (Et_{CO_2}) monitoring be of particular use in a patient with TOF/PS?
3. What is near-infrared spectroscopy (NIRS) and what does it measure?
4. What are the important management issues during creation of a palliative shunt?
5. What is the effect of inhalation anesthetics on airway reflexes, myocardial contractility, systemic vascular resistance (SVR), and pulmonary vascular resistance (PVR) in children?
6. What are the anesthetic goals pre-cardiopulmonary bypass (pre-CPB) for a patient undergoing definitive surgical correction of TOF/PS?
7. What interventions reliably reduce PVR?
8. How does heparin administration and activated coagulation time (ACT) monitoring for CPB differ in children when compared to adults?
9. How is the effect of unfractionated heparin reversed?
10. What is the incidence of protamine reactions in children?

11. What is the role of transesophageal echocardiography (TEE) in this patient?
12. What effect would a residual ventricular septal defect (VSD) have on this patient following separation from CPB?

D. Postoperative Management

1. How should postoperative ventilation be managed in this patient following placement of a transannular patch for TOF/PS?
2. What $Sa{O_2}$ is expected following complete repair of TOF/PS in the infant?
3. What $Sa{O_2}$ is expected following placement of a modified Blalock-Taussig shunt (MBTS) for TOF/PS in the infant?
4. What is junctional ectopic tachycardia (JET)?

A. Medical Disease and Differential Diagnosis

A.1. What is TOF?

TOF is a complex of anatomic malformations consisting of a large malaligned conoventricular VSD, rightward and anterior displacement of the aorta such that it overrides the VSD, and a variable degree of subvalvular RVOT obstruction due to anterior, superior, and leftward deviation of the conal (infundibular) ventricular septum. It was first characterized in 1888 by the French physician Étienne-Louis Arthur Fallot who described a congenital heart defect with four characteristics: (1) large VSD, (2) right ventricular (RV) outflow obstruction, (3) overriding aorta, and (4) right ventricle hypertrophy (RVH). In addition, RV abnormalities in the septal and parietal bands of the crista supraventricularis exacerbate the infundibular RVOT obstruction. RVH is the result of chronic RVOT obstruction. The most common associated lesion is a right aortic arch with mirror image arch vessel branching that occurs in 25% of patients with TOF. In this lesion, the innominate artery gives rise to the left carotid and left subclavian arteries and the right carotid and subclavian arteries arise separately. TOF/PS and TOF with pulmonary atresia are two broad subsets of TOF. A third rare variant of TOF occurs when the pulmonary valve is absent.

Tetralogy of Fallot With Pulmonary Stenosis

TOF/PS is a form of tetralogy of Fallot where RV outflow tract obstruction is primarily due to varying degrees of valvular PS. At one end of the spectrum, the pulmonary valve annulus is mildly hypoplastic with minimal fusion of the pulmonary valve leaflets (**Figure 38.1A**). At the other end of the spectrum, the pulmonary annulus is very small and the pulmonary valve leaflets are nearly fused. The RVOT from valvular PS is fixed, whereas the coexisting subvalvular component of RVOT obstruction is dynamic. If left uncorrected, compensatory RVH from valvular or subvalvular components of the RVOT increases the mass of the RV and the infundibulum and worsens subvalvular obstruction. The anatomy of TOF/PS can usually be definitively delineated by two-dimensional transthoracic echocardiography, so further imaging with cardiac catheterization is rarely necessary or indicated.

Tetralogy of Fallot With Pulmonary Atresia

TOF with pulmonary atresia has the features of TOF with infundibular and pulmonary valvular atresia in conjunction with varying degrees of pulmonary artery (PA) atresia. TOF with pulmonary atresia is divided into four groups based on the degree of PA atresia. *Group 1* patients have isolated infundibular and pulmonary valve atresia with main PA and branch PAs of near-normal size and architecture. In some of these patients, the main PA extends to the atretic infundibulum. In others, atresia involves a short segment of the main PA (**Figure 38.2**). Patients in this group have pulmonary blood flow supplied from a patent ductus arteriosus (PDA). In *group 2* patients, the main PA is absent, but the left and right PAs are in continuity and supplied by a PDA. *Group 3* patients have severely hypoplastic native PAs, and the left and right PAs might not be in continuity. Pulmonary blood flow is from collateral vessels from the aorta to the PAs, known as major aortopulmonary collateral arteries (MAPCAs). A PDA can be present as well. Some segments of lung can be perfused from MAPCAs, some only by the native PAs, and others by both sources (**Figure 38.3**). *Group 4* patients have no native PAs, and all pulmonary blood flow is derived entirely from MAPCAs.

The anatomy of MAPCAs in TOF with pulmonary atresia can almost never be clearly delineated by two-dimensional transthoracic echocardiography alone. Cardiac catheterization and/or magnetic resonance imaging or magnetic resonance angiography are usually necessary to delineate collateral anatomy and determine Q_P:Q_S.

Jonas RA. Tetralogy of Fallot with Pulmonary Atresia. In: Jonas RA, ed. *Comprehensive Surgical Management of Congenital Heart Disease*. 2nd ed. CRC Press; 2014:585-602.

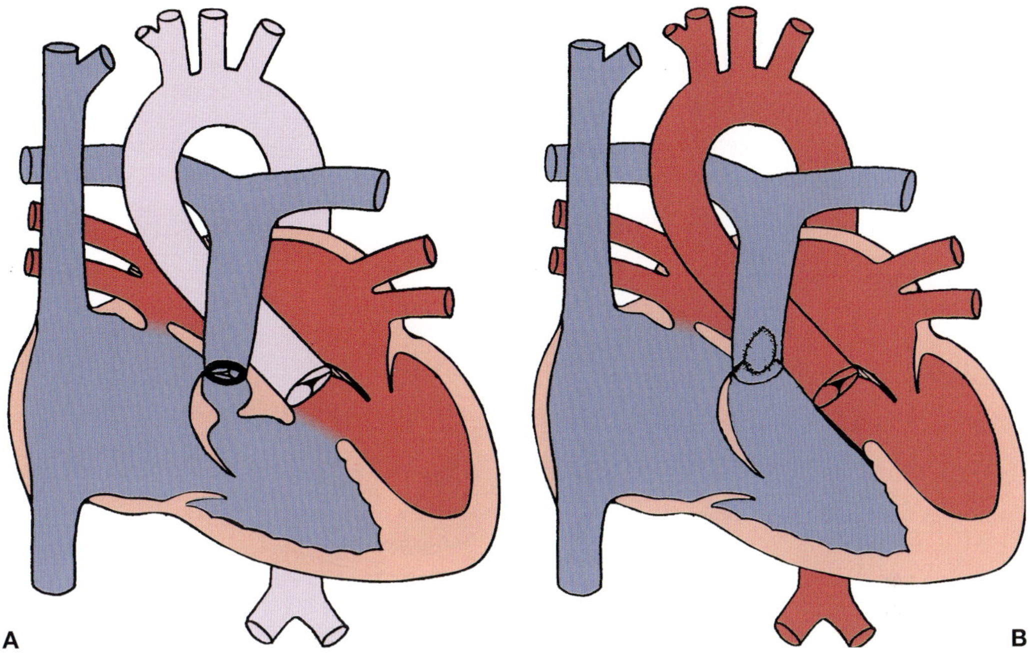

FIGURE 38.1. Tetralogy of Fallot with pulmonary stenosis. A. Uncorrected tetralogy of Fallot with pulmonary stenosis (TOF/PS) demonstrating malalignment ventricular septal defect (VSD) with aortic override, valvular, and subvalvular (dynamic) PS. There is a left aortic arch. **B.** Definitively repaired TOF/PS with VSD closure creating left ventricle to aortic continuity, resection of subvalvular muscle bundles and deviated conal septum, and creation of a transannular patch (with pulmonary valvectomy) creating pulmonary insufficiency. A small atrial-level communication has been left.

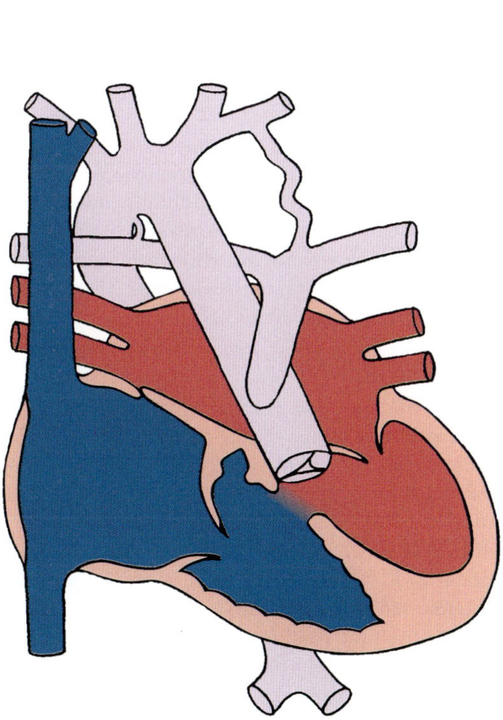

FIGURE 38.2. Illustration of tetralogy of Fallot with pulmonary atresia group 1 with short segment pulmonary artery (PA), good-sized PAs in continuity supplied by a right-sided patent ductus arteriosus, and one major aortopulmonary collateral artery from the left subclavian artery. There is a right aortic arch with mirror image arch vessel branching.

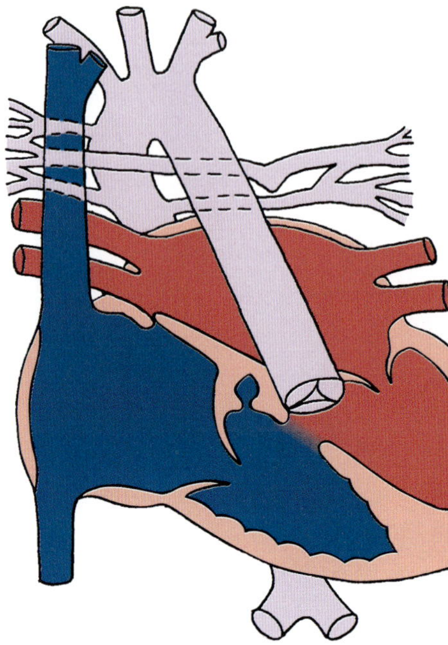

FIGURE 38.3. Illustration of tetralogy of Fallot with pulmonary atresia group 3 with no main pulmonary artery (PA), small branch PAs in continuity supplied by major aortopulmonary collateral arteries (MAPCAs). Some lung segments are supplied by the native PAs, whereas others are supplied directly by MAPCAs. There is a right aortic arch with mirror image arch vessel branching.

Nasr VG, DiNardo JA. Tetralogy of fallot. In: Nasr VG, DiNardo JA, eds. *The Pediatric Cardiac Anesthesia Handbook*. 2nd ed. Wiley; 2025.

Nasr VG, DiNardo JA. Tetralogy of fallot pulmonary atresia. In: Nasr VG, DiNardo JA, eds. *The Pediatric Cardiac Anesthesia Handbook*. 2nd ed. Wiley; 2025.

Nasr VG, DiNardo JA. Tetralogy of fallot absent pulmonary valve. In: Nasr VG, DiNardo JA, eds. *The Pediatric Cardiac Anesthesia Handbook*. 2nd ed. Wiley; 2025.

Tetralogy of Fallot With Absent Pulmonary Valve

TOF with absent pulmonary valve is the least common variant of TOF, accounting for only 3% to 6% of cases of TOF. These patients have a displaced infundibulum, VSD, and varying degrees of RVOT obstruction as well as aneurysmal dilation of the main and branch PAs from pulmonary regurgitation in utero. The pathophysiology of TOF is complicated by symptoms of tracheobronchial compression that are similar to those caused by an anterior mediastinal mass. These patients usually must be positioned on their sides even when mechanically ventilated.

A.2. What is the pathophysiology of TOF/PS?

The pathophysiology of TOF/PS is characterized by the presence of an intracardiac right-to-left shunt through an interventricular defect with varying degrees of RV outflow obstruction caused by RV infundibular and valvular stenosis. The shunt is defined as complex because resistance to RV outflow is a combination of the resistance from the obstructive lesions and the pulmonary vasculature. If resistance from the RV obstructive lesions is high, changes in PVR have little effect on shunt magnitude and direction. Most patients with TOF/PS have a fixed (valvular) and dynamic (variations in caliber of the RV infundibulum) component to RVOT obstruction. In addition, because the aorta overrides the VSD and the RV, desaturated systemic venous blood tends to stream out of the RV directly to the aorta, even in the presence of mild RVOT obstruction, resulting in further systemic desaturation.

The degree of cyanosis is related to the percentage of desaturated hemoglobin. A markedly hypoxemic child with baseline arterial saturations in the 70% range who is anemic might appear less cyanotic than another child with similar oxygen saturation and a hematocrit of 65%. The Sao_2 is determined by the relative volumes and saturations of recirculated systemic venous blood and the effective systemic blood flow that has mixed and reached the aorta. This is summarized in the following equation:

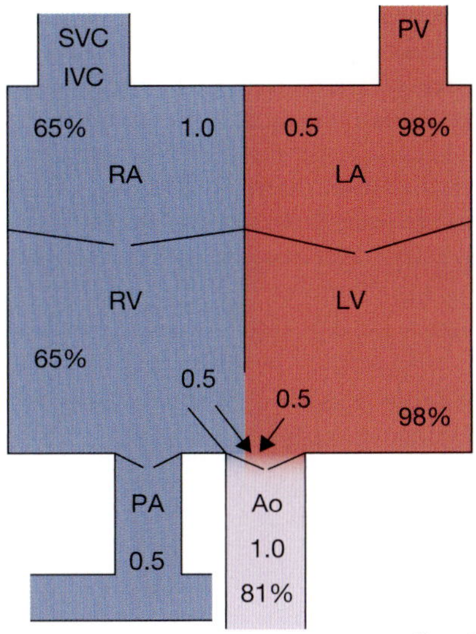

$$Q_p : Q_s = 0.5 : 1$$

$$SaO_2 = \frac{(98)(0.5) + (65)(0.5)}{1.0} = 81$$

FIGURE 38.4. Chamber oxygen saturations and relative flows for a patient with uncorrected tetralogy of Fallot with pulmonary stenosis (TOF/PS). Arterial oxygen saturation (Sao_2) and Q_P:Q_S are shown. Ao, aorta; IVC, inferior vena cava; LA, left atrium; LV, left ventricle; PA, pulmonary artery; PV, pulmonary vein; RA, right atrium; RV, right ventricle; SVC, superior vena cava.

$$\text{Aortic } Sao_2 = \frac{[(\text{pulmonary venous } O_2 \text{ saturation} \times \text{effective systemic blood flow}) + (\text{systemic venous } O_2 \text{ saturation} \times \text{recirculated systemic venous blood flow})]}{(\text{total systemic blood flow})}$$

This is demonstrated in Figure 38.4. Notice that the patient has a Q_P:Q_S = 0.5:1.

A.3. What is shunting, and how is Q_P:Q_S calculated?

Shunting is the process where venous return from one circulatory system is recirculated into the arterial outflow of the same circulatory system. Flow of blood from the systemic venous atrium (right atrium) to the aorta produces a physiologic right-to-left (R-L) shunt with recirculation of systemic venous blood. Flow of blood from the pulmonary venous atrium (left atrium) to the PA produces a physiologic left-to-right (L-R) shunt with recirculation of pulmonary venous blood. A physiologic R-L or L-R shunt is usually caused by a communication (orifice) at the level of the cardiac chambers or great vessels; however, physiologic shunts can exist in the absence of an anatomic shunt; transposition physiology is the best example.

Effective blood flow is the quantity of venous blood from one circulatory system reaching the arterial system of the other circulatory system. Effective pulmonary blood flow is the volume of systemic venous blood reaching the pulmonary circulation, whereas effective systemic blood flow is the volume of pulmonary venous blood reaching the systemic circulation. Effective pulmonary and effective systemic blood flows are always equal, no matter how complex the lesions. Effective blood flow usually is the result of a normal pathway through the heart, but it can occur as the result of an anatomic R-L or L-R shunt.

Total pulmonary blood flow (Q_P) is the sum of effective pulmonary blood flow and recirculated pulmonary blood flow. Total systemic blood flow (Q_S) is the sum of effective systemic blood flow and recirculated systemic blood flow. Total pulmonary blood flow and total systemic blood flow do not have to be equal because the amount of recirculated systemic or pulmonary venous blood do not have to be equal. Q_S (systemic cardiac output) tends to remain constant to maintain end-organ blood supply, even in the presence of a physiologic R-L shunt (systemic venous recirculation), although the Sao_2 will be lower. Conversely, a physiologic L-R shunt (pulmonary recirculation) causes pulmonary volume overload.

The calculation of Q_P:Q_S can be made by the Fick equation, where the pulmonary and systemic blood flows (Q_P and Q_S) are calculated individually by dividing the rate of oxygen extraction by the change in oxygen content in the arterial and venous side of each circulation. The rate of oxygen extraction is the same as effective systemic or pulmonary blood flow and must be equal, so these numbers cancel out in the equation. The calculation of oxygen content is simplified when the determination is made using low inspired concentrations of oxygen (fraction of inspired oxygen [F_{IO_2}]), the contribution of oxygen carried in solution ($P_{O_2} \times 0.003$) can be ignored, so calculation of Q_P:Q_S can be simplified using oxygen saturations. Failure to account for the contribution of oxygen carried in solution, when calculation oxygen content of blood, will introduce substantial error.

$$(S_{A}O_2 - S_{SVC}O_2)/(S_{PV}O_2 - S_{PA}O_2)$$

where A = arterial, SVC = superior vena cava, PV = pulmonary vein that can be assumed to be 98% in the absence of significant pulmonary disease, and PA = pulmonary artery.

Kussman BD, McGowan FX, Powell, AJ, DiNardo JA. Anesthesia for congenital heart surgery. In: Davis PJ, Cladis FP, eds. *Smith's Anesthesia for Infants and Children*. 10th ed. Elsevier; 2022:732-831.

A.4. What is the pathophysiology of TOF with pulmonary atresia?

The pathophysiology of TOF with pulmonary atresia is characterized as single ventricle physiology because there is a VSD and little or no antegrade flow from the RV. In single ventricle physiology, there is complete mixing of pulmonary venous and systemic venous blood at the atrial or ventricular level and the ventricle(s) distributes output to both the systemic and pulmonary vascular beds. As a result of this physiology, the following are observed:

- Ventricular output is the sum of pulmonary blood flow (Q_P) and systemic blood flow (Q_S).
- Distribution of systemic and pulmonary blood flow is dependent on the relative resistances to flow (both intracardiac and extracardiac) into the two parallel circuits.
- Oxygen saturations are the same in the aorta and the PA.

Single ventricle physiology can exist with one hypoplastic ventricle and one well-developed ventricle or with two well-formed anatomic ventricles when there is atresia or near atresia of outflow from one of the ventricles.

Examples include the following:

- TOF with pulmonary atresia where pulmonary blood flow is supplied through a large PDA or MAPCAs
- Truncus arteriosus
- Severe neonatal aortic stenosis and interrupted aortic arch; in both lesions, a substantial portion of systemic blood flow is supplied through a PDA.
- Heterotaxy syndrome

Patients with a single anatomic ventricle have complete or near-complete obstruction to inflow and/or outflow from the hypoplastic ventricle so there must be an alternate source of either systemic or pulmonary blood flow to ensure postnatal survival. An example of an alternate source of blood flow is in ductal-dependent circulation where a PDA forms a direct connection between the aorta and is the only source of systemic blood flow in hypoplastic left heart syndrome or of pulmonary blood flow in PA with intact ventricular septum. In other instances of a single anatomic ventricle, intracardiac pathways provide both systemic and pulmonary blood flow as in tricuspid atresia with normally related great vessels, a nonrestrictive VSD and minimal or absent PS.

Kussman BD, McGowan FX, Powell, AJ, DiNardo JA. Anesthesia for congenital heart surgery. In: Davis PJ, Cladis FP, eds. *Smith's Anesthesia for Infants and Children*. 10th ed. Elsevier; 2022:732-831.

A.5. How is Sa_{O_2} determined in single ventricle physiology?

The Sa_{O_2} is determined by the relative volumes and saturations of pulmonary venous and systemic venous blood flows that have mixed and reached the aorta. This is summarized in the following equation:

$$\text{Aortic } O_2 \text{ saturation} = \frac{[(\text{systemic venous saturation})(\text{total systemic venous blood flow}) + (\text{pulmonary venous saturation})(\text{total pulmonary venous blood flow})]}{(\text{total systemic blood flow} + \text{total pulmonary venous blood flow})}$$

The primary goal in the management of patients with single ventricle physiology is optimization of systemic oxygen delivery and perfusion pressure to prevent end-organ (myocardial, renal, hepatic, splanchnic) dysfunction, so the systemic and pulmonary circulations must be balanced. The term balanced circulation is used because both laboratory and clinical evaluations have demonstrated that maximal systemic oxygen delivery (the product of systemic oxygen content and systemic blood flow) is achieved for single ventricle lesions when Q_P:Q_S is at or just below 1:1. Increases in Q_P:Q_S in excess of 1:1 are associated with a progressive decrease in systemic oxygen delivery because the subsequent increase in systemic oxygen content is more than offset by the progressive decrease in systemic blood flow and by diastolic hypotension due to runoff into the pulmonary circulation. Decreases in Q_P:Q_S below 0.7 to 0.8:1 are associated with a precipitous decrease in systemic oxygen delivery because the subsequent increase in systemic blood flow is more than offset by the dramatic decrease in systemic oxygen content.

Kussman BD, McGowan FX, Powell, AJ, DiNardo JA. Anesthesia for congenital heart surgery. In: Davis PJ, Cladis FP, eds. *Smith's Anesthesia for Infants and Children*. 10th ed. Elsevier; 2022:732-831.

A.6. What is a "pink Tet"?

The term pink Tet refers to any patient with TOF/PS or TOF with pulmonary atresia who is not cyanotic despite having a normal hemoglobin concentration. In these patients, Q_P:Q_S is sufficiently high (usually >0.8:1 in the presence of a normal mixed venous saturation and pulmonary vein saturations) to maintain deoxyhemoglobin concentration less than 5 g/dL with Sao_2 generally greater than 80%. Examples are TOF/PS patients with minimal valvular and subvalvular PS and all patients with TOF with pulmonary atresia where pulmonary blood flow is supplied from a large PDA and/or MAPCAs.

DiNardo JA, Zvara DA. Congenital heart disease. In: DiNardo JA, Zvara DA, eds. *Anesthesia for Cardiac Surgery*. 3rd ed. Blackwell; 2008:167-251.

A.7. What are hypercyanotic spells? How are they treated?

Hypercyanotic or "Tet spells" are sudden episodes of profound cyanosis in patients with TOF that can be life-threatening. These spells occur more frequently in patients who are severely cyanotic at baseline but can occur in any patient with TOF. The peak frequency of spells is between 2 and 3 months of age. The onset of spells usually prompts urgent surgical intervention, so anesthesiologists might care for infants who is at great risk for spells during the perioperative period. The etiology of Tet spells is not completely understood, but acute infundibular spasm that acutely decreases flow through the RV outflow tract and increased magnitude of the R-L shunt through the VSD is thought to be causal. Crying, defecation, feeding, fever, and awakening from sleep all can be precipitating events. During a Tet spell, the infant appears pale and limp secondary to poor cardiac output leading to syncope, convulsions or death.

Paroxysmal hyperpnea is often the initial finding of a Tet spell. Hyperpnea maintains and worsens hypoxic spells by increasing both the work of breathing and oxygen consumption, and in spontaneously ventilated patients by decreasing mean intrathoracic pressure and increasing systemic venous return which increase the magnitude of the R-L shunt and the degree of cyanosis because of the increase in RV volume and pressure. Hypoxemia further increases the magnitude of the R-L shunt and the degree of cyanosis by reducing SVR. Treatment of a "Tet spell" is focused on increasing pulmonary blood flow and decreasing the magnitude of the R-L shunt and includes:

- Administration of 100% oxygen
- Compression of the femoral arteries or placing the patient in a knee-chest position to transiently increase SVR and reduce the magnitude of the R-L shunt.
- Manual compression of the abdominal aorta to increase SVR and reduce the R-L shunt. This maneuver is particularly effective in the anesthetized patient. A cardiac surgeon can manually compress the ascending aorta to increase impedance to left ventricle (LV) ejection and reduce the R-L shunt.
- Administration of morphine sulfate (0.05-0.1 mg/kg IV) for sedation reduces oxygen demand and reduces hyperpnea by depressing the respiratory drive.
- Administration of 15 to 30 mL/kg of a crystalloid solution IV. Increasing preload to the heart increases the diameter of the RVOT and reduces dynamic RVOT obstruction.
- Administration of sodium bicarbonate to treat the severe metabolic acidosis can be seen during a spell. Correction of the metabolic acidosis helps normalize SVR and reduce hyperpnea. Empiric administration of sodium bicarbonate (1-2 mEq/kg IV) in the absence of a blood gas determination should be considered during a spell.
- Phenylephrine (5-10 μg/kg IV or 2-5 μg/kg/min as an infusion) can be used to increase SVR and reduce R-L shunting. In the presence of severe RV outflow obstruction, phenylephrine-induced increases of PVR have little or no effect on RV outflow resistance. Treatment with phenylephrine increases SVR and can decrease R-L shunting across the VSD and augment preload by decreasing unstressed venous volume, but the underlying cause of the spell is not treated.

- β-Adrenergic agonists are absolutely contraindicated. By increasing contractility, they can cause further narrowing of the stenotic infundibulum.
- Administration of β-adrenergic antagonists such as propranolol (0.1 mg/kg IV) or esmolol (0.5 mg/kg IV followed by an infusion of 50-300 μg/kg/min) can reduce infundibular spasm by depressing contractility. In addition, slowing of heart rate can increase preload by improving diastolic filling, increasing heart size, and the diameter RV outflow tract. Caution is warranted when administering β-adrenergic agonists after administering α-adrenergic agonists because the LV might not tolerate the increased SVR after β-adrenergic antagonist-mediated reduction in contractility.
- Extracorporeal membrane oxygenation resuscitation is another alternative in refractory episodes when immediate operative intervention is not possible.

Nasr VG, DiNardo JA. Tetralogy of fallot. In: Nasr VG, DiNardo JA, eds. *The Pediatric Cardiac Anesthesia Handbook.* 2nd ed. Wiley; 2025.

A.8. What palliative surgical procedures are available for treating patients with TOF/PS?

Palliative surgical systemic-to-pulmonary artery (L-R) shunts increase pulmonary blood flow and improve cyanosis when surgical anatomy or institutional practice precludes definitive repair at the time of presentation. These shunts create a volume load on the LV that parallels the increase in pulmonary blood flow. Note that the pathophysiology of TOF is unchanged, so the hypertrophy of the body and infundibulum of the RV progresses, and RV outflow tract obstruction worsens in the interval from shunt placement to definitive repair. The shunts can be summarized as follows:

Waterston shunt: a side-to-side anastomosis between the ascending aorta and the right PA. This procedure is performed through a right thoracotomy without CPB.

Potts shunt: a side-to-side anastomosis between the descending aorta and the left PA. This procedure is performed through a left thoracotomy without CPB.

Waterston and Potts shunts are of historic interest only. These shunts were difficult to size—too small of an orifice overly restricted pulmonary blood flow, whereas too large an orifice resulted in pulmonary overperfusion and congestion and predisposed the patient to unilateral pulmonary vascular obstructive disease. Furthermore, these shunts were difficult to take down and frequently distorted PA anatomy making definitive repair more difficult.

Central shunt: a synthetic tube graft between the ascending aorta and the main or branch PA. This shunt can be performed with or without CPB through a thoracotomy or median sternotomy. It is usually only used when prior shunt procedures have failed.

Blalock-Taussig shunt (BTS): an end-to-side anastomosis of the right or left subclavian artery to the ipsilateral branch PA. Currently, a modification of this procedure known as the modified Blalock-Taussig (MBT) shunt is performed where a Gore-Tex tube graft (usually 3.5-4.0 mm diameter in infants) is interposed between the subclavian or innominate artery and the branch PA. These shunts usually are performed on the side opposite the aortic arch through a thoracotomy without CPB (**Figure 38.5**).

Nasr VG, DiNardo JA. Tetralogy of fallot. In: Nasr VG, DiNardo JA, eds. *The Pediatric Cardiac Anesthesia Handbook.* 2nd ed. Wiley; 2025.

A.9. What palliative catheter-based procedures are available for patients with TOF?

A catheter-based palliative RVOT stent is an alternative to a systemic-to-pulmonary artery shunt in patients who are not candidates for a complete repair at clinical presentation. These patients are usually symptomatic low-birth weight infants with multiple comorbidities or infants with small PAs or other anatomy unfavorable for primary repair. The procedure is performed in the cardiac catheterization lab or an operating room with biplane fluoroscopy. The stent is placed through a femoral vein or using a hybrid perventricular approach where the apex of the RV is approached through a subxiphoid incision. The indications for the procedure are not clearly defined and vary from institution to institution. Results including early morbidity, time to complete repair, and rate of PA growth have been encouraging when compared to an MBT shunt.

Ghaderian M, Ahmadi A, Sabri MR, et al. Clinical outcome of right ventricular outflow tract stenting versus Blalock-Taussig shunt in tetralogy of Fallot: a systematic review and meta-analysis. *Curr Probl Cardiol.* 2021; 46:100643.

Quandt D, Ramchandani B, Penford G, et al. Right ventricular outflow tract stent versus BT shunt palliation in tetralogy of Fallot. *Heart.* 2017;103:1985-1991.

A.10. What definitive surgical procedures are available for treating patients with TOF/PS?

Most patients with TOF/PS have an elective full anatomic repair between the ages of 2 and 10 months. Definitive repair for TOF/PS in the neonatal period is done in some centers if favorable anatomy is

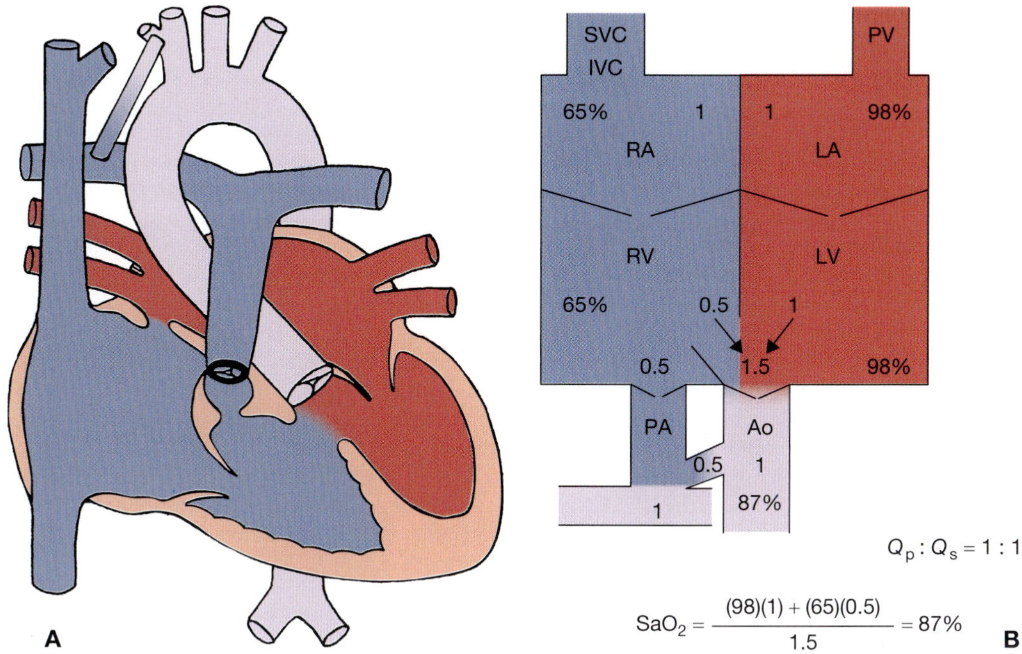

FIGURE 38.5. Modified Blalock-Taussig shunt. A. Palliative modified Blalock-Taussig shunt (MBTS) for tetralogy of Fallot with pulmonary stenosis (TOF/PS). Shunt connects the innominate artery to the right pulmonary artery (PA). This patient has a left aortic arch. **B.** Chamber oxygen saturations and relative flows for a patient with MBTS and TOF/PS. Arterial oxygen saturation (Sao_2) and Q_P:Q_S are illustrated. Ao, aorta; IVC, inferior vena cava; LA, left atrium; LV, left ventricle; PV, pulmonary vein; RA, right atrium; RV, right ventricle; SVC, superior vena cava.

present, whereas other centers delay surgery as long as possible until cyanotic episodes require urgent repair. Surgery is aimed at relieving the RV outflow obstruction by resection of the hypertrophied muscles that obstruct the RVOT and enlargement of the RVOT with a pericardial patch. A valve sparing technique is possible if the pulmonary annulus is near-normal in size and the pulmonary valve stenosis is mild and can be dilated intraoperatively, otherwise a transannular pericardial patch is placed across the pulmonary valve annulus and into the main PAs. A transannular patch is avoided if possible because the patch renders the pulmonary valve insufficient resulting in free pulmonary regurgitation requiring valve repair or replacement later in life. The pericardial patch can be extended beyond the bifurcation of the PAs to relieve distal obstruction. In neonates, the VSD is closed through the right ventriculotomy that was created for resection of the RVOT obstruction and placement of the transannular patch. In infants and older children, the VSD can be closed through the right atrium and the tricuspid valve.

An important surgical consideration for patients with TOF/PS is the presence of coronary artery abnormalities. Approximately 8% of patients have either the left main coronary artery or the left anterior descending artery as a branch of the right coronary artery. In these cases, a right ventriculotomy to enlarge the RVOT could endanger the left coronary artery, so an extracardiac conduit (RV to main PA) may be necessary to bypass the outflow tract obstruction and avoid injury to the coronary artery.

Jonas RA. Early primary repair of tetralogy of Fallot. *Semin Thorac Cardiovasc Surg Pediatr Card Surg Annu.* 2009; 12:39-47.

Jonas RA. Tetralogy of Fallot with Pulmonary Atresia. In: Jonas RA, ed. *Comprehensive Surgical Management of Congenital Heart Disease.* 2nd ed. CRC Press; 2014:347-368.

Nasr VG, DiNardo JA. Tetralogy of fallot. In: Nasr VG, DiNardo JA, eds. *The Pediatric Cardiac Anesthesia Handbook.* 2nd ed. Wiley; 2025.

SECTION 10

A.11. What palliative and definitive surgical procedures are available for patients with TOF with pulmonary atresia?

Patients with TOF with pulmonary atresia in groups 1 and 2 are dependent on prostaglandin E_1 (PGE_1) to maintain pulmonary blood flow through a PDA, so surgery to establish a reliable source of pulmonary blood flow must be performed in the neonatal period. These patients can undergo a palliative shunt procedure or a definitive procedure. A definitive procedure includes placement of an RV to PA conduit and closure of the VSD, usually through the ventriculotomy used for the proximal attachment of the RV to PA conduit.

Patients in groups 3 and 4 are more challenging to manage. These patients have single ventricle physiology with a tendency toward excessive pulmonary blood flow (Q_P:Q_S > 2 to 3:1) as the PVR drops in the neonatal period. In group 3 patients, neonatal repair with placement of an RV to PA conduit is undertaken to place the PAs in continuity with the RV to promote native PA growth. In this circumstance, the VSD is left open as a source of R-L shunting and delivery of desaturated blood to the systemic circulation in case the RV cannot deliver an adequate cardiac output to the left atrium across the hypoplastic pulmonary vascular bed. These infants undergo multiple cardiac catheterization procedures to dilate and stent the hypoplastic native PAs to increase the size of the pulmonary vascular bed and promote antergrade flow across the RVOT and to occlude major aortopulmonary collateral arteries (MAPCAs) that provide competitive pulmonary blood flow to lung segments supplied by the native PAs. MAPCAs that provide pulmonary blood flow to segments of lung not supplied by native PAs must be unifocalized to the proximal pulmonary circulation. Unifocalization involves removal of the collateral vessel from the aorta with anastomosis to the RV to PA conduit or a proximal PA branch. This establishes antegrade blood flow from the RV to the pulmonary vascular bed. Usually, 80% to 90% of the pulmonary vascular bed or about 10 to 12 bronchopulmonary segments must be in direct continuity with the RV to ensure that adequate cardiac output can cross the pulmonary bed so the VSD can be closed. In group 4 patients, the initial intervention might be to create an RV to PA conduit and unifocalize several large collaterals to the distal end of conduit from the RV. Alternatively, several large collaterals can be unifocalized to an MBTS or central shunt. These procedures serve to promote pulmonary vascular growth, prevent the development of pulmonary vascular obstructive disease, and control the Q_P:Q_S.

Bauser-Heaton H, Borquez A, Han B, et al. Programmatic approach to management of tetralogy of Fallot with major aortopulmonary collateral arteries: a 15-year experience with 458 patients. *Circ Cardiovasc Interv*. 2017;10:e004952.

Hofferberth SC, Esch JJ, Zurakowski D, et al. Pulmonary atresia with ventricular septal defect and major aortopulmonary collaterals: collateral vessel disease burden and unifocalisation strategies. *Cardiol Young*. 2018;28:1091-1098.

A.12. What are the long-term outcomes of patients with TOF/PS?

Overall long-term transplant-free survival after complete repair of TOF/PS is excellent with survival rates of 98.6%, 97.8%, 97.1%, 95.5%, and 94.5% at 1-year, 5-year, 10-year, 20-year, and 25-year follow-up, respectively. Factors that adversely affect long-term survival include older age at initial repair, initial palliative procedures, and presence of residual PS and/or pulmonary regurgitation. RV dysfunction from chronic pressure and volume overload as well as the development of ventricular dysrhythmias can prompt pulmonary valve repair or replacement. Most patients are largely asymptomatic and RV dysfunction may only be evident on echocardiography and exercise stress testing.

Geva T. Indications for pulmonary valve replacement in repaired tetralogy of Fallot: the quest continues. *Circulation*. 2013;128:1855-1857.

Smith CA, McCracken C, Thomas AS, et al. Long-term outcomes of tetralogy of Fallot: a study from the pediatric cardiac care consortium. *JAMA Cardiol*. 2019;4:34-41.

B. Preoperative Evaluation and Preparation

B.1. What preoperative history and physical examination information do you need for this patient?

The medical history and review of systems should include an assessment of ability to perform age-appropriate activities. This will help in the evaluation of cardiac function and reserve. The observation by a parent that the patient cannot keep the same pace as siblings is often a reliable clinical sign that cyanosis or congestive heart failure is worsening. Symptoms of low cardiac reserve that include sweating, dyspnea, and circumoral cyanosis might first occur during feeding, which is a strenuous activity for a newborn. Interpretation of vital signs must be age specific. Growth curves also are useful because congestive heart failure will inhibit age-appropriate gains in weight, height, and head circumference. It is not unusual for patients with severe congestive heart failure to weigh less at 3 or 4 months of age than at birth. Interestingly, cyanotic children often do not manifest this failure to thrive.

It is often difficult to differentiate signs and symptoms of congestive heart failure from a mild upper respiratory tract infection in infants and children, so surgery might need to proceed even when the diagnosis is not clear. Children and infants with increased pulmonary blood flow are predisposed to multiple respiratory tract infections so surgery is needed in these patients to reduce pulmonary blood flow and the propensity for chronic lung infections.

Physical examination might reveal cyanosis, clubbing, or signs of congestive heart failure similar to those seen in adults, such as hepatomegaly, ascites, edema, or tachypnea. Some manifestations of congestive heart failure such as râles might not be heard in infants and children, so the severity of heart failure can be more reliably assessed by the signs and symptoms outlined previously.

Physical examination should include evaluation of the potential limitations to vascular access and monitoring sites imposed by previous surgeries. A child who has undergone a BT or MBT palliative shunt procedure might have a diminished pulse or unobtainable blood pressure in the ipsilateral arm, preventing accurate blood pressure and pulse oximetry measurements in that extremity. Venous access should also be assessed preoperatively because this can affect the mode of induction of anesthesia.

Nasr VG, DiNardo JA. Tetralogy of fallot. In: Nasr VG, DiNardo JA, eds. *The Pediatric Cardiac Anesthesia Handbook.* 2nd ed. Wiley; 2025.

B.2. Which other abnormalities need to be considered in this patient?

About 8% of children with congenital heart disease have other congenital abnormalities. Patients with TOF/PS or TOF with pulmonary atresia have a higher incidence of 22q11.2 deletion syndrome. Different phenotypes of this syndrome include DiGeorge syndrome, velocardiofacial syndrome, and conotruncal anomaly face syndrome. These syndromes are characterized by hypocalcemia, immunodeficiency, facial dysmorphia, palate anomalies, velopharyngeal dysfunction, renal anomalies, tracheoesophageal fistula as well as speech, feeding, neurocognitive, behavioral, and psychiatric disorders. Many of these defects can complicate airway management.

McDonald-McGinn DM, Sullivan KE, Marino B, et al. 22q11.2 deletion syndrome. *Nat Rev Dis Primers.* 2015;1:15071.

Nasr VG, DiNardo JA. Tetralogy of fallot. In: Nasr VG, DiNardo JA, eds. *The Pediatric Cardiac Anesthesia Handbook.* 2nd ed. Wiley; 2025.

B.3. What premedication will you give to a child with congenital heart disease?

Premedication alleviates anxiety and eases separation of children from parents. In infants, premedication facilitates placement of an intravenous catheter for induction of anesthesia, alone or in combination with inhaled anesthesia. Midazolam (1 mg/kg PO) might be sufficient in infants and young children, but addition of ketamine (3-5 mg/kg PO) is sometimes necessary in older children with heightened anxiety or in patients who are tolerant to benzodiazepines from previous procedures. Intramuscular ketamine (2-3 mg/kg) and glycopyrrolate (10 μg/kg) alone or in combination with midazolam (0.1 mg/kg) works well in children who will not take oral medications.

Kussman BD, McGowan FX, Powell, AJ, DiNardo JA. Anesthesia for congenital heart surgery. In: Davis PJ, Cladis FP, eds. *Smith's Anesthesia for Infants and Children.* 10th ed. Elsevier; 2022:732-831.

C. Intraoperative Management

C.1. How will you induce anesthesia in this patient if intravenous access cannot be obtained?

Induction of anesthesia with ketamine (3-5 mg/kg IM), succinylcholine (5 mg/kg IM), and glycopyrrolate (10 μg/kg IM) is an alternative to intravenous induction in infants and neonates with difficult peripheral intravenous access. Glycopyrrolate is an important adjunct to reduce airway secretions associated with ketamine administration and to prevent bradycardia associated with succinylcholine. This technique provides prompt induction of anesthesia, allowing immediate control of the airway with tracheal intubation. This is useful in circumstances where it is anticipated that initial intravenous access will have to be obtained through the external jugular vein, femoral vein, or internal jugular vein. Rocuronium (1 mg/kg IM) can be substituted for succinylcholine, but the time to adequate intubating conditions and duration of action may vary.

Kussman BD, McGowan FX, Powell, AJ, DiNardo JA. Anesthesia for congenital heart surgery. In: Davis PJ, Cladis FP, eds. *Smith's Anesthesia for Infants and Children.* 10th ed. Elsevier; 2022:732-831.

C.2. Why would end-tidal carbon dioxide ($Etco_2$) monitoring be of particular use in a patient with TOF/PS?

$Etco_2$ monitoring is particularly helpful in patients with congenital heart disease because the difference between arterial CO_2 and alveolar CO_2 reflects physiologic dead space ventilation which is indicative of changes in lung perfusion. Acute reduction in pulmonary blood flow caused by a reduction in cardiac output, pulmonary embolus, or increased intracardiac R-L shunting increases this gradient. In a patient with TOF/PS, a gradual reduction in $Etco_2$ often precedes a decrease in Sao_2 as the first manifestation of increased R-L intracardiac shunting during a "Tet spell."

Levy RJ. Anesthesia for congenital heart surgery. In: Jonas RA, ed. *Comprehensive Surgical Management of Congenital Heart Disease*. 2nd ed. CRC Press; 2014:19-36.

C.3. What is near-infrared spectroscopy (NIRS) and what does it measure?

NIRS is a real-time monitor of cerebral tissue oxygenation. This technology is based on the physical principle that light of an appropriate wavelength passing through a solution of a colored compound (chromophore) is absorbed by the compound. The intensity of the light emerging from the solution will be lower than the intensity of light projected into the solution. The Beer-Lambert equation ($\log [I_O/I] = c\,\alpha\,d$) allows quantification of the concentration (c) of a chromophore if the emergent light intensity (I) is measured and the following are known:

- Extinction coefficient (α), a constant that describes the absorption characteristics of a particular chromophore at a given wavelength of light
- Thickness (path length) of the solution (d)
- Incident light intensity (I_O)

NIRS technology is particularly suited to use in neonates and infants because the thin skull and small head allow light to be transmitted through one side of the head and detected on the other side, a technique known as *transmission spectrometry*. Cerebral oxygen saturation (Sco_2) as measured by all NIRS technology is the combined oxygen saturation of an uncertain mix of arterioles, capillaries, and venules. Traditional pulse oximetry differs in this respect from NIRS because it can isolate and measure the arteriolar component by gating measurements to arterial pulsatility. It has been assumed that Sco_2 represented contributions of cerebral arterial and venous blood in a ratio of 25:75, with the contribution of capillary blood felt to be negligible. More recent data suggest that in children, the average ratio is 15:85. The issue is further complicated by the fact that there is significant variability in the ratio (from 0:100 to 40:60) between patients.

Ferradal SL, Yuki K, Vyas R, et al. Non-invasive assessment of cerebral blood flow and oxygen metabolism in neonates during hypothermic cardiopulmonary bypass: feasibility and clinical implications. *Sci Rep*. 2017;7:44117.

Kussman BD, McGowan FX, Powell, AJ, DiNardo JA. Anesthesia for congenital heart surgery. In: Davis PJ, Cladis FP, eds. *Smith's Anesthesia for Infants and Children*. 10th ed. Elsevier; 2022:732-831.

C.4. What are the important management issues during creation of a palliative shunt?

- Unilateral lung retraction is required for surgical exposure if a thoracotomy approach is used. The resulting atelectasis can severely compromise ventilation and worsen oxygenation and CO_2 elimination.
- The main or branch PAs must be partially occluded by a clamp to allow creation of the distal anastomosis for all palliative systemic to PA shunts. The resulting increase in physiologic dead space and $Paco_2$ and $Etco_2$ gradients can compromise oxygenation and CO_2 removal. Efforts to optimize ventilation, reduce PVR, and increase pulmonary blood flow should be initiated before PA occlusion.
- Partial occlusion of the aorta with a clamp will be necessary during creation of Waterston, Potts, and central shunts. The resulting increase in LV afterload can compromise LV systolic function, and inotropic support might need to be initiated.
- All the palliative shunts impose a volume load on the LV. Inotropic support might be necessary to ensure systemic and shunt perfusion after shunt creation.
- Palliative shunts are mildly restrictive simple shunts. It is important to maintain SVR and reduce PVR to maintain pulmonary blood flow in these patients.
- Be prepared to treat episodes of hypercyanosis.

Nasr VG, DiNardo JA. Tetralogy of fallot. In: Nasr VG, DiNardo JA, eds. *The Pediatric Cardiac Anesthesia Handbook*. 2nd ed. Wiley; 2025.

C.5. What is the effect of inhalation anesthetics on airway reflexes, myocardial contractility, systemic vascular resistance (SVR), and pulmonary vascular resistance (PVR) in children?

Sevoflurane, isoflurane, and desflurane dose-dependently reduce cardiac output and SVR with mild depression of contractility at 1 and 1.5 times the minimal alveolar concentration (MAC). At these concentrations, sevoflurane and isoflurane do not alter the ratio of PVR to SVR enough to change the Q_P:Q_S.

Isoflurane and desflurane are not good choices for inhalational induction because their pungency is responsible for a high incidence of airway complications in children. Sevoflurane has cardiovascular effects similar to isoflurane and is a good agent for inhalational induction.

Laird TH, Stayer SA, Rivenes SM, et al. Pulmonary-to-systemic blood flow ratio effects of sevoflurane, isoflurane, halothane, and fentanyl/midazolam with 100% oxygen in children with congenital heart disease. *Anesth Analg.* 2002; 95:1200-1206.

Nasr VG, DiNardo JA. Intraoperative Management. In: Nasr VG, DiNardo JA, eds. *The Pediatric Cardiac Anesthesia Handbook.* 2nd ed. Wiley; 2025.

C.6. What are the anesthetic goals pre-cardiopulmonary bypass (pre-CPB) for a patient undergoing definitive surgical correction of TOF/PS?

- Maintain heart rate, contractility, and preload to maintain cardiac output. Maintaining euvolemia is important to prevent exacerbation of dynamic RVOT obstruction from hypovolemia and reflex increases in heart rate and contractility.
- Avoid increases in the PVR:SVR ratio. Increases in PVR relative to SVR and decreases in SVR relative to PVR will increase R-L shunting, reduce pulmonary blood flow, and produce or worsen cyanosis. This effect is more pronounced when the RV outflow obstruction is not severe.
- Maintain or increase SVR. This is particularly important when RV outflow obstruction is severe, and changes in PVR will have little or no effect on shunt magnitude and direction.
- Treat episodes of hypercyanosis.
- Maintain contractility. Depression of contractility, particularly in the face of severe RV outflow obstruction, can produce RV afterload mismatch and drastically reduce pulmonary blood flow. The exception to this is a patient in whom the dynamic component of infundibular obstruction is active. Reducing contractility in these patients can reduce RV outflow obstruction through relaxation of the infundibulum.

Nasr VG, DiNardo JA. Tetralogy of fallot. In: Nasr VG, DiNardo JA, eds. *The Pediatric Cardiac Anesthesia Handbook.* 2nd ed. Wiley; 2025.

C.7. What interventions reliably reduce PVR?

Increase Po$_2$. High inspired O_2 fraction reduces elevated PVR, whereas alveolar hypoxia and arterial hypoxemia induce pulmonary vasoconstriction. Arterial O_2 tension less than 50 mm Hg increases PVR over a wide range of arterial pH values. This effect is most pronounced when pH is less than 7.40.

Reduce Pco$_2$. Consistent reductions in PVR and increases in pulmonary blood flow and Po$_2$ are seen in children with R-L shunts who are hyperventilated to a Pco$_2$ near 30 mm Hg and a pH near 7.50. Hypocarbia reduces PVR through production of respiratory alkalosis, but hypercarbia increases PVR independent of changes in arterial pH. Patients with preoperative pulmonary hypertension who are hyperventilated post-CPB to Pco$_2$ of 30 to 35 mm Hg and pH of 7.50 to 7.56 have a reduction in PVR compared to ventilation that produces normocarbia or hypercarbia.

Reduce pH. Both respiratory and metabolic alkalosis reduce PVR, whereas respiratory and metabolic acidosis increase PVR.

Variation in lung volumes. At small lung volumes, atelectasis compresses extra-alveolar vessels, whereas at high lung volumes, hyperinflation of alveoli compresses intra-alveolar vessels. Therefore, PVR is normally lowest at lung volumes at/or near the functional residual capacity. Positive end-expiratory pressure (PEEP) can increase PVR by increasing alveolar pressure through hyperinflation. However, a decrease in PVR is generally seen in situations in which PEEP works to recruit atelectatic alveoli and increase arterial Po$_2$.

Vasodilator agents. PGE$_1$, prostaglandin I$_2$ (PGI$_2$), nitroglycerin, sodium nitroprusside, and tolazoline are intravenous drugs that induce pulmonary vasodilation as well as systemic vasodilation. There is no intravenous drug that selectively acts as a pulmonary vasodilator. Inhaled nitric oxide, PGE$_1$, and PGI$_2$ are the only specific pulmonary vasodilators available.

Nasr VG, DiNardo JA. Important Concepts in Congenital Heart Disease. In: Nasr VG, DiNardo JA, eds. *The Pediatric Cardiac Anesthesia Handbook.* 2nd ed. Wiley; 2025.

C.8. How does heparin administration and activated coagulation time (ACT) monitoring for CPB differ in children when compared to adults?

Adequate anticoagulation, usually defined as an ACT more than 400 seconds, is necessary before cannulation and commencement of CPB. Most of the evidence for assessing adequacy of anticoagulation in

SECTION 10

children during heart surgery has been extrapolated from the adult literature. The ACT will overestimate the antifactor IIa and Xa effects of heparin in children because the ACT is also prolonged by hypothermia, hemodilution, platelet dysfunction, and low coagulation factor levels. These factors are more significant in children than in adults during CPB because of their small size relative to the CPB circuits.

Most institutions use an age- or weight-based protocol to administer the initial pre-CPB dose of heparin. An example of a simple weight-based protocol is all patients weighing less than 30 kg receive 300 IU heparin per kg and patients weighing more than 30 kg receive 400 IU per kg. The large circuit prime volume to blood volume ratio in infants and children is expected to decrease plasma heparin levels with initiation of CPB unless an appropriate quantity of heparin is added to the CPB prime. Most institutions add heparin to the CPB prime: 3.0 IU heparin per milliliter of CPB prime for patients weighing less than 30 kg and 2.5 IU heparin per milliliter of CPB prime for patients weighing more than 30 kg.

Heparin should always be given into a central line through which venous return can be demonstrated easily or directly into the heart by the surgeon. This is necessary to ensure that the heparin dose has reached the central circulation. An ACT can be drawn within minutes of heparin administration as peak arterial ACT prolongation occurs within 30 seconds and peak venous ACT prolongation within 60 seconds.

Matte GS. The bypass plan. In: Matte GS, ed. *Perfusion for Congenital Heart Surgery: Notes on Cardiopulmonary Bypass for a Complex Patient Population*. Wiley; 2015:33-65.

Matte GS, DiNardo JA. Cardiopulmonary Bypass for Pediatric and Congenital Cardiac Surgery. In: Gravlee GP, Davis RF, Hammon JW, Kussman BD, eds. *Cardiopulmonary Bypass and Mechanical Support: Principles and Practice*. 5th ed. Wolters Kluwer; 2024:655-695.

C.9. How is the effect of unfractionated heparin reversed?

The effect of unfractionated heparin is reversed with protamine, a polyvalent cation that irreversibly chelates unfractionated heparin. There are several approaches to neutralization of heparin with protamine, all with reportedly good clinical results. Some centers titrate the amount of protamine to the amount of heparin determined to exist at the termination of CPB using the in vitro protamine-heparin neutralization ratio of 1.3:1.0. This method had been criticized because the amount of heparin present post-CPB is calculated based on the ACT, and the ACT can be affected by factors other than the concentration of heparin, such as CPB-induced platelet dysfunction, hypothermia, and hemodilution. This can result in overestimation of the heparin present at the termination of CPB with a larger than necessary calculated protamine dose. Other centers administer a fixed dose of protamine based on patient weight (3-4 mg/kg IV) regardless of the ACT or heparin dose administered, whereas others administer 1.0 to 1.3 mg of protamine for each 100 units of heparin administered prior to and during CPB.

Protamine is administered to reverse the effect of unfractionated heparin once adequacy of the surgical repair has been determined after termination of CPB. The heparinized CPB circuit must be protected from protamine reversal so that CPB can be used emergently if necessary. This is usually accomplished by discontinuing cardiotomy suction and removal of arterial and venous canulae before protamine reversal.

Matte GS. The bypass plan. In: Matte GS, ed. *Perfusion for Congenital Heart Surgery: Notes on Cardiopulmonary Bypass for a Complex Patient Population*. Wiley; 2015:33-65.

Matte GS, DiNardo JA. Cardiopulmonary Bypass for Pediatric and Congenital Cardiac Surgery. In: Gravlee GP, Davis RF, Hammon JW, Kussman BD, eds. *Cardiopulmonary Bypass and Mechanical Support: Principles and Practice*. 5th ed. Wolters Kluwer; 2024:655-695.

C.10. What is the incidence of protamine reactions in children?

The incidence of protamine reactions in children following cardiac surgery is substantially lower than in adults. Acute reactions to protamine can be mild with transient erythema and hypotension or severe with bronchoconstriction, PA hypertension, and cardiovascular collapse. The mechanism has not been fully characterized. A retrospective analysis of 1,249 children showed the incidence of hypotension (defined as a 25% decrease in mean arterial pressure) following protamine administration to be 1.76% to 2.88%, depending on the stringency of criteria linking the hypotensive episode to protamine administration. No episodes of pulmonary hypertension or RV dysfunction were noted. Clinical experience indicates that pulmonary hypertensive episodes in children following protamine administration are very rare.

Matte GS, DiNardo JA. Cardiopulmonary Bypass for Pediatric and Congenital Cardiac Surgery. In: Gravlee GP, Davis RF, Hammon JW, Kussman BD, eds. *Cardiopulmonary Bypass and Mechanical Support: Principles and Practice*. 5th ed. Wolters Kluwer; 2024:655-695.

Seifert H, Jobes DR, Ten Have T, et al. Adverse events after protamine administration following cardiopulmonary bypass in infants and children. *Anesth Analg*. 2003;97:383-389.

C.11. What is the role of transesophageal echocardiography (TEE) in this patient?

TEE has a major impact on post-CPB decision-making in children, such as return to CPB to repair residual lesions in approximately 15% of cases when it is used nonselectively. In the subset of patients undergoing valve repair and outflow tract reconstruction (such as this patient), the impact of TEE would be expected to be greater by providing immediate assessment of the adequacy of the operative procedure and directing the revision, if necessary. Although detection of retained intracardiac air is facilitated by using intraoperative TEE, it remains to be determined what role TEE plays in improving cardiac de-airing algorithms, particularly in neonates/infants.

TEE can be used to detect residual VSDs following repair of both simple and complex defects. Residual defects less than 3 mm are detectable by TEE but generally do not require immediate reoperation because they are hemodynamically insignificant. The majority (75%) of these small defects are not present at the time of hospital discharge as determined by transthoracic echocardiography. Residual defects greater than 3 mm detected by TEE require immediate reoperation only when intraoperative assessment suggests that the defect will be hemodynamically significant. Examples of concerning findings are elevated left atrial pressure and/or PA pressure in the presence of good ventricular function, right atrium to PA oxygen saturation step-up with F_{IO_2} less than or equal to 0.50, and oximetric measurement of $Q_P:Q_S$ greater than 1.5.

Yang SG, Novello R, Nicolson S, et al. Evaluation of ventricular septal defect repair using intraoperative transesophageal echocardiography: frequency and significance of residual defects in infants and children. *Echocardiography*. 2000;17: 681-684.

C.12. What effect would a residual ventricular septal defect (VSD) have on this patient following separation from CPB?

A residual VSD is usually poorly tolerated in patients with repaired TOF/PS. There is potential for a large L-R shunt through a residual VSD because RVOT obstruction will be completely or near completely eliminated post repair and the PVR is likely to be low and the pulmonary vasculature very compliant. This will acutely place a large volume load on both the LV and RV. The RV is not likely to tolerate the volume load because the RV compliance is reduced from the preoperative concentric hypertrophy, and function might be impaired post-CPB and from the ventriculotomy. Low cardiac output in this circumstance is described as low cardiac output syndrome and is characterized by tachycardia, elevated left atrial pressure, and elevated PA pressure.

Nasr VG, DiNardo JA. Tetralogy of fallot. In: Nasr VG, DiNardo JA, eds. *The Pediatric Cardiac Anesthesia Handbook*. 2nd ed. Wiley; 2025.

D. Postoperative Management

D.1. How should postoperative ventilation be managed in this patient following placement of a transannular patch for TOF/PS?

The inspiratory phase of mechanical positive pressure ventilation should be adjusted to minimize mean airway pressure. The inspiratory phase of mechanical positive pressure ventilation increases impedance to RV ejection and RV afterload by elevating alveolar pressure and creating more West zone I (alveolar pressure greater than arterial and venous pressure) and West zone II (alveolar pressure greater than venous pressure) lung segments. This is directly related to the duration of inspiration (respiratory rate and inspiratory-to-expiratory [I:E] ratio) and to mean airway pressure. Increasing RV afterload impedes antegrade pulmonary blood flow and exacerbates the extent of pulmonary insufficiency induced by the transannular patch. RV afterload is increased by elevations in PVR.

As discussed in Section C.7, ventilation and gas mixture should be adjusted to minimize PVR. This is usually accomplished with a tidal volume of 10 to 15 mL/kg, 3 to 5 mm Hg of PEEP, and a respiratory rate and I:E ratio adjusted to minimize mean airway pressure.

Nasr VG, DiNardo JA. Tetralogy of fallot. In: Nasr VG, DiNardo JA, eds. *The Pediatric Cardiac Anesthesia Handbook*. 2nd ed. Wiley; 2025.

D.2. What Sa_{O_2} is expected following complete repair of TOF/PS in the infant?

The Sa_{O_2} should be 100% following complete repair of TOF/PS if there are no residual lesions or intrapulmonary shunts. The surgeon might choose to leave a patent foramen ovale or create a small 3- to

4-mm atrial-level communication in infants and small children. The atrial-level communication allows intracardiac R-L shunting that augments systemic cardiac output at the expense of systemic oxygen saturation in the setting of RV dysfunction or pulmonary hypertension by allowing direct delivery of desaturated venous blood to the left atrium across the atrial communication. This is particularly important in patients with restrictive RV dysfunction from the surgical ventriculotomy, extensive RV hypertrophy, or pulmonary insufficiency. In these patients, Pa_{O_2} of 40 to 50 mm Hg and Sa_{O_2} of 70% to 80% are acceptable until RV function improves over the course of days.

Nasr VG, DiNardo JA. Tetralogy of fallot. In: Nasr VG, DiNardo JA, eds. *The Pediatric Cardiac Anesthesia Handbook*. 2nd ed. Wiley; 2025.

D.3. What Sa_{O_2} is expected following placement of a modified Blalock-Taussig shunt (MBTS) for TOF/PS in the infant?

As illustrated in **Figure 38.5B**, the expected Sa_{O_2} is 80% to 90% in the presence of some antegrade pulmonary blood flow. In the absence of antegrade pulmonary blood flow, single ventricle physiology exists and Sa_{O_2} of 70% to 80% is expected. Sa_{O_2} is determined by the relative volumes and saturations of recirculated systemic venous blood and effective systemic blood flows that have mixed and reached the aorta. This is summarized in **Figure 38.5B** and in the following equation:

$$\text{Aortic } Sa_{O_2} = \frac{\begin{array}{c}[(\text{pulmonary venous saturation} \times \text{effective systemic blood flow}) + \\ (\text{systemic venous saturation} \times \text{recirculated systemic venous blood flow})]\end{array}}{(\text{total systemic blood flow})}$$

Three variables ultimately affect Sa_{O_2}:

1. *The ratio of total pulmonary to total systemic blood flow* (Q_P:Q_S). A greater proportion of the arterial blood will consist of saturated blood (pulmonary venous blood) than of desaturated blood (systemic venous blood) when Q_P:Q_S is greater than or equal to 1:1. Q_P:Q_S will be increased when systemic arterial blood pressure is high and PVR is low.
2. *Systemic venous saturation*. For a given Q_P:Q_S and pulmonary venous saturation, a decrease in systemic venous saturation will decrease arterial saturation. Decreases in systemic venous saturation occur as a result of decreases in systemic oxygen delivery or increases in systemic oxygen consumption. Recall that systemic oxygen delivery is the product of systemic blood flow and arterial oxygen content. Arterial oxygen content, in turn, depends on hemoglobin concentration and arterial saturation. Efforts should be made to increase hematocrit 40% to 45%, increase cardiac output with inotropes, and reduce systemic O_2 consumption with sedation/anesthesia and neuromuscular block if necessary.
3. *Pulmonary venous saturation*. For any given systemic venous saturation and Q_P:Q_S, a reduction in pulmonary venous saturation results in decreased arterial saturation. In the absence of large intrapulmonary shunts and/or $\dot{V}/\dot{Q}$ mismatch, pulmonary venous saturation should be close to 100% when breathing room air. In the presence of pulmonary parenchymal disease, pulmonary venous saturation can be reduced. The mismatched component of pulmonary venous desaturation is largely eliminated with an FI_{O_2} of 1.0, whereas the intrapulmonary shunt contribution is not eliminated.

Nasr VG, DiNardo JA. Important concepts in congenital heart disease. In: Nasr VG, DiNardo JA, eds. *The Pediatric Cardiac Anesthesia Handbook*. 2nd ed. Wiley; 2025.

D.4. What is junctional ectopic tachycardia (JET)?

JET is a transient tachyarrhythmia due to abnormal automaticity around the atrioventricular (AV) node or proximal His bundle that can occur in the first 72 hours following congenital heart surgery. The incidence of JET following TOF/PS repair can be as high as 20% and is felt to be secondary to ischemia and trauma around the AV node from surgical retraction that is necessary to expose the VSD and RVOT from across the tricuspid valve. Patients who develop JET have a higher-than-average incidence of postoperative AV block. A rare form of congenital tachycardia presents in the first 6 months of life with persistent tachycardia associated with gene mutations that cause enhanced automaticity around the AV node.

JET typically manifests with a junctional rate only slightly faster than the sinus node rate. It is the only narrow complex tachycardia in which the atrial rate is less than the ventricular rate (A:V ratio <1:1). In less than 10% of cases of JET, there can be retrograde activation of the atrium with inverted P waves and an A:V ratio of 1:1. Cardiac output is reduced because there is a loss of AV synchrony which reduces the contribution of the atrial transport factor or "atrial kick" to cardiac output. In many instances, this arrhythmia is well tolerated, but JET with heart rate greater than 170 beats per minute is associated with hemodynamic instability and increased postoperative mortality. Restoring AV by pacing the atria at a rate slightly faster than the junctional rate can be helpful unless the junctional rate is greater than 160 to 170 beats per minute, where the hemodynamic benefits of reinitiating AV synchrony are offset by the dramatic reduction in diastolic filling seen at heart rates greater than 170 beats per minute.

Treatment of postoperative JET is multimodal and aims to terminate JET or reduce the rate to a point where atrial pacing can be initiated and AV synchrony restored. Cardioversion and adenosine are not effective since the mechanism of JET is abnormal automaticity of the myocardium and not AV nodal reentry. JET requiring aggressive treatment prolongs postoperative ventilation times and intensive care unit stay.

The following treatment modalities are usually applied in this order:

- Fever is aggressively treated with antipyretics.
- Sedation and hemodynamics are optimized.
- Doses of inotropic agents are reduced because most of these agents have positive chronotropic effects. This can be difficult in the setting of hemodynamic instability and low cardiac output syndrome.
- Mild systemic hypothermia is initiated. A cooling blanket and icepacks are used to reduce patient temperature to 32 °C (89.6 °F) to 35 °C (95 °F). This usually requires sedation and paralysis to prevent shivering.
- Procainamide or amiodarone therapy is initiated.

Walsh EP. Automatic atrial and junctional tachycardias. In: Walsh EP, Saul JP, Triedman JK, eds. *Cardiac Arrhythmias in Children and Young Adults with Congenital Heart Disease*. Lippincott Williams & Wilkins; 2001:115-135.

39 Transposition of the Great Arteries

David Whiting and James A. DiNardo

A 3-day-old, full-term, 3.4-kg male is scheduled for an arterial switch operation (ASO). Shortly after birth, he demonstrated reverse differential cyanosis with right arm arterial saturation (Sao_2) of 40% and lower extremity Sao_2 of 60%, despite initiation of prostaglandin E_1 therapy. A bedside balloon atrial septostomy was performed with resolution of reverse differential cyanosis and improvement of systemic Sao_2 to 75%. Prostaglandin E_1 was discontinued 4 hours after the septostomy. He is breathing spontaneously with 0.5 L/min of supplemental oxygen through a nasal cannula. His arterial Sao_2 is 75%, blood pressure 63/37 mm Hg, pulse 145 beats per minute, and respiration 46 breaths per minute.

A. Medical Disease and Differential Diagnosis

1. What defines the cardiac situs?
2. What is dextro-transposition of the great arteries (D-TGA)?
3. What additional cardiac lesions are associated with D-TGA?
4. What is the natural history of D-TGA?
5. What is the pathophysiology of D-TGA?
6. What determines the oxygen saturation (Sao_2) in patients with D-TGA?
7. Why did this infant have reverse differential cyanosis?
8. What are the preoperative issues pertaining to the coronary arteries in D-TGA?
9. What are the clinical subsets of D-TGA?
10. What is the differential diagnosis of D-TGA and how is the diagnosis made?
11. What preoperative interventions can help stabilize a patient with D-TGA?
12. What are the surgical options for repair? Why is one chosen over the others?

B. Preoperative Evaluation and Preparation

1. What information is important to prepare for this case?
2. What are the anesthetic goals before cardiopulmonary bypass (CPB)?
3. What is the plan for glucose management in this patient?

C. Intraoperative Management

1. How would you monitor this infant?
2. What is the best way to induce and maintain general anesthesia in this patient?
3. How is CPB in infants and children different from adults?
4. What is modified ultrafiltration (MUF)?
5. Briefly describe the surgical techniques of the Mustard/Senning, ASO, and Rastelli procedures.
6. What is hypothermia, and how is it classified? What is low-flow CPB? What is deep hypothermic circulatory arrest (DHCA)?
7. Why is hypothermia beneficial to the brain during low-flow CPB and DHCA?
8. Explain the difference between α-stat and pH-stat blood gas management.
9. What are the immediate post-CPB issues following ASO?

D. Postoperative Management

1. How is myocardial ischemia addressed in the intensive care unit (ICU) following the ASO?
2. What immediate postoperative problems would be anticipated following the Rastelli procedure?
3. What intermediate- and long-term surgical problems are seen after ASO?

4. What are the long-term outcomes after ASO?
5. What are the long-term outcomes after Rastelli repair for patients with D-TGA with left ventricular outflow tract (LVOT) obstruction?
6. What is the long-term neurologic outcome like after ASO?

A. Medical Disease and Differential Diagnosis

A.1. What defines the cardiac situs?

Cardiac situs refers to the orientation of the morphologic right atrium (RA). Cardiac situs is "solitus" if the RA is to the right of the midline, "inversus" if the morphologic RA is to the left of the midline, or "ambiguous" when the situs is indeterminate. Cardiac structures may not be in the expected location, so echocardiography can help characterize the anatomy of the atria, atrioventricular (AV) valves, ventricles, ventriculoarterial (VA) valves, and great arteries. A few anatomic characteristics are consistent. The RA receives the vena cava and coronary sinus. There is always concordance between the AV valves and the ventricle, so the tricuspid valve is always the inflow valve for the right ventricle (RV), and the mitral valve is the inflow valve for the left ventricle (LV). The muscular conus arteriosus (infundibulum) always separates the tricuspid AV and pulmonary VA valves of the RV, and the mitral AV and aortic VA valves of the LV are always in fibrous continuity.

Kloesel B, DiNardo JA, Body SC. Cardiac embryology and molecular mechanisms of congenital heart disease: a primer for anesthesiologists. *Anesth Analg*. 2016;123:551-569.

Williams GD, Feng A. Heterotaxy syndrome: implications for anesthesia management. *J Cardiothorac Vasc Anesth*. 2010;24:834-844.

A.2. What is dextro-transposition of the great arteries (D-TGA)?

D-TGA is a common congenital heart lesion accounting for 5% to 7% of all congenital cardiac defects, second in frequency only to isolated ventricular septal defects (VSDs). In D-TGA, there is a concordance of the AV connections and discordance of the VA connections. The segmental anatomy is {*S, D, D*} with atrial situs *S*olitus, *D*-loop ventricles, and *D*-loop great arteries. A right-sided RA connects through a right-sided tricuspid valve and RV to a right-sided and anterior aorta. A left-sided LA connects through a left-sided mitral valve and LV to a left-sided and posterior pulmonary artery (PA). As a result, there is fibrous continuity between the mitral and pulmonic valves with a lack of fibrous continuity (conus) between the tricuspid and aortic valves. The combination of AV concordance (RA to RV and LA to LV) and VA discordance (RV to aorta and LV to PA) results in parallel systemic and pulmonary circulation that is incompatible with life, rather than a normal series circulation.

Kussman BD, McGowan FX, Powell AJ, DiNardo JA. Anesthesia for congenital heart surgery. In: Davis PJ, Cladis FP, ed. *Smith's Anesthesia for Infants and Children*. 10th ed. Elsevier; 2022:732-831.

A.3. What additional cardiac lesions are associated with D-TGA?

The commonly associated cardiac anomalies are persistent patent foramen ovale (PFO), patent ductus arteriosus (PDA), VSD, and subpulmonic stenosis resulting in LVOT obstruction. Approximately 50% of patients with D-TGA present with a PDA before initiation of prostaglandin E_1 therapy and diagnosis of D-TGA. There is almost always a PFO, but a true secundum atrial septal defect (ASD) exists in approximately 5% of patients. Angiographically detectable VSDs occur in 30% to 40% of patients, but only approximately 30% of these defects are hemodynamically significant. Therefore, for practical purposes, 75% of patients have an intact ventricular septum. LVOT obstruction is present in approximately 30% of patients with VSD and is most often due to an extensive subpulmonic fibromuscular ring or posterior malposition of the outlet portion of the ventricular septum.

Qureshi AM, Justino H, Heinle JS. Transposition of the great arteries. In: Shaddy RE, Penny DJ, Feltes TF, et al, eds. *Moss & Adams' Heart Disease in Infants, Children, and Adolescents*. 10th ed. Wolters Kluwer; 2022:1122-1144.

A.4. What is the natural history of D-TGA?

Forty-five percent of patients with D-TGA will die within the first month without intervention, and 90% will die within the first year of life. Survival in the neonatal period is dependent on sufficient mixing of the parallel systemic and pulmonary circulations at the atrial, ventricular, or arterial level. Patency of the ductus arteriosus can be maintained with prostaglandin E_1, allowing for mixing at the arterial level. An emergent Rashkind-Miller balloon atrial septostomy can be performed to increase mixing at the atrial level in those infants who do not have adequate mixing through the PDA or VSD. Following stabilization as a neonate, infants with favorable anatomy undergo the definitive ASO, while those with unfavorable anatomy undergo palliative procedures.

Hypoxia and intractable congestive heart failure (CHF) are the two primary causes of death in infants without intervention who survive the neonatal period. Infants with D-TGA are at particular risk for early-onset accelerated pulmonary artery hypertension (PAH). The etiology is most likely related to systemic hypoxemia, the presence of bronchopulmonary collaterals (which deliver deoxygenated blood to the precapillary pulmonary arterioles), polycythemia, and platelet aggregation. Infants with D-TGA and a large VSD without LVOT obstruction are at the highest risk for the early development of PAH due to exposure of the pulmonary vascular bed to systemic pressures with unrestricted flow. Advanced, nonreversible pulmonary hypertension reduces the corrective surgical options available to the patient.

Kussman BD, McGowan FX, Powell AJ, DiNardo JA. Anesthesia for congenital heart surgery. In: Davis PJ, Cladis FP, eds. *Smith's Anesthesia for Infants and Children*. 10th ed. Elsevier; 2022: 732-831.

A.5. What is the pathophysiology of D-TGA?

The pathophysiology of D-TGA is characterized by parallel systemic and pulmonary circulations with varying degrees of intercirculatory mixing. Transposition physiology is defined as any circumstance where the PA oxygen saturation is greater than the aortic oxygen saturation. Deoxygenated systemic venous blood recirculates through the systemic circulation (a physiologic right-to-left shunt), and oxygenated pulmonary venous blood recirculates through the pulmonary circulation (a physiologic left-to-right shunt). The physiologic shunt fraction or the percentage of venous blood from one system that recirculates in the arterial outflow of the same system is 100% for both circuits in parallel. This is why there must be a connection at the atrial, ventricular, or arterial level to allow for any survival, even in the neonatal period.

The sites for intercirculatory mixing in D-TGA can be intracardiac (PFO, ASD, and VSD) or extracardiac (PDA, bronchopulmonary collaterals). The number, size, and position of anatomic communications are factors that affect the amount of intercirculatory mixing. One large nonrestrictive communication will provide better mixing than two or three restrictive communications. The position of the communication is also important because poor mixing can occur with large anterior muscular VSDs if their orientation is not favorable. Reduced ventricular compliance and elevated systemic vascular resistance (SVR) and pulmonary vascular resistance (PVR) tend to reduce intercirculatory mixing by impeding flow across the anatomic communications. In the presence of anatomically adequate intercirculatory mixing sites, mixing is directly related to total pulmonary blood flow. Patients with reduced pulmonary blood flow secondary to subpulmonic stenosis or PAH will have reduced intercirculatory mixing.

Kussman BD, McGowan FX, Powell AJ, DiNardo JA. Anesthesia for congenital heart surgery. In: Davis PJ, Cladis FP, eds. *Smith's Anesthesia for Infants and Children*. 10th ed. Elsevier; 2022:732-831.

A.6. What determines the oxygen saturation (Sao_2) in patients with D-TGA?

Sao_2 is determined by the relative volumes and saturations of the recirculated systemic and effective systemic blood flows reaching the aorta. This is summarized in the following equation:

$$\text{Arterial saturation} = \frac{([(\text{systematic venous saturation})(\text{recirculated systemic blood flow})] + [(\text{pulmonary venous saturation})(\text{effective systemic blood flow})])}{(\text{total systemic blood flow})}$$

The anatomic left-to-right shunt produces effective systemic blood flow equal to the volume of pulmonary venous blood reaching the systemic circulation. The anatomic left-to-right shunt is the result of intercirculatory mixing at the atrial, ventricular, and arterial levels and must equal the amount of the right-to-left shunt at the same sites. Greater effective systemic blood flow is the result of greater intercirculatory mixing relative to the recirculated systemic blood flow. The Sao_2 depends on the amount of effective systemic blood flow from intercirculatory mixing relative to total systemic blood flow. For a given amount of total systemic blood flow, a decrease in systemic venous or pulmonary venous saturation will result in a decrease in Sao_2. Total systemic blood flow is the sum of recirculated systemic venous blood plus effective systemic blood flow. Likewise, total pulmonary blood flow is the sum of recirculated pulmonary venous blood plus

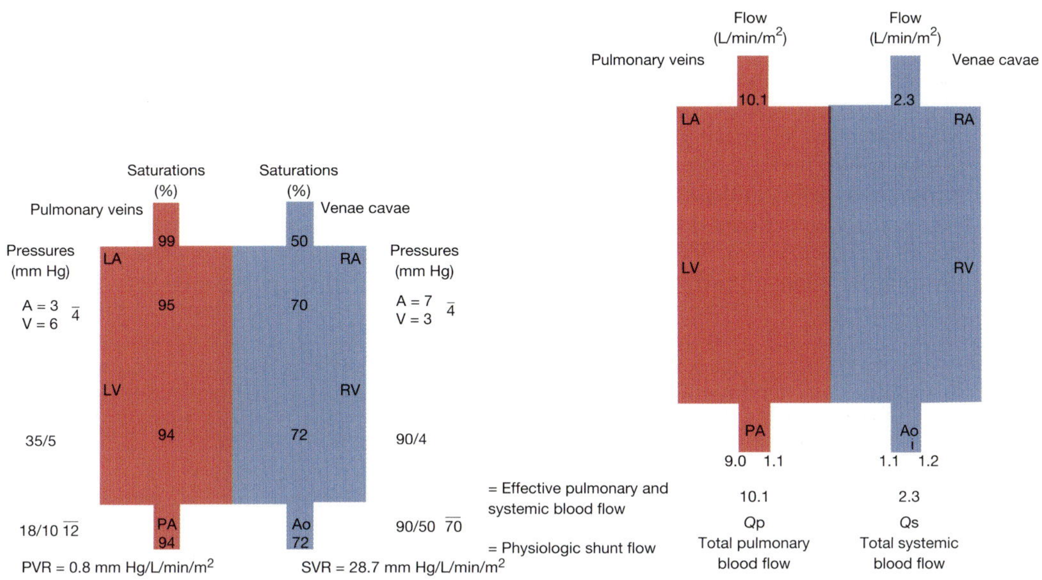

FIGURE 39.1. Oxygen saturations, blood pressures, and blood flows in complete transposition of the great vessels with intercirculatory mixing at the atrial level and a small left ventricular outflow tract gradient. Total pulmonary blood flow (10.1 L/min/m^2) is almost 5 times the total systemic blood flow (2.3 L/min/m^2). Effective pulmonary and effective systemic blood flow are equal (1.1 L/min/m^2) and are the result of an anatomic shunt at the atrial level. The physiologic left-to-right shunt is 9 L/min/m^2; this represents blood recirculated from the pulmonary veins to the pulmonary artery (PA). The physiologic right-to-left shunt is 1.2 L/min/m^2; this represents blood recirculated from the systemic veins to the aorta. In this depiction, pulmonary vascular resistance is low (~1/35 of systemic vascular resistance), and there is a small (17 mm peak-to-peak) gradient from the left ventricle to the PA. These findings are compatible with the high pulmonary blood flow depicted. A, artery; Ao, aorta; LA, left atrium; LV, left ventricle; LVOT, left ventricular outflow tract; PVR, pulmonary vascular resistance; *Qp*, total pulmonary blood flow; *Qs*, total systemic blood flow; RA, right atrium; RV, right ventricle; SVR, systemic vascular resistance; V, vein. (Modified with permission from Freed MO, Keane JF. Profiles in congenital heart disease. In: Grossman W, ed. *Cardiac Catheterization and Angiography*. Lea & Febiger; 1986:463.)

effective pulmonary blood flow. Recirculated blood makes up the largest portion of total pulmonary and systemic blood flow, with effective blood flows contributing only a small portion of the total flow. This is particularly true in the pulmonary circuit, where the total pulmonary blood flow and the volume of the pulmonary circuit (LA, LV, and PA) are 3 to 4 times larger than the total systemic blood flow and the volume of the systemic circuit (RA, RV, and aorta). The net result is transposition physiology, where the PA oxygen saturation is greater than the aortic oxygen saturation. Figure 39.1 further elucidates these concepts. The equation below describes the SaO2 for the conditions shown in the figure.

$$Sao_2 = [(50)(1.2)] + [(99)(1.1)]/2.3 = 72\%$$

Kussman BD, McGowan FX, Powell AJ, DiNardo JA. Anesthesia for congenital heart surgery. In: Davis PJ, Cladis FP, eds. *Smith's Anesthesia for Infants and Children*. 10th ed. Elsevier; 2022:732-831.

A.7. Why did this infant have reverse differential cyanosis?

Reverse differential cyanosis describes the phenomenon in transposition physiology where the preductal right upper extremity oxygen saturation is lower than the postductal left upper and lower extremity oxygen saturation. This occurs when there is pulmonary hypertension and the PA pressure is higher than the aortic pressure. Oxygenated blood is shunted across the PDA to the left upper and lower extremities. The right upper extremity is perfused by antegrade flow from the PA that is partially oxygenated from bidirectional intracardiac shunts.

The dynamics of intercirculatory mixing in D-TGA with intact ventricular septum are complex. The anatomic mixing sites are usually a PDA and a PFO. Anatomic shunting at the atrial level is ultimately determined by the size of the atrial communication and the cyclic pressure variations between the left and right atria. These cyclic pressure variations are influenced by the volume and compliance of the atria, ventricles, and vascular beds in each circuit as well as the heart rate and the hemodynamic effects of respiratory phase variation. Shunting is from the RA to the LA during diastole as the result of the reduced ventricular and vascular compliance of the systemic circuit (RV and systemic arterial circuit). In systole, the shunt is from the LA to the RA primarily because of the large volume of blood returning to the LA as a result of the high volume of recirculated pulmonary blood flow.

The direction of shunting across the PDA largely depends on the PVR and the size of the intra-atrial communication. When the PVR is low and the intra-atrial communication is nonrestrictive, shunting is predominantly from the aorta to the PA through the PDA (effective pulmonary blood flow) and predominantly from the LA to RA across the atrial septum (effective systemic blood flow). When PVR is elevated, shunting across the PDA is likely to be bidirectional, which in turn encourages bidirectional shunting across the atrial septum. When PVR is high and PA pressure exceeds aortic pressure, shunting at the PDA will be predominantly from the PA to the aorta. This will create reverse differential cyanosis wherein the preductal arterial saturation (right arm) is lower than the postductal arterial saturation (legs). This physiology is usually the result of restrictive atrial communication producing left atrial hypertension and is associated with poor intercirculatory mixing, low effective systemic blood flow, and hypoxemia. A balloon atrial septostomy can be lifesaving in this setting. Decompression of the LA promotes mixing at the atrial level and reduces PVR and PA pressure promoting mixing at the PDA. Other causes of reverse differential cyanosis to be considered in D-TGA are the presence of an interrupted aortic arch or severe aortic coarctation.

Kussman BD, McGowan FX, Powell AJ, DiNardo JA. Anesthesia for congenital heart surgery. In: Davis PJ, Cladis FP, eds. *Smith's Anesthesia for Infants and Children*. 10th ed. Elsevier; 2022:732-831.

A.8. What are the preoperative issues pertaining to the coronary arteries in D-TGA?

Anatomic variations of the coronary arteries in D-TGA affect the way the coronary arteries are reimplanted and can increase the risk of postoperative ischemia. The coronary arteries in D-TGA arise from the aortic sinuses that face the PA. In normally related vessels, these sinuses are located on the anterior portion of the aorta, whereas in D-TGA, they are located posteriorly. In about 70% of patients with D-TGA, the right sinus is the origin of the right coronary artery and the left sinus is the origin of the left main coronary artery. In the remainder of cases, there is considerable variability, with the most common variations being shown in **Figure 39.2**.

Most patients with D-TGA have coronary artery anatomy that is suitable for reimplantation on the neoaorta. This is a critical step of the ASO, as distortion of the coronary ostia or coronary artery during reimplantation increases the risk for postoperative myocardial ischemia and early mortality. Examples of challenging coronary artery anatomy include the presence of a single coronary artery or an anomalous origin of one or both coronary arteries with an intramural course. Patients with intramural coronaries generally require resuspension of the posterior leaflet of the neopulmonary valve when the coronary arteries are excised prior to reimplantation. The presence of a single coronary artery or intramural coronary arteries is a risk factor for early mortality, and this risk has persisted over the last two decades despite improvements in surgical technique.

Kussman BD, McGowan FX, Powell AJ, DiNardo JA. Anesthesia for congenital heart surgery. In: Davis PJ, Cladis FP, eds. *Smith's Anesthesia for Infants and Children*. 10th ed. Elsevier; 2022:732-831.

Pasquali SK, Hasselblad V, Li JS, et al. Coronary artery pattern and outcome of the arterial switch operation for transposition of the great arteries: a meta-analysis. *Circulation*. 2002;106:2575-2580.

A.9. What are the clinical subsets of D-TGA?

The four clinical subsets of D-TGA are characterized by differences in anatomy, amount of pulmonary blood flow, and sites of intercirculatory mixing, as summarized in **Table 39.1**.

A.10. What is the differential diagnosis of D-TGA and how is the diagnosis made?

Figure 39.3 delineates the differential diagnosis for D-TGA in the cyanotic newborn.

D-TGA can be associated with either cyanosis or CHF. Cyanosis is severe in patients with limited intercirculatory mixing. Infants with a large quantity of intercirculatory mixing have increased pulmonary blood flow, mild cyanosis, and symptoms of CHF.

Chest radiographs in patients with D-TGA show the classic radiologic triad of an enlarged egg-shaped heart, narrow superior mediastinum, and increased pulmonary vascular markings. These findings are prominent at birth in infants with D-TGA with VSD without LVOT obstruction but might not be seen in the first few weeks of life in infants with D-TGA and intact ventricular septum until the PVR falls and RA and RV enlargement develop.

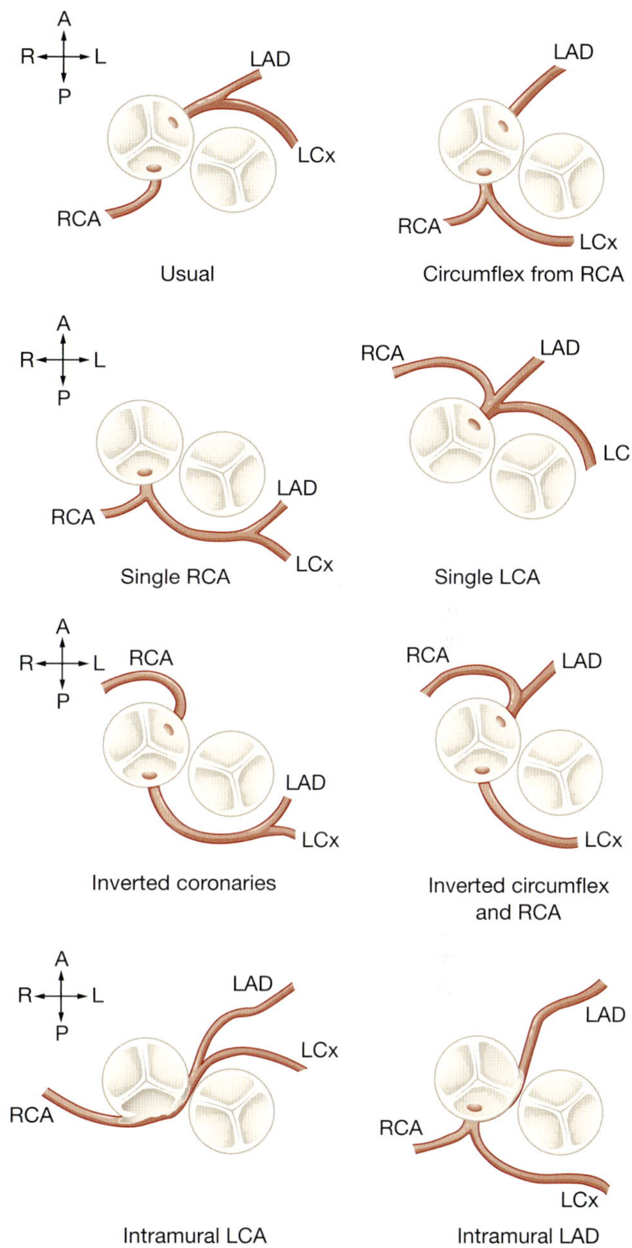

FIGURE 39.2. The most common coronary artery patterns in transposition of the great vessels. The aorta is depicted anterior and to the right of the pulmonary artery. LAD, left anterior descending coronary artery; LCA, left coronary artery; LCx, left circumflex coronary artery; RCA, right coronary artery. (Adapted with permission from Mayer JE Jr, Sanders SP, Jonas RA, et al. Coronary artery pattern and outcome of arterial switch operation for transposition of the great arteries. *Circulation*. 1990; 82:144.)

TABLE 39.1 Clinical Subsets of Transposition of Great Arteries

Anatomy	Pulmonary Blood Flow	Intercirculatory Mixing
D-TGA with intact ventricular septum	Increased	Small
D-TGA with intact ventricular septum, nonrestrictive atrial septum, or PDA	Increased	Large
D-TGA with VSD	Increased	Large
D-TGA with VSD and LVOT obstruction	Reduced	Small
D-TGA with PAH	Reduced	Small

D-TGA, dextro-transposition of great arteries; LVOT, left ventricular outflow tract; PAH, pulmonary artery hypertension; PDA, patent ductus arteriosus; VSD, ventricular septal defect.

Reprinted with permission from DiNardo JA. Transposition of the great vessels. In: Lake CL, Booker PD, eds. *Pediatric Cardiac Anesthesia*. 4th ed. Lippincott Williams & Wilkins; 2005:357-380.

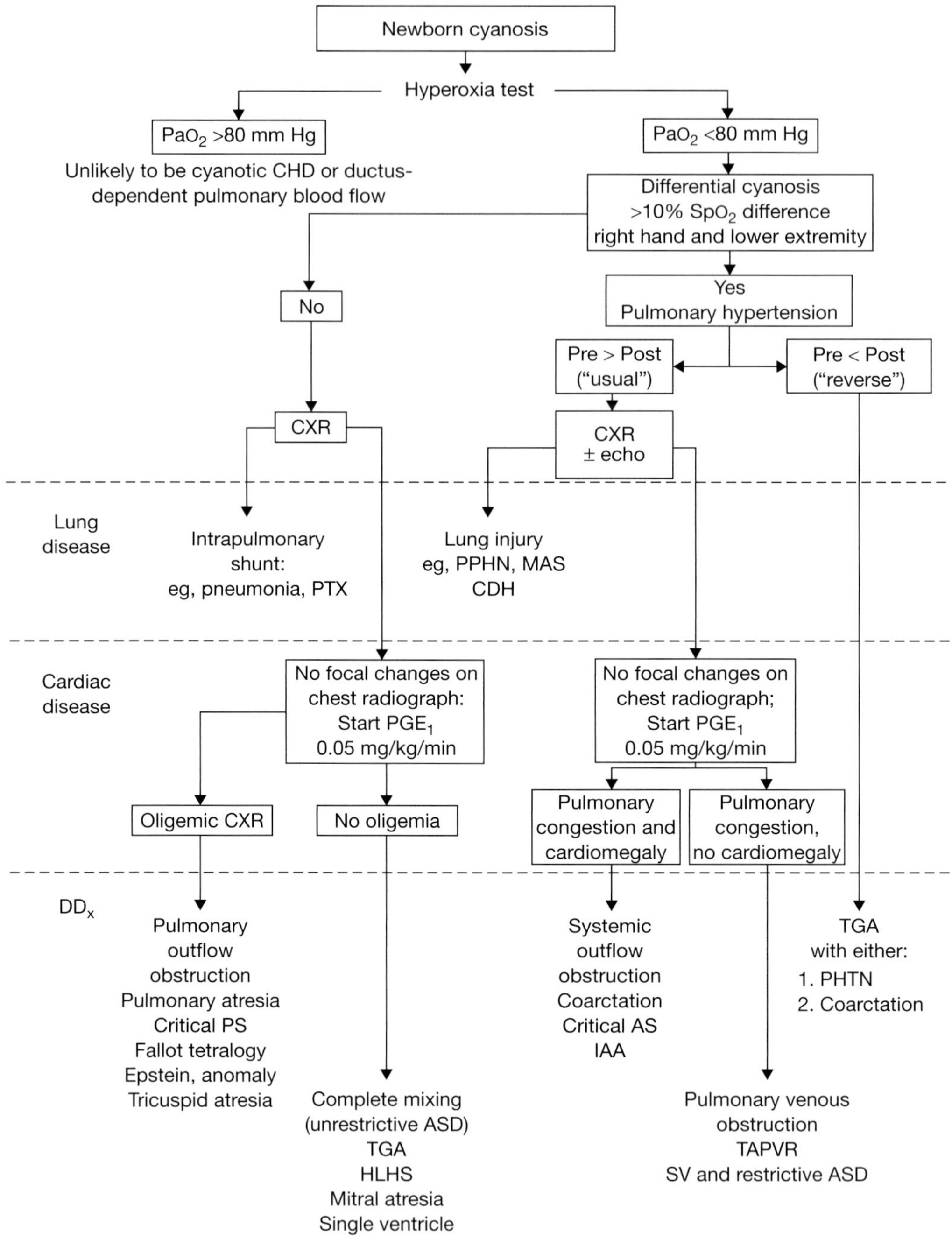

FIGURE 39.3. Differential diagnosis of transposition of the great arteries. AS, aortic stenosis; ASD, atrial septal defect; CDH, congenital diaphragmatic hernia; CHD, congenital heart disease; CXR, chest radiograph; DD_x, differential diagnosis; HLHS, hypoplastic left heart syndrome; IAA, interrupted aortic arch; MAS, meconium aspiration syndrome; PGE_1, prostaglandin E_1; PHTN, pulmonary hypertension; PPHN, persistent pulmonary hypertension of the newborn; PS, pulmonary stenosis; PTX, pneumothorax; Spo_2, peripheral oxygen saturation; SV, single ventricle; TAPVR, total anomalous pulmonary venous return; TGA, transposition of great arteries.

Electrocardiographic (ECG) findings in infants with D-TGA with intact ventricular septum prior to repair include right axis deviation and right ventricular hypertrophy, whereas ECG findings in infants with D-TGA and VSD are right axis deviation, LV hypertrophy, and RV hypertrophy.

Two-dimensional transthoracic echocardiography (TTE) is the diagnostic modality of choice in the diagnosis and assessment of infants with D-TGA. It accurately establishes the diagnosis of D-TGA and reliably identifies associated abnormalities, such as VSD, mitral valve, and tricuspid valve abnormalities, and LVOT obstruction. It also reliably delineates coronary artery anatomy. Echocardiographic analysis of the intact ventricular septum position or LV geometry is also used to noninvasively assess the LV to RV pressure ratio and IV mass in neonates with D-TGA and intact ventricular septum who are being evaluated as candidates for an ASO.

In institutions with high-level TTE, a comprehensive cardiac catheterization is no longer routinely performed in neonates with D-TGA. A limited catheterization can be performed in conjunction with a balloon atrial septostomy. In the rare instance where coronary anatomy cannot be clearly delineated by echocardiography, coronary angiography might be indicated. During catheterization of infants with PAH, a trial of a fraction of inspired oxygen (F_{IO_2}) of 1.0 can be used to determine whether PVR is fixed or remains responsive to oxygen-induced pulmonary vasodilation.

Kussman BD, McGowan FX, Powell AJ, DiNardo JA. Anesthesia for congenital heart surgery. In: Davis PJ, Cladis FP, eds. *Smith's Anesthesia for Infants and Children*. 10th ed. Elsevier; 2022:732-831.

A.11. What preoperative interventions can help stabilize a patient with D-TGA?

Intact Ventricular Septum

Most neonates with D-TGA and intact ventricular septum will be in extremis shortly after birth without intervention. Findings may include Sa_{O_2} less than 60%, Pa_{O_2} less than 20 mm Hg, hypercarbia, and an evolving metabolic acidosis secondary to severely reduced effective pulmonary and systemic blood flow with low tissue oxygen delivery immediately following birth without intervention. Prostaglandin E_1 (0.01-0.05 μg/kg/min) is administered to dilate and maintain the patency of the ductus arteriosus. This is effective in increasing effective pulmonary and systemic blood flow and in improving Pa_{O_2} and tissue oxygen delivery *if* (1) PVR is less than SVR and (2) there is a nonrestrictive or minimally restrictive atrial septal communication. Prostaglandin E_1 therapy is associated with apnea, pyrexia, fluid retention, and platelet dysfunction.

An emergent balloon atrial septostomy is performed in the catheterization laboratory utilizing angiography or in the ICU utilizing echocardiography if prostaglandin E_1 does not improve tissue oxygen delivery. This increases the amount of intercirculatory mixing at the atrial level and increases effective systemic and pulmonary blood flow.

For a given amount of intercirculatory mixing and total systemic blood flow, an increase in pulmonary venous or systemic venous saturation results in an increase in arterial saturation. Pulmonary venous saturation is increased by tracheal intubation and mechanical ventilation with oxygen. This also reduces $\dot{V}/\dot{Q}$ mismatch and reduces PVR through the induction of respiratory alkalosis. Sedation and paralysis reduce oxygen consumption, thereby increasing mixed venous oxygen saturation and arterial saturation.

In some centers, all neonates stabilized on prostaglandin E_1 undergo a balloon atrial septostomy to enlarge the atrial septal communication and increase effective systemic and pulmonary blood flow enough that prostaglandin E_1 therapy can be discontinued, with surgery scheduled on a semi-elective basis.

In rare instances, the combination of prostaglandin E_1, an atrial septostomy, and mechanical ventilation with sedation and paralysis is ineffective. In this circumstance, extracorporeal membrane oxygenation (either venoarterial or venovenous) support to improve tissue oxygenation and to reverse end-organ insult and lactic acidosis before surgery is an alternative approach to emergent surgery in a critically ill neonate.

Ventricular Septal Defect

Infants in this subset are mildly cyanotic with symptoms of CHF. Pulmonary blood flow is elevated, and there is extensive intercirculatory mixing. Reducing PVR to further augment pulmonary blood flow and intercirculatory mixing will not greatly influence systemic oxygenation. Reducing PVR in these patients might increase the recirculated volume in the pulmonary circuit by increasing the compliance of the pulmonary circulation. Maintaining systemic blood flow necessitates increased cardiac output from a heart that is already volume overloaded. That said, these patients are usually stable enough not to require an immediate surgical or catheterization laboratory procedure, but ASO needs to be performed before intractable CHF or advanced PAH develops.

Ventricular Septal Defect and Left Ventricular Outflow Tract Obstruction

LVOT obstruction reduces pulmonary blood flow and intercirculatory mixing and protects the pulmonary vasculature from pressure and volume loads that accelerate the development of PAH. The degree of cyanosis depends on the degree of LVOT obstruction. Efforts to increase pulmonary blood flow by decreasing PVR are less effective when LVOT obstruction is severe. These infants can be severely cyanotic and develop erythrocytosis. They might require a palliative aortopulmonary shunt to increase pulmonary blood flow prior to definitive repair. The Rastelli, LeCompte, and Nikaidoh procedures are performed for D-TGA with LVOT obstruction.

Pulmonary Artery Hypertension

PAH is the long-term consequence of volume and pressure loads to the pulmonary system seen as a complication of unrepaired D-TGA. The goal of diagnosis and treatment of infants with D-TGA is to intervene surgically before the development of PAH. As PAH progresses, patients become progressively cyanotic and polycythemic. Efforts to reduce PVR increase pulmonary blood flow and intercirculatory mixing in infants where PVR is not fixed. Infants with advanced PAH (PVR >10 Wood units; histologic grade 4) are generally candidates only for palliative therapy. Closure of a VSD in the presence of advanced PAH has a high mortality rate owing to the afterload mismatch and resultant pulmonary ventricle (LV) dysfunction. These patients are candidates for a palliative intra-atrial physiologic repair (Mustard or Senning procedure) without closure or with fenestrated closure (4- to 5-mm hole in the center of the VSD patch) of the VSD.

Kussman BD, McGowan FX, Powell AJ, DiNardo JA. Anesthesia for congenital heart surgery. In: Davis PJ, Cladis FP, eds. *Smith's Anesthesia for Infants and Children*. 10th ed. Elsevier; 2022:732-831.

A.12. What are the surgical options for repair? Why is one chosen over the others?

Arterial Anatomic Repair: Arterial Switch (Jatene) Operation

The ASO anatomically corrects the discordant VA connections and is the procedure of choice for patients with D-TGA. Following repair, the RV is connected to the PA and the LV to the aorta. Clinical success with the ASO, summarized in **Figure 39.4**, was achieved in 1975. For the ASO to be successful, the

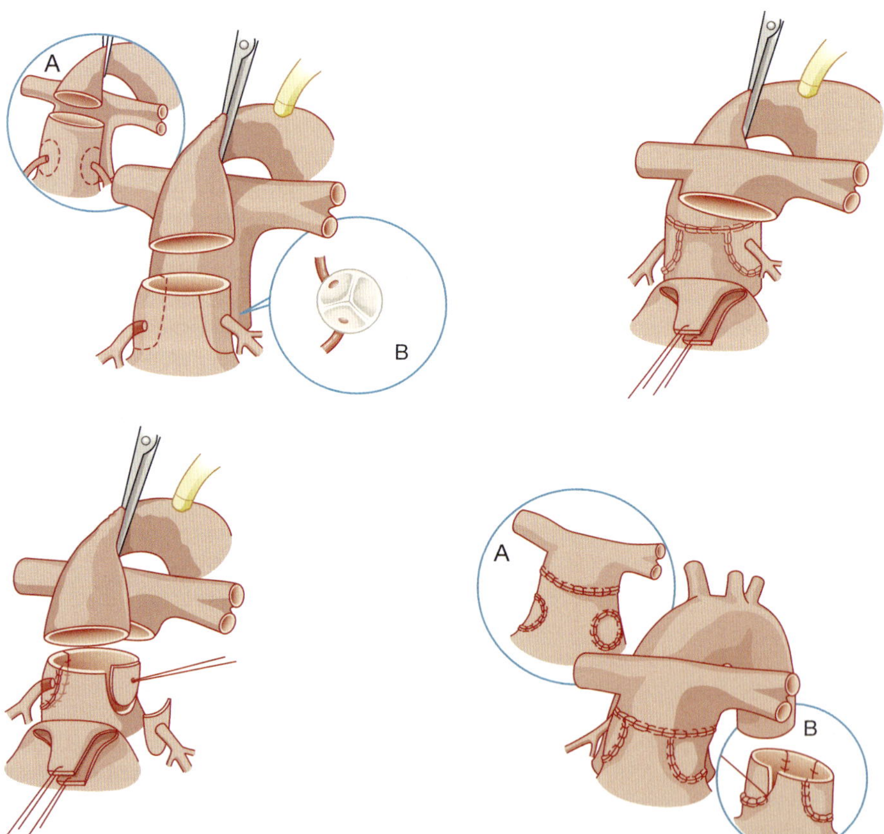

FIGURE 39.4. Details of the arterial switch procedure. Upper left. Aorta is transected and the left and right main coronary arteries are excised using either the button of the aortic wall **(A)** or a segment of the aortic wall **(B)** extending from the rim of the aorta. **Lower left.** An equivalent segment of the pulmonary arterial wall is excised, and coronary arteries are sutured to PA. **Upper right.** Distal PA is brought anterior to the ascending aorta (LeCompte maneuver), and proximal PA is anastomosed to the distal aorta. **Lower right.** Sites of coronary explantation are repaired using either a patch of prosthetic material **(A)** or a segment of pericardium **(B)**. Finally, the proximal aorta is sutured to distal PA. (Adapted from Castaneda AR, Norwood WI, Jonas RA, et al. Transposition of the great arteries and intact ventricular septum: anatomical repair in the neonate. *Ann Thorac Surg.* 1984;38:438-443. Copyright © 1984 The Society of Thoracic Surgeons. With permission.)

original pulmonary ventricle (LV) must have sufficient mass to be capable of functioning as the systemic ventricle following the ASO. Patient selection and the timing of the surgical procedure are important variables in determining success. The ASO was originally described in patients with D-TGA and a large VSD or a large PDA. In these patients, the pulmonary ventricle (LV) remains exposed to systemic pressures, and the LV mass remains sufficient to support systemic circulation. For this subset of patients, the ASO is generally performed within the first 2 to 3 months of life before intractable CHF or irreversible PAH develops.

Patients with D-TGA and intact ventricular septum have a progressive reduction in LV mass over the first 3 or 4 weeks of life as the afterload of the anatomic LV falls as the physiologic PAH present at birth resolves. Adequate mass to support the systemic circulation reliably exists in these patients only for the first 3 or 4 weeks of life, so a primary ASO must be performed in this period. Most are performed in the first few days of life. Historically, favorable candidates for a primary ASO in the neonatal period were identified by cardiac catheterization with an LV to an RV pressure ratio of at least 0.6. Currently, two-dimensional echocardiography is used to noninvasively assess the LV to RV pressure ratio. Three types of ventricular septal geometry have been described. Patients in whom the ventricular septum bulges to the left (type 3), indicating a low pressure in the pulmonary ventricle (LV), are not candidates for a neonatal ASO. Patients with septal bulging to the right (type 1), indicating a high pressure in the pulmonary ventricle (LV), and those patients with an intermediate septal position (type 2) are considered good candidates. Most neonates with D-TGA and intact ventricular septum who are suitable candidates for an ASO have type 2 septal geometry.

The staged ASO for D-TGA with intact ventricular septum is used for those neonates in whom surgery cannot be performed in the first month of life secondary to events such as prematurity, sepsis, low birth weight (<1.0 kg), or late referral. The first step of a staged procedure retrains the LV to accept the systemic workload and usually involves the creation of a nonrestrictive atrial septum (if it does not already exist), placement of a PA band, and creation of an aortopulmonary shunt with entry to the PA distal to the band. The PA band must be tight enough to increase pressure in the pulmonary ventricle (LV) to approximately one-half to two-thirds of that in the systemic ventricle (RV). This will increase the afterload sufficiently to stimulate an increase in LV mass. Previously, a PA band was left on for 3 to 6 months, after which the band was removed, the shunt taken down, and an ASO was performed. Currently, a rapid two-stage repair is favored where the ASO is performed as early as 1 week after preparatory PA banding, often during the same hospitalization. This approach is possible because the LV mass usually doubles after 1 week of PA banding. Establishing the appropriate tightness of the band can be challenging, and the PA band as well as the systemic to PA shunt can distort the PA, making the ASO difficult. Intraoperative echocardiography is useful in guiding the placement of the PA band. The band is tightened enough to flatten the intact ventricular septum by shifting it toward the RV.

Jonas RA, Giglia TM, Sanders SP, et al. Rapid, two-stage arterial switch for transposition of the great arteries and intact ventricular septum beyond the neonatal period. *Circulation*. 1989;80:I203-I208.

Intra-Atrial Physiologic Repairs: Mustard and Senning Procedures

The Mustard and the Senning procedures are atrial switch procedures that surgically create discordant AV connections so that there is a physiologic correction of the VA discordance. Systemic venous blood is routed to the anatomic LV and the PA, whereas pulmonary venous blood is routed to the anatomic RV and the aorta. This is not an anatomic correction because the RV becomes the systemic ventricle. These atrial switch procedures are primarily of historic interest, as the ASO is nearly universally performed for D-TGA.

Vejlstrup N, Sørensen K, Mattsson E, et al. Long-term outcome of Mustard/Senning correction for transposition of the great arteries in Sweden and Denmark. *Circulation*. 2015;132:633-638.

Rastelli, LeCompte, and Nikaidoh Procedures

These procedures are used to correct D-TGA with VSD and LVOT (subpulmonic and/or pulmonic) obstruction. In the Rastelli procedure, the subpulmonic LVOT obstruction is resected, and the LVOT is baffled to the aorta with the patch used to close the VSD. An RV-PA conduit is created. The LeCompte procedure involves resecting the LV outlet septum, closing the VSD to route the LV blood to the aorta, and bringing the PAs anteriorly to be anastomosed to the RV. The Nikaidoh procedure is an aortic translocation procedure where the aortic root and coronary arteries are resected and anastomosed to the RV after the outlet septum has been resected. The right ventricular outflow (RVOT) is reconstructed with a pericardial patch or homograft. The ASO is not performed when there is subpulmonic and/or pulmonic LVOT since the infant would be left with residual neoaortic or subneoaortic LVOT obstruction.

Bautisa-Hernandez V, Marx GR, Bacha EA, et al. Aortic root translocation plus arterial switch for transposition of great arteries with left ventricular outflow tract obstruction: intermediate-term results. *J Am Coll Cardiol.* 2007;49: 485-490.

Honjo O, Kotani Y, Bharucha T, et al. Anatomical factors determining surgical decision-making in patients with transposition of the great arteries with left ventricular outflow tract obstruction. *Eur J Cardiothorac Surg.* 2013;44:1085-1094.

Martins P, Castela E. Transposition of the great arteries. *Orphanet J Rare Dis.* 2008;3:27.

B. Preoperative Evaluation and Preparation

B.1. What information is important to prepare for this case?

The preoperative evaluation should begin with a careful history and physical examination including gestational age, birth history, family history, and other medical problems. A comprehensive airway evaluation and any previously used tracheal tube sizes and leak pressures should be noted. Sites for arterial and intravenous access should be assessed. A blood sample must be sent to the blood bank to ensure an adequate supply of red blood cells, and blood component therapies are available in the operating room.

The preoperative ECG, chest radiograph, and echocardiograms should be reviewed. Particular attention should be paid to septal geometry, biventricular function, coronary anatomy, and adequacy of mixing at the atrial septal and ductal levels. The ductus arteriosus can remain patent even if prostaglandin E_1 has been discontinued.

Laboratory data should include a complete blood count, electrolytes, platelet count, arterial blood gas, calcium, blood urea nitrogen, creatinine, liver function tests, and blood glucose. Given that this infant presented with severe hypoxemia, end-organ dysfunction must be ruled out. Liver function tests and creatinine should be normal; if they are elevated, consideration should be given to further medical optimization. A head ultrasonographic examination should be performed to rule out intraventricular hemorrhage.

Kussman BD, McGowan FX, Powell AJ, DiNardo JA. Anesthesia for congenital heart surgery. In: Davis PJ, Cladis FP, eds. *Smith's Anesthesia for Infants and Children.* 10th ed. Elsevier; 2022:732-831.

B.2. What are the anesthetic goals before cardiopulmonary bypass (CPB)?

- Optimize heart rate (HR), contractility, and preload to maintain cardiac output. A reduction in cardiac output decreases systemic venous saturation with a resultant fall in arterial saturation.
- Maintain ductal patency with prostaglandin E_1 (0.01-0.05 μg/kg/min) in ductus-dependent patients.
- Avoid increases in PVR relative to SVR. Increases in PVR decrease pulmonary blood flow and reduce intercirculatory mixing. In patients with PAH, ventilatory interventions should be used to reduce PVR. Pulmonary blood flow and intercirculatory mixing are increased unless restricted by severe LVOT obstruction.
- Reductions in SVR relative to PVR should be avoided. Reducing SVR increases the recirculation of systemic venous blood and decreases arterial oxygen saturation.
- In patients with D-TGA and VSD with symptoms of CHF, ventilatory interventions to reduce PVR are not warranted because they will produce only small improvements in arterial saturation at the expense of a reduction in systemic perfusion.

Kussman BD, McGowan FX, Powell AJ, DiNardo JA. Anesthesia for congenital heart surgery. In: Davis PJ, Cladis FP, eds. *Smith's Anesthesia for Infants and Children.* 10th ed. Elsevier; 2022:732-831.

B.3. What is the plan for glucose management in this patient?

Maintenance for caloric requirements in the awake neonate/infant is 100 kcal/kg/d or 4 kcal/kg/h. This caloric requirement can be met with glucose 25 g/kg/d or 1 g/kg/h. From a practical point of view, this can be met with 10% dextrose (100 mg/mL) run at the maintenance volume replacement rate of 4 mL/kg/h. Half this rate (2 mL/kg/h) is usually sufficient to meet the caloric requirements of an anesthetized infant while avoiding both hyperglycemia and hypoglycemia, which can be detrimental to neurologic outcome, particularly following DHCA. Dextrose infusions should be discontinued before the commencement of CPB because the associated neuroendocrine response to CPB generally produces mild hyperglycemia without the need for supplementation. Some infants receive nutritional support as part of medical stabilization before surgery. High-calorie total parenteral nutrition and lipid therapy should be discontinued and replaced with a 10% dextrose infusion several hours before transport to the operating room. Continued administration of high-calorie parenteral nutrition infusions can make intraoperative serum glucose management challenging, and higher dextrose infusion rates might be necessary pre-CPB to avoid rebound hypoglycemia once they are discontinued.

Kussman BD, McGowan FX, Powell AJ, DiNardo JA. Anesthesia for congenital heart surgery. In: Davis PJ, Cladis FP, eds. *Smith's Anesthesia for Infants and Children*. 10th ed. Elsevier; 2022:732-831.

C. Intraoperative Management

C.1. How would you monitor this infant?

Standard American Society of Anesthesiologists monitors including pre- and postductal pulse oximetry and existing invasive monitors are monitored before the induction of general anesthesia. Noninvasive blood pressure is measured frequently until arterial blood pressure can be continuously monitored by an upper or lower extremity arterial catheter. The plan for central venous access is discussed with the surgical team and will likely include some combination of an existing umbilical venous line, an internal jugular central venous line, or a surgically placed atrial line. Core body temperature is measured with rectal, esophageal, or bladder temperature probes, and nasopharyngeal temperature is measured as an estimate of brain temperature during CPB. Most small infants are too small for a transesophageal echocardiogram probe placement, so the surgery and cardiology team perform an epicardial echocardiogram to assess the heart before and after repair.

Kussman BD, McGowan FX, Powell AJ, DiNardo JA. Anesthesia for congenital heart surgery. In: Davis PJ, Cladis FP, eds. *Smith's Anesthesia for Infants and Children*. 10th ed. Elsevier; 2022:732-831.

C.2. What is the best way to induce and maintain general anesthesia in this patient?

There is no single best way to induce and maintain general anesthesia in this (or any) patient. The current clinical status of the patient determines which anesthesia technique is indicated. A high-dose opioid technique is particularly useful in sick neonates and infants since anesthetic levels of synthetic opioids maintain hemodynamic stability, blunt reactive pulmonary hypertension, and do not suppress myocardial function. A high-dose opioid technique for this case would require 25 to 100 μg/kg fentanyl or 2.5 to 10 μg/kg sufentanil for the entire case supplemented as tolerated with low inhaled concentrations of a volatile anesthetic or a benzodiazepine. A low- or moderate-dose opioid technique would require higher concentrations of volatile anesthetic or higher doses of a benzodiazepine to induce and maintain general anesthesia with a higher likelihood of hemodynamic instability.

Infants born with D-TGA have usually been stabilized in the ICU so peripheral or central intravenous access and possibly invasive arterial monitoring would have been established.

Kussman BD, McGowan FX, Powell AJ, DiNardo JA. Anesthesia for congenital heart surgery. In: Davis PJ, Cladis FP, eds. *Smith's Anesthesia for Infants and Children*. 10th ed. Elsevier; 2022:732-831.

C.3. How is CPB in infants and children different from adults?

The major differences between adult and pediatric CPB are summarized in **Table 39.2**.

Flows of 2.0 to 2.5 L/min/m^2 are commonly used for infants, children, and adults during mild to moderate systemic hypothermia. Flow rates (expressed in mL/kg/min) are substantially higher in neonates than in adults because of age-related differences in surface area-to-weight ratios. The recommended full flow rates for pediatric CPB are summarized in **Table 39.3**.

Most operative procedures in children require the use of either total CPB or DHCA. Arterial and venous cannulation can be particularly challenging in neonates and infants. Venous cannulation for DHCA is usually accomplished with a single large venous cannula in the RA. Once cooling is complete, CPB flow rates are reduced to zero and the venous cannula is removed to allow for maximum surgical exposure. In cases requiring total CPB, the superior and inferior venae cavae and other sources of systemic venous return are cannulated, and surgical tourniquets or tapes are passed around the external circumference of the vessels. When these tapes are tightened around the cannulae, the right heart can be isolated completely and opened without entrainment of air into the venous circuit or obscuration of the surgical field by venous blood. At least one tape must be left untightened during delivery of antegrade cardioplegia to allow egress of cardioplegia solution from the

TABLE 39.2 Major Differences Between Adult and Pediatric Cardiopulmonary Bypass

Parameter	Adult	Pediatrics
Temperature	Rarely below 25 °C-32 °C	Commonly 15° C-20 °C
Use of total circulatory arrest	Rare	Common
Pump prime		
Dilution effects on blood volume	25%-33%	200%-300%
Additional additives in pediatric primes		Blood, albumin
Perfusion pressures	50-80 mm Hg (Some centers accept 30 mm Hg.)	20-50 mm Hg
Influence of pH management strategy	Minimal at moderate hypothermia	Marked at deep hypothermia
Measured $Paco_2$ differences	30-45 mm Hg	20-80 mm Hg
Glucose regulation		
Hypoglycemia	Rare—Requires significant hepatic injury	Common—Reduced hepatic glycogen stores
Hyperglycemia	Frequent—Generally easily controlled with insulin	Less common—Rebound hypoglycemia may occur.

coronary sinus without distension of the RA. The superior vena cava (SVC) is larger than the inferior vena cava (IVC) in neonates and infants, so the larger venous cannula is usually placed in the SVC. The opposite is true in older children, where two-thirds of systemic venous return is from the IVC.

Aortic cannulation in children can be complicated by a hypoplastic ascending aorta or aortic arch, as in patients with hypoplastic left heart syndrome. In these cases, systemic circulation is ductus dependent, so it might be necessary to establish systemic perfusion through the ductus arteriosus by cannulating the PA. If the aortic arch is interrupted, cannulation of the aorta proximal and distal to the interruption is necessary. In infants and children, the arterial cannula is large relative to the size of the aorta, so constant vigilance is necessary to avoid complete or partial obstruction of the aorta by the cannula. Signs of this include dampening of the arterial pressure tracing, distension of the systemic ventricle, and an increase in the aortic line pressure during placement or manipulation of the aortic cannula. The surgeon must reposition the line to ensure adequate perfusion. Some centers utilize near-infrared spectroscopy and transcranial Doppler ultrasonography as adjunctive methods to assess cerebral blood flow during CPB.

Kussman BD, McGowan FX, Powell AJ, DiNardo JA. Anesthesia for congenital heart surgery. In: Davis PJ, Cladis FP, eds. *Smith's Anesthesia for Infants and Children*. 10th ed. Elsevier; 2022:732-831.

Matte GS, DiNardo JA. Pediatric cardiopulmonary bypass. In: Gravlee GP, Davis RF, Hammon JW, et al, eds. *Cardiopulmonary Bypass and Mechanical Support: Principles and Practice*. 4th ed. Wolters Kluwer; 2015:655-695.

C.4. What is modified ultrafiltration (MUF)?

MUF is a technique used to ultrafiltrate blood after weaning from CPB while maintaining the integrity of the bypass circuit. Ultrafiltration removes excess fluid from blood by hydrostatic pressure across a

TABLE 39.3 Recommended Full Flow Rates for Pediatric Cardiopulmonary Bypass

Patient Weight (kg)	Full CPB Flow Rates (mL/kg/min)
<3	150-200
3-10	125-175
10-15	120-150
15-30	100-120
30-50	75-100
>50	50-75

CPB, cardiopulmonary bypass.

semipermeable membrane. The devices are the same as those used in hemodialysis, but no dialysate is used. When used in conjunction with CPB, they are commonly called hemoconcentrators because they produce an increase in hematocrit by removing excess fluid. These devices consist of a core of microporous hollow fibers made of polysulfone, polyamide, or polyacrylonitrile material arranged in a bundle, with a pore size of 0.30 to 0.40 µm. Blood inflow must be from the arterial side of the CPB circuit because of the pressure gradient needed for blood to flow through the hemoconcentrator unless a separate roller pump is used to flow into the hemoconcentrator. Outflow is diverted to the cardiotomy reservoir or venous reservoir. The composition of the ultrafiltrate is similar to a glomerular filtrate and is collected in a container connected to a vacuum source and discarded.

The rate at which ultrafiltrate is produced depends on the transmembrane pressure (TMP) gradient, which is determined by the arterial inlet pressure (P_a), the venous outlet pressure (P_v), the absolute value of applied suction at the outlet (P_n), the oncotic pressure at the inlet (P_i), and the oncotic pressure at the outlet (P_o):

$$\text{TMP} = \frac{P_a + P_v}{2} + P_n - \frac{P_i + P_o}{2}$$

P_n is increased by adjusting the regulated vacuum source connected to the outlet of the device. TMP should not exceed 500 mm Hg.

MUF can be performed using either an arteriovenous or venovenous system. In the arteriovenous system, blood flows from the aortic cannula through a separate circuit and roller pump to the inflow of the hemoconcentrator before returning to the RA. Blood volume is kept constant as ultrafiltrate is lost by replacing the ultrafiltrate volume with blood from the venous reservoir of the CPB circuit, which also passes through the hemoconcentrator circuit before returning to the RA. In this way, the patient's blood as well as the CPB circuit blood is hemoconcentrated and the CPB circuit remains primed. In the venovenous system, blood passes from the IVC cannula through a separate circuit and roller pump to the inflow of the hemoconcentrator before returning to the patient through the SVC cannula. Blood volume is also kept constant in this system by replacing ultrafiltrate volume with blood from the CPB circuit, which also passes through the ultrafiltrator before returning to the patient. The end point for termination of MUF following CPB varies from institution to institution, with institutions terminating MUF after a set time interval (15-20 minutes), a set hematocrit (40%), or a set volume removed (750 mL/m^2). Heparin anticoagulation must be maintained during MUF, with protamine reversal of heparin initiated after termination of MUF.

Neonates and infants are the patients who benefit most from MUF because the volume of the CPB circuit is large relative to their blood volume. Hemoconcentration increases the hematocrit and concentration of coagulation factors and reduces total body water. MUF may be an effective method of attenuating the deleterious consequences of using large asanguinous primes, particularly in neonates and infants. In studies comparing MUF to no ultrafiltration, a large asanguinous pump prime was usually defined as a 400- to 900-mL prime with packed red blood cells added to reach a hematocrit of 15% to 20%.

Continuous ultrafiltration is a similar MUF, except it can occur only during CPB and only when there is sufficient volume in the CPB circuit. MUF and continuous ultrafiltration are indistinguishable in their effect on hematocrit, mean arterial pressure, HR, and LV shortening fraction when equal volumes of fluid are removed.

Matte GS, DiNardo JA. Cardiopulmonary bypass for pediatric and congenital cardiac surgery. In: Gravlee GP, Davis RF, Hammon JW, Kussman BD, eds. *Cardiopulmonary Bypass and Mechanical Support: Principles and Practice.* 5th ed. Wolters Kluwer; 2024:655-695.

Whiting D, Yuki K, DiNardo JA. Cardiopulmonary bypass in the pediatric population. *Best Pract Res Clin Anaesthesiol.* 2015;29:241-256.

Williams GD, Ramamoorthy C, Chu L, et al. Modified and conventional ultrafiltration during pediatric cardiac surgery: clinical outcomes compared. *J Thorac Cardiovasc Surg.* 2006;132:1291-1298.

C.5. Briefly describe the surgical techniques of the Mustard/Senning, ASO, and Rastelli procedures.

Intra-Atrial Physiologic Repairs: Mustard and Senning Procedures

The Mustard and Senning procedures are *atrial* switch procedures where the interatrial septum is excised, and a baffle is used to redirect pulmonary and systemic venous blood. In the Mustard procedure, the baffle is made of native pericardium or synthetic material. The Senning procedure uses autologous tissue from the right atrial wall and interatrial septum. In both procedures, the pulmonary blood flows over the baffle and is directed across the tricuspid valve into the RV and aorta, and the systemic venous blood flows on the underside of the baffle and is directed across the mitral valve into the LV and out the PA. This results in a physiologic but not anatomic correction of D-TGA because the morphologic RV functions as the systemic ventricle. These procedures are performed with total hypothermic CPB, bicaval cannulation, aortic cross-clamping during cardioplegic arrest, and sometimes low-flow CPB.

Arterial Anatomic Repair: Arterial Switch (Jatene) Operation

The *ASO* is an anatomic and physiologic repair of D-TGA where the great arteries are divided above the semilunar valves and switched so that VA concordance is restored. The PA and the aorta are transected distal to their respective valve, and then the coronary arteries are explanted from the ascending aorta with 3 to 4 mm of surrounding tissue and reimplanted into the proximal PA (neoaorta). The explant sites are repaired either with pericardium or synthetic material. The distal PA is brought anterior to the aorta (LeCompte maneuver) to be reanastomosed to the old proximal aorta (RVOT), and the distal aorta is reanastomosed to the old proximal PA (left ventricular outflow) and the pulmonary valve becomes the neoaortic valve. The ASO is done using total hypothermic CPB with aortic cross-clamping and cardioplegic arrest. Intervals of low-flow CPB are used, and a short interval of DHCA might be employed to close the atrial septum or VSD if a single venous cannula rather than bicaval venous cannulation is used. Closure of a VSD is preferentially done with a transatrial approach through the tricuspid valve to avoid a ventriculotomy that could contribute to postoperative RV dysfunction.

Jatene AD, Fontes VF, Paulista PP, et al. Anatomic correction of transposition of the great vessels. *J Thorac Cardiovasc Surg*. 1976;72:364-370.

Kussman BD, McGowan FX, Powell AJ, DiNardo JA. Anesthesia for congenital heart surgery. In: Davis PJ, Cladis FP, eds. *Smith's Anesthesia for Infants and Children*. 10th ed. Elsevier; 2022:732-831.

Rastelli Procedure

The Rastelli procedure is a physiologic repair for D-TGA with VSD and subpulmonic stenosis, where the LV and aorta are brought into continuity with a patch tunnel that also closes the VSD. The PA is transected and ligated, and the RV and proximal PA are brought into continuity with a valved conduit or homograft. The VSD may have to be enlarged in some cases to prevent subaortic stenosis. The patch tunnel that connects the LV to the aorta bypasses subpulmonic and pulmonic stenosis. This procedure is performed under similar conditions as the ASO, with total hypothermic CPB, bicaval cannulation, aortic cross-clamping during cardioplegic arrest, and intervals of low-flow CPB.

Historically, most of these patients had a palliative systemic to PA shunt placed in the newborn period and then returned for the Rastelli procedure and takedown of the shunt at 2 to 3 years of age. The delay was felt necessary to avoid performing a right ventriculotomy in infants with immature myocardium and limited contractile elements and to allow adequate growth of the RV and PAs to permit placement of an RV to PA conduit. In the current era, with improvements in myocardial protection, CPB technology, and surgical technique, this procedure can be performed as a primary procedure in the neonatal period.

Jatene AD, Fontes VF, Paulista PP, et al. Anatomic correction of transposition of the great vessels. *J Thorac Cardiovasc Surg*. 1976;72:364-370.

Kussman BD, McGowan FX, Powell AJ, DiNardo JA. Anesthesia for congenital heart surgery. In: Davis PJ, Cladis FP, eds. *Smith's Anesthesia for Infants and Children*. 10th ed. Elsevier; 2022:732-831.

C.6. What is hypothermia, and how is it classified? What is low-flow CPB? What is deep hypothermic circulatory arrest (DHCA)?

The levels of systemic hypothermia employed during CPB are generally defined as follows: mild (35 °C [95.0 °F] to 32 °C [89.6 °F]), moderate (31 °C [87.8 °F] to 26 °C [78.8 °F]), deep (25 °C [77 °F] to 20 °C [68 °F]), and profound (<20 °C [68 °F]). It is not uncommon for temperatures less than 20 °C (68 °F) used in conjunction with pediatric cardiac surgery to be called deep hypothermia. Low-flow CPB in neonates/infants conducted in conjunction with temperatures of 18 °C (64.4 °F) to 25 °C (77 °F) is generally defined as flow rates of 50 to 70 mL/kg/min or approximately 1.0 to 1.5 L/min/m^2.

Profound hypothermic circulatory arrest, commonly referred to as DHCA, is conducted at temperatures of 18 °C (64.4 °F) to 20 °C (68 °F) and allows cessation of CPB, venous and arterial cannula removal, and exsanguination of the patient into the venous reservoir of the CPB circuit. This technique is used to improve exposure of intracardiac defects and to facilitate aortic arch reconstruction in infants and children. There has been substantial refinement of the technique of DHCA since its successful inception in the 1970s. In the current era, DHCA is used selectively and for short intervals. It is utilized primarily for the aortic arch reconstruction component of the Norwood procedure, repair of interrupted aortic arch, neonatal repair of total anomalous pulmonary venous connection, and complicated intracardiac repairs such as complete AV canal defects in small (<2.0 kg) neonates and infants.

Matte GS. *Perfusion for Congenital Heart Surgery: Notes on Cardiopulmonary Bypass for a Complex Patient Population.* Wiley-Blackwell; 2015:33-65.

Matte GS, DiNardo JA. Cardiopulmonary bypass for pediatric and congenital cardiac surgery. In: Gravlee GP, Davis RF, Hammon JW, Kussman BD, eds. *Cardiopulmonary Bypass and Mechanical Support: Principles and Practice.* 5th ed. Wolters Kluwer; 2024:655-695.

Whiting D, Yuki K, DiNardo JA. Cardiopulmonary bypass in the pediatric population. *Best Pract Res Clin Anaesthesiol.* 2015;29:241-256.

C.7. Why is hypothermia beneficial to the brain during low-flow CPB and DHCA?

Hypothermia is arguably the most important component of low-flow CPB and DHCA. The hypothermia-induced reduction in cerebral metabolic rate for oxygen ($CMRO_2$) slows the rate of depletion of high-energy phosphates and the development of intracellular acidosis and delays or prevents the neuronal energy failure that leads to terminal membrane depolarization and subsequent neuronal injury or death during an ischemic episode.

Q_{10} defines the ratio of organ oxygen consumption at a defined temperature to the oxygen consumption at a temperature 10 °C (18 °F) lower. The cerebral Q_{10} is approximately 3.65 in children and 2.3 in adults. The cerebral metabolic rate will still be approximately 10% to 15% of its normothermic baseline at 15 °C (59 °F). If it is assumed that 3 to 5 minutes of cerebral ischemia can be tolerated at 37 °C (98.6 °F) and the Q_{10} is 3.0, 9 to 15 minutes of ischemia can be tolerated at 27 °C (80.6 °F) and 27 to 45 minutes can be tolerated at 17 °C (62.6 °F).

In addition to reducing $CMRO_2$, hypothermia serves to ameliorate some of the sequelae of neuronal ischemia when instituted before the ischemic insult. Specifically, hypothermia markedly reduces the release of the excitatory neurotransmitters glutamate, aspartate, and glycine that accompany cerebral ischemia and subsequent reperfusion. In energy-deprived cells, glutamate is neurotoxic in part due to the role it plays in inducing massive calcium influx through *N*-methyl-D-aspartic acid receptors. Hypothermia also blunts the inhibitory effect of hypoxia on nitroxidergic (postganglionic parasympathetic nerve where nitric oxide is the neurotransmitter)-induced cerebral vasodilation. In addition, there is evidence that hypothermia attenuates neutrophil migration into ischemic tissue.

Matte GS, DiNardo JA. Pediatric cardiopulmonary bypass. In: Gravlee GP, Davis RF, Hammon JW, et al, eds. *Cardiopulmonary Bypass and Mechanical Support: Principles and Practice.* 4th ed. Wolters Kluwer; 2015:655-695.

McCullough JN, Zhang N, Reich DL, et al. Cerebral metabolic suppression during hypothermic circulatory arrest in humans. *Ann Thorac Surg.* 1999;67:1895-1899.

C.8. Explain the difference between α-stat and pH-stat blood gas management.

pH-Stat and α-stat are acid-base management strategies that address the temperature-induced differences in blood pH, oxygen solubility, and CO_2 solubility. These management strategies directly influence blood flow to the brain and other organs during hypothermic CPB or DHCA. The difference between these two strategies becomes marked if the patient's temperature progressively decreases below 37 °C (98.6 °F) but is not clinically relevant until the patient's temperature is less than 30 °C (86 °F). At normothermia (37 °C [98.6 °F]), there is no difference between pH-stat and α-stat management.

Although pH-stat and α-stat acid-base management are commonly mentioned in association with temperature-corrected and temperature-uncorrected interpretation of blood gases, these are entirely different concepts. The method of blood gas interpretation (corrected or uncorrected) does not dictate the method of acid-base management (pH-stat or α-stat). α-Stat or pH-stat management is possible with the use of both temperature-corrected and temperature-uncorrected blood gases.

When a blood gas sample is drawn from a hypothermic patient at 25 °C (77 °F), the sample is warmed to 37 °C (98.6 °F) before measurement. Values obtained at 37 °C (98.6 °F) are temperature-uncorrected values. These values are converted to temperature-corrected values using a nomogram. The nomogram accounts for temperature-induced changes in pH, oxygen solubility, and CO_2 solubility in a closed-blood system. When blood in a closed system is cooled to a lower temperature, the electrochemically neutral pH is higher and the associated Pco_2 is lower than in a closed-blood system at 37 °C (98.6 °F). Therefore, electrochemical neutrality is maintained by keeping pH alkalotic in temperature-corrected blood gases and normal in temperature-uncorrected gases. This is known as *α-stat regulation*. For practical purposes, it is easier to use uncorrected gases and keep pH and Pco_2 in the range considered normal at 37 °C (98.6 °F). Cerebral blood flow and oxygen consumption are appropriately coupled when α-stat regulation is used. Deep hypothermia in the presence of α-stat regulation produces loss of cerebral autoregulation such that cerebral blood flow varies directly with arterial pressure.

pH-Stat regulation refers to maintaining pH and Pco_2 at normal values for blood at 37 °C (98.6 °F), regardless of actual blood temperature. With this strategy, a blood sample will have a normal pH and Pco_2 when temperature-corrected gases are used and have acidotic pH and Pco_2 values when temperature-uncorrected gases are used. For practical purposes, pH-stat is maintained by adding CO_2 to the ventilating gas during hypothermic CPB to increase Pco_2 and decrease the pH. In contrast to α-stat regulation, in which total CO_2 content is kept constant, pH-stat regulation results in an increase in total CO_2 content. The cerebral vasculature maintains vasomotor responses to varying Pco_2 during hypothermic CPB during both moderate and deep hypothermia even though deep hypothermia induces loss of cerebral blood flow autoregulation. When pH-stat regulation is used with moderate hypothermic CPB, there is uncoupling of cerebral blood flow and metabolism and loss of cerebral autoregulation. As a result, cerebral blood flow varies linearly with arterial blood pressure, and cerebral hyperperfusion exists with cerebral blood flow far in excess of that dictated by cerebral metabolic rate. This hyperperfusion state is the result of (1) reduced cerebral oxygen consumption induced by hypothermia and (2) cerebral vasodilation resulting from a disproportionately high Pco_2 for the degree of hypothermia present. The potential danger of the hyperperfused state is that it could increase the delivery of microemboli into the cerebral circulation.

Matte GS. *Perfusion for Congenital Heart Surgery: Notes on Cardiopulmonary Bypass for a Complex Patient Population.* Wiley-Blackwell; 2015:33-65.

Matte GS, DiNardo JA. Cardiopulmonary bypass for pediatric and congenital cardiac surgery. In: Gravlee GP, Davis RF, Hammon JW, Kussman BD, eds. *Cardiopulmonary Bypass and Mechanical Support: Principles and Practice.* 5th ed. Wolters Kluwer; 2024:655-695.

C.9. What are the immediate post-CPB issues following ASO?

Hemorrhage from the extensive suture lines can require emergent surgical repair on CPB or can be caused by post-CPB coagulopathy. Temporarily reducing arterial blood pressure with vasodilating agents can be helpful. Aggressive blood component therapy is often required and can require 1 to 2 units of platelets (0.25-0.5 units per kilogram) to obtain a therapeutic platelet count increase in neonates. Because platelets are suspended in fresh frozen plasma, a platelet transfusion of this size usually results in a fresh frozen plasma transfusion of 10 to 15 mL/kg. Cryoprecipitate transfusion is sometimes necessary to restore fibrinogen levels to presurgical levels. Point-of-care assessment and characterization of coagulopathy using thromboelastography or rotational thromboelastometry can be helpful (see Chapter 31).

Myocardial ischemia following reimplantation of the coronary arteries is a potential problem following the ASO. Epicardial or transesophageal echocardiography is helpful to assess the patency of the reimplanted coronary arteries and to prevent coronary artery air emboli by ensuring adequate removal of air from the LA and LV before termination of CPB. Maintenance of high perfusion pressures on CPB after aortic cross-clamp removal will facilitate the distal migration of air emboli. In other instances, kinking of the reimplanted artery or compromise of the implanted coronary ostia may require immediate surgical intervention. Kinking of the reimplanted coronary arteries can also be caused by LA hypertension, with resolution of ischemia following correction of the LA hypertension. Pharmacologic intervention with traditional therapies to improve the balance of myocardial oxygen demand and delivery such as nitroglycerin and β-blockade is never a long-term alternative to prompt surgical revision of the appropriate anastomosis.

Despite comprehensive preoperative evaluation, the LV of patients undergoing an ASO can be limited in its ability to support systemic circulation in the post-CPB period. This can occur as the result of myocardial ischemia, inadequate LV mass, poor protection of the LV during aortic cross-clamping, or a combination. Echocardiography is useful in identifying and continuously evaluating both global and regional LV systolic dysfunction. It also detects mitral regurgitation, which can occur secondary to papillary muscle dysfunction or to dilation of the mitral valve annulus. Inotropic support of the LV and afterload reduction can be necessary to terminate CPB.

Kussman BD, McGowan FX, Powell AJ, DiNardo JA. Anesthesia for congenital heart surgery. In: Davis PJ, Cladis FP, eds. *Smith's Anesthesia for Infants and Children.* 10th ed. Elsevier; 2022:732-831.

Whiting D, DiNardo JA. TEG and ROTEM: technology and clinical applications. *Am J Hematol.* 2014;89:228-232.

D. Postoperative Management

D.1. How is myocardial ischemia addressed in the intensive care unit (ICU) following the ASO?

Myocardial ischemia in the ICU following an ASO is usually heralded by ST-segment/T-wave changes or by atrial or ventricular arrhythmias. Myocardial ischemia is usually mechanical in nature until proven otherwise. Thrombin-soaked absorbable gelatin pads are sometimes used for hemostasis around the coronary anastomoses and can compress the coronary ostia, as can adjacent thrombi. Surgical reexploration is indicated and likely to be immediately therapeutic.

LV dilation can initiate and exacerbate myocardial ischemia in patients following an ASO. Myocardial ischemia, afterload mismatch, or overzealous volume infusion can result in LV distension and LA hypertension. This is more likely if there is mitral insufficiency from either papillary muscle dysfunction or dilation of the mitral valve annulus. LV distension can result in stretching or kinking of the coronary reanastomoses, causing a cycle of worsening myocardial ischemia and LV dilation. LA hypertension produces elevations in PA pressure and distension of the PA and can compress or place tension on the coronary ostia because the LeCompte maneuver brings the distal PA anterior to the ascending aorta. The resulting myocardial ischemia produces further LV dilation, progressive elevations in LA and PA pressures, and continuing compromise of coronary blood flow. Attempts to induce coronary vasodilation with nitroglycerin are unlikely to be beneficial in this setting, although reduction in preload and afterload can be beneficial. Afterload reduction with milrinone might also be helpful.

Kussman BD, McGowan FX, Powell AJ, DiNardo JA. Anesthesia for congenital heart surgery. In: Davis PJ, Cladis FP, eds. *Smith's Anesthesia for Infants and Children*. 10th ed. Elsevier; 2022:732-831.

D.2. What immediate postoperative problems would be anticipated following the Rastelli procedure?

Right (pulmonary) ventricular dysfunction related to the ventriculotomy used to close the VSD and create the new pulmonary outflow tract can occur, as can heart block, given the proximity of the VSD to the intraventricular conduction pathways. A residual VSD following repair is possible, as is LV outflow tract obstruction around the tunnel used to create LV and aortic continuity.

Kreutzer C, De Vive J, Oppido G, et al. Twenty-five-year experience with Rastelli repair for transposition of the great arteries. *J Thorac Cardiovasc Surg*. 2000;120:211-223.

Kussman BD, McGowan FX, Powell AJ, DiNardo JA. Anesthesia for congenital heart surgery. In: Davis PJ, Cladis FP, eds. *Smith's Anesthesia for Infants and Children*. 10th ed. Elsevier; 2022:732-831.

D.3. What intermediate- and long-term surgical problems are seen after ASO?

Supravalvular pulmonary stenosis is the most common complication of ASO. This is usually caused by retraction of the tissue used to repair the PA in the area of the explanted coronaries, but in most patients is not extensive enough to result in valvular pulmonary stenosis. Series with long-term follow-up (15 years) confirm that the incidence of supravalvular stenosis severe enough to require reoperation (generally a gradient >50-60 mm Hg) is approximately 4% to 8%.

The second most common complication of ASO is aortic insufficiency, which occurs in approximately 10% to 15% of patients at long-term follow-up, with the majority (96%) graded as trivial or mild. This is a rare source of morbidity or indication for reoperation following the ASO.

Early concerns for the long-term patency and growth potential of the reimplanted coronary arteries following the ASO have not materialized on a large scale.

Kussman BD, McGowan FX, Powell AJ, DiNardo JA. Anesthesia for congenital heart surgery. In: Davis PJ, Cladis FP, eds. *Smith's Anesthesia for Infants and Children*. 10th ed. Elsevier; 2022:732-831.

Villafañe J, Lantin-Hermoso MR, Bhatt AB, et al. D-transposition of the great arteries: the current era of the arterial switch operation. *J Am Coll Cardiol*. 2014;64:498-511.

D.4. What are the long-term outcomes after ASO?

Actuarial survival in experienced centers at 1 year is 90% for patients with D-TGA and intact ventricular septum and 83% for patients with D-TGA and VSD. A review of 470 patients from one institution experienced in the ASO revealed a 1-year survival of 92% and an 8-year survival of 91% for patients with both D-TGA and intact ventricular septum and D-TGA and VSD. A similar review of 1,200 patients from another experienced institution revealed a 1- and 15-year survival of 92% for patients with D-TGA and intact ventricular septum, and 1- and 15-year survival of 81% and 80% for D-TGA and VSD, respectively. A recent multi-institution review of 631 patients with D-TGA and 167 patients with D-TGA and VSD revealed similar initial and long-term (15-year) outcomes. Freedom from adverse cardiovascular events has recently been shown to be 93% at 25 years.

A recent single-center retrospective study of 844 patients with biventricular circulation who underwent an ASO showed excellent late survival and functional status after 25 years. Freedom from overall reintervention was 77%, freedom from reoperation on the neoaortic root valve was 92%, freedom from coronary reoperation was 99%, and LV function was normal in 98% of patients, but clinically significant aortic regurgitation (AR) with the need for neoaortic valve replacement occurred in 15% of survivors after 25 years.

In all, 90% to 97% of patients with D-TGA have normal-sized, patent coronary arteries as assessed by coronary angiography. A recent study of a large cohort demonstrated that survival without coronary events (death from myocardial infarction, sudden death, and reoperation for coronary stenosis) is 92.7% at 1 year and 88.2% at 15 years. The incidence of coronary events is bimodal with a high early and low late event rate. Eighty-nine percent of all coronary events occurred in the first 3 months after ASO. The event rate did not increase again until 6 years after ASO. Abnormal coronary, specifically a single coronary artery origin or two coronaries originating close to each other at a facing commissure were risk factors for a coronary event.

One of the potential advantages of the ASO over the atrial switch procedure is the use of the native LV as the systemic ventricle. Long-term follow-up indicates that patients who have undergone an ASO have higher systemic ventricular ejection fractions than do patients who have undergone atrial switch procedures. In fact, patients who had D-TGA and intact ventricular septum repaired in infancy and patients who had D-TGA and VSD repaired later have LV end-diastolic dimensions and contractile indices similar to infants born with structurally normal hearts. Myocardial contractility in patients having undergone a rapid or traditional two-stage arterial switch is mildly depressed as compared to patients having undergone a primary arterial switch. No progression of this ventricular dysfunction has been noted at either intermediate- or long-term follow-up.

Fricke TA, Buratto E, Weintraub RG, et al. Long-term outcomes of the arterial switch operation. *J Thorac Cardiovasc Surg*. 2022;163:212-219.

Khairy P, Clair M, Fernandes SM, et al. Cardiovascular outcomes after the arterial switch operation for D-transposition of the great arteries. *Circulation*. 2013;127:331-339.

Kussman BD, McGowan FX, Powell AJ, DiNardo JA. Anesthesia for congenital heart surgery. In: Davis PJ, Cladis FP, eds. *Smith's Anesthesia for Infants and Children*. 10th ed. Elsevier; 2022:732-831.

Villafañe J, Lantin-Hermoso MR, Bhatt AB, et al. D-transposition of the great arteries: the current era of the arterial switch operation. *J Am Coll Cardiol*. 2014;64:498-511.

D.5. What are the long-term outcomes after Rastelli repair for patients with D-TGA with left ventricular outflow tract (LVOT) obstruction?

The outcome following the Rastelli procedure for TGA with VSD and LVOT obstruction is good, with a near 100% early survival rate. A recent series reports survival to be 93% at 5, 10, and 20 years. The need for reintervention (either surgical or catheterization) increases over time. Intervention to relieve RVOT (RV to PA conduit) obstruction accounts for 75% of all interventions, with pacemaker insertion and relief of LVOT obstruction (aortic outflow) accounting for most of the remaining interventions. In an effort to reduce the need to intervene again for LVOT obstruction associated with the Rastelli procedure, some institutions are making greater use of the LeCompte and Nikaidoh procedures.

Brown JW, Ruzmetov M, Huynh D, et al. Rastelli operation for transposition of the great arteries with ventricular septal defect and pulmonary stenosis. *Ann Thorac Surg*. 2011;91:188-194.

Emani SM, Beroukhim R, Zurakowski D, et al. Outcomes after anatomic repair for d-transposition of the great arteries with left ventricular outflow tract obstruction. *Circulation*. 2009;120:S53-S58.

Hazekamp MG, Gomez AA, Koolbergen DR, et al. Surgery for transposition of the great arteries, ventricular septal defect and left ventricular outflow tract obstruction: European Congenital Heart Surgeons Association multicentre study. *Eur J Cardiothorac Surg*. 2010;38:699-706.

D.6. What is the long-term neurologic outcome like after ASO?

The best assessment of neurologic outcome following ASO is from the Boston Circulatory Arrest Trial. In this trial, 171 infants undergoing ASO for D-TGA with intact ventricular septum or VSD were randomized to either DHCA or low-flow CPB using α-stat pH management. Infants in the DHCA group underwent an average of 52 minutes of DHCA, whereas those in the low-flow CPB group underwent 14 minutes of DHCA.

Children in this cohort had overall physical and psychosocial health status similar to the general population. However, at age 8 years, parents of children in both groups reported more problems with attention, learning, speech, and developmental delay than parents of children in a normative sample. There was no association between physical and psychosocial scores and the presence or absence of a VSD or the use of low-flow CPB versus DHCA. Neurodevelopmental outcome in this cohort was generally not adversely affected unless the duration of DHCA exceeded 41 minutes. Beyond 41 minutes, there was a nonlinear (steadily worsening) outcome with increasing duration of DHCA.

Eight-year and 16-year data from the trial also demonstrated that neurologic status, IQ, academic achievement, memory, problem-solving, and visual-motor integration did not differ between the DHCA and low-flow CPB groups. Nonetheless, DHCA was associated with greater functional deficiencies in motor function, visual-motor tracking, phonic awareness, and speech apraxia, whereas patients in the low-flow CPB exhibited more impulsive behavior and worse behavior in school as rated by teachers.

Marelli A, Miller SP, Marino BS, et al. Brain in congenital heart disease across the lifespan: the cumulative burden of injury. *Circulation*. 2016;133:1951-1962.

Mebius MJ, Kooi EMW, Bilardo CM, et al. Brain injury and neurodevelopmental outcome in congenital heart disease: a systematic review. *Pediatrics*. 2017;140:e20164055.

40

Pyloric Stenosis

Aarti Sharma and Roshan Patel

A 3-week-old first-born male infant had projectile vomiting, which contained the ingested formula but no bile. His body weight was 2.5 kg; serum electrolytes were: K^+, 2.2 mM; Cl^-, 86 mM; and venous [?] blood pH, 7.68. This infant was also noted to have a systolic murmur heard best at the second intercostal space along the left sternal border, which was assessed by a cardiologist and diagnosed as a ventricular septal defect (VSD).

A. Medical Disease and Differential Diagnosis

1. What is the diagnosis in this patient?
2. What is the differential diagnosis of pyloric stenosis?
3. What are the metabolic problems in this newborn secondary to his disease?
4. What are the adverse effects of metabolic alkalosis?
5. How would you treat this infant?
6. How would you determine fluid replacement in a newborn, and what fluids would you use?
7. How would you correct the metabolic alkalosis?
8. What causes a cardiac murmur?

B. Preoperative Evaluation and Preparation

1. How would you evaluate this patient preoperatively?
2. How would you evaluate a heart murmur?
3. How would you differentiate between functional and pathologic murmur?
4. What are the types of VSD? What type of shunt do they cause?
5. What are the risks of surgery and anesthesia in a patient with VSD?
6. How would you prepare this patient rapidly for emergency surgery? Is surgical intervention an acute emergency in this case?
7. How would you prepare this patient for anesthesia?

C. Intraoperative Management

1. What induction-intubation sequence would you use?
2. What are the anatomic characteristics of the airway in the newborn and how do they differ from those in the adult?
3. How do you determine the size of a tracheal tube in a pediatric patient?
4. What anesthesia system would you use and why?
5. What are the advantages and the disadvantages of commonly employed nonrebreathing systems?
6. How would you monitor this patient intraoperatively?
7. What factors affect the measurement of oxygen saturation by pulse oximetry?
8. What are some of the pain management considerations in this patient?

D. Postoperative Management

1. What are the complications that can occur in the postanesthesia recovery period?
2. How would you treat postextubation "croup" in this infant?

A. Medical Disease and Differential Diagnosis

A.1. What is the diagnosis in this patient?

The most likely diagnosis in this patient is pyloric stenosis. The factors that favor the diagnosis are:

- Age of 3 weeks (average age at onset; range 5 days to 5 months)
- Boy (boy-to-girl ratio = 4:1)
- Projectile vomiting (characteristic)
- Vomitus consisting of ingested formula with no bile

The resultant biochemical abnormalities in this patient are hypokalemia, hypochloremia, metabolic alkalosis.

Pyloric stenosis occurs in 3 of 1,000 infants born in the United States; its incidence might be increasing. It is more common in Whites of Northern European ancestry, less common in Blacks, and rare in Asians. Reduced nitric oxide in pyloric tissue might contribute to the pathogenesis of pyloric stenosis.

Singh A, Liacouras CS. Pyloric Stenosis and Other Congenital Anomalies of the Stomach. In: Kliegman RM, St. Geme JW, Blum NJ, et al. eds. *Nelson Textbook of Pediatrics*. 22nd ed. Elsevier; 2025.

A.2. What is the differential diagnosis of pyloric stenosis?

Pyloric stenosis can be distinguished from other congenital anomalies that cause obstruction of the alimentary tract in the newborn. The other anomalies include achalasia of the esophagus, hiatal hernia, duodenal atresia, jejunal atresia, ileal atresia, pancreatic annulus, malrotation of the gut, intra-abdominal hernias, and Meckel diverticulum. Pathognomonic features of pyloric stenosis include absence of bile staining of the vomitus and visible gastric peristaltic waves on abdominal examination along with palpable pyloric mass. The diagnosis is commonly made clinically. An "olive" is sometimes palpated in the epigastrium just to the right of the midline. The diagnosis can be confirmed by abdominal ultrasound. Occasionally, an upper gastrointestinal (GI) series with barium is necessary.

Singh A, Liacouras CS. Pyloric Stenosis and Other Congenital Anomalies of the Stomach. In: Kliegman RM, St. Geme JW, Blum NJ, et al. eds. *Nelson Textbook of Pediatrics*. 22nd ed. Elsevier; 2025.

A.3. What are the metabolic problems in this newborn secondary to his disease?

Metabolic changes secondary to protracted vomiting characteristically include hypokalemic, hypochloremic alkalosis, as evident in this infant. Hyponatremia, although present, might not be manifested in serum value determinations because of severe dehydration. Compensatory respiratory acidosis is a frequent finding; this results from hypoventilation that can be marked and associated with periods of apnea. In severe dehydration leading to circulatory shock, the lack of adequate perfusion coupled with impaired renal and hepatic function can produce an entirely different picture of metabolic acidosis with hyperventilation, resulting in respiratory alkalosis. Therefore, depending on the severity and duration of vomiting and the type of fluid replenishment, one can encounter wide variations in arterial blood gas and electrolyte determinations. However, the most frequent findings are hypokalemia, hyponatremia, hypochloremia, and primary metabolic alkalosis with secondary respiratory acidosis. The renal response to vomiting is 2-fold. Initially, serum pH is maintained by excretion of alkaline urine with sodium and potassium loss. Then, after the depletion of these electrolytes, the kidneys secrete acidic urine (paradoxical acidosis), which exacerbates the metabolic alkalosis. These findings are summarized in **Table 40.1**.

Singh A, Liacouras CS. Pyloric Stenosis and Other Congenital Anomalies of the Stomach. In: Kliegman RM, St. Geme JW, Blum NJ, et al. eds. *Nelson Textbook of Pediatrics*. 22nd ed. Elsevier; 2025.

Whitaker EE, Williams RK, Lauro HV, Chaudhry R, Davis PJ. Anesthesia for General Abdominal, Urologic Surgery. In: Davis PJ, Cladis FP, eds. *Smith's Anesthesia for Infants and Children*. 10th ed. Elsevier; 2022:885-916.e7.

SECTION 10

TABLE 40.1 Metabolic Findings in the Newborn Secondary to Pyloric Stenosis

	Arterial Blood Gases				Serum Electrolytes			
Severity of Dehydration	**pH**	**P_{CO_2}**	**CO_2**	**P_{O_2}**	**Na^+**	**K^+**	**Cl^-**	**HCO_3^-**
Mild	↑	↑	↑	↔	↓↔	↓	↓↓	↑
Moderate	↑↑	↑↑	↑↑	↔	↓	↓↓	↓↓↓	↑↑
Severe	↓↓	↓	↓↓	↓	↓	↓↓	↓↓↓	↓↓

↔, no change; ↑/↓, slight change; ↑↑/↓↓, moderate change; ↑↑↑/↓↓↓, marked change.

A.4. What are the adverse effects of metabolic alkalosis?

An increase in pH results in a shift of the hemoglobin oxygen-dissociation curve to the left, leading to tighter binding of oxygen to hemoglobin and reduced offloading of oxygen at the tissue level. This phenomenon assumes even more importance in newborns because, at 3 weeks, they still have up to 70% fetal hemoglobin with an already low P50 (ie, 20-22 mm Hg).

Respiratory compensation is affected by hypoventilation with increased potential for atelectasis as well as periods of apnea.

There is also a reduction in ionized calcium, and an increased potential for seizures.

Singh A, Liacouras CS. Pyloric stenosis and other congenital anomalies of the stomach. In: Kliegman RM, St. Geme JW, Blum NJ, et al. eds. *Nelson Textbook of Pediatrics*. 22nd ed. Elsevier; 2025.

A.5. How would you treat this infant?

Medical management of pyloric stenosis is acutely urgent. The principles of management can be grouped under the following three categories: supportive therapy to stabilize the patient, diagnostic tests to confirm the diagnosis and monitor therapy, and surgery as the corrective therapy.

Supportive Therapy

- Circulatory support
- Correction of electrolyte imbalance
- Prevention of aspiration

Fluids

Infants with pyloric stenosis are hypovolemic and dehydrated secondary to persistent vomiting. Dehydration severity can vary from mild hypovolemia to circulatory shock. The following parameters are good indicators of dehydration severity:

- Physical appearance—skin turgor, parched mucous membranes, sunken fontanels, sunken eyeballs
- Blood pressure—decreased
- Pulse rate—increased
- Urine output—decreased
- Weight loss (birth to present)

Quantitative assessment of these parameters gives a fair estimate of the amount of total body fluid depletion. A wide-bore intravenous (IV) cannula should be placed and an infusion should be started immediately to correct the deficits and provide maintenance fluids.

Electrolytes

The patient is alkalotic, hypokalemic, hypochloremic, and hyponatremic and must be provided with necessary ions to replenish this deficit. Albumin or Ringer lactate can be used to first treat the shock. Next, the deficit should be corrected with 0.45% to 0.9% saline in 5% to 10% dextrose (D-glucose). Potassium (usually 40 mEq/L) must be added to this to correct hypokalemia and aid in the correction of alkalosis. However, potassium infusion should be withheld until satisfactory renal function is established. Fluid therapy should be continued until the infant is rehydrated and serum bicarbonate concentration is less than 30 mM, which implies that the alkalosis has been corrected.

Prevention of Aspiration

A nasogastric tube should be inserted to thoroughly empty the stomach, and the upper airway reflexes should be preserved.

Diagnostic Tests

To assess the severity of fluid and electrolyte derangement and to monitor therapy, the following should be evaluated: complete blood count, serum electrolytes, arterial blood gases, blood urea nitrogen (BUN), electrocardiogram (ECG) (for marked hypokalemia).

To confirm the diagnosis: barium swallow, ultrasound imaging

Surgery

Pyloromyotomy is the definitive treatment for these infants. Ramstedt pyloromyotomy through a right upper quadrant transverse incision has been the traditional treatment for hypertrophic pyloric stenosis. Recently, laparoscopic and circumumbilical approaches have been introduced as alternative methods to improve cosmesis, but concerns about greater operative times, costs, and complications remain. Surgery should be carried out early but only after the patient has been stabilized satisfactorily.

Schwartz MZ. Hypertrophic pyloric stenosis. In: Coran AG, Caldamone A, Adzick NS, Krummel TM, Laberge JM, Shamberger R, eds. *Pediatric Surgery*. 7th ed. Elsevier Saunders; 2012:1021-1028.

Singh A, Liacouras CS. Pyloric stenosis and other congenital anomalies of the stomach. In: Kliegman RM, St. Geme JW, Blum NJ, et al. eds. *Nelson Textbook of Pediatrics*. 22nd ed. Elsevier; 2025.

A.6. How would you determine fluid replacement in a newborn, and what fluids would you use?

The general principles of fluid therapy are based on fluid maintenance, correction of deficits, and replacement of losses.

Maintenance Fluids

In the newborn, maintenance fluids are:

- First 48 hours of life—75 mL/kg/d or 3 mL/kg/h
- 2 days to 1 month—150 mL/kg/d or 6 mL/kg/h
- 1 month onward (up to 10 kg)—100 mL/kg/d or 4 mL/kg/h

Estimation of the degree of dehydration in a newborn is shown in **Table 40.2**.

Maintenance fluids take into account the fluid losses occurring normally via the kidneys, bowel, skin, and lungs. At birth, the kidneys are still undergoing maturation, and what may be called "a glomerular imbalance" exists. What it implies is that some mature glomeruli can be connected to the immature tubules and *vice versa*. Hence, the kidney is functionally limited at birth but undergoes rapid maturation during the first week of life.

Electrolytes

The newborn is an obligate sodium loser and does not tolerate excessive sodium overload. Maintenance electrolytes are:

- Sodium—3 to 5 mEq/kg/d
- Potassium—2 to 3 mEq/kg/d
- Chloride—1 to 3 mEq/kg/d

Correction of Deficits

Deficits take into account previous unreplaced losses because of a period of no intake by mouth and dehydration resulting from increased losses (eg, from vomiting, diarrhea, and increased body temperature). The magnitude of the deficit can be assessed by physical examination (**Table 40.2**), change in body weight, and hematocrit.

Replacement of Losses

Replacing losses covers ongoing abnormal losses not covered by maintenance fluids. Intraoperatively, it covers evaporative losses from the operative site, "third spacing" or extravascular compartments, and losses from the lungs if dry gases are used in nonrebreathing circuits (**Table 40.3**).

The younger and more physically immature the patient, the greater the skin permeability, the ratio of body surface area to weight, and the metabolic demand. In addition, the use of radiant warmers and phototherapy increases insensible water loss.

Vutskits L, Davidson A, Soriano SG. Pediatric anesthesia. In: Gropper MA, Cohen NH, Eriksson LI, Fleisher LA, Johnson-Akeju S, Leslie K, eds. *Miller's Anesthesia*. 10th ed. Elsevier; 2025:2266-2299.e7.

A.7. How would you correct the metabolic alkalosis?

To correct the metabolic alkalosis in this patient, the underlying electrolyte derangements (hyponatremia, hypokalemia, and hypochloremia) must be corrected. Correct the deficits by using calculated volumes of 5% dextrose in normal saline or Ringer lactate solution, which helps to restore sodium and chloride. Dextrose, 5%, with one-fourth strength normal saline can be used to provide maintenance fluids. Once renal function is established, potassium supplements are added to the infusion. Depending on the deficit,

SECTION 10

TABLE 40.2 Estimation of the Degree of Dehydration in a Newborn

	Mild	Moderate	Severe
Percentage fluid loss	5	10	15-20
Skin turgor	Poor	Very poor	Flaccid
Mucous membrane and tongue	Dry	Dry	Parched
Fontanel and eyes	Normal	Sunken fontanel	Sunken eyes
Urine	Concentrated oliguria	Oliguria	Oliguria, anuria
Pulse	Normal	Tachycardia	Marked tachycardia, weak
Blood pressure	Normal	Hypotension	Marked hypotension, shock

TABLE 40.3 Fluid Requirement to Replace Intraoperative Fluid Losses (Except Blood Loss) in the Newborn

	Fluid Replacement (mL/kg/h)
Minor surgery (eg, herniorrhaphy)	1-3
Moderate surgery (eg, pyloromyotomy)	3-5
Major surgery (eg, intestinal)	5-7
Respiratory water loss due to dry gases	2

this therapy can require from 12 to 72 hours. In patients with severe alkalosis, HCl (hydrochloric acid) and NH_4Cl (ammonium chloride) have been used to correct the derangement. However, this is rarely necessary.

Archibald T, Peramunage DS, Barnes CR. Acid–base, fluids, and electrolytes. In: Cullen BF, Stock MC, Ortega R, et al, eds. *Barash, Cullen, and Stoelting's Clinical Anesthesia*. 9th ed. Wolters Kluwer; 2024:362-397.

Mukkamala SG, Long JB. Neonatal anesthesia. In: Cullen BF, Stock MC, Ortega R, et al, eds. *Barash, Cullen, and Stoelting's Clinical Anesthesia*. 9th ed. Wolters Kluwer; 2024:1143-1182.

Stafford-Smith M, Pollak AL, Kuhn CM, Privratsky JR. The renal system and anesthesia for urologic surgery. In: Cullen BF, Stock MC, Ortega R, et al, eds. *Barash, Cullen, and Stoelting's Clinical Anesthesia*. 9th ed. Wolters Kluwer; 2024:1349-1389.

A.8. What causes a cardiac murmur?

Cardiac murmurs are caused by turbulent blood flow across cardiac valves or septal defects, and are audible sound waves in the range of 20 to 2,000 Hz. Most murmurs in pediatric patients are normal or innocent occurring in approximately 50% of all school-age children, but these must be distinguished from murmurs associated with significant structural heart disease. Auscultation is critically important in diagnosing these murmurs; however, echocardiography remains the gold standard.

Driscoll D. History and physical evaluation. In: Shaddy RE, Penny DJ, Feltes TF, et al, eds. *Moss & Adams' Heart Disease in infants, Children, and Adolescents: Including the Fetus and Young Adult*. 10th ed. Wolters Kluwer; 2022:243-250.

B. Preoperative Evaluation and Preparation

B.1. How would you evaluate this patient preoperatively?

The following information is necessary in evaluating this patient:

History

Onset of illness, frequency and amount of vomiting, last feeding, diarrhea, urine output, activity of the newborn (active or lethargic), and birth weight

Physical Examination

Present and birth body weight (to determine weight loss), temperature, signs of dehydration (skin turgor, mucous membranes, fontanels, eyeballs, blood pressure, pulse, color, and volume of urine), muscle tone, and level of consciousness

Laboratory Findings

Complete blood count, electrolytes, BUN and blood sugar, urinalysis, and arterial blood gases. Based on the available data, one can determine the fluid and electrolyte status of the patient and correct these accordingly to stabilize the patient for surgery and anesthesia.

B.2. How would you evaluate a heart murmur?

Heart murmurs can be innocent or due to structural heart disease. By definition, innocent murmurs occur in the absence of structural or physiologic cardiac disease. The clinical diagnosis of a normal or innocent murmur should occur in the setting of an otherwise normal history, physical examination, and appearance. The presence of a family history of hypertrophic cardiomyopathy, congenital cardiac disease, or unexplained infant, childhood, or early adult death is particularly worrisome. The perinatal history of prematurity, maternal diabetes mellitus, drug or toxin ingestion, fetal distress, or clearly definable chromosomal disorders has particular cardiorespiratory relevance.

The initial approach to the evaluation of the cardiovascular system should include assessment of cardiorespiratory system function as a pump and delivery system. An index of exercise or play capacity should be sought as a component of assessing growth and development. History should include exercise tolerance, shortness of breath, cyanotic episodes, growth (because congestive heart failure can manifest as failure to thrive), and symptoms of congestive heart failure.

Driscoll D. History and physical evaluation. In: Shaddy RE, Penny DJ, Feltes TF, et al, eds. *Moss & Adams' Heart Disease in infants, Children, and Adolescents: Including the Fetus and Young Adult*. 10th ed. Wolters Kluwer; 2022:243-250.

B.3. How would you differentiate between functional and pathologic murmur?

Normal murmurs of childhood are composed of five systolic and two continuous types but never solely diastolic (**Table 40.4**). A functional murmur is usually soft, 1/6 or 2/6, and never associated with palpable thrill. Pathologic murmurs are usually louder, 3/6 or greater, and are associated with other pathologic cardiovascular features.

Park MK, Salamat M. Physical Examination. In: Park MK, Salamat M, eds. *Park's Pediatric Cardiology for Practitioners*. 7th ed. Elsevier; 2021:6-30.

B.4. What are the types of VSD? What type of shunt do they cause?

A common classification of VSD is based on anatomic location.

- Type I defects or supracristal defects (5% of all VSDs) are outflow defects located above the crista supraventricularis just under the annulus of the aorta.
- Type II defects or infracristal defects (80% of all VSDs) are lower in membranous septum beneath the crista supraventricularis.
- Type III defects or canal type (11% incidence) are inlet VSDs that accompany complete atrioventricular (AV) canal defects. They result from failure of the endocardial cushions to fuse.
- Type IV or muscular defects (2%-7% incidence) probably result from excessive resorption of septal tissue during the muscular septal formation. They can be located anywhere in the muscular septum and can be multiple (also known as the Swiss cheese defect).

Pathophysiologic effects of VSD include left-to-right shunting, pulmonary hypertension, and heart failure resulting from volume overload.

Cohen MS, Lopez L. Ventricular septal defects. In: Shaddy RE, Penny DJ, Feltes TF, et al, eds. *Moss & Adams' Heart Disease in infants, Children, and Adolescents: Including the Fetus and Young Adult*. 10th ed. Wolters Kluwer; 2022:746-763.

B.5. What are the risks of surgery and anesthesia in a patient with VSD?

Infective endocarditis is a complication of most congenital cardiac anomalies, so the patient requires antibiotic prophylaxis. There is also risk of increasing the shunt flow or reversing the flow of the shunt, resulting from decreases in pulmonary vascular resistance causing hypoxemia and congestive heart failure or acute and persistent increases in systemic vascular resistance. Right ventricular infundibular hypertrophy can be present with a VSD. Normally, this is a beneficial change because it increases the resistance to right ventricular ejection, leading to decrease in magnitude of the left-to-right shunt (see Chapter 39: Transposition of the Great Arteries). Nevertheless, perioperative events that exaggerate this obstruction to right ventricular outflow, such as increased myocardial contractility or hypovolemia, must be minimized. Therefore, these patients are often anesthetized with a volatile anesthetic to take advantage of their negative inotropic properties. Intravascular fluid volume should be maintained by prompt replacement of blood loss. Normal end-tidal carbon dioxide (CO_2) should be maintained and precautions against introduction of intravascular air bubbles should be taken.

TABLE 40.4 Innocent Murmurs of Childhood

Systolic Murmurs	Continuous Murmurs
Vibratory still murmur	Venous hum
Pulmonary flow murmur	Mammary arterial souffle
Peripheral pulmonary artery stenosis murmur	
Supraclavicular systolic murmur	
Aortic systolic murmur	

Diu MW, Walker KK. Pediatric diseases. In: Hines RL, Jones SB, eds. *Stoelting's Anesthesia and Co-Existing Disease*. 8th ed. Elsevier; 2022:663-696.

Steppan J, Wadia RS. Congenital heart disease. In: Hines RL, Jones SB, eds. *Stoelting's Anesthesia and Co-Existing Disease*. 8th ed. Elsevier; 2022:135-154.

B.6. How would you prepare this patient rapidly for emergency surgery? Is surgical intervention an acute emergency in this case?

Hypertrophic pyloric stenosis is a medical emergency and not a surgical emergency. Therefore, no newborn should be subjected to the additional risks of anesthesia and surgery until stabilized medically.

Singh A, Liacouras CS. Pyloric stenosis and other congenital anomalies of the stomach. In: Kliegman RM, St. Geme JW, Blum NJ, et al. eds. *Nelson Textbook of Pediatrics*. 22nd ed. Elsevier; 2025.

B.7. How would you prepare this patient for anesthesia?

Fluid and electrolyte replacement should be accomplished satisfactorily, which can take from 12 to 72 hours depending on severity. The next step is to empty the stomach through a wide-bore nasogastric tube, lavaging the gastric contents and any leftover barium. Alternatively, an orogastric approach allows for passage of a tube with wider lumen that ensures better stomach emptying. Premedication is usually atropine (0.01-0.02 mg/kg) IV or intramuscular if the patient does not have IV catheter (unlikely in this case).

Whitaker EE, Williams RK, Lauro HV, Chaudhry R, Davis PJ. Anesthesia for general abdominal, urologic surgery. In: Davis PJ, Cladis FP, eds. *Smith's Anesthesia for Infants and Children*. 10th ed. Elsevier; 2022:885-916.e7.

C. Intraoperative Management

C.1. What induction-intubation sequence would you use?

The patient should arrive to the operating room with IV access. Standard monitors are placed. The stomach is emptied by inserting an orogastric tube (atropine can be used as premedication) to reduce the chance of regurgitation during induction. Because the stomach might not be completely emptied, a rapid sequence induction and intubation with cricoid pressure is highly recommended to minimize the risk of aspiration. Awake intubation can be accomplished in skillful hands in a lethargic neonate or in a critically sick infant. In most cases, however, neonates presenting for this procedure are fit and do not require awake intubation, which can be more traumatic.

Whitaker EE, Williams RK, Lauro HV, Chaudhry R, Davis PJ. Anesthesia for general abdominal, urologic surgery. In: Davis PJ, Cladis FP, eds. *Smith's Anesthesia for Infants and Children*. 10th ed. Elsevier; 2022:885-916.e7.

Jöhr M. Anesthesia for the child with full stomach. *Curr Opin Anaesthesiol*. 2007;20:201-203.

C.2. What are the anatomic characteristics of the airway in the newborn and how do they differ from those in the adult?

The special characteristics of the upper airway in the newborn are:

- Nasopharynx—narrow nasal passages, obligate nasal breathers
- Oropharynx—large tongue, long and pendulous epiglottis
- Larynx—the distinctive features are shown in **Table 40.5**

TABLE 40.5 Comparative Anatomy of the Larynx and Trachea in the Newborn and the Adult

Anatomic Features	Newborn	Adult
Size	4 cm	10-13 cm
Shape	Funnel	Cylindrical
Position of the glottis	C3-C4	C6
Narrowest point	1 cm below vocal cords	At vocal cords
Vocal cords	Slanting anteriorly	Transverse or slightly Slanting posteriorly
Mucous membranes	Loose (swells easily)	More firm

Newborns, who have low respiratory reserve, can develop airway obstruction easily. The infant can present problems during intubation and tolerate airway trauma poorly.

Comparative anatomy of the larynx and trachea in the newborn and the adult is shown in **Table 40.5**.

Kovatsis PG, Peyton J, Cooper EB, Davis PJ. Normal and difficult airway management. In: Davis PJ, Cladis FP, eds. *Smith's Anesthesia for Infants and Children*. 10th ed. Elsevier; 2022:382-404.e4.

C.3. How do you determine the size of a tracheal tube in a pediatric patient?

The two parameters of tracheal tube sizes are the tube length and diameter, depending on the age of the child (**Table 40.6**). However, these are approximate sizes and one must have one size bigger and one size smaller available when selecting any size tube. A simple way to remember these numbers is to know the sizes for a newborn, 6 months, and 1 year. Between 2 and 12 years, the following guide can be used:

- Tube length from tip to incisor teeth (cm) = 11 + age in years
- Tube internal diameter (mm) = 4 + age/4
- French size (French) = 18 + age
- External circumference (French) = ID (mm) × 4 + 2

French size means external circumference (mm), or π (3.14) times external diameter.

Kovatsis PG, Peyton J, Cooper EB, Davis PJ. Normal and difficult airway management. In: Davis PJ, Cladis FP, eds. *Smith's Anesthesia for Infants and Children*. 10th ed. Elsevier; 2022:382-404.e4.

C.4. What anesthesia system would you use and why?

A circle system with a light circuit is typical. A circle system is advantageous because it maintains heat and humidification better and offers the freedom of choosing varying gas flows. The controversy about the increased resistance in the adult system is reduced since respiration is assisted or controlled intraoperatively. Newer anesthesia machines use valves with less resistance than older models. Dead space in these systems is no more than that of Mapleson circuits.

Dorsch JA, Dorsch SE, eds. Breathing systems. In: *A Practical Approach to Anesthesia Equipment*. Lippincott Williams & Wilkins; 2011:109-162.

C.5. What are the advantages and the disadvantages of commonly employed nonrebreathing systems?

Commonly used nonrebreathing systems include the Bain breathing circuit (Mapleson D system) and Jackson-Rees modification of Ayre's T-piece. They offer the following advantages and disadvantages:

Advantages

- Minimal dead space
- No valves, low resistance
- Lightweight
- Reservoir bag to assist ventilation
- Good appreciation of respiratory exchange

Disadvantages

- High flow of fresh gases is required.
- Low flows can allow rebreathing of gases without CO_2 absorption.

TABLE 40.6 Tracheal Tube Size for Pediatric Patient

Age	Length	Internal Diameter (mm)	French Size
Newborn	10	3.0	14
6 mo	12	3.5	16
1 y	14	4.0	18
2 y	15	4.5	20
4 y	16	5.0	22
6 y	17	5.5	24
8 y	18	6.0	26
10 y	19	6.5	28
12 y	20	7.0	30

- Loss of heat and humidity because of high flow of cold, dry gases (Bain circuit allows some heating of inspired gases by surrounding fresh gas flow tubing with expired gas tubing).
- Scavenging of waste gases is a problem.

Dorsch JA, Dorsch SE, eds. Breathing systems. In: *A Practical Approach to Anesthesia Equipment*. Lippincott Williams & Wilkins; 2011:109-162.

C.6. How would you monitor this patient intraoperatively?

Monitoring should include blood pressure, ECG, central temperature, pulse oximetry, and end-tidal CO_2. Patients with known significant cardiac history might warrant invasive hemodynamic monitoring with arterial line placement.

C.7. What factors affect the measurement of oxygen saturation by pulse oximetry?

Dysfunctional hemoglobin, such as carboxyhemoglobin, sulfhemoglobin, and methemoglobin, can affect the accuracy of oximetry. Intravascular dyes, such as indocyanine green and methylene blue, can also interfere with accuracy. Skin color, tissue thickness, venous blood, light intensity, and ambient light can affect accuracy in rare cases.

Barker SJ. Pulse Oximetry. In: Ehrenwerth J, Eisenkraft JB, Berry JM, eds. *Anesthesia Equipment: Principles and Applications*. 3rd ed. Elsevier; 2021:253-270.

C.8. What are some of the pain management considerations in this patient?

Opioids, specifically with this patient population, should be used with caution. Infants who are hypoventilating from their baseline compensatory respiratory acidosis can progress to apnea. While there is regional variability in opioid use for pyloromyotomy, postoperative opioid use is associated with prolonged hospital stay. Nonopioid analgesia should strongly be considered. This can include parenteral medications such as intravenous acetaminophen, as well as regional techniques such as ultrasound-guided rectus sheath blocks or administration of local anesthetic at laparoscopic port insertion sites.

Breschan C, Jost R, Stettner H, et al. Ultrasound-guided rectus sheath block for pyloromyotomy in infants: a retrospective analysis of a case series. *Paediatr Anaesth*. 2013;23:1199.

McLaughlin C, Squillaro AI, Ourshaliman S, et al. The association between opioid use and outcomes in infants undergoing pyloromyotomy. *Clin Ther*. 2019;41:1690.

D. Postoperative Management

D.1. What are the complications that can occur in the postanesthesia recovery period?

The patient should be carefully observed for signs of respiratory depression and periods of apnea secondary to the combination of metabolic alkalosis, general anesthesia, and decreased body temperature. However, these infants do not appear to be at increased risk of postoperative apnea. Hypoventilation predisposes to atelectasis. These patients should be awake and responsive to avoid pulmonary aspiration. Severe hypoglycemia resulting from depletion of liver glycogen has been reported 2 to 3 hours after surgery. Postextubation "croup" is a potentially dangerous complication in this age group.

Whitaker EE, Williams RK, Lauro HV, Chaudhry R, Davis PJ. Anesthesia for general abdominal, urologic surgery. In: Davis PJ, Cladis FP, eds. *Smith's Anesthesia for Infants and Children*. 10th ed. Elsevier; 2022:885-916.e7.

D.2. How would you treat postextubation "croup" in this infant?

Treatment of potentially catastrophic postextubation laryngeal edema should be immediate, vigorous, and carried out under direct observation of the anesthesiologist. It consists of the following:

- Increasing inspired oxygen concentration (50%-60%)
- Humidification of inspired gases
- Adequate hydration using parenteral fluids
- Light sedation to calm the patient and allow for cooperation in therapy
- Avoidance of significant respiratory depression
- Epinephrine through handheld nebulizer and mask, 50 μg/kg/min of active isomer
- Racemic epinephrine (2.25%) 0.05 mL/kg diluted in 5 mL saline solution delivered over 10 minutes

Treatment should be given over 10 minutes and can be repeated every 30 minutes, as necessary. Recurrence can be expected approximately 2 hours after cessation of this therapy.

- Corticosteroids—dexamethasone, 0.5 to 1 mg/kg IV
- Reintubation—if signs of deterioration or hypoxemia appear
- Tracheostomy, if necessary—rarely, subglottic edema can be so rapid and so severe that tracheostomy is necessary.

The age group most likely to manifest this complication is 1 to 4 years. Infants younger than 1 year are at risk because of the size of their airway. Fortunately, an infant of this age is most amenable to early and vigorous intervention and should always be treated as an emergency requiring continued presence and evaluation by a physician who is adept at securing the airway for the child.

Whitaker EE, Williams RK, Lauro HV, Chaudhry R, Davis PJ. Anesthesia for general abdominal, urologic surgery. In: Davis PJ, Cladis FP, eds. *Smith's Anesthesia for Infants and Children*. 10th ed. Elsevier; 2022:885-916.e7.

41 Infectious Respiratory Disease in Infants and Children: Laryngotracheobronchitis

Miles Dinner and Albert C. Yeung

A 3-year-old boy was brought to the emergency room because of respiratory distress. He was noted to have stridor with substernal retractions and excessive drooling. He complained of a sore throat and had a fever of 39.5 °C (103.1 °F).

A. Medical Disease and Differential Diagnosis

1. Which part of the airway is affected in the croup syndrome and why?
2. What is stridor?
3. How does stridor correlate with anatomic location?
4. Define croup. What is the clinical presentation of laryngotracheitis?
5. What is the differential diagnosis of acute upper airway obstruction in children?
6. What is bacterial tracheitis?
7. What congenital problems can mimic features of croup?
8. How is the severity of croup assessed?
9. What is the medical management of croup? Does this have implications for the anesthesiologist?
10. What is epiglottitis? What are its common causes? What is the incidence?
11. What are the clinical manifestations of epiglottitis?
12. How is the diagnosis of epiglottitis made?
13. What is postextubation croup? How is it managed?
14. What are the nonacute causes of partial airway obstruction in children?
15. What are the clinical manifestations of severe COVID-19 in infants and children?
16. What is human metapneumovirus and how does it cause disease in the pediatric population?

B. Preoperative Evaluation and Preparation

1. Is tracheal intubation always required in children with epiglottitis?
2. Why is general anesthesia administered to a child with epiglottitis?
3. How would you prepare the patient for anesthesia?

C. Intraoperative Management

1. How is the airway of the child with epiglottitis best secured?
2. How would you induce general anesthesia?
3. Should a child with epiglottitis undergo a rapid sequence induction of anesthesia?
4. Is awake tracheal intubation a practical alternative to secure the patient's airway?
5. What would you do if the airway cannot be secured by tracheal intubation?
6. Should this patient have a nasotracheal or orotracheal tube placed?
7. Shortly after intubation, frothy secretions were obtained on suctioning the endotracheal tube. What is the reason for this? How can this be treated?

D. Postoperative Management

1. How long should this patient remain intubated? What criteria determine extubation time?
2. How would you make this patient comfortable during the course of intubation?
3. What outcome can one expect for a child with acute epiglottitis?

A. Medical Disease and Differential Diagnosis

A.1. Which part of the airway is affected in the croup syndrome and why?

The subglottis is typically involved in infants and children presenting with croup. The subglottis is defined as the segment of the upper airway directly below the vocal cords fusing with the upper trachea. It contains pseudostratified columnar respiratory epithelium, which is loosely adherent and prone to swelling. Because this segment is fully cartilaginized in childhood, it lacks the ability to expand and thus can produce early symptoms in response to even a small degree of inflammation.

Bruins BB, Ross PA, Kilbaugh TJ. Pediatric and neonatal critical care. In: Gropper MA, Eriksson LI, Fleisher LA, Cohen NH, Leslie K, Johnson-Akeju O, eds. *Miller's Anesthesia*. 10th ed. Elsevier; 2025:2411-2482.

Eskander A, de Almeida JR, Irish JC. Acute upper airway obstruction. *N Engl J Med*. 2019;381:1940-1949.

Murto K, Carr MM, Lerman J. Otorhinolaryngologic procedures. In: Cote CJ, Lerman J, Anderson BJ, eds. *A Practice of Anesthesia for Infants and Children*. 7th ed. Elsevier Saunders; 2024:841-899.

A.2. What is stridor?

Stridor is a high-pitched adventitious sound produced in the respiratory cycle by the turbulent flow of respiratory gases through a segmental narrowing in the airway. It can be biphasic, inspiratory, or expiratory, depending on the anatomic location.

Bruins BB, Ross PA, Kilbaugh TJ. Pediatric and neonatal critical care. In: Gropper MA, Eriksson LI, Fleisher LA, Cohen NH, Leslie K, Johnson-Akeju O, eds. *Miller's Anesthesia*. 10th ed. Elsevier; 2025:2411-2482.

Murto K, Carr MM, Lerman J. Otorhinolaryngologic procedures. In: Cote CJ, Lerman J, Anderson BJ, eds. *A Practice of Anesthesia for Infants and Children*. 7th ed. Elsevier Saunders; 2024:841-899.

A.3. How does stridor correlate with anatomic location?

Inspiratory stridor is characteristic of laryngeal or supraglottic obstruction. Conditions such as laryngeal papillomatosis, laryngeal web, laryngomalacia, and vocal cord paresis produce inspiratory stridor. Expiratory stridor is usually typical of intrathoracic processes such as extrinsic tracheal compression by a vascular ring or mass, tracheomalacia, or bronchotracheitis. Biphasic stridor is indicative of lesions or infections involving both the larynx and subglottis, such as the croup syndrome, subglottic stenosis, or intralaryngeal masses.

Murto K, Carr MM, Lerman J. Otorhinolaryngologic procedures. In: Cote CJ, Lerman J, Anderson BJ, eds. *A Practice of Anesthesia for Infants and Children*. 7th ed. Elsevier Saunders; 2024:841-899.

A.4. Define croup. What is the clinical presentation of laryngotracheitis?

Croup is the constellation of inspiratory stridor, barking cough, and possible respiratory distress due to subglottic mucosal edema. The majority of croup cases is infectious and is termed laryngotracheobronchitis for the structures involved. Spasmodic croup is considered an allergic reaction to viral antigens. Patients with spasmodic croup are afebrile, lack severe laryngeal inflammation, and are typically managed as outpatients with supportive care. Infectious croup is caused by a number of viruses, including human rhinovirus, *Haemophilus parainfluenzae* virus types 1, 2, and 3, respiratory syncytial virus, influenza virus, or human coronavirus. It commonly affects children 6 months to 3 years of age, with a median age of 18 months.

Most cases of infectious croup occur during the colder months, and there is a 1:1 male-to-female prevalence. It manifests subacutely as an exacerbation of cold symptoms with low fever, barking cough, noisy breathing, and hoarseness. Exudative inflammation of the upper airway can cause dyspnea, and in extreme cases, lead to exhaustion and frank hypoxemia. In most cases, it is self-limited and benign.

Bruins BB, Ross PA, Kilbaugh TJ. Pediatric and neonatal critical care. In: Gropper MA, Eriksson LI, Fleisher LA, Cohen NH, Leslie K, Johnson-Akeju O, eds. *Miller's Anesthesia*. 10th ed. Elsevier; 2025:2411-2482.

Florin TA, Plint AC, Zorc JJ. Viral bronchiolitis. *Lancet*. 2017;389:211-224.

Johnson DW. Croup. *BMJ Clin Evid*. 2014;2014:0321.

Murto K, Carr MM, Lerman J. Otorhinolaryngologic procedures. In: Cote CJ, Lerman J, Anderson BJ, eds. *A Practice of Anesthesia for Infants and Children*. 7th ed. Elsevier Saunders; 2024:841-899.

A.5. What is the differential diagnosis of acute upper airway obstruction in children?

A full differential for this condition involves a host of infectious causes. Among the most important are bacterial tracheitis, diphtheria (which is accompanied by the formation of a false membrane in the pharynx), retropharyngeal abscess, peritonsillar abscess, measles, and Epstein-Barr viral infection. Other causes to be considered are thermal burns, foreign body aspiration, laryngeal fractures, angioneurotic edema, vocal cord paralysis, and uvulitis.

Mandal A, Kabra SK, Lodha R. Upper airway obstruction in children. *Indian J Pediatr.* 2015;82:737-744.

Murto K, Carr MM, Lerman J. Otorhinolaryngologic procedures. In: Cote CJ, Lerman J, Anderson BJ, eds. *A Practice of Anesthesia for Infants and Children.* 7th ed. Elsevier Saunders; 2024:841-899.

A.6. What is bacterial tracheitis?

Bacterial tracheitis is a severe and potentially fatal disease of infectious nature occurring as a consequence of infection with *Staphylococcus aureus*, various streptococcal species, and *H. influenzae*. It occurs in colder weather in young children as a secondary complication of viral laryngotracheitis. Although presenting with the same symptoms as epiglottitis, it tends not to evolve as rapidly, and generally does not have odynophagia and drooling, two characteristic signs of epiglottitis. Most of these children require intubation for thick and difficult-to-clear secretions, and during endoscopy, subglottic edema with mucosal ulceration is seen.

Casazza G, Graham ME, Nelson D, Chaulk D, Sandweiss D, Meier J. Pediatric bacterial tracheitis—a variable entity: case series with literature review. *Otolaryngol Head Neck Surg.* 2019;160:546-549.

Mandal A, Kabra SK, Lodha R. Upper airway obstruction in children. *Indian J Pediatr.* 2015;82:737-744.

A.7. What congenital problems can mimic features of croup?

A host of anatomic problems can share similar signs and symptoms with the infectious agents causing airway compromise. These are distinguished from croup by the absence of fever and the chronicity of the illness. Vocal cord paralysis, vascular anomalies, laryngeal webs, laryngomalacia, subglottic masses (hemangiomas), and airway stenosis can all cause airway compromise.

Johnson DW. Croup. *BMJ Clin Evid.* 2014;2014:0321.

A.8. How is the severity of croup assessed?

The following parameters are evaluated in assessing severity of the illness: (1) Work of breathing: is there tachypnea or retractions? (2) Chest wall motion: is the tidal volume adequate with inspiration? (3) Overall appearance: is the child cyanotic, obtunded, or comfortable? (4) Vocal quality: is there stridor, diminished voice, or cry? Severe croup unresponsive to medical therapy can require tracheal intubation. Once the diagnosis of croup has been established, the child is given a croup score, which helps determine therapy (**Table 41.1**).

Johnson DW. Croup. *BMJ Clin Evid.* 2014;2014:0321.

Murto K, Carr MM, Lerman J. Otorhinolaryngologic procedures. In: Cote CJ, Lerman J, Anderson BJ, eds. *A Practice of Anesthesia for Infants and Children.* 7th ed. Elsevier Saunders; 2024:841-899.

TABLE 41.1 The Westley Croup Score

	0	1	2	3	4	5
Cyanosis	None	—	—	—	With agitation	At rest
Level of consciousness	Normal, including sleep	—	—	—	—	Disoriented
Stridor	None	With agitation	At rest	—	—	—
Air entry	Normal	Decreased	Markedly decreased	—	—	—
Retractions	None	Mild	Moderate	Severe	—	—

Mild croup has a score less than 2, moderate is between 3 and 7, and severe has a score greater than 8.

Derived from Sizar O, Carr B. Croup. In: *StatPearls* [Internet]. StatPearls Publishing; 2025. Updated July 24, 2023. https://www.ncbi.nlm.nih.gov/books/NBK431070/

A.9. What is the medical management of croup? Does this have implications for the anesthesiologist?

Most cases of croup resolve with minimal intervention and less than 10% of patients require hospitalization. Mild croup is treated with inspired gas humidification, hydration, and oxygen to improve the attendant hypoxemia. Steroids and racemic epinephrine are the main therapies.

If the patient has moderate retractions and appears dyspneic, 0.5 mL of a 2.25% racemic epinephrine solution in 2.5 mL of normal saline can be administered via nebulizer every 1 to 2 hours. Airway resistance can be high due to the presence of reactive transudation and intraluminal narrowing. By vasoconstricting the arterioles of the mucosal vasculature, racemic epinephrine relieves edema. Racemic epinephrine is a 1:1 mixture of the levo (L) and dextro (D) isomers to limit cardiac stimulation because only the L form is an active component. Patients often improve markedly within 30 minutes, but edema can recur due to epinephrine's brief duration of action. Racemic epinephrine should be avoided in children with glaucoma and ventricular outflow obstruction.

Dexamethasone and budesonide when given early in viral croup can be beneficial in reducing inflammation and alleviating symptoms but can require hours for onset. The pediatric dose of dexamethasone is 0.5 to 1 mg/kg orally or intramuscularly. Clinical evaluation of topical steroids such as budesonide has shown improvement, especially with laryngeal edema. Nebulized budesonide has been shown to be as effective as dexamethasone for treatment. The role of Heliox (helium-oxygen mixture) has yet to be defined but might be helpful in severe croup.

Aregbesola A, Tam CM, Kothari A, Le ML, Ragheb M, Klassen TP. Glucocorticoids for croup in children. *Cochrane Database Syst Rev*. 2023;1:CD001955.

Bjornson C, Russell K, Vandermeer B, et al. Nebulized epinephrine for croup in children. *Cochrane Database Syst Rev*. 2013:CD006619.

Moraa I, Sturman N, McGuire TM, van Driel ML. Heliox for croup in children. *Cochrane Database Syst Rev*. 2021;8:CD006822.

Rodrigues KK, Roosevelt GE. Acute inflammatory upper airway obstruction (croup, epiglottitis, laryngitis, and bacterial tracheitis). In: Kliegman R, St. Geme J, Blum N, Schuh A, Tasker RC, Mack CL, Wilson K, eds. *Nelson Textbook of Pediatrics*. 22nd ed. Elsevier; 2025:2568-2572.

A.10. What is epiglottitis? What are its common causes? What is the incidence?

Epiglottitis is an inflammation of the epiglottis usually secondary to an infectious process. It can involve other supraglottic structures such as the arytenoids, false cords, and posterior tongue leading to obstruction of the airway. Progression of swelling can rapidly lead to complete airway occlusion and death. **Table 41.2** contrasts epiglottitis with croup.

Epiglottitis is most often bacterial in origin. The causative agent used to be mainly *H. influenzae* type B, but the *H. influenzae* type B vaccine has resulted in a remarkable decline in incidence, although epiglottis can still occur in vaccinated individuals. *Streptococcus pneumoniae* also has been infrequently associated with epiglottitis, and recently, group A β-hemolytic streptococci cases have been on the increase. Burn injury, neoplastic infiltration, caustic ingestion, lymphoproliferative disease, and angioneurotic edema are other causes. The incidence has declined to 1.8 per 10,000 admissions at the Children's Hospital of Philadelphia after the *H. influenzae* type B vaccine.

A 2010 retrospective review reaffirms that epiglottitis remains a significant problem in the United States, with nearly 4,000 admissions in 2006. The demographics of the disease have shifted away from

TABLE 41.2 Characteristics of Croup and Epiglottitis

	Croup	Epiglottitis
Etiology	Parainfluenza virus	*Haemophilus influenzae*
Age	4 mo to 2 y	2-5 y
Onset	Subacute exacerbation of preexistent URI	Acute
Temperature	Low-grade fever	High fever
Course	Usually mild, stridor may worsen at night	Rapid progress of symptoms
Symptoms	Barky cough, stridor	Dysphagia, sore throat Dysphonia, respiratory distress

URI, upper respiratory infection.

that of predominantly pediatric nature to one of adulthood. Surprisingly, the mean age in the study period from 1998 to 2006 was 45 years, and mortality was 36%. In a 2021 study evaluating trends in mortality from acute epiglottitis from 1979 to 2017, mortality decreased after the widespread adoption of *H. influenzae* type B vaccine, with adults now more likely than children to die of acute epiglottitis.

Allen M, Meraj TS, Oska S, Spillinger A, Folbe AJ, Cramer JD. Acute epiglottitis: analysis of U.S. mortality trends from 1979 to 2017. *Am J Otolaryngol.* 2021;42:102882.

D'Agostino J. Pediatric airway nightmares. *Emerg Med Clin North Am.* 2010;28:119-126.

Shah RK, Roberson DW, Jones DT. Epiglottitis in the *Hemophilus influenzae* type B vaccine era: changing trends. *Laryngoscope.* 2004;114:557-560.

Shah RK, Stocks C. Epiglottitis in the United States: national trends, variances, prognosis, and management. *Laryngoscope.* 2010;120:1256-1262.

A.11. What are the clinical manifestations of epiglottitis?

Epiglottitis presents acutely in otherwise healthy children 2 to 5 years of age with fever as high as 40 °C. Within a few hours, epiglottic inflammation progresses, and the child becomes dyspneic. The child sits forward to use the accessory muscles of respiration and complains of a fullness and pain in the throat. Speech sounds are muffled, known as a "hot potato voice." Salivation is characteristic and swallowing is difficult. The child appears anxious and concentrates only on breathing. The barking cough of croup usually is absent. The older child will assume a tripod posture with the neck extended to maximize air entry. As the child fatigues, cyanosis leading to complete asphyxia can ensue without intervention. Inspiratory effort is maximal with severe airway compromise, and thoracoabdominal asynchrony, otherwise known as paradoxical breathing, can be observed in the supine position: the abdomen protrudes and the chest wall retracts due to upper airway obstruction. Negative-pressure pulmonary edema can occur. Chest auscultation can reveal decreased breath sounds.

Bruins BB, Ross PA, Kilbaugh TJ. Pediatric and neonatal critical care. In: Gropper MA, Eriksson LI, Fleisher LA, Cohen NH, Leslie K, Johnson-Akeju O, eds. *Miller's Anesthesia.* 10th ed. Elsevier; 2025:2411-2482.

Murto K, Carr MM, Lerman J. Otorhinolaryngologic procedures. In: Cote CJ, Lerman J, Anderson BJ, eds. *A Practice of Anesthesia for Infants and Children.* 7th ed. Elsevier Saunders; 2024:841-899.

Rodrigues KK, Roosevelt GE. Acute inflammatory upper airway obstruction (croup, epiglottitis, laryngitis, and bacterial tracheitis). In: Kliegman R, St. Geme J, Blum N, Schuh A, Tasker RC, Mack CL, Wilson K, eds. *Nelson Textbook of Pediatrics.* 22nd ed. Elsevier; 2025:2568-2572.

A.12. How is the diagnosis of epiglottitis made?

Acute epiglottitis is a dire emergency, and any child whose clinical presentation warrants the diagnosis of epiglottitis must be evaluated promptly in a hospital. Although epiglottitis and croup have similar features, the presence of drooling and absence of coughing are sensitive and specific signs of epiglottitis, whereas the absence of drooling and the presence of coughing are sensitive and specific signs of croup.

Pharyngoscopy to visualize the inflamed epiglottis should not be attempted in an office setting because this can stimulate upper airway reflexes and lead to increasing dyspnea. All medical centers should have in place a management protocol that standardizes the approach to this rapidly progressive and potentially fatal disease and that involves a team of physicians and nurses from the specialties of pediatrics, otolaryngology, and anesthesiology. A logical approach includes:

- The child is kept calm with a parent in attendance at all times. Supplementary oxygen, a sitting position, and reassurance are essential.
- If the patient clinically conforms to a classical presentation of epiglottitis, the operating room is alerted and the child is taken there immediately for tracheal intubation.
- With other diagnostic considerations, such as a foreign body in the upper airway, retropharyngeal abscess, congenital anomalies, and croup, the child can be escorted to radiology. The time taken for the radiologic examination should be avoided in the critically ill child. A physician skilled in airway management should accompany the child with all necessary resuscitation equipment available.
- The classic "thumb sign" on a lateral radiograph is an aptly named shape seen with epiglottic enlargement. However, the absence of this sign does not eliminate the diagnosis of epiglottitis. Croup is distinguished by the "steeple sign" representing a uniform narrowing of the subglottic airway by inflammation.
- Laboratory evidence is nonspecific, although a high white count with bands and polymorphonuclear leukocytes is more suggestive of epiglottitis than of croup.

- Fiberoptic pharyngoscopy can be effective if performed gently by a skilled examiner; it immediately confirms or eliminates the diagnosis. Do not perform laryngoscopy (direct or video assisted) if anxiety is increased by the procedure and hence exacerbates airway obstruction.

Rodrigues KK, Roosevelt GE. Acute inflammatory upper airway obstruction (croup, epiglottitis, laryngitis, and bacterial tracheitis). In: Kliegman R, St. Geme J, Blum N, Schuh A, Tasker RC, Mack CL, Wilson K, eds. *Nelson Textbook of Pediatrics*. 22nd ed. Elsevier; 2025:2568-2572.

Tibballs J, Watson T. Symptoms and signs differentiating croup and epiglottitis. *J Paediatr Child Health*. 2011;47:77-82.

A.13. What is postextubation croup? How is it managed?

Anesthesiologists are often in the position of treating patients with postextubation airway edema, which resembles croup in its symptomatology.

Pediatric patients undergoing general endotracheal anesthesia can mimic many of the physical signs of the croup syndrome following extubation. The tracheal and subglottic mucosa have become irritated by the tracheal tube, which initiates an inflammatory response, causing airway luminal narrowing. Because airway resistance is inversely proportional to the fourth power of the tracheal radius (with turbulent flow, this increases to the fifth power), the pediatric airway is especially compromised by edema. Halving the lumen diameter increases laminar airflow resistance by 16-fold.

Postextubation croup can manifest more frequently in a patient who has received large quantities of fluid or transfusion, maintained unusual or strained lateral head positioning, has a history of smoke inhalation, restrictive congenital anomalies such as a tracheoesophageal fistula, or acquired subglottic stenosis secondary to prolonged intubation as a neonate, has coexistent upper respiratory infection (URI), especially bronchitis, or has a cuffed or uncuffed endotracheal tube with a high (>25 cm H_2O) leak pressure. The air leak test, which gauges the pressure needed to generate an audible leak in the presence of an endotracheal tube, can be predictive of postextubation stridor in children over 7 years of age. Ensuring an adequate air leak can decrease the risk of postextubation croup.

Management involves reducing airway constriction by administering nebulized racemic epinephrine, steroids, and humidification of inspired gases. On occasion, reintubating with a soft tracheal tube one-half to one size smaller than previously used is necessary until the inflammation subsides. Topical lidocaine ointment can have vasodilatory actions and should not be used in patients with postextubation croup.

Kimura S, Ahn JB, Takahashi M, Kwon S, Papatheodorou S. Effectiveness of corticosteroids for post-extubation stridor and extubation failure in pediatric patients: a systematic review and meta-analysis. *Ann Intensive Care*. 2020;10:155.

Mhanna MJ, Zamel YB, Tichy CM, et al. The air leak test around the endotracheal tube as a predictor of post extubation stridor is age dependent in children. *Crit Care Med*. 2002;30:2639-2643.

Murto K, Carr MM, Lerman J. Otorhinolaryngologic procedures. In: Cote CJ, Lerman J, Anderson BJ, eds. *A Practice of Anesthesia for Infants and Children*. 7th ed. Elsevier Saunders; 2024:841-899.

Suominen P, Taivainen T, Tuominen N, et al. Optimally fitted tracheal tubes decrease the probability of postextubation adverse events in children undergoing general anesthesia. *Paediatr Anaesth*. 2006;16:641-647.

A.14. What are the nonacute causes of partial airway obstruction in children?

Several congenital anomalies are associated with respiratory difficulties. These can be subdivided into intrinsic and extrinsic causes.

Extrinsic Causes

- Cystic hygroma—a proliferation or expansion of lymphatic channels, usually in the cervical region, that can compress the airway and lead to enlargement of the tongue
- Vascular anomalies—abnormalities of the aortic arch usually caused by aberrant vessels lead to compression of the airway. This is often position dependent and can cause coughing and wheezing when the patient is supine.
- Neoplastic compression of the trachea by lymphoma, hemangioma, neurofibromatosis, rhabdomyosarcoma, and other neural tumors in the mediastinum can enlarge or compress airway structures.

Intrinsic Causes

- Subglottic stenosis—especially acquired as previously intubated neonates. This form of airway narrowing occurs below the vocal cords, and can lead to marked airway obstruction with respiratory infections. The congenital form might not be appreciated until an URI is present when stridor can occur.

- Vocal cord paralysis—considered the second most common laryngeal anomaly in children, and is associated with the Arnold-Chiari malformation.
- Laryngeal structural anomalies—webs, laryngoceles, and cysts

Weiner DL, Deanehan JK. Respiratory distress. In: Shaw KN, Bachur RG, eds. *Fleisher & Ludwig's Textbook of Pediatric Emergency Medicine*. 8th ed. Wolters Kluwer; 2021:478-490.

A.15. What are the clinical manifestations of severe COVID-19 in infants and children?

The spectrum of pediatric COVID-19 is wide ranging from asymptomatic seroconversion to complex multisystem involvement. Asymptomatic infection ranges widely in different series. A meta-review of over 80,000 health records in a pediatric population showed that 66% were asymptomatic, 27% had mild COVID-19 symptoms, 5% had moderate symptoms (characterized as pneumonia and/or gastroenteritis), and 2% were considered severe requiring intensive care unit (ICU) admission (with or without the need for mechanical ventilation). The ICU category shared overlapping symptomatology with severe influenza pneumonitis. In general, respiratory involvement manifests with cough, fever, chills, nasal congestion, headache, sneezing, sore throat, and croup-like syndromes. In its severe form, when respiratory involvement leads to severe bronchospasm, pneumonia, and pleural effusion, anesthesiology assistance to secure the airway has been necessary especially with intervening dyspnea, hypoxemia, and cardiovascular instability.

Forest CB, Burrows ER, Mejias A, et al. Severity of acute COVID-19 in children <18 years old March 2020 to December 2021. *Pediatrics*. 2022;149.

Venn AMR, Schmidt JM, Mullan PC. Pediatric croup with COVID-19. *Am J Emerg Med*. 2021;43;287.e1.

A.16. What is human metapneumovirus and how does it cause disease in the pediatric population?

Human metapneumovirus (HMPV) is an RNA virus first isolated in 2001 and now responsible for the second highest incidence of lower respiratory illness in infants and young children after respiratory syncytial virus (RSV). It is recurrent and seasonal usually appearing in winter and early spring. Approximately 10% of respiratory illness in children is related to HMPV and up to 15% of those patients will go on to develop both lower and upper respiratory infections with bronchiolitis, bronchitis, and pneumonia.

Jartti T, van den Hoogen B, Garofalo RP, et al. Metapneumovirus and acute wheezing in children. *Lancet*. 2002;360;1393.

Williams JV, Harris PA, Tollefson SJ, et al. Human metapneumovirus and lower respiratory tract disease in otherwise healthy infants and children. *N Engl J Med*. 2004;350:443-450.

B. Preoperative Evaluation and Preparation

B.1. Is tracheal intubation always required in children with epiglottitis?

Adult patients often can be managed by vigilant observation provided that there is no impending danger of obstruction. However, contemporary practice warrants establishing an airway with an endotracheal tube in the vast majority of infants and children. Nasotracheal intubation is most often used for ease of maintaining comfort and safety. Endoscopic evaluation using appropriate fiberoptic airway endoscopy is a major advance in the management of epiglottitis.

Acevedo JL, Lander L, Choi S, et al. Airway management in pediatric epiglottis: a national perspective. *Otolaryngol Head Neck Surg*. 2009;140:548-551.

Murto K, Carr MM, Lerman J. Otorhinolaryngologic procedures. In: Cote CJ, Lerman J, Anderson BJ, eds. *A Practice of Anesthesia for Infants and Children*. 7th ed. Elsevier Saunders; 2024:841-899.

Weiner DL, Deanehan JK. Respiratory distress. In: Shaw KN, Bachur RG, eds. *Fleisher & Ludwig's Textbook of Pediatric Emergency Medicine*. 8th ed. Wolters Kluwer; 2021:478-490.

B.2. Why is general anesthesia administered to a child with epiglottitis?

General anesthesia facilitates a thorough examination of the supraglottic anatomy, which would be impossible and dangerous in the awake child. In addition, tracheal intubation can be accomplished under controlled, relaxed conditions without trauma and laryngospasm. Intubation can be difficult because of the swelling and deformation of paraepiglottic tissues. Clinicians who have no experience with this unusual appearance will find it easier to visualize landmarks and secure the airway when the patient is in a surgical plane of anesthesia.

Murto K, Carr MM, Lerman J. Otorhinolaryngologic procedures. In: Cote CJ, Lerman J, Anderson BJ, eds. *A Practice of Anesthesia for Infants and Children*. 7th ed. Elsevier Saunders; 2024:841-899.

B.3. How would you prepare the patient for anesthesia?

Expedience is crucial. Once the diagnosis is made and the operating room alerted, the child is transported accompanied by parents and a physician with airway supportive equipment. An intravenous line can be placed more easily under anesthesia without upsetting the child. Anything that causes the child to cry will potentially worsen obstruction and interfere with breathing. The child should, therefore, be kept calm and reassured. Nasal prong or face tent oxygen should be provided, and portable pulse oximetry should be used.

Airway equipment including a suitable mask and tracheal tubes up to two sizes smaller than normally expected should be available. Lidocaine, succinylcholine, atropine, and ketamine in appropriate dilutions should be ready. A cricothyrotomy tray should be available as a precaution.

The parent should accompany the child into the operating room. Before induction of anesthesia, the parent is instructed about their role in comforting the child, encouraging compliance with mask breathing, and gently holding the child when inhalation induction commences. When parents can provide their assistance in an emotionally controlled, supportive way, a smooth, safe anesthetic induction via mask can be accomplished.

Murto K, Carr MM, Lerman J. Otorhinolaryngologic procedures. In: Cote CJ, Lerman J, Anderson BJ, eds. *A Practice of Anesthesia for Infants and Children*. 7th ed. Elsevier Saunders; 2024:841-899.

C. Intraoperative Management

C.1. How is the airway of the child with epiglottitis best secured?

There is little debate over the safety and efficacy of tracheal intubation when supportive staff is readily available. The tracheal tube should be downsized by 0.5 or 1.0 mm due to the inherent swelling and to protect against postextubation complications. Thick, copious secretions must be cleared frequently to prevent obstruction, and the child must be sedated to tolerate the endotracheal tube and to keep it secure in place.

Charles R, Fadden M, Brook J. Acute epiglottitis. *BMJ*. 2013;347:f5235.

Murto K, Carr MM, Lerman J. Otorhinolaryngologic procedures. In: Cote CJ, Lerman J, Anderson BJ, eds. *A Practice of Anesthesia for Infants and Children*. 7th ed. Elsevier Saunders; 2024:841-899.

Weiner DL, Deanehan JK. Respiratory distress. In: Shaw KN, Bachur RG, eds. *Fleisher & Ludwig's Textbook of Pediatric Emergency Medicine*. 8th ed. Wolters Kluwer; 2021:478-490.

C.2. How would you induce general anesthesia?

Verbal assurance is given continuously. The child is seated on the parent's lap in the operating room and preoxygenated. Sevoflurane is a good choice for induction agent because it is less pungent and irritant than desflurane and is usually well tolerated; halothane (if available) can be used if sevoflurane is not available. The volatile anesthetic should be initiated in low concentration and slowly increased as tolerated. As the child becomes sedated, they are placed in the supine position. The patient might undergo a brief period of excitation during which care is taken not to be overzealous with ventilation. Spontaneous, unassisted ventilation should continue as an intravenous line is placed. Glycopyrrolate 0.01 mg/kg is given IV as an anti-sialagogue. A crystalloid fluid bolus of 20 to 40 mL/kg should be administered to treat dehydration. Ventilation can be assisted but not controlled. End-tidal gas is monitored continuously, and the airway is adjusted to provide maximal tidal volume exchange. Sevoflurane concentration is increased as tolerated to 8%, provided cardiovascular stability is maintained, to achieve an adequate depth of anesthesia. Airway obstruction will decrease ventilation and anesthetic uptake, requiring a longer induction time.

When the patient is in a deep plane of anesthesia (minimal alveolar concentration of sevoflurane in children is higher than in adults), a careful laryngoscopy is carried out. Paralysis is unnecessary in this deep plane of anesthesia. However, if several attempts are required with the possibility of the patient becoming light and reactive, a small dose of a neuromuscular blocker (eg, rocuronium 0.4 mg/kg) can provide stable intubating conditions. This should be given only after it has been shown that the patient can be ventilated with a bag and mask.

Murto K, Carr MM, Lerman J. Otorhinolaryngologic procedures. In: Cote CJ, Lerman J, Anderson BJ, eds. *A Practice of Anesthesia for Infants and Children*. 7th ed. Elsevier Saunders; 2024:841-899.

Spalding MB, Ala-Kokko TI. The use of inhaled sevoflurane for endotracheal intubation in epiglottitis. *Anesthesiology*. 1998;89:1025-1026.

C.3. Should a child with epiglottitis undergo a rapid sequence induction of anesthesia?

In a child with a full stomach, a mask induction leaves the airway unprotected from aspiration of gastric contents. However, a rapid sequence induction can predispose the patient to severe hypoxemia and hypoventilation should the clinician not be able to intubate the trachea expediently. Because the supraglottic landmarks are distorted by erythema and edema, recognition of the glottic inlet is obscured. In the spontaneously breathing patient, small air movements and the resultant bubbling of secretions can highlight the glottic opening. Paralysis in no way assures the ability to ventilate.

If the patient must be manually ventilated, it is possible to encounter complete obstruction secondary to invagination of the swollen supraglottic tissues into the laryngeal introitus. In such a case, positive end-expiratory pressure or a jaw-thrust maneuver can fail to correct the airway obstruction.

Should the child be too agitated to cooperate with an inhalational induction, an intramuscular dose of ketamine (2-3 mg/kg) will accomplish sedation and preserve ventilation. However, it can accentuate airway reflexes, and the clinician should be aware of laryngospasm. Videolaryngoscopy is the optimal choice whenever available.

Murto K, Carr MM, Lerman J. Otorhinolaryngologic procedures. In: Cote CJ, Lerman J, Anderson BJ, eds. *A Practice of Anesthesia for Infants and Children*. 7th ed. Elsevier Saunders; 2024:841-899.

Nagler J, Bachur RG. Advanced airway management. *Curr Opin Pediatr*. 2009;21:299-305.

Weiner DL, Deanehan JK. Respiratory distress. In: Shaw KN, Bachur RG, eds. *Fleisher & Ludwig's Textbook of Pediatric Emergency Medicine*. 8th ed. Wolters Kluwer; 2021:478-490.

C.4. Is awake tracheal intubation a practical alternative to secure the patient's airway?

Awake tracheal intubation is not generally recommended even though some authors have suggested awake intubation with topical anesthesia in the past. Risks of difficult visualization, agitation, trauma, worsening of epiglottic edema, and compromised ventilation far outweigh the benefits. Unless one has acquired great skill at awake pediatric intubation in the child with a normal airway, this technique should be avoided in these patients. In the adult, awake intubation using either a GlideScope or McGrath videolaryngoscope has been reported with success.

Rosenstock CV, Thogersen B, Afshari A, Christensen AL, Eriksen C, Gatke MR. Awake fiberoptic or awake video laryngoscopic tracheal intubation in patients with anticipated difficult airway management: a randomized clinical trial. *Anesthesiology*. 2012;116:1210-1216.

Sinofsky AH, Milo SP, Scher C. The awake Glidescope intubation: an additional alternative to the difficult intubation. *Middle East J Anesthesiol*. 2010;20:743-746.

C.5. What would you do if the airway cannot be secured by tracheal intubation?

Preemptive preparation is critical, and an otorhinolaryngologist should be present. In the event when the airway is lost, percutaneous transtracheal ventilation can be performed. This involves inserting a needle through the cricothyroid membrane as follows. Localize the cricothyroid membrane and topically cleanse the area with antiseptic. Anesthetize the skin with lidocaine (if time permits) and then insert a 16-gauge catheter (attached to needle) in the midline in the inferior portion of the cricothyroid membrane and directed caudally. Attach a 3-mL syringe to the needle barrel applying negative pressure. If the syringe contains a few milliliters of saline, air bubbles will be apparent when the trachea is entered. Following entry, advance the catheter into the trachea. Depending on the hub size, a 3.0- or 3.5-mm tracheal tube adapter can be inserted into the catheter to interface with an Ambu bag. Alternatively, a 6.5- or 7.0-mm tracheal tube adapter can be inserted into a 3-mL syringe barrel without the plunger to interface with an Ambu bag or anesthesia circuit (**Figure 41.1**). Jet ventilation can also be applied with high-pressure tubing keeping careful observation of respiratory dynamics and saturation. A tracheotomy in skilled hands can also be performed.

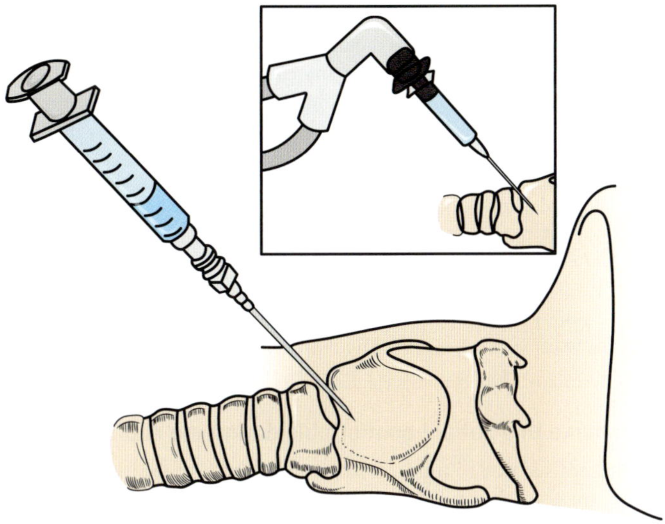

FIGURE 41.1. An emergency cricothyrotomy can be performed by passing a 14- to 16-gauge intravenous catheter through the cricothyroid membrane into the trachea. A 3-mL syringe with the plunger removed will accept a 15-mm tracheal tube adapter that allows attachment of an oxygen-delivery system. (Reprinted with permission from Mecca RS. Postoperative recovery. In: Barash PG, Cullen BF, Stoelting RK, eds. *Clinical Anesthesia*. 5th ed. Lippincott Williams & Wilkins; 2001:Figure 54.4.)

Delaney WA, Kaiser RE Jr. Percutaneous transtracheal jet ventilation made easy. *Anesthesiology*. 1991;74:952.

Watters KF. Tracheostomy in infants and children. *Respir Care*. 2017;62:799-825.

C.6. Should this patient have a nasotracheal or orotracheal tube placed?

The patient will better tolerate a nasal endotracheal tube for prolonged intubation. Oropharyngeal toilet will also be easier in the setting of nasotracheal intubation. However, because the intubation can be difficult with epiglottitis and can predispose to the problems listed in Section C.4, the orotracheal route is easier and safer. Once the airway is secured orally, a nasotracheal tube can be inserted with laryngoscopic guidance.

C.7. Shortly after intubation, frothy secretions were obtained on suctioning the endotracheal tube. What is the reason for this? How can this be treated?

About 7% of these patients develop pulmonary edema after intubation. This phenomenon relates to the transudation into the alveoli during periods of increased transpulmonary pressure. This occurs especially during obstructed inspiration. If the obstruction is complete, it is referred to as the "Müller" maneuver. The high negative pressures are buffered by the decreased venous return during exhalation. However, relief of the airway obstruction facilitates the extravasation of fluid for an increased venous return.

Treatment of negative-pressure pulmonary edema requires positive end-expiratory pressure. Diuretics and fluid restriction are not required because this condition generally is self-correcting. This can be administered by nasal bilevel means, mask continuous pressure, or intubation.

Davis HW, Gartner JC, Galvis AG, et al. Acute upper airway obstruction: croup and epiglottitis. *Pediatr Clin North Am*. 1981;28:859-880.

Silva PS, Monteiro Neto H, Andrade MM, et al. Negative-pressure pulmonary edema: a rare complication of upper airway obstruction in children. *Pediatr Emerg Care*. 2005;21:751-754.

D. Postoperative Management

D.1. How long should this patient remain intubated? What criteria determine extubation time?

Earlier studies have shown a mean intubation duration of 36 hours in 23 patients with a range of 19 to 67 hours. These patients were treated with ampicillin or chloramphenicol, and the epiglottis was visualized before extubation. The current antibiotic regimen is cefazolin 75 to 100 mg/kg/d in three divided doses or clindamycin 30 to 40 mg/kg/d in three divided doses with the addition of a third-generation cephalosporin such as cefotaxime or ceftriaxone.

Criteria for tracheal extubation include increased air leak around the endotracheal tube as well as decreased erythema and edema. However, instrumentation and examination of the child might be unnecessary, and extubation at 36 to 48 hours can be accomplished easily in all patients. Flexible fiberoptic laryngoscopy can be used to visualize the epiglottis and determine extubation time.

Charles R, Fadden M, Brook J. Acute epiglottitis. *BMJ*. 2013;347:f5235.

Damm M, Eckel HE, Jungehülsing M, et al. Airway endoscopy in the interdisciplinary management of acute epiglottitis. *Int J Pediatr Otorhinolaryngol*. 1996;38:41-51.

Hopkins RL. Extubation in epiglottitis. *Anesth Analg*. 1984;63:468.

Murto K, Carr MM, Lerman J. Otorhinolaryngologic procedures. In: Cote CJ, Lerman J, Anderson BJ, eds. *A Practice of Anesthesia for Infants and Children*. 7th ed. Elsevier Saunders; 2024:841-899.

Vernon DD, Sarnaik AP. Extubation in epiglottitis. *Anesth Analg*. 1984;63:469-470.

D.2. How would you make this patient comfortable during the course of intubation?

The child must be kept sedated to minimize movement, to prevent inadvertent extubation, and to provide anxiolytics. There are several options. Midazolam (0.075 mg/kg) as a starting dose titrated upward to effect followed by a continuous infusion of 0.04 to 0.1 mg/kg/h will be effective, often in combination with a fentanyl infusion of 1 to 3 μg/kg/h. Alternatively, a short infusion of propofol can be given, taking care to monitor for propofol-related infusion syndrome. Dexmedetomidine is also an effective adjunct. A bilateral superior laryngeal nerve block in experienced hands can allow for better tolerance of the endotracheal tube.

Appropriate respiratory care, humidification, suctioning, and secretion mobilization should be provided.

Charles R, Fadden M, Brook J. Acute epiglottitis. *BMJ*. 2013;347:f5235.

Murto K, Carr MM, Lerman J. Otorhinolaryngologic procedures. In: Cote CJ, Lerman J, Anderson BJ, eds. *A Practice of Anesthesia for Infants and Children*. 7th ed. Elsevier Saunders; 2024:841-899.

D.3. What outcome can one expect for a child with acute epiglottitis?

Residual airway problems are unusual in the vast majority of children. Most children who are diagnosed in time and intubated go on to a full recovery without sequelae. Complications are related to securing the airway and include associated pneumonia, respiratory failure, hypoxemia, cardiac arrest, and death.

Charles R, Fadden M, Brook J. Acute epiglottitis. *BMJ*. 2013;347:f5235.

Rodrigues KK, Roosevelt GE. Acute inflammatory upper airway obstruction (croup, epiglottitis, laryngitis, and bacterial tracheitis). In: Kliegman R, St. Geme J, Blum N, Schuh A, Tasker RC, Mack CL, Wilson K, eds. *Nelson Textbook of Pediatrics*. 22nd ed. Elsevier; 2025:2568-2572.

Cleft Palate

Shona M. Lee and Aarti Sharma

42

A 3-month-old male infant is scheduled for repair of a cleft lip and palate. According to his pediatrician, the infant was born at full term and has no other medical problems.

A. Medical Disease and Differential Diagnosis

1. Describe the anatomic defects of a cleft palate and a cleft lip.
2. What is the cause of an orofacial cleft?
3. What is the incidence of an orofacial cleft?
4. Discuss the pathophysiology of cleft lip and palate in neonates and in children older than 5 years.
5. What other conditions are associated with orofacial clefts?
6. What is Pierre Robin syndrome?
7. What is Treacher Collins syndrome?
8. What kind of specialized team care would these patients need?
9. Discuss indications and timing of closure of cleft lip and palate.
10. What is velopharyngeal incompetence, and how can it be diagnosed?
11. What is the relation of tonsillectomy and adenoidectomy to velopharyngeal incompetence and postoperative obstructive breathing episodes?

B. Preoperative Evaluation and Preparation

1. What information do you need before closure of a cleft lip and palate?
2. What preoperative orders are needed?
3. What airway equipment would you prepare in the operating room?

C. Intraoperative Management

1. What monitors will you need for cheiloplasty and palatoplasty?
2. Discuss the induction and management of anesthesia for cleft lip and palate in this nonsyndromic, otherwise healthy infant.
3. What positioning is recommended for cleft palate repair surgery?
4. What are the reported complications of this type of surgery and anesthesia?
5. Briefly describe the surgical techniques used to repair cleft defects.
6. How does a pharyngeal flap affect anesthetic management or any subsequent anesthetic administered to this patient?
7. What is an Abbe flap? What are its anesthetic implications?
8. What are the crucial anesthetic concerns for cleft palate repair? What are the unique considerations of this surgical repair?
9. What is laryngospasm? How would you make a diagnosis of laryngospasm?
10. How would you manage the patient with laryngospasm?

D. Postoperative Management

1. What complications of cleft lip and cleft palate surgery can be seen in the recovery room?
2. How do you protect the airway postoperatively?
3. How would you control postoperative pain in patients following a cleft lip and cleft palate repair? Describe a multimodal analgesic plan including regional anesthesia options.

A. Medical Disease and Differential Diagnosis

A.1. Describe the anatomic defects of a cleft palate and a cleft lip.

Congenital clefts of the upper lip occur because of failed fusion of the maxillary, medial, and lateral nasal processes. They vary from a notch in the upper lip to a partial cleft through the lip and the floor of the nose involving the alveolar ridge, or they can be complete cleft of the lip and the palate.

The cleft palate is divided into prepalatal and postpalatal clefts. The incisive foramen marks the boundary between the two, and each arises differently during embryologic development. A prepalatal cleft involves the anterior palate, alveolus, lip, nostril floor, and ala nasi. Postpalatal clefts can extend anywhere from the soft and hard palate to the incisive foramen. A submucosal cleft exists when a bone defect is present without a mucosal defect. The most common cleft of the palate is a left-sided, complete cleft of the prepalatal and palatal structures. The second most common is a midline cleft of the entire soft palate and part of the hard palate without involvement of the prepalatal area. Various degrees of the cleft palate and lip are shown in **Figure 42.1**.

Ganske IM, Rogers-Vizena CR. Cleft lip and palate: principles and treatment. In: Chung KC, ed. *Grabb and Smith's Plastic Surgery*. 9th ed. Wolters Kluwer; 2025:183-196.

Schafer S, Card E, Liao EC. Cleft lip and palate: embryology and genetics. In: Chung KC, ed. *Grabb and Smith's Plastic Surgery*. 9th ed. Wolters Kluwer; 2025:197-208.

Schindler E, Martini M, Messing-Jünger M. Anesthesia for Plastic and Craniofascial Surgery. In: Andropoulous DB & Gregory GA, ed. *Gregory's Pediatric Anesthesia*. 6th ed. Wiley-Blackwell; 2020: 904-905.

A.2. What is the cause of an orofacial cleft?

Major components of the face develop between 4 and 7 weeks in utero. There are three mesodermal islands, one central and two lateral. Prepalatal clefts are caused by failure of these mesodermal elements to develop and fuse. Palatal clefts are caused when the palatal ridges fail to migrate medially, contact, and fuse (**Figure 42.1**).

Ganske IM, Rogers-Vizena CR. Cleft lip and palate: principles and treatment. In: Chung KC, ed. *Grabb and Smith's Plastic Surgery*. 9th ed. Wolters Kluwer; 2025:183-196.

Schafer S, Card E, Liao EC. Cleft lip and palate: embryology and genetics. In: Chung KC, ed. *Grabb and Smith's Plastic Surgery*. 9th ed. Wolters Kluwer; 2025:197-208.

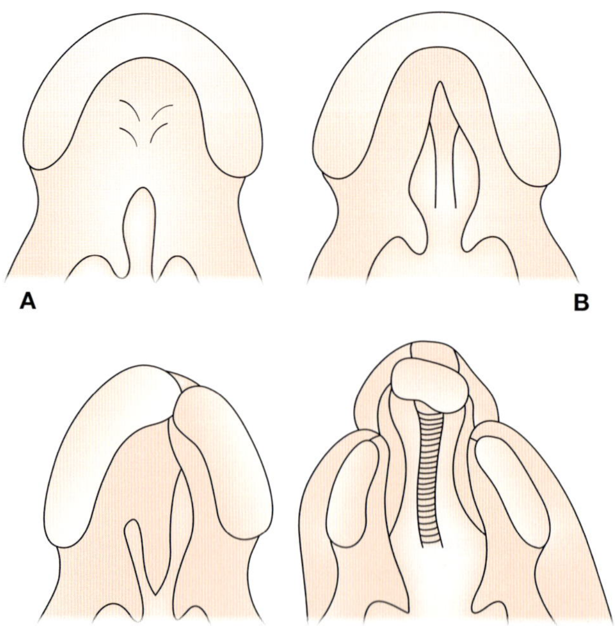

FIGURE 42.1. Various degrees of cleft palate and cleft lip. A. Cleft of the soft palate only. **B.** Cleft of the soft and hard palate as far forward as the incisive foramen. **C.** Complete unilateral alveolar cleft, usually involving the lip. **D.** Complete bilateral alveolar cleft, usually associated with bilateral clefts of the lip. (Modified from McCarthy JG, Cutting CB, Jogan VM. Introduction to Facial Clefts. In: McCarthy JG, ed. *Plastic Surgery. Vol. 4: Cleft Lip and Palate and Craniofacial Abnormalities.* WB Saunders; 1990: 2443.)

A.3. What is the incidence of an orofacial cleft?

Cleft lip and cleft palate can occur together or separately. A cleft lip with or without a cleft palate is more common in males, whereas an isolated cleft palate is more common in females. In a large, international perinatal database, the overall prevalence of cleft lip with or without cleft palate was 9.92 per 10,000. The prevalence of cleft lip was 3.28 per 10,000, and that of cleft lip and palate was 6.64 per 10,000. Of 10,000 cases, there were 5,918 cases (76.8%) that were isolated, 1,224 (15.9%) had malformations in other systems, and 562 (7.3%) occurred as part of recognized syndromes. Cases with greater dysmorphology of the cleft lip with or without cleft palate were more likely to include malformations of other systems.

The highest incidence of a cleft lip and a cleft palate occurs among Asians (1.61:1,000 births), whereas the lowest incidence is in African Americans (0.3:1,000 births). The incidence in Whites is intermediate (0.9:1,000 births).

IPDTOC Working Group. Prevalence at birth of cleft lip with or without cleft palate: data from the International Perinatal Database of Typical Oral Clefts (IPDTOC). *Cleft Palate Craniofac J*. 2011;48:66-81.

Samanich J. Cleft palate. *Pediatr Rev*. 2009;30:230-232.

A.4. Discuss the pathophysiology of cleft lip and palate in neonates and in children older than 5 years.

A cleft palate is responsible for some major physiologic disorders. The pharynx communicates extensively with the nasal fossae and the oral cavity. The complex mechanisms of swallowing, breathing, hearing (through the eustachian tube), and speech are therefore impaired.

The presence of a cleft lip and palate results in neonatal feeding difficulties. The neonate cannot suck because the cleft makes the creation of a negative pressure seal difficult. Breastfeeding can be impossible, and bottle-feeding is challenging. Without intervention, affected children suffer from growth difficulties or failure to thrive.

Children with a cleft palate have middle ear disease because abnormal anatomy of the nasopharynx adversely affects eustachian tube function. Chronic middle ear effusion produces varying degrees of conductive hearing loss and recurrent otitis. Nasal septation between food and air is absent, creating a nonphysiologic mixing chamber in the nasopharynx. Frequently, this is associated with chronic rhinorrhea which must be distinguished preoperatively from infection.

Secondary defects of tooth development, growth of the ala nasi, and velopharyngeal function (contact between the soft palate and the posterior pharynx for speech and swallowing) can also occur. Speech is typically nasal with an inability to generate the so-called plosives (*p*/*k*/*d*/*t*) and fricatives (*s*/*f*).

The detrimental impact of orofacial clefts is seen at both the individual and societal levels, with high economic burden and increased morbidity and mortality at all ages, particularly in association with other syndromes. Psychological problems can be considerable as children approach school age and peer association.

Kosowski TR, Weathers WM, Wolfswinkel EM, et al. Cleft palate. *Semin Plast Surg*. 2012;26:164-169.

Shkoukani MA, Lawrence LA, Liebertz DJ, Svider PF. Cleft palate: a clinical review. *Birth Defects Res C Embryo Today*. 2014;102:333-342.

A.5. What other conditions are associated with orofacial clefts?

Associated anomalies occur 30 times more frequently in the patient with an isolated cleft palate than in the noncleft population. The most common nonsyndromic abnormalities are umbilical hernias, clubfoot, limb, and ear deformities. The most common syndromes associated with cleft lip and cleft palate are:

- Velocardiofacial (Shprintzen) syndrome
- van der Woude syndrome
- Stickler syndrome
- Pierre Robin syndrome (PRS)
- Fetal alcohol syndrome
- Goldenhar syndrome (facio-auriculo-vertebral syndrome or hemifacial microsomia)
- Treacher Collins syndrome
- Nager syndrome
- Down syndrome

Calzolari E, Pierini A, Astolfi G, et al. Associated anomalies in multi-malformed infants with cleft lip and palate: an epidemiologic study of nearly 6 million births in 23 EUROCRAT registries. *Am J Med Genet A*. 2007;143A:528-537.

A.6. What is Pierre Robin syndrome?

This syndrome is characterized by retrognathia or micrognathia, glossoptosis, and a soft palate cleft. The presumed inciting factor is mandibular micrognathia before 9 weeks in utero causing glossoptosis (posterior-inferior displacement of the tongue) which mechanically impairs the union of the palatal shelves. This forms the classic U-shaped or high-arched cleft, which is incomplete in approximately 50% of these patients.

This anatomy results in airway obstruction that is magnified during inspiration, relaxation, and sleep. Crying or straining can often keep the airway open. Because of these respiratory problems and increased energy expenditure, feeding can become exceedingly difficult. If left untreated, this vicious cycle can lead to hypoxemia, exhaustion, failure to thrive, cerebral impairments, cardiac failure (cor pulmonale), and ultimately death.

The Pierre Robin sequence is a rare disease with a birth incidence ranging from 1:8,500 to 1:30,000. This wide range derives from variable clinical presentations, particularly in those with mild symptoms that can go unrecognized, as well as inconsistent diagnostic and reporting in studies of heterogeneous populations. In 38% of cases, it occurs in other normal individuals.

Cladis F, Kumar A, Grunwaldt L, Otteson T, Ford M, Losee JE. Pierre Robin sequence: a perioperative review. *Anesth Analg*. 2014;119:400-412.

Giudice A, Barone S, Belhous K, et al. Pierre Robin sequence: A comprehensive narrative review of the literature over time. *J Stomatol Oral Maxillofac Surg*. 2018;119:419-428.

Jones KL, Jones MC, del Campo M. Facial Defects as Major Feature. *Smith's Recognizable Patterns of Human Malformation*. 8th ed. WB-Saunders; 2021: 334.

A.7. What is Treacher Collins syndrome?

Treacher Collins syndrome is highly complex disease process consisting of the following:

- Hypoplastic cheeks, zygomatic arches, and mandible
- Microtia with possible hearing loss
- High-arched or cleft palate
- Macrostomia (abnormally large mouth)
- Antimongoloid slant to the eyes
- Coloboma (notching of the outer portion of the lower eyelid)
- Increased anterior facial height
- Malocclusion (anterior open bite)
- Small oral cavity and airway with normal-sized tongue
- Pointed nasal prominence

Mutations in the *TCOF1* gene account for the majority of cases and have autosomal dominant inheritance. Critical airway issues after birth (occurring in up to 20% of patients with the syndrome), feeding difficulties, obstructive sleep apnea, and hearing and vision loss should all be addressed.

Jones KL, Jones MC, del Campo M. Facial Defects as Major Feature. Treacher Collins Syndrome. *Smith's Recognizable Patterns of Human Malformation*. 8th ed. WB-Saunders; 2021: 362-363.

A.8. What kind of specialized team care would these patients need?

These patients require a multidisciplinary approach with a pediatrician to maintain their overall health, an otolaryngologist in conjunction with reconstructive or maxillofacial surgeons, and an anesthesiologist. Patients should be carefully monitored for early respiratory failure and intervention, potentially with a surgical airway or tracheostomy. Plans for a possible difficult airway are crucial.

A speech therapist can work closely with an occupational therapist to prevent or overcome speech and feeding deficiencies, and an orthodontist can help develop and maintain relatively normal bite and dentition. A comprehensive care team also includes a geneticist, pediatric dentist, prosthodontist, psychologist, medical social worker, and a public health nurse.

Rozzelle A & Arneja J. Cleft Lip and Cleft Palate. In: Adam HM, Campbell DE, DeWitt TG, Foy JM & McInerny TK, ed. *American Academy of Pediatrics Textbook of Pediatric Care*. 2nd ed. American Academy of Pediatrics; 2016: 1849 – 1852.

A.9. Discuss indications and timing of closure of cleft lip and palate.

Functional goals of cleft palate surgery are normal speech, hearing, and maxillofacial growth. It is thought that speech and hearing are improved by early cleft palate repair (before 24 months of age). This is balanced against delayed closure (after 4 years), which is associated with less retardation of midfacial growth. There is no absolute consensus on the timing of lip and palate closure. These variations likely reflect the anatomic variabilities in different patients, as well as the personal preferences of the surgeon. An early two-stage palate repair is advocated in the management of these patients. The recommended sequence involves closure of the soft palate at 3 to 6 months of age with secondary closure of the residual hard palate at 15 to 18 months of age. This sequence takes advantage of the early physiology and growth that occurs in the soft palate, which is vital in the development of speech. Furthermore, it avoids the potential pitfalls of the growth disturbance related to early periosteal undermining of palatal and vomerine tissue. This repair sequence also provides total palatal closure before speech evolves. If the soft palate is repaired at the time of lip repair, an additional anesthetic is avoided.

Thiele OC, Kreppel M, Dunsche A. et al. Current concepts in cleft care: a multicenter analysis. *J Craniomaxillofac Surg*. 2018;46:705-708.

A.10. What is velopharyngeal incompetence, and how can it be diagnosed?

Velopharyngeal incompetence is the inability of the soft palate to fulfill its role in closing the nasopharynx, which seriously affects phonation. To produce plosive sounds (*p/k/t/d*) or the sibilants (*s/sh*), the soft palate must touch the posterior pharyngeal wall to close the nasal passage. Failure of closure seriously affects phonation and competent speech, resulting in the typical hypernasal speech.

The most common cause of velopharyngeal incompetence is cleft palate, but patients with congenitally short palates can also have this typical speech pattern. The diagnosis of velopharyngeal incompetence can be suggested by the child's speech. More objective diagnosis can be obtained by direct visualization of the soft palate while the child is pronouncing certain keywords (*kah, kah*), by fogging of a hand mirror placed under the nose during phonation, and from cinefluorographic films.

Treatment consists of surgical lengthening of the palate by the "pushback" operation with or without pharyngeal flap. In patients with velopharyngeal incompetence, videofluoroscopy and nasopharyngoscopy can provide information that will help select the appropriate procedure, either pharyngoplasty or posterior pharyngeal flap.

Dudas JR, Deleyiannis FW, Ford MD, et al. Diagnosis and treatment of velopharyngeal insufficiency: clinical utility of speech evaluation and videofluoroscopy. *Ann Plast Surg*. 2006;56:511-517.

Sullivan SR, Taylor HOB, Stiles E, Nuss RC, Balkin DM, Mulliken JB. Videofluoroscopy versus nasopharyngoscopy of lateral pharyngeal wall movement for assessment of velopharyngeal insufficiency. *J Craniofac Surg*. 2023;34:40-44.

A.11. What is the relation of tonsillectomy and adenoidectomy to velopharyngeal incompetence and postoperative obstructive breathing episodes?

There is often a considerable mass of tonsillar and adenoidal tissue at the age when orofacial cleft surgery is performed. In fact, adenotonsillar hypertrophy is the leading cause of obstructive sleep disordered breathing in young children and the leading indication for adenotonsillectomy. Children with cleft palate are already prone to development of obstructive sleep apnea due to a narrow airway. Furthermore, bulky tonsils can hinder retrodisplacement of the soft palate or block airflow by obstructing the cavum, which has already been reduced in volume by the retrodisplacement and presence of the flap after palate repair. In addition to the latent danger of infection, the flap used in pharyngoplasty creates an obstruction that seriously complicates plans for subsequent adenotonsillectomy. Therefore, it might be preferable to remove the tonsils and adenoids a few months before pharyngoplasty if indicated. Small studies have advocated for adenotonsillectomy and cleft palate repair in one surgical procedure, reporting lower obstructive respiratory events postoperatively without negative speech effects.

Parents might question the logic behind adenotonsillectomy if they received information that adenoid removal in the case of a cleft palate might create or aggravate velar insufficiency by removing the adenoid tissue's compensation for a short or poorly mobile palate. However, once velar inadequacy is confirmed, these precautions are no longer justified. In fact, tonsillar hypertrophy can impair velopharyngeal closure due to impingement of its upper pole between the palate and the posterior pharyngeal wall. Therefore, tonsillectomy can improve speech. During tonsillectomy, it is important to leave the tonsillar pillars intact because their muscle structure has a vital physiologic role.

Abdel-Aziz M, El-Tahan AR, Abdel-Wahid A, Kamel A. Concomitant adenotonsillectomy and cleft palate repair in one sitting. *Eur Arch Otorhinolaryngol*. 2020;277:1133-1137.

Milczuk HA. Effects of oropharyngeal surgery on velopharyngeal competence. *Curr Opin Otolaryngol Head Neck Surg*. 2012;20:522-526.

B. Preoperative Evaluation and Preparation

B.1. What information do you need before closure of a cleft lip and palate?

The preoperative anesthetic evaluation provides the necessary information regarding the patient's general health, and includes the pertinent birth (if age appropriate) and medical history along with physical examination with relevant laboratory data. A baseline hemoglobin level, which is often low in very young infants (physiologic anemia of infancy reaches a nadir of 10-11 g/dL around 6-9 months), should be obtained.

A thorough airway history and exam should identify obstructive symptoms and predictors of difficult intubation. If Treacher Collins or Pierre Robin syndrome is suspected, a radiograph of the mandible can be helpful. The examination also offers a good opportunity to assess the family dynamics because parental cooperation is essential for proper postoperative care.

Periosteoplasty with cleft lip repair is a less extensive surgery than cleft palate repair, and is typically performed as soon as the segments are in alignment. The "Rule of 10s" was introduced in the 1960s, with modifications in 1976, as a set of criteria to mitigate risk in young infants regarding timing of repair. It was posited that a violation of any patient characteristics would confer an increased rate of postoperative complications from 7.6 to over 38%. Thresholds for surgical candidacy were:

- *Weight*—Greater than 10 lb
- *Hemoglobin*— Greater than 10 g/dL
- *White blood cell count*—Less than 10,000/μL
- *Age*—Greater than 10 weeks

Since the initial recommendation over 50 years ago, considerable advances have been made in the anesthetic, surgical, and perioperative care of pediatric patients. More recent studies show that of the original metrics, only weight below 10 lb (4.5 kg) at the time of surgery was identified as an independent predictor of overall complications in cleft patients, which has led to a shift toward earlier cleft lip repair. Nonetheless, preoperative screening is essential in patients with cleft lip and palate, as underlying cardiac abnormalities dramatically increase the risk of perioperative morbidity. If a cleft occurs as part of a syndrome, an echocardiogram should be performed, especially if a murmur is present. Other independent risk factors for increased complications include decreasing weight and preoperative ventilator dependence.

General health, growth, reflux, feeding difficulties, and recent infection must be considered. With an open cleft palate, it is common to have crusting and low-grade infection of the nasopharynx because of food and fluid regurgitation through the cleft. It is impossible to eliminate this completely. Unless an acute inflammatory process is present, this does not lead to further complications.

Chow I, Purnell CA, Hanwright PJ, Gosain AK. Evaluating the rule of 10s in cleft lip repair: do data support dogma? *Plast Reconstr Surg*. 2016;138:670-679.

Ganske IM, Rogers-Vizena CR. Cleft lip and palate: principles and treatment. In: Chung KC, ed. *Grabb and Smith's Plastic Surgery*. 9th ed. Wolters Kluwer; 2025:183-196.

Schafer S, Card E, Liao EC. Cleft lip and palate: embryology and genetics. In: Chung KC, ed. *Grabb and Smith's Plastic Surgery*. 9th ed. Wolters Kluwer; 2025:197-208.

B.2. What preoperative orders are needed?

Preoperative fasting is a prerequisite for elective surgery to reduce the risk of perioperative pulmonary aspiration. Fasting guidelines for infants and children in the United States follow the American Society of Anesthesiologists Guidelines (**Table 42.1**). It is important to avoid prolonged fasting times which lead to increased patient discomfort, caregiver dissatisfaction, and other adverse outcomes (dehydration, metabolic disturbances, hypoglycemia, difficult vascular access, arterial hypotension with induction, nausea, and vomiting).

TABLE 42.1 Minimum Fasting Period for Pediatric Patients

Clear fluids	2 h
Breast milk	4 h
Formula/Nonhuman milk/Light meal (eg, toast)	6 h
Solids (eg, fried or fatty foods)	8 h

Because multiple operations can be required, the emotional trauma of each hospital experience must be minimized. The most common premedication in pediatric patients is oral midazolam at doses from 0.25 to 0.5 mg/kg orally. Children younger than 8 months rarely require premedication. Children with anticipated difficulty in airway management and those with a propensity toward airway obstruction are safer without premedication.

The anesthesiologist might consider topical (eutectic mixture of local anesthetics, cream) or subcutaneous local anesthetic prior to peripheral venous access in patients with an expected difficult airway or for infants less than 6 months old if prolonged fasting is anticipated. This allows for the expeditious administration of emergency medications in the former and hydration with dextrose-containing fluids to avoid hypoglycemia in the latter.

Special orders include antibiotics if the infant or child has associated congenital heart disease and typing and crossmatching of blood for palatal surgery.

Practice guidelines for preoperative fasting and the use of pharmacologic agents to reduce the risk of pulmonary aspiration: application to healthy patients undergoing elective procedures: an updated report by the American Society of Anesthesiologists Task Force on preoperative fasting and the use of pharmacologic agents to reduce the risk of pulmonary aspiration. *Anesthesiology.* 2017;126:376-393.

Wright M and Sury M. Anxiety, Psychological Preparation, Awareness, and Behavior Change. In: Andropoulous DB & Gregory GA, ed. *Gregory's Pediatric Anesthesia.* 6th ed. Wiley-Blackwell; 2020: 298-305

B.3. What airway equipment would you prepare in the operating room?

A plan for challenging mask ventilation and tracheal intubation should be made. Airway adjuvants, including nasal and oropharyngeal airways, an intubating laryngeal mask airway, a fiberoptic bronchoscope, and a videolaryngoscope should be in the operating room and prepared for use.

C. Intraoperative Management

C.1. What monitors will you need for cheiloplasty and palatoplasty?

Heart rate (electrocardiogram), noninvasive blood pressure (NIBP), pulse oximetry, end-tidal carbon dioxide ($EtCO_2$), and temperature (choice of nasal/rectal/axillary) are monitored at all times. Once the surgery has begun, the anesthesiologist no longer has easy direct access to the airway. Therefore, the use of pulse oximetry and end-tidal CO_2 monitors is indispensable. A warming blanket should be used to avoid hypothermia. Blood loss determination should be made by a calibrated catchment trap in the suction line and by weighing sponges. Blood loss rarely exceeds 10% of circulating blood volume; however, properly crossmatched and screened blood should be available but used only if necessary.

C.2. Discuss the induction and management of anesthesia for cleft lip and palate in this nonsyndromic, otherwise healthy infant.

After suitable monitors are attached, anesthesia is induced with 100% oxygen and an inhalational agent, most commonly sevoflurane (or halothane in countries where sevoflurane is not available). Once the patient is unresponsive, an intravenous line is established, and appropriate intravenous fluids are started. Spontaneous ventilation should be maintained if any possibility of difficulty with tracheal intubation exists until the glottic opening is visualized. Otherwise, intubation can be facilitated with a nondepolarizing neuromuscular blocking agent.

Laryngoscopy in patients with cleft lip is generally straightforward, but the cleft palate has the capability to trap and immobilize a straight blade. Should this occur, the anesthesiologist must first recognize the problem and then consider inserting a gauze pack or a dental roll in the cleft before laryngoscopy.

To achieve a cosmetic repair, symmetry is essential, so the endotracheal tube (ETT) should exit the mouth in the midline without facial distortion from either the ETT or the securing tape. Some surgeons prefer to suture the ETT to the lower gum.

An orogastric tube should be passed to empty the stomach of gas and secretions, and removed before preparation of the surgical field.

A pharyngeal pack of moistened ribbon gauze is inserted for cleft lip repair; for cleft palate repair, the surgeon inserts the gag before insertion of the pharyngeal pack. Following the gag and pack insertion, ventilation should be reassessed because tube compression may have occurred. To avert eye injury, an ocular lubricant is placed, and the upper eyelids are secured closed with tape.

The recommended maximal dose of lidocaine from surgical infiltration for palate or lip surgery is 5 mg/kg and of epinephrine 10 μg/kg. This epinephrine dose is for hypocarbic or normocarbic patients.

During the surgery, it is necessary to have good communication and cooperation between the surgeon and the anesthesiologist due to the very small yet important shared space.

Schindler E, Martini M, Messing-Jünger M. Anesthesia for Plastic and Craniofacial Surgery. In: Andropoulous DB & Gregory GA, ed. *Gregory's Pediatric Anesthesia*. 6th ed. Wiley-Blackwell; 2020: 923 – 924.

C.3. What positioning is recommended for cleft palate repair surgery?

Correct positioning of the child is important for the plastic surgeon, who sits at the head of the operating table. Head extension must be maximal for cleft palate surgery. The entire body is raised with a thick foam mat or folded blanket, allowing the head to drop back hyperextended into a head support. Not only does this position provide good surgical exposure, but it also allows blood to flow away from larynx and toward the nasopharynx so it can be removed by suction.

C.4. What are the reported complications of this type of surgery and anesthesia?

Anesthetic complications include obstruction of the ETT, inadvertent extubation during the procedure or positioning (neck extension), and cardiac arrest. Postanesthetic complications include airway obstruction, bleeding with or without aspiration, and pneumonia. Complications unrelated to anesthetic management include wound healing, diarrhea, and otitis media. The mortality rate has been reported to be less than 0.5%.

Schindler E, Martini M, Messing-Jünger M. Anesthesia for Plastic and Craniofacial Surgery. In: Andropoulous DB & Gregory GA, ed. *Gregory's Pediatric Anesthesia*. 6th ed. Wiley-Blackwell; 2020: 924 – 925.

C.5. Briefly describe the surgical techniques used to repair cleft defects.

The Furlow procedure is the most common technique for cleft palate closure. It involves opposing Z-plasties of the mucosa and the musculature of the soft palate. The goal is to separate the nonfunctioning attachments from the posterior border of the hard palate and to displace the mucosa and the musculature posteriorly. Other basic surgical techniques include the von Langenbeck technique, the Schweckendiek technique, the two-flap technique, and the three-flap/V-Y technique. Although most of the repairs do not involve repairing the muscular sling, doing so allows better palatal and eustachian tube function.

Sadove AM, van Aalst JA, Culp JA. Cleft palate repair: art and issues. *Clin Plast Surg*. 2004;31:231-241.

C.6. How does a pharyngeal flap affect anesthetic management or any subsequent anesthetic administered to this patient?

In the early postoperative period after the "pushback" and pharyngeal flap operation (pharyngoplasty), significant airway obstruction can occur, with sleeping pulse oximetry demonstrating hemoglobin desaturation in the first 48 to 72 hours. The degree of obstruction is related to the width of the flap. For subsequent procedures, knowledge of prior surgical interventions is essential. The pharyngoplasty makes nasotracheal intubation (and other transnasal procedures such as insertion of a nasogastric tube) more difficult (eg, for orthognathic or dental surgeries typically requiring a nasal ETT). Traumatic rupture of this flap secondary to attempted nasotracheal intubation could produce bleeding, aspiration, and laryngospasm. While it is generally avoided, methods such as fiberoptic assistance or a Seldinger technique over a well-lubricated red rubber catheter with direct visualization have been utilized. One should consider nasal endoscopy evaluation in the otolaryngoscopy clinic to assess the size, position, and shape of the velopharyngeal port in all patients who underwent a pharyngoplasty and are scheduled to have a nasotracheal intubation. This might be difficult in younger, uncooperative patients.

Traumatic rupture of soft palate can also occur from placement of a laryngeal mask airway, most likely during insertion or if a rotational technique is used.

Cohen MD, Ahmed Z, Zestos M, Hildebrand J. A novel approach to nasotracheal intubation in pediatric patients with prior palate or pharyngeal surgery. Accessed March 26, 2025. https://www2.pedsanesthesia.org/meetings/2007winter/pdfs/CR68.pdf

Dearlove O, Perkins RJ, Briggs G. Anaesthesia after cleft palate repair. *Anaesthesia*. 2004;59:1032.

Somerville NS, Fenlon S, Boorman J, et al. Disruption of cleft palate repair following the use of the laryngeal mask airway. *Anaesthesia*. 2004;59:401-403.

C.7. What is an Abbe flap? What are its anesthetic implications?

An Abbe flap is a full-thickness pedicle flap taken from the lower lip and rotated on its own artery to a position in the upper lip to replace a tissue deficit resulting from any cause, such as surgical excision of malignancy or loss of tissue in a bilateral cleft lip. The lips must remain closed until the flap "takes" to allow for neovascularization. Then, it can be detached from its blood supply. Usually, this operation is performed in older children under local anesthesia, but it occasionally requires general anesthesia if the patient is young. All the problems of a closed mouth, such as the possibility of vomiting and aspiration, are encountered in addition to those associated with preservation of the flap.

Koshy JC, Ellsworth WA, Sharabi SE, et al. Bilateral cleft lip revisions: the Abbe flap. *Plast Reconstr Surg.* 2010;126:221-227.

C.8. What are the crucial anesthetic concerns for cleft palate repair? What are the unique considerations of this surgical repair?

Establishment, maintenance, and protection of the airway are the crucial goals of anesthesia for palate surgery. Failure to achieve these aims can result in tachypnea, hypercarbia, hypoxemia, increased bleeding, hypovolemia, arrhythmia, cardiac arrest, and death. The major cause of cardiac arrest in infants and children is hypoxemia.

Positioning of the patient is usually supine with the table rotated 90° to 180°. A preformed oral RAE (Ring-Adair-Elwyn) or reinforced ETT extends down the midline of the jaw taped to the chin. This type of ETT allows for easier visualization of the airway and decreased risk of inadvertent kinking intraoperatively. The mouth gag that is used for surgical exposure can be released intermittently to allow tongue reperfusion. However, each manipulation can affect positioning of the ETT. Blood that collects in the oropharynx should be carefully suctioned at the end of the procedure without disrupting the suture line. Residual blood and secretions in the oropharyngeal cavity can irritate the larynx and cause laryngospasm.

Schendel SA, Yi Sun N, Agarwal R, Furukawa LK. Surgery for craniofacial malformations. In: Jaffe RA, Schmiesing CA, Golianu B, eds. *Anesthesiologist's Manual of Surgical Procedures.* 6th ed. Wolters Kluwer; 2020:1597-1628.

C.9. What is laryngospasm? How would you make a diagnosis of laryngospasm?

Laryngospasm is defined as glottic closure resulting from a reflex constriction of the laryngeal muscles. It is much more common in pediatric than adult patients. In the pediatric patient, oxygen consumption is greater and inversely correlated with age, so the consequences of laryngospasm are more serious.

Laryngospasm can occur during anesthesia for two main reasons: a lack of inhibition of glottic reflexes because of central nervous system depression, and an increased number of triggering stimuli such as manipulation of the airway, secretions or blood irritating the vocal cords, and stimulation of visceral nerve endings at an inadequate depth of anesthesia. Airway complications are further increased in children with upper respiratory tract infections.

Fiadjoe J, Stricker P, Litman R. Pediatric Airway Management. In: Andropoulous DB & Gregory GA, ed. *Gregory's Pediatric Anesthesia*. 6th ed. Wiley-Blackwell; 2020: 340-341.

C.10. How would you manage the patient with laryngospasm?

Laryngospasm can be partial or complete. Partial laryngospasm can be diagnosed by a characteristic stridulous noise and a mismatch between respiratory effort and the small movements of the reservoir bag.

Methods of overcoming laryngospasm include applying continuous positive pressure to the airway with 100% inspired oxygen, deepening the level of anesthesia, and administering neuromuscular blockers or a bolus of propofol. A bolus of propofol works quickly, without the side effects of succinylcholine, by increasing the depth of anesthesia or a direct effect on the glottis.

When there is complete laryngospasm, there is no air movement or breath sounds. The application of positive pressure might not be helpful in this circumstance and indeed could make the situation worse by forcing the false cords against the tightly closed true cords. It is much better to relax the cords before hypoxemia becomes severe. A small dose of succinylcholine can be given intramuscularly or intravenously to relax laryngospasm.

Fiadjoe J, Stricker P, Litman R. Pediatric Airway Management. In: Andropoulous DB & Gregory GA, ed. *Gregory's Pediatric Anesthesia*. 6th ed. Wiley-Blackwell; 2020: 340-341.

D. Postoperative Management

D.1. What complications of cleft lip and cleft palate surgery can be seen in the recovery room?

The most important issue for the anesthesiologist is maintenance of an airway. Postextubation obstruction is more likely due to a combination of a closed palate, a small mandible pushing the tongue into a small pharynx, swelling (hypopharyngeal, subglottic, or flap edema), blood, and the residual effects of anesthesia. There could also be swelling of the tongue due to mouth gag placement during surgery. In the case of a pushback procedure with or without a pharyngeal flap, the obstruction is due to the new posterior position of the palate and the pharyngeal flap.

The anesthesiologist must also be aware of potential problems such as bleeding, neurosensory disturbances, increased oral secretions, a retained throat pack, and hypothermia. Blood loss is not an anesthetic complication, but its replacement is an anesthesiologist's responsibility, as is prevention of aspiration. Patients can experience paresthesias in the cheek after surgery. Very rarely, the sensory disturbance can be permanent. Hypothermia delays emergence and can produce metabolic acidosis and respiratory and myocardial depression.

Cladis F, Grunwaldt L, Losee J. Anesthesia for Plastic Surgery. In: Davis PJ & Cladis, FP, ed. *Smith's Anesthesia for Infants and Children*. 10th ed. Elsevier; 2021: 957-963.

Goldstein JA, Baker SB. Rodriguez ED, Losee JE, Neligan PC. Cleft and craniofacial orthognathic surgery. *Plastic Surgery. Craniofacial, Head and Neck Surgery and Pediatric Plastic Surgery*. Vol 3. 4th ed. Elsevier; 2018:660-677.

D.2. How do you protect the airway postoperatively?

Following palatoplasty, the pharynx and nasopharynx are carefully suctioned before tracheal extubation. Some anesthesiologists advocate that this should be done with the aid of the laryngoscope to ensure removal of any mucus, blood, or clots. If suctioning is done before removing the Dingman gag, the laryngoscope might not be necessary. The infant should be as awake as possible. A long traction suture is placed through the tongue, tied loosely, and taped to the outside cheek for easy access. Traction on the suture stimulates respiration and clears the airway. Neither an oral nor a nasal airway should be inserted unless absolutely necessary; either one could disrupt the sutures and undo the surgical repair. The traction suture is removed when the infant leaves the recovery room.

Following palate surgery, the infant is placed in a prone or lateral position with the head dependent, turned to the side, and extended. This position can be achieved with a jack placed under the foot of the crib or by placing a bulky bath blanket under the hips of the infant. Any blood or mucus will accumulate in the dependent cheek or drain out of the mouth.

Following cleft lip surgery, a Logan bow is frequently used to take the tension off the newly sutured lip. The infant can still be placed in the lateral position. Elbow restraints are applied before leaving the operating room. A high-humidity atmosphere is recommended postoperatively to reduce the incidence of tracheitis, but benefit has not been clearly demonstrated.

Cladis F, Grunwaldt L, Losee J. Anesthesia for Plastic Surgery. In: Davis PJ & Cladis, FP, ed. *Smith's Anesthesia for Infants and Children*. 10th ed. Elsevier; 2021: 957-963.

D.3. How would you control postoperative pain in patients following a cleft lip and cleft palate repair? Describe a multimodal analgesic plan including regional anesthesia options.

Cleft lip and cleft palate repairs are painful procedures that can lead to patient distress and adverse physiologic consequences if not appropriately managed. No child should be discharged from the postanesthesia care unit with uncontrolled pain, and this management continues to the pediatric intensive care unit or ward bed.

Nerve blocks can provide analgesia with less perioperative consumption of opioids and its associated adverse outcomes, such as airway complications (respiratory depression, airway obstruction, and desaturation), postoperative nausea, vomiting, and delayed oral intake.

The infraorbital nerve block can be used for cleft lip repair. This nerve is a branch of the maxillary nerve (pure sensory nerve), which is the second division (V2) of the trigeminal nerve. It exits the infraorbital foramen then supplies sensation to the upper lip, lower eyelid, nasal ala, and the maxillary process. It may be blocked by either the extraoral or intraoral approach, with the latter being more common. The procedure involves everting the upper lip and injecting a small volume (0.5 mL) of local anesthetic into the sulcus of the buccal mucosa opposing the second bicuspid tooth. The needle is directed superiorly and parallel to the second bicuspid until it is palpated externally near the foramen. Several small studies favor the infraorbital nerve block over placebo, local infiltration, and intravenous analgesics due to lower pain scores, time to first rescue analgesic, and shorter time to first feeding without significant adverse events, while others demonstrate conflicting results. Larger, multicenter trials with more rigorous methodology are needed to identify optimal technique and dosing.

For cleft palate repair, nasopalatine and palatine nerve blocks provide palatal hard and soft tissue anesthesia. In infants, the greater palatine foramen is typically located behind the posterior molar. This regional procedure involves a syringe directed into the mouth from the opposite side at a right angle to

TABLE 42.2 Recommended Opioid Analgesics for Pediatric Patients

Drugs	Dosage	Form
Fentanyl	1 μg/kg	IV
Morphine	0.05-0.1 mg/kg	IV
Meperidine	1 mg/kg	IV
Oxycodone	0.15 mg/kg	PO: 5-mg tablets; syrup 5 mg/mL

IV, intravenous; PO, by mouth.

the target with the needle bevel toward the palatal soft tissue. The greater palatine nerve block anesthetizes the palatal mucosa and hard palate from the first premolar anteriorly to the posterior part of the hard palate. The lesser palatine nerve block is similar and provides analgesia to the soft palate. The nasopalatine nerve block is performed at the incisive foramen. It cannot be performed in complete clefts where the premaxilla is not developed or is malformed.

Suprazygomatic maxillary nerve blocks can also be used for effective pain relief of cleft palate repair by anesthetizing the entire sensory distribution of the maxillary nerve and its terminal branches. The needle is inserted perpendicularly at the angle formed by the superior edge of the zygomatic arch below and the posterior orbital rim forward. The needle is advanced perpendicularly to the skin until it reaches the greater wing of the sphenoid (~2 cm), then withdrawn and reoriented in an anterior/caudal direction (toward the nasolabial fold) and advanced further to 3.5 to 4.5 cm to reach the pterygopalatine fossa. Local anesthetic (0.1-0.15 mL/kg/side) is slowly injected after negative aspiration. Real-time, ultrasound guidance, with the transducer placed in the infrazygomatic area, allows visualization of the pterygopalatine fossa, identification of the maxillary artery, needle tip localization, and visualization of spread within the pterygopalatine fossa.

All these techniques have been shown to have very minimal adverse side effects and can be performed safely in anesthetized patients.

Opioid analgesics that can be used postoperatively are shown in **Table 42.2**.

Nonopioid analgesics that can be used postoperatively are shown in **Table 42.3**. Dexmedetomidine can be used for both analgesic properties and to decrease emergence excitation.

Chiono J, Raux O, Bringuier S, et al. Bilateral suprazygomatic maxillary nerve block for cleft palate repair in children: a prospective, randomized, double-blind study versus placebo. *Anesthesiology*. 2014;120:1362-1369.

Cho HK, Yoon HY, Jin HJ, Hwang SH. Efficacy of dexmedetomidine for perioperative morbidities in pediatric tonsillectomy: a metaanalysis. *Laryngoscope*. 2018;128:E184-E193.

Feriani G, Hatanaka E, Torloni MR, da Silva EMK. Infraorbital nerve block for postoperative pain following cleft lip repair in children. *Cochrane Database Syst Rev*. 2016;4:CD011131.

Lonnqvist PA, Morton NS. Paediatric day-case anaesthesia and pain control. *Curr Opin Anaesthesiol*. 2006;19:617-621.

Nardi NM, Alvarado AC, Schaefer TJ. *Infraorbital Nerve Block*. StatPearls Publishing; 2022.

TABLE 42.3 Recommended Nonopioid Analgesics for Pediatric Patients

Drug	Dosage	Forms Available
Acetaminophen (Tylenol)	10-15 mg/kg PO maximum 2,600 mg/d	Tablets: 80 mg Syrup: 325 mg/5 mL Suppositories: 120, 325, 650 mg
Ibuprofen (Motrin)	10-20 mg/kg PO q6h	Tablets: 300, 400 mg Syrup: 100 mg/5 mL
Ketorolac (Toradol)	0.5 mg/kg IV to load (maximum dose 30 mg) 0.5 mg/kg q8h intramuscularly or intravenously (limit use to 48 h)	Parenteral form used IM/IV
Dexmedetomidine	0.3-1 μg/kg IV	IV

IV, intravenous; PO, by mouth.

43 Congenital Heart Disease With a Cervical Mass in Infancy

Miles Dinner and Elizabeth Starker Pealy

A 1-week-old male infant was diagnosed shortly after birth with an interrupted aortic arch (IAA). The workup revealed the child to have a 22q11 deletion syndrome (formerly known as *DiGeorge syndrome*). An enlarging cervical mass was noted, and the child was brought to the operating room for exploration.

A. Medical Disease and Differential Diagnosis

1. What is 22q11 deletion syndrome?
2. What are the associated cardiovascular defects in 22q11 deletion syndrome?
3. What are the metabolic and endocrine abnormalities in patients with 22q11 deletion syndrome and the attendant manifestations?
4. What are the immunologic findings in 22q11 deletion syndrome?
5. What is the differential diagnosis of cervical masses in infancy?
6. What is a cystic hygroma? What are the complications? What is the treatment?
7. What is the IAA anomaly?
8. What is the pathophysiology of the IAA syndrome?
9. How is ductal patency maintained?
10. What are the side effects of prostaglandin infusion?
11. What is the hyperoxia test?

B. Preoperative Evaluation and Preparation

1. What preoperative studies should be obtained to evaluate the neck mass?
2. How would you categorize the difficult airway in children?
3. What features of the difficult airway can be noted on physical examination?
4. How would you preoperatively optimize the ability to secure the airway in the operating room?
5. What laboratory studies are necessary before surgery?
6. What are the causes of heart failure (HF) in this infant? How would you assess this infant in your preoperative evaluation for signs of HF?
7. How would you optimize the preoperative treatment of HF?
8. How would you premedicate this infant?
9. When is premedication useful in infants and children?
10. Before the planned surgery, the infant is scheduled for a magnetic resonance imaging (MRI) scan. You are asked to ensure that the baby remains immobile for 20 minutes to perform the scan adequately. How would you accomplish this?

C. Intraoperative Management

1. What anesthesia equipment, circuit, and monitors would you use?
2. Describe techniques other than direct laryngoscopy that would be useful for securing the airway in this baby.
3. How would you monitor blood loss in this patient?
4. What anesthetic technique should be used in a patient who may experience severe loss of blood intraoperatively?
5. How would you induce and maintain anesthesia?
6. Intraoperatively, the surgeon must dissect the tumor in the anterior mediastinum and needs to have a quiet surgical field. How would you accomplish this?

D. Postoperative Management

1. How would you manage this patient postoperatively?

A. Medical Disease and Differential Diagnosis

A.1. What is 22q11 deletion syndrome?

The 22q11 deletion syndrome is one of the most common multiple anomaly syndromes in humans and has historically been referred to as velocardiofacial syndrome, DiGeorge sequence, conotruncal anomalies face syndrome, CATCH 22, and Sedlackova syndrome, all different names describing the same disorder. This syndrome has an expansive phenotype with more than 180 clinical features that can involve every organ and system. The syndrome is caused by a microdeletion of chromosome 22 at the q11.2 band. The syndrome has a prevalence of approximately 1 in 3,000 to 6,000 live births in the United States. About 6% to 10% of cases are inherited, while the remainder are due to de novo mutations.

The majority of patients have a constellation of abnormalities resulting from an embryogenic disruption in the formation of the third and fourth aortic arches. The common clinical features are hypocalcemia, immunodeficiency, dysmorphic facial features, palatal and velopharyngeal dysfunction, renal anomalies, congenital heart disease (CHD), and intellectual disability. The DiGeorge variant is characterized by thymic and parathyroid aplasia or hypoplasia, cardiovascular defects, and dysmorphic facies. Depending on the extent of the thymic hypoplasia, clinical manifestations can range from frequent upper respiratory tract infections to severe immunodeficiency that can only be corrected with T-cell-replete hematopoietic stem cell transplantation (HSCT) or thymus transplantation.

Bartik LE, Hughes SS, Tracy M, et al. 22q11.2 duplications: expanding the clinical presentation. *Am J Med Genet A.* 2022;188:779-787.

Campbell IM, Sheppard SE, Crowley TB, et al. What is new with 22q? An update from the 22q and You Center at the Children's Hospital of Philadelphia. *Am J Med Genet A.* 2018;176:2058-2069.

Cirillo A, Lioncino M, Maratea A, et al. Clinical manifestations of 22q11.2 deletion syndrome. *Heart Fail Clin.* 2022;18:155-164.

Goldmuntz E. 22q11.2 deletion syndrome and congenital heart disease. *Am J Med Genet C Semin Med Genet.* 2020;184:64-72.

A.2. What are the associated cardiovascular defects in 22q11 deletion syndrome?

Congenital heart defects are found in 60% to 80% of patients with 22q11 deletion syndrome. Most of these patients have conotruncal defects with additional anomalies of the aortic arch, pulmonary arteries, infundibular septum, and semilunar valves. The most common abnormalities include tetralogy of Fallot, pulmonary atresia with ventricular septal defect (VSD), truncus arteriosus (TA), IAA, isolated anomalies of the aortic arch, and VSD. These defects arise during the crucial developmental stages of the truncoconal parts of the heart from the pharyngeal pouch derivatives. The American Heart Association now recommends screening fetal, pediatric, and adult patients for 22q11.2 deletion syndrome if the patient is diagnosed with the specific cardiac anomalies listed earlier. Echocardiography, computed tomography (CT), and cardiac MRI are important in defining the cardiac and associated anatomy in detail. These modalities can provide an invaluable understanding of the anatomy required for presurgical planning.

Cirillo A, Lioncino M, Maratea A, et al. Clinical manifestations of 22q11.2 deletion syndrome. *Heart Fail Clin.* 2022;18:155-164.

Friedman K. Preoperative physiology, imaging, and management of interrupted aortic arch. *Semin Cardiothorac Vasc Anesth.* 2018;22:265-269.

Goldmuntz E. 22q11.2 deletion syndrome and congenital heart disease. *Am J Med Genet C Semin Med Genet.* 2020;184:64-72.

A.3. What are the metabolic and endocrine abnormalities in patients with 22q11 deletion syndrome and the attendant manifestations?

Because of errors in embryogenesis of the third and fourth pharyngeal arches, parathyroid hypoplasia or aplasia is common and results in hypocalcemia. The prevalence of hypocalcemia in this patient population ranges from 32% to 80%. Hypocalcemia can be transient in neonates or can be permanent, requiring calcium and vitamin D supplementation. Because hypocalcemia can be difficult to detect in the neonate, a high index of suspicion is necessary if a neonate exhibits irritability, jitteriness, twitching, seizure activity, failure to thrive, tachycardia, and hypotension. Stridor (which needs to be differentiated from laryngeal web, which is also prevalent in 22q11 deletion syndrome) and carpopedal spasm can also occur. It is important to remember that in patients with this syndrome, hypocalcemia can be precipitated by the stress of surgery and by increased needs during puberty or pregnancy. Chronic hypocalcemia can result in poor dentition that is prone to caries.

The prevalence of thyroid disease is significantly higher in the pediatric population with 22q11 deletion syndrome than in the general pediatric population. Some sources suggest that screening for thyroid disease, including blood tests for thyroid function and immunity, as well as a thyroid ultrasound, should be added to the routine medical management of these children.

Lin HY, Tsai WY, Tung YC, et al. Endocrine and growth disorders in Taiwanese children with 22q11.2 deletion syndrome. *Front Endocrinol (Lausanne)*. 2022;13:771100.

Ricci S, Sarli WM, Lodi L, et al. Characterization of autoimmune thyroid disease in a cohort of 73 paediatric patients affected by 22q11.2 deletion syndrome: longitudinal single-centre study. *Genes (Basel)*. 2022;13:1552.

Root AW. Disorders of Mineral Metabolism: Normal homeostasis. In: Sperling MA, ed. *Pediatric Endocrinology*. 5th ed. Elsevier Health Sciences; 2021:220-278.

A.4. What are the immunologic findings in 22q11 deletion syndrome?

Patients with this syndrome demonstrate marked variability in their immune system, ranging from complete thymic aplasia to reduced T-cell counts and function. The majority of patients (~75%) have a decrease in the total number of T cells, and approximately 1.5% of patients have complete thymic aplasia requiring transplant. Reduced levels of immunoglobulin A (IgA) and immunoglobulin M (IgM) also occur more frequently compared to the general population. Almost all patients have a tendency toward infection, particularly of the respiratory tract. As long as there is a working thymus, patients with 22q11 deletion syndrome can be immunized and generate a good antibody response because humoral immunity is usually intact. However, poor vaccine-specific antibody responses have been described. Neonatal diagnosis historically relied on fluorescence in situ hybridization (FISH) testing and phenotype recognition. However, T-cell receptor excision circles (TRECs) and polymerase chain reaction (PCR) testing are now included in the newborn screening panel for severe combined immunodeficiency (SCID). This allows for early identification of 22q11.2 deletion syndrome patients with severe T-cell lymphopenia. In addition, cell-free DNA from maternal serum might help identify these patients in utero. Autoimmune conditions are found in up to a third of patients, the most common being juvenile chronic arthritis, autoimmune thrombocytopenia, hemolytic anemia, Raynaud phenomena, and autoimmune thyroid disease.

Kuo CY, Signer R, Saitta SC. Immune and genetic features of chromosome 22q11.2 deletion (DiGeorge syndrome). *Curr Allergy Asthma Rep*. 2018;18:75.

Sullivan KE. Chromosome 22q11.2 deletion syndrome and DiGeorge syndrome. *Immunol Rev*. 2019;287:186-201.

Urschel D, Hernandez-Trujillo VP. Spectrum of genetic T-cell disorders from 22q11.2DS to CHARGE. *Clin Rev Allergy Immunol*. 2022;63:99-105.

A.5. What is the differential diagnosis of cervical masses in infancy?

Neck masses can originate from a congenital anatomic anomaly, infection, or neoplasm. Congenital anomalies consist of branchial and thyroglossal duct cysts and failed thymic descents. In the embryo, branchial cysts arise from the thymic stalk or the pharyngeal pouch and can be present at birth or develop later. They lie beneath the sternocleidomastoid muscle and can bulge out from its anterior border. The branchial cysts can become infected and enlarge to the extent that they compress the airway or upper esophagus. Thyroglossal duct cysts are spherical, midline masses that can extend back to the base of the tongue and represent all of the neonate's thyroid tissue. In the embryo, the thymus gland arises high in the neck and descends into the anterior mediastinum. If there is any interruption of this caudal movement, the thymus can appear as a soft, compressible mass anywhere along the anterior border of the sternocleidomastoid muscle.

Infectious masses can be due to tuberculosis, Epstein-Barr viral infection, cellulitic facial infections (Ludwig angina), and subacute regional lymphadenitis (cat scratch disease). Noninfectious causes include Kawasaki disease, sarcoidosis, Rosai-Dorfman disease, and histiocytic necrotizing lymphadenitis.

Neoplastic masses in the cervical region can be teratomas, hemangiomas, neurofibromas, lymphomas, goiters, or cystic hygromas. Teratomas are firm, midline masses arising adjacent to the thyroid isthmus. Hemangiomas may be extensive, consequently compressing vital structures. Neurofibromas may arise individually or as a consequence of neurofibromatosis (von Recklinghausen disease) and can be very large. Goiters are enlarged thyroid glands that present as a hypothyroid, hyperthyroid, or euthyroid state. Ultrasound, CT, and MRI are the imaging modalities used most often to determine the nature of a neonatal neck mass.

Levine MC, Arroyo A, Likourezos A, Homel P, Dickman E. The use of point of care ultrasound in the evaluation of pediatric soft tissue neck masses. *Am J Emerg Med.* 2019;37:1466-1469.

Thorell EA. Cervical lympadenitis and neck infections. In: Long SS, Prober CG, Fischer M, eds. *Principles and Practice of Pediatric infectious Diseases.* 6th ed. Elsevier; 2023:142-153.

A.6. What is a cystic hygroma? What are the complications? What is the treatment?

Cystic hygroma is a developmental malformation of the lymphatic system found most often in the posterior triangle of the neck and axilla of children. They are divided into suprahyoid and subhyoid masses. They are compressible masses that are most often found in infants younger than 1 year and can intermittently enlarge. Suprahyoid masses can be extremely difficult to manage because of the associated obstructive symptoms, feeding difficulties, and potential for infection, which can compromise airway patency. Surgical removal is the treatment of choice, but complete surgical removal of these masses is often impossible. Repeat debulking is sometimes the only treatment. The mortality of a prenatally diagnosed cystic hygroma remains high, due to other comorbidities and the risk of airway obstruction. Therefore, tracheal intubation at delivery while maintaining uninterrupted maternal-fetal circulation until the airway is secured (ex utero intrapartum treatment [EXIT] procedure) has been performed to prevent the fatal consequences of immediate postnatal airway obstruction. Other treatment modalities include radiofrequency ablation, CO_2 laser therapy, and percutaneous sclerotherapy. Bleomycin, doxycycline, OK432, and tetracycline have been used as sclerosing agents with favorable results.

Behera S, Bawa M, Kanojia RP, Saha PK, Singh T, Samujh R. Outcome of antenatally diagnosed cystic hygroma—lessons learnt. *Int J Pediatr Otorhinolaryngol.* 2020;138:110227.

Boruga VM, Szilagyi DN, Prodea M, et al. Cystic hygroma of the neck-case report. *Rom J Morph Embryol.* 2021;62:845-848.

Damaskos C, Garmpis N, Manousi M, et al. Cystic hygroma of the neck: single center experience and literature review. *Eur Rev Med Pharmacol Sci.* 2017;21:4918-4923.

Laje P, Tharakan SJ, Hedrick HL. Immediate operative management of the fetus with airway anomalies resulting from congenital malformations. *Semin Fetal Neonatal Med.* 2016;21:240-245.

Levine MC, Arroyo A, Likourezos A, Homel P, Dickman E. The use of point of care ultrasound in the evaluation of pediatric soft tissue neck masses. *Am J Emerg Med.* 2019;37:1466-1469.

A.7. What is the IAA anomaly?

An IAA anomaly is extremely rare and represents approximately 1% of CHD. In IAA, there is complete aorta atresia somewhere along its arch, which is usually associated with a VSD and other complex cardiovascular anomalies. This defect is categorized into three types depending on where the atresia occurs. Left untreated, it is uniformly lethal within 1 week of life as a result of closure of the ductus arteriosus. In type A (30%), the aorta is interrupted between the left subclavian artery and the aortic isthmus. In type B (the most common, 65%-70%), the interruption lies between the left common carotid and the left subclavian arteries. With type C (least common type, <1%), the arch is interrupted between the innominate and the left common carotid arteries. About 50% of patients with IAA have the 22q11.2 deletion, which is usually associated with a more proximal location of the arch interruption (type B).

Friedman, K. Preoperative physiology, imaging, and management of interrupted aortic arch. *Semin Cardiothorac Vasc Anesth.* 2018;22:265-269.

Goldmuntz E. 22q11.2 deletion syndrome and congenital heart disease. *Am J Med Genet C Semin Med Genet.* 2020;184:64-72.

Ron HA, Crowley TB, Liu Y, et al. Improved outcomes in patients with 22q11.2 deletion syndrome and diagnosis of interrupted aortic arch prior to birth hospital discharge, a retrospective study. *Genes.* 2023;14:1-11.

Sanchez Mejia AA, Cambronero N, Dongarwar D, et al. Hospital outcomes among infants with interrupted aortic arch with simple and complex associated heart defects. *Am J Cardiol.* 2022;166:97-106.

A.8. What is the pathophysiology of the IAA syndrome?

IAA is a neonatal medical emergency. It warrants immediate infusion of prostaglandin E_1 (PGE_1) to maintain ductal patency as well as stabilization of coexisting HF. Due to the discontinuity between the descending aorta and the arch, blood flow to the descending aorta and its tributaries cannot occur unless

SECTION 10

the ductus arteriosus stays open. After medical stabilization, surgical correction should occur as soon as possible because of the risk of mortality in untreated IAA. Although there is no difference in mortality between patients with isolated TA malformations and TA-IAA, TA-IAA patients undergo surgery earlier and have a longer hospital length of stay.

The cause of death is usually a combination of greatly increased left-to-right shunt with increased pulmonary blood flow (which results in biventricular failure and pulmonary edema), ductal stenosis, the sequelae of renal failure, and metabolic acidosis. Pulse oximetry will reveal normal saturation in the right arm, with a decreased saturation in the lower extremities. If there is inadequate perfusion to the lower body because of ductal closure, death quickly ensues from the combination of increased left-to-right shunt with increased pulmonary blood flow via the VSD, biventricular congestive heart failure (CHF), pulmonary edema, renal insufficiency, severe metabolic acidosis, and shock. Symptoms of ductal closure include tachypnea, lethargy, and poor feeding. Transthoracic echocardiography is diagnostic. Cardiac CT, MRI, and catheterization are also utilized in the diagnosis of IAA.

Burbano-Vera N, Zaleski KL, Latham GJ, et al. Perioperative and anesthetic considerations of interrupted aortic arch. *Semin Cardiothorac Vasc Anesth.* 2018;22:270-277.

Friedman, K. Preoperative physiology, imaging, and management of interrupted aortic arch. *Semin Cardiothorac Vasc Anesth.* 2018;22:265-269.

Goldmuntz E. 22q11.2 deletion syndrome and congenital heart disease. *Am J Med Genet C Semin Med Genet.* 2020;184:64-72.

Jones BA, Conaway MR, Spaeder MC, Dean PN. Hospital survival after surgical repair of truncus arteriosus with interrupted aortic arch: results from a multi-institutional database. *Pediatr Cardiol.* 2021;42:1058-1063.

Bernstein D. Epidemiology and genetic basis of congenital heart disease. In: Kliegman RM, St. Geme JW, eds. *Nelson Textbook of Pediatrics.* 22nd ed. Elsevier; 2024:2763-2773.

A.9. How is ductal patency maintained?

The ductus arteriosus is kept open by infusion of PGE_1. Both PGE_1 and PGE_2 are produced endogenously in the ductus and metabolized in the lungs. Among the endogenous prostaglandins, PGE_2 is the most important. Postnatally, levels fall dramatically secondary to increased metabolism, resulting from the increase in pulmonary blood flow. A prostaglandin infusion will delay the natural closure of the ductus and improve systemic arterial perfusion and oxygenation. Less acidosis will also be seen in arterial blood gases compared to those obtained prior to PGE_1 infusion administration. In the case of an IAA, circulation to the lower body is completely dependent on the patency of the ductus; therefore, PGE_1 must be continuously infused to keep the infant alive. Of note, the PGE_1 infusion has a relatively long half-life; its inadvertent discontinuation will not acutely cause ductal closure, but it should be maintained until surgical repair is complete.

Burbano-Vera N, Zaleski KL, Latham GJ, et al. Perioperative and anesthetic considerations of interrupted aortic arch. *Semin Cardiothorac Vasc Anesth.* 2018;22:270-277.

Kliegman RM, St. Geme JW, Blum NG et al. Acyanotic congenital heart disease: obstructive lesions. In: Kliegman RM, St. Geme JW eds. *Nelson Textbook of Pediatrics.* 22nd ed. Elsevier; 2024:2787-2796.

Ron HA, Crowley TB, Liu Y, et al. Improved outcomes in patients with 22q11.2 deletion syndrome and diagnosis of interrupted aortic arch prior to birth hospital discharge, a retrospective study. *Genes.* 2023;14:1-11.

A.10. What are the side effects of prostaglandin infusion?

Prostaglandin has a wide array of side effects including fever, seizure-like activity, hypotension, flushing, and edema. Platelet aggregation can be reduced, and apnea with associated bradycardia can occur. This is most often seen in neonates weighing less than 2 kg at birth and usually appears during the first hour of initiating the drug infusion. Therefore, respiratory status should be monitored throughout treatment with mechanical ventilation as a consideration. It is recommended that a prostaglandin infusion be continuously administered via a separate intravenous line that can be monitored for any disruptions in flow.

Kliegman RM, St. Geme JW, Blum NJ, et al. Cyanotic congenital heart disease: lesions associated with increased pulmonary blood flow. In: Kliegman RM, St. Geme JW eds. *Nelson Textbook of Pediatrics.* 22nd ed. Elsevier; 2024:2811-2826.

A.11. What is the hyperoxia test?

In the past, the hyperoxia test was performed to distinguish pulmonary causes from cardiac causes of cyanosis. The patient is first administered 100% oxygen for 10 minutes. A preductal arterial blood gas is then taken from the patient's right arm. In patients with pulmonary disease, this supplemental oxygen significantly augments systemic oxygenation, which is not the case in cyanotic congenital heart defects.

However, in some pulmonary conditions, the oxygen tension might not rise significantly. In these patients, a chest radiograph is invaluable for affirming pulmonary pathology. In some congenital heart lesions with mixing (ie, TA), the supplemental oxygen decreases the pulmonary vascular resistance, which results in an increase in oxygen tension but rarely greater than 150 mm Hg. Although useful in differentiating pulmonary and cardiac causes of cyanosis, this test requires arterial blood sampling, which is invasive and difficult in neonates. In 2009, the American Academy of Pediatrics and the American Heart Association recommended pulse oximetry screening for improved critical CHD detection. Current guidelines recommend that infants be screened with pulse oximetry on the right hand and one foot at 24 hours of life, with a saturation of 95% or greater considered negative.

Geggel RL, Fulton DR. History, physical examination, oximetry, chest radiograph, and other baseline testing. In: Walsh EP, Mayer JE, Teele SA et al. *Nadas' Pediatric Cardiology*. 3rd ed. Elsevier; 2025:75-91.

Martin GR, Ewer AK, Gaviglio A, et al. Updated strategies for pulse oximetry screening for critical congenital heart disease. *Pediatrics*. 2020;146:1-10.

B. Preoperative Evaluation and Preparation

B.1. What preoperative studies should be obtained to evaluate the neck mass?

Because cervical masses have a variable nature and the potential for airway compression, studies must be done preoperatively. Flexible neonatal bronchoscopy can define extrinsic compressive deformations of the airway. Ultrasound, CT, and MRI of the head and neck can define the nature of the cystic hygroma and elucidate the degree of airway compression. These cysts are known to invade the anterior mediastinum and can cause extrinsic distortion of the lower airway anywhere from the cricoid ring to the carina. If a neoplastic lesion is suspected, nuclear medicine studies can be utilized to gain functional assessment and staging. Once diagnostic imaging is obtained, interventional radiology can be consulted for minimally invasive procedures. Under sonographic guidance, cystic fluid can be aspirated to reduce the size of the mass and potentially relieve compressive symptoms. Rarely, there is invasion into the pericardium and displacement of the lung. If the mass is suprahyoid, radiologic studies can reveal the degree of laryngeal compression and retropharyngeal involvement, which are vital to know prior to intubation.

Ho ML. Pediatric neck masses: imaging guidelines and recommendations. *Radiol Clin North Am*. 2022;60:1-14.

B.2. How would you categorize the difficult airway in children?

Children with difficult airways can be grouped into four main groups. The first group includes children who have congenital anomalies affecting the airway, such as vascular rings, laryngomalacia, micrognathia, or neurofibromatosis. The second group includes patients with an acutely acquired obstruction of the airway, such as trauma or foreign body. The third group includes infectious etiologies such as retropharyngeal abscess, laryngotracheobronchitis, or peritonsillar abscess. The fourth group includes children without known congenital or anatomic abnormalities who have unanticipated difficulty with intubation secondary to glottic visualization problems on direct laryngoscopy such that videolaryngoscopy is indicated.

Huang AS, Hajduk J, Rim C, Coffield S, Jagannathan N. Focused review on management of the difficult paediatric airway. *Indian J Anaesth*. 2019;63:428-436.

Stein ML, Park RS, Kovatsis PG. Emerging trends, techniques, and equipment for airway management in pediatric patients. *Paediatr Anaesth*. 2020;30:269-279.

Disma N, Asai T, Cools E, et al. Airway management in neonates and infants: European Society of Anaesthesiology and Intensive Care and British Journal of Anaesthesia joint guidelines. *Eur J Anaesthesiol*. 2024;41:3-23.

B.3. What features of the difficult airway can be noted on physical examination?

Many anatomic abnormalities can be noted simply by performing a thorough airway exam. Visual inspection of the size of the mouth can alert the anesthesiologist to a constricted oral opening that can be seen in conditions such as scleroderma, epidermolysis bullosa, or congenital microstomia, which could prevent insertion of a laryngoscope. Micrognathia or maxillary protrusion often accompanies an anterior larynx, making glottic visualization during direct laryngoscopy impossible. This is seen in children with craniofacial syndromes, such as Pierre Robin sequence, Treacher Collins syndrome, Apert syndrome, or Crouzon syndrome. Macroglossia as a consequence of certain metabolic storage diseases (ie, Hurler syndrome,

Hunter syndrome), cystic abnormalities, and hamartomatous tumors of the tongue (Goltz syndrome) can also make effective laryngoscopy impossible. Assessing the temporomandibular joint can reveal signs of ankylosis, which can occur in patients with juvenile rheumatoid arthritis and other autoimmune processes that can prevent adequate mouth opening. A narrow, high-arched palate can also suggest difficult tracheal intubation. One should evaluate a range of motion of the neck to reveal decreased neck extension, which can accompany some neuromuscular disorders, arthritic conditions, trauma, Klippel-Feil syndrome, or Goldenhar syndrome. Lastly, one should attempt to palpate the neck to assess for tracheal deviation. A preoperative chest radiograph might better serve to note tracheal deviation, as well as provide a baseline for the state of the lungs.

Huang AS, Hajduk J, Rim C, Coffield S, Jagannathan N. Focused review on management of the difficult paediatric airway. *Indian J Anaesth*. 2019;63:428-436.

Oliveira CRD. Pediatric syndromes with noncraniofacial anomalies impacting the airways. *Paediatr Anaesth*.2020;30:304-310.

B.4. How would you preoperatively optimize the ability to secure the airway in the operating room?

Because there are inherent risks in inducing anesthesia and securing the airway in this neonate, one would prepare for a combined supraglottic airway-fiberoptic intubation. The infant bronchoscope is so small in diameter that it does not accommodate a suction port, and visualization can be impaired by excessive secretions. An antisialagogue should be given at least 15 to 20 minutes before beginning the fiberoptic intubation to facilitate recognition of the anatomy. Glycopyrrolate (0.01 mg/kg intravenously [IV] or intramuscularly [IM]) will limit secretions without causing the excessive tachycardia that can occur with atropine. In this neonate with cardiac compromise, unnecessary stress on the heart should be avoided. In addition to a fiberoptic bronchoscope and appropriate laryngeal mask airway (LMA) being available, a videolaryngoscope and equipment trays for an emergency cricothyrotomy should also be ready. Having a pediatric otolaryngologist present for induction of anesthesia as well as a rigid infant bronchoscope with video imaging capability should also be considered. The rigid bronchoscope cannot only facilitate visualization of the laryngeal inlet, but it can also provide a route to temporarily ventilate the patient and hold the endotracheal tube as an introducing stylet to facilitate intubation. Passive oxygenation should also be utilized during intubation attempts to prolong the time to desaturation.

Apfelbaum JL, Hagberg CA, Connis RT, et al. 2022 American Society of Anesthesiologists practice guidelines for management of the difficult airway. *Anesthesiology*. 2022;136:31-81.

Stein ML, Park RS, Kovatsis PG. Emerging trends, techniques, and equipment for airway management in pediatric patients. *Paediatr Anaesth*. 2020;30:269-279.

B.5. What laboratory studies are necessary before surgery?

Serum calcium should be measured because of the strong association of 22q11 deletion syndrome with hypocalcemia. Serum glucose and sodium levels should be reviewed, as the infant will have been started on total parenteral nutrition due to the inability of oral feeding from dysphagia caused by the cystic hygroma. Because there is also the potential for severe metabolic acidosis secondary to inadequate perfusion of the lower body as a result of the IAA, serum pH and bicarbonate concentrations must be obtained. The $Paco_2$ will indicate baseline adequacy of ventilation in the face of a potentially obstructing mass, and the Pao_2 will serve as a guide in assessing the degree of CHF, pulmonary insufficiency, and central shunting. Because the surgery can be extensive with a significant loss of blood, a baseline complete blood count with hematocrit, as well as a type and screen, should be obtained. Prothrombin time and partial thromboplastin time should be obtained before surgery because of the possibility of baseline immaturity in coagulation factor production and the inherent bleeding potential from the large dissection that will be done.

B.6. What are the causes of heart failure (HF) in this infant? How would you assess this infant in your preoperative evaluation for signs of HF?

The causes of HF in this infant can be divided into five major areas:

- Cardiac rhythm disturbances (heart block and supraventricular tachycardia)
- Volume overload (anemia, sepsis, and VSD)
- Systolic ventricular dysfunction (myocarditis, malnutrition, and dilated cardiomyopathy)
- Pressure overload (aortic stenosis and coarctation)
- Diastolic ventricular dysfunction (pericardial tamponade and restrictive cardiomyopathy)

HF occurs either in response to an excessive volume or pressure load or as a consequence of myocardial muscle impairment. Volume overload is due to factors causing a large increase in cardiac output (eg, large VSD or ductus arteriosus). In these circumstances, there must be a sufficiently large left-to-right shunt to cause severe strain on the heart. In the normal newborn, these lesions do not usually produce HF until 1 to 2 months of age because it takes longer than usual for the pulmonary vascular resistance to fall. Elevated pulmonary vascular resistance protects the left ventricle from the stress of overcirculation. This is not true in premature neonates who do not manifest the same degree of pulmonary arteriolar constriction; therefore, they are susceptible to large left-to-right shunts early and show HF more readily.

Regurgitant valvular lesions can also lead to HF. In complex CHD (ie, TA or tricuspid atresia with transposition), the additional stress of hypoxemia or univentricular overload can herald the early onset of HF. Large arteriovenous malformations can also occur intracranially and cause HF. Excessive pressure loads are seen in obstruction to cardiac output from aortic stenosis, aortic coarctation, and aortic interruption.

In the immediate newborn period, right-sided HF is seen with greater frequency because of severe pulmonary hypertension. Pulmonary hypertension has many causes including intrinsic lung parenchymal insufficiency or pathology (ie, diaphragmatic hernia, meconium aspiration, or hyaline membrane disease), chronic hypoxemia, hypervolemia, and polycythemia.

Primary myocardial failure is unusual and rare in the newborn. If it occurs, it is likely due to endocardial fibroelastosis and anomalous coronary circulation. Nonetheless, the myocardium in the infant is susceptible to depression from metabolic derangements such as hypoglycemia, hypocalcemia, hypoxemia, and hypercarbia. Also, severe anemia with the associated decreases in systemic and myocardial oxygen supply forces an increase in myocardial work that can lead to HF.

Infants are different from adults in their manifestations of HF. Signs of cardiac dilation can be absent because of decreased systemic venous return from the elevated intrathoracic pressure as a consequence of coexisting lung disease in premature infants. Although immature, the carotid baroreceptors still initiate an increase in sympathetic outflow in response to reduced perfusion. The increased α-adrenergic stimulation impairs blood flow to the systemic arteriolar beds, resulting in cold, underperfused extremities and diminished splanchnic perfusion. Fatigue, loss of appetite, and failure to thrive quickly follow. Tachycardia from β-adrenergic receptor stimulation occurs. Generalized sweating results from sympathetic cholinergic fiber stimulation. Extracellular water increases because of decreased renal excretion of sodium due to a decreased glomerular filtration rate; however, peripheral pitting edema is much less common in infants compared to older children and adults. The venous system in infants is extremely distensible, so much so that elevated right atrial pressures might not show jugular venous engorgement. The most prominent manifestation of HF in the infant is tachypnea. Because pulmonary venous pressure is elevated from left ventricular failure, the lung compliance decreases because of the augmented interstitial fluid. Breathing becomes rapid and shallow, further increasing oxygen requirements, which leads to a cyclic dependency to maintain both tachycardia and tachypnea. It is common to see subcostal retractions due to the increase in respiratory effort in infants with HF.

Infants have a greater lymphatic drainage capacity compared to adults and can clear interstitial fluid more readily. Therefore, rales are less often appreciated in infants with HF, as opposed to adults with HF. The bronchial mucosa can become swollen because of engorgement of the bronchial venous system, resulting in narrowing of the airway lumen. This can produce an audible wheeze that is often seen in infantile HF. Lastly, hepatomegaly is a cardinal sign of right ventricular failure in infants.

Kannan BR. Clinical diagnostic approach to congenital acyanotic congenital heart disease in infants and children. *Indian J Pediatr*. 2020;87:381-384.

Watanabe K, Shih R. Update of pediatric heart failure. *Pediatr Clin North Am*. 2020;67:889-901.

SECTION 10

B.7. How would you optimize the preoperative treatment of HF?

The typical manifestations of CHF in infants (ie, tachycardia, tachypnea, subcostal retractions, and rhonchi) are also cardinal signs of pulmonary infection in this age group. They can be difficult to distinguish. Often, they coexist, and treatment must address both conditions. In this patient, the structural abnormality of the IAA needs surgical correction; however, correction must be deferred until the neck mass is resected. In this infant, CHF is caused by pressure overload from the IAA, and the hypocalcemia is due to parathyroid hormone insufficiency. Calcium must be normalized by intravenous infusion. If glucose is low, as would be expected in an infant who is unable to feed by mouth, has glycogen depletion from the stress of illness, has an immature liver that is unable to generate sufficient gluconeogenesis, and has an increased utilization from a baseline higher metabolic rate (compared to adults), a glucose source should be continuously provided by slow intravenous administration. Myocardial work is compromised by the presence of metabolic acidosis, which occurs as a consequence of the increased lactic acid production during anaerobic metabolism, resulting from lower body hypoperfusion. The pH should be normalized with sodium bicarbonate.

With the guidance of a pediatric cardiologist, myocardial function should be optimized with angiotensin converting enzyme (ACE) inhibitors, β-blockers, and digoxin in infants with HF. A catecholamine (eg, epinephrine, dopamine, or dobutamine) can be infused to boost contractility. Pulmonary symptoms should be treated with antibiotics and positive pressure ventilation (ie, high-flow nasal cannula, nasal continuous positive airway pressure [CPAP]) with oxygen titrated to arterial blood gas measurements. Intubation and mechanical ventilation might be necessary in many infants with HF. Diuresis with furosemide, in conjunction with fluid restriction, will promote restoration of pulmonary compliance by decreasing lung water.

Burstein DS, Rossano JW. Heart failure. In: Kliegman RM, St. Geme JW eds. *Nelson Textbook of Pediatrics*. 22nd ed. Elsevier;2024:2893-2902.

Kannan BR. Clinical diagnostic approach to congenital acyanotic congenital heart disease in infants and children. *Indian J Pediatr*. 2020;87:381-384.

Watanabe K, Shih R. Update of pediatric heart failure. *Pediatr Clin North Am*. 2020;67:889-901.

B.8. How would you premedicate this infant?

Infants younger than 2 years do not routinely require preoperative anxiolytics or opioids. An infant with a compromised airway and abnormal circulation cannot tolerate any degree of respiratory depression; therefore, no sedative premedication should be given. Because a fiberoptic intubation is planned, glycopyrrolate should be given preoperatively for its antisialagogue activity.

B.9. When is premedication useful in infants and children?

Patients with dynamically responsive cyanotic CHD (ie, tetralogy of Fallot) benefit from premedication before coming to the operating room. In these children, the inherent anxiety of transfer to unfamiliar surroundings, change in temperature, and parental separation can trigger infundibular spasm and reduce pulmonary blood flow, thereby leading to a "tet spell." This transient increase in pulmonary vascular resistance dramatically decreases pulmonary blood flow and increases the flow of desaturated blood to the body via VSD. Acute hypoxemia is not an optimal state in which to initiate induction of anesthesia. Therefore, sedation with oral midazolam or nasal dexmedetomidine is useful to allay preoperative anxiety and reduce the risk of provoking a hypoxemic spell. Premedication can make the perioperative experience for a child less frightening, produce variable degrees of amnesia, and decrease the risk of emergence delirium. Pharmacologic premedication is one of many tools a pediatric anesthesiologist has to ensure a positive perioperative experience for the patient and their family. Studies have shown promising results with nonpharmacologic interventions including handheld video games, low sensory stimulation, and virtual reality.

Freriksen JJM, van der Zanden TM, Holsappel IGA, et al. Best evidence-based dosing recommendations for dexmedetomidine for premedication and procedural sedation in pediatrics: outcome of a risk-benefit analysis by the Dutch Pediatric Formulary. *Paediatr Drugs*. 2022;24:247-257.

Heikal S, Stuart G. Anxiolytic premedication for children. *BJA Educ*. 2020;20:220-225.

McPherson C, Grunau RE. Pharmacologic analgesia and sedation in neonates. *Clin Perinatol*. 2022;49:243-265.

Wang E, Thomas JJ, Rodriguez ST. Virtual reality for pediatric periprocedural care. *Curr Opin Anaesthesiol*. 2021;34:285-291.

Wise-Faberowski L, Asija R, McElhinney DB. Tetralogy of Fallot: everything you wanted to know but were afraid to ask. *Paediatr Anaesth*. 2019;29:475-482.

B.10. Before the planned surgery, the infant is scheduled for a magnetic resonance imaging (MRI) scan. You are asked to ensure that the baby remains immobile for 20 minutes to perform the scan adequately. How would you accomplish this?

Because this neonate has a severely compromised airway while awake, the safest anesthetic plan to ensure immobility and adequate ventilation is to perform general anesthesia with an endotracheal tube. Any form of sedation without an endotracheal tube puts this patient at risk for complete airway obstruction. If the neonate has demonstrated a postprandial sleep cycle and can take oral fluids, it might be worth an attempt to perform the MRI scan while the neonate is swaddled in a warm baby blanket sucking on a pacifier filled with dextrose solution ("Sweetie Soother pacifier") such that the patient remains "motionless" from the inherent feeling of comfort of being able to feed and bundled in a warm blanket.

Dong SZ, Zhu M, Bulas D. Techniques for minimizing sedation in pediatric MRI. *J Magn Reson Imaging*. 2019;50:1047-1054.

Salerno S, Granata C, Trapenese M, et al. Is MRI imaging in pediatric age totally safe? A critical reprisal. *Radiol Med*. 2018;123:695-702.

C. Intraoperative Management

C.1. What anesthesia equipment, circuit, and monitors would you use?

This patient is especially susceptible to infection because of baseline depressed cellular immunity. As with every patient, strict attention must be paid to maintaining a sterile technique during the central line placement. The anesthesiologist must wear a sterile gown and gloves to protect the neonate. Sterility of the disposable circle system, mask, endotracheal tube, and airway equipment should be ensured. Routine monitors for all surgery on infants include pulse oximetry, electrocardiogram, blood pressure, capnograph, spirometer, and temperature probe. Multiple pulse oximeters should be available to offer flexibility in the event of monitor dysfunction. In this neonate, the IAA precludes saturation data from the lower body and left arm. End-tidal expired gas concentrations should be recorded for anesthetic gases, nitrogen, and oxygen. Accurate capnography in small infants can be hampered by sidearm gas sampling resulting from the relatively high gas flows relative to the expired gas flow from the infant.

In this procedure, an arterial line should be inserted in the right upper extremity because the IAA will not allow accurate blood pressure determination on the left side. Because there is potential for significant blood loss, a central line should be placed under ultrasound guidance at the best available site (ie, internal jugular, subclavian, or femoral). Obtaining central access in such a small patient with distorted anatomy can be very difficult. If an internal jugular or subclavian central line is placed, a chest radiograph should be obtained after placement and reviewed for correct positioning and to rule out pneumothorax before proceeding with this complicated case. Catheter length must be taken into consideration during placement to avoid inadvertently inserting the central line inside the right atrium or across the tricuspid valve, leading to arrhythmias and misleading right ventricular pressures. The arterial line and central venous pressure (CVP) transducers should be placed at the approximate level of the right atrium and adjusted accordingly as the table height is changed. Cerebral and somatic oximetry is useful in providing early recognition of intraoperative hypoperfusion to the brain and body.

Burbano-Vera N, Zaleski KL, Latham GJ, et al. Perioperative and anesthetic considerations of interrupted aortic arch. *Semin Cardiothorac Vasc Anesth*. 2018;22:270-277.

Modestini M, Hoffmann L, Niezen C, Armocida B, Vos JJ, Scheeren TWL. Cerebral oxygenation during pediatric congenital cardiac surgery and its association with outcome: a retrospective observational study. *Can J Anaesth*. 2020;67:1170-1181.

C.2. Describe techniques other than direct laryngoscopy that would be useful for securing the airway in this baby.

It is highly unlikely that glottic visualization could be accomplished in this neonate with direct laryngoscopy alone. The following alternative forms of securing the airway can be used when direct laryngoscopy is not expected to provide easy visualization of the glottis.

Infant Videolaryngoscope

The various forms of this device on the market allow for excellent glottic visualization and facilitation of intubation if the mouth opening is large enough to accommodate the blade and can provide superior visualization compared to conventional direct laryngoscopy in some patients.

Intubation Through a Laryngeal Mask Airway

Securing the airway with an LMA and demonstrating that one can ventilate through it can add an extra margin of safety when performing an anticipated difficult pediatric intubation. The LMA is then used as a conduit for the insertion of the fiberoptic-guided endotracheal tube into the glottis.

Retrograde Cricothyroid Wire

This technique is not ideal for this patient for many reasons. First, the size of the patient would make it technically difficult. Second, the large cystic hygroma distorts the external anatomy landmarks that facilitate this type of intubation. Given newer developments in pediatric airway management, this approach is rarely used.

Blind Nasal Intubation

Although very successful in adult patients, the blind nasal intubation technique can be very challenging in infants or small children. Performing an awake sedated intubation in this manner mandates giving adequate topical anesthesia to a less-than-cooperative infant. In addition, the smaller endotracheal tubes used in pediatrics are far more compliant than adult-sized tubes, especially when warmed with nasopharyngeal respiratory gases, which makes it difficult to maintain the anterior curve on the tube to enter the larynx.

Nasal Intubation With Laryngoscope and Magill Forceps

If the larynx cannot be visualized by direct laryngoscopy, an anesthetized, spontaneously breathing nasal intubation with laryngoscopic assistance can be carried out in some patients. In this case, great care is taken to ensure that the patient continues to maintain spontaneous and adequate ventilatory exchange during the inhalational induction. Sevoflurane is used for pediatric inhalational inductions because it is less pungent and more easily tolerated than other agents. The pediatric anesthesiologist should be mindful that total airway obstruction can happen at any point during the inhalation induction due to the relaxation of pharyngeal tone and other airway abnormalities. If spontaneous breathing can be maintained, intubation should be attempted after a surgical plane of anesthesia is achieved. The laryngoscope is then used to visualize the epiglottis. Using Magill forceps, the tip of the endotracheal tube is aligned with the subepiglottic region and slowly advanced. Capnographic monitoring during this maneuver can help verify the direction of the endotracheal tube tip.

Fiberoptic Intubation

Fiberoptic intubation is most successful when it is carried out as the initial maneuver before the airway is traumatized from previous attempts at intubation. It can be nearly impossible to use after several unsuccessful attempts because the upper airway becomes hypersecretory and bloody. The appropriate fiberoptic technology is not widely available unless one is practicing at a tertiary pediatric hospital with a wide range of airway devices (including the smallest, "ultrathin" 2.2 mm in diameter fiberoptic scope necessary for this neonate). Due to their small size, pediatric bronchoscopes lack a suction port and need to be lubricated to facilitate the sliding of the endotracheal tube off the scope once it is through the glottis.

In older patients, three specialized fiberoptic methods can be useful in intubating pediatric patients with difficult airways. First, the clinician can pass a guidewire through the suction port of the larger instrument to serve as a stylet for the endotracheal tube. Second, the scope can be used to visualize and guide a nasal endotracheal tube inserted into the opposite nostril. Finally, a 4.5-mm tube can be placed at the laryngeal orifice to be used as a stent for inserting a small guidewire, which can in turn be used to place a smaller endotracheal tube.

Combined Videolaryngoscopy and Fiberoptic Intubation

A common pitfall with the use of videolaryngoscopes is identifying a view of the larynx but being unable to pass the tracheal tube, especially in a patient with an anterior airway. To avoid this pitfall, a combined technique of videolaryngoscopy and fiberoptic intubation can be utilized. First, a videolaryngoscope is inserted into the oropharynx to obtain a view of the vocal cords. A tracheal tube is placed over a flexible fiberoptic scope, inserted into the oropharynx, and dually guided through the vocal cords with visualization from both the videolaryngoscope and fiberoptic scope. This technique allows for an increased range of motion with the fiberoptic scope as well as displacement of the tongue and soft tissue with the videolaryngoscope to angle the tracheal tube through the laryngeal inlet.

Transtracheal Jet Ventilation

For this technique, a 16-gauge intravenous catheter is placed through the cricothyroid membrane, and jet ventilation with 100% oxygen is provided. A second intravenous catheter is placed through the cricothyroid membrane, and a guidewire (0.021-in. diameter J-tip) is introduced with cephalad angulation. Jet ventilation continues, as the guidewire is threaded through the nose and connected to the working part of a fiberoptic scope. The scope is then advanced through the laryngeal inlet, and a tube is threaded over the scope and then the guidewire is removed. Sedation can be provided with a remifentanil infusion

(0.1-0.2 μg/kg/min) or dexmedetomidine infusion (0.5-1 μg/kg/h). Because patient safety is the foremost consideration in any technique for inserting an artificial airway, an anesthesiologist or otolaryngologist should be immediately available to perform an emergent cricothyrotomy in case of life-threatening loss of airway.

In a pediatric patient with a known difficult airway, a preemptive collaborative approach of securing the airway with a pediatric otolaryngologist can greatly increase the degree of safety and minimize harm. Pediatric surgeons can also be consulted in case ECMO is required during acute decompensation during difficult airway management. Passive oxygenation and supplemental oxygen should be utilized during every attempt with the airway to prolong the time to desaturation. When performing an emergency cricothyrotomy, a longitudinal incision is made in the skin and fascia above the cricothyroid membrane, after which the cricothyroid membrane is punctured and entered with a small endotracheal tube. Another technique utilizes an 18-gauge angiocatheter (or larger), which is inserted into the cricothyroid membrane. Intratracheal location is verified by the loss of resistance with an attached syringe and the aspiration of air. The catheter is attached to a 3-mL syringe (without plunger), which is then connected to the Y-piece of the anesthesia circuit by an adapter from a 3.0-mm internal diameter endotracheal tube.

Dhanyee AS, Pillai R, Sahajanandan R. Wire guided fibreoptic retrograde intubation in a case of glottic mass. *Indian J Anaesth*. 2016;60:219-221.

Sohn L, Peyton J, von Ungern-Sternberg BS, Jagannathan N. Error traps in pediatric difficult airway management. *Paediatr Anaesth*. 2021;31:1271-1275.

Stein ML, Park RS, Kovatsis PG. Emerging trends, techniques, and equipment for airway management in pediatric patients. *Paediatr Anaesth*. 2020;30:269-279.

Tsao M, Vargas AA, Hajduk J, et al. Pediatric airway management devices: an update on recent advances and future directions. *Expert Rev Med Devices*. 2018;15:911-927.

C.3. How would you monitor blood loss in this patient?

In many of these procedures, blood loss can be significant and easily exceed calculated blood volume. It is difficult to accurately measure blood loss when it is lost under the drapes or irrigated away. Meticulous weighing of the sponges and observation of suction canisters are important, but blood loss can be continuous from the time of skin incision and seems relentless for an inexperienced clinician. Absolute changes in CVP are a relative guide to the volume in the central compartment, but no one isolated value correlates with a known blood volume. A steady decrease in CVP in association with a downward trend in mean arterial pressures (MAPs) during periods of surgical intervention known to produce significant bleeding should be treated aggressively with crystalloid (20 mL/kg) or colloid (ie, 5% albumin) replacement first, followed by a vasopressor as necessary. Ideally, with an arterial line in place and point-of-care testing, one can follow the trend in hemoglobin prior to initiation of blood transfusion. Persistent hypotension with a normal hematocrit could be due to hypocalcemia, either from parathyroid hormone insufficiency or from citrate (used as an anticoagulant in blood products), which binds ionized calcium if the patient was recently transfused.

C.4. What anesthetic technique should be used in a patient who may experience severe loss of blood intraoperatively?

Blood loss should be replaced to prevent falling behind in intravascular volume. It is wise to choose an anesthetic technique that produces a relatively stable blood pressure throughout the surgery, so new downward trends in blood pressure can be easily attributable to blood loss and not to pharmacologic action. For instance, if a steady level of desflurane or sevoflurane is given at 1.25 minimal alveolar concentration (MAC) with MAP 15% lower than awake, further dips in MAP during surgical intervention can be taken as intravascular volume depletion secondary to bleeding and replaced accordingly. This interpretation would be obscured if there were frequent anesthetic interventions associated with MAP changes, such as intermittent opioids or titration of hypotension-inducing agents. An important clue to the blood volume loss is the blood pressure at 1 MAC of anesthesia. If a stable pressure is established at a given dose of inhalational agent, a lower-than-expected blood pressure at this dose is almost always indicative of hypovolemia and therefore calls for fluid or blood replacement. Another anesthetic technique for this procedure on a neonate is to use a high-dose opioid technique with paralysis, which will lessen the impact of inhalational agents on MAP. Serial hematocrit determinations drawn throughout the case should guide management. It is most unusual in an otherwise healthy infant to produce hypotension with intravascular overload unless there are other attendant problems.

C.5. How would you induce and maintain anesthesia?

After securing the airway and verifying bilateral breath sounds, opioid titration with fentanyl should be given in repeated doses. This neonate might be sensitive to any anesthetic agent because of their cardiovascular anomalies; therefore, titrating fentanyl to arterial blood pressure via the arterial line decreases the chance of inadvertent drops in perfusion. Because the neonate is not going to be extubated, fentanyl can be dosed safely at 50 μg/kg or higher to allow for dense analgesia. Neuromuscular blocking agents such as rocuronium and cisatracurium can be given and redosed at regular intervals to facilitate surgical dissection. If tolerated, small concentrations of 0.5% to 4% desflurane or sevoflurane 0.25% to 1.5% can be administered to synergize with the opioid. The prostaglandin infusion should be maintained throughout the surgery.

C.6. Intraoperatively, the surgeon must dissect the tumor in the anterior mediastinum and needs to have a quiet surgical field. How would you accomplish this?

Double-lumen tubes are not used in the neonatal age group because of the exceedingly small lumen and the technical difficulties of securing both lungs. Instead, a single-lumen endotracheal tube can be advanced into the right or left mainstem bronchus or an extraluminal bronchial blocker placed to allow for one-lung ventilation. This can be fraught with consequences in this infant with an IAA, but it can still be attempted. Keep in mind that hypoxic pulmonary vasoconstriction might not occur readily in the neonate and excessive shunting can occur. In addition, having an infant on one-lung ventilation can lead to excessive hypercarbia or hypoxemia. During one-lung ventilation in infants, $\dot{V}/\dot{Q}$ mismatch occurs due to compression of the dependent lung as a result of a less rigid cartilaginous rib cage and abdominal pressure, causing reduced compliance and ventilation. In addition, there is a decrease in shunting of blood away from the nondependent lung to the dependent lung, which also worsens $\dot{V}/\dot{Q}$ mismatch.

Lazar A, Chatterjee D, Templeton TW. Error traps in pediatric one-lung ventilation. *Paediatr Anaesth.* 2022;32:346-353.

Templeton TW, Piccioni F, Chatterjee D. An update on one-lung ventilation in children. *Anesth Analg.* 2021;132:1389-1399.

D. Postoperative Management

D.1. How would you manage this patient postoperatively?

Multiple factors mandate that this neonate remain intubated or have a tracheostomy placed at the end of the case. This surgery involves an extensive dissection of the patient's neck and upper thorax that will result in a tremendous amount of upper airway and neck edema. Consequently, this would make extubation life threatening. High-dose opioids and neuromuscular blocking agents have been used, which also hamper safe extubation. The neonate should continue to remain well narcotized and paralyzed to facilitate effective mechanical ventilation. Artificial ventilation and oxygen supplementation should be titrated to serial arterial blood gases. In addition, the prostaglandin drip must be continued to ensure ductal patency. Generous opioid supplementation will ensure that the pulmonary vascular resistance stays low. At 24 hours postoperatively, a leak test can be performed to assess residual vocal cord and airway edema. Fiberoptic visualization of the laryngeal inlet can provide useful information about the state of the laryngeal inlet in anticipation of extubation.

Anatomic airway factors aside, the IAA and associated HF will make extubation more challenging. Assuming all other factors are under control, the following ventilatory parameters should be met prior to extubation: normal arterial blood gases with satisfactory oxygenation on 28% oxygen, spontaneous tidal volume greater than 5 mL/kg, and an inspiratory force greater than 12 cm H_2O. One needs to be vigilant for early signs of airway obstruction and be ready to reintubate or perform an emergent tracheostomy if airway obstruction and desaturation occur.

44

Patent Ductus Arteriosus and Prematurity

Albert C. Yeung

A 2-week-old male infant weighing 900 g is scheduled for ligation of patent ductus arteriosus (PDA). He was born at week 27 of gestation as part of a triplet pregnancy complicated by preterm labor. Immediately after delivery, his trachea was intubated because of respiratory distress. He was given indomethacin prophylactically because of his prematurity and presumed PDA. A transthoracic echocardiogram (TTE) confirmed the patency of the ductus arteriosus and demonstrated its closure after one course of indomethacin. His respiratory function was gradually improving with ventilatory support until 2 weeks later when his oxygenation and ventilation suddenly worsened. A murmur was heard over his chest. A repeat TTE demonstrated left-to-right shunting through the ductus arteriosus. Another course of indomethacin was administered, but the ductus remained patent. His blood pressure was 50/20 mm Hg, and his heart rate was 165 beats per minute. The laboratory data were as follows: white blood cell (WBC) count, 17,000/μL; hemoglobin, 11 g/dL; hematocrit, 34%; urine specific gravity, 1.005; protein, 1+; sugar, 1+; serum calcium, 6.0 mg/dL; blood glucose, 60 mg/dL; arterial blood gases: pH, 7.30; $Paco_2$, 60 mm Hg; Pao_2, 49 mm Hg on fraction of inspired oxygen (Fio_2) 50%; inspiratory pressure, 19/6 cm H_2O; and ventilation rate, 40 breaths per minute.

A. Medical Disease and Differential Diagnosis

1. How would you classify prematurity? What are the common problems associated with prematurity?
2. What are the survival rates of preterm infants?
3. What are the incidence and survival rates of respiratory distress syndrome (RDS)? Discuss its pathophysiology.
4. What is bronchopulmonary dysplasia (BPD)? How would you treat it?
5. What are apnea spells? What are the possible causes of apneic spells?
6. Discuss the incidence and pathophysiology of PDA in preterm infants.
7. How would you make a diagnosis of PDA? Describe its treatment.
8. Would you give digitalis to treat congestive heart failure in preterm infants? Why?
9. How does indomethacin help in the closure of the ductus? What are the adverse effects of indomethacin? What are other pharmacologic options?
10. When is surgical closure indicated? What are the complications associated with surgical ligation? What other interventional procedures are available?
11. What is retinopathy of prematurity (ROP)? Discuss its etiology, pathophysiology, prognosis, prevention, and treatment.
12. Define neutral and critical temperatures. What are these values in the preterm neonate, in the term neonate, and in the adult? Discuss temperature regulation in the neonate.

B. Preoperative Evaluation and Preparation

1. How would you evaluate this patient preoperatively?
2. What are the normal values of arterial blood gases and pH in neonates and infants?
3. Interpret the arterial blood gases: pH, 7.30; $Paco_2$, 60 mm Hg; Pao_2, 49 mm Hg; HCO_3^-, 20 mEq/L on 50% oxygen; and 6 cm H_2O of positive end-expiratory pressure (PEEP). How would you improve them?
4. What are the normal values of arterial blood pressure, heart rate, and respiratory rate for preterm infants?

5. What are the normal values of WBC, red blood cells (RBCs), hemoglobin, glucose, electrolytes, calcium, blood urea nitrogen, and creatinine for preterm infants?
6. Would you transfuse blood to this patient preoperatively?
7. How would you interpret the urinalysis: specific gravity, 1.005; sugar, 1+; and protein, 1+?
8. Would you correct a serum calcium level of 6.0 mg/dL? What other information would you like to have? Which contains more calcium, 10 mL of 10% calcium chloride or 10 mL of 10% calcium gluconate? Could you hyperventilate this child safely?
9. How would you premedicate this patient?

C. Intraoperative Management

1. Should this procedure be performed in the neonatal intensive care unit (NICU) or the operating room?
2. What monitors would you use for this child during surgery?
3. What levels of arterial oxygen saturation would you like to keep during surgery?
4. How would you maintain the patient's body temperature?
5. How do the anesthetic requirements of the preterm infant differ from those of the adult?
6. What size endotracheal tube would you have used if the patient had not been intubated?
7. How would you have induced anesthesia if the patient had not been intubated?
8. How would you maintain anesthesia?
9. How would you ventilate the patient? What tidal volume, respiratory rates, and FIO_2 would you set for the infant?
10. Discuss blood and fluid therapy in this preterm infant.
11. During dissection of the ductus arteriosus, the arterial oxygen saturation decreased from 92% to 80% and the heart rate decreased from 140 beats per minute to 80 beats per minute. What could be the likely causes and how would you treat them?

D. Postoperative Management

1. Would you reverse the neuromuscular blockade and extubate the patient at the end of surgery?
2. How can one minimize the risk of transporting the patient to the NICU after surgery?
3. The patient's respiratory status deteriorated in the days following surgery, with chest radiography demonstrating evidence of continued congestive failure. Physical examination revealed a persistent cardiac murmur. What was the possible diagnosis?

A. Medical Disease and Differential Diagnosis

A.1. How would you classify prematurity? What are the common problems associated with prematurity?

Live-born infants delivered before 37 weeks from the first day of the last menstrual period are termed premature by the World Health Organization. Preterm infants can be classified into three groups, as shown in **Table 44.1**. Infants of borderline prematurity usually require no special care, but they should be observed closely for 24 to 48 hours in the newborn nursery because of their susceptibility to RDS. Furthermore, those with a poor suck reflex may require gavage feedings. Infants classified as moderately premature require intense neonatal care, and neonatal mortality correlates inversely with gestational age. Neonates of extreme prematurity constitute only 1% of all preterm infants; however, mortality in this group is extremely high, accounting for more than 70% of all neonatal deaths. Furthermore, morbidity in surviving infants is substantial, often secondary to irreversible neurologic or respiratory insult.

Brandsma E, Christ LA, Duncan AF. The high-risk infant. In: Kliegman RM, St. Geme JW III, eds. *Nelson Textbook of Pediatrics*. 22nd ed. Elsevier; 2025:1038-1050.

Gregory GA. Anesthesia for premature infants. In: Gregory GA, Andropoulos DB, eds. *Gregory's Pediatric Anesthesia*. 6th ed. Wiley-Blackwell; 2020:505-512.

Sparth JP, Lam JE. The extremely premature infant (micropremie) and common neonatal emergencies. In: Coté C, Lerman J, Anderson B, eds. *A Practice of Anesthesia for Infants and Children*. 7th ed. Elsevier; 2024:953-981.

A.2. What are the survival rates of preterm infants?

The survival rates of preterm infants depend mainly on their maturity or birth weights. Because of the advances in neonatal care, survival rates have continued to improve for extremely premature infants. Survival has increased for infants born at 23 to 24 weeks' gestation, and survival without major comorbidities increased for infants born at 25 to 28 weeks. In a 2022 observational study looking at the survival of extremely premature infants born in the United States from 2013 to 2018, rates of

TABLE 44.1 Classification of Prematurity

	Borderline Prematurity	Moderate Prematurity	Extreme Prematurity
Gestational age (weeks)	36-37	31-35	24-30
Percentage live births	16%	6%-7%	<1%
Weight (g)	2,500-3,200	1,500-2,500	500-1,500
Associated problems	Poor suck	Poor suck	Poor suck
	RDS	RDS	RDS
	Temperature regulation	Temperature regulation	Temperature regulation
		Sepsis	Sepsis
		Intracranial hemorrhage	Intracranial hemorrhage
			Necrotizing enterocolitis
			Congestive heart failure
			Birth asphyxia
Level of care	Careful observation in newborn nursery	Neonatal ICU	Neonatal ICU

ICU, intensive care unit; RDS, respiratory distress syndrome.

survival to hospital discharge or 1 year of age of infants born at 22, 23, 24, 25, and 26 weeks' gestation were 11%, 50%, 70%, 78%, and 88%, respectively.

Bell EF, Hintz SR, Hansen NI, et al. Mortality, in-hospital morbidity, care practices, and 2-year outcomes for extremely preterm infants in the US, 2013-2018. *JAMA*. 2022;327:248-263.

Brandsma E, Christ LA, Duncan AF. The high-risk infant. In: Kliegman RM, St. Geme JW III, eds. *Nelson Textbook of Pediatrics*. 22nd ed. Elsevier; 2025:1038-1050.

A.3. What are the incidence and survival rates of respiratory distress syndrome (RDS)? Discuss its pathophysiology.

RDS, formerly called hyaline membrane disease, is common in preterm infants. RDS is a life-threatening condition associated with 50% to 75% of all deaths of premature infants. The incidence of RDS is inversely related to gestational age and birth weight. RDS occurs in 60% to 80% of infants born at less than 28 weeks' gestational age and 15% to 30% of infants between 32 and 36 weeks. The risk increases with maternal diabetes, multiple gestation, cesarean delivery, and precipitous delivery.

Survival depends on the infant's size and gestational age. Survival is 80% for those weighing less than 750 g, 85% for those weighing less than 1,000 g, and greater than 95% for those weighing 1,500 to 2,500 g. Maternal corticosteroid administration and administration of exogenous surfactant into the lungs of neonates of less than 28 weeks' gestation at birth has been associated with an increase in survival and a decrease in the severity of RDS.

Deficiency of the alveolar phospholipid surfactant is thought to be the cause of RDS. The surfactant is produced by the type II alveolar cells and is necessary for the maintenance of alveolar stability. Surfactant production is usually inadequate before 35 weeks of gestational age. In its absence, alveolar collapse and a decrease in functional residual capacity (FRC) occur, with consequent right-to-left shunting, arterial hypoxemia, and metabolic acidosis. Administration of betamethasone to females 48 hours before the delivery of fetuses less than 34 weeks' gestation significantly reduces the incidence, mortality, and morbidity of RDS.

Physical examination of the infant with RDS will likely reveal cyanosis, tachypnea, intercostal retractions, and bilateral rales that fail to clear with suctioning. An arterial blood gas sample will demonstrate hypoxemia, metabolic acidosis, and respiratory alkalosis; a chest radiograph will show diffuse, hazy ("ground glass") infiltrates. RDS causes a decrease in lung volume and lung compliance, which may pose a problem for the anesthesiologist if these patients require surgery. Ventilation with high positive pressures and large volumes increases the likelihood of pneumothorax and lung injury.

Diu MW, Walker KK. Pediatric diseases. In: Hines RL, Jones SB, eds. *Stoelting's Anesthesia and Co-Existing Disease.* 8th ed. Elsevier; 2022:667

Gregory GA. Anesthesia for premature infants. In: Gregory GA, Andropoulos DB, eds. *Gregory's Pediatric Anesthesia.* 6th ed. Wiley-Blackwell; 2020:505-512.

Spreacher AJ, Acharya KK, Cohen SS. Respiratory distress syndrome (hyaline membrane disease). In: Kliegman RM, St. Geme JW III, eds. *Nelson Textbook of Pediatrics.* 22nd ed. Elsevier; 2025:1077-1083.

A.4. What is bronchopulmonary dysplasia (BPD)? How would you treat it?

Bronchopulmonary dysplasia is a chronic lung disease of prematurity. BPD is defined as an oxygen requirement at 28 days of life, with the severity dependent on the required level of supplemental oxygen and ventilatory support at specific time points of postconceptual age. BPD is thought to be a result of mechanical ventilation, oxygen toxicity, infection, or a combination of these factors that cause a lung injury–induced increase in cytokine production. Lung injury in the premature infant disrupts pulmonary maturation that normally occurs around 36 weeks' gestation, resulting in larger but fewer alveoli, decreased surface area for pulmonary gas exchange, and abnormal muscularization of peripheral pulmonary vessels. Infants with BPD may have interstitial fibrosis, lobar emphysema, and components of reactive airway disease. BPD results in a mismatch of ventilation and perfusion, resulting in hypoxemia and hypercarbia. With progressive disease, it may lead to pulmonary hypertension and right heart failure.

The treatment for BPD is supportive ventilatory and medical therapies. Ventilatory goals include avoidance of intubation and hyperoxia if possible and the use of smaller tidal volumes with permissive hypercapnia to avoid barotrauma. Medical therapies include diuretics to decrease pulmonary edema, bronchodilators to reduce airway resistance, corticosteroids, and inotropes as needed to support cardiac contractility.

Diu MW, Walker KK. Pediatric diseases. In: Hines RL, Jones SB, eds. *Stoelting's Anesthesia and Co-Existing Disease.* 8th ed. Elsevier; 2022:667.

Gregory GA. Anesthesia for premature infants. In: Gregory GA, Andropoulos DB, eds. *Gregory's Pediatric Anesthesia.* 6th ed. Wiley-Blackwell; 2020:505-512.

Spreacher AJ, Acharya KK, Cohen SS. Bronchopulmonary dysplasia. In: Kliegman RM, St. Geme JW III, eds. *Nelson Textbook of Pediatrics.* 22nd ed. Elsevier; 2025:1084-1087.

A.5. What are apnea spells? What are the possible causes of apneic spells?

Apnea spells are defined as cessation of breathing lasting greater than 20 seconds or greater than 10 seconds and produce oxygen desaturation and bradycardia. Apneic spells are common in preterm infants, especially after the first week of life, and almost universal in infants who are less than 1,000 g at birth. Failure to breathe (central apnea) or failure to maintain a patent airway (obstructive apnea) can both be present. The causes are multiple and include the following:

- Hypothermia or hyperthermia
- Hypoglycemia or hyperglycemia
- Hypocalcemia or hypercalcemia
- Hypovolemia or hypervolemia
- Anemia
- Decreased FRC
- PDA
- Constipation
- Hypothyroidism
- Immature brainstem function
- Lack of type I muscle fibers in the diaphragm
- Excessive handling
- Sepsis
- Gastroesophageal reflux disease

Repeated apnea increases the likelihood of central nervous system damage because of repeated episodes of hypoxemia. Infants who have apneic spells may not breathe during anesthesia; therefore, they should be ventilated throughout anesthesia, including the induction phase. Inhaled and intravenous anesthetics affect the control of breathing and contribute to upper airway obstruction, thereby increasing the likelihood of apnea during the postoperative period, especially in preterm infants less than 60 weeks postconception age.

Finer NN, Higgins R, Kattwinkel J, Martin RJ. Summary proceedings from the apnea-of-prematurity group. *Pediatrics.* 2006;117:S47-S51.

Gregory GA. Anesthesia for premature infants. In: Gregory GA, Andropoulos DB, eds. *Gregory's Pediatric Anesthesia.* 6th ed. Wiley-Blackwell; 2020:505-512.

Sparth JP, Lam JE. The extremely premature infant (micropremie) and common neonatal emergencies. In: Coté C, Lerman J, Anderson B, eds. *A Practice of Anesthesia for Infants and Children*. 7th ed. Elsevier; 2024:953-981.

A.6. Discuss the incidence and pathophysiology of PDA in preterm infants.

In term infants, the ductus arteriosus closes soon after birth in response to the increased arterial oxygen tension. Closure is delayed in preterm infants, with the ductus remaining open on day 7 after birth in 2% of infants born at 30 through 37 weeks' gestation, 65% of those born at 25 through 29 weeks' gestation, and 87% of those born at 24 weeks' gestation. Compared to term infants, the ductus arteriosus in preterm infants has a thinner, more poorly contractile muscular layer with diminished responsiveness to the increasing oxygen levels after birth. In addition, preterm infants often suffer from hypoxemia because of RDS so that there are both a reduced stimulus to and a reduced response to physiologic closure. Shunting from the systemic to the pulmonary circulation results in pulmonary vascular overload and ultimately left heart failure. Pulmonary congestion worsens respiratory failure, resulting in further hypoxemia and carbon dioxide (CO_2) retention. Prolonged patency is associated with increased mortality, BPD, pulmonary hemorrhage, necrotizing enterocolitis, and intraventricular hemorrhage.

Hamrick SEG, Sallmon H, Rose AT, et al. Patent ductus arteriosus of the preterm infant. *Pediatrics*. 2020;146:e20201209.

Kussman BD, McGowan FX, Powell AJ, DiNardo JA. Anesthesia for congenital heart disease. In: Davis PJ, Cladis FP, eds. *Smith's Anesthesia for Infants and Children*. 10th ed. Elsevier; 2022:754-756

A.7. How would you make a diagnosis of PDA? Describe its treatment.

The diagnosis of PDA in preterm infants may be suspected when there is a sudden increase in respiratory failure, tachycardia, tachypnea, and widened pulse pressure. The classic continuous or machinery murmur of PDA is usually not present in this population, but a systolic murmur, sometimes extending into diastole, and a hyperdynamic precordium are nearly always present. The diagnosis is confirmed by echocardiography to assess PDA diameter, shunt pattern, and shunt volume. Continuous-wave Doppler can detect abnormal flow in the pulmonary artery. Color Doppler can visualize the jet of abnormal flow.

The treatment of PDA in preterm infants includes conservative management with fluid restriction and administration of diuretics, pharmacologic closure using cyclooxygenase (COX) inhibitors, prophylactic COX inhibitor therapy, and surgical or catheter-based closure. There is a trend toward less aggressive treatment of PDA in preterm infants, but there are no large randomized controlled trials comparing the strategies. At many centers, management begins with conservative treatment with subsequent pharmacologic or surgical interventions for symptomatic infants.

Gregory GA. Anesthesia for premature infants. In: Gregory GA, Andropoulos DB, eds. *Gregory's Pediatric Anesthesia*. 6th ed. Wiley-Blackwell; 2020:505-512.

Kussman BD, McGowan FX, Powell AJ, DiNardo JA. Anesthesia for congenital heart disease. In: Davis PJ, Cladis FP, eds. *Smith's Anesthesia for Infants and Children*. 10th ed. Elsevier; 2022:754-756.

Hamrick SEG, Sallmon H, Rose AT, et al. Patent ductus arteriosus of the preterm infant. *Pediatrics*. 2020;146:e20201209.

A.8. Would you give digitalis to treat congestive heart failure in preterm infants? Why?

Although digitalis was once a mainstay in the treatment of congestive heart failure in both children and adults, there is controversy over digitalis use, as newer therapies with fewer potential toxicities have been introduced. Digitalis should not be given to small preterm infants because it does not effectively improve stroke volume or ventricular emptying. However, it does decrease the heart rate, resulting in a detrimental decrease in cardiac output. Digitalis toxicity increases mortality in preterm infants.

Berman W Jr, Dubynsky O, Whitman V, Friedman Z, Maisels MJ. Digoxin therapy in low-birth-weight infants with patent ductus arteriosus. *J Pediatr*. 1978;93:652-655.

Burstein DS, Rossano JW. Heart failure. In: Kliegman RM, St. Geme JW III, eds. *Nelson Textbook of Pediatrics*. 22nd ed. Elsevier; 2025:2893-2902.

A.9. How does indomethacin help in the closure of the ductus? What are the adverse effects of indomethacin? What are other pharmacologic options?

The ductus arteriosus functionally closes shortly after birth in term infants when the vascular smooth muscle contracts. The muscular contraction of the ductus is initiated by the increased oxygen content and is influenced by other factors, such as the release of vasoactive substances, the relative resistances in the aorta and pulmonary artery, and the differences in sensitivity of the vessel to oxygen. Prostaglandins, including prostaglandin E_2 (PGE_2), relax the smooth muscle of the ductus and keep the ductus patent. The circulating levels of PGE_2 in the newborn decrease after birth due to separation from the placenta and increased pulmonary clearance.

COX enzymes catalyze the first two steps in the biosynthesis of prostaglandins. Indomethacin is a potent nonselective inhibitor of COX. Therefore, indomethacin decreases the synthesis of prostaglandins, potentially resulting in the closure of the ductus. Adverse effects of indomethacin include decreased mesenteric, renal, and cerebral blood flow.

Ibuprofen is another nonselective COX inhibitor that can be used effectively to treat PDA and has less side effects on organ blood circulation than indomethacin. When the agents were compared with each other, no differences were observed in the rate of PDA closure, neonatal outcomes, or adverse effects. Acetaminophen, which inhibits prostaglandin synthetase, is a pharmacologic option for cases in which COX inhibitors are contraindicated.

Clyman RI. Ontogeny of the ductus arteriosus response to prostaglandins and inhibitors of their synthesis. *Semin Perinatol.* 1980;4:115-124.

Hamrick SEG, Sallmon H, Rose AT, et al. Patent ductus arteriosus of the preterm infant. *Pediatrics.* 2020;146:e20201209.

A.10. When is surgical closure indicated? What are the complications associated with surgical ligation? What other interventional procedures are available?

Surgical ligation is indicated for infants with hemodynamically significant PDA where medical treatment has failed and the infant is unable to be weaned from respiratory support. Recently, the role of surgical ligation has come under scrutiny because of associations with adverse neonatal and neurodevelopmental outcomes. Systematic reviews have found that surgical ligation is associated with higher morbidity with lower mortality. Complications associated with surgical ligation include pneumothorax, chylothorax, vocal cord palsy, postligation cardiac syndrome, and abnormal neurodevelopmental outcome.

Percutaneous transcatheter occlusion of PDA in a cardiac catheterization setting is becoming increasingly common. In 2019, the US Food and Drug Administration approved the Amplatzer Piccolo Occluder device for PDA closure in premature infants weighing greater than or equal to 700 g. A meta-analysis in 2021 concluded that percutaneous transcatheter closure is feasible in infants weighing less than or equal to 1.5 kg with an 8% rate of major adverse events. Currently, such procedures are confined to institutions with the required facilities and expertise, and additional long-term outcome studies are needed.

Bischoff AR, Jasani B, Sathanandam SK, Backes C, Weisz DE, McNamara PJ. Percutaneous closure of patent ductus arteriosus in infants 1.5 kg or less: a meta-analysis. *J Pediatr.* 2021;230:84-92.e14.

Hamrick SEG, Sallmon H, Rose AT, et al. Patent ductus arteriosus of the preterm infant. *Pediatrics.* 2020;146:e20201209.

Jain A, Shah PS. Diagnosis, evaluation, and management of patent ductus arteriosus in preterm neonates. *JAMA Pediatr.* 2015;169:863-872.

A.11. What is retinopathy of prematurity (ROP)? Discuss its etiology, pathophysiology, prognosis, prevention, and treatment.

ROP is a retinal disorder affecting preterm infants that can result in blindness if untreated. Some degree of ROP occurs in approximately 50% of infants weighing 1,000 to 1,500 g at birth, 78% of those weighing 750 to 999 g, and greater than 90% of those weighing less than 750 g. ROP is thought to be initiated by oxygen-induced retinal vasoconstriction with retinal vascular obliteration, which is followed by increased vascularity, hemorrhage, cicatrization, and finally retinal detachment. ROP refers to all stages of the disease and its sequelae. Retrolental fibroplasia (RLF), the term previously used for this disease, described only the cicatricial stages.

The factors that cause ROP and determine its outcome are not fully known, but prematurity, the degree of retinal immaturity at birth, and days on supplemental oxygen therapy are major factors. Other contributing factors include respiratory distress, apnea, bradycardia, heart disease, infection, hypoxia, hypercarbia, acidosis, anemia, and the need for transfusion. Generally, the lower the birth weight and the sicker the infant, the greater the risk for ROP.

The retinal vasculature in the developing fetus spreads outward from the optic disc, reaching the nasal side of the retinal periphery by 36 weeks' gestational age and the temporal side at 40 weeks. Classically, it was postulated that hyperoxia constricts the retinal arterioles, resulting in swelling and degeneration of the endothelium. This causes paradoxical retinal ischemia despite systemic hyperoxia. When normoxic conditions are restored, vascularization resumes in an aberrant manner, leading to retinal detachment and blindness.

ROP is divided into five stages:

- *Stage 1*: A thin, white line separates the posterior vascularized portion of the retina from the anterior avascular retina.
- *Stage 2*: The demarcation line increases in volume and elevates. At this point, it is known as the "ridge." The changes in stage 1 and 2 regress in 80% of patients. Between 5% and 10% of premature infants with stage 1 and 2 disease progress to stage 3.
- *Stage 3*: Tissue proliferation develops from the ridge, usually posteriorly. Stage 3 can be mild, moderate, or severe, depending on the volume of the extraretinal tissue.
- *Stage 4*: Partial retinal detachment occurs with the macula still attached (stage 4a). The macula is detached in stage 4b.
- *Stage 5*: Total retinal detachment occurs.

Eighty-five percent of ROP cases undergo spontaneous recovery. Mild ROP regresses in 2 to 3 months, and moderate ROP in 6 months. The most severe ROP usually results in blindness or limited vision.

It is unclear what level of $Pa{O_2}$ causes ROP, but a $Pa{O_2}$ of 150 mm Hg for as short a time as 1 to 2 hours can do so. In addition, it is possible that ROP will develop at lower $Pa{O_2}$ levels because infants of this age are normally exposed to a much lower $Pa{O_2}$ (30-40 mm Hg) in utero than the levels found during the neonatal period. To reduce the possibility of ROP, a $Pa{O_2}$ level between 50 and 70 mm Hg or oxygen saturation ($Sp{O_2}$) between 87% and 92% for premature infants less than 44 weeks' gestation should be maintained.

However, prevention of ROP ultimately depends on the prevention of premature birth and its attendant problems. Oxygen alone is neither sufficient nor necessary to produce ROP, and no safe level of oxygen has yet been determined. Therefore, each infant must be treated with whatsoever is necessary to sustain life and neurologic function. Treatment of ROP includes cryotherapy and laser photocoagulation for moderate disease and scleral buckling surgery and vitrectomy for severe disease.

Diu MW, Walker KK. Pediatric diseases. In: Hines RL, Jones SB, eds. *Stoelting's Anesthesia and Co-Existing Disease*. 8th ed. Elsevier; 2022:667.

Gregory GA. Anesthesia for premature infants. In: Gregory GA, Andropoulos DB, eds. *Gregory's Pediatric Anesthesia*. 6th ed. Wiley-Blackwell; 2020:505-512.

Olitsky SE, Marsh JD. Disorders of the retina and vitreous. In: Kliegman RM, St. Geme JW III, eds. *Nelson Textbook of Pediatrics*. 22nd ed. Elsevier; 2025:3955-3963.

Sparth JP, Lam JE. The extremely premature infant (micropremie) and common neonatal emergencies. In: Coté C, Lerman J, Anderson B, eds. *A Practice of Anesthesia for Infants and Children*. 7th ed. Elsevier; 2024:953-981.

A.12. Define neutral and critical temperatures. What are these values in the preterm neonate, in the term neonate, and in the adult? Discuss temperature regulation in the neonate.

Neutral temperature is the ambient temperature that results in minimal oxygen consumption. Critical temperature is the ambient temperature below which an unclothed, unanesthetized individual cannot maintain a normal core temperature (**Table 44.2**).

Normally, body heat is lost by conduction, convection, radiation, and evaporation. The neonate is particularly susceptible to heat loss owing to a large surface-to-volume ratio, lack of insulating fat, and naturally flaccid and open posture. When stressed by a cold environment, vasoconstriction occurs, but the neonate is unable to shiver and relies on nonshivering thermogenesis. Cold stress stimulates norepinephrine release, promoting the exothermic metabolism of brown fat deposits to maintain core temperature. However, under anesthesia, nonshivering thermogenesis appears to be inhibited. Hypothermia can result in bradycardia, apnea, hypoglycemia, or metabolic acidosis and is a risk factor for infant mortality.

When the infant's rectal temperature reaches 36.6 °C (97.88 °F) to 37.3 °C (99.14 °F), dilation of peripheral vessels occurs. The term neonate will perspire at 37.2 °C (98.96 °F) to maintain a normal core temperature, whereas those infants born before 37 weeks' gestation are unable to sweat.

Gregory GA. Anesthesia for premature infants. In: Gregory GA, Andropoulos DB, eds. *Gregory's Pediatric Anesthesia*. 6th ed. Wiley-Blackwell; 2020:505-512.

Sparth JP, Lam JE. The extremely premature infant (micropremie) and common neonatal emergencies. In: Coté C, Lerman J, Anderson B, eds. *A Practice of Anesthesia for Infants and Children*. 7th ed. Elsevier; 2024:953-981.

TABLE 44.2 Neutral and Critical Temperature

	Neutral Temperature (°C)	Critical Temperature (°C)
Preterm neonate	34	28
Term neonate	32	23
Adults	28	1

SECTION 10

B. Preoperative Evaluation and Preparation

B.1. How would you evaluate this patient preoperatively?

The preoperative evaluation of preterm infants should be based on a clear understanding of the pathophysiology of prematurity. The preoperative evaluation of this patient should begin with a careful review of the medical record, followed by a systematic physical examination and laboratory evaluation, specifically:

- *History*—birth trauma, asphyxia, maternal drug history, respiratory, cardiovascular, and fluid status
- *Physical examination*—evaluation of the airway, cardiopulmonary system, fluid status (skin texture, turgor, mucous membranes, and fontanelles), and abdominal examination
- *Laboratory data*—WBC count, hemoglobin and hematocrit, serum electrolytes, serum coagulation profile, including prothrombin time, partial thromboplastin time, and platelet count; serum calcium and serum protein, arterial blood gases, urinalysis and urine specific gravity, and chest and abdominal radiographs

B.2. What are the normal values of arterial blood gases and pH in neonates and infants?

The normal blood gas and pH values for pediatric patients are shown in **Table 44.3**. The normal pH and $Paco_2$ values for pediatric patients are similar to those for adults, whereas the normal Pao_2 values are lower in pediatric patients than in adult patients.

Andropoulos DB. Appendix B: Pediatric normal laboratory values. In: Gregory GA, Andropoulos DB, eds. *Gregory's Pediatric Anesthesia*. 6th ed. Wiley-Blackwell; 2020:1265-1266.

B.3. Interpret the arterial blood gases: pH, 7.30; $Paco_2$, 60 mm Hg; Pao_2, 49 mm Hg; HCO_3^-, 20 mEq/L on 50% oxygen; and 6 cm H_2O of positive end-expiratory pressure (PEEP). How would you improve them?

The blood gases show respiratory and metabolic acidosis. The Pao_2 of 49 mm Hg is low but acceptable for preterm infants with chronic lung disease. To prevent ROP, Pao_2 between 50 and 70 mm Hg should be maintained. $Paco_2$ of 60 mm Hg indicates hypoventilation, which can be corrected by increasing respiratory rate or tidal volume. To avoid pulmonary oxygen toxicity, Fio_2 should be lowered to less than 40% by increasing levels of PEEP. Mild metabolic acidosis can be corrected by improving fluid balance and circulation.

B.4. What are the normal values of arterial blood pressure, heart rate, and respiratory rate for preterm infants?

The blood pressure is related to the size of infants, as shown in **Table 44.4**. The heavier the birth weight, the higher the blood pressure is. The normal heart rate is 120 to 160 beats per minute. The respiratory rate is normally between 30 and 60 breaths per minute. However, it can increase to 100 to 150 breaths per minute depending on how severely the lung compliance is decreased.

Coté CJ, Anderson BJ, Lerman J. Growth and development. In: Coté CJ, Lerman J, Anderson BJ, eds. *A Practice of Anesthesia for Infants and Children*. 7th ed. Elsevier; 2024:1-21.

Versmold HT, Kitterman JA, Phibbs RH, et al. Aortic blood pressure during the first 12 hours of life in infants with birth weight 610 to 4,220 grams. *Pediatrics*. 1981;67:607-613.

B.5. What are the normal values of WBC, red blood cells (RBCs), hemoglobin, glucose, electrolytes, calcium, blood urea nitrogen, and creatinine for preterm infants?

The WBC count usually ranges from 9,000 to 30,000/μL at birth and decreases to 5,000 to 20,000/μL during the fifth week of life.

The normal RBC and hemoglobin are $5.1 \pm 1.0 \times 10^6$/μL and 19.5 ± 5.0 g/dL, respectively, at birth and decrease to $4.5 \pm 0.7 \times 10^6$/μL and 12.2 ± 2.3 g/dL, respectively, at 3 months of age. At birth, most

TABLE 44.3 Normal Values of Arterial Blood Gases and pH in Pediatric Patients

Age	Preterm	Term	1 Mo	1 Y
pH	7.37 ± 0.03	7.40 ± 0.02	7.41 ± 0.04	7.39 ± 0.02
Pao_2 (mm Hg)	60 ± 8	70 ± 11	95 ± 8	93 ± 10
$Paco_2$ (mm Hg)	37 ± 6	39 ± 7	40 ± 6	41 ± 7

TABLE 44.4 Normal Blood Pressure of Infants Weighing Between 1,000 and 4,000 g

	Weight (g)			
	1,000	2,000	3,000	4,000
Systolic BP (mm Hg)	50	55	60	70
Diastolic BP (mm Hg)	25	30	35	40
Mean BP (mm Hg)	35	40	45	50

BP, blood pressure.

of the hemoglobin is fetal hemoglobin, which has a greater affinity for oxygen. Therefore, the oxygen saturation (and content) of blood for a given $Pa{O_2}$ is higher. By 7 months of age, the circulating hemoglobin is of the adult type.

The normal blood glucose level is between 45 and 90 mg/dL. A glucose level less than 40 mg/dL is common in preterm infants. It should be corrected with a bolus of 10% to 20% glucose (2-5 g/kg) given over 5 minutes, followed by a continuous infusion of glucose. Severe hypoglycemia (<10 mg/dL) can cause brain damage.

The serum calcium concentration of preterm infants is normally lower than that of term infants because preterm infants have decreased serum proteins. Normal calcium level is over 8.0 mg/dL.

The normal values of sodium, potassium, and chloride are 135 to 145, 3.0 to 5.0, and 105 to 115 mEq/L, respectively.

The creatinine levels of term infants at birth are 0.6 to 1.2 mg/dL but, within 1 month, fall to levels of 0.1 to 0.2 mg/dL. Preterm infants have relatively high serum creatinine levels compared with term infants. They are 0.8 to 1.8 mg/dL at birth and fall to 0.2 to 0.8 mg/dL in 1 month.

The normal blood urea nitrogen level is 10 to 20 mg/dL in term infants, whereas it is 16 to 28 mg/dL in preterm infants.

Andropoulos DB. Appendix B: Pediatric normal laboratory values. In: Gregory GA, Andropoulos DB, eds. *Gregory's Pediatric Anesthesia*. 6th ed. Wiley-Blackwell; 2020:1265-1266.

B.6. Would you transfuse blood to this patient preoperatively?

The patient has a hemoglobin of 11 g/dL; a transfusion is not indicated. To ensure oxygen-carrying capacity, most clinicians agree that a hemoglobin of 10 g/dL is the lowest acceptable level if cardiorespiratory disease exists. If infants are well, a hemoglobin level of greater than 7.0 g/dL is usually acceptable.

Adams TL, Kanmanthreddy S, Eisses MJ, Bender MA, Lantham GJ. Essentials of hematology. In: Coté CJ, Lerman J, Anderson BJ, eds. *A Practice of Anesthesia for Infants and Children*. 7th ed. Elsevier; 2024:236-260.

Downey LA, Rollins MR, Miller BE. Coagulation, bleeding, and blood transfusion. In: Gregory GA, Andropoulos DB, eds. *Gregory's Pediatric Anesthesia*. 6th ed. Wiley-Blackwell; 2020:266-269.

B.7. How would you interpret the urinalysis: specific gravity, 1.005; sugar, 1+; and protein, 1+?

Normal urine specific gravity is 1.001 to 1.035. A higher specific gravity may be suggestive of dehydration. Mild glucosuria may be present in preterm infants, likely due to decreased renal tubular reabsorption of glucose. Albumin is normally filtered by the glomerulus and is completely reabsorbed. However, because of tubular immaturity, preterm infants have mild proteinuria.

Handoko R. Nephrology. In: Kleinman K, McDaniel L, Molloy M, eds. *The Harriet Lane Handbook*. 22nd ed. Elsevier; 2021:473-474.

B.8. Would you correct a serum calcium level of 6.0 mg/dL? What other information would you like to have? Which contains more calcium, 10 mL of 10% calcium chloride or 10 mL of 10% calcium gluconate? Could you hyperventilate this child safely?

Normally, the serum calcium is maintained at 8.0 mg/dL; however, in the preterm infant, a level of 7.0 mg/dL is acceptable. This child's serum calcium is 6.0 mg/dL. Therefore, supplementation with 30 to 100 mg/kg of calcium gluconate or 10 to 20 mg/kg of calcium chloride is appropriate.

Hypocalcemia in neonates is defined as serum calcium less than 3.5 mEq/L or serum ionized calcium less than 1.5 mEq/L. When evaluating the serum calcium levels, it is important to know the serum protein concentration; neonatal hypocalcemia is usually due to hypoproteinemia. It is also important to determine the ionized calcium concentration (usually 45% of the total calcium concentration) because this is the calcium immediately available at the cellular level. The chloride molecule is approximately one-third the weight of the gluconate molecule. For this reason, approximately 3 times more calcium is effectively available when the same volume of calcium chloride is administered instead of 10% calcium gluconate. Respiratory alkalosis following hyperventilation will reduce serum ionized calcium levels and, for this reason, should be avoided in this infant.

Gregory GA. Anesthesia for premature infants. In: Gregory GA, Andropoulos DB, eds. *Gregory's Pediatric Anesthesia.* 6th ed. Wiley-Blackwell; 2020:505-512.

Moritz ML, Ellis D. Regulation of fluids and electrolytes. In: Davis PJ, Cladis FP, eds. *Smith's Anesthesia for Infants and Children.* 10th ed. Elsevier; 2022:150-152.

B.9. How would you premedicate this patient?

Children under 1 year of age do not usually need sedation or anxiolysis. However, atropine, 0.01 to 0.02 mg/kg, may be given to attenuate the vagal response to a host of different stimuli.

Sivak EL, Hall-Burton DM. Anesthetic adjuncts. In: Davis PJ, Cladis FP, eds. *Smith's Anesthesia for Infants and Children.* 10th ed. Elsevier; 2022:279-280.

C. Intraoperative Management

C.1. Should this procedure be performed in the neonatal intensive care unit (NICU) or the operating room?

Surgical ligation of the PDA can be performed either in the operating room or in the NICU. The decision is frequently institution dependent. Studies have demonstrated the safety of PDA ligation in the NICU setting when performed by an experienced team. Advantages of performing ligation in the NICU include minimizing transport, continuity of care, and maintenance of NICU interventions such as specialized ventilator settings or nitric oxide. Advantages of performing ligation in the operating room include familiarity with the operating room environment for the surgical and anesthesia teams, availability of familiar equipment, potential for improved sterility, and proximity to other surgical and anesthesia personnel.

Jenkins IA, Kelly Ugarte LR, Mancuso TJ. Where should we operate on the preterm neonate? *Paediatr Anaesth.* 2014;24:127-136.

Lee LK, Woodfin MY, Vadi MG, et al. A comparison of postoperative outcomes with PDA ligation in the OR versus the NICU: a retrospective cohort study on the risks of transport. *BMC Anesthesiol.* 2018;18:199.

C.2. What monitors would you use for this child during surgery?

Proper monitoring of this child for safe administration of anesthesia includes the following:

- *Respiratory*—precordial or esophageal stethoscope, end-tidal CO_2, inspiratory oxygen monitor, pulse oximeter, arterial blood gases, inspiratory pressure gauge
- *Cardiovascular*—precordial or esophageal stethoscope, electrocardiogram, blood pressure cuff, and urinary catheter
- *Thermoregulatory*—esophageal or axillary temperature probe

Pulse oximetry and blood pressure monitoring in both the upper and lower extremities can assist in detecting inadvertent ligation of the descending aorta. An increase in diastolic blood pressure from the elimination of pulmonary runoff during diastole can be observed once the PDA has been successfully ligated.

If the patient has an umbilical artery catheter in place, it is useful for the measurement of blood pressure and arterial blood gases. However, in the absence of severe coexisting disease, it is probably unnecessary to establish an arterial line for the surgery alone because invasive monitoring in this age group is not without risk.

Walker SG. Anesthesia for left-to-right shunt lesions. In: Andropoulos DB, Mossad EB, Gottlieb EA, eds. *Anesthesia for Congenital Heart Disease.* 4th ed. John Wiley & Sons; 2023:205, 627-628.

C.3. What levels of arterial oxygen saturation would you like to keep during surgery?

Safe anesthesia practice requires the monitoring of arterial oxygen saturation in all patients to prevent hypoxia. However, in ex-premature infants less than 44 weeks' postconceptional age, it is also vital to guard against hyperoxia, which may cause ROP. The arterial oxygen saturation should be kept between 90% and 95% during the neonatal period.

Barnes SS, Davis PJ, Brett C. Anesthesia for general surgery in neonates. In: Davis PJ, Cladis FP, eds. *Smith's Anesthesia for Infants and Children.* 10th ed. Elsevier; 2022:675.

Purohit DM, Ellison RC, Zierler S, Miettinen OS, Nadas AS. Risk factors for retrolental fibroplasia: experience with 3,025 premature infants. National collaborative study on patent ductus arteriosus in premature infants. *Pediatrics*. 1985;76:339-344.

C.4. How would you maintain the patient's body temperature?

Hypothermia greatly increases the metabolic rate and oxygen consumption of preterm infants. The preterm infant is particularly susceptible to heat loss because of a large surface-to-volume ratio, lack of insulating fat, and a naturally flaccid and open posture. In addition, the preterm infant often has impaired thermal regulatory ability; therefore, all precautions must be taken to ensure normothermia. The patient should be transported to the operating room in a heated isolette. If unavailable, the infant should be covered with a plastic sheet or warm blanket, and a cap should be put on the head to prevent heat loss. The operating room should be warmed to greater than 27 °C (80 °F) and a servo-controlled infrared heater placed over the operating table. A water-circulating heating blanket or forced air warmer should be used. All extremities should be covered if possible. All intravenous fluids and inspired gases should be warmed and humidified to help maintain the patient's body temperature. If the appropriate setup and equipment are available, then in very low-birth-weight infants, the procedure can be done at the bedside using the ICU ventilator for airway management. This helps minimize the risks associated with transportation and avoid hypothermia.

Gregory GA. Anesthesia for premature infants. In: Gregory GA, Andropoulos DB, eds. *Gregory's Pediatric Anesthesia*. 6th ed. Wiley-Blackwell; 2020:505-512.

Ohliger S, Cronin J, Deutsch N. Induction, maintenance, and recovery. In: Davis PJ, Cladis FP, eds. *Smith's Anesthesia for Infants and Children*. 10th ed. Elsevier; 2022:447.

C.5. How do the anesthetic requirements of the preterm infant differ from those of the adult?

Achieving proper anesthetic depth in the preterm infant presents a unique challenge to the anesthesiologist. Anesthetic requirements (as determined by minimal alveolar concentration) are decreased in the preterm infant as compared with the adult, possibly due to immaturity of the central nervous system and increased circulating concentrations of progesterone and β-endorphins. Cardiovascular sensitivity is greatly pronounced because of greater myocardial depression and a reduced peripheral response to catecholamines. Furthermore, the baroreceptor reflex that maintains blood pressure is often poorly developed in the preterm infant and can be abolished by even light levels of inhalation anesthesia. Therefore, the preterm infant is extremely susceptible to anesthetic overdose, which produces cardiovascular depression leading to hypotension or cardiovascular collapse.

Unfortunately, an inadequate depth of anesthesia is also uniquely hazardous in the neonate. Because there is a lack of cerebral autoregulation, systemic hypertension from inadequate depth of anesthesia may be transmitted directly to the cerebral circulation, resulting in intraventricular hemorrhage.

For these reasons, it is essential to carefully tailor anesthetic depth to surgical conditions because the therapeutic margin between underdose and overdose is extremely narrow.

Gregory GA. Anesthesia for premature infants. In: Gregory GA, Andropoulos DB, eds. *Gregory's Pediatric Anesthesia*. 6th ed. Wiley-Blackwell; 2020:505-512.

Sparth JP, Lam JE. The extremely premature infant (micropremie) and common neonatal emergencies. In: Coté C, Lerman J, Anderson B, eds. *A Practice of Anesthesia for Infants and Children*. 7th ed. Elsevier; 2024:953-981.

Lou HC, Lassen NA, Friis-Hansen B. Impaired autoregulation of cerebral blood flow in the distressed newborn infant. *J Pediatr*. 1979;94:118-121.

C.6. What size endotracheal tube would you have used if the patient had not been intubated?

The larynx of a full-term neonate usually accommodates a 3.0-mm or 3.5-mm endotracheal tube, whereas infants weighing less than 3,500 g will require a 3.0-mm or smaller tube. In infants weighing less than 1,500 g, a 2.5-mm tube is usually recommended. The endotracheal tube diameter should be large enough to allow easy ventilation but small enough to permit the leaking of gas between the tube and trachea when the lung is ventilated with 15 to 20 cm H_2O pressure. Excessive pressure on the tracheal mucosa from an inappropriately large endotracheal tube can lead to tracheal stenosis from tissue injury. However, a higher leak pressure of 25 to 35 cm H_2O may be necessary if high peak inspiratory pressures are required during anesthesia, such as during a thoracotomy or an upper laparotomy or if the patient has decreased pulmonary compliance.

Fiadjoe JE, Stricker PA, Litman RS. Pediatric airway management. In: Gregory GA, Andropoulos DB, eds. *Gregory's Pediatric Anesthesia*. 6th ed. Wiley-Blackwell; 2020:336-337.

Sparth JP, Lam JE. The extremely premature infant (micropremie) and common neonatal emergencies. In: Coté C, Lerman J, Anderson B, eds. *A Practice of Anesthesia for Infants and Children*. 7th ed. Elsevier; 2024:953-981.

C.7. How would you have induced anesthesia if the patient had not been intubated?

Preterm infants require adequate anesthesia and analgesia for painful procedures. Although the use of premedication for intubation in the NICU may be institution dependent, studies have demonstrated that premedication in the newborn improves intubating conditions, decreases the time and number of attempts to secure airway, decreases potential intubation-related airway injury, and attenuates the physiologic responses to laryngoscopy and intubation. After preoxygenation with 100% oxygen and premedication with fentanyl 1 to 4 μg/kg, rocuronium 0.6 to 1.2 mg/kg can be used to facilitate intubation. After intubation, breath sounds should be checked bilaterally to ensure that the tube is properly positioned.

Alternatively, anesthesia may be induced in the operating room with an inhalation anesthetic such as sevoflurane followed by paralysis with rocuronium before intubation.

Foglia EE, Ades A, Sawyer T, et al. Neonatal intubation practice and outcomes: an International Registry Study. *Pediatrics*. 2019;143:e20180902.

Kumar P, Denson SE, Mancuso TJ; Committee on Fetus and Newborn, Section on Anesthesiology and Pain Medicine. Premedication for nonemergency endotracheal intubation in the neonate. *Pediatrics*. 2010;125:608-615.

C.8. How would you maintain anesthesia?

Because preterm infants are extremely sensitive to cardiovascular depression from volatile anesthetics, an intravenous anesthetic technique using opioids such as fentanyl and a neuromuscular blocker can be used for the maintenance of anesthesia. Increments of fentanyl, 3 to 5 μg/kg are titrated to maintain hemodynamic stability. A bolus injection of high-dose fentanyl, 30 to 50 μg/kg, often causes hypotension because the infant is usually dehydrated due to fluid restriction and diuretic therapy for congestive heart failure from PDA.

Neuromuscular blockers commonly used in children, such as cisatracurium, vecuronium, or rocuronium, can be administered to maintain immobility. Pancuronium is an attractive choice for small infants because it causes mild tachycardia and the infant's blood pressure is dependent on heart rate. However, pancuronium has become unavailable in many parts of the world.

McEwan A, Rolo VL. Anesthesia for children undergoing heart surgery. In: Coté CJ, Lerman J, Anderson BJ, eds. *A Practice of Anesthesia for Infants and Children*. 7th ed. Elsevier; 2024:433-467.

Walker SG. Anesthesia for left-to-right shunt lesions. In: Andropoulos DB, Mossad EB, Gottlieb EA, eds. *Anesthesia for Congenital Heart Disease*. 4th ed. John Wiley & Sons; 2023:205, 628.

C.9. How would you ventilate the patient? What tidal volume, respiratory rates, and F_{IO_2} would you set for the infant?

Controlled ventilation should be employed because preterm infants do not breathe well under anesthesia. One option is hand ventilation with a Jackson-Rees device. This technique potentially allows for instantaneous compensation for changes in pulmonary compliance and resistance, especially during thoracotomy. It also permits the use of PEEP. However, manual ventilation may be unreliable for sensing changes in compliance. Mechanical ventilation, preferably with a pediatric bellows or NICU ventilator, may be used to ventilate the infant.

During spontaneous respiration, normal tidal volume is 7 mL/kg for all ages. However, ventilator tidal volumes based on body weight for adult patients, such as 6 to 8 mL/kg, might not be applicable for pediatric patients, especially small infants. A ventilator-delivered tidal volume may be lost from the leak around an uncuffed endotracheal tube. Older anesthesia ventilators were not designed to deliver small tidal volumes accurately, but modern ventilators can compensate for the compliance of the breathing system. However, most modern anesthesia ventilators have a minimal tidal volume of 20 mL, which might not be appropriate for the smallest patients. In cases where a leak cannot be eliminated, such as with an uncuffed tube, or the desired tidal volumes are below the limitations of the ventilator, pressure control ventilation is appropriate. Usually, the peak inspiratory pressures are set between 15 and 25 cm H_2O, depending on the patient's respiratory condition, to ensure adequate chest expansion.

The respiratory rates and inspiratory pressures are adjusted as needed to maintain the Pa_{CO_2} between 35 and 40 mm Hg or the end-tidal CO_2 between 30 and 35 mm Hg. The F_{IO_2} is adjusted to keep the Pa_{O_2} between 50 and 70 mm Hg or the arterial oxygen saturation between 87% and 95%.

Feldman JM. Optimal ventilation of the anesthetized pediatric patient. *Anesth Analg*. 2015;120:165-175.

Gregory GA. Anesthesia for premature infants. In: Gregory GA, Andropoulos DB, eds. *Gregory's Pediatric Anesthesia*. 6th ed. Wiley-Blackwell; 2020:505-512.

C.10. Discuss blood and fluid therapy in this preterm infant.

Fluid therapy should be aimed at correcting the preoperative deficit, providing maintenance fluid, and replacing intraoperative evaporative, third-space, and surgical blood losses.

Intraoperative blood loss must be carefully estimated by weighing the sponges and using small-calibrated suction bottles in plain view of the anesthesiologist. The preterm infant's blood volume is only 85 to 100 mL/kg; therefore, even a 10-mL blood loss can be critical. Despite these precautions, estimation of blood loss is inevitably inaccurate because of the unmeasured loss in the drapes and tissues. For this reason, it is recommended that 125% to 150% of measured blood loss be replaced. Each 1 mL of estimated blood loss is replaced with 3 mL of Ringer lactate or 1 mL of 5% albumin in saline. If the hematocrit is low (<30%) to begin with, blood losses are replaced with packed RBC.

Maintenance fluids consisting of 5% dextrose in one-fourth strength normal saline are given at 4 mL/kg/h, whereas evaporative and third-space losses are replaced with a balanced crystalloid solution at 8 to 12 mL/kg/h for abdominal or thoracic procedures. The adequacy of blood and fluid therapy may be evaluated by the maintenance of stable blood pressure, normal central venous pressure (over 3 cm H_2O), and adequate urine output of greater than 0.75 mL/kg/h with a specific gravity of less than 1.010. In addition, the infant's fontanel should be above the inner table of the skull if there is no volume depletion.

Gregory GA. Anesthesia for premature infants. In: Gregory GA, Andropoulos DB, eds. *Gregory's Pediatric Anesthesia*. 6th ed. Wiley-Blackwell; 2020:505-512.

Jones CT, McClain CD, McManus ML. Fluid management. In: Coté CJ, Lerman J, Anderson BJ, eds. *A Practice of Anesthesia for Infants and Children*. 7th ed. Elsevier; 2024:216-235.

C.11. During dissection of the ductus arteriosus, the arterial oxygen saturation decreased from 92% to 80% and the heart rate decreased from 140 beats per minute to 80 beats per minute. What could be the likely causes and how would you treat them?

Young infants, especially preterm infants, develop hypoxemia quickly after hypoventilation because they have high metabolism (increased oxygen demand) and low FRC. FRC in awake young infants is dynamically determined by inspiratory muscle tone, diaphragmatic activity, alterations in glottic diameter during the respiratory cycle, and respiratory rate. These variables that sustain FRC are lost with general anesthesia and muscle relaxation.

During dissection of the ductus arteriosus, the ipsilateral lung is retracted and compressed by the surgeon. Therefore, pulmonary resistance increases and pulmonary compliance decreases. Consequently, the delivered tidal volume to the patient decreases, and the gas leak around the endotracheal tube increases if the inspiratory pressures remain unchanged. Decreasing tidal volume causes hypoventilation, resulting in hypoxemia and CO_2 retention. In addition, compressing the lung tissue increases intrapulmonary shunt, which causes further hypoxemia. In pediatric patients, the most common cause of bradycardia is hypoxemia. During dissection of the ductus arteriosus, surgical manipulation of the vagus nerve and lung tissue may initiate a vagal reflex, with resultant bradycardia.

The infant should be manually ventilated with 100% oxygen to correct hypoxemia and bradycardia. If bradycardia persists, atropine, 0.01 to 0.02 mg/kg, should be given. The surgical manipulation should be stopped and the collapsed lung reexpanded. Blood loss or hypovolemia should also be corrected.

When the hemodynamic status and oxygenation are stabilized, the FIO_2 and respiratory pressures should be adjusted to ensure adequate ventilation and oxygenation.

Motoyama EK, Finder JD. Respiratory physiology. In: Davis PJ, Cladis FP, eds. *Smith's Anesthesia for Infants and Children*. 10th ed. Elsevier; 2022:49-53.

D. Postoperative Management

D.1. Would you reverse the neuromuscular blockade and extubate the patient at the end of surgery?

No. Postoperative ventilatory support would be necessary for this preterm infant with RDS; therefore, reversal of muscle relaxation and extubation are not indicated.

D.2. How can one minimize the risk of transporting the patient to the NICU after surgery?

The anesthesiologist's responsibilities do not end with the successful completion of the operative procedure. Removal of the surgical drapes must be done with caution to prevent inadvertent extubation

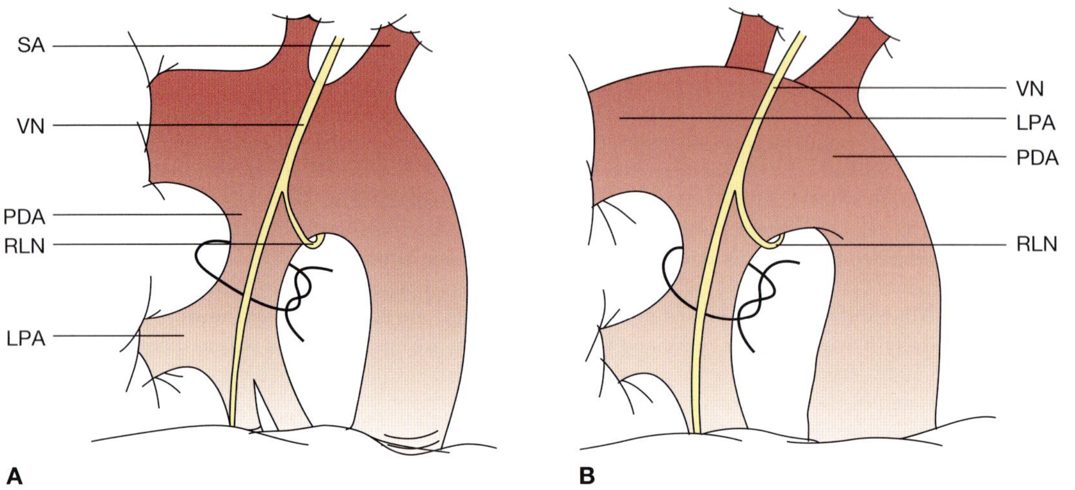

FIGURE 44.1. **A.** Anatomically, atypical patent ductus arteriosus (PDA) arising proximal to the left subclavian artery (SA). **B.** Large patent ductus arteriosus sweeping into the descending aorta and appearing to be the arch. The ductus overlies the arch and hides it from view. A large distal left pulmonary artery is misinterpreted as the patent ductus (encircled by ligature). LPA, left pulmonary artery; RLN, recurrent laryngeal nerve; VN, vagus nerve. (Adapted from Pontius RG, Danielson GK, Noonan JA, et al. Illusions leading to surgical closure of the distal left pulmonary artery instead of the ductus arteriosus. *J Thorac Cardiovasc Surg.* 1981;82:107-113. Copyright © 1981 Elsevier. With permission.)

or removal of the arterial or venous cannula. Transportation of the infant to the NICU is an extremely hazardous transition and requires watchful vigilance.

Arrangements must be made in advance so that elevators are waiting and the nursery is ready to accept the patient. The anesthesiologist must accompany the child until satisfied that care has been appropriately transferred to the NICU staff.

The same monitors that were employed for surgery must be used in transport, including electrocardiogram and monitors for arterial blood pressure and oxygen saturation. Ventilation should be maintained by hand with a Jackson-Rees device or by a battery-operated transport ventilator. A precordial stethoscope is especially helpful to monitor the adequacy of respiration and heart sounds. Every effort to ensure thermal stability must be made, including the use of a heated isolette, plastic sheet, warm blankets, and a cap on the infant's head.

Gregory GA. Anesthesia for premature infants. In: Gregory GA, Andropoulos DB, eds. *Gregory's Pediatric Anesthesia.* 6th ed. Wiley-Blackwell; 2020:505-512.

D.3. The patient's respiratory status deteriorated in the days following surgery, with chest radiography demonstrating evidence of continued congestive failure. Physical examination revealed a persistent cardiac murmur. What was the possible diagnosis?

Complications from surgical closure of a PDA include bleeding, chylothorax, injury to the recurrent laryngeal nerve, pneumothorax, recurrent PDA, and inadvertent ligation of the left pulmonary artery or descending aorta. A large ductus arteriosus arising from the aortic arch proximal to the subclavian artery can create the illusion of the arch, leading to surgical closure of the distal left pulmonary artery instead of ductus arteriosus (**Figure 44.1**). A sign of successful PDA ligation is an increase in diastolic blood pressure from the elimination of pulmonary runoff during diastole. To help identify the ductus, some surgeons place a temporary clip on what they believe is the ductus and observe whether the diastolic pressure increases correspondingly.

In this case, the ductus arteriosus was not ligated; therefore, the ductus murmur persisted. Inadvertent ligation of the distal left pulmonary artery resulted in pulmonary ischemia distal to the ligation. Meanwhile, the right lung was further flooded with the shunted blood through the unligated PDA. The resultant ventilation/perfusion mismatch caused further hypoxemia and CO_2 retention in this infant. The patient should be brought to the operating room for repair of the left pulmonary artery and ligation of the ductus arteriosus.

Rosen DA, Rosen KR. Anomalies of the aortic arch and valve. In: Lake CL, Booker PD, eds. *Pediatric Cardiac Anesthesia*. 4th ed. Lippincott Williams & Wilkins; 2005:381-425.

Pontius RG, Danielson GK, Noonan JA, Judson JP. Illusions leading to surgical closure of the distal left pulmonary artery instead of the ductus arteriosus. *J Thorac Cardiovasc Surg*. 1981;82:107-113.

45 Post-Tonsillectomy Hemorrhage

Dana L. Gurvitch, Shona M. Lee, and Hugh C. Hemmings Jr.

The patient is a 10-year-old male with a history of diagnosed obstructive sleep apnea (apnea-hypopnea index [AHI] of 27) who presents to the emergency department with bleeding in the posterior oropharynx 7 days following tonsillectomy. On physical exam, the patient is lethargic with pallor and decreased capillary refill. His vital signs are significant for tachycardia to 140 beats per minute, hypotension with blood pressure of 70/40 mm Hg, and tachypnea with a respiratory rate of 25 breaths per minute. His oxygen saturation is 97%. The patient is accompanied by his mother, who states that the bleeding started 2 hours ago after the child ate a sandwich.

A. Medical Disease and Differential Diagnosis

1. Approximately how many pediatric tonsillectomies are performed in the United States each year? What are the indications for tonsillectomy?
2. What is the differential diagnosis for this patient?
3. What is the treatment for a patient with von Willebrand disease?
4. Describe the vascular anatomy of the tonsils and the stages of healing post-tonsillectomy.
5. What is the incidence of post-tonsillectomy hemorrhage?
6. What are the risk factors for post-tonsillectomy hemorrhage? Does age matter?
7. Describe the morbidity and mortality of post-tonsillectomy hemorrhage.

B. Preoperative Evaluation and Preparation

1. What is your approach to assessing this patient?
2. What will you set up in the operating room for this patient? How will your preparation be different from a routine general anesthetic setup?
3. Should you plan to use vasopressors?
4. The patient seems anxious. Will you administer a sedative to calm the patient down?
5. How do you plan on interpreting this patient's laboratory results?
6. What are your expectations of the surgeon, specifically as it relates to induction of anesthesia?

C. Intraoperative Management

1. What is your plan for induction of anesthesia? During the initial procedure, this patient underwent an uneventful inhalational induction, with postinduction intravenous (IV) placement. Would you perform an inhalational induction again? Why or why not?
2. What is your plan for management of blood in the oropharynx?
3. What is your plan for airway management?
4. Laryngoscopy and intubation prove challenging due to blood in the airway. What options do you have now?
5. What is your plan for maintenance of anesthesia? What other medications might you want to give?
6. Assuming the surgical intervention is successful, what is your plan for emergence and extubation?

D. Postoperative Management

1. Is postoperative management in the pediatric intensive care unit (PICU) indicated? If this was an uncomplicated adenotonsillectomy, what are the suggested criteria for planned admission?
2. What would you require for safe transport from the operating room to the PICU?
3. Discuss potential postoperative complications for this patient. What are other morbidities associated with pediatric tonsillectomy?

4. What is the overall incidence of mortality after pediatric tonsillectomy? What are the clinical predictors of post-tonsillectomy mortality?
5. What discharge instructions should be given post-tonsillectomy?

A. Medical Disease and Differential Diagnosis

A.1. Approximately how many pediatric tonsillectomies are performed in the United States each year? What are the indications for tonsillectomy?

Despite a declining incidence in recent years, approximately 289,000 tonsillectomies are performed in the United States annually in children less than 15 years of age, making it the second most common pediatric ambulatory procedure (behind myringotomy tube insertion).

The two most common indications for tonsillectomy in children are obstructive sleep-disordered breathing (OSDB) and infection. OSDB exists on a continuum, with the mildest end being snoring. Obstructive sleep apnea syndrome (OSAS), due to partial or complete airway obstruction during sleep, represents the severe end of the spectrum and is now the most common indication for surgery. The severity of OSAS can be evaluated via polysomnography. Results of polysomnography are graded by the AHI (the average number of apneic and hypopneic episodes per hour). The AHI allows OSAS to be classified as mild ($1 < \text{AHI} \leq 5$), moderate ($5 < \text{AHI} \leq 10$), or severe ($\text{AHI} > 10$). Patients with OSDB can exhibit delayed growth, enuresis, daytime sleepiness or hyperactivity, poor concentration, aggression, anxiety, depression, and other behavioral disorders. In addition, patients with OSDB can have a lower intelligence quotient (IQ) and quality of life. Less robust pediatric data show evidence of cardiometabolic disease, which is highly correlated with OSAS in adults.

A second indication for tonsillectomy in children is infection. This can include recurrent tonsillitis, chronic tonsillitis, or peritonsillar abscess. The American Academy of Otolaryngology-Head and Neck Surgery recommends watchful waiting over tonsillectomy if there has been fewer than seven infections in the past year, fewer than five infections per year for the last 2 years, or fewer than three infections per year for at least 3 years (also known as the Paradise Criteria), with documentation of either temperature greater than 38.3 °C, cervical adenopathy, tonsillar exudates/erythema, or a positive test for Group A β-hemolytic *Streptococcus*.

In general, the natural history of tonsillitis episodes diminishes in frequency over time. In addition, many advantages seen in tonsillectomy patients (decreased infection recurrence, missed school days, and health care utilization) over control groups, decrease after 1 year. Therefore, caregiver education and a discussion on the benefits of tonsillectomy versus potential harm should be carefully considered. Modifying factors, such as multiple antibiotic allergies, PFAPA (periodic fever, aphthous stomatitis, pharyngitis, and adenitis), or a history of more than one peritonsillar abscess can be exceptions to these criteria.

Dehlink E, Tan HL. Update on paediatric obstructive sleep apnoea. *J Thorac Dis*. 2016;8:224-235.

Hall MJ, Schwartzman A, Zhang J, Liu X. Ambulatory Surgery Data from Hospitals and Ambulatory Surgery Centers: United States, 2010. *Natl Health Stat Report*. 2017:1-15.

Mitchell RB, Archer SM, Ishman SL, et al. Clinical practice guideline: tonsillectomy in children (update). *Otolaryngol Head Neck Surg*. 2019;160:S1-S42.

Paradise JL, Bluestone CD, Bachman RZ, et al. Efficacy of tonsillectomy for recurrent throat infection in severely affected children. Results of parallel randomized and nonrandomized clinical trials. *N Engl J Med*. 1984;310:674-683.

Vanderhoek, SM, Dalesio, NM, & Schwengel, DA. Anesthesia for Otorhinolaryngologic Surgery. In: Davis PJ & Cladis, FP, ed. *Smith's Anesthesia for Infants and Children*. 10th ed. Elsevier; 2021:922-924.

A.2. What is the differential diagnosis for this patient?

Blood in the posterior oropharynx could have several etiologies, and it is important to start with a broad differential. Given this patient's recent tonsillectomy, postoperative bleeding from the surgical site is the most likely diagnosis. However, other possible causes of bleeding include trauma, underlying coagulopathy, vascular malformation, or it may be spontaneous. Bleeding from the tonsillar bed is the most likely cause of this patient's surgical bleeding. However, damage to nearby structures, including the uvula, should not be overlooked. Epistaxis secondary to trauma, and possibly unrelated to the prior surgery, can also be a cause of bleeding into the posterior pharynx. Additionally, underlying coagulopathies, such as von Willebrand disease (incidence of 1% in the general population), can be a cause for continued bleeding following surgery. Finally, spontaneous hemorrhage from vessel erosion secondary to infection is a rare event since the advent of antibiotics.

Centers for Disease Control and Prevention. Data and statistics on von Willebrand disease. *Von Willebrand Disease (VWD)*. Published May 22, 2024. Accessed April 1, 2025. https://www.cdc.gov/von-willebrand/data/index.html

Salem A, Healy S, Pau H. Management of spontaneous tonsillar bleeding: review. *J Laryngol Otol*. 2010;124:470-473.

A.3. What is the treatment for a patient with von Willebrand disease?

To combat the dual defects on hemostasis (abnormal coagulation due to low levels of expressed factor VIII and abnormal platelet adhesion), there are three main treatment options:

- Desmopressin (raises endogenous factor VIII and von Willebrand factor levels)
- von Willebrand factor concentrate
- Transfusion therapy with blood products

Eighty percent of patients with von Willebrand disease have type 1 von Willebrand disease, which is responsive to desmopressin. In patients with type 2 or type 3 von Willebrand disease, desmopressin is not effective, and plasma concentrates containing factor VIII and von Willebrand factor concentrate must be used.

Mannucci PM. Treatment of von Willebrand's disease. *N Engl J Med*. 2004;351:683-694.

Von Willebrand disease (VWD): treatment of minor bleeding, use of DDAVP, and routine preventive care. Published July 8, 2024. Accessed April 1, 2025. https://www.uptodate.com/contents/von-willebrand-disease-vwd-treatment-of-minor-bleeding-use-of-ddavp-and-routine-preventive-care

A.4. Describe the vascular anatomy of the tonsils and the stages of healing post-tonsillectomy.

The arterial blood supply of the tonsils comes from several branches of the external carotid artery, including the ascending pharyngeal artery, descending palatine artery, ascending palatine artery, facial artery branches, and dorsal lingual artery (**Figure 45.1**). The internal carotid artery can have an aberrant course, allowing it to run close to the tonsillar bed. Venous return is to the peritonsillar plexus, the lingual vein, and the pharyngeal plexus. Sources of tonsillar bleeding can be arterial, venous (most commonly), or involve vascular anomalies.

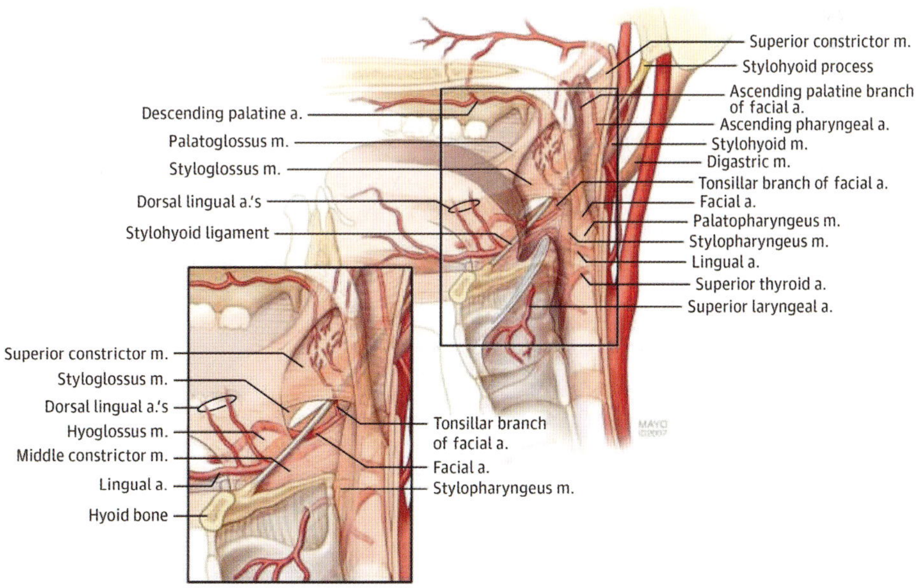

FIGURE 45.1. Blood supply to the lateral oropharynx. a, artery; m, muscle. (From Van Abel KM, Moore EJ. Surgical management of the base of tongue. *Oper Tech Otolaryngol*. 2013;24:74-85. Used with permission of Mayo Foundation for Medical Education and Research. All rights reserved.)

SECTION 10

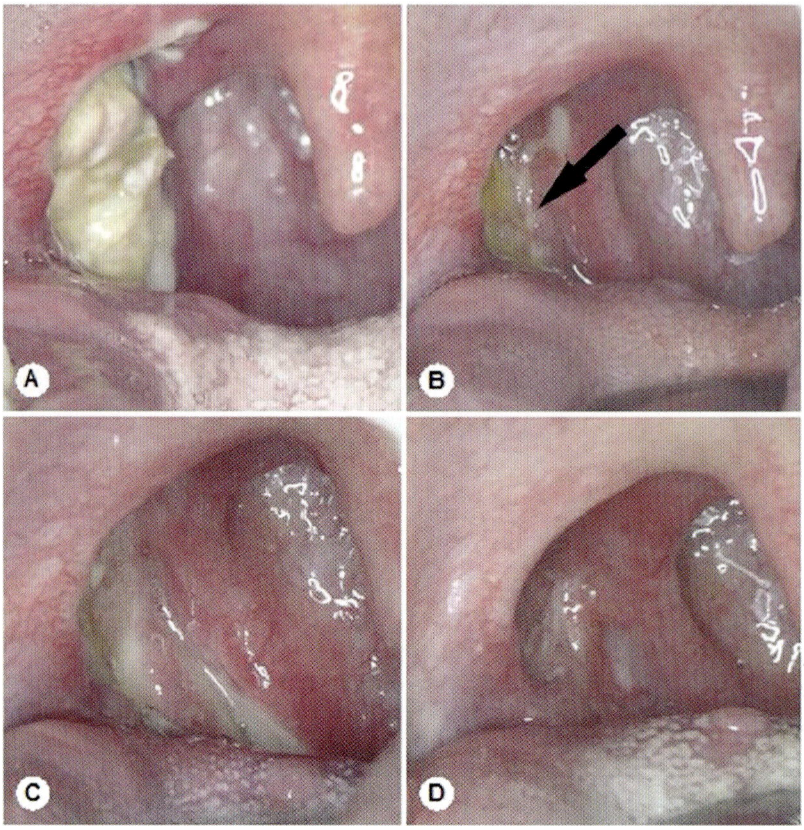

FIGURE 45.2. Stages of tonsillectomy healing. A. Postoperative day (POD) 5: Exudative fibrin clot fills tonsillar fossa, protruding beyond tonsillar pillars. **B.** POD 7: Fibrin clot has separated from tonsillar fossa. New stroma lines the tonsillar fossa. Initial ingrowth of posterior pillar epithelium is discernible (*arrow*). **C.** POD 9: Bridge of epithelium has widened, advancing laterally across stromal bed. **D.** POD 17: Tonsillar fossa is covered by layer of epithelium. Initial epithelium bridge has thickened and resembles normal mucosa. (Reprinted with permission from Isaacson G. Tonsillectomy healing. *Ann Otol Rhinol Laryngol.* 2012;121:645–649. Copyright © 2012 SAGE Publications.)

Stages of tonsillectomy healing are shown in **Figure 45.2**.

Isaacson G. Tonsillectomy healing. *Ann Otol Rhinol Laryngol.* 2012;121:645-649.

Paulsen F, Tillmann B, Christofides C, Richter W, Koebke J. Curving and looping of the internal carotid artery in relation to the pharynx: frequency, embryology and clinical implications. *J Anat.* 2000;197:373-381.

Strandring S. Pharynx. In: Stranding S, ed. *Gray's Anatomy: The Anatomical Basis of Clinical Practice.* 42nd ed. Elsevier; 2021:702-716.

A.5. What is the incidence of post-tonsillectomy hemorrhage?

Post-tonsillectomy hemorrhage is the most serious risk of the procedure, varying from blood-tinged mucus to life-threatening hemorrhage. Post-tonsillectomy hemorrhage occurs in 2% to 4.5% of patients and can be a surgical emergency. Primary bleeding occurs within 24 hours of surgery, in 0.2% to 2.2% of patients with tonsillectomy. Secondary bleeding occurs more than 24 hours after surgery (usually between postoperative days 5 through 7), with a range of 0.1% to 4.8%. Primary hemorrhage is usually a result of inadequate surgical hemostasis, whereas secondary hemorrhage occurs when the fibrin clot, or eschar, sloughs off the tonsillar bed.

Francis DO, Fonnesbeck C, Sathe N, McPheeters M, Krishnaswami S, Chinnadurai S. Postoperative bleeding and associated utilization following tonsillectomy in children. *Otolaryngol Head Neck Surg.* 2017;156:442-455.

Lee AC, Haché M. Pediatric anesthesia management for post-tonsillectomy bleed: current status and future directions. *Int J Gen Med.* 2022;15:63-69.

Windfuhr JP, Chen YS, Remmert S. Hemorrhage following tonsillectomy and adenoidectomy in 15,218 patients. *Otolaryngol Head Neck Surg.* 2005;132:281-286.

A.6. What are the risk factors for post-tonsillectomy hemorrhage? Does age matter?

Risk factors for post-tonsillectomy hemorrhage include age, male sex, history of recurrent infection, and, in rare cases, underlying coagulopathy (such as von Willebrand disease). There are also rare cases of unsuspected vascular anomalies. The incidence of post-tonsillectomy bleeding increases with age, particularly after 12 years of age, when patients can experience up to 6 times the odds of post-tonsillectomy hemorrhage compared to younger patients. Age over 6 years is associated with higher surgical intervention rates to achieve hemostasis. Despite early concerns that perioperative steroid administration might increase the risk of post-tonsillectomy hemorrhage, this concern appears to be unfounded.

Arora R, Saraiya S, Niu X, Thomas RL, Kannikeswaran N. Post tonsillectomy hemorrhage: who needs intervention? *Int J Pediatr Otorhinolaryngol.* 2015;79:165-169.

Chorney SR, Weinberger R, Weintraub AY, Buzi A. Post-tonsillectomy hemorrhage and the diagnosis of occult pediatric coagulopathies. *Laryngoscope.* 2021;131:E2069-E2073.

Lee WT, Witsell DL, Parham K, et al. Tonsillectomy bleed rates across the CHEER practice research network: pursuing guideline adherence and quality improvement. *Otolaryngol Head Neck Surg.* 2016;155:28-32.

Titirungruang C, Seresirikachorn K, Kasemsuwan P, Hirunwiwatkul P. The use of steroids to reduce complications after tonsillectomy: a systematic review and meta-analysis of randomized controlled studies. *Eur Arch Otorhinolaryngol.* 2019;276:585-604.

Tomkinson A, Harrison W, Owens D, Harris S, McClure V, Temple M. Risk factors for postoperative hemorrhage following tonsillectomy. *Laryngoscope.* 2011;121:279-288.

A.7. Describe the morbidity and mortality of post-tonsillectomy hemorrhage.

Efficient and early intervention and resuscitation should be implemented in the face of active bleeding post-tonsillectomy to prevent hypovolemia, decreased cardiac output, and airway obstruction. Morbidity and mortality occur secondary to aspiration, laryngospasm, and hemorrhagic shock. Mortality rates range from 1 in 10,000 to 1 in 35,000.

Windfuhr JP, Schloendorff G, Baburi D, Kremer B. Lethal outcome of post-tonsillectomy hemorrhage. *Eur Arch Otorhinolaryngol.* 2008;265:1527-1534.

B. Preoperative Evaluation and Preparation

B.1. What is your approach to assessing this patient?

The preoperative assessment must be focused and efficient, with emphasis on the airway, vital signs, and cardiovascular status. Important questions to ask yourself during preoperative assessment include the following:

- Is the patient alert and maintaining their airway?
- Is the bleeding active?
- Bleeding characteristics: volume, duration, number of episodes, last episode
- Has the patient been adequately resuscitated?

Patients with active bleeding, oozing, or clot formation in the oropharynx are typically managed surgically. Inadequate volume resuscitation, anemia, swallowing of blood (which increases the risk of aspiration and can lead to underestimation of reported blood loss), and compromised airway visualization are all critical issues. As the patient continues to manifest hypotension and tachycardia, aggressive volume resuscitation should be employed. Laboratory values will help identify the severity of anemia (and thus the need for preoperative transfusion), coagulation issues (platelet count, prothrombin time, partial thromboplastin time, international normalized ratio values), and the need to order clotting factors or platelets. Additionally, laboratory values can help determine acidosis and volume contraction necessitating additional crystalloid administration. Nil per os (NPO) status should be determined and maintained during evaluation and observation (although no recent oral intake does not preclude full-stomach considerations due to the likelihood that an unknown volume of blood has been swallowed).

Fields R, Gencorelli F, Litman R. Anesthetic management of the pediatric bleeding tonsil. *Paediatr Anaesth.* 2010;20:982-986.

Randall DA, Hoffer ME. Complications of tonsillectomy and adenoidectomy. *Otolaryngol Head Neck Surg.* 1998;118:61-68.

Vanderhoek, SM, Dalesio, NM, & Schwengel, DA. Anesthesia for Otorhinolaryngologic Surgery. In: Davis PJ & Cladis, FP, ed. *Smith's Anesthesia for Infants and Children.* 10th ed. Elsevier; 2021:922-924.

Wall JJ, Tay KY. Postoperative tonsillectomy hemorrhage. *Emerg Med Clin North Am.* 2018;36:415-426.

Windfuhr JP, Schloendorff G, Sesterhenn AM, Prescher A, Kremer B. A devastating outcome after adenoidectomy and tonsillectomy: ideas for improved prevention and management. *Otolaryngol Head Neck Surg.* 2009;140: 191-196.

B.2. What will you set up in the operating room for this patient? How will your preparation be different from a routine general anesthetic setup?

Along with standard operating room equipment, additional items to be prepared in the procedure room include the following:

- Blood transfusion tubing along with a fluid warmer
- Double suction setup with Yankauer suction tips, as one may become occluded with blood clots
- Multiple sizes of styleted cuffed endotracheal tubes
- Backup laryngoscope blades and handles
- Emergency airway equipment (McGrath videolaryngoscope, GlideScope, fiberoptic intubation equipment)
- Resuscitation medications
- Ultrasound or intraosseous access equipment in cases of difficult intravenous access
- A tracheostomy set in the unlikely need of an emergency surgical airway

The temperature in the operating room should also be increased to minimize heat loss in the patient.

Fields R, Gencorelli F, Litman R. Anesthetic management of the pediatric bleeding tonsil. *Paediatr Anaesth.* 2010;20:982-986.

Lee AC, Haché M. Pediatric anesthesia management for post-tonsillectomy bleed: current status and future directions. *Int J Gen Med.* 2022;15:63-69.

Vanderhoek, SM, Dalesio, NM, & Schwengel, DA. Anesthesia for Otorhinolaryngologic Surgery. In: Davis PJ & Cladis, FP, ed. *Smith's Anesthesia for Infants and Children.* 10th ed. Elsevier; 2021:922-924.

B.3. Should you plan to use vasopressors?

If the patient is hemodynamically unstable, vasopressors can be titrated until the patient is able to be adequately volume resuscitated. A blood type and crossmatch should be done, laboratory tests should be sent, and the patient should be given fluids and/or blood products in the operating room. Vasopressors should also be considered if the patient has a cardiac history, pulmonary hypertension, or if there is a need to manage the blood pressure tightly. It should be noted that circulatory compensation can mask the true volume of blood loss until more than 40% of blood volume is lost.

Lee AC, Haché M. Pediatric anesthesia management for post-tonsillectomy bleed: current status and future directions. *Int J Gen Med.* 2022;15:63-69.

B.4. The patient seems anxious. Will you administer a sedative to calm the patient down?

The decision to administer preoperative sedation should be weighed against the patient's increased risk for regurgitation and aspiration as well as the potential for respiratory depression. Thus, preoperative sedation in this patient is likely not a wise decision.

Park RS, Peyton JM. Anesthesia for otolaryngologic surgery. In: Cullen BF, Stock MC, Ortega R, et al, eds. *Barash, Cullen, and Stoelting's Clinical Anesthesia.* 9th ed. Wolters Kluwer; 2024:1304-1329.

B.5. How do you plan on interpreting this patient's laboratory results?

The need for blood transfusion should be based on hemoglobin/hematocrit assessment and ongoing blood loss. Although recognizing optimal oxygen-carrying capacity is imperative, the threshold for transfusion should be addressed and discussed with the parents and surgical team preoperatively.

B.6. What are your expectations of the surgeon, specifically as it relates to induction of anesthesia?

The surgeon should be gowned and gloved with a headlight on when the patient enters the operating room. The surgeon should have a rigid bronchoscope and a tracheotomy set ready in addition to the standard surgical equipment.

Windfuhr JP, Schloendorff G, Sesterhenn AM, Prescher A, Kremer B. A devastating outcome after adenoidectomy and tonsillectomy: ideas for improved prevention and management. *Otolaryngol Head Neck Surg.* 2009;140: 191-196.

C. Intraoperative Management

C.1. What is your plan for induction of anesthesia? During the initial procedure, this patient underwent an uneventful inhalational induction with postinduction intravenous (IV) placement. Would you perform an inhalational induction again? Why or why not?

Adequate preoxygenation is essential to ensuring maximal oxygen reserves in the functional residual volume in the unlikely event of an airway issue. Regardless of the actual NPO time, a rapid sequence induction (RSI) should be performed using IV propofol if the patient is hemodynamically stable, or etomidate or ketamine if the patient is unstable. High-dose rocuronium or succinylcholine can be administered for rapid paralysis. If succinylcholine is deemed appropriate and safe, an anticholinergic, such as glycopyrrolate, should be administered prior to succinylcholine to minimize vagal response.

Classical (apneic) RSI with cricoid pressure (Sellick maneuver) versus a controlled (gentle mask ventilation after induction using less than 12 cm H_2O) RSI is debated. Downsides of cricoid pressure include incorrect cartilage location and/or excessive force causing airway distortion, increased intubation time, and greater difficulty. Recent studies support a trend toward a controlled RSI, demonstrating less severe hypoxemia and better views on direct laryngoscopy than the classical RSI group. The risk of aspiration was not increased and remains low in both groups.

Curley GF. Rapid sequence induction with rocuronium—a challenge to the gold standard. *Crit Care*. 2011;15:190.

Lee AC, Haché M. Pediatric anesthesia management for post-tonsillectomy bleed: current status and future directions. *Int J Gen Med*. 2022;15:63-69.

Vanderhoek, SM, Dalesio, NM, & Schwengel, DA. Anesthesia for Otorhinolaryngologic Surgery. In: Davis PJ & Cladis, FP, ed. *Smith's Anesthesia for Infants and Children*. 10th ed. Elsevier; 2021:922-924.

C.2. What is your plan for management of blood in the oropharynx?

There should be two large-bore suction catheters ready prior to anesthesia induction and intubation. Suctioning should be done carefully, as disruption of formed clots can cause exacerbation of the bleeding. If suctioning is needed, the suction catheter should be directed into the midline of the oropharynx, avoiding the tonsillar fossa. Once the bleeding is surgically controlled, suctioning of the stomach can be done carefully and with direct visualization of the oropharynx.

Olutoyin O, Arvind Chandrakantan A, & Watcha M. Otolaryngological and Dental Surgery. In: Andropoulous DB & Gregory GA, ed. *Gregory's Pediatric Anesthesia*. 6th ed. Wiley-Blackwell; 2020:865.

C.3. What is your plan for airway management?

Airway management must proceed with a plan. Two direct laryngoscopes should be readily available in case one of them fails. A Macintosh-blade videolaryngoscope can be used for direct visualization if blood obscures the video function or for indirect visualization if soiling is minimal and the direct view is suboptimal. A fiberoptic bronchoscope and multiple styleted, cuffed endotracheal tubes should also be in the operating room. Additionally, a double suction set up, a backup anesthesiologist, and an ear, nose, and throat (ENT) surgeon should be present.

Fields R, Gencorelli F, Litman R. Anesthetic management of the pediatric bleeding tonsil. *Paediatr Anaesth*. 2010;20:982-986.

Weiss M, Dullenkopf A. Cuffed tracheal tubes in children: past, present and future. *Expert Rev Med Devices*. 2007;4:73-82.

C.4. Laryngoscopy and intubation prove challenging due to blood in the airway. What options do you have now?

Gently pressing on the chest to simulate respiration can create air bubbles at the glottic opening to guide placement of the endotracheal tube. Simultaneous suctioning of blood in the oropharynx by a second anesthesia provider can also help the laryngoscopist focus on intubation.

Olutoyin O, Arvind Chandrakantan A, & Watcha M. Otolaryngological and Dental Surgery. In: Andropoulous DB & Gregory GA, ed. *Gregory's Pediatric Anesthesia*. 6th ed. Wiley-Blackwell; 2020:865.

C.5. What is your plan for maintenance of anesthesia? What other medications might you want to give?

Maintenance of the anesthesia will depend both on the patient's hemodynamic status and surgical cessation of bleeding. Inhalational anesthetics are appropriate for maintenance. Given the usual brevity of these procedures, it is important to exercise caution when choosing to administer IV opioids as this can prolong respiratory depression, especially in patients with OSAS. Other opioid side effects, such as nausea and constipation, can make a smooth recovery more challenging. If opioids are utilized, they should be carefully titrated with dose reduction.

A multimodal, opioid-sparing regimen with caregiver education and expectation management is important. Acetaminophen (10-15 mg/kg), dexmedetomidine (0.3-1 μg/kg), and dexamethasone (0.15-0.5 mg/kg) might be considered a better alternative for analgesia. In addition to analgesic properties, dexmedetomidine decreases emergence agitation.

Antiemetics, such as ondansetron (0.15 mg/kg) and dexamethasone (0.15 mg/kg), and adequate hydration, should also be administered to prevent postoperative nausea and vomiting (PONV), which is a major cause of morbidity in these patients and occurs in more than 70% of children without prophylaxis. Of note, higher dose steroids have not been associated with increased risk of bleeding. In fact, The American Academy of Otolaryngology-Head and Neck Surgery strongly recommends a single dose of dexamethasone after tonsillectomy to decrease PONV, pain scores, and time to first oral intake.

Baugh RF, Archer SM, Mitchell RB, et al. Clinical practice guideline: tonsillectomy in children. *Otolaryngol Head Neck Surg*. 2011;144:S1-S30.

Cho HK, Yoon HY, Jin HJ, Hwang SH. Efficacy of dexmedetomidine for perioperative morbidities in pediatric tonsillectomy: a metaanalysis. *Laryngoscope*. 2018;128:e184-e193.

Mitchell RB, Archer SM, Ishman SL, et al. Clinical practice guideline: tonsillectomy in children (update). *Otolaryngol Head Neck Surg*. 2019;160:S1-S42.

C.6. Assuming the surgical intervention is successful, what is your plan for emergence and extubation?

Once hemostasis and hemodynamic stability are achieved, and the decision is made to extubate, gastric contents should be suctioned, adequate reversal of neuromuscular blockage should be confirmed by a quantitative (ideally) neuromuscular monitor, and the patient should be awake and responsive with laryngeal reflexes.

Fields R, Gencorelli F, Litman R. Anesthetic management of the pediatric bleeding tonsil. *Paediatr Anaesth*. 2010;20:982-986.

Thilen SR, Weigel WA, Todd MM, et al. 2023 American Society of Anesthesiologists Practice Guidelines for monitoring and antagonism of neuromuscular blockade: a report by the American Society of Anesthesiologists Task Force on neuromuscular blockade. *Anesthesiology*. 2023;138:13-41.

Tomkinson A, Harrison W, Owens D, Fishpool S, Temple M. Postoperative hemorrhage following adenoidectomy. *Laryngoscope*. 2012;122:1246-1253.

D. Postoperative Management

D.1. Is postoperative management in the pediatric intensive care unit (PICU) indicated? If this was an uncomplicated adenotonsillectomy, what are the suggested criteria for planned admission?

Deciding whether to admit patients to the PICU status post-tonsillectomy hemorrhage should be jointly determined by the anesthesiologist and surgeon. In a patient without significant comorbidities who had an uneventful intraoperative course, admission to the postanesthesia care unit (PACU) is appropriate and safe for management until discharge criteria are met and the patient is ready to go home (**Table 45.1**).

Planned admission criteria after uncomplicated adenotonsillectomy typically include patients less than 3 years of age without comorbid conditions, patients over 3 years of age with comorbidities, and patients with severe OSA, or with an AHI greater than or equal to 10. Comorbid conditions include cardiac conditions from OSAS, Down syndrome, failure to thrive, neuromuscular disorders, craniofacial anomalies, active or recent respiratory infection, and morbid obesity (body mass index [BMI] >95th percentile for age/sex) without polysomnography results. These patients are at higher risk of perioperative respiratory adverse events. Children with poor predicted oral intake (eg, behavioral factors) or difficult to manage postoperative pain should also be admitted.

The location for monitoring (general floor vs step-down unit vs PICU) varies based on hospital capabilities and the discretion of the surgeon and anesthesiologist. PICU admission is encouraged for very

TABLE 45.1 Postanesthesia Care Unit (PACU) Discharge Criteria for the Pediatric Patients

Infant <1 Y			
Optimal pain relief achieved	☐ YES	☐ NO	
1. BP within pre-op value/age-specific range	☐ YES	☐ NO	
2. HR 120-160	☐ YES	☐ NO	
A. Unchanged from pre-op rhythm?	☐ YES	☐ NO	☐ N/A
3. Level of consciousness: Awake or at pre-op baseline	☐ YES	☐ NO	
4. Temp 36 °C-38 °C	☐ YES	☐ NO	
5. Respiratory rate 30-60	☐ YES	☐ NO	
A. O_2 sat ≥94% or at pre-op baseline (if <94%)	☐ YES	☐ NO	
6. Dressing dry	☐ YES	☐ NO	☐ N/A
7. Urinary output adequate for size	☐ YES	☐ NO	☐ N/A
Age 1-5 Y			
Optimal pain relief achieved	☐ YES	☐ NO	
1. BP within pre-op value/Age-specific range	☐ YES	☐ NO	
2. HR 80-150	☐ YES	☐ NO	
A. Unchanged from pre-op rhythm?	☐ YES	☐ NO	☐ N/A
3. Level of consciousness: Awake or at pre-op baseline	☐ YES	☐ NO	
4. Temp 36 °C-38 °C	☐ YES	☐ NO	
5. Respiratory rate 20-30	☐ YES	☐ NO	
A. O_2 sat ≥94% or at pre-op baseline (if <94%)	☐ YES	☐ NO	
6. Dressing dry	☐ YES	☐ NO	☐ N/A
7. Urinary output adequate for size	☐ YES	☐ NO	☐ N/A
Age 6-12 Y			
Optimal pain relief achieved	☐ YES	☐ NO	
1. BP within pre-op value/age-specific range	☐ YES	☐ NO	
2. HR 60-130	☐ YES	☐ NO	
A. Unchanged from pre-op rhythm?	☐ YES	☐ NO	☐ N/A
3. Level of consciousness: Awake or at pre-op baseline	☐ YES	☐ NO	
4. Temp 36 °C-38 °C	☐ YES	☐ NO	
5. Respiratory rate 12-20	☐ YES	☐ NO	
A. O_2 sat ≥94% or at pre-op baseline (if ≤94%)	☐ YES	☐ NO	
6. Dressing dry	☐ YES	☐ NO	☐ N/A
7. Urinary output adequate for size	☐ YES	☐ NO	☐ N/A

Courtesy of NewYork-Presbyterian/Weill Cornell Medical Center Perioperative Nursing Postanesthesia Record.

SECTION 10

severe OSA (AHI >30 and/or oxygen nadir <80%), associated desaturation events, and comorbidities with a known difficult airway or a syndrome predisposing patients to postoperative airway obstruction.

Lescanne E, Chiron B, Constant I, et al. Pediatric tonsillectomy: clinical practice guidelines. *Eur Ann Otorhinolaryngol Head Neck Dis*. 2012;129:264-271.

McKeon M, Kirsh E, Kawai K, Roberson D, Watters K. Risk factors for multiple hemorrhages following tonsil surgery in children. *Laryngoscope*. 2019;129:2765-2770.

Mitchell RB, Archer SM, Ishman SL, et al. Clinical practice guideline: tonsillectomy in children (update). *Otolaryngol Head Neck Surg*. 2019;160:S1-S42.

Windfuhr JP. Lethal post-tonsillectomy hemorrhage. *Auris Nasus Larynx*. 2003;30:391-396.

D.2. What would you require for safe transport from the operating room to the PICU?

Positioning the patient in the left or right lateral position can reduce the risk of airway obstruction. Supplemental oxygen, emergency airway equipment, and emergency medications are essential for safe transport. If transport over a long distance is required, monitoring equipment should also be employed.

Randall DA, Hoffer ME. Complications of tonsillectomy and adenoidectomy. *Otolaryngol Head Neck Surg*. 1998;118:61-68.

D.3. Discuss potential postoperative complications for this patient. What are other morbidities associated with pediatric tonsillectomy?

Potential postoperative complications include fever, intravascular volume depletion, airway edema, coagulopathy, anemia, electrolyte disturbances, and perioperative respiratory adverse events ranging from oxygen desaturation to apnea requiring ventilatory support. Although rare, a rebleed may also occur. Risk factors for a rebleed include older age (≥12 years) and high BMI for age (≥85%). If stridor is present postextubation, humidified oxygen and nebulized racemic epinephrine (0.25 mL of 2.25% solution diluted to 3 mL with normal saline) should be promptly administered.

Guida RA, Mattucci KF. Tonsillectomy and adenoidectomy: an inpatient or outpatient procedure? *Laryngoscope*. 1990;100:491-493.

Katz SL, Monsour A, Barrowman N, et al. Predictors of postoperative respiratory complications in children undergoing adenotonsillectomy. *J Clin Sleep Med*. 2020;16:41-48.

Leach J, Manning S, Schaefer S. Comparison of two methods of tonsillectomy. *Laryngoscope*. 1993;103:619-622.

D.4. What is the overall incidence of mortality after pediatric tonsillectomy? What are the clinical predictors of post-tonsillectomy mortality?

Mortality in otherwise healthy children is low. The overall 30-day mortality is reported as 1 in 55,000 patients, primarily from respiratory failure/arrest with fewer deaths secondary to bleeding. Pediatric patients with complex medical comorbidities experience a higher rate of death (117 per 100,000 tonsillectomies, representing 44% of overall deaths) than those without comorbidities (4 per 100,000). Of those with chronic, complex comorbidities, children with underlying neurologic disorders are at especially increased risk. Neither age under 3 years nor OSDB is significantly associated with mortality, though these patients may require increased postoperative monitoring.

Edmonson MB, Zhao Q, Francis DO, et al. Association of patient characteristics with postoperative mortality in children undergoing tonsillectomy in 5 US states. *JAMA*. 2022;327:2317-2325.

Johnson RF, Mitchell RB. Mortality risk after pediatric tonsillectomy. *JAMA*. 2022;327:2292-2293.

D.5. What discharge instructions should be given post-tonsillectomy?

After discharge criteria are met, patients (and their parents) should be instructed to visit the nearest emergency room in the event of ongoing bleeding. In addition, patients should be encouraged to hydrate and add soft solids to their diet as tolerated. The most common morbidity after post-tonsillectomy is oropharyngeal pain, which can lead to decreased oral intake, dehydration, behavioral issues, and hospital readmission. It is important to educate caregivers to frequently reassess and manage pain. Pharmacologic interventions for pain management are determined on an individual basis but should aim to optimize the use of nonopioid analgesics such as acetaminophen and nonsteroidal anti-inflammatories (NSAIDs) on a set, alternating schedule. Recommended prescribing of acetaminophen is 10 to 15 mg/kg/dose every 4 to 6 hours, with a maximum dose of 75 mg/kg/d or 4 g, whichever is less. For ibuprofen, it is 5 to 10 mg/kg/dose every 6 to 8 hours. Several large studies support that NSAIDs are not associated with increased risk of bleeding.

Baugh RF, Archer SM, Mitchell RB, et al. Clinical practice guideline: tonsillectomy in children. *Otolaryngol Head Neck Surg*. 2011;144:S1-S30.

Mitchell RB, Archer SM, Ishman SL, et al. Clinical practice guideline: tonsillectomy in children (update). *Otolaryngol Head Neck Surg*. 2019;160:S1-S42.

Pfaff JA, Hsu K, Chennupati SK. The use of ibuprofen in posttonsillectomy analgesia and its effect on posttonsillectomy hemorrhage rate. *Otolaryngol Head Neck Surg*. 2016;155:508-513.

46

Brachial Plexus Block

Shelby Badani and Tiffany R. Tedore

A 72-year-old male presents with a right proximal humeral fracture after a fall. He has hypertension and chronic obstructive pulmonary disease (COPD) with a 30 pack-year smoking history. His only other remarkable history is a report of several episodes of fainting over the last 3 years. Recent pulmonary function tests 6 months before admission include a forced vital capacity (FVC) of 1.4 L (33% predicted). The patient's routine medications include atenolol and chlorthalidone. Hydromorphone 1 mg was administered intravenously in the emergency room.

A. Medical Disease and Differential Diagnosis

1. What are the presenting problems in this patient?
2. What additional medical history would you want to obtain?
3. What implications does the use of atenolol have on the patient's coexisting medical condition?
4. Why is immobilization of the arm important following humeral fracture?
5. Which nerves are at risk of injury from a displaced humeral fracture?

B. Preoperative Evaluation and Preparation

1. What testing would be helpful to elucidate the cause of this patient's fainting spells?
2. Given the potential for periprocedural complications, how would you approach a patient when obtaining consent for a regional block?
3. What premedication would you order?
4. What are the respiratory effects of benzodiazepines?

C. Intraoperative Management

1. What anesthetic technique would you use?
2. Describe the relevant anatomy of the brachial plexus.
3. What relevant anatomic structures in the neck and below the neck can be injured or injected accidentally during brachial plexus block?
4. What regional technique would you choose to block the brachial plexus in this patient?
5. What are the advantages and disadvantages of the following blocks?
    a. Interscalene block
    b. Supraclavicular block
    c. Infraclavicular block
    d. Axillary block
6. Describe the landmarks and procedures for nerve stimulator and ultrasound-guided interscalene block.
7. Describe the landmarks and procedures for supraclavicular block.
8. Describe the landmarks and procedures for infraclavicular block.
9. Describe the landmarks and procedures for axillary block.
10. The patient requests to have the brachial plexus block performed after you administer general anesthesia. Would you agree to this request?

11. What relevant respiratory complications or side effects are you concerned about in this patient?
12. What is the incidence of hemidiaphragmatic paresis following interscalene brachial plexus block? Can this complication be avoided by decreasing the volume or concentration of local anesthetic injected or by using ultrasound-guided supraclavicular block?
13. Describe the pulmonary function changes that occur after interscalene brachial plexus block.
14. What would you do if the patient complained of dyspnea after you performed an interscalene or supraclavicular block?
15. The surgeon prefers to perform the surgical procedure in the sitting position or "beach chair." What are the advantages and disadvantages of this position compared to the lateral position in this patient?
16. Which nerves are most commonly missed with axillary brachial plexus block? With interscalene block? With all brachial plexus blocks?
17. What is the expected duration of brachial plexus block with 30 mL of 1.5% mepivacaine with 5 μg/mL epinephrine?
18. What is the maximum safe dose of local anesthetic for brachial plexus block?

D. Postoperative Management

1. What regimen would you suggest for postoperative pain management?
2. In the postanesthesia care unit, the patient complains of dyspnea. How would you evaluate and manage this?
3. On the third postoperative day after removal of the brachial plexus catheter, the patient complains of persistent numbness and paresthesia in the ulnar nerve distribution. What would you tell the patient? How would you manage neurologic dysfunction after brachial plexus block that persists for 1 week?

A. Medical Disease and Differential Diagnosis

A.1. What are the presenting problems in this patient?

The patient presented for urgent surgery for a proximal humeral fracture and potential internal bleeding. The patient has significant COPD, most likely secondary to his long cigarette smoking history, and has a history of multiple fainting episodes in the past. He also has chronic hypertension.

A.2. What additional medical history would you want to obtain?

It is important to know if the patient's fall was a syncopal episode or if it was simply a mechanical fall. A thorough history should be obtained about any additional trauma that might have occurred at the time of the fall. Has the patient's history of fainting been evaluated in the past? Does the patient have any known cardiac problems? Does he have any history of stroke or carotid disease?

A.3. What implications does the use of atenolol have on the patient's coexisting medical condition?

The patient's use of atenolol could exacerbate COPD, especially if there is a reversible component of his airway disease. It would be useful to determine whether the atenolol is being taken for the treatment of hypertension or syncope. Although β-blockers have been commonly used for vasovagal reflex syncope, large long-term controlled trials do not support their efficacy. The American College of Cardiology/American Heart Association/Heart Rhythm Society (ACC/AHA/HRS) and the European Society of Cardiology (ESC) guidelines do not recommend their use. There is some evidence that in adults over 42 years of age, β-blockers can be protective with regard to development of severe bradycardia or sudden asystole during surgical procedures performed in the "beach chair" or head-up position.

Brignole M, Moya A, de Lange FJ, et al. 2018 ESC guidelines for the diagnosis and management of syncope. *Eur Heart J*. 2018;39:1883-1948.

Shen WK, Sheldon RS, Benditt DG, et al. 2017 ACC/AHA/HRS guideline for the evaluation and management of patients with syncope: a report of the American College of Cardiology/American Heart Association Task Force on Clinical Practice Guidelines and the Heart Rhythm Society. *Circulation*. 2017;136:e60-e122.

A.4. Why is immobilization of the arm important following humeral fracture?

Immobilization of the arm following humeral fracture is important to avoid injury to the brachial plexus or its terminal branches.

A.5. Which nerves are at risk of injury from a displaced humeral fracture?

The axillary nerve is at greatest risk from a proximal humerus fracture, and the radial nerve is at risk with midshaft humeral fracture. Following proximal humeral fracture, the shoulder can be dislocated, and malpositioning can cause stretching or pressure on components of the brachial plexus, especially the axillary nerve. To this extent, it is important to verify and document preexisting neurologic findings on examination, especially if a brachial plexus block is being considered.

B. Preoperative Evaluation and Preparation

B.1. What testing would be helpful to elucidate the cause of this patient's fainting spells?

Syncope is defined as a transient, sudden, and complete loss of consciousness accompanied by a loss of postural tone with a complete and spontaneous recovery. The major categories of syncope include reflex or neurally mediated syncope (vasovagal, situational, carotid sinus), orthostatic syncope (autonomic failure, drug-induced, hypovolemia), and cardiac syncope (arrhythmia, drug-induced, structural disease). Syncope is common, affecting approximately 11% of the population. Vasovagal syncope is the most frequent cause, accounting for 21% of syncopal episodes. Most affected patients experience a first episode between the ages of 10 and 30 years; only 5% of patients experience their first episode after the age of 40. The incidence of syncope increases with age, peaking after the age of 65.

The workup of syncope should include a detailed history and physical examination, including a measurement of orthostatic blood pressure and an electrocardiogram. An echocardiogram is indicated if the history or physical exam is suggestive of cardiac disease. Tilt-table testing or a neurologic workup might also be appropriate depending on the history and physical exam.

This patient had a prior evaluation that documented an abnormal response to head-up tilt-table testing during isoproterenol infusion and received a diagnosis of reflex (vasovagal) syncope. He has managed this conservatively with physical maneuvers (sitting, leg crossing) when feeling faint and has not experienced a complete loss of consciousness for over 20 years.

Brignole M, Moya A, de Lange FJ, et al. 2018 ESC guidelines for the diagnosis and management of syncope. *Eur Heart J*. 2018;39:1883-1948.

Shen WK, Sheldon RS, Benditt DG, et al. 2017 ACC/AHA/HRS guideline for the evaluation and management of patients with syncope: a report of the American College of Cardiology/American Heart Association Task Force on Clinical Practice Guidelines and the Heart Rhythm Society. *Circulation*. 2017;136:e60-e122.

Soteriades ES, Evans JC, Larson MG, et al. Incidence and prognosis of syncope. *N Engl J Med*. 2002;347:878-885.

B.2. Given the potential for periprocedural complications, how would you approach a patient when obtaining consent for a regional block?

Essential elements to informed consent include disclosure, understanding, and shared decision-making. Prior to any elective procedure, a discussion should be had with the patient or with the appropriate patient representative regarding the risks and benefits of the procedure. Benefits can include avoidance of general anesthesia and improved perioperative pain control, the importance of which tends to increase based on the patient's preferences and comorbidities. The risks of peripheral never blocks include common and uncommon events, both of which must be considered when evaluating a patient for a regional technique. While uncommon, postoperative neurologic injury is often multifactorial and may have surgical and patient contributing factors. Ensuring that a patient understands and accepts the additional risk of a peripheral nerve block is crucial. These risks include structural damage to local vessels or organs, and also bleeding or infection as a result of this injury. Other uncommon complications include nerve injury resulting in temporary or permanent deficits in sensory or motor function. The incidence of block-related neurologic symptoms is low (as discussed above) which is often helpful in reassuring patients when discussing risks.

Brull R, McCartney CJ, Chan VW, El-Beheiry H. Neurological complications after regional anesthesia: contemporary estimates of risk. *Anesth Analg*. 2007;104:965-974.

Gerancher JC, Grice SC, Dewan DM, Eisenach J. An evaluation of informed consent prior to epidural analgesia for labor and delivery. *Int J Obstet Anesth*. 2000;9:168-173.

B.3. What premedication would you order?

This patient has already received a recent significant intravenous dose of hydromorphone in the emergency room, and might not require any additional medication. If the patient is anxious, and assuming that a careful history rules out any significant problems or other drug intake, intravenous midazolam can be carefully administered in the operating room while the patient is monitored with pulse oximetry in the presence of the anesthesia practitioner. Additional opioids can be avoided if he is not in pain.

B.4. What are the respiratory effects of benzodiazepines?

Although benzodiazepines cause a dose-related, centrally mediated respiratory depression, overall respiratory depression is not nearly as profound as with the administration of intravenous opioids. The combination of benzodiazepines with opioids produces synergistic respiratory depression. Use of carefully administered smaller therapeutic doses of midazolam is usually well tolerated, without significant respiratory depression. Use of benzodiazepines has been shown to elevate the seizure threshold during local anesthetic administration.

Arcangeli A, Antonelli M, Mignani V, Sandroni C. Sedation in PACU: the role of benzodiazepines. *Curr Drug Targets*. 2005;6:745-748.

C. Intraoperative Management

C.1. What anesthetic technique would you use?

Both interscalene and supraclavicular brachial plexus blocks provide excellent operating conditions and allow for postoperative analgesia. Interscalene block can provide better coverage if arthrotomy is required. Concomitant intravenous sedation and oxygen via nasal cannula might be appropriate; laryngeal mask airway or endotracheal intubation might be preferable depending on the surgical positioning and access to the airway.

C.2. Describe the relevant anatomy of the brachial plexus.

The brachial plexus supplies the nerves to the upper limb. It is formed by the ventral primary divisions of the fifth to the eighth cervical (C5-C8) and the first thoracic (T1) nerve roots, with possible contributions from the fourth cervical (C4) and second thoracic (T2) nerve roots. The roots join to form the superior, middle, and inferior trunks, which divide into anterior and posterior divisions (Figure 46.1). The three posterior divisions form the posterior cord, whose major branches are the radial and axillary nerves.

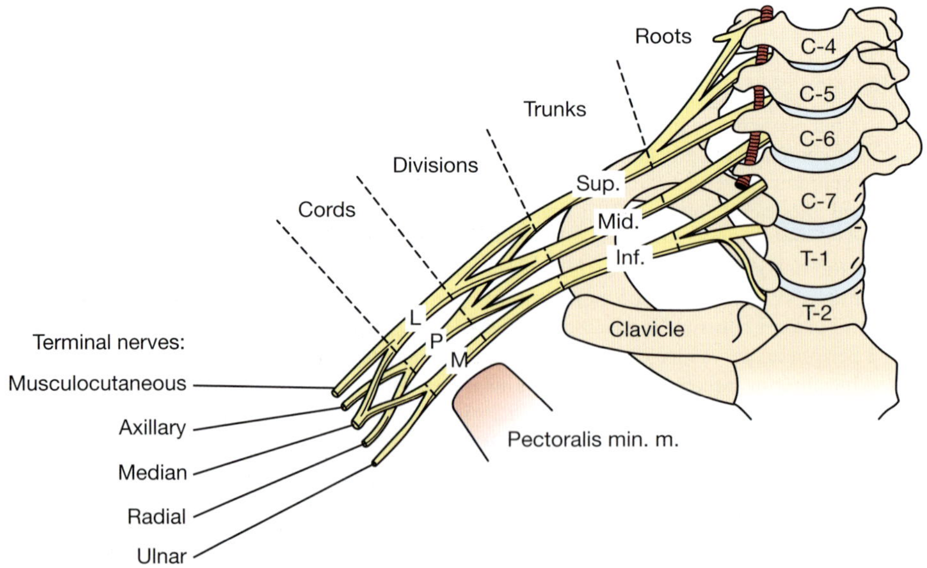

FIGURE 46.1. The brachial plexus. The roots join to form the superior (Sup.), middle (Mid.), and inferior (Inf.) trunks, which divide into anterior and posterior divisions. L, lateral; M, medial; P, posterior.

The upper two anterior divisions form the lateral cord, whose major branches are the musculocutaneous nerve and the lateral root of the median nerve. The lowest anterior division forms the medial cord, which gives the medial root to the median nerve and terminates as the ulnar nerve. The sympathetic contributions to the brachial plexus are derived from the middle cervical ganglion and the stellate ganglion.

The brachial plexus begins at the level of the nerve roots, usually at C5-T1. It is at this level that the interscalene brachial plexus block, first described by Winnie, is performed. Injections at this level result in a block with central characteristics, much like a one-sided neuraxial block. Resulting sensory block at this level is characterized by a dermatomal pattern of analgesia. If the block is incomplete, the typical cause is inadequate spread of local anesthetic to certain nerve roots. For example, the C8-T1 nerve roots are often spared during interscalene block anesthesia because local anesthetic distribution fails to include the lower, most caudal, nerve roots of the brachial plexus ("ulnar-sparing" block). As the brachial plexus courses more peripherally from the neck to the axilla, the nerve roots transform to trunks, divisions, and cords and finally form fully differentiated peripheral nerves. At the level of the axilla, where axillary block is performed, the plexus is composed of terminal nerves that include the median, radial, ulnar, and musculocutaneous nerves. At this level, an incomplete block typically spares sensory or motor blockade in the distribution of a given peripheral nerve, for example, the lateral antebrachial cutaneous nerve (the terminal sensory branch of the musculocutaneous nerve), which exits the surrounding fascia high in the brachial plexus. At this level, the nerves are spread out anatomically around the axillary artery and, depending upon the location of the needle tip during injection and the volume of local anesthetic, any of the four nerves could be spared. This has resulted in the description of multiple injection techniques for axillary block to ensure complete brachial plexus anesthesia.

At the level of the nerve roots or trunks, the brachial plexus is simply a neural plexus, being devoid of major consistently identifiable blood vessels. At this level, brachial plexus identification (ie, needle tip location) relies on a neural response (paresthesia or motor response to electrical nerve stimulation) or direct imaging (eg, using ultrasonographic guidance) of the neural tissue itself. At the level of the clavicle and first rib, the plexus is adjacent to the subclavian artery, which continues as the axillary artery. At this level or below, one can use the blood vessels as landmarks by palpation, Doppler flow guidance, or ultrasonographic guidance to assist in the performance of brachial plexus block.

Mian A, Chaudhry I, Huang R, et al. Brachial plexus anesthesia: a review of the relevant anatomy, complications, and anatomical variations. *Clin Anat.* 2014;27:210-221.

Neal JM, Gerancher JC, Hebl JR, et al. Upper extremity regional anesthesia: essentials of our current understanding, 2008 [published correction appears in *Reg Anesth Pain Med.* 2010;35:407]. *Reg Anesth Pain Med.* 2009;34:134-170.

Urmey WF. Pulmonary complications. In: Neal JM, Rathmell J, eds. *Complications in Regional Anesthesia and Pain Medicine.* Saunders; 2007:147-156.

Winnie AP. Interscalene brachial plexus block. *Anesth Analg.* 1970;49:455-466.

C.3. What relevant anatomic structures in the neck and below the neck can be injured or injected accidentally during brachial plexus block?

The brachial plexus in the neck has multiple significant anatomic relationships that include the phrenic nerve, subarachnoid space, epidural space, spinal cord, proximal nerve roots, vertebral artery, jugular veins, and the apex of the lung. Errant needle passes can hit any one of these, and in fact, there are case reports of complications from needle injury or local anesthetic injection for each of these anatomic structures. Below the neck, the major relevant structures are the blood vessels in the neurovascular plexus, which include the subclavian artery and vein, which more distally become the axillary artery and vein, as well as the parietal pleural, visceral pleural, and lung.

Mian A, Chaudhry I, Huang R, et al. Brachial plexus anesthesia: a review of the relevant anatomy, complications, and anatomical variations. *Clin Anat.* 2014;27:210-221.

C.4. What regional technique would you choose to block the brachial plexus in this patient?

Interscalene block provides the most complete anesthetic block for shoulder surgery. While the interscalene approach has historically had a concerning high rate of phrenic nerve block, newer studies have shown that this can be reduced with a decrease in the total volume used without altering postoperative analgesia. Extrafascial injection (injecting local anesthetic outside of the brachial plexus sheath) has also been shown to reduce phrenic involvement compared to intrafascial injection. However, none of these modifications eliminate the possibility of phrenic spread of local anesthetic from the interscalene approach.

The supraclavicular block has not historically been used for shoulder surgery due to the concern that it can spare the supraclavicular (C3-C4) and suprascapular (C5-C6) nerves and thus not provide anesthesia to the entire shoulder joint and skin over the cape of the shoulder. Recent experience suggests that at higher volumes of local anesthetic (50 mL), supraclavicular block provides equivalent anesthetic conditions to interscalene block. The supraclavicular block can also have a decreased incidence of phrenic nerve blockade compared to interscalene block when lower volumes of local anesthetic (20 mL) are used. Blockade of the upper trunk of the brachial plexus has also been shown to provide coverage of the shoulder with a reduction in phrenic nerve blockade. If coverage of the shoulder cape is a concern with the use of lower volumes of local anesthetic, the supraclavicular nerves can be anesthetized separately with a superficial cervical plexus block.

Analgesic alternatives to interscalene block and supraclavicular block for shoulder surgery include the combination of posterior suprascapular block and distal axillary nerve block. This approach seeks to provide analgesia by targeting the peripheral nerves innervating the shoulder where they are anatomically more removed from the phrenic nerve.

Eckmann MS, Bickelhaupt B, Fehl J, et al. Cadaveric study of the articular branches of the shoulder joint. *Reg Anesth Pain Med.* 2017;42:564-570.

Liu SS, Gordon MA, Shaw PM, Wilfred S, Shetty T, Yadeau JT. A prospective clinical registry of ultrasound-guided regional anesthesia for ambulatory shoulder surgery. *Anesth Analg.* 2010;111:617-623.

Neal JM, Gerancher JC, Hebl JR, et al. Upper extremity regional anesthesia: essentials of our current understanding, 2008 [published correction appears in *Reg Anesth Pain Med.* 2010;35:407]. *Reg Anesth Pain Med.* 2009;34:134-170.

Renes SH, Spoormans HH, Gielen MJ, Rettig HC, van Geffen GJ. Hemidiaphragmatic paresis can be avoided in ultrasound-guided supraclavicular brachial plexus block. *Reg Anesth Pain Med.* 2009;34:595-599.

Tran DQ, Layera S, Bravo D, Cristi-Sanchéz I, Bermudéz L, Aliste J. Diaphragm-sparing nerve blocks for shoulder surgery, revisited. *Reg Anesth Pain Med.* 2019:rapm-2019-100908.

C.5. What are the advantages and disadvantages of the following blocks?

Interscalene Block

One advantage of the interscalene block is a superficial location that makes it easily accessible by paresthesia, nerve stimulation, or ultrasonographic guidance techniques. Injection of an adequate volume of local anesthetic at the interscalene level results in reliably complete anesthesia or analgesia for surgery on or about the shoulder, including proximal humeral surgery. A single injection results in success rates approaching 100%. A catheter can be easily placed at this site. This technique blocks the axillary nerve to the deltoid and the musculocutaneous nerve to the biceps brachialis derived from the C5-C6 nerve roots and therefore guarantees reliable relaxation of the deltoid and biceps muscles. This block also reliably anesthetizes the distribution of the supraclavicular nerve (C3-C4) which supplies sensory innervation to the cape of the shoulder, as well as the suprascapular (C5-C6) and lateral pectoral nerves (C5-C7), which innervate the shoulder joint, adjacent ligaments, and soft tissues. This allows optimal surgical exposure and facilitates dislocation of the humeral head from the glenoid socket. If performed properly, it is unlikely to cause a pneumothorax with an appropriate-sized needle using this approach.

Disadvantages include the close proximity of the phrenic nerve, or perhaps nerve root marginalization of those fibers contributing to phrenic nerve formation, which has rarely resulted in injury to these structures and reported cases of permanent phrenic nerve palsy. Interscalene block with a volume of local anesthetic adequate for surgery results in 100% incidence of ipsilateral hemidiaphragmatic paresis.

Supraclavicular Block

The supraclavicular block is used for surgeries distal to and including the shoulder, although this block may spare the supraclavicular nerve (C3-C4) supplying sensation to the skin over the top of the shoulder, as well as the suprascapular nerve (C5-C6), which innervates the shoulder joint and adjacent ligaments and soft tissues. If being performed for shoulder surgery, the supraclavicular block can be supplemented with a superficial cervical plexus block and/or a suprascapular block. The supraclavicular block is most commonly performed using ultrasound guidance. Advantages of ultrasound-guided supraclavicular block include superficial location of the artery and plexus that allow for easy imaging and perivascular block. Also, one is able to visualize two-dimensional local anesthetic distribution and can avoid inadvertent puncture or injection into the vessels. Disadvantages include the intimate proximity to the apex of the lung with a risk of pneumothorax. Supraclavicular block is associated with a variable incidence of diaphragmatic paresis, reported in the literature as 0% to 100% depending on injection location and volume. Overall, however, the supraclavicular block is thought to be associated with a lower incidence of phrenic nerve blockade than the interscalene block, especially when smaller volumes of local anesthetic are used.

Infraclavicular Block

The infraclavicular block is used for procedures distal to the shoulder. It can be performed with nerve stimulation or ultrasound guidance. One advantage of the ultrasound-guided infraclavicular block is the visualization of the artery, which facilitates imaging for perivascular brachial plexus block. The block does not require positioning of the upper extremity. It is easy to place a catheter at a central location of the plexus via this approach. Disadvantages are related to the depth of the plexus at this level. This can cause more discomfort during placement as the needle must pass through both the pectoralis major and minor muscles.

Axillary Block

The axillary block is utilized for anesthesia distal to the elbow. This block is characterized by the major advantage of the superficial location of the individual terminal branches of the brachial plexus. Thus, one can target the fully differentiated terminal nerves by using either nerve stimulation, paresthesia, or ultrasound-guided techniques. Disadvantages include the need to locate more than one nerve to guarantee successful brachial plexus block at this level. The musculocutaneous nerve is often located relatively distant to the other terminal nerves, lying within the body of the coracobrachialis muscle or between the coracobrachialis and biceps muscles and usually requires a separate injection.

Neal JM, Gerancher JC, Hebl JR, et al. Upper extremity regional anesthesia: essentials of our current understanding, 2008. *Reg Anesth Pain Med.* 2009;34:134-170. Erratum in: *Reg Anesth Pain Med.* 2010;35:407.

Neal JM, Moore JM, Kopacz DJ, Liu SS, Kramer DJ, Plorde JJ. Quantitative analysis of respiratory, motor, and sensory function after supraclavicular block. *Anesth Analg.* 1998;86:1239-1244.

Petrar SD, Seltenrich ME, Head SJ, Schwarz SK. Hemidiaphragmatic paralysis following ultrasound-guided supraclavicular versus infraclavicular brachial plexus blockade: a randomized clinical trial. *Reg Anesth Pain Med.* 2015;40:133-138.

Renes SH, Spoormans HH, Gielen MJ, Rettig HC, van Geffen GJ. Hemidiaphragmatic paresis can be avoided in ultrasound-guided supraclavicular brachial plexus block. *Reg Anesth Pain Med.* 2009;34:595-599.

Soares LG, Brull R, Lai J, Chan VW. Eight ball, corner pocket: the optimal needle position for ultrasound-guided supraclavicular block. *Reg Anesth Pain Med.* 2007;32:94-95.

Tedore TR, Lin HX, Pryor KO, et al. Dose-response relationship between local anesthetic volume and hemidiaphragmatic paresis following ultrasound-guided supraclavicular brachial plexus blockade. *Reg Anesth Pain Med.* 2020;45:979-984.

Urmey WF. Pulmonary complications. In: Neal JM, Rathmell J, eds. *Complications in Regional Anesthesia and Pain Medicine.* Saunders; 2007:147-156.

C.6. Describe the landmarks and procedures for nerve stimulator and ultrasound-guided interscalene block.

For interscalene block by electrical nerve stimulation, the patient's head is turned away from the side of the block by about 45° to the surface of the bed or table. The interscalene groove (between the anterior and middle scalene muscles) is located by palpation just posterior to the lateral border of the sternocleidomastoid muscle. The electrically shielded stimulating needle is introduced in a dorsal, medial, and caudal direction until an appropriate motor response is elicited. Because of the orientation of the nerve roots in a cephalocaudad plane, a response from C5-C6 nerve roots is most frequently obtained first. The C5-C6 motor response is characterized by deltoid, biceps, or brachioradialis muscle contractions. Reduction of electrical current amplitude below 0.5 mA at a pulse duration of 0.1 ms results in a success rate with single injection close to 100%.

For interscalene block by ultrasonographic guidance (**Figures 46.2-46.4**), either an in-plane or out-of-plane approach can be used, depending on the experience and preference of the operator. For an in-plane approach, the needle is inserted in a posterolateral to anteromedial direction along the long axis of a high-frequency linear array transducer with the needle shaft and tip visualized. The middle and anterior scalene muscles should be visualized, and the hypoechoic nerve roots are usually stacked in a somewhat cephalocaudad arrangement. Injection should be made so that real-time spread of anesthetic can be visualized within the brachial plexus sheath spreading the cross-sectional nerve roots apart.

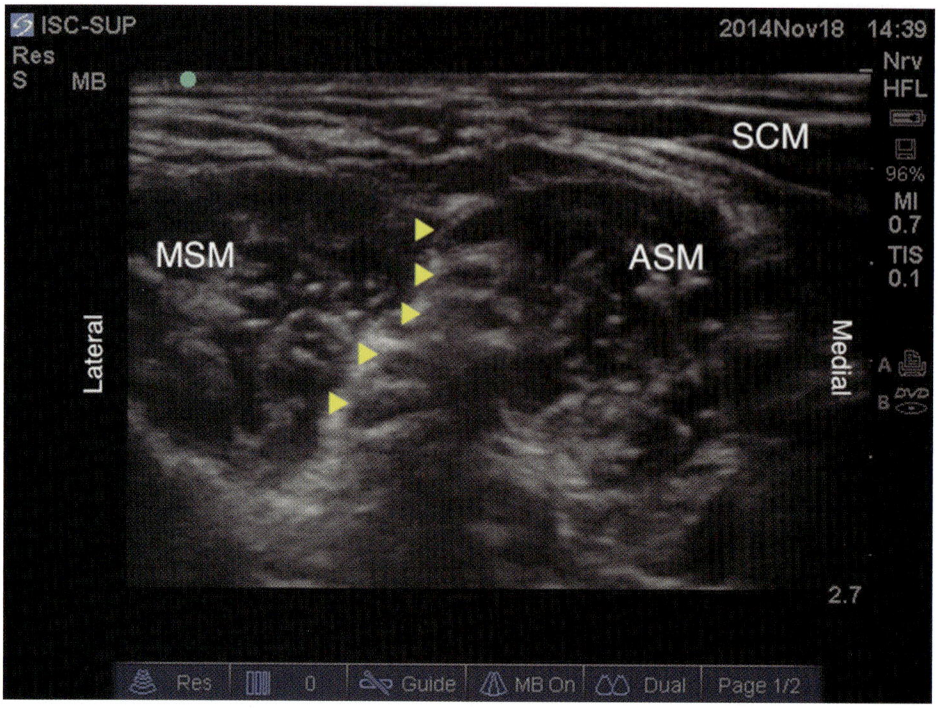

FIGURE 46.2. Ultrasound image of interscalene groove. The hypoechoic nerve roots of the brachial plexus (*yellow arrowheads*) can be seen between the anterior scalene muscle (ASM) and middle scalene muscle (MSM). SCM, sternocleidomastoid muscle.

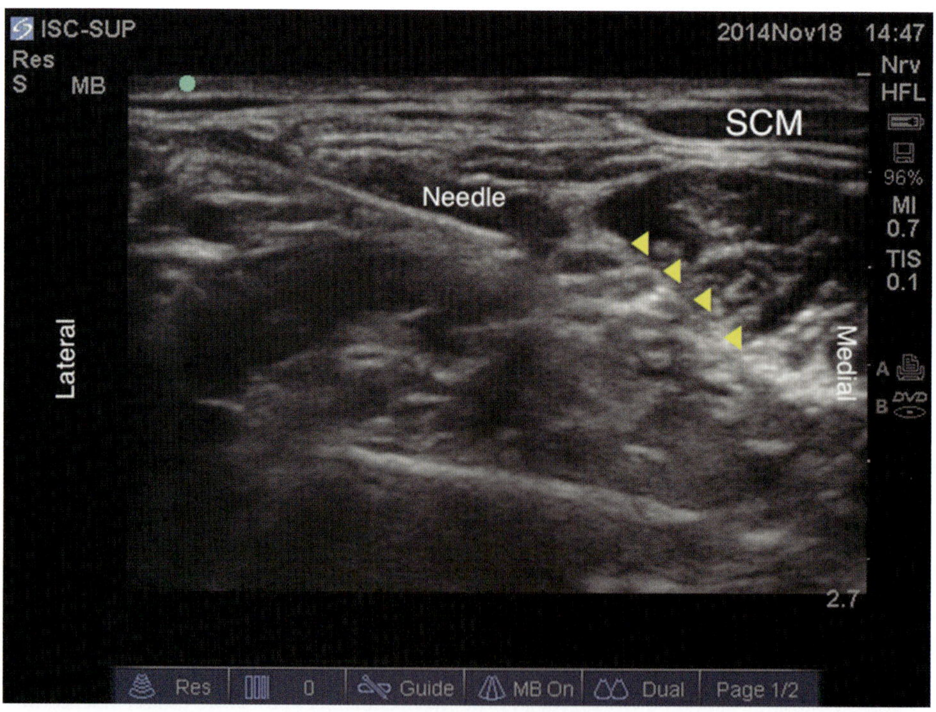

FIGURE 46.3. Ultrasound-guided interscalene block. The needle can be seen approaching the nerve roots (*yellow arrowheads*) in the interscalene groove from lateral to medial. SCM, sternocleidomastoid muscle.

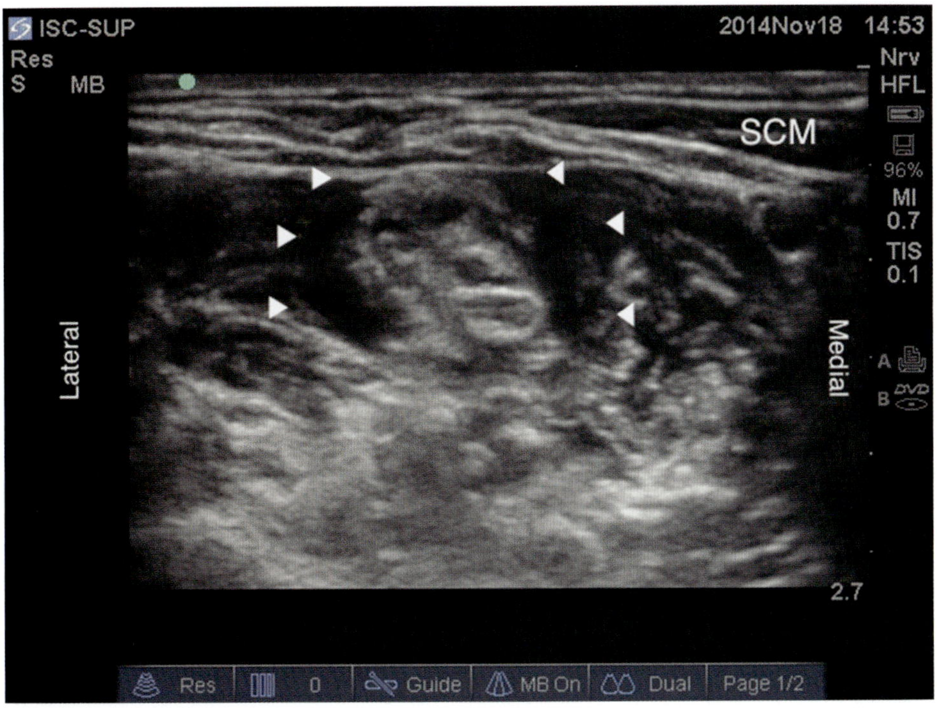

FIGURE 46.4. Ultrasound-guided interscalene block. Hypoechoic local anesthetic (*white arrowheads*) can be seen surrounding the brachial plexus in the interscalene groove. SCM, sternocleidomastoid muscle.

For an out-of-plane approach, the high-frequency linear array transducer is placed just caudal to the conventional interscalene block injection point and just above the clavicle. The longitudinal axis of the transducer is oriented in a posterolateral to anteromedial direction, with the center of the probe overlying the interscalene space and the image of the nerve roots, which again will be hypoechoic in cross-section. The needle is introduced in a slightly dorsal, medial, and caudal direction, as originally described in the conventional technique by Winnie. It is technically challenging to observe the needle tip when using the out-of-plane approach. Tissue movement as seen on the ultrasound image can be used to guide needle placement, as can intermittent injection of small volumes of local anesthetic. Nerve stimulation can also be used to confirm position of the needle tip within the brachial plexus.

Chan V. *A Practical Guide to Ultrasound Imaging for Regional Anesthesia: Part 2- Upper Limb Blocks.* Version 1.1. Toronto Center for Ultrasound Education; 2013:17-41.

Goutier PE, Vandepitte C, Lopez AM. Ultrasound-guided interscalene block. In: Hadzic A, ed. *Hadzic's Textbook of Regional Anesthesia and Acute Pain Management.* 2nd ed. McGraw-Hill; 2017:558-567.

Kapral S, Greher M, Huber G, et al. Ultrasonographic guidance improves the success rate of interscalene brachial plexus blockade. *Reg Anesth Pain Med.* 2008;33:253-258.

Winnie AP. Interscalene brachial plexus block. *Anesth Analg.* 1970;49:455-466.

C.7. Describe the landmarks and procedures for supraclavicular block.

The divisions of the brachial plexus in the supraclavicular area are located cephaloposterior to the subclavian artery and superior to the first rib. Due to the high risk of subclavian artery puncture and pneumothorax with the perivascular and "plumb-bob" techniques, this block is predominately performed using ultrasound guidance. A high-frequency linear array transducer is placed just above and parallel to the clavicle in the supraclavicular fossa (**Figures 46.5** and **46.6**). In the resulting ultrasound image, the plexus can be visualized superior and lateral to the subclavian artery and directly above the first rib. The dome of the lung can be seen medial to the first rib. An in-plane posterolateral to anteromedial technique is generally used, making sure that the needle tip and shaft are visualized throughout manipulation of the

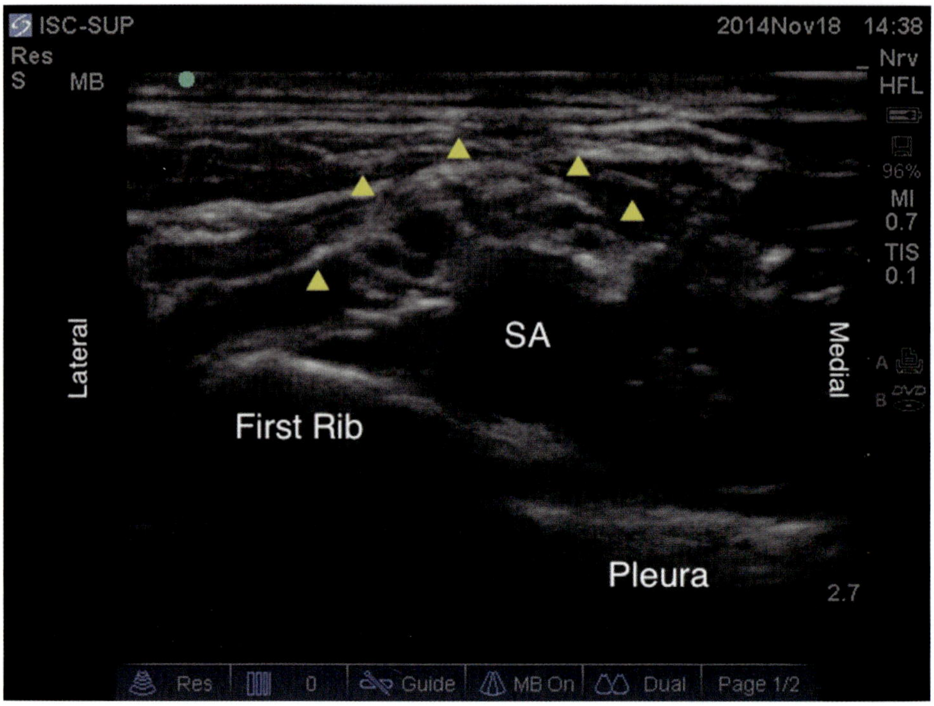

FIGURE 46.5. Ultrasound image of the supraclavicular fossa. The hypoechoic divisions of the brachial plexus (*yellow arrowheads*) can be seen superior and lateral to the subclavian artery (SA).

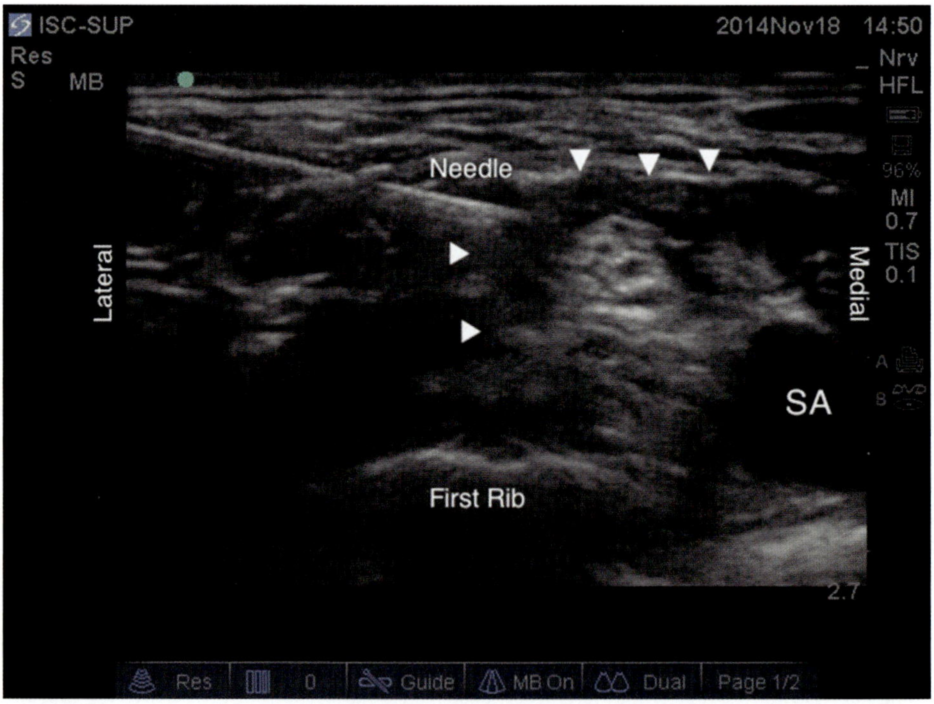

FIGURE 46.6. Ultrasound-guided supraclavicular block. The needle is positioned just superior and lateral to the brachial plexus. Hypoechoic local anesthetic (*white arrowheads*) can be seen surrounding the plexus. SA, subclavian artery.

needle and that the pleura is clearly seen. Local anesthetic is deposited at the superior aspect of the plexus for proximal procedures (shoulder, humerus) and in the "eight ball, corner pocket" between the subclavian artery, first rib, and brachial plexus for distal procedures (forearm, hand).

Bendtsen TF, et al. Ultrasound-guided supraclavicular brachial plexus block. In: Hadzic A, ed. *Hadzic's Textbook of Regional Anesthesia and Acute Pain Management*. 2nd ed. McGraw-Hill Education; 2017. https://accessanesthesiology-mhmedical-com.ezproxy.med.cornell.edu/content.aspx?bookid=2070&sectionid=157602146

Farag E, Mounir-Soliman L. *Brown's Atlas of Regional Anesthesia*. 7th ed. Elsevier Inc.; 2025:63-66.

Soares LG, Brull R, Lai J, Chan VW. Eight ball, corner pocket: the optimal needle position for ultrasound-guided supraclavicular block. *Reg Anesth Pain Med*. 2007;32:94-95.

C.8. Describe the landmarks and procedures for infraclavicular block.

The infraclavicular block is performed at the cord level of the brachial plexus near the second portion of the axillary artery. For the nerve stimulator approach, the patient is placed supine with the arm to be blocked abducted 90° at the elbow. The coracoid process is palpated, and the needle insertion site is located 2 cm medial and 2 cm caudad to the process. The needle is inserted in a vertical parasagittal plane until a distal upper extremity motor response is elicited. The needle can be redirected in a cephalocaudad arc if a response is not elicited on the initial attempt. The depth of the brachial plexus can vary from 3 to 10 cm depending on patient size.

The ultrasound-guided infraclavicular block (**Figure 46.7**) is usually performed with the patient supine and with the arm either adducted at the side or abducted 90°. The ultrasound probe is placed in the deltopectoral groove just medial to the coracoid process. There is a large amount of variation in the precise location of the cords, but in this position, the lateral cord is most often located cephalad, the posterior cord posterior, and the medial cord caudad to the axillary artery. The medial cord can lie between the axillary artery and vein. Abduction of the arm to 90° can improve visualization of the cords and will pull the clavicle down and away from the needle insertion site. A 10-cm needle is inserted in-plane and cephalad to the long axis of the probe, and the tip is positioned posterior to the axillary artery near the posterior cord. The steep insertion angle required and the depth of the brachial plexus at this level often results in poor visualization of the needle. The use of a small curvilinear probe and an echogenic needle can enhance

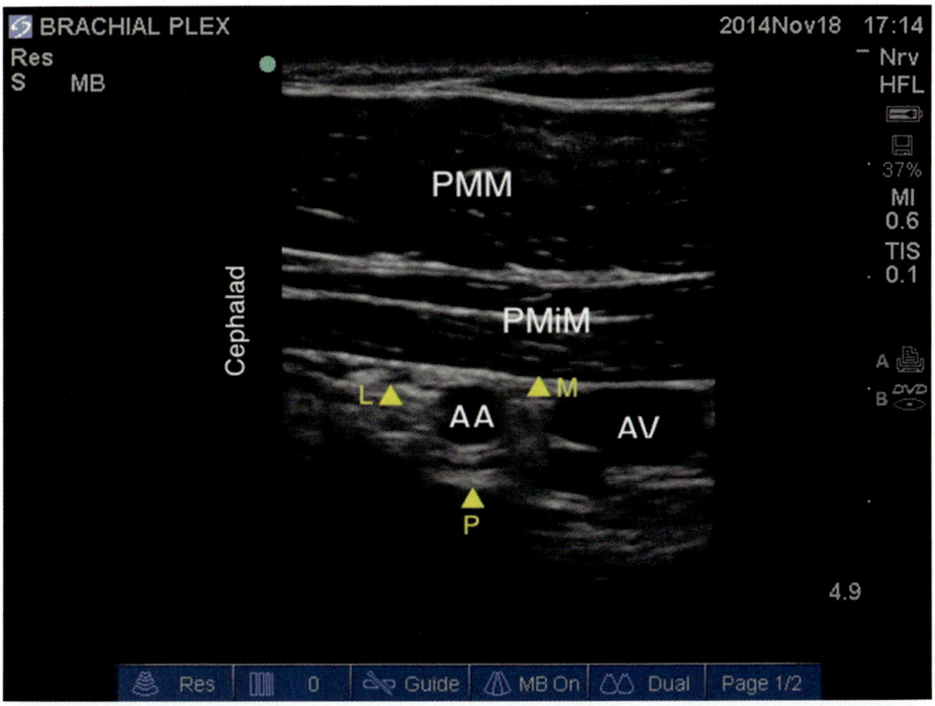

FIGURE 46.7. Ultrasound image of the infraclavicular region using a high-frequency linear probe. The lateral (L), posterior (P), and medial (M) cords can be seen surrounding the axillary artery (AA). AV, axillary vein; PMiM, pectoralis minor muscle; PMM, pectoralis major muscle.

SECTION 11

needle visualization. The curvilinear probe allows greater room for needle entry and a wide sector view of the involved structures at the expense of reduced resolution when compared to a high-frequency linear probe. If all three cords are not easily identifiable, deposition of a ring of local anesthetic surrounding the axillary artery is associated with an effective block in 95% of cases. It might be necessary to reposition the needle and give multiple injections in order to surround all three cords.

Atchabahian A, et al. Ultrasound-guided infraclavicular brachial plexus block. In: Hadzic A, ed. *Hadzic's Textbook of Regional Anesthesia and Acute Pain Management*. 2nd ed. McGraw-Hill Education; 2017. https://accessanesthesiology-mhmedical-com.ezproxy.med.cornell.edu/content.aspx?bookid=2070&sectionid=157602188

Chan V. *A Practical Guide to Ultrasound Imaging for Regional Anesthesia: Part 2- Upper Limb Blocks*. Version 1.1. Toronto Center for Ultrasound Education; 2013:63-84.

Farag E, Mounir-Soliman L. *Brown's Atlas of Regional Anesthesia*. 7th ed. Elsevier Inc.; 2025:73-82.

Ootaki C, Hayashi H, Amano M. Ultrasound-guided infraclavicular brachial plexus block: an alternative technique to anatomical landmark-guided approaches. *Reg Anesth Pain Med*. 2000;25:600-604.

C.9. Describe the landmarks and procedures for axillary block.

In the axilla, the median, ulnar, and radial nerves lie close to the axillary artery and are surrounded by the biceps, triceps, and coracobrachialis muscles. The radial nerve generally lies between the axillary artery and the humerus. The musculocutaneous nerve separates from the lateral cord proximal to the axilla and is often found between the biceps and coracobrachialis muscles.

For the nerve stimulator technique, the patient is positioned supine and the arm is abducted to 90° and bent at the elbow. The patient's axillary artery is palpated, and a small-gauge electrically shielded stimulating needle is introduced just below the artery to elicit motor response from the radial nerve (deep to the artery) or ulnar nerve (medial to the artery; ie, immediately below with the arm in this position). The needle is repositioned and advanced superficially to the artery for a median nerve motor response. Highest success rate correlates with at least two motor responses in which one response is from radial nerve stimulation. By insisting on current amplitude levels of 0.5 mA or below, at short pulse duration (0.1 ms), success rates in the 95% to 100% range can be expected.

The ultrasound-guided axillary block (Figure 46.8) is performed with the patient in the same position as for the nerve stimulator technique. The ultrasound probe is placed along the axillary crease in order to

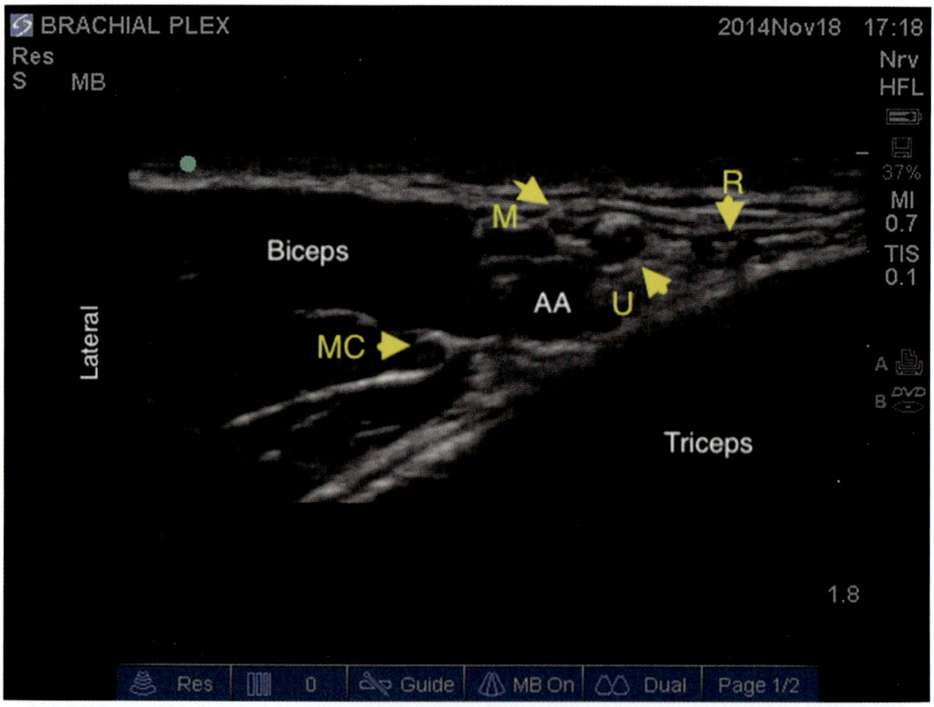

FIGURE 46.8. Ultrasound image of the axilla. The median (M), radial (R), and ulnar (U) nerves can be seen surrounding the axillary artery (AA). The musculocutaneous nerve (MC) lies between the body of the biceps and the coracobrachialis muscles.

obtain a transverse view of the vessels and nerves. Care should be taken to identify the location of axillary veins because even slight pressure from the ultrasound transducer can collapse these vessels and obscure their identification. The nerves will appear hyperechoic with a honeycomb-like texture and can be traced distally in the arm to confirm their identification. The block is usually performed in-plane with a 5-cm needle oriented from lateral to medial, or out-of-plane with the needle oriented perpendicular to the long axis of the transducer. A shallow needle angle is utilized due to the superficial location of the nerves in the axilla and generally results in a clear image of the needle. If an out-of-plane technique is used, injections of small amounts of local anesthetic during needle advancement can assist in identifying the location of the needle tip. If the individual radial, median, and ulnar nerves are difficult to identify, a perivascular ring of local anesthetic surrounding the axillary artery usually ensures a successful block of these nerves.

Chan V. *A Practical Guide to Ultrasound Imaging for Regional Anesthesia: Part 2- Upper Limb Blocks*. Version 1.1. Toronto Center for Ultrasound Education; 2013:85-102.

Neal JM, Gerancher JC, Hebl JR, et al. Upper extremity regional anesthesia: essentials of our current understanding, 2008. *Reg Anesth Pain Med*. 2009;34:134-170. Erratum in: *Reg Anesth Pain Med*. 2010;35:407.

Vandepitte C, et al. Ultrasound-guided axillary brachial plexus block. In: Hadzic A, ed. *Hadzic's Textbook of Regional Anesthesia and Acute Pain Management*. 2nd ed. McGraw-Hill Education; 2017. https://accessanesthesiology-mhmedical-com.ezproxy.med.cornell.edu/content.aspx?bookid=2070&sectionid=157602228

C.10. The patient requests to have the brachial plexus block performed after you administer general anesthesia. Would you agree to this request?

In a landmark publication, Benumof reported four cases of permanent injury to the cervical spinal cord resulting from interscalene block performed during general anesthesia. Imaging of the cervical spinal cord showed vacuolization of the cord or the presence of a syrinx. Intraneural injection of local anesthetic under pressure has been found to spread along the longitudinal axis along the nerve during experimental studies. Thus, theoretically, injection into a proximal nerve root can spread and disrupt the cervical spinal cord.

Performance of regional anesthesia in the anesthetized patient does not allow the patient to report painful paresthesia or other sensations. Sudden severe pain on injection during peripheral nerve block is a concerning signal that neural tissue is endangered and that the needle should be promptly withdrawn and repositioned. Needle contact with the nerve is often not associated with the ability to elicit a motor response during electrical stimulation. Reports of accidental intraneural injection during ultrasonographic needle guidance have been published. Therefore, no available modality can ensure against this complication and hence the caution that regional blocks not be performed in patients who are heavily sedated or following induction of general anesthesia. There are certain important exceptions to this rule where children and adults who suffer from dementia, developmental delay, or for other reasons are unable to tolerate regional block under only minimal sedation.

Auroy Y, Benhamou D, Bargues L, et al. Major complications of regional anesthesia in France: the SOS regional anesthesia hotline service. *Anesthesiology*. 2002;97:1274-1280. Erratum in: *Anesthesiology*. 2003;98:595. Mercier Frédéric [corrected to Mercier Frédéric J].

Benumof JL. Permanent loss of cervical spinal cord function associated with interscalene block performed under general anesthesia. *Anesthesiology*. 2000;93:1541-1544.

Hadzic A, Dilberovic F, Shah S, et al. Combination of intraneural injection and high injection pressure leads to fascicular injury and neurologic deficits in dogs. *Reg Anesth Pain Med*. 2004;29:417-423.

Neal JM, Barrington MJ, Brull R, et al. The second ASRA practice advisory on neurologic complications associated with regional anesthesia and pain medicine: executive summary 2015. *Reg Anesth Pain Med*. 2015;40:401-430.

Urmey WF, Stanton J. Inability to consistently elicit a motor response following sensory paresthesia during interscalene block administration. *Anesthesiology*. 2002;96:552-554.

C.11. What relevant respiratory complications or side effects are you concerned about in this patient?

Ipsilateral hemidiaphragmatic paresis is a consistent side effect associated with interscalene block. It occurs with an incidence of 100% when using local anesthetic volumes of 20 mL or greater. It is also a variable side effect of supraclavicular block. This expected side effect takes on added importance if the patient has respiratory comorbidities, including contralateral phrenic or diaphragmatic pathology, severe chronic obstructive cardiopulmonary disease, neuromuscular disorders in which a 25% reduction in FVC would not be tolerated, or conditions that restrict rib cage motion such as ankylosing spondylitis. If these conditions are present, significant atelectasis or respiratory failure can occur. With proper technique and needle size, the risk of pneumothorax is minimal. Introduction of a catheter, nevertheless, could theoretically reach the apex of the lung.

El-Boghdadly K, Chin KJ, Chan VWS. Phrenic nerve palsy and regional anesthesia for shoulder surgery: anatomical, physiologic, and clinical considerations. *Anesthesiology.* 2017;127:173-191. PMID: 28514241.

Urmey WF, Talts KH, Sharrock NE. One hundred percent incidence of hemidiaphragmatic paresis associated with interscalene brachial plexus anesthesia as diagnosed by ultrasonography. *Anesth Analg.* 1991;72:498-503.

C.12. What is the incidence of hemidiaphragmatic paresis following interscalene brachial plexus block? Can this complication be avoided by decreasing the volume or concentration of local anesthetic injected or by using ultrasound-guided supraclavicular block?

Hemidiaphragmatic paresis cannot be reliably avoided by reducing the volume of local anesthetic injected. Volumes as low as 5 mL (which is inadequate for surgical anesthesia) have been associated with a 45% incidence of hemidiaphragmatic paresis. Similarly, reductions in local anesthetic concentration do not avoid this side effect, with concentrations of bupivacaine as low as 0.125% being associated with 100% incidence of hemidiaphragmatic paresis. Use of ultrasound-guided supraclavicular blocks can reduce the incidence of hemidiaphragmatic paresis from 100% but will still be expected to be associated with a variable incidence. Blocks above the clavicle are associated with spread of local anesthetic into the cervical plexus. The mechanism for phrenic nerve paresis is motor blockade of the C3-C5 nerve roots before forming the phrenic nerve. The main nerve root contributing to the formation of the phrenic nerve is the C4 nerve root. Any block causing sensory blockade of C5, C4, or C3 would be expected to have associated phrenic paresis. A recent publication suggests that with careful deposition of lower volumes of local anesthetic by ultrasonographic guidance at the intersection of the first rib and subclavian artery, hemidiaphragmatic paresis can be avoided during supraclavicular block.

Kang RA, Chung YH, Ko JS, Yang MK, Choi DH. Reduced hemidiaphragmatic paresis with a "Corner Pocket" technique for supraclavicular brachial plexus block: single-center, observer-blinded, randomized controlled trial. *Reg Anesth Pain Med.* 2018;43:720-724.

Renes SH, Spoormans HH, Gielen MJ, Rettig HC, van Geffen GJ. Hemidiaphragmatic paresis can be avoided in ultrasound-guided supraclavicular brachial plexus block. *Reg Anesth Pain Med.* 2009;34:595-599.

Riazi S, Carmichael N, Awad I, Holtby RM, McCartney CJ. Effect of local anaesthetic volume (20 vs 5 ml) on the efficacy and respiratory consequences of ultrasound-guided interscalene brachial plexus block. *Br J Anaesth.* 2008;101:549-556.

Sinha SK, Abrams JH, Barnett JT, et al. Decreasing the local anesthetic volume from 20 to 10 mL for ultrasound-guided interscalene block at the cricoid level does not reduce the incidence of hemidiaphragmatic paresis. *Reg Anesth Pain Med.* 2011;36:17-20.

Urmey WF, Gloeggler PJ. Pulmonary function changes during interscalene brachial plexus block: effects of decreasing local anesthetic injection volume. *Reg Anesth.* 1993;18:244-249.

Urmey WF, Talts KH, Sharrock NE. One hundred percent incidence of hemidiaphragmatic paresis associated with interscalene brachial plexus anesthesia as diagnosed by ultrasonography. *Anesth Analg.* 1991;72:498-503.

C.13. Describe the pulmonary function changes that occur after interscalene brachial plexus block.

Pulmonary function (such as FVC and forced expiratory volume in 1 second) reductions of 25% to 30% occur routinely. These changes are usually complete within 15 minutes of completion of the injection. Increased upper rib cage expansion and ipsilateral paradoxical inward motion of the hemiabdomen have been reported. The combined effect of these changes is a reduced ability to cough and clear secretions, which can be poorly tolerated by a patient with severe COPD.

Hortense A, Perez MV, Amaral JL, Oshiro AC, Rossetti HB. Interscalene brachial plexus block. Effects on pulmonary function. *Rev Bras Anestesiol.* 2010;60:130-137, 174-178. English, Portuguese, Spanish.

Melton MS, Monroe HE, Qi W, et al. Effect of interscalene brachial plexus block on the pulmonary function of obese patients: a prospective, observational cohort study. *Anesth Analg.* 2017;125:313-319.

Urmey WF, McDonald M. Hemidiaphragmatic paresis during interscalene brachial plexus block: effects on pulmonary function and chest wall mechanics. *Anesth Analg.* 1992;74:352-357.

C.14. What would you do if the patient complained of dyspnea after you performed an interscalene or supraclavicular block?

The patient should be reassured and observed. Most patients complaining of dyspnea will have more than adequate pulmonary function for normal respiration. Symptoms of dyspnea can be relieved by placing the patient in the upright or sitting position as tolerated. This position optimizes diaphragmatic geometry and function and increases functional residual capacity. Auscultation often reveals diminished or silent breath sounds on the side of the block. Chest radiography may be obtained if pneumothorax is suspected. Application of a face mask to assess ventilation or end-tidal carbon dioxide, and assisted or controlled ventilation can be used if necessary. Endotracheal intubation should be performed if clinically indicated.

C.15. The surgeon prefers to perform the surgical procedure in the sitting position or "beach chair." What are the advantages and disadvantages of this position compared to the lateral position in this patient?

As discussed earlier, the seated position optimizes chest wall mechanics. The sitting position also allows easier access to the airway and is more comfortable for the patient if sedation is preferred over general anesthesia. However, placing the patient in the seated position is associated with hypotensive bradycardic episodes (HBE), in which severe bradycardia or asystole can occur. It is suggested that these events occur as a result of the Bezold-Jarisch reflex (paradoxical cardiac inhibition and bradycardia in response to decreased ventricular volume resulting from venous pooling in sitting position). The sitting position can be considered a variation of the tilt-table test. This patient would be at particular risk for developing intraoperative bradycardia in the sitting position because of the history of syncopal episodes and positive findings on the tilt test. The use of β-blockers to decrease the likelihood of HBEs advocated on basis of observational studies has not been corroborated by large randomized studies. Ephedrine appears to be the drug of choice for HBEs. Epinephrine, atropine, α-agonists, and intravenous fluids are effective treatments for hypotension and bradycardia. Vigilance and rapid response are of critical importance.

In case reports, the seated position has been associated with stroke and neurologic deficit following shoulder surgery. There is some evidence to suggest improved cerebral perfusion when spontaneous, rather than positive pressure, ventilation is used for shoulder procedures in the upright position.

Gold BS, Weitz SR, Lurie KG. Intraoperative "syncope": evaluation with tilt-table testing. *Anesthesiology*. 1992;76:635-637.

Kinsella SM, Tuckey JP. Perioperative bradycardia and asystole: relationship to vasovagal syncope and the Bezold-Jarisch reflex. *Br J Anaesth*. 2001;86:859-868.

Pohl A, Cullen DJ. Cerebral ischemia during shoulder surgery in the upright position: a case series. *J Clin Anesth*. 2005;17:463-469.

Sheldon R, Connolly S, Rose S, et al. Prevention of Syncope Trial (POST): a randomized, placebo-controlled study of metoprolol in the prevention of vasovagal syncope. *Circulation*. 2006;113:1164-1170.

Weiner MM, Fischer GW, Rosenblatt MA. The beach-chair position and general anesthesia. *Reg Anesth Pain Med*. 2012;37:120.

Yadeau JT, Casciano M, Liu SS, et al. Stroke, regional anesthesia in the sitting position, and hypotension: a review of 4169 ambulatory surgery patients. *Reg Anesth Pain Med*. 2011;36:430-435.

C.16. Which nerves are most commonly missed with axillary brachial plexus block? With interscalene block? With all brachial plexus blocks?

Axillary brachial plexus block commonly misses the musculocutaneous nerve, which arises from C5-C6 nerve roots and exits the plexus above the axilla. The interscalene block commonly spares the ulnar nerve, which is formed by the C8-T1 nerve roots at the lower extent of the brachial plexus. The intercostobrachial nerve is a branch of the second thoracic nerve root and is not anesthetized by brachial plexus blocks. A separate injection is required for procedures involving the medial upper arm or axilla, or if a tourniquet will be inflated for extended periods on the upper arm.

Mian A, Chaudhry I, Huang R, et al. Brachial plexus anesthesia: a review of the relevant anatomy, complications, and anatomical variations. *Clin Anat*. 2014;27:210-221.

Neal JM, Gerancher JC, Hebl JR, et al. Upper extremity regional anesthesia: essentials of our current understanding, 2008. *Reg Anesth Pain Med*. 2009;34:134-170. Published correction appears in *Reg Anesth Pain Med*. 2010;35:407.

C.17. What is the expected duration of brachial plexus block with 30 mL of 1.5% mepivacaine with 5 μg/mL epinephrine?

Such an injection typically lasts 4 to 5 hours for surgical anesthesia.

C.18. What is the maximum safe dose of local anesthetic for brachial plexus block?

There is no absolute maximum safe dose of local anesthetic. The brachial plexus is characterized by relatively low systemic absorption compared to that of other blocks, such as epidural or intercostal nerve block. Absorption of local anesthetic following regional anesthetic injection is site specific. The American Society of Regional Anesthesia and Pain Medicine has published guidelines for local anesthetic toxicity. Recent publications describe the efficacy of intravenous infusion of lipid emulsion in reversing local anesthetic–induced cardiac toxicity in animals and in multiple case reports. Background information as well as advice concerning resuscitation equipment and procedure, including recommended dosing of lipid emulsion, can be obtained by accessing lipidrescue.org.

Neal JM, Barrington MJ, Fettiplace MR, et al. The Third American Society of Regional Anesthesia and Pain Medicine Practice Advisory on local anesthetic systemic toxicity: executive summary 2017. *Reg Anesth Pain Med.* 2018;43:113-123.

Rosenberg PH, Veering BT, Urmey WF. Maximum recommended doses of local anesthetics: a multifactorial concept. *Reg Anesth Pain Med.* 2004;29:564-575; discussion 524.

D. Postoperative Management

D.1. What regimen would you suggest for postoperative pain management?

Patient-controlled regional analgesia with a continuous infusion of local anesthetic is superior to intravenous patient-controlled analgesia for the treatment of pain after major shoulder surgery. It also results in a faster time to discharge and increased patient satisfaction when used as part of a multimodal pain regimen. A supraclavicular or interscalene infusion of 0.2% ropivacaine at 4 to 8 mL/h with patient-administered boluses of 2 to 4 mL every 20 to 30 minutes is a good starting point. This can be combined with standing acetaminophen, cyclooxygenase-2 (COX-2) selective nonsteroidal anti-inflammatory drugs, and oral or intravenous opioids as needed.

Alternatively, if a peripheral nerve catheter is logistically challenging or undesirable, additives can extend the duration of the block. Dexamethasone can add up to several hours of analgesia to a block. Other additives used include epinephrine (to extend the duration but also as a marker of intravascular injection), dexmedetomidine, and clonidine.

Extended-release formulations of local anesthetics, such as liposomal bupivacaine, have also added an additional agent by which peripheral nerve blockade can be extended. A block utilizing liposomal bupivacaine can extend analgesia similar to plain bupivacaine with perineural dexamethasone.

Borgeat A, Tewes E, Biasca N, Gerber C. Patient-controlled interscalene analgesia with ropivacaine after major shoulder surgery: PCIA vs PCA. *Br J Anaesth.* 1998;81:603-605.

Grosh T, Elkassabany NM. Enhanced recovery after shoulder arthroplasty. *Anesthesiol Clin.* 2018;36:417-430.

Herrick MD, Liu H, Davis M, et al. Regional anesthesia decreases complications and resource utilization in shoulder arthroplasty patients. *Acta Anaesthesiol Scand.* 2018;62:540-547.

Ilfeld BM, Vandenborne K, Duncan PW, et al. Ambulatory continuous interscalene nerve blocks decrease the time to discharge readiness after total shoulder arthroplasty: a randomized, triple-masked, placebo-controlled study. *Anesthesiology.* 2006;105:999-1007.

Kim DH, Liu J, Beathe JC, et al. Interscalene brachial plexus block with liposomal bupivacaine versus standard bupivacaine with perineural dexamethasone: a noninferiority trial. *Anesthesiology.* 2022;136:434-447. Erratum in: *Anesthesiology.* 2023;138:233.

Prabhakar A, Lambert T, Kaye RJ, et al. Adjuvants in clinical regional anesthesia practice: a comprehensive review. *Best Pract Res Clin Anaesthesiol.* 2019;33:415-423.

D.2. In the postanesthesia care unit, the patient complains of dyspnea. How would you evaluate and manage this?

The patient's vital signs should be monitored, including oxygen saturation. Duration of hemidiaphragmatic paresis following brachial plexus block with mepivacaine or bupivacaine with added epinephrine is

3 to 4 hours or 9 to 18 hours, respectively. If a catheter has been placed, it should be checked using imaging to ascertain that it is not in the cervical plexus. Chest radiography should be performed to rule out pneumothorax or significant atelectasis. Patients experiencing symptomatic hemidiaphragmatic paresis should be supported with placement in the sitting position and oxygen as needed. Noninvasive ventilation through bilevel positive airway pressure (BiPaP) or continuous positive airway pressure (CPAP) can provide ventilatory assistance and augmentation for patients who are particularly weak from a respiratory standpoint until the local anesthetic effect begins to wear off. Rarely, particularly tenuous patients might require intubation and mechanical ventilation.

El-Boghdadly K, Chin KJ, Chan VWS. Phrenic nerve palsy and regional anesthesia for shoulder surgery: anatomical, physiologic, and clinical considerations. *Anesthesiology*. 2017;127:173-191.

Mehta S, Hill NS. Noninvasive ventilation. *Am J Respir Crit Care Med*. 2001;163:540-577.

D.3. On the third postoperative day after removal of the brachial plexus catheter, the patient complains of persistent numbness and paresthesia in the ulnar nerve distribution. What would you tell the patient? How would you manage neurologic dysfunction after brachial plexus block that persists for 1 week?

Postoperative neurologic symptoms can be due to the block, the surgery, or to patient-related factors. Causes unrelated to the brachial plexus block can include restrictive casts, compartment syndrome, or surgical causes such as tourniquet or traction injuries. The incidence of peripheral nerve injury after general anesthesia is approximately 0.04%. The incidence of block-related neurologic symptoms in the first several postoperative days ranges from 0.9/1,000 to 3/100 (0.18%-3%). The incidence of symptoms lasting longer than 6 months ranges from 0.14 to 0.9/1,000 (0.014%-0.09%).

It is appropriate to reassure the patient that these symptoms will likely resolve over time. If the symptoms persist for more than 1 week, a neurologist should be consulted to evaluate for neuropathy or brachial plexopathy. Electromyography (EMG) studies provide information on the location and degree of injury. It can take up to 4 weeks for an injury to cause sufficient Wallerian degeneration of axons to result in muscle denervation. EMG testing immediately after the injury can help define any preexisting neurologic injury but should be repeated after 3 to 4 weeks. Serial testing can help assess the evolution or recovery of the initial injury. Magnetic resonance imaging (MRI) is also considered a standard tool for the workup of neurologic injuries. It is especially suited to image the brachial plexus, where injuries often present with enhancement. The diagnostic ability of MRI is limited due to the fact that abnormalities seen on MRI can be nonspecific. Consultation with a pain management specialist is warranted if the symptoms include dysesthesias or pain.

Aminoff MJ. Electrophysiologic testing for the diagnosis of peripheral nerve injuries. *Anesthesiology*. 2004;100:1298-1303.

Auroy Y, Benhamou D, Bargues L, et al. Major complications of regional anesthesia in France: the SOS regional anesthesia hotline service. *Anesthesiology*. 2002;97:1274-1280. Erratum in: *Anesthesiology*. 2003;98:595. Mercier Frédéric [corrected to Mercier Frédéric J].

Barrington MJ, Morrison W, Sutherland T, Tay VS, Watson JC. Case scenario: postoperative brachial plexopathy associated with infraclavicular brachial plexus blockade: localizing postoperative nerve injury. *Anesthesiology*. 2014;121:383-387.

Barrington MJ, Watts SA, Gledhill SR, et al. Preliminary results of the Australasian Regional Anaesthesia Collaboration: a prospective audit of more than 7000 peripheral nerve and plexus blocks for neurologic and other complications. *Reg Anesth Pain Med*. 2009;34:534-541.

Brull R, McCartney CJ, Chan VW, El-Beheiry H. Neurological complications after regional anesthesia: contemporary estimates of risk. *Anesth Analg*. 2007;104:965-974.

Sites BD, Taenzer AH, Herrick MD, et al. Incidence of local anesthetic systemic toxicity and postoperative neurologic symptoms associated with 12,668 ultrasound-guided nerve blocks: an analysis from a prospective clinical registry. *Reg Anesth Pain Med*. 2012;37:478-482.

Welch MB, Brummett CM, Welch TD, et al. Perioperative peripheral nerve injuries: a retrospective study of 380,680 cases during a 10-year period at a single institution. *Anesthesiology*. 2009;111:490-497.

Acknowledgment

We gratefully acknowledge the contributions of previous edition author, William Urmey, MD, as portions of those chapters have been retained in this revision.

47

Nerve Blocks of the Lower Extremity

Marissa M. Weber and Tiffany R. Tedore

A 60-year-old male was struck by a car while crossing a street. Upon arrival in the emergency room (ER), he complained of severe right lower extremity pain. His Glasgow Coma Score was 13: he was slightly confused and only opened his eyes to speech. His past medical history was significant for paroxysmal atrial fibrillation and chronic low back pain. Prior surgeries included a right anterior cruciate ligament (ACL) repair 4 years ago and an L4-S1 fusion. His medications include dabigatran (Pradaxa), methadone 15 mg every 6 hours, and oxycodone 15 to 30 mg every 6 hours as needed for breakthrough pain. His heart rate is irregular at a rate of 85 beats per minute, and his blood pressure is 130/70 mm Hg. An electrocardiogram shows atrial fibrillation. Head computed tomography (CT) scan in the ER reveals a small subdural hematoma. He has lacerations of the skin on both the medial and the lateral aspects of his right ankle, and plain film radiographs show a high right ankle fracture of the tibia and fibula. The consulting neurosurgical service has determined that the patient does not require immediate intervention and will be followed with close observation. The orthopedic surgery team wants to take the patient for an open reduction and internal fixation (ORIF) of his ankle as soon as medical conditions allow.

A. Preoperative Evaluation

1. What is the Glasgow Coma Scale and its significance in this patient?
2. Should surgery be allowed to proceed in this patient who has a subdural hematoma?
3. Does the patient's atrial fibrillation need to be addressed prior to surgery, and if so, how?

B. Preoperative Preparation

1. What is dabigatran (Pradaxa)? How is its effect measured? How far in advance of elective surgery should it be stopped? Can its effect be reversed?
2. What concerns do you have regarding neuraxial anesthesia in this patient who has a subdural hematoma?
3. What concerns do you have regarding neuraxial anesthesia in this patient who had prior back surgery?
4. The surgeon is willing to wait a few days prior to surgery while the swelling around the injury decreases. When would it be safe to proceed with surgery in this patient?

C. Intraoperative Management

The patient presents to the operating room (OR) 72 hours after his injury. He was medically cleared for the ORIF of his right ankle. You have decided to proceed with a regional nerve block anesthetic technique.

1. What two nerve plexuses need to be blocked in this case? What nerve roots contribute to each plexus? Name the major nerves that come from each plexus.
2. What is the innervation to the medial and lateral aspects of the ankle? What nerves need to be blocked for this surgery?
3. What nerves are blocked with an ankle block? Would you do an ankle block in this case?
4. Explain the posterior landmark technique to blocking the lumbar plexus. What motor response would be elicited with a nerve stimulator? At what stimulation level would it be safe to inject the patient? Why not at a lower level of stimulation? Can ultrasound guidance be utilized for this injection?

5. What is a fascia iliaca block (three-in-one block)?
6. What is the pericapsular nerve group (PENG) block? Is it relevant for this case?
7. Describe the different ultrasound-guided approaches to blocking the saphenous nerve above the knee.
8. What benefits might a saphenous nerve block above the knee provide compared to a femoral nerve block?
9. How would pain from a midthigh tourniquet dictate which peripheral nerve blocks to use in this patient? Describe the landmark technique of sciatic nerve block in the gluteal region. What is seen while performing an ultrasound-guided technique to block the sciatic nerve?
10. Why does a popliteal nerve block have a high failure rate if performed too proximal to the popliteal fossa when using a landmark/nerve stimulator technique? Describe how this can be avoided when using ultrasound-guided popliteal block.
11. What is the iPACK block? In what situations would this block be useful?

D. Postoperative Pain Management

1. Describe compartment syndrome and how that risk would influence your postoperative plan for peripheral regional analgesia.
2. How would the addition of dexamethasone to local anesthetic influence the duration of the blocks placed in the OR?
3. What is liposomal bupivacaine?
4. What benefit would a peripheral nerve catheter provide over a long-acting local anesthetic? Are there any downsides?
5. You were able to perform a continuous spinal epidural (CSE) at L3-L4 and used 0.125% bupivacaine via the epidural catheter for postoperative pain control. The patient reports that he is comfortable regarding both his back pain and his ankle pain. What benefit would continuing methadone confer in this case?
6. How can regional analgesia aid in fast-track postoperative care?

A. Preoperative Evaluation

A.1. What is the Glasgow Coma Scale and its significance in this patient?

The Glasgow Coma Scale (Score) was developed as a practical structured assessment of consciousness in patients following acute brain trauma. The scale, first described in 1974 and later revised in 1979, scores three different components of responsiveness for a range of 3 to 15. The levels of response include eye opening (none, to pressure, to speech, spontaneous), verbal response (none, sounds, words, confused, oriented), and best motor response (none, extension, abnormal flexion, normal flexion or withdrawal, localizing, obeying commands), with the worse response receiving a lower number. Generally, scores of 13 to 15 signify mild head injury, 9 to 12 as moderate, and 8 and below as severe. Components of the scale and the overall score seem to strongly correlate with outcome after acute brain injury. A baseline score should be established on patient presentation, with a revised and more predictive score on stabilization of respiratory, circulatory, and metabolic abnormalities.

Teasdale G, Maas A, Lecky F, et al. The Glasgow Coma Scale at 40 years: standing the test of time. *Lancet Neurol.* 2014;13:844-854.

A.2. Should surgery be allowed to proceed in this patient who has a subdural hematoma?

Although the patient suffered acute brain trauma and appears stable, he remains at risk for sudden deterioration secondary to increased hematoma formation or cerebral edema. Following acute brain trauma, preservation of normal intracranial pressures and avoiding hypotension while maintaining cerebral perfusion pressure between 60 and 70 mm Hg are essential to decrease poor outcomes. Subdural hematomas are the result of bleeding from bridging veins into the space between the dura and the arachnoid. These can develop over the course of a few days and can often result from a seemingly benign injury or spontaneously. Patients complain of a headache and often appear drowsy or obtunded. The diagnosis is by head CT scan, and the patient can be managed conservatively or with surgical evacuation. Assuming the patient's medical condition does not change over the course of 24 to 48 hours, it would then be safe to proceed with repair of the ankle fracture.

Carney N, Totten AM, O'Reilly C, et al. Guidelines for the management of severe traumatic brain injury, fourth edition. *Neurosurgery*. 2017;80:6-15.

Huner Guevara LR, Pasternak JJ. Diseases affecting the brain. In: Hines RL, Jones SB, eds. *Stoelting's Anesthesia and Co-Existing Disease*. 8th ed. Elsevier; 2021:273-308.

A.3. Does the patient's atrial fibrillation need to be addressed prior to surgery, and if so, how?

This patient has preexisting paroxysmal atrial fibrillation. Prior to surgery, he should be asked if he knows when his last episode of atrial fibrillation was; if he has symptoms; when they occur; if he is typically rate controlled; if he has ever taken medications for rate control; and if he ever required a cardioversion or ablation. Because these patients are more likely to have cardiac disease, a preoperative transthoracic echocardiogram in nonemergent cases is helpful in evaluating cardiac and valvular functions. Although this patient's heart rate is controlled, consider the addition of a β-blocker or calcium channel blocker of not rate controlled, as tolerated by blood pressure. For patients on chronic β-blocker therapy, resumption of medications by the end of postoperative day 1 is associated with a lower incidence of postoperative atrial fibrillation in those undergoing noncardiac, nonthoracic, and nonvascular surgeries compared to those who delay restarting their medication beyond postoperative day 1. In addition to inquiring about the last dabigatran (Pradaxa) use, discuss with the surgical team the plan for possible perioperative anticoagulation as this can affect the anesthetic and analgesic plan, particularly if neuraxial block is being considered.

Horlocker TT, Vandermeulen E, Kopp SL, et al. Regional anesthesia in the patient receiving antithrombotic or thrombolytic therapy: American Society of Regional Anesthesia and Pain Medicine evidence-based guidelines (fourth edition). *Reg Anesth Pain Med.* 2018;43:263-309.

January CT, Wann LS, Calkins H, et al. 2019 AHA/ACC/HRS focused update of the 2014 AHA/ACC/HRS guideline for the management of patients with atrial fibrillation: a report of the American College of Cardiology/American Heart Association Task Force on Clinical Practice Guidelines and the Heart Rhythm Society. *J Am Coll Cardiol.* 2019;74:104-132.

Khanna AK, Naylor DF, Naylor AJ, et al. Early resumption of β blockers is associated with decreased atrial fibrillation after noncardiothoracic and nonvascular surgery. *Anesthesiology.* 2018;129:1101-1110.

Schleifer JW, Ramakrishna H. Perioperative atrial fibrillation: a systematic review of evolving therapeutic options in pharmacologic and procedural management. *Ann Card Anaesth.* 2015;18:565-570.

B. Preoperative Preparation

B.1. What is dabigatran (Pradaxa)? How is its effect measured? How far in advance of elective surgery should it be stopped? Can its effect be reversed?

Patients with atrial fibrillation will often take an oral anticoagulant to reduce their risk of stroke. Dabigatran etexilate (Pradaxa) is a direct thrombin (factor IIa) inhibitor that is among a group of drugs known as direct oral anticoagulants (DOACs). Unlike warfarin, DOACs are generally easier to manage and do not require laboratory monitoring, but until recently, specific reversal agents for these drugs did not exist. Thrombin activates factors V, VIII, and IX, converts fibrinogen to fibrin, and stimulates platelet aggregation. Dabigatran inhibits both free and clot-bound thrombin. It is a prodrug that is hydrolyzed by serum esterases into its active form. Peak plasma level occurs within 0.5 to 2 hours of administration, and its half-life is 12 to 17 hours in healthy patients and up to 28 hours in patients with end-stage renal disease. Eighty percent of the medication is excreted unchanged via the kidneys. In patients with normal renal function, the medication should be stopped 24 hours prior to low-risk surgery and 48 hours prior to high-risk surgery. These time intervals are extended up to 4 times with renal impairment. In terms of anesthetic management, it is recommended that dabigatran be discontinued 120 hours (5 days) prior to neuraxial block.

Prothrombin time (PT) and international normalized ratio (INR) cannot be used reliably to determine anticoagulation status in patients receiving dabigatran. Although activated partial thromboplastin time (aPTT) is correlated nonlinearly to dabigatran plasma levels and can be used to provide some qualitative measure of anticoagulation status in emergency situations, there remains considerable variability between patients. The most sensitive assays to monitor quantitative dabigatran activity are thrombin time (TT) and dilute thrombin time (dTT), but the availability of these specialized tests is limited. Idarucizumab (Praxbind) is a monoclonal antibody fragment that binds to dabigatran and can be used for emergency reversal of life-threatening bleeding in patients on dabigatran. The recommended dose is 5 g via intravenous infusion. If idarucizumab is not available, activated prothrombin complex concentrate (PCC) or unactivated three-factor or four-factor PCC has been suggested for reversal of dabigatran associated bleeding. In addition, gastric lavage with activated charcoal within 2 hours of administration can be attempted. Dialysis can remove the anticoagulant effects of dabigatran.

Doherty JU, Gluckman TJ, Hucker WJ, et al. 2017 ACC expert consensus decision pathway for periprocedural management of anticoagulation in patients with nonvalvular atrial fibrillation: a report of the American College of Cardiology Clinical Expert Consensus Document Task Force. *J Am Coll Cardiol.* 2017;69:871-898.

Horlocker TT, Vandermeulen E, Kopp SL, et al. Regional anesthesia in the patient receiving antithrombotic or thrombolytic therapy: American Society of Regional Anesthesia and Pain Medicine evidence-based guidelines (fourth edition). *Reg Anesth Pain Med.* 2018;43:263-309.

Pollack CV Jr, Reilly PA, van Ryn J, et al. Idarucizumab for dabigatran reversal—full cohort analysis. *N Engl J Med.* 2017;377:431-441.

Schulman S, Carrier M, Lee AY, et al. Perioperative management of dabigatran: a prospective cohort study. *Circulation.* 2015;132:167-173.

Tomaselli GF, Mahaffey KW, Cuker A, et al. 2020 ACC expert consensus decision pathway on management of bleeding in patients on oral anticoagulants: a report of the American College of Cardiology Solution Set Oversight Committee. *J Am Coll Cardiol.* 2020;76:594-622.

B.2. What concerns do you have regarding neuraxial anesthesia in this patient who has a subdural hematoma?

Given that this patient has already developed a subdural hematoma, neuraxial anesthesia would need to be undertaken carefully. The sheering of bridging veins, generally at their thinnest point in the subdural space, is the likely etiology of subdural hematomas associated with trauma and those associated with postdural puncture headache and low cerebrospinal fluid (CSF) pressure. A review documented 46 cases of subdural hematoma that developed following intentional dural puncture during spinal procedures or unintentional violation of the dura mater during epidural catheter placement.

Edlow JA, Caplan LR, O'Brien K, et al. Diagnosis of acute neurological emergencies in pregnant and post-partum women. *Lancet Neurol.* 2013;12:175-185.

Zeidan A, Farhat O, Maaliki H, et al. Does postdural puncture headache left untreated lead to subdural hematoma? Case report and review of the literature. *Int J Obstet Anesth.* 2006;15:50-58.

B.3. What concerns do you have regarding neuraxial anesthesia in this patient who had prior back surgery?

Neuraxial anesthesia should be considered with caution in this patient with a history of a lumbar fusion at L4-S1. Neuraxial anesthesia can be challenging due to abnormalities of the usual landmarks, scar formation, presence of hardware, and bone grafts. These patients are at higher risk for false loss of resistance, inability to access the epidural or subarachnoid space, patchy and failed blocks, unintentional dural puncture, and traumatic needle placement. In a retrospective review of 937 patients with a history of spinal stenosis and/or lumbar disc disease, prior spinal surgery in 207 of the patients did not affect block success rate or frequency of complications. However, of the 207 patients, only 5 had prior spinal fusion. Care should be taken to confirm that the fusion is at the level that the patient reports. If available, imaging of the patient's spine should be reviewed to identify relevant anatomy, deformity, or surgical implants. In addition, ultrasound can be helpful in determining the best interspace, correct level, midline, and epidural space depth.

Hebl JR, Horlocker TT, Kopp SL, et al. Neuraxial blockade in patients with preexisting spinal stenosis, lumbar disk disease, or prior spine surgery: efficacy and neurologic complications. *Anesth Analg.* 2010;111:1511-1519.

Neal JM, Barrington MJ, Brull R, et al. The second ASRA practice advisory on neurologic complications associated with regional anesthesia and pain medicine: executive summary 2015. *Reg Anesth Pain Med.* 2015;40:401-430.

B.4. The surgeon is willing to wait a few days prior to surgery while the swelling around the injury decreases. When would it be safe to proceed with surgery in this patient?

After assessing the patient's current medical status and prior medical history, an anesthetic plan of general, regional, or neuraxial should be considered. If choosing an anesthetic plan of neuraxial anesthesia or one involving deep regional blocks, the anticoagulation status of the patient must be considered. The most recent guidelines from the American Society of Regional Anesthesia and Pain Medicine (ASRA) recommend waiting 120 hours from the last dose of dabigatran prior to neuraxial block. However, these guidelines also suggest that patients with stable renal function, creatinine clearance of 80 mL/min or greater, and no other risk factors for bleeding need only wait 72 hours prior to neuraxial block. Otherwise, for a general anesthetic or superficial peripheral nerve block, surgery can proceed once stable from a neurosurgical perspective, usually after 24 to 48 hours, assuming that the atrial fibrillation is stable with preserved cardiac function.

Doherty JU, Gluckman TJ, Hucker WJ, et al. 2017 ACC expert consensus decision pathway for periprocedural management of anticoagulation in patients with nonvalvular atrial fibrillation: a report of the American College of Cardiology Clinical Expert Consensus Document Task Force. *J Am Coll Cardiol.* 2017;69:871-898.

Horlocker TT, Vandermeulen E, Kopp SL, et al. Regional anesthesia in the patient receiving antithrombotic or thrombolytic therapy: American Society of Regional Anesthesia and Pain Medicine evidence-based guidelines (fourth edition). *Reg Anesth Pain Med.* 2018;43:263-309.

Schulman S, Carrier M, Lee AY, et al. Perioperative management of dabigatran: a prospective cohort study. *Circulation.* 2015;132:167-173.

C. Intraoperative Management

The patient presents to the operating room (OR) 72 hours after his injury. He was medically cleared for the ORIF of his right ankle. You have decided to proceed with a regional nerve block anesthetic technique.

C.1. What two nerve plexuses need to be blocked in this case? What nerve roots contribute to each plexus? Name the major nerves that come from each plexus.

Peripheral regional anesthesia for almost all major orthopedic surgery of the lower extremity involves blocking the whole or branches of both the lumbar and the lumbosacral plexuses. In broad terms, the lumbar plexus innervates the ventral aspect of the lower extremity, whereas the sacral plexus innervates the dorsal aspect. The lumbar plexus is made up of the ventral rami of L1-L3, part of L4, and, in 50% of patients, a branch from T12. The plexus is located within the psoas muscle, anterior to the transverse processes of the lumbar vertebra. The plexus gives off the iliohypogastric (T12-L1), ilioinguinal (L1), genitofemoral (L1-L2), lateral femoral cutaneous (L2-L3), femoral (L2-L4), and obturator nerves (L2-L4) (**Figure 47.1**).

The lumbosacral trunk is formed from ventral rami of L4 and L5 and the anterior branch of S1. The sacral plexus is composed of the union of the lumbosacral trunk with S1-S3 and occasionally, S4. The sciatic nerve contains the tibial nerve, which is made up of the anterior divisions of the ventral rami of L4, L5, and S1-S3 and the common peroneal nerve, which is made up of the dorsal branches of the same nerve roots. The sciatic nerve splits into the tibial and common peroneal nerves in the popliteal

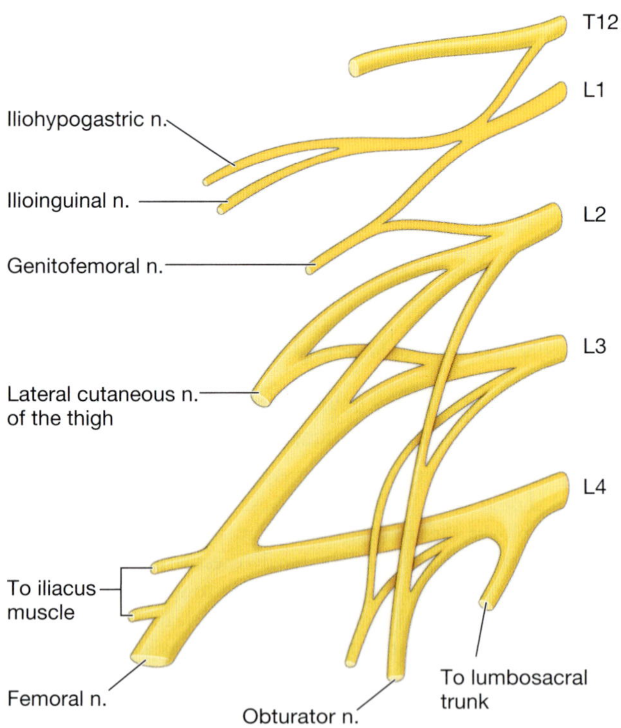

FIGURE 47.1. Lumbar plexus. (From Drake RL, Vogl AW, Mitchell AWM. Lower limb. In: Drake RL, Vogl AW, Mitchell AWM, eds. *Gray's Atlas of Anatomy.* 6th ed. Elsevier; 2025:293-384., with permission.)

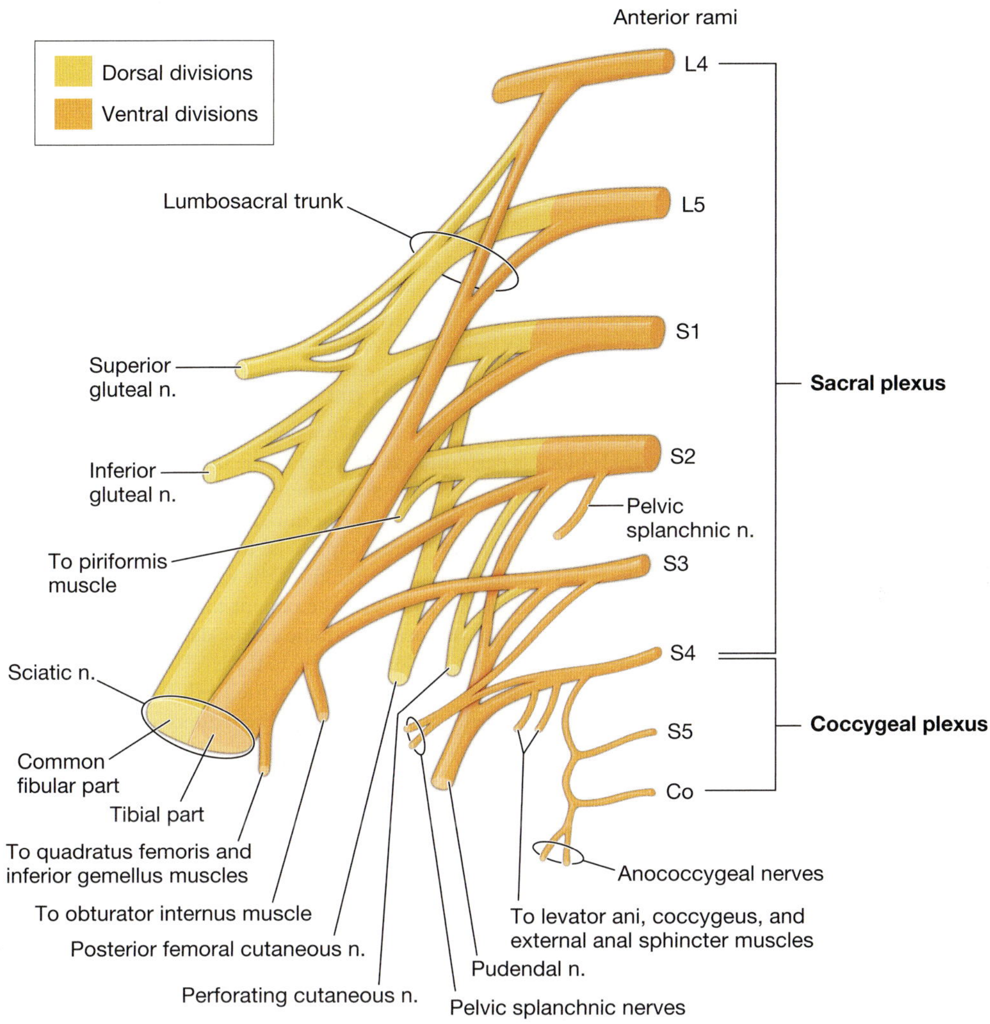

FIGURE 47.2. Sacral plexus.

fossa. The common peroneal nerve branches into the superficial and deep tibial nerves. The tibial nerve branches into the medial plantar, calcaneal, and sural (with contribution from communicating superficial peroneal branches) nerves. Other nerves from the lumbosacral plexus include the superior gluteal (L4-S1), inferior gluteal (L5-S2), posterior femoral cutaneous (S1-S3), piriformis (S1-S2), obturator internus (L5, S1-S2), and quadratus femoris (L4-L5, S1) (**Figure 47.2**).

Drake RL. Lower extremity block anatomy. In: Farag E, Mounir-Soliman L, eds. *Brown's Atlas of Regional Anesthesia*. 7th ed. Elsevier; 2025:115-126.

Johnson RL, Kopp SL, Kessler J, Gray AT. Peripheral nerve blocks and ultrasound guidance for regional anesthesia. In: Gropper MA, Evered LA, Hemmings HC, et al, eds. *Miller's Anesthesia*. 10th ed. Elsevier; 2025:1305-1330.e3.

Lopez A. Ankle block. In: Hadzic A, ed. *Hadzic's Textbook of Regional Anesthesia and Acute Pain Management*. 3rd ed. McGraw-Hill; 2021:217-321.

Singh M, Awad IT, McCartney CJL. Ultrasound-guided nerve blocks of the lower limb. In: Narouze SN, ed. *Atlas of Ultrasound-Guided Procedures in Interventional Pain Management*. 2nd ed. Springer; 2018:201-216.

C.2. What is the innervation to the medial and lateral aspects of the ankle? What nerves need to be blocked for this surgery?

Below the knee, the saphenous nerve provides innervation to the medial aspect of the lower extremity. The lateral aspect is innervated by the common peroneal nerve, with the tibial nerve providing innervation in the posterior aspect. The superficial peroneal nerve innervates the dorsal aspect of the foot, whereas the deep peroneal nerve provides innervation to the deep dorsal structures and the web space between the first and second digits. The sural nerve innervates the lateral aspect of the foot, whereas the calcaneal and medial plantar nerves innervate the plantar aspect of the foot.

In this case, to provide effective surgical anesthetic peripheral nerve blockade, both the medial and the lateral aspects of the ankle would need to be anesthetized. Thus, the tibial, common peroneal, and the saphenous branch of the femoral nerve would require surgical blockade.

Drake RL. Lower extremity block anatomy. In: Farag E, Mounir-Soliman L, eds. *Brown's Atlas of Regional Anesthesia.* 7th ed. Elsevier; 2025:115-126.

Johnson RL, Kopp SL, Kessler J, Gray AT. Peripheral nerve blocks and ultrasound guidance for regional anesthesia. In: Gropper MA, Evered LA, Hemmings HC, et al, eds. *Miller's Anesthesia.* 10th ed. Elsevier; 2025:1305-1330.e3.

Singh M, Awad IT, McCartney CJL. Ultrasound-guided nerve blocks of the lower limb. In: Narouze SN, ed. *Atlas of Ultrasound-Guided Procedures in Interventional Pain Management.* 2nd ed. Springer; 2018:201-216.

C.3. What nerves are blocked with an ankle block? Would you do an ankle block in this case?

The posterior tibial, deep and superficial peroneal, sural, and saphenous nerves require blockade for anesthesia of the foot. Typically, an ankle block is performed at the level of the medial and lateral malleoli. The posterior tibial nerve is blocked by inserting a fine needle along the medial aspect of the Achilles tendon at the level of the medial malleolus and advanced until the posterior tibia/medial malleolus is contacted (**Figure 47.3**). Three to 5 mL of local anesthetic is deposited superficial to the periosteum. The deep peroneal nerve at the level of the malleoli lies deep between the tendons of the tibialis anterior and the extensor hallucis longus (EHL). These tendons are identified by asking the patient to dorsiflex the big toe (EHL) and the foot (tibialis anterior). Another 2 to 3 mL of local anesthetic can be deposited here just superficial to the periosteum. The deep peroneal nerve can also be blocked distal to the level of the malleoli on the dorsum of the foot by injecting local anesthetic deep to the fascia lateral to the EHL and medial to the dorsalis pedis artery (**Figure 47.4**). At the level of the malleoli, the needle can be redirected to block the branches of the superficial peroneal and saphenous nerves by making a subcutaneous ring across the dorsum of the foot using 5 to 10 mL of the anesthetic solution. The sural nerve can be blocked by inserting a needle lateral to the Achilles tendon at the level of the lateral malleolus. The needle is advanced until the periosteum is contacted, and another 3 to 5 mL of local anesthetic is deposited superficial to the periosteum.

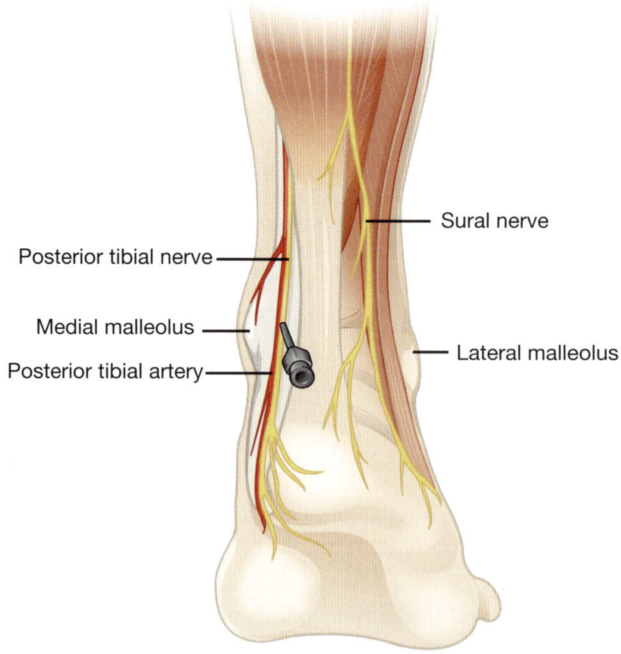

FIGURE 47.3. **The posterior tibial nerve block.**

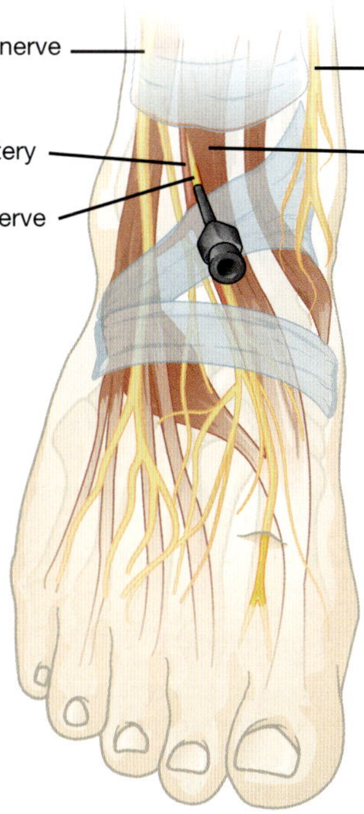

FIGURE 47.4. The deep peroneal nerve block.

This patient would require anesthesia cephalad to the level of the malleoli, given that he has sustained a high ankle fracture. Thus, an ankle block would likely not provide adequate surgical anesthesia and should not be employed as the primary anesthetic in this case.

Drake RL. Lower extremity block anatomy. In: Farag E, Mounir-Soliman L, eds. *Brown's Atlas of Regional Anesthesia*. 7th ed. Elsevier; 2025:115-126.

Sharrock NE, Waller JF, Fierro LE. Midtarsal block for surgery of the forefoot. *Br J Anaesth*. 1986;58:37-40.

C.4. Explain the posterior landmark technique to blocking the lumbar plexus. What motor response would be elicited with a nerve stimulator? At what stimulation level would it be safe to inject the patient? Why not at a lower level of stimulation? Can ultrasound guidance be utilized for this injection?

The posterior approach to the lumbar plexus block, also known as a psoas compartment block, is performed by injecting 20 to 40 mL of local anesthetic into a lumbar paravertebral location. For this injection, the patient should be in the lateral decubitus position. The classic approach was described by Winnie et al at the L4 level using a paresthesia technique that can be modified with the use of a nerve stimulator. The point of puncture is at the intersection of the intercristal line (line joining the iliac crests) and a caudad-cephalad line that passes through the posterior superior iliac spine (PSIS) and is parallel to the spinal column. If the lumbar plexus is not located, the needle should be directed more medially. Mannion et al recommended a medial needle redirection of no more than 15° to reduce the risk of bilateral spread. Capdevila et al described a modification of this approach by using a point of puncture at the lateral two-thirds of the distance between the spinous process and the PSIS and 1 cm above the intercristal line. The needle should be advanced in a perpendicular plane and contact made with the L4 transverse process. The needle should then be redirected caudally, until a quadriceps femoris twitch is obtained, usually at the depth of another 18 mm.

With the widespread availability of ultrasonography for peripheral nerve blocks, it can similarly be utilized to image the relevant anatomy and to guide needle placement in the lumbar plexus block. An ultrasound-guided technique allows the visualization of the lumbar paravertebral region, which includes the psoas major muscle, erector spinae muscle, and quadratus lumborum muscle. For most techniques, the block needle is advanced under ultrasound guidance to the posterior aspect of the psoas muscle. Because the lumbar plexus nerves cannot always be delineated within the psoas muscle, ultrasound-guided approaches are often combined with nerve stimulation.

Although inadvertent spinal anesthesia, intravascular injections, incorrect catheter placement, and renal and psoas hematoma have all been reported, the most common complication of a lumbar plexus block is inadvertent epidural anesthesia and bilateral spread. Motor stimulation should be elicited between 0.5 and 1.0 mA, as twitches evoked at lower currents can indicate needle placement in a dural sleeve, which might increase the risk of epidural or spinal spread.

Capdevila X, Coimbra C, Choquet O. Approaches to the lumbar plexus: success, risks, and outcome. *Reg Anesth Pain Med.* 2005;30:150-162.

Capdevila X, Macaire P, Dadure C, et al. Continuous psoas compartment block for postoperative analgesia after total hip arthroplasty: new landmarks, technical guidelines, and clinical evaluation. *Anesth Analg.* 2002;94:1606-1613.

Karmakar MK, Li JW, Kwok WH, et al. Ultrasound-guided lumbar plexus block using a transverse scan through the lumbar intertransverse space: a prospective case series. *Reg Anesth Pain Med.* 2015;40:75-81.

Kirchmair L, Entner T, Kapral S, et al. Ultrasound guidance for the psoas compartment block: an imaging study. *Anesth Analg.* 2002;94:706-710.

Lopez A. Ankle block. In: Hadzic A, ed. *Hadzic's Textbook of Regional Anesthesia and Acute Pain Management.* 3rd ed. McGraw-Hill; 2021:217-321.

Mannion S, O'Callaghan S, Walsh M, et al. In with the new, out with the old? Comparison of two approaches for psoas compartment block. *Anesth Analg.* 2005;101:259-264.

Winnie AP, Ramamurthy S, Durrani Z, et al. Plexus blocks for lower extremity surgery: new answers to old problems. *Anesthesiol Rev.* 1974;1:1-6.

C.5. What is a fascia iliaca block (three-in-one block)?

The femoral, lateral femoral cutaneous, and obturator nerves can be blocked separately (**Figure 47.5**). The three-in-one block is a large-volume block, first described by Winnie et al, intended as an anterior approach to block all three nerves with one needle. The intention is to provide analgesia to the anterior and lateral thigh, as opposed to only the anterior thigh, by blocking the femoral and lateral cutaneous nerves, which lie together under the iliacus fascia, as they travel through the pelvis. The fascia iliaca block has been shown to provide good pain relief in older patients with hip fractures, in post-hip surgery patients, and in anterior thigh and knee surgery.

Anatomically, the nerves of the lumbar plexus run posterior to the iliacus fascia. The fascia iliaca is continuous with the posterior aspect of the inguinal ligament, passes behind the femoral vessels, and laterally attaches to the anterior superior iliac spine. It is covered by the fascia lata and forms the top

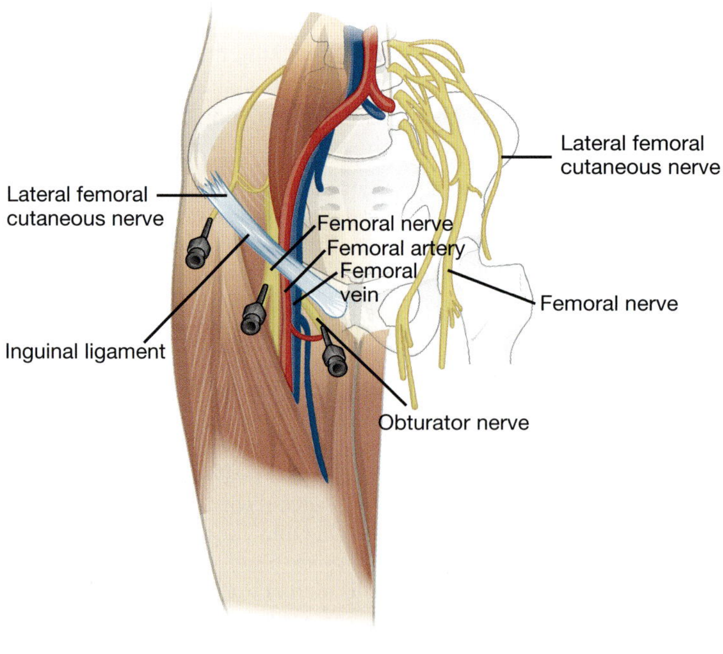

FIGURE 47.5. **The femoral nerve block, lateral femoral cutaneous nerve block, and obturator nerve block.**

of a fat-filled space called the lacuna musculorum (lateral to the lacuna vasorum; the femoral vessels sheath). Using the landmark-based technique, a line, mimicking the inguinal ligament, is drawn from the pubic bone to the anterior superior iliac spine. The puncture site is 0.5 cm caudal to a point at the lateral two-thirds of that line. The anesthetic is injected on the second "give" or loss of resistance as the needle passes through the fascia lata and fascia iliaca, with pressure caudad to the needle.

Although the landmark-based technique is quick and easy to perform, complete sensory block of the anterior, medial, and lateral aspects of the thigh increased from 47% with the loss of resistance technique to 82% using ultrasound guidance.

One technique to an ultrasound-guided fascia iliaca block utilizes placement of the ultrasound probe in the transverse position, similarly to the standard ultrasound-guided femoral nerve block. Once the femoral artery is located, the hyperechoic femoral nerve is identified lateral to that with the fascia iliaca running above it (**Figure 47.6**). The probe is moved laterally, tracing the fascia iliaca until the sartorius muscle is identified (**Figure 47.7**). The needle is passed in plane under the fascia iliaca, and local anesthetic is injected while the distal femoral sheath is compressed. For the second technique, the probe is placed in the sagittal plane above the iliac bone, located where the sartorius muscle and the external oblique muscle come together above the iliacus (**Figure 47.8**). Injecting the local anesthetic under the fascia iliaca with the needle in plane in a cephalad direction at this location theoretically results in a more proximal spread of the anesthetic in the direction of the lumbar plexus. The obturator nerve is not blocked reliably using either approach.

Dolan J, Williams A, Murney E, et al. Ultrasound guided fascia iliaca block: a comparison with the loss of resistance technique. *Reg Anesth Pain Med.* 2008;33:526-531.

Drake RL. Lower extremity block anatomy. In: Farag E, Mounir-Soliman L, eds. *Brown's Atlas of Regional Anesthesia.* 7th ed. Elsevier; 2025:115-126.

Kransingh S, Salti A. Fascia iliaca block. In: Hadzic A, ed. *Hadzic's Peripheral Nerve Blocks and Anatomy for Ultrasound-Guided Regional Anesthesia.* 3rd ed. McGraw-Hill; 2021:229-237.

Kumar D, Hooda S, Kiran S, et al. Analgesic efficacy of ultrasound guided FICB in patients with hip fracture. *J Clin Diagn Res.* 2016;10:UC13-UC16.

Winnie AP, Ramamurthy S, Durrani Z. The inguinal paravascular technic of lumbar plexus anesthesia: the "3-in-1 block." *Anesth Analg.* 1973;52:989-996.

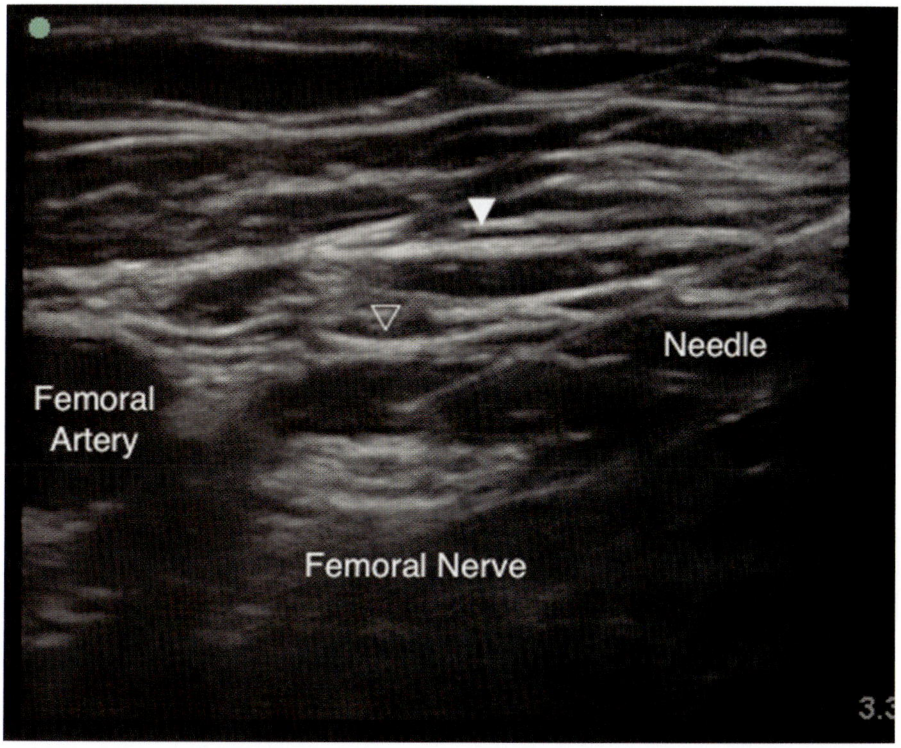

FIGURE 47.6. Perineural femoral nerve block. Fascia lata indicated by *solid triangle* and fascia iliaca by *blank triangle.*

SECTION 11

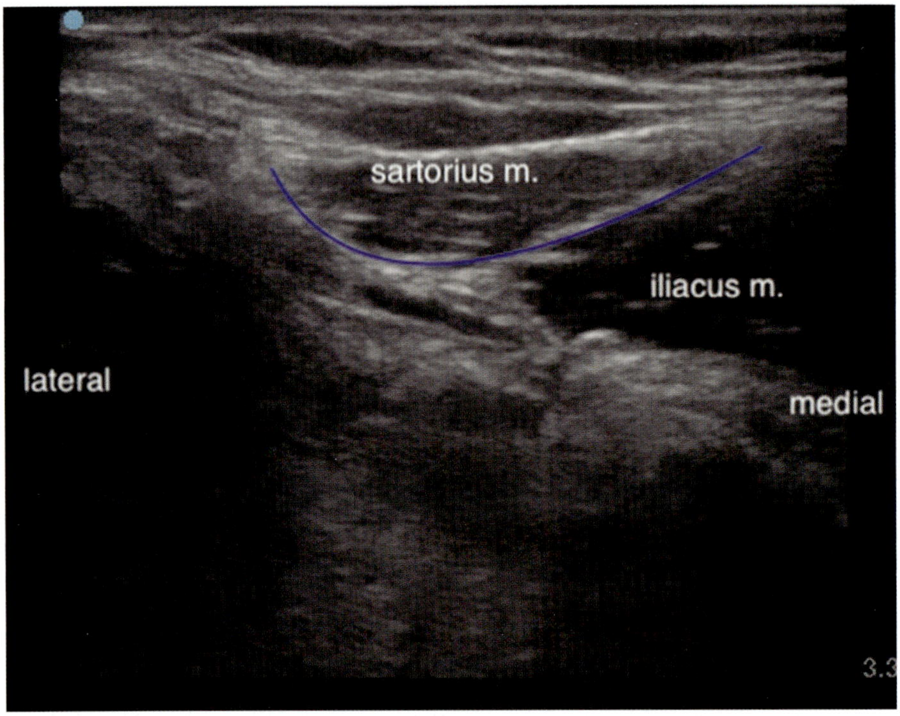

FIGURE 47.7. Fascia iliaca-infrainguinal fascia iliaca block, transverse approach. Blue curved line indicates fascia iliaca.

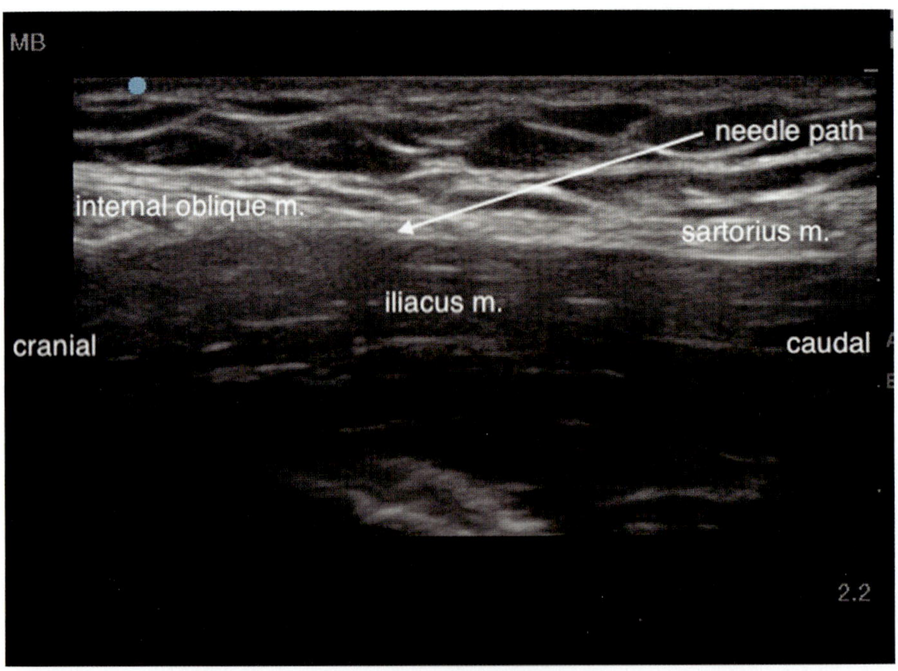

FIGURE 47.8. Suprainguinal fascia iliaca block, sagittal approach.

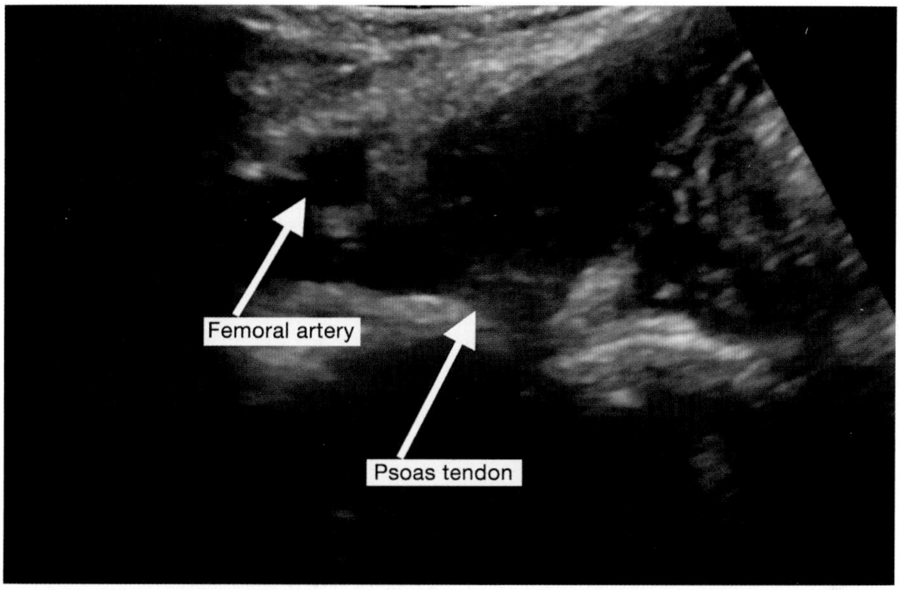

FIGURE 47.9. Pericapsular nerve group (PENG) block anatomy.

C.6. What is the pericapsular nerve group (PENG) block? Is it relevant for this case?

The PENG was described in 2018 as a technique to provide analgesia for patients with hip fracture (**Figure 47.9**). The fascia iliaca and femoral nerve blocks have been used to provide analgesia for hip fracture; however, the obturator nerve is not reliably blocked with these techniques. As the anterior hip capsule is innervated by the obturator nerve, accessory obturator nerve, and femoral nerve, the PENG block was proposed as a more reliable alternative for providing analgesia for patients. Because the high articular branches from the femoral nerves and accessory obturator nerves are found along the anterior inferior iliac spine (AIIS) and iliopubic eminence (IPE) while the obturator nerve is often along the inferomedial acetabulum, the PENG block is performed in the musculofascial plane between the psoas tendon anteriorly and pubic ramus posteriorly. A curvilinear low-frequency ultrasound probe is placed in the transverse plane over the AIIS and aligned with the pubic ramus, ensuring the IPE, ilipsoas muscle and tendon, femoral artery, and pectineus muscle are observed. Then, a needle is inserted laterally to medially toward the plane between the psoas tendon and the bone, injecting 20 mL of local anesthetic. At least one study comparing the PENG block to femoral blocks has shown superior analgesia with motor-sparing benefits. A separate study comparing the PENG block to the fascia iliaca block found a motor benefit with no difference in patient analgesia after surgery.

As the PENG block anesthetizes articular branches in the hip joint, it would not be of benefit in this patient with a distal lower extremity fracture.

Aliste J, Layera S, Bravo D, et al. Randomized comparison between pericapsular nerve group (PENG) block and suprainguinal fascia iliaca block for total hip arthroplasty. *Reg Anesth Pain Med.* 2021;46:874-878.

Girón-Arango L, Peng PWH, Chin KJ, Brull R, Perlas A. Pericapsular nerve group (PENG) block for hip fracture. *Reg Anesth Pain Med.* 2018;43:859-863.

Lin DY, Morrison C, Brown B, et al. Pericapsular nerve group (PENG) block provides improved short-term analgesia compared with the femoral nerve block in hip fracture surgery: a single-center double-blinded randomized comparative trial. *Reg Anesth Pain Med.* 2021;46:398-403.

C.7. Describe the different ultrasound-guided approaches to blocking the saphenous nerve above the knee.

The saphenous nerve is a sensory branch of the femoral nerve, which when blocked in combination with a sciatic nerve block, provides anesthesia for surgeries distal to the knee. Previously, this nerve was blocked by a subcutaneous wheel of local anesthetic from the medial aspect of the tibial tuberosity to the anterior aspect of the tibia. The nerve runs lateral to the femoral artery while exiting the femoral triangle and then crosses over the roof of the adductor canal (subsartorial canal) and runs medial to the artery at

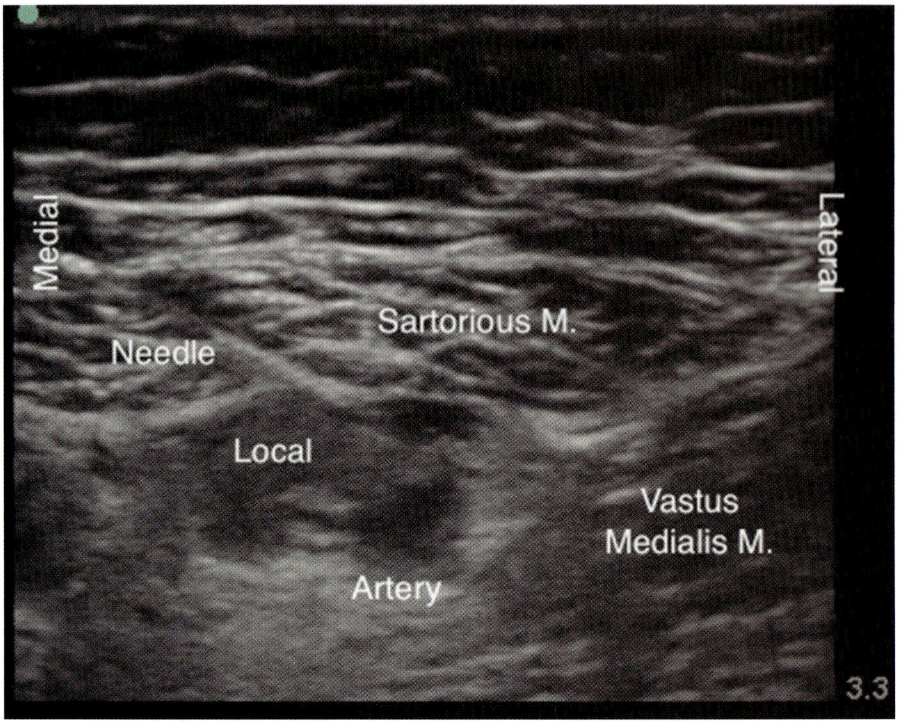

FIGURE 47.10. Post-periarterial saphenous nerve injection in the adductor canal.

the distal aspect of the adductor canal. The canal is bound anterolaterally by the vastus medialis muscle, anteriorly by the sartorius muscle, and posteromedially by the adductor magnus muscle. The saphenous nerve emerges from the adductor canal with the saphenous branch of the descending genicular artery and divides into the infrapatellar and sartorial branches. The sartorial branch courses through the fascia between the sartorius and gracilis muscles and emerges subcutaneously below the knee. Studies have shown ultrasound-guided techniques to be reliable and effective in blocking this nerve, as the saphenous nerve emerges from the adductor canal. Just above the level of the knee, the nerve can be blocked between the sartorius and gracilis muscles in close proximity to the saphenous branch of the descending genicular artery. The saphenous nerve can be blocked about 5 to 7 cm proximal to the popliteal crease, in the vastoadductor membrane (facial plane adjacent to the vastus medialis) deep to the sartorius muscle, or more proximally in the distal adductor canal deep to the sartorius and anteromedial to the femoral artery (**Figures 47.10** and **47.11**).

Horn JL, Pitsch T, Salinas F, et al. Anatomic basis to the ultrasound-guided approach for saphenous nerve blockade. *Reg Anesth Pain Med.* 2009;34:486-489.

Johnson RL, Kopp SL, Kessler J, Gray AT. Peripheral nerve blocks and ultrasound guidance for regional anesthesia. In: Gropper MA, Evered LA, Hemmings HC, et al, eds. *Miller's Anesthesia.* 10th ed. Elsevier; 2025:1305-1330.e3.

Krombach J, Gray AT. Sonography for saphenous nerve block near the adductor canal. *Reg Anesth Pain Med.* 2007;32:369-370.

Manickam B, Perlas A, Duggan E, et al. Feasibility and efficacy of ultrasound-guided block of the saphenous nerve in the adductor canal. *Reg Anesth Pain Med.* 2009;34:578-580.

Saranteas T, Anagnostis G, Paraskeuopoulos T, et al. Anatomy and clinical implications of the ultrasound-guided subsartorial saphenous nerve block. *Reg Anesth Pain Med.* 2011;36:399-402.

C.8. What benefits might a saphenous nerve block above the knee provide compared to a femoral nerve block?

Femoral and saphenous nerve blocks have been shown to provide effective analgesia at the level of the knee and below. However, as a femoral nerve block provides analgesia to all the branches of the femoral nerve, it confers significant motor blockade to the quadriceps and has been associated with a small risk of falls during postoperative ambulation. Ideally, in cases where early ambulation and mobilization are

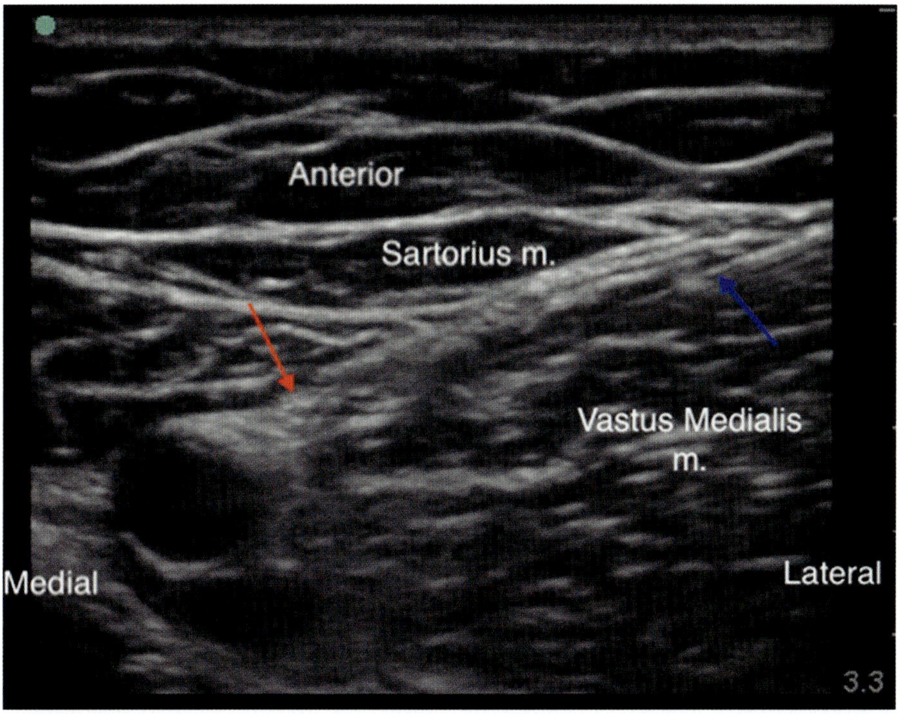

FIGURE 47.11. Saphenous nerve block: view of the lower adductor canal. Note the sartorius muscle tracking medially. *Blue arrow* indicates needle. Red arrow indicates saphenous nerve.

desired, such as fast-track joint replacements, an analgesic block with motor preservation would be advantageous. Studies have shown that adductor canal saphenous nerve block provides equivalent analgesia compared to femoral block with improved quadriceps function in cases of knee arthroscopy, as well as ACL repair. In a group of healthy volunteers, a saphenous nerve block in the adductor canal reduced quadriceps strength 8% from baseline, whereas a femoral nerve block caused a 49% reduction from baseline. Although 100% could mobilize after a saphenous nerve block, only about 50% were mobile following a femoral nerve block. A possible basis for improved strength is that analgesia decreases centrally mediated inhibition of voluntary muscle contraction. Although a midthigh saphenous nerve block in the adductor canal often spreads to the nerve to the vastus medialis (sensory and motor), there is less reduction in quadriceps muscle strength compared to a femoral nerve block.

Grevstad U, Mathiesen O, Valentiner LS, et al. Effect of adductor canal block versus femoral nerve block on quadriceps strength, mobilization, and pain after total knee arthroplasty: a randomized, blinded study. *Reg Anesth Pain Med.* 2015;40:3-10.

Jaeger P, Nielsen ZJ, Henningsen MH, et al. Adductor canal block versus femoral nerve block and quadriceps strength: a randomized, double-blind, placebo-controlled, crossover study in healthy volunteers. *Anesthesiology.* 2013;118:409-415.

Kim DH, Lin Y, Goytizolo EA, et al. Adductor canal block versus femoral nerve block for total knee arthroplasty: a prospective, randomized, controlled trial. *Anesthesiology.* 2014;120:540-550.

Xerogeanes JW, Premkumar A, Godfrey W, et al. Adductor canal vs. femoral nerve block in anterior cruciate ligament reconstruction: a randomized controlled trial. *Orthop J Sports Med.* 2017;5:2325967117S00277.

C.9. How would pain from a midthigh tourniquet dictate which peripheral nerve blocks to use in this patient? Describe the landmark technique of sciatic nerve block in the gluteal region. What is seen while performing an ultrasound-guided technique to block the sciatic nerve?

A midthigh tourniquet will have implications in determining what blocks should be performed for lower extremity surgery. Although a tourniquet is used to decrease intraoperative blood loss, it occasionally has the unintended consequence of causing considerable pain in the thigh. The tourniquet is wrapped entirely around the leg and can affect both the femoral and sciatic nerves. Thus, it is important to block these nerves more proximally than at the adductor canal or the popliteal fossa. The mechanism of tourniquet

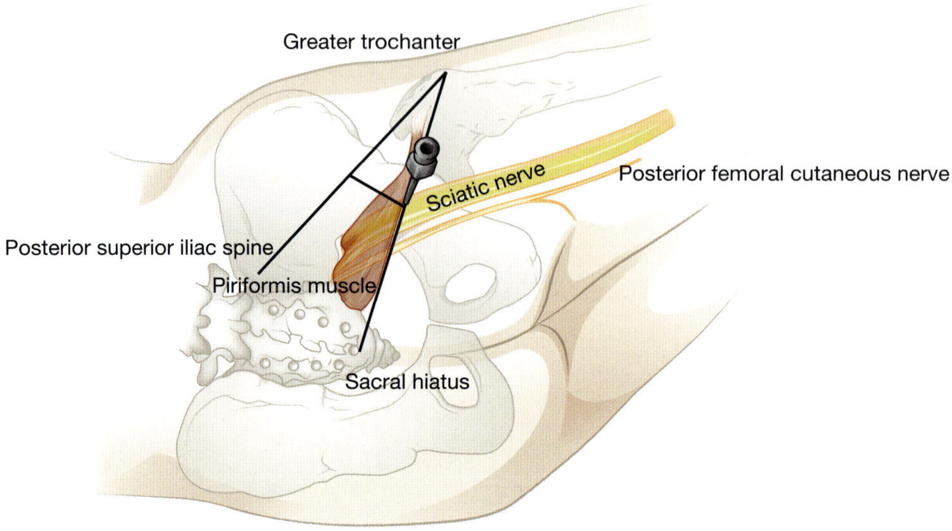

FIGURE 47.12. Sciatic nerve block. The Labat approach.

pain is more complex than just secondary to pressure from the tourniquet and involves both unmyelinated C fibers and myelinated A fibers. The C fibers are more resistant to local anesthetic blockade, so when either neuraxial anesthesia or a regional block begins to wear off, or if they are incomplete to begin with, the C fibers can conduct, resulting in the sensation of dull pain. This dull pain is experienced even with an "adequate" sensory block of the A fibers. C fibers are more readily blocked during general anesthesia, offering the lowest likelihood of tourniquet pain.

To perform a transgluteal sciatic nerve block with the landmark technique, the patient should be positioned in the lateral decubitus position with the leg to be blocked uppermost and flexed at the hip and knee. The landmarks are the greater trochanter and the PSIS. The distance between the greater trochanter and the PSIS is measured, and the skin at 4 cm distal to the midpoint is marked as the insertion site. Alternatively, that point lies on a line from the greater trochanter to the sacral hiatus (**Figure 47.12**). Once this site is located and the skin prepped, the block needle is introduced at 90° to the skin. Using a nerve stimulator, muscle twitches of the gluteal muscles are initially seen, and with further advancement, hamstring or calf twitches are seen. Ideally, the twitch remains at about 0.2 to 0.5 mA, indicating appropriate closeness to the nerve. When negative aspiration is confirmed, the local anesthetic of choice can then be injected.

When utilizing an ultrasound-guided subgluteal approach, the nerve can be visualized between the ischial tuberosity and the greater trochanter. The patient is positioned in the prone or lateral decubitus position; again, the leg and knee are flexed. Once the skin is cleaned, the curved transducer probe is placed over the skin. The nerve will be visualized between the two osseous structures, frequently described as being in a "hammock" under the gluteus muscle. The local anesthetic solution will usually push the nerve away and actually improve the visualization of the nerve.

Johnson RL, Kopp SL, Kessler J, Gray AT. Peripheral nerve blocks and ultrasound guidance for regional anesthesia. In: Gropper MA, Evered LA, Hemmings HC, et al, eds. *Miller's Anesthesia*. 10th ed. Elsevier; 2025:1305-1330.e3.

Langenaeken A, Louage S. Popliteal sciatic block. In: Hadzic A, ed. *Hadzic's Peripheral Nerve Blocks and Anatomy for Ultrasound-Guided Regional Anesthesia*. 3rd ed. McGraw-Hill; 2021:291-298.

Sharma JP, Salhotra R. Tourniquets in orthopedic surgery. *Indian J Orthop*. 2012;46:377-383.

C.10. Why does a popliteal nerve block have a high failure rate if performed too proximal to the popliteal fossa when using a landmark/nerve stimulator technique? Describe how this can be avoided when using ultrasound-guided popliteal block.

The landmark technique for performing a popliteal fossa block involves delineating the biceps femoris tendon, the semitendinosus and semimembranosus tendons, as well as the popliteal fossa crease. Needle insertion is at a point 7 cm above the popliteal crease at the midpoint between the lateral and medial tendons. Although this technique will work for a large majority of patients, a high failure rate does occur as a significant proportion of the population has variant anatomy, where the division of the sciatic nerve into the common peroneal nerve and the tibial nerve occurs more proximal to the level of the needle insertion

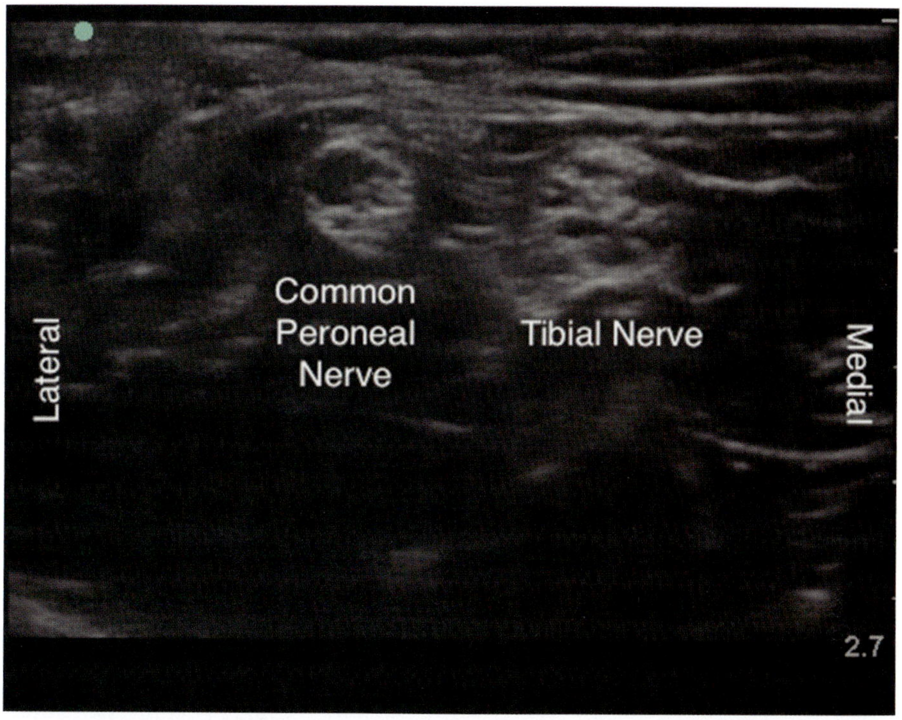

FIGURE 47.13. Popliteal fossa block showing local anesthetic surrounding nerves distal to nerve bifurcation.

point (**Figure 47.13**). Thus, an incomplete blockade could occur if only one branch of the sciatic nerve is effectively blocked. The use of an ultrasound-guided technique allows for visualization of the nerve and the exact location of the division, helping prevent such failure (**Figure 47.14**).

Adibatti M, Sangeetha V. Study on variant anatomy of sciatic nerve. *J Clin Diagn Res*. 2014;8:AC07-AC09.

Langenaeken A, Louage S. Popliteal sciatic block. In: Hadzic A, ed. *Hadzic's Peripheral Nerve Blocks and Anatomy for Ultrasound-Guided Regional Anesthesia*. 3rd ed. McGraw-Hill; 2021:291-298.

C.11. What is the iPACK block? In what situations would this block be useful?

iPACK stands for infiltration between the popliteal artery and the capsule of the knee. The iPACK block provides analgesia to the posterior compartment of the knee by anesthetizing the sensory articular branches of the sciatic nerve while sparing the motor branches. It is typically performed under ultrasound guidance by first identifying the popliteal artery just proximal to the level of the femoral condyles (**Figure 47.15**). The needle is placed between the popliteal artery and the femur in close proximity to the periosteum, and 20 to 25 mL of local anesthetic is infiltrated in the area (**Figure 47.16**).

The iPACK block is increasingly being used in conjunction with an adductor canal block to provide pain control after total knee arthroplasty (TKA) in the setting of fast-track recovery protocols. Although a sciatic block can also provide analgesia to the posterior knee, it is associated with significant motor block of the foot and ankle, delaying early mobilization after surgery and potentially masking a surgical injury to the peroneal nerve, which is not uncommon after TKA. Therefore, much like the adoption of the saphenous nerve block over the femoral nerve block, the iPACK block is increasingly incorporated as a motor-sparing peripheral nerve block to enhance recovery after TKA. In a randomized trial of 86 patients undergoing TKA, addition of the iPACK and adductor canal block significantly improved postoperative analgesia and reduced opioid consumption compared to periarticular injection by the surgeon alone.

Kim DH, Beathe JC, Lin Y, et al. Addition of infiltration between the popliteal artery and the capsule of the posterior knee and adductor canal block to periarticular injection enhances postoperative pain control in total knee arthroplasty: a randomized controlled trial. *Anesth Analg*. 2019;129:526-535.

Sinha SK, Abrams JH, Arumugam S, et al. Femoral nerve block with selective tibial nerve block provides effective analgesia without foot drop after total knee arthroplasty: a prospective, randomized, observer-blinded study. *Anesth Analg*. 2012;115:202-206.

SECTION 11

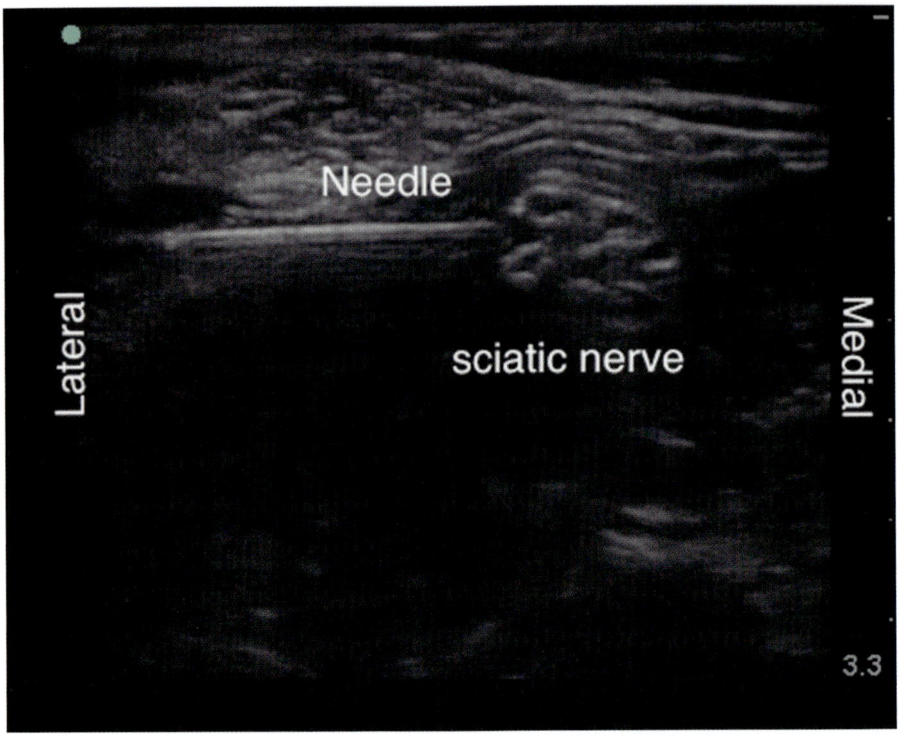

FIGURE 47.14. Popliteal fossa block just proximal to bifurcation.

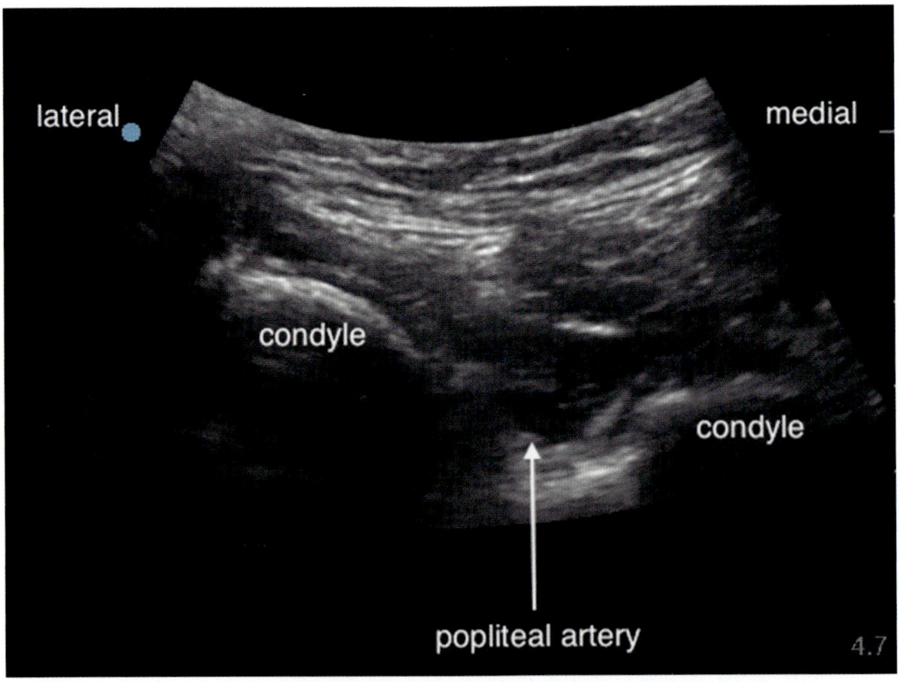

FIGURE 47.15. iPACK block. Scanning at the level of the femoral condyles.

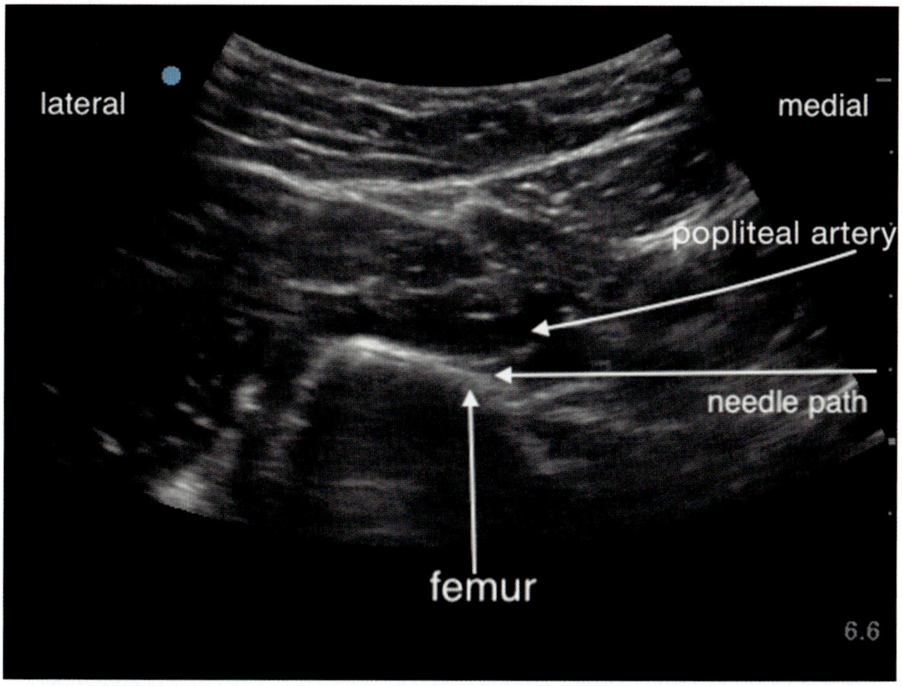

FIGURE 47.16. iPACK injection. Location of iPACK injection between the popliteal artery and the femur, proximal to the femoral condyles.

D. Postoperative Pain Management

D.1. Describe compartment syndrome and how that risk would influence your postoperative plan for peripheral regional analgesia.

Compartment syndrome develops when there is an increase in pressure within a fixed compartment. Patients often have a collection of signs and symptoms, including pain that is out of proportion to the injury, paresthesia, pallor, decreased sensation, weakness, and a late finding of paralysis. It is typically seen after trauma, especially long bone fractures, and after any injury that increases the volume of a compartment of limited size. Tibial fractures are the most common cause, with an incidence of 1% to 10%. The pathophysiology has been described as cellular anoxia due to the inability of the blood flow in an injured area to meet the metabolic demands of the tissue. The resultant swelling and obstruction to venous outflow further decreases the arteriovenous gradient.

Use of regional anesthesia in patients at risk for compartment syndrome remains controversial. Neuraxial blockade can prevent recognition of an acute compartment syndrome. Case reports have shown that signs and symptoms of acute compartment syndrome were present in patients given high concentrations of local anesthetic for neuraxial analgesia but that the significance of the symptoms were not appropriately recognized. Other case reports have demonstrated that patients with dense motor and sensory blocks who were later diagnosed with acute compartment syndrome still reported severe pain in the distribution of the peripheral nerve block. A recent systematic review article concluded that regional anesthesia does not increase the risk of delayed diagnosis of compartment syndrome. Still, one should consider the risks of compartment syndrome, the location of the fracture, positioning during surgery, and the benefits of a regional anesthetic in this patient, taking into account his chronic pain issues.

Driscoll E, Maleki AH, Jahromi L, et al. Regional anesthesia or patient-controlled analgesia and compartment syndrome in orthopedic surgical procedures: a systematic review. *Local Reg Anesth.* 2016;9:65-81.

Elliot KG, Johnstone AJ. Diagnosing acute compartment syndrome. *J Bone Joint Surg Br.* 2003;85:625-632.

Johnson RL, Kopp SL, Kessler J, Gray AT. Peripheral nerve blocks and ultrasound guidance for regional anesthesia. In: Gropper MA, Evered LA, Hemmings HC, et al, eds. *Miller's Anesthesia.* 10th ed. Elsevier; 2025:1305-1330.e3.

Kucera TJ, Boezaart AP. Regional anesthesia does not consistently block ischemic pain: two further cases and a review of the literature. *Pain Med.* 2014;15:316-319.

Mannion S, Capdevila X. Acute compartment syndrome and the role of regional anesthesia. *Int Anesthesiol Clin.* 2010;48:85-105.

SECTION 11

D.2. How would the addition of dexamethasone to local anesthetic influence the duration of the blocks placed in the OR?

The addition of dexamethasone to local anesthetic for peripheral nerve blockade can increase the duration of blockade. When dexamethasone is added to bupivacaine or ropivacaine 0.5%, the duration of sensory block increases from approximately 12 to 24 hours. There is some evidence that giving an equivalent dose of intravenous dexamethasone concomitant to the block can prolong the duration of the sensory block to 24 hours. A meta-analysis has shown that perineural dexamethasone prolongs analgesia by 3.8 hours with a slight decrease of opioid consumption when compared with intravenous dexamethasone while providing a similar duration of prolonged motor blockade.

Chong MA, Berbenetz NM, Lin C, et al. Perineural versus intravenous dexamethasone as an adjuvant for peripheral nerve blocks: a systematic review and meta-analysis. *Reg Anesth Pain Med.* 2017;42:319-326.

De Oliveira GS Jr, Castro Alves LJ, Nader A, et al. Perineural dexamethasone to improve postoperative analgesia with peripheral nerve blocks: a meta-analysis of randomized control trials. *Pain Res Treat.* 2014;2014:179029.

Desmet M, Braems H, Reynvoet M, et al. I.V. and perineural dexamethasone are equivalent in increasing the analgesic duration of a single-shot interscalene block with ropivacaine for shoulder surgery: a prospective, randomized, placebo-controlled study. *Br J Anaesth.* 2013;111:445-452.

D.3. What is liposomal bupivacaine?

Liposomal bupivacaine is a slow-release form of the local anesthetic bupivacaine that has US Food and Drug Administration (FDA) approval for local infiltration, interscalene brachial plexus block, sciatic nerve block in the popliteal fossa, and adductor canal block for postoperative pain control. It consists of bupivacaine encapsulated within multivesicular liposomes, which is gradually released as the liposomes are broken down. The routine use of liposomal bupivacaine for peripheral nerve blocks has been controversial due to conflicting evidence about its efficacy and its cost when compared to plain bupivacaine or ropivacaine. A recent narrative review of published randomized control trials of liposomal bupivacaine concluded that the current evidence does not support the routine use of liposomal bupivacaine in place of standard long-acting local anesthetics for treating postoperative pain. A systematic review and meta-analysis also found that liposomal bupivacaine offered a statistically significant but clinically unimportant improvement in the area-under-the-curve (AUC) of postoperative pain scores when compared to standard local anesthetics.

Hussain N, Brull R, Sheehy B, et al. Perineural liposomal bupivacaine is not superior to nonliposomal bupivacaine for peripheral nerve block analgesia: a systematic review and meta-analysis. *Anesthesiology.* 2021;134:147-164.

Ilfeld BM, Eisenach JC, Gabriel RA. Clinical effectiveness of liposomal bupivacaine administered by infiltration or peripheral nerve block to treat postoperative pain. *Anesthesiology.* 2021;134:283-344.

McCann ME. Liposomal bupivacaine: effective, cost-effective, or (Just) costly? *Anesthesiology.* 2021;134:139-142.

D.4. What benefit would a peripheral nerve catheter provide over a long-acting local anesthetic? Are there any downsides?

Peripheral nerve catheters are a proven method for prolonging postoperative pain control with decreased intravenous or oral opioid use and hence their related side effects. They have also been shown to decrease the incidence and/or severity of chronic postsurgical pain syndromes. A peripheral nerve catheter gives patients the ability to have some control over their own pain management. Compared with long-lasting single-shot injections with additives, a catheter technique could provide analgesia beyond the first 24 hours, which is the limit of duration of a single-shot block. As compared to a long-lasting single-shot injection, peripheral catheters can be stopped or removed if needed. Peripheral nerve catheters are increasingly used in the ambulatory and outpatient settings, with patients being discharged to home with an infusing peripheral nerve catheter in place. Large studies continue to show a low-risk profile with the use of at-home patient management of catheters.

Some limitations to the placement of peripheral nerve catheters include the risk of infection, technical challenges inherent in their placement, time of placement, and the need for management and supervision by anesthesiologists and other health care providers. Other risks of peripheral nerve catheters include damage to the nerve itself from direct contact or nerve entrapment, damage to nearby structures, and intravascular placement and migration. Although these risks are recognized and need to be monitored, a recent comprehensive review article reports them to be exceedingly rare.

Ilfeld BM. Continuous peripheral nerve blocks: an update of the published evidence and comparison with novel, alternative analgesic modalities. *Anesth Analg.* 2017;124:308-335.

Merritt CK, Mariano ER, Kaye AD, et al. Peripheral nerve catheters and local anesthetic infiltration in perioperative analgesia. *Best Pract Res Clin Anaesthesiol.* 2014;28:41-57.

D.5. You were able to perform a continuous spinal epidural (CSE) at L3-L4 and used 0.125% bupivacaine via the epidural catheter for postoperative pain control. The patient reports that he is comfortable regarding both his back pain and his ankle pain. What benefit would continuing methadone confer in this case?

Use of chronic opioid regimens for patients suffering from chronic nonmalignant pain has increased dramatically over the past two decades. Acute postoperative pain control in patients who are taking maintenance opioids for addiction and dependence presents a challenge for health care providers. These patients require opioid doses that are multiples of the doses needed by patients not exposed to opioids chronically. Aside from tolerance to opioids, these patients often exhibit increased pain to surgical stimuli compared to an opioid-naive population. This can be secondary to increased anxiety and depression, development of opioid-induced hyperalgesia, and changes in the endogenous opioid system. Multimodal analgesia, including regional techniques and nonopioid adjuvants, such as ketamine, nonsteroidal anti-inflammatory drugs, gabapentinoids, and acetaminophen, greatly aid in controlling their pain postoperatively. Nonetheless, continuation of maintenance opioids (50%-100%) is essential to avoid withdrawal symptoms. Approaches to maintaining opioid levels include continuation of the same preoperative opioid and route, changing the route of administration while continuing the same opioid or using an equianalgesic conversion to a different opioid with a likely dose reduction secondary to lack of 100% cross tolerance. In addition, patients should generally receive their usual dose of opioids prior to surgery. Signs of withdrawal from methadone can present 12 to 24 hours after the last doses, whereas withdrawal from medications such as morphine occurs within 6 to 18 hours. Withdrawal syndrome can present with agitation, diaphoresis, hypertension, diarrhea, nausea, emesis, abdominal cramps, and seizures.

Hadi I, Morley-Forster PK, Dain S, et al. Brief review: perioperative management of the patient with chronic non-cancer pain. *Can J Anaesth.* 2006;53:1190-1199.

Mehta V, Langford R. Acute pain management for opioid dependent patients. *Anaesthesia.* 2006;61:269-276.

Richebé P, Beaulieu P. Perioperative pain management in the patient treated with opioids: continuing professional development. *Can J Anaesth.* 2009;56:969-981.

D.6. How can regional analgesia aid in fast-track postoperative care?

Fast-track programs are used to help decrease morbidity by decreasing perioperative hospitalization. Both neuraxial and peripheral blockade can be utilized as an effective modality to aid in fast-track programs. Regional anesthesia can attenuate the inflammatory, endocrine, and metabolic responses to surgical stress and thus decrease perioperative complications. Blockade of the sympathetic response helps with improved blood flow, decreased thromboembolic events, and decreased blood loss. It also tempers the shivering response, which can potentially prolong postanesthetic care unit stays. Regional techniques can be used to minimize inhalational agents, neuromuscular blocking agents, and opioids with a resultant earlier emergence from general anesthesia or complete avoidance of general anesthesia. It improves immediate postoperative analgesia and has been shown to decrease the risk of infection. In addition, there is often earlier return of bowel function. For lower extremity surgery, regional anesthesia can improve patient satisfaction with decreasing time to home readiness, opioid consumption, pain scores, time to ambulation, and postoperative nausea and vomiting. Regional anesthesia is the cornerstone of the new movement toward total joint replacement in the ambulatory setting.

Aasvang EK, Luna IE, Kehlet H. Challenges in postdischarge function and recovery: the case of fast-track hip and knee arthroplasty. *Br J Anaesth.* 2015;115:861-866.

Carli F, Kehlet H, Baldini G, et al. Evidence basis for regional anesthesia in multidisciplinary fast-track surgical care pathways. *Reg Anesth Pain Med.* 2011;36:63-72.

Memtsoudis SG, Sun X, Chiu YL, et al. Perioperative comparative effectiveness of anesthetic technique in orthopedic patients. *Anesthesiology.* 2013;118:1046-1058.

Acknowledgments

We gratefully acknowledge the contributions of previous edition author(s), Roniel Weinberg, Melvin La, and Danielle Gluck, as portions of those chapters have been retained in this revision.

48 Complex Regional Pain Syndromes

Rohan Jotwani, Philip A. Petrou , and Neel D. Mehta

A 35-year-old female complains of diffuse burning pain in the left arm and hand for the last 6 months. She recalls spraining her left wrist while playing volleyball. Her left hand feels colder than the right, and her fingertips are blue. She is a recently divorced high-profile executive.

A. Medical Disease and Differential Diagnosis

1. What is the differential diagnosis of pain in this patient?
2. What is complex regional pain syndrome (CRPS)?
3. What are the two types of CRPS?
4. What are the diagnostic criteria for CRPS? What is its incidence?
5. Define allodynia, hyperalgesia, hyperesthesia, and dysesthesia.
6. What are the stages of CRPS?
7. What are the possible etiologies of CRPS?
8. Explain the pathophysiology of the development of CRPS.
9. Define sympathetically maintained pain (SMP) and sympathetically independent pain (SIP).
10. How does CRPS differ from neuralgia?
11. What is central pain? How will you differentiate central pain from CRPS?
12. Is the social history of this patient relevant to the development of chronic pain syndrome?

B. Pain Management

1. How will you work up CRPS types I and II?
2. Describe the sympathetic nerve supply to the arm?
3. Where is the stellate ganglion located?
4. What are the anatomic landmarks used in the stellate ganglion block?
5. What are the clinical signs of stellate ganglion block?
6. What is Horner syndrome?
7. After a stellate ganglion block, this patient reports no significant change in the degree of pain despite developing Horner syndrome. Is the pain psychogenic?
8. What types of nerve fibers are interrupted in stellate ganglion block?
9. What is differential block?
10. What are the two major classes of local anesthetics? Describe the major differences in their clinical pharmacology.
11. What factors determine the onset, potency, and duration of local anesthetic block?
12. How does the addition of epinephrine to commercially available premixed solutions affect the efficacy of local anesthetics?
13. How will you treat this patient?
14. What is the pharmacologic management of CRPS?
15. What is the role of intravenous regional block (Bier block) in diagnosis and treatment of CRPS?
16. Compare and contrast the mechanisms of action of ketamine and methadone.
17. What roles does ketamine infusion play in the treatment of CRPS? Is there a guideline for ketamine infusion in treating CRPS?
18. What is neuromodulation? What is the role of stimulation-based therapies in treating CRPS?
19. What is the role of surgical sympathectomy?

20. What role does intrathecal (IT) therapy play in managing CRPS?
21. If opioids are prescribed as treatment for patients with CRPS, what is the Centers for Disease Control and Prevention (CDC) guideline on chronic opioid therapy?

C. Complications

1. What are the complications of stellate ganglion block?
2. What is the systemic toxicity of local anesthetics?
3. How do you treat systemic toxicity of local anesthetic drugs?
4. What are the possible complications of spinal cord stimulation (SCS)?
5. What are the possible complications of IT therapy?

A. Medical Disease and Differential Diagnosis

A.1. What is the differential diagnosis of pain in this patient?

Pain accompanied by abnormal sudomotor, vasomotor, and sensory changes is most likely due to CRPS. The differential diagnosis also includes the following:

1. Peripheral neuropathy
2. Soft tissue injury
3. Vascular insufficiency (Raynaud disease)
4. Nerve entrapment syndrome (carpal tunnel syndrome)
5. Brachial plexopathy

Over the years, CRPS has been referred to as *reflex sympathetic dystrophy* (RSD), causalgia, sympathetically maintained pain (SMP), algodystrophy, Sudeck atrophy and chronic peripheral pain syndrome. The term *CRPS* was introduced in 1994 by the International Association for the Study of Pain subcommittee on taxonomy. It is subdivided into CRPS type I (formerly described as *RSD*) and CRPS type II (formerly described as *causalgia*).

Shim H, Rose J, Halle S, Shekane P. Complex regional pain syndrome: a narrative review for the practising clinician. *Br J Anaesth*. 2019;123:e424-e433.

Stanton-Hicks MD. CRPS: what's in a name? Taxonomy, epidemiology, neurologic, immune, and autoimmune considerations. *Reg Anesth Pain Med*. 2019;44:376-387.

A.2. What is complex regional pain syndrome (CRPS)?

CRPS is characterized by pain associated with sensory, autonomic, trophic, and motor abnormalities. CRPS is triggered by *noxious stimuli* (type I) or by *nerve injury* (type II). It is characterized by autonomic dysfunction not limited to the distribution of a single peripheral nerve or dermatomal distribution, usually affects a distal limb, and is disproportionate to the inciting event.

RSD, causalgia, algodystrophy, Sudeck atrophy, and various other conditions are all grouped under CRPS. This diagnosis better describes the wide range of clinical signs and symptoms and the complexity of the pathophysiology responsible for the clinical picture.

Shim H, Rose J, Halle S, Shekane P. Complex regional pain syndrome: a narrative review for the practising clinician. *Br J Anaesth*. 2019;123:e424-e433.

Stanton-Hicks MD. CRPS: what's in a name? Taxonomy, epidemiology, neurologic, immune, and autoimmune considerations. *Reg Anesth Pain Med*. 2019;44:376-387.

A.3. What are the two types of CRPS?

CRPS-I is defined as a clinical syndrome triggered by a *noxious stimulus* that is not limited to the distribution of a single peripheral nerve; no nerve lesion can be identified. CRPS-II is defined as a clinical syndrome that is due to a *nerve injury* and is mostly limited to the distribution of the injured nerve. The diagnostic criteria are the same for CRPS-I and II.

Marinus J, Moseley GL, Birklein F, et al. Clinical features and pathophysiology of complex regional pain syndrome. *Lancet Neurol*. 2011;10:637-648.

Taylor SS, Noor N, Urits I, et al. Complex regional pain syndrome: a comprehensive review. *Pain Ther*. 2021;10:875-892.

A.4. What are the diagnostic criteria for CRPS? What is its incidence?

The diagnosis of CRPS is a clinical diagnosis and can be made in the following context: a history of trauma to the affected area associated with pain that is disproportionate to the inciting event plus one or more of the following as defined by the Budapest Criteria, International Association for the Study of Pain, or Veldman Criteria. Similar elements across these scales include:

- Abnormal function of the sympathetic nervous system (vasomotor changes, skin color changes, temperature changes)
- Swelling
- Movement disorder
- Increased sudomotor activity
- Changes in tissue growth (dystrophy and atrophy)
- Sensory disturbances (hyperalgesia or allodynia)

The main features include pain that is continuous, burning in nature, independent of type and severity of injury, and not limited to a dermatomal distribution. Patients complain of allodynia, dysesthesia, or hyperalgesia. Movement or stress exacerbates the pain. Edema is usually present. Abnormal sudomotor activity, limb discoloration, and local temperature changes are common but inconsistent.

Specifically, the Budapest Criteria require that a patient report one symptom in three of the following four categories: sensory, vasomotor, sudomotor/edema, and motor/trophic. The patient must display signs and symptoms (at the time of evaluation) in at least two of the following four categories: sensory, vasomotor, sudomotor, and motor. In addition, the patient must report a history of a noxious event or trauma that preceded the onset of symptoms and have no other diagnosis that more clearly explains the signs or symptoms. These criteria have been developed to improve the accuracy and consistency of CRPS diagnosis and to ensure that patients receive appropriate treatment for their condition.

The incidence of CRPS has been reported to be approximately 5 to 6 cases per 100,000 in the United States, with females approximately 3 times more likely to be diagnosed. This syndrome follows as many as 5% of all traumatic injuries, with the arms affected in approximately 60% to 70% of cases and the legs approximately 30% to 40%.

Mesaroli G, Hundert A, Birnie KA, Campbell F, Stinson J. Screening and diagnostic tools for complex regional pain syndrome: a systematic review. *Pain*. 2021;162:1295.

Shim H, Rose J, Halle S, Shekane P. Complex regional pain syndrome: a narrative review for the practising clinician. *Br J Anaesth*. 2019;123:e424-e433.

Turk DC, Robinson JP. Multidisciplinary assessment of patients with chronic pain. In: Ballantyne JC, Fishman SM, Rathmell JP, eds. *Bonica's Management of Pain*. 5th ed. Wolters Kluwer; 2018:313-328.

A.5. Define allodynia, hyperalgesia, hyperesthesia, and dysesthesia.

- *Allodynia*: pain caused by a stimulus that normally does not provoke pain (ie, light touch with a cotton swab)
- *Hyperalgesia*: an increased response to a stimulus that is normally painful (ie, increased response to pinprick)
- *Hyperesthesia*: increased sensitivity to a stimulus either due to a diminished threshold or an increased response to stimuli that are normally recognized. Hyperesthesia includes both allodynia and hyperalgesia.
- *Dysesthesia*: an abnormal sensation that is unpleasant to the patient. It may be either spontaneous or evoked (ie, lumbar radiculopathy).

Turk DC, Robinson JP. Multidisciplinary assessment of patients with chronic pain. In: Ballantyne JC, Fishman SM, Rathmell JP, eds. *Bonica's Management of Pain*. 5th ed. Wolters Kluwer; 2018:313-328.

A.6. What are the stages of CRPS?

Stage I

- Onset of severe pain limited to the site of injury
- Increased sensitivity of skin to touch and light pressure (hyperesthesia)
- Localized swelling
- Muscle cramps
- Stiffness and limited mobility

At the onset, the skin is usually warm, red, and dry; it can change to blue (cyanotic) in appearance and become cold and sweaty.

- Increased sweating (hyperhidrosis)
- In mild cases, this stage lasts a few weeks and then subsides spontaneously or responds rapidly to treatment.

Stage II

- Pain becomes even more severe and more diffuse.
- Swelling tends to spread and can change from a soft to a hard (brawny) type.
- Hair can become coarse, then scant; nails can grow faster and become brittle, cracked, and heavily grooved.
- Spotty wasting of bone (osteoporosis) occurs early but can become severe and diffuse.
- Muscle wasting begins.

Stage III

- Marked wasting of tissue (atrophic) eventually becomes irreversible.
- For many patients, the pain becomes intractable and can involve the entire limb.
- A small percentage of patients develop generalized CRPS affecting the entire body.

Similarly, a CRPS Severity Score (CSS) was developed to better quantify the disease and progression based on self-reported and observed physical findings. Higher scores were associated with significantly higher pain intensity, distress, and functional impairments, as well as greater bilateral temperature asymmetry and thermal perception abnormalities.

Patient reported symptoms include:

- Allodynia
- Temperature, skin color, sweating, trophic, or motor changes
- Restricted range of motion
- Edema

Examination findings:

- Hyperpathia to pinprick
- Allodynia
- Temperature change
- Skin color or sweating asymmetry

Harden RN, Bruehl S, Perez RS. Development of a severity score for CRPS. *Pain.* 2010;151:870-876.

Turk DC, Robinson JP. Multidisciplinary assessment of patients with chronic pain. In: Ballantyne JC, Fishman SM, Rathmell JP, eds. *Bonica's Management of Pain.* 5th ed. Wolters Kluwer; 2018:313-328.

A.7. What are the possible etiologies of CRPS?

CRPS can follow relatively minor trauma with or without nerve injury. Causes leading to CRPS include the following:

- Injuries to peripheral tissues (eg, fractures, dislocations, and surgery)
- Inflammatory conditions (eg, fasciitis, tendonitis, bursitis, and arthritis)
- Immobilization as a result of injury or cast application
- Peripheral nerve injury resulting from direct compression or ischemia (eg, brachial plexopathy, postherpetic neuralgia, and nerve root injury)
- Central nervous system insults (eg, head injury, ischemia, and brain tumor)
- Spinal cord lesions
- Idiopathic

Turk DC, Robinson JP. Multidisciplinary assessment of patients with chronic pain. In: Ballantyne JC, Fishman SM, Rathmell JP, eds. *Bonica's Management of Pain.* 5th ed. Wolters Kluwer; 2018:313-328.

A.8. Explain the pathophysiology of the development of CRPS.

Several hypotheses have been postulated, but none can explain all the findings and the varying responses to treatment in these patients. Hypotheses include:

- Abnormal discharges in sympathetic and nociceptive afferents produced by trauma
- Sensitization of peripheral sensory receptors produced by sympathetic hyperactivity
- Formation of ephapses (artificial synapses) after peripheral nerve injury

- Spontaneous neuronal ectopy at the site of demyelination or axonal injury
- Central reorganization of pain processing (central sensitization)

More than one sequence of events likely take place in a patient, giving rise to a mixed clinical picture. A dynamic change in the physiology and structure of central pain projecting neurons can be mediated through the *N*-methyl-D-aspartate (NMDA) receptor. Injury initiates and maintains a state of central sensitization in the central pain pathways, resulting in a lower threshold to fire pain transmission neurons and an increase in their receptive fields. This might involve disinhibition of spinal and trigeminal nociceptive neurons and often precedes thermal and mechanical allodynia and spontaneous pain. Finally, the psychological component and neuromodulation cannot be discernibly separated.

Binder A, Baron R. Complex regional pain syndromes. In: McMahon SB, Koltzenburg M, Tracey I, et al, eds. *Wall and Melzack's Textbook of Pain*. 6th ed. Churchill Livingstone; 2013:961-977.

Knudsen LF, Terkelsen AJ, Drummond PD, et al. Complex regional pain syndrome: a focus on the autonomic nervous system. *Clin Auton Res*. 2019;29:457-467.

Lam CM, Chadwick AL, Hurley RW. Evaluation and treatment of neuropathic pain syndromes. In: Benzon H, Rathmell JP, Wu CL, et al, eds. *Practical Management of Pain*. 6th ed. Mosby; 2023:479-499.

A.9. Define sympathetically maintained pain (SMP) and sympathetically independent pain (SIP).

Pain that is maintained by sympathetic innervation or circulating catecholamines is defined as SMP. It describes a pain mechanism, not a clinical syndrome. Therefore, by definition, patients with CRPS who report pain relief after a sympathetic block (eg, stellate ganglion block) have SMP. Conversely, pain conditions that show features of sympathetic overactivity, yet fail to respond to sympathetic blocks, are described as SIP.

Turk DC, Robinson JP. Multidisciplinary assessment of patients with chronic pain. In: Ballantyne JC, Fishman SM, Rathmell JP, eds. *Bonica's Management of Pain*. 5th ed. Wolters Kluwer; 2018:313-328.

A.10. How does CRPS differ from neuralgia?

The chronic pain seen in neuralgia is usually paroxysmal in nature and follows the distribution of the nerve. The pain is sharp and shooting without associated vasomotor or sudomotor changes. The chronic pain syndrome of CRPS is a sustained, diffuse, burning pain that is independent of nerve distribution and associated with vasomotor and sudomotor changes, edema, allodynia or hyperalgesia, and changes in skin color.

Lam CM, Chadwick AL, Hurley RW. Evaluation and treatment of neuropathic pain syndromes. In: Benzon H, Rathmell JP, Wu CL, et al, eds. *Practical Management of Pain*. 6th ed. Mosby; 2023:479-499.

Taylor SS, Noor N, Urits I, et al. Complex regional pain syndrome: a comprehensive review. *Pain Ther*. 2021;10:875-892.

A.11. What is central pain? How will you differentiate central pain from CRPS?

Central pain is regional pain initiated or caused by a primary lesion or dysfunction in the central nervous system; it is usually associated with abnormal sensitivity to temperature and to noxious stimulus. Central pain, also referred to as *deafferentation pain*, is a difficult pain syndrome to treat because the pathophysiology is not well understood. Regional pain not relieved by peripheral nerve blocks, either sympathetic or somatic, is more likely to be central pain. Central pain can be associated with various neurologic symptoms and signs such as monoparesis, hemiparesis, or paraparesis. Central pain conditions typically include partial or complete loss of sensation, involvement of spinothalamic functions, and development of hypersensitivity in body parts that have lost normal somatosensory feedback as a result of a central nervous system lesion.

Jensen TS, Finnerup NB. Central pain. In: McMahon SB, Koltzenburg M, Tracey I, et al, eds. *Wall and Melzack's Textbook of Pain*. 6th ed. Churchill Livingstone; 2013:990-1002.

A.12. Is the social history of this patient relevant to the development of chronic pain syndrome?

In patients with CRPS, the disproportionate pain and dysfunction and the absence of clear pathogenesis and pathophysiology have led to examination of potential psychological factors. As the CRPS progresses, patients' personality measures such as Minnesota Multiphasic Personality Inventory (MMPI) profiles tend to resemble those of patients experiencing chronic pain and psychological distress as evidenced by hypochondriasis, depression, and hysteria scales. Certainly, stress has been implicated in increasing sympathetic outflow. The presence of psychological disorders, particularly anxiety and depression, can predispose to the development of CRPS. However, a large case-control study reported no differences in psychological variables between those with CRPS and those without CRPS after controlling for age, sex, and trauma. Furthermore, anxiety and stress can augment nociception, and, therefore, antidepressive treatments can be useful.

Jensen TS, Finnerup NB. Central pain. In: McMahon SB, Koltzenburg M, Tracey I, et al, eds. *Wall and Melzack's Textbook of Pain*. 6th ed. Churchill Livingstone; 2013:990-1002.

Knudsen LF, Terkelsen AJ, Drummond PD, et al. Complex regional pain syndrome: a focus on the autonomic nervous system. *Clin Auton Res*. 2019;29:457-467.

Scarff JR. Managing psychiatric symptoms in patients with complex regional pain syndrome. *Innov Clin Neurosci*. 2022;19:56-59.

B. Pain Management

B.1. How will you work up CRPS types I and II?

CRPS is diagnosed clinically with a detailed history and physical examination. Because it is a clinical diagnosis of exclusion, other specific conditions that could account for the degree of pain and dysfunction must be ruled out. Objective signs are variable but almost universally include loss of function of the affected part due to pain. Allodynia and hyperalgesia are extremely common. Change in temperature and sweating vary depending on the stage of the disease.

Several diagnostic studies aid in the diagnosis of CRPS but are seldom definitive. A quantitative sweat test can show excessive sweating, and thermography can demonstrate abnormal heat regulation and disparity in temperature between affected and normal regions. Radiologic studies can reveal patchy osteoporosis in early stages. Triple-phase bone scintigraphy using technetium-99m can show increased periarticular uptake in the affected extremity illustrated by unilateral hyperperfusion in the perfusion and blood pool phases. Negative triple-phase bone scan results do not rule out CRPS. Thermographic, radiologic, or scintigraphic findings can be nonspecific and should be correlated with clinical findings. Positive diagnostic sympathetic blocks can confirm the sympathetically mediated component of CRPS.

Magnetic resonance neurography using high contrast and spatial resolution techniques to highlight pathologic anatomic and physiologic changes in the nerves and tissues can be helpful for suspected CRPS-II with sensory or motor dysfunction. Magnetic resonance neurography can be helpful in cases where the spine MRI is normal, but nerve injury is suspected, such as in tumor, lesions, trauma, or entrapment. Magnetic resonance neurography imaging challenges include the small size of peripheral nerves, low sensitivity, difficulty of limiting the area of interest undergoing scanning, and inexperience of radiologists. Nerve injury or inflammation can appear as increased T2 signal intensity in whole nerve or individual fascicles, a size change of the whole nerve or individual fascicles, epineurial thickening, secondary muscle changes including edema and atrophy (due to decreased nerve growth factors), or a path detour (eg, Hairpin turns at the joint).

Jensen TS, Finnerup NB. Central pain. In: McMahon SB, Koltzenburg M, Tracey I, et al, eds. *Wall and Melzack's Textbook of Pain*. 6th ed. Churchill Livingstone; 2013:990-1002.

Johnson EM, Yoon D, Biswal S, et al. Characteristics of patients with complex limb pain evaluated through an interdisciplinary approach utilizing magnetic resonance neurography. *Front Pain Res (Lausanne)*. 2021;2:689402.

Stanton-Hicks MD. CRPS: what's in a name? Taxonomy, epidemiology, neurologic, immune and autoimmune considerations. *Reg Anesth Pain Med*. 2019;44:376-387.

B.2. Describe the sympathetic nerve supply to the arm?

The preganglionic sympathetic outflow to the upper extremity is derived from T2-T9. These fibers synapse with postganglionic neurons in the stellate ganglion. Therefore, a stellate ganglion block interrupts sympathetic outflow to the upper extremity.

Huygen FJPM. Evaluation and treatment of complex regional pain syndrome. In: Benzon H, Rathmell JP, Wu CL, et al, eds. *Practical Management of Pain*. 6th ed. Mosby; 2023:500-506.

B.3. Where is the stellate ganglion located?

The stellate ganglion is formed by the fusion of the inferior cervical and the first thoracic ganglia. It usually measures $2.5 \times 1.5 \times 0.5$ cm and lies between the base of the transverse process of the seventh cervical vertebra and the neck of the first rib. It is situated behind the carotid sheath, ventral to the longus

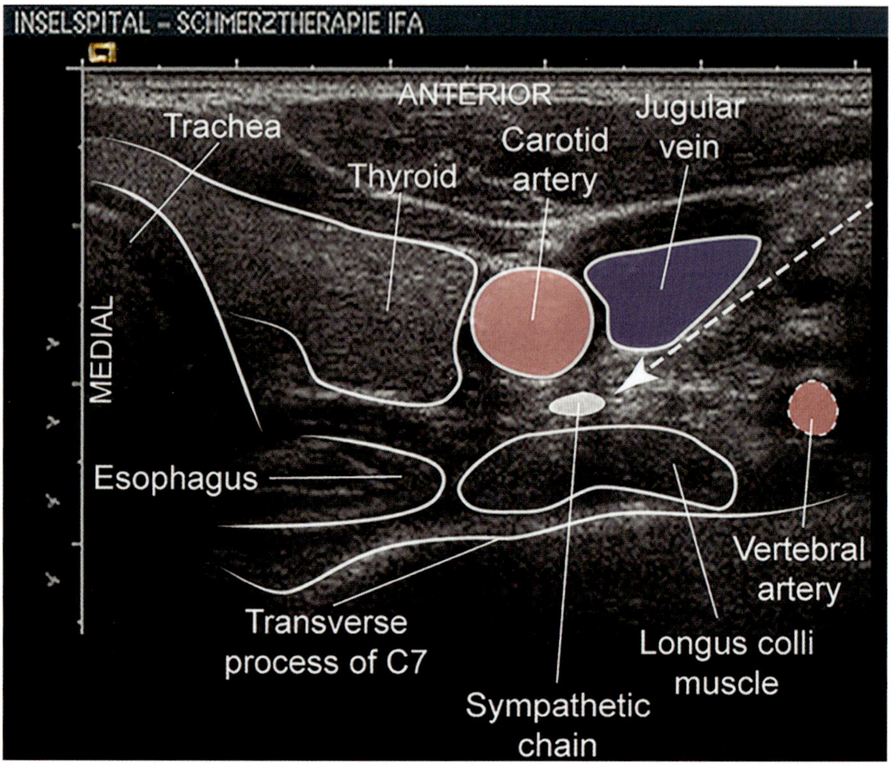

FIGURE 48.1. Stellate ganglion block. Note that the vertebral artery can be seen anterior to the echogenic transverse process at the level of C7. The vertebral artery cannot be seen clearly at the C6 level on ultrasound, as it lies posterior to the echogenic transverse process within the foramen transversarium. At the level of C7, the superior margin of the thyroid is seen just lateral to the trachea. The *dashed arrow* indicates the optimal trajectory for placing a needle using an in-plane approach, for example, placing the needle in a lateral to medial direction with the shaft in the transverse plane of the ultrasound image. (Ultrasound image courtesy of Urs Eichenberger MD, PhD, University Department of Anesthesiology and Pain Therapy, University Hospital of Bern, Bern, Switzerland, 2011.)

colli muscle, behind the vertebral artery, and lateral to the body of the vertebra (**Figure 48.1**). The vertebral, subclavian, inferior thyroid, and the first intercostal arteries are in close proximity to the ganglion, as is the recurrent laryngeal nerve. The left pleura is 1 to 2 cm below it, whereas the right pleura is in closer proximity.

Huygen FJPM. Evaluation and treatment of complex regional pain syndrome. In: Benzon H, Rathmell JP, Wu CL, et al, eds. *Practical Management of Pain*. 6th ed. Mosby; 2023:500-506.

Tsui B, Suresh S. Regional anesthesia in children. In: Gropper MA, Cohen NH, Eriksson LI, et al, eds. *Miller's Anesthesia*. 10th ed. Elsevier; 2025:2354-2410.e8.

B.4. What are the anatomic landmarks used in the stellate ganglion block?

The landmarks used in the stellate ganglion block are the jugular notch of the sternum, the sternocleidomastoid muscle, the cricoid cartilage, and Chassaignac tubercle. In a supine patient with the neck extended, a mark placed approximately 3.5 cm from the midline along the jugular notch and the same distance above the clavicle should overlie the transverse process of the seventh vertebra and the medial border of the sternocleidomastoid muscle. This marking is further confirmed by palpating the cricoid cartilage, which lies at the level of the sixth cervical vertebra, and the anterior tubercle on the vertebral transverse process, which is the most prominent tubercle in the neck (Chassaignac tubercle).

Huygen FJPM. Evaluation and treatment of complex regional pain syndrome. In: Benzon H, Rathmell JP, Wu CL, et al, eds. *Practical Management of Pain*. 6th ed. Mosby; 2023:500-506.

B.5. What are the clinical signs of stellate ganglion block?

Stellate ganglion block results in the following ipsilateral signs:

- *Eye*: ptosis, narrowing of the palpebral fissure, miosis, enophthalmos, conjunctival injection, and lacrimation

- *Face and neck*: anhidrosis, elevated local temperature, and nasal stuffiness
- *Arm*: increased temperature and plethysmographic evidence of improved cutaneous blood flow

Tsui B, Suresh S. Regional anesthesia in children. In: Gropper MA, Cohen NH, Eriksson LI, et al, eds. *Miller's Anesthesia*. 10th ed. Elsevier; 2025:2354-2410.e8.

B.6. What is Horner syndrome?

Horner syndrome is a clinical entity characterized by ptosis, miosis, anhidrosis, and enophthalmos. It is usually seen with disease processes involving the cervical sympathetic nerves, and is the classic sign of a successful stellate ganglion block.

Tsui B, Suresh S. Regional anesthesia in children. In: Gropper MA, Cohen NH, Eriksson LI, et al, eds. *Miller's Anesthesia*. 10th ed. Elsevier; 2025:2354-2410.e8.

B.7. After a stellate ganglion block, this patient reports no significant change in the degree of pain despite developing Horner syndrome. Is the pain psychogenic?

Not necessarily. Horner syndrome indicates only interruption of sympathetic supply to the head and neck. Unless it is accompanied by objective changes in the arm, it does not indicate a sympathetic nerve block of the upper extremity. Furthermore, SMP will respond to sympathectomy, whereas SIP will not.

Jensen TS, Finnerup NB. Central pain. In: McMahon SB, Koltzenburg M, Tracey I, et al, eds. *Wall and Melzack's Textbook of Pain*. 6th ed. Churchill Livingstone; 2013:990-1002.

B.8. What types of nerve fibers are interrupted in stellate ganglion block?

Stellate ganglion block results in interruption of the preganglionic, thinly myelinated type B fibers as well as the postganglionic, unmyelinated type C fibers.

Casale R, Glynn CJ, Buonocore M. Autonomic variations after stellate ganglion block: are they evidence of an autonomic afference? *Funct Neurol*. 1990;5:245-246.

B.9. What is differential block?

The variable effect of local anesthetics on fibers performing different functions is referred to as *differential block*. The diagnostic distinction can be made by selectively blocking the function of these nerve fibers. Differential block is best explained by fiber size and myelination because these factors determine different sensitivities of nerve fibers to local anesthetics. By using different concentrations of local anesthetic, sympathetic or somatic fibers can be selectively blocked (eg, using bupivacaine 0.25% for a sensory peripheral nerve block versus bupivacaine 0.5% for a combined motor and sensory peripheral nerve block). A differential block can be helpful in differentiating somatic versus sympathetic pain and peripheral versus central pain.

B.10. What are the two major classes of local anesthetics? Describe the major differences in their clinical pharmacology.

The two major classes of clinically employed local anesthetics are esters and amides. The esters are hydrolyzed in the plasma by pseudocholinesterase; the amides are biotransformed in the liver. Although infrequent, local anesthetic toxicity is encountered more commonly in the ester group because of the para-aminobenzoic acid moiety. True allergic reactions to amides are rare and in most instances are caused by preservatives in the solution. Each of the two groups of local anesthetics contains drugs with varying rate of onset, duration of neural blockade, potency, and toxicity.

Huygen FJPM. Evaluation and treatment of complex regional pain syndrome. In: Benzon H, Rathmell JP, Wu CL, et al, eds. *Practical Management of Pain*. 6th ed. Mosby; 2023:500-506.

B.11. What factors determine the onset, potency, and duration of local anesthetic block?

- Onset correlates with pK_a.
- Potency correlates with lipid solubility.
- Duration correlates with degree of protein binding.

The commonly used local anesthetics are weakly basic tertiary amines that are lipid soluble and unstable in water. They are prepared as acidic salts because the ionized form, which is soluble in water, is stable. Therefore, the aqueous solution contains the ionized (cation) form of the local anesthetic in dissociation equilibrium, with the unionized (free base) form depending on the pH of the medium.

$$\underset{\text{Cation}}{R \equiv NH^+} \rightleftharpoons \underset{\text{Base}}{R \equiv N} + H^+$$

TABLE 48.1 Physiochemical Properties of Commonly Used Local Anesthetics

Local Anesthetic	pK_a	Protein Binding (%)
Esters		
Procaine	8.9	5.8
Chloroprocaine	8.7	—
Tetracaine	8.5	75.6
Amides		
Lidocaine	7.9	64.3
Mepivacaine	7.6	77.5
Bupivacaine	8.1	95.6
Ropivacaine	8.07	94.0
Etidocaine	7.7	94.0

When injected into the body, the relative rise in pH allows the local anesthetic to convert to the uncharged base. The free base, being lipid soluble, can diffuse across the neural membrane and is responsible for neural blockade. With the exception of procaine and chloroprocaine, the commonly employed local anesthetics are highly protein bound and are therefore longer acting (**Table 48.1**).

Huygen FJPM. Evaluation and treatment of complex regional pain syndrome. In: Benzon H, Rathmell JP, Wu CL, et al, eds. *Practical Management of Pain*. 6th ed. Mosby; 2023:500-506.

B.12. How does the addition of epinephrine to commercially available premixed solutions affect the efficacy of local anesthetics?

The addition of epinephrine to a local anesthetic increases the duration and intensity of a block. However, in commercially available premixed solutions containing epinephrine, antioxidants are added to preserve epinephrine, and the result is a lower buffered pH of the solution. This lower pH can result in decreased efficacy. Best results are achieved by adding the desired concentration of epinephrine to the local anesthetic solution just before injection.

Huygen FJPM. Evaluation and treatment of complex regional pain syndrome. In: Benzon H, Rathmell JP, Wu CL, et al, eds. *Practical Management of Pain*. 6th ed. Mosby; 2023:500-506.

B.13. How will you treat this patient?

Early diagnosis and aggressive physical therapy with pharmacologic control of pain form the foundation of treatment for CRPS. Physical therapy is recommended and accepted as a first line of treatment. Treatment of CRPS will differ depending on whether the pain is SMP or SIP. Sympathetic blocks have been shown effective in treating and evaluating for the extent of SMP in CRPS. A multidisciplinary approach including physical and occupational therapies, medication management, interventional therapies, and symptom-specific psychological treatments (eg, biofeedback and hypnosis) can be beneficial. Many patients have a component of both SMP and SIP, and a combination of sympathectomy and analgesic treatment is recommended. However, no single treatment is consistently successful. Therefore, the treatment plan should be individualized.

Jensen TS, Finnerup NB. Central pain. In: McMahon SB, Koltzenburg M, Tracey I, et al, eds. *Wall and Melzack's Textbook of Pain*. 6th ed. Churchill Livingstone; 2013:990-1002.

Shim H, Rose J, Halle S, Shekane P. Complex regional pain syndrome: a narrative review for the practising clinician. *Br J Anaesth*. 2019;123:e424-e433.

B.14. What is the pharmacologic management of CRPS?

Sympathetically mediated pain of CRPS is treated with drugs that deplete norepinephrine from sympathetic nerve terminals. Oral sympatholytic agents include phenoxybenzamine, prazosin, and terazosin. Topical clonidine, a selective α_2-agonist, has been successfully used to treat SMP. Tricyclic antidepressants are effective in about half of patients and have been recommended as first-line agents. Other drugs that have been successfully used to treat CRPS are anticonvulsants (eg, gabapentin, pregabalin, carbamazepine, and topiramate), local anesthetics such as lidocaine and mexiletine, calcitonin, corticosteroids, bisphosphonates, and low-dose naltrexone. Corticosteroids can be most helpful in the early/acute phase of CRPS (within 1 year of initial injury) to decrease posttraumatic inflammation; however, no optimal dose has been reported. Harmful effects from high doses of corticosteroids include mood swings, sleep disturbances, as well as reduced bone-healing if used too early (within 6-8 weeks post surgery). Bisphosphonates are also likely to decrease CRPS-associated inflammation and are most effective in early/acute phase. The highest efficacy occurs in those with documented osteopenia, as determined by imaging. Patients are advised to limit dental work while on bisphosphonates due to risk of jaw necrosis. Nonsteroidal anti-inflammatory drugs have also been used successfully. Low-dose naltrexone antagonizes the Toll-like receptor 4 (TLR4) of microglial cells involved in pain transmission, leading to an anti-inflammatory effect that might reduce the pain and other symptoms of CRPS.

Giusti A, Bianchi G. Treatment of complex regional pain syndrome type I with bisphosphonates. *RMD Open.* 2015;1:e000056.

Taylor SS, Noor N, Urits I, et al. Complex regional pain syndrome: a comprehensive review. *Pain Ther.* 2021;10:875-892.

B.15. What is the role of intravenous regional block (Bier block) in diagnosis and treatment of CRPS?

Intravenous regional block with guanethidine, reserpine, bretylium, and phentolamine has been used to achieve temporary sympatholytic effect and relieve SMP of CRPS. Intravenous guanethidine and reserpine have been reported to relieve pain in >50% of patients as compared with a control group in one study. However, guanethidine and reserpine are not commercially available in the USA. The combination of bretylium and lidocaine is more effective than lidocaine alone. α-Adrenergic blockade with intravenous phentolamine is a sensitive test to identify patients with SMP. Phentolamine has been used as a predictive agent before more invasive sympathetic blocks.

Blanchard J, Ramamurthy S, Walsh N, et al. Intravenous regional sympatholysis: a double-blind comparison of guanethidine, reserpine, and normal saline. *J Pain Symptom Manage.* 1990;5:357-361.

Hord AH, Rooks MD, Stephens BO, et al. Intravenous regional bretylium and lidocaine for treatment of reflex sympathetic dystrophy: a randomized, double-blind study. *Anesth Analg.* 1992;74:818-821.

Raja SN, Treede RD, Davis KD, et al. Systemic alpha-adrenergic blockade with phentolamine: a diagnostic test for sympathetically maintained pain. *Anesthesiology.* 1991;74:691-698.

B.16. Compare and contrast the mechanisms of action of ketamine and methadone.

Methadone is a long-acting opioid analgesic, whereas ketamine is a dissociative anesthetic. Methadone is used as an opioid but also has mild NMDA receptor antagonist properties, the only strong opioid that has this quality. Ketamine is used in oral preparations, intravenous delivery systems, in skin preparations, and other delivery methods, including being compounded in various percentages. These medications can block NMDA glutamate receptors and decrease the windup pain and central sensitization typical of chronic intractable pain. Windup causes an amplification of the incoming pain signal at the level of second-degree neurons in the dorsal horn of the spinal cord. By blocking these receptors, not only is windup pain decreased but also tolerance to opioid medications can be decreased. Ketamine has the added effect of blocking sodium channels.

Corriger A, Voute M, Lambert C, et al. Ketamine for refractory chronic pain: a 1-year follow-up study. *Pain.* 2022;163:690-701.

Huygen FJPM. Evaluation and treatment of complex regional pain syndrome. In: Benzon H, Rathmell JP, Wu CL, et al, eds. Practical Management of Pain. 6th ed. Mosby; 2023:500-506.

B.17. What roles does ketamine infusion play in the treatment of CRPS? Is there a guideline for ketamine infusion in treating CRPS?

Although ketamine has more than one mechanism of action, the basis for using it to treat CRPS might reside in its ability to block NMDA receptors. Ketamine is the only potent NMDA-blocking drug currently available for clinical use. An appropriately prolonged infusion of ketamine appears to maintain a level of ketamine in the central nervous system long enough to reverse the effects of the sensitization process and associated pain.

Currently, three methods of ketamine administration have been used for treatment: outpatient low-dose ketamine administration; low-dose awake inpatient administration; and a ketamine "coma" technique, which is a controversial treatment not currently allowed in the United States. Although studies are continuing, ketamine therapy can be effective for relief of pain CRPS-I; to date, no adverse cognitive effects of extended ketamine infusion treatment have occurred. Side effects can occur in the high-dose setting; infusion can be associated with significant risks, including chronic catheterization, need for parenteral nutrition, and endotracheal intubation. The outpatient therapy requires the patient to return for a 10-day period and often loses effectiveness after 6 to 12 weeks.

The guideline currently available for ketamine infusion is focused on chronic neuropathic pain. Although there is moderate evidence showing ketamine infusion can provide effective short-term relief of CRPS-I pain, there is no consensus on the role of ketamine infusion in its long-term management.

Cohen SP, Bhatia A, Buvanendran A, et al. Consensus guidelines on the use of intravenous ketamine infusions for chronic pain from the American Society of Regional Anesthesia and Pain Medicine, the American Academy of Pain Medicine, and the American Society of Anesthesiologists. *Reg Anesth Pain Med.* 2018;43:521-546.

Goldberg ME, Torjman MC, Schwartzman RJ, et al. Pharmacodynamic profiles of ketamine (R)- and (S)- with 5-day inpatient infusion for the treatment of complex regional pain syndrome. *Pain Physician.* 2010;13:379-387.

Kiefer RT, Rohr P, Ploppa A, et al. Complete recovery from intractable complex regional pain syndrome, CRPS-type I, following anesthetic ketamine and midazolam. *Pain Pract.* 2007;7:147-150.

Sigtermans MJ, van Hilten JJ, Bauer MC, et al. Ketamine produces effective and long-term pain relief in patients with complex regional pain syndrome type 1. *Pain.* 2009;145:304-311.

Zhao J, Wang Y, Wang D. The effect of ketamine infusion in the treatment of complex regional pain syndrome: a systemic review and meta-analysis. *Curr Pain Headache Rep.* 2018;22:12.

B.18. What is neuromodulation? What is the role of stimulation-based therapies in treating CRPS?

Neuromodulation, according to the International Neuromodulation Society definition, is "the alteration of nerve activity through the delivery of electrical stimulation or chemical agents to targeted sites of the body." Neuromodulatory therapies come in several forms, including, but not limited to, central (spinal cord or dorsal root) stimulation or peripheral nerve stimulation (PNS). Ongoing research shows multiple potential mechanisms of actions for efficacy of electrical stimulation-based therapies from alterations in pain signaling due to the Gate Theory of Pain to neurohormonal changes in cerebrospinal fluid. Randomized controlled studies support the efficacy of spinal cord stimulation (SCS) in treating the pain of CRPS, and SCS has been shown to be superior to conventional medication management. Neurostimulation Appropriateness Consensus Committee (NACC) guidelines suggest use of SCS for treating both CRPS-I and CRPS-II (evidence I, recommend strength A).

While the effectiveness and efficiency of different SCS stimulation modes are being investigated, dorsal root ganglion (DRG) stimulation has also significantly improved management of CRPS and been proven to be noninferior in managing the pain of CRPS, with less paresthesia in undesired body locations. PNS has also been reported to successfully achieve analgesia in patients with CRPS. PNS requires that the injured nerve(s) be known and identifiable for targeted stimulation but offers a smaller and less invasive option for patients.

Deer TR, Krames E, Mekhail N, et al. The appropriate use of neurostimulation: new and evolving neurostimulation therapies and applicable treatment for chronic pain and selected disease states. Neuromodulation Appropriateness Consensus Committee. *Neuromodulation.* 2014;17:599-615.

Deer TR, Mekhail N, Provenzano D, et al. The appropriate use of neurostimulation of the spinal cord and peripheral nervous system for the treatment of chronic pain and ischemic diseases: the Neuromodulation Appropriateness Consensus Committee. *Neuromodulation.* 2014;17:515-550.

Deer TR, Pope JE, Lamer TJ, et al. The neuromodulation appropriateness consensus committee on best practices for dorsal root ganglion stimulation. *Neuromodulation.* 2019;22:1-35.

Herschkowitz D, Kubias J. Wireless peripheral nerve stimulation for complex regional pain syndrome type I of the upper extremity: a case illustration introducing a novel technology. *Scand J Pain.* 2018;18:555-560.

Sokal P, Harat M, Zieliński P, et al. Tibial nerve stimulation with a miniature, wireless stimulator in chronic peripheral neuropathic pain. *J Pain Res.* 2017;10:613-619.

B.19. What is the role of surgical sympathectomy?

Surgical, chemical, or radiofrequency sympathectomy produces short-term pain relief, but long-term results are poor and inconsistent. Delayed failure of sympathectomy can be due to regeneration of ipsilateral nerves or reinnervation from the contralateral sympathetic nerves.

Kumar K, Nath RK, Toth C. Spinal cord stimulation is effective in the management of reflex sympathetic dystrophy. *Neurosurgery.* 1997;40:503-508.

Rocco AG. Radiofrequency lumbar sympatholysis. The evolution of a technique for managing sympathetically maintained pain. *Reg Anesth.* 1995;20:3-12.

B.20. What role does intrathecal (IT) therapy play in managing CRPS?

As a form of neuraxial analgesia, IT therapy bypasses first-pass metabolism and the blood-brain barrier, allowing lower effective doses and decreased systemic adverse effects. It is usually achieved through an IT drug delivery system/device and should be considered only as a salvage approach after failing high doses of systemic opioids. Polyanalgesic Consensus Conference (PACC) guidelines recommend both morphine (evidence level IIIB) and ziconotide (evidence level IA) as first-line IT monotherapy for either cancer- or non-cancer-related chronic pain, including CRPS; however, each medication has specific limitations and thus requires monitoring. PACC guidelines recommend trialing before a permanent device is placed, and that the pros and cons of the therapy must be thoroughly discussed with patients before initiating the treatment.

Deer TR, Pope JE, Hanes MC, et al. Intrathecal therapy for chronic pain: a review of morphine and ziconotide as firstline options. *Pain Med.* 2019;20:784-798.

Deer TR, Pope JE, Hayerk SM, et al. The Polyanalgesic Consensus Conference (PACC): recommendations on intrathecal drug infusion systems best practices and guidelines. *Neuromodulation.* 2017;20:96-132.

B.21. If opioids are prescribed as treatment for patients with CRPS, what is the Centers for Disease Control and Prevention (CDC) guideline on chronic opioid therapy?

In 2016, CDC published a guideline to address the (1) timing, (2) strategies, and (3) risk–benefit assessment of prescribing opioids for chronic pain other than cancer treatment, palliative care, or end-of-life care. Other resources, including checklist, fact sheets, and mobile application, are also available.

CDC guidelines also recommend thoroughly discussing risks and benefits with patients before starting therapy, initiating therapy with immediate-release opioids after considering and trialing nonopioid-based therapies, and reevaluating benefits and harms frequently. Also, offer treatment for opioid use disorder when aberrant behavior of opioid use is perceived.

An update to these guidelines was published by the CDC in 2022, which continues to reinforce judicious use of opioid therapies for chronic nonmalignant pain. These newer guidelines advise clinicians on the importance of weighing the risks and benefits of tapering opioid medications and stresses the importance of avoiding abrupt discontinuation or rapid decreases of chronic opioid medications.

Dowell D, Haegerich TM, Chou R. CDC guideline for prescribing opioids for chronic pain—United States, 2016. *MMWR Recomm Rep.* 2016;65:1-49.

Dowell D, Ragan KR, Jones CM, Baldwin GT, Chou R. CDC clinical practice guideline for prescribing opioids for pain—United States, 2022. *MMWR Recomm Rep.* 2022;71:1-95.

C. Complications

C.1. What are the complications of stellate ganglion block?

Although complications appear infrequently, the more common complications of stellate ganglion block include:

- Intra-arterial injection: seizure and hematoma
- Recurrent laryngeal nerve paralysis: hoarseness
- Brachial plexus block: motor weakness
- Accidental epidural or subarachnoid injection
- Esophageal injury
- Pneumothorax: respiratory distress

To avoid complications, aspiration of the needle should be performed before, during, and after administration of local anesthetics to look for (1) air, (2) blood, and (3) cerebrospinal fluid.

Huygen FJPM. Evaluation and treatment of complex regional pain syndrome. In: Benzon H, Rathmell JP, Wu CL, et al, eds. *Practical Management of Pain.* 6th ed. Mosby; 2023:500-506.

Tsui B, Suresh S. Regional anesthesia in children. In: Gropper MA, Cohen NH, Eriksson LI, et al, eds. *Miller's Anesthesia.* 10th ed. Elsevier; 2025:2354-2410.e8.

C.2. What is the systemic toxicity of local anesthetics?

The toxic systemic effects of local anesthetics are related to drug levels in the blood and are manifested mainly in the central nervous system and the cardiovascular system. The central nervous system effects usually, but not always, precede the cardiovascular toxic manifestations.

Central Nervous System Effects

Central nervous system effects include light-headedness, dizziness, tinnitus, visual disturbances, drowsiness, disorientation, slurred speech, muscle twitching, generalized grand mal seizures, and electroencephalographic changes. Blood levels of local anesthetics associated with central nervous system changes in humans are:

- Procaine: 20 μg/mL
- Lidocaine, mepivacaine, and prilocaine: 5 to 10 μg/mL
- Tetracaine, bupivacaine, and etidocaine: 1.5 to 4 μg/mL
- Lowering the $Paco_2$ by hyperventilation decreases the convulsive threshold dose of local anesthetics.

Cardiovascular Effects

Ventricular arrhythmias are reported with intravenous bupivacaine only. Cardiac resuscitation is extremely difficult in patients with bupivacaine-induced cardiac arrhythmias. Ropivacaine is less toxic than bupivacaine but more toxic than lidocaine. The mechanism of enhanced cardiotoxicity in pregnant patients is not well understood; nevertheless, 0.75% bupivacaine is no longer recommended in pregnant patients (**Table 48.2**).

Huygen FJPM. Evaluation and treatment of complex regional pain syndrome. In: Benzon H, Rathmell JP, Wu CL, et al, eds. *Practical Management of Pain*. 6th ed. Mosby; 2023:500-506.

Tsui B, Suresh S. Regional anesthesia in children. In: Gropper MA, Cohen NH, Eriksson LI, et al, eds. *Miller's Anesthesia*. 10th ed. Elsevier; 2025:2354-2410.e8.

C.3. How do you treat systemic toxicity of local anesthetic drugs?

The principles of treatment for local anesthetic systemic toxicity (LAST) include:

- Secure and maintain the airway.
- Ensure adequate oxygenation and ventilation.
- Treat hypotension and bradycardia promptly.

Current guidelines are available at www.asra.com/news-publications/asra-updates/blog-landing/guidelines/2020/11/01/checklist-for-treatment-of-local-anesthetic-systemic-toxicity.

For patients in cardiac arrest or with severe, refractory arrhythmias, intravenous fat emulsion should be given. The suggested bolus dose is 1.5 mL/kg of 20% fat emulsion (Intralipid) over 1 minute followed by a continuous infusion at 0.25 mL/kg/min. If there is no clinical improvement, the bolus dose should be repeated, and the infusion should be increased to 0.5 mL/kg/min. The infusion should be continued for at least 10 minutes after hemodynamic stability is restored but discontinued within an hour.

- Perform immediate cardiopulmonary resuscitation for profound cardiovascular collapse.
- Perform electrical cardioversion for ventricular tachycardia or fibrillation.
- Control seizures with diazepam, 0.1 to 0.2 mg/kg intravenously

Huygen FJPM. Evaluation and treatment of complex regional pain syndrome. In: Benzon H, Rathmell JP, Wu CL, et al, eds. *Practical Management of Pain*. 6th ed. Mosby; 2023:500-506.

Tsui B, Suresh S. Regional anesthesia in children. In: Gropper MA, Cohen NH, Eriksson LI, et al, eds. *Miller's Anesthesia*. 10th ed. Elsevier; 2025:2354-2410.e8.

TABLE 48.2 Cardiovascular Effects of Lidocaine

Blood Level (μg/mL)	Electrocardiographic Changes	Hemodynamic Effects
<5	—	—
5-10	↑ PR interval ↑ QRS duration Sinus bradycardia	↓ Myocardial contractility ↓ Cardiac output Vasodilation
>10	↑ PR interval ↑ QRS duration Sinus bradycardia Atrioventricular block Asystole	↓ Myocardial contractility ↓ Cardiac output Circulatory collapse

↑, increase; ↓, decrease.

C.4. What are the possible complications of spinal cord stimulation (SCS)?

Epidural SCS is a simple procedure and carries low morbidity. The majority of complications are associated with the implants involving electron fracture or lead migration, which are correctable. Other more serious complications include epidural hematoma, epidural abscess, permanent neurologic deficits, or serious spinal cord injury; however, the risk of these adverse events is less than for spine surgery.

Deer TR, Krames E, Mekhail N, et al. The appropriate use of neurostimulation: new and evolving neurostimulation therapies and applicable treatment for chronic pain and selected disease states. Neuromodulation Appropriateness Consensus Committee. *Neuromodulation*. 2014;17:599-615.

Deer TR, Mekhail N, Provenzano D, et al. The appropriate use of neurostimulation of the spinal cord and peripheral nervous system for the treatment of chronic pain and ischemic diseases: the neuromodulation appropriateness consensus committee. *Neuromodulation*. 2014;17:515-550.

Deer TR, Pope JE, Lamer TJ, et al. The neuromodulation appropriateness consensus committee on best practices for dorsal root ganglion stimulation. *Neuromodulation*. 2019;22:1-35.

C.5. What are the possible complications of IT therapy?

There are five classes of potential intrathecal therapy complications, including mechanical system, pharmacologic, surgical, patient-specific, and refill complications. The severity of the results range from local hygroma to life-threatening anaphylaxis, respiratory depression, or arrest. Ziconotide can cause adverse neuropsychiatric effects and is contraindicated in patients with preexisting history of psychosis or suicidal ideation.

Bottros MM, Christo PJ. Current perspectives on intrathecal drug delivery. *J Pain Res*. 2014;7:615-626.

Deer TR, Pope JE, Hanes MC, et al. Intrathecal therapy for chronic pain: a review of morphine and ziconotide as firstline options. *Pain Med*. 2019;20:784-798.

Acknowledgments

We gratefully acknowledge the contributions of previous edition author(s), Mohammad M. Piracha, Sudhir A. Diwan, and Vinod Malhotra, as portions of those chapters have been retained in this revision.

49 Cancer Pain

Daniel Pak and Philip A. Petrou

A 44-year-old male was referred to the pain clinic for evaluation and management of abdominal pain. He was recently diagnosed with adenocarcinoma of the pancreas with retroperitoneal lymph nodes in the para-aortic region. His pain is localized in the epigastric region, and is worse at night and decreased during the day. He is taking sustained-release morphine sulfate (MS Contin) 100 mg orally every 8 hours and immediate-release morphine sulfate, 30 mg orally every 3 hours as needed for breakthrough pain. The patient reports inadequate pain control, nausea, vomiting, and constipation.

A. Medical Disease and Differential Diagnosis

1. What is the definition of pain?
2. How significant is the problem of pain in patients with cancer?
3. How does the pain contribute to the suffering of patients with cancer?
4. How do psychological factors affect pain in patients with cancer?
5. What are the causes of pain in patients with cancer?
6. What are the characteristics of pancreatic cancer pain?
7. How do you assess pain in patients with cancer?
8. What is the differential diagnosis of abdominal pain?

B. Pharmacologic Treatment of Pain

1. What is the World Health Organization stepladder approach for cancer pain management?
2. What class of drugs does morphine sulfate belong to?
3. What is the difference between morphine and synthetic opioids?
4. How does a mixed opioid agonist/antagonist differ from an opioid agonist?
5. Describe the role of methadone in the management of cancer pain.
6. What are the advantages and disadvantages of methadone?
7. What is the mechanism of action of opioids?
8. What are the side effects of opioid therapy?
9. Define tolerance and physical dependence.
10. How would you treat the side effects of opioid therapy?
11. What is tramadol? Is it an opioid?
12. When would you consider adjuvant analgesics as part of the treatment plan?
13. The patient and his family are worried about addiction. How would you approach this problem?
14. Describe the different routes of opioid administration.
15. Describe advantages and complications of patient-controlled analgesia (PCA). What is the minimum effective analgesic concentration (MEAC)?
16. What is meperidine? How is it different from other opioids?
17. What is opioid rotation? When would you consider rotation of opioids?

C. Invasive Therapy

1. Describe the role of peripheral nerve blocks in cancer pain management.
2. Describe the role of celiac plexus block in cancer pain management.
3. What are the complications of celiac plexus block?
4. Would you consider neuraxial opioid infusion in this patient? Discuss complications of this procedure.

5. Which medications can be used intrathecally? What is ziconotide?
6. What is a Personal Therapy Manager (PTM), and what role does it play in neuraxial pain relief?
7. Would you consider neuraxial neurolysis in this patient to manage his pain? Discuss advantages and disadvantages of these blocks.
8. Which neuroablative procedures can be considered in the terminal stage of pancreatic cancer?
9. Describe the role of radiation therapy in cancer pain.

D. Nonpharmacologic Management

1. What are the various nonpharmacologic techniques of cancer pain management?
2. What physical modalities have been successful in cancer pain management?
3. Describe the role of neuromodulation in cancer pain management.
4. What psychological techniques have been promoted for comfort care and pain relief?
5. What are distraction and reframing techniques? What is the role of hypnosis in cancer pain?

A. Medical Disease and Differential Diagnosis

A.1. What is the definition of pain?

According to the International Association for the Study of Pain, pain is defined as "an unpleasant, sensory and emotional experience associated with actual or potential tissue damage or described in terms of such damage." It is a complex phenomenon that can vary in intensity, duration, and quality. It can deeply impact one's physical abilities and quality of life.

Williams and Craig proposed another definition in light of the new understanding of pain, noting that "pain is a distressing experience associated with actual or potential tissue damage with sensory, emotional, cognitive and social components."

Raja SN, Carr DB, Cohen M, et al. The revised International Association for the Study of Pain definition of pain: concepts, challenges, and compromises. *Pain*. 2020;161:1976-1982.

Williams AC, Craig KD. Updating the definition of pain. *Pain*. 2016;157:2420-2423.

A.2. How significant is the problem of pain in patients with cancer?

An estimated 1.9 million new cases of cancer were diagnosed in 2022 with roughly 600,000 deaths, making it the second leading cause of death in the United States. Thirty percent of patients with cancer have pain at the time of diagnosis, 65% to 85% of patients with cancer have pain at advanced stages, and 36% have pain severe enough to impair their ability to function.

Van den Beuken-van Everdingen and colleagues demonstrated in a pooled meta-analysis of 52 studies that the prevalence of pain was more than 50% in all cancer types, with the highest prevalence in patients with head and neck cancer at 70%. Furthermore, more than one-third of all cancer patients graded their pain as moderate or severe.

Daut and Cleeland found pain to be an early symptom of cancer in 48% to 50% of patients with cancer of the breasts, ovary, prostate, colon, and rectum and in 20% of patients with uterine and cervical cancer.

American Cancer Society, Inc. Cancer facts & figures 2023. 2022. Accessed January 15, 2025. https://www.cancer.org/research/cancer-facts-statistics/all-cancer-facts-figures/2023-cancer-facts-figures.html

Bruera E, Kim HN. Cancer pain. *JAMA*. 2003;290:2476-2479.

Daut RL, Cleeland CS. The prevalence and severity of pain in cancer. *Cancer*. 1982;50:1913-1918.

van den Beuken-van Everdingen M, de Rijke J, Kessels A, et al. Prevalence of pain in patients with cancer: a systematic review of the past 40 years. *Ann Oncol*. 2007;18:1437-1449.

A.3. How does the pain contribute to the suffering of patients with cancer?

Pain can have many downstream effects that contribute to the suffering of patients with cancer. Pain can cause physical limitations in those with cancer, reducing the ability to perform activities of daily living independently and impacting quality of life. Patients with cancer also often identify pain as an indicator of disease progression.

Patients worry about the social impact of their disease, particularly if they are concerned about the burden it might have on their loved ones. Pain can contribute to feelings of anxiety, depression, and helplessness as patients have difficulty engaging in activities that they previously enjoyed or maintaining social connections. Spiritually, pain can also impact one's own sense of meaning and purpose, leading to existential distress.

Tang ST, Chang WC, Chen JS, Su YC, Hsieh CH, Wen FH. The impact of pain on the quality of life and the unmet needs of cancer patients: a qualitative study. *J Pain Symptom Manage*. 2015;50:368-378.

A.4. How do psychological factors affect pain in patients with cancer?

Pain and psychological well-being impact each other bidirectionally. Chronic pain has been associated with anxiety, depression, and other mood disorders. Twenty-five percent of patients with cancer meet criteria for major depressive syndromes at some point in their illness, with an overall prevalence of 53% in hospitalized patients with cancer. Other downstream effects of chronic pain include irritability, sleep disorders, slowness in motor response, and an overall sense of hopelessness. Moreover, preexisting psychological factors such as stress and anxiety can increase muscle tension and affect pain regulation, thereby increasing the perception of pain intensity and duration. A recent meta-analysis demonstrated that depression predicts mortality, but not progression, in patients with cancer.

Hagen NA. Epidemiology, prevalence, and cancer pain syndromes. In: Ballantyne JH, Fishman SM, Rathmell JPC, eds. *Bonica's Management of Pain*. 5th ed. Wolters Kluwer; 2019:599-620.

Satin JR, Linden W, Phillips MJ. Depression as a predictor of disease progression and mortality in cancer patients: a meta-analysis. *Cancer*. 2009;115:5349-5361.

Speigel D, Giese-Davis J. Depression and cancer: mechanisms and disease progression. *Biol Psychiatry*. 2003;54:269-282.

A.5. What are the causes of pain in patients with cancer?

Pain in patients with cancer can be due to:

- Presence and progression of the tumor itself. For example, bone involvement, viscus obstruction, and nerve compression
- Indirect effect of the tumor. For example, metabolic imbalance, infection, and venous/lymphatic obstruction
- Consequence of cancer treatment, such as chemotherapy, radiation therapy, or surgery

Grond and colleagues found in a prospective study of 2,266 patients with cancer that 30% had one pain syndrome, 39% had two pain syndromes, 31% had three pain syndromes, 85% due to the cancer itself (bone, 35%; soft tissue, 45%; and visceral, 34%), and 17% due to cancer treatment.

Grond S, Zech D, Diefenbach C, et al. Assessment of cancer pain: a prospective evaluation in 2266 cancer patients referred to a pain service. *Pain*. 1996;64:107-114.

Hagen NA. Epidemiology, prevalence, and cancer pain syndromes. In: Ballantyne JH, Fishman SM, Rathmell JPC, eds. *Bonica's Management of Pain*. 5th ed. Wolters Kluwer; 2019:599-620.

Mantyh PW. Bone cancer pain: from mechanism to therapy. *Curr Opin Support Palliat Care*. 2014;8:83-90.

A.6. What are the characteristics of pancreatic cancer pain?

Pancreatic cancer affects roughly 12 patients per 100,000 in the Western world. In 2023, an estimated 64,000 new cases of pancreatic cancer were projected in the United States. If the cancer is detected at an early stage, when surgical removal is possible, the 5-year survival rate is 37.4%. Roughly 10% of people are diagnosed at this stage. If the cancer has spread to surrounding tissues or organs, the 5-year survival rate is 12%. For the 53% of people who are diagnosed after the cancer has spread to a distant part of the body, the 5-year survival rate is 3%.

About 30% to 60% of patients present with pain, and 80% of patients with advanced cancer report pain. Patients typically complain of diffuse epigastric pain radiating to the back that is increased with lying down and improved with sitting. About 90% of pancreatic tumors are adenocarcinoma. Cancer in the head of the pancreas usually invades the stomach, duodenum, gall bladder, and peritoneum, whereas tumors in the pancreatic body spread to the liver, spleen, lymph nodes, and adrenal glands.

American Cancer Society, Inc. Cancer facts & figures 2023. 2022. Accessed January 15, 2025. https://www.cancer.org/research/cancer-facts-statistics/all-cancer-facts-figures/2023-cancer-facts-figures.html

Howlader N, Noone AM, Krapcho M, et al, eds. *SEER Cancer Statistics Review*, 1975-2018. National Cancer Institute; Bethesda, MD. Based on November 2020 SEER data submission. Posted to the SEER website April 2021. https://seer.cancer.gov/csr/1975_2018

Siegel RL, Miller KD, Jemal A. Cancer statistics, 2019. *CA Cancer J Clin*. 2019;69:7-34.

A.7. How do you assess pain in patients with cancer?

A stepwise approach is required for the assessment of pain. It includes history, physical examination, and review of diagnostic imaging. Assessment involves identifying features of pain, such as location, intensity, quality, timing, exacerbating/relieving factors, response to previous analgesics, and disease-modifying treatments; effects of pain on daily activities and psychological state; associated symptoms; prognosis and goals of care.

Hagen NA. Epidemiology, prevalence, and cancer pain syndromes. In: Ballantyne JH, Fishman SM, Rathmell JPC, eds. *Bonica's Management of Pain.* 5th ed. Wolters Kluwer; 2019:599-620.

A.8. What is the differential diagnosis of abdominal pain?

Although abdominal pain can arise from different structures within the peritoneal cavity, the retroperitoneal organs can cause similar pain syndromes. Location and radiation of the pain can give important clues to make the diagnosis. Retroperitoneal structures present with dull or sharp back pain that is increased on lying down and relieved with sitting. Abdominal tumors are frequently characterized by colicky pain associated with nausea that is worse after eating. Abdominal pain can be referred to distant areas like shoulder, neck, or back depending on the organ involved. Tumors of the small bowel or large bowel can present with symptoms of obstruction (eg, abdominal distention, nausea, and bilious vomiting), hematemesis, or melena. Other common causes of abdominal pain include omental metastasis, volvulus of the intestine, infectious peritonitis, radiation enteritis, and peritoneal carcinomatosis. Mesenteric ischemia presents with diffuse pain that is increased with meals and weight loss.

Nonmalignant causes of abdominal pain such as appendicitis, cholecystitis, and pancreatitis can occur in patients with cancer coincidentally, which can complicate the diagnostic process.

Hagen NA. Epidemiology, prevalence, and cancer pain syndromes. In: Ballantyne JH, Fishman SM, Rathmell JPC, eds. *Bonica's Management of Pain.* 5th ed. Wolters Kluwer; 2019:599-620.

B. Pharmacologic Treatment of Pain

B.1. What is the World Health Organization stepladder approach for cancer pain management?

The World Health Organization advocated a stepladder approach to manage cancer pain exclusively with oral medications depending on the pain intensity and, to some extent, the pain mechanism (**Figure 49.1**).

- Step 1. Manage the pain by nonopioid medications with or without adjuvants.
- Step 2. If pain is persisting or increasing, add weak opioids to nonopioid analgesics and adjuvants.

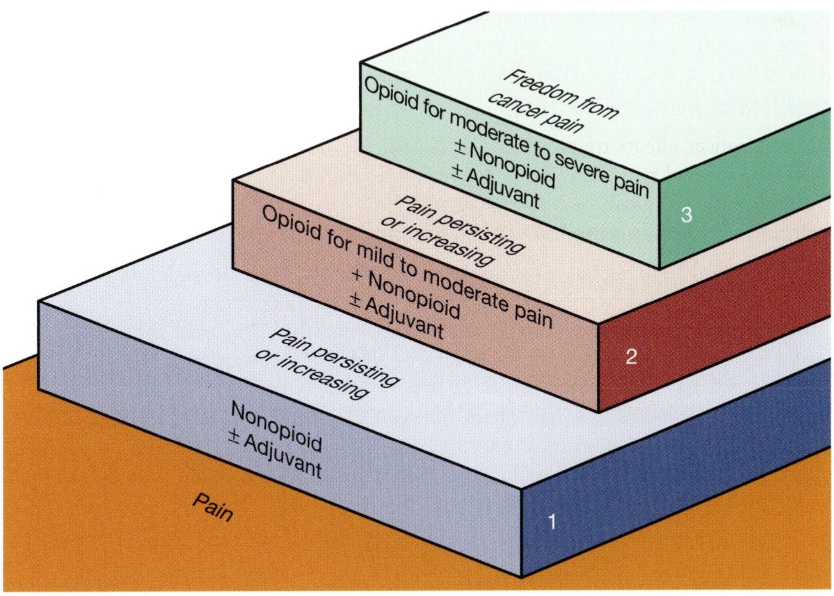

FIGURE 49.1. World Health Organization—advocated stepladder approach to management of cancer pain.

SECTION 11

- Step 3. Strong opioids are used with nonopioid analgesics and adjuvants until the patient achieves complete analgesia.

Noninvasive routes of drug delivery should be maintained as long as possible because of its simplicity, convenience, and cost. A fourth step has been added for patients who still have significant pain despite maximum medical management. At this point, interventional procedures including neuromodulation, drug delivery systems, and/or neurolysis should be employed.

Cuomo A, Bimonte S, Forte CA, et al. Multimodal approaches and tailored therapies for pain management: the trolley analgesic model. *J Pain Res.* 2019;12:711-714.

van den Beuken-van Everdingen MH, Hochstenbach LM, Joosten EA, et al. Update on prevalence of pain in patients with cancer: systematic review and meta-analysis. *J Pain Symptom Manage.* 2016;51:1070-1090.

B.2. What class of drugs does morphine sulfate belong to?

Morphine is classified as a μ-opioid receptor (MOR) agonist because of its high specificity for activation of μ-opioid receptors. An ideal opioid agonist would have a high specificity for receptors producing desirable effects (analgesia) and minimal or no specificity for other receptors that cause side effects.

Murphy PB, Patel P, Barrett MJ. Morphine. In: *StatPearls.* StatPearls Publishing; 2025. https://www.ncbi.nlm.nih.gov/books/NBK526115/

B.3. What is the difference between morphine and synthetic opioids?

Morphine is the principal phenanthrene alkaloid present in opium. It is highly ionized and water soluble. The most active molecule of morphine is the levorotatory isomer. The synthetic opioids contain the phenanthrene nucleus of morphine and are manufactured by synthesis, rather than chemical modification. Clinically, histamine release by morphine differentiates it from the synthetic opioids. This can cause histamine-induced urticaria, allergic reactions, and hemodynamic instability, particularly in patients with depleted volume.

Hagen NA. Epidemiology, prevalence, and cancer pain syndromes. In: Ballantyne JH, Fishman SM, Rathmell JPC, eds. *Bonica's Management of Pain.* 5th ed. Wolters Kluwer; 2019:599-620.

B.4. How does a mixed opioid agonist/antagonist differ from an opioid agonist?

The mixed-action opioids bind to μ-opioid receptors as partial agonists or competitive antagonists. Antagonistic properties of these drugs can attenuate the efficacy of subsequently administered opioid agonists and cause withdrawal symptoms in patients already receiving full opioid agonists. The advantages of these drugs include low potential for respiratory depression and physical dependence. Their use is limited because of a ceiling effect, whereby progressive escalation in dose does not increase analgesia as with pure opioid agonists.

Webster L, Gudin J, Raffa RB, et al. Understanding buprenorphine for use in chronic pain: expert opinion. *Pain Med.* 2020;21:714-723.

B.5. Describe the role of methadone in the management of cancer pain.

The efficient oral and rectal absorption with prolonged duration of analgesic action of methadone makes it a highly effective and attractive drug for cancer pain management.

Methadone is a synthetic opioid with a unique agonist/antagonist action. Methadone is a μ-opioid receptor agonist and an *N*-methyl-D-aspartate (NMDA) receptor antagonist. Activation of NMDA receptors is involved in the development of hypersensitivity and central sensitization in neuropathic pain and tolerance to opioids. Because of the antagonistic effect at the NMDA receptor site, methadone is effective in neuropathic pain secondary to cancer-related pathology and therapeutic interventions. The same antagonistic action of methadone minimizes the development of tolerance to opioids.

Chou R, Cruciani RA, Fiellin DA, et al. Methadone safety: a clinical practice guideline from the American Pain Society and College on Problems of Drug Dependence, in collaboration with the Heart Rhythm Society. *J Pain.* 2014;15:321-337.

Mercadante S, Bruera E. Methadone as a first-line opioid in cancer pain management: a systematic review. *J Pain Symptom Manage.* 2018;55:998-1003.

Nicholson AB, Watson GR, Derry S, et al. Methadone for cancer pain. *Cochrane Database Syst Rev.* 2017;2:CD003971.

B.6. What are the advantages and disadvantages of methadone?

Methadone has several advantages, including oral and rectal absorption with bioavailability to 95%, high potency, high lipid solubility, low cost, and no active metabolites. Methadone has a long half-life, and its analgesic effect lasts 6 to 8 hours. Because methadone has been used for patients with opioid use disorder as treatment for detoxification and maintenance, it carries a social stigma, which can interfere with adequate pain management. Methadone has an irregular elimination half-life with interindividual variation between 20 and 60 hours. The cumulative effect of methadone causes sedation, makes titration difficult, and has led to the concept of individualization of methadone dosing.

Glue P, Cape G, Tunnicliff D, et al. Switching opioid-dependent patients from methadone to morphine: safety, tolerability, and methadone pharmacokinetics. *J Clin Pharmacol.* 2016;56:960-965.

Fitzgibbon D. Cancer pain: principles of management and pharmacotherapy. In: Ballantyne JH, Fishman SM, Rathmell JPC, eds. *Bonica's Management of Pain.* 5th ed. Wolters Kluwer; 2019:676-710.

Mercadante S, Bruera E. Methadone as a first-line opioid in cancer pain management: a systematic review. *J Pain Symptom Manage.* 2018;55:998-1003. doi:10.1016/j.jpainsymman.2017.10.017

B.7. What is the mechanism of action of opioids?

Opioids act as agonists at stereoselective opioid receptors that are normally activated by endogenous ligands known as endorphins in the brainstem and spinal cord. Binding of opioids to the receptor inhibits adenylyl cyclase activity and causes hyperpolarization of neurons, which results in suppression of spontaneous discharge and evoked potential. Opioids also interfere with transmembrane transport of calcium ions and with the release of neurotransmitters such as acetylcholine, dopamine, norepinephrine, and substance P.

Che T, Roth BL. Molecular basis of opioid receptor signaling. *Cell.* 2023;186:5203-5219.

Inturrisi CE, Craig DS, Lipman AG. Opioid analgesics. In: Ballantyne JH, Fishman SM, Rathmell JPC, eds. *Bonica's Management of Pain.* 5th ed. Wolters Kluwer; 2019:1333-1351.

B.8. What are the side effects of opioid therapy?

Sedation and respiratory depression, like analgesia, are mediated by μ-opioid receptor activation. Tolerance to these side effects is developed within a very short period of treatment. The dysphoric reaction is due to activation of κ-opioid receptors. Psychotomimetic and depersonalization reactions are due to activation of σ-opioid receptors. Nausea and vomiting are caused by direct stimulation of the chemoreceptor trigger zone (CTZ). Increased intrabiliary pressure is due to spasm of the sphincter of Oddi. Other side effects commonly observed are constipation, pruritus, and myoclonus. Almost all side effects diminish with time, except constipation and myoclonus. Patients with cancer who develop constipation secondary to opioid therapy are advised to be on a regular bowel regimen to avoid subsequent serious consequences. In patients with compromised renal function, metabolites of morphine (M3G, M6G) cause excessive sedation, and metabolites of meperidine (normeperidine) lower the seizure threshold. The most commonly reported adverse events in the MERITO clinical trial of the analgesic effect and tolerability of oral morphine in patients with cancer were somnolence (24% of patients), constipation (22%), vomiting (13%), nausea (10%), and confusion (7%).

De Conno F, Ripamonti C, Fagnoni E, et al; MERITO Study Group. The MERITO study: a multicentre trial of the analgesic effect and tolerability of normal-release oral morphine during 'titration phase' in patients with cancer pain. *Palliat Med.* 2008;22:214-221.

Fukuda K. Opioids. In: Gropper MA, Cohen NH, Eriksson LI, et al, eds. *Miller's Anesthesia.* 10th ed. Elsevier; 2025:555-622.e14.

B.9. Define tolerance and physical dependence.

Tolerance occurs with the development of the need to gradually escalate the dose to achieve equivalent pain control and can be seen in as early as 2 to 3 weeks following medication administration. Tolerance does not indicate abuse or addiction, but it is commonly associated with increasing pain or disease progression. Physical dependence develops after chronic use of opioids; it is characterized by the development of a withdrawal syndrome after administration of an opioid antagonist or abrupt discontinuation of the medication. The potential for tolerance is an effect of opioid agonists.

Canfield MC, Keller CE, Frydrych LM, et al. Prescription opioid use among patients seeking treatment for opioid dependence. *J Addict Med.* 2010; 4:108-113.

Inturrisi CE, Craig DS, Lipman AG. Opioid analgesics. In: Ballantyne JH, Fishman SM, Rathmell JPC, eds. *Bonica's Management of Pain.* 5th ed. Wolters Kluwer; 2019:1333-1351.

B.10. How would you treat the side effects of opioid therapy?

Oversedation and respiratory depression are treated with a specific μ-opioid receptor antagonist, naloxone, as well as supplemental oxygen. Naloxone, in a 1 to 4 μg/kg intravenous bolus, promptly reverses sedation, respiratory depression, and analgesia. Continuous intravenous infusion at 2 to 4 μg/kg/h reverses side effects without reversing analgesia. Nausea and vomiting should be managed by antiemetics. Constipation should be treated with a regular bowel regimen of laxatives and stool softener. Peripherally acting μ-opioid receptor antagonists (PAMORA; methylnaltrexone, naloxegol, naldemedine) and a chloride channel activator (lubiprostone) improve opioid-induced bowel dysfunction without reversing analgesia. Generalized pruritus can respond to one or more doses of an antihistamine; however, pruritus might not be related to histamine release.

De Conno F, Ripamonti C, Fagnoni E, et al. The MERITO Study: a multicentre trial of the analgesic effect and tolerability of normal-release oral morphine during 'titration phase' in patients with cancer pain. *Palliat Med.* 2008;22:214-221.

Slatkin N, Thomas J, Lipman AG, et al. Methylnaltrexone for treatment of opioid-induced constipation in advanced illness patients. *J Support Oncol.* 2009;7:39-46.

Viscusi ER. Clinical overview and considerations for the management of opioid-induced constipation in patients with chronic noncancer pain. *Clin J Pain.* 2019;35:174-188.

Wiffen PJ, Wee B, Derry S, et al. Opioids for cancer pain—an overview of Cochrane reviews. *Cochrane Database Syst Rev.* 2017;7:CD012592.

B.11. What is tramadol? Is it an opioid?

Tramadol (Ultram) is a nonopioid synthetic analgesic with weak μ-opioid receptor agonist activity. Its analgesic effects also involve inhibition of norepinephrine and serotonin reuptake. It should be started at 50 to 100 mg every 6 to 8 hours. It can exhibit μ-opioid receptor–related clinical side effects such as respiratory depression and constipation. Prolonged use can lead to physical and psychological dependence. Tramadol was made Drug Enforcement Administration schedule IV effective 2014.

Tapentadol is a centrally acting pain reliever, with agonist activity at the μ-opioid receptor and inhibition of norepinephrine reuptake. Compared to oxycodone IR, tapentadol has reduced gastrointestinal side effects, specifically nausea, constipation, and vomiting. Tapentadol should be administered first in the 50-mg strength and can be increased to 100 mg every 4 to 6 hours as needed. It can also cause respiratory depression due to its μ-opioid agonist activity.

Both tramadol and tapentadol can cause life-threatening serotonin syndrome with the use of other serotonin-norepinephrine reuptake inhibitors, selective serotonin reuptake inhibitors, tricyclic antidepressants, or monoamine oxidase inhibitors. They should be used with caution in patients on these medications.

There is limited evidence from randomized controlled trials that demonstrates efficacy of tramadol for adults with cancer pain and no evidence for children.

Drug Enforcement Administration, U.S. Department of Justice. Schedule of controlled substances: placement of tramadol into schedule IV. Final rule. *Fed Regist.* 2014;79:37623-37630.

Grond S, Sablotzki A. Clinical pharmacology of tramadol. *Clin Pharmacokinet.* 2004;43:879-923.

Jutkiewicz EM, Traynor JR. Opioid analgesics. In: Brunton LL, Knollmann BC, eds. *Goodman & Gilman's: The Pharmacological Basis of Therapeutics.* 14th ed. McGraw-Hill Education; 2023:443-470.

B.12. When would you consider adjuvant analgesics as part of the treatment plan?

In cancer pain management, adjuvant agents are considered to enhance pain relief. The adjuvant analgesics are a heterogeneous group of medications originally developed for purposes other than pain relief. These drugs are useful in a multimodal approach to treat pain and for concomitant psychological disturbances such as insomnia, anxiety, depression, and psychosis. The most useful adjuvants used clinically to manage cancer pain are:

- Corticosteroids
- Tricyclic antidepressants (eg, amitriptyline)
- Anticonvulsants (eg, gabapentin)
- Amphetamines
- NMDA receptor antagonists (eg, methadone, ketamine)
- α_2-Adrenergic receptor agonists (eg, clonidine)
- Antihistamines
- Phenothiazines

Haywood A, Good P, Khan S, et al. Corticosteroids for the management of cancer-related pain in adults. *Cochrane Database Syst Rev.* 2015:CD010756.

Inturrisi CE, Craig DS, Lipman AG. Opioid analgesics. In: Ballantyne JH, Fishman SM, Rathmell JPC, eds. *Bonica's Management of Pain.* 5th ed. Wolters Kluwer; 2019:1333-1351.

Oosterling A, te Boveldt N, Verhagen C, et al. Neuropathic pain components in patients with cancer: prevalence, treatment, and interference with daily activities. *Pain Pract.* 2016;16:413-421.

B.13. The patient and his family are worried about addiction. How would you approach this problem?

It can be difficult to differentiate between drug abuse and the deterioration in physical or psychosocial functioning caused by the disease and its treatment. For example, questionable drug-related behaviors might be difficult to recognize in a patient who develops social withdrawal or cognitive changes following brain irradiation for metastases.

Addiction is defined as a persistent pattern of dysfunctional use of opioids that can involve adverse consequences associated with continued use, loss of control over use, compulsive use, craving for the drug, and typical drug-seeking behavior. Patients with chronic pain who are using opioids are not at higher risk of addiction than the general population. The goals of treatment, including palliation of pain and improvement in quality of life, must be clearly defined and explained to the patient and his relatives. At no time should patients with cancer pain be undertreated because of the fear of addiction. The patient and his family should be educated about the common misconception that addiction is a common outcome of opioid therapy.

Opioid analgesic therapy must be tailored to monitor all patients in order to minimize misuse and abuse, as every patient is at some degree of risk for opioid misuse. This is affected by the disease progression, tolerance, changes in pain quality, mental health, comorbidities, other drug therapies, and changes in the patient's lifestyle.

Benyamin R, Trescot AM, Datta S, et al. Opioid complications and side effects. *Pain Physician.* 2008;11:S105-S120.

Byker GL, Leskuski D. Nonpharmacological management of pain. In: Berger A, Shuster J, Von Roenn J, eds. *Principles and Practice of Palliative Care and Supportive Oncology.* 4th ed. Lippincott Williams & Wilkins; 2014:42-54.

Pergolizzi JV, Gharibo C, Passik S, et al. Dynamic risk factors in the misuse of opioid analgesics. *J Psychosom Res.* 2012;72:443-451.

B.14. Describe the different routes of opioid administration.

Oral medications should be used as the first-line approach in most patients with cancer pain who are receiving opioid analgesics. **Table 49.1** outlines the routes of opioid administration and available opioid preparations.

The rectal or transdermal route should be chosen before considering invasive therapy for cancer pain. The sublingual route is limited by the inability to deliver large doses. The intramuscular route is not preferred for long-term administration because it requires repeated painful injections and offers no pharmacodynamic advantages. Intravenous administration provides quick onset and is ideal for painful crises in patients with cancer as patient-controlled analgesia (PCA). The equianalgesic doses of opioids used orally and parenterally are listed in **Table 49.2**.

Caraceni A, Hanks G, Kaasa S, et al. Use of opioid analgesics in the treatment of cancer pain: evidence-based recommendations from the EAPC. *Lancet Oncol.* 2012;13:e58-e68.

Jutkiewicz EM, Traynor JR. Opioid analgesics. In: Brunton LL, Knollmann BC, eds. *Goodman & Gilman's: The Pharmacological Basis of Therapeutics.* 14th ed. McGraw-Hill Education; 2023:443-470.

TABLE 49.1 Routes of Opioid Administration

Route of Administration	Available Opioid Preparation
Oral	Morphine Hydromorphone (Dilaudid) Methadone (Dolophine) Oxycodone, hydrocodone Codeine, meperidine Levorphanol
Rectal	Suppositories containing morphine, hydromorphone, oxycodone
Transdermal	Fentanyl patch
Sublingual	Fentanyl, methadone, buprenorphine
Intramuscular/subcutaneous	Morphine, hydromorphone, methadone Meperidine, levorphanol
Intravenous	Morphine, meperidine, methadone, fentanyl Hydromorphone, oxymorphone
Epidural/intrathecal	Morphine, methadone, hydromorphone Fentanyl, sufentanil, meperidine

Knotkova H, Fine PG, Portenoy RK. Opioid rotation: the science and the limitations of the equianalgesic dose table. *J Pain Symptom Manage*. 2009;38:426-439.

Mercadante S. The patient with difficult cancer pain. *Cancers (Basel)*. 2019;11:E565.

B.15. Describe advantages and complications of patient-controlled analgesia (PCA). What is the minimum effective analgesic concentration (MEAC)?

Intravenous PCA is advantageous because it allows patients to self-administer medication and find their personal comfort zone between side effects and pain control within limits set by the providers. The PCA device is a programmable portable pump with the capability of storage and retrieval of data by a microprocessor. The pump is programmed for three modes of drug delivery: (1) continuous rate infusion only, which is preset by the physician; (2) continuous infusion with boluses for breakthrough pain, boluses controlled by the patient; and (3) boluses with lockout time in minutes set by the physician and that the patient can control. If required, the physician or nurse can deliver extra boluses. Intermittent rescue doses for breakthrough pain, along with continuous infusion, decrease the total requirement of opioids. However, continuous-delivery mode carries risks of oversedation and respiratory depression. PCA can also be provided by subcutaneous, epidural, or intrathecal routes.

Functional impairment of excretory organs is common in the older people; thus, the half-life of the active drug and metabolites is increased in the older people and in patients with renal dysfunction, except

TABLE 49.2 Opioids Used Orally or Parenterally to Treat Cancer Pain

	Equianalgesic Dose (mg)[a]	
Drug	**Oral**	**Parental**
Morphine	30	10
Hydromorphone	6	2
Oxycodone	20-30	NA
Methadone	10[b]	10[b]
Levorphanol	2-3[b]	2[b]
Codeine	130[c]	75

NA, not available in the United States.
[a]Suggested doses are guidelines only. Doses are based on chronic opioid use.
[b]Particular care with titration is recommended because doses might need to be reduced significantly when steady-state levels are reached after 2 to 3 days.
[c]Codeine doses greater than 65 mg may be associated with significant constipation.

for buprenorphine. Therefore, doses should be reduced and a longer time interval between doses. Creatinine clearance should be monitored.

MEAC is the lower limit of the therapeutic window.

Alarcón MDL, Estévez FV, Cabezón-Gutiérrez L, et al. Expert consensus on the management of breakthrough cancer pain in older patients. A Delphi study. *J Geriatr Oncol.* 2019;10:643-652.

Fitzgibbons D. Assessment and diagnosis of the cancer patient with pain. In: Ballantyne JH, Fishman SM, Rathmell JPC, eds. *Bonica's Management of Pain.* 5th ed. Wolters Kluwer; 2019:621-675.

Jutkiewicz EM, Traynor JR. Opioid analgesics. In: Brunton LL, Knollmann BC, eds. *Goodman & Gilman's: The Pharmacological Basis of Therapeutics.* 14th ed. McGraw-Hill Education; 2023:443-470.

Mercadante S. The patient with difficult cancer pain. *Cancers (Basel).* 2019;11:E565.

B.16. What is meperidine? How is it different from other opioids?

Meperidine is a synthetic opioid that pharmacologically resembles morphine. Meperidine is not an ideal drug for chronic pain because of its short duration of action and its high potential for abuse. The by-product, normeperidine, is excreted exclusively by the renal system with an elimination half-life of 36 to 40 hours. In patients with compromised renal function, metabolite accumulation has been associated with central nervous system toxicity, including myoclonus, tremulousness, hallucinations, and seizures. Meperidine possesses anticholinergic activity similar to atropine, causing mydriasis, orthostatic hypotension, and tachycardia. Compared with other opioids, meperidine rarely causes pruritus when given neuraxially. It is effective in the treatment of postoperative shivering. Meperidine also demonstrates local anesthetic actions. It is contraindicated in patients who are receiving monoamine oxidase inhibitors because of the risk of serotonin syndrome.

Jutkiewicz EM, Traynor JR. Opioid analgesics. In: Brunton LL, Knollmann BC, eds. *Goodman & Gilman's: The Pharmacological Basis of Therapeutics*. 14th ed. McGraw-Hill Education; 2023:443-470.

B.17. What is opioid rotation? When would you consider rotation of opioids?

The sequential trial of changing one opioid to another when either treatment-limiting toxicity or poor responsiveness develops has become known as *opioid rotation*. The variable response from opioid to opioid in an individual has led to this approach; changing to an alternative opioid can yield a better balance between side effects and analgesia.

For those patients who experience inadequate pain control and who have intolerable side effects, different strategies are implemented to improve analgesia. Opioid rotation is a simple strategy that almost all physicians can implement. Depending on equianalgesic potency ratio guidelines, a switch is made to other opioids such as methadone or transdermal fentanyl patch. This should be done under close supervision and preferably in an inpatient environment.

Afsharimani B, Kindl K, Good P, et al. Pharmacological options for the management of refractory cancer pain-what is the evidence? *Support Care Cancer*. 2015;23:1473-1481.

Caraceni A, Hanks G, Kaasa S, et al. Use of opioid analgesics in the treatment of cancer pain: evidence-based recommendations from the EAPC. *Lancet Oncol*. 2012;13:e58-e68.

Fitzgibbons D. Assessment and diagnosis of the cancer patient with pain. In: Ballantyne JH, Fishman SM, Rathmell JPC, eds. *Bonica's Management of Pain*. 5th ed. Wolters Kluwer; 2019:621-675.

Kotlinska-Lemieszek A. Rotation, partial rotation (semi-switch), combining opioids, and titration. Does "opioid plus opioid" strategy make a step forward on our way to improving the outcome of pain treatment? *J Pain Symptom Manage*. 2010;40:e10-e12.

C. Invasive Therapy

C.1. Describe the role of peripheral nerve blocks in cancer pain management.

Many patients experience inadequate pain control despite more conservative treatments such as medication management. Interventional techniques can significantly reduce the level of pain, allowing for a significant decrease in analgesic requirements. Common peripheral nerve blocks that can be considered depending on the location of thoracic or abdominal pain and the involvement of viscera are:

Upper abdomen, thorax:

- Intercostal nerve blocks
- Splanchnic nerve blocks

- Celiac plexus block
- Paravertebral blocks

Lower abdomen, pelvis:

- Superior hypogastric plexus block
- Ganglion impar block
- Pudendal nerve block
- Paravertebral blocks

Peripheral nerve blocks are performed at anatomic sites away from the central neuraxis. More distal blocks have greater chances of incomplete analgesia due to spatial distribution, overlap of nerve innervation, and difficulty in blocking multiple branches of arborizing nerves.

Patients who receive only short-term benefit from nerve blocks can be considered for chemical (phenol or alcohol) or thermal neurolysis (cyro-ablation).

Swarm RA, Abernethy AP, Anghelescu DL, et al. Adult cancer pain. *J Natl Compr Canc Netw*. 2013;11:992-1022.

Thapa D, Rastogi V, Ahuja V. Cancer pain management-current status. *J Anaesthesiol Clin Pharmacol*. 2011;27:162-168.

Waldman SD. Celiac plexus block: single-needle retrocrural technique. In: Waldman SD, ed. *Atlas of Interventional Pain Management*. 5th ed. Elsevier; 2020:451.

C.2. Describe the role of celiac plexus block in cancer pain management.

Diagnostic celiac plexus block with a local anesthetic is performed to differentiate sympathetically mediated abdominal pain and localize retroperitoneal or upper abdominal pain. A positive result of the diagnostic block is an indication for more definitive neurolysis in chronic cancer pain. Success rates of celiac plexus neurolysis are lower in patients suffering from chronic nonmalignant abdominal pain compared to those suffering from abdominal pain due to neoplasms.

Neurolysis with alcohol or phenol is commonly performed under fluoroscopic guidance or computed tomography (CT) guidance using the following approaches: single- or two-needle periaortic technique, single-needle transaortic technique, single-needle anterior technique, or endoscopic ultrasound (EUS)–guided technique. Individual skills of the treating physician, available facilities, patient condition, and extent of disease should be considered in determining the best technique to use. CT guidance typically provides superior visibility of tumor, lymph nodes, and the celiac plexus.

Celiac plexus neurolysis commonly necessitates up to 40 mL of 50% to 70% alcohol or 6% to 10% phenol. Smaller volumes are recommended for absolute alcohol and higher concentrations of phenol. Neurolysis with phenol is generally less painful because of its local anesthetic action, whereas alcohol neurolysis should be pretreated with a local anesthetic.

A meta-analysis of celiac plexus neurolysis for abdominal pain associated with unresectable pancreatic cancer demonstrated its efficacy for managing abdominal pain at 4 weeks post procedure compared to conventional medication management. While there are limitations associated with neurolytic procedures, they can be considered in patients who have had minimal benefit with medications alone.

Okita M, Otani K, Gibo N, Matsui S. Systematic review and meta-analysis of celiac plexus neurolysis for abdominal pain associated with unresectable pancreatic cancer. *Pain Pract*. 2022;22:652-661.

Rosland JH, Geitung JT. CT guided neurolytic blockade of the coeliac plexus in patients with advanced and intractably painful pancreatic cancer. *Scand J Pain*. 2018;18:247-251.

Waldman SD. Celiac plexus block: single-needle retrocrural technique. In: Waldman SD, ed. *Atlas of Interventional Pain Management*. 5th ed. Elsevier; 2020:451.

Wong GY, Carns PE, de Leon-Casasola OA. Neurolytic celiac plexus block. In: de Leon-Casasola OA, ed. *Cancer Pain: Pharmacological, Interventional and Palliative Care Approaches*. Saunders; 2006:401-416.

C.3. What are the complications of celiac plexus block?

Hypotension and increased gastrointestinal motility from the abdominal visceral sympathectomy induced by the procedure are the most common complications of this block. Neurologic complications include subarachnoid or epidural injection and lumbar nerve root injury. A potentially severe complication can occur as a result of accidental injection into the nutrient artery of the spinal cord (artery of Adamkiewicz), causing paraplegia. Injury to the kidney can cause temporary hematuria that is typically treated conservatively without additional intervention. Other complications have been reported due to proximity of other vital structures, including pneumothorax, chylothorax, intradiscal injection, and retroperitoneal hematoma.

Brogan SE, Sindt J, Viswanathan A. Interventional pain therapies. In: Ballantyne JH, Fishman SM, Rathmell JPC, eds. *Bonica's Management of Pain.* 5th ed. Wolters Kluwer; 2019:711-731.

Hadad CS, Pak DJ. Pancreatic cancer. In: Pak DJ, Yong RJ, Shah KB, eds. *Interventional Management of Chronic Visceral Pain Syndromes.* Elsevier; 2021:77-84

C.4. Would you consider neuraxial opioid infusion in this patient? Discuss complications of this procedure.

In properly selected patients, epidural, intrathecal (subarachnoid), or intraventricular infusions of opioids have the advantage of producing profound analgesia without motor, sensory, or autonomic blockade. This is achieved with preservative-free medications when pain is not adequately controlled with less invasive (oral, subcutaneous, or intravenous) routes and escalation of doses is limited by intolerable side effects. The potency ratio of epidural to oral morphine is 1:30, and that from intrathecal to oral morphine is 1:300, thereby reducing the potential side effects with potential superior pain control. Fixed or flexible doses of medications can be delivered by intrathecal pumps. Morphine is the most commonly used drug. Other medications that can be used include local anesthetics, ziconotide, and α_2-adrenergic agonists.

Implementation of neuraxial therapies requires an experienced clinician as well as sufficient home and facility support for close monitoring and follow-ups. These procedures are reversible but involve an initial expense for specialized care. Intraspinal opioids can produce the same side effects of nausea, mental clouding, and sedation as in oral and parenteral dosing. Infection (eg, meningitis and epidural abscess) and hematoma are potentially devastating complications that can cause permanent neurologic deficits if not dealt with on a timely basis. Pruritus and urinary retention are more common than with oral or parenteral administration.

Deer TR, Pope JE, Hayek SM, et al. The Polyanalgesic Consensus Conference (PACC): recommendations on intrathecal drug infusion systems best practices and guidelines. *Neuromodulation.* 2017;20:96-132.

Hadad CS, Pak DJ. Pancreatic cancer. In: Pak DJ, Yong RJ, Shah KB, eds. *Interventional Management of Chronic Visceral Pain Syndromes.* Elsevier; 2021:77-84.

Stearns L, Boortz-Marx R, Du Pen S, et al. Intrathecal drug delivery for the management of cancer pain: a multidisciplinary consensus of best clinical practices. *J Support Oncol.* 2005;3:399-408.

C.5. Which medications can be used intrathecally? What is ziconotide?

Morphine is the most commonly used opioid for intrathecal drug delivery. Other opioids such as hydromorphone, fentanyl, and sufentanil can also be used intrathecally. In addition, other agents, local anesthetics, α_2-adrenergic agonists such as clonidine, and baclofen can be used as recommended by the Polyanalgesic Consensus Conference.

Ziconotide (Prialt), a synthetic equivalent of a naturally occurring peptide found in marine snails, can be effective in pain relief when used intrathecally. It is a selective voltage-gated calcium channel blocker that inhibits release of glutamate, calcitonin, and substance *P* in the brain and spinal cord to provide analgesia. Side effects include dizziness, nausea, confusion, and psychosis. Therefore, patients trialed on ziconotide should be monitored for cognitive impairment, hallucinations, or changes in mood.

It is important to note that only morphine, baclofen, and ziconotide have been approved by the US Food and Drug Administration (FDA) for intrathecal delivery.

Bhatia G, Lau ME, Koury KM, et al. Intrathecal drug delivery (ITDD) systems for cancer pain. *F1000Res.* 2014;2:96.

Deer TR, Pope JE, Hayek SM, et al. The Polyanalgesic Consensus Conference (PACC): recommendations on intrathecal drug infusion systems best practices and guidelines. *Neuromodulation.* 2017;20:96-132.

Stearns L, Boortz-Marx R, Du Pen S, et al. Intrathecal drug delivery for the management of cancer pain: a multidisciplinary consensus of best clinical practices. *J Support Oncol.* 2005;3:399-408.

Williams J, Day M, Heavner J. Ziconotide: an update and review. *Expert Opin Pharmacother.* 2008;9:1575-1583.

C.6. What is a Personal Therapy Manager (PTM), and what role does it play in neuraxial pain relief?

PTM enables the patient to activate delivery of physician-programmed supplemental doses of intrathecal medication (PTM, Medtronics Neurological). This is especially useful for patients experiencing intermittent pain of severe intensity that cannot be adequately managed with a simple continuous infusion.

It is also effective for patients who have an unpredictable need for varying doses of drug or those who experience inadequate pain relief or intolerable side effects from supplemental systemic breakthrough pain medications. Nevertheless, risk of sedation, respiratory depression, and other adverse effects can occur, and, therefore, caution and careful programming should be ensured.

Ilias W, le Polain B, Buchser E, et al. Patient-controlled analgesia in chronic pain patients: experience with a new device designed to be used with implanted programmable pumps. *Pain Pract.* 2008;8:164-170.

Stearns L, Boortz-Marx R, Du Pen S, et al. Intrathecal drug delivery for the management of cancer pain: a multidisciplinary consensus of best clinical practices. *J Support Oncol.* 2005;3:399-408.

White C, Rajagopal A. Intraspinal therapy. In: de Leon-Casasola OA, ed. *Cancer Pain: Pharmacological, Interventional and Palliative Care Approaches.* Saunders; 2006:417-429.

C.7. Would you consider neuraxial neurolysis in this patient to manage his pain? Discuss advantages and disadvantages of these blocks.

Due to the physical separation of motor and sensory nerve roots in the spinal canal and intrathecal space, chemical neurolytic procedures can allow for sensory blockade without loss of motor function. Inadequate pain control with intolerable side effects of other systemic therapies makes this patient a candidate for neuraxial neurolysis; however, complications of the procedure should be weighed against benefits. Epidural or intrathecal (subarachnoid) neurolytic blocks are considered for severe, intractable pain from advanced cancer as an adjuvant to relieve pain and suffering. These blocks are primarily effective in relieving pain of somatic origin and less effective for visceral and neuropathic pain.

In selected patients in whom pain relief is not achieved by less invasive measures, these blocks can provide rapid analgesia and allow dosage (and side effect) reduction of systemic drugs. However, risks of postural hypotension, bowel/bladder incontinence, and motor/sensory deficits in the lower extremities need to be considered. These blocks are irreversible and require a skilled clinician to perform the procedure.

McHugh ME, Miller-Saultz D, Wuhrman E, et al. Interventional pain management in the palliative care patient. *Int J Palliat Nurs.* 2012;18:426-428, 430-433.

Plancarte-Sanchez R, Guajardo-Rosas J, Guillén-Nuñez MDR. Neurolytic techniques for cancer pain management. In: de Leon-Casasola OA, ed. *Cancer Pain: Pharmacological, Interventional and Palliative Care Approaches.* Saunders; 2006:501-507.

C.8. Which neuroablative procedures can be considered in the terminal stage of pancreatic cancer?

Based on the location/type of pain (somatic, visceral, deafferentation), the general condition of the patient, stage of disease, life expectancy, and the expertise available, the following neurosurgical procedures could be considered:

- Peripheral neurectomy
- Dorsal rhizotomy
- Anterolateral cordotomy (spinal tractotomy)
- Commissural myelotomy
- Hypophysectomy

Grannan NL, Hadzipasic M, Eskandar EN. Ablative neurosurgical procedures for chronic pain. In: Ballantyne JC, Fishman SM, Rathmell JP, eds. *Bonica's Management of Pain.* 5th ed. Wolters Kluwer; 2019:1698-1707.

C.9. Describe the role of radiation therapy in cancer pain.

Radiation therapy can be curative or palliative to relieve pain from metastasis and symptoms from local extension of disease. Radiation therapy is complementary to chemotherapy, surgery, and analgesic drug therapies to enhance the effectiveness of pain control. Radiation therapy can palliate when disease cannot be controlled. It is most commonly used for bone metastasis. The radiation dosage should be administered in the fewest fractions possible to promote pain control during and after treatment.

Johnstone C, Lutz ST. The role of hypofractionated radiation in the management of non-osseous metastatic or uncontrolled local cancer. *Ann Palliat Med.* 2014;3:291-303.

McQuay HJ, Collins SL, Carroll D, et al. Radiotherapy for the palliation of painful bone metastases. *Cochrane Database Syst Rev.* 2000:CD001793.

D. Nonpharmacologic Management

D.1. What are the various nonpharmacologic techniques of cancer pain management?

Eisenberg and colleagues demonstrated that cancer and other chronic pain syndromes can benefit from alternative modalities. Practicing physical activity improves fatigue and quality of life and reduces symptoms of depression. The common therapies offered are:

- Physical therapy
- Physical activity and sports
- Relaxation and massage
- Chiropractic manipulation
- Spiritual healing
- Biofeedback and hypnosis
- Magnetic and low-power laser therapy
- Transcutaneous electrical nerve stimulation (TENS)
- Homeopathy
- Acupuncture
- Prayer

Bouillet T, Bigard X, Brami C, et al. Role of physical activity and sport in oncology: scientific commission of the National Federation Sport and Cancer CAMI. *Crit Rev Oncol Hematol.* 2015;94:74-86.

Bradley LA, McKendree-Smith NL, Cianfrini LR. Cognitive-behavioral therapy interventions for pain associated with chronic illness: evidence for their effectiveness. *Semin Pain Med.* 2003;1:44-54.

Eisenberg DM, Kessler RC, Foster C, et al. Unconventional medicine in the United States. Prevalence, costs, and patterns of use. *N Engl J Med.* 1993;328:246-252.

Pinell XA, Kirkpatrick SH, Hawkins K, et al. Manipulative therapy of secondary lymphedema in the presence of locoregional tumors. *Cancer.* 2008;112:950-954.

D.2. What physical modalities have been successful in cancer pain management?

Physical modalities can be useful in conjunction with conventional systemic and interventional treatments used to control cancer-related pain, especially in patients with movement-associated pain. Physical modalities can help decrease stiffness, increase blood flow, relax the patient, and reduce the dose of analgesics. They include cutaneous stimulation, superficial heat and cold therapy, massage, vibration, and pressure. Cold therapy (cryotherapy) causes vasoconstriction, reduces inflammation, and decreases muscle spasm. Superficial application of heat (thermotherapy) acts through conduction or convection to increase blood flow to the skin and superficial organs. Heat also decreases joint stiffness and increases muscle flexibility. Physical therapy and exercise help to strengthen weak muscles, mobilize stiff joints, and restore coordination. Weight-bearing exercises are avoided if an impending fracture is suspected.

Bouillet T, Bigard X, Brami C, et al. Role of physical activity and sport in oncology: scientific commission of the National Federation Sport and Cancer CAMI. *Crit Rev Oncol Hematol.* 2015;94:74-86.

Cheville AL, Basford JR. Role of rehabilitation medicine and physical agents in the treatment of cancer-associated pain. *J Clin Oncol.* 2014;32:1691-1702.

Fitzgibbon D, Hsu M. Evaluation and treatment of cancer-related pain. In: Benzon H, Rathmell JP, Wu CL, et al, eds. *Practical Management of Pain.* 6th ed. Mosby; 2023:461-478.

D.3. Describe the role of neuromodulation in cancer pain management.

Neuromodulation techniques like spinal cord stimulation have not been popular in cancer pain management because of incompatibility with magnetic resonance imaging (MRI). But this therapy is now being used more frequently since the availability of MRI compatible spinal cord stimulator systems. Neuromodulation techniques have variable outcome results with success rates of 18% to 80% depending on the study and disease. Much of the literature is about chronic nonmalignant pain syndromes.

TENS and acupuncture are believed to activate endogenous pain-relieving pathways. Low-voltage stimulation to large myelinated peripheral nerves via cutaneous electrodes can significantly reduce pain. Spinal cord stimulation is a promising therapy for intractable cancer pain and can offer relief of neuropathic pain, which is present in 15% to 40% of patients with cancer pain. Recently, high-frequency spinal cord stimulation, burst stimulation, dorsal root ganglion stimulation, and MRI compatible spinal cord stimulation systems could increase the role of this therapy in patients with cancer. Studies have shown significant pain relief in postthoracotomy pain, back pain, leg pain, groin pain, and testicular pain related to carcinoma.

Burchiel KJ, Raslan AM. Contemporary concepts of pain surgery. *J Neurosurg*. 2019;130:1039-1049.

Yakovlev AE, Resch BE. Spinal cord stimulation for cancer-related low back pain. *Am J Hosp Palliat Care*. 2012;29:93-97.

Yakovlev AE, Resch BE, Karasev SA. Treatment of cancer-related chest wall pain using spinal cord stimulation. *Am J Hosp Palliat Care*. 2010;27:552-556.

D.4. What psychological techniques have been promoted for comfort care and pain relief?

Psychological distress impacts pain. Depression, anxiety, anger, and mood disturbances have been correlated with higher levels of perceived cancer pain. Moreover, there has been an increase in the number of people surviving with cancer, as a result of advances in cancer treatment, who are suffering from intractable pain. Psychological interventions are an important part of a multimodal approach to pain management in patients with cancer. Some techniques that are used are relaxation, biofeedback, hypnosis, imagery, and cognitive-behavioral therapy. They help patients gain a sense of control over pain. Cognitive and behavioral techniques are designed to influence the interpretation of events and bodily sensations. Cognitive techniques help patients think differently about their pain and its management. Behavioral techniques help patients develop skills to cope with pain and help modify their reactions to pain. Patients who undergo psychotherapy report less pain. Relaxation therapy is a well-established modality in managing cancer pain. Several variations of relaxation strategies and techniques have been widely practiced in patients suffering from advanced cancer and have proven effective. Relaxation and imagery are used to achieve a state of mental and physical relaxation, thereby relieving anxiety and muscle tension. Relaxation strategies like deep breathing, muscle relaxation, and imagery are recommended for the promotion of comfort and relief of pain in hospitalized patients.

Patients with higher levels of social support have reported lower intensity of cancer pain. These interventions have medium-size effects on both pain severity and interference per meta-analysis by Gorin. Therefore, quality controlled psychosocial interventions should be part of a multimodal approach to managing pain in patients with cancer.

Byker GL, Leskuski D. Nonpharmacological management of pain. In: Berger A, Shuster J, Von Roenn J, eds. *Principles and Practice of Palliative Care and Supportive Oncology*. 4th ed. Lippincott Williams & Wilkins; 2014:42-54.

Eccleston C, Morley SJ, Williams AC. Psychological approaches to chronic pain management: evidence and challenges. *Br J Anaesth*. 2013;111:59-63.

National Institutes of Health. *National Institutes of Health State-of-the-Science Conference Statement: Symptom Management in Cancer: Pain, Depression, and Fatigue*. National Institute of Health; 2002.

Sheinfeld Gorin S, Krebs P, Badr H, et al. Meta-analysis of psychosocial interventions to reduce pain in patients with cancer. *J Clin Oncol*. 2012;30:539-547.

D.5. What are distraction and reframing techniques? What is the role of hypnosis in cancer pain?

Distraction and reframing techniques encourage focused attention on stimuli other than pain. Reframing helps monitor and evaluate negative thoughts and images while encouraging positive thoughts and behavior. Hypnosis by a skilled person decreases pain and anxiety in patients who have difficulty managing their pain. It also increases coping skills. This technique allows heightened awareness and focused concentration to manipulate perception of pain and has been effective in the management of cancer-related pain syndromes.

Devine EC. Meta-analysis of the effect of psychoeducational interventions on pain in adults with cancer. *Oncol Nurs Forum*. 2003;30:75-89.

Ong AD, Zautra AJ, Reid MC. Chronic pain and the adaptive significance of positive emotions. *Am Psychol*. 2015;70:283-284.

Sheinfeld Gorin S, Krebs P, Badr H, et al. Meta-analysis of psychosocial interventions to reduce pain in patients with cancer. *J Clin Oncol*. 2012;30:539-547.

Acknowledgments

We gratefully acknowledge the contributions of previous edition author(s), Shakil Ahmed and Sudhir A. Diwan, as portions of those chapters have been retained in this revision.

50

Low Back Pain and Sciatica

David Y. Wang

A 57-year-old former factory worker was injured on the job 8 years ago. He experienced severe low back and right leg pain after lifting a heavy piece of equipment, and was found to have a herniated L4-L5 intervertebral disc with compression of the right L5 nerve root. He underwent a lumbar laminectomy and decompression surgery, but has continued to complain of back pain and right sciatica.

A. Medical Disease and Differential Diagnosis

1. How significant is the issue of low back pain in the general population?
2. What is the prevalence of low back pain?
3. What is the societal cost of low back pain?
4. What causes low back pain?
5. What are the risk factors for low back pain?
6. What are the potential sources of pain in the spine?
7. What is the anatomy of the intervertebral discs? What is the mechanism of pain from herniated discs?
8. What is the anatomy of spinal facets? How do the facet joints cause pain?
9. What are the important findings through history and physical examination?
10. What are the appropriate diagnostic studies for low back pain?
11. What is the differential diagnosis of low back pain?
12. What are the causes of persistent back pain after multiple spine surgeries?

B. Management of Low Back Pain and Sciatica

1. What are the noninterventional treatments available?
2. What interventional treatments are available and how should they be used?
3. What are some of the recent safety improvements recommended for lumbar epidural steroid injection?
4. What are some of other approaches in minimally invasive interventions?
5. What are the concerns about magnetic resonance imaging (MRI) safety in patients with a spinal cord stimulator (SCS)?
6. When should surgery be considered?
7. What surgical options are available for the treatment of disc disease or lumbar spinal stenosis?

A. Medical Disease and Differential Diagnosis

A.1. How significant is the issue of low back pain in the general population?

Disorders of the lumbosacral spine cause pain, suffering, public health issues, disability, and socioeconomic issues. Most adults will experience several episodes of low back pain during their lifetime. It is estimated that 80% of workers will lose work time because of this complaint. Based on primary diagnosis only, a National Ambulatory Medical Care Survey from 1989 to 1990 ranked low back pain as the fifth most frequent reason for adults to visit an office-based medical practice. In 2010, low back pain was ranked third behind ischemic heart disease and chronic obstructive pulmonary disease in causing poor health and mortality burden in the

United States. Low back pain has been ranked the greatest cause of disability and fifth in the overall burden per the Global Burden of Disease 2010 study. In the past, it was estimated that 1 in 4 adults suffered from chronic lower back pain, and that in 40% of those affected, pain radiated to the leg. More recent data from 2019 revealed that 39% of adults (aged 18 years and over) had back pain, 36.5% had lower limb pain, and 30.7% had upper limb pain in the past 3 months according to Center for Disease Control and Prevention (CDC)/National Center for Health Statistics (NCHS).

Hart LG, Deyo RA, Cherkin DC. Physician office visits for low back pain. Frequency, clinical evaluation, and treatment patterns from a U.S. national survey. *Spine (Phila Pa 1976)*. 1995;20:11-19.

Hoy D, March L, Brooks P, et al. The global burden of low back pain: estimates from the Global Burden of Disease 2010 study. *Ann Rheum Dis.* 2014;73:968-974.

Lucas JW, Connor EM, Bose J. Back, lower limb, and upper limb pain among U. S. adults, 2019. *NCHS Data Brief.* 2021; 415:1-7.

National Institute of Neurological Disorders and Stroke. *Low Back Pain Fact Sheet*. National Institute of Neurological Disorders and Stroke; 2014:1-50. NIH publication 15-5161.

A.2. What is the prevalence of low back pain?

Recent global statistics demonstrated point prevalence of low back pain was 8.2% (377.5 million people) in 1990 and 7.5% in 2017 (577 million people). It increased with age, peaked between 80 and 89 years of age, and then decreased slightly. It was also higher in females than in males. The years lived with disability (YLDs) were also higher in females and increased initially with age, peaked at 35 to 39 years of age in 1990, peaked at 45 to 49 years of age in 2017, before decreasing. In 2020, low back pain affected 619 million people globally and it is estimated to reach 843 million by 2050. Thus, as the population ages and expands over the coming decades, the number of individuals with low back pain is likely to increase substantially.

Low back pain can be acute (lasting 4-6 weeks), subacute (6-12 weeks), or chronic (over 12 weeks). An acute episode of low back pain usually resolves within 6 weeks. More persistent pain lasting beyond 3 to 6 months occurred in only 5% to 10% of cases. The US Agency for Health Care Policy and Research reported that 90% of patients with acute low back pain recover their usual activity tolerance within 4 to 6 weeks of injury. The remaining 10% of patients who do not recover with time or routine therapy go on to develop chronic symptoms and secondary problems. After 1 year, the incidence of acute back pain converting to chronic back pain is 20%. Recurrences of low back pain are also common, with the percentage of subsequent low back pain episodes ranging from 20% to 44% within 1 year for working populations to lifetime recurrences of up to 85%.

Ferreira MI, Luca K, Haile LM, et al. Global, regional, and national burden of low back pain, 1990-2020, its attributable risk factors, and projections to 2050: a systematic analysis of the Global Burden of Disease Study 2021. *Lancet Rheumatol.* 2023;5:e316-e329.

National Institute of Neurological Disorders and Stroke. *Low Back Pain Fact Sheet*. National Institute of Neurological Disorders and Stroke; 2014:1-50. NIH publication 15-5161.

Wu A, March L, Zheng X, et al. Global lower back pain prevalence and years lived with disability from 1990 to 2017: estimates from the Global Burden of Disease Study 2017. *Ann Transl Med.* 2020;8:299.

A.3. What is the societal cost of low back pain?

The costs of low back pain include functional impairment, activity limitations, reduced quality of life, disability, underemployment, reduced work productivity, and direct medical cost. It appears that the societal perception of disability has changed dramatically over time. This has resulted in an increased rate and cost of disability and overutilization of medical care, including surgical treatments. Based on data from the Medical Expenditure Panel Survey (MEPS) in 1998, patients suffering from back pain consumed $90.7 billion annually in health care expenses, with approximately $26.3 billion of that amount directly attributable to treating the back pain. Their results demonstrated the enormous economic impact of back pain. The $90 billion spent in 1998 represented 1% of the US gross domestic product (GDP), and the $26 billion in direct back pain costs accounted for 2.5% of all health care expenditures for that year. The team found that 25.9 million adults reported back pain in 1998, with 172.7 million reporting no back pain. On average, individuals with back pain incurred health care expenditures about 60% higher than individuals without back pain ($3,498 vs $2,178) in 1998.

Total health care spending has increased from an estimated 1.4 trillion, or $5,295 per person, 13.3% of GDP in 1996 to an estimated $ 3.1 trillion, or $9,655 per person, about 17.9% of the US GDP in 2016. The top three expenditures are $380.9 billion in musculoskeletal disorders as the highest; $309.1 billion in diabetes mellitus, urogenital, blood and endocrine diseases as 2nd highest; and $255.1 billion in cardiovascular diseases as the 3rd highest expenditure. In 2016, Americans spent an estimated $380 billion on lower back and neck pain, as well as on joint and limb pain, and other musculoskeletal disorders. Of the above, the combination of lower back and neck pain alone generated the highest expenditures at $134.5 billion, which was 0.78% of GDP. On average, low back pain occurs at a rate roughly twice that of neck pain, with some variation across different age groups.

Dagenais S, Caro J, Haldeman S. A systemic review of low back pain cost of illness studies in the United States and internationally. *Spine J.* 2008;8:8-20.

Dieleman JL, Cao J, Chapin A, et al. US health care spending by payer and health condition, 1996-2016. *JAMA.* 2020;323: 863-884.

Luo X, Pietrobon R, Sun SX, et al. Estimates and patterns of direct health care expenditures among individuals with back pain in the United States. *Spine (Phila Pa 1976).* 2004;29:79-86.

Ricci JA, Stewart WF, Chee E, et al. Back pain exacerbations and lost productive time cost in United States workers. *Spine (Phila Pa 1976).* 2006;31:3052-3060.

A.4. What causes low back pain?

Low back pain can be classified as nonspecific (90%, no known pathoanatomic cause) or specific (10%, accounted for by an underlying disease such as cancer, infection, tissue damage, or pathologic changes). Specific low back pain is mechanical in nature caused by injury, compression, tears, and bone and disc degeneration. Common causes include the following:

- Intervertebral disc degeneration/internal disc disruption (IDD)
- Disc displacements (diffuse: disc bulge, annular bulge *vs* focal [herniations]: protrusion, extrusion, extrusion with sequestration)
- Radiculopathy
- Spondylosis/facet joint arthrosis
- Facet cyst/synovial cyst (most commonly at the L4-L5 level)
- Ligamentum flavum thickness or hypertrophy/ligamentum flavum infoldings
- Spondylolisthesis (Grade I/II/III/IV and spondyloptosis)
- Spinal stenosis/lateral recess stenosis (subarticular recess stenosis/foraminal stenosis)
- Spinal epidural lipomatosis (SEL)
- Baastrup's disease (kissing spine syndrome)
- Bertolotti syndrome (lower back pain associated with lumbosacral transitional vertebra)
- Skeletal irregularity (scoliosis, kyphosis)
- Traumatic injury/compression fracture/end plate fracture
- Cluneal nerve entrapment (superior and middle cluneal nerves)
- Sacroiliac joint dysfunction
- Other underlying conditions
  - Infection
  - Tumor
  - Abdominal aortic aneurysm
  - Kidney stones
  - Endometriosis
  - Fibromyalgia

Baastrup disease (kissing spine syndrome) is a term referring to close approximation of adjacent spinous processes due to degenerative changes of the spine. It happens most commonly at the lumbar spine, usually at L4-L5. Contact of adjacent spinous processes results in edema, sclerosis, flattening, and enlargement. Symptoms include back pain with midline distribution that worsens during extension. On the other hand, the presence of a lumbosacral transitional vertebra (LSTV) is variable between 4% and 30%; however, it is considered an uncommon cause of chronic lower back pain. Bertolotti syndrome is only diagnosed when the cause of pain is attributed to this transitional anatomy.

Alonzo F, Cobar A, Cahueque M, et al. Bertolotti's syndrome: an underdiagnosed cause for lower back pain. *J Surg Case Rep.* 2018;10:1-4.

Crane J, Cragon R, O'Neill J, et al. A comprehensive update of the treatment and management of Bertolotti's syndrome: a best practice review. *Orthop Rev.* 2021;13:1-8.

Filippiadis, DK, Mazioti, A, Argentos S, et al. Baastrup's disease (kissing spines syndrome): a pictorial review. *Insights Imaging.* 2015, 6:123-128.

Maher C, Underwood M, Buchbinder R. Non-specific low back pain. *Lancet* 2017:389:736-747.

National Institute of Neurological Disorders and Stroke. *Low Back Pain Fact Sheet*. National Institute of Neurological Disorders and Stroke; 2014:1-50. NIH publication 15-5161.

Sergiy VK, Glushko T, Jarraya M, et al. ABC of the degenerative spine. *Insights Imaging*. 2018, 9:253-274.

A.5. What are the risk factors for low back pain?

It is widely believed that heavy physical jobs that required high-energy demand caused significant stress and strain on the spine, whereas light jobs required low-energy demand. Contrary to popular belief, many low-energy jobs are static which is an inherent risk factor for low back pain. Low back pain, degenerative disc disease, and disc herniation are associated with the following:

- Repetitive heavy lifting (the weight of the load and the number of lifts)
- Static work posture (prolonged sitting or standing)
- Frequent twisting and bending
- Vibration (operation of motor vehicle or industrial device)
- Fatigue of the abdominal and paraspinal muscles has been demonstrated when subjected to 30 minutes of vibration. In the absence of this support, the spine is further susceptible to injury.
- Cigarette smoking is linked to low back pain, sciatica, and lumbar disc herniation. In an animal model, cigarette smoking significantly affects the vasculature outside the intervertebral disc, where the most pronounced effect is the reduction of solute-exchange capacity, cellular uptake, and metabolism within the disc.
- Cross-country skiing. In a study of skiing and spinal trauma, the diagonal body position required for cross-country skiing was the most common back pain–inducing stance, whereas no skier experienced back pain when only downhill skiing.
- Body weight increase
- Psychological stress (anxiety and depression)

A meta-analysis of 17 studies revealed that whole-body vibration is associated with an increased risk of low back pain, sciatica, and lumbar intervertebral disc disorders. The common vibration of construction vehicles and industrial devices ranges in frequency from 3.5 to 8.9 Hz. Low-frequency vibration, especially around 5 Hz, in conjunction with a prolonged seated position is associated with spine problems.

The "oxidative stress hypothesis of aging" theory proposed that enhancement of oxygen consumption resulting from increased physical activity may accelerate disc degeneration. On the other hand, strenuous exercises can contribute to positive nutritional effect by facilitating the transport of small solutes into and out of the disc. Generally, people who are physically fit or who maintain a balanced exercise program appear to have a lower risk for chronic low back pain and a more rapid recovery after an episode of acute back pain. Back pain was estimated to be present in 23.5% of never-smokers, 33.1% of former smokers, and 36.9% of current smokers by a study published in 2016. Regarding the relationship between low back pain and the change in body weight for people over 50 years of age, the adjusted odds ratio (OR) was 1.24 times higher for the 3 to 6 kg increase group, and 1.42 times higher in those who gained 6 kg or more compared to the group without weight gain.

Lee CA, Jang HD, Moon JE, et al. The relationship between change of weight and chronic lower back pain in population over 50 years of age: a nationwide cross-sectional study. *Int J Environ Res Public Health*. 2021;18:1-9.

Parreira P, Maher CG, Steffens D, et al. Risk factors for low back pain and sciatica: an umbrella review. *Spine J*. 2018;18:1715-1721.

Wilder DG, Woodworth BB, Frymoyer JW, et al. Vibration and the human spine. *Spine (Phila Pa 1976)*. 1982;7:243-254.

A.6. What are the potential sources of pain in the spine?

The potential sources of low back and radicular pain include the bony structure of vertebrae, muscles attached to the spine and hips, fasciae, ligaments, discs, facet joints, meninges, vessels, nerve roots, dorsal root ganglion (DRG), and nerves in the surrounding areas. The spine can be anatomically categorized into three compartments: anterior, middle, and posterior.

The anterior compartment consists of the vertebral body and intervertebral disc. The anterior unit is bound together by cephalocaudal ligaments: anterior longitudinal ligament and posterior longitudinal ligament (PLL). The anterior longitudinal ligament is anatomically much broader and stronger than the PLL. The PLL is intact throughout the length of the vertebral column until it reaches the lumbar vertebrae. From L1 downwards, a gradual reduction in PLL width is observed, culminating in a 50% decrease by L5-S1. This anatomic feature contributes to an inherent structural weakness in the lumbar spine. Hence, the lower lumbar spine is the region subjected to the greatest static stress and most spinal movement resulting in the greatest kinetic strain.

The middle (neuraxial) compartment contains all of the structures within the bony and ligamentous boundaries of the spinal canal. This includes the PLL, epidural space, meninges, spinal cord, dorsal and ventral nerve roots, root sleeves, dorsal root ganglia, and ligamentum flavum.

The posterior compartment contains the facet joints, laminae, vertebral arches, and structures posterior to the plane of the transverse processes and innervated by the dorsal rami of the spinal nerves. The ligaments are extremely important in stabilizing the vertebral column. The ligamentum flavum ("yellow ligament" due to high content of yellow elastin), which connects the laminae of adjacent vertebrae, is the thickest and strongest ligament in the lumbar region. It can contribute to spinal stenosis by folding inward during an upright posture, extension of the back, and hypertrophying. Thickening of the ligamentum flavum is also correlated with disc degeneration and herniation.

The sinuvertebral nerve (also known as recurrent meningeal nerve) originates lateral to the neural foramina and enters the spinal canal anterior to the DRG. It is a branch of the somatic ventral nerve root and the sympathetic gray ramus communicans. This specific nerve, the nerve of Luschka, innervates the outer one-third of the disc annulus, PLL, epidural membranes, and dura at the segmental level of origin and adjacent levels. Therefore, it transmits pain signals from a problematic disc to the brain. It is important to note that central low back pain, with or without referred pain to the buttocks, can derive from the irritation of the outer part of the annulus fibrosus or the PLL.

The natural wear and tear on the discs and facet joints results in microtrauma and degeneration. This can induce the release of neurohumoral mediators, such as phospholipase A_2, serotonin, H^+, substance P, prostaglandin E_2, and so on, to produce inflammation of the nerve roots or meninges and to sensitize local nociceptors. Furthermore, material from the nucleus pulposus, protected from the immune system by the annulus fibrosus, might act as a foreign protein and trigger an autoimmune reaction. The demonstration of an activated immunocompetent cellular response at the epidural interface of the herniation of the nucleus pulposus supports the concept of the immunogenic capacity of the nucleus pulposus.

Tissue injury or inflammation can cause a barrage of nociceptive input to the spinal cord. This can lead to a phenomenon called *central sensitization* or *windup* of neurons in the dorsal horn of the spinal cord. The release of excitatory amino acids and neuropeptides in the dorsal horn is thought to be the mechanism underlying the phenomenon of central sensitization. At the cellular level, there is an increase in spontaneous discharge and an expansion of neural receptive fields of wide dynamic range (WDR) neurons located in Rexed lamina V of the spinal cord. Clinically, this is characterized by sensation of pain when exposed to nonnoxious stimuli (allodynia), a significantly increased response to painful input (hyperalgesia), and an increased response to repetitive stimulation (hyperpathia).

Cavanaugh JM. Neural mechanisms of lumbar pain. *Spine (Phila Pa 1976)*. 1995;20:1804-1809.

Kang JD, Georgescu HI, McIntyre-Larkin L, et al. Herniated lumbar intervertebral discs spontaneously produce matrix metalloproteinases, nitric oxide, interleukin-6, and prostaglandin E2. *Spine (Phila Pa 1976)*. 1996;21:271-277.

King W, Bogduk N. Chronic low back pain. In: Ballantyne JC, Fishman SM, Rathmell JP, eds. *Bonica's Management of Pain*. 5th ed. Wolters Kluwer; 2018:1259-1282.

Saal JS. The role of inflammation in lumbar pain. *Spine (Phila Pa 1976)*. 1995;20:1821-1827.

Sergiy VK, Glushko T, Jarraya M, et al. ABC of the degenerative Spine. *Insights Imaging*. 2018;9:253-274.

Vorobeychik Y, Bogduk N. Intradiscal therapies for low back Pain. In: Ballantyne JC, Fishman SM, Rathmell JP, eds. *Bonica's Management of Pain*. 5th ed. Wolters Kluwer; 2018:1643-1652.

A.7. What is the anatomy of the intervertebral discs? What is the mechanism of pain from herniated discs?

The intervertebral disc is a ring-like structure composed of a centrally located well-hydrated pliable proteoglycan matrix, the nucleus pulposus, which comprises two-thirds of the surface area of the disc. Surrounding the nucleus is a fibrocartilaginous ring composed predominantly of type I collagen, the annulus fibrosus, which makes up the remaining one-third of the surface area of the disc. The annulus fibrosus is stronger anteriorly but often defective posteriorly. As a self-contained fluid system, the disc absorbs shock, permits transient compression, and allows movement. It provides a cushion between the vertebral bodies and allows for greater flexibility.

With age, the number of viable cells in the nucleus pulposus decreases, and the proportion of cells that exhibit necrotic changes from 2% in infancy to 50% in young adults and 80% in older adults. The water content in the young disc is 80% to 90% in the nucleus pulposus. With aging, the discs lose up to

70% of their water content. As the nucleus pulposus further dehydrates, it becomes more fibrous and less compliant. A disc will usually herniate under strain and pressure. Under excessive pressure, it tends to protrude along in the path of least resistance, typically in a posterolateral direction. This can cause direct mechanical pressure on the nerve roots resulting in radiculopathy.

Normally, only the outer third of the annulus fibrosus is innervated. In the degenerative or disrupted disc, small unmyelinated nerve fibers grow into the inner third of the annulus fibrosus and even into the nucleus pulposus. IDD is a condition characterized by a degenerated nucleus pulposus with radial fissures extending into the peripheral annulus fibrosus. Upon rupture of the disc, the release of irritative material near the meninges can induce radiculitis and symptoms of radiculopathy without actual herniated disc material compressing the nerve roots. Under such circumstances, significant disc herniation might not be visualized on MRI or computed tomography (CT) scan. In brief, the proposed mechanisms of radiculopathy include direct pressure on nerve fibers due to compression injury and indirect impact through impairment of microcirculation, chemical irritation and inflammation, immune reaction, edema formation secondary to permeability changes of the intraneural capillaries, and impairment of the nutritional transport to the nerve root.

Compression of the nerve roots depends on the effective space available within the neural foramina, the osseous structures surrounding the neural foramina, and the tethering effects of the intraspinal and extraspinal ligaments. Posterolateral disc herniations can impinge on the lumbar dorsal root, which then initiates electrical discharges for as long as 25 minutes after the mechanical stimulus has been removed. Radiculopathy can be produced by either biochemical or mechanical stimulation of a swollen, stretched, or compressed nerve root. From 3% to 12% of all lumbar disc herniations occur laterally and extend into or beyond the foraminal zone; in this setting, patients complain of sudden and severe radicular pain, often with dysesthesia. On the other hand, discogenic pain resulting from a central disc bulge or herniation stimulates several lumbar tissues such as the outer layer of the annulus fibrosus or PLL. Clinically, this is manifested as central low back pain without radicular symptoms.

Devlin VJ, ed. *Spine Secret Plus*. 2nd ed. Elsevier Mosby; 2012:332-336.

Freemont AJ, Peacock TE, Goupille P, et al. Nerve ingrowth into diseased intervertebral disc in chronic back pain. *Lancet*. 1997;350:178-181.

Takebayashi T, Cavanaugh JM, Cüneyt Ozaktay A, et al. Effect of nucleus pulposus on the neural activity of dorsal root ganglion. *Spine (Phila PA 1976)*. 2001;26:940-945.

Vorobeychik Y, Bogduk N. Intradiscal therapies for low back pain. In: Ballantyne JC, Fishman SM, Rathmell JP, eds. *Bonica's Management of Pain*. 5th ed. Wolters Kluwer; 2018: 1643-1652.

A.8. What is the anatomy of spinal facets? How do the facet joints cause pain?

The facet (zygapophyseal) joints consist of two arthrodial joints both superiorly and inferiorly, are each lined with synovium, lubricated by synovial fluid, and contained within a joint capsule. These synovial joints enhance spinal stability and flexibility. In the upper part of the lumbar spine (L1-L3), the facet planes lie in a generally vertical sagittal plane and permit flexion and extension but prevent lateral flexion or bending in the lordotic curve. The lumbosacral facet joints at the level of L5-S1 depart the farthest from the sagittal plane, allowing some rotation of the lower part of the lumbar spine. With slight forward flexion, the facets of the other lumbar vertebrae separate and permit a modest degree of lateral movement and rotation. Facet loading, if of a repetitive nature, may play a role in the degeneration of the facet joint. After repeated wear and tear, these joints are susceptible to osteoarthritis and associated synovial cyst (facet cyst) formation. Hypertrophic facet joints or cysts can encroach on the spinal canal or the intervertebral foramina and contribute to the development of central spinal, lateral recess, or foraminal stenosis. These abnormalities can result in lower back pain with or without radiculopathy.

Devlin VJ, ed. *Spine Secret Plus*. 2nd ed. Elsevier Mosby; 2012:332-336.

Du R, Xu G, Bai X, et al. Facet joint syndrome: pathophysiology, diagnosis, and treatment. *J Pain Res*. 2022;15:3689-3710.

Sergiy VK, Glushko T, Jarraya M, et al. ABC of the degenerative spine. *Insights Imaging*. 2018, 9:253-274.

A.9. What are the important findings through history and physical examination?

A problem-focused pain history should include onset, location, intensity (eg, pain scale 0-10), characteristics (achy, dull, sharp, spasmodic, stabbing, burning, shooting, tingling, pins-and-needles sensation, etc), and duration plus aggravating and alleviating factors. The essential purpose in the initial evaluation is to differentiate patients with serious underlying pathology from those with mild-to-moderate problems.

TABLE 50.1 Differentiating Spinal Shock, Upper Motor Neuron Lesions, and Lower Motor Neuron Lesions

Disease State	Deep Tendon Reflex	Pathologic Reflex (Plantar Response)	Superficial Reflex (Normal)
Spinal shock	Absent	Absent	Absent
Upper motor neuron disease	Increased; rarely may be decreased in the acute setting	Positive/extensor Babinski sign + Oppenheim sign +	Decreased or absent For example, cremasteric reflex −
Lower motor neuron disease	Decreased	Negative/flexor	Present (but L1-L2 lesion will have cremasteric reflex −)

+, positive; −, negative.

Patients with a disc problem usually experience an exacerbation of their symptoms with spinal flexion, which increases intradiscal pressure. By contrast, in the setting of spinal stenosis, standing or walking exacerbates back and leg pain, whereas some forward flexion may alleviate these symptoms. In moderate-to-severe spinal stenosis, extension of the spine may cause radicular pain.

Patients with compression fractures typically present with severe back pain, often intense with minimal lateral rotation or with flexion and relieved by rest. A history of bladder, bowel, or sexual dysfunction may indicate compression of the cauda equina or conus medullaris. Unlike sciatica, often with its unilateral nerve root involvement, patients with cauda equina syndrome usually have bilateral involvement. Although motor function can be normal (with pain being uncommon) in those with conus lesions, patients often have abnormalities of sensation in a saddle distribution, feeling touch or dysesthesia, but neither pain nor temperature. Causes of these symptoms can be a fracture of L1 or L2, tumor, large central disc herniations, or intramedullary cysts affecting the conus. Surgical emergencies of this nature require immediate evaluation and consultation with a surgical expert.

The physical examination should include Lasègue sign (the straight leg raising test), Bragard test (dorsiflexion of the ankle with elevation of the leg), and the crossover test. These clinical tests are considered positive when sciatica is reproduced with elevation of the leg between 30° and 60°. If testing the uninvolved leg produces contralateral symptoms, disc disease should be considered. A positive crossover sign occurs when straight leg raising of the patient's contralateral leg elicits pain on the affected side. It is usually a strong indication of nerve root irritation or compression. Extension of the knee while in a seated position, also known as *distracted straight leg raise*, can test sciatic nerve tension too. The patient with significant nerve root irritation tends to complain of increased pain or lean backward to reduce tension on the nerve. The differential diagnosis of spinal shock, upper motor neuron lesions, and lower neuron lesions is shown in **Table 50.1**. The nerve root signs are shown in **Table 50.2**.

Benzon HT, Rathmell JP, Wu CL, et al, eds. *Practical Management of Pain*. 5th ed. St. Mosby Elsevier; 2014:151-161.

Waldman SD, ed. *Pain Management*. Saunders Elsevier; 2007:762-764.

A.10. What are the appropriate diagnostic studies for low back pain?

In the absence of signs of serious medical disease, there is no need for special studies because 90% of patients recover spontaneously within 4 weeks of the onset of pain. Waiting for 4 weeks before considering special tests allows these patients to recover spontaneously and avoid unneeded procedures.

TABLE 50.2 Nerve Root Signs

Root Level	Reflex Decrease	Sensory Defect	Motor Weakness
L4	Knee jerk	Anterior thigh, knee, and shin	"Single squat and rise test"; quadriceps (mostly L4)
L5	No easily elicited reflex	Lateral leg and middle dorsal foot	"Heel-walking test"; dorsiflexion of foot and toes (L5 and some L4); especially big toe, extensor hallucis longus (EHL)
S1	Ankle jerk	Posterior calf and sole	"Toe-walking test"; gastrocnemius/soleus; "toe flexors"

When pain persists beyond 4 to 6 weeks (or shorter if it is severe), plain radiographs of the spine should be considered. Pertinent findings include the height of the intervertebral spaces and vertebral bodies, and bony changes in the end plates. With oblique views, the facet joint space and any spondylolysis can be revealed. The lateral view can help estimate the severity of spondylolisthesis. If there is symptom of vague flank pain with or without hematuria that marks the onset of renal colic pain, a kidney, ureter, and bladder (KUB) radiograph can help to identify stones. A CT scan can show a herniated disc or fragment in the spinal canal. It can help identify early epidural hematoma. With contrast, it can help further differentiate tumors, abscesses, and granuloma in the central nervous system. MRI provides excellent anatomic definition of the disc and its hydration status; it can also show the anatomy of the surrounding soft tissues. MRI with intravenous gadolinium is indicated for distinguishing between a recurrent disc herniation and recent postoperative scar tissue. It is particularly useful when distinguishing intrinsic from extramedullary or epidural spinal cord lesions. When MRI is contraindicated, a myelogram might reveal a filling defect at the level of posterior bulging discs. The myelogram in conjunction with a CT scan enables axial imaging of the spinal cord and subarachnoid space. A bone scan is helpful in the diagnosis of bone or bony fractures that might not be visible by radiography or CT scan, or whenever metastatic disease is suspected.

King W, Bogduk N. Chronic low back pain. In: Ballantyne JC, Fishman SM, Rathmell JP, eds. *Bonica's Management of Pain*. 5th ed. Wolters Kluwer; 2018:1259-1282.

Wheeler SG, Wipf JE, Staiger TO, et al. *Evaluation of Low Back Pain in Adults—UpToDate*. Wolters Kluwer; 2022:1-37.

A.11. What is the differential diagnosis of low back pain?

In general, there are numerous diagnostic labels used to describe low back pain, for example, lumbosacral sprain, lumbar discogenic syndrome, mechanical low back pain, spinal stenosis, spondylosis, spondylolisthesis, osteoarthritis/facet joint syndrome, myofascial pain syndrome, unstable low back, discitis, and failed back surgery syndrome (FBSS). Each of these labels suggests the underlying pathology. It is also helpful to review causes of low back pain that are described in Section A.4.

Acute lumbosacral sprain, by far the most common cause of new-onset low back pain, is often only associated with the presence of postural back pain. It frequently results from reflex muscle spasms secondary to local irritation of structures in the back. When muscle spasms occur, the normal anatomy can be disturbed, and undue force is applied to surrounding tissues and structures.

Clinically, the following five tests are most commonly requested by spinal surgeons for further differential diagnosis. Discography/discogram/discomanometry (discometry) is a specialized diagnostic test specifically indicated to help diagnose discogenic pain. The presence of pain fibers in the outer third of the annulus fibrosus can explain back pain in some individuals with an annulus tear or IDD. The test involves an intradiscal puncture and instillation of contrast into the disc nucleus. It provides direct confirmation of nuclear morphology and the integrity of the vertebral end plate and annulus. Provocative discography, a test for presumptive discogenic pain in the lumbar spine, has become less common due to false positive results and potential further disc degeneration after this procedure. Selective nerve root block with local anesthetic is performed to determine if a specific spinal nerve is the source of pain. Either facet joint block (intra-articular injection) or medial branches block can help differentiate between axial discogenic pain and facet joint pain syndrome. Sacroiliac joint injection can help to rule out pain resulting from sacroiliac joint dysfunction. Electromyography (EMG) and nerve conduction studies (NCS) can help diagnose neuromuscular abnormalities and disorders. In every case, a careful history, physical examination, and the appropriate diagnostic studies can help elucidate the "pain generator."

Benzon HT, Rathmell JP, Wu CL, et al, eds. *Practical Management of Pain*. 5th ed. Mosby Elsevier; 2014:312-327.

Cuellar JM, Stauff MP, Herzog RJ. Does provocative discography cause clinically important injury to the lumbar intervertebral disc? A 10-year matched cohort study. *Spine J*. 2016;16:273-280.

Schwarzer AC, Aprill CN, Bogduk N. The sacroiliac joint in chronic low back pain. *Spine (Phila Pa 1976)*. 1995;20:31-37.

A.12. What are the causes of persistent back pain after multiple spine surgeries?

Persistent back or leg pain after one or more spinal surgeries is called FBSS or post-laminectomy syndrome (PLS), and implies persistent radicular symptoms or neuropathic complaints after previous surgery, most commonly in the lumbar spine. The cause is usually a combination of both nociceptive and neuropathic pain. Over time, a strong psychological component can develop with progressive disability as treatments fail.

When pain persists or recurs in a patient after spinal surgery, the most common causes are those of foraminal stenosis, discogenic disorder, and recurrent disc herniation. Epidural fibrosis and scarring are less common. Patients with this condition often report constant dull, aching, poorly localized low back pain with intermittent sharp episodes. They can also report pain or abnormal sensations with neuropathic characteristics such as burning, shooting, throbbing, stabbing, or pulling. The exact source of these complaints is unclear, although scar tissue or arachnoiditis is frequently implicated. When reoperation is performed for the purpose of neurolysis only, transient improvement of sciatica can be seen, but it usually recurs within the first postoperative year. Success rates for reoperating on patients with FBSS are highly variable, ranging from 25% to 80%. These patients are perhaps the most challenging. They deserve a comprehensive multidisciplinary evaluation, including orthopedic and neurosurgical consultations. Furthermore, surgical intervention should be avoided in the absence of a clear indication. Repeated imaging studies add to health care expenses and interventions that might not have a great therapeutic yield.

Benzon HT, Rathmell JP, Wu CL, et al, eds. *Practical Management of Pain*. 5th ed. Mosby Elsevier; 2014:312-327.

Petraglia WF III, Farber SH, Thomas SM, et al. Increasing rates of imaging in failed back surgery syndrome (FBSS) patients: a 10 year perspective. *Neurosurgery*. 2015;62:200-201.

Schofferman J. Failed back surgery. In: Ballantyne JC, Fishman SM, Rathmell JP, eds. *Bonica's Management of Pain*. 5th ed. Wolters Kluwer; 2018:1288-1297.

B. Management of Low Back Pain and Sciatica

B.1. What are the noninterventional treatments available?

The cornerstone of treatment for low back pain and mild sciatica caused by a herniated lumbar disc is conservative care, which includes bed rest, medications, and physical therapy. Treatments for nonspecific low back pain include physical therapy, psychological and social support, reducing strain during physical work, and lifestyle changes including more physical activity, healthy diet, and good sleep habits. For specific low back pain, treatments focus on the underlying condition causing the pain. The main components of acute nonspecific low back pain management consist of education, reassurance, and analgesic medicines (NSAIDs with or without muscle relaxants) as first-line care. Among those who receive high-quality first-line care, approximately 50% recover completely within 2 to 3 weeks. Thus, nonpharmacologic therapies such as manual therapy, exercise, massage, and acupuncture can be deferred as they might be unnecessary and wasteful of health care resources.

Both clinical and epidemiologic data suggest that the longer the back pain and work loss persist, the less likely there will be improvement of the pain. An early return to activity seems to be associated with a better outcome than prolonged bed rest (greater than 4 days).

In December 1994, the Agency for Health Care Policy and Research announced the following guidelines for the care of acute low back:

- A brief period of rest
- Over-the-counter pain relievers
- Trunk-strengthening exercises
- A single spinal manipulation

More recently, the contemporary view is that bed rest, in most cases, should be avoided. The patient should remain as active as possible and either continue or gradually resume their normal activity level, and if possible, remain at work.

The role of medications in the treatment of low back pain is to control pain, facilitate rehabilitation, restore normal sleep patterns, and improve mood and motivation. Nonsteroidal anti-inflammatory drugs (NSAIDs) are an essential part of the treatment of patients with inflammatory back pain, such as that associated with spondylitis. Muscle relaxants are often used to decrease muscle spasms and assist in promoting rest for patients with severe pain. These are usually indicated for short-term treatment and acute relief. Although there is evidence of effectiveness of NSAIDs and muscle relaxants, any potential benefits should be weighed against the risk of harm. Short-term therapy with opioid analgesics might be needed to promote rest as well as maintain activity in the acute phase of low back pain. Long-term use of these medications is generally discouraged. When recovery does not occur within 4 to 6 weeks and no additional pathology is detected, physical therapy is indicated. Patients should be encouraged to increase activities by degrees. Patients limited by back pain symptoms can minimize the stress of lifting by keeping any lifted object close to the body at the level of the navel. Activities such as bending, twisting, and reaching while lifting can also increase stress on lumbar disc or back. This is well-demonstrated by Nachemson's studies of total load on the L3 disk in different body positions. His pioneering studies of disc pressure measurements are still quoted extensively in many textbooks.

Prolonged sitting can aggravate back symptoms in patients with discogenic pain because of the progressive increase in pressure at specific points in the abnormal lumbar disc. Body weight optimization and a program that teaches good posture and body mechanics are very important. Neuromuscular reconditioning must be included to ensure a function-specific, task-oriented program. The exercise training shall be designed as a step-by-step program to improve function and optimize neutral spine posture. These programs include core muscles enhancement and stabilization training to attain adequate dynamic control of their lumbar spine forces and eliminate repetitive injury. Soft tissue flexibility, joint mobility, abdominal muscle strengthening, and aerobic exercise are also important factors. Spinal manipulation is controversial and is neither recommended in patients with radiculopathy pain nor is it wise in those for whom a diagnosis has not been established.

Benzon HT, Rathmell JP, Wu CL, et al, eds. *Practical Management of Pain*. 5th ed. Mosby Elsevier; 2014:312-327.

Maher C, Underwood M, Buchbinder R. Non-specific low back pain. *Lancet*. 2017:389:736-747.

Nachemson A. The load on lumbar disks in different positions of the body. *Clin Orthop Relat Res*. 1966;45:107-122.

B.2. What interventional treatments are available and how should they be used?

Common interventional treatments include:

- Trigger point injection
- Epidural steroid injection (interlaminar or caudal approach)
- Transforaminal epidural steroid injection (transforaminal approach)
- Facet joint intra-articular joint injection or medial branch block with the option of a radiofrequency procedure
- Cluneal neuralgia injection
- Sacroiliac joint injection with the option of a radiofrequency procedure

Interventional techniques such as trigger point injections and local infiltration are used to provide pain relief of short duration, especially in acute phase, so that other activities and physical therapy that might otherwise be severely limited by pain can be pursued.

Corticosteroids play an important role against inflammation and reduction of edema. Steroids injected into the epidural space have been used for treating low back pain and radiculopathy for decades. Despite widespread use, the results of epidural steroid injection are still in question because studies evaluating effectiveness have been small, poorly controlled, and lacking good long-term follow-up. The effectiveness of epidural steroid injections varies from 18% to 90%. Epidural steroid injections can be performed through the interlaminar route, the caudal canal, or the intervertebral foramina. The spread of solution in both caudal and interlaminar injection is less controllable because of inconsistent lateral flow into the ventral compartment. This renders the medication less effective as it is diverted away from the compartment, depending on the tightness of the lateral recess (eg, lateral recess stenosis) and the size of the dural sac. In normal volunteers, the transforaminal approach showed good ventral flow, whereas the interlaminar approach showed predominantly dorsal flow, which was far from the usual site of impingement.

Patients who suffer from lumbar facet arthropathy can have symptoms including band-like low back pain and associated hip, groin, or thigh pain. Pain rarely radiates below the knee in this condition. Blockade of the medial branch of the dorsal ramus of the spinal nerve or intra-articular facet joint injections of the lumbar facets can be effective in short-term alleviation of this type of pain. Radiofrequency ablation (RFA) procedures use radiofrequency energy to disrupt or denature medial branch nerves that innervate to painful facet joint. The transmission of pain from problematic facet joints can be limited or reduced for several months (4-6 months). A cooled RFA technique was developed to generate a larger lesion to compensate for variable nerve locations. The bipolar RFA technique might provide even better result. With this technique, the pain might return 4 to 6 months later after axons regenerate; repeating the procedure is then indicated.

In advanced facet joint degeneration, a synovial cyst can form by herniation of the synovium through the facet capsule (up to 80% at the L4-L5 level). Due to the location of the nearby lateral recess, it can cause radiculopathy or symptomatic spinal stenosis. Percutaneous puncture of facet joint cyst (synovial cyst) can be done either by fluoroscopy or CT guidance with intra-articular facet joint, interlaminar toward cyst, or transforaminal approach depending on the location of the cyst.

Low back pain, buttock, and even leg pain can result from superior cluneal nerve (SCN) and middle cluneal nerve (MCN) entrapment or dysfunction. These nerves are cutaneous branches of the lateral branches of the dorsal rami of T11-S4. Multiple branches of the SCN can be entrapped where they pierce the thoracolumbar fascia over the iliac crest whereas the MCN can be entrapped where it passes under or through the long posterior sacroiliac ligament. Cluneal neuralgia or cluneal nerve syndrome is characterized by pain, tender points, and relief with local anesthetic injection. If pain relief from the diagnostic injection is complete but only temporary, longer lasting modalities such as cryoneuroablation, radiofrequency lesioning, and chemical neurolysis can be considered. Other options include peripheral nerve stimulation or surgery.

Among patients with low back pain, 15% to 30% were found to have pain arising from the sacroiliac (S-I) joint. The joint is innervated by L5-S2 ventrally and L5-S4 dorsally. A cadaveric study of the posterior S-I joint innervation revealed contribution from L5 (8%), S1 and S2 (100%), S3 (88%), and S4 (4%). About 40% of patients with post-lumbar fusion had pain that was derived from S-I joint, and 75% showed S-I joint degenerative changes on CT scan at 5 years follow-up. Block of the S-I joint serves as a diagnostic procedure to determine if it is the source of the patient's pain. In most studies, radiofrequency (monopolar, cooled monopolar, peri-foraminal bipolar, or multielectrode probe) targets of treatment included the S1-3 sacral lateral branches and the L5 dorsal ramus.

Chazen JL, Leeman K, Singh JR et al. Percutaneous CT-guided facet joint synovial cyst rupture: success with refractory cases and technical considerations. *Clin Imaging*. 2018;49:7-11.

DePalma MJ, Ketchum JM, Saullo TR. Etiology of chronic low back pain in patients having undergone lumbar fusion. *Pain Med.* 2011;12:732-739.

Karl HW, Helm S, Trescot AM. Superior and middle cluneal nerve entrapment: a cause of low back and radicular pain. *Pain Physician*. 2022;25:E503-E521.

Liliang PC, Lu K, Liang CL, et al. Sacroiliac joint pain after lumbar and lumbosacral fusion: findings using dual sacroiliac joint blocks. *Pain Med.* 2011;12:565-570.

Thawrani DP, Agabegi SS, Asghar F. Diagnosing sacroiliac joint pain. *J Am Acad Orthop Surg*. 2019;27:85-93.

Yang AJ, Wagner G, Burnham T, et al. Radiofrequency ablation for chronic posterior sacroiliac joint complex pain: a comprehensive review. *Pain Med.* 2021;22:S9-13.

B.3. What are some of the recent safety improvements recommended for lumbar epidural steroid injection?

An expert working group with facilitation from the US Food and Drug Administration (FDA) Safe Use Initiative (SUI) and advising national organizations (representatives from leading specialty societies) unanimously agreed that epidural injections of steroid were rarely associated with serious complications due to injuries of the central nervous system. They agreed that transforaminal injections are associated with a risk of catastrophic neurovascular complications and that particulate steroids appear to be inordinately represented in case reports of these complications. Clinical considerations improving technical aspects of the procedures included use of appropriate image-guided views (**Figures 50.1** and **50.2**), injection of contrast under real-time fluoroscopy, review of prior imaging studies, use of face mask and sterile gloves, use of extension tubing, and avoidance of heavy sedation. Although digital subtraction imaging (DSI) can help detect vascular uptake (**Figure 50.3**), the sensitivity was 60% in one study as compared to aspiration sensitivity of 20%.

Due to allergic reactions to iodinated contrast agent such as Omnipaque (iohexol), gadolinium-based contrast agent (GBCA) has been used as an alternative for years. However, encephalopathy or devastating side effects are reported with unintentional intrathecal gadolinium injections during neuraxial procedures such as epidural steroid injection (ESI). Interventional pain physicians should take precautions when using GBCAs during interlaminar ESI.

Chauhan G, Upadhyay A. Gadolinium-based contrast agent-induced neurotoxicity: seeing is believing. *BMJ Case Rep*. 2021;14:e241372.

Lee MH, Yang KS, Kim YH, et al. Accuracy of live fluoroscopy to detect intravascular injection during lumbar transforaminal epidural injections. *Korean J Pain*. 2010;23:18-23.

Rathmell JP, Benzon HT, Dreyfuss P, et al. Safeguards to prevent neurologic complications after epidural steroid injections: consensus opinions from a multidisciplinary working group and national organizations. *Anesthesiology*. 2015;122:974-984.

Zhai J, Zhang L, Li M, et al. Epidural injection with or without steroid in managing chronic low back and lower extremity pain: a meta-analysis of ten randomized controlled trials. *Int J Clin Exp Med*. 2015;8:8304-8316.

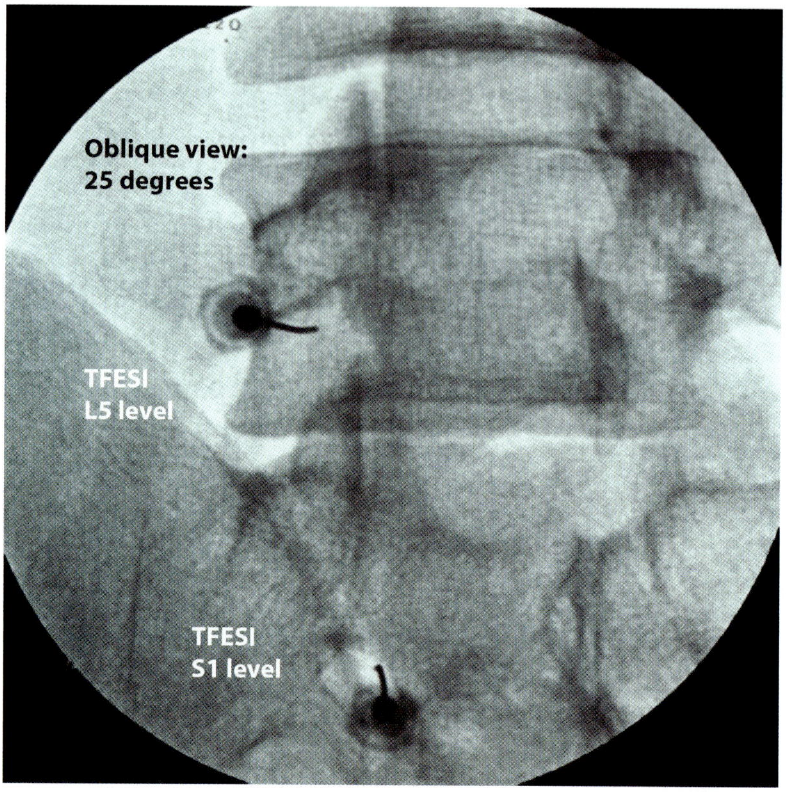

FIGURE 50.1. Transforaminal epidural steroid injection (TFESI) at L5 and S1 levels, oblique view at 25°.

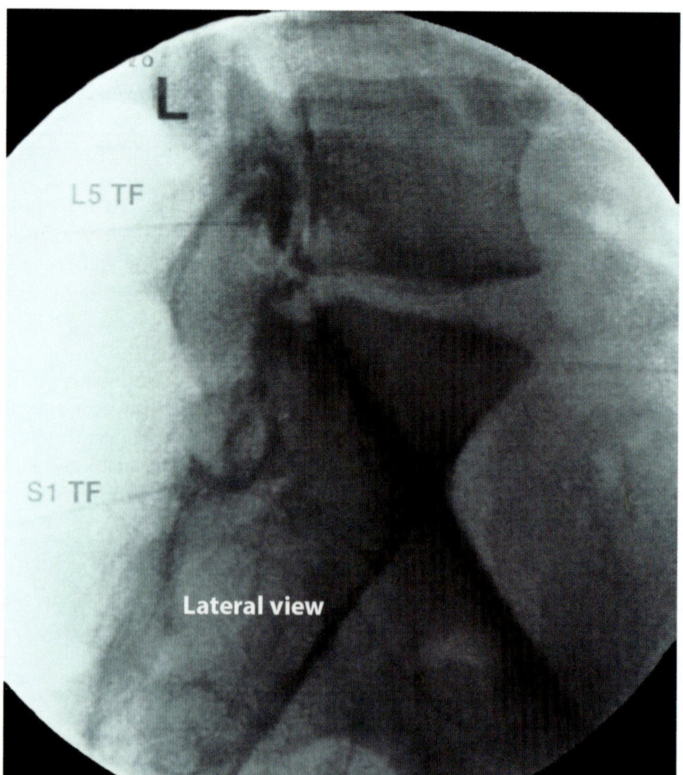

FIGURE 50.2. Transforaminal epidural steroid injection at L5 and S1 levels, lateral view.

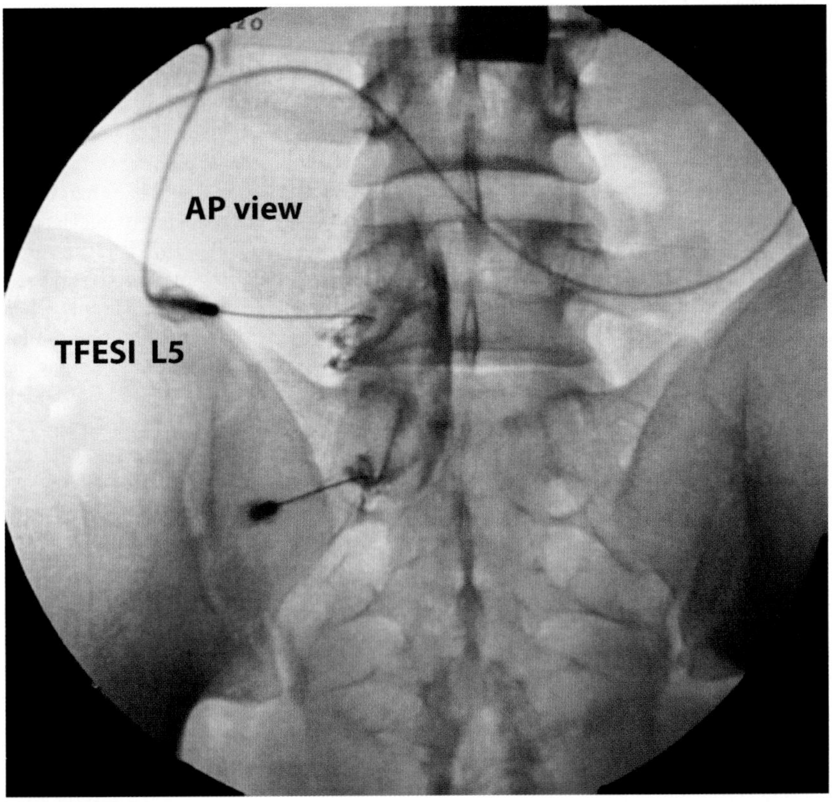

FIGURE 50.3. Transforaminal epidural steroid injection (TFESI) at L5 and S1 levels, anterior-posterior (AP) view (after digital subtraction image checking).

B.4. What are some of other approaches in minimally invasive interventions?

There are different interventional techniques for management of low back pain and sciatica that can be applied to appropriately selected patients. These include:

- Epidural neuroplasty or epidural adhesiolysis
- Epiduroscopy (spinal canal endoscopy)
- Automated percutaneous discectomy (APD) or percutaneous automated discectomy (PAD) or percutaneous automated nucleotomy (PAN)
- Percutaneous laser disc decompression (PLDD)
- Intradiscal electrothermal therapy (IDET)
- Percutaneous disc decompression using nucleoplasty
- Percutaneous lumbar discectomy using the Dekompressor probe
- Minimally invasive lumbar decompression (MILD) procedure
- SCS versus DRG stimulation
- Intrathecal drug delivery
- Percutaneous vertebroplasty (PV) and percutaneous kyphoplasty (PK)

Epidural neuroplasty or epidural adhesiolysis is done with hypertonic saline and hyaluronidase to lyse epidural adhesions. This involves placing a rigid catheter into the epidural space, with manipulation of the catheter to physically release the adhesions and applying local anesthetic, steroid, hypertonic saline (10%), and hyaluronidase over several days.

Epiduroscopy (or spinal canal endoscopy) allows direct visualization of the epidural space using a flexible fiberoptic catheter. Adhesions are lysed with the catheter under direct vision; thereafter, better delivery of medications to the target area can be achieved.

Percutaneous manual nucleotomy was first presented in 1975 as a method of preventing perineural and epidural scar formation by avoidance of entry into the spinal canal. Thereafter, APD or PAD or PAN was designed as a procedure using a "nucleotome" (reciprocating suction-cutting probe) for intradiscal decompression in 1985. The cannula requires a sizable annular incision to reach the nucleus. Its success rate is 70% to 80%.

PLDD, introduced in 1987, uses neodymium:yttrium-aluminum-garnet (Nd:YAG) laser to vaporize a small portion of the nucleus pulposus in an attempt to decompress the involved disc. The inner pressure of the nucleus pulposus drops significantly after disc ablation with a success rate of approximately 78%. After 4 to 6 months from this treatment, one-third of repeat MRI scans showed a modest-to-moderate decrease in the size of disc herniation. There is concern, nevertheless, that the technique is potentially hazardous to bone and nerve tissue because of the significant rise in temperature resulting from thermal energy transfer.

IDET or annuloplasty has been shown to be effective in managing discogenic pain. It is a minimally invasive procedure in which a catheter is inserted into the nucleus pulposus through which an electrode is passed so that a controlled level of heat at a temperature of 90 °C (194 °F) can be applied to a broad section of the affected disc's inner wall. This thermal therapy is postulated to alleviate discogenic pain by shrinking collagen at a target temperature of 65 °C (149 °F) to 75 °C (167 °F). Another proposed mechanism is denervation of exposed nociceptor endings in the outer disc annulus starting at 45 °C (113 °F).

Percutaneous disc decompression with nucleoplasty is used for those patients whose symptoms are attributed to radiographically contained discs, that is, a disc with an intact outer annulus. Since 2000, by combining tissue removal with thermal treatment, disc decompression has been achieved. It applies a focused "coblation" technique, ablating while coagulating (by using bipolar radiofrequency) to reach the level of 40 °C (104 °F) to 70 °C (158 °F). At this temperature, molecular dissociation is achieved and thought to minimize the potential for surrounding tissue damage.

Percutaneous disc decompression using a Dekompressor probe is another option for those patients whose symptoms are attributed to radiographically contained discs. It provides objective evidence that disc was removed, the cellular character of that material, and provides a qualitative and quantitative measure.

MILD is a procedure that involves limited percutaneous laminotomy and thinning of the ligamentum flavum in order to increase the critical diameter of the stenosed spinal canal.

For SCS, electrodes are passed into the posterior epidural space. Electrical stimulation of the spinal cord is effective in the management of certain neuropathic pain syndromes and PLSs. The mechanism by which pain relief is achieved remains controversial. A systematic review of the literature reported level II evidence for the use of SCS for FBSS on a long-term basis. Newer advances in spinal stimulation include high-frequency (10 kHz), burst, and DRG stimulation. High-frequency stimulation preferentially blocks larger diameter fibers and concomitantly recruits medium and small fibers. Burst stimulation involves delivering closely spaced, high-frequency stimuli to the spinal cord as opposed to the usual low-frequency tonic stimulation, which is constant. Therefore, it can provide a benefit by breaking through the physiologic tolerance issue derived from tonic stimulation. The DRG contains the primary sensory neurons that transmit pain signals from peripheral nerves to the brain, and can modulate or filter the transmission of peripheral painful signals. A recent study showed that DRG stimulation induced pain relief in patients with failed back pain syndrome. These reductions in pain were also associated with improvements in quality of life and disability. An analysis in 2023 of 13 studies with a combined total of 669 participants reported that although mean function was slightly better and opioid use was 15% lower with the addition of SCS to medical management, current evidence indicates that SCS does not have sustained clinical benefit that would outweigh the cost and risks of this surgical intervention.

Intrathecal drug delivery directly into the cerebrospinal fluid through an implanted catheter and pump can be used to treat intractable pain from a variety of causes, both nociceptive and neuropathic. A variety of medications and combinations can be used depending on the type and location of symptoms. This is known as *intrathecal polyanalgesia*, and is indicated when increasing doses of opioid are required to achieve pain relief but at the expense of disabling side effects. The dose is effectively reduced to approximately 1/300, for example, when converting an oral dose of morphine to its equipotent equivalent delivered intrathecally.

PV and PK are both advanced techniques used in the treatment of painful compression fracture. In the United States, compression fractures occur in approximately 700,000 patients per year, and 80% of these fractures occur in females. Conventional management includes bed rest, analgesics, and bracing. PV was a technique developed in 1984 for the treatment of painful vertebral hemangiomas. It has since become popular for treatment of osteoporotic vertebral body compression fracture. It involves application of liquid cement (polymethylmethacrylate), tobramycin, and barium powder (as nonionic contrast) through a special metal needle inserted under fluoroscopy. Cement provides vertebral solidification and buttresses the compressed bone within the vertebral body. The procedure usually takes 45 to 60 minutes, and the patient can be discharged several hours later. Some risks are involved, such as leakage of cement into surrounding areas (ie, disc, spinal cord, and nerve roots), infection, bleeding, worsened pain, embolism, and paralysis. Overall, over 80% of treated patients had moderate to marked pain relief.

PK, approved by the FDA in 1998, is similar to PV and involves the additional application of an inflatable balloon inside the collapsed vertebral body. The compressed fracture is thus expanded, the lost height of the vertebral body is restored, and an inner space or cavity is created for the cement. A significant reconstitution of the curvature of the spine can be seen following kyphoplasty. In 70% of the collapsed vertebral bodies, the kyphoplasty restored 47% of lost height. This newer technique offers the additional advantage of realigning the spinal column and restoring height to the fractured vertebrae.

Benzon HT, Rathmell JP, Wu CL, et al, eds. *Practical Management of Pain*. 5th ed. Mosby Elsevier; 2014:312-327.

Heavner JE, Racz GB, Raj P. Percutaneous epidural neuroplasty: prospective evaluation of 0.9% NaCl versus 10% NaCl with or without hyaluronidase. *Reg Anesth Pain Med*. 1999;24:202-207.

Kallewaard JW, Nijhuis H, Huygen F, et al. Prospective cohort analysis of DRG stimulation for failed back surgery syndrome pain following lumbar discectomy. *Pain Pract*. 2019;19:204-210.

Peh WC, Gilula LA, Peck DD. Percutaneous vertebroplasty for severe osteoporotic vertebral body compression fractures. *Radiology*. 2002;223:121-126.

Saal JS, Saal JA. Management of chronic discogenic low back pain with a thermal intradiscal catheter. *Spine (Phila Pa 1976)*. 2000;25:382-388.

Schmidt GL. The use of spinal cord stimulation/neuromodulation in the management of chronic pain. *J Am Acad Orthop Surg*. 2019;27:e401-e407.

Traeger AC, Gilbert SE, Harris IA, et al. Spinal cord stimulation for low back pain. *Cochrane Database Syst Rev*. 2023;3: CD014789.

Vorobeychik Y, Bogduk N. Intradiscal Therapies for Low Back Pain. In: Ballantyne JC, Fishman SM, Rathmell JP, eds. *Bonica's Management of Pain*. 5th ed. Wolters Kluwer; 2018: 1643-1652.

B.5. What are the concerns about magnetic resonance imaging (MRI) safety in patients with a spinal cord stimulator (SCS)?

MRI safety recommendations vary between models of SCS devices. Recent updates reveal that multiple models from different companies are more compatible with MRI full body scan (eg, Prime Advanced SureScan, Restore Advanced SureScan, Restore Sensor SureScan and Intellis platform from Medtronic, Proclaim Elite SCS system from Abbott, Precision Montage from Boston Scientific, and Senza I from Nevro). Other models might be compatible with just head or "head and extremity" only MRI scans. In addition, each company's SCS has specific parameters and limitations including MRI system type (1.5 T), radiofrequency coil type, radiofrequency power specific absorption rate (SAR), gradient slew rate, spatial gradient, patient position, total active scan time limits (30 minutes on per 30 minutes off vs 30 minutes on per 60 minutes off), and others.

Before an MRI is performed, it is imperative to ascertain that the system is intact, without any lead breaks or low impedances because these can result in heating of the SCS and injury to the patient. With an SCS, there is a risk of thermal injury to the patient at any point along the course of the device because of induction of current by the magnetic fields during the MRI.

During these scans, there is potential for heating or discomfort, and the patient must be advised to communicate with the technicians should this occur. The devices are also at risk for permanent malfunction after MRI, which would require surgical replacement. Magnetic pull could result in torque or rotation movement of the device with potential destruction of surrounding tissues. After the scan, the device must be interrogated for device damage or failure and turned back on. Ultimately, these devices have specific conditions under which MRI can be performed, and physicians must consult the manual for the specific implanted device before ordering MRI scans.

Harned ME, Gish B, Zuelzer A, et al. Anesthetic considerations and perioperative management of spinal cord stimulators: literature review and initial recommendations. *Pain Physician*. 2017;20:319-329.

Rubino S, Adepoju A, Kumar V, et al. MRI conditionality in patients with spinal cord stimulation devices. *Stereotact Funct Neurosurg*. 2016;94:254-258.

Walsh KM, Machado AG, Krishnaney AA. Spinal cord stimulation: a review of the safety literature and proposal for perioperative evaluation and management. *Spine J*. 2015;15:1864-1869.

B.6. When should surgery be considered?

Several surgeries are indicated for low back pain and sciatica. These include laminotomy, laminectomy, microdiscectomy, foraminotomy, intervertebral body insertion, spinal fusion, and others. Long-term results appear to be no different between the surgical or nonsurgical group in the case of low back pain. If the following situations occur, surgery should be considered:

- Failure to respond to conservative management for at least 3 months
- A profound or progressing neurologic defect such as a complete foot drop
- Recurring episodes of intractable sciatica involving the same segment, mainly to avoid the cumulative disability of repeated events

Muscle weakness is a dubious indication for surgery if the paresis is of unknown duration. If the pressure on the nerve root can be relieved immediately after the appearance of the paresis, surgery has been regarded as the therapy of choice. Unfortunately, most patients are unaware of the subtle loss of motor function. The greatest concern and complaints are largely centered on pain, paresthesia, and immobility.

Within the first 3 months of acute low back symptoms, surgery is considered only when serious spinal pathology or nerve root dysfunction resulting from an obviously herniated lumbar disc is detected. Nerve root decompression can be considered for a patient if all of the following criteria exist:

- Sciatica is both severe and disabling.
- Symptoms of sciatica persist without improvement for longer than 4 weeks or with extreme progression.
- There is strong physiologic evidence of dysfunction of a specific nerve root with intervertebral disc herniation confirmed ipsilaterally at the corresponding level by imaging.

Patients with acute low back pain alone, without findings of serious conditions or significant nerve root compression, rarely benefit from a surgical consultation. With or without surgery, more than 80% of patients with obvious surgical indications eventually recover. On the other hand, Atlas et al found that surgically treated patients with a herniated lumbar disc had more complete relief of leg pain and improved function and satisfaction compared with nonsurgical treated patients over 10 years. Nevertheless, improvement in the patient's predominant symptom and work and disability outcomes were similar regardless of treatment received.

Atlas SJ, Keller RB, Wu YA, et al. Long-term outcomes of surgical and nonsurgical management of sciatica secondary to a lumbar disc herniation: 10 year results from the maine lumbar spine study. *Spine (Phila Pa 1976)*. 2005;20:927-935.

Benzon HT, Rathmell JP, Wu CL, et al, eds. *Practical Management of Pain*. 5th ed. Mosby Elsevier; 2014:162-184, 312-327, 328-334.

Slipman CW, Derby R, Simeone FS, et al, eds. *Interventional Spine: An Algorithmic Approach*. Saunders Elsevier; 2008:939-966.

B.7. What surgical options are available for the treatment of disc disease or lumbar spinal stenosis?

- Artificial disc replacement (ADR) or total disc replacement (TDR)
- Interspinous process decompression system (X-STOP in 2005 and Coflex device in 2012)
- Annular closure device
- Decompression (laminotomy, laminectomy, and/or discectomy) or decompression with fusion

Since its development by German orthopedic surgeons in the mid-1980s, a metal and plastic prosthesis known as the *SB CHARITÉ* disc has been in use. The design of artificial discs for the lower back are still evolving and improving. When compared to spinal fusion surgery with two vertebrae locked in place, putting additional stress on discs above and below the fusion site which can result in adjacent segment degeneration (ASD), ADR, or TDR is intended to duplicate the function level of a normal, healthy disc and retain motion in the spine. ASD can develop at approximately 3% per year (or 16.5% at 5 years, 36.1% at 10 years).

In October 2004, the CHARITÉ artificial disc became the first to be approved for disc replacement in the United States. It is composed of two metallic end plates and a polyethylene core that moves between them (**Figures 50.4-50.7**). Other lumbar prosthetic discs are available (eg, ProDisc-L one level

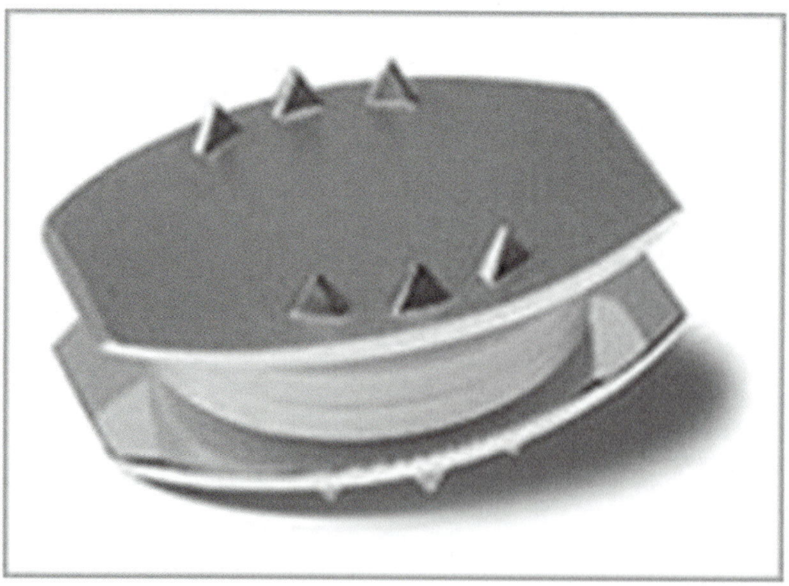

FIGURE 50.4. CHARITÉ disc. (Courtesy of DePuy Spine, a Johnson & Johnson company.)

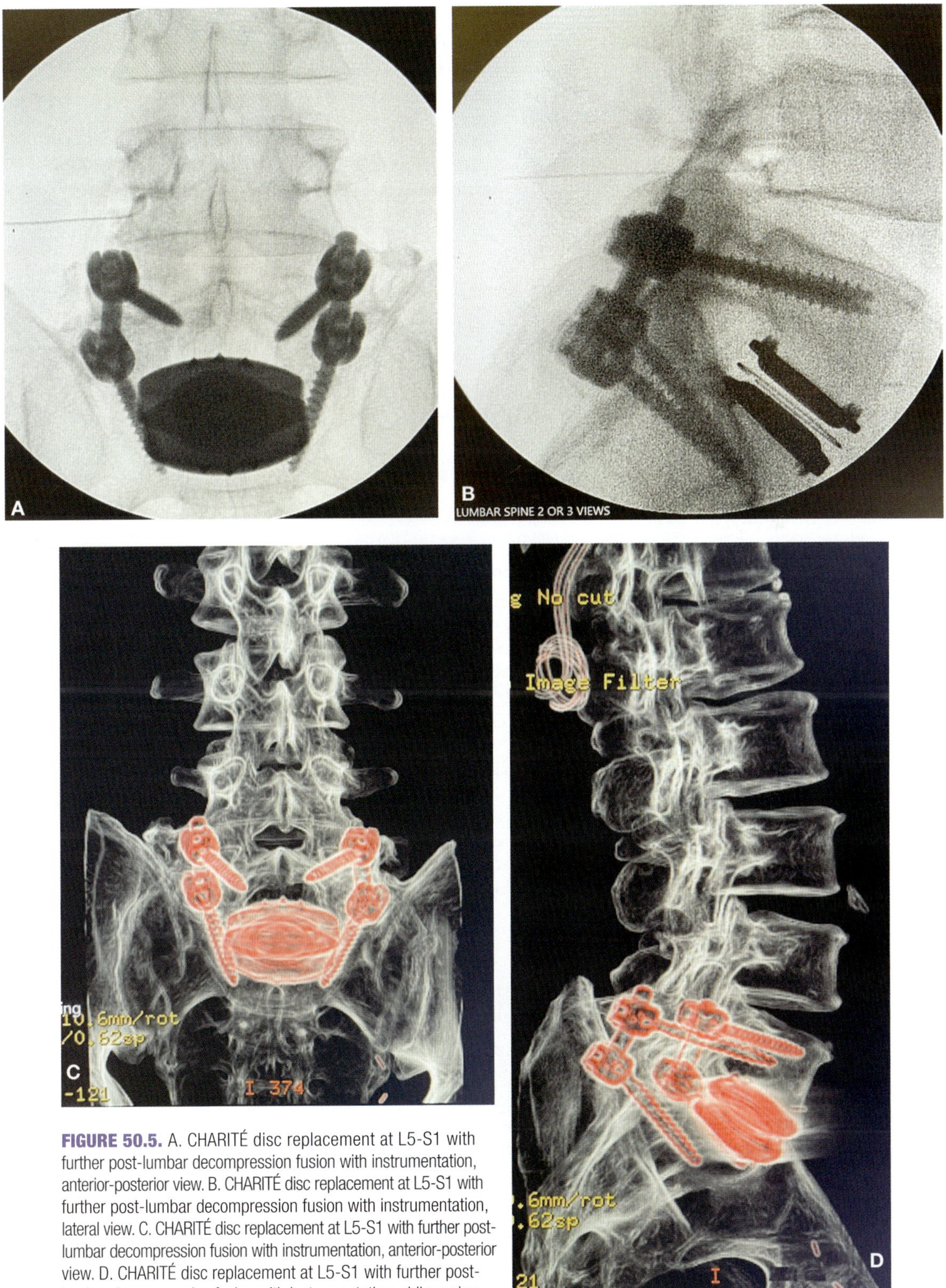

FIGURE 50.5. A. CHARITÉ disc replacement at L5-S1 with further post-lumbar decompression fusion with instrumentation, anterior-posterior view. B. CHARITÉ disc replacement at L5-S1 with further post-lumbar decompression fusion with instrumentation, lateral view. C. CHARITÉ disc replacement at L5-S1 with further post-lumbar decompression fusion with instrumentation, anterior-posterior view. D. CHARITÉ disc replacement at L5-S1 with further post-lumbar decompression fusion with instrumentation, oblique view.

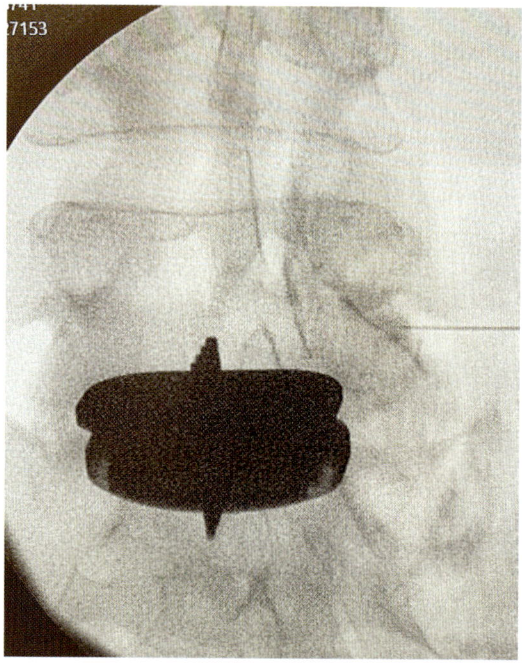

FIGURE 50.6. L5-S1 ProDisc-L ADR, fluoroscopic anterior-posterior view.

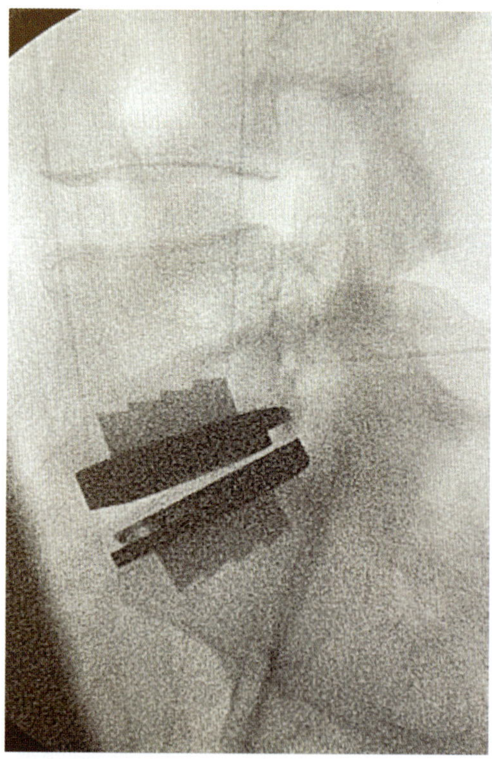

FIGURE 50.7. L5-S1 ProDisc-L ADR, fluoroscopic lateral view.

in 2006 and two-level in 2020, Maverick in 2002, FlexiCore, Kineflex and activ-L in 2015) and many more among cervical artificial discs (eg, ProDisc-C in 2007, Secure-C in 2012, Mobi-C in 2013, Prestig LP in 2016, M6 in 2019, Simplify for 1-level in 2020, and 2 level in 2021). The potential disadvantage of ADR is limited durability or implant wear due to polyethylene debris and the biologic sequelae which have been shown to cause osteolysis and aseptic loosening in total hip and knee replacement. For younger people with herniated discs (those in their 20s, 30s, or 40s), revision surgery could become an issue after decades if artificial discs deteriorate. Revision ADR can be very challenging because of scar tissue from the original surgery and nearby vascular structures. In addition, there is a 1% to 3% incidence of the complication of retrograde ejaculation in males from spinal ADR surgery.

Based on the systemic review of overlapping meta-analyses, the best available evidence indicated that TDR or ADR compared with fusion for lumbar degenerative disc disease (LDDD) had statistically, but not clinically, significant superiority regarding disability, pain relief, and quality of life in a selected group of patients in the short term. Therefore, considering that disadvantages may appear after years, spine surgeons should be cautious about performing TDR on a large scale. Another similar meta-analysis result in 2019 suggests that TDR could be alternative treatment for LDDD, because it yielded better clinical success and patient satisfaction, shorter hospital stays and operative time, less pain, and lower complication rates than did lumbar fusion.

In a retrospective study of ADR in 2017, overall clinical failure (one level operations performed at L4-L5 or L5-S1) occurred in 26% of patients at 2-year follow-up including Maverick (28%), Charité (39%), and Kineflex (14%). It implied that overall clinical success might be improved most by patient selection and implant type. For example, patients with facet joint arthrosis, spondylolisthesis, segmental autofusion (eg, ankylosing spondylitis), and poor bone quality are contraindications for TDR. With the advent of new generation implants, TDR has reemerged, more in cervical than lumbar spine, and has shown favorable outcomes compared to fusion surgery. The biggest challenge for TDR surgery is optimization of the available implants to minimize wear (implant wear) and extend longevity.

The interspinous process decompression system (X-STOP) is a titanium metal implant made to fit between the lumbar spinous processes of the vertebrae (**Figures 50.8**). It is designed to relieve narrowing

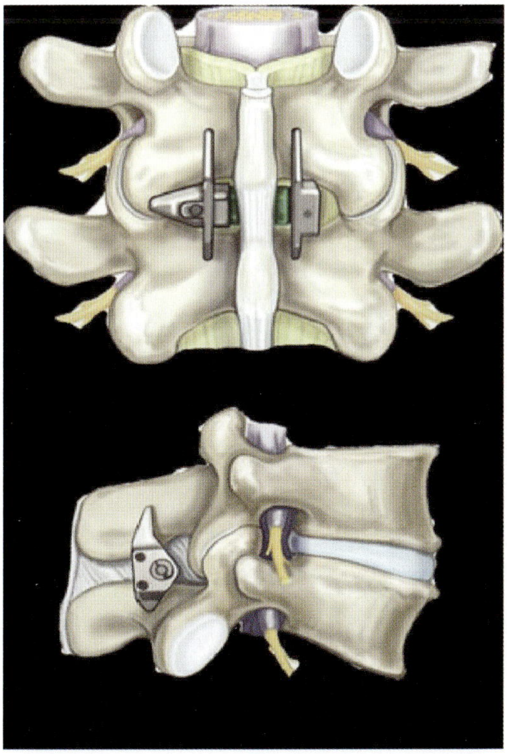

FIGURE 50.8. Interspinous process decompression system in place. (From Kondrashov DG, Hannibal M, Hsu KY, Zucherman JF. Interspinous process decompression with the X-STOP device for lumbar spinal stenosis: a 4-year follow-up study. *J Spinal Disord Tech.* 2006 Jul;19:323-7. Figure 2.)

of the spinal canal and neural foramen during extension, thereby reducing the symptoms of neurogenic intermittent claudication. The indications include spinal stenosis and degenerative lumbar spondylolisthesis. A Norwegian study in 2015 revealed that the higher cost of X-STOP is mainly due to implant cost and the higher reoperation rate (33%) when compared to minimally invasive decompression surgery in patients with symptomatic lumbar spinal stenosis.

In 2012, the FDA approved the Coflex interlaminar stabilization device, a small U-shaped titanium implant that provides spinal stability without the invasiveness and loss of mobility associated with spinal fusion. It is indicated for patients with moderate-to-severe lumbar spinal stenosis (LSS) who have undergone at least 6 months of nonoperative treatment. The surgery involves two steps including lumbar spine decompression first and then placement of Coflex device for interlaminar stabilization. It is intended to keep spine stable while maintaining normal height and motion. In 2022, a biomechanical effect study revealed both Coflex and X-stop spacers at the L4-L5 level can effectively decrease the range of motion (ROM) and intradiscal pressure in extension, without affecting the adjacent levels. A meta-analysis of 26 studies in 2023 showed that the Coflex device group had shorter operation time, less intraoperative blood loss, shorter hospital stays, lower VAS pain scores, lower complication rate, lower ASD, and higher ROM when compared to posterior lumbar fusion group for spinal stenosis. However, there was no significant difference in reoperation rate and internal fixation problem rate.

Surgical treatment options for lumbar disc herniation include microdiscectomy, lumbar fusion, TDR, and other minimally invasive applications. Microdiscectomy procedures are the most utilized techniques; however, they leave a defect in annulus fibrosus, which, if left untreated, can contribute to high reherniation rates (7%-18%) and changes in the biomechanics of the lumbar spine. A large defect in the annulus fibrosus after surgery is a major risk factor for reherniation. In 2022, a multicenter randomized clinical trial study revealed that annular closure with a bone-anchored implant (Barricaid, Intrinsic therapy) lowers the risk of symptomatic recurrence and reoperation over 5 years of follow-up in patients who are at high risk for recurrent disc herniation following microdiscectomy (Figures 50.9 and 50.10).

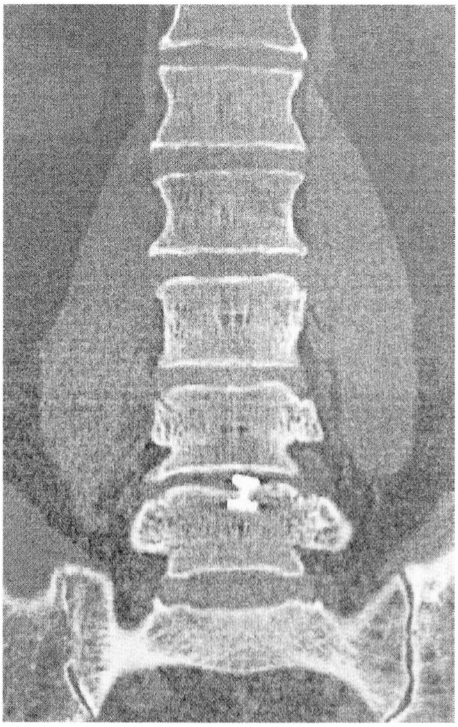

FIGURE 50.9. L4-L5 Annular closure device (Barricaid), computed tomography anterior-posterior view.

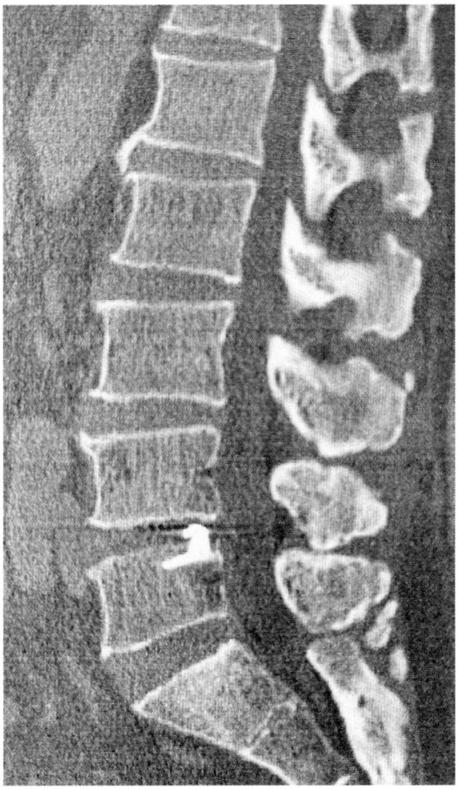

FIGURE 50.10. L4-L5 Annular closure device (Barricaid bvcfd), computed tomography lateral view.

Spinal surgery often involves direct decompression, where the pressure is reduced or removed from the nerve; it can include laminotomy, laminectomy, foraminotomy, or discectomy. These surgeries can be done by either a traditional open approach or a minimally invasive technique/minimally invasive surgery (MIS). The latter can avoid separation of muscles and preserve stabilizing structures. It has many surgical advantages such as less muscle trauma, minimal postoperative back pain, earlier mobilization, shorter hospital stays, and faster recovery. The MIS decompression technique can be done by using a microscopic, tubular (using tubular retractors), or endoscopic decompression technique such as percutaneous transforaminal endoscopic discectomy (PTED).

Degenerative spondylolisthesis in the lumbar spine occurs when the cephalad vertebral body slips relative to the caudal body. Symptoms can result from spinal stenosis and nerve root compression. Surgical management of this condition entails decompression of the spinal canal followed by posterolateral fusion with or without an interbody fusion. The additional anterior stabilization of the vertebral column with an interbody fusion reduces the incidence of nonunion, degree of slippage, and recurrence of deformity in patients with degenerative spondylolisthesis. Additional anterior stabilization can be accomplished by using different approaches such as anterior lumbar interbody fusion (ALIF), posterior lumbar interbody fusion (PLIF), transforaminal lumbar interbody fusion (TLIF), or eXtreme lateral interbody fusion (XLIF).

Symptomatic LSS is characterized by pain and discomfort in the lower back and the lower extremities, impaired walking ability (intermittent neurogenic claudication), and functional disability. Imaging shows a narrowing of the lumbar spinal canal. The surgical procedure for LSS is the most frequently performed procedure in the adult lumbar spine. A randomized clinical trial that compared three minimally invasive surgical techniques (unilateral laminotomy with crossover, bilateral laminotomy, and spinous process osteotomy) for LSS revealed no differences in clinical outcomes or complication rates.

Guo A, Liu G, Wang L, et al. Biomechanical effect of Coflex and X-stop spacers on the lumbar spine: a finite element analysis. *Am J Transl Res.* 2022;14:5155-5163.

Hermansen E, Austevoll IM, Hellum C, et al. Comparison of 3 different minimally invasive surgical techniques for lumbar spinal stenosis. *JAMA Netw Open.* 2022;5:e224291.

Lee CW, Yoon KJ, Ha SS. Comparative analysis between three different lumbar decompression techniques (microscopic, tubular, and endoscopic) in lumbar canal and lateral recess stenosis: preliminary report. *Biomed Res Int.* 2019;2019:6078469.

Li T, Yan J, Ren Q et al. Efficacy and safety of lumbar dynamic stabilization device coflex for lumbar spinal stenosis: a systemic review and meta-analysis. *World Neurosurg.* 2023;170:7-20.

Othman YA, Verma R, Qureshi SA. Artificial disc replacement in spine surgery. *Ann Transl Med.* 2019;7:S170.

Pettine K, Ryu R, Techy F. Why lumbar artificial disk replacement (LADRs) fail. *Clin Spine Surg.* 2017;30:E743-E747.

Thome C, Kursumovic A, Klassen PD, et al. Effectiveness of an annular closure device to prevent recurrent lumbar disc herniation. A secondary analysis with 5 years of follow-up. *JAMA Netw Open.* 2021;4:e2136809.

Perioperative Pain Management and Multimodal Pain Management

51

Mohammad M. Piracha, Anuj Malhotra, and Vinod Malhotra

A 70-year-old female is scheduled for nonemergent surgery for right hip fracture after a fall. The patient was very dissatisfied with postoperative pain management after a prior surgery done under general anesthesia 3 months earlier.

A. Perioperative Pain Management for Inpatient Surgery

1. What is your advice to this patient for the planned open reduction and internal fixation (ORIF) of her right hip and postoperative pain relief?
2. How will you decide about the choice of anesthetic technique?
3. What is chronic postsurgical pain (CPSP)?
4. What would be your perioperative analgesic strategy?
5. Does the choice of analgesic technique influence postoperative outcome?
6. Does the choice of drugs influence the efficacy or safety of epidural analgesia?
7. What are the usual doses and concentrations of the anesthetic combinations commonly employed in epidural analgesia?
8. If accidental dural puncture occurs during placement of the epidural needle, what steps should be taken?
9. What are the alternatives to epidural analgesia?
10. What is the usual clinical regimen for intravenous patient-controlled analgesia (IV-PCA) and is special patient monitoring required during its use?
11. What are the side effects and complications of epidural analgesia?
12. What recommendations for placement and removal of the epidural catheter would you make if this patient is on antiplatelet or anticoagulant therapy or if thromboprophylaxis is planned?

A 27-year-old male presents for elective shoulder arthroscopy. Preoperative evaluation reveals a history of OUD being treated with buprenorphine/naloxone 8/2 mg sublingual tablets twice daily with treatment initiated within the last 60 days.

B. Perioperative Pain Management and Medications for Opioid Use Disorder (OUD)

1. What are the unique pharmacologic aspects of buprenorphine?
2. What are the considerations if a patient is taking buprenorphine for chronic pain versus medication treatment for opioid use disorder (OUD)?
3. What are the management strategies for perioperative pain control in a patient taking buprenorphine for OUD?
4. What issues need to be considered before discharging a patient taking buprenorphine for OUD?
5. What can be done if a patient is identified with untreated OUD perioperatively?
6. What are the legal ramifications of buprenorphine prescribing?

A. Perioperative Pain Management for Inpatient Surgery

A.1. What is your advice to this patient for the planned open reduction and internal fixation (ORIF) of her right hip and postoperative pain relief?

It is essential that patients undergoing any surgery be informed about what to expect postoperatively because realistic expectations of pain and rehabilitation can promote recovery and return to normal activity. It is also important that providers identify patients with preoperative pain and those at risk for severe acute postoperative pain as these are known risk factors for chronic postsurgical pain (CPSP) if perioperative analgesia is not managed appropriately.

Different modalities can be used to manage pain intraoperatively, immediately following surgery, within the first few postoperative days, and for discharge home, and each of these should be discussed. Pain management for these cases often involves a step-down approach from neuraxial or regional analgesia to intravenous opioids to oral medications. The following issues should be addressed:

- Information should be given on how pain will be assessed, for example, the use of visual analog or numerical rating scores.
- Patients require a realistic expectation of the intensity and duration of postoperative pain.
- Pain management techniques that require patient involvement (IV-PCA, PCEA) need to be properly explained in advance with confirmation that the patient can participate in their care.
- Resources for chronic pain management should be discussed in case the pain goes beyond the expected duration.

Johnson RL, Kopp SL, Kessler J, et al. Peripheral nerve blocks and ultrasound guidance for regional anesthesia; Hurley RW, Elkassabany NM, Wu CL. Acute postoperative pain; Castro De Oliveira BM, Vazquez R. Anesthesia for orthopedic surgery. In: Gropper MA, Eriksson LI, Fleisher LA, et al, eds. *Miller's Anesthesia*. 10th ed. Elsevier; 2023:1305–1330; 1458–1475; 1952–1983.

Tetsunaga T, Sato T, Shiota N, et al. Comparison of continuous epidural analgesia, patient-controlled analgesia with morphine, and continuous three-in-one femoral nerve block on postoperative outcomes after total hip arthroplasty. *Clin Orthop Surg*. 2015;7:164-170.

Zaccagnino MP, Bader AM, Sang CN, et al. The perioperative surgical home: a new role for the acute pain service. *Anesth Analg*. 2017;125:1394-1402.

A.2. How will you decide about the choice of anesthetic technique?

The decision about which anesthetic technique to use for an individual patient is based on a review of their overall medical condition and any medications that they are taking along with discussion with the surgeon. Surgical considerations include potential blood loss, hypotension, need for fluid restriction, and invasiveness of surgery. Anesthetic options include regional or neuraxial anesthesia, general anesthesia, or both. A combined spinal-epidural (CSE) technique is commonly used for ORIF of the hip. This technique allows for sufficient intraoperative anesthesia from the spinal anesthetic along with the ability to supplement anesthesia intraoperatively if needed and continued infusion postoperatively via the epidural catheter for postoperative pain control. Intraoperative epidural use prior to emergence has the benefit of ensuring epidural catheter function and can facilitate a more comfortable transition to the immediate postoperative period. Other factors such as surgeon preference, anesthesiologist experience and practice, desire for postoperative ambulation, need for perioperative anticoagulation or deep venous thrombosis (DVT) prophylaxis, and institutional protocols for postoperative pain relief also influence the choice of technique.

Use of lumbar epidural analgesia has become one option for management of pain associated with many lower extremity surgeries, including hip ORIF. Clinical studies have shown that lumbar epidural analgesia via infusion can have effects far beyond pain relief, including decreased opioid consumption, reduced risk of nausea and vomiting, improved bowel recovery, and a significant reduction in the incidence of myocardial infarction. More recently, peripheral nerve blocks have become more widely used over epidural analgesia for hip surgery due to several key factors that offer distinct advantages for both patients and clinicians.

Firstly, peripheral nerve blocks, such as the PENG block (pericapsular nerve group block), fascia iliaca block, and femoral block, provide targeted pain relief. These blocks specifically target the nerves innervating the hip region, leading to effective analgesia without the widespread sensory and motor block associated with epidurals. This targeted approach reduces the risk of complications such as hypotension, urinary retention, and motor block, which can impede early mobilization and rehabilitation.

Secondly, peripheral nerve blocks have a better safety profile compared to epidural analgesia. Epidurals carry risks such as dural puncture, epidural hematoma, and infection, which can lead to serious complications. Peripheral nerve blocks, being less invasive, have a lower incidence of these complications, making them a safer option for many patients.

Thirdly, peripheral nerve blocks allow for easier management in the perioperative period. They can be administered quickly and do not require the same level of postprocedure monitoring as epidural analgesia. This ease of administration and management is particularly beneficial in busy surgical settings where efficiency and patient throughput are critical.

Lastly, the advent of ultrasound guidance has significantly improved the precision and efficacy of peripheral nerve blocks. Ultrasound allows for real-time visualization of anatomic structures, ensuring accurate placement of the local anesthetic around the target nerves. This increased accuracy translates to more reliable pain relief and fewer complications.

Chou R, Gordon DB, de Leon-Casasola OA, et al. Management of postoperative pain: a clinical practice guideline from the American Pain Society, the American Society of Regional Anesthesia and Pain Medicine, and the American Society of Anesthesiologists' Committee on Regional Anesthesia, Executive Committee, and Administrative Council. *J Pain*. 2016;17:131-157.

Guay J, Parker MJ, Gajendragadkar PR, Kopp S. Anaesthesia for hip fracture surgery in adults. *Cochrane Database Syst Rev*. 2016;2:CD000521.

Johnson RL, Kopp SL, Kessler J, et al. Peripheral nerve blocks and ultrasound guidance for regional anesthesia; Hurley RW, Elkassabany NM, Wu CL. Acute postoperative pain; Castro De Oliveira BM, Vazquez R. Anesthesia for orthopedic surgery. In: Gropper MA, Eriksson LI, Fleisher LA, et al, eds. *Miller's Anesthesia*. 10th ed. Elsevier; 2023:1305–1330; 1458–1475; 1952–1983.

A.3. What is chronic postsurgical pain (CPSP)?

CPSP is defined as pain that recurs or persists at least 2 months after surgery and is not related to ongoing tissue injury such as recurrence of tumor, wound dehiscence, or infection. The incidence of CPSP can vary greatly based on the surgery and has been quoted to range from as low as 5% to as high as 30%. CPSP often has a neuropathic component that differentiates it from usual postsurgical pain, but not always and there can be a mixed picture. Several studies suggest that severe perioperative pain is a predictor for development of CPSP, and thus aggressive management of early postoperative pain might be important to prevent this transition.

Johnson RL, Kopp SL, Kessler J, et al. Peripheral nerve blocks and ultrasound guidance for regional anesthesia; Hurley RW, Elkassabany NM, Wu CL. Acute postoperative pain; Castro De Oliveira BM, Vazquez R. Anesthesia for orthopedic surgery. In: Gropper MA, Eriksson LI, Fleisher LA, et al, eds. *Miller's Anesthesia*. 10th ed. Elsevier; 2023:1305–1330; 1458–1475; 1952–1983.

Lu Y, Hu B, Dai H, Wang B, Yao J, Yao X. Predictors of chronic postsurgical pain in elderly patients undergoing hip arthroplasty: a multi-center retrospective cohort study. *Int J Gen Med*. 2021;14:7885-7894.

Thapa P, Euasobhon P. Chronic postsurgical pain: current evidence for prevention and management. *Korean J Pain*. 2018;31:155-173.

A.4. What would be your perioperative analgesic strategy?

The analgesic plan should consider the entire perioperative period and ideally be determined in advance. A multimodal approach would be preferable to account for the multiple pathways by which nociceptive input is conveyed to the central nervous system, the number of pharmacologically distinct mechanisms of modulating this input, the need for effective analgesia throughout the perioperative period and after discharge, and the importance of minimizing side effects by avoiding higher dosing of any one agent (particularly opioids).

Epidural analgesia is the main recommended therapy for reasons discussed in the previous section. Contraindications to an epidural include patient refusal, coagulopathy, thrombocytopenia, therapeutic anticoagulation, previous lumbar spine surgery at the level of intended epidural placement, and local infection over the entry site. When epidural catheters fail intraoperatively or have patchy coverage, femoral nerve block or fascia iliaca nerve block can supplement or replace epidural analgesia.

Nonsteroidal anti-inflammatory drugs (NSAIDs) are useful for treating joint pain secondary to surgical trauma. A concern with NSAIDs is platelet dysfunction; however, their efficacy and lack of respiratory side effects make them an optimal choice for adjunct analgesia when possible. Cyclooxygenase-2

(COX-2) inhibitors have more limited effects on platelet aggregation and comparable efficacy to traditional NSAIDs and thus can be of use in this setting. Adverse cardiac side effects are unlikely with short-term perioperative dosing unless preexisting heart failure is present. Regular administration of paracetamol or acetaminophen (APAP) is also useful for treating postoperative pain. Topical lidocaine patch or use of gabapentinoids can have a role in select patients. Other options for procedural hip analgesia that have become the predominant options over epidural analgesia include the PENG block, fascia iliaca block, and femoral block. Each of these plays a distinct role in managing pain following hip fracture and hip arthroplasty.

The PENG block is a relatively new block specifically designed for pain management in hip fractures and surgery. It targets the articular branches of the femoral nerve, accessory obturator nerve, and obturator nerve which innervate the hip capsule to provide effective analgesia for hip pain. This block is advantageous because it can provide targeted pain relief without causing significant motor block, which is beneficial for early mobilization and rehabilitation.

The fascia iliaca block is commonly used for pain management in hip fracture and hip surgery. It involves the injection of local anesthetic underneath the fascia iliaca, spreading to block the femoral, obturator, and lateral femoral cutaneous nerves. This results in analgesia for the anterior and lateral hip, thigh, and knee. This block is relatively easy to perform and has a low risk of complications. It provides good pain relief, improving patient comfort and facilitating early mobilization and rehabilitation.

The femoral block, or femoral nerve block, is also used to provide analgesia for hip fracture, particularly in the preoperative and postoperative periods. It involves the injection of local anesthetic around the femoral nerve, resulting in anesthesia of the anterior thigh and knee, as well as partial anesthesia of the hip joint. This block can provide significant pain relief for patients with hip fracture, reducing the need for systemic opioids and their associated side effects. However, it can cause motor block of the quadriceps muscle, which can affect mobility.

Choi JV, Cheung RM, Mozel MR, Merchant RN, Lee SM. Perioperative outcomes after preoperative epidural analgesia in patients with hip fracture undergoing surgical repair: a systematic review. *Pain Med.* 2022;23:234-245.

Fahey A, Cripps E, Ng A, Sweeny A, Snelling PJ. Pericapsular nerve group block for hip fracture is feasible, safe and effective in the emergency department: a prospective observational comparative cohort study. *Emerg Med Australas.* 2022;34:884-891.

Gola W, Bialka S, Owczarek AJ, Misiolek H. Effectiveness of fascia iliaca compartment block after elective total hip replacement: a prospective, randomized, controlled study. *Int J Environ Res Public Health.* 2021;18:4891.

Min BW, Kim Y, Cho HM, et al. Perioperative pain management in total hip arthroplasty: Korean hip society guidelines. *Hip Pelvis.* 2016;28:15-23.

Muse IO, Deiling B, Grinman L, Hadeed MM, Elkassabany N. Peripheral nerve blocks for hip fractures. *J Clin Med.* 2024;13:3457.

Scala VA, Lee LSK, Atkinson RE. Implementing regional nerve blocks in hip fracture programs: a review of regional nerve blocks, protocols in the literature, and the current protocol at the Queen's Medical Center in Honolulu, HI. *Hawaii J Health Soc Welf.* 2019;78:11-15.

A.5. Does the choice of analgesic technique influence postoperative outcome?

Evidence from multiple studies suggests that epidural analgesia is associated with lower rates of perioperative morbidity, particularly fewer pulmonary and cardiac complications. Mortality might also be reduced, as indicated by a meta-analysis of patients receiving epidural analgesia versus PCA after surgery requiring general anesthesia, which demonstrated decreased mortality in the epidural group. However, there is less evidence supporting its use for less invasive procedures. The benefits of epidural analgesia are more pronounced in large open abdominal and thoracic surgeries. Compared with systemic opioids, epidural opioids decrease the incidence of postoperative atelectasis, hypoxemia, and overall pulmonary complications. Postoperative myocardial infarction rate is also reduced when epidural analgesia is incorporated into anesthesia and extended for at least 24 hours postoperatively. The cardioprotective mechanism of epidural analgesia is believed to be related to its sympatholytic effects.

Epidural analgesia also provides superior postoperative analgesia compared with IV-PCA in certain surgical cases. As discussed, better postoperative pain relief can reduce the likelihood of developing CPSP.

Guay J, Choi P, Suresh S, Albert N, Kopp S, Pace NL. Neuraxial blockade for the prevention of postoperative mortality and major morbidity: an overview of Cochrane systematic reviews. *Cochrane Database Syst Rev.* 2014;2014:CD010108.

Pöpping DM, Elia N, Van Aken HK, et al. Impact of epidural analgesia on mortality and morbidity after surgery: systematic review and meta-analysis of randomized controlled trials. *Ann Surg.* 2014;259:1056-1067.

Salicath JH, Yeoh EC, Bennett MH. Epidural analgesia versus patient-controlled intravenous analgesia for pain following intra-abdominal surgery in adults. *Cochrane Database Syst Rev*. 2018;8:CD010434.

Thapa P, Euasobhon P. Chronic postsurgical pain: current evidence for prevention and management. *Korean J Pain*. 2018;31:155-173.

A.6. Does the choice of drugs influence the efficacy or safety of epidural analgesia?

Effective postoperative pain control can be achieved by delivering an opioid, local anesthetic, or a combination of both into the epidural space. Combinations are most commonly used because synergy between opioids and local anesthetics enables balance between analgesia and minimizing blockade of motor function and sympatholysis. Common components include opioids, such as morphine, fentanyl, or hydromorphone, and local anesthetics, such as bupivacaine, levobupivacaine, or ropivacaine. Systemic absorption effects (eg, sedation) tend to be more common with the lipophilic opioids, such as fentanyl, presumably because of increased absorption into the epidural fat. Hydrophilic opioids, such as morphine, produce a wider dermatomal band of analgesia with less systemic absorption. Of the three commonly used local anesthetics, bupivacaine possesses the least favorable cardiac safety profile but is also the least expensive and most readily available. Ropivacaine offers the potential advantage of differential dose-dependent sensory and motor blockade; however, when used in dilute concentrations, it is unlikely that an advantage of one agent over the other will be apparent.

Garimella V, Cellini C. Postoperative pain control. *Clin Colon Rectal Surg*. 2013;26:191-196.

Ramdev B, Gopal T, Sharma DK. Safety and efficacy of patient controlled epidural analgesia versus conventional epidural analgesia in lower limb orthopedic surgeries: a prospective randomized study. *Ain-Shams J Anesthesiol*. 2023;15:46.

Rodgers A, Walker N, Schug S, et al. Reduction of postoperative mortality and morbidity with epidural or spinal anaesthesia: results from overview of randomised trials. *BMJ*. 2000;321:1493.

Tetsunaga T, Sato T, Shiota N, et al. Comparison of continuous epidural analgesia, patient-controlled analgesia with morphine, and continuous three-in-one femoral nerve block on postoperative outcomes after total hip arthroplasty. *Clin Orthop Surg*. 2015;7:164.

A.7. What are the usual doses and concentrations of the anesthetic combinations commonly employed in epidural analgesia?

Before the initiation of PCEA, a test dose of 3 mL of 1.5% lidocaine with epinephrine 1:200,000 is usually administered with the patient awake to rule out intrathecal or intravascular catheter placement. Once malposition is ruled out, a bolus is usually administered though the catheter (as allowed by hemodynamic status) prior to beginning continuous infusion.

Commonly employed combinations of epidural drugs vary. However, in the interest of patient safety, sterility, compliance, auditing, and quality assurance, standardization within the institution is recommended. Mixtures can later be titrated to achieve the desired effect or to avoid side effects, for example, increasing or decreasing local anesthetic concentration to change block density, increasing or decreasing volume infused to vary spread, and adding or subtracting opioids to increase analgesia or decrease opioid side effects such as itching, nausea, or sedation.

The following drugs and drug combinations are often used at a starting infusion rate of 4 to 6 mL/h with a demand bolus of 2 to 3 mL as needed and a lock out period between boluses. This clinical dosing is consistent with fluoroscopic epidurography that shows vertebral spread of 6 to 8 levels with a 2.5 to 5 mL bolus.

- Bupivacaine 0.0625% to 0.1% with fentanyl 5 μg/mL with a lockout period of 10 to 20 minutes
- Bupivacaine 0.0625% to 0.1% plain with a lockout period of 20 minutes
- Fentanyl 5 to 10 μg/mL plain with a lockout period of 10 to 20 minutes
- Bupivacaine 0.0625% to 0.1% with hydromorphone 100 μg/mL with a lockout period of 20 minutes (see sample order form, **Figure 51.1**)

Hong J, Jung SW. Fluoroscopically guided interlaminar epidural injection: a comparative epidurography study using 2.5 mL and 5 mL of contrast dye. *Pain Physician*. 2016;19:E1013-E1018.

A.8. If accidental dural puncture occurs during placement of the epidural needle, what steps should be taken?

If accidental dural puncture occurs during placement of the Tuohy needle, the general practice is to remove the needle and place the epidural catheter at an adjacent intervertebral space. The likelihood of intrathecal spread should be carefully assessed with the test dose. Epidural infusion can be started at the usual

NewYork-Presbyterian
The University Hospital of Columbia and Cornell

45171

EPIDURAL ANALGESIA ORDER SHEET
PAIN MANAGEMENT

IF NO PLATE, PRINT NAME, SEX AND MEDICAL RECORD NO.

DATE: / / TIME: am/pm	ORDER POSTED	CHECKED BY RN
1) Analgesia by epidural infusion (using the PCA infuser).		
2) The patient **MUST NOT** receive any supplemental narcotics, sedatives and/or antiemetics while receiving Epidural Analgesic unless orders are written by the Pain Management Service.		
3) Narcotic (Specify drug, # of mgs, volume, and diluent and concentration):		
4) Initial Bolus given by Pain Service M.D. (Dose given ________________) ml		
5) Initial Machine Settings: **Epidural Mode** (circle one) Continuous/Bolus/Both Program in ml. a) **Program in ml.** b) Bolus/Demand Dose _________ ml per attempt. c) Bolus/Demand Lockout ________ minutes. d) Continuous Rate ____________ ml per hour. e) Limit ______________________ ml per four hours.		
6) If pain is not controlled at the above settings (pain ≥ 6), the nurse may administer a PRN rescue/loading dose ____________ ml every 10 minutes until the patient is comfortable. The maximum rescue / loading dose is __________ ml Increase pump settings to: a) Bolus/Demand Dose _________ ml per attempt. b) Bolus/Demand Lockout ________ minutes. c) Continuous Rate ____________ ml per hour. d) Limit ______________________ ml per four hours.		
7) A) For oversedation (sedation scale ≥ 4/R4) and respiratory rates 10–14 minutes, notify Acute Pain Service, and decrease pump settings to: a) Bolus/Demand Dose _________ ml per attempt. b) Bolus/Demand Lockout________ minutes c) Continuous Rate ____________ ml per hour. d) Limit ______________________ ml per four hours B) For respiratory rate less than 10/minute, stop infusion and call the Acute Pain Service (X-66700, beeper 16664). C) For respiratory rate less than 8/minute, obtain naloxone (0.4 mg/ml) and administer 0.1 mg (0.25 ml) IV bolus q2 minutes until respiratory rate is 8/minute or greater, stop Infusion, and notify Pain Management Service (X-66700, beeper 16664).		
8) Upon initiation and after every loading dose, obtain BP, pulse, respiratory rates, sedation scale and sensory motor function (q30 min · 2 hours then q1 h · 2 then q4 hours. Pain analog q4 hours, Temp q12 hours).		
9) If no maintenance IV solution is ordered, IV to med lock.		
10) For Nausea (Specify drug and dosing):		
11) For Sleep (Specify drug and dosing):		
12) Activity level per surgical/medical orders.		
13) For questions or problems, call the Pain Management Service at X-62960 or page: X-66700, beeper 16664.		
14) Please call Unit Coordinator when the pump is discontinued.		

M.D Signature Print Name Code Beeper Number

50306 (6/01)

FIGURE 51.1. Epidural analgesia order sheet. BP, blood pressure; IV, intravenous; PCA, patient-controlled analgesia; PRN, as needed; RN, registered nurse. (Courtesy of NewYork-Presbyterian/Weill Cornell Medical Center.)

rate. Frequent monitoring for sensory and sympathetic block should continue in a controlled setting until the efficacy and safety of the epidural analgesia is established. In addition, the patient should be assessed for symptoms of nerve pain relevant to the level attempted. The patient should be informed of the dural puncture and the potential for postdural puncture headache, although this is less frequent in older patients.

Kwak KH. Postdural puncture headache. *Korean J Anesthesiol.* 2017;70:136-143.

Thummala V, Nageswararao L, Swetha D, Sriharitha S, Mounica U. Accidental dural puncture-perioperative management. *Indian J Anaesth.* 2020;64:425-427.

Weji BG, Obsa MS, Melese KG, Azeze GA. Incidence and risk factors of postdural puncture headache: prospective cohort study design. *Perioper Med (Lond).* 2020;9:32.

A.9. What are the alternatives to epidural analgesia?

There are times when for technical, medical, or other reasons, epidural catheter placement is unsuccessful, undesirable, or not possible. Alternatives to epidural analgesia include femoral nerve block, fascia iliaca block, intrathecal opioids, local anesthetic infiltration, lumbar plexus blocks, and systemic analgesia. Femoral nerve block or fascia iliaca plane block can be performed percutaneously using anatomic or ultrasound-guided techniques or under direct vision intraoperatively, using single injections or placement of a catheter. Although often initially effective, unpredictable spread of local anesthetic and rapid local anesthetic absorption by surrounding vessels make these techniques less effective than epidural analgesia when catheters are used to prolong duration. Additionally, percutaneous positioning and securing of catheters can be technically problematic. Lumbar plexus block for hip ORIF has some advantages over an epidural catheter including less hypotension, but placement is more challenging due to difficulty with visualization using an ultrasound-guided technique and less reliable placement with anatomic or stimulator-based placement. A single preoperative bolus of preservative free spinal morphine can be considered in order to decrease the need for systemic opioids. Similarly, direct local anesthetic wound infiltration can be used intraoperatively, but must be combined with longer acting strategies to provide adequate pain control throughout the perioperative period. Although systemic opioids can reduce postsurgical pain, their adverse respiratory effects after general anesthesia, even using patient-controlled delivery systems, and their inability to provide optimal dynamic pain relief favor regional anesthetic techniques when possible. Systemic analgesics are best suited as adjuncts to these techniques and should become the mainstay of analgesic therapy only when regional or neuraxial approaches are discontinued, lose effect, or are otherwise contraindicated.

Amiri HR, Zamani MM, Safari S. Lumbar plexus block for management of hip surgeries. *Anesth Pain Med.* 2014;4:e19407.

Dangle J, Kukreja P, Kalagara H. Review of current practices of peripheral nerve blocks for hip fracture and surgery. *Curr Anesthesiol Rep.* 2020;10:259-266.

Tyagi A, Salhotra R. Total hip arthroplasty and peripheral nerve blocks: limited but salient role? *J Anaesthesiol Clin Pharmacol.* 2018;34:379-380.

A.10. What is the usual clinical regimen for intravenous patient-controlled analgesia (IV-PCA) and is special patient monitoring required during its use?

Clinical regimens for IV-PCA vary among institutions with the most commonly used opioids being fentanyl, morphine, and hydromorphone. Continuous delivery, or basal infusion, is commonly avoided to decrease the likelihood of respiratory depression. For patients who are opioid-naive, boluses of fentanyl of 10 to 15 μg, morphine sulfate 1 to 2 mg, or hydromorphone 0.2 to 0.3 mg are given per demand with a lockout period of 8 to 10 minutes. Incremental boluses can be given\if pain is not controlled. The dose can be decreased or the opioid discontinued if respiratory depression occurs. Close monitoring and rescue strategies must be in place to ensure patient safety, particularly for patients who are at risk, including central monitoring of oxygenation and ventilation and availability of opioid reversal agents (see sample order form, **Figure 51.2**).

A workshop of the Anesthesia Patient Safety Foundation (APSF) looked at the issue of dangers of postoperative opioids to identify patient populations who are at risk. The observed incidence of respiratory depression overall was 0.1% to 1.0% and increased to 3.2% in those older than 80 years. Patients with obstructive sleep apnea and older patients are at a higher risk for opioid-induced respiratory depression, but there is also a low and unpredictable incidence of life-threatening respiratory depression in young, healthy patients without identifiable risk factors. The workshop highlighted the argument that in the

NewYork-Presbyterian
The University Hospital of Columbia and Cornell

45171

PATIENT CONTROLLED ANALGESIA (PCA) ADULT ORDER SHEET

IF NO PLATE, NAME, SEX AND MEDICAL RECORD NO.

DATE: / / TIME: am/pm	ORDERED POSTED	CHECKED BY RN
1) Analgesia by Patient Controlled Analgesia (PCA).		
2) The patient **MUST NOT** receive any supplemental narcotics, sedatives and/or antiemetics while receiving PCA unless approved the Pain Management Service or House Officer		
3) Narcotics (Specify drug, # of mgs, volume, and diluent)		
4) Initial Loading: Dose______________mg every 5 minutes until the patient is comfortable. Maximum total load________mg.		
5) Initial Machine Settings: **PCA Mode** (circle one) Continuous / PCA / Both a) **Program in mg.** b) Continuous Rate___________mg per hour. c) PCA Dose______________mg per demand. d) PCA Lockout_____________minutes. e) Limit___________________mg per four hours.		
6) If pain is not controlled at the above settings (pain ≥ 6), the nurse may administer a PRN recue / loading dose_________every 5 minutes until the patient is comfortable. The maximum rescue / loading dose is_______mg. Increase pump settings to: a) PCA Dose______________mg per demand. b) Continuous Rate___________mg per hour. c) PCA Lockout_____________minutes. d) Limit___________________mg per four hours.		
7) For over sedation (sedation ≥ 4/R4) and respiratory rate < 14, decrease pump settings to: a) PCA Dose______________mg per demand. b) Continuous Rate___________mg per hour. c) PCA Lockout_____________minutes. d) Limit___________________mg per four hours. For respiratory rate of 10 or lower, stop the pump and call the Pain Management Service (X66700, beeper 16664) or House Officer.		
8) Upon initiation, and after every loading dose given, obtain respiratory rate, heart rate and blood pressure. Repeat qh X 2, q4h X 3, and then heart rate and blood pressure per unit routine or as otherwise ordered. Monitor respiratory rate, pain analog and sedation scale q4h.		
9) Note: For patients who receive intrathecal/Epidural Morphine intraoperatively and have PCA initiated within 12 hours, monitor blood pressure, pulse, respiratory rate, pain analog/sedation q30minutes X 2h, qh X2 and then q4 hours X3, Then, BP per unit routine, Monitor respiratory rate, pain analog/sedation of 4hr.		
10) If no maintenance IV is ordered, infuse D5 1/2NS at 40 ml/h via PCA Extension Set.		
11) For Nausea (Specify drug and dosing):		
12) For Sleep (Specify drug and dosing):		
13) For questions or problems, call the Pain Management Service at X62960 or page X66700, beeper 16664		
14) Please call the Unit Coordinator when the pump is discontinued. 15)		

M.D. Signature Print Name Code Beeper Number

50305 (6/01)

FIGURE 51.2. PCA adult order sheet. BP, blood pressure; IV, intravenous. (Courtesy of NewYork-Presbyterian/Weill Cornell Medical Center.)

United States, The Joint Commission emphasis on pain as the "fifth vital sign" has had the unintended consequence of creating an expectation among patients that they will have little to no pain after surgery. As a result, more patients are receiving inappropriate amounts of opioids to meet this expectation. The conclusions of the APSF workshop were that continuous monitoring of oxygenation and ventilation can prevent patient harm; any monitoring system should be centrally linked so that a health care professional can be summoned in a timely manner; programs should be instituted to educate providers and patients about the risks of opioid-induced life-threatening respiratory depression; and that while treatment of postoperative, opioid-induced respiratory depression is an important consideration; prevention is the more effective strategy.

Johnson RL, Kopp SL, Kessler J, et al. Peripheral nerve blocks and ultrasound guidance for regional anesthesia; Hurley RW, Elkassabany NM, Wu CL. Acute postoperative pain; Castro De Oliveira BM, Vazquez R. Anesthesia for orthopedic surgery. In: Gropper MA, Eriksson LI, Fleisher LA, et al, eds. *Miller's Anesthesia*. 10th ed. Elsevier; 2023:1305–1330; 1458–1475; 1952–1983.

Weinger MB. Dangers of postoperative opioids. APSF workshop and white paper address prevention of postoperative respiratory complications. *APSF Newsletter*. 2006-2007;21:61-67.

A.11. What are the side effects and complications of epidural analgesia?

Epidural analgesia interferes with sympathetic outflow and can produce hypotension through cardiodepressant actions (blockade of cardiac accelerator fibers, occurring only if very high spread of local anesthetic) and a reduction in systemic vascular resistance (blockade of sympathetic chain, occurring more commonly with lumbar placement). The use of dilute local anesthetic solutions has led to less significant motor blockade while maintaining adequate sensory block, although some muscle weakness can still be observed.

Opioid-related side effects include sedation, nausea and vomiting, pruritus, delayed gastrointestinal motility, urinary retention, and respiratory depression, all at lower rates than with systemic administration. The incidence of delayed respiratory depression after administration of epidural opioids is very low, and epidural opioid analgesia can be used safely on most hospital units, with the caveat if intrathecal morphine was coadministered there can be a biphasic peak in respiratory depression out to 24 hours. All patients who receive epidural analgesia should have standard orders for the treatment of breakthrough pain and side effects.

The overall catheter-related complication rate is low and includes dural puncture and associated postdural puncture headache, transient paresthesia, and more rarely, sustained neurologic injury. The most commonly documented complication is unsuccessful placement, reported in 5% to 10% of cases. Nerve injury associated with epidural analgesia results from direct trauma, epidural hematoma, or less commonly from epidural abscess. The potentially catastrophic complications of epidural or intrathecal hematoma are best prevented by realization that motor blockade should not occur with dilute local anesthetic solutions and that unexpected or progressive postoperative motor weakness should trigger immediate imaging evaluation (CT or MRI) and neurosurgical consultation. Clearly, if there are significant concerns about coagulopathy or local overlying infection prior to placement of an epidural catheter, risks and benefits should be considered in advance and might preclude neuraxial analgesia altogether, or at least warrant additional vigilance.

Pöpping DM, Elia N, Van Aken HK, et al. Impact of epidural analgesia on mortality and morbidity after surgery: systematic review and meta-analysis of randomized controlled trials. *Ann Surg*. 2014;259:1056-1067.

Wu CL, Murphy JD. Epidural anesthesia-analgesia and patient outcomes: a perspective. *Adv Anesth*. 2014;2014:1-5.

A.12. What recommendations for placement and removal of the epidural catheter would you make if this patient is on antiplatelet or anticoagulant therapy or if thromboprophylaxis is planned?

Recommendations vary based on the particular medication, indication, dose, dosing schedule, and patient factors such as renal function. In general, most antiplatelet or anticoagulant agents should be discontinued five half-lives in advance of placement and can be resumed after a period of time following removal of the neuraxial catheter, though there are some exceptions where therapy can be resumed prior to catheter removal (eg, warfarin). For complete discussion of individual agents, it is best to reference the 4th consensus statement for Regional Anesthesia in the Patient Receiving Antithrombotic or Thrombolytic Therapy developed by the American Society of Regional Anesthesia and Pain Medicine (ASRA), available online and via a phone-based application.

Horlocker TT, Vandermeulen E, Kopp SL, Gogarten W, Leffert LR, Benzon HT. Regional anesthesia in the patient receiving antithrombotic or thrombolytic therapy: ASRA and Pain Medicine evidence-based guidelines: Erratum. *Reg Anesth Pain Med.* 2018;43:566.

B. Perioperative Pain Management and Medications for Opioid Use Disorder (OUD)

B.1. What are the unique pharmacologic aspects of buprenorphine?

Buprenorphine is a partial mu-opioid receptor (MOR) agonist with high binding affinity for the receptor. As a result of only partial activation of the opioid receptor, it has a ceiling-effect for analgesia, euphoria, and respiratory depression that makes it a desirable choice for treatment of both chronic pain and addiction. Simply because it is a partial agonist does not make buprenorphine a weak analgesic; it is more potent per milligram than morphine. However, because of its high receptor binding affinity and long half-life, buprenorphine can decrease receptor availability for full agonist opioids and even displace them, which can result in inadequate analgesia or precipitate withdrawal in the perioperative period.

Coe MA, Lofwall MR, Walsh SL. Buprenorphine pharmacology review: update on transmucosal and long-acting formulations. *J Addict Med.* 2019;13:93-103.

Shulman M, Wai JM, Nunes EV. Buprenorphine treatment for opioid use disorder: an overview. *CNS Drugs.* 2019;33:567-580.

Walsh SL, Preston KL, Stitzer ML, et al. Clinical pharmacology of buprenorphine: ceiling effects at high doses. *Clin Pharmacol Ther.* 1994;55:569-580.

B.2. What are the considerations if a patient is taking buprenorphine for chronic pain versus medication treatment for opioid use disorder (OUD)?

Buprenorphine is FDA approved for treatment of outpatient chronic pain in milligram formulations, either as a transdermal weekly patch or buccal film taken 1 to 2 times daily. It is also available in intravenous and oral formulations for inpatient use. At these low doses, usually 0.5 to 2 mg total per day, there is significant remaining opioid receptor availability, and the medication can generally be continued in the perioperative period with little effect on perioperative analgesia conferred by full agonist opioids.

Buprenorphine for OUD is combined with naloxone unless administered as a subdermal injection or implant. The inclusion of naloxone is intended as an abuse deterrent, as it becomes bioavailable only if attempts are made to inject the drug combination intravenously, in which case, the full opioid antagonist naloxone blocks even the partial opioid-agonist effect of buprenorphine. Buprenorphine/naloxone combinations are available as sublingual tablets or buccal films taken daily. Extended-release subdermal buprenorphine is given as a once-monthly treatment. The most common treatment dose for OUD is an equivalent of 16 mg buprenorphine daily but doses can be as high as 24 to 32 mg/d. At these doses, opioid receptor availability is estimated to be less than 20% and as low as 2%.

Greenwald MK, Comer SD, Fiellin DA. Buprenorphine maintenance and mu-opioid receptor availability in the treatment of opioid use disorder: implications for clinical use and policy. *Drug Alcohol Depend.* 2014;144:1-11.

Mattick RP, Breen C, Kimber J, et al. Buprenorphine maintenance versus placebo or methadone maintenance for opioid dependence. *Cochrane Database Syst Rev.* 2014:CD002207.

Raffa RB, Haidery M, Huang HM, et al. The clinical analgesic efficacy of buprenorphine. *J Clin Pharm Ther.* 2014;39:577-583.

B.3. What are the management strategies for perioperative pain control in a patient taking buprenorphine for OUD?

Management recommendations for patients with OUD in the perioperative setting have changed substantially in the last 20 years. Initially, cessation of buprenorphine in advance of surgery was advised based on a 2004 US Center for Substance Abuse Treatment statement that "administration of buprenorphine be discontinued while patients are taking full mu-opioid agonists." This guidance was not specific to the perioperative period but was bolstered by case reports of hospitalized patients taking buprenorphine for OUD who experienced poor pain control when treated for acute injury or surgery. However, discontinuing buprenorphine for OUD is not without risks, as doing so can precipitate withdrawal, require bridging with a short-acting opioid, or result in relapse, particularly in patients who are newly abstinent.

With additional experience caring for patients taking buprenorphine, improved regional/neuraxial techniques, and more extensive use of multimodal analgesia, recommendations for management have moved away from cessation toward tapering of buprenorphine preoperatively, and most recently to continuing buprenorphine throughout the perioperative period without tapering in most cases (**Figure 51.3**). Supplemental analgesia is suggested by splitting the maintenance buprenorphine dose into 2 to 3 times daily dosing, using additional buprenorphine doses for breakthrough pain, or by adding short-acting opioids with high receptor affinity (fentanyl, hydromorphone) for the shortest duration required.

Recommendations for Postoperative Management

Clinical Pearl: Buprenorphine home dose should not be routinely discontinued or tapered perioperatively

All surgery types (elective, urgent, emergent)

Buprenorphine Management

Mild/Moderate Pain:
- Home buprenorphine dose can be split into 2 times per day/3 times per day dosing to provide an analgesic effect.

Severe Pain:
- Home buprenorphine dose can be split into 3 times per day dosing to provide improved analgesic effect.
- Consider increasing dose of buprenorphine to 24-32 mg given in divided doses or using buprenorphine intravenous 0.3 mg every 6 hours PRN.
- Consider close monitoring if increasing or adding opiate for pain.

Acute Pain With Other Opioids

- Maximize non opioid strategies.
- Treat acute pain with high affinity additional opioids as indicated in patients with OUD, avoid the opioid of past misuse.
- Fentanyl derivatives and hydromorphone likely to be most effective due to high receptor affinity
- Consider close monitoring if increasing or adding opiate for pain.

Nonopioid Pharmacologic Management

- Regional anesthesia (epidural catheter, transversus abdominus plane block, peripheral nerve blocks with or without catheters including but not limited to erector spinae plane blocks, paravertebral block, femoral/adductor canal block, etc.)
- Local infiltration by surgical team
- Intraoperative or postoperative ketamine/lidocaine/magnesium infusions
- Consider dexmedetomidine if Intravenous sedation used postoperatively.
- Topical agents (eg, ice, lidocaine ointment or patches)
- NSAIDs when indicated (eg, ketorolac, ibuprofen, etc.)
- Intravenous vs oral acetaminophen when indicated
- Antineuropathic agents when indicated or if comorbid anxiety (eg, gabapentinoids, antidepressants such as TCAs, SNRIs, etc.)
- Muscle relaxants as indicated (eg, baclofen, tizanidine, cyclobenzaprine; avoid benzodiazepines or carisoprodol)

Non-pharmacologic Management

- Ice to surgical site
- Position change
- Relaxation strategies and mindfulness techniques for pain (eg, guided "apps" such as the free app "Calm")
- Peer recovery support
- Distraction aligned with interests (eg, reading, music, family and social support, etc.)

Postoperative Disposition

- Post anesthesia care unit
- Discharge home if satisfactory pain control, coordinate buprenorphine dosing plan with prescriber
- Inpatient floor admission as applicable
- Consider ICU admission if uncontrolled pain and respiratory concerns

FIGURE 51.3. Recommendations for perioperative buprenorphine management. ICU, intensive care unit; NSAIDs, nonsteroidal anti-inflammatory drugs; OUD, opioid use disorder; PRN, as needed; SNRIs, serotonin and norepinephrine reuptake inhibitors; TCAs, tricyclic antidepressants. (From Kohan L, Potru S, Barreveld AM, et al. Buprenorphine management in the perioperative period: educational review and recommendations from a multisociety expert panel. *Reg Anesth Pain Med.* 2021;46:840-859. Figure 1, with permission from BMJ Publishing Group Ltd.)

Center for Substance Abuse Treatment. Clinical Guidelines for the Use of Buprenorphine in the Treatment of Opioid Addiction. Treatment improvement protocol (TIP) series 40. DHHS publication No. (SMA) 04-3939. Substance Abuse and Mental Health Services Administration (US); 2004.

Goel A, Azargive S, Lamba W. The perioperative patient on buprenorphine: a systematic review of perioperative management strategies and patient outcomes. *Can J Anaesth.* 2019;66:201-217.

Kohan L, Potru S, Barreveld AM, et al. Buprenorphine management in the perioperative period: educational review and recommendations from a multisociety expert panel. *Reg Anesth Pain Med.* 2021;46:840-859.

Lembke A, Ottestad E, Schmiesing C. Patients maintained on buprenorphine for opioid use disorder should continue buprenorphine through the perioperative period. *Pain Med.* 2019;20:425-428.

Warner NS, Warner MA, Cunningham JL, et al. A practical approach for the management of the mixed opioid agonist-antagonist buprenorphine during acute pain and surgery. *Mayo Clin Proc.* 2020;95:1253-1267.

B.4. What issues need to be considered before discharging a patient taking buprenorphine for OUD?

When a patient taking buprenorphine leaves the hospital, there are two issues to address. The first is reestablishing care with the patient's outpatient provider for continued management of OUD. It is advised that the continuity provider be consulted and aware of the planned surgery in advance if at all possible. In most cases, the patient should be discharged on their chronic medication, and follow-up with their prescriber is suggested within 1 week of discharge. The second consideration is discontinuation of opioids for acute postoperative pain. This is best accomplished through a preplanned taper with additional oral buprenorphine or a short-acting full agonist for a defined amount of time based on the specific surgery. For patients at risk for relapse, small daily prescriptions might be required until the planned end-date is reached.

Joo SS, Hunter OO, Tamboli M, et al. Implementation of a patient-specific tapering protocol at discharge decreases total opioid dose prescribed for 6 weeks after elective primary spine surgery. *Reg Anesth Pain Med.* 2020;45:474-478.

Kohan L, Potru S, Barreveld AM, et al. Buprenorphine management in the perioperative period: educational review and recommendations from a multisociety expert panel. *Reg Anesth Pain Med.* 2021;46:840-859.

Tamboli M, Mariano ER, Gustafson KE, et al. A multidisciplinary patient-specific opioid prescribing and tapering protocol is associated with a decrease in total opioid dose prescribed for six weeks after total hip arthroplasty. *Pain Med.* 2020;21:1474-1481.

B.5. What can be done if a patient is identified with untreated OUD perioperatively?

Substance misuse is common in hospitalized patients, and persistent opioid use is well-documented after surgery. Patients can be identified using a screening tool such as the Opioid Risk Tool (ORT), Screener and Opioid Assessment for Patients with Pain (SOAPP), or Current Opioid Misuse Measure (COMM). Studies indicate that nearly half of patients with OUD express interest in medical treatment. Some states have even mandated treatment if opioid misuse is discovered in the hospital setting. The perioperative period can thus serve as an opportunity to identify and treat these patients, and several protocols have been proposed for initiating treatment perioperatively, most involving discontinuation of full agonist opioids for 3 to 6 hours followed by induction with 2 mg buprenorphine every 1 to 2 hours until resolution of withdrawal symptoms using a Clinical Opioid Withdrawal Scale (COWS). Arranging follow-up with a community provider within 1 week (a list can be found on the Substance Abuse and Mental Health Services Administration [SAMHSA] website) and a bridge prescription until follow-up or a loading dose of oral buprenorphine up to 32 mg (based on the patient's tolerance and inpatient requirement) prior to discharge are key to facilitating continued treatment.

Brummett CM, Waljee JF, Goesling J, et al. New persistent opioid use after minor and major surgical procedures in US adults. *JAMA Surg.* 2017;152:e170504.

Englander H, Weimer M, Solotaroff R, et al. Planning and designing the improving addiction care team (impact) for hospitalized adults with substance use disorder. *J Hosp Med.* 2017;12:339-342.

Patel N, Schwenk ES, Ferd P, et al. An anesthesiologist-led inpatient buprenorphine initiative. *Pain Pract.* 2021;21:692-697.

US Department of Health & Human Services: Substance Abuse and Mental Health Services Administration. Millions of Americans have mental and substance use disorders. Find treatment here. FindTreatment.gov. Accessed February 22, 2023. https://findtreatment.gov/

B.6. What are the legal ramifications of buprenorphine prescribing?

Buprenorphine can be ordered in microgram formulations for inpatient or outpatient chronic pain without restriction other than the usual state and Drug Enforcement Administration (DEA) licensing requirements inclusive of schedule III controlled-substance prescribing. Inpatient administration of milligram formulations of buprenorphine for OUD has also long been allowed as an incidental adjunct to medical or surgical care for other conditions. Outpatient prescribing of buprenorphine for OUD has been more limited in scope due to a required X-waiver, which can be obtained after completing 8 hours of training for primary providers and 24 hours of training for advanced practice providers. To improve access in light of the opioid epidemic, SAMHSA provided this training free and allowed an exception to the requirement if treating less than 30 patients at a time, but this still required a submission of a Notice of Intent (NOI) waiver in advance. For urgent situations, a "good faith" waiver was available on a case-by-case basis. As of January 2023, Section 1262 of the Consolidated Appropriations Act, also known as the Mainstreaming Addiction Treatment Act, removed the federal requirement for a waiver to prescribe buprenorphine for any indication in order to increase access for patients and ease provider burden. As of June 27th, 2023, prescribers renewing or registering a new DEA license are required to attest to completion of 8 hours of self-directed training on the "management of patients with opioid or other substance use disorders" as mandated by the Medication Access and Training Expansion (MATE) Act.

Federal Register. Practice guidelines for the administration of buprenorphine for treating opioid use disorder. Accessed February 22, 2023. https://www.federalregister.gov/documents/2021/04/28/2021-08961/practice-guidelines-for-the-administration-of-buprenorphine-for-treating-opioid-use-disorder

GovInfo. Title 21 Code of Federal Regulations (CFR) §1306.07—Administering or dispensing of narcotic drugs. Accessed February 22, 2023. https://www.govinfo.gov/app/details/CFR-2022-title21-vol9/CFR-2022-title21-vol9-sec1306-07

US Department of Health & Human Services: Substance Abuse and Mental Health Services Administration. HHS releases new buprenorphine practice guidelines, expanding access to treatment for opioid use disorder. Accessed February 22, 2023. https://www.samhsa.gov/newsroom/press-announcements/202104270930

US Department of Health & Human Services: Substance Abuse and Mental Health Services Administration. Removal of DATA waiver (X-waiver) requirement. Accessed February 22, 2023. https://www.samhsa.gov/medications-substance-use-disorders/removal-data-waiver-requirement

52 Acupuncture

Yuan-Chi Lin

A 67-year-old female with a history of osteoarthritis was scheduled for arthroscopic surgery of her right knee. She experienced severe postoperative nausea and vomiting (PONV) in the postanesthesia care unit. Despite the use of conventional therapies, her nausea and vomiting persisted. Her past medical history was significant including knee osteoarthritis for 10 years, mastectomy 5 years ago for breast cancer, anxiety disorder, chronic headaches, chronic neck and back pain, peptic ulcer disease, and an allergy to lidocaine. What role can acupuncture therapy play in her care?

A. Acupuncture as a Complementary Medical Therapy

1. What is acupuncture?
2. How is acupuncture practiced?
3. What are the mechanisms of acupuncture analgesia?
4. What were the conclusions of the National Institutes of Health Consensus Conference on acupuncture?
5. Can acupuncture serve as a novel complementary nonopioid pain therapy?

B. Acupuncture for the Treatment of Medical Conditions

1. What are the rationales for integrating acupuncture in the treatment of PONV?
2. Can acupuncture be used to treat chemotherapy-induced nausea and vomiting?
3. Can acupuncture be used to ease postoperative pain?
4. How effective is acupuncture in managing chronic headache?
5. Can acupuncture be used to treat chronic neck and back pain?
6. Can acupuncture be used to treat osteoarthritis?
7. What role can acupuncture play in the care of patients with cancer?
8. Can acupuncture or acupressure be used to reduce anxiety?
9. What is ear acupuncture or acupressure? Can it be useful for alleviating anxiety and pain?

C. Complications

1. What are the potential complications of acupuncture treatment?

A. Acupuncture as a Complementary Medical Therapy

A.1. What is acupuncture?

Acupuncture is one of the treatment modalities in comprehensive traditional Chinese medicine (TCM). The word *acupuncture* is derived from the Latin words *acus*, meaning "needle," and *punctura*, meaning "a pricking." The original Chinese term for acupuncture is *Jin Jiao*, which describes the practice of "acupuncture and moxibustion." Moxibustion involves the burning of moxa (*Artemisia vulgaris*) near acupuncture points.

The Yellow Emperor's Classic of Internal Medicine from the fourth century BC described the practice of puncturing the body for pain relief. TCM is a system of thoughts and practices that is based on the investigations of nature, causes, and effects. It incorporates principles of realism and ethics to prevent diseases and promote healing. Sir William Osler in his book *The Principles and Practice of Medicine* advocated for the use of acupuncture for conditions such as sciatica and lumbago.

The concept of *yin and yang* underlies the theoretical framework of acupuncture. Yin and yang represent two opposite dynamics that cannot exist in isolation and are in a constant state of dynamic balance.

Imbalances between yin and yang are believed to contribute to illnesses. The human body is regulated by a vital force called *Qi* ("chee"). *Qi* circulates throughout the body and defends its various parts. The body contains 365 identified acupuncture points, which are located along 12 principal meridians and 8 extra meridians. Qi is believed to flow through these meridians. The mechanism of acupuncture is to unblock the Qi flow, facilitate its movement, and to restore balance to Yin and Yang.

A.2. How is acupuncture practiced?

Acupuncture utilizes a technique of inserting fine thread-thin needles into specific points in the body called *acupuncture points*. Acupuncture needles vary from 36 to 42 gauge and 0.5 to 5 inches in length. There are a variety of needles available for use. In *The Yellow Emperor's Classic of Internal Medicine* by Ling Shu, nine different shapes of acupuncture needles are described. The current standard for acupuncture treatment is use of sterile, disposable stainless steel acupuncture needles. Once the site of the needle insertion on the skin is cleaned, the acupuncture needle is inserted a few millimeters into the epidermis. After the needle is placed, the acupuncture point can be manually stimulated or electrically stimulated using low-voltage electrodes, a technique called *electroacupuncture*.

Each acupuncture point has a specific depth of insertion. Manual techniques include lifting and thrusting or twisting and twirling the needle. Proper acupuncture needle placement typically elicits a sensation called *De-Qi*. Patients describe this sensation as a feeling of soreness, numbness, warmth, heaviness, or pressure around the area where the needle is inserted. Many practitioners consider this sensation to be crucial in achieving the effects of acupuncture. Electroacupuncture achieves a similar effect by using high- or low-frequency electrical current.

Acupuncture is generally associated with minimal pain or discomfort. For certain conditions, multiple acupuncture treatment sessions over an extended period are necessary to achieve optimal effectiveness. The frequency and number of acupuncture treatments can vary among providers. However, most practitioners agree that more than one treatment is usually necessary to experience the full benefits of acupuncture.

Auricular, hand, and scalp acupuncture can be used as microsystems within acupuncture. For instance, auricular acupuncture (**Figure 52.1**) focuses on manipulating specific regions of the external ear to alleviate conditions in corresponding areas of the body. Auricular acupuncture can also be utilized for preoperative anxiety control.

Chernyak GV, Sessler DI. Perioperative acupuncture and related techniques. *Anesthesiology*. 2005;102:1031-1049.

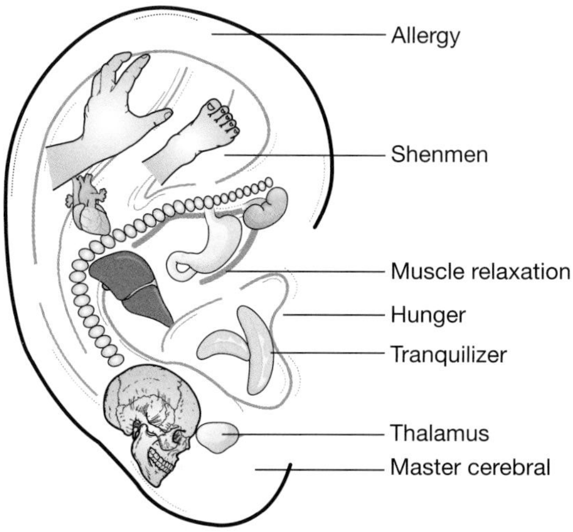

FIGURE 52.1. Auricular acupuncture. (From Wang SM. Acupuncture for Adult and Pediatric Pain. In: Urman RD, Vadivelu N, eds. *Pocket Pain Medicine*. Wolters Kluwer; 2012:18-1-18-3. Figure 18.1.)

A.3. What are the mechanisms of acupuncture analgesia?

Acupuncture inhibits the transmission of pain according to the gate control theory. It appears to act by stimulating sensory A-β fibers, thereby directly inhibiting the spinal transmission of pain by smaller A-δ and C fibers.

Acupuncture also stimulates the endorphin system to increase endorphins and enkephalins, and by activating the endogenous descending inhibitory pathways. Analysis of cerebrospinal fluid showed elevated levels of serotonin, endorphins, and enkephalins following acupuncture treatments. Acupuncture analgesia is achieved by activating the endogenous antinociceptive system to modulate pain transmission and pain response. Low-frequency (2 Hz) and high-frequency (100 Hz) electrical acupunctures selectively induce release of enkephalins and dynorphins in both experimental animals and humans. Acupuncture analgesia can be reversed by naloxone.

Functional magnetic resonance imaging (fMRI) has been used to investigate the effect of acupuncture in normal volunteers. Acupuncture needle manipulation on the LI4 (He Gu) point (**Figure 52.2**) modulates activity of the limbic system and subcortical regions. There is individual variation in cortical activation patterns elicited by electrical acupuncture stimulation. Actual acupuncture elicited greater activation than sham acupuncture in the hypothalamus, primary somatosensory and motor cortex, and deactivation in the rostral segment of anterior cingulate cortex.

Han JS. Acupuncture and endorphins. *Neurosci Lett*. 2004;361:258-261.

Hui KK, Liu J, Makris N, et al. Acupuncture modulates the limbic system and subcortical gray structures of the human brain: evidence from fMRI studies in normal subjects. *Hum Brain Mapp*. 2000;9:13-25.

Wu MT, Sheen JM, Chuang KH, et al. Neuronal specificity of acupuncture response: an fMRI study with electroacupuncture. *Neuroimage*. 2002;16:1028-1037.

Zhang R, Lao L, Ren K, et al. Mechanisms of acupuncture-electroacupuncture on persistent pain. *Anesthesiology*. 2014;120:482-503.

A.4. What were the conclusions of the National Institutes of Health Consensus Conference on acupuncture?

A National Institutes of Health Consensus Conference concluded that acupuncture is an effective therapeutic intervention widely practiced in the United States. Promising results have emerged supporting the efficacy of acupuncture in adult postoperative and chemotherapy-related nausea and vomiting as well as postoperative dental pain. Acupuncture can also be useful as an adjunct treatment or as an acceptable alternative in other conditions such as addiction, stroke rehabilitation, headache, menstrual cramps, tennis elbow, fibromyalgia, myofascial pain, osteoarthritis, low back pain, carpal tunnel syndrome, and asthma, when included in a comprehensive management program. Further research is expected to uncover additional areas in which acupuncture interventions can be beneficial.

National Institutes of Health Consensus Conference. Acupuncture. *JAMA*. 1998;280:1518-1524.

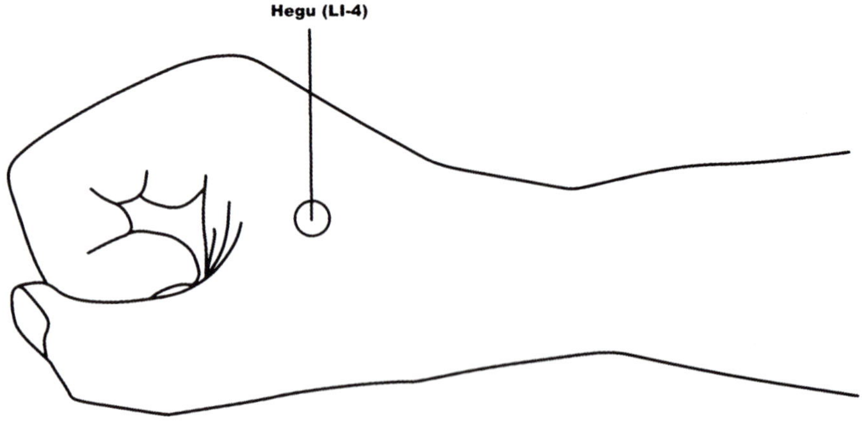

FIGURE 52.2. The location of the LI4 (He Gu) acupoint. The LI4 acupoint is positioned on the dorsum of the hand, at the midpoint of the second metacarpal bone and close to its radial border. LI4 = large Intestine 4. (From Wang FL, Chu JM, Yu J, et al. Acupuncture at Hegu point (LI4) for myofascial temporomandibular disorders. A case report. *Med Case Rep Study Protoc*. 2022;3:e0263. Figure 2.)

A.5. Can acupuncture serve as a novel complementary nonopioid pain therapy?

Opioid analgesics have been used in the management of acute and chronic pain. However, the use of opioids is associated with adverse effects and potential for addiction, particularly with chronic use. Increasing reliance on opioids for chronic pain can further contribute to the ongoing opioid crisis. As a result, there is a growing emphasis on exploring novel nonopioid therapies. Acupuncture, as an integrative medicine approach to pain management, can play a significant role in reducing the frequency and dose of opioid use. Acupuncture has demonstrated strong positive evidence in pain management and can be routinely integrated into pain management protocols.

Lin YC, Wan L, Jamison RL. Using integrative medicine in pain management: an evaluation of current evidence. *Anesth Analg*. 2017;125:2081-2093.

Volkow ND, Collins FS. The role of science in addressing the opioid crisis. *N Engl J Med*. 2017;377:391-394.

B. Acupuncture for the Treatment of Medical Conditions

B.1. What are the rationales for integrating acupuncture in the treatment of PONV?

PONV frequently occur following surgery and should be avoided whenever possible. Acupuncture is a commonly utilized therapy for managing these symptoms. Stimulation of the acupuncture PC6 points (also known as *Nei Guan acupuncture point*, meaning *gate of the internal organ* in Chinese) using acupuncture needles, electrical devices, pressure, or magnets is employed to alleviate nausea and vomiting. The PC6 acupuncture point is located approximately 2.5 inches or three fingerbreadths above the transverse crease of the wrist, between the tendons of the muscle palmaris longus and muscle flexor carpi radialis. (**Figure 52.3**).

Studies support the use of acupuncture for treatment of PONV. A systemic review of 33 randomized controlled trials of acupuncture or acupressure showed positive results in 27 of these trials. A randomized controlled trial involving pediatric patients undergoing tonsillectomy demonstrated a significant reduction in PONV compared to sham and control groups. The efficacy of acupuncture in preventing PONV is comparable to that of commonly prescribed pharmacotherapies. In a double-blind, randomized, placebo-controlled study, hand acupressure was found to be an effective method for reducing PONV in children after strabismus repair.

PC6 acupressure, a noninvasive method, can serve as prophylactic antiemetic therapy during gynecologic surgery. A prospective randomized controlled trial of acupressure for the prevention of PONV in females undergoing general anesthesia for elective gynecologic surgery showed positive results. A comparison of PC6 acupoint stimulation with six antiemetics for pharmacoprophylaxis (metoclopramide, cyclizine, prochlorperazine, droperidol, ondansetron, and dexamethasone) revealed no differences in PONV or need for rescue antiemetics.

Alkaissi A, Evertsson K, Johnsson VA, et al. P6 acupressure may relieve nausea and vomiting after gynecological surgery: an effectiveness study in 410 women. *Can J Anaesth*. 2002;49:1034-1039.

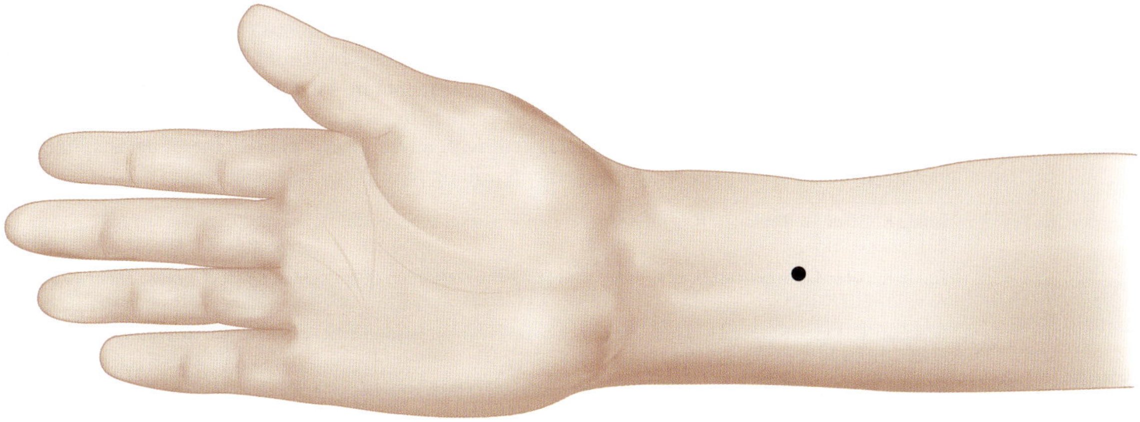

FIGURE 52.3. The PC6 (Nei Guan) acupuncture point is located three fingerbreadths, or about 2.5 inches, above the transverse crease of the wrist, between the tendons of the muscle palmaris longus and muscle flexor capri radialis.

Frey UH, Scharmann P, Löhlein C, et al. P6 acustimulation effectively decreases postoperative nausea and vomiting in high-risk patients. *Br J Anaesth*. 2009;102:620-625.

Gan TJ, Belani KG, Bergese S, et al. Fourth consensus guidelines for the management of postoperative nausea and vomiting. *Anesth Analg*. 2020;131:441-448.

B.2. Can acupuncture be used to treat chemotherapy-induced nausea and vomiting?

Acupuncture or acupressure at the PC6 acupuncture point has been shown to have a protective effect in chemotherapy-induced nausea and vomiting. A review of 11 randomized controlled trials of the effectiveness of acupuncture-point stimulation on chemotherapy-induced nausea and vomiting revealed that electroacupuncture reduced chemotherapy-induced acute vomiting.

Ezzo JM, Richardson MA, Vickers A, et al. Acupuncture-point stimulation for chemotherapy-induced nausea or vomiting. *Cochrane Database Syst Rev*. 2006;CD002285.

B3. Can acupuncture be used to ease postoperative pain?

Postoperative pain management remains a significant challenge for perioperative clinicians. In a systemic review of 15 randomized controlled trials involving 1,166 patients, 608 patients received acupuncture and related techniques as adjunct analgesia for acute postoperative pain. The effectiveness of acupuncture and related techniques was assessed by analyzing variables such as cumulative opioid consumption, postoperative pain intensity, and incidence of opioid-related side effects. The findings suggested that perioperative acupuncture might serve as a beneficial adjunct for managing acute postoperative pain. Another systemic review and meta-analysis, encompassing 11 trials, revealed that patients who underwent treatment with acupuncture or related techniques experienced less pain and required lower opioid doses on the first day following surgery compared to those in the control group. Acupuncture and related techniques have the potential to play a valuable role in reducing postoperative pain and minimizing the reliance on opioid analgesics.

Sun Y, Gan TJ, Dubose JW, et al. Acupuncture and related techniques for postoperative pain: a systematic review of randomized controlled trials. *Br J Anaesth*. 2008;101:151-160.

Wu MS, Chen KH, Chen IF, et al. The efficacy of acupuncture in post-operative pain management: a systematic review and meta-analysis. *PLoS One*. 2016;11:e0150367.

B.4. How effective is acupuncture in managing chronic headache?

Acupuncture therapy for migraine headaches has been reported to be effective in several studies in adults. In a randomized controlled trial of 160 females with migraines, acupuncture was adequate for migraine prophylaxis. Compared to flunarizine, acupuncture exhibited greater efficacy in the first months of therapy and better patient tolerance. A systemic review of 22 trials including 1,042 patients suggested that acupuncture has a role in the treatment of recurrent headaches. In a randomized controlled trial of 401 patients with chronic migraine headaches, at 12 months of follow-up acupuncture was relatively cost-effective. Compared with patients in the control groups, patients receiving acupuncture used 15% less medication, made 25% fewer visits to general practitioners, and took 15% fewer sick days from work.

A Cochrane systematic review of 11 trials of 2,317 patients with episodic or chronic tension-type headache suggested that acupuncture can be a valuable nonpharmacologic tool for patients with frequent episodic or chronic tension-type headaches. Regarding acupuncture for migraine prophylaxis, a meta-analysis of 22 trials with 4,419 participants showed acupuncture to be at least as effective as, and possibly more effective than, prophylactic drug treatment with fewer adverse effects. Therefore, acupuncture should be considered a treatment option for patients willing to undergo this treatment.

Linde K, Allais G, Brinkhaus B, et al. Acupuncture for tension-type headache. *Cochrane Database Syst Rev*. 2016;CD007587.

Linde K, Allais G, Brinkhaus B, et al. Acupuncture for the prevention of episodic migraine. *Cochrane Database Syst Rev*. 2016;CD001218.

Melchart D, Linde K, Fischer P, et al. Acupuncture for recurrent headaches: a systematic review of randomized controlled trials. *Cephalalgia*. 1999;19:779-786.

Vickers AJ, Rees RW, Zollman CE, et al. Acupuncture for chronic headache in primary care: large, pragmatic, randomized trial. *BMJ*. 2004;328:744.

B.5. Can acupuncture be used to treat chronic neck and back pain?

In a randomized controlled trial of 177 patients with chronic neck pain, the effectiveness of acupuncture, massage, and sham laser acupuncture were compared. Patients in the acupuncture group received up to 15 acupuncture sessions over 3 months. Reported neck pain levels and disability scores of the members of the acupuncture group improved compared to those in the control group. Treatment success was followed and maintained for 6 months.

A large German clinical study involving 1,162 patients with chronic low back pain indicated that both "real" and "sham" acupuncture treatment were significantly better than conventional therapy for at least 6 months. Another large German study of 1,549 patients with chronic low back pain showed that acupuncture plus routine care was associated with marked clinical improvements in patients with chronic low back pain and was cost-effective. A systemic review involving 23 trials of 6,359 patients with low back pain revealed that acupuncture can be a useful supplement to other forms of conventional therapy for nonspecific low back pain.

Haake M, Müller HH, Schade-Brittinger C, et al. German Acupuncture Trials (GERAC) for chronic low back pain: randomized, multicenter, blinded, parallel-group trial with 3 groups. *Arch Intern Med.* 2007;167:1892-1898.

Irnich D, Behrens N, Molzen H, et al. Randomised trial of acupuncture compared with conventional massage and "sham" laser acupuncture for treatment of chronic neck pain. *BMJ.* 2001;322:1574-1578.

Witt CM, Jena S, Brinkhaus B, et al. Acupuncture for patients with chronic neck pain. *Pain.* 2006;125:98-106.

Yuan J, Purepong N, Kerr DP, et al. Effectiveness of acupuncture for low back pain: a systematic review. *Spine.* 2008;33:887-900.

B.6. Can acupuncture be used to treat osteoarthritis?

Evidence exists for the efficacy of acupuncture in reducing pain and dysfunction in osteoarthritis. In a study of 300 patients with chronic osteoarthritis of the knee, participants were randomly assigned to acupuncture, minimal acupuncture, or a wait-list control group. After 8 weeks of treatment, acupuncture resulted in greater improvements in pain and joint function compared to minimal or no acupuncture. In a randomized controlled trial of 570 patients with osteoarthritis of the knee, the acupuncture group received 23 true acupuncture sessions over 26 weeks. Acupuncture was shown to be beneficial in improving function and providing pain relief as an adjunctive therapy for knee osteoarthritis when compared to credible sham acupuncture and education control groups.

In a trial of 30 patients with symptomatic osteoarthritis of the knee, participants were randomly assigned to one of three treatment groups. One group received acupuncture alone, another group received acupuncture along with their symptomatic medication, and the third group used their symptomatic medication for the first 5 weeks followed by a course of acupuncture. The patients receiving acupuncture underwent treatment twice a week for over 5 weeks. Both manual and electroacupuncture led to significant improvement in the symptoms of osteoarthritis of the knee, either as standalone treatment or as an adjunct therapy, with no loss of benefit observed after 1 month.

Current evidence supports the use of acupuncture for managing osteoarthritis. A systemic review evaluating the role of acupuncture in osteoarthritis pain management demonstrated a reduction in pain intensity and improvement in functional mobility and quality of life.

Berman BM, Lao L, Langenberg P, et al. Effectiveness of acupuncture as adjunctive therapy in osteoarthritis of the knee: a randomized, controlled trial. *Ann Intern Med.* 2004;141:901-910.

Manyanga T, Froese M, Zarychanski R, et al. Pain management with acupuncture in osteoarthritis: a systemic review and meta-analysis. *BMC Complement Altern Med.* 2014;14:312-320.

Tukmachi E, Jubb R, Dempsey E, et al. The effect of acupuncture on the symptoms of knee osteoarthritis—an open randomized controlled study. *Acupunct Med.* 2004;22:14-22.

Witt C, Brinkhaus B, Jena S, et al. Acupuncture in patients with osteoarthritis of the knee: a randomized trial. *Lancet.* 2005;366:136-143.

B.7. What role can acupuncture play in the care of patients with cancer?

A randomized controlled trial involving 90 patients with cancer pain demonstrated clear benefits from auricular acupuncture, even when their analgesic treatment was stable. Therefore, it is reasonable to consider using acupuncture for the management of chronic cancer-related pain management. Additionally, acupuncture can be utilized to effectively control chemotherapy-related nausea and vomiting.

Alimi D, Rubino C, Pichard-Léandri E, et al. Analgesic effect of auricular acupuncture for cancer pain: a randomized, blinded, controlled trial. *J Clin Oncol.* 2003;21:4120-4126.

Ezzo JM, Richardson MA, Vickers A, et al. Acupuncture-point stimulation for chemotherapy-induced nausea or vomiting. *Cochrane Database Syst Rev.* 2006;CD002285.

B.8. Can acupuncture or acupressure be used to reduce anxiety?

Acupuncture or acupressure applied to the Yin-Tang acupuncture point is effective in inducing sedation. The Yin-Tang acupuncture point is located on the forehead, at the midway between the medial ends of the two eyebrows (**Figure 52.4**). A prospective, randomized, single-blind, controlled study involving 52 patients who received either acupuncture on the Yin-Tang or sham acupuncture showed that bispectral index (BIS) values in the acupuncture group were significantly lower than those in the sham group. A study of 50 patients who were randomly assigned to acupuncture of the Yin-Tang point or a control point showed that acupuncture applied to the Yin-Tang point significantly reduced the BIS value compared to the control group, further supporting the sedative effects of acupuncture at this specific point.

Acar HV, Cuvaş O, Ceyhan A, et al. Acupuncture on Yintang point decreases preoperative anxiety. *J Altern Complement Med.* 2013;19:420-424.

Paraskeva A, Melemeni A, Petropoulos G, et al. Needling of the extra 1-point decreases BIS values and preoperative anxiety. *Am J Chin Med.* 2004;32:789-794.

B.9. What is ear acupuncture or acupressure? Can it be useful for alleviating anxiety and pain?

Auricular acupressure has been identified as an effective treatment for anxiety during ambulance transport. In a study involving 36 patients who required ambulance transport to medical facilities, patients randomly assigned to receive auricular acupressure at the relaxation point or at a sham point reported lower levels of anxiety compared to patients in the sham group. Furthermore, in a randomized controlled trial involving 38 patients with acute hip fracture, patients receiving auricular acupressure during ambulance transport exhibited less pain, anxiety, and tachycardia upon arrival at the hospital compared with sham acupressure.

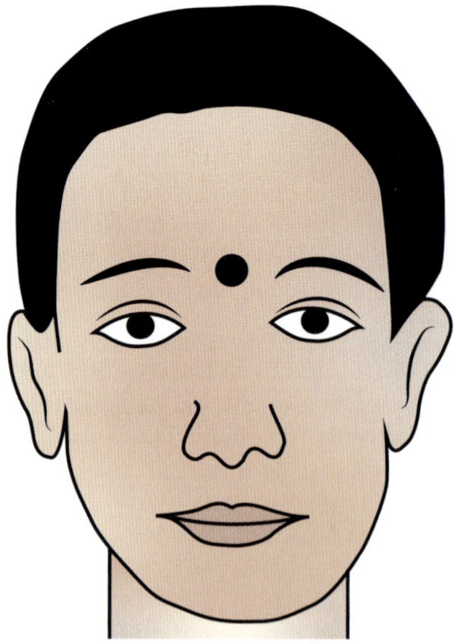

FIGURE 52.4. The Yin-Tang acupuncture point is located on the forehead, midway between the medial ends of the two eyebrows.

To produce auricular acupuncture for a longer duration, ear seeds or ear tacks can be utilized. Ear seeds can be small seeds derived from the dry *Vaccaria* plant or can be made from stainless steel, and are affixed to the ear using a small piece of adhesive tape.

Barker R, Kober A, Hoerauf K, et al. Out-of-hospital auricular acupressure in elder patients with hip fracture: a randomized double-blinded trial. *Acad Emerg Med.* 2006;13:19-23.

Kober A, Scheck T, Schubert B, et al. Auricular acupressure as a treatment for anxiety in prehospital transport settings. *Anesthesiology.* 2003;98:1328-1332.

C. Complications

C.1. What are the potential complications of acupuncture treatment?

Acupuncture is an extremely safe practice. In rare cases, a patient can experience minor bruising at an acupuncture site, which typically resolves quickly. The main risk associated with acupuncture is infection, which can be minimized by using disposable sterile acupuncture needles and ensuring proper needle insertion. Rare incidents of vasovagal syncope have been reported. Additionally, there have been documented case reports of pneumothorax caused by improper insertion of acupuncture needles.

A study on adverse effects of 34,000 acupuncture consultations in the UK found that the most common adverse events were bleeding, needling pain, and temporary worsening of symptoms. None of these events were considered serious. Similarly, a review of nine surveys indicated that the most common adverse events were needle pain, fatigue, and minor bleeding. Feelings of lightheadedness and faintness were uncommon. Notably, up to 86% of patients reported feelings of relaxation following acupuncture treatment.

Pneumothorax is one of the rare complications when needling the chest acupuncture points. To minimize the risk of pneumothorax, techniques such as using shorter acupuncture needles, grasping the skin to retract soft tissue away from the chest wall, and inserting needles at an oblique angle can be employed. Clinicians should remain vigilant for symptoms like chest pain or shortness of breath during or after acupuncture treatment.

In a study that involved a prospective review of treatments performed by 1,848 professional acupuncturists in the UK over 4 weeks, 43 minor adverse events were reported, resulting in a rate of 1.3 per 1,000 treatments. The reported events included instances of severe nausea, fainting, prolonged worsening of symptoms, pain, and bruising. Overall, the frequency of acupuncture-related adverse events is exceptionally low, and prospective studies have consistently shown that even minor adverse events are uncommon.

When acupuncture is applied appropriately by a competent practitioner, it is considered a very safe intervention, and the occurrence of adverse effects is particularly rare.

Ernst E, White A. Prospective studies of the safety of acupuncture: a systemic review. *Am J Med.* 2001;110:481-485.

MacPherson H, Thomas K, Walters S, et al. The York acupuncture safety study: prospective survey of 34,000 treatments by traditional acupuncturists. *BMJ.* 2001;323:486-487.

Ochi JW. Pneumothorax after acupuncture: medicolegal consequences and prevention. *Med Acupunct.* 2023;35:9-12.

von Riedenauer WB, Baker MK, Brewer RJ. Video-assisted thoracoscopic removal of migratory acupuncture needle causing pneumothorax. *Chest.* 2007;131:899-901.

53 Myasthenia Gravis

James B. Eisenkraft and Marc A. Sherwin

A 35-year-old female with a history of generalized anxiety disorder and morbid obesity presents for emergent exploratory laparotomy for perforated sigmoid colon. She was diagnosed 3 years ago with myasthenia gravis (MG) after developing progressive diplopia, dysphagia, and proximal muscle weakness. She underwent a transcervical thymectomy 1 year ago with improvement of symptoms. Her medications are pyridostigmine (Mestinon) 60 mg three times a day (TID) and diazepam 5 mg/day. Vital signs are as follows: pulse rate, 95 beats per minute; blood pressure, 105/65 mm Hg; respiratory rate, 20 breaths per minute; and Spo_2, 97% breathing room air. She is 160 cm tall, weighs 95 kg, and her body mass index (BMI) is 37 kg/m^2.

A. Medical Disease and Differential Diagnosis

1. What is MG?
2. What is the etiology and pathophysiology of MG?
3. Describe the clinical classification of MG.
4. How is the diagnosis of MG made?
5. What should be considered in the differential diagnosis?
6. How does myasthenic syndrome (Lambert-Eaton syndrome) differ from MG?
7. What treatments are available for a patient with MG?

B. Preoperative Evaluation and Preparation

1. Describe the preoperative evaluation of this patient.
2. What preoperative laboratory data are required?
3. How should the patient's medications be managed preoperatively?

C. Intraoperative Management

1. What are your considerations in the choice of anesthetic technique?
2. How should this patient be monitored intraoperatively?
3. What anesthetic regimen would you choose for this patient?
4. Can neuromuscular blocking drugs be used safely in a patient with MG?
5. Should the patient with MG who is in remission (symptom free without treatment) be managed differently?

D. Postoperative Management

1. What factors will help you predict this patient's need for continued tracheal intubation or other postoperative ventilatory support?
2. How will you determine if this patient's trachea can be safely extubated?
3. How will you manage postoperative analgesia?
4. How will you define and manage postextubation ventilatory failure in this patient?

A. Medical Disease and Differential Diagnosis

A.1. What is MG?

MG is a disorder of the neuromuscular junction and, therefore, of great significance to the anesthesiologist. It is a chronic disorder characterized by fluctuating, painless weakness and fatigability of voluntary muscles. It is made worse by exertion and improves following rest. The onset is usually slow and insidious; any skeletal muscle or muscle group can be affected. The most common onset is ocular, presenting with ptosis and diplopia. MG is confined to the ocular muscles in 20% of cases, but in 75% of cases, it is generalized to other skeletal muscles. Proximal muscles are more commonly involved than distal muscles. Peripheral muscle weakness can manifest as clumsiness, difficulty holding up the head, or in ambulating. Respiratory muscle weakness can cause dyspnea, a decrease in the ability to cough, and therefore to clear secretions.

MG is the most common neuromuscular junction disorder. The incidence of MG is between 4.1 and 30 cases per million person-years, and the prevalence rate ranges from 150 to 200 cases per million. The incidence is bimodal. In females, it peaks around 30 to 50 years old, while in males it steadily increases with age, and is highest over age 60 years. Females are more commonly affected than males before age 40, but after the age of 50, males are more likely to be affected. MG affects people of all races.

Daum P, Smelt J, Ibrahim IR. Perioperative management of myasthenia gravis. *BJA Educ.* 2021;21:414-419.

Dresser L, Wlodarski R, Rezania K, Soliven B. Myasthenia gravis: epidemiology, pathophysiology and clinical manifestations. *J Clin Med.* 2021;10:2235.

Spillane J, Higham E, Kullmann DM. Myasthenia gravis. *BMJ.* 2013;346:36e9.

A.2. What is the etiology and pathophysiology of MG?

In normal neuromuscular transmission, acetylcholine released from the motor nerve terminal stimulates postsynaptic nicotinic receptors at the motor end plate to generate an action potential, leading to depolarization of the membrane and contraction of the motor unit. The normal neuromuscular junction has a very large number of postsynaptic acetylcholine receptors (AChRs), such that muscle weakness only becomes apparent when 70% or more of the receptors are blocked. This excess of receptors has been termed the "margin of safety of neuromuscular transmission." Patients with MG have a significant decrease in the number of postsynaptic AChRs at muscle end plates of affected muscles, resulting in a decreased margin of safety of neuromuscular transmission.

MG is an autoimmune disorder, and about 80% of affected patients have detectable circulating antibodies to the nicotinic AChR. These anti-AChR antibodies can cause complement-mediated lysis of the postsynaptic membrane, directly block AChRs, or modulate receptor turnover, such that the rate of degradation exceeds the rate of resynthesis. Studies of the motor end plate show loss of synaptic folds and a widening of the synaptic cleft. About 10% of patients with MG have antibodies to muscle-specific tyrosine kinase (MuSK). These MuSK antibody-positive patients with MG often develop prominent oculobulbar muscle weakness.

The cause of MG is unknown but appears to be related in some way to the thymus gland. It has been suggested that thymic T cells are stimulated to produce antibodies following sensitization by a protein similar to the AChR. MG has recently been found to be a rare adverse effect of novel cancer immunotherapies, including pembrolizumab and other immune checkpoint inhibitors, while D-penicillamine might cause a drug-induced form of the disease. Patients with MG also have a higher incidence of other autoimmune diseases including thyroid, lupus, and rheumatoid.

Blichfeldt-Lauridsen L, Hansen BD. Anesthesia and myasthenia gravis. *Acta Anaesthesiol Scand.* 2012;56:17-22.

Paton WD, Waud DR. The margin of safety of neuromuscular transmission. *J Physiol.* 1967;191:59-90.

Rodriguez Cruz PM, Cossins J, Beeson D, et al. The neuromuscular junction in health and disease: molecular mechanisms governing synaptic formation and homeostasis. Review article. *Front Mol Neurosci.* 2020;13:1-22.

A.3. Describe the clinical classification of MG.

The Medical Scientific Advisory Board of the Myasthenia Gravis Foundation of America Clinical Classification describes five main classes and several subclasses of MG:

- Class I: any ocular muscle weakness; can have weakness of eye closure; all other muscle strength is normal.

- Class II: mild weakness affecting other than ocular muscles; can also have ocular muscle weakness of any severity
  - Class IIa: predominantly affecting limb, axial muscles, or both; can also have lesser involvement of oropharyngeal muscles
  - Class IIb: predominantly affecting oropharyngeal, respiratory muscles, or both; can also have lesser or equal involvement of limb, axial muscles, or both
- Class III: moderate weakness affecting other than ocular muscles; can also have ocular muscle weakness of any severity
  - Class IIIa: predominantly affecting limb, axial muscles, or both; can also have lesser involvement of oropharyngeal muscles
  - Class IIIb: predominantly affecting oropharyngeal, respiratory muscles, or both; can also have lesser or equal involvement of limb, axial muscles, or both
- Class IV: severe weakness affecting other than ocular muscles; can also have ocular muscle weakness of any severity
  - Class IVa: predominantly affecting limb, axial muscles, or both; can also have lesser involvement of oropharyngeal muscles
  - Class IVb: predominantly affecting oropharyngeal, respiratory muscles, or both; can also have lesser or equal involvement of limb, axial muscles, or both; use of a feeding tube without intubation
- Class V: defined by the need for intubation, with or without mechanical ventilation, except when used during routine postoperative management

Jaretzki A III, Barohn RJ, Ernstoff RM, et al. Myasthenia gravis: recommendations for clinical research standards. Task Force of the Medical Scientific Advisory Board of the Myasthenia Gravis Foundation of America. *Neurology.* 2000;55:16-23.

A.4. How is the diagnosis of MG made?

The diagnosis of MG is suspected from the history and confirmed by clinical, electrophysiologic, pharmacologic, or immunologic testing. Typically, the patient cannot sustain or repeat muscular contraction. Clinical tests of fatigability include maintaining an upward gaze, holding out an affected limb, and respiratory function testing (vital capacity, maximum breathing capacity).

Initial testing should include antibody testing and thyroid function tests. Antibodies to the nicotinic AChR are detectable in 80% of patients with MG. If studies for anti-AChR antibodies are negative, anti-MuSK and anti-LRP4 antibodies should be tested. Seronegative patients should undergo electrophysiologic studies.

The electrophysiologic counterpart of fatigability is a decrement in the compound muscle action potentials evoked by repetitive stimulation of a motor nerve. Supramaximal stimulation of a peripheral nerve at 2 Hz is applied; a decrement in the size of the fourth or fifth response compared to the first is diagnostic. This is the most specific of the nerve tests for MG, but it can be performed only on certain muscles, which might not be the ones affected in an individual patient. A more sensitive electrophysiologic test is single-fiber electromyography (EMG), where an increase in jitter is found.

Pharmacologic testing is based on the administration of a short-acting anticholinesterase, such as edrophonium, and observing a rapid improvement in function. Mechanical and electrophysiologic (eg, EMG) decrements improve with 2 to 10 mg of intravenous edrophonium (Tensilon test). Patients with MG are characteristically sensitive to nondepolarizing neuromuscular blocking agents (NMBAs), but these tests are now rarely performed. Finally, patients with MG should undergo CT or MRI of the mediastinum to detect thymoma.

Blichfeldt-Lauridsen L, Hansen BD. Anesthesia and myasthenia gravis. *Acta Anaesthesiol Scand.* 2012;56:17-22.

Dresser L, Wlodarski R, Rezania K, Soliven B. Myasthenia gravis: epidemiology, pathophysiology and clinical manifestations. *J Clin Med.* 2021;10:2235.

A.5. What should be considered in the differential diagnosis?

Several disorders can mimic MG and should be included in the initial differential diagnosis.

Thyrotoxicosis can present with generalized weakness and abnormal thyroid function. Patients with neurasthenia characteristically have weakness, which disappears when individual muscle groups are tested. Progressive external ophthalmoplegia; restrictive cardiomyopathies; muscular dystrophies; brain tumors; amyotrophic lateral sclerosis; myasthenic polymyopathy with hypersensitivity to neostigmine;

and drugs such as D-penicillamine, aminoglycosides, quinine, procainamide, and calcium channel blockers can also cause myasthenia-like symptoms.

Gilhus NE, Nacu A, Andersen JB, et al. Myasthenia gravis and risks for comorbidity. *Eur J Neurol.* 2015;22:17-23.

A.6. How does myasthenic syndrome (Lambert-Eaton syndrome) differ from MG?

Myasthenic syndrome (Lambert-Eaton syndrome) is a very rare immune-mediated disorder of neuromuscular transmission associated with antibodies to presynaptic voltage-gated calcium channels. The prevalence is estimated to be about 1 per 100,000. It is associated with small cell carcinoma of the lung in 50% to 60% of cases. Complaints of weakness can be mistaken for MG, but in Lambert-Eaton syndrome, the main difference is that strength improves with activity. Furthermore, the symptoms do not respond to administration of anticholinesterases or steroids. The defect in this condition is prejunctional, is associated with diminished release of acetylcholine from nerve terminals, and is improved by facilitating agents such as 4-aminopyridine that increase repetitive firing. Affected patients are particularly sensitive to the effects of all NMBAs, which should be used with great caution or avoided entirely. The possibility of Lambert-Eaton syndrome should be considered in all patients with known malignant disease and those patients undergoing diagnostic procedures for suspected carcinoma of the lung. Anesthesia considerations in these patients are essentially the same as for those with MG.

Keogh M, Sedehizadeh S, Maddison P. Treatment for Lambert-Eaton myasthenic syndrome. *Cochrane Database Syst Rev.* 2011;2011:CD003279.

Petty R. Lambert Eaton myasthenic syndrome. *Pract Neurol.* 2007;7:265-267.

Weingarten TN, Araka CN, Mogensen ME, et al. Lambert-Eaton myasthenic syndrome during anesthesia: a report of 37 patients. *J Clin Anesth.* 2014;26:648-653.

A.7. What treatments are available for a patient with MG?

Medical Therapy

Medications available to treat MG fall into the categories of anticholinesterase inhibitors and immunosuppressive agents. Walker was the first physician to report the similarity between the symptoms and signs of MG and curare poisoning and to use an anticholinesterase to treat MG. Anticholinesterases are the most commonly used therapy and prolong the action of acetylcholine at the postsynaptic membrane. No randomized controlled trial has been conducted on the use of acetylcholinesterase inhibitors in patients with MG because the response in observational studies is so obvious that a placebo group could not be justified. Acetylcholinesterase medication should be titrated to optimum effect (**Table 53.1**). Acetylcholinesterase overdosage causes muscarinic effects of acetylcholine and can cause a cholinergic crisis. Muscarinic adverse effects can be controlled with oral anticholinergic drugs, including propantheline and mebeverine. Cholinergic crisis can be treated with atropine. Underdosage causes weakness or a myasthenic crisis. To distinguish between the two types of crises, a Tensilon test can be performed or examination of pupil size, which will be large (mydriatic) in a myasthenic crisis but small (miotic) in a cholinergic crisis.

Pyridostigmine is the anticholinesterase drug most used to treat MG and has fewer muscarinic side effects than neostigmine. Its onset of action following oral administration is 15 to 30 minutes, with peak effect at 1 to 2 hours, and duration of action of 3 to 4 hours. Daily dosage is typically 30 to 120 mg given orally in divided doses. For patients who are weak on awakening in the morning, a long-acting formulation of 180 mg is available and can be taken at bedtime.

The immunologic basis of MG has led to the use of short- and long-term immunosuppressive drugs. Corticosteroids are used to complement anticholinesterase therapy and for short-term immunosuppression. Prolonged use of steroids can produce unwanted effects, such as peptic ulcers and osteoporosis. Steroids often produce initial deterioration before improvement. The usual regimen is prednisone 1 mg/kg

TABLE 53.1 Anticholinesterase Drugs Used to Treat Myasthenia Gravis (Dose in mg)

Drug	Oral	IV	IM	Efficacy
Pyridostigmine (Mestinon)	60	2	2-4	1
Neostigmine (Prostigmin)	1.5	0.5	0.7-1.0	1

IM, intramuscular; IV, intravenous.

on alternate days. For long-term therapy, azathioprine, cyclophosphamide, cyclosporine, methotrexate, mycophenolate mofetil, rituximab, and tacrolimus have been used. Rapid short-term immunomodulation has been achieved in acute exacerbations or to improve muscle strength prior to surgery. Plasma exchange or plasmapheresis can produce dramatic but transient improvements in muscle strength with decreases in anti-AChR and anti-MuSK titers, as well as other inflammatory mediators. Plasma exchange is usually reserved for severe MG and has been shown to improve respiratory function in both operated and nonoperated patients with MG. Plasmapheresis can decrease circulating levels of antibodies in patients in severe crisis or prior to surgery. It usually produces a rapid but short-lived improvement. Plasmapheresis also causes a decrease in plasma cholinesterase levels, which can prolong the effect of drugs such as succinylcholine that are metabolized by cholinesterase.

Surgical Therapy

Long-term immunomodulation is achieved by surgical thymectomy with the goal of achieving a remission or at least a reduction in the dosage of medications. Abnormalities are found in 75% of thymus glands removed from patients with MG (85% show hyperplasia, 15% show thymoma). After thymectomy, about 75% of patients either go into remission or show some improvement. Thymectomy is always indicated in patients with thymoma and is now considered the treatment of choice in most patients with MG, except for those with only ocular myasthenia. Response to thymectomy is best if it is performed within the first 3 years following diagnosis. Thymectomy is also recommended for patients with anti-AChR antibodies without a thymoma if under the age of 45 years, as it can reduce corticosteroid requirements and induce remission. Clinical outcome from thymectomy is equivalent whether performed via a transsternal (open) or video-assisted transcervical (minimally invasive) approach. A report describing anesthesia concerns in 17 patients who underwent robotic-assisted thoracoscopic thymectomy suggested that refinements of the surgical technique and positioning are required.

Daum P, Smelt J, Ibrahim IR. Perioperative management of myasthenia gravis. *BJA Educ*. 2021;21:414-419.

Kumar V, Kaminski HJ. Treatment of myasthenia gravis. *Curr Neurol Neurosci Rep*. 2011;11:89-96.

Maurizi G, D'Andrilli A, Sommella L, et al. Transsternal thymectomy. *Thorac Cardiovasc Surg*. 2015;63:178-186.

Mehndiratta MM, Pandey S, Kuntzer T. Acetylcholinesterase inhibitor treatment for myasthenia gravis. *Cochrane Database Syst Rev*. 2011;CD006986.

Sathasivam S. Current and emerging treatments for the management of myasthenia gravis. *Ther Clin Risk Manag*. 2011;7:313-323.

Walker MB. Case showing the effect of prostigmin on myasthenia gravis. *Proc R Soc Med*. 1935;28:759-761.

B. Preoperative Evaluation and Preparation

B.1. Describe the preoperative evaluation of this patient.

Several problems must be considered: history of MG, open abdominal procedure in Trendelenburg position, obesity, and anxiety state. The preoperative interview should be used to identify factors that suggest the need for postoperative ventilation. Factors that have been associated with an increased need for postoperative ventilation include concomitant chronic obstructive pulmonary disease, BMI greater than 28 kg/m^2, disease duration for more than 2 years, symptoms of generalized weakness or bulbar and respiratory symptoms, history of previous myasthenic crises, pyridostigmine dose greater than 750 mg/d, vital capacity less than 2 L, serum AChR antibody concentrations greater than 100 nmol/mL, surgeries with intraoperative blood loss greater than 1 L, and lung resection. This information can guide the anesthesiologist in formulating the anesthetic plan, selecting of preoperative medications, and arranging for postoperative care. When possible, patients with MG should be scheduled for elective surgery while in remission. Both physical and emotional states should be optimized regarding the patient's anxiety. Current drug therapy should be reviewed, and possible drug interactions considered. The patient should be informed of the possible need for postoperative tracheal intubation and ventilation. A thorough airway exam and evaluation for obstructive sleep apnea should be completed, given her morbid obesity.

Daum P, Smelt J, Ibrahim IR. Perioperative management of myasthenia gravis. *BJA Educ*. 2021;21:414-419.

B.2. What preoperative laboratory data are required?

Laboratory studies should be individualized to the patient. In addition to routine preoperative laboratory data, electrolyte abnormalities, particularly hypokalemia which can exacerbate weakness, should be ruled out. Given that this case is an emergency, studies might not be required before proceeding to surgery.

If the patient is receiving or has recently taken corticosteroids, blood glucose levels should be checked. Preoperative arterial blood gas analysis and pulmonary function tests can be helpful in knowing baseline lung function; however, this should not be done if it would cause a delay in this emergency case. A respiratory therapist should educate the patient about breathing exercises and the use of an incentive spirometer.

Blichfeldt-Lauridsen L, Hansen BD. Anesthesia and myasthenia gravis. *Acta Anaesthesiol Scand.* 2012;56:17-22.

B.3. How should the patient's medications be managed preoperatively?

Management of anticholinesterase medication preoperatively should be individualized to the patient. Anticholinesterase therapy should be continued if the patient is physically or psychologically dependent on it. For elective cases, the practice is to withhold pyridostigmine therapy on the morning of surgery so that the patient is weak on arrival to the operating room. This avoids interactions with other drugs used in the operating room. For emergency cases such as this one, there might not be time or opportunity to alter pyridostigmine therapy perioperatively, and therefore, considerations need to be made for dosing of medications intraoperatively. For example, anticholinesterase inhibits both plasma cholinesterase and acetylcholinesterase, so the metabolism of succinylcholine will be slowed. Others recommend continuing pyridostigmine, including an oral dose just before induction (**Table 53.1**). Anxiolysis is satisfactorily achieved with a benzodiazepine. Opioids are usually avoided because of the potential for causing respiratory depression. Ideally, patients with MG should be scheduled to be the first case of the day in the operating room, as muscle function is at its best then.

Blichfeldt-Lauridsen L, Hansen BD. Anesthesia and myasthenia gravis. *Acta Anaesthesiol Scand.* 2012;56:17-22.

Daum P, Smelt J, Ibrahim IR. Perioperative management of myasthenia gravis. *BJA Educ.* 2021;21:414-419.

C. Intraoperative Management

C.1. What are your considerations in the choice of anesthetic technique?

Although regional and neuraxial anesthetic techniques have been used successfully, general anesthesia is the better choice in this patient for this surgery for several reasons:

- Open abdominal procedure with a patient with obesity in Trendelenburg position would likely make spontaneous ventilation difficult.
- Any weakness would exacerbate ventilatory difficulty.
- Anxiety might require the administration of sedatives that could depress respiration and can be contraindicated if the patient is not NPO (nothing by mouth) for surgery.
- In the event of an ascending (neuraxial) block level causing respiratory muscle weakness, emergent tracheal intubation and ventilation would become necessary. Securing the airway at the outset would be preferable, given her morbid obesity and risk of difficult airway.

C.2. How should this patient be monitored intraoperatively?

Standard American Society of Anesthesiologists (ASA) basic monitors must be used. In addition, an arterial line might be useful to draw arterial blood samples for gas analysis intra- and postoperatively. A peripheral nerve stimulator, and ideally a means to quantify responses to stimulation (eg, EMG, accelerometer, and kinemyography), should be used from the beginning even if NMBAs will be avoided. Potent inhaled anesthetics also depress neuromuscular transmission, and monitoring of recovery from this effect is similarly needed. Once the patient is asleep, baseline recordings should be made before any potent inhaled or NMBA is administered. Subsequent responses may then be quantitatively compared to baseline. In MG, fade-in response to train-of-four and tetanic stimulation occurs in the affected muscles at baseline. If a total intravenous anesthesia (TIVA)-based anesthetic is used, a bispectral index electroencephalogram (EEG) is helpful to evaluate the depth of anesthesia.

Daum P, Smelt J, Ibrahim IR. Perioperative management of myasthenia gravis. Review article. *BJA Educ.* 2021;21:414-419.

Blichfeldt-Lauridsen L, Hansen BD. Anesthesia and myasthenia gravis. *Acta Anaesthesiol Scand.* 2012;56:17-22.

C.3. What anesthetic regimen would you choose for this patient?

For the reasons given earlier, the safest approach is general tracheal anesthesia. Maintenance of anesthesia in the intubated, ventilated patient can be achieved with an inhalational anesthetic, a balanced technique, or TIVA.

If the preoperative evaluation does not predict a difficult airway, tracheal intubation can be performed with the patient asleep rather than awake. Prior to induction of anesthesia, the patient should be preoxygenated by breathing 100% oxygen until the end-tidal oxygen is greater than 90%. Ideally, it should be 95%, the other 5% of the exhaled gas mixture being carbon dioxide and water vapor. Induction of anesthesia is readily achieved with propofol or etomidate. This patient should have a rapid-sequence induction, given the risk for pulmonary aspiration. Effects of NMBAs can be unpredictable and come with risks in reversal with anticholinesterases, and thus, they should ideally be avoided if possible. Propofol and remifentanil can provide satisfactory conditions for tracheal intubation and can be used for maintenance to try to avoid NMBAs. If paralysis is required, succinylcholine might not be reliable for rapid sequence since patients with MG can be resistant to succinylcholine due to decreased AChR density at the neuromuscular junction. Patients with MG are profoundly sensitive to NMBAs, but this might be the agent of choice in this case, given that a 1.2-mg/kg bolus of rocuronium will provide adequate and fast relaxation to aid in rapid tracheal intubation.

Patients with MG are more sensitive than normal patients to the neuromuscular depressant effects of potent inhaled agents. In patients with MG, isoflurane at 1.9 minimum alveolar concentration (MAC) end-tidal concentration induced a neuromuscular block of 30% to 50%, whereas halothane at 1.8 MAC induced a block of 10% to 20%. Both agents produced fade in the train-of-four ratio of 41% and 28%, respectively. The less-soluble inhaled agents, sevoflurane and desflurane, are even more rapidly taken up and eliminated; they are now the most commonly used anesthetic drugs for patients with MG. Whichever agent is used, at the end of the procedure, the inhaled agent is discontinued and recovery of neuromuscular function begins.

Blichfeldt-Lauridsen L, Hansen BD. Anesthesia and myasthenia gravis. *Acta Anaesthesiol Scand.* 2012;56:17-22.

Daum P, Smelt J, Ibrahim IR. Perioperative management of myasthenia gravis. Review article. *BJA Educ.* 2021;21:414-419.

Nilsson E, Muller K. Neuromuscular effects of isoflurane in patients with myasthenia gravis. *Acta Anaesthesiol Scand.* 1990;34:126-131.

Nitahara K, Sugi Y, Higa K, et al. Neuromuscular effects of sevoflurane in myasthenia gravis patients. *Br J Anaesth.* 2007;98:337-341.

Troy AM, Hutchinson RC, Easy WR, Kenny GN. Tracheal intubating conditions using propofol and remifentanil target-controlled infusions. *Anaesthesia.* 2002;57:1204-1207.

C.4. Can neuromuscular blocking drugs be used safely in a patient with MG?

If the patient cannot tolerate the depth of anesthesia needed to produce relaxation with the potent inhaled agent or TIVA, NMBAs can be used, titrating dose against the monitored effect. Patients with MG are sensitive (ie, show a decrease in ED50 and ED95 when compared with patients without MG) to nondepolarizing NMBAs because of the decreased number of postsynaptic receptors at the motor end plate. All nondepolarizing NMBAs have been successfully and uneventfully used with careful monitoring in patients with MG. Because the sensitivity of any individual MG patient is unknown, these drugs should be titrated in 1/10 of the usual dose. Before use of sugammadex, cisatracurium was preferred because of its short elimination half-life, small volume of distribution, lack of cumulative effect, and high clearance. However, rocuronium is a good choice since it can be rapidly and reliably reversed with sugammadex and avoid the need for anticholinesterases. Several case reports and series have shown the effective use of sugammadex in patients with MG and demonstrated superiority to neostigmine for reversing moderate-to-deep neuromuscular block, likely reducing the risk of perioperative myasthenic crises.

Patients with MG are resistant to the neuromuscular blocking effects of succinylcholine due to the decrease in the number of postsynaptic receptors at the motor end plate. The ED95 is 2.6 times normal in these patients (0.8 vs 0.3 mg/kg). Clinically, the use of succinylcholine has been without incident, with the usual clinical doses producing adequate paralysis for tracheal intubation and a normal recovery time, despite occasionally reported early onset of phase II block. Doses of 0.2 to 1.0 mg/kg have been used in a number of patients with MG, and most did not show fasciculation before becoming paralyzed. Fade in response to train-of-four stimulation was observed in some patients during recovery, but recovery was not delayed. Prior administration of an anticholinesterase complicates the response to succinylcholine by delaying its metabolism.

Baraka AS, Taha SK, Kawkabani NI. Neuromuscular interaction of sevoflurane—cisatracurium in a myasthenic patient. *Can J Anaesth.* 2000;47:562-565.

Carron M, De Cassai A, Linassi F. Sugammadex in the management of myasthenic patients undergoing surgery: beyond expectations. *Ann Transl Med.* 2019;7:307.

Daum P, Smelt J, Ibrahim IR. Perioperative management of myasthenia gravis. *BJA Educ.* 2021;21:414-419.

de Boer HD, Shields MO, Booij LH. Reversal of neuromuscular blockade with sugammadex in patients with myasthenia gravis: a case series of 21 patients and review of the literature. *Eur J Anaesthesiol.* 2014;31:715-721.

Eisenkraft JB, Book WJ, Mann SM, et al. Resistance to succinylcholine in myasthenia gravis: a dose-response study. *Anesthesiology.* 1988;69:760-763.

Eisenkraft JB, Book WJ, Papatestas AE. Sensitivity to vecuronium in myasthenia gravis: a dose-response study. *Can J Anaesth.* 1990;37:301-306.

Kiss G, Lacour A, D'Hollander A. Fade of train-of-four ratio despite administration of more than 12 mg.kg^{-1} sugammadex in a myasthenia gravis patient receiving rocuronium. *Br J Anaesth.* 2013;110:854-855.

Kopman AF. Sugammadex: a revolutionary approach to neuromuscular antagonism. *Anesthesiology.* 2006;104:631-633.

Unterbuchner C, Fink H, Blobner M. The use of sugammadex in a patient with myasthenia gravis. *Anaesthesia.* 2010;65:302-305.`

C.5. Should the patient with MG who is in remission (symptom free without treatment) be managed differently?

Although it is well established that patients with MG are sensitive to nondepolarizing and resistant to depolarizing NMBAs, there is no consensus on the response to these drugs during a remission. It is therefore prudent to manage the patient who is in remission as if they had active disease and titrate nondepolarizing NMBAs to effect while monitoring the responses.

Abel M, Eisenkraft JB, Patel N. Response to suxamethonium in a myasthenic patient during remission. *Anaesthesia.* 1991;46:30-32.

Basaranoglu G, Erden V, Delatioglu H. Anesthesia of a patient with cured myasthenia gravis. *Anesth Analg.* 2003;96:1842-1843.

Wainwright AP, Brodrick PM. Suxamethonium in myasthenia gravis. *Anaesthesia.* 1987;42:950-957.

D. Postoperative Management

D.1. What factors will help you predict this patient's need for continued tracheal intubation or other postoperative ventilatory support?

MG places patients at an increased risk of respiratory failure after general anesthesia. Several studies have attempted to identify specific characteristics of patients undergoing surgery that could help predict the increased likelihood of postoperative respiratory failure patients with MG (see Section B.1). These predictors are based on patient factors (coexisting diseases, vital capacity, and BMI), disease factors (duration, symptoms, history of crises, antibody concentrations, and pyridostigmine dose), and surgery factors (blood loss >1 L and lung resection). Although a definitive risk stratification system has not yet been validated, it is important to assess each patient on a case-by-case basis and engage in frank preoperative discussions regarding the risk of postoperative myasthenic crisis and the possible need for prolonged ventilatory support.

Daum P, Smelt J, Ibrahim IR. Perioperative management of myasthenia gravis. *BJA Educ.* 2021;21:414-419.

Eisenkraft JB, Papatestas AE, Kahn CH, et al. Predicting the need for postoperative mechanical ventilation in myasthenia gravis. *Anesthesiology.* 1986;65:79-82.

Leuzzi G, Meacci E, Cusumano G, et al. Thymectomy in myasthenia gravis: proposal for a predictive score of postoperative myasthenic crisis. *Eur J Cardiothorac Surg.* 2014;45:e76-e88.

Mori T, Yoshioka M, Watanabe K, et al. Changes in respiratory condition after thymectomy for patients with myasthenia gravis. *Ann Thorac Cardiovasc Surg.* 2003;9:93-97.

D.2. How will you determine if this patient's trachea can be safely extubated?

Postoperative weakness is the greatest contributing factor to perioperative respiratory failure in patients with MG. As such, it is important to establish that the patient is fully awake and alert prior to attempting extubation and that any residual neuromuscular blockade has been completely reversed. Adequate respiratory effort should be confirmed by the ability to generate a negative inspiratory pressure of at least −20 cm H_2O. Following extubation, it is essential to monitor closely for signs of fatigue, weakness, or evidence of deteriorating respiratory status (hypercarbia, hypoxemia, tachypnea). If the patient was taking pyridostigmine preoperatively, oral dosing should be reestablished as soon as possible after extubation; if necessary, alternative anticholinesterase medications, such as neostigmine or edrophonium, can be used as a bridging measure. The dosage equivalents are shown in **Table 53.1**.

Care should be taken to ensure that somnolence related to opioid administration does not place the patient at increased risk of hypoventilation. In addition, vigilance is required to ensure that impending myasthenic crisis is not masked by intraoperative reversal agents whose effect may wear off in the postanesthesia care unit.

Blichfeldt-Lauridsen L, Hansen BD. Anesthesia and myasthenia gravis. *Acta Anaesthesiol Scand.* 2012;56:17-22.

Daum P, Smelt J, Ibrahim IR. Perioperative management of myasthenia gravis. Review article. *BJA Educ.* 2021;21:414-419.

D.3. How will you manage postoperative analgesia?

Patients with MG are especially sensitive to the central respiratory depressive effects of parenteral opioid administration. On the other hand, inadequately treated pain related to surgery can inhibit ventilatory effort and thus can also worsen respiratory status. Nonopioid pain regimens should be considered whenever possible, including regional and neuraxial anesthesia where appropriate, because of a greatly reduced total dose of opioid compared to parenteral administration. Truncal nerve blocks or thoracic epidural analgesia would be preferred in this open abdominal case. Intravenous nonsteroidal anti-inflammatory drugs (NSAIDs) and acetaminophen regimens have also been effective in controlling pain without causing respiratory depression. If oral or parenteral opioids are used, the dose should be reduced for patients receiving anticholinesterase therapy because these medications have been reported to increase the efficacy of opioids.

Blichfeldt-Lauridsen L, Hansen BD. Anesthesia and myasthenia gravis. *Acta Anaesthesiol Scand.* 2012;56:17-22.

Su C, Su Y, Chou CW, et al. Intravenous flurbiprofen for post-thymectomy pain relief in patients with myasthenia gravis. *J Cardiothorac Surg.* 2012;7:98.

D.4. How will you define and manage postextubation ventilatory failure in this patient?

The postsurgical state is uniquely perilous to the patient with MG for respiratory decompensation after extubation; indeed, cases have been reported in which previously undetected MG was diagnosed as a result of unexpected respiratory failure in the postoperative period. Suggested criteria for reintubation have included tachypnea (respiratory rate >40 breaths per minute), respiratory acidosis not due to opioids, or vital capacity less than or equal to 8 mL/kg.

In the patient with MG experiencing postoperative respiratory distress, it is crucial to differentiate cholinergic crisis from myasthenic crisis because the precipitating events and appropriate therapies are different. Each can present as muscle weakness, salivation, and sweating. Although myasthenic crisis is thought to result from surgical stress leading to decreased responsiveness to anticholinesterase therapy, cholinergic crisis results from an overdose of anticholinergic drugs. The two conditions can be differentiated using the Tensilon test: 10 mg of edrophonium IV. The patient in myasthenic crisis will respond with an improvement in respiratory muscle strength, whereas the patient in cholinergic crisis will exhibit no change or a worsening of symptoms. The treatment for myasthenic crisis is anticholinesterase therapy titrated to effect; in contrast, the treatment for cholinergic crisis can incorporate antimuscarinic drugs to treat salivation and sweating but is mostly supportive and can require mechanical ventilation until the crisis resolves.

Antevil JL, Carroll CG, Roberts PF, et al. Myasthenia gravis—an unexpected cause of respiratory failure and reversible left ventricular dysfunction after cardiac surgery. *J Card Surg.* 2010;25:662-664.

Cheng S, Liu S, Chou C, et al. An uncommon cause of postthyroidectomy respiratory failure. *Thyroid.* 2009;19:1129-1130.

Gorback MS, Moon RE, Massey JM. Extubation after transsternal thymectomy for myasthenia gravis: a prospective analysis. *South Med J.* 1991;84:701-706.

Acknowledgments

We gratefully acknowledge the contributions of previous edition author, Bryan S. Carter, as portions of those chapters have been retained in this revision.

54

Malignant Hyperthermia

Adam D. Lichtman, Henry Rosenberg,
Harvey K. Rosenbaum, and Vinod Malhotra

A healthy 27-year-old male is scheduled for ambulatory laparoscopic repair of an inguinal hernia under general anesthesia. Previous anesthetic history includes an uneventful anesthetic as a child for a tonsillectomy. However, he did note that his uncle had to be "packed in ice" when had had surgery many years ago, and several of his male cousins from the Midwest have had "bad reactions" to anesthesia, but could not elaborate on exactly what happened. On further questioning, the patient noted that he has muscle cramps and heat intolerance during the summer.

A. Medical Disease and Differential Diagnosis

1. What is the problem of concern in this case?
2. What is malignant hyperthermia (MH)?
3. What are the clinical features of a patient with MH susceptibility?
4. Does the history of previous uneventful general anesthesia reasonably exclude the patient's susceptibility to MH?
5. What are the clinical features of MH?
6. What are the laboratory findings during an acute MH crisis?
7. What is the incidence of MH?
8. What is the mode of inheritance of MH? Does it "skip" generations?
9. What genetic disorders result in MH susceptibility?
10. What is the pathophysiology of MH syndrome?
11. What laboratory tests can be used to diagnose MH susceptibility?
12. What is neuroleptic malignant syndrome (NMS)? What is serotonin syndrome?

B. Preoperative Evaluation and Preparation

1. How would you prepare this patient for anesthesia and surgery?
2. Is dantrolene prophylaxis indicated?
3. What laboratory tests would you obtain before surgery?
4. Is outpatient surgery appropriate for this patient?
5. If general anesthesia is needed, what preparations would you make?

C. Intraoperative Management

1. What anesthetic techniques and agents would you employ?
2. Should body (core) temperature be monitored during general anesthesia lasting more than 30 minutes?
3. What anesthetic agents are contraindicated in MH?
4. If the surgeon wants to use local anesthesia for a procedure, what local anesthetics will you recommend?
5. What is the significance of masseter muscle rigidity occurring after succinylcholine administration?
6. Twenty minutes into the procedure with sevoflurane anesthesia, the patient develops increasing tachycardia with ventricular premature beats and mottled skin. What emergency measures should you take?
7. What modalities would you monitor closely during management of the crisis?
8. What steps should be taken to avoid major morbidity from MH?
9. How does the new formulation of dantrolene (Ryanodex) compare with the previous formulations of dantrolene (Dantrium or Revonto)?

D. Postoperative Management

1. What are the potential complications that can follow an MH event?
2. How should you follow-up in this case?
3. What would you advise the patient and the family?
4. What precautions should a patient with MH susceptibility take outside of the operating room?
5. What is the relationship between MH and exertional heat stroke (EHS)?

A. Medical Disease and Differential Diagnosis

A.1. What is the problem of concern in this case?

The report of several family members having "bad reactions" to anesthesia is of concern, but without specific information no conclusions can be drawn. The addition of the uncle's history of having to be "packed in ice" raises the concern for a family history of MH. This strong suspicion has supported a history of multiple family members with reported adverse reactions to anesthesia, the geographic location that family members are from, and the patient's report of heat intolerance and muscle cramps. There is a 2:1 male:female predominance of MH, and there is a high density of families susceptible to MH in Michigan, Nebraska, West Virginia, and Wisconsin.

Litman RS, Griggs SM, Dowling JJ, et al. Malignant hyperthermia susceptibility and related diseases. *Anesthesiology*. 2018;128:159-167.

Rodrigues G, de Andrade PV, Dos Santos JM, et al. Impact of a digital manual for guidance on malignant hyperthermia: patient education. *Orphanet J Rare Dis*. 2022;17:265.

A.2. What is malignant hyperthermia (MH)?

MH, first described by Denborough and Lovell in 1960, is a potentially fatal inherited pharmacogenetic disorder characterized by hypermetabolism. For MH to occur, it is generally accepted that a patient with MH susceptibility receives an agent or "trigger," that is, potent inhalation anesthetic agents or succinylcholine, to cause MH. This can occur on introduction of one of these agents or on subsequent exposure. There have been reports of MH occurring without classic triggers. Signs and symptoms of MH include elevated core temperature (hyperpyrexia), tachycardia, tachypnea, hypercarbia, rigidity, acidosis, and hyperkalemia. These are all signs of a hypermetabolic state. However, not all signs appear in all cases, and MH can appear in humans in the absence of anesthetic agents (see A.5). The underlying abnormality is an uncontrolled elevation of intracellular calcium in skeletal muscle. This activation of muscle contractile elements causes hypermetabolism and usually death if untreated. Dantrolene is the specific pharmacologic agent used to treat MH.

Denborough MA, Lovell RRH. Anesthetic deaths in a family. *Lancet*. 1960;2:45.

Litman RS, Griggs SM, Dowling JJ, et al. Malignant hyperthermia susceptibility and related diseases. *Anesthesiology*. 2018;128:159-167.

A.3. What are the clinical features of a patient with MH susceptibility?

A family history, if present, particularly in a first-degree relative, or the presence of certain musculoskeletal disorders is a strong indicator of MH susceptibility. However, most patients susceptible to MH do not have obvious family histories or known musculoskeletal disorders. Epidemiologic studies have demonstrated that certain comorbidities such a scoliosis and muscle disorders are more frequent in patients with MH susceptibility. There are several myopathic disorders that are associated with MH susceptibility. They include central core disease, King-Denborough syndrome, multiminicore disease, congenital myopathy with cores and rods, nemaline rod myopathy, idiopathic hyperCKemia, and Native American myopathy. Hypokalemic periodic paralysis has been rarely associated with MH susceptibility (**Table 54.1**). Patients who have Duchenne or Becker muscular dystrophy should not be anesthetized with MH trigger agents, not due to MH susceptibility but because hyperkalemia and rhabdomyolysis can result.

Biesecker LG, Dirksen RT, Girard T, et al. Genomic screening for malignant hyperthermia susceptibility. *Anesthesiology*. 2020;133:1277-1282.

Larach MG, Gronert GA, Allen GC, et al. Clinical presentation, treatment, and complications of malignant hyperthermia in North America from 1987 to 2006. *Anesth Analg*. 2010;110:498-507.

Litman RS, Griggs SM, Dowling JJ, et al. Malignant hyperthermia susceptibility and related diseases. *Anesthesiology*. 2018;128:159-167.

Rosenberg H, Pollock N, Schiemann A, et al. Malignant hyperthermia: a review. *Orphanet J Rare Dis*. 2015;10:93.

TABLE 54.1 Associated Musculoskeletal Disorders and Signs in Patients Susceptible to Malignant Hyperthermia

Scoliosis
Hypotonia
Exercise-induced rhabdomyolysis
Strabismus
Central core disease
Multiminicore disease
King-Denborough syndrome
Congenital myopathy with cores and rods
Nemaline rod myopathy
Idiopathic hyperCKemia
Native American myopathy
Hypokalemic periodic paralysis (rarely associated with malignant hyperthermia susceptibility)

A.4. Does the history of previous uneventful general anesthesia reasonably exclude the patient's susceptibility to MH?

No, it does not. Cases can occur during subsequent anesthetics with the third exposure being the most common.

Heytens L, Forget P, Scholtès JC, et al. The changing face of malignant hyperthermia: less fulminant, more insidious. *Anaesth Intensive Care*. 2015;43:506-511.

Larach MG, Gronert GA, Allen GC, et al. Clinical presentation, treatment, and complications of malignant hyperthermia in North America from 1987 to 2006. *Anesth Analg*. 2010;110:498-507.

Rosenbaum HK. Malignant hyperthermia: diagnosis and management of acute crisis. In: Post T, ed. *UpToDate*. UpToDate; 2019. Accessed May, 2023. https://www.uptodate.com/contents/malignant-hyperthermia-diagnosis-and-management-of-acute-crisis

Urman RD, Rajan N, Belani K, et al. Malignant hyperthermia-susceptible adult patient and Ambulatory Surgery Center: Society for Ambulatory Anesthesia and Ambulatory Surgical Care Committee of the American Society of Anesthesiologists Position Statement. *Anesth Analg*. 2019;129:347-349.

A.5. What are the clinical features of MH?

The clinical features of MH are the result of an uncontrolled, exaggerated, hypermetabolic state triggered by potent inhalation anesthetic agents or succinylcholine. Common manifestations include:

Specific for MH

- Increase in end-tidal carbon dioxide (CO_2) during constant ventilation (the most sensitive and specific sign). Use of CO_2 during laparoscopic surgery can increase end-tidal CO_2 in the absence of MH. Deliberate hyperventilation during laparoscopic surgery can obscure an initial rise in end-tidal CO_2, however, the rate of CO_2 production can outpace changes in minute ventilation.
- Generalized rigidity (extremely high specificity); when due to MH, it does NOT improve with administration of neuromuscular blocking agents or increasing anesthetic depth.
- Masseter muscle rigidity (MMR)

Nonspecific

- Tachycardia (the earliest and most consistent clinical sign, however, not specific)
- Tachypnea; patients with incomplete paralysis under general anesthesia can attempt to over breathe the ventilator settings.
- Hyperthermia (hyperpyrexia), which can exceed 40 °C
- Cardiac arrhythmias
- Skin mottling
- Profuse sweating
- Labile hemodynamics: hypotension or hypertension

Hyperthermia (hyperpyrexia) is an important sign of MH, but it is nonspecific. Iatrogenic overheating can cause intraoperative hyperthermia. However, intraoperative hypothermia is much more common than hyperthermia in the operating room due to environmental conditions, so development of hyperthermia should raise concern. The reliable measurement of patient temperatures requires accurate devices used at representative locations. Examples include measurements of core temperature from the esophagus, tympanic membrane, or bladder. The measurement of skin temperature is unreliable and can give falsely low readings. Failure to measure core temperature or reliance on inaccurate temperature monitors is associated with increased mortality from an MH episode.

Hyperkalemic Cardiac Arrest

Sudden hyperkalemic cardiac arrest has been reported after administration of MH triggering agents in children with undiagnosed myopathy, especially the dystrophinopathies, for example, Duchenne or Becker muscular dystrophy. This response is due to acute muscle membrane destruction leading to hyperkalemia. The pathway leading to the abnormal response to potent inhalational anesthetics is not clear. Fulminant MH can also result in hyperkalemic cardiac arrest associated with severe acidosis, rhabdomyolysis, and hyperthermia. Treatment of hyperkalemia includes glucose and insulin, calcium chloride or gluconate, and hyperventilation.

Gurnaney H, Brown A, Litman RS. Malignant hyperthermia and muscular dystrophies. *Anesth Analg.* 2009;109:1043-1048.

Larach MG, Brandom BW, Allen GC, et al. Malignant hyperthermia deaths related to inadequate temperature monitoring, 2007-2012: a report from the North American malignant hyperthermia registry of the Malignant Hyperthermia Association of the United States. *Anesth Analg.* 2014;119:1359-1366.

Larach MG, Gronert GA, Allen GC, et al. Clinical presentation, treatment, and complications of malignant hyperthermia in North America from 1987 to 2006. *Anesth Analg.* 2010;110:498-507.

Larach MG, Rosenberg H, Gronert GA, et al. Hyperkalemic cardiac arrest during anesthesia in infants and children with occult myopathies. *Clin Pediatr (Phila).* 1997;36:9-16.

Nathan A, Ganesh A, Godinez RI, et al. Hyperkalemic cardiac arrest after cardiopulmonary bypass in a child with unsuspected Duchenne muscular dystrophy. *Anesth Analg.* 2005;100:672-674.

A.6. What are the laboratory findings during an acute MH crisis?

Laboratory values reflect the hypermetabolic state and muscle tissue damage (**Table 54.2**). Hence, hypercarbia, respiratory and metabolic acidosis, hyperkalemia, elevated creatine kinase (CK), and myoglobinemia

TABLE 54.2 Laboratory Findings in Acute Malignant Hyperthermia

Metabolic and Respiratory Acidosis
Arterial blood gases
↓↓ pH
↑↑ P_{CO_2}
Mild decreases in P_{O_2}
Electrolytes
↑ K
Later decreased serum calcium
↑ Mg
Serum
↑ Lactate
↑ Pyruvate
↑ Creatine kinase
↑ Lactate dehydrogenase
↑ Aldolase
↑ Myoglobin
Increased INR, increased FSP, increased PT/PTT
Thrombocytopenia if DIC develops

DIC, disseminated intravascular coagulation; FSP, fibrin split products; INR, international normalized ratio; K, potassium; Mg, magnesium; P_{CO_2}, partial pressure of carbon dioxide; P_{O_2}, partial pressure of oxygen; PT/PTT, prothrombin time/partial thromboplastin time.

are common findings. If the hyperthermia is extreme, coagulopathy is common. In the early stage of an MH episode, metabolic acidosis, hyperkalemia, and CK elevation might be absent. The presence of a mixed respiratory and metabolic acidosis is both specific and highly sensitive as a marker of MH.

Larach MG, Gronert GA, Allen GC, et al. Clinical presentation, treatment, and complications of malignant hyperthermia in North America from 1987 to 2006. *Anesth Analg*. 2010;110:498-507.

A.7. What is the incidence of MH?

The incidence of clinical MH is difficult to measure because many clinical syndromes resemble MH and often the anesthetic management is altered when initial signs suggesting MH are detected. The incidence also depends on the prevalence in a population of genetic mutations causal for MH as well as the prevalence of use of MH trigger agents. For most conditions, the incidence is determined by coded diagnoses in the medical record. However, in the case of MH, because many clinicians are not familiar with the disorder, some cases of high fever with bad patient outcome are labeled generically as "malignant hyperthermia." In one small study based on such coded diagnoses, only 25% of cases coded as MH were determined to represent clinical episodes of MH by an expert panel.

One of the earliest epidemiologic studies of MH was conducted in Denmark where an estimate of the incidence of fulminant MH was 1 in 260,000 general anesthetics and 1 in 60,000 anesthetics where succinylcholine was used. The incidence was even higher, that is, 1 in 5,000 anesthetics, when such signs as MMR, unexplained tachycardia, and unexplained fever were included. Two recent studies of coded hospital discharge data showed that the prevalence of MH was 1 in 100,000 hospital discharges for adults and 4 per 100,000 discharges for children.

In Quebec, Canada, the prevalence of MH was calculated as 0.2% of the population based on a detailed genealogic study of families with MH susceptibility. Genetic studies have suggested that the prevalence of MH-causative mutations is 1 in 2,000 people in France and Japan. Incomplete penetrance results in an incidence of MH episodes far lower than anticipated by mutation prevalence. However, mortality from acute MH ranges from 6% to 10%.

Brady J, Sun L, Rosenberg H, et al. Prevalence of malignant hyperthermia due to anesthesia in New York State, 2001-2005. *Anesth Analg*. 2009;109:1162-1166.

Li G, Brady JE, Rosenberg H, et al. Excess comorbidities associated with malignant hyperthermia diagnosis in pediatric hospital discharge records. *Paediatr Anaesth*. 2011;21:958-963.

Monnier N, Krivosic-Horber R, Payen JF, et al. Presence of two different genetic traits in malignant hyperthermia families: implication for genetic analysis, diagnosis, and incidence of malignant hyperthermia susceptibility. *Anesthesiology*. 2002;97:1067-1074.

Pinyavat T, Rosenberg H, Lang B, et al. Accuracy of malignant hyperthermia diagnoses in hospital discharge records. *Anesthesiology*. 2015;122:55-63.

Riazi S, Kraeva N, Hopkins PM. Malignant hyperthermia in the post-genomics era: new perspectives on an old concept. *Anesthesiology*. 2018;128:168-180.

Rosero EB, Adesanya AO, Timaran CH, et al. Trends and outcomes of malignant hyperthermia in the United States, 2000 to 2005. *Anesthesiology*. 2009;110:89-94.

van den Bersselaar LR, Hellblom A, Gashi M, et al. Referral indications for malignant hyperthermia susceptibility diagnostics in patients without adverse anesthetic events in the era of next-generation sequencing. *Anesthesiology*. 2022;136:940-953.

A.8. What is the mode of inheritance of MH? Does it "skip" generations?

MH inheritance in humans is autosomal dominant with reduced penetrance and variable expressivity. MH is heterogeneic with up to seven gene loci implicated, but only three are confirmed: *RYR1*, *CACNA1S*, and *STAC3*. A missense mutation in *STAC3* is associated with Native American myopathy and MH susceptibility; the disorder displays autosomal recessive transmission. *STAC3*-related myopathy has been described in other ethnic groups and has not been described in heterozygous family members.

The vast majority (over 70%) of MH cases are linked to the skeletal muscle ryanodine receptor gene *RYR1* located on chromosome 19. Less than 2% of MH cases are associated with mutations in the calcium voltage-gated channel α1 subunit of the dihydropyridine receptor (*CACNA1S)* gene. Over 400 variants have been found in *RYR1* with 48 documented as causal mutations for the syndrome.

Because MH is usually inherited in an autosomal dominant manner, susceptibility to MH does not "skip" generations. However, because of the low penetrance, not all those with MH mutations display the syndrome on exposure to trigger agents. De novo mutations have also been described. Some patients with MH susceptibility with overt myopathy are homozygous or compound heterozygous for *RYR1* mutations that are causal or potentially causal for MH. Nonmyopathic family members might also be MH susceptible.

Biesecker LG, Dirksen RT, Girard T, et al. Genomic screening for malignant hyperthermia susceptibility. *Anesthesiology*. 2020;133:1277-1282.

McCarthy TV, Healey JM, Jeffron JJ, et al. Localization of the malignant hyperthermia susceptibility locus to human chromosome 19q12-13.2. *Nature*. 1990;343:562-563.

Riazi S, Kraeva N, Hopkins PM. Malignant hyperthermia in the post-genomics era: new perspectives on an old concept. *Anesthesiology*. 2018;128:168-180.

Sambuughin N, Holley H, Muldoon S, et al. Screening of the entire ryanodine receptor type 1 coding region for sequence variants associated with malignant hyperthermia susceptibility in the North American population. *Anesthesiology*. 2005;102:515-521.

Stewart SL, Hogan K, Rosenberg H, et al. Identification of the Arg1086His mutation in the alpha subunit of the voltage-dependent calcium channel (CACNA1S) in a North American family with malignant hyperthermia. *Clin Genet*. 2001;59:178-184.

A.9. What genetic disorders result in MH susceptibility?

In most cases, patients with MH susceptibility have a mutated RYR1 ryanodine receptor, which is located in the membrane of the sarcoplasmic reticulum (SR) of skeletal muscle. This channel is closely associated with many other proteins, such as the dihydropyridine calcium channel that mediates transfer of voltage change to the RYR1 receptor. Other proteins associated with the ryanodine receptor include triadin, STAC3, DHPR subunit $\beta 1\alpha$, and FKB-12 binding protein. Mutations or potentially pathogenic variants in the *RYR1* gene are found in approximately 70% of patients with MH susceptibility and their families. Hundreds of additional *RYR1* variants have yet to be characterized as to effects on calcium movements. One reason for the slow progress in deciphering the significance of these many mutations is that, unlike many other conditions, there are many unique mutations that predispose to MH. No single mutation accounts for more than 10% of MH cases. The dihydropyridine receptor gene, also involved in intracellular calcium control, is associated with MH susceptibility in 1% to 2% of families with MH susceptibility.

The *STAC3* gene encodes a T-tubule protein that is essential for excitation-contraction coupling. Native American myopathy is an autosomal recessive disorder caused by a specific *STAC3* mutation and is associated with MH susceptibility.

There are probably mutations in other genes that contribute to MH susceptibility. A recent estimate suggests that up to 23% of families with MH susceptibility do not have mutations in *RYR1*, *CACNA1S*, or *STAC3*.

Mutations associated with central core disease and multiminicore disease, two myopathies that also predisposes to MH, are located on the *RYR1* gene as well. In central core disease, the SR is depleted of calcium to a significant extent due to the increased permeability of the ryanodine receptor. With depletion of calcium, muscle contraction is weakened when the muscle is activated.

Genetically engineered mice have been developed that include one or more of the mutations causal for MH in the mouse genome. The mouse displays signs typical of MH during exposure to MH trigger agents and also on exposure to raised environmental temperature.

Beam TA, Loudermilk EF, Kisor DF. Pharmacogenetics and pathophysiology of CACNA1S mutations in malignant hyperthermia. *Physiol Genomics*. 2017;49:81-87.

Horstick EJ, Linsley JW, Dowling JJ, et al. Stac3 is a component of the excitation-contraction coupling machinery and mutated in Native American myopathy. *Nat Commun*. 2013;4:1952.

Litman RS, Griggs SM, Dowling JJ, et al. Malignant hyperthermia susceptibility and related diseases. *Anesthesiology*. 2018;128:159-167.

Lopez JR, Kaura V, Diggle CP, et al. Malignant hyperthermia, environmental heat stress, and intracellular calcium dysregulation in a mouse model expressing the p.G2435R variant of RYR1. *Br J Anaesth*. 2018;121:953-961.

Miller DM, Daly C, Aboelsaod EM, et al. Genetic epidemiology of malignant hyperthermia in the UK. *Br J Anaesth*. 2018;121:944-952.

Sambuughin N, Holley H, Muldoon S, et al. Screening of the entire ryanodine receptor type 1 coding region for sequence variants associated with malignant hyperthermia susceptibility in the North American population. *Anesthesiology*. 2005;102:515-521.

A.10. What is the pathophysiology of MH syndrome?

The MH syndrome results from abnormal and uncontrolled elevation of intracellular calcium levels in skeletal muscle. The normal process of calcium release from the SR normally begins with depolarization of the sarcolemma, which is transmitted via the T-tubules to the dihydropyridine receptor that in turn activates the calcium channel termed the ryanodine receptor to release calcium. Elevated calcium removes the inhibition of actin and myosin interaction that leads to mechanical force generation. Reuptake of calcium returns the intracellular cytoplasmic concentration of calcium to normal and muscle relaxation takes place. Reuptake is mediated via sarcoplasmic/endoplasmic reticulum calcium ATPase (SERCA) pumps. The control of calcium release is highly regulated because when muscle contraction takes place, a variety of energy-consuming steps are required resulting in adenosine triphosphate (ATP) breakdown and heat production.

There are a variety of intermediate proteins that also regulate the concentration of calcium in SR such as calsequestrin, a calcium-binding protein. Genetically engineered mice that do no express calsequestrin develop clinical signs of MH on exposure to trigger anesthetics. It is believed that in the absence of the calcium buffer, intracellular calcium levels increase significantly but only on exposure to MH triggers. Association of variants in the calsequestrin gene with human MH has not been observed.

During an MH episode, the ryanodine receptor calcium channel is locked in an open position leading to uncontrolled leak or release of calcium. In addition, there is increased entry of extracellular calcium, with an elevation of intracytoplasmic calcium levels, and continuous muscle activation with ATP breakdown. As a result of this uncontrolled calcium release, the SR calcium pump is unable to sufficiently resequester the calcium. ATP breakdown during this process aggravates heat production further.

Further, energy-consuming processes take place through glycolysis as well as oxidative phosphorylation. Eventually, due to low ATP levels, sarcolemmal integrity is impaired causing release of intracellular contents, for example, potassium, myoglobin, and CK leading to hyperkalemia, myoglobinuria, and other metabolic sequelae of MH.

Eltit JM, Ding X, Pessah IN, et al. Nonspecific sarcolemmal cation channels are critical for the pathogenesis of malignant hyperthermia. *FASEB J*. 2013;27:991-1000.

Gillies RL, Bjorksten AR, Du Sart D, et al. Analysis of the entire ryanodine receptor type 1 and alpha 1 subunit of the dihydropyridine receptor (CACNA1S) coding regions for variants associated with malignant hyperthermia in Australian families. *Anaesth Intensive Care*. 2015;43:157-166.

Kraeva N, Zvaritch E, Frodis W, et al. CASQ1 gene is an unlikely candidate for malignant hyperthermia susceptibility in the North American population. *Anesthesiology*. 2013;118:344-349.

Protasi F, Paolini C, Dainese M. Calsequestrin-1: a new candidate gene for malignant hyperthermia and exertional/environmental heat stroke. *J Physiol*. 2009;587:3095-3100.

A.11. What laboratory tests can be used to diagnose MH susceptibility?

Two types of test can be used to diagnose MH susceptibility. They are functional tests using a skeletal muscle exposed to a trigger and molecular genetic tests to identify known mutations that cause MH. The most accurate diagnostic test for MH is the halothane-caffeine contracture test. In this test, about 2 g of skeletal muscle is harvested from a suspected patient's thigh under regional anesthesia, or a nontriggering general anesthesia in the case of a child at least 8 years old. Strips or fascicles of muscle weighing 100 to 200 mg are suspended in a water bath at 37 °C, and exposed to halothane, caffeine, ryanodine, or chlorocresol in graded concentrations. Isometric contracture, not contraction, of the muscle is measured by strain gauge following specific guidelines. If the contracture threshold and strength exceed specific values, a diagnosis of MH is made.

The test is highly sensitive, close to 100%, but with about 20% false positives. Nevertheless, the value of the test resides in ruling out MH susceptibility. Patients with MH-causal mutations and MH nonsusceptible (MHN) contracture tests have been described. Although these might be false-negative contracture tests, it is possible that the patient is MHN due to unknown genetic or epigenetic factors that counteract the causal mutation. Caution dictates that such patients would nonetheless be treated as MH susceptible.

There are only four testing centers in North America (https://www.mhaus.org/testing/muscle-biopsy-chct/chct-muscle-biopsy-testing-centers/) and 20 in Europe. The test is invasive, costly, and requires strict adherence to specific requirements. There are slight differences in the ways that tests are performed between North American and Europe. The main difference is in the concentration of drugs used during exposure of the muscle and the threshold for determining a positive response. The patient and their history must be carefully evaluated by the biopsy center director prior to recommending the test in order to enhance its positive predictive value.

Molecular Genetic Testing for MH Susceptibility

The era of DNA testing for MH susceptibility began in 1990 when a single missense mutation in the *RYR1* gene was shown to be causal for MH in pigs. In humans, several genes are associated with MH;

however, the *RYR1* gene is probably responsible for most cases of MH. At present, at least 48 mutations in the *RYR1* gene have been found in humans that are causal for MH based on strict criteria related to in vitro calcium release or clinical MH in several generations and families. Unfortunately, no mutation accounts for more than a small percentage of all patients with MH susceptibility. All that is required for genetic testing is a blood sample that can be sent to a reference laboratory. The sensitivity of genetic testing is less than 75% and there are frequent findings of variants of unknown significance in both *RYR1* and *CACNA1S*. Undoubtedly, the sensitivity will improve as more mutations are identified and tested for their ability to alter the structure and function of the ryanodine receptor.

Patients should consider genetic testing if:

1. They have had a positive contracture test.
2. A family member has had a positive contracture test.
3. They have suffered a convincing MH episode but have not had a contracture test.
4. A family member has been found to have a causal mutation.

Patients with a causal mutation identified are then considered MH susceptible (high specificity). The absence of a confirmed or probable pathogenic variant does ***not*** rule out MH susceptibility as they might harbor an as yet undescribed mutation.

At present, there are four clinical testing laboratories in the United States that perform molecular genetic testing for patients suspected to be MH susceptible (https://www.mhaus.org/testing/genetic-testing/genetic-testing-centers/). The decision to undergo genetic testing is complex because the test for examining *RYR1* and *CACNA1S* costs approximately $2,000. However, once a mutation is discovered, the cost for screening additional family members is approximately $200 each. This compares to the cost of approximately $6,000 for the caffeine-halothane contracture test. The pros and cons of MH testing should be discussed with either an MH expert or a genetic counselor.

Allen GC, Larach MG, Kunselman AR. The sensitivity and specificity of the caffeine-halothane contracture test: a report from the North American Malignant Hyperthermia Registry. The North American Malignant Hyperthermia Registry of MHAUS. *Anesthesiology*. 1998;88:579-588.

European Malignant Hyperthermia Group. Diagnostic mutations. Accessed April 15, 2023. https://www.emhg.org/diagnostic-mutations

European Malignant Hyperthermia Group. Testing for MH. Accessed April 15, 2023. https://www.emhg.org/testing-for-mh

Gaburjakova J, Gaburjakova M. Molecular aspects implicated in Dantrolene selectivity with respect to ryanodine receptor isoforms. *Int J Mol Sci*. 2023;24:5409.

Malignant Hyperthermia Association of the United States. CHCT—muscle biopsy testing centers. Accessed April 15, 2023. https://www.mhaus.org/testing/muscle-biopsy-chct/chct-muscle-biopsy-testing-centers/

Malignant Hyperthermia Association of the United States. Genetic testing centers. Accessed April 15, 2023. https://www.mhaus.org/testing/genetic-testing/genetic-testing-centers/

Miller DM, Daly C, Aboelsaod EM, et al. Genetic epidemiology of malignant hyperthermia in the UK. *Br J Anaesth*. 2018;121:944-952.

Riazi S, Kraeva N, Hopkins PM. Malignant hyperthermia in the post-genomics era: new perspectives on an old concept. *Anesthesiology*. 2018;128:168-180.

Rosenberg H, Sambuughin N, Riazi S, et al. Malignant hyperthermia susceptibility. In: Adam MP, Mirzaa GM, Pagon RA, eds. *GeneReviews®* [Internet]. University of Washington, Seattle; 2003:1993-2023. Updated January 16, 2020.

A.12. What is neuroleptic malignant syndrome (NMS)? What is serotonin syndrome?

The NMS is a constellation of symptoms that can mimic MH. Symptoms include acidosis, hyperthermia, altered mental status, rigidity, rhabdomyolysis, and tachycardia. Unlike MH, NMS is precipitated by a variety of neuroleptic drugs including butyrophenones (droperidol and haloperidol), phenothiazines (promethazine and chlorpromazine), the atypical antipsychotics, and other centrally acting drugs.

This syndrome differs from MH in that central dopamine antagonism or depletion is thought responsible for the clinical picture, although NMS is an idiosyncratic reaction. Other factors such as antimuscarinic effect, acute inflammation, and hypovolemia are often associated with NMS. If a patient with NMS requires tracheal intubation and mechanical ventilation, nondepolarizing neuromuscular blockers usually result in partial or complete resolution of rigidity, unlike in MH. The mainstays of treatment are supportive care, benzodiazepines, and, if necessary, a dopamine agonist such as bromocriptine. Patients also respond symptomatically to dantrolene. A recent report identified *RYR1* mutations in a small percentage of patients manifesting NMS. Anesthesiologists can encounter NMS in patients who are sedated with haloperidol in the intensive care unit (ICU) and on infrequent occasions when patients are given dopamine antagonist agents such as metoclopramide and promethazine.

Serotonin syndrome, like NMS, can mimic MH. Unlike NMS, serotonin toxicity is responsible for serotonin syndrome, and despite some similarities to MH (hyperthermia), specific signs such as hyperreflexia differentiate it from MH Illicit agents such as ecstasy, and other methylenedioxymethamphetamine (MDMA) agonists are often implicated in serotonin syndrome. Administration of a monoamine oxidase (MAO)-A inhibitor, such as intravenous methylene blue to a patient chronically receiving a selective serotonin reuptake inhibitor (SSRI) antidepressant, or administration of a medication with SSRI activity, such as meperidine, to a patient taking an MAO-A or nonspecific MAO inhibitor can cause serotonin syndrome.

Baldo BA, Rose MA. The anaesthetist, opioid analgesic drugs, and serotonin toxicity: a mechanistic and clinical review. *Br J Anaesth*. 2020;124:44-62.

Caroff SN, Roberts CB, Rosenberg H, et al. Intravenous dantrolene in hypermetabolic syndromes: a survey of the U.S. Veterans Health Administration database. *BMC Anesthesiol*. 2022;22:298.

Gillman PK. Neuroleptic malignant syndrome: mechanisms, interactions, and causality. *Mov Disord*. 2010;25:1780-1790.

Horseman M, Panahi L, Udeani G, et al. Drug-induced hyperthermia review. *Cureus*. 2022;14:e27278.

Perry PJ, Wilborn CA. Serotonin syndrome vs neuroleptic malignant syndrome: a contrast of causes, diagnoses, and management. *Ann Clin Psychiatry*. 2012;24:155-162.

Strawn JR, Keck PE Jr, Caroff SN. Neuroleptic malignant syndrome. *Am J Psychiatry*. 2007;164:870-876.

B. Preoperative Evaluation and Preparation

B.1. How would you prepare this patient for anesthesia and surgery?

Preoperative preparation should include a detailed family and medical history, assessment of the physical status, evaluation of laboratory findings including CK (if a clinical myopathy is suspected), and specific investigations to determine the susceptibility of the patient to MH if available. Three possible scenarios are:

1. The caffeine-halothane contracture test result is normal. In this case, the patient should not be considered MH susceptible and there are no restrictions to the anesthetic.
2. The caffeine-halothane contracture test is abnormal or a mutation associated with MH or a probable pathogenic *RYR1* variant is identified. This implies MH susceptibility, and in this case, a trigger-free anesthetic should be employed and preparations should be made to treat MH if it develops.
3. Most commonly, the caffeine-halothane contracture test or genetic testing is not available. In such situations, the patient should be treated as MH susceptible, and all appropriate steps should be followed.

Frei D, Stowell KM, Langton EE, et al. Administration of anaesthetic triggering agents to patients tested malignant hyperthermia normal and their relatives in New Zealand: an update. *Anaesth Intensive Care*. 2017;45:611-618.

Rosenberg H, Pollock N, Schiemann A, et al. Malignant hyperthermia: a review. *Orphanet J Rare Dis*. 2015;10:93.

B.2. Is dantrolene prophylaxis indicated?

If a nontriggering anesthetic is administered with appropriate monitoring to a patient with MH susceptibility, dantrolene prophylaxis is *not* indicated. With the judicious use of trigger-free anesthetics, MH is extremely unlikely. However, patients with MH susceptibility that exhibit a history of symptomatic myopathies might benefit from oral dantrolene (see D.5).

Dantrolene has side effects, such as nausea, vomiting, pain at the injection site, thrombophlebitis, and depression of the twitch response. In patients with preexisting muscle weakness, dantrolene can cause respiratory insufficiency in the postoperative period.

Carr AS, Lehman J, Cunliffe M, et al. Incidence of malignant hyperthermia reactions in 2,214 patients undergoing muscle biopsy. *Can J Anaesth*. 1995;42:281-286.

Ibarra Moreno CA, Kraeva N, Zvaritch E, et al. Oral dantrolene for myopathic symptoms in malignant hyperthermia-susceptible patients: a 25-year retrospective cohort study of adverse effects and tolerability. *Anesth Analg*. 2023;136:569-577.

B.3. What laboratory tests would you obtain before surgery?

There are no routine laboratory tests required for patients suspected of MH. Preoperative work up is dictated by the underlying conditions. If a clinical myopathy is present or suspected a baseline serum CK should be obtained.

B.4. Is outpatient surgery appropriate for this patient?

With the use of a trigger-free anesthetic and appropriate monitoring, outpatient surgery is acceptable. In the event that a patient with MH susceptibility will have surgery in an office-based or ambulatory setting, the entire perioperative team should be informed well in advance. This ensures preparedness to care for a patient with MH susceptibility. Even when planning a trigger-free anesthetic, sufficient dantrolene for treatment of an acute MH episode should be available. Postoperative admission to the hospital solely on the basis of MH susceptibility is not warranted. When MH occurs, it is usually in the immediate postoperative period and usually not beyond 2 hours postoperatively. Therefore, it is appropriate to keep the patient longer than usual in the postanesthesia care unit (PACU) in a monitored setting and longer in the ambulatory discharge area. The discharge plan should include instructions and contact phone numbers in the rare event of delayed MH reaction.

All ambulatory surgery and office-based surgery settings should have a plan for managing an MH episode. This includes how to initiate transfer of the patient to a hospital while continuing to assess and treat the episode, and communicating key items to the receiving emergency department (ED) or ICU team.

Larach MG. A primer for diagnosing and managing malignant hyperthermia susceptibility. *Anesthesiology*. 2018;128:8-10.

Larach MG, Dirksen SJ, Belani KG, et al. Special article: creation of a guide for the transfer of care of the malignant hyperthermia patient from ambulatory surgery centers to receiving hospital facilities. *Anesth Analg*. 2012;114:94-100.

Litman RS, Joshi GP. Malignant hyperthermia in the ambulatory surgery center: how should we prepare? *Anesthesiology*. 2014;120:1306-1308.

Pollock N, Langton E, McDonnell N, et al. Malignant hyperthermia and day stay surgery. *Anaesth Intensive Care*. 2006;34:40-45.

B.5. If general anesthesia is needed, what preparations would you make?

If general anesthesia is used, preparation for this patient should include measures to prevent and treat an acute crisis of MH. The following steps should be taken and equipment should be available.

Equipment

- Remove vaporizers. Place a conspicuous warning on the anesthesia workstation that the patient is MH susceptible. For a patient undergoing cardiac surgery, the vaporizer should be removed from the cardiopulmonary bypass machine in addition to the anesthesia machine.
- Use a fresh airway circuit, reservoir bag, and CO_2 absorber.
  - Flush the anesthesia machine and ventilator by flowing 10 L oxygen per minute for at least 10 minutes.
  - For newer anesthesia work stations, the washout period can take up to 60 minutes. The manufacturers' guidelines for machine preparation should be followed.
  - Use of activated charcoal filters greatly reduces the length of time required to prepare an anesthetic workstation for a patient with MH susceptibility. After a 90-second flush with high flow oxygen, placement of activated charcoal filters on the inspiratory port immediately reduces residual breathing circuit vapor concentration to less than 5 ppm (**Figure 54.1**).
- Use routine American Society of Anesthesiologists (ASA) monitors including:
  - Pulse oximeter
  - Capnometer
  - Core temperature monitoring using one of the following sites: esophagus or nasopharynx. For procedures where the patient will have a bladder catheter, bladder temperature can be monitored. Avoid using skin temperature probes as they can be unreliable.
  - ECG and blood pressure monitors as indicated by the medical history.

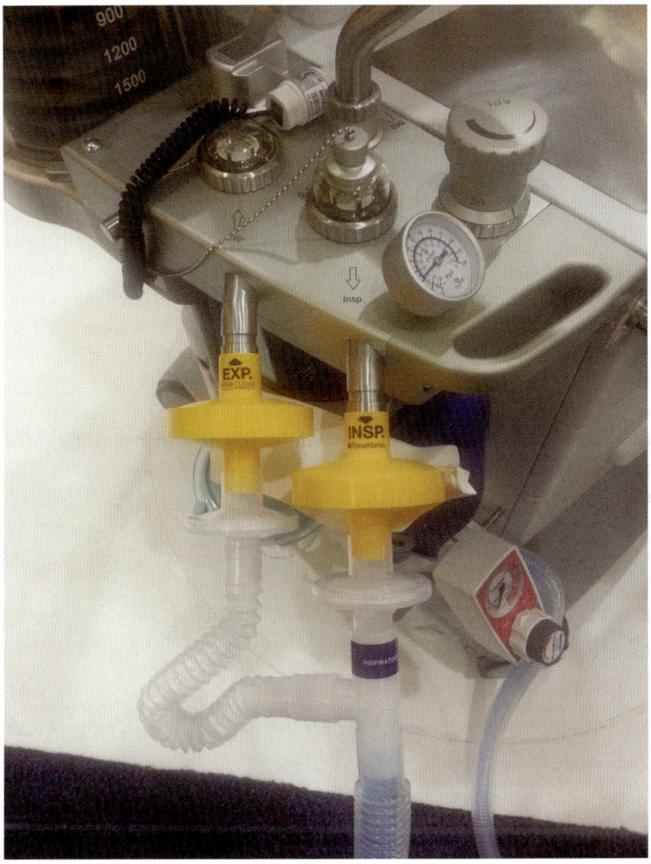

FIGURE 54.1. Vapor-Clean Charcoal Filters. (© Copyright 2023, Dynasthetics.)

Items to Have Available

Cooling aids

- Hypothermia blanket
- Crushed ice
- Cold 0.9% saline for intravenous infusion (eg, 30 mL/kg): This is the most rapid, reliable technique of lowering body temperature if the temperature is more than 39 °C or rapidly increasing.
- Point-of-care laboratory testing devices, that is, blood gas and electrolytes (if available)

Medications

- Dantrolene (intravenous), sterile water, sodium bicarbonate, mannitol, furosemide, calcium chloride, insulin, 50% dextrose, and medications for advanced cardiac life support, for example, antiarrhythmic drugs.

Bilmen JG, Hopkins PM. The use of charcoal filters in malignant hyperthermia: have they found their place? *Anaesthesia*. 2019;74:13-16.

Birgenheier N, Stoker R, Westenskow D, et al. Activated charcoal effectively removes inhaled anesthetics from modern anesthesia machines. *Anesth Analg*. 2011;112:1363-1370.

Heiderich S, Thoben C, Dennhardt N, et al. Preparation of Dräger Atlan A350 and General Electric Healthcare Carestation 650 anesthesia workstations for malignant hyperthermia susceptible patients. *BMC Anesthesiol*. 2021;21:315.

Kim TW, Nemergut ME. Preparation of modern anesthesia workstations for malignant hyperthermia-susceptible patients: a review of past and present practice. *Anesthesiology*. 2011;114:205-212.

Larach MG, Brandom BW, Allen GC, et al. Malignant hyperthermia deaths related to inadequate temperature monitoring, 2007-2012: a report from the North American malignant hyperthermia registry of the malignant hyperthermia association of the United States. *Anesth Analg*. 2014;119:1359-1366.

C. Intraoperative Management

C.1. What anesthetic techniques and agents would you employ?

Potent inhalation agents (excluding nitrous oxide) and succinylcholine **MUST** be avoided. Local, regional, or neuraxial anesthesia with intravenous sedation as needed is preferable if the surgeon and the anesthesiologist are confident with these techniques. If required, general anesthesia can be induced with propofol, benzodiazepines, or other intravenous hypnotics. Fentanyl or other opioids can be added for analgesia, and intermediate-acting nondepolarizing neuromuscular blocking agents can be used to facilitate intubation. Anesthetic maintenance is achieved using oxygen with or without nitrous oxide, an opioid, and a nondepolarizing neuromuscular blocking agent as required. Total intravenous anesthesia (TIVA) with a continuous infusion of propofol and boluses or infusions of analgesics are most often employed for nontriggering general anesthetics expected to last over 30 minutes. Vital signs are monitored with very close attention to capnography.

C.2. Should body (core) temperature be monitored during general anesthesia lasting more than 30 minutes?

Definitely. Although temperature elevation is often not the first sign of MH, it is one of the common early signs. Therefore, core temperature, esophageal, rectal, urinary bladder, or nasopharyngeal temperature should be monitored for all procedures lasting more than about 30 minutes. Temperature monitoring is also important in detecting hypothermia.

Sessler DI. Temperature monitoring and perioperative thermoregulation. *Anesthesiology*. 2008;109:318-338.

C.3. What anesthetic agents are contraindicated in MH?

The anesthetic agents to be avoided include **all potent inhalation agents** and **the depolarizing neuromuscular blocking agent succinylcholine**. Of the agents commonly employed today, the following have been implicated in triggering MH:

- Inhalation agents: halothane, enflurane, isoflurane, desflurane, and sevoflurane
- Neuromuscular blocking agents: succinylcholine

Larach MG. A primer for diagnosing and managing malignant hyperthermia susceptibility. *Anesthesiology*. 2018;128:8-10.

Litman RS, Rosenberg H. Malignant hyperthermia: update on susceptibility testing. *JAMA*. 2005;293:2918-2924. doi:10.1001/jama.293.23.2918.

C.4. If the surgeon wants to use local anesthesia for a procedure, what local anesthetics will you recommend?

Both ester and amide local anesthetics are considered safe for use in patients with MH susceptibility.

D'Ambrosio J, Adragna MG. Guidelines for the use of local anesthetics in the dental treatment of patients who are susceptible to malignant hyperthermia. *Spec Care Dentist*. 1988;8:61-63.

Maccani RM, Wedel DJ, Melton A, et al. Femoral and lateral femoral cutaneous nerve block for muscle biopsies in children. *Paediatr Anaesth*. 1995;5:223-227.

Murray C, Sasaki SS, Berg D. Local anesthesia and malignant hyperthermia: review of the literature and recommendations for the dermatologic surgeon. *Dermatol Surg*. 1999;25:626-630.

C.5. What is the significance of masseter muscle rigidity occurring after succinylcholine administration?

Rigidity of the jaw muscles after administration of succinylcholine is referred to as MMR or trismus. MMR presages clinical MH in up to 30% of cases. Even in the absence of clinical MH, myoglobinuria following succinylcholine-induced MMR is common postoperatively. MMR can occur in individuals of all ages; however, MMR is more common in children, particularly following volatile anesthesia induction.

MMR has been reported in 1% of children after halothane/succinylcholine induction and in adults after succinylcholine administration. Should MMR occur, elective surgery should be postponed, the patient observed in a monitored setting for 24 hours, serial CK levels obtained, and the patient observed for myoglobinuria or early signs of MH. The patient should be followed until CK levels normalize.

In emergency surgery in a patient that develops MMR, the anesthetic should be converted to a "non-triggering" technique (along with steps listed above to "clean the anesthesia machine"), and the patient observed for early signs of MH. Dantrolene and other MH treatment procedures should be made ready. The patient or family should be advised to be evaluated for MH susceptibility.

The incidence of MMR in children has decreased as a result of recommendations that the use of succinylcholine in children be reserved for emergency situations and the overall decrease in the use of succinylcholine.

Other causes of succinylcholine-induced MMR include any form of myotonia or periodic paralysis.

Hudig K, Pollock N, Bulger T, et al. Masseter muscle rigidity and the role of DNA analysis to confirm malignant hyperthermia susceptibility. *Anaesth Intensive Care*. 2019;47:60-68.

Litman RS, Smith V, Larach MG, et al. Consensus statement of the Malignant Hyperthermia Association of the United States on unresolved clinical questions concerning the management of patients with malignant hyperthermia. *Anesth Analg*. 2019;128:652-659.

Parness J, Bandschapp O, Girard T. The myotonias and susceptibility to malignant hyperthermia. *Anesth Analg*. 2009;109:1054-1064.

C.6. Twenty minutes into the procedure with sevoflurane anesthesia, the patient develops increasing tachycardia with ventricular premature beats and mottled skin. What emergency measures should you take?

This constitutes an emergency. Although tachycardia can arise from other more common causes, such as a light plane of anesthesia or hypovolemia, its association with dysrhythmias in this patient with MH susceptibility raises suspicion that an MH crisis might be beginning. End-expiratory CO_2 should be monitored, and if rising despite increasing minute ventilation, the diagnosis of MH should be **strongly** considered. Because time is of the essence, the following steps should be taken immediately (use of a cognitive aid such as a checklist or poster is highly recommended):

- Stop all potent inhalational anesthetics and surgery (if possible).
- Hyperventilate with 100% oxygen using a high fresh gas flow. It is recommended to increase minute ventilation if using mechanical ventilation, particularly in settings of limited manpower.
- Call for help. When time and manpower permit, contact the MH hotline of the Malignant Hyperthermia Association of the United States (MHAUS): 1-800-MH-HYPER.
- Administer dantrolene sodium early while muscle perfusion is still present. An initial intravenous dose of 2.5 mg/kg should be followed by repeated doses of 1 to 2 mg/kg to a total of 10 mg/kg depending on the response. More dantrolene may be administered if clinically indicated.
- If available, place activated charcoal filters on the inspiratory and expiratory ports of the breathing circuit (**Figure 54.1**).
- Initiate aggressive cooling immediately for rapidly increasing temperatures and for those with temperature more than 39 °C. Methods for rapid cooling include surface cooling (cooling blankets, ice packs) and administration of cold intravenous 0.9% saline or Plasmalyte A (avoid Lactated Ringer's). To prevent inadvertent hypothermia (after drop), cooling should be discontinued when the patient's temperature decreases to less than 38 °C.
- An arterial catheter and an indwelling urinary catheter should be inserted in all cases of fulminant MH. Central venous access should be considered in all patients but especially for unstable patients.
- Treat metabolic acidosis with sodium bicarbonate (2 mEq/kg initial dose and titrate as necessary). Consider increasing minute ventilation to counteract rise in end-tidal CO_2 from sodium bicarbonate administration and hypermetabolic state.
- Treat hyperkalemia with intravenous calcium chloride or calcium gluconate, hyperventilation, sodium bicarbonate, insulin, and 50% dextrose; in severe cases, consider emergent hemodialysis.
- Treat cardiac arrhythmias with standard antiarrhythmic drugs. **Avoid intravenous verapamil or diltiazem for treatment of arrhythmias during an MH episode** because of interaction with dantrolene possibly resulting in cardiac arrest. In a patient taking oral verapamil or diltiazem who is suspected of having an acute MH episode, do ***NOT*** withhold dantrolene treatment.
- If hyperkalemia is suspected, do not administer lidocaine or procainamide.
- Maintain urine output (1-2 ml/kg/h) with mannitol or furosemide. Each 20 mg bottle of Dantrium or Revonto contains 3 g mannitol. In comparison, each 250 mg bottle of Ryanodex contains only 125 mg mannitol. If Ryanodex is used, additional mannitol might be required.
- Follow CK levels every 12 hours. CK levels can be higher if succinylcholine was administered.

- Monitor and track electrolytes, hemoglobin/hematocrit, platelet count, and coagulation parameters, and urine and serum myoglobin levels. Blood and urine cultures should be sent to rule out sepsis.
- After the MH episode, register the patient and the event with the North American MH Registry (https://anest.ufl.edu/namhr/).

Hardy JB, Gouin A, Damm C, et al. The use of a checklist improves anaesthesiologists' technical and non-technical performance for simulated malignant hyperthermia management. *Anaesth Crit Care Pain Med.* 2018;37:17-23.

Stanford Anesthesia Cognitive Aid Program, Goldhaber-Fiebert SN, Austin Net al. Emergency manual: cognitive aids for perioperative crises, Version 4, 2021. See http://emergencymanual.stanford.edu for latest version. Creative Commons BY-NC-ND (https://creativecommons.org/licenses/by-nc-nd/4.0/legalcode).

C.7. What modalities would you monitor closely during management of the crisis?

The modalities that should be monitored closely include:

- End-tidal CO_2 and minute ventilation
- Arterial blood gases, electrolytes, coagulation tests
- Core temperature

The following should be monitored for ongoing evaluation and management:

- CK levels
- Myoglobin levels (urine and serum)
- Urine output

C.8. What steps should be taken to avoid major morbidity from MH?

All sites where triggering agents are administered should have 36 vials of dantrolene or 3 bottles of Ryanodex available within about 10 minutes.

All patients undergoing general anesthesia for more than 30 minutes should have core temperature monitored.

It is highly recommended that ORs and procedural areas where general anesthesia is employed conduct an MH drill each year. This drill should involve all perioperative staff and include, defining individual roles, mechanisms for alerting the team in the event of an MH crisis, obtaining all necessary equipment, obtaining and mixing dantrolene (expired dantrolene can be used), simulating venous and arterial blood draws, cooling the patient, and discussing the episode with family members. Practicing clinical skills is less important than simulating crisis management, roles, workflows, and logistics.

In addition, nonhospital sites should ensure that there is a transport plan to a hospital that is designated to receive a patient who is experiencing an MH episode. The plan should include who will accompany the patient and what medications and monitors will accompany the transport personnel. The plan should also include that the designated hospital has dantrolene as well as familiarity with treating MH.

C.9. How does the new formulation of dantrolene (Ryanodex) compare with the previous formulations of dantrolene (Dantrium or Revonto)?

Current formulations of dantrolene (Dantrium and Revonto) are lyophilized and dispensed as 20 mg of dantrolene sodium in a 70-mL vial with 3,000 mg of mannitol. It should be reconstituted with 60 mL of sterile water without a bacteriostatic agent, and the vial should be shaken until the dantrolene is fully dissolved. As the solution is fairly viscous, warming the sterile water to 40 °C immediately prior to mixing can accelerate the solubilization process and aid in drawing the drug into a syringe. From 4 to 7 vials of Dantrium or Revanto are required to begin treatment, and up to 36 vials in an adult requiring the maximum dose. Mixing the medication can be a tedious and time-consuming process. Enlisting dedicated help such as pharmacists to mix the medication allows clinicians to focus on patient care.

Ryanodex is a recent formulation of dantrolene that is a nanocrystalline dantrolene sodium suspension which allows a much larger dose of 250 mg to be dispensed in a vial that requires only 5 mL of sterile water to dissolve it in solution. It offers the advantage of rapid reconstitution and administration. In an animal study, the time for preparation (<60 seconds) was 10- to 15-fold shorter compared with dantrolene sodium (658-1,062 seconds), and the time taken to inject was a 100-fold faster. As Ryanodex contains only 125 mg of mannitol per vial, additional mannitol needs to be administered separately. Due to the small amount of diluent required compared with older preparations, the risk of fluid overload is less significant especially in pediatric patients.

The cost of Ranodex (required supply of three vials) is currently approximately $7,000 in the United States, with a shelf life of 24 months. Dantrolene sodium has a shelf life of 36 months and costs less than half as much (for the required supply of 36 vials). The cost can be substantially reduced when purchased for several locations within the same organization. Despite the difference in cost, the ease of use, especially in locations with limited manpower, makes Ryanodex an attractive option.

Larach MG, Dirksen SJ, Belani KG, et al.. Special article: Creation of a guide for the transfer of care of the malignant hyperthermia patient from ambulatory surgery centers to receiving hospital facilities. *Anesth Analg*. 2012;114:94-100.

Rosenberg H, Pollock N, Schiemann A, et al. Malignant hyperthermia: a review. *Orphanet J Rare Dis*. 2015;10:93.

Schütte JK, Becker S, Burmester S, et al. Comparison of the therapeutic effectiveness of a dantrolene sodium solution and a novel nanocrystalline suspension of dantrolene sodium in malignant hyperthermia normal and susceptible pigs. *Eur J Anaesthesiol*. 2011;28:256-264.

Zavilla CM, Skledar S, Lang MB, et al. Implementation of a new dantrolene formulation across a multifacility health system. *Am J Health Syst Pharm*. 2016;73:463-467.

D. Postoperative Management

D.1. What are the potential complications that can follow an MH event?

Death and neurologic injury are the most feared complication. Disseminated intravascular coagulation syndrome is another major complication of MH especially when the temperature exceeds 41 °C. Other complications include rhabdomyolysis, compartment syndrome, hyperkalemia, cardiac arrest, and renal failure. As a result of massive muscle breakdown, patients can be weak for days and complain of muscle cramps and pain.

Brandom BW, Larach MG, Chen MS, et al. Complications associated with the administration of dantrolene 1987 to 2006: a report from the North American Malignant Hyperthermia Registry of the Malignant Hyperthermia Association of the United States. *Anesth Analg*. 2011;112:1115-1123.

Rosenberg H, Pollock N, Schiemann A, et al. Malignant hyperthermia: a review. *Orphanet J Rare Dis*. 2015;10:93.

D.2. How should you follow-up in this case?

The vigorous therapies begun in the OR should be continued in the immediate postoperative period into the PACU or ICU. Dantrolene administration should be continued for at least 24 hours after an MH episode with 1 mg/kg administered every 4 to 6 hours titrated to signs of MH. Serum CK should be followed until consistently trending downward.

Other laboratory tests that should be monitored until normalized include:

- Arterial blood gases
- Electrolytes
- Coagulation profile

Body temperature should be monitored along with other vital signs. Recrudescence of MH occurs in about 20% of treated cases and therefore the patient should be observed in an ICU setting for at least 36 hours following an MH episode.

Burkman JM, Posner KL, Domino KB. Analysis of the clinical variables associated with recrudescence after malignant hyperthermia reactions. *Anesthesiology*. 2007;106:901-906.

D.3. What would you advise the patient and the family?

The patient and family should be counseled as to the dangerous nature of this syndrome and should be advised to wear a medical alert identification band at all times. Genetic counseling should be obtained, and the pedigree of the family should be prepared. Family members should be investigated for susceptibility to this syndrome and issued medical identification bands if susceptible. While not changing his future anesthetic management, molecular genetic testing would be recommended for this patient. If an MH-causal mutation is discovered, this will facilitate noninvasive confirmation of MH susceptibility in other family members.

In addition, the patient and family should consult with one of the MH diagnostic centers or with a MHAUS hotline consultant to discuss further evaluation. A complete listing is available through MHAUS. The patient should be registered with the North American MH Registry. The website for the North American MH Registry is https://anest.ufl.edu/namhr/; the phone number is 888-274-7899. The Registry is located at the University of Florida.

D.4. What precautions should a patient with MH susceptibility take outside of the operating room?

In general, patients with MH susceptibility should be cognizant of their response to heat and exercise. As for any patient, excess exposure to heat and humidity, especially with exercise should be limited or avoided. At present, there is no way to predict which previously asymptomatic patients might have an adverse response to environmental conditions. Even family members with the same MH-causal mutation can respond differently to vigorous exercise, heat, or infection.

Litman RS, Smith V, Larach MG, et al. Consensus statement of the Malignant Hyperthermia Association of the United States on unresolved clinical questions concerning the management of patients with malignant hyperthermia. *Anesth Analg*. 2019;128:652-659.

Zvaritch E, Gillies R, Kraeva N, et al. Fatal awake malignant hyperthermia episodes in a family with malignant hyperthermia susceptibility: a case series. *Can J Anaesth*. 2019;66:540-545.

D.5. What is the relationship between MH and exertional heat stroke (EHS)?

"Awake MH" or nonanesthetic triggered cases of MH have been described. In these cases, patients have developed hyperpyrexia and a hypermetabolic state (including muscle cramping) when precipitated by environmental factors such as exercise or high ambient temperature causing heat stress. Follow-up testing has often revealed an *RYR1* MH-causative variant. These events can be self-limited upon removal of environmental factors, a reduction in body temperature, or after self-administered oral dantrolene. However, in some cases, hyperkalemia, rhabdomyolysis and death have resulted. Athletes or military service members with a history of "heat intolerance," severe heat cramps, rhabdomyolysis, or other signs of MH when exposed to heat stress should be considered MH susceptible and warrant an MH workup including a detailed family history. A history of MH is disqualifying for military service, however, without a prior documented MH event or family history, individuals can be at risk without knowing.

Laitano O, Murray KO, Leon LR. Overlapping mechanisms of exertional heat stroke and malignant hyperthermia: evidence vs. conjecture. *Sports Med*. 2020;50:1581-1592.

Lavezzi WA, Capacchione JF, Muldoon SM, et al. Case report: death in the emergency department: an unrecognized awake malignant hyperthermia-like reaction in a six-year-old. *Anesth Analg*. 2013;116:420-423.

Lichtman AD, Oribabor C. Malignant hyperthermia following systemic rewarming after hypothermic cardiopulmonary bypass. *Anesth Analg*. 2006;1022:372-375.

Tobin JR, Jason DR, Challa VR, et al. Malignant hyperthermia and apparent heat stroke. *JAMA*. 2001;286:168-169.

Zvaritch E, Gillies R, Kraeva N, et al. Fatal awake malignant hyperthermia episodes in a family with malignant hyperthermia susceptibility: a case series. *Can J Anaesth*. 2019;66:540-545.

Suggested Resources

The Malignant Hyperthermia Association of the United States (MHAUS) has been active since 1981 and offers current information and advice on patient management as well as identification bracelets and a variety of material for health care professionals. The following are some useful contact information:

Emergency hotline: 1-800-MH-HYPER
Address: MHAUS, 39 East State Street, P.O. Box 1609, Sherburne, NY 13815
Phone: 1-800-98-MHAUS
Internet: www.mhaus.org
Website of the Neuroleptic Malignant Syndrome Information Service: www.nmsis.org
Website of the European MH Group: www.emhg.org

55 Postoperative Residual Neuromuscular Weakness and Prolonged Apnea

Danielle McCullough and Mary So

A healthy 35-year-old, 65-kg female was scheduled for an elective abdominal hysterectomy. Anesthesia was induced with propofol (2.0 mg/kg) and rocuronium (1.2 mg/kg). Anesthesia, which lasted 90 minutes, was maintained with desflurane 6.0% end-tidal and was supplemented with fentanyl as needed. No reversal of neuromuscular blockade (NMB) was given at the end of surgery because tidal volumes were deemed adequate. The train-of-four (TOF) count using facial nerve stimulation was 4, with no detectable fade. Upon arrival in the postanesthesia care unit (PACU), the patient was tachypneic, with uncoordinated, floppy arm movements, and appeared to be agitated and in distress. Oxygen saturation by pulse oximetry (Spo_2) on room air was 89%.

A. Medical Diseases and Differential Diagnosis

1. What is the differential diagnosis for postoperative hypoventilation?
2. How is residual NMB diagnosed?
3. What is the order of recovery of voluntary muscle groups from nondepolarizing neuromuscular blocking agents (NMBAs)?
4. What is the mechanism of action of succinylcholine, and how is it metabolized? What are the side effects of succinylcholine?
5. If succinylcholine were the only NMBA used during the case and the patient did not exhibit a response to TOF stimulation, what is the likely diagnosis? How would you confirm it?
6. What are acetylcholinesterase and plasma cholinesterase? What is the clinical significance of heterozygosity for atypical pseudocholinesterase (PChE)?
7. What is the incidence of atypical cholinesterase activity?
8. What are some factors that can lower PChE levels?

B. Intraoperative Management

1. How is the choice of NMBA made?
2. What factors can alter sensitivity to nondepolarizing NMBAs?
3. What are the characteristics of nondepolarizing neuromuscular block?
4. What is a TOF stimulus?
5. Why is the TOF ratio of clinical importance?
6. How do we define adequate recovery of neuromuscular function?
7. Are clinical tests of neuromuscular recovery reliable?
8. How accurate are qualitative estimates of the TOF ratio, and what purpose do peripheral nerve stimulator (PNS) monitors serve?
9. What is double burst stimulation (DBS)?
10. What is the posttetanic count (PTC)?
11. How can the TOF ratio be measured quantitatively?
12. What are the limitations of acetylcholinesterase antagonists?
13. Is it appropriate to administer neostigmine when the train-of-four count (TOFC) is less than 3?
14. Is reversal of NMB always necessary?
15. Is there any way to rapidly antagonize a profound nondepolarizing block?

C. Postoperative Management

1. What is the incidence of residual NMB in the PACU?
2. Does an undetected postoperative residual neuromuscular block (PORB) have clinical consequences?

A. Medical Diseases and Differential Diagnosis

A.1. What is the differential diagnosis for postoperative hypoventilation?

The differential diagnosis for postoperative hypoventilation includes the following:

- Residual anesthetic agent effect
- Residual opioid effect
- Residual NMB
- Hypercarbia
- Occurrence of a medical complication during anesthesia, such as stroke or embolism

Renew JR, Fuchs-Buder T. Neuromuscular monitoring. In: Gropper MA, Cohen NH, Eriksson LI, et al, eds. *Miller's Anesthesia*. 10th ed. Elsevier; 2025:1209-1226.

A.2. How is residual NMB diagnosed?

When residual NMB is clinically suspected, it is diagnosed by testing the TOFC using a PNS. This patient showed clear signs of residual neuromuscular weakness upon arrival in the PACU. TOF stimulation at the ulnar nerve showed a TOFC of only 2 at the adductor pollicis (thumb). A diagnosis of residual NMB was made, and the patient received neostigmine 0.05 mg/kg plus an appropriate dose of glycopyrrolate (0.01 mg/kg). Seven minutes later, the TOFC was 4 with no evidence of fade on palpation of the thumb, and all signs of residual block had abated. Alternatively, a dose of 2 to 4 mg/kg sugammadex could have been given to reverse blockade by forming tight, water-soluble complexes with steroidal NMBAs.

Renew JR, Fuchs-Buder T. Neuromuscular monitoring. In: Gropper MA, Cohen NH, Eriksson LI, et al, eds. *Miller's Anesthesia*. 10th ed. Elsevier; 2025:1209-1226.

Naguib M. Sugammadex: another milestone in clinical neuromuscular pharmacology. *Anesth Analg*. 2007;104:575-581.

A.3. What is the order of recovery of voluntary muscle groups from nondepolarizing neuromuscular blocking agents (NMBAs)?

Onset and recovery of muscular blockade depend on blood supply to the muscle group in question. Peripheral muscles (eg, adductor pollicis) tend to have lower relative perfusion compared to central muscles (eg, diaphragm), leading to a slower onset and offset of NMBA effect. Muscles of the upper airway and pharynx are an exception. They exhibit a fast onset of blockade but are slower to recover than peripheral muscles. When the TOFC at the orbicularis oculi or corrugator supercilii muscles shows recovery from nondepolarizing block, the response at the adductor pollicis can be almost nonexistent. Thus, facial nerve stimulation can give the clinician a false sense of security about the adequacy of neuromuscular recovery at the end of a case.

Similarly, in the intubated patient breathing spontaneously, a normal tidal volume and maintenance of an acceptable P_{CO_2} do not necessarily indicate adequate neuromuscular recovery. The diaphragm is the first muscle to recover from the nondepolarizing block and requires significantly higher plasma levels of NMBA to maintain paralysis. The muscles that protect the upper airway are far more sensitive to nondepolarizing NMBAs and cannot be clinically tested in the intubated patient. Thus, a patient who is able to maintain adequate respiratory exchange while intubated can experience airway obstruction due to inadequate pharyngeal muscle recovery when extubated.

Donati F. Neuromuscular monitoring: more than meets the eye. *Anesthesiology*. 2012;117:934-936.

Donati F, Bejan DR. Not all muscles are the same. *Br J Anaesth*. 1992;68:235-236.

McGrath CD, Hunter JM. Monitoring of neuromuscular block. *Contin Educ Anaesth Crit Care Pain*. 2006;6:7-12.

Thilen SR, Hansen BE, Ramaiah R, et al. Intraoperative neuromuscular monitoring site and residual paralysis. *Anesthesiology*. 2012;117:964-972.

A.4. What is the mechanism of action of succinylcholine, and how is it metabolized? What are the side effects of succinylcholine?

Succinylcholine is a depolarizing neuromuscular blocker. Its structure is essentially two acetylcholine (ACh) molecules linked via the acetyl groups, which are capable of binding to ACh receptor agonist binding sites. This activates the receptor, depolarizing the membrane and causing the characteristic fasciculations (ie, muscle contractions) seen when using this drug. Succinylcholine is metabolized by plasma cholinesterase, also known as butyrylcholinesterase (BChE) or PChE.

The most common untoward side effect seen after succinylcholine administration is muscle pain occurring in the first 24 to 48 hours postoperatively. Females and patients undergoing ambulatory surgery appear most susceptible. The reported incidence of succinylcholine-induced myalgia is variable but probably occurs in 25% to 50% of patients. Discomfort is typically characterized as being similar to the muscle soreness that occurs after heavy or unusual exercise. It has been postulated that the etiology of the phenomenon is related to muscle damage caused by asynchronous contractions during the initial muscle depolarization that precedes paralysis. Defasciculating doses of nondepolarizing NMBAs (10% of the ED_{95}) given 2 to 5 minutes prior to succinylcholine have been shown to reduce the incidence of myalgia by as much as 50%. Pretreatment with nonsteroidal anti-inflammatory drugs can also reduce the incidence of muscle pain following succinylcholine administration.

Succinylcholine can also be associated with various cardiac dysrhythmias, including bradycardia, tachycardia, and junctional and ventricular dysrhythmias. Stimulation of nicotinic receptors at sympathetic and parasympathetic ganglia and muscarinic receptors at the sinus node is believed to be involved in this phenomenon. Infants and children are more likely to manifest clinically significant bradycardia following succinylcholine administration secondary to their relatively high degree of resting vagal tone as compared to adults; however, pretreatment with atropine is no longer recommended in this patient population. Junctional rhythms following succinylcholine administration are also relatively common. The postulated mechanism of action is muscarinic stimulation of the sinus node that results in diminished sinus activity and subsequent emergence of the atrioventricular node as the dominant pacemaker. Various mechanisms have been postulated to explain ventricular dysrhythmias that sometimes occur after succinylcholine administration, including potassium release from skeletal muscle, succinylcholine-mediated sensitization to catecholamines, and profound sinus and atrioventricular node slowing.

The most serious complication associated with succinylcholine administration is severe and potentially lethal levels of hyperkalemia in at-risk individuals. When succinylcholine is administered to an otherwise healthy patient during the induction of anesthesia, plasma potassium levels typically increase by 0.5 mM as potassium ions move from the intracellular to the extracellular space. The increase is transient and is typically tolerated well by most patients. In at-risk patients, however, the efflux of potassium from the intracellular space can be in excess of 3.5 mM, enough to induce malignant dysrhythmias and cardiac arrest. The list of susceptible patients includes those with congenital muscular dystrophies, upper or lower motor neuron defects, prolonged chemical denervation (eg, neuromuscular blockers, magnesium, clostridial neurotoxins), direct muscle trauma or inflammation, extensive burns, and disuse atrophy. In the event that succinylcholine is inadvertently given to an at-risk patient and an exaggerated hyperkalemic response is suspected, prompt intravenous treatment with calcium chloride (1-2 g), hyperventilation, sodium bicarbonate (1 mEq/kg), regular insulin, and dextrose should be initiated to prevent severe dysrhythmias and cardiac arrest.

Succinylcholine also causes increases in intraocular, intragastric, and intracranial pressures (ICPs). The increase in intraocular pressure (IOP) caused by succinylcholine begins rapidly after drug administration. Peak pressures rise as much as 5 to 15 mm Hg before returning to baseline levels about 6 minutes after drug dosing. The etiology of this phenomenon is unclear, but detachment of the intraocular muscles from the globe fails to prevent the pressure rise, which is suggestive of an intraocular mechanism. It has been suggested that succinylcholine use should be avoided in the setting of open-eye injuries, although there is scant evidence that its administration has led to the extrusion of intraocular contents or blindness. The increase in intragastric pressure (IGP) caused by succinylcholine is likely related to fasciculations of the abdominal skeletal musculature. A defasciculating dose of a nondepolarizing NMBA given prior to succinylcholine administration can prevent increases in IGP.

Succinylcholine can also cause a transient increase in ICP. The increase in ICP after succinylcholine administration correlates with muscle fasciculations, increased electroencephalogram (EEG) activity, and elevated cerebral blood flow. Prior administration of a nondepolarizing NMBA can attenuate or even prevent this pressure increase. The use of succinylcholine in the setting of intracranial hypertension is probably best limited to emergency situations where the benefits of rapid airway control outweigh the risks of a transient increase in ICP.

Lastly, succinylcholine is a potent trigger of malignant hyperthermia (MH; see Chapter:54). Its use should be restricted to settings where prompt recognition and treatment of MH are possible.

Appiah-Ankam J, Hunter JM. Pharmacology of neuromuscular blocking drugs. *Contin Educ Anaesth Crit Care Pain.* 2004;4:2-7.

Brull SJ, Meistelman C, Nemes R, et al. Pharmacology of neuromuscular blocking drugs and antagonists (reversal agents). In: Gropper MA, Cohen NH, Eriksson LI, et al, eds. *Miller's Anesthesia*. 10th ed. Elsevier; 2025:676-741.

Kelly RE, Dinner M, Turner LS, et al. Succinylcholine increases intraocular pressure in the human eye with the extraocular muscles detached. *Anesthesiology*. 1993;79:948-952.

Martyn JA, Richtsfeld M. Succinylcholine-induced hyperkalemia in acquired pathologic states: etiologic factors and molecular mechanisms. *Anesthesiology*. 2006;104:158-169.

A.5. If succinylcholine were the only NMBA used during the case and the patient did not exhibit a response to TOF stimulation, what is the likely diagnosis? How would you confirm it?

The most likely diagnosis is atypical plasma cholinesterase. In this patient, stimulation of the ulnar nerve with a PNS resulted in no response of the muscles of the hand, confirming the diagnosis of prolonged response to succinylcholine. Extreme prolongation in the duration of effect is usually a manifestation of an atypical cholinesterase genotype. Following a dose of 1.0 mg/kg of succinylcholine, patients homozygous for the most common atypical genotypes will exhibit apnea for an hour or more; it can take as much as 3 hours for adequate respiratory efforts to return. However, the duration of apnea is highly dependent on the cholinesterase variant in question and can be shorter or longer than this.

Traditionally, the identification of the human cholinesterase variant has been performed by biochemical analysis. These tests, which have been used for decades, consist of the measurement of plasma cholinesterase activity with different substrates and of testing the degree of inhibition with a well-known inhibitor, such as dibucaine, fluoride, or R02-0683. These tests have identified multiple genes that can reside at the same allelic site, such as atypical, silent, fluoride-resistant, J, K, H, and Newfoundland variants. However, biochemical testing often leads to equivocal results. More recently, molecular biologic techniques have been applied to identifying a patient's exact genotype.

Brull SJ, Meistelman C, Nemes R, et al. Pharmacology of neuromuscular blocking drugs and antagonists (reversal agents). In: Gropper MA, Cohen NH, Eriksson LI, et al, eds. *Miller's Anesthesia*. 10th ed. Elsevier; 2025:676-741.

A.6. What are acetylcholinesterase and plasma cholinesterase? What is the clinical significance of heterozygosity for atypical pseudocholinesterase (PChE)?

Acetylcholinesterase is a relatively specific enzyme that hydrolyzes ACh faster than it does other choline esters. It is found in red blood cells, the central nervous system, and at the neuromuscular junction. It is responsible for hydrolyzing and inactivating the ACh produced during normal neuromuscular transmission. It does not hydrolyze succinylcholine.

Plasma cholinesterase, also called *cholinesterase*, *PChE*, *BChE*, and *nonspecific cholinesterase*, hydrolyzes many choline esters, including succinylcholine. It is found in many human tissues but not in red blood cells. It is synthesized in the liver. Its physiologic function is unknown, but it can hydrolyze choline esters, such as propionylcholine and butyrylcholine, which can be formed by bacterial action in the gut and by the enzyme systems responsible for the formation of ACh.

A patient who is heterozygous for atypical PChE can exhibit a prolonged response to succinylcholine. Sedation should be terminated only after a strong, sustained response to indirect tetanic stimulation at the wrist and an attempt is made to wean the patient off controlled ventilation. Once the diagnosis of an atypical response to succinylcholine is ascertained, treatment is entirely supportive and symptomatic. Because the duration of the residual block is hard to predict, the patient should remain intubated, artificially ventilated, and sedated.

Patients recovering from a prolonged succinylcholine-induced block usually exhibit a "dual" or "phase II" block during recovery (fade on repetitive stimulation). Although neostigmine or edrophonium can, under certain circumstances, antagonize this block, this approach is risky when dealing with prolonged succinylcholine apnea. If significant plasma levels of succinylcholine are still present, administration of an acetylcholinesterase inhibitor can be counterproductive.

The patient should be informed that she had a prolonged episode of muscular weakness and that the presumptive cause was an atypical reaction to succinylcholine. She should also be encouraged to have this diagnosis confirmed through laboratory testing. If an atypical genotype is confirmed, she should encourage her family members to be tested as well. Finally, the patient should be assured that this diagnosis has no adverse health consequences, but that in the future, when surgery is planned, her anesthesiologist needs to be informed of this diagnosis.

The dibucaine number (DN) is the percentage of BChE enzyme activity that is inhibited by dibucaine. The "normal" variant of BChE is 80% inhibited by dibucaine; therefore, a "normal" DN is 80. Together, the DN and the BChE enzyme activity results can help identify individuals at risk for prolonged

TABLE 55.1 Relation Between Dibucaine Number and Duration of Succinylcholine Neuromuscular Blockade

Type of Pseudocholinesterase	Genotype	Frequency	Dibucaine Number[a]	Response to Succinylcholine or Mivacurium
Homozygous typical	EuEu	Normal	70-80	Normal
Heterozygous	EuEa	1/480	50-60	Slightly prolonged
Homozygous atypical	EaEa	1/3,200	20-30	Markedly prolonged

[a]The dibucaine number indicates the percentage of enzyme inhibited.

paralysis following the administration of succinylcholine. Decreased BChE enzyme activity in conjunction with a DN less than 30 suggests a high risk for prolonged paralysis. Normal to decreased BChE enzyme activity in conjunction with a DN 30 to 79 suggests variable risk. The relation between the DN and the duration of succinylcholine NMB is shown in **Table 55.1**.

Brull SJ, Meistelman C, Nemes R, et al. Pharmacology of neuromuscular blocking drugs and antagonists (reversal agents). In: Gropper MA, Cohen NH, Eriksson LI, et al, eds. *Miller's Anesthesia*. 10th ed. Elsevier; 2025:676-741.

Cerf C, Mesguish M, Gabriel I, et al. Screening patients with prolonged neuromuscular blockade after succinylcholine and mivacurium. *Anesth Analg*. 2002;94:461-466.

Levano S, Ginz H, Siegemund M, et al. Genotyping the butyrylcholinesterase in patients with prolonged neuromuscular block after succinylcholine. *Anesthesiology*. 2005;102:531-535.

Levano S, Keller D, Schobinger E, et al. Rapid and accurate detection of atypical and Kalow variants in the butyrylcholinesterase gene using denaturing high performance liquid chromatography. *Anesth Analg*. 2008;106:147-151.

Pantuck EJ. Plasma cholinesterase: gene and variations. *Anesth Analg*. 1993;77:380-386.

Taylor P, Schumacher M, MacPhee-Quingley K, et al. The structure of acetylcholinesterase: relationship to its function and cellular disposition. *Trends Neurosci*. 1987;10:93-95.

A.7. What is the incidence of atypical cholinesterase activity?

The incidence of atypical cholinesterase activity varies with the population studied, but is about 1 in 2,800 in the general population of the United States with a 1:1 male/female ratio.

Brull SJ, Meistelman C, Nemes R, et al. Pharmacology of neuromuscular blocking drugs and antagonists (reversal agents). In: Gropper MA, Cohen NH, Eriksson LI, et al, eds. *Miller's Anesthesia*. 10th ed. Elsevier; 2025:676-741.

A.8. What are some factors that can lower PChE levels?

Reduced PChE activity can be associated with the following:

- Abnormal genotype
- Normal physiologic variation (eg, pregnancy). However, until BChE activity is reduced to less than 30% of normal, only modest increases in the duration of succinylcholine are to be expected.
- Liver disease
- Malnutrition
- End-stage renal disease
- Burns
- Plasmapheresis
- Noncompetitive cholinesterase inhibitors (eg, pesticides, certain nerve gases)
- Other drugs including neostigmine, oral contraceptives, monoamine oxidase inhibitors, echothiophate, cytotoxic drugs, tetrahydroaminacrine, metoclopramide, and hexafluorenium

Brull SJ, Meistelman C, Nemes R, et al. Pharmacology of neuromuscular blocking drugs and antagonists (reversal agents). In: Gropper MA, Cohen NH, Eriksson LI, et al, eds. *Miller's Anesthesia*. 10th ed. Elsevier; 2025:676-741.

Davis L, Britten JJ, Morgan M. Cholinesterase. Its significance in anaesthetic practice. *Anaesthesia*. 1997;52:244-260.

B. Intraoperative Management

B.1. How is the choice of NMBA made?

An NMBA can be chosen based on onset characteristics, duration of action, and method of metabolism (**Table 55.2**). NMBAs can be characterized as short, intermediate, and long duration. Metabolism can depend on liver and kidney function (eg, patients with hepatic dysfunction can have PChE deficiency) or

TABLE 55.2 Characteristics of Commonly Used Neuromuscular Blocking Agents

Drug	ED_{95} Under N_2O/O_2 (mg/kg)	Dose for Intubation (mg/kg)	Intubation Time (s)	Clinical Duration (min)	Metabolism (%)	Elimination Kidney (%)	Elimination Liver (%)
Ultrashort acting							
Succinylcholine	0.5	1.0	60	5-10	Plasma cholinesterase (98-99)	<2	0
Short acting							
Mivacurium	0.08	0.2-0.25	120	12-15	Plasma cholinesterase (95-99)	<5	0
Intermediate acting							
Vecuronium	0.05	0.1-0.2	120	45-60	Liver (30-40)	40-50	50-60
Rocuronium	0.3	0.6-1.0	90	45-55	None	<10	>70
Cisatracurium	0.05	0.15-0.2	120	45-60	Hofmann elimination (77)	16	—
Long acting							
α-Tubocurarine	0.5	0.5-0.6	150	100-120	None	80	20
Pancuronium	0.07	0.08-0.12	150	100-120	Liver (10-20)	85	15
Pipecuronium	0.05	0.08-0.10	180	100-120	10	>90	<10
Doxacurium	0.025	0.05-0.08	240	120-150	None	>90	<10

From Renew JR, Fuchs-Buder T. Neuromuscular monitoring. In: Gropper MA, Cohen NH, Eriksson LI, et al, eds. *Miller's Anesthesia*. 10th ed. Elsevier; 2025:1209-1226.

not. When surgical relaxation is not necessary, an NMBA can be given solely to provide optimal tracheal intubating conditions by paralyzing the larynx, pharynx, and muscles of the jaw. Succinylcholine is useful for its rapid onset and recovery times, especially when performing a rapid-sequence induction or facilitating motor nerve monitoring during the procedure.

If a rapid-sequence induction is indicated, either succinylcholine or rocuronium can be used as NMBA. Succinylcholine has a more rapid onset and is usually the preferred agent if there are no contraindications (eg, immobility, history of MH, hyperkalemia). In patients with hepatic or renal dysfunction, one can consider using cisatracurium. This nondepolarizing NMBA undergoes Hofmann elimination and, therefore, is not affected by renal or hepatic dysfunction.

Brull SJ, Meistelman C, Nemes R, et al. Pharmacology of neuromuscular blocking drugs and antagonists (reversal agents). In: Gropper MA, Cohen NH, Eriksson LI, et al, eds. *Miller's Anesthesia*. 10th ed. Elsevier; 2025:676-741.

B.2. What factors can alter sensitivity to nondepolarizing NMBAs?

In any group of healthy patients, there exists a wide variability in sensitivity to the effects of NMBAs. The potency of these drugs is expressed as ED_{50} or ED_{95} (ie, the dose that will produce 50% or 95% depression of a single twitch [T1] in an average individual). The coefficient of variation (the standard deviation as a percentage of the mean value) for the ED_{50} of most NMBAs approximates 20% to 25%. Thus, if the ED_{95} for drug X is 1.0 mg/kg, in 5% of normal individuals, the ED_{95} will be less than 0.60 mg/kg. Because of the shape of the dose-response curve of nondepolarizing NMBAs, this modest difference in drug requirement can have large consequences on the depth of block. In these individuals, a plasma level that produces only a 50% block of T1 in the average subject can produce a block that is greater than 90%.

Similarly, the duration of the effect of NMBAs is quite variable between patients. For example, following a 1.2-mg/kg dose, the clinical duration of rocuronium (time to 25% T1 recovery) in a sample size of only 12 averaged 67 minutes; however, the range in responses was from 39 to 118 minutes. Following a dose 2 times the ED_{95} of a blocker of intermediate duration (eg, vecuronium), 30% of individuals still need pharmacologic antagonism 2 hours later.

In older patients or in patients with renal or hepatic disease, this variability is even more pronounced. This is especially true of aminosteroid NMBAs, such as vecuronium or rocuronium, when compared to the benzylisoquinolinium NMBAs atracurium or cisatracurium.

Arain SR, Kern S, Ficke DJ, et al. Variability of duration of action of neuromuscular-blocking drugs in elderly patients. *Acta Anaesthesiol Scand.* 2005;49:312-315.

Heier T, Feiner JR, Wright PM, et al. Sex-related differences in the relationship between acceleromyographic adductor pollicis train-of-four ratio and clinical manifestations of residual neuromuscular block: a study in healthy volunteers during near steady-state infusion of mivacurium. *Br J Anaesth.* 2012;108:444-451.

Kopman AF, Kahn NA, Neuman GG. Precurarization and priming: a theoretical analysis of safety and timing. *Anesth Analg.* 2001:93:1253-1256.

B.3. What are the characteristics of nondepolarizing neuromuscular block?

The distinguishing feature of a nondepolarizing block is fade on repetitive stimulation. For example, consider a situation in which the amplitude of twitch height (T1) is reduced by 50% with a nondepolarizing blocker when stimuli are delivered at 0.10 Hz (1 every 10 seconds). If the rate of stimulation is increased to 1 Hz, the height of T1 may fall to less than 20% of control, and at 2 Hz to about 10% of control. This fade is most easily appreciated subjectively when tetanic stimuli (rates ≥30 Hz) are delivered.

Kopman AF. Surrogate endpoints and neuromuscular recovery. *Anesthesiology.* 1997;87:1029-1031.

Naguib M, Brull SJ, Johnson KB. Conceptual and technical insights into the basis of neuromuscular monitoring. *Anaesthesia.* 2017;72:16-37.

B.4. What is a TOF stimulus?

A "train-of-four" consists of four stimuli delivered at 0.5-second intervals (2 Hz). The TOF ratio is the height of the fourth indirectly elicited response divided by the amplitude of the first response. This ratio in unparalyzed individuals normally approximates a value of 1.0 when measured by mechanomyography (MMG), electromyography (EMG), or kinemyography, but can exceed 1.10 when measured by acceleromyography (AMG) (see Section B.11). As the depth of the block increases, this ratio becomes smaller, and eventually the fourth, the third, and so on, responses "drop out." Two responses to a TOF stimulus are referred to as a TOF count of 2.

Kopman AF. Surrogate endpoints and neuromuscular recovery. *Anesthesiology.* 1997;87:1029-1031.

Naguib M, Brull SJ, Johnson KB. Conceptual and technical insights into the basis of neuromuscular monitoring. Review article. *Anaesthesia.* 2017;72:16-37.

B.5. Why is the TOF ratio of clinical importance?

The TOF fade is a far more sensitive index of residual block than single-twitch depression. In addition, the TOF ratio is useful because each TOF sequence serves as its own control. It is not necessary to know the amplitude of the evoked response prior to the administration of an NMBA or to worry about baseline drift over time. TOF ratio is measured at the hand by noting the response of thumb adduction to stimulation of the ulnar nerve. Although clinicians are much more interested in the neuromuscular function of the diaphragm, masseter, and laryngeal adductors, correlation with adductor pollicis muscle function has served as a useful clinical surrogate.

Kopman AF. Surrogate endpoints and neuromuscular recovery. *Anesthesiology.* 1997;87:1029-1031.

Naguib M, Brull SJ, Johnson KB. Conceptual and technical insights into the basis of neuromuscular monitoring. Review article. *Anaesthesia.* 2017;72:16-37

B.6. How do we define adequate recovery of neuromuscular function?

Once the TOF ratio at the adductor pollicis has recovered to 0.70, tests of mechanical respiratory reserve, such as vital capacity and peak expiratory flow rate, have usually recovered to within 90% of control. Clinically, this means that a patient can exhibit spontaneous respiration but require pressure support or have upper airway obstruction when extubated.

Studies done in the 1970s suggested that a TOF ratio of 0.70 was synonymous with adequate neuromuscular recovery, and this was the accepted standard for the next two decades. However, by the late 1990s, this assumption was questioned. Work in awake volunteers demonstrated that at a TOF ratio of 0.70, grip strength was decreased by more than 40%. At a TOF ratio of 0.70, the vast majority of subjects had difficulty apposing their incisor teeth and could not sip water from a straw because they could not make a tight seal around the straw with their lips. All individuals had double vision at a TOF ratio less than 0.90. It was clear that these healthy volunteers were not "street ready" until their TOF ratios reached or exceeded a value of 0.90. In addition, other volunteer studies revealed even more alarming data. At a

TOF ratio of 0.70, there is a decreased ventilatory response to hypoxemia (via a mechanism at the carotid body), and the swallowing mechanism is disorganized. Partial paralysis (TOF of 0.70) causes pharyngeal dysfunction, and there is an increased risk for aspiration with mechanical adductor pollicis TOF ratios less than 0.90. Pharyngeal function is not normalized until an adductor pollicis TOF ratio of greater than 0.90 is reached. Thus, the current standard for adequate neuromuscular recovery is a TOF of 0.90 or better.

Heier T, Caldwell JE, Feiner JR, et al. Relationship between normalized adductor pollicis train-of-four ratio and manifestations of residual neuromuscular block: a study using acceleromyography during near steady-state concentrations of mivacurium. *Anesthesiology*. 2010;113:825-832.

Kopman AF, Yee PS, Neuman GG. Relationship of the train-of-four fade ratio to clinical signs and symptoms of residual paralysis in awake volunteers. *Anesthesiology*. 1997;86:765-771.

Naguib M, Brull SJ, Johnson KB. Conceptual and technical insights into the basis of neuromuscular monitoring. Review article. *Anaesthesia*. 2017;72:16-37.

Renew JR, Fuchs-Buder T. Neuromuscular monitoring. In: Gropper MA, Cohen NH, Eriksson LI, et al, eds. *Miller's Anesthesia*. 10th ed. Elsevier; 2025:1209-1226.

B.7. Are clinical tests of neuromuscular recovery reliable?

The first commercially available PNS did not appear until the mid-1960s, and units capable of delivering TOF stimuli did not arrive for another decade. Even today, devices that can quantify or measure the TOF ratio in real time are not widely distributed. Thus, clinicians have been reluctant to abandon clinical tests of neuromuscular recovery first suggested half a century ago, including tidal volume, negative inspiratory force, grip strength, 5-second head lift, ability to protrude the tongue, and others. Unfortunately, most of these tests share one fundamental weakness: they require an awake and cooperative patient. Ideally, we would like to know the state of neuromuscular recovery prior to awakening the patient and certainly prior to tracheal extubation.

The most widely cited test, the 5-second head lift, is not a sensitive test of residual block. At a TOF ratio of 0.50, the majority of patients can still pass this test. Other widely discussed tests are no better and can be very misleading. Traditional "bedside" tests of residual muscle weakness lack sensitivity and are considered unreliable.

Heier T, Caldwell JE, Feiner JR, et al. Relationship between normalized adductor pollicis train-of-four ratio and manifestations of residual neuromuscular block: a study using acceleromyography during near steady-state concentrations of mivacurium. *Anesthesiology*. 2010;113:825-832.

Renew JR, Fuchs-Buder T. Neuromuscular monitoring. In: Gropper MA, Cohen NH, Eriksson LI, et al, eds. *Miller's Anesthesia*. 10th ed. Elsevier; 2025:1209-1226.

Thilen SR, Weigel WA, Todd MM, et al. 2023 American Society of Anesthesiologists Practice Guidelines for monitoring and antagonism of neuromuscular blockade: a report by the American Society of Anesthesiologists Task Force on Neuromuscular Blockade. *Anesthesiology*. 2023;138:13-41.

B.8. How accurate are qualitative estimates of the TOF ratio, and what purpose do peripheral nerve stimulator (PNS) monitors serve?

Visual or tactile estimations of the TOF ratio are notoriously inaccurate. Once the TOF ratio exceeds a value of 0.40 to 0.50, a majority of experienced anesthesiologists are unable to detect the presence of any fade at all. Thus, failure to detect fade can indicate a true value anywhere from 0.50 to 1.0. Accurate assessment of the TOF ratio requires an objective or quantitative monitor.

Because subjective qualitative estimates of the TOF ratio are so unreliable, one may ask does intraoperative TOF stimulation serve any purpose. The answer is a resounding yes. The only satisfactory method of determining the degree of neuromuscular block is to stimulate a motor nerve with an electric current and observe the contraction of the muscles innervated by that nerve. The TOFC (eg, the number of evoked responses at the thumb that can be detected) gives a useful estimate of the depth of neuromuscular block. A rough guide is as follows: TOFC of 1 = 5% recovery, TOFC of 2 = 15% recovery, TOFC of 3 = 25% recovery, and TOFC of 4 (with fade) = ≥35% recovery. This information allows the clinician to guide further dosing and to determine whether the patient can be given reversal and the appropriate dose.

Kopman AF. Tactile evaluation of train-of-four count as an indicator of reliability of antagonism from vecuronium- or atracurium-induced neuromuscular blockade. *Anesthesiology*. 1991;75:588-593.

Thilen SR, Weigel WA, Todd MM, et al. 2023 American Society of Anesthesiologists Practice Guidelines for monitoring and antagonism of neuromuscular blockade: a report by the American Society of Anesthesiologists Task Force on Neuromuscular Blockade. *Anesthesiology*. 2023;138:13-41.

B.9. What is double burst stimulation (DBS)?

Because of the limitations in the subjective interpretation of TOF fade, other patterns of stimulation have been investigated. A somewhat more sensitive test is the response to DBS; however, this test should not replace more quantitative measures of neuromuscular function recovery. This sequence consists of a very brief tetanic pulse (three stimuli at 50 Hz), a 0.75-second pause, and another brief tetanic pulse. The observer feels two strong twitches. Most observers lose the ability to detect DBS fade at a TOF ratio of about 0.60.

Naguib M, Brull SJ, Johnson KB. Conceptual and technical insights into the basis of neuromuscular monitoring. Review article. *Anaesthesia*. 2017;72:16-37.

Thilen SR, Weigel WA, Todd MM, et al. 2023 American Society of Anesthesiologists Practice Guidelines for monitoring and antagonism of neuromuscular blockade: a report by the American Society of Anesthesiologists Task Force on Neuromuscular Blockade. *Anesthesiology*. 2023;138:13-41.

B.10. What is the posttetanic count (PTC)?

As the level of NMB is progressively increased, the TOFC eventually falls to zero. Because posttetanic potentiation is a prominent feature of nondepolarizing block, it is still possible to get additional information about the depth of block once the TOF response disappears. The following sequence is employed: a 5-second 50-Hz tetanus, a 3-second pause, and then 20 single-twitch stimuli at 1 Hz. The number of responses elicited is referred to as the PTC. Generally, when the count approximates 10, the first response to TOF stimulation appears.

Naguib M, Brull SJ, Johnson KB. Conceptual and technical insights into the basis of neuromuscular monitoring. Review article. *Anaesthesia*. 2017;72:16-37.

Thilen SR, Weigel WA, Todd MM, et al. 2023 American Society of Anesthesiologists Practice Guidelines for monitoring and antagonism of neuromuscular blockade: a report by the American Society of Anesthesiologists Task Force on Neuromuscular Blockade. *Anesthesiology*. 2023;138:13-41.

B.11. How can the TOF ratio be measured quantitatively?

Prior to the current decade, the vast bulk of clinical research on neuromuscular function was done by measuring either evoked mechanical force (MMG) or summated electrical action potentials (EMG) at the adductor pollicis. Although these techniques represent gold standards for reliability, they are unfortunately cumbersome to use in daily practice. In addition, at present, there are no commercially available free-standing MMG or EMG monitors designed for use in the operating room. However, using a different method of measurement, AMG, it is now possible to obtain a real-time display of the TOF ratio using a small device, which is relatively easy to set up and has a user-friendly interface. The rationale for AMG is based on Newton's second law of motion, which states that force is equal to mass times acceleration. Since the mass of the thumb remains constant, acceleration is directly proportional to force. For measurement of acceleration, a piezoelectric ceramic wafer is fixed to the thumb. When an evoked mechanical response of the thumb is elicited, an electrical signal proportional to the acceleration is generated in the ceramic transducer. This signal can then be digitized, processed, and electronically displayed in real time. Thus, it is now possible for the clinician to accurately and easily determine the extent of neuromuscular block (the TOF ratio) in real time. An excellent review of the pros, cons, and limitations of AMG can be found in the following references.

Claudius C, Viby-Mogensen J. Acceleromyography for use in scientific and clinical practice: a systematic review of the evidence. *Anesthesiology*. 2008;108:1117-1140.

Fuchs-Buder T, Schreiber JU, Meistelman C. Monitoring neuromuscular block: an update. *Anaesthesia*. 2009;64:82-89.

Hemmerling TM, Le N. Brief review: neuromuscular monitoring: an update for the clinician. *Can J Anaesth*. 2007;54:58-72.

Loughnan T, Loughnan AJ. Overview of the introduction of neuromuscular monitoring to clinical anaesthesia. *Anaesth Intensive Care*. 2013;41:19-24.

Stewart PA, Freelander N, Liang S, et al. Comparison of electromyography and kinemyography during recovery from non-depolarising neuromuscular blockade. *Anaesth Intensive Care*. 2014;42:378-384.

B.12. What are the limitations of acetylcholinesterase antagonists?

Nondepolarizing NMBAs are competitive in nature. Molecules of the NMBA compete with molecules of ACh for access to binding sites on receptors at the neuromuscular junction. The duration of NMBA-receptor or ACh receptor binding is evanescent (milliseconds). Thus, the relative concentration of NMBA versus ACh determines which molecule is most likely to succeed for receptor access. Anticholinesterases such as neostigmine affect antagonism by preventing ACh hydrolysis and thus increase the concentration of ACh in the synaptic cleft. However, there is a ceiling to this effect. Once the cholinesterase enzyme is completely inhibited, the addition of additional neostigmine or edrophonium has no further effect. In contrast, there is no limit to the concentration of NMBA that can exist at the receptor if excessive doses of NMBA are administered. In practical terms, the maximum depth of block that can be rapidly antagonized by anticholinesterases corresponds approximately to the reappearance of the fourth response to TOF stimulation. To achieve rapid (within 10 minutes) reversal to a TOF ratio of 0.7 in more than 87% of patients, three or four tactile responses should be present at the time of neostigmine administration. It is not possible within 30 minutes to achieve a TOF ratio of 0.9 in all patients, regardless of the number of tactile responses present at neostigmine administration.

Beemer GH, Goonetilleke PH, Bjorksten AR. The maximum depth of an atracurium neuromuscular block antagonized by edrophonium to effect adequate recovery. *Anesthesiology*. 1995;82:852-858.

Kirkegaard H, Heier T, Caldwell JE. Efficacy of tactile-guided reversal from cisatracurium-induced neuromuscular block. *Anesthesiology*. 2002;96:45-50.

B.13. Is it appropriate to administer neostigmine when the TOFC is less than 3?

When the TOFC is only 1 or 2, anticholinesterases cannot reliably achieve satisfactory reversal in a timely manner. The peak effect of the antagonist is followed by a plateau phase that represents the balance between diminishing anticholinesterase activity and spontaneous recovery. The latter becomes the major determinant at profound levels of NMB. However, even at a TOFC of 1 to 2, it might be possible to achieve a TOF ratio greater than 0.40 within 10 minutes. The problem for the clinician is that further recovery can be quite slow, and unless an objective monitor of neuromuscular function is being used, the clinician is likely to have the false impression that adequate recovery has been achieved, as subjective detection of fade at TOF ratios greater than 0.40 is highly unreliable.

Kopman AF, Kopman DJ, Ng J, et al. Antagonism of profound cisatracurium and rocuronium block: the role of objective assessment of neuromuscular function. *J Clin Anesth*. 2005;17:30-35.

Naguib M, Brull SJ, Johnson KB. Conceptual and technical insights into the basis of neuromuscular monitoring. *Anaesthesia*. 2017;72:16-37.

Thilen SR, Weigel WA, Todd MM, et al. 2023 American Society of Anesthesiologists Practice Guidelines for monitoring and antagonism of neuromuscular blockade: a report by the American Society of Anesthesiologists Task Force on Neuromuscular Blockade. *Anesthesiology*. 2023;138:13-41.

B.14. Is reversal of NMB always necessary?

If a quantitative monitor of neuromuscular function is used, the answer to this question is simple. If the TOF ratio approximates a value of 0.90 or better, anticholinesterase administration is pointless and is best avoided. Neostigmine, edrophonium, atropine, and so on, all have their own side effects and should not be administered unnecessarily. Similarly, if the TOFC is less than 4 or 4 with obvious fade, then anticholinesterase administration is indicated. However, objective monitors are still not widely available. What should be done when the TOFC is 4 with no detectable fade?

Many clinicians base the decision of whether to reverse or not on the time interval since the last dose of NMBA. Unfortunately, this is an unreliable approach. Two hours after a single dose of an intermediate-duration NMBA, 30% of individuals have TOF ratios less than 0.90, and 10% will still not have returned to a value of 0.70. Therefore, in the absence of objective evidence that the TOF ratio is greater than 0.90, a reversal agent should be administered. However, when no fade to TOF stimulation can be subjectively detected, the dose of neostigmine can be safely reduced to only 0.02 mg/kg.

Fuchs-Buder T, Meistelman C, Alla F, et al. Antagonism of low degrees of atracurium-induced neuromuscular blockade: dose-effect relationships for neostigmine. *Anesthesiology*. 2010;112:34-40.

Thilen SR, Weigel WA, Todd MM, et al. 2023 American Society of Anesthesiologists Practice Guidelines for monitoring and antagonism of neuromuscular blockade: a report by the American Society of Anesthesiologists Task Force on Neuromuscular Blockade. *Anesthesiology*. 2023;138:13-41.

B.15. Is there any way to rapidly antagonize a profound nondepolarizing block?

A relatively new approach to reversal presented itself with the introduction of sugammadex. This drug was approved by the US Food and Drug Administration in 2015 for use to reverse the effects of NMB induced by rocuronium bromide and vecuronium bromide. Sugammadex is a γ-cyclodextrin (**Figure 55.1**).

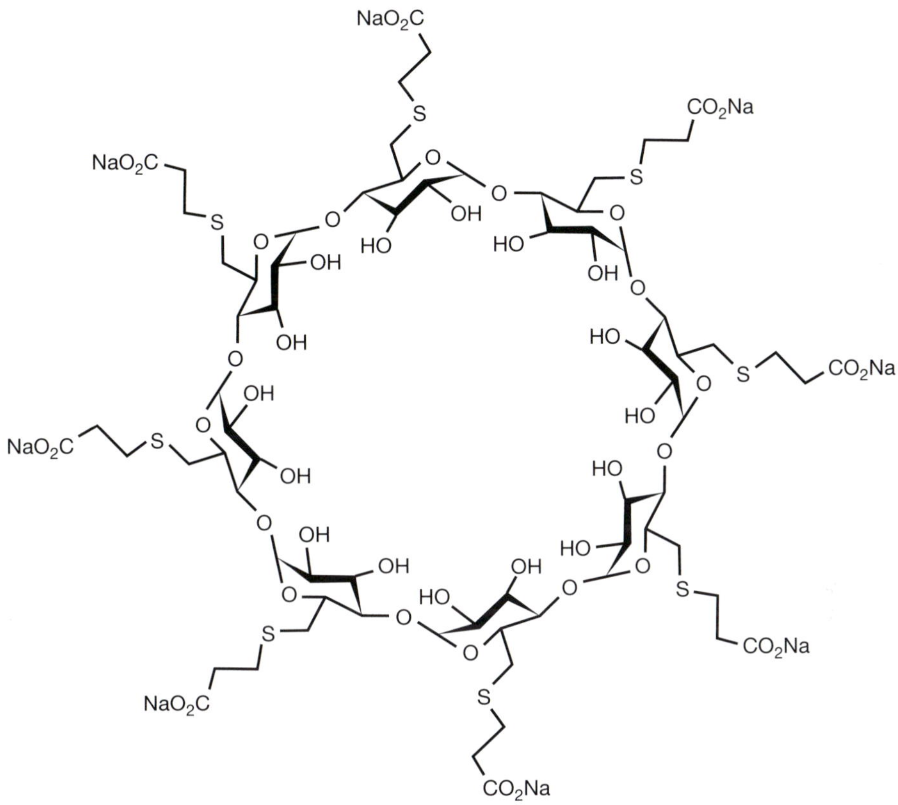

FIGURE 55.1. Structure of sugammadex, a synthetic γ-cyclodextrin. (Reprinted with permission from Naguib MMB. Sugammadex: another milestone in clinical neuromuscular pharmacology. *Anesth Analg*. 2007;104:575-581.)

Sugammadex has a three-dimensional (3D) appearance similar to a doughnut with a hydrophobic interior and hydrophilic exterior. The hydrophobic core acts by strongly binding with monoquaternary aminosteroid blocking agents (eg, rocuronium and vecuronium), thus "trapping" the drug (**Figure 55.2**). The resulting sugammadex-rocuronium complex is water soluble and excreted renally. The complex formed creates a concentration gradient for molecules in the neuromuscular junction to move out and be further excreted. It forms a high-affinity bond utilizing hydrogen bonds, van der Waals forces, and hydrophobic interactions, so molecule dissociation from the "trap" is not a concern. Sugammadex is not an effective antagonist of benzylisoquinolinium NMBAs such as cisatracurium.

Sugammadex can be used to rapidly reverse intubating doses of steroidal NMBAs in "cannot intubate, cannot ventilate" situations or when surgery concludes more quickly than anticipated. A dose of 16 mg/kg

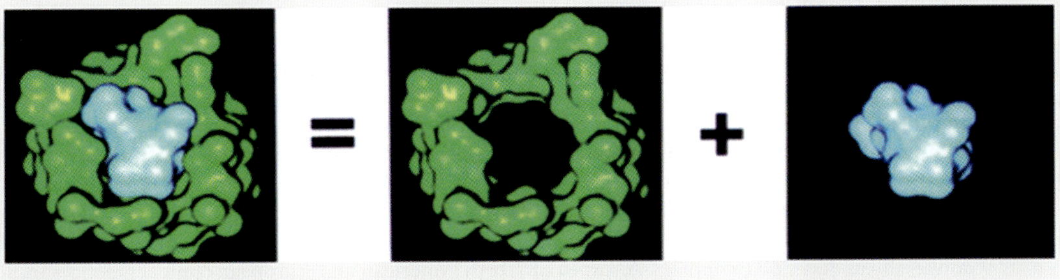

FIGURE 55.2. X-ray crystal structure of sugammadex (*green*) and rocuronium (*blue*) with encapsulation of a rocuronium molecule by a sugammadex molecule at a ratio of 1:1. (Reprinted with permission from Gijsenbergh F, Ramael S, Houwing N, et al. First human exposure of Org 25969, a novel agent to reverse the action of rocuronium bromide. *Anesthesiology*. 2005;103:695-703.)

SECTION 12

is recommended for the rapid reversal of steroidal NMBAs when there are no posttetanic twitches. After sugammadex is given, it takes approximately 4 minutes to fully recover from a 1.2-mg/kg dose of rocuronium. This is faster than spontaneous recovery following succinylcholine, which takes approximately 7 minutes. Recommended doses are 4 mg/kg when there are one to two posttetanic twitches and 2 mg/kg when there are more than two twitches. Randomized controlled trials have shown that TOFC recovery with a similar density of blockade is faster with sugammadex than with neostigmine-glycopyrrolate or edrophonium-atropine. Sugammadex dose is determined by actual body weight, even in the patient who is morbidly obese. Hepatic dysfunction does not alter drug kinetics as the molecular complex is cleared by the kidneys.

Since sugammadex does not affect acetylcholinesterase, anticholinergic drugs are avoided as are their side effects. The most common side effects associated with sugammadex include postoperative nausea and vomiting (PONV), dry mouth, headache, hypotension, and parosmia (abnormal smell). Rare but significant side effects include anaphylaxis and severe bradycardia. Sugammadex also sequesters (oral) hormonal contraceptives, and patients need to be advised to use alternative forms of contraception for 7 days after sugammadex administration. Sugammadex has not been widely used in pregnancy due to concerns about possible progesterone binding and its theoretical potential for interference with the maintenance of the pregnancy. A small case series of sugammadex use in nonobstetrical and obstetrical surgeries during pregnancy has been published, but avoidance of the drug in pregnant patients is still generally practiced due to its unknown safety profile. One notable clinical exception in the use of sugammadex in pregnant patients is in the difficult airway algorithm. In emergency "cannot intubate, cannot ventilate" situations, sugammadex can be a necessary lifesaving choice even in the pregnant patient.

de Boer H, Driessen JJ, Marcus MA, et al. Reversal of rocuronium-induced (1.2 mg/kg) profound neuromuscular block by sugammadex: a multicenter, dose-finding and safety study. *Anesthesiology*. 2007;107:239-244.

Geldner G, Niskanen M, Laurila P, et al. A randomised controlled trial comparing sugammadex and neostigmine at different depths of neuromuscular blockade in patients undergoing laparoscopic surgery. *Anaesthesia*. 2012;67:991-998.

Lemmens HJ, El-Orbany MI, Berry J, et al. Reversal of profound vecuronium-induced neuromuscular block under sevoflurane anesthesia: sugammadex versus neostigmine. *BMC Anesthesiol*. 2010;10:15.

Naguib MMB. Sugammadex: another milestone in clinical neuromuscular pharmacology. *Anesth Analg*. 2007;104:575-581.

Naguib MMB, Brull SJ. Sugammadex: a novel selective relaxant binding agent. *Expert Rev Clin Pharmacol*. 2009;2:37-53.

Richardson MG, Raymond BL. Sugammadex administration in pregnant women and in women of reproductive potential: a narrative review. *Anesth Analg*. 2020;130:1628-1637.

Sacan O, White PF, Tufanogullari B, et al. Sugammadex reversal of rocuronium-induced neuromuscular blockade: a comparison with neostigmine-glycopyrrolate and edrophonium-atropine. *Anesth Analg*. 2007;104:569-574.

C. Postoperative Management

C.1. What is the incidence of residual NMB in the PACU?

Numerous reports since 2000 make it clear that even with NMBAs of intermediate duration, undetected residual weakness in the postoperative period is not a rare event. Large studies from Europe, where routine reversal with cholinesterase inhibitors was not practiced, report that 20% to 40% of patients arrived in the PACU with TOF values less than 0.70.

As might be expected when a TOF ratio of 0.90 is set as the standard of adequate antagonism, the incidence of PORB approaches 40%. The incidence of PORB is highly variable from institution to institution and very dependent on individual practice patterns. Diligent intraoperative monitoring and routine antagonism of residual block can result in dramatic reductions in the incidence of PORB. In a study from France, between 1995 and 2004, quantitative measurement and reversal of neuromuscular block in the operating room of one institution increased from 2% to 60% and from 6% to 42%, respectively. During the same time, the incidence of residual neuromuscular block, defined as a TOF ratio less than 0.9, decreased from 62% to 3%. Unfortunately, the lessons vividly demonstrated by these authors are far from universally understood or applied. A survey of North American and European clinical practices indicates that even in 2009, 10% of clinicians rarely or never monitored neuromuscular function with even the simplest of PNS, and the routine administration of antagonists was even less common.

Naguib M, Kopman AF, Lien CA, et al. A survey of current management of neuromuscular block in the United States and Europe. *Anesth Analg*. 2010;111:110-119.

Todd MM, Hindman BJ, King BJ. The implementation of quantitative electromyographic neuromuscular monitoring in an academic anesthesia department. *Anesth Analg*. 2014;119:323-331.

Yip PC, Hannam JA, Cameron AJ, et al. Incidence of residual neuromuscular blockade in a post-anaesthetic care unit. *Anaesth Intensive Care*. 2010;38:91-95.

C.2. Does an undetected postoperative residual neuromuscular block (PORB) have clinical consequences?

In North America, an excess of 20 million patients each year receive an anesthetic. The size of the subgroup that receives a nondepolarizing NMBA is unknown but still numbers in the millions. As indicated previously, the incidence of PORB varies greatly from institution to institution. Nonetheless, even if it is as low as 5% overall (highly optimistic), the number of individuals who arrive in the PACU with suboptimal neuromuscular recovery is substantial. The majority of patients who arrive in the PACU with TOF ratios less than 0.90 do not experience complications. However, not all individuals are so fortunate. Undetected PORB is clearly associated with potentially adverse respiratory events and increased morbidity. A recent prospective case-controlled study of critical respiratory events (CREs) (eg, episodes of hypoxemia, signs of airway obstruction, need for reintubation) in a university hospital PACU is instructive. Sixty-one patients with CREs were identified. Their mean TOF ratio, as measured by AMG, was 0.62. The TOF value in 42 matched controls was 0.98. The same authors, in a separate study, demonstrated a lower frequency of residual NMB in the PACU (4.5%; TOF ratio ≤0.9) in cases where intraoperative AMG was employed compared with the cases where conventional PNS was used (30%). During transport to the PACU, fewer AMG patients developed oxygen saturation values, measured by pulse oximetry, of less than 90% (0%) or airway obstruction (0%) compared with subjective monitoring (21.1% and 11.1%, respectively). The incidence, severity, and duration of hypoxemic events during the first 30 minutes of PACU admission were less in the AMG group (all $P < .0001$). These findings add credence to the concept that incomplete neuromuscular recovery is an important contributing factor in the development of adverse respiratory events in the PACU.

Brull SJ, Murphy GS. Residual neuromuscular block: lessons unlearned. Part II: methods to reduce the risk of residual weakness. *Anesth Analg*. 2010;111:129-140.

Butterly A, Bittner EA, George E, et al. Postoperative residual curarization from intermediate-acting neuromuscular blocking agents delays recovery room discharge. *Br J Anaesth*. 2010;105:304-309.

Kopman AF, Brull SJ. Is postoperative residual neuromuscular block associated with adverse clinical outcomes? What is the evidence? *Curr Anesthesiol Rep*. 2013;3:114-121.

Kumar GV, Nair AP, Murthy HS, et al. Residual neuromuscular blockade affects postoperative pulmonary function. *Anesthesiology*. 2012;117:1234-1244.

Murphy GS, Brull SJ. Residual neuromuscular block: lessons unlearned. Part I: definitions, incidence, and adverse physiologic effects of residual neuromuscular block. *Anesth Analg*. 2010;111:120-128.

Murphy GS, Szokol JW, Marymount JH, et al. Intraoperative acceleromyographic monitoring reduces the risk of residual neuromuscular blockade and adverse respiratory events in the postanesthesia care unit. *Anesthesiology*. 2008;109:389-398.

Thilen SR, Weigel WA, Todd MM, et al. 2023 American Society of Anesthesiologists Practice Guidelines for monitoring and antagonism of neuromuscular blockade: a report by the American Society of Anesthesiologists Task Force on Neuromuscular Blockade. *Anesthesiology*. 2023;138:13-41.

56 Burns

Shreyajit R. Kumar and Anup Pamnani

A 48-year-old female incurred a flame injury while attempting to light a gas grill. She has 40% second- and third-degree burns over her face, neck, chest, and upper extremities. She had a history of hypertension, angina, and angioplasty of the right coronary artery 1 year ago. She has smoked three packs of cigarettes per day for 20 years and drinks alcohol daily. She is scheduled for tangential excision of eschar on the third postburn day. Her blood pressure is 190/100 mm Hg with a heart rate of 120 beats per minute, and she weighs 110 kg.

A. Medical Disease and Differential Diagnosis

1. How do you classify the burn injury?
2. How do you express the extent of burn injury?
3. Should the "rule of nines" be used in children?
4. What are the functions of the skin?
5. What pathophysiologic changes accompany major thermal injury?
6. What is the prognosis for this patient? What major factors affect her prognosis?
7. What are the common causes of death in burn patients?
8. Does this patient have a smoke inhalation injury? How do you make the diagnosis?
9. What is carbon monoxide poisoning? How do you diagnose and treat carbon monoxide poisoning?
10. What resuscitative measure would you institute immediately in this patient with 40% burns?
11. What fluid formula would you use?
12. What cardiovascular changes typify the burn injury?
13. What changes occur in hepatic function? What are the anesthetic implications of such changes?
14. What are Curling ulcers? How can they be prevented?
15. What complications are associated with electrical burns?

B. Preoperative Evaluation and Preparation

1. What preoperative preparations would you order? What are the principal concerns in this patient?
2. What are the various operative and management options available for severely burned patients?
3. What are the advantages and disadvantages of early tangential excision split-thickness skin grafting (TE/STSG)?
4. What is this patient's mean arterial blood pressure? How is it calculated?
5. Are you concerned about this patient's blood pressure and heart rate? What treatment would you institute?
6. This patient was ventilated with respirator settings of tidal volume 800 mL, respiratory rate 20 breaths per minute, fraction of inspired oxygen (F_{IO_2}) 60%, and positive end-expiratory pressure 10 cm H_2O. Arterial blood gas analyses showed pH 7.24, Pa_{O_2} 56 mm Hg, Pa_{CO_2} 60 mm Hg, and oxygen saturation 80%. How would you interpret these results? What are the possible causes of high Pa_{CO_2} and low Pa_{O_2}?
7. How do you calculate oxygen content and oxygen delivery? What factors govern oxygen delivery to the tissues?

C. Intraoperative Management

1. What monitors would you use intraoperatively?
2. What information can be obtained from an arterial catheter and a pulmonary artery catheter? How are these calculations performed?

3. If the patient had not been intubated, how would you proceed with induction of anesthesia?
4. Why is awake tracheal intubation considered the safest?
5. What anesthetic agents would you use? Discuss inhalation versus intravenous agents.
6. Why are you concerned about the patient's body temperature? What is normothermia for a burned patient?
7. How is temperature best maintained?
8. What derangements occur with hypothermia?
9. What neuromuscular blocking agent would you use?
10. Why is succinylcholine contraindicated in burned patients? For how long should it be avoided?
11. What other adverse effects are associated with succinylcholine?
12. How does burn injury affect the dosing of nondepolarizing neuromuscular blocking agents?
13. How are neuromuscular blocking agents, such as succinylcholine, atracurium, cisatracurium, vecuronium, pancuronium, rocuronium, and curare, metabolized and eliminated? Which have significant histamine release?

D. Postoperative Management

1. How would you monitor this patient during transport?
2. What is meant by diffusion hypoxia? How do you prevent it?
3. Why do patients often shiver in the recovery room on emergence from general anesthesia?
4. Discuss the causes of oliguria in PACU.

A. Medical Disease and Differential Diagnosis

A.1. How do you classify the burn injury?

Burns classification is based on both the degree of tissue injury and depth. First-degree burns are confined to epidermal injury and characterized as superficial. Second-degree burns are partial-thickness burns and involve the epidermis and dermis, and third-degree burns involve irreversible destruction of all dermal and epidermal elements, noted as full thickness. Fourth-degree burns involve injury to underlying tissue structures: muscle, fascia, tendon, and bone (**Table 56.1**).

MacLennan N, Heimbach DM, Cullen BF. Anaesthesia for major thermal injury. *Anesthesiology*. 1998;89:749-770.

Townsend CM Jr, Beauchamp D, Evers MB, et al, eds. Burns. In: *Sabiston Textbook of Surgery: The Biological Basis of Modern Surgical Practice*. 21st ed. Elsevier Saunders; 2022:484-506.

TABLE 56.1 Classification of Burn Depth

Classification	Burn Depth	Outcome
Superficial		
First degree	Confined to epidermis	Heals spontaneously
Partial thickness		
Second degree		
Superficial dermal burn	Epidermis and upper dermis	Heals spontaneously
Deep dermal burn	Epidermis and deep dermis	Requires excision and grafting for rapid return of function
Full thickness		
Third degree	Destruction of the epidermis and dermis	Wound excision and grafting required Some limitation of function and scar formation
Fourth degree	Muscle, fascia, bone	Complete excision required, limited function

Reprinted with permission from MacLennan N, Heimbach DM, Cullen BF. Anesthesia for major thermal injury. *Anesthesiology.* 1998;89:749-779.

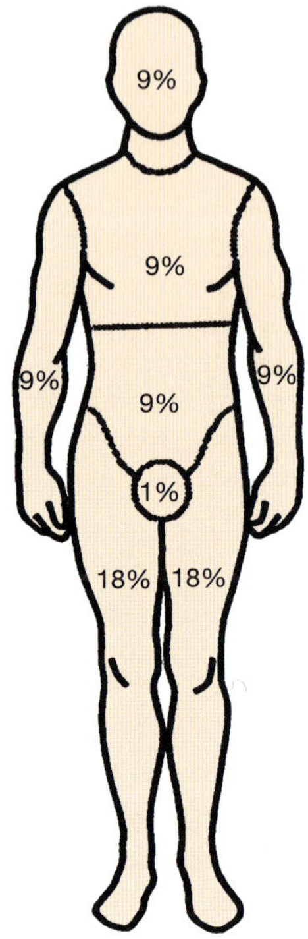

FIGURE 56.1. The rule of nines for determining the percentage of body surface area burned in adults. (Adapted with permission from MacLennan N, Heimbach DM, Cullen BF. Anesthesia for major thermal injury. *Anesthesiology*. 1998;89:749-770.)

A.2. How do you express the extent of burn injury?

The extent of burn injury is expressed as total body surface area (TBSA) percentage. Burn size is estimated by the "rule of nines" (**Figure 56.1**). In adults, each upper extremity and the head and neck approximates 9% of TBSA. Each of the lower extremities, anterior trunk, and posterior trunk accounts for 18%, and the perineum accounts for approximately 1% of the TBSA. Burn proportions are additive, yielding a TBSA burn.

MacLennan N, Heimbach DM, Cullen BF. Anesthesia for major thermal injury. *Anesthesiology*. 1998;89:749-770.

Townsend CM Jr, Beauchamp D, Evers MB, et al, eds. Burns. In: *Sabiston Textbook of Surgery: The Biological Basis of Modern Surgical Practice*. 21st ed. Elsevier Saunders; 2022:484-506.

A.3. Should the "rule of nines" be used in children?

The "rule of nines" will not estimate TBSA burns in children because of their different relative proportions compared to adults. A child's head and neck comprise a relatively larger portion of the body surface area and a smaller surface area in the lower extremities. The Lund and Browder chart represents a precise method, accounting for the changing proportions of TBSA from infancy to adulthood (**Figure 56.2**).

MacLennan N, Heimbach DM, Cullen BF. Anesthesia for major thermal injury. *Anesthesiology*. 1998;89:749-770.

Townsend CM Jr, Beauchamp D, Evers MB, et al, eds. Burns. In: *Sabiston Textbook of Surgery: The Biological Basis of Modern Surgical Practice*. 21st ed. Elsevier Saunders; 2022:484-506.

A.4. What are the functions of the skin?

The skin is the largest organ of the body by surface area and is the primary immune barrier, protecting against microorganisms. The skin provides thermal regulation, fluid and electrolyte homeostasis, vitamin D metabolism, and sensation (touch, temperature, and pain).

Herndon DN, ed. *Total Burn Care*. 6th ed. Saunders Elsevier; 2025.

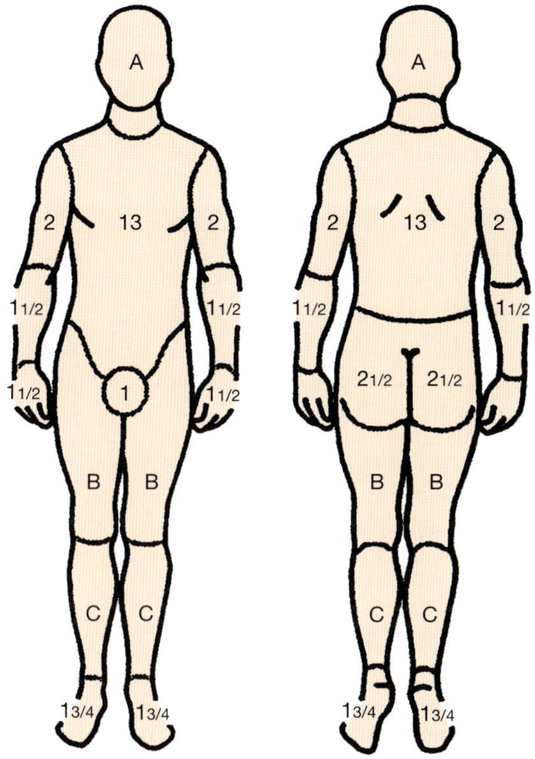

Relative percentages of areas affected by growth

	AGE IN YEARS					
AREA	**0**	**1**	**5**	**10**	**15**	**Adult**
A: half of head	9½	8½	6½	5½	4½	3½
B: half of thigh	2¾	3¼	4	4¼	4½	4¾
C: half of leg	2½	2½	2¾	3	3¼	3½

FIGURE 56.2. Diagram and table for determining the percentage of body surface area burned in children. (Adapted with permission from MacLennan N, Heimbach DM, Cullen BF. Anesthesia for major thermal injury. *Anesthesiology.* 1998;89:749-770.)

A.5. What pathophysiologic changes accompany major thermal injury?

The pathophysiologic alterations that accompany major thermal injury are complex. Destruction of the skin has a profound systemic impact. Thermal regulation, fluid and electrolyte homeostasis, and protection against bacterial infection are all affected. Inflammatory mediators released from burn injury result in a leaky capillary syndrome; fluid and albumin are sequestered from the intravascular compartment into the burn wound, causing hemoconcentration and hypoalbuminemia. Increased secretion of antidiuretic hormone can cause oliguria or anuria.

Metabolic rate is markedly increased after burn injury. Depending on burn size, the increase in metabolic rate can be doubled or tripled, with concomitant increases in oxygen consumption and carbon dioxide production. This hypermetabolic state persists for weeks or months until full tissue repair is complete.

Cardiac output (CO) is often decreased in patients with major burns. This decrease results from a rapid reduction in circulating blood volume as well as the upregulation of myocardial depressant factor.

Changes in vascular integrity occur in areas remote from the injury site. The entire vascular compartment becomes increasingly permeable, manifesting as edema. Severe pulmonary edema is devastating, and airway edema is the impetus for early tracheal intubation.

Pulmonary function is significantly altered, with a reduction of functional residual capacity, lung capacity, and chest wall compliance. Increases occur in the alveolar-arterial oxygen gradient (P_{AO_2}-Pa_{O_2}) and minute ventilation (as high as 40 L/min; normal 6 L/min).

Anderson JH, Mandell SP, Gibran NS. Burns. In: Brunicardi FC, Andersen DK, Billiar TR, eds. *Schwartz's Principles of Surgery*. 11th ed. McGraw-Hill; 2019:251-271.

Herndon DN, ed. *Total Burn Care*. 6th ed. Saunders Elsevier; 2025.

MacLennan N, Heimbach DM, Cullen BF. Anesthesia for major thermal injury. *Anesthesiology*. 1998;89:749-770.

A.6. What is the prognosis for this patient? What major factors affect her prognosis?

The prognosis for this patient is very poor. Statistical survival based on TBSA alone predicts survival less than 50%. Other factors that affect her prognosis are age, size and depth of burn, associated pulmonary injury, and preexisting medical disease. In this patient with a history of angioplasty for coronary artery disease, hypertension, heavy smoking, and obesity, the risk of myocardial infarction is greatly increased.

A.7. What are the common causes of death in burn patients?

The major early cause of death is asphyxia. The most common cause of long-term mortality is septic complications.

A.8. Does this patient have a smoke inhalation injury? How do you make the diagnosis?

This patient probably sustained a smoke inhalation injury. Smoke inhalation should be suspected in patients who were burned in an enclosed space, received burns on the face, were burned while under the influence of alcohol or drugs, or lost consciousness at the time of the accident.

A patient with smoke inhalation often exhibits a "lucid period" of no physical signs or symptoms during the first 24 hours after the burn. Early symptoms and signs of respiratory tract injury include burned nasal mucosa, lips and mouth, singed nasal hair, and soot in the sputum. The posterior pharynx can appear red and edematous. Radiographic findings are usually unremarkable immediately after injury. Laboratory tests include blood gas analysis, carboxyhemoglobin concentration, xenon scans, and fiberoptic bronchoscopy.

Anderson JH, Mandell SP, Gibran NS. Burns. In: Brunicardi FC, Andersen DK, Billiar TR, eds. *Schwartz's Principles of Surgery*. 11th ed. McGraw-Hill; 2019:251-271.

Herndon DN, ed. *Total Burn Care*. 6th ed. Saunders Elsevier; 2025.

A.9. What is carbon monoxide poisoning? How do you diagnose and treat carbon monoxide poisoning?

Carbon monoxide is the leading cause of hypoxia in survivors of burn injuries; it is liberated from the incomplete combustion of carbon-containing fuels (wood, coal, and gasoline). Carbon monoxide has a 250 times greater affinity for hemoglobin than oxygen, displacing oxygen from its hemoglobin-binding sites. Carbon monoxide oximetry is necessary for the diagnosis of carbon monoxide poisoning; arterial blood gas Pao_2 will be falsely normal.

Expeditious oxygen therapy will displace carbon monoxide from hemoglobin. The half-life of carbon monoxide elimination is 4 to 6 hours at room air. This reduces to 40 to 80 minutes with 100% oxygen and 15 to 30 minutes with hyperbaric oxygen therapy.

Anderson JH, Mandell SP, Gibran NS. Burns. In: Brunicardi FC, Andersen DK, Billiar TR, eds. *Schwartz's Principles of Surgery*. 11th ed. McGraw-Hill; 2019:251-271.

Herndon DN, ed. *Total Burn Care*. 6th ed. Saunders Elsevier; 2025.

A.10. What resuscitative measure would you institute immediately in this patient with 40% burns?

Early and aggressive fluid resuscitation will combat distributive hypovolemia. Liberal fluid administration ensures end-organ perfusion and adequate urine output. If an upper airway burn is involved, tracheal intubation helps prevent edematous airway compromise.

A.11. What fluid formula would you use?

The Parkland formula guides initial resuscitation in hypovolemic shock after burn injury. It has been adopted as the standard of practice at most burn centers due to its simplicity, reduced cost, and equivalent outcome when compared to other calculations for fluid administration. Other formulas differ widely in the colloid:crystalloid ratio and in the rate of fluid administration. Research supports the need for both crystalloid and colloid solutions (**Table 56.2**) and calculation using the Parkland formula as a resuscitation "starting point." Urine output of 0.5 to 1.0 mL/kg/h should guide resuscitation.

Parkland Formula

First 24 hours

- *Electrolyte solution (lactated Ringer)*: 4 mL/kg/percentage of body area with second- and third-degree burns
- *Administration rate*: half the solution given in the first 8 hours, one-quarter in the second 8 hours, and one-quarter in the third 8 hours

TABLE 56.2 Fluid Resuscitation for Adults With Major Burns

Crystalloid Regimens		
Parkland	Lactated Ringer	4 mL/kg/% burn
Modified Brooke	Lactated Ringer	2 mL/kg/% burn
Colloid Regimens		
Evans	Normal saline	1 mL/kg/% burn
	Colloid	1 mL/kg/% burn
	5% Dextrose	2,000 mL/24 h
Brooke	Lactated Ringer	1.5 mL/kg/% burn
	Colloid	0.5 mL/kg/% burn
	5% Dextrose	2,000 mL/24 h

- *Urine output*: maintain at 0.5 to 1.0 mL/kg/h.

Second 24 hours

- *Glucose in water*: to replace evaporated water losses and maintain a serum sodium concentration of 140 mM
- *Colloid solutions (eg, albumin)*: amount proportional to burn
- *30% to 50% burn*: 0.3 mL/kg/percentage of burn
- *50% to 70% burn*: 0.4 mL/kg/percentage of burn
- *Larger than 70% burn*: 0.5 mL/kg/percentage of burn
- *Urine output*: maintain at 0.5 to 1.0 mL/kg/h.

Anderson JH, Mandell SP, Gibran NS. Burns. In: Brunicardi FC, Andersen DK, Billiar TR, eds. *Schwartz's Principles of Surgery*. 11th ed. McGraw-Hill; 2019:251-271.

Blumetti J, Hunt JL, Arnoldo BD, et al. The Parkland formula under fire: is the criticism justified? *J Burn Care Res*. 2008;29:180-186.

Herndon DN, ed. *Total Burn Care*. 6th ed. Saunders Elsevier; 2025.

A.12. What cardiovascular changes typify the burn injury?

Microvascular disruption of capillary membranes results in acute fluid sequestration from intravascular compartment to interstitial spaces. Decreased plasma volume leads to depressed CO and hypotension. Catecholamine release triggers vasoconstriction, which further compromises tissue perfusion. Ventricular dysfunction is attributed to myocardial depressant factor.

Herndon DN, ed. *Total Burn Care*. 6th ed. Saunders Elsevier; 2025.

Townsend CM Jr, Beauchamp D, Evers MB, et al, eds. Burns. In: *Sabiston Textbook of Surgery: The Biological Basis of Modern Surgical Practice*. 21st ed. Elsevier Saunders; 2022:484-506.

A.13. What changes occur in hepatic function? What are the anesthetic implications of such changes?

Decreased circulating volume during the initial burn phase can result in shock to the liver and restrict hepatic detoxification capacity. Albumin levels can fall, which can increase the free fraction of benzodiazepines and phenytoin. In contrast, a rise in the acute phase reactant α_1-acid-glycoprotein increases the binding of positively charged basic drugs such as lidocaine, propranolol, and neuromuscular blocking agents.

Herndon DN, ed. *Total Burn Care*. 6th ed. Saunders Elsevier; 2025.

Jeevendra Martin JA, Fukushima Y, Chon JY, et al. Muscle relaxants in burns, trauma, and critical illness. *Int Anesthesiol Clin*. 2006;44:123-143.

A.14. What are Curling ulcers? How can they be prevented?

A Curling ulcer is a gastric or duodenal stress ulcer resulting from a systemic thermal injury. Without treatment, the incidence is as high as 80%. Atrophy of the small bowel mucosa occurs within 12 hours of injury and is proportional to burn extent. Additional decreases in intestinal blood flow exacerbate the gastric injury. Curling ulcers can be prevented prophylactically with antacids, H_2-antagonists, and early enteral feeding.

Townsend CM Jr, Beauchamp D, Evers MB, et al, eds. Burns. In: *Sabiston Textbook of Surgery: The Biological Basis of Modern Surgical Practice*. 21st ed. Elsevier Saunders; 2022:484-506.

A.15. What complications are associated with electrical burns?

Electrical burns result in small area of skin necrosis, with extensive damage to deep tissue structures including muscles, tendons, blood vessels, and nerves. Fluid losses are greater than predicted from the Parkland calculation. The total injury is determined by the duration of current flow, the resistance of the tissue, and the area of contact. Muscle necrosis can cause myoglobinuria and acute tubular necrosis. Thrombotic phenomena can occur. Cardiac conduction abnormalities, ectopy, and congestive heart failure can occur secondary to electrical injury.

Herndon DN, ed. *Total Burn Care*. 6th ed. Saunders Elsevier; 2025.

B. Preoperative Evaluation and Preparation

B.1. What preoperative preparations would you order? What are the principal concerns in this patient?

A thorough medical history and physical examination should focus on the patient's salient risk factors. Her hypertension, ischemic heart disease, left main coronary artery angioplasty, and history of heavy smoking and heavy alcohol consumption are of particular concern. The following laboratory tests should be ordered: complete blood count, basic metabolic profile, lactate, coagulation profile, liver function tests, electrocardiogram (ECG), urinalysis, chest radiograph, and arterial blood gas analysis. Cardiac enzymes will reflect any acute sequelae of her left main coronary artery disease. Tenuous cardiac status should prompt cardiologist evaluation.

B.2. What are the various operative and management options available for severely burned patients?

Early tangential excision of burn tissue and early wound closure, primarily by skin grafting, have significantly improved mortality among the severely burned population. Eschar, or burned skin, is an active medium for bacterial propagation, and topical antibiotic cream such as silver sulfadiazine should be applied. Early removal of injured tissue prevents wound infection and decreases systemic inflammatory response. A widely adopted strategy involves a 48-hour period of initial resuscitation to achieve hemodynamic stability, followed by early tangential TE/STSG. The extent of escharotomy is limited to 20% of TBSA and repeated every 2 days until excision is complete.

Anderson JH, Mandell SP, Gibran NS. Burns. In: Brunicardi FC, Andersen DK, Billiar TR, eds. *Schwartz's Principles of Surgery*. 11th ed. McGraw-Hill; 2019:251-271.

Townsend CM Jr, Beauchamp D, Evers MB, et al, eds. Burns. In: *Sabiston Textbook of Surgery: The Biological Basis of Modern Surgical Practice*. 21st ed. Elsevier Saunders; 2022:484-506.

B.3. What are the advantages and disadvantages of early tangential excision split-thickness skin grafting (TE/STSG)?

Expeditious escharotomy (within 2 days) will reduce bacterial load and risk of bacteremia and sepsis and shorten the recovery phase and overall hospital length of stay. Very early excision (within 24 hours) has the disadvantage of major operative stress during the resuscitative phase of injury; the patient is not optimized and incurs anesthetic risk.

Herndon DN, ed. *Total Burn Care*. 6th ed. Saunders Elsevier; 2025.

Townsend CM Jr, Beauchamp D, Evers MB, et al, eds. Burns. In: *Sabiston Textbook of Surgery: The Biological Basis of Modern Surgical Practice*. 21st ed. Elsevier Saunders; 2022:484-506.

B.4. What is this patient's mean arterial blood pressure? How is it calculated?

This patient's mean arterial pressure (MAP) can be calculated from her blood pressure of 190/100 mm Hg as MAP = two-thirds of diastolic pressure + one-third of the systolic pressure. An equivalent calculation is MAP = diastolic pressure + one-third of the pulse pressure or 130 mm Hg in this case; the pulse pressure is the difference between systolic and diastolic pressures.

B.5. Are you concerned about this patient's blood pressure and heart rate? What treatment would you institute?

We are concerned with this patient's extremely high blood pressure, given her history of angina and coronary disease requiring left main coronary angioplasty. Our goal is to maintain normotension. β-Blockers (labetalol, metoprolol), calcium channel blockers (nicardipine), angiotensin converting enzyme inhibitors (enalapril), and hydralazine are all intravenous vasodilators that can be employed.

Her tachycardia (heart rate 120 beats per minute) would benefit from β-blockade with labetalol or metoprolol. Reduction of afterload and tachycardia will decrease overall myocardial oxygen demand and reduce the risk of myocardial infarction.

Adequacy of volume resuscitation should be assessed. Urine output, central venous pressure (CVP), pulmonary artery occlusion pressure (PAOP), CO, and cardiac index will all guide fluid resuscitation.

B.6. This patient was ventilated with respirator settings of tidal volume 800 mL, respiratory rate 20 breaths per minute, fraction of inspired oxygen (F_{IO_2}) 60%, and positive end-expiratory pressure 10 cm H_2O. Arterial blood gas analyses showed pH 7.24, Pa_{O_2} 56 mm Hg, Pa_{CO_2} 60 mm Hg, and oxygen saturation 80%. How would you interpret these results? What are the possible causes of high Pa_{CO_2} and low Pa_{O_2}?

Arterial blood gas analysis shows uncompensated respiratory acidosis with a substantial Alveolar-arterial (A-a) oxygen gradient. This patient was being hypoventilated, reflected in the elevated Pa_{CO_2} of 60 mm Hg (normal is 35-45 mm Hg). The etiology of her hypercapnia could be a hypermetabolic state with a marked increase in CO_2 production.

The most common cause of hypoxemia with an increased A-a gradient is $\dot{V}/\dot{Q}$ mismatch. Atelectasis, pneumonia, pulmonary edema, or malposition of the tracheal tube with single-lung ventilation increases dead space or shunt fraction, resulting in $\dot{V}/\dot{Q}$ mismatch.

B.7. How do you calculate oxygen content and oxygen delivery? What factors govern oxygen delivery to the tissues?

The oxygen content of arterial blood (Ca_{O_2}) is the sum of two components, the oxygen dissolved in plasma and the oxygen bound to hemoglobin (Hgb). Ca_{O_2} is expressed as:

$$Ca_{O_2}\ (\text{mL/dL}) = 1.31 \times \text{Hgb (g/dL)} \times Sa_{O_2}\ (\%) + 0.003 \times Pa_{O_2}$$

Normal arterial oxygen content: Ca_{O_2} = 20.73 mL/dL
Oxygen delivery (DO_2) is directly proportional to CO and arterial oxygen content:

$$DO_2 = \text{CO} \times Ca_{O_2} = \text{CO} \times ([1.31 \times \text{Hgb (g/dL)} \times Sa_{O_2}\ (\%)] + 0.003 \times Pa_{O_2}).$$

Thus, the three main factors that govern oxygen delivery to the tissues are CO, hemoglobin, and arterial oxygen saturation.

Criner GJ, Barnette RE, D'Alonzo GE, eds. *Critical Care Study Guide: Text and Review*. 2nd ed. Springer; 2010:493-494.

C. Intraoperative Management

C.1. What monitors would you use intraoperatively?

Standard monitors, including noninvasive blood pressure, ECG (leads II and V_5), pulse oximetry, capnography, and temperature, should be used in this patient. A Foley catheter will assess urine output and indirectly volume status. An arterial catheter, pulmonary artery catheter, and CVP monitoring will be beneficial in this severely burned patient with ischemic heart disease.

C.2. What information can be obtained from an arterial catheter and a pulmonary artery catheter? How are these calculations performed?

The transduced arterial catheter displays continuous blood pressure measurements. This is most useful in fluctuating hypotensive or hypertensive situations. During dysrhythmias such as atrial fibrillation or ventricular tachycardia, variations in ventricular response or blood pressure can be recognized instantly.

The morphology of the waveform provides information about arterial resistance (ie, a narrow waveform is suggestive of both a reduced stroke volume and an increased systemic vascular resistance), stroke volume (area under the curve), and preload (pulse pressure variation and its response to positive pressure ventilation). In addition, it serves as vascular access for blood sampling (eg, arterial blood gas analysis, electrolytes, hematocrit, and blood glucose levels).

A pulmonary artery catheter allows measurement of PAOP, a surrogate of left atrial pressure. Left atrial pressure reflects left ventricular end-diastolic pressure, the preload of the left ventricle. CVP, although useful as a rough estimate of preload, does not correlate with left ventricular end-diastolic pressure when either isolated right-sided or left-sided cardiac dysfunction occurs. Multi-lumen pulmonary artery catheters are capable of measuring CVP and CO via the thermodilution method. It also permits the sampling of mixed venous blood. These measurements allow the calculation of many hemodynamic variables.

$$\text{Cardiac index (CI)} = \frac{\text{CO}}{\text{Body surface area}} \text{ (normal 2.8-4.2 L/min/m}^2\text{).}$$

$$\text{Stroke volume (SV)} = \frac{\text{CO}}{\text{Heart rate}} \text{ (normal 60-80 mL/beat).}$$

$$\text{Stroke index (SI)} = \frac{\text{CI}}{\text{Heart rate}} \text{ (normal 40-65 mL/beat/m}^2\text{).}$$

$$\text{Systematic vascular resistance (SVR)} = \frac{\text{Mean BP} - \text{CVP}}{\text{CO}} \times 80 \text{ (normal 900-1,400 dynes/sec/cm}^5\text{).}$$

$$\text{Pulmonary vascular resistance (PVR)} = \frac{\text{Mean BP} - \text{CVP}}{\text{CO}} \times 80 \text{ (normal 150-250 dynes/sec/cm}^5\text{).}$$

Mixed venous blood samples are needed for shunt calculations:

$$\frac{Q_s}{Q_t} = \frac{(CcO_2 - CaO_2)}{(CcO_2 - C\bar{v}O_2)}$$

Cco_2= pulmonary capillary oxygen content

Cao_2= artery oxygen content

$C\bar{v}o_2$= mixed venous oxygen content

A low mixed venous oxygen (<30 mm Hg) is suggestive of inadequate tissue perfusion.

Bittner EA, Martyn JA, Sjoberg F. Burn management. In: Gropper MA, Eriksson LI, Fleisher LA, Cohen NH, Leslie K, Johnson-Akeju O, eds. *Miller's Anesthesia*. 10th ed. Elsevier; 2025:2746-2773.

C.3. If the patient had not been intubated, how would you proceed with induction of anesthesia?

This patient has a facial burn, which portends a difficult intubation. Burns on the face can cause severe airway and facial edema; careful assessment of the mouth opening, pharynx, and larynx is warranted. The safest way to secure the airway is to perform awake tracheal intubation with topical anesthesia and mild sedation achieved by either direct or fiberoptic-guided intubation. If prolonged postoperative intubation is anticipated, the nasotracheal route is more easily secured, provides better patient comfort, and permits better oral hygiene. Phenylephrine drops can achieve nasal mucosa vasoconstriction. Alternatively, a tracheostomy should be considered early in patients with acute lung injury who will require prolonged mechanical ventilation.

C.4. Why is awake tracheal intubation considered the safest?

Awake intubation is the safest approach to secure an airway because spontaneous breathing retains protective airway reflexes, lowers the risk of upper airway obstruction, maintains oxygen saturation, and lends more time for laryngoscopy. Identifying the passage of air from the glottis can be helpful in blind intubation. An awake patient precludes the need for mask ventilation and avoids the risk of stomach distention.

C.5. What anesthetic agents would you use? Discuss inhalation versus intravenous agents.

For the severely burned patient, once the airway is secured, a high-dose opioid technique would be preferred. This confers intraoperative hemodynamic stability and optimal postoperative analgesia.

Opioids such as morphine, meperidine (Demerol), fentanyl, or sufentanil do not depress myocardial contractility; potent inhalation agents depress myocardial function. If inhalation agents are chosen, the concentration should be carefully titrated to prevent hemodynamic impact.

C.6. Why are you concerned about the patient's body temperature? What is normothermia for a burned patient?

Massive burn injury with loss of skin integrity can lead to considerable evaporative fluid losses and risks profound intraoperative hypothermia. This is exacerbated by the vasodilatory effects of general anesthesia and by the cool, dry operating room air. The infusion of large volumes of intravenous fluids at room temperature also contributes to the development of hypothermia.

Normothermia for a burned patient is approximately 38.5 °C. The stress of thermal injury results in a resetting of the hypothalamic thermostat.

Anderson JH, Mandell SP, Gibran NS. Burns. In: Brunicardi FC, Andersen DK, Billiar TR, eds. *Schwartz's Principles of Surgery*. 11th ed. McGraw-Hill; 2019:251-271.

Herndon DN, ed. *Total Burn Care*. 6th ed. Saunders Elsevier; 2025.

Townsend CM Jr, Beauchamp D, Evers MB, et al, eds. Burns. In: *Sabiston Textbook of Surgery: The Biological Basis of Modern Surgical Practice*. 21st ed. Elsevier Saunders; 2022:484-506.

C.7. How is temperature best maintained?

Hypothermia is a chief concern from the loss of the insulator effect of the skin. Heat losses occur through convection, conduction, evaporation, and radiation. Methods to maintain normothermia involve active warming and prevention of heat loss. Crystalloid and blood transfusions must be administered through a blood- and/or fluid-warming device. A prewarmed forced air mattress is placed under a single-layer sterile sheet on the operating table. Warming the operating room to temperatures between 24 °C (75.2 °F) and 27 °C (80.6 °F) with a relative humidity higher than 50% is particularly effective. The nonsurgical areas of the patient's body must be covered. Heated, humidified airway circuits are most effective in minimizing heat loss from ventilation with cold anesthetic gases.

C.8. What derangements occur with hypothermia?

Hypothermia causes many physiologic changes. Hypothermia decreases metabolism, heart rate, CO, and blood pressure. At temperatures less than 28 °C (82.4 °F), atrial pacing becomes irregular, and ventricular ectopy increases. Ventricular fibrillation occurs between 25 °C (77 °F) and 30 °C (86 °F).

Bittner EA, Martyn JA, Sjoberg F. Burn management. In: Gropper MA, Eriksson LI, Fleisher LA, Cohen NH, Leslie K, Johnson-Akeju O, eds. *Miller's Anesthesia*. 10th ed. Elsevier; 2025:2746-2773.

C.9. What neuromuscular blocking agent would you use?

A nondepolarizing neuromuscular blocking agent should be used; depolarizing agents should be avoided. In general, the choice of neuromuscular blocking agent should be based on the duration of the operation and the presence of any coexisting diseases affecting drug elimination. Agents without histamine release are preferred, such as vecuronium and rocuronium.

C.10. Why is succinylcholine contraindicated in burned patients? For how long should it be avoided?

Succinylcholine is contraindicated in burned patients because it can cause a significant, transient increase in plasma potassium concentration (as high as 13 mEq/L), resulting in ventricular fibrillation and cardiac arrest. This hyperkalemic response begins 5 to 15 days after the burn and persists for 2 to 3 months or longer, irrespective of the degree and size of the burn injury.

The mechanism responsible for this response is not known. It is hypothesized that the abrupt release of potassium is from the hypersensitive muscle with extrajunctional nicotinic acetylcholine receptors in burned patients. Stimulation of these receptors can mediate a potentially lethal efflux of intracellular potassium.

The exact time for this hypersensitivity is unclear. Most advocate against succinylcholine use from 24 to 48 hours after the burn injury until complete recovery has occurred. A hyperkalemic response has been reported in a patient after 480 days. The recommended limit is now extended to 2 years after the burned skin has healed.

Bittner EA, Martyn JA, Sjoberg F. Burn management. In: Gropper MA, Eriksson LI, Fleisher LA, Cohen NH, Leslie K, Johnson-Akeju O, eds. *Miller's Anesthesia*. 10th ed. Elsevier; 2025:2746-2773.

Gronert GA. Succinylcholine hyperkalemia after burns. *Anesthesiology*. 1999;91:320-322.

TABLE 56.3 Metabolism, Elimination, and Histamine Release of Neuromuscular Blocking Agents

	Elimination			
Agent	**Kidney (%)**	**Liver (%)**	**Plasma Metabolism (%)**	**Histamine Release**
Succinylcholine	<2	0	98	Slight
Atracurium	10-40	0	60-90	Slight
Cisatracurium	16	7	77	None
Vecuronium	40	60	0	None
Pancuronium	85	15	0	None
Rocuronium	25	70	0	None
D-Tubocurarine	80	20	0	Moderate

From Gropper MA, Cohen NH, Eriksson LI, et al, eds. *Miller's Anesthesia.* 9th ed. Elsevier; 2020:2746-2773.

Jeevendra Martyn JA. Succinylcholine hyperkalemia after burns. *Anesthesiology.* 1999;91:321-322.

Schaner P Brown RL, Kirksey TD, et al. Succinylcholine-induced hyperkalemia in burned patients - 1. *Anesth Analg.* 1969;48:764-770.

C.11. What other adverse effects are associated with succinylcholine?

The many adverse effects of succinylcholine include:

- Hyperkalemia, particularly following burns, spinal cord injuries, and generalized major trauma.
- Increased intracranial and intraocular pressure, the clinical significance of which is controversial.
- Increased intragastric pressure, counterbalanced by an increase in lower esophageal pressure, which reduces the increased risk of regurgitation.
- Myalgia, more likely to concern the patient with minor injuries who ambulates soon after surgery.
- Prolonged paralysis in patients with atypical plasma cholinesterase.
- Cardiac arrhythmias, particularly bradycardia after repeated doses.
- Trigger for malignant hyperthermia.

Bittner EA, Martyn JA, Sjoberg F. Burn management. In: Gropper MA, Eriksson LI, Fleisher LA, Cohen NH, Leslie K, Johnson-Akeju O, eds. *Miller's Anesthesia.* 10th ed. Elsevier; 2025:2746-2773.

C.12. How does burn injury affect the dosing of nondepolarizing neuromuscular blocking agents?

Burn patients can show resistance to the nondepolarizing neuromuscular blocking agents. Martyn et al first reported that burn patients required a 5 times higher plasma concentration of D-tubocurarine to attain a given percentage of twitch depression compared with healthy subjects. The dose of pancuronium was increased by 2.5-fold. This increased requirement appears secondary to the upregulation of an altered affinity of junctional receptors. The burn patient also has increased plasma protein binding of nondepolarizing neuromuscular blocking agents.

Bittner EA, Martyn JA, Sjoberg F. Burn management. In: Gropper MA, Eriksson LI, Fleisher LA, Cohen NH, Leslie K, Johnson-Akeju O, eds. *Miller's Anesthesia.* 10th ed. Elsevier; 2025:2746-2773.

Martyn JA, Fukushima Y, Chon JY, et al. Muscle relaxants in burns, trauma, and critical illness. *Int Anesthesiol Clin.* 2006;44:123-143.

C.13. How are neuromuscular blocking agents, such as succinylcholine, atracurium, cisatracurium, vecuronium, pancuronium, rocuronium, and curare, metabolized and eliminated? Which have significant histamine release?

See **Table 56.3**.

Bittner EA, Martyn JA, Sjoberg F. Burn management. In: Gropper MA, Eriksson LI, Fleisher LA, Cohen NH, Leslie K, Johnson-Akeju O, eds. *Miller's Anesthesia.* 10th ed. Elsevier; 2025:2746-2773.

D. Postoperative Management

D.1. How would you monitor this patient during transport?

This patient was most likely intubated, paralyzed, apneic, and still under the influence of general anesthetics. Monitoring should be directed toward respiration, oxygenation, and hemodynamics. These can be achieved by utilizing a transport monitor capable of monitoring ECG, blood pressure, and pulse oximetry.

During transport, ventilation should be controlled with positive pressure ventilation via a self-inflating bag valve mask (Ambu bag) with supplemental oxygen.

D.2. What is meant by diffusion hypoxia? How do you prevent it?

Fink et al first reported diffusion hypoxemia during recovery from nitrous oxide-oxygen anesthesia. A mild degree of hypoxemia can develop after cessation of nitrous oxide-oxygen anesthesia if the patient is breathing room air. The arterial oxygen saturation can fall 5% to 10% and often reaches values less than 90% (Pao_2 <60 mm Hg). This desaturation occurs upon rapid elimination of nitrous oxide, which is 35 times more soluble in blood than nitrogen. Alveolar oxygen is diluted by the high nitrous oxide concentration diffusing from blood. Diffusion hypoxia can be prevented by the administration of a high fraction of inspired oxygen for several minutes.

Bittner EA, Martyn JA, Sjoberg F. Burn management. In: Gropper MA, Eriksson LI, Fleisher LA, Cohen NH, Leslie K, Johnson-Akeju O, eds. *Miller's Anesthesia*. 10th ed. Elsevier; 2025:2746-2773.

Fink R. Diffusion anoxia. *Anesthesiology*. 1955;16:511-519.

Fink R, Carpenter SL, Holiday DA, et al. Diffusion anoxia during recovery from nitrous oxide-oxygen anesthesia. *Fed Proc*. 1954;13:354.

D.3. Why do patients often shiver in the recovery room on emergence from general anesthesia?

Postanesthetic shivering is commonly observed in the recovery room after emergence from inhalational general anesthesia. It is postulated that inhalation agents inhibit central hypothalamic thermoreceptors. Shivering is a thermoregulatory response to intraoperative heat loss, as it generates energy to maintain normothermia. Secondarily, tremors can be the result of anesthetic-induced disinhibition of descending spinal reflexes. Similar nonthermoregulatory tremors have been seen in females during labor after neuraxial anesthesia.

Bittner EA, Martyn JA, Sjoberg F. Burn management. In: Gropper MA, Eriksson LI, Fleisher LA, Cohen NH, Leslie K, Johnson-Akeju O, eds. *Miller's Anesthesia*. 10th ed. Elsevier; 2025:2746-2773.

D.4. Discuss the causes of oliguria in PACU.

Oliguria is arbitrarily defined as the production of less than 400 mL of urine in 24 hours. It is the functional manifestation of renal dysfunction, including *acute renal failure* (ARF). The syndrome of ARF may be classified into three groups:

- *Prerenal ARF (hypovolemic)*: A reduction of renal blood flow decreases both glomerular filtration rate (GFR) and overall urine output. There is no structural damage to the kidney. Prerenal azotemia is reversible with volume expansion. However, if untreated, it can progress to the ischemic form of acute tubular necrosis.
- *Renal ARF (acute tubular necrosis)*: Ischemia or nephrotoxic substances result in structural damage to the renal tubules.
- *Postrenal ARF (obstruction of urinary outflow)*: Obstruction occurs distal to the kidney, at the level of the ureter, bladder, or urethra. Pus, tubular debris, blood clots, nephrolithiasis, tumor burden, prostatic hypertrophy, or a nonfunctioning Foley catheter can cause mechanical cessation of urinary flow.

Determining the underlying cause of oliguria is essential, as management varies greatly. To identify the cause of oliguria, one must assess urinary sediment. The presence of renal tubular cells, renal tubular cell casts, and pigmented granular casts supports acute tubular necrosis. Normal urinary sediment is consistent with prerenal azotemia. CVP and PAOP provide insight into the state of hydration. Postrenal etiologies of ARF are supported by bladder ultrasonography (demonstrating an enlarged and distended bladder) or elevated pressure on bladder manometry (supporting intraabdominal hypertension).

Perazella MA, Coca SG, Kanbay M, et al. Diagnostic value of urine microscopy for differential diagnosis of acute kidney injury in hospitalized patients. *Clin J Am Soc Nephrol*. 2008;3:1615-1619.

57 Trauma

Rohan K. Panchamia, Jaideep K. Malhotra, and
Ralph L. Slepian

A 31-year-old male sustained multiple stab wounds to the left upper quadrant of the abdomen and to the left hemithorax. Vital signs were blood pressure, 85/60 mm Hg; heart rate (HR), 130 beats per minute; respiratory rate, 32 breaths per minute; and temperature, 34.5 °C (94.1 °F). His hematocrit was 27%. He was emergently brought to the operating room for exploratory laparotomy and possible thoracotomy.

A. Medical Disease and Differential Diagnosis

1. How is trauma classified?
2. What injuries are associated with thoracic trauma?
3. What injuries are associated with cardiac trauma?
4. What is the pathophysiology of acute pericardial tamponade?
5. What are the anesthetic implications of cardiac tamponade?
6. What is the definition of massive hemothorax? What are the signs and symptoms of hemothorax?
7. What are the indications for thoracotomy to treat hemothorax?
8. How are pneumothoraces categorized?
9. What is an occult pneumothorax?
10. If the patient has a widened mediastinum on the chest radiograph, what are your concerns?
11. What is focused abdominal sonography for trauma (FAST) examination?
12. Define shock.
13. What are the four types of shock?
14. What are the signs and symptoms of hypovolemic shock?
15. What is the pathophysiology of hypovolemic shock?
16. How is hemorrhage classified?
17. What is the initial treatment of hemorrhagic shock?
18. Would you choose crystalloid, colloid, or blood products to treat hemorrhagic shock?

B. Preoperative Evaluation and Preparation

1. What premedication would you order?
2. What preoperative testing would you order?

C. Intraoperative Management

1. How would you monitor this patient?
2. How would you induce general anesthesia?
3. What technique could you use if one-lung ventilation was indicated?
4. What agents would you choose to maintain anesthesia?
5. What neuromuscular blocking agent would you choose?
6. What can be done to decrease the incidence of accidental intraoperative awareness?
7. Five minutes after tracheal intubation, the peak airway pressure increased from 20 to 40 cm H_2O. What are the possible causes?
8. How would you make a diagnosis of tension pneumothorax?
9. What is the treatment of tension pneumothorax?
10. The patient's blood loss continued, and the hematocrit was 18%. What type of blood would you give if the type and crossmatch were not completed?
11. What are the complications associated with any blood transfusion?

12. What is considered a massive transfusion (MT)? What scoring systems can be used to predict the need for massive transfusion protocol (MTP) in patients with trauma?
13. What is acute coagulopathy of trauma (ACT)?
14. What are the complications associated with MT?
15. Can the shift of the oxygen-hemoglobin dissociation curve be quantified?
16. How is hypothermia defined? How can it be prevented and treated?
17. What are the adverse effects of hypothermia?
18. What are the guidelines for the ratio of plasma/platelet transfusion to packed red blood cells (pRBCs) in MT?
19. If a patient were a member of the Jehovah's Witness religious group, would you give a blood transfusion?
20. If a child is a Jehovah's Witness and has hemorrhagic shock, what would you do?
21. What concentrated factors and hemostatic agents are available for bleeding patients?
22. What is thromboelastometry? How can it guide transfusion?

D. Postoperative Management

1. What is acute respiratory distress syndrome (ARDS)? What is acute lung injury?
2. How is ARDS treated?
3. You are called to see this patient in the postanesthesia care unit (PACU) because of oliguria. How would you evaluate and treat this patient?
4. If this patient had a crush injury and low urine output, what other concerns might you have? What if the patient has dark or "tea-colored" urine?

A. Medical Disease and Differential Diagnosis

A.1. How is trauma classified?

Trauma is usually separated into penetrating and blunt trauma. Both can disrupt the vascular, visceral, musculoskeletal, and nervous systems.

A.2. What injuries are associated with thoracic trauma?

Penetrating injuries associated with thoracic trauma are typically associated with stab wounds and gunshot wounds. The latter causes far more damage because of the large amount of kinetic energy transferred to the thoracic cavity from the impact of the bullet. As a result, gunshot wounds to the thorax are diffuse and much more likely to be fatal compared to stab wounds.

Blunt injuries to the chest are far more common than penetrating injuries. The most common causes of blunt injuries are deceleration injuries (as a result of motor vehicle accidents) and crush injuries. These range from relatively minor injuries such as rib fractures to more severe injuries such as lung contusions, tracheobronchial tears, flail chest, pneumothorax, hemothorax, injuries to the great vessels, and traumatic rupture of the esophagus or diaphragm.

A.3. What injuries are associated with cardiac trauma?

Penetrating cardiac injuries often lead to immediate cardiovascular collapse, and patients rarely survive to reach the operating room. Injuries associated with penetrating cardiac trauma include pericardial tamponade, cardiac perforation, rupture of a chamber, and fistula formation.

Blunt cardiac injuries (BCI) include cardiac contusion (most common), pericardial rupture, rupture of a chamber, valvular tears, coronary artery injuries, and ventricular aneurysms. Screening for BCI includes an electrocardiogram (ECG) and troponin I level; echocardiography is reserved for those with new ECG changes, elevated troponin I levels, hypotension, and/or arrhythmias. At the very least, patients with abnormal cardiac studies should be admitted for monitoring.

Bellister SA, Dennis BM, Guillamondegui OD. Blunt and penetrating cardiac trauma. *Surg Clin North Am.* 2017;97:1065-1076.

Clancy K, Velopulos C, Bilaniuk J, et al. Screening for blunt cardiac injury: an Eastern Association for the Surgery of Trauma practice management guideline. *J Trauma.* 2012;73:S301-S306.

Howes BL, Shapiro ML. Thoracic trauma management. In: Barbeito A, Shaw AD, Grichnik K, eds. *Thoracic Anesthesia.* McGraw-Hill; 2012:379–402.

A.4. What is the pathophysiology of acute pericardial tamponade?

Acute pericardial tamponade represents a rapid increase in intrapericardial pressure exceeding intracardiac pressures, resulting in impaired venous return and diastolic filling. If pericardial pressure is high enough, cardiac chamber collapse can occur, leading to decreased cardiac output and systemic hypoperfusion, which can result in cardiopulmonary arrest. Physical exam findings associated with pericardial tamponade include Beck triad (hypotension, distended neck veins, and muffled heart sounds), tachycardia, and pulsus paradoxus (decrease in systolic blood pressure [SBP] >10 mm Hg during inspiration). Some of these signs can be easily missed in a hypovolemic trauma patient who could be in a low-pressure tamponade state with low central venous pressure. Diagnosis of cardiac tamponade can be aided with transthoracic echocardiography, demonstrating key findings including the presence of a pericardial effusion, dilated inferior vena cava (IVC), right-sided chamber collapse during diastole, exaggerated respirophasic transvalvular flow velocities (pulse wave pulsus paradoxus), respirophasic septal shift, and a swinging heart. The hemodynamic effects of pericardial effusion depend on the change in ventricular diastolic function in response to increased intracardiac pressure and not the size of the effusion per se. If a diagnosis of acute pericardial tamponade is made and the patient is unstable, immediate evacuation of the pericardium by pericardiocentesis or pericardial window is required (see Chapter 12: Cardiac Tamponade).

A.5. What are the anesthetic implications of cardiac tamponade?

The main anesthetic goal for patients with acute cardiac tamponade is to maintain intrinsic sympathetic tone. These patients are extremely dependent on their intrinsic sympathetic activity, so maintenance of HR (likely compensatory tachycardia) and preload are of utmost importance in the setting of limited diastolic filling and stroke volume. An arterial catheter and large-bore intravenous access are essential. Inotropes such as epinephrine should be readily available and can be given in small doses to avoid bradycardia and hypotension. Positive pressure ventilation can precipitate hemodynamic collapse, but if tracheal intubation is necessary, rapid-sequence induction with succinylcholine or awake intubation can be performed. Ketamine and etomidate are considered appropriate agents for sedation and induction of anesthesia. Anesthesia should be induced and the trachea intubated only after prepping and draping the patient for a pericardial window have been completed in the event the patient suddenly becomes hemodynamically unstable and requires immediate drainage of the effusion (see Chapter 12: Cardiac Tamponade).

Alerhand S, Carter JM. What echocardiographic findings suggest a pericardial effusion is causing tamponade? *Am J Emerg Med.* 2019;37:321-326.

Appleton C, Gillam L, Koulogiannis K. Cardiac tamponade. *Cardiol Clin.* 2017;35:525-537.

Argulian E, Messerli F. Misconceptions and facts about pericardial effusion and tamponade. *Am J Med.* 2013;126:858-861.

A.6. What is the definition of massive hemothorax? What are the signs and symptoms of hemothorax?

A massive hemothorax is defined as a rapid accumulation of greater than 11.5 L of blood in the thoracic cavity. It is usually caused by rib fractures (intercostal or internal mammary vessel bleeding), lung injury, great vessel injury, cardiac injury, or diaphragmatic injury. The signs and symptoms of hemothorax include diminished breath sounds on the affected side, hypoxemia, hypotension, mediastinal shift, and respiratory distress.

A.7. What are the indications for thoracotomy to treat hemothorax?

Hemothorax, if severe enough, can lead to hemorrhagic shock. Therefore, timely diagnosis and treatment are paramount. After a chest tube is placed, if drainage of blood is greater than 1.5 L or one-third of blood volume, or if drainage is greater than 200 mL/h for over 2 to 4 hours, a thoracotomy is indicated. Alternatively, if the patient is older than 60 years and drainage is greater than 100 mL/h for over 4 hours, a thoracotomy is also indicated. If the patient does not meet these criteria but is still hemodynamically unstable or if ventilation is difficult, emergent surgery should be performed.

A.8. How are pneumothoraces categorized?

Pneumothoraces are categorized as simple, open, or tension pneumothorax. The principal physiologic changes are hypoxemia due to reduced vital capacity, alveolar hypoventilation, and impaired venous return secondary to increased intrathoracic pressure.

Simple pneumothorax can result from both blunt and penetrating chest trauma. It is defined as the presence of air in the pleural space without an open chest wound or evidence of tension pneumothorax.

Diagnosis can be made radiographically, by chest radiography or computed tomography, although in many trauma situations, the patient's condition precludes obtaining conventional imaging. In such cases, diagnosis can be made by lung ultrasound. The lack of pleural sliding, lung pulse, and vertical artifacts over the anterior chest wall, coupled with the presence of a lung point, are highly sensitive and specific findings for pneumothorax. Recent studies have demonstrated that using lung ultrasound can be a faster and more sensitive test than a supine anterior-posterior chest radiography. Definitive treatment is the placement of a chest tube or pleural pigtail if the patient is experiencing cardiopulmonary instability, and/or if the pneumothorax is sizable, that is greater than 10% of the pleural cavity. Of note, pigtail catheters have been shown to be equally as effective as chest tubes with decreased complications.

Open pneumothorax is the result of an open wound in the thoracic cavity that favors constant entrainment of air through the wound. Treatment entails placing an occlusive dressing on three sides over the wound, to create a "flutter valve" and allow egress of air but not entrainment of air, followed by chest tube placement.

Tension pneumothorax is the rapid buildup of air within the pleural space that cannot escape, causing an acute rise in airway pressures with resulting mediastinal shift and obstructive shock. Management is immediate decompression of the thoracic cavity by needle thoracentesis or finger thoracostomy followed by chest tube insertion.

Capan LM, Sutin KM, Miller S. Thoracic trauma. In: Reed AP, Yudkowitz FS, eds. *Clinical Cases in Anesthesia*. 4th ed. Elsevier Saunders; 2014:395–410.

Chang SH, Kang YN, Chiu HY, et al. A systematic review and meta-analysis comparing pigtail catheter and chest tube as the initial treatment for pneumothorax. *Chest*. 2018;153:1201-1212.

Kruisselbrink R, Chan V, Cibinel GA, et al. I-AIM (Indication, acquisition, interpretation, medical decision-making) framework for point of care lung ultrasound. *Anesthesiology*. 2017;127:568-582.

Mowery NT, Gunter OL, Collier BR, et al. Practice management guidelines for management of hemothorax and occult pneumothorax. *J Trauma*. 2011;70:510-518.

Wilkerson RG, Stone MB. Sensitivity of bedside ultrasound and supine anteroposterior chest for the identification of pneumothorax after blunt trauma. *Acad Emerg Med*. 2010;17:11-17.

A.9. What is an occult pneumothorax?

An occult pneumothorax is seen on CT but was not identified previously on chest radiography, comprising as many as 50% of all pneumothoraces, with an overall incidence of 5% in patients with trauma. In many cases, this type of pneumothorax is managed conservatively with serial imaging and resolves over time, without requiring the placement of a chest tube. However, decompression should be considered if the patient is symptomatic, hemodynamically unstable, or has a pneumothorax greater than 10% in size. Another indication for decompression, although controversial, is the delivery of positive pressure ventilation. Whether these patients should have a chest tube or pigtail placed preemptively is up for debate; for now, the decision should be made on a case-by-case basis.

Ball CG, Kirkpatrick AW, Feliciano DV. The occult pneumothorax: what have we learned? *Can J Surg*. 2009;52:E173-E179.

Ouellet JF, Trottier V, Kmet L, et al. The OPTICC trial: a multi-institutional study of occult pneumothoraces in critical care. *Am J Surg*. 2009;197:581-586.

A.10. If the patient has a widened mediastinum on the chest radiograph, what are your concerns?

A chest radiograph revealing a widened mediastinum can indicate the presence of a thoracic aortic injury; other radiographic features suggestive of aortic injury include abnormal mediastinal contour, hemothorax, pleural cap, and tracheal deviation. A contrast-enhanced CT of the chest is indicated for further evaluation.

These injuries are often life threatening, necessitating immediate identification and intervention. Blunt aortic injury is associated with high-speed deceleration and is the second leading cause of death in patients with trauma, accounting for 16% of all trauma-related deaths. Open surgical repair requires a double-lumen tube (DLT), one-lung ventilation, and clamping of the proximal aorta while taking measures to protect the spinal cord. In patients with coexisting conditions, such as increased intracranial pressure, profound bleeding, or hypoxemia, this procedure is extremely high risk and might be contraindicated. The mainstay of treatment of aortic transection includes control of blood pressure and ventricular ejection force (dP/dt) with β-blocker infusions and/or mixed β-blocker/α-antagonist medications, followed by endovascular repair. At high-volume centers, endovascular repair is associated with a higher survival benefit and decreased incidence of complications, especially paraplegia, compared to open surgical repair.

Demetriades D, Velmahos GC, Scalea TM, et al. Operative repair or endovascular stent graft in blunt traumatic thoracic aortic injuries: results of an American Association for the Surgery of Trauma multicenter study. *J Trauma.* 2008;64:561-571.

Fox N, Schwartz D, Salazar JH, et al. Evaluation and management of blunt traumatic aortic injury: a practice management guideline from the Eastern Association for the Surgery of Trauma. *J Trauma Nurs.* 2015;22:99-110.

Neschis DG, Scalea TM, Flinn WR, et al. Blunt aortic injury. *N Engl J Med.* 2008;359:1708-1716.

A.11. What is focused abdominal sonography for trauma (FAST) examination?

The FAST exam is a rapid ultrasonography examination that is routinely performed in the setting of blunt or penetrating torso trauma. It is designed to evaluate for free fluid (blood until proven otherwise) in the peritoneum, pleural space, and around the heart. Four areas are interrogated with ultrasound: the subxiphoid, right upper quadrant, left upper quadrant, and pelvis/suprapubic areas. The most dependent space (most likely to collect fluid) in supine adult patients is the hepatorenal space (Morison pouch) which is therefore usually the first space to be assessed; however, the order of the FAST exam can be changed depending on the mechanism of injury.

A downside to the FAST exam is the fact that usually 200 to 250 mL of fluid needs to accumulate before it can be visualized sonographically. Furthermore, it cannot evaluate the retroperitoneum and misses solid organ injuries. The utility of FAST resides in the bedside examination of the hemodynamically unstable patient with trauma, determining operative management versus considering other potential sources of shock. It has largely replaced deep peritoneal lavage as the initial screening tool for intra-abdominal injury. An extended version of the FAST exam (E-FAST) incorporates the thoracic window to allow detection of pneumothorax as a potential cause of hemodynamic instability.

Austin S, Haase D, Hamera J. Advances in trauma ultrasound. *Emerg Med Clin North Am.* 2023;41:131-142.

Hoff WS, Holevar M, Nagy KK, et al. Practice management guidelines for the evaluation of blunt abdominal trauma: the East Practice Management Guidelines Work Group. *J Trauma.* 2002;53:602-615.

Richards JR, McGahan JP. Focused assessment with sonography in trauma (FAST) in 2017: what radiologist can learn. *Radiology.* 2017;283:30-48.

Rozycki GS, Root HD. The diagnosis of intraabdominal visceral injury. *J Trauma.* 2010;68:1019-1023.

A.12. Define shock.

Shock is defined as circulatory dysfunction or failure leading to inadequate organ perfusion and tissue oxygenation. End-organ hypoperfusion is the final common denominator in all forms of shock.

A.13. What are the four types of shock?

Shock is classified according to its cause:

- *Hypovolemic (hemorrhagic) shock*: characterized by a loss of circulatory blood and plasma volumes
- *Cardiogenic shock*: characterized by an inability of the myocardium to pump blood
- *Distributive (neurogenic, septic) shock*: characterized by reduced systemic vascular resistance
- *Obstructive*: characterized by impairment in cardiac function due to direct cardiac compression or decreased venous return

Reynolds BR, Watson GA. Resuscitation from hemorrhagic shock. In: Tisherman SA, Forsythe RM, eds. *Trauma Intensive Care.* Oxford University Press; 2013:63–72.

Smith SG, Schreiber MA. Shock, electrolytes, and fluid. In: Townsend CM Jr, Beauchamp RD, Evers BM, Mattox KL, eds. *Sabiston Textbook of Surgery: The Biological Basis of Modern Surgical Practice.* 21st ed. Elsevier; 2021:44–94.

A.14. What are the signs and symptoms of hypovolemic shock?

Tachycardia, hypotension, decreased capillary refill, reduced pulse pressure, pallor, cool extremities, low end-tidal CO_2, agitation, and loss of consciousness are manifestations of life-threatening hypovolemic shock. With the exhaustion of the compensatory mechanism, hypotension tends to be a late finding; however, its absence does not rule out shock.

A.15. What is the pathophysiology of hypovolemic shock?

Cardiovascular Derangements

Several hemodynamic and neurohormonal responses occur in the setting of hypovolemic shock. Initially, a sympathoexcitatory response to hemorrhagic shock predominates. An acute decrease in circulating blood volume activates arterial baroreceptors within the aortic arch and carotid sinus, inducing reflex tachycardia and peripheral vasoconstriction. Stimulation of the sympathetic nervous system leads to catecholamine release from the adrenal gland; α-adrenergic agonism is responsible for peripheral vasoconstriction, shunting blood away from metabolically active organs to preserve flow to the coronary and cerebral circulations. Vasopressin and the renin-angiotensin-aldosterone system contribute to renal water retention, sodium and chloride resorption, and peripheral vasoconstriction. If hemorrhage progresses, a sympathoinhibitory phase occurs, characterized by activation of cardiac C-fiber afferents, resulting in bradycardia and vasodilation.

Various immunologic mediators, such as tissue necrosis factor-α and nitric oxide, are released in response to tissue injury. These proinflammatory mediators can cause myocardial depression, inappropriate vasodilatation, and end-organ dysfunction. Administration of vasopressors, such as norepinephrine and arginine vasopressin, to decrease systemic venous compliance, increase mean systemic filling pressures, and ultimately improve flow to end-organs, has been associated with mixed outcomes.

Acid-Base Disturbances

Metabolic acidosis is almost always seen in association with a shock state. As a result of tissue hypoperfusion, oxygen delivery to vital organs is reduced, resulting in tissue hypoxia and oxygen debt. At the cellular level, there is a change from aerobic to anaerobic metabolism. This switch leads to the production of anaerobic metabolites, such as lactic acid. Sequelae include hypotension, decreased myocardial contractility, arrhythmias, encephalopathy, and worsening end-organ function.

A.16. How is hemorrhage classified?

Classification of hemorrhage based on blood loss is as follows:

Class I: blood loss of up to 15% of blood volume—normal pulse and blood pressure

Class II: blood loss of up to 30% of blood volume—tachycardia, decreased urine output, and mild anxiety

Class III: blood loss of up to 40% of blood volume—significant tachycardia and hypotension with narrow pulse pressure; oliguria; development of a base deficit; and declining Glasgow Coma Scale score

Class IV: blood loss of more than 40% of blood volume—profound tachycardia and hypotension; delayed capillary refill; tachypnea; anuria; worsening base deficit; and confusion or lethargy

Galvagno SM Jr, Nahmias JT, Young DA. Advanced Trauma Life support update 2019: management and applications for adults and special populations. *Anesthesiol Clin*. 2019;37:13-32.

A.17. What is the initial treatment of hemorrhagic shock?

The initial approach to resuscitation of traumatic hemorrhagic shock entails (1) restoring intravascular volume with a high ratio of blood products to maintain oxygen delivery and tissue perfusion, (2) treating the coagulopathy, and (3) managing complications related to shock and MT, including metabolic acidosis and hypothermia. For more than a decade, trauma centers have adapted the practice of initial resuscitation with hemostatic components, such as plasma and platelets. This strategy for treating massive hemorrhage was pioneered from experience and knowledge gained during combat in Afghanistan and Iraq; it involves limiting the total volume of crystalloid administered and replacing intravascular volume with pRBCs and plasma in a ratio approaching 1:1. The overall goal is to provide fluids with oxygen-carrying capacity and hemostatic capabilities while avoiding the acute coagulopathy associated with major trauma and blood loss, which has been shown to increase mortality rates. Permissive hypotension is a resuscitation strategy at some trauma centers to minimize further bleeding at the site of injury. The goal is to not "pop the clot" by tolerating a low mean arterial pressure. Further studies are needed to validate the clinical benefits of this approach.

Leech C, Turner J. Shock in Trauma. *Emerg Med Clin North Am*. 2023;41:1-17.

Puskarich MA, Jones AE. Shock. In: Walls RM, Hockberger RS, Gausche-Hill M, Erickson TB, Wilcox SR, eds. *Rosen's Emergency Medicine: Concepts and Clinical Practice*. 10th ed. Elsevier; 2022:34–41.e1.

Reynolds BR, Watson GA. Resuscitation from hemorrhagic shock. In: Tisherman SA, Forsythe RM, eds. *Trauma Intensive Care*. Oxford University Press; 2013:63–72.

Richards JE, Harris T, Dünser MW, et al. Vasopressors in trauma: a never event? *Anesth Analg*. 2021;133:68-79.

Smith SG, Schreiber MA. Shock, electrolytes, and fluid. In: Townsend CM Jr, Beauchamp RD, Evers BM, Mattox KL, eds. *Sabiston Textbook of Surgery: The Biological Basis of Modern Surgical Practice*. 21st ed. Elsevier; 2021:44–94.

A.18. Would you choose crystalloid, colloid, or blood products to treat hemorrhagic shock?

Isotonic crystalloid solutions can sustain hemodynamic function and deliver adequate oxygenation in healthy patients who have lost as much as 30% of their total blood volume. Still, controversy remains over the use of crystalloid or colloid therapy for the initial therapy of hypovolemic shock.

Proponents of crystalloid therapy argue that both intravascular and interstitial fluid losses occur in hypovolemic shock and that these can be readily replaced with crystalloids. Another benefit of crystalloids is the decrease in blood viscosity that might enhance perfusion. A particular advantage to lactated Ringer solution is that lactate is metabolized to bicarbonate, which can help buffer the acidosis. Finally, the cost of crystalloid is much less than that of colloid. Because crystalloid leaves the intravascular space and enters the interstitial space, large quantities are needed, and some feel that these quantities lead to both pulmonary and peripheral edema, although studies have not confirmed this.

Proponents of colloid therapy argue that much less volume is needed to counteract hypovolemic shock and that early colloid therapy can prevent the complications associated with large-volume crystalloid resuscitation such as dilutional coagulopathy, hyperchloremic acidosis, and edema. Colloids maintain oncotic pressure and hold fluids in the intravascular space, which can possibly prevent pulmonary edema. If leaky alveolar-capillary membranes are seen within the lung, colloids might worsen pulmonary edema. Despite the potential benefits of colloid administration, there is a lack of quality evidence showing a decreased mortality among patients who receive colloid for hypovolemic shock.

The best resuscitative fluid to treat hemorrhagic shock is whole blood. It provides a balanced resuscitation, reversing shock and coagulopathy, by containing all components of blood: hematocrit of 38% to 50%, plasma clotting factors, fibrinogen, and 150 to 400 $10^3/\mu L$ platelets. A major advantage whole blood possesses over crystalloid and colloid is that it does not promote dilutional coagulopathy. From a logistical standpoint, it requires limited processing. In terms of its safety profile, administration of uncrossmatched, cold-stored, low-titer (low levels of anti-A and anti-B immunoglobulins M), type O whole blood is well tolerated, without causing hemolysis or transfusion reactions.

Annane D, Siami S, Jaber S, et al. Effects of fluid resuscitation with colloids vs crystalloids on mortality in critically Ill patients presenting with hypovolemic shock: the CRISTAL randomized trial. *JAMA.* 2013;310:1809-1817.

Choi PT, Yip G, Quinonez LG, et al. Crystalloids vs. colloids in fluid resuscitation: a systematic review. *Crit Care Med.* 1999;27:200-210.

Griffee MJ, Deloughery TG, Thorborg PA. Coagulation management in massive bleeding. *Curr Opin Anaesthesiol.* 2010;23:263-268.

Orlinsky M, Shoemaker W, Reis ED, et al. Current controversies in shock and resuscitation. *Surg Clin North Am.* 2001;81:1217-1262.

Seheult JN, Bahr M, Anto V, et al. Safety profile of uncrossmatched, cold-stored, low-titer, group O+ whole blood in civilian trauma patients. *Transfusion.* 2018;58:2280-2288.

Sihler KC, Napolitano LM. Complications of massive transfusion. *Chest.* 2010;137:209-220.

B. Preoperative Evaluation and Preparation

B.1. What premedication would you order?

None. This is a critically ill patient who is coming to the operating room for emergency surgery. Opioids and sedatives are contraindicated because they could worsen an already tenuous hemodynamic state.

B.2. What preoperative testing would you order?

Because of the emergent nature of the trauma setting, preoperative tests and imaging studies are frequently limited. If the patient is hemodynamically unstable, preoperative evaluation is aborted and the patient is taken directly to the operating room.

If the patient is stable, a portable chest radiograph, arterial blood gas analysis, complete blood count, and FAST can be done in a relatively short period in the resuscitation bay before surgery. Often, these tests are obtained while the patient is being prepared for emergency surgery. This information is then combined with other primary survey adjuncts, such as oxygen saturation and ECG, to evaluate the patient and formulate an appropriate management strategy. Although it is usually not possible to clinically clear the cervical spine before surgery, it is important to know the results of any radiologic studies that have been done (eg, in order to rule out an unstable cervical spine fracture) and to adjust the anesthetic plan accordingly.

C. Intraoperative Management

C.1. How would you monitor this patient?

Routine noninvasive monitoring would include ECG, blood pressure cuff, pulse oximetry, end-tidal carbon dioxide, esophageal stethoscope, temperature probe, and Foley catheter.

Invasive monitors include an arterial catheter and a central venous catheter. An arterial catheter is useful for serial blood sampling and continuous arterial blood pressure monitoring. There is a low threshold to place a central venous line to assist with resuscitation efforts. A pulmonary artery catheter is indicated if the patient has a history of heart failure, myocardial dysfunction, mixed shock picture, and/or poor response to resuscitation.

C.2. How would you induce general anesthesia?

In the deteriorating trauma patient who is exsanguinating but spontaneously ventilating and able to protect their airway, it is reasonable to perform basic airway management and delay intubation until resuscitation efforts, such as blood product administration, have been initiated. The rationale behind this approach is to preserve the remaining physiologic reserve and compensatory mechanisms while avoiding further decompensation from induction of anesthesia, paralysis, and positive pressure ventilation until definitive surgical care can be provided in the operating room. Once in the operating room, the best way to protect the patient's airway is to perform a rapid-sequence induction while maintaining inline cervical spine immobilization if the patient is in a cervical collar. For the patient with a suspected difficult airway, one could perform awake, topicalized tracheal intubation; however, awake intubation can be difficult because patients can be confused, uncooperative, and even combative.

If tolerated, the patient should be preoxygenated for 3 to 5 minutes. Next, ketamine 0.5 to 2 mg/kg, depending on the patient's physiology, can be given followed by succinylcholine 1.5 mg/kg. Ketamine was chosen in this case because of its hemodynamically favorable profile. Etomidate (0.15-0.2 mg/kg) would be another appropriate choice for an induction agent.

If the patient is comatose, in severe shock, or in full arrest on admission to the resuscitation room, no drugs other than oxygen and possibly a neuromuscular blocking agent are required until the blood pressure and HR sufficiently rebound so that anesthetics can be titrated.

Brown CVR, Inaba K, Shatz DV, et al. Western trauma association critical decisions in trauma: airway management in adult trauma patients. *Trauma Surg Acute Care Open*. 2020;5:e000539.

C.3. What technique could you use if one-lung ventilation was indicated?

If the patient does not already have a secure airway, the airway should be secured as mentioned previously. One-lung ventilation is indicated in this situation if the patient is bleeding from one lung and protection of the other lung is required or to improve surgical exposure (lower priority). Once the airway is secured, there are several ways to obtain one-lung ventilation. The easiest and safest technique would be to place a bronchial blocker (BB) through the endotracheal tube and direct it to the affected lung with fiberoptic bronchoscopy before inflating the distal cuff. A limitation to the use of a BB is the inability to adequately suction the isolated lung.

Another method of obtaining one-lung ventilation would be to change the endotracheal tube to a DLT using a Cook exchange catheter. The major disadvantages of DLT placement are losing a previously secured airway and aspiration occurring while attempting to change the tube; improper DLT size selection; and iatrogenic tracheobronchial injury during insertion.

Kanellakos GW, Slinger P. Intraoperative one-lung ventilation for trauma anesthesia. In: Smith CE, ed. *Trauma Anesthesia*. 2nd ed. Cambridge University Press; 2015:555-568.

C.4. What agents would you choose to maintain anesthesia?

As the patient stabilizes and the hemodynamics improve, other anesthetic agents can be carefully titrated to prevent hypotension, as follows:

- Sedatives or amnestics should be added to the anesthetic as soon as tolerated. Start with small doses and check the response between doses.
- Opioids should be titrated to control the hemodynamic response to surgery.

- Nitrous oxide is best avoided since it can accumulate in closed airspaces and expand an occult pneumothorax which is very likely in this patient.
- Inhalational anesthetics can be used in low concentrations if the patient's hemodynamics are not compromised.

C.5. What neuromuscular blocking agent would you choose?

Vecuronium, rocuronium, and cisatracurium are acceptable agents that are free of cardiovascular side effects and have an intermediate duration of action. Pancuronium is a long-acting agent that can be deleterious due to its vagolytic properties.

C.6. What can be done to decrease the incidence of accidental intraoperative awareness?

The incidence of accidental awareness under general anesthesia is commonly cited as approximately 0.2% which is probably an overestimation. According to other sources, the incidence of traumatic intraoperative recall associated with pain is less than 0.03%. The American Society of Anesthesiologists Closed Claims database states that claims associated with recall during anesthesia constitute 1.5% of claims. An increased relative risk for recall is seen in certain types of surgery, including cardiac surgery, cesarean delivery, and trauma surgery; this most likely represents intentional light anesthesia during varying levels of surgical stimulation. The Anesthesia Patient Safety Foundation recommends maintaining an inhaled anesthetic concentration of 0.7 MAC whenever a neuromuscular blocking agent is given to avoid intraoperative awareness, and if this is not possible, to use a processed electroencephalogram (EEG) monitor such as bispectral index to help monitor and assure adequate depth of anesthesia.

Bispectral index monitoring can be useful, but the application of these monitors during trauma resuscitation might not be easily accomplished. Patients with a bispectral index value of 50 were able to respond to verbal commands less than 10% of the time.

APSF Committee on Technology. The APSF Committee on Technology. APSF endorsed statement on revising recommendations for patient monitoring during anesthesia. *APSF Newsl.* 2022;37:7-8.

Johansen JW. Update on bispectral index monitoring. *Best Pract Res Clin Anaesthesiol.* 2006;20:81-99.

Rampil IJ. Monitoring depth of anesthesia. *Curr Opin Anaesthesiol.* 2001;14:649-653.

C.7. Five minutes after tracheal intubation, the peak airway pressure increased from 20 to 40 cm H_2O. What are the possible causes?

Possible causes of increased peak airway pressure in this patient are:

- Tension pneumothorax.
- Bronchospasm.
- Endobronchial intubation.
- Pulmonary edema.
- Secretions.
- Kink in the anesthesia circuit or endotracheal tube.

Manning HL. Peak airway pressure: why the fuss? *Chest.* 1994;105:242-247.

Woods BD, Sladen RN. Perioperative considerations for the patient with asthma and bronchospasm. *Br J Anaesth.* 2009;103:i57-i65.

C.8. How would you make a diagnosis of tension pneumothorax?

Clinical signs concerning tension pneumothorax include tachycardia, hypotension, and tachypnea; absence of breath sounds on the affected side; neck vein distension; asymmetric chest movement; and tracheal deviation. Any patient who deteriorates under anesthesia while being mechanically ventilated and has wounds to the upper abdomen, lower neck, or ribs should be assumed to have a tension pneumothorax until proven otherwise.

C.9. What is the treatment of tension pneumothorax?

Immediate decompression of the chest is mandatory for tension pneumothorax; otherwise, the patient's hemodynamics will deteriorate. The diagnosis is made clinically and not by a chest radiograph. A long (at least 5 cm) 16- or 18-gauge angiocath can be placed into pleural space at the fifth intercostal space along the midaxillary plane. After air escapes confirming the diagnosis and the tension pneumothorax is converted to an open pneumothorax, a chest tube should be placed.

American College of Surgeons. *Advanced Trauma Life Support*. 10th ed. American College of Surgeons; 2018:65-67.

C.10. The patient's blood loss continued, and the hematocrit was 18%. What type of blood would you give if the type and crossmatch were not completed?

This patient needs immediate blood transfusion. Type O uncrossmatched red blood cells can be given until type-specific blood is available; in this case, type O Rh-positive red blood cells would be appropriate if there is no prior history of a blood transfusion reaction. Type O Rh-negative blood is typically reserved for populations, for example, females of childbearing age, at a higher risk of developing alloimmunization. In the setting of massive hemorrhage protocol, switching over to type-specific blood should happen as soon as possible, regardless of the number of group O units administered.

Trudeau JD, Dawe P, Shih AW. Chapter 11: Massive hemorrhage and emergency transfusion. In: Clarke G, Chargé S, eds. *Clinical Guide to Transfusion* [Internet]. Canadian Blood Services; 2021. Accessed April 15, 2023. professionaleducation.blood.ca

C.11. What are the complications associated with any blood transfusion?

Complications associated with blood transfusion are:

Transfusion Reactions

- Transfusion-related acute lung injury (TRALI) is characterized by the onset of hypoxemia and bilateral pulmonary edema within 6 hours of a transfusion, in the absence of other causes such as heart failure. It is attributed to donor plasma human leukocyte antigen class I and II antibodies activating recipient neutrophils, leading to a lung immune response. In 2006, US blood collection agencies instituted a male-only plasma donor policy because multiparous females are more likely to carry the offending antibodies. The TRALI rate decreased to about one-third of its previous level. TRALI is now the leading cause of transfusion-related mortality. Treatment of this noncardiogenic pulmonary edema is aggressive supportive care.
- Transfusion-associated circulatory overload (TACO) occurs in 1% to 6% of transfused patients and can cause pulmonary edema secondary to fluid overload. Large amounts of plasma transfused during MT or coagulopathy correction increase the likelihood of TACO.
- Transfusion-related immunomodulation (TRIM) is a risk with allogeneic red blood cell transfusion. Although incompletely understood, there is a decrease in immunity with an increased incidence of nosocomial infection, postoperative infection, and cancer recurrence.
- Febrile reactions occur in approximately 1% of all transfusions. In an awake patient, this is usually no more than an annoyance that requires antipyretics and decreasing the infusion rate. Leukoreduction decreases the likelihood of a febrile reaction.
- Allergic (nonanaphylactic/nonanaphylactoid) nonhemolytic reactions to properly crossmatched blood manifest as an increase in temperature, pruritus, and urticaria. This can be difficult to diagnose in the anesthetized patient. Treatment consists of the administration of antihistamines and discontinuation of the transfusion.
- Hemolytic reactions occur when incompatible blood is administered. The risk of an ABO-incompatible transfusion is 1:33,500 for red blood cell transfusion. Mortality remains high at approximately 40%. Caused by activation of the complement system, hemolytic reactions can be life threatening. In the awake patient, fever, chills, dyspnea, and substernal and lumbar pain are seen in addition to hypotension. Under general anesthesia, the only sign that is not masked is hypotension. Free hemoglobin detected in the plasma or urine is indicative of a transfusion reaction. Substances released by the hemolyzed cells can lead to disseminated intravascular coagulation (DIC) and acute renal failure (ARF). Treatment consists of immediate discontinuation of the transfusion. Hypotension should be treated with hydration, vasopressors, and inotropic agents if needed. Urinary output must be maintained by adequate hydration. Although its value is uncertain, sodium bicarbonate has been used to alkalinize the urine to improve the solubility of the hemoglobin degradation products.
- Other reactions include posttransfusion purpura, microchimerism, and graft-versus-host disease.

Transmission of Disease

- Human immunodeficiency virus (HIV), hepatitis B virus, hepatitis C virus, and cytomegalovirus can all be transmitted by transfusion of blood products. Because the risk of disease transmission increases with each unit of blood or its components given, they must be carefully scrutinized before being administered. Currently, the incidence of posttransfusion HIV 1 and 2 infection is 1:1,476,000 per transfused unit of blood, similar to the risk of hepatitis C transmission, which is 1:1,149,000 per unit transfused. In comparison, the risk of hepatitis B transmission is higher, approximately 1 per 350,000 units. Nevertheless, cytomegalovirus remains the most common viral agent transmitted by transfusion; it produces clinically important infections only in patients with immunosuppression. Laboratory testing done to detect these viruses includes enzyme immunoassays and nucleic acid testing.
- Malaria, syphilis, Lyme disease, Chagas disease, West Nile virus, Creutzfeldt-Jakob disease, and other diseases can also be transmitted through transfusion of blood.
- Bacterial infection occurs in 1:75,000 transfusions. As new nonhemoglobin solutions appear on the market, less blood will be transfused and disease transmission will diminish.

Microembolization

Microembolization can occur from the transfusion of blood or its components. Stored blood forms microaggregates that are too small to be removed by standard 170-µm blood filters. Smaller filters have been developed to remove these particles. When using blood filters in the 20- to 40-µm range, the rate of transfusion is dramatically decreased because of the increased resistance of the filters. Some early reports suggested that these microaggregates lead to pulmonary dysfunction, but this has never been proven.

Blumberg N, Refaai MA, Heal JM. Transfusion-induced immunomodulation. In: Murphy MF, Roberts DJ, Yazer MH, Dunbar NM, eds. *Practical Transfusion Medicine*. 6th ed. Wiley-Blackwell; 2022:153–167.

Chestnut DH, Wong CA, Tsen LC, et al, eds. *Chestnut's Obstetric Anesthesia: Principles and Practice*. 6th ed. Elsevier; 2020:920-921, 1291.

Steurer MP, Sikorski RA, Richards JE, Galvagno SM. Anesthesia for trauma. In: Gropper MA, Cohen NH, Eriksson LI, Fleisher LA, Johnson-Akeju S, Leslie K, eds. *Miller's Anesthesia*. 10th ed. Elsevier; 2024:2000–2043.

Virk MS, Pandey S, Andrews J. Transfusion medicine. In: Means RT, Arber DA, Glader BE, et al, eds. *Wintrobe's Clinical Hematology*. 15th ed. Wolters Kluwer; 2024:558-598.

C.12. What is considered a massive transfusion (MT)? What scoring systems can be used to predict the need for massive transfusion protocol (MTP) in patients with trauma?

MT refers to a situation where a patient receives 5 or more units of pRBCs in 4 hours or 10 or more units of pRBCs in 24 hours. Nevertheless, this definition is considered arbitrary without clear-cut clinical implications; furthermore, it fails to identify those at an increased risk for hemorrhagic death. In contrast, the critical administration threshold (CAT) definition of 3 or more units in 1 hour has a stronger association with mortality compared to MT; it can serve as an activation trigger for initiating an MTP, a system created to facilitate rapid administration of large-volume transfusions to patients in hemorrhagic shock.

The ABC score is a validated, nonlaboratory scoring system, designed to identify patients who will require MTP. It looks at four parameters: (1) penetrating mechanism, (2) positive FAST, (3) arrival SBP less than or equal to 90 mm Hg, and (4) arrival HR greater than or equal to 120. A score of 2 (positive cutoff) or greater was 75% sensitive and 86% specific for predicting MT. Shock index (SI) is another scoring system; it is calculated as initial HR divided by initial SBP. An SI greater than or equal to 0.8 to 1 is often used as the cutoff to predict the need for MTP. Schroll et al found that SI was a more sensitive predictor of MTP and required less skill to calculate.

Nunez TC, Voskresensky IV, Dossett LA, et al. Early prediction of massive transfusion in trauma: simple as ABC (assessment of blood consumption)? *J Trauma*. 2009;66:346-352.

Savage SA, Zarzaur BL, Croce MA, et al. Redefining massive transfusion when every second counts. *J Trauma Acute Care Surg*. 2013;74:396-402.

Schroll R, Swift D, Tatum D, et al. Accuracy of shock index versus ABC score to predict need for massive transfusion in trauma patients. *Injury*. 2018;49:15-19.

C.13. What is acute coagulopathy of trauma (ACT)?

An ACT is characterized by a disrupted equilibrium between procoagulant, anticoagulant, and fibrinolytic systems, triggered by the upregulation and release of endogenous mediators. Early on, the ACT phenotype is one of a hypercoagulable state that is often exacerbated by acidosis, hypothermia, and dilution of procoagulants with aggressive crystalloid/colloid resuscitation. With ongoing tissue injury and shock, DIC and fibrinolysis can occur; therefore, prompt treatment of hypoperfusion is essential for survival.

Brohi K, Singh J, Heron M, et al. Acute traumatic coagulopathy. *J Trauma*. 2003;54:1127-1130.

Moore EE, Moore HB, Kornblith LZ, et al. Trauma-induced coagulopathy. *Nat Rev Dis Primers*. 2021;7:30.

C.14. What are the complications associated with MT?

In addition to coagulopathy, other complications of MT include hypothermia, hypocalcemia, hyperkalemia, hypokalemia, acid-base imbalance, and impaired hemoglobin function.

- Hypothermia is a consequence of exposure, impaired thermoregulation, and the rapid transfusion of cold, banked blood. It is recommended that the room temperature be increased, and all fluids and blood pass through fluid warmers, in order to prevent hypothermia.
- Hypocalcemia can result from blood loss and inadequate citrate metabolism. Sodium citrate is present in stored blood to bind calcium and prevent clotting. With a high rate of transfusion, ionized calcium can be chelated by citrate, resulting in decreased levels of circulating free calcium. Consequences of hypocalcemia include bradycardia and ST segment prolongation, hypotension due to decreased myocardial contractility, and worsening coagulopathy from impaired coagulation (calcium is clotting factor IV). It is recommended to administer 1 to 2 gm of IV calcium chloride with every round of MTP.
- Hyperkalemia can occur in the massively transfused patient. Potassium concentrations in pRBCs can range from 7 to 77 mEq/L, in part due to inactivation of the red blood cell membrane Na, K-ATPase pump. Although the likelihood of life-threatening sequelae from hyperkalemia is low during MTP, in the shock state with hypoperfusion and acidemia, dangerous manifestations of hyperkalemia, such as cardiac arrhythmias, become more evident.
- Hypokalemia is also a possibility after MTP. Citrate is metabolized to bicarbonate by the liver, inducing a metabolic alkalosis that can lead to hypokalemia. Furthermore, transfused red blood cells take up potassium, with reactivation of the membrane Na, K-ATPase pump, which could potentiate hypokalemia.
- Acid-base imbalance is a problem during MTP. Donor blood pH has a low of 6.8 with prolonged storage. However, alkalosis rather than acidosis is more commonly seen during MTP due to the metabolism of citrate to bicarbonate. The presence of acidosis can usually be attributed to shock, which is often reversible with restoration of normal perfusion. In general, supplemental bicarbonate should not be given based on an arbitrary number of units transfused. Nevertheless, if metabolic acidosis persists, sodium bicarbonate might be warranted, especially in the setting of renal failure and severe muscle damage.
- Impaired hemoglobin function is possible after MTP. The 2,3-diphosphoglycerate levels are decreased in banked blood, shifting the oxygen-hemoglobin dissociation curve to the left. A leftward shift causes oxygen to be held onto more tightly by the hemoglobin molecule with a potential of limiting oxygen release to the tissues. However, no studies have documented any clinical adverse effects related to this phenomenon.

Ditzel RM Jr, Anderson JL, Eisenhart WJ, et al. A review of transfusion- and trauma-induced hypocalcemia: is it time to change the lethal triad to the lethal diamond? *J Trauma Acute Care Surg*. 2020;88:434-439.

Drummond JC, Petrovitch CT. The massively bleeding patient. *Anesthesiol Clin North Am*. 2001;19:633-649.

Sihler KC, Napolitano LM. Complications of massive transfusion. *Chest*. 2010;137:209-220.

C.15. Can the shift of the oxygen-hemoglobin dissociation curve be quantified?

Yes, the shift of the oxygen-hemoglobin dissociation curve is quantified by means of the P_{50} value (the oxygen tension at which hemoglobin is 50% saturated). The normal P_{50} value of blood is 27 mm Hg. Decreased levels of 2,3-diphosphoglycerate (normal 4.8 mmol/mL of erythrocytes) cause a leftward shift of the curve, lowering the P_{50} value and reducing oxygen unloading at the tissues.

Lumb A, Thomas C. Hypoxia. In: *Nunn and Lumb's Applied Respiratory Physiology*. 9th ed. Elsevier; 2020:273–278.

C.16. How is hypothermia defined? How can it be prevented and treated?

Hypothermia is defined as a core body temperature of less than 35 °C (95 °F). Prolonged exposure to a cold operating room, evaporative heat loss from the respiratory tract, infusions of cold fluids, and loss of heat production secondary to shock cause decreased core temperatures in most patients with trauma.

Strategies to reduce the risk of hypothermia include covering skin surfaces that are not in the surgical field with warm forced air blankets (to reduce convective and radiant heat loss), humidifying inspired gases (to reduce evaporative heat loss from the lungs), using a warming device for fluids and blood, and increasing the room temperature.

C.17. What are the adverse effects of hypothermia?

- Shivering-induced increase in oxygen consumption by as much as 400%
- A leftward shift in the oxygen-hemoglobin dissociation curve
- Decreased blood clotting ability (10% reduction in coagulation factor activity for every 1 °C drop in body temperature)
- Increased epinephrine and norepinephrine levels, causing vasoconstriction
- As hypothermia becomes severe, possible decreases in both HR and blood pressure
- Cardiac arrhythmias that can progress to ventricular fibrillation

Lester ELW, Fox EE, Holcomb JB, et al. The impact of hypothermia on outcomes in massively transfused patients. *J Trauma Acute Care Surg*. 2019;86:458-463.

Petrosoniak A, Pavenski K, da Luz LT, et al. Massive hemorrhage protocol: a practical approach to the bleeding trauma patient. *Emerg Med Clin North Am*. 2023;41:51-69.

Sihler KC, Napolitano LM. Complications of massive transfusion. *Chest*. 2010;137:209-220.

C.18. What are the guidelines for the ratio of plasma/platelet transfusion to packed red blood cells (pRBCs) in MT?

Most trauma centers have implemented MTPs that use the strategy of "hemostatic resuscitation." These protocols are highly variable but largely involve minimizing aggressive crystalloid use, delivering early resuscitation with a ratio of blood products that approximates whole blood, and providing early administration of fresh frozen plasm (FFP) and platelets.

At present, the optimal ratio of blood product transfusion is not known. Although more studies are required, current literature shows an association toward increased survival when a ratio of FFP to pRBCs is 1:2 or higher during MT. The Pragmatic, Randomized Optimal Platelets and Plasma Ratios study randomized 680 severely injured patients with trauma to receive FFP:platelets:RBCs in a 1:1:1 or 1:1:2 fashion. The 1:1:1 cohort was found to be noninferior to 1:1:2, as there was no significant difference in mortality or adverse events between the groups.

Griffee MJ, Deloughery TG, Thorborg PA. Coagulation management in massive bleeding. *Curr Opin Anaesthesiol*. 2010;23:263-268.

Holcomb JB, Tilley BC, Baraniuk S, et al. Transfusion of plasma, platelets, and red blood cells in a 1:1:1 vs a 1:1:2 ratio and mortality in patients with severe trauma: the PROPPR randomized clinical trial. *JAMA*. 2015;313:471-482.

Ketchum L, Hess JR, Hiippala S. Indications for early fresh frozen plasma, cryoprecipitate, and platelet transfusion in trauma. *J Trauma*. 2006;60:S51-S58.

Teixeira PG, Inaba K, Shulman I, et al. Impact of plasma transfusion in massively transfused trauma patients. *J Trauma*. 2009;66:693-697.

C.19. If a patient were a member of the Jehovah's Witness religious group, would you give a blood transfusion?

Most Jehovah's Witnesses believe human blood is sacred and would not accept transfused blood. In the otherwise competent adult with capacity, courts have ruled that physicians cannot be held liable for complying with a patient's directive and withholding life-saving blood administration after providing specific and detailed informed consent of the consequences of such an omission of treatment. The right of a Jehovah's Witness to refuse a blood transfusion is absolute and has been upheld in legal cases. Clinical providers should be aware that many Jehovah's Witnesses carry a medical alert card that states their wishes regarding transfusion therapies. It is crucial that an open and honest avenue of communication exists between the patient, surgeon, and anesthesiologist in making clinical decisions.

Jehovah's Witnesses will generally refuse transfusion of whole blood, packed red blood cells, white blood cells, plasma, and platelets; however, they may allow the use of cardiopulmonary bypass, dialysis, or similar equipment, as well as intraoperative blood salvage, in which the extracorporeal circulation is uninterrupted. Their religious understanding does not absolutely prohibit albumin, immune globulins, or hemophilia therapies; those products must be decided on an individual basis. They generally accept all nonblood replacements, including nonblood colloids, crystalloids, dextrans, and oxygen-carrying blood substitutes.

An anesthesiologist can refuse to care for any patient when a procedure is elective. In an emergency, legal and ethical requirements apply. The issue of providing blood products becomes clouded when patients are deemed incompetent, are unconscious, or are minors.

C.20. If a child is a Jehovah's Witness and has hemorrhagic shock, what would you do?

Care of minors presents the greatest concern and often leads to legal action against the parents under child-neglect status. Such actions are questioned by Jehovah's Witnesses, who do seek good medical care for their children while claiming that consideration be given to their families' religious beliefs. Doctors can appeal to the court for permission to transfuse blood to children who are underage. In an emergency, blood can be given without consulting the court.

Dasen KR, Niswander DG, Schlenker RE. Autologous and allogenic blood products for unanticipated massive blood loss in a Jehovah's Witness. *Anesth Analg*. 2000;90:553-555.

Lawson T, Ralph C. Perioperative Jehovah's Witnesses: a review. *Br J Anaesth*. 2015;115:676-687.

Waters JH, Potter PS. Cell salvage in the Jehovah's Witness patient. *Anesth Analg*. 2000;90:229-230.

C.21. What concentrated factors and hemostatic agents are available for bleeding patients?

Recombinant Activated Factor VII (rFVIIa, NovoSeven)

NovoSeven is approved in the United States for prophylaxis and treatment of hemorrhage in hemophiliacs with inhibitors of factor VIII, IX, or congenital factor VII deficiency. Despite its limited approval, it has been used off-label in patients with refractory traumatic hemorrhage. Although NovoSeven is extremely effective at stopping uncontrolled bleeding, it might not provide a survival benefit versus a placebo, as suggested by the CONTROL study. Moreover, there have been reports linking it to thromboembolic adverse events, such as an increased risk of stroke.

Four-Factor Prothrombin Complex Concentrate

Four-factor prothrombin complex concentrate (4F-PCC) contains plasma-derived, vitamin-dependent factors II, VII, IX, and X in their inactivated forms, as well as low amounts of the anticoagulant factors protein C, protein S, antithrombin III, and heparin. It has the advantages of requiring significantly less volume for infusion compared with plasma, achieving a more rapid reversal of the international normalized ratio (INR), and almost eliminating the risk of TRALI. PCC has US Food and Drug Administration (FDA) approval for the reversal of vitamin K antagonists, for example, warfarin, in patients with acute major bleeding, but has also shown promise in treating acute coagulopathy in trauma (off-label indication). In fact, its administration is recommended by European trauma guidelines in managing patients with evidence of delayed thrombin generation. Zeeshan and colleagues performed the largest retrospective analysis to date on the use of 4F-PCC in trauma. Their study suggests that 4F-PCC can be a useful adjustment to FFP for the control of posttrauma hemorrhage when used early.

Fibrinogen Concentrates

Fibrinogen is usually the first coagulation factor or protein to reach critically low levels in patients with trauma requiring MTP. Decreased fibrinogen levels in trauma are related to multiple factors, including blood loss, consumption of clotting factors and platelets, decreased fibrinogen synthesis due to hypothermia, dilution by fluids, and fibrinolysis. Fibrinogen concentrate is a pasteurized collection from human plasma that is FDA approved for the treatment of clinically significant bleeding in patients with congenital hypofibrinogenemia or dysfibrinogenemia, so its administration during trauma-related massive hemorrhage is considered off-label. Compared to FFP and cryoprecipitate, it has a minimal risk of infection transmission, the dosing is accurate and consistent, and it can be rapidly administered since it does not require thawing or crossmatching. A Cochrane Review by Wikkelsø et al found no differences in outcomes in terms of adverse events, bleeding, or recovery between fibrinogen concentrate and blood products. The bulk of studies that examine fibrinogen concentrate's role in trauma resuscitation are observational or retrospective cohort studies, and they do not offer strong evidence in favor of its use in severe trauma.

Tranexamic Acid

Tranexamic acid (TXA) is an antifibrinolytic that blocks the interaction of plasminogen with fibrin, effectively preventing clot breakdown and lysis. It can be used to treat hyperfibrinolysis in trauma, which is an independent predictor of mortality in patients with trauma. The CRASH-2 trial, an international randomized study of over 20,000 patients with trauma, found TXA was associated with a significant reduction in all-cause mortality compared with placebo (14.5% vs 16%, $P = .035$). Subsequent analyses revealed the greatest benefit of TXA was seen only when given less than 3 hours from injury, supporting early administration in trauma.

Hauser CJ, Boffard K, Dutton R, et al. Results of the CONTROL trial: efficacy and safety of recombinant activated factor VII in the management of refractory traumatic hemorrhage. *J Trauma*. 2010;69:489-500.

Mengoli C, Franchini M, Marano G, et al. The use of fibrinogen concentrate for the management of trauma-related bleeding: a systematic review and meta-analysis. *Blood Transfus*. 2017;15:318-324.

Napolitano LM, Cohen MJ, Cotton BA, et al. Tranexamic acid in trauma: how should we use it? *J Trauma Acute Care Surg*. 2013;74:1575-1586.

Rossaint R, Bouillon B, Cerny V, et al. The European guideline on management of major bleeding and coagulopathy following trauma: fourth edition. *Crit Care*. 2016;20:100.

Shakur H, Roberts I, Bautista R, et al. Effects of tranexamic acid on death, vascular occlusive events, and blood transfusion in trauma patients with significant haemorrhage (CRASH-2); a randomized, placebo-controlled trial. *Lancet*. 2010;376:23-32.

Wikkelsø A, Lunde J, Johansen M, et al. Fibrinogen concentrate in bleeding patients. *Cochrane Database Syst Rev*. 2013;CD008864.

Zeeshan M, Hamidi M, Feinstein AJ, et al. Four-factor prothrombin complex concentrate is associated with improved survival in trauma-related hemorrhage: A nationwide propensity-matched analysis. *J Trauma Acute Care Surg*. 2019;87:274-281.

C.22. What is thromboelastometry? How can it guide transfusion?

Rotational thromboelastography (ROTEM) and thromboelastography (TEG) are point-of-care viscoelastic hemostatic assays (VEAs) used to assess clot kinetics. Both tests employ a suspended pin that sits in a conical cup containing whole blood. As a clot forms with the addition of an activator, the change in resistance is detected by VEA and plotted as a thromboelastogram. Results can then be used to tailor transfusion therapy in trauma resuscitation by goal-directed coagulation therapy; nevertheless, VEA has not been shown to improve mortality.

Rotation Thromboelastography

ROTEM uses a rotating pin in a stationary cup to detect increases in tensile force as a clot forms. It determines several different clotting parameters:

- INTEM—intrinsic pathway of the coagulation cascade
- HEPTEM—the intrinsic pathway of the coagulation cascade with the addition of heparinase, which removes the effects of heparin from the results
- EXTEM—the extrinsic pathway of the coagulation cascade
- FIBTEM—extrinsic pathway of the coagulation cascade with the addition of cytochalasin D, which inhibits the effects of platelets on clot formation
- APTEM—extrinsic pathway with the addition of aprotinin to block fibrinolysis

These tests generate images based on the coagulation status, which can be used to guide transfusion therapy (**Figures 57.1-57.6**). Algorithms have been developed to guide therapy based on ROTEM results (**Figure 57.7**).

Thromboelastography

TEG is based on the same principles as ROTEM except that instead of having a mobile pin in a stationary cup, TEG has a stationary pin in a mobile cup (**Figure 57.8**). TEG values can be compared to ROTEM values (**Table 57.1**). Some examples of the effect of different coagulation states on TEG (**Figure 57.9**) and a guideline for transfusion therapy (**Figure 57.10**) are shown.

Baksaas-Aasen K, Gall LS, Stensballe J, et al. Viscoelastic haemostatic assay augmented protocols for major trauma haemorrhage (ITACTIC): a randomized, controlled trial. *Intensive Care Med*. 2021;47:49-59.

Bolliger D, Seeberger MD, Tanaka KA. Principles and practice of thromboelastography in clinical coagulation management and transfusion practice. *Transfus Med Rev*. 2012;26:1-13.

Jackson GN, Ashpole KJ, Yentis SM. The TEG vs the ROTEM thromboelastography/thromboelastometry systems. *Anaesthesia*. 2009;64:212-215.

Johansson PI, Stissing T, Bochsen L, et al. Thrombelastography and thromboelastometry in assessing coagulation in trauma. *Scand J Trauma Resusc Emerg Med*. 2009;17:45.

Ogawa S, Szlam F, Chen EP, et al. A comparative evaluation of rotation thromboelastometry and standard coagulation tests in hemodilution-induced coagulation changes after cardiac surgery. *Transfusion*. 2012;52:14-22.

TEM Systems. Result interpretation. Accessed April 15, 2023. http://www.rotem-usa.com/methodology/result-interpretation/

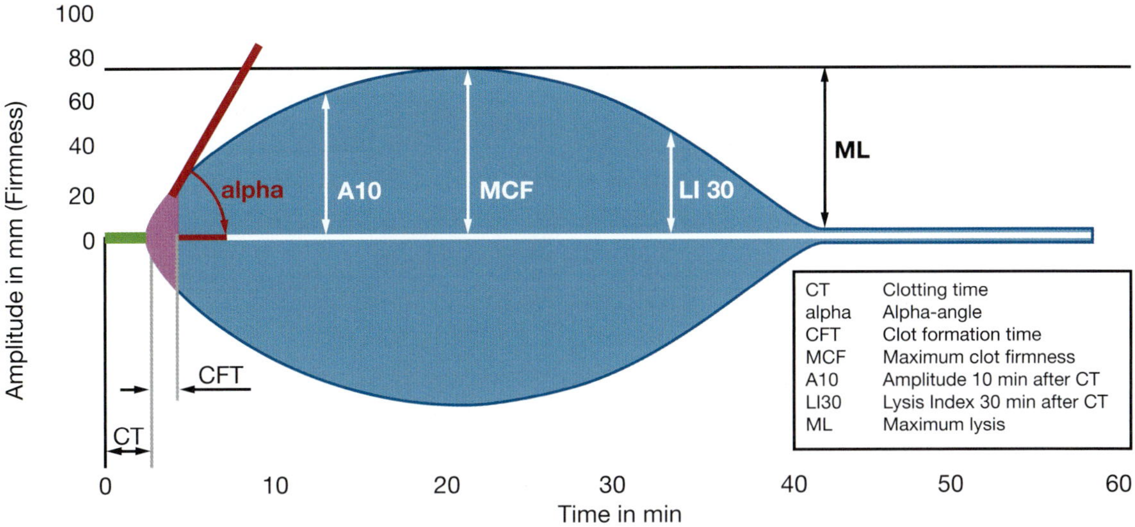

FIGURE 57.1. Basic ROTEM thromboelastogram. Clotting time (CT): the measured time until clot formation starts; affected by clotting factors and anticoagulants. Clot formation time (CFT): a measure of the initial rate of clot formation, the time from clot formation until the clot forms to an amplitude of 20 mm; depends on platelets and fibrinogen. α Angle: a measure of the initial rate of clot formation. Maximum clot firmness (MCF): the maximum tensile strength of the clot; describes the quality of the clot and is dependent on platelets, fibrinogen, factor XIII, and fibrinolysis. Maximum lysis (ML): reduction of clot firmness during measurement; abnormality in the ML at 30 minutes indicated fibrinolysis. Amplitude: A5/A10/A15 is the amplitude of the clot at 5, 10, and 15 minutes.

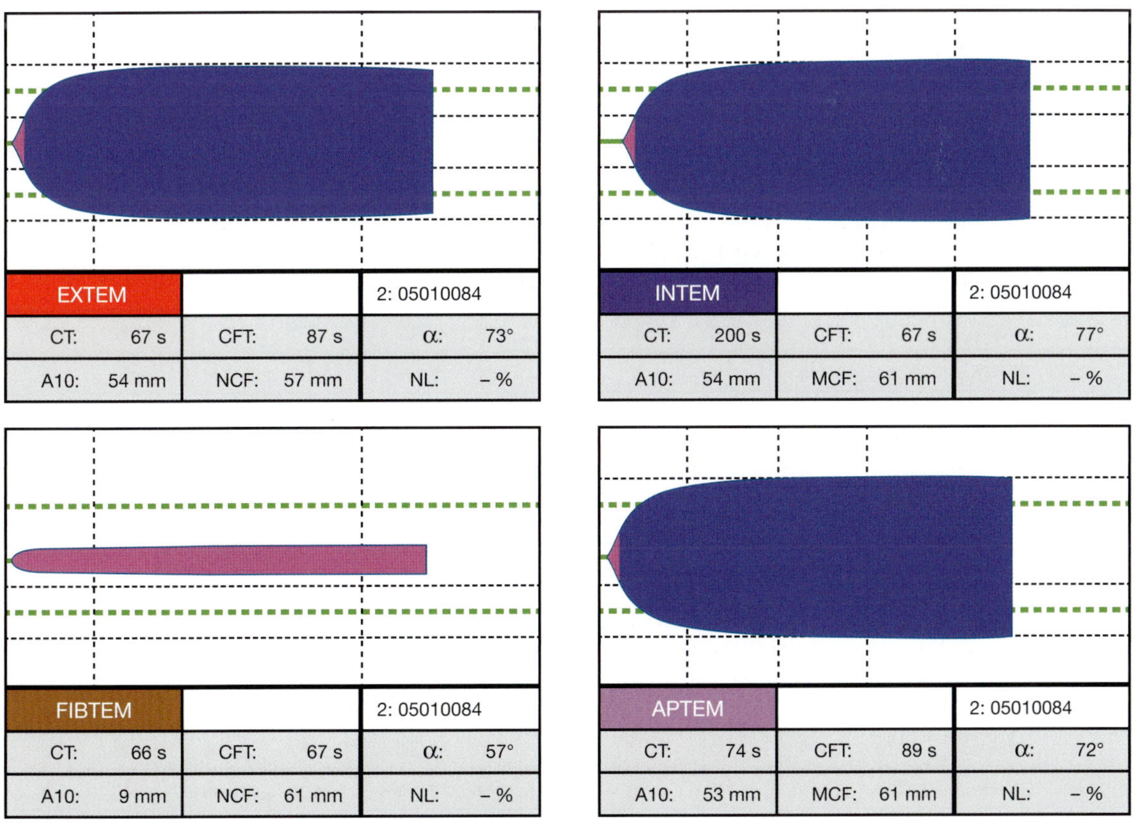

FIGURE 57.2. ROTEM in a patient with normal coagulation parameters.

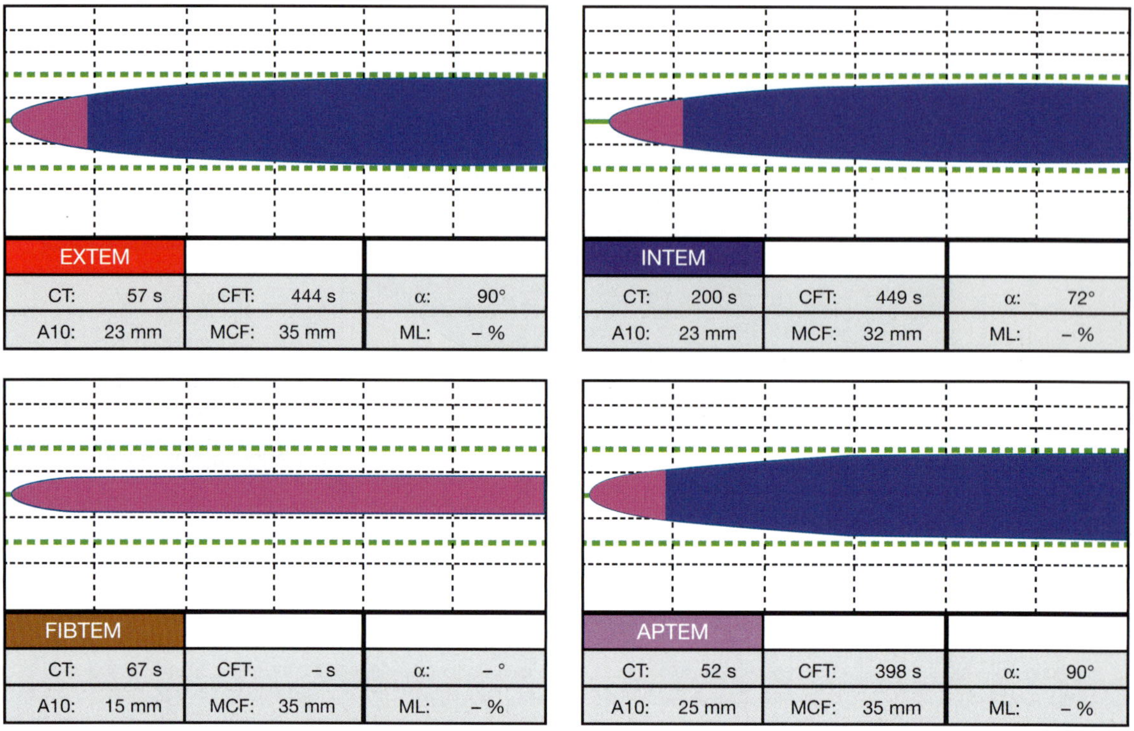

FIGURE 57.3. ROTEM in a patient with a platelet deficiency.

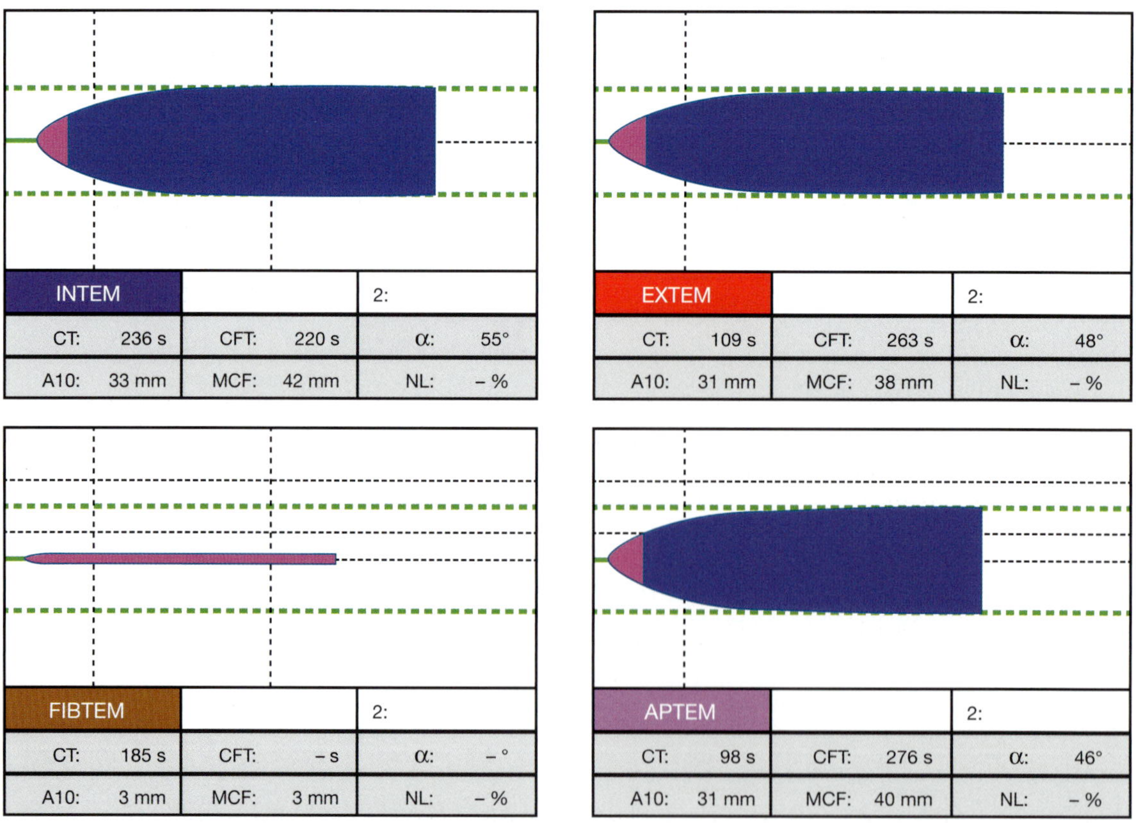

FIGURE 57.4. ROTEM in a patient with a fibrinogen deficiency.

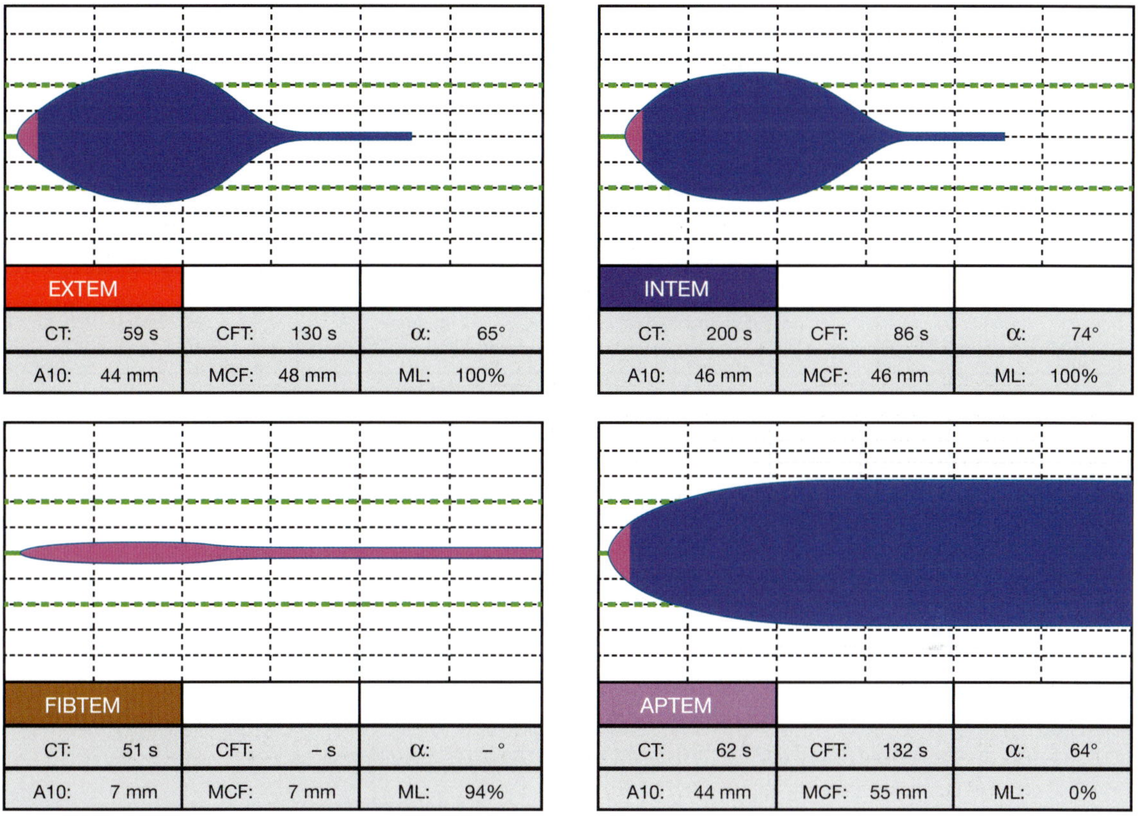

FIGURE 57.5. **ROTEM in a patient with hyperfibrinolysis.**

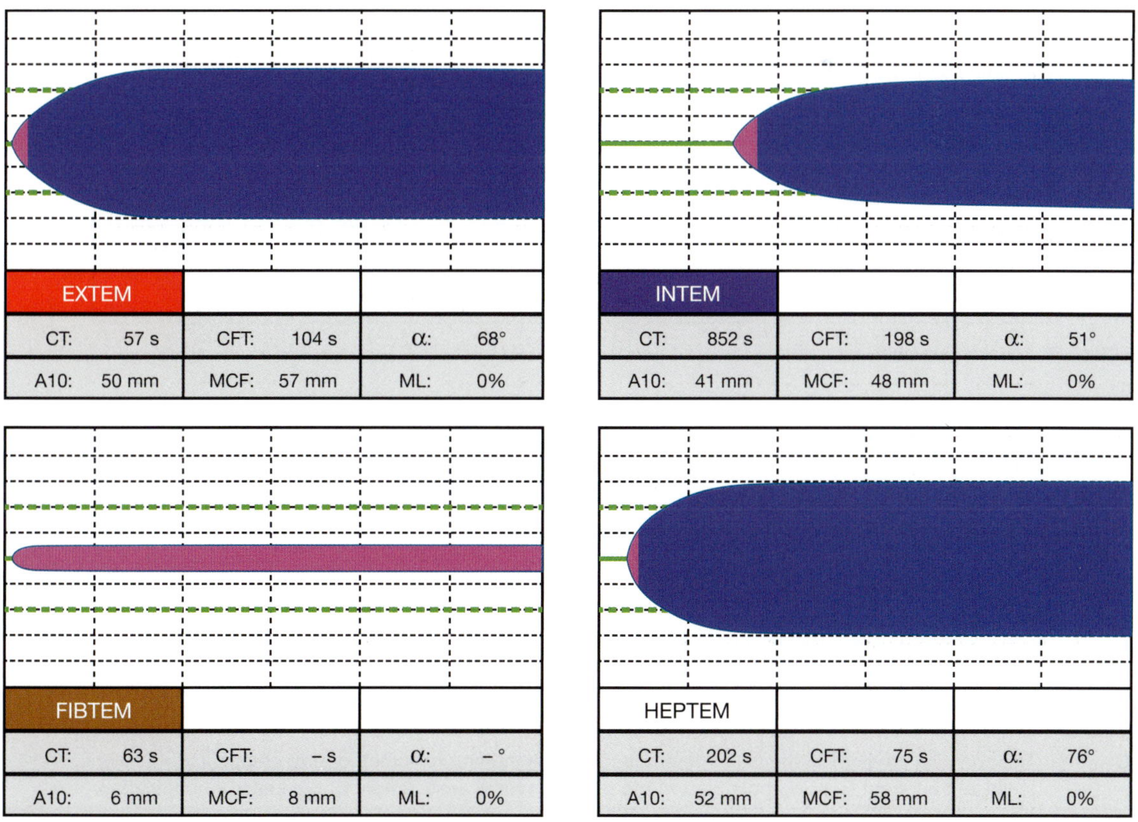

FIGURE 57.6. **ROTEM in a patient with heparin influence.**

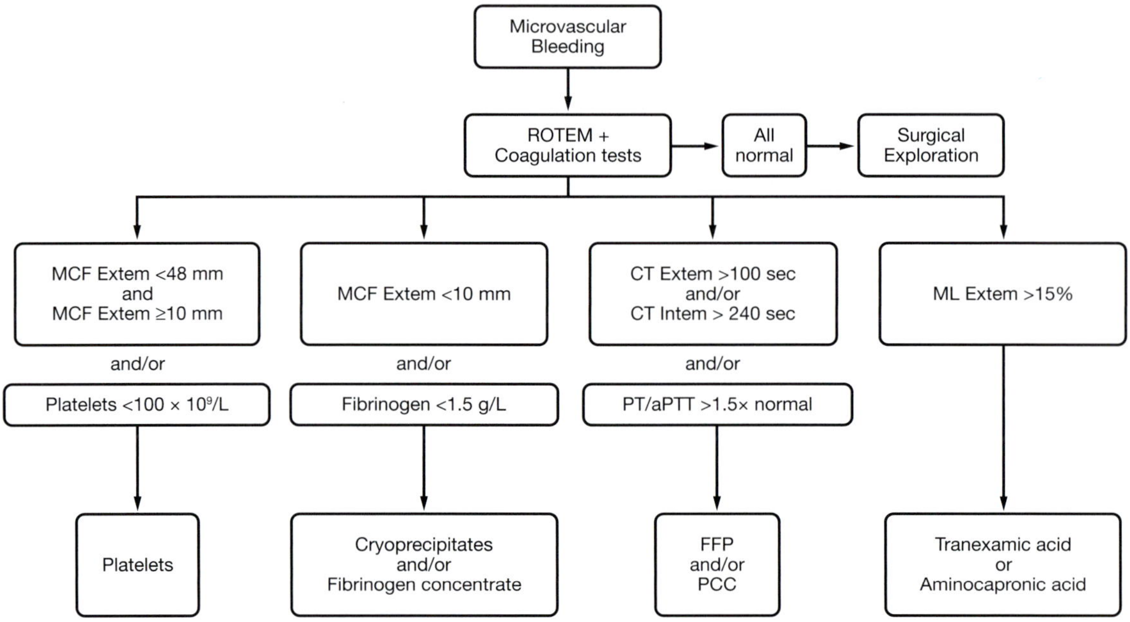

FIGURE 57.7. Guide to therapy based on ROTEM results. aPTT, activated partial thromboplastin time; CT, computed tomography; FFP, fresh frozen plasma; MCF, maximum clot firmness; ML, maximum lysis; PCC, prothrombin complex concentrate; PT, prothrombin time. (Reprinted from Bolliger D, Seeberger MD, Tanaka KA. Principles and practice of thromboelastography in clinical coagulation management and transfusion practice. *Transfus Med Rev.* 2012;26:1-13. Copyright © 2012 Elsevier. With permission.)

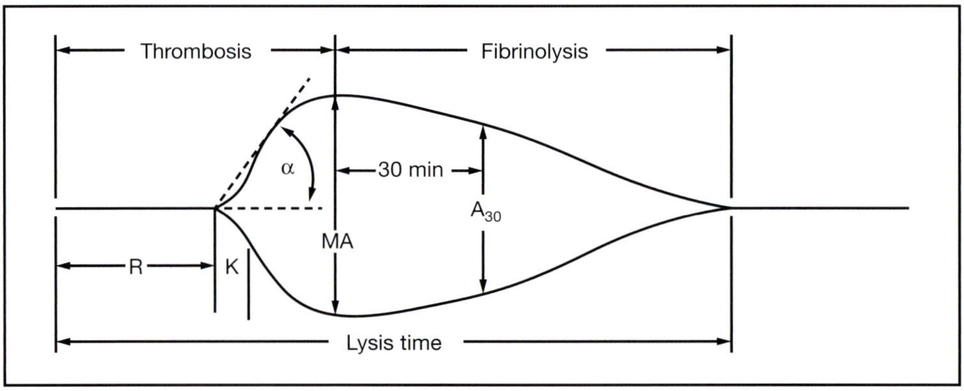

FIGURE 57.8. Basic thromboelastogram.

TABLE 57.1 Thromboelastography (TEG) Values Compared to Their Rotational Thromboelastometry (ROTEM) Equivalents

TEG	Measures	ROTEM Equivalent
R time	Time to 2 mm amplitude	CT
K time	Time from 2 to 20 mm	CFT
α Angle	The slope between R and K	α Angle
MA	Maximum amplitude of clot	MCF
LY30	Percentage of clot lysis at 30 min after MA	ML
A30	Size of a clot at 30 min after MA	A10
G	Clot elasticity	MCE
CI	The coagulation index is the value determined by a manufacturer-created mathematical formula which takes into account R, K, α angle, and MA to give an overall assessment of the state of coagulation.	

CFT, clot formation time; CI, coagulation index; CT, clotting time; K, kinetics; MA, maximum amplitude; MCE, maximum clot elasticity; MCF, maximum clot firmness; ML, maximum lysis; R, reaction time.

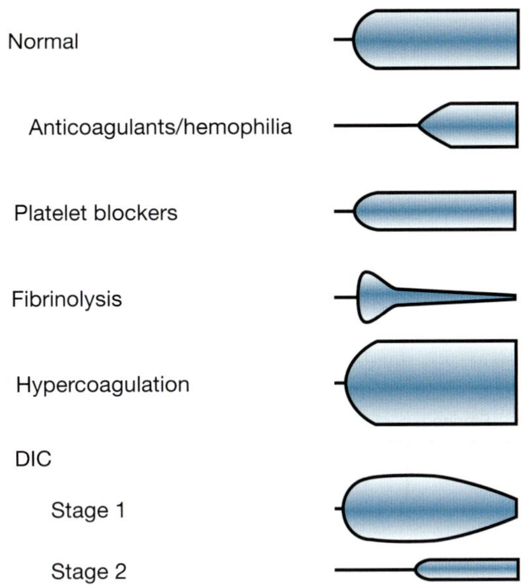

FIGURE 57.9. Effects of different coagulation states on TEG results. DIC, disseminated intravascular coagulation; TEG, thromboelastography.

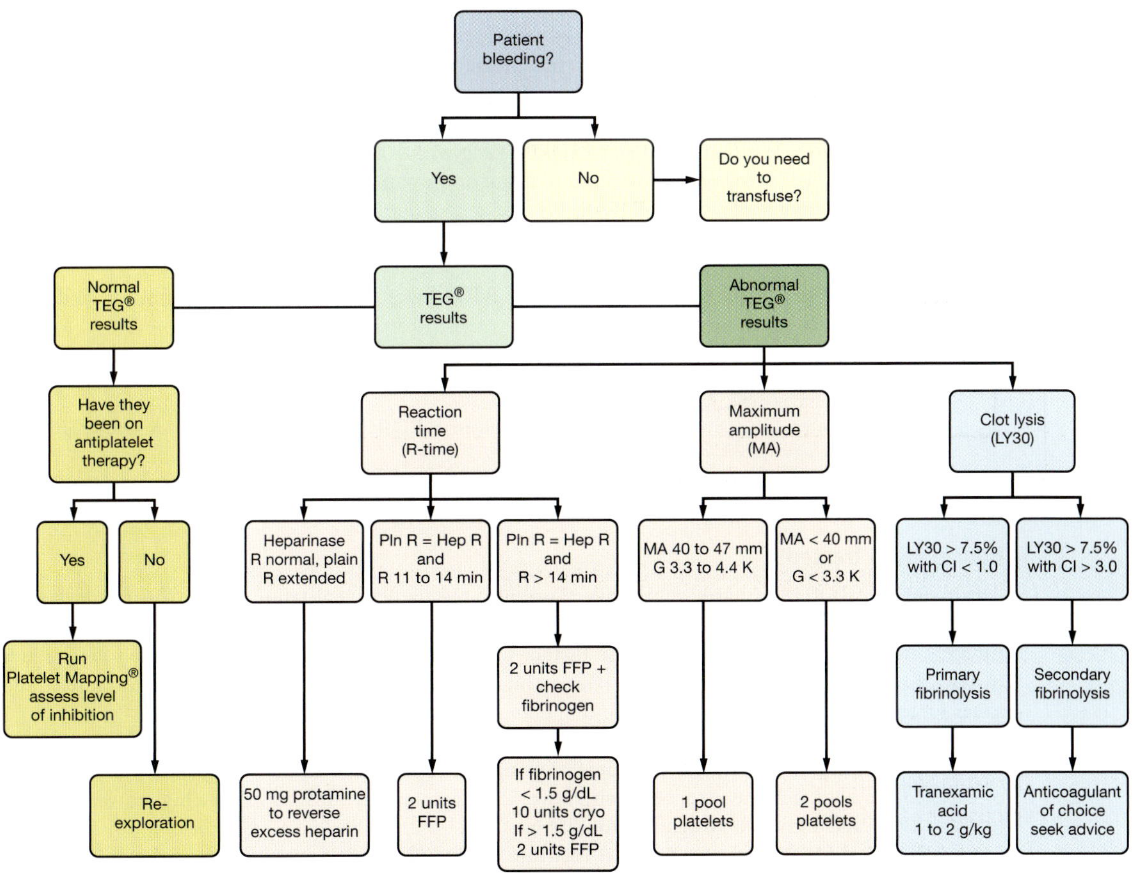

FIGURE 57.10. A guideline for transfusion based on TEG results. CI, coagulation index; FFP, fresh frozen plasma; G, clot elasticity; K, kinetics; MA, maximum amplitude; Pln, plain; TEG, thromboelastography.

D. Postoperative Management

D.1. What is acute respiratory distress syndrome (ARDS)? What is acute lung injury?

ARDS is a type of acute respiratory failure seen after direct (eg, aspiration, infection) or indirect (eg, severe trauma) lung injury. Initially, when this clinical syndrome was thought to be related to the underlying shock state and its resuscitation, names such as "shock lung" and "traumatic wet lung" were applied to the subsequent acute respiratory insufficiency. It is now recognized that many types of insults result in damage to the alveolar-capillary membrane, resulting in leakage of proteinaceous fluid into the alveolar space. This injury, with its resulting interstitial and alveolar edema, produces a clinical picture ranging from mild to severe pulmonary dysfunction that can be fatal.

ARDS was formerly defined as:

- Acute onset of respiratory failure.
- Bilateral infiltrates on chest radiography.
- PaO_2/fraction of inspired oxygen (FIO_2) ratio of 200 or less.
- Pulmonary capillary wedge pressure less than 18 mm Hg.

However, this definition was reevaluated in 2012 secondary to concerns regarding its accuracy. First, the diagnosis of bilateral infiltrates on chest radiograph had wide interobserver variability and thus was inconsistent. Next, the PaO_2/FIO_2 ratio varied greatly based on ventilator status and needed to be refined. Third, patients with heart failure with elevated left atrial pressures can have ARDS, so high pulmonary capillary wedge pressures are not enough to rule out the diagnosis of ARDS. Finally, the definition was found to have low specificity when compared to autopsy results of patients with diffuse alveolar damage.

For these reasons, the Berlin definition was established, which characterizes ARDS by the following:

Oxygenation

- Mild—PaO_2/FIO_2 less than 200 mm Hg or less than or equal to 300 mm Hg with positive end-expiratory pressure (PEEP) or continuous positive airway pressure (CPAP) greater than or equal to 5 cm H_2O
- Moderate—PaO_2/FIO_2 less than or equal to 100 mm Hg or less than or equal to 200 mm Hg with PEEP greater than or equal to 5 cm H_2O
- Severe—PaO_2/FIO_2 less than or equal to 100 mm Hg with PEEP greater than or equal to 5 cm H_2O

Timing—onset within 1 week of a known clinical insult or the patient has worsening respiratory symptoms

Chest radiograph—demonstrates opacities bilaterally that are not due to pleural effusions, atelectasis, or nodules

Origin of edema—respiratory insufficiency that is not solely caused by cardiogenic causes, that is, left heart failure or volume overload

Acute lung injury—a term for a less severe form of ARDS was removed from the definition and is no longer used.

Fanelli V, Vlachou A, Ghannadian S, et al. Acute respiratory distress syndrome: new definition, current and future therapeutic options. *J Thorac Dis*. 2013;5:326-334.

Faugno AJ, Epstein SK. Acute respiratory failure. In: Kellerman RD, Heidelbaugh JJ, Lee EM, eds. *Conn's Current Therapy*. 1st ed. Elsevier; 2025:913–918.

Hallman MR. Critical care medicine. In: Cullen BF, Stock MC, Ortega R, et al, eds. *Barash, Cullen, and Stoelting's Clinical Anesthesia*. 9th ed. Wolters Kluwer; 2024:1539-1565.

D.2. How is ARDS treated?

Treatment of ARDS is primarily supportive. Currently, mechanical ventilation is the mainstay of therapy for ARDS. The principal goal of mechanical ventilation is to allow time for the lungs to heal. Unfortunately, mechanical ventilation can cause further lung injury, known as ventilator-induced lung injury (VILI). Excessive alveolar volumes (volutrauma), high mean and peak airway pressures (barotrauma), and shear forces caused by frequent collapse and opening of alveolar units contribute to VILI.

Investigators have looked at protective ventilator strategies in patients with ARDS. Amato et al used a strategy to limit peak inspiratory pressures by using low tidal volumes (<6 mL/kg) and the institution of PEEP. Their approach was associated with lower 28-day mortality (38% vs 71%), a higher weaning rate (66% vs 29%), and a lower barotrauma rate (7% vs 42%).

The National Heart, Lung, and Blood Institute ARDS Network reported improved survival with a low tidal volume strategy (6 vs 12 mL/kg). Moreover, there was a decrease in mortality of approximately 25% in the intervention group compared with the control group.

Amato MB, Barbas CS, Medeiros DM, et al. Effect of a protective-ventilation strategy on mortality in the acute respiratory distress syndrome. *N Engl J Med*. 1998;338:347-354.

Brower RG, Ware LB, Berthiaume Y, et al. Treatment of ARDS. *Chest*. 2001;120:1347-1367.

Faugno AJ, Epstein SK. Acute respiratory failure. In: Kellerman RD, Heidelbaugh JJ, Lee EM, eds. *Conn's Current Therapy*. 1st ed. Elsevier; 2025:913–918.

Thomson BT, Bernard GR. ARDS Network (NHLBI) studies: successes and challenges in ARDS clinical research. *Crit Care Clin*. 2011;27:459-468.

D.3. You are called to see this patient in the postanesthesia care unit (PACU) because of oliguria. How would you evaluate and treat this patient?

Oliguria is a decrease in urinary output to less than 0.3 to 0.5 mL/kg/h. ARF is a syndrome characterized by a rapid (hours to weeks) decline in glomerular filtration rate (GFR) and retention of waste products such as urea. Most cases of ARF are reversible, as the kidney is remarkable in its ability to recover from almost complete loss of function. ARF is associated with major in-hospital morbidity and mortality. The diagnosis of ARF usually hinges on changes in serum creatinine, GFR, and urine output.

Causes of renal failure can be grouped into three categories:

Prerenal

Prerenal failure is the most common cause of ARF. It is usually caused by a low flow state, such as hypovolemia or cardiac failure. Evaluation begins with reviewing hemodynamic trends, fluid balance, and relevant studies (eg, echocardiogram). If hypovolemia is suspected, treatment would consist of a fluid bolus. If cardiac output is inadequate, then inotropic support and/or diuretics could be administered. Severe renal hypoperfusion can cause ischemic acute tubular necrosis (ATN); therefore, prerenal azotemia and ischemic ATN are part of a spectrum of manifestations of renal hypoperfusion.

Renal

Intrinsic renal failure is generally due to toxic injury or ischemia resulting in glomerular and tubular damage. Ischemic ATN, unlike prerenal azotemia, is associated with injury to renal parenchyma and does not typically resolve immediately on restoration of renal perfusion. In its more extreme form, renal hypoperfusion can result in bilateral renal cortical necrosis and irreversible renal failure. Urinalysis can show cells or casts that are indicative of ARF. Intrinsic renal failure can be minor and short lived, or it can progress to chronic renal failure, depending on the severity of the insult.

Postrenal

Urinary tract obstruction accounts for less than 5% of cases of ARF. Urinary tract obstruction must be sought and corrected to treat possible causes of postrenal oliguria. This usually requires irrigation or changing of the Foley catheter. Consider the possibility of an intraoperative mishap causing postrenal obstruction.

Okusa MD, Portilla D. Pathophysiology of acute kidney injury. In: Yu ASL, Chertow GM, Luyckx VA, Marsden PA, Skorecki K, Taal MW, eds. *Brenner and Rector's The Kidney*. 11th ed. Elsevier; 2019:906–939.

D.4. If this patient had a crush injury and low urine output, what other concerns might you have? What if the patient has dark or "tea-colored" urine?

Leakage of myoglobin from muscle and damaged tissue secondary to a crush injury can result in rhabdomyolysis. Myoglobin at high concentrations precipitates in the nephron, appearing pigmented and causing acute renal injury. The urine can look suspicious for hematuria or have a "tea-colored" appearance. Rhabdomyolysis can be diagnosed by the presence of myoglobinuria, electrolyte disorders, isolated elevated aspartate aminotransferase, and/or increased serum creatine kinase levels. Preventing ARF in these patients is essential because the development of ARF is associated with increased mortality. Treatment in patients with hypovolemia and euvolemia is hydration with large volumes of isotonic crystalloid, resulting in goal urine output as high as 100 to 300 mL/h. In addition, alkalization of the urine, with agents such as isotonic sodium bicarbonate, can help by decreasing the rate of precipitation. Mannitol has also been used to induce osmotic diuresis and flush the myoglobin through the kidneys. The evidence for the utility of bicarbonate and mannitol in the management of rhabdomyolysis is weak. Electrolyte abnormalities, including hyperkalemia, hyperphosphatemia, and hypocalcemia, mimicking a tumor lysis pattern, can develop with crush injury, so this should be monitored.

Bosch X, Poch E, Grau JM. Rhabdomyolysis and acute kidney injury. *N Engl J Med*. 2009;361:62-72.

Gonzalez D. Crush syndrome. *Crit Care Med*. 2005;33:S34-S41.

Lee GX, Duong DK. Rhabdomyolysis: evidence-based management in the emergency department. *Emerg Med Pract*. 2020;22:1-20.

Okusa MD, Portilla D. Pathophysiology of acute kidney injury. In: Yu ASL, Chertow GM, Luyckx VA, Marsden PA, Skorecki K, Taal MW, eds. *Brenner and Rector's The Kidney*. 11th ed. Elsevier; 2019:906–939.

58 Major and Complex Spine Surgery

Seyed A. Safavynia

A 51-year-old male (68.6 kg, body mass index [BMI] 20.7) has a past medical history significant for a motor vehicle accident resulting in a T10-11 fracture with bilateral lower extremity paralysis and neurogenic bladder and bowel. He has since had multiple spine surgeries, including T7-T12 Harrington rod placement, T12-L3 fusion, C4-6 laminoplasty, and T12 to S1 fusion. He uses a wheelchair and has contractures and muscular atrophy of his lower extremities. His home medications include tapentadol, tramadol, baclofen, diazepam, acetaminophen, and nonsteroidal anti-inflammatory drugs (NSAIDs) as needed. He now presents with worsening back pain despite medical interventions and multiple epidural steroid injections.

The patient is scheduled for an L4-S1 anterior lumbar interbody fusion (ALIF), posterior removal of L2-iliac rods, and posterior revision of T12-S1 fusion with plastic surgery closure. The procedure will be performed with intraoperative computed tomography (CT) and intraoperative neuromonitoring. He is also scheduled to be placed on an enhanced recovery after surgery (ERAS) protocol, which recommends a 600-mg dose of preoperative gabapentin, intraoperative methadone, and subanesthetic ketamine infusion during anesthetic maintenance.

A. Pathophysiology and Differential Diagnosis

1. What is the differential diagnosis for the evaluation of back pain?
2. What are the nonsurgical treatment options for back pain?
3. What are the major anatomic landmarks of the vertebral column? Where does the spinal cord terminate, and where do the nerve roots exit the spine? What is the blood supply to the spinal cord?
4. How are minor, major, and complex spine surgeries classified?

B. Preoperative Evaluation and Preparation

1. What aspects of the patient's history and physical exam are most important in formulating your anesthetic plan?
2. What is the pathophysiology of neurogenic bladder/bowel? What conditions can cause neurogenic bladder/bowel?
3. What is autonomic hyperreflexia? Is autonomic hyperreflexia a concern in this patient?
4. What aspects of the patient's history and proposed surgical intervention are concerning for potentially large intraoperative blood loss? How would you prepare for potentially large intraoperative blood loss?
5. How will the details of the surgical procedure influence anesthetic management?
6. How would you counsel the patient for his risk of complications during the procedure?

C. Intraoperative Management

1. How would you manage this patient's airway?
2. How will the surgical considerations affect your anesthetic plan for this patient?
3. What is your analgesic plan?
4. What neuromonitoring techniques are used in major spine surgery to minimize neurologic complications? How does the location of the surgical procedure affect the choice of neuromonitoring technique?
5. How are somatosensory evoked potentials (SSEPs) and motor evoked potentials (MEPs) administered? How are they interpreted? What will you see behaviorally during SSEP/MEP monitoring? What additional precautions should you take during MEP monitoring?

6. Shortly after incision, the neurophysiologist indicates that the patient is getting "light" despite there being no change in anesthetic dose or processed electroencephalography (EEG) index. How is this determination being made?
7. The anterior portion of the case is uneventful; however, shortly after prone positioning, the neurophysiologist reports a loss of upper extremity MEPs/SSEPs. What factors can affect spinal cord neuromonitoring?
8. Point-of-care testing at the start of the posterior portion of the case reveals a hemoglobin and hematocrit (Hb/Hct) of 11.1/33. Two hours into the posterior portion, Hb/Hct is 7.8/23. Would you transfuse? What are your thresholds for blood transfusion?
9. Two hours later, estimated blood loss (EBL) is approximately 2 L and the patient has been resuscitated with 3 units of packed red blood cells (pRBCs), 229 mL intraoperative cell salvage (cell saver), and 500 mL albumin in addition to 4 L crystalloid. The surgeon says the field is still "oozy" and there is ongoing blood loss. What are your concerns for resuscitation moving forward? How will you guide your resuscitation?
10. You decide to use rotational thromboelastometry (ROTEM) to guide your resuscitation efforts. After 20 minutes, the results of the ROTEM are normal; however, the field is still bloody. The surgeon suggests tranexamic acid (TXA) for the patient. What is TXA and what is its mechanism of action? Is TXA effective at reducing blood loss in major spine surgery? What are the risks of TXA administration? Is TXA an appropriate choice in this patient?
11. What is transfusion-related acute lung injury (TRALI)? How is it differentiated from transfusion-associated circulatory overload (TACO)?

D. Postoperative Anesthetic Management

1. Hemostasis is achieved, and the surgeon prepares for a staple closure. By this time, the patient has received a total of 7.5 L of Plasma-Lyte, 1 L of albumin, 5 units of pRBCs, 2 units of fresh frozen plasma (FFP), and 229 mL of cell salvage with 1.6 L of urine output. Total case time is 14 hours with a prone time of 10 hours. How would you decide whether to extubate the patient's trachea?
2. Given the nature of the case and difficulties in neuromonitoring, the surgeon asks for a wake-up test before supinating the patient and leaving the operating room. How is a wake-up test performed? Are there any contraindications to performing a wake-up test?
3. What are the major postoperative complications following spinal surgery, and which patients are at the highest risk?
4. What strategies can be used to minimize the risk of postoperative visual loss (POVL)?
5. What is an ERAS pathway? How has it been applied to the recovery of patients undergoing major spine surgery?
6. What is the evidence regarding the efficacy and utility of perioperative gabapentinoids, intraoperative methadone, and subanesthetic ketamine in postoperative recovery as recommended in ERAS protocols?

A. Pathophysiology and Differential Diagnosis

A.1. What is the differential diagnosis for the evaluation of back pain?

Back pain is a common diagnosis, affecting up to 39% of the population and 46% of people over age 65 years. Aside from nonspinal causes (eg, referred pain, vascular ischemia), the most common etiology of nonspecific back pain (~90%) is muscular in nature, has a good prognosis, and does not require further intervention. More severe back pain that has a radicular or spinal component warrants imaging and may reveal either mechanical impingement of nerve roots (radiculopathy) or the spinal cord (spinal stenosis). This is due to pathologies affecting the vertebral discs or the vertebral column, which can be acquired, congenital, or neoplastic (see **Table 58.1** for a full differential). Other etiologies include inflammatory conditions with or without mechanical nerve impingement and infectious etiologies.

Lucas JW, Connor EM, Bose J. *Back, Lower Limb, and Upper Limb Pain Among U.S. Adults, 2019* [NCHS Data Brief No. 415]. National Center for Health Statistics; 2021.

Traeger A, Buchbinder R, Harris I, Maher C. Diagnosis and management of low-back pain in primary care. *CMAJ*. 2017;189:E1386-E1395.

TABLE 58.1 Differential Diagnosis of Back Pain

Muscular causes
- Muscular strain/sprain
- Myofascial pain syndrome

Conditions causing neural mechanical impingement
- Acquired
  - Degenerative disc disease
  - Herniated/ruptured nucleus pulposus
  - Spondylolysis
  - Spondylolisthesis
  - Vertebral fracture
  - Cauda equina syndrome
- Congenital
  - Scoliosis
  - Kyphosis
- Neoplastic
  - Primary tumor
  - Metastatic disease
  - Multiple myeloma

Inflammatory conditions with or without mechanical impingement
- Ankylosing spondylitis
- Inflammatory arthritis
- Cauda equina syndrome

Infectious etiologies
- Osteomyelitis
- Vertebral discitis
- Arachnoiditis
- Epidural abscess

A.2. What are the nonsurgical treatment options for back pain?

Nonsurgical options should be exhausted before initiating surgical treatment of back pain, as they are less invasive, have a better safety profile, and present less risk to the patient. Moreover, surgical treatments may not be definitive in relieving back pain; indeed, failed back syndrome (or postlaminectomy syndrome) is described by recurrent back pain following surgical intervention. Though failed back syndrome may be caused by an incomplete or inappropriate procedure (eg, residual disc protrusion, inadequate surgical exposure), it often occurs when surgeries are performed with a more equivocal surgical indication. Surgical interventions for back pain are most effective when there is a specific anatomic deformity with functional correlation, such as spondylolisthesis. However, even in the presence of obvious anatomic structural abnormalities, fusions of spinal segments change the loading of adjacent vertebrae, transmitting stress and strain forces to neighboring vertebrae and propagating symptoms to adjacent nerve root distributions.

Conservative nonsurgical treatment options for back pain are rest, massage, and physical therapy (PT). These options are most effective for mild, local musculoskeletal problems without a neuropathic component (eg, muscular strain/sprain without radiculopathy). Pharmacologic options are tried next: Anti-inflammatory approaches include NSAIDs and corticosteroid therapy (either systemic or via injection). Muscle relaxants are used to relieve the pain associated with muscular spasticity (baclofen), spasm (tizanidine, diazepam), or both (cyclobenzaprine), though their therapeutic profiles may be limited due to their sedative properties. Similarly, the anticonvulsant medication gabapentin is US Food and Drug Administration (FDA) approved for neuropathic pain, though it may not be well tolerated due to significant sedative effects. Opioids may also be used but should be prescribed more sparingly due to their side effect profiles (respiratory depression, constipation) and the potential for tolerance and addiction.

More invasive nonsurgical treatment options are focused on neuromodulation. Patients can undergo directed nerve blocks and/or nerve ablations; however, these procedures may have variable efficacy, have several side effects (eg, numbness in nerve distribution), and are often only temporary. Other newer neuromodulatory therapies include acupuncture, electrical nerve stimulation, and biofeedback, though they are also temporary and confer mixed results.

Sonntag VR, Hadley MN. Surgical approaches to the thoracolumbar spine. *Clin Neurosurg*. 1990;36:168-185.

Traeger A, Buchbinder R, Harris I, Maher C. Diagnosis and management of low-back pain in primary care. *CMAJ*. 2017;189:E1386-E1395.

A.3. What are the major anatomic landmarks of the vertebral column? Where does the spinal cord terminate, and where do the nerve roots exit the spine? What is the blood supply to the spinal cord?

The spine is a complex structure that provides support for the body and houses and protects the spinal cord. The vertebrae of the spine are divided into four sections: cervical (C1-7), thoracic (T1-12), lumbar (L1-5), and sacral (S1-5). Apart from the sacral vertebrae that fuse by adulthood, each vertebra is in articulation with adjacent vertebrae. Further, C2-S1 vertebrae are separated by an intervertebral disc.

The anatomy of a lumbar vertebra is shown in **Figure 58.1**. Except for the atlas (C1) and axis (C2), a vertebra is comprised of a vertebral body anteriorly, a spinous process posteriorly, and transverse processes laterally. The transverse processes are connected to the vertebral bodies via a pair of pedicles and connected to the spinous processes via a pair of laminae. Collectively, the pedicles, laminae, and spinous process form the vertebral arch, and with the vertebral body form a central vertebral foramen. The lumbar vertebral bodies are larger and thicker to support the weight of the body, while the cervical vertebrae have larger vertebral foramina to accommodate the larger diameter of the cervical spinal cord. Notably, the transverse processes of the cervical vertebrae also have foramina that house the vertebral arteries.

Apart from the atlantoaxial joint between C1 and C2, cervical, thoracic, and lumbar vertebrae have intervertebral discs between them that provide cushioning to the spine and help facilitate movement along the spinal column. Further, each vertebra has superior and inferior processes that articulate with adjacent processes, forming the synovial facet joints bilaterally (**Figure 58.1**). The interlocking structure of the individual vertebrae creates bilateral intervertebral foramina.

The spinal cord sits within the vertebral foramen and tapers caudally until it terminates at the conus medullaris at L1-L2 in adults (L3 in children). Caudal to the conus medullaris, the nerve roots of the lumbosacral plexus form the cauda equina. Nerve roots exit the spinal column via the intervertebral foramina: cervical nerve roots C1-C7 exit superior to cervical vertebrae, with C8 exiting between C7 and T1. Thoracic, lumbar, and sacral roots exit inferior to their correspondingly named vertebrae.

The spinal cord is supplied anteriorly by a single anterior spinal arteries and posteriorly by a pair of posterior spinal arteries. The ASA is formed from the bilateral vertebral arteries inferior to the formation

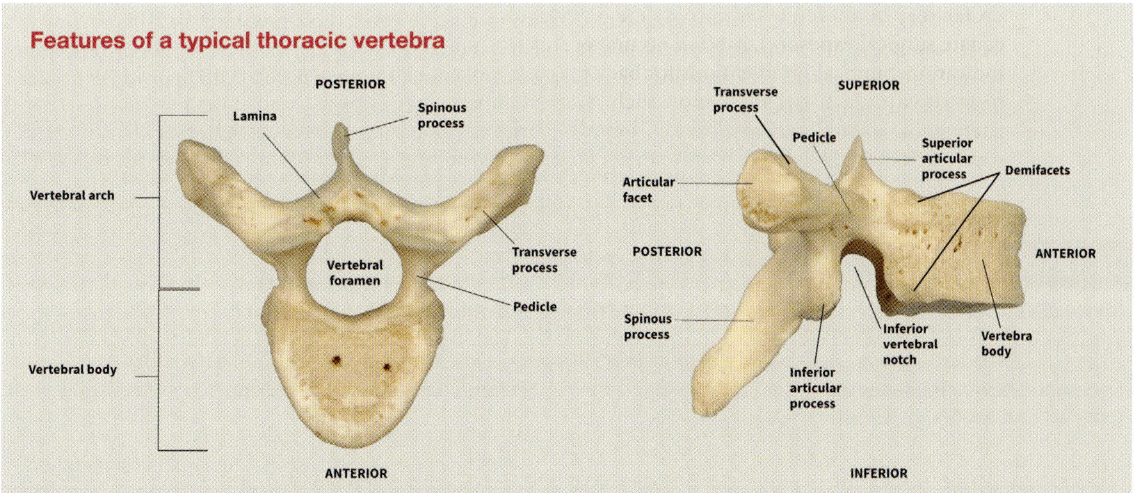

FIGURE 58.1. Anatomy of a typical thoracic vertebra. (Reprinted with permission from Bazira PJ. Clinical applied anatomy of the vertebral column. *Surgery [Oxford]*. 2024;42:355-363. Figure 2.)

of the basilar artery. The PSAs come off directly from the vertebral arteries without joining. Spinal cord blood flow is further augmented by a series of segmental medullary arteries, the most dominant being the artery of Adamkiewicz, which typically arises between T9 and L2.

Bazira PJ. Clinical applied anatomy of the vertebral column. *Surgery (Oxford)*. 2021;39:315-323.

Gerlach R, Seifert V, Espinosa de Rueda Ruiz M, et al. The spine and spinal cord: basics. In: Lumenta CB, Di Rocco C, Haase J, Mooij JJA, eds. *Neurosurgery*. 1st ed. Springer; 2010:339-351.

A.4. How are minor, major, and complex spine surgeries classified?

There is no formal or standardized classification of minor, major, and complex spine surgery. Documented classification schemes in the literature are broadly defined, have overlapping criteria, and can be institution specific. In general, procedures meeting various criteria for major and/or complex surgery are those that involve multiple levels, fusion of multiple vertebrae, reoperations, and multiple approaches (eg, combined anterior/posterior procedures). A risk-based stratification based on the amount of EBL during a procedure is useful for the anesthesiologist, as it can help guide anesthetic and/or resuscitation plans (**Table 58.2**).

Minor spine surgeries are less invasive and carry a low risk of blood loss (EBL < 100 mL). These include small segment (1-2) procedures on intervertebral discs (minimally invasive discectomy, microdiscectomy, nucleoplasty, artificial disc replacement), removal of part or all of the vertebral lamina (laminotomy, laminectomy, cervical laminoplasty), and procedures relieving nerve root impingement as they pass through the intervertebral foramina (foraminotomy, partial or complete facetectomy). These procedures do not require additional stabilization of the spine and thus preserve a range of motion over the involved vertebral segments.

As the number and/or the proportion of the vertebrae removed increase, the spine may need to be stabilized via interbody fusion. In a fusion procedure, the intervertebral disc is removed and replaced with either bone autograft/allograft or an interbody fusion cage, a radiolucent metal or carbon fiber space filled with bone fragments. Compared to bone graft, cages can provide better intervertebral and foraminal height and more effectively contain bone graft. More modern cages can also expand after placement, minimizing the space necessary for cage placement; however, overexpansion may cause recurrence of symptoms. In all cases, the bone fragments help provide a scaffolding matrix for osteogenesis in the intervertebral space, completing the fusion. A variety of screws and rods are placed to immobilize and support the spine while ossification ensues.

Procedures involving interbody fusion are more invasive, require larger surgical fields, and carry an increased risk of intraoperative blood loss. As such, most fusion procedures meet the criteria for major or complex spine surgery (**Table 58.2**). These procedures can be performed via an anterior approach (anterior cervical discectomy and fusion [ACDF], ALIF), a posterior approach (posterior cervical discectomy and fusion [PCDF], posterior lumbar interbody fusion [PLIF]) or with a paramedian or lateral approach (transforaminal interbody fusion [TLIF], extreme lateral interbody fusion [XLIF]). In general, anterior approaches allow for the creation of larger interbody spaces; however, these procedures are in proximity to large vessels and are commonly performed in collaboration with a vascular surgeon. Posterior procedures require cutting through erector spinae muscles and can be much more painful. Both approaches confer a high level of spinal stability.

Chakravarthy VB, Yokoi H, Coughlin DJ, et al. Development and implementation of a comprehensive spine surgery enhanced recovery after surgery protocol: the Cleveland clinic experience. *Neurosurg Focus*. 2019;46:E11.

TABLE 58.2 Classification Scheme for Spine Surgery

Minor (EBL < 100 mL)	Major (EBL 100-1,000 mL)	Complex (EBL > 1,000 mL)
ACDF/PCDF	<3-level ALIF/TLIF/XLIF	Pedicle subtraction osteotomy
Decompression or microdiscectomy without fusion ≤2 levels	≤2-level anterior/posterior fusion	Tumor corpectomy/debulking
		≥3 levels anterior/posterior fusion/instrumentation

ACDF, anterior cervical discectomy and fusion; ALIF, anterior lumbar interbody fusion; EBL, estimated blood loss; PCDF, posterior cervical discectomy and fusion; TLIF, transforaminal lumbar interbody fusion; XLIF, extreme lateral interbody fusion.
Modified from Chakravarthy VB, Yokoi H, Coughlin DJ, et al. Development and implementation of a comprehensive spine surgery enhanced recovery after surgery protocol: the Cleveland clinic experience. *Neurosurg Focus*. 2019;46:E11.

Lenz M, Mohamoud K, Bredow J, et al. Comparison of different approaches in lumbosacral spinal fusion surgery: a systematic review and meta-analysis. *Asian Spine J.* 2022;16:141-149.

Lewandrowski K, Ferrara L, Cheng B. Expandable interbody fusion cages: an editorial on the surgeon's perspective on recent technological advances and their biomechanical implications. *Int J Spine Surg.* 2020;14:S56-S62.

Nunna RS, Khalid S, Chiu R, et al. Anterior vs posterior approach in multilevel cervical spondylotic myelopathy: a nationwide propensity-matched analysis of complications, outcomes, and narcotic use. *Int J Spine Surg.* 2022;16:88-94.

B. Preoperative Evaluation and Preparation

B.1. What aspects of the patient's history and physical exam are most important in formulating your anesthetic plan?

In approaching patients presenting for spine surgery, it is imperative to evaluate baseline neurologic function to formulate an appropriate anesthetic plan and to put the postoperative neurologic exam in context. Here, the patient has had severe prior neurologic injury with autonomic manifestations, contractures and muscle atrophy, and a history of multiple spine procedures concerning for a technically difficult procedure. The patient should undergo a full neurologic assessment, with attention to symptom location, quality, and radiation.

Second, any patient with cervical spinal disease or previous cervical spinal surgery should undergo a detailed airway evaluation, including a careful assessment of neck range of motion that the patient can perform comfortably, eliciting any symptoms at the limits of their range of motion. One must exercise caution to mitigate any neck manipulations beyond these safe limits, which often requires multiple potential plans to manage the airway, including the prospect of an awake fiberoptic intubation or a surgical airway. Note that an awake fiberoptic intubation requires a calm and cooperative patient; it is thus imperative to counsel the patient on the procedure preoperatively and establish expectations.

Lastly, patients presenting for spine surgery commonly have complex pain management regimens, and it is important to understand baseline medication consumption to tailor an anesthetic and analgesic plan. One should conduct a careful history of opioid use, as patients with chronic opioid use will have higher intraoperative and postoperative opioid requirements. Additionally, patients taking medications with sedative properties (eg, baclofen, diazepam, gabapentin) can have lower or higher anesthetic requirements based on their overall level of sedation or tolerance due to these drugs, respectively. Thus, a thorough evaluation of a patient's level of sedation while taking these medications is useful in tailoring an anesthetic plan.

Artime CA, Parotto M, Hagberg CA. Airway management in the adult. In: Gropper MA, ed. *Miller's Anesthesia.* 10th ed. Elsevier; 2025:1227-1266.

Lemkuil BP, Drummond JC, Patel PM, et al. Anesthesia for neurologic surgery and neurointerventions. In: Gropper MA, ed. *Miller's Anesthesia.* 10th ed. Elsevier; 2025:1740-1783.

B.2. What is the pathophysiology of neurogenic bladder/bowel? What conditions can cause neurogenic bladder/bowel?

Normally, the neural control of urination and defecation is provided by multiple coordinated neural circuits in the cerebral cortex, brainstem, and spinal cord. Most caudally, parasympathetic efferents from S2 to S4 stimulate bladder contraction via the pelvic nerves and are responsible for gut motility in the distal colon (the vagus nerve modulates gastrointestinal transit proximal to the transverse colon). Both processes are balanced by sympathetic efferents, originating from T11 to 12 for micturition and T9 to L2 for defecation. Voluntary control of the external urethral sphincter and external anal sphincter is achieved via the pudendal nerve. Patients with spinal cord injuries above S1 will have a variable degree of atonic bladder requiring regular catheterization and bowel incontinence with constipation.

Clinically, neurogenic bladder and bowel are manifest in conditions that impinge sacral nerve roots. Though both are commonly associated with spinal cord injuries, more commonly they arise from nontraumatic causes including multiple sclerosis and cauda equina syndrome due to herniated discs, spinal stenosis, and or mass effect from tumor. Other causes of nontraumatic injury include vascular or infectious etiologies. Neurogenic bladder and bowel can also be seen in patients with moderate to severe Parkinson disease, for which the pathophysiology is related to dystonia of pelvic floor and external anal sphincter muscles.

Bulloch L, Thompson K, Spector L. Cauda equina syndrome. *Orthop Clin North Am.* 2022;53:247-254.

Preziosi G, Emmanuel A. Neurogenic bowel dysfunction: pathophysiology, clinical manifestations and treatment. *Expert Rev Gastroenterol Hepatol.* 2009:3:417-423.

Taweel WA, Seyam R. Neurogenic bladder in spinal cord injury patients. *Res Rep Urol.* 2015;7:85-99.

B.3. What is autonomic hyperreflexia? Is autonomic hyperreflexia a concern in this patient?

Autonomic hyperreflexia is a neurologic disorder that occurs in patients after a spinal cord injury, following the resolution of the initial spinal shock and return of spinal cord reflexes. In this condition, afferent sympathetic impulses below the level of spinal injury are still transmitted to the spinal cord; however, cortical modulation of sympathetic activity is lost. As a result, a painful sensory input (as seen in response to a surgical stimulus) can cause aberrant activation of the sympathetic nervous system below the level of injury, resulting in severe, unmodulated vasoconstriction and hypertension. Above the level of injury, where cortical modulation of sympathetic activity is preserved, the surge of sympathetic activity causes reflex parasympathetic activation, resulting in vasodilation and bradycardia. Treatment for this condition involves alpha-adrenergic antagonists, direct-acting vasodilators (eg, nitroglycerin), and deep general anesthesia (with a minimum alveolar concentration [MAC] sufficient to blunt autonomic responses [MAC-BAR]).

Though autonomic hyperreflexia can be seen in patients with spinal cord lesions as low as T10, it usually occurs in patients with lesions above T7, affecting approximately 85% of patients with lesions above T6. This is because the greater splanchnic ganglion receives innervation from T5 to T9 and can partially blunt the sympathetic response when intact.

Cowan H, Lakra C, Desai M. Autonomic dysreflexia in spinal cord injury. *BMJ*. 2020;371:m3596.

Eldahan KC, Rabchevsky AG. Autonomic dysreflexia after spinal cord injury: systemic pathophysiology and methods of management. *Auton Neurosci*. 2018;209:59-70.

B.4. What aspects of the patient's history and proposed surgical intervention are concerning for potentially large intraoperative blood loss? How would you prepare for potentially large intraoperative blood loss?

The proposed revision of prior major spine surgery spanning multiple levels and an anterior component all raise concerns for potential large-volume blood loss. Revisions of procedures (or "re-ops") are technically challenging due to the amount of scar tissue and/or spinal adhesions in the surgical field. Similarly, the more spinal levels involved, the larger the surgical field will need to be, increasing the potential for vascular injury. In anterior procedures, the iliac arteries are in close proximity to the surgical field, and if injured can produce rapid and catastrophic blood loss.

The potential for large-volume blood loss necessitates a resuscitation-oriented anesthetic plan and a careful discussion with the patient. Multiple, large-bore intravenous (IV) access should be established and verified before surgical start. In cases of difficult IV access, there should be a low threshold to place a large-bore central introducer for resuscitation. An arterial catheter should be placed for real-time hemodynamic monitoring and early identification of coagulopathy. Cell salvage should be utilized if available, and multiple blood products should be in the operating room or immediately available for resuscitation. A thorough discussion with the patient on the need for blood products should take place, identifying individual products (pRBCs, FFP, and platelets) that the patient would agree to receive. Risks and benefits of blood transfusion should be discussed with the patient. If there are significant concerns regarding the patient's ability to tolerate the procedure, it is fair to discuss staging with the surgeon.

Chakravarthy VB, Yokoi H, Coughlin DJ, et al. Development and implementation of a comprehensive spine surgery enhanced recovery after surgery protocol: the Cleveland clinic experience. *Neurosurg Focus*. 2019;46:E11.

Ongaigui C, Fiorda-Diaz J, Dada O, et al. Intraoperative fluid management in patients undergoing spine surgery: a narrative review. *Front Surg*. 2020;7:45.

B.5. How will the details of the surgical procedure influence anesthetic management?

In addition to a resuscitation plan, there are several surgical considerations in major spine surgery, including the need for neuromonitoring, prone positioning and position changes, and limited patient access.

Intraoperative neuromonitoring is commonly utilized in spine surgery. A variety of modalities exist, including evoked potentials, electromyography (EMG), and EEG, which provide a quantitative baseline description of neurologic integrity and can offer consistent, real-time feedback to guide the surgeon during their approach and intervention. Neuromonitoring modalities that assess neuromuscular transmission (MEPs, EMGs) preclude the use of paralysis during monitoring. This can be accomplished using succinylcholine for induction or a single intubation dose of a nondepolarizing neuromuscular blocking agent with subsequent reversal (if necessary). Evoked potentials (MEPs, SSEPs) are degraded in the presence of volatile anesthetics, rendering it difficult to evaluate intraoperative changes in neurologic integrity. To mitigate this problem, total intravenous anesthesia (TIVA) should be employed when patients are receiving evoked potential monitoring, and excessive levels of anesthesia should be avoided.

Care should be taken with positioning the patient (especially while prone) to maintain patency of the airway and avoid compression and neurologic injury. When positioned prone, the neck should be in a neutral position; shoulder bolsters should be placed in a way to preserve adequate space between the chest and chin, keeping the airway free of external pressure. The tracheal tube should be free of kinking, and peak airway pressures should be noted upon prone positioning. The eyes should be free of pressure, and the head should be at or above the level of the heart to avoid visual injury. In cases involving the cervical spine, the head is often fixed in pins, alleviating pressure on the face and allowing the tracheal tube to hang freely; however, one should always ensure that the circuit is not under tension that might dislodge the tracheal tube.

The superposition of surgical, neuromonitoring, and radiographic imaging (ie, fluoroscopy, intraoperative CT) in a prone patient presents several access challenges for the anesthesiologist. Arterial and venous lines should have ample tubing to prevent tension and accidental removal, and line patency should be established regularly and with all position changes.

Bustillo MA, Lien CA, Mack PF, et al. Optimizing patient access during an emergency while using intraoperative computed tomography. *World Neurosurg*. 2019;121:274-278.

Lemkuil BP, Drummond JC, Patel PM, et al. Anesthesia for neurologic surgery and neurointerventions. In: Gropper MA, ed. *Miller's Anesthesia*. 10th ed. Elsevier; 2025:1740-1783.

B.6. How would you counsel the patient for his risk of complications during the procedure?

As with any patient undergoing major spine surgery, in addition to discussing the risks of cardiopulmonary complications, he should be informed of the risk of further neurologic injury at the operative site as well as the occurrence of neurologic symptoms at adjacent spinal levels. The patient can be reassured that these risks are greatly mitigated using intraoperative neuromonitoring and/or intraoperative radiographic guidance. If likely, the possibility of a wake-up test should be discussed with the patient to set expectations, though this discussion should be nuanced to avoid heightening preoperative anxiety. In addition to a discussion about the transfusion of blood products as discussed previously, the patient should be counseled on the need to remain intubated postoperatively in the setting of large-volume resuscitation and prone positioning. Lastly, with prolonged prone positioning, he should be counseled on his potential risk of visual loss, which will be mitigated by good hemodynamic management.

American Society of Anesthesiologists Task Force on Perioperative Visual Loss; North American Neuro-Ophthalmology Society; Society for Neuroscience in Anesthesiology and Critical Care. Practice advisory for perioperative visual loss associated with spine surgery 2019: an updated report by the American Society of Anesthesiologists Task Force on Perioperative Visual Loss, the North American Neuro-Ophthalmology Society, and the Society for Neuroscience in Anesthesiology and Critical Care. *Anesthesiology*. 2019;130:12-30.

Cotter S, Yen A, Fleisher LA. Risk of anesthesia. In: Gropper MA, ed. *Miller's Anesthesia*. 10th ed. Elsevier; 2025: 782-807.

C. Intraoperative Management

C.1. How would you manage this patient's airway?

This patient's previous cervical spinal surgery warrants attention. A thorough airway evaluation is warranted, though the absence of cervical fusion with his C4-6 laminoplasty is reassuring from a neck mobility standpoint. Even with a normal neck exam, videolaryngoscopy is preferred for tracheal intubation, as it offers excellent visualization of the airway with less cervical displacement compared to direct laryngoscopy. If the patient's neck range of motion is severely limited, or if he has a concomitant airway abnormality such as limited mouth opening, fiberoptic intubation should be considered. If there is no concern with the ability to ventilate the patient, a fiberoptic intubation can be performed asleep or with sedation; however, if there are any concerns regarding the ability to ventilate, awake fiberoptic intubation should be performed with a spontaneously breathing patient. Note that awake fiberoptic intubation is also required in patients with unstable cervical spines or in cases where positioning during intubation could potentially cause injury to the spine. If a patient requires awake intubation but is unable to cooperate with the procedure, one can consider a surgical airway in concert with the surgical team.

Bebawy JPF, Hemmer LB, Pasternak JJ. Anesthesia for neurosurgery. In: Cullen BF, Stock CM, Ortega R, et al, eds. *Barash, Cullen and Stoelting's Clinical Anesthesia*, 9th ed. Wolters Kluwer; 2023:979-1002.

Paik H, Park HP. Randomized crossover trial comparing cervical spine motion during tracheal intubation with a Macintosh laryngoscope versus a C-MAC D-blade videolaryngoscope in a simulated immobilized cervical spine. *BMC Anesthesiol.* 2020;20:201.

C.2. How will the surgical considerations affect your anesthetic plan for this patient?

In addition to standard ASA monitoring, the potential for large-volume intraoperative blood loss necessitates a resuscitation plan. The patient should have a baseline Hb/Hct for estimation of transfusion needs, with type and cross-matched pRBCs in the room at the start of surgery. Large-bore IV access should be obtained before surgical start, with a central introducer sheath as backup if peripheral access cannot be obtained. Cell salvage should be discussed with the surgeon and utilized for the case. A postinduction arterial catheter should be placed for hemodynamic monitoring and frequent blood sampling, with a target mean arterial pressure (MAP) greater than 80 mm Hg to preserve spinal cord perfusion.

The need for intraoperative neuromonitoring in this patient will preclude the use of volatile anesthetic and necessitate a TIVA without neuromuscular blockade. EEG is useful for depth-of-anesthesia monitoring for TIVA. Though succinylcholine is preferred during induction, given this patient's long-standing immobility, a nondepolarizing neuromuscular blocking agent such as rocuronium is a better choice to avoid succinylcholine-induced hyperkalemia. The neuromuscular blockade should be fully reversed before neuromonitoring commences.

Positioning this patient can be challenging in the setting of limb contractures, especially in the prone position. Ensure that any bolsters are not compressing soft tissues and that the patient is pressure free from all lines, ports, and wires. The patient might require extra bolsters and support to ensure that pressure points are appropriately padded. Consider a wire-reinforced tracheal tube to prevent kinking while in the prone position; however, if there is a high likelihood of remaining intubated postoperatively with sedation, there is a risk of occlusion with tracheal tube manipulation and patient movement (eg, biting down on tube).

Khan SA, James ML. Anesthetic Considerations. In: Husain AM, ed. *A Practical Approach to Neurophysiologic Intraoperative Monitoring*. 2nd ed. Demos Medical; 2015:76-84.

Ongaigui C, Fiorda-Diaz J, Dada O, et al. Intraoperative fluid management in patients undergoing spine surgery: a narrative review. *Front Surg.* 2020;7:45.

Lemkuil BP, Drummond JC, Patel PM, et al. Anesthesia for neurologic surgery and neurointerventions. In: Gropper MA, ed. *Miller's Anesthesia*. 10th ed. Elsevier; 2025:1740-1783.

C.3. What is your analgesic plan?

Given the patient's history of chronic pain and multimodal pain regimen at baseline, he will likely need higher levels of analgesia in the perioperative period. A multimodal analgesic approach can augment analgesia while limiting his opioid burden.

Despite the utility of a multimodal analgesic plan, opioids remain the mainstay. A long-acting opioid such as methadone given on induction (0.1-0.2 mg/kg bolus for opioid-naive patients; 0.2-0.3 mg/kg bolus for opioid-tolerant patients) will last through the immediate postoperative period. Intraoperative methadone 0.1 to 0.25 mg/kg has been shown to improve pain scores and reduce further opioid consumption for up to 72 hours after surgery in meta-analysis. However, one should be careful not to overdose on methadone, as respiratory depression will be long lasting and could result in the need to administer naloxone or leave the patient intubated (both unfavorable outcomes). The long-acting effects of methadone are well tempered with a short-acting intraoperative agent like remifentanil, which is also beneficial for maintaining a stable plane of anesthesia in the setting of surgical dynamics and neuromonitoring. Alternatively, sufentanil can be used alone as a bolus (induction dose 0.5 μg/kg with 5-10 μg bolus dose as needed) or as part of an infusion (bolus dose 0.2 μg/kg, infusion dose 0.1-0.2 μg/kg/h). Because of the longer duration of action of sufentanil compared to remifentanil, the infusion should be decreased throughout the case and stopped about 1 hour before emergence.

Nonopioid analgesic options include acetaminophen (orally [PO] or IV; ideally patients should receive oral acetaminophen just prior to surgery with intraoperative redosing after 6 hours not to exceed 4,000 mg/d) and subanesthetic ketamine (maximum bolus 0.35 mg/kg with infusion 5-10 μg/kg/min [or 0.5 mg/kg/h]; maximum infusion 1 mg/kg/h). Note that ketamine and methadone may have additive effects, as both are N-methyl D-aspartate (NMDA)-receptor antagonists. A randomized controlled trial of 130 spinal surgery patients given intraoperative methadone with intraoperative and postoperative ketamine infusion *versus* intraoperative methadone alone demonstrated a decrease in opioid requirements at postoperative days 1 to 3 in the methadone and ketamine group. For posterior procedures, erector spinae blocks can further inhibit nociception from dorsal and ventral rami in the affected segments. This is performed by injecting local anesthetic between the transverse process and the erector spinae muscles via ultrasound or anatomic landmarks. Erector spinae blocks are easily learned and safely performed; moreover, they have been shown to reduce opioid consumption and postoperative nausea and vomiting. In patients with complicated pain management regimens, an acute pain consult can be useful, ideally established preoperatively to ensure a good trajectory throughout the postoperative period.

Liu MJ, Zhou XY, Yao YB, et al. Postoperative analgesic efficacy of erector spinae plane block in patients undergoing lumbar spinal surgery: a systematic review and meta-analysis. *Pain Ther*. 2021;10:333-347.

Machado FC, Vieira JE, de Orange FA, et al. Intraoperative methadone reduces pain and opioid consumption in acute postoperative pain: a systematic review and meta-analysis. *Anesth Analg*. 2019;129:1723-1732.

Murphy GS, Avram MJ, Greenberg SB, et al. Perioperative methadone and ketamine for postoperative pain control in spinal surgical patients: a randomized, double-blind, placebo-controlled trial. *Anesthesiology*. 2021;134:697-708.

Schwenk ES, Viscusi ER, Buvanendran A, et al. Consensus guidelines on the use of intravenous ketamine infusions for acute pain management from the American Society of Regional Anesthesia and Pain Medicine, the American Academy of Pain Medicine, and the American Society of Anesthesiologists. *Reg Anesth Pain Med*. 2018;43:456-466.

C.4. What neuromonitoring techniques are used in major spine surgery to minimize neurologic complications? How does the location of the surgical procedure affect the choice of neuromonitoring technique?

Intraoperative neuromonitoring techniques are used in spine surgery to ensure the integrity of neural pathways in the setting of the surgical procedure, which helps guide the surgeon in their approach and helps identify neuronal injury. The major neuromonitoring techniques employed in major and complex spine surgery include evoked potentials or "cord monitoring" (SSEPs, MEPs), EMG, and EEG. Together, neuromonitoring modalities can greatly reduce the risk of neural complications. SSEP monitoring has a sensitivity of 92% and a specificity of 98.9% for identifying neural insults, and MEP monitoring has a sensitivity of up to 100% with a specificity of 97%.

Evoked potentials (SSEPs, MEPs) are utilized in surgical procedures on vertebral segments that house the spinal cord (above L1). SSEPs monitor the integrity of the dorsal (posterior) columns, while MEPs monitor the integrity of the anterior cord. Major and complex spine surgeries commonly have a posterior approach; here, SSEPs are useful because it is the posterior cord that is most exposed and more likely to be compromised. Moreover, SSEPs are safer than MEPs, as direct cortical stimulation for MEPs can cause seizure. However, as discussed earlier, the anterior and posterior cords have separate blood supplies, and the anterior cord is more sensitive to ischemia. Though anterior and posterior injuries often occur in tandem during spine surgery, there are case reports of postoperative limb paralysis in the setting of normal intraoperative SSEPs. Thus, SSEP/MEP monitoring is usually performed together, with appropriate precautions.

Below the termination of the spinal cord (L1-2), there only exist peripheral nerves of the cauda equina. In these cases, EMG can be used to record muscle activation freely via indwelling or surface electrodes. When peripheral nerves are irritated via surgical manipulation, EMG activity of the affected muscle increases, which allows the surgeon to identify and avoid nerve roots during the procedure.

Charalampidis A, Jiang F, Wilson JRF, et al. The use of intraoperative neurophysiological monitoring in spine surgery. *Global Spine J*. 2020;10:104S-114S.

Gonzalez AA, Shilian P. Somatosensory Evoked Potentials. In: Husain AM, ed. *A Practical Approach to Neurophysiologic Intraoperative Monitoring*. 2nd ed. Demos Medical; 2015:18-32.

Gutierrez-Hernandez S, Ritzl EK. Motor Evoked Potentials. In: Husain AM, ed. *A Practical Approach to Neurophysiologic Intraoperative Monitoring*. 2nd ed. Demos Medical; 2015:33-45.

C.5. How are somatosensory evoked potentials (SSEPs) and motor evoked potentials (MEPs) administered? How are they interpreted? What will you see behaviorally during SSEP/MEP monitoring? What additional precautions should you take during MEP monitoring?

For SSEPs, an electrical stimulus is sent to the peripheral nerve, and responses are recorded in the somatosensory cortex (**Figure 58.2**). The amount of current needed to produce an SSEP is low, and the resulting evoked potentials are of low amplitude, so SSEPs are performed frequently during a surgical procedure and are averaged across multiple (50-100) trials for interpretation. In contrast, for MEPs, the

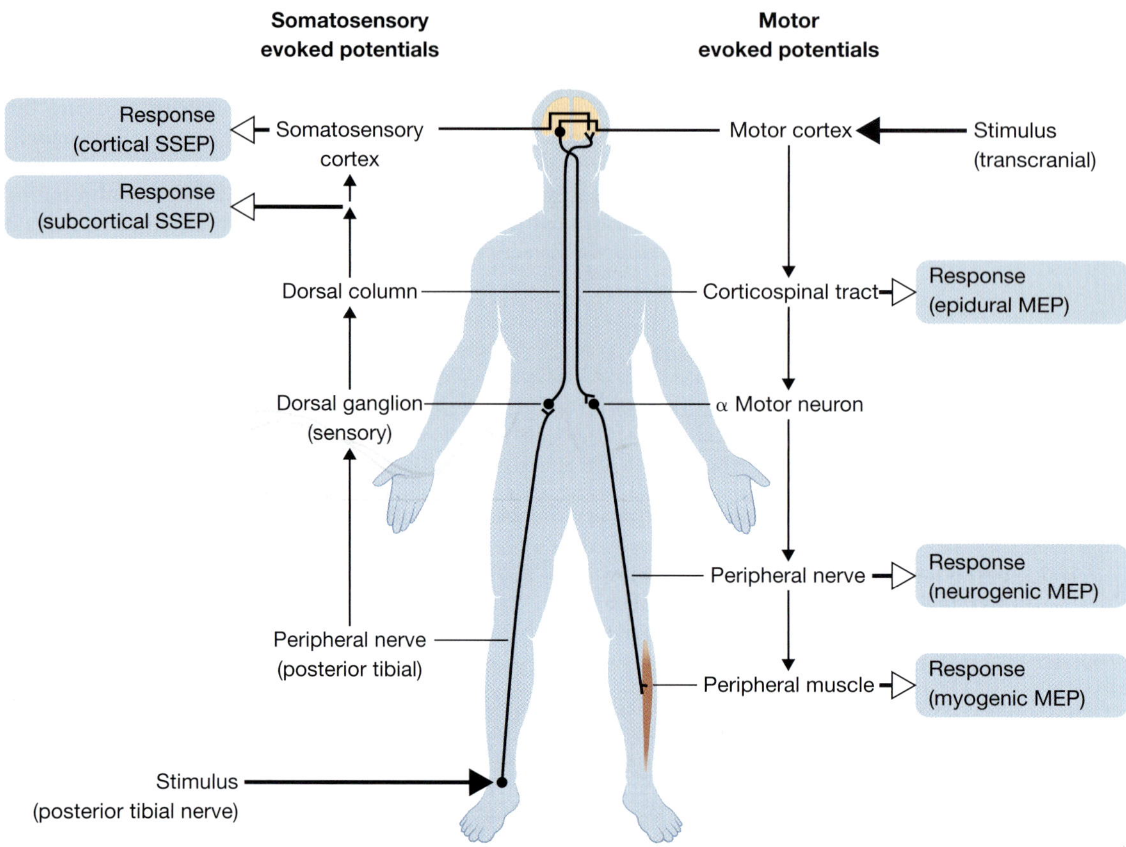

FIGURE 58.2. Outline of pathways involved in somatosensory evoked potential (SSEP) and motor evoked potential (MEP) monitoring. (From de Haan P, Kalkman CJ. Spinal cord monitoring: somatosensory- and motor-evoked potentials. *Anesthesiol Clin North Am.* 2001;19:923-945. Copyright © 2001 Elsevier. With permission.)

motor cortex is directly stimulated from scalp electrodes (or rarely epidural electrodes), and responses are measured in a variety of locations in the periphery (**Figure 58.2**). The broad, direct cortical electrical stimulation can cause aberrant cortical excitation and seizure; EEG is always recorded with cortical MEPs for early seizure identification.

Both SSEPs and MEPs are interpreted in terms of the amplitude and latency of responses from a controlled stimulus. In the case of SSEPs, cortical somatosensory neurons exhibit characteristic waveforms with well-defined positive and negative deflections in response to peripheral stimuli (**Figure 58.3**, bottom trace). The amplitude and latency of these deflections are recorded at baseline, with a decrease in amplitude of greater than 50% or an increase in latency of greater than 10% concerning for neural compromise. For MEPs, cortical stimulation is increased (within safe levels) until peripheral motor responses are observed via indwelling EMG electrodes (**Figure 58.4**). As latency of motoneurons is primarily affected by the degree of myelination, which is not expected to acutely change intraoperatively, the interpretation of MEPs is largely focused on amplitude, with a decrement of greater than 80% representing a clinically significant change.

Behaviorally, during SSEP monitoring, one can observe small distal limb movements (ie, wrist/ankle flexion/extension). This is due to retrograde activation of motor units through mixed peripheral nerves. MEPs are generated from broad cortical activation, behaviorally resulting in whole-body muscular contraction. The most common complication from MEP monitoring is tongue laceration from jaw clenching; thus, it is important to place large, sturdy bite blocks bilaterally to protect the tongue. Seizure from cortical activation is rare but can be detrimental, necessitating EEG monitoring for early identification.

Amlong C, Fallahian W, Becker A, et al. Monitoring techniques: somatosentory-evoked potentials. In: Seubert CN, Balzer JR, eds, *Koht, Sloan, Toleikis's Monitoring the Nervous System for Anesthesiologists and Other Health Care Professionals.* 3rd ed. Springer; 2023:3-19.

TABLE 58.3 Effects of Inhaled and Intravenous Anesthetics on Evoked Potentials

	SSEP		MEP	
Agent	**Latency**	**Amplitude**	**Latency**	**Amplitude**
Inhaled anesthetics				
Isoflurane	↑	↓	↑	↓
Sevoflurane	↑	↓	↑	↓
Desflurane	↑	↓	↑	↓
Nitrous oxide	0	↓	↑	↓
Barbiturates				
Low dose	0	0	↑	↓
High dose	↑	↓	↑	↓
Benzodiazepines	↑	↓	↑	↓
Opioids	↑	↓	0	0
Etomidate	↑	↑	0	0
Propofol	↑	↓	↑	↓
Ketamine	↑	↑	0	0

↑, increase; ↓, decrease; 0, no change; MEP, motor evoked potential; SSEP, somatosensory evoked potential.
Modified with permission from Husain AM, ed. *A Practical Approach to Neurophysiologic Intraoperative Monitoring*. 2nd ed. Demos Medical; 2015.

In addition to anesthetic choice and dose, several other factors can cause a decrement or loss of evoked potentials and should be promptly investigated. Hypotension can result in spinal ischemia and can be due to decreased systemic vascular resistance from medication, blood loss, or inadequate resuscitation. Other causes include hypoxemia due to inadequate oxygen supply (eg, F_{IO_2}) or inadequate oxygen delivery (eg, anemia, alkalosis), poor positioning causing local or regional impingement on peripheral vessels and nerves, or scalp edema.

If spinal monitoring becomes abnormal, all attempts should be made to address the problem and correct the underlying cause. The anesthetic regimen should be checked and optimized to avoid excessive anesthesia; hypotension should be corrected with judicious fluid management and restoration of peripheral vascular resistance; arterial oxygen tension should be optimized and anemia corrected; arterial P_{CO_2} should be normalized and hyperventilation corrected; positioning should be checked to limit pressure points that can compromise peripheral vessels and nerves; and surgeons should investigate surgical causes (eg, distraction).

Khan SA, James ML. Anesthetic Considerations. In: Husain AM, ed. *A Practical Approach to Neurophysiologic Intraoperative Monitoring*. 2nd ed. Demos Medical; 2015:76-84.

Rabai F, Sloan TB, Seubert CN. From techniques to the operating room: general considerations. Optimization of intraoperative neurophysiological monitoring through anesthetic management. In: Seubert CN, Balzer JR, eds. *Koht, Sloan, Toleikis's Monitoring the Nervous System for Anesthesiologists and Other Health Care Professionals*. 3rd ed. Springer; 2023:361-392.

Seubert CN, Sung-Jin Ok M. Neurophysiologic monitoring. In: Gropper MA, ed. *Miller's Anesthesia*. 10th ed. Elsevier; 2025:1099-1132.

C.8. Point-of-care testing at the start of the posterior portion of the case reveals a hemoglobin and hematocrit (Hb/Hct) of 11.1/33. Two hours into the posterior portion, Hb/Hct is 7.8/23. Would you transfuse? What are your thresholds for blood transfusion?

There is no consensus in guiding hemostatic therapies in the setting of major and complex spine surgery. Traditionally, intraoperative transfusion thresholds are set to a goal Hb greater than 7 g/dL, but given the consequences of inadequate spinal perfusion (ie, paresis/paralysis) during spine surgery, it is fair to set a higher Hb goal to avoid spinal ischemia. A meta-analysis of studies investigating transfusion thresholds in spine surgery showed that patients with an intraoperative Hb nadir above 9 g/dL had better postoperative outcomes than those with lower thresholds; indeed, many centers target intraoperative Hb greater than 8 to 8.5 g/dL. Moreover, the resuscitation should be proactive, considering the rate of expected and ongoing blood loss. Notably, lowering MAP to limit blood loss in these scenarios should be discussed and employed sparingly on a case-by-case basis, as the risks of spinal ischemia greatly outweigh the risks of greater blood loss and increased transfusion.

Barrie U, Youssef CA, Pernik MN, et al. Transfusion guidelines in adult spine surgery: a systematic review and critical summary of currently available evidence. *Spine J.* 2022;22:238-248.

Ongaigui C, Fiorda-Diaz J, Dada O, et al. Intraoperative fluid management in patients undergoing spine surgery: a narrative review. *Front Surg.* 2020;7:45.

C.9. Two hours later, estimated blood loss (EBL) is approximately 2 L and the patient has been resuscitated with 3 units of packed red blood cells (pRBCs), 229 mL intraoperative cell salvage (cell saver), and 500 mL albumin in addition to 4 L crystalloid. The surgeon says the field is still "oozy" and there is ongoing blood loss. What are your concerns for resuscitation moving forward? How will you guide your resuscitation?

At this point, the patient has lost roughly 40% of his blood volume, approaching the criteria for massive transfusion (loss of >50% of blood volume in 4 hours). Additionally, his blood loss has been replaced solely with pRBCs and cell salvage without replenishment of plasma and platelets. Though the patient has not yet met the criteria for massive transfusion, he might have a clinically significant coagulopathy with an "oozy" field and ongoing blood loss. Thus, it is necessary to replace other blood components and correct the underlying coagulopathy.

In situations of large blood loss due to trauma, massive transfusion protocols recommend a 1:1:1 ratio for administration of pRBCs:FFP:platelets. A balanced empiric intraoperative administration of 1:1 FFP:pRBCs has been shown to have better 30-day mortality than ratios of 1:2 or 1:4 and has been validated in large randomized clinical trials. Alternatively, more targeted replacement therapy can be useful in situations with less severe blood loss, which can mitigate the risks associated with blood product administration. The mainstay of targeted replacement therapy is to identify coagulopathy and correct it, restoring hemostatic pathways, known as goal-directed therapy. Identification of coagulopathy can be achieved by a panel of laboratory tests (prothrombin time, partial thromboplastin time, platelet count, platelet function assay, fibrinogen level, fibrinolysis assay) or by newer techniques that evaluate clot formation (thromboelastography [TEG], ROTEM). Thrombocytopenia and defects in platelet functioning can be corrected with platelet administration. Broad defects in intrinsic/extrinsic coagulation pathways can be corrected with FFP; coagulation defects believed to be due to vitamin K antagonists (eg, warfarin) can be corrected using two- or three-factor prothrombin complex concentrate (PCC). Inadequate fibrinogen can be replaced by fibrinogen concentrate or cryoprecipitate (which contains fibrinogen, von Willebrand factor, FVIII, and FXIII). Defects in fibrinolysis can be corrected with antifibrinolytic agents, such as TXA or ε-aminocaproic acid (EACA).

Any patient with ongoing bleeding and resuscitation with blood product administration should be monitored for hypocalcemia. pRBCs, FFP, and platelets all contain citrate in their formulations to prevent clotting during storage. Citrate binds calcium ions (clotting factor IV), and free citrate can further bind endogenous calcium stores, causing hypotension via decreased myocardial contractility and decreased systemic vascular resistance.

American Society of Anesthesiologists Task Force on Perioperative Blood Management. Practice guidelines for perioperative blood management: an updated report by the American Society of Anesthesiologists Task Force on Perioperative Blood Management. *Anesthesiology.* 2015;122:241-275.

Holcomb JB, Tilley BC, Baraniuk S, et al. Transfusion of plasma, platelets, and red blood cells in a 1:1:1 vs a 1:1:2 ratio and mortality in patients with severe trauma: the PROPPR randomized clinical trial. *JAMA.* 2015;313:471-482.

Kietaibl S, Ahmed A, Afshari A, et al. Management of severe peri-operative bleeding: guidelines from the European Society of Anaesthesiology and Intensive Care. Second update 2022. *Eur J Anesthesiol.* 2023;40:226-304.

Patil V, Shetmahajan M. Massive transfusion and massive transfusion protocol. *Indian J Anaesth.* 2014;58:590-595.

Wikkelso A, Wetterslev J, Moller AM, et al. Thromboelastography (TEG) or rotational thromboelastometry (ROTEM) to monitor haemostatic treatment in bleeding patients: a systematic review with meta-analysis and trial sequential analysis. *Anaesthesia.* 2017;72:519-531.

C.10. You decide to use rotational thromboelastometry (ROTEM) to guide your resuscitation efforts. After 20 minutes, the results of the ROTEM are normal; however, the field is still bloody. The surgeon suggests tranexamic acid (TXA) for the patient. What is TXA and what is its mechanism of action? Is TXA effective at reducing blood loss in major spine surgery? What are the risks of TXA administration? Is TXA an appropriate choice in this patient?

TXA is a lysine analogue that prevents fibrinolysis by binding to plasminogen and preventing its activation to plasmin. It is the most extensively used antifibrinolytic to reduce bleeding and transfusion requirements in orthopedic surgery, cardiac surgery, and spine surgery.

In 2010, the CRASH-2 trial found that TXA administration in patients with trauma was associated with a reduction in blood loss, transfusion requirements, and 28-day mortality. More recently, in large randomized controlled clinical trials, TXA administration has been shown to reduce mortality in postpartum hemorrhage and to reduce major hemorrhage and transfusion requirements in coronary artery bypass surgery. In major and complex spine surgery, meta-analyses have shown that TXA reduces blood loss (mean difference ~250 mL) and results in higher postoperative Hb concentrations. However, evidence that TXA reduces transfusion requirements in complex spine surgery is inconclusive, which might be due in part to the absence of a single "best" dosing strategy.

Venous thromboembolism (VTE) is the primary risk of therapy with TXA and other fibrinolytics, though rates of VTE and pulmonary embolism were not significantly higher in the CRASH-2 and WOMAN trials. The risks of TXA administration have not been explored extensively in prophylactic and nontraumatic settings. In spine surgery, VTE is unlikely, but only a few studies have specifically investigated thromboembolic events, and these studies had a small sample size with coagulopathy as an exclusion criterion.

There is also concern that TXA might increase the risk of convulsive seizures. As a lysine analogue, TXA can antagonize both γ-aminobutyric acid (GABA) and glycine receptors, decreasing inhibitory neurotransmission and potentially causing cortical hyperexcitability. Similar to VTE, however, seizure is not uniformly reported, and seizure reports range from electrographic seizure on EEG to nonspecific findings such as twitching. Studies reporting increased seizure risk with TXA commonly use high doses (≥100 mg/kg), suggesting a dose-dependent effect, which is corroborated in animal models. As a result, absolute and relative contraindications for TXA based on expert consensus (**Table 58.4**) center on patients who are at increased risk for thromboembolic events or seizures.

This patient might be an appropriate candidate for careful TXA administration with vigilance for adverse events. Though the ROTEM is normal at 20 minutes, hyperfibrinolysis remains a possibility and should be evaluated between 30 and 60 minutes. Further, the patient is actively being transfused, so the potential risks of TXA administration are outweighed by the benefits of mitigating ongoing bleeding in an oozy field. The patient does not have any absolute or relative contraindications to TXA administration.

CRASH-2 Trial Collaborators; Shakur H, Roberts I, et al. Effects of tranexamic acid on death, vascular occlusive events and blood transfusion in trauma patients with significant haemorrhage (CRASH-2): a randomized, placebo-controlled trial. *Lancet*. 2010;376:23-32.

Lecker I, Wang DS, Whissell PD, et al. Tranexamic acid-associated seizures: causes and treatment. *Ann Neurol*. 2016;79:18-26.

Lu VM, Ho YT, Nambiar M, et al. The perioperative efficacy and safety of antifibrinolytics in adult spinal fusion surgery: a systematic review and meta-analysis. *Spine (Phila Pa 1976)*. 2018;43:E949-E958.

Myles PS, Smith JA, Forbes A, et al. Tranexamic acid in patients undergoing coronary-artery surgery. *N Engl J Med*. 2017;376:136-148.

Rahmani R, Singleton A, Fulton Z, Pederson JM, Andreshak T. Tranexamic acid dosing strategies and blood loss reduction in multilevel spine surgery: a systematic review and network meta-analysis: tranexamic acid for multilevel spine surgery. *N Am Spine Soc J*. 2021;8:100086.

WOMAN Trial Collaborators. Effect of early tranexamic acid administration on mortality, hysterectomy, and other morbidities in women with post-partum haemorrhage (WOMAN): an international, randomized, double-blind, placebo-controlled trial. *Lancet*. 2017;389:2105-2116.

C.11. What is transfusion-related acute lung injury (TRALI)? How is it differentiated from transfusion-associated circulatory overload (TACO)?

TRALI is noncardiogenic pulmonary edema that occurs 1 to 6 hours following transfusion of any blood product containing plasma, most commonly platelets. It is clinically indistinguishable from adult acute respiratory distress syndrome, and in intubated patients, it can resemble negative pressure pulmonary

TABLE 58.4 Contraindications to Tranexamic Acid Administration in Spine Surgery

Absolute Contraindications	Relative Contraindications
Preexisting active thromboembolic disorder	Patients at high risk for venous/arterial thrombosis
Disseminated intravascular coagulation/consumptive coagulopathy	Seizure disorder
Renal failure	Renal dysfunction
Coronary or vascular stent placed within past 6 mo-1 y	Preexisting coagulopathy (liver disease, malignancy)
Acute subarachnoid hemorrhage	

edema with copious, pink, and frothy fluid in the endotracheal tube. Although the exact mechanism of TRALI remains unknown, pathologic leukocyte antibodies in donor plasma might cause white blood cell agglutination on pulmonary endothelium, causing increased permeability. Therapy is supportive, and the chest radiograph and arterial oxygen saturation typically return to baseline within 72 hours.

TACO is a result of increased hydrostatic pressure in pulmonary capillaries causing pulmonary edema. The clinical features and radiologic findings are similar, and the two are difficult to distinguish. A thorough understanding of the patient's fluid status, cardiovascular function, and the amount and type of blood products transfused is helpful in identifying the cause.

Alvarez P, Carrasco R, Romero-Kapueto C, et al. (TRALI): current concepts. *Open Respir Med J.* 2015;9:92-96.

Gajic O, Gropper MA, Hubmayr RD. Pulmonary edema after transfusion: how to differentiate transfusion-associated circulatory overload from transfusion-related acute lung injury. *Crit Care Med.* 2006;34:S109-S113.

Skeate RC, Eastlund T. Distinguishing between transfusion related acute lung injury and transfusion associated circulatory overload. *Curr Opin Hematol.* 2007;14:682-687.

D. Postoperative Anesthetic Management

D.1. Hemostasis is achieved, and the surgeon prepares for a staple closure. By this time, the patient has received a total of 7.5 L of Plasma-Lyte, 1 L of albumin, 5 units of pRBCs, 2 units of fresh frozen plasma (FFP), and 229 mL of cell salvage with 1.6 L of urine output. Total case time is 14 hours with a prone time of 10 hours. How would you decide whether to extubate the patient's trachea?

As with any patient, tracheal extubation should only be performed at the end of the case if the patient is in a stable condition and has the ability to protect their airway following extubation. This patient underwent large-volume resuscitation: hemostasis should be achieved and Hb measurements should be stable. These data should be incorporated with any acid-base disturbances or vasopressor requirements to formulate an extubation plan.

Increased capillary permeability from the long surgical and anesthetic time with reduced oncotic pressure from large-volume fluid resuscitation is concerning for laryngeal edema and postextubation airway obstruction. One can assess the potential safety of extubation by performing a cuff leak test. The endotracheal tube cuff is deflated while listening for air movement around the tube when ventilating with positive pressure not to exceed 20 cm H_2O. The presence of breath sounds is reassuring that there is adequate laryngeal opening, though if there are signs of fluid overload and peripheral edema, immediate extubation can be risky, as there can be dynamic fluid shifts in the immediate postoperative period.

Lemkuil BP, Drummond JC, Patel PM, et al. Anesthesia for neurologic surgery and neurointerventions. In: Gropper MA, ed. *Miller's Anesthesia.* 10th ed. Elsevier; 2025:1740-1783.

Ongaigui C, Fiorda-Diaz J, Dada O, et al. Intraoperative fluid management in patients undergoing spine surgery: a narrative review. *Front Surg.* 2020;7:45.

D.2. Given the nature of the case and difficulties in neuromonitoring, the surgeon asks for a wake-up test before supinating the patient and leaving the operating room. How is a wake-up test performed? Are there any contraindications to performing a wake-up test?

A wake-up test is used to assess motor function intraoperatively and is implemented when neuromonitoring techniques are either equivocal or unavailable. The behavioral response provides feedback to the surgeon, and hardware adjustments can be made in real time to improve the patient's motor function. Logistically, the level of anesthesia is reduced to the point where the patient can cooperate and move their extremities on command; however, given the nature of spine surgery, the wake-up test is often performed while the patient is prone, and potentially in head pins. This presents several challenges for the anesthesiologist. High-risk patients should be counseled preoperatively for the possibility of a wake-up test to set expectations and allay anxiety. Analgesia should be ensured to tolerate the presence of the endotracheal tube and any fixation devices. This can be achieved with a short-acting and titratable opioid infusion such as remifentanil. There are no absolute contraindications to performing a wake-up test, but the procedure requires a cooperative and responsive patient, which might not be practical in some settings (eg, trauma, altered mental status).

Bebawy JPF, Hemmer LB, Pasternak JJ. Anesthesia for neurosurgery. In: Cullen BF, Stock CM, Ortega R, et al. eds. *Barash, Cullen and Stoelting's Clinical Anesthesia,* 9th ed. Wolters Kluwer; 2023:979-1002.

D.3. What are the major postoperative complications following spinal surgery, and which patients are at the highest risk?

Spinal cord or nerve root injury is a feared complication of all spine surgeries, with the risk of injury increasing with the number of vertebral levels affected and the technical difficulty of the procedure. Use of neuromonitoring techniques allows for real-time evaluation of intraoperative function and has greatly mitigated this risk, though no modality is both 100% sensitive and specific. The risk of injury is greater if baseline evoked potentials are of poor quality, as it is difficult to assess intraoperative changes in these settings.

Another feared complication of spine surgery is POVL, which has an incidence of 0.03% among all spinal fusion cases. POVL is related to occlusion of blood flow supplying the optic nerve; the regions of the optic nerve that have a comparatively sparse vascular supply are more susceptible to ischemia, especially in the setting of decreased venous drainage. An analysis of 93 spine surgery cases with POVL from the American Society of Anesthesiologists (ASA) showed that posterior ischemic optic neuropathy was more common (60%) than anterior ischemic optic neuropathy (29%) or central retinal artery occlusion (11%). Risk factors for POVL include settings that compromise optic nerve blood flow and increase venous pressure, including prone positioning, direct orbital pressure from positioning devices, prolonged procedures, obesity, high intraoperative blood loss, preoperative anemia, vascular risk factors (previous stroke, carotid artery stenosis), and male sex, though cases of POVL have been documented in the supine position with the head suspended in pins. Interstitial edema from inflammation, capillary leak, and suboptimal fluid management can increase intercapillary distance and further reduce oxygen delivery, increasing the risk of ischemia.

Other rare but severe complications include fat and air embolism, cerebrospinal fluid (CSF) leak from a dural tear, and infection. Fat embolism can be caused by extrusion of marrow or bone fragments into the venous circulation. Dural tears are possible, especially in revision surgery due to scar tissues. Intraoperatively, the surgeon might request a Valsalva maneuver (sustained inspiration at 30-40 cm H_2O) to check for a CSF leak. Infection is possible in all surgical procedures, but can have serious consequences when involving the central nervous system.

American Society of Anesthesiologists Task Force on Perioperative Visual Loss; North American Neuro-Ophthalmology Society; Society for Neuroscience in Anesthesiology and Critical Care. Practice advisory for perioperative visual loss associated with spine surgery 2019: an updated report by the American Society of Anesthesiologists Task Force on Perioperative Visual Loss, the North American Neuro-Ophthalmology Society, and the Society for Neuroscience in Anesthesiology and Critical Care. *Anesthesiology*. 2019;130:12-30.

Nickels TJ, Manlapaz MR, Farag E. Perioperative visual loss after spine surgery. *World J Orthop*. 2014;5:100-106.

Ongaigui C, Fiorda-Diaz J, Dada O, et al. Intraoperative fluid management in patients undergoing spine surgery: a narrative review. *Front Surg*. 2020;7:45.

D.4. What strategies can be used to minimize the risk of postoperative visual loss (POVL)?

The ASA practice advisory recommendations to minimize the risk of POVL center on maintaining adequate ocular perfusion. Baseline blood pressure should be assessed, and systemic blood pressure should be continually monitored in high-risk patients. MAP should be maintained at higher levels in patients who are hypertensive at baseline to prevent end-organ damage. Deliberate hypotension should be avoided if possible and the necessity discussed with the surgeon on a case-by-case basis. Hb/Hct should be periodically monitored in high-risk patients with substantial blood loss, transfusing as deemed appropriate (usually Hb > 8-8.5 g/dL), and using crystalloids and colloids in combination for resuscitation. Though comparative studies are insufficient to evaluate the effects of high-dose adrenergic agonists on POVL, the ASA recommends using adrenergic agonists on a case-by-case basis only when necessary. The patient's head should be higher than the rest of the body when possible to promote venous return, and direct pressure on the eye should be avoided with periodic checking of eye position. Postoperatively, high-risk patients should undergo ophthalmologic assessment, and an urgent ophthalmology consult should be placed if there is any concern regarding potential visual loss. As with intraoperative management, careful optimization of hemodynamic status and oxygen delivery is critical to ensure retinal and optic nerve perfusion and mitigate ischemic events.

American Society of Anesthesiologists Task Force on Perioperative Visual Loss; North American Neuro-Ophthalmology Society; Society for Neuroscience in Anesthesiology and Critical Care. Practice advisory for perioperative visual loss associated with spine surgery 2019: an updated report by the American Society of Anesthesiologists Task Force on Perioperative Visual Loss, the North American Neuro-Ophthalmology Society, and the Society for Neuroscience in Anesthesiology and Critical Care. *Anesthesiology*. 2019;130:12-30.

Nickels TJ, Manlapaz MR, Farag E. Perioperative visual loss after spine surgery. *World J Orthop*. 2014;5:100-106.

Ongaigui C, Fiorda-Diaz J, Dada O, et al. Intraoperative fluid management in patients undergoing spine surgery: a narrative review. *Front Surg*. 2020;7:45.

D.5. What is an ERAS pathway? How has it been applied to the recovery of patients undergoing major spine surgery?

ERAS protocols are a set of evidence-based, multimodal perioperative strategies to mitigate postoperative complications and promote accelerated functional recovery. They are widely employed and encompass several strategies including patient education, prehabilitation, fluid management, multimodal analgesia, and early mobility. Although they are informed by the literature, they are heterogeneous and often institution specific. Several ERAS protocols have been developed for major and complex spine surgery to reduce the protracted recovery period; however, ERAS outcomes data in spine surgery are inconclusive, likely due to the heterogeneity in patient population and protocol specifics. In 2021, the ERAS Society reviewed 22 ERAS items for lumbar fusion to develop consensus guidelines; among these, the Society offered a strong recommendation for 19 elements, though the level of evidence was high for only 9 of these elements. For spine surgery, the elements with high-grade evidence include risk assessment and prophylaxis for postoperative nausea and vomiting, local anesthetic techniques for pain management, maintaining normothermia, allowing clear fluids up to 2 hours before surgical time, administration of a broad-spectrum antibiotic with *Staphylococcus aureus* coverage, and skin preparation with an alcohol-based iodine or chlorhexidine solution.

Debono B, Wainwright TW, Wang MY, et al. Consensus statement for perioperative care in lumbar spinal fusion: Enhanced Recovery After Surgery (ERAS®) Society recommendations. *Spine J*. 2021;21:729-752.

Dietz N, Sharma M, Adams S, et al. Enhanced Recovery After Surgery (ERAS) for spine surgery: a systematic review. *World Neurosurg*. 2019;130:415-426.

D.6. What is the evidence regarding the efficacy and utility of perioperative gabapentinoids, intraoperative methadone, and subanesthetic ketamine in postoperative recovery as recommended in ERAS protocols?

The gabapentinoids gabapentin and pregabalin are structural analogues of GABA that block the α_2-δ subunit of voltage-gated calcium channels and readily cross the blood-brain barrier. They are FDA approved for postherpetic neuralgia and as an adjunct therapy for partial seizures; their use in surgical pain is off-label. Although gabapentinoids have been associated with lower postoperative pain intensity up to 48 hours postoperatively, the observed effects for either gabapentin or pregabalin were not clinically significant. Pregabalin has been shown to reduce 24-hour morphine consumption; however, its use is also associated with serious adverse events, including hospital readmission, prolonged hospital stay, postponed operation due to sedation, stroke, pulmonary embolus, myocardial infarction, pneumonia, bleeding, and death.

Ketamine is an NMDA antagonist that is used as a general anesthetic at high doses (~2 mg/kg IV) and an analgesic at low doses (0.25-1 mg/kg/h). Consensus guidelines from the American Society of Regional Anesthesia and Pain Medicine, the American Academy of Pain Medicine, and the ASA recommend considering subanesthetic ketamine infusions for thoracic, abdominal, and orthopedic surgery (Grade B evidence), with Grade B contraindications including pregnancy and active psychosis and Grade C contraindications including poorly controlled cardiovascular disease, cirrhosis, and elevated intracranial pressure.

Methadone is a racemic opioid: the R enantiomer is a μ-opioid receptor agonist, while the S enantiomer is an NMDA-receptor antagonist. It has a plasma half-life of approximately 35 hours when large (0.2-0.3 mg/kg) doses are administered at anesthetic induction. Methadone also inhibits the reuptake of serotonin and norepinephrine, which can precipitate serotonin syndrome and is contraindicated in patients taking monoamine oxidase inhibitors (MAOIs). In a meta-analysis, methadone reduces total opioid consumption, opioid-related side effects, and postoperative pain scores, and improves patient satisfaction. It is effective and safe in a monitored setting.

Fabritius ML, Strom C, Koyuncu S, et al. Benefit and harm of pregabalin in acute pain treatment: a systematic review with meta-analyses and trial sequential analyses. *Br J Anaesth*. 2017;119:775-791.

Machado FC, Vieira JE, de Orange FA, et al. Intraoperative methadone reduces pain and opioid consumption in acute postoperative pain: a systematic review and meta-analysis. *Anesth Analg*. 2019;129:1723-1732.

Schwenk ES, Viscusi ER, Buvanendran A, et al. Consensus guidelines on the use of intravenous ketamine infusions for acute pain management from the American Society of Regional Anesthesia and Pain Medicine, the American Academy of Pain Medicine, and the American Society of Anesthesiologists. *Reg Anesth Pain Med.* 2018;43(5):456-466.

Verret M, Lauzier F, Zarychanski R, et al. Perioperative use of gabapentinoids for the management of postoperative acute pain: a systematic review and meta-analysis. *Anesthesiology.* 2020;133:265-279.

Acknowledgments

We gratefully acknowledge the contributions of previous edition author(s), Jordan M. Ruby and Victor M. Zayas, as portions of those chapters have been retained in this revision.

59 Hypoxia and Equipment Failure

James B. Eisenkraft and Cesar A. Rodriguez-Diaz

A 68-year-old African American female with a past medical history of hypertension and type 2 diabetes is to undergo an emergency exploratory laparotomy for small bowel obstruction. Breathing supplemental oxygen at 3 L/min via a nasal cannula, her pulse oximeter saturation reading (Spo_2) is 94%. The airway examination reveals a Mallampati 3 view, small (<3 cm) mouth-opening, and limited jaw protrusion. An awake fiberoptic tracheal intubation with topical anesthesia is planned. During the awake intubation, the patient vomited gastric content that was promptly suctioned. After induction of anesthesia, her Spo_2 is 99% on 100% oxygen. About 20 minutes later, the Spo_2 decreases to 85% on the same ventilator settings, with no change in end-tidal carbon dioxide.

A. Medical Disease and Differential Diagnosis

1. What is hypoxia, and what is hypoxemia?
2. What are the general causes of hypoxia?
3. What is the alveolar gas equation?
4. Is the partial pressure of oxygen in arterial blood (Pao_2) related to age?
5. Was this patient hypoxemic before the procedure?
6. What is an A-a difference?
7. What Fio_2 values do a nasal cannula, a facemask, and a nonrebreather mask provide?
8. What is the difference between shunt, ventilation/perfusion ($\dot{V}/\dot{Q}$) mismatch, and dead space?
9. How will you determine whether the hypoxia is due to hypoventilation, $\dot{V}/\dot{Q}$ mismatch, shunt, or impaired alveolar diffusion?
10. What is a pulse oximeter, and what is a hemoximeter?
11. How does a two-wavelength pulse oximeter work?
12. How is a two-wavelength pulse oximeter calibrated?
13. What can affect the accuracy of a two-wavelength pulse oximeter?
14. Does skin pigmentation affect the accuracy of the pulse oximeter?
15. How do the dyshemoglobins, methemoglobin (metHb), and carboxyhemoglobin (Hbco) affect Spo_2 readings?
16. What is the treatment for methemoglobinemia and carboxyhemoglobinemia?
17. What is capnography? Of what value is it in patient monitoring?
18. What is meant by the term end-tidal carbon dioxide ($Etco_2$)?
19. What is the appearance of a normal capnogram, and what is its significance?
20. What are mainstream and sidestream capnometers?
21. Show some common capnograms and provide a differential diagnosis of each event.
22. What is the arterial-end tidal difference in carbon dioxide (CO_2)?
23. What are some of the important safety features of the contemporary anesthesia workstation?
24. What are the common sites for gas leakage?
25. How is the anesthesia machine checked for leaks?

B. Preoperative Evaluation and Preparation

1. What should be included in the equipment checkout in preparation for anesthesia?
2. What emergency equipment should be readily available?

C. Intraoperative Management

1. How should this patient be monitored?
2. After the Spo_2 decreases to 85%, what acute diagnostic and therapeutic interventions would you perform?
3. An arterial blood gas shows a Pao_2 of 250 mm Hg and a hemoglobin saturation (Sao_2) of 85%. How would you treat this?

D. Postoperative Management

1. What criteria would you use for tracheal extubation?
2. Postoperatively, the patient developed hypoxia and pulmonary edema. What is the differential diagnosis of pulmonary edema? What is the most likely cause of pulmonary edema in this patient?
3. How should the ventilator be set if mechanical ventilation is required postoperatively?
4. If this patient had acute respiratory distress syndrome (ARDS) secondary to aspiration, besides low-tidal volume ventilation, what other changes in routine therapy should be considered?
5. What therapies routinely administered by the anesthesiologist can cause acute lung injury?
6. What methods of oxygen administration can be used postoperatively?

A. Medical Disease and Differential Diagnosis

A.1. What is hypoxia, and what is hypoxemia?

Hypoxia is defined as the reduction of oxygen supply to tissue below physiologic levels. Hypoxemia is defined as deficient oxygenation of the blood. From the anesthesiologist's perspective, hypoxia is usually considered to be decreased oxygen tension (Po_2) inside the body at the tissue level or outside the body (eg, hypoxic gas mixture), and hypoxemia is decreased oxygen tension in the arterial blood (Pao_2).

Dorland WAN. *Dorland's Illustrated Medical Dictionary*. 33rd ed. 2019.

Hess DR, Kacmarek RM. Monitoring respiratory function. In: Longnecker DE, Newman MF, Zapol WM, et al, eds. *Anesthesiology*. 3rd ed. McGraw Hill; 2018:411-424.

Hypoxemia vs. hypoxia. *N Engl J Med.* 1966;274:908-909.

A.2. What are the general causes of hypoxia?

Etiologies of hypoxia can be grouped into five major categories:

Hypoxemic Hypoxia: Low oxygen tension in the arterial blood (Pao_2) is due to the inability of the lungs to properly oxygenate the blood. Causes include low-inspired oxygen concentration ($P{\small IO}_2$), hypoventilation, impaired alveolar diffusion, pulmonary shunting, and $\dot{V}/\dot{Q}$ mismatch.

Circulatory Hypoxia: The heart is unable to pump enough blood to meet metabolic demands; therefore, oxygen delivery is impaired.

Demand Hypoxia: Increased metabolic states such as fever or thyrotoxicosis

Anemic Hypoxia: A decrease in oxygen-carrying capacity due to low hemoglobin leading to inadequate oxygen delivery

Histotoxic Hypoxia (Dysoxia): Cells are unable to utilize oxygen effectively. The best example of this is cyanide poisoning, which inhibits the enzyme cytochrome C oxidase in the mitochondria, blocking the use of oxygen to make ATP.

Butterworth JF, Mackey DC, Wasnick JD. Inhalation therapy & mechanical ventilation in the PACU & ICU. In: Butterworth JF, Mackey DC, Wasnick JD, eds. *Morgan & Mikhail's Clinical Anesthesiology*. 7th ed. McGraw Hill; 2022:1359-1382.

A.3. What is the alveolar gas equation?

$$Pao_2 = [(P{\small IO}_2 - PAco_2)/R].$$

For clinical purposes, $Paco_2$ is used as an estimate of $PAco_2$. $P{\small IO}_2$ at sea level is calculated as $F{\small IO}_2 \times$ (atmospheric pressure − water vapor pressure). Water vapor pressure at 37 °C is approximately 47 mm Hg. *R* is the respiratory exchange quotient (ratio of carbon dioxide production to oxygen consumption; a typical value for *R* is 0.8). Thus, a patient breathing room air is estimated to have an alveolar gas partial pressure of $0.21 \times (760 - 47) - 40/0.8 = 99.7$ mm Hg.

The alveolar gas equation is used to estimate alveolar-arterial (A-a) oxygen differences for clinical purposes. Lack of steady-state breathing and the use of an assumed rather than measured R can limit the accuracy of the A-a oxygen difference in clinical situations. The A-a oxygen difference is often inappropriately referred to as a "gradient," thereby incorrectly suggesting that a physical difference in oxygen tension between alveoli and their associated end-capillary blood exists.

Bhakta NR, Kaminsky DA. Pulmonary function testing: physiologic and technical principles. In: Courtney Broaddus V, Ernst JD, King TE Jr, et al, eds. *Murray & Nadel's Textbook of Respiratory Medicine*. 7th ed. Elsevier; 2021:424-438.

David W. Kaczka DW, Chitilian HV, Vidal-Melo MF. Respiratory monitoring. In: Gropper MA, Cohen NH, Eriksson LI, et al, eds. *Miller's Anesthesia*. 10th ed. Elsevier; 2025:1153-1194.

A.4. Is the partial pressure of oxygen in arterial blood (Pao_2) related to age?

Yes. There is an age-dependent decrease in the Pao_2 as described by Sorbini et al for subjects breathing room air:

$$\text{Mean } Pao_2 \text{ in mm Hg} = 109 - 0.43 \text{ (age in years) mm Hg.}$$

About this regression line, there are 95% confidence limits (2 standard deviations [SDs]) of 10 mm Hg.

According to Cerveri et al, Pao_2 in normal nonsmoking subjects aged 40 to 90 years was related to age in subjects between 40 and 74 years with the following reference equation:

$$Pao_2 \text{ (mm Hg)} = 143.6 - (0.39 \times \text{age in years}) - (0.56 \times \text{body mass index [BMI]}) - (0.57 \times Paco_2).$$

For subjects 75 years and older, there was no correlation with age.

Cerveri I, Zoia MC, Fanfulla F, et al. Reference values of arterial oxygen tension in the middle-aged and elderly. *Am J Respir Crit Care Med*. 1995;152:934-941.

Marshall BE, Wyche MQ. Hypoxemia during and after anesthesia. *Anesthesiology*. 1972;37:178-209.

Sorbini CA, Grassi V, Solinas E, et al. Arterial oxygen tension in relation to age in healthy subjects. *Respiration*. 1968;25:3-13.

A.5. Was this patient hypoxemic before the procedure?

No. The Spo_2 reading of 94% does not signify hypoxemia when the age of the patient is taken into consideration. Using Sorbini et al's equation for expected Pao_2:

$$Pao_2 = 109 - (0.43 \times 60) = 83 \text{ mm Hg.}$$

Assuming normal adult hemoglobin, temperature, and pH, this Pao_2 corresponds to a hemoglobin oxygen saturation of approximately 94% on the normal hemoglobin oxygen saturation versus Po_2 curve.

Although the definitions of hypoxemia given in sections A.1 and A.2 must take age into consideration, from a practical point of view, hypoxemia (in the absence of anemia) is generally considered to exist when the Pao_2 is less than 60 mm Hg, which is equivalent to a hemoglobin oxygen saturation of 90%.

Lumb AB. Oxygen. In: Lumb AB. *Nunn's Applied Respiratory Physiology*. 8th ed. Elsevier; 2017:169-202.

A.6. What is an A-a difference?

Given the alveolar gas equation and a correction for age, an estimated Pao_2 for a patient can be calculated. The first step in evaluating the hypoxia is to calculate the A-a difference of oxygen. This is the difference in the amount of oxygen between the alveoli "A" and the amount of oxygen in the arterial blood "a." In other terms, the A-a oxygen difference = $PAo_2 - Pao_2$.

Pao_2 can be obtained from an arterial blood gas analysis. PAo_2 is calculated using the alveolar gas equation:

The A-a difference changes with age, and thus it is corrected for age using this equation:

$$\text{A-a difference} = 2.5 + (0.21 \times \text{age}) \text{ mm Hg.}$$

The current patient would have an expected A-a difference of $2.5 + (0.21 \times 68) = 16.8$ mm Hg.

If the A-a difference is normal, the cause of hypoxia is low oxygen content in the alveoli, either due to low oxygen content in the air (low F_{IO_2}, as in the high altitude) or more commonly due to hypoventilation such as from central nervous system (CNS) depression, obesity, hypoventilation syndrome, or obstructed airways as in an exacerbation of chronic obstructive pulmonary disease (COPD).

If the A-a difference is greater than normal, the cause of hypoxia is either due to a diffusion defect or a perfusion defect ($\dot{V}/\dot{Q}$ mismatch or a shunt). Administration of 100% oxygen can help differentiate the two, as the oxygenation will improve in $\dot{V}/\dot{Q}$ mismatch in contrast to situations where shunt pathology is present.

David W. Kaczka DW, Chitilian HV, Vidal-Melo MF. Respiratory monitoring. In: Gropper MA, Cohen NH, Eriksson LI, et al, eds. *Miller's Anesthesia*. 10th ed. Elsevier; 2025:1153-1194.

Sparling JL, Vidal Melo MF. Pulmonary Pathophysiology and Lung mechanics in Anesthesiology. In: Cohen E, ed. *Cohen's Comprehensive Thoracic Anesthesia*. Elsevier; 2021:66-87.

A.7. What F_{IO_2} values do a nasal cannula, a facemask, and a nonrebreather mask provide?

A nasal cannula delivering oxygen at a flow rate of 6 L/min can provide an F_{IO_2} of up to 45%. Advantages are ease of use, patient comfort, and comfort for the patient. Disadvantages are dry mucous membranes if the oxygen is not humidified and less benefit when the patient is mouth-breathing. The following formula can be used to approximate the F_{IO_2}:

$$F_{IO_2} = 20\% + (4 \text{ times oxygen flow in L/min}).$$

A facemask at an oxygen flow rate of 10 L/min can provide an F_{IO_2} of 50%. Advantages are that it is well tolerated by patients, even when mouth-breathing. Disadvantages include the need for a high flow rate to wash out CO_2, dry mucous membranes if the oxygen is not humidified, and interference with activities such as eating and drinking.

A nonrebreather mask has an attached 500-mL reservoir bag and two one-way valves. At a flow rate of 15 L/min, it can provide an F_{IO_2} of 90%.

Bhakta NR, Kaminsky DA. Pulmonary function testing: physiologic and technical principles. In: Courtney Broaddus V, Ernst JD, King TE Jr, et al, eds. *Murray & Nadel's Textbook of Respiratory Medicine*. 7th ed. Elsevier; 2021:424-438.

A.8. What is the difference between shunt, ventilation/perfusion ($\dot{V}/\dot{Q}$) mismatch, and dead space?

The relative quantity of perfusion and ventilation defines these terms. A normal lung has a small portion in which perfusion and ventilation are perfectly matched. Two extreme conditions exist at either end of the spectrum of perfectly matched perfusion and ventilation: shunt and dead space ventilation.

In a shunt, the alveolus is perfused, but it is not ventilated. The physiologic result is hypoxemia. This is characterized by a failure of the Pa_{O_2} to increase despite an increase in the F_{IO_2}. Hypoxemia caused by small amounts of shunted blood (<20% of cardiac output) is easily overcome by increasing the F_{IO_2}. This is because the blood that is not shunted will contain enough "extra" dissolved oxygen to make up for the deficit that the shunted blood contributes to the combined total blood oxygen content. Once the shunt fraction approaches 0.3 (30%), increasing the F_{IO_2} even to 100% will not be effective in preventing hypoxemia. The term venous admixture is often used synonymously for shunt.

In dead space ventilation, the alveolus is ventilated, but not perfused. The physiologic result is hypercarbia. This is characterized by a failure to maintain a normal Pa_{CO_2} despite an increase in minute ventilation (tidal volume × respiratory rate).

Ventilation/perfusion ($\dot{V}/\dot{Q}$) mismatch is the term applied to any condition that is not a perfect match, complete shunt, or complete dead space ventilation. The physiologic result is a variable combination of hypoxemia and hypercarbia. The resultant degree of hypoxemia and hypercarbia depends on the relative contributions of partial shunt and dead space ventilation.

Lumb AB. Distribution of Pulmonary Ventilation and Perfusion. In: Lumb AB. *Nunn's Applied Respiratory Physiology*. 8th ed. Elsevier; 2017:109-135.

A.9. How will you determine whether the hypoxia is due to hypoventilation, $\dot{V}/\dot{Q}$ mismatch, shunt, or impaired alveolar diffusion?

1. Hypoventilation presents with an increased Pa_{CO_2} with a normal A-a difference.
2. Low-inspired oxygen presents with a normal Pa_{CO_2} plus normal A-a difference.

3. Shunting presents with a normal $Paco_2$ and increased A-a difference that does not correct with the administration of 100% oxygen.
4. $\dot{V}/\dot{Q}$ mismatch presents with a normal $Paco_2$ and increased A-a difference that corrects with administration of 100% oxygen.
5. Impaired alveolar diffusion presents with normal to increased $Paco_2$ and increased A-a difference that modestly improves with administration of 100% oxygen.

Chang M, Horvath R. The postanesthesia care unit. In: Gropper MA, Cohen NH, Eriksson LI, et al, eds. *Miller's Anesthesia*. 10th ed. Elsevier; 2025:2484-2511.

A.10. What is a pulse oximeter, and what is a hemoximeter?

The pulse oximeter is a noninvasive device that provides a real-time estimate (designated the Spo_2%) of arterial hemoglobin saturation with oxygen. It is a transmission oximeter in which the patient's fingertip (or other probe site; eg, earlobe) serves as the path through which light at two different wavelengths is transmitted.

If one requires an accurate determination of the arterial hemoglobin saturation with oxygen, an arterial blood sample must be drawn and analyzed in a laboratory co-oximeter, sometimes called a *hemoximeter*. The laboratory co-oximeter is a transmission oximeter that uses numerous wavelengths of light (eg, the radiometer co-oximeter uses 128 wavelengths of light) to measure total hemoglobin (HbTOT), oxygenated hemoglobin (Hbo_2), deoxygenated ("reduced") hemoglobin (RHb), metHb, Hbco, and other dyshemoglobins, such as sulfhemoglobin. Because each species of hemoglobin has a characteristic absorbance spectrum (absorbance vs wavelength), examination of a blood sample using multiple wavelengths permits identification and quantification of each hemoglobin species. Conventional pulse oximeters use only two wavelengths of light; therefore, they are unable to determine all different hemoglobin species and assume that only Hbo_2 and RHb are present. *Fractional saturation* (*Hbo_2%*) is defined as Hbo_2/(Hbo_2 + RHb + Hbco + metHb), that is, Hbo_2 per total Hb. *Functional saturation (Sao_2)* is defined as Hbo_2/(Hbo_2 + RHb). Note that dyshemoglobins are absent from the denominator in the definition of Sao_2.

Barker SJ. Pulse oximetry. In: Ehrenwerth J, Eisenkraft JB, Berry JM, eds. *Anesthesia Equipment: Principles and Applications*. 3rd ed. Elsevier; 2021:253-270.

A.11. How does a two-wavelength pulse oximeter work?

The pulse oximeter combines spectrophotometry and optical plethysmography. In the pulse oximeter probe, light-emitting diodes transmit red light at a wavelength of 660 nm and infrared light at a wavelength of 940 nm through the fingertip or other probe site. Light that passes through the probe site is sensed by a single photodetector and expressed as absorbance at each wavelength. The spectrophotometric ratio of absorbances 660/940 nm is related to the hemoglobin saturation with oxygen. Detection of pulsatile flow is by optical plethysmography. With each pulse of arterial blood, the probe site (eg, fingertip) increases in volume, the path length of the transmitted light increases, and the absorbance of light at 660 and 940 nm increases. This *pulse-added* absorbance is considered to be due to the pulsatile flow of arterial blood at the probe site, so that the ratio of pulse-added absorbances (660/940 nm) can be used to provide an estimate of hemoglobin oxygen saturation in arterial blood.

Barker SJ. Pulse oximetry. In: Ehrenwerth J, Eisenkraft JB, Berry JM, eds. *Anesthesia Equipment: Principles and Applications*. 3rd ed. Elsevier; 2021:253-270.

Pologe JA. Pulse oximetry: technical aspects of machine design. *Int Anesthesiol Clin*. 1987;25:137-153.

A.12. How is a two-wavelength pulse oximeter calibrated?

Each pulse oximeter manufacturer creates an empiric calibration algorithm based on observations in human volunteers. The algorithm relates the average ratio of pulse-added absorbances at 660 and 990 nm to the actual hemoglobin oxygen saturation in arterial blood samples drawn simultaneously and analyzed in a laboratory hemoximeter. Observations are made with the volunteers breathing varying Fio_2 values so that data for saturations as low as 70% are obtained. The calibration algorithm that is created relates the ratio (R) of pulse-added absorbances at 660 and 990 nm to the laboratory hemoximeter readings of Hbo_2 or Sao_2% (depending on the pulse oximeter manufacturer). The calibration algorithm is then stored in the software of the pulse oximeter as a "lookup" table. Therefore, the pulse oximeter merely measures R, consults its lookup table, and displays the corresponding saturation reading as Spo_2. The pulse oximeter does not actually measure saturation; it infers it from R, and therefore, it predicts what the laboratory hemoximeter would read if an arterial sample drawn at that moment were analyzed.

A high value for R corresponds to a low Spo_2 reading; $R = 1$ corresponds to an Spo_2 reading of 85%, and a low value for R corresponds to a high Spo_2 reading. When the Spo_2 reading is approximately 85%, one should consider the possibility of a spurious reading as a result of the "$R = 1$" phenomenon. This is commonly due to malpositioning of the probe on the fingertip.

The pulse oximeter (Spo_2) reading is usually specified by the manufacturer to have an SD of ±2%. Assuming a normal distribution, for an Spo_2 reading of 96%, there is a 68% likelihood that the true saturation (as measured by a hemoximeter) is 96% ± 2% (±1 SD) and a 95% likelihood that the true saturation is 96% ± 4% (±2 SD).

Guan Z, Baker K, Sandberg WS. Misalignment of disposable pulse oximeter probes results in false saturation readings that influence anesthetic management. *Anesth Analg*. 2009;109:1530-1533.

Kelleher JF, Ruff RH. The penumbra effect: vasomotion-dependent pulse oximeter artifact due to probe malposition. *Anesthesiology*. 1989;71:787-791.

A.13. What can affect the accuracy of a two-wavelength pulse oximeter?

The two-wavelength pulse oximeter is most accurate when the conditions of its clinical use most closely resemble those of its calibration. Spurious readings or failure can occur during patient movement (eg, shivering, peripheral nerve stimulation, "twitching"), intense ambient light (low signal:noise ratio), electrocautery use, administration of intravenous dyes with absorbance peaks at 660 nm (eg, methylene blue), presence of dyshemoglobins (eg, metHb, Hbco, and sulfhemoglobin), certain colors of nail polish, poor pulsatile flow at the probe site (eg, hypotension, vasoconstriction, Raynaud disease), and venous pulsations (eg, tricuspid regurgitation or earlobe placement of the probe in a patient who is in a head-down position).

Improvements in pulse oximetry technology include paradigms to increase the signal:noise ratio, thereby permitting motion artifact reduction and increased sensitivity to pulsatile flow. Modern pulse oximeters have significantly lower failure rates during patient movement (such as in the postanesthesia care unit) and during conditions of low flow (eg, hypothermia).

Barker SJ. Pulse oximetry. In: Ehrenwerth J, Eisenkraft JB, Berry JM, eds. *Anesthesia Equipment: Principles and Applications*. 3rd ed. Elsevier; 2021:253-270.

Barker SJ. "Motion-resistant" pulse oximetry: a comparison of new and old models. *Anesth Analg*. 2002; 95:967-972.

A.14. Does skin pigmentation affect the accuracy of the pulse oximeter?

Poor circulation, certain skin pigmentation, skin thickness, skin temperature, current tobacco use, and use of fingernail polish can affect the ability of a pulse oximeter to predict oxygen saturation accurately. However, it was not until the COVID-19 pandemic that the inaccuracy of pulse oximetry in darker-skinned people drew widespread publicity and attention. In 2020, Sjoding et al reported a comparison of pulse oximetry in self-identified Black and White patients in the critical care setting. The frequency of clinically significant "occult hypoxemia" ($Sao_2 < 88\%$ despite $Spo_2 > 92\%$) was about three times higher in Black (11.4%) than in White (3.6%) patients. In 2021, Wong et al reported the incidence of "hidden hypoxemia" ($Sao_2 < 88\%$ when the $Spo_2 > 88\%$) in self-identified race/ethnicity as Black 6.9%; Hispanic 6.0%; Asian 4.9%; and White 4.9%, which was associated with greater organ dysfunction and higher in-hospital mortality (Black patient mortality 21.1% vs White patient mortality 15.0%). In February 2021, the U.S. Food and Drug Administration (FDA) issued a warning that skin pigmentation and other factors could impact pulse oximeter readings, as these devices were being widely utilized for triage during the COVID-19 pandemic. Therefore, if there is any question about the true hemoglobin saturation in a dark-skinned patient or if the Spo_2 might be unreliable as an estimate of arterial hemoglobin saturation with oxygen, an arterial blood sample should be drawn for analysis and measurement of Sao_2.

Barker SJ, Wilson WC. Racial effects on Masimo pulse oximetry: a laboratory study. *J Clin Monit Comput*. 2023;37:567-574.

Burnett GW, Stannard B, Wax DB, et al. Self-reported race/ethnicity and intraoperative occult hypoxemia: a retrospective cohort study. *Anesthesiology*. 2022;136:688-696.

Gottlieb ER, Ziegler J, Morley K, Rush B, Celi LA. Assessment of racial and ethnic differences in oxygen supplementation among patients in the intensive care unit. *JAMA Intern Med*. 2022;182:849-858.

Henry NR, Hanson AC, Schulte PJ, et al. Disparities in hypoxemia detection by pulse oximetry across self-identified racial groups and associations with clinical outcomes. *Crit Care Med.* 2022;50:204-211.

Sjoding MW, Dickson RP, Iwashyna TJ, Gay SE, Valley TS. Racial bias in pulse oximetry measurement. *N Engl J Med.* 2020;383:2477-2478.

Wong AK, Charpignon M, Kim H, et al. Analysis of discrepancies between pulse oximetry and arterial oxygen saturation measurements by race and ethnicity and association with organ dysfunction and mortality. *JAMA Netw Open.* 2021;4:e2131674.

A.15. How do the dyshemoglobins, methemoglobin (metHb), and carboxyhemoglobin (Hbco) affect Spo_2 readings?

In metHb, iron in the heme moiety is oxidized (such as by dapsone, benzocaine, nitric oxide, and prilocaine) to the Fe^{3+} state from the normal Fe^{2+} state. MetHb cannot carry oxygen and creates a physiologic anemia. The absorbance spectrum for metHb has similar absorbances to light at 660 and 940 nm. Therefore, the more metHb is present, the more R tends toward 1 and the Spo_2 reading toward 85%. In the presence of metHb, the Spo_2 reading overestimates the Hbo_2% and underestimates the Sao_2.

In carbon monoxide (CO) poisoning, CO combines with hemoglobin to create a physiologic hypoxemia. Hbco has a similar absorbance to Hbo_2 at 660 nm but a very low absorbance at 940 nm. In the presence of Hbco, the Spo_2 overestimates Hbo_2% and underestimates functional saturation. Although blood that is poisoned with CO appears "cherry red" to the naked eye, and therefore can look like it is fully saturated with oxygen, the ratio of absorbances at 660 and 940 nm will suggest that the Spo_2 is in the 90s. In a subject breathing an Fio_2 of 100% (when functional saturation is 100%), as the level of Hbco increases, Spo_2 decreases from close to 100% to approximately 91%.

If the presence of dyshemoglobins is suspected, arterial blood must be drawn and analyzed in a laboratory hemoximeter to obtain accurate measurements of saturation.

Pulse oximetry technology continues to evolve. Multiwavelength pulse oximeters, called pulse co-oximeters, are now clinically available. They use more than seven wavelengths of light (Masimo Rainbow SET Pulse CO-Oximetry, Masimo Company), similar to a laboratory hemoximeter. This technology makes it possible to estimate carboxyhemoglobin (Spco), methemoglobin (SpMet), and total hemoglobin (SpHbt), all noninvasively and in real time.

Although continuous noninvasive total hemoglobin measurement provides information in real time, it can have a wide limit of agreement when compared to traditional invasive laboratory measurements. Thus, patients who have low SpHbTOT on a noninvasive monitor should have confirmation by sending a blood sample to the laboratory for analysis.

Barker SJ, Curry J, Redford D, et al. Measurement of carboxyhemoglobin and methemoglobin by pulse oximetry: a human volunteer study. *Anesthesiology.* 2006;105:892-897.

Kim SH, Lilot M, Murphy LS, et al. Accuracy of continuous noninvasive hemoglobin monitoring: a systematic review and meta-analysis. *Anesth Analg.* 2014;119:332-346.

Miller RD, Ward TA, Shiboski SC, et al. A comparison of three methods of hemoglobin monitoring in patients undergoing spine surgery. *Anesth Analg.* 2011;112:858-863.

Shamir MY, Avramovich A, Smaka T. The current status of continuous noninvasive measurement of total, carboxy, and methemoglobin concentration. *Anesth Analg.* 2012;114:972-978.

A.16. What is the treatment for methemoglobinemia and carboxyhemoglobinemia?

Methemoglobinemia

The normal erythrocyte maintains methemoglobin levels at 1% or less by the methemoglobin reductase enzyme system. The methemoglobin oxyhemoglobin dissociation curve is shifted markedly to the left, and it therefore delivers little oxygen to the tissues. Methemoglobin levels less than 30% of total Hb content can cause no compromise in tissue oxygenation. However, levels between 30% and 50% cause symptoms and signs of oxygen deprivation, and levels greater than 50% can result in coma and death.

It is recommended that patients who cannot tolerate a reduction in oxygen-carrying capacity be treated when methemoglobin levels reach 10%, regardless of the presence or absence of symptoms. Treatment entails withdrawal of the causative agent, supportive treatment, and intravenous methylene blue at a dose of 1 to 2 mg/kg infused over 3 to 5 minutes. A single treatment is usually effective but might need to be repeated after 30 minutes. Methylene blue acts through the methemoglobin reductase system and requires the activity of glucose-6-phosphate dehydrogenase (G6PD). Patients who are G6PD deficient and patients severely affected by methemoglobin might require an exchange transfusion. Increasing levels of methemoglobin cause the two-wavelength pulse oximeter reading to trend toward 85%. Administration of methylene blue causes a spuriously low Spo_2 reading because it absorbs light at 660 nm. Thus, the Spo_2 reading that is low due to methemoglobin transiently decreases further as the methemoglobin percentage decreases and methylene blue is diluted and excreted.

Carboxyhemoglobinemia

Carboxyhemoglobin level is normally between 0% and 10% in heavy smokers. At 10% to 20%, symptoms of nausea and headache are present. At 20% to 30%, drowsiness and lethargy are experienced. Levels greater than 50% are fatal. Treatment is stopping exposure to CO and administration of 100% oxygen with a nonrebreather facemask, which displaces CO from hemoglobin much faster than atmospheric oxygen. The half-life of Hbco is 4 to 6 hours when patients are breathing room air and 1 hour at an F_{IO_2} of 1. Hyperbaric oxygen can reduce the half-life of carboxyhemoglobin to 23 minutes. Patients with carboxyhemoglobin levels greater than 25% to 30% have had clinically significant exposure to combustion products and should be mechanically ventilated. Hyperbaric oxygen is recommended for patients with carboxyhemoglobin levels greater than 40%, myocardial ischemia, cardiac dysrhythmias, or central neurologic abnormalities. Hyperbaric oxygen is also recommended for pregnant patients and young children with carboxyhemoglobin levels greater than or equal to 15%.

Feiner JR, Rollins MD, Sall J, Eilers H, Au P, Bickler PE. Accuracy of carboxyhemoglobin detection by pulse CO-oximetry during hypoxemia. *Anesth Analg*. 2013;117:847.

Oprea AD. Hematologic disorders. In: Hines RL, Jones SB, eds. *Stoelting's Anesthesia and Co-existing Disease*. 8th ed. Elsevier; 2022:465-496.

A.17. What is capnography? Of what value is it in patient monitoring?

A capnometer is a device that measures the tension of CO_2 in units of millimeters of mercury (mm Hg) or kilopascals (kPa), or concentration in volume%, in the gas in the vicinity of the patient's airway throughout the respiratory cycle. Capnography is the graphic display of the CO_2 concentration on the y-axis against time on the x-axis.

Capnometry may be achieved using different technologies that can monitor CO_2. Most capnometers now use infrared spectroscopy to measure the Pco_2 (ie, CO_2 partial pressure in mm Hg). A built-in barometer measures barometric pressure (P_B) so that CO_2 can also be displayed as a percentage ($Pco_2 \times 100/P_B = \%CO_2$).

Capnography is one of the American Society of Anesthesiologists' standards for basic anesthetic monitoring (ie, "Continual monitoring for the presence of expired CO_2 shall be performed unless invalidated by the nature of the patient, procedure or equipment."). It is the "gold standard" for establishing the presence of ventilation.

American Society of Anesthesiologists. Standards for basic anesthetic monitoring. American Society of Anesthesiologists; Published 2010. Last affirmed December 13, 2020. Accessed April 25, 2025. https://www.asahq.org/standards-and-practice-parameters/standards-for-basic-anesthetic-monitoring

Gravenstein N, Jaffe MB. Capnography. In: Ehrenwerth J, Eisenkraft JB, Berry JM, eds. *Anesthesia Equipment: Principles and Applications*. 3rd ed. Elsevier; 2021:239-252.

A.18. What is meant by the term end-tidal carbon dioxide ($Etco_2$)?

$Etco_2$ is the concentration of CO_2 in the exhaled gas at the end of an exhalation, usually displayed in units of mm Hg. Because this gas originates from the alveoli, it is considered to represent the CO_2 tension in the alveolar gas ($Paco_2$). The $PETco_2$ results from the combination of gases coming from ideal alveoli, where ventilation and perfusion are perfectly matched and the CO_2 concentration is the same as arterial ($Paco_2$) and alveolar dead space (alveoli that are ventilated but not perfused) where CO_2 concentration is the same as inspired (P_{ICO_2}) and is normally zero.

The presence of a normal capnogram and $Etco_2$ depends on (1) the production of CO_2 by the tissues, (2) cardiac output and pulmonary blood flow to carry CO_2 to the lungs, and (3) ventilation. Monitoring of $Etco_2$ can be used to adjust mechanical ventilation and monitor ventilation as well as to detect ventilator malfunctions and breathing system problems, such as leaks, incompetent unidirectional valves, exhausted CO_2 absorbent, metabolic problems (eg, malignant hyperthermia), and gas embolism.

Gravenstein N, Jaffe MB. Capnography. In: Ehrenwerth J, Eisenkraft JB, Berry JM, eds. *Anesthesia Equipment: Principles and Applications*. 3rd ed. Elsevier; 2021:239-252.

Lumb AB. Carbon Dioxide. In: Lumb AB. *Nunn's Applied Respiratory Physiology*. 8th ed. Elsevier; 2017:151-167.

A.19. What is the appearance of a normal capnogram, and what is its significance?

A typical normal capnogram (Pco_2 vs time) is shown in **Figure 59.1**. Four phases have been described. *Phase I.* This is the expiratory baseline. During exhalation, CO_2-free gas from the mechanical (apparatus) dead space (eg, flexible or "goose-neck" connector) and anatomic dead space (large conducting airways) flows past the CO_2 sampling port.

Phase II. This is the expiratory upstroke. It is due to CO_2 from alveoli mixed with anatomic dead space gas passing the gas sampling port and is usually a steep upslope.

Phase III. This is the expiratory or alveolar plateau and is due to alveolar CO_2.

In patients with healthy lungs, it is nearly horizontal, but in patients with obstructive airway disease, there is a more pronounced upward slope. The maximum expired CO_2 is usually considered as the $Etco_2$.

Phase IV. This is the inspiratory downstroke. During the commencement of inspiration, fresh (ie, CO_2-free) gas is inhaled past the sensor, and the capnogram falls sharply to baseline.

The angle between the upstroke of phase II and the plateau of phase III is referred to as the α *angle*. The angle between phases III and IV is the β *angle*. An increase in the α angle and slope of phase III is seen commonly in acute bronchospasm. The angle usually decreases with the treatment of the bronchospasm.

Gravenstein N, Jaffe MB. Capnography. In: Ehrenwerth J, Eisenkraft JB, Berry JM, eds. *Anesthesia Equipment: Principles and Applications*. 3rd ed. Elsevier; 2021:239-252.

Lumb AB. Carbon Dioxide. In: Lumb AB. *Nunn's Applied Respiratory Physiology*. 8th ed. Elsevier; 2017:151-167.

A.20. What are mainstream and sidestream capnometers?

In a mainstream or nondiverting capnometer, the gas analyzer sensor is brought to the airway itself, and no gas is removed from the breathing system. A cuvette with a quartz window is placed between the breathing system Y-piece and the tracheal tube connector. As respired gases flow past the window in the cuvette, a beam of infrared light (wavelength 4.3 μm) is directed through the window, and absorbance at 4.3 μm is used to measure Pco_2. Advantages of the nondiverting analyzer are rapid response time, accurate waveform, and no need to scavenge gases. Disadvantages are that this additional device in the airway can be a site for a disconnect, needs sterilization (or replacement of a disposable single-use cuvette) between cases, needs to be heated because water vapor condensing on the window causes error, and can be blocked by secretions or blood on its window.

A sidestream or diverting gas analyzer aspirates gas from the breathing circuit through a sampling adapter placed by the airway. The sampled gas passes through a sampling catheter (usually 6-10 ft in length) to reach the gas analyzer. Advantages of diverting analyzers are that the breathing circuit adapter is disposable. The analyzer, being remote from the airway, can be more versatile and incorporate several technologies in one "box" to analyze multiple gases (eg, infrared analysis for CO_2, nitrous oxide, anesthetic agents; paramagnetic sensor or fuel cell for oxygen). Disadvantages of sidestream sampling analysis are slower response times, the possibility of sampling leaks, errors resulting from the length of the gas

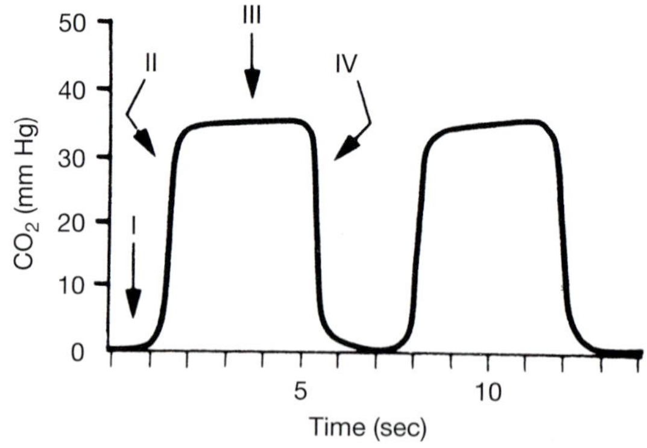

FIGURE 59.1. Phases of the normal capnogram. (*Phase I*) Inspiratory baseline. (*Phase II*) Expiratory upstroke. (*Phase III*) Expiratory plateau. (*Phase IV*) Inspiratory downstroke.

sampling tube, the need to scavenge gases from the analyzer after analysis, and susceptibility of the sampling tube to becoming clogged by water or secretions. Because of their versatility in regard to gas monitoring, most anesthetizing locations now use sidestream sampling analyzers.

Jaffe MB, Eisenkraft JB, Orr J. Respiratory gas monitoring. In: Ehrenwerth J, Eisenkraft JB, Berry JM, eds. *Anesthesia Equipment: Principles and Applications*. 3rd ed. Elsevier; 2021:195-217.

A.21. Show some common capnograms and provide a differential diagnosis of each event.

Elevated baseline equals the amount of CO_2 present in inspired gas (**Figure 59.2A**).

- Capnometer not properly calibrated to zero
- Delivery of CO_2 to breathing system through fresh gas inflow
- Incompetent unidirectional valves
- Failure of CO_2 absorber (channeling, exhaustion, bypass)

Prolonged expiratory plateau and expiratory upstroke (**Figure 59.2B**)

- Mechanical obstruction to exhalation
- COPD
- Bronchospasm

Dips in expiratory plateau (**Figure 59.2C[1]**)

- Patient making spontaneous inspiratory effort
- "Curare cleft"

Cardiogenic oscillations if synchronized with electrocardiogram (**Figure 59.2C[2]**)

- Ventilator pressure relief valve perturbations

Elevated expiratory plateau (**Figure 59.2D**)

- Incorrect calibration
- Increased CO_2 production/delivery versus laparoscopic CO_2 gas insufflation
- Decreased CO_2 removal
- Hypoventilation
- Leak

Decreased expiratory plateau (**Figure 59.2E**)

- Incorrect calibration

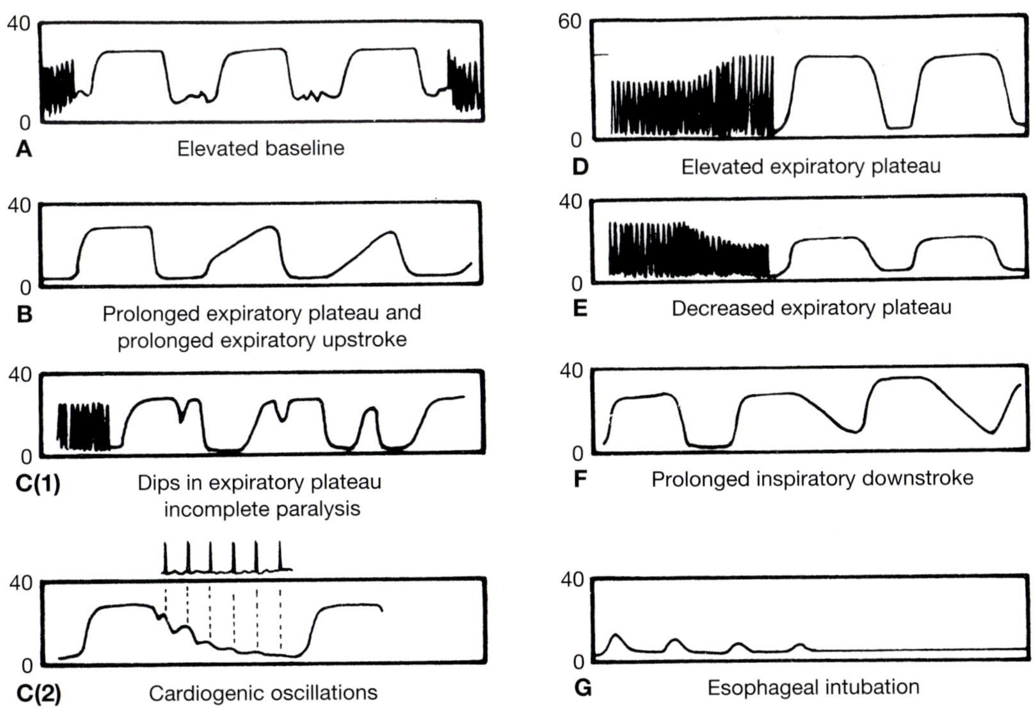

FIGURE 59.2. Abnormal capnograms.

- Air leak into gas sampling system
- Hyperventilation
- Decreased CO_2 production (hypothermia)
- Increased arterial-alveolar CO_2 gradient (ventilation/perfusion mismatch pulmonary embolus)

Prolonged inspiratory downstroke and raised baseline (**Figure 59.2F**)

- Incompetent or missing inspiratory unidirectional valve
- Inspiratory obstruction to gas flow (eg, kinked tracheal tube)

Esophageal intubation (**Figure 59.2G**)

- As CO_2 that has been insufflated into the stomach during bag-mask ventilation or produced as a result of ingestion of a carbonated beverage is washed out during esophageal ventilation, the CO_2 waveform disappears within a few breaths.

Berry JM, Eisenkraft JB. Monitoring ventilation. In: Ehrenwerth J, Eisenkraft JB, Berry JM, eds. *Anesthesia Equipment: Principles and Applications*. 3rd ed. Elsevier; 2021:239-252.

A.22. What is the arterial-end tidal difference in carbon dioxide (CO_2)?

The arterial-alveolar difference in CO_2 is usually expressed as the difference between the arterial and $Etco_2$ tensions. In an ideal alveolus, the $Paco_2$ equals the $PAco_2$ and the $Paco_2$-$PAco_2$ difference is zero. Ventilation of unperfused alveoli leads to alveolar dead space or wasted alveolar ventilation. Because the $Etco_2$ comprises gas from both ideal and dead space alveoli, the $Paco_2$-$PAco_2$ difference is a measure of alveolar dead space ventilation. For example,

$$\text{Tidal volume} = 500 \text{ mL, anatomic dead space} = 150 \text{ mL}$$

$$Paco_2 = 40 \text{ mm Hg, } Etco_2 = 36 \text{ mm Hg}$$

$$\text{Alveolar tidal volume} = (500 - 150) = 350 \text{ mL}$$

$$\text{Ratio of (alveolar dead space/alveolar tidal volume)} = (Paco_2 - Etco_2)/Paco_2 = (40 - 36)/40 = 10\%$$

Therefore, 350 mL × 10% = 35 mL of wasted ventilation from each alveolar tidal volume.
Ideal alveolar ventilation = (350 − 35) = 315 mL per breath.
In this example, physiologic dead space = anatomic + alveolar = 150 + 35 = 185 mL per breath.
Physiologic dead space/tidal volume = 185/500 = 37%.

Therefore, $Paco_2$-$Etco_2$ measures alveolar dead space ventilation as a percentage of total *alveolar* ventilation. The alveolar dead space is increased by ventilation in excess of perfusion or a decrease in perfusion, such as occurs with pulmonary embolism. Shunt has minimal effect on the $Paco_2$-$Etco_2$ difference.

The $Paco_2$-$Etco_2$ difference is normally 3 to 5 mm Hg in the patient under general anesthesia, but it is not constant. Therefore, although one commonly uses $Etco_2$ to noninvasively estimate $Paco_2$, only analysis of an arterial blood sample in a blood gas analyzer can provide an accurate measure of $Paco_2$, and this should be measured when knowledge of it is critical, such as during neurosurgical anesthesia.

Lumb AB. Carbon Dioxide. In: Lumb AB. *Nunn's Applied Respiratory Physiology*. 8th ed. Elsevier; 2017:151-167.

A.23. What are some of the important safety features of the contemporary anesthesia workstation?

Because most problems with anesthesia machines are due to user error, safety design of the contemporary workstation is at four levels.

Features Intended to Prevent Human Error

The medical gas pin index and diameter index safety systems ensure that medical gas connections are made correctly. Therefore, one cannot attach a nitrous oxide cylinder to an oxygen hanger yoke or connect a nitrous oxide hose to the oxygen pipeline inlet of the machine.

The "fail-safe" valve is a pressure-sensitive device that interrupts flow of all hypoxic gases on the machine to their flow control valves if the supply pressure of oxygen in the intermediate-pressure system (ie, components downstream of the first stage oxygen regulator that reduces the high pressure in the tank to 45 lb psi, and upstream of the oxygen flow control needle valve) falls below a threshold (~20 psi in GE machines; 12 psig in Dräger machines).

When the pressure of oxygen in the intermediate-pressure system falls below 30 psig, an oxygen supply pressure failure alarm is annunciated. In older machines, the oxygen flow control knob is "touch coded"; that is, it is fluted and larger in diameter than the other gas flow control knobs and is normally located on the right of all other gas flow control valves. In the Dräger Fabius GS workstation, the gas flow controls are arranged vertically, with the oxygen flow control knob as the lowest. Modern anesthesia machines are fully electronic with integrated alarms.

Key-fill systems for anesthesia vaporizers are safety features that also decrease the likelihood of atmospheric contamination during vaporizer filling. The most important of such systems is the Safe-T-Fill system used on desflurane bottles and desflurane vaporizers because filling a vaporizer specific for another agent with desflurane could result in a lethal overdose of desflurane.

A pressure relief valve built into the machine's common gas outlet, breathing system, or ventilator provides some protection against positive pressure barotrauma.

Features to Correct for User Error

Gas flow proportioning systems ensure a minimum oxygen concentration of 25% when nitrous oxide and oxygen are being used. Therefore, if the anesthesiologist were to accidentally attempt to increase the flow of nitrous oxide, either the oxygen flow would be increased automatically or the flow of nitrous oxide would be limited according to the flow of oxygen that was set.

On older machines, during use of the anesthesia ventilator, changes in fresh gas flow, inspiratory-expiratory (I:E) ratio, or respiratory rate result in changes in delivered tidal volume that might result in overventilation, underventilation, or even barotrauma. On modern systems (eg, GE workstations that incorporate a ventilator with the Smart Vent feature; Dräger Fabius GS, and Dräger Apollo workstations), once the ventilation parameters have been set, they are maintained because the ventilator or circuit automatically compensates for changes in fresh gas flow. In the GE workstations with Smart Vent, tidal volume is monitored continually by a computer. If the measured tidal volume changes from that set to be delivered, the computer adjusts the volume delivered by the ventilator bellows. Dräger workstations use fresh gas decoupling to maintain a constant tidal volume. In this system, during the inspiratory phase, a decoupling valve closes so that fresh gas entering the breathing system is directed into the reservoir bag and only gas from the ventilator is delivered to the patient. During exhalation, the ventilator chamber refills from the fresh gas flow and the fresh gas that was collected in the reservoir bag during the previous inspiration.

A vaporizer interlock system prevents the unintentional simultaneous use of more than one vaporizer.

Monitoring Systems

A monitor of oxygen in the gas delivered to the patient is always enabled, and the low oxygen concentration alarm is activated whenever the anesthesia workstation is capable of delivering an anesthetic gas mixture into the breathing system. Other monitors in the anesthesia workstation include pressure, volume, flow, and gas composition. Some also incorporate airway gas flow monitoring. The breathing system low-pressure monitor alarm is automatically enabled when the ventilator is turned on.

Alarm Systems

Contemporary workstations incorporate an integrated prioritized alarm system with visible and audible alerts when set parameter limits are exceeded.

An important safety feature of all modern machines/workstations is the checkout prior to its use. In 1993, FDA published anesthesia apparatus checkout recommendations. The machine should be checked by an educated user. Item 1 on the FDA checklist is that an alternative means to ventilate the patient's lungs should be present and functioning. If a problem arises with the machine, the patient's lungs can be ventilated using a self-inflating resuscitation bag (eg, Ambu bag). If a machine problem arises and the cause and remedy are not immediately obvious, one should instinctively reach for the self-inflating resuscitation bag and call for help. A recent analysis of the American Society of Anesthesiologists Closed Claims Project data found that 35% of adverse outcomes were likely preventable if a proper prior checkout had been performed.

In 2008, recognizing that not all of the FDA 1993 checkout recommendations can be applied to many of the contemporary anesthesia workstations, the American Society of Anesthesiologists published guidelines applicable to all anesthesia delivery systems so that individual departments can develop their own workstation-specific preanesthesia checkout that can be performed consistently and expeditiously. The 2008 guidelines are intended to provide a template for developing checkout procedures that are appropriate for each individual anesthesia machine design and practice setting. They discuss which systems and components should be checked, the checkout interval (eg, before first case vs before every case), and who is responsible for performing each checkout procedure: the anesthesiologist, other anesthesia provider, or technician (**Table 59.1**).

Feldman JM, Olympio MA, Martin D, Striker A. New guidelines available for pre-anesthesia checkout. APSF Newsletter. 2008;23. https://www.apsf.org/article/new-guidelines-available-for-pre-anesthesia-checkout/

Goyal VK, Venticinque S. Machine checkout and quality assurance. In: Ehrenwerth J, Eisenkraft JB, Berry JM, eds. *Anesthesia Equipment: Principles and Applications*. 3rd ed. Elsevier; 559-583.

TABLE 59.1 Preanesthesia Equipment Checkout Procedures

To Be Completed Daily		Responsible Party
Item to Be Completed		
Item 1	Verify auxiliary oxygen cylinder and self-inflating manual ventilation device are available and functioning.	Provider and Tech
Item 2	Verify patient suction is adequate to clear the airway.	Provider and Tech
Item 3	Turn on anesthesia delivery system and confirm that AC power is available.	Provider and Tech
Item 4	Verify availability of required monitors, including alarms.	Provider and Tech
Item 5	Verify that pressure is adequate on the spare oxygen cylinder mounted on the anesthesia machine.	Provider and Tech
Item 6	Verify that the piped gas pressures are ≥50 psi.	Provider and Tech
Item 7	Verify that vaporizers are adequately filled and, if applicable, that the filler ports are tightly closed.	Provider and Tech
Item 8	Verify that there are no leaks in the gas supply lines between the flowmeters and the common gas outlet.	Provider and Tech
Item 9	Test scavenging system function.	Provider and Tech
Item 10	Calibrate, or verify calibration of, the oxygen. Monitor and check the low oxygen alarm.	Provider and Tech
Item 11	Verify carbon dioxide absorbent is not exhausted.	Provider and Tech
Item 12	Breathing system pressure and leak testing	Provider and Tech
Item 13	Verify that gas flows properly through the breathing circuit during both inspiration and exhalation.	Provider and Tech
Item 14	Document completion of checkout procedures.	Provider and Tech
Item 15	Confirm ventilator settings and evaluate readiness to deliver anesthesia care. (ANESTHESIA TIME OUT)	Provider
To Be Completed Prior to Each Procedure		**Responsible Party**
Item to Be Completed		
Item 2	Verify patient suction is adequate to clear the airway.	Provider and Tech
Item 4	Verify availability of required monitors, including alarms.	Provider or Tech
Item 7	Verify that vaporizers are adequately filled and, if applicable, that the filler ports are tightly closed.	Provider
Item 11	Verify carbon dioxide absorbent is not exhausted.	Provider or Tech
Item 12	Breathing system pressure and leak testing	Provider and Tech
Item 13	Verify that gas flows properly through the breathing circuit during both inspiration and exhalation.	Provider and Tech
Item 14	Document completion of checkout procedures.	Provider and Tech
Item 15	Confirm ventilator settings and evaluate readiness to deliver anesthesia care. (ANESTHESIA TIME OUT)	Provider

Mehta SP, Eisenkraft JB, Posner KL, et al. Patient injuries from anesthesia gas delivery equipment: a closed claims update. *Anesthesiology*. 2013;119:788-795.

U.S. Food and Drug Administration. Anesthesia apparatus checkout recommendations, 1993. Updated April 20, 2006. Accessed May 1, 2023. http://vam.anest.ufl.edu/FDApreusecheck.pdf

A.24. What are the common sites for gas leakage?

Because gas can leak from numerous points in the anesthesia workstation and breathing system, anesthetists must be able to trace the flow of gases from the supply and storage sources through the system components. Most commonly, leaks occur in the breathing system and low-pressure parts of the machine (components downstream of the gas flow control valves). For the breathing system, trace the flow of gas from the common gas outlet (if accessible), through the antidisconnect fitting and hose, to the breathing circuit fresh gas inlet. Trace the flow of gas past the inspiratory valve, inspiratory limb, gas sampling connector, elbow adapter, to the tracheal tube or airway device. Common sites for leaks include a partially deflated tracheal tube cuff or a disconnection of the sidestream sampling gas analyzer sampling line. Check flow back down the expiratory limb, spirometer, expiratory valve, absorber, pressure gauge, pressure sampling lines, and any user-added components such as filters, humidifiers, condensers, and positive end-expiratory pressure (PEEP) valves. Check both the bag and the ventilator circuits for leaks.

Leaks in the machine's low-pressure system can occur because of cracked rotameter flow tubes, incorrectly mounted vaporizers, vaporizer leak around agent filling device, or fracture in the gas piping. Leaks in the high-pressure and intermediate-pressure systems usually result from defective valves, connectors, and hanger yokes.

Palaniappa NC, Weston SD. Inhaled anesthetic delivery systems. In: Gropper MA, Cohen NH, Eriksson LI, et al, eds. *Miller's Anesthesia*. 10th ed. Elsevier; 2025:457-511.

Raphael DT, Weller RS, Doran DJ. A response algorithm for the low-pressure alarm condition. *Anesth Analg*. 1988;67:876-883.

A.25. How is the anesthesia machine checked for leaks?

Leaks in the machine's low-pressure system should be tested according to the manufacturer's specific recommendations for that brand and model. In general, older model Dräger machines (Narkomed 2, 3, 4) are tested using a positive pressure leak check. The inspiratory and expiratory connections on the absorber are connected by a short length of 22-mm diameter tubing (ie, the circle breathing system tubing is removed). The reservoir bag (usually 3 L) is removed, and a test terminal is connected to the bag mount. A short piece of plastic tubing and a sphygmomanometer bulb are connected to the test terminal. With no gases flowing and with the pop-off valve closed, the system is pressurized to 50 cm H_2O by squeezing the sphygmomanometer bulb. Pressure should not decrease by more than 20 cm H_2O in 30 seconds. In this test, the pressure is applied to all the rigid components of the breathing system and through the fresh gas hose into the machine's low-pressure system all the way back to the flow control valves. This test is then repeated with each vaporizer turned on in turn to test for leaks in each vaporizer.

Some anesthesia machines (eg, GE Excel) have a one-way outlet check valve just upstream of the common gas outlet. Other models have no outlet check valve. The presence of an outlet check valve precludes the application of a positive pressure leak check. If such a valve is present, a negative pressure leak test can be used to check the low-pressure system. In this test, a suction bulb (negative pressure leak-check device) is connected to the common gas outlet. With all gas flows turned off and vaporizers off, the bulb is squeezed empty (to create a negative pressure of −65 mm Hg) and then connected to the common gas outlet of the workstation. Expansion of the bulb should not occur in less than 30 seconds. The test is repeated with each vaporizer turned on in turn to check for leaks in the vaporizers. The FDA 1993 preanesthesia checkout recommendations for use of the negative pressure (bulb) leak-check device state that the bulb should not refill within 10 seconds.

The newer electronic anesthesia workstations incorporate a partially automated checkout to test for leaks. The user of the workstation must understand what the automated checkout is designed to check and, more importantly, what it does not check. Even with an automated preanesthesia checkout, some steps must be performed manually as prompted and directed by the checkout screen.

Eng TS, Durieux MR. Automated machine checkout leaves an internal gas leak undetected: the need for complete checkout procedures. *Anesth Analg*. 2012;114:144-146.

Myers JA, Good ML, Andrews JJ. Comparison of tests for detecting leaks in the low pressure system of anesthesia gas machines. *Anesth Analg*. 1997;84:179-184.

U.S. Food and Drug Administration. Anesthesia apparatus checkout recommendations, 1993. Updated April 20, 2006. Accessed May 1, 2023. http://vam.anest.ufl.edu/FDApreusecheck.pdf

B. Preoperative Evaluation and Preparation

B.1. What should be included in the equipment checkout in preparation for anesthesia?

In 1993, the FDA published its *14-Step Anesthesia Apparatus Checkout Recommendations* (accessible at http://vam.anest.ufl.edu/fdacheckout.html). It is worthwhile to review the steps in this checkout, recognizing that in contemporary computerized workstations, many of the steps have been automated. The preamble to the FDA 1993 recommendations states that:

This checkout, or a reasonable equivalent, should be conducted before administration of anesthesia. These recommendations are valid only for an anesthesia system that conforms to the then current (1993) and relevant standards and includes an ascending bellows ventilator and at least the following monitors: capnograph, pulse oximeter, oxygen analyzer, respiratory volume monitor (spirometer), and breathing system pressure monitor with high- and low-pressure alarms. This is a guideline that users are encouraged to modify to accommodate differences in equipment design and variations in local clinical practice. Such local modifications should have appropriate peer review. Users should refer to the operator's manual for the manufacturer's specific procedures and precautions, especially the manufacturer's low-pressure leak test (Step 5).

Emergency Ventilation Equipment

Step 1. Verify backup ventilation equipment is available and functioning.

High-Pressure System

Step 2. Check oxygen cylinder supply.

- Open oxygen cylinder and verify at least half full (~1,000 psig).
- Close cylinder.

Step 3. Check central pipeline supplies.

- Check that hoses are connected and pipeline gauges read approximately 50 psig.

Low-Pressure Systems

Step 4. Check initial status of the low-pressure system.

- Close flow control valves and turn vaporizers off.
- Check fill level and tighten vaporizer filler caps.

Step 5. Perform leak check of machine low-pressure system.

- Verify that the machine master switch and flow control valves are off.
- Attach "suction bulb" to common fresh gas outlet.
- Squeeze the bulb repeatedly until it is fully collapsed.
- Verify that the bulb stays fully collapsed for at least 10 seconds.
- Open one vaporizer at a time and repeat the tests as discussed earlier.
- Remove suction bulb and reconnect fresh gas hose.

Step 6. Turn on machine master switch and all other necessary electrical equipment.

Step 7. Test flowmeters.

- Adjust flow of all gases through their full range, checking for smooth operation of floats and undamaged flow tubes (for older machines).
- Attempt to create a hypoxic oxygen/nitrous oxide mixture and verify correct changes in flow and/or alarm.

Scavenging System

Step 8. Adjust and check scavenging system.

- Ensure proper connections between the scavenging system and both the adjustable-pressure limit (APL or "pop-off") valve and ventilator relief valve.
- Adjust waste gas vacuum (if possible).
- Fully open APL valve and occlude Y-piece.
- With minimum oxygen flush activated, allow the scavenger reservoir bag to distend fully and then verify that the absorber pressure gauge reads less than 10 cm H_2O.

Breathing System

Step 9. Calibrate oxygen monitor.

- Ensure monitor reads 21% in room air.
- Verify low oxygen alarm is enabled and functioning.

- Reinstall sensor in circuit and flush the breathing system with oxygen.
- Verify that monitor now reads more than 90%.

Step 10. Check initial status of the breathing system.

- Set selector switch to "bag" mode.
- Check that the breathing circuit is complete, undamaged, and unobstructed.
- Verify that CO_2 absorbent is adequate.[1]
- Install breathing circuit accessory equipment (eg, humidifier, PEEP valve) to be used during the case.

Step 11. Perform leak check of the breathing system.

- Set all gas flows to zero (or minimum).
- Close APL (pop-off) valve and occlude Y-piece.
- Pressurize the breathing system to approximately 30 cm H_2O with oxygen flush.
- Ensure that pressure remains fixed for at least 10 seconds.
- Open APL (pop-off) valve and ensure that pressure decreases to zero.

Manual and Automatic Ventilation Systems

Step 12. Test ventilation systems and unidirectional valves.

- Place a second breathing bag on the Y-piece.
- Set appropriate ventilator parameters for the next patient.
- Switch to automatic ventilation ("ventilator") mode.
- Fill bellows and breathing bag with oxygen flush and then turn the ventilator on.
- Set oxygen flow to minimum and other gas flows to zero.
- Verify that during inspiration, bellows deliver appropriate tidal volume, and that during expiration, bellows fill completely.
- Set fresh gas flow to approximately 5 L/min.
- Verify that the ventilator bellows and simulated lungs fill and empty appropriately without sustained pressure at end expiration.
- Check for proper action of unidirectional valves.
- Exercise breathing circuit accessories to ensure proper function.
- Turn ventilator off and switch to manual ventilation ("bag/APL") mode.
- Ventilate manually, and ensure inflation and deflation of artificial lungs and appropriate feel of system resistance and compliance.
- Remove second breathing bag from the Y-piece.

Monitors

Step 13. Check, calibrate, and/or set alarm limits for all monitors.

- Capnometer
- Pulse oximeter
- Oxygen analyzer
- Respiratory volume monitor (spirometer)
- Pressure monitor
- High- and low-airway alarms

Final Position

Step 14. Check final status of machine.

- Vaporizers off
- APL valve open
- Selector switch to "bag"
- All flowmeters to zero
- Patient suction level adequate
- Breathing system ready to use

[1]Note that in step 10, checking adequacy of the CO_2 absorbent should include changing or hydrating it if there is any possibility that it may have become desiccated. This is because desiccated soda lime can react with desflurane, enflurane (obsolete), and isoflurane, and sevoflurane to produce high levels of CO in the breathing system. Also be aware that the color of the absorbent, Amsorb, changes to violet when it is desiccated and when it is exhausted.

The preanesthesia equipment checkout procedures are shown in **Table 59.1**. Although many modern anesthesia machines have automated many of the steps described earlier, it is important to understand the principles of each step of a preanesthesia checkout procedure.

American Society of Anesthesiologists. Summary of American Society of Anesthesiologists 2008 checkout recommendations by frequency and responsible party. Recommendations for pre-anesthesia checkout procedures. American Society of Anesthesiologists; 2008. https://www.apsf.org/article/new-guidelines-available-for-pre-anesthesia-checkout/

Loeb RG, Gravenstein N. Simultaneous color change at opposite ends of carbon dioxide absorbent canisters. *Anesthesiology*. 2018;129:1170.

B.2. What emergency equipment should be readily available?

In checking the anesthesia machine, step 1 on the FDA 1993 checklist and the 2008 American Society of Anesthesiologists' guidelines is to verify that backup ventilation equipment is available and functioning. This means a self-inflating resuscitation bag appropriate for patient size (adult vs pediatric) is present and tested. Emergency airway management equipment must be available.

One method for having emergency airway management equipment available and accessible is to have a "difficult airway cart" for the "cannot intubate, cannot ventilate" scenario. This cart should include supraglottic airways such as a laryngeal mask airway, nasal trumpets, or oral airways, as well as supplies for a needle cricothyrotomy and jet ventilation.

Other emergency equipment includes a working flashlight, a backup battery for electricity-dependent workstations, an oxygen tank and regulator, a malignant hyperthermia cart, a "code" cart and defibrillator, a difficult airway cart, a fire extinguisher, knowledge of appropriate response to a fire, and an evacuation plan.

Apfelbaum JL, Caplan RA, Barker SJ, et al. Practice advisory for the prevention and management of operating room fires: an updated report by the American Society of Anesthesiologists Task Force on Operating Room Fires. *Anesthesiology*. 2013;118:271-290.

ECRI Institute. New clinical guide to surgical fire prevention. Patients can catch fire—here's how to keep them safer. *Health Devices*. 2009;38:314-332.

C. Intraoperative Management

C.1. How should this patient be monitored?

The "Standards for Basic Anesthetic Monitoring" are established by the American Society of Anesthesiologists and were last amended in October 2010 and affirmed in December 2020.

American Society of Anesthesiologists. Standards for basic anesthetic monitoring. American Society of Anesthesiologists; 2010. Last affirmed December 13, 2020. Accessed April 25, 2025. https://www.asahq.org/standards-and-practice-parameters/standards-for-basic-anesthetic-monitoring

They are as follows:

- *Standard I*: Qualified anesthesia personnel shall be present in the room throughout the conduct of all general anesthetics, regional anesthetics, and monitored anesthesia care.
- *Standard II*: During all anesthetics, the patient's oxygenation, ventilation, circulation, and temperature shall be continually evaluated.

Oxygenation

- *Inspired gas*: During every administration of general anesthesia using an anesthesia machine, the concentration of oxygen in the patient's breathing system shall be measured by an oxygen analyzer with a low oxygen concentration limit alarm in use.*
- *Blood oxygenation*: During all anesthetics, a quantitative method of assessing oxygenation such as pulse oximetry shall be employed.* When the pulse oximeter is utilized, the variable pitch pulse tone and the low threshold alarm shall be audible to the anesthesiologist or the anesthesia care team personnel.* Adequate illumination and exposure of the patient are necessary to assess color.*

Ventilation

- Every patient receiving general anesthesia shall have adequacy of ventilation continually evaluated. Qualitative clinical signs such as chest excursion, observation of the reservoir breathing bag, and auscultation of breath sounds are useful. Continual monitoring for the presence of expired CO_2 shall be performed unless invalidated by the nature of the patient, procedure, or equipment. Quantitative monitoring of the volume of expired gas is strongly encouraged.*

- When an endotracheal tube or laryngeal mask is inserted, its correct positioning must be verified by clinical assessment and by identification of CO_2 in the expired gas. Continual $Etco_2$ analysis, in use from the time of endotracheal tube/laryngeal mask placement until extubation/removal or initiating transfer to a postoperative care location, shall be performed using a quantitative method such as capnography, capnometry, or mass spectroscopy.* When capnography or capnometry is utilized, the $Etco_2$ alarm shall be audible to the anesthesiologist or the anesthesia care team personnel.*
- When ventilation is controlled by a mechanical ventilator, there shall be in continuous use a device that is capable of detecting disconnection of components of the breathing system. The device must give an audible signal when its alarm threshold is exceeded.
- During regional anesthesia and monitored anesthesia care, the adequacy of ventilation shall be evaluated by continual observation of qualitative clinical signs and/or monitoring for the presence of exhaled CO_2.

Circulation

- Every patient receiving anesthesia shall have the electrocardiogram continuously displayed from the beginning of anesthesia until preparing to leave the anesthetizing location.*
- Every patient receiving anesthesia shall have arterial blood pressure and heart rate determined and evaluated at least every 5 minutes.*
- Every patient receiving general anesthesia shall have, in addition to earlier, circulatory function continually evaluated by at least one of the following: palpation of a pulse, auscultation of heart sounds, monitoring of a tracing of intra-arterial pressure, ultrasound peripheral pulse monitoring, or pulse plethysmography or oximetry.

Body Temperature

- Every patient receiving anesthesia shall have temperature monitored when clinically significant changes in body temperature are intended, anticipated, or suspected.

The American Society of Anesthesiologists' website includes the most recent version of the standards: https://www.asahq.org/standards-and-guidelines/standards-for-basic-anesthetic-monitoring.*Under extenuating circumstances, the responsible anesthesiologist may waive the requirements marked with an asterisk (*); it is recommended that when this is done, it should be so stated (including the reasons) in a note in the patient's medical record.

C.2. After the Spo_2 decreases to 85%, what acute diagnostic and therapeutic interventions would you perform?

It should be immediately determined whether the tracheal tube is in the trachea. Visualization of the tube passing between the vocal cords, visualization of bilateral chest rise, equal breath sounds bilaterally by auscultation, and sustained end-tidal CO_2 are rapid methods for confirming endotracheal placement of the tube.

The differential diagnosis for hemoglobin desaturation is shown in **Table 59.2**.

In this patient, the presence of bilateral breath sounds and the quality of those breath sounds must be ascertained. The Fio_2, $Etco_2$, heart rate, and blood pressure also need to be checked.

Therapeutically, the Fio_2 should be increased immediately to 1 (100% oxygen), and a change to manual ventilation should be initiated. If unilateral breath sounds are heard, potential causes include

TABLE 59.2 Differential Diagnosis of Low Spo_2

Cause	Examples
Hypoxic gas mixture	Low Fio_2, altitude
Hypoventilation	Airway obstruction, splinting associated with chest or abdominal surgery, bronchospasm
Right-to-left shunt	Atelectasis, mainstem bronchial intubation, mucous plug, intracardiac shunt, pulmonary edema
Ventilation/perfusion mismatch	Chronic obstructive pulmonary disease, pulmonary embolism, pneumonia, pulmonary edema
Diffusion impairment	Interstitial lung disease
Spurious reading	Sensor not properly applied to extremity causing penumbra effect; methemoglobinemia

Fio_2, fraction of inspired oxygen.

endobronchial intubation, mucous plug, bronchospasm, or pneumothorax. Suctioning the tube and possibly bronchoscopy should be performed if there is no rapid improvement after switching to manual ventilation. The tube should be gently withdrawn if a main stem intubation is suspected or confirmed with bronchoscopy. Attention should be paid to not extubate the trachea accidentally. After these maneuvers, obtaining an arterial blood gas would help in the differential diagnosis of hypoxemia. A portable chest radiograph can also help with the diagnosis.

Chang M, Horvath R. The Postanesthesia care unit. In: Gropper MA, Cohen NH, Eriksson LI, et al, eds. *Miller's Anesthesia*. 10th ed. Elsevier; 2025:2484-2511.

Postanesthesia Care. In: Butterworth JF IV, Mackey DC, Wasnick JD, eds. *Morgan & Mikhail's Clinical Anesthesiology*. 7th ed. McGraw Hill Education; 2022:1313-1332.

C.3. An arterial blood gas shows a Pao_2 of 250 mm Hg and a hemoglobin saturation (Sao_2) of 85%. How would you treat this?

The arterial blood gas reveals a large A-a difference and a low Sao_2 that does not correlate with the Pao_2. Given the clinical scenario of aerosolized local anesthetic administration for an awake fiberoptic intubation, methemoglobinemia should be considered, along with a pulmonary pathologic process arising from aspiration of gastric contents. An arterial blood gas analysis by co-oximetry will show the percentage of methemoglobin. The treatment for methemoglobinemia is intravenous methylene blue. Administration of methylene blue will cause a transient decrease in the Spo_2 reading because this dye is a strong absorber at 660 nm.

Oprea AD. Hematologic disorders. In: Hines RL, Jones SB, eds. *Stoelting's Anesthesia and Co-existing Disease*. 8th ed. Elsevier; 2022:465-496.

D. Postoperative Management

D.1. What criteria would you use for tracheal extubation?

In the operating room, traditional extubation criteria fall into two categories: general and respiratory. General criteria include return of consciousness, demonstration of ability to protect the airway, adequate reversal of residual neuromuscular blockade, absence of hypothermia, and presence of a normal metabolic milieu (eg, no significant anemia, acidosis, and electrolyte abnormality). Commonly applied respiratory criteria are a vital capacity greater than 15 mL/kg, tidal volume greater than or equal to 6 mL/kg, and predicted Spo_2 greater than 90% while breathing an Fio_2 less than 0.40.

Patients with respiratory compromise and the need for postoperative mechanical ventilation in the postanesthesia care unit or intensive care unit will be assessed using additional and more stringent criteria. The ratio of respiratory rate to tidal volume is widely used and commonly referred to as the *rapid shallow breathing index* (RSBI). Slow, deep breathing during minimal respiratory support predicts successful extubation while rapid, shallow breathing predicts probable failure. To determine this ratio, the patient is observed breathing from a T-piece or a low level of pressure support (usually ~5 cm H_2O); this is referred to as a spontaneous breathing trial (SBT). The following is then calculated:

$$\text{RSBI} = \text{respiratory rate (breaths per minute)/tidal volume (L).}$$

An RSBI greater than 100 is rapid, shallow breathing, and predicts that the patient will likely fail an extubation attempt. When the RSBI is less than 100, it is predicted that the patient will breathe at a rate and tidal volume that can be easily maintained after extubation and will be able to adequately maintain a normal Pao_2 and $Paco_2$. It does not, however, rule out the possibility of an upper airway obstruction. If during the period of observation while breathing from a T-piece or with pressure support, the patient develops signs of distress such as diaphoresis, agitation, tachycardia, bradycardia, hypertension, hypotension, hypoxemia, or hypercarbia, the trial is abandoned and the patient is said to have had a "weaning" or "SBT" failure.

Although more sophisticated measurements might be helpful, including measurement of maximum negative inspiratory force, vital capacity, elastance index, and so on, routine application of this basic and easy-to-reproduce measurement has stood the test of time, and certainly for most patients who are intubated and mechanically ventilated for less than 7 to 10 days, it should be a daily routine.

Ghiani A, Paderewska J, Sainis A, Crispin A, Walcher S, Neurohr C. Variables predicting weaning outcome in prolonged mechanically ventilated tracheotomized patients: a retrospective study. *J Intensive Care*. 2020;8:19.

Torrini F, Gendreau S, Morel J, et al. Prediction of extubation outcome in critically ill patients: a systematic review and meta-analysis. *Cri Care*. 2021;25:1-2.

Trivedi V, Chaudhuri D, Jinah R, et al. The usefulness of the rapid shallow breathing index in predicting successful extubation: a systematic review and meta-analysis. *Chest*. 2022;161:97-111.

Xie J, Cheng G, Zheng Z, Luo H, Ooi OC. To extubate or not to extubate: risk factors for extubation failure and deterioration with further mechanical ventilation. *J Card Surg*. 2019;34:1004-1011.

D.2. Postoperatively, the patient developed hypoxia and pulmonary edema. What is the differential diagnosis of pulmonary edema? What is the most likely cause of pulmonary edema in this patient?

Pulmonary edema is categorized into cardiac or noncardiac in etiology. The differential diagnosis of pulmonary edema is shown in **Table 59.3**.

Conditions that physiologically result from an increase in the pressure within the vessel that causes transudation of fluid from inside the vessel (intravascular) to outside the vessel (extravascular) are termed congestive heart failure (CHF). CHF is associated with a diminution of cardiac function (eg, ejection fraction) and an increase in the left ventricular end-diastolic pressure.

A decrease in extravascular pressure can also result in the net movement of fluid from inside to outside the vessel. A classic example is negative pressure pulmonary edema, a condition seen in patients who inspire against a closed glottis and generate a large net negative force, which acutely draws fluid into the alveoli, leading to pink frothy sputum and hypoxemia almost instantaneously.

A change in the permeability of the vessel wall is the major cause of pulmonary edema seen in ARDS. Diagnosis of ARDS requires a history of exposure to a risk factor within 1 week, the development of bilateral infiltrates on chest radiography, decreased oxygenation, and respiratory failure not explained by cardiac failure or volume overload. Diagnostic criteria for ARDS are listed in **Table 59.4**.

Risk factors for ARDS include aspiration, long bone fracture, transfusion-related acute lung injury (TRALI), pancreatitis, inhalational injury, and sepsis.

Aspiration pneumonitis leading to ARDS is most likely to develop in this patient, who had gastric secretions in the posterior pharynx and an unprotected airway.

ARDS Definition Task Force. Acute respiratory distress syndrome: the Berlin definition. *JAMA*. 2012;307:2526-2533.

Kacmarek RM, Hess DR. Mechanical Ventilation for the Surgical Patient. In: Longnecker DE, Newman MF, Zapol WM, et al, eds. *Anesthesiology*. 3rd ed. McGraw Hill; 2018:1333-1335.

TABLE 59.3 Differential Diagnosis of Pulmonary Edema

Condition	Pathophysiology	Sample Cause
Congestive heart failure	↑ Filling pressure, ↓ cardiac output	Myocardial infarction
Negative pressure pulmonary edema	↑ Outside-inside pressure gradient	Laryngospasm
Acute respiratory distress syndrome	↑ Permeability	Sepsis, aspiration, fat embolus, TRALI

↓, decrease; ↑, increase; TRALI, transfusion-related acute lung injury.

TABLE 59.4 Diagnostic Criteria for Acute Respiratory Distress Syndrome

Timing	Within 1 week of clinical insult or new or worsening respiratory symptoms
Imaging	Bilateral infiltrates on chest radiography
Origin of edema	Respiratory failure not explained by cardiac failure or volume overload
Decreased oxygenation	*Mild:* $Pao_2/Fio_2 \leq 300$ mm Hg with PEEP or CPAP ≥ 5 cm H_2O *Moderate:* $Pao_2/Fio_2 \leq 200$ mm Hg with PEEP ≥ 5 cm H_2O *Severe:* $Pao_2/Fio_2 \leq 100$ mm Hg with PEEP ≥ 5 cm H_2O

CPAP, continuous positive airway pressure; Fio_2, fraction of inspired oxygen; Pao_2, partial pressure of oxygen in arterial blood; PEEP, positive end-expiratory pressure.

D.3. How should the ventilator be set if mechanical ventilation is required postoperatively?

Parameters that must be set include the mode, respiratory rate, tidal volume, PEEP, and F_{IO_2}.

Patients with an acute need for mechanical ventilation should be given full support with the mode set as volume control (sometimes also known as *assist control*) or pressure control, so that all the breaths are delivered by the ventilator, even those initiated by the patient. Other modes to be considered as the patient improves include synchronized intermittent mandatory ventilation (SIMV), pressure support ventilation (PSV), and combinations of SIMV and PSV.

Tidal volume was usually set at 10 mL/kg. Normally, during spontaneous ventilation, the respiratory rate is 12 to 16 breaths per minute, and the tidal volume is 6 mL/kg. However, during spontaneous ventilation, there are yawns and sighs that prevent atelectasis. Yawns and sighs are not administered during routine mechanical ventilation. Therefore, standard mechanical ventilation settings developed more than 50 years ago use a lower respiratory rate and higher tidal volume than spontaneous values, resulting in the same minute ventilation and no need for sigh (150% of tidal volume) breaths.

More recently, traditional mechanical ventilation utilizing a tidal volume of 10 mL/kg has been recognized as a potential cause of morbidity and mortality when applied to injured lungs and might even have adverse consequences when applied routinely in the operating room. The excessive tidal volume is associated with alveolar injury and worsened pulmonary function (ie, volutrauma). This should be distinguished from the more easily recognized concern of pneumothorax, resulting from ventilation of stiff lungs with high inflation pressures, commonly referred to as barotrauma. Hence, the current recommendation in ARDS is that the tidal volume be set at 6 mL/kg of premorbid weight. Additionally, peak inspiratory pressure should ideally be less than 35 cm H_2O. This can result in CO_2 retention, but if the pH is greater than 7.25, no intervention is necessary. If CO_2 retention is severe and the pH is less than 7.25 after increasing respiratory rate to as high as 20 breaths per minute, administration of sodium bicarbonate can be considered. To maximize oxygenation and limit exposure to potentially toxic concentrations of oxygen (ie, $F_{IO_2} = 1$), usually a PEEP of 10 cm H_2O is set.

In addition to standard monitoring, prolonged mechanical ventilation in ARDS requires arterial line placement to facilitate frequent arterial blood gas determinations. A daily chest radiograph is also required to follow cardiopulmonary changes.

The Acute Respiratory Distress Syndrome Network. Ventilation with lower tidal volumes as compared with traditional tidal volumes for acute lung injury and the acute respiratory distress syndrome. *N Engl J Med.* 2000;342:1301-1308.

Umbrello M, Formenti P, Bolgiaghi L, et al. Current concepts of ARDS: a narrative review. *Int J Mol Sci.* 2016;18:64.

Zhang Z, Spieth PM, Chiumello D, et al. Declining mortality in patients with acute respiratory distress syndrome: an analysis of the acute respiratory distress syndrome network trials. *Crit Care Med.* 2019;47:315-323.

D.4. If this patient had acute respiratory distress syndrome (ARDS) secondary to aspiration, besides low-tidal volume ventilation, what other changes in routine therapy should be considered?

Other management strategies include efforts at minimizing lung water and usual standard intensive care unit measures aimed at deep venous thrombosis (DVT) prophylaxis, gastrointestinal aspiration prophylaxis, daily sedation breaks, and early mobility. Conservative administration of intravenous fluids originated in a National Institutes of Health–sponsored study; excessive administration of fluid is harmful, whereas minimizing intravenous fluids appears to be safe and not associated with other organ insufficiency or failure.

Banavasi H, Nguyen P, Osman H, Soubani AO. Management of ARDS–What works and what does not. *Am J Med Sci.* 2021;362:13-23.

Peck TJ, Hibbert KA. Recent advances in the understanding and management of ARDS. *F1000Res.* 2019;8:F1000 Faculty Rev-1959.

Wiedemann HP, Wheeler AP, Bernard GR, et al; National Heart, Lung, and Blood Institute Acute Respiratory Distress Syndrome (ARDS) Clinical Trials Network. Comparison of two fluid-management strategies in acute lung injury. *N Engl J Med.* 2006;354:2564-2575.

D.5. What therapies routinely administered by the anesthesiologist can cause acute lung injury?

TRALI was a leading cause of transfusion-related morbidity and mortality in the United States. This injury is almost always recognized during or shortly after transfusion and is diagnosed by the absence of cardiac failure and fluid overload. Although any blood product can cause this injury, transfusion of fresh frozen plasma and platelets, especially those donated by females who were previously pregnant, is most often responsible. This injury can be seen even after the transfusion of a single blood product unit, and "massive" transfusion is not, as previously thought, a prerequisite. Changes in the blood supply have reduced this complication by favoring male donors for plasma transfusions.

Alam A, Huang M, Yi QL, et al. Perioperative transfusion-associated lung injury: the Canadian Blood Service experience. *Transfus Apher Sci.* 2014;50:392-398 .

D.6. What methods of oxygen administration can be used postoperatively?

Most postoperative patients who are prone to develop hypoxemia can be managed with nasal cannula or face mask. Nasal cannulas are inexpensive and comfortable, but regardless of flow rates, they cannot achieve an FIO_2 of greater than 0.30 unless special high-flow devices are used. Face masks can deliver a range of precise FIO_2 levels of up to 1.

Occasionally, a patient requires more aggressive oxygen therapy than can be provided by nasal cannula or face mask, but less invasive than tracheal intubation and mechanical ventilation. Noninvasive positive pressure ventilation should be considered. Continuous positive airway pressure, bilevel positive airway pressure (BiPAP), or high-flow nasal cannula can be applied. Single-use high-flow nasal positive airway pressure devices such as SuperNO_2VA can also be used intraoperatively or postoperatively. These modes can be used in patients who either have previously used these devices at home or who are on the verge of requiring tracheal intubation and mechanical ventilation but have conditions thought to be rapidly resolving (eg, CHF and COPD exacerbation). These patients usually do not require an arterial catheter for blood sampling but do need frequent assessment of their respiratory effort, particularly their respiratory rate and use of accessory muscles, as well as continuous SpO_2 monitoring. A respiratory therapist should be involved to achieve the best mask fit and patient comfort possible. If noninvasive ventilation fails, preparation to emergently intubate the trachea must always be maintained.

Chaudhuri D, Granton D, Wang DX, et al. High-flow nasal cannula in the immediate postoperative period: a systematic review and meta-analysis. *Chest.* 2020;158:1934-1946.

Chawla R, Dixit SB, Zirpe KG, et al. ISCCM guidelines for the use of non-invasive ventilation in acute respiratory failure in adult ICUs. *Indian J Crit Care Med.* 2020;24:S61-S81.

Landoni G, Likhvantsev V, Kuzovlev A, Cabrini L. Perioperative noninvasive ventilation after adult or pediatric surgery: a comprehensive review. *J Cardiothorac Vasc Anesth.* 2022;36:785-793.

60 Electroconvulsive Therapy

Patricia Fogarty Mack and Janine Limoncelli

A 72-year-old male with major depressive disorder who has failed medication therapy and psychotherapy is scheduled for electroconvulsive therapy (ECT). His past medical history reveals significant coronary artery disease after three-vessel coronary bypass surgery 5 years ago. He also has chronic atrial fibrillation. He had a transient ischemic attack (TIA) 2 years previously after which he underwent left carotid endarterectomy. In addition, he has sleep apnea and gastroesophageal reflux disease (GERD). The patient has had a nonproductive cough for 4 weeks. The patient weighs 115 kg and is 5 ft 3 in tall and has a Mallampati class 2 airway. Medications include venlafaxine, rivaroxaban, atenolol, and esomeprazole.

A. Medical Disease and Differential Diagnosis

1. What are the indications for ECT?
2. Are there any contraindications to ECT?
3. What is the mechanism of action of ECT?

B. Preoperative Evaluation and Preparation

1. How would you assess the cardiac status of this patient?
2. How should his anticoagulation be managed during ECT?
3. What implications do his history of sleep apnea have on management of ECT?
4. How does his history of TIA and carotid endarterectomy impact your preoperative evaluation?
5. Is ECT contraindicated in a patient with a permanent pacemaker or implantable cardioverter-defibrillator?
6. Are there any psychiatric medications he is taking that would impact your anesthetic care?
7. How does his cough impact your anesthetic plan?

C. Intraoperative Management

1. Describe the hemodynamic and cardiac response to ECT in a typical patient.
2. Is an arterial line warranted in this patient?
3. By what means would you attempt to maximize hemodynamic stability?
4. Describe the cerebral hemodynamic effects of ECT.
5. How would you proceed with an induction of anesthesia for this procedure?
6. How do you intend to manage his airway during each treatment?
7. How might the management of a patient with recent COVID-19 or another viral respiratory virus be adjusted for patient and staff safety?

D. Postoperative Management

1. The patient is extremely agitated upon emergence. Discuss the risk factors for postictal agitation (PIA) as well as the therapeutic options.
2. After three consecutive uneventful inpatient treatments, the psychiatrist asks if the patient can undergo ECT as an outpatient. Would you agree to this plan?
3. What alternative therapies are available for patients in whom ECT is relatively contraindicated?

A. Medical Disease and Differential Diagnosis

A.1. What are the indications for ECT?

For centuries, it had been noted that psychosis did not tend to occur in those people with epilepsy. Since the 16th century, patients with severe mental illness were treated with various agents, such as camphor, to induce seizures (pharmacoconvulsive therapy). ECT was first instituted in the late 1930s. The addition of curare followed in 1951 by succinylcholine greatly diminished fractures due to the convulsions. Finally, the advent of methohexital, which ensured unconsciousness without significantly diminishing seizure initiation, led to the acceptance of ECT as an efficacious and safe treatment.

From the mid-1970s to the 1980s, many new drug treatments for psychiatric illness were developed and found to be efficacious. ECT fell into disfavor as it was perceived to be a "barbaric treatment" when compared to pharmacotherapy. In the past three decades, the pendulum has again swung back in favor of ECT as a safe and effective treatment for drug-resistant major depressive disorder and bipolar disorder.

Specific indications for ECT include, but are not limited to, major depressive disorder and bipolar disorder, acute schizophrenia (especially with affective or catatonic symptoms), and schizoaffective disorder. Although usually reserved as a second-line therapy for those who are resistant to pharmacologic treatment, ECT has, in some circumstances, been recommended as a first-line therapy, especially if a rapid response is urgently required as in patients with severe suicidal potential, malnutrition and dehydration, and catatonia. Finally, ECT has been recommended in patients who are unable to tolerate pharmacotherapeutic agents for any reason, including during pregnancy.

American Psychiatric Association. Indications for the use of electroconvulsive therapy. In: *The Practice of Electroconvulsive Therapy: Recommendations for Treatment, Training, and Privileging (A Task Force Report of the American Psychiatric Association)*. 3rd ed. Elsevier; 2025:6-25.

Joung KW, Park DH, Jeong CY, Yang HS. Anesthetic care for electroconvulsive therapy. *Anesth Pain Med (Seoul)*. 2022;17:145-156.

Kellner CH. ECT: patient selection and preparation. In: Kellner CH, ed. *Handbook of ECT: A Guide to Electroconvulsive Therapy for Practitioners*. Cambridge University Press; 2019:19-21.

A.2. Are there any contraindications to ECT?

There is no absolute contraindication to ECT. There is significantly increased risk in patients with intracranial space occupying lesions, any condition associated with intracranial hypertension, recent myocardial infarction with diminished ventricular function, severe hypertension, especially associated with pheochromocytoma, evolving stroke, retinal detachment, and American Society of Anesthesiologists physical status 4 or 5.

American Psychiatric Association. *The Practice of Electroconvulsive Therapy: Recommendations for Treatment, Training, and Privileging (A Task Force Report of the American Psychiatric Association)*. 3rd ed. Springer; 2025:6-25.

Joung KW, Park DH, Jeong CY, Yang HS. Anesthetic care for electroconvulsive therapy. *Anesth Pain Med (Seoul)*. 2022;17:145-156.

Kellner CH. ECT: patient selection and preparation. In: Kellner CH, ed. *Handbook of ECT: A Guide to Electroconvulsive Therapy for Practitioners*. Cambridge University Press; 2019:25-35.

A.3. What is the mechanism of action of ECT?

The mechanism of ECT is unknown. There are many neurochemical, neuroendocrine, electrophysiologic, and neuropsychological hypotheses regarding the mechanism of ECT (**Table 60.1**).

Although it was long assumed that a generalized seizure of adequate duration is sufficient for effective treatment, research has shown that barely suprathreshold stimulation, especially with unilateral ECT, is also efficacious. The cognitive impairment associated with ECT can be reduced by utilizing an "ultrabrief" stimulus, marked by a shorter pulse width of electrical stimulation, apparently without sacrificing efficacy.

Cognitive impairment, primarily short-term memory deficits, after ECT has been extensively investigated. Confounding this issue, though, is the observation that the major depressive state itself is associated with a decline in cognition. Although acute confusion and amnesia, both anterograde and retrograde, can occur as a result of ECT, verbal memory shows greater improvement in depressed patients treated with ECT compared to controls.

TABLE 60.1 Mechanisms of Action of Electroconvulsive Therapy

Neurophysiologic
Anticonvulsant (changes in seizure threshold)
Cerebral blood flow and metabolic rate change
Increased slow-wave electroencephalographic activity
Antidelirium/sleep mechanisms
Neuroendocrine
Prolactin release
Neuropeptide release
Melatonin
Neurochemical
Stimulation of β-receptors, changes in receptor binding and neurotransmitter reuptake
Monoamine release including norepinephrine, epinephrine, and dopamine
Modulation of serotonin
Neuropeptide/Neurotrophic
Neuropeptide Y, glutamate
Brain-derived neurotrophic factor (BDNF)
Increased endorphins
Epigenetic Changes
Induction of multiple genes encoding for neurogenesis, neuroplasticity, and increased neuronal connectivity
Neurotropic
Increased gray matter volume and cortical thickness (proliferation of neurons) in amygdala, hippocampus, and other brain areas
Inactivation of multiple apoptotic factors
Immune Modulation
Reduction in pro-inflammatory cytokines and activated immune cells noted in depression

In addition, there is no increased risk of dementia for patients with major depression who are treated with ECT *versus* patients who did not receive ECT.

Biedermann SV, Bumb JM, Demiracka T, et al. Improvement in verbal memory performance in depressed in-patients after treatment with electroconvulsive therapy. *Acta Psychiatr Scand*. 2016;134:461-468.

Joung KW, Park DH, Jeong CY, Yang HS. Anesthetic care for electroconvulsive therapy. *Anesth Pain Med (Seoul)*. 2022;17:145-156.

Kellner CH. Basic concepts of ECT. In: Kellner CH, ed. *Handbook of ECT: A Guide to Electroconvulsive Therapy for Practitioners*. Cambridge University Press; 2019:1-11.

Loo CK, Katalinic K, Smith DJ, et al. A randomized controlled trial of brief and ultrabrief pulse right unilateral electroconvulsive therapy. *Int J Neuropsychopharmacol*. 2014;18:pyu145.

Osler M, Rozing MP, Christensen GT, et al. Electroconvulsive therapy and risk of dementia in patients with affective disorders: a cohort study. *Lancet Psychiatry*. 2018;5:348-356.

Singh A, Kar SK. How electroconvulsive therapy works?: understanding the neurobiological mechanisms. *Clin Psychopharmacol Neurosci*. 2017;15:210-221.

B. Preoperative Evaluation and Preparation

B.1. How would you assess the cardiac status of this patient?

The cardiac status of the patient needs to be assessed as it would for any other general anesthetic procedure. Because there can be periods of significant tachycardia and hypertension following seizure induction, it would be useful to ensure that there is no significant myocardium at risk for ischemia and that systolic function is not compromised. If this information cannot be obtained from patient history and assessment of his functional status, it might be useful to obtain a cardiac consult to determine if a stress test and echocardiogram are warranted. Bear in mind that it can be difficult to get an accurate history of functional status from patients who are psychotic or severely depressed.

American Psychiatric Association. Pre-ECT evaluation of the patient. In: *The Practice of Electroconvulsive Therapy: Recommendations for Treatment, Training, and Privileging (A Task Force Report of the American Psychiatric Association).* 3rd ed. American Psychiatric Association; 2025:70-81

Halvorsen S, Mehilli J, Cassese S, et al. 2022 ESC guidelines on cardiovascular assessment and management of spatients undergoing noncardiac surgery. *Eur Heart J.* 2022;43:3826-3924.

Thompson A, Fleishmann KE, Smilowitz N et al. 2024 AHA/ACC/ASNC/HRS/SCA/SCCT/SCMR/SVM Guideline for Perioperative Cardiovascular Management for Noncardiac Surgery: A Report of the American College of Cardiology/American Heart Association Joint Committee on Clinical Practice Guidelines. *Circulation.* 2024;150:e351-e442.

B.2. How should his anticoagulation be managed during ECT?

Anticoagulation for atrial fibrillation should be continued throughout his course of therapy, maintaining an international normalized ratio (INR) between 2.0 and 3.0. Although intracerebral hemorrhage is a potential concern, a retrospective study suggests that ECT can be safely performed in patients on warfarin therapy. Although the safety of newer anticoagulants has not been formally investigated in ECT, case series do not report hemorrhagic complications in patients receiving either dabigatran or rivaroxaban. Finally, if a patient has drug-eluting arterial stents, aspirin and clopidogrel or any alternative antiplatelet maintenance medication should be continued throughout treatment.

American Psychiatric Association. Pre-ECT evaluation of the patient. In: *The Practice of Electroconvulsive Therapy: Recommendations for Treatment, Training, and Privileging (A Task Force Report of the American Psychiatric Association).* 3rd ed. American Psychiatric Association; 2025:70-81.

Joglar JA, Chung MK, Armbruster AL, et al. 2023 ACC/AHA/ACCP/HRS guideline for the diagnosis and management of atrial fibrillation: a report of the American College of Cardiology/American Heart Association Joint Committee on Clinical Practice Guidelines. *Circulation.* 2024;149:e1-e156.

Mehta V, Mueller PS, Gonzalez-Arriaza HL, et al. Safety of electroconvulsive therapy in patients receiving long-term warfarin therapy. *Mayo Clin Proc.* 2004;79:1396-1401.

Schmidt ST, Lapid MI, Sundsted KK, et al. Safety of electroconvulsive therapy in patients receiving dabigatran therapy. *Psychosomatics.* 2014;55:400-403.

Shuman M, Hieber R, Moss L, et al. Rivaroxaban for thromboprophylaxis in a patient receiving electroconvulsive therapy. *J ECT.* 2015;31:e19-e20.

B.3. What implications do his history of sleep apnea have on management of ECT?

A history of sleep apnea is important because suboptimal management of respiratory function can reduce efficacy of treatment and increase complications. Hypocarbia is sometimes required to ensure adequate seizure duration. Additionally, after onset of seizure activity, oxygen consumption is increased dramatically as is carbon dioxide (CO_2) production. Hypercarbia can exacerbate the tachycardia and hypertensive responses to seizure. Therefore, adequate mask ventilation is required to ensure optimal respiratory status. Use of a supraglottic airway device might be required to ensure adequate ventilation in this patient.

Finally, if the patient uses continuous positive airway pressure (CPAP) or bilevel positive airway pressure (BiPAP) machine at home, it might be useful to have that device, or a nasal positive airway pressure system or similar noninvasive ventilation option, available to the patient in the postprocedure period when postanesthetic and postictal somnolence might compromise his ability to maintain a patent airway.

Saito S. Anesthesia management for electroconvulsive therapy: hemodynamic and respiratory management. *J Anesth.* 2005;19:142-149.

Trakada G, Velentza L, Konsta A, et al. Complications of anesthesia during electroconvulsive therapy due to undiagnosed obstructive sleep apnea: a case study. *Respir Med Case Rep.* 2017;20:145-149.

B.4. How does his history of TIA and carotid endarterectomy impact your preoperative evaluation?

A history of TIA or stroke is an indication for magnetic resonance imaging (MRI) of the head before their first course of ECT. Additionally, this can be utilized to rule out an organic cause for depression. Although a comprehensive neurologic examination before ECT is routinely recommended by the

American Psychiatric Association, in this patient, more sophisticated neuropsychological testing might be useful in documenting subtle deficits and establishing a true baseline. Finally, if the patient has not had a follow-up carotid Doppler ultrasound examination, it might be useful to ensure that there has not been restenosis or that no new plaques have formed. This is particularly important in view of the fact that the rate pressure product can be increased by as much as 400% in the sympathetic phase of the cardiac response.

American Psychiatric Association. Pre-ECT evaluation of the patient. In: *The Practice of Electroconvulsive Therapy: Recommendations for Treatment, Training, and Privileging (A Task Force Report of the American Psychiatric Association)*. 3rd ed. American Psychiatric Association; 2025:70-81.

B.5. Is ECT contraindicated in a patient with a permanent pacemaker or implantable cardioverter-defibrillator?

In short, there have been no reports of pacemaker or automatic implantable cardioverter-defibrillator (AICD) dysfunction related to ECT. The site of electrical activity, be it electrocautery or ECT, needs to be 6 in (15 cm) from the implanted cardiac device. See Chapter 8: Cardiac Implantable Electronic Devices, Section C.11.

B.6. Are there any psychiatric medications he is taking that would impact your anesthetic care?

Medications for depression can have many serious side effects. In fact, one of the indications for ECT is that the patient has had an inadequate response to pharmacologic therapy. Furthermore, there are many possible drug interactions between antidepressant medications and anesthetic agents as well as other medications that might be administered in the course of an anesthetic. The most common of these side effects and interactions are shown in **Table 60.2**.

B.7. How does his cough impact your anesthetic plan?

Medical or pulmonary evaluation should be considered in the case of chronic cough, and pulmonary status optimized in terms of treatment for asthma, bronchitis, or respiratory infection. ECT is generally contraindicated if a patient has COVID-19 or any respiratory infection, both due to the risks to the patient in receiving general anesthesia as well as droplet spread and aerosolization of virus particles due to airway management. The only time when ECT should be performed on a patient who has an active infection is when the patient is either catatonic or has failed other therapies and the procedure is considered lifesaving.

Espinoza RT, Kellner CH, McCall WV. ECT during COVID-19: an essential medical procedure-maintaining service viability and accessibility. *J ECT*. 2020;78-79.

Fink M, Kellner CH, McCall WV. The role of ECT in suicide prevention. *J ECT*. 2014:30:5-9.

C. Intraoperative Management

C.1. Describe the hemodynamic and cardiac response to ECT in a typical patient.

A parasympathetic discharge occurs within a few seconds of application of the electrical stimulus. This can result in bradycardia, which can be profound and even progress to asystole. Hypotension is a concern as patients are likely to be hypovolemic as they are NPO (nothing by mouth) prior to the procedure (which can be exacerbated by poor oral intake); hypotension can be further compounded by psychotropic medications and anesthetic induction agents. Sympathetic activation due to the seizure results in tachycardia (and at times dysrhythmias) as well as hypertension to up to 150% of baseline values. Hypertension usually lasts for 2 to 5 minutes. If the patient is not adequately ventilated, hypercarbia can add to the hypertension. During the first ECT treatment, the electrical stimulus can often be titrated upward until a generalized seizure occurs. When a generalized seizure does not follow the electrical stimulation, the parasympathetic response predominates and the patient can experience a sustained bradycardia.

With such a dramatic increase in heart rate and blood pressure, the rate pressure product, an indicator of myocardial oxygen demand, is significantly elevated. This can lead to electrocardiographic ischemia as well as regional wall motion abnormalities on echocardiography.

Messina AG, Paranicas M, Katz B, et al. Effect of electroconvulsive therapy on the electrocardiogram and echocardiogram. *Anesth Analg*. 1992;75:511-514.

Saito S. Anesthesia management for electroconvulsive therapy: hemodynamic and respiratory management. *J Anesth*. 2005;19:142-149.

TABLE 60.2 The Most Common Side Effects and Anesthetic Interactions of Common Psychiatric Medications

Drug Group	Examples of Drug	Mechanism	Side Effects/ Toxicities	Perioperative Concerns	Potential Interactions	Alternative Medications	Preoperative Continuation
SSRI/SNRI	Venlafaxine, fluoxetine	Presynaptic inhibition of SER/NE	Nausea, vomiting Sexual dysfunction Headache Agitation SIADH (rare) Cytochrome P450 inhibition	Prolonged/ increased action of β-blockers, benzodiazepines, barbiturates, anticholinergics	Serotonin syndrome: MAOIs, meperidine, and highly protein-bound drugs (lidocaine, midazolam, fentanyl, linezolid, methylene blue)	Reduce dose of cytochrome P450 metabolized drugs. Avoid serotonin crisis precipitants.	Continue
Bupropion		SNRI/dopamine reuptake antagonist	Dry mouth, nausea, tremor	Theoretically reduced seizure threshold, prolonged seizure	May interact with medications that increase or decrease dopamine		Some recommend discontinuing prior to ECT.
Lithium	Lithium	Unclear	Sinus node dysfunction AV block Bradycardia Nephrogenic diabetes insipidus	Prolongation of nondepolarizing muscle relaxants Reducing MAC	Toxicity with drugs that decrease renal function: NSAIDs, angiotensin-converting enzyme inhibitors, etc.	Careful dose titration	Discontinue 24 h before surgery.
TCAs	Amitriptyline, imipramine	Presynaptic inhibition of SER uptake	Conduction deficits (wide QRS, prolonged QT) Postural hypotension Anticholinergic symptoms Sedation	Muscarinic, histaminergic, and α_1-adrenergic blocking effects	MAC increased and increased likelihood of dysrhythmia Hypertensive crisis caused by indirect sympathomimetic drugs Atropine/scopolamine increased emergence delirium, increased muscarinic activity Pancuronium may cause tachyarrhythmia.	Phenylephrine Glycopyrrolate Other nondepolarizing muscle relaxant	Discontinue

(continued)

TABLE 60.2 The Most Common Side Effects and Anesthetic Interactions of Common Psychiatric Medications (*continued*)

Drug Group	Examples of Drug	Mechanism	Side Effects/ Toxicities	Perioperative Concerns	Potential Interactions	Alternative Medications	Preoperative Continuation
MAOIs	Phenelzine, tranylcypromine	Inhibit breakdown of NE and SER by MAO enzyme	Hypertension Nausea Dizziness Headache Sleep disturbance Severe hypertension with tyramine-containing foods Thrombocytopenia and anemia	Avoid indirect acting sympathomimetics. Avoid serotonin crisis precipitants.	Indirect sympathomimetic: hypertensive crisis Serotonergic syndrome from meperidine, dextromethorphan, etc. Inhibiting acetylcholinesterase Increasing MAC	Avoid indirect acting sympathomimetics. Avoid serotonin crisis precipitants. Use fentanyl. Use nondepolarizing muscle relaxants. Titration	Irreversible MAOI—discontinue 2 wk before surgery Reversible MAOI—discontinue on day of procedure
Antipsychotics	Prochlorperazine, chlorpromazine	Block D2 dopamine receptors Atypical antipsychotics also block some serotonin receptors. Also block histamine and α_1-adrenergic receptors	Hypotension Tachycardia, prolonged QT interval Extrapyramidal symptoms Tremor Tardive dyskinesia Neuroleptic malignant syndrome Muscle rigidity, hyperthermia, autonomic dysfunction		Hypertension with halogenated agents Anticholinergic effects with atropine and scopolamine	Careful titration/ TIVA Glycopyrrolate	Continue

Serotonin syndrome: hyperreflexia, agitation, hyperthermia.

AV, atrioventricular; ECT, electroconvulsive therapy; MAC, minimal alveolar concentration; MAO, monoamine oxidase; MAOI, monoamine oxidase inhibitor; NE, norepinephrine; NSAIDs, nonsteroidal anti-inflammatory drugs; SER, serotonin; SIADH, syndrome of inappropriate antidiuretic hormone secretion; SNRI, serotonin-norepinephrine reuptake inhibitor; SSRI, selective serotonin reuptake inhibitor; TCAs, tricyclic antidepressants; TIVA, total intravenous anesthesia.

C.2. Is an arterial line warranted in this patient?

Arterial catheter is not warranted; in spite of the potential dramatic perturbations in heart rate and blood pressure, these responses are predictable and can be attenuated by judicious use of anticholinergic and antihypertensive drugs. Atropine (0.4 mg) or glycopyrrolate (0.2 mg) are used to prevent the bradycardia associated with parasympathetic discharge. The tachycardia and hypertension seen as part of the sympathetic response can be prevented and treated with short-acting β-blockade, nitroglycerin, or even remifentanil, administered just at the beginning of the sympathetic stimulation. Pretreatment with dexmedetomidine can also ameliorate the tachycardia and hypertension that occurs immediately after the seizure.

Patients can have transient electrocardiogram changes or a transient decrease in left ventricular function following ECT. Rarely, takotsubo cardiomyopathy occurs. Although severe cardiac complications during ECT have been thought to be very rare, even in patients with underlying coronary disease, a meta-analysis reported a rate of cardiac event as frequent as 1 out of 50 patients or 1 in 200 ECT treatments; a separate meta-analysis indicated a mortality of 1 in 200,000 treatments.

Cristancho MA, Sattherwaite TD, O'Reardon JP. Cardiac complications of ECT: myocardial stunning syndrome and Takotsubo cardiomyopathy after ECT: different names for the same phenomenon. *J ECT*. 2010;26:146-147.

Duma A, Maleczek M, Panjikaran B, et al. Major adverse cardiac events and mortality associated with electroconvulsive therapy: a systematic review and meta-analysis. *Anesthesiology*. 2019;130:83-91.

Fuenmayor AJ, el Fakih Y, Moreno J, et al. Effects of electroconvulsive therapy on cardiac function in patients without heart disease. *Cardiology*. 1997;88:254-257.

Joung KW, Park DH, Jeong CY, Yang HS. Anesthetic care for electroconvulsive therapy. *Anesth Pain Med (Seoul)*. 2022;17:145-156.

McCully RB, Karon BL, Rummans TA, et al. Frequency of left ventricular dysfunction after electroconvulsive therapy. *Am J Cardiol*. 2003;91:1147-1150.

Messina AG, Paranicas M, Katz B, et al. Effect of electroconvulsive therapy on the electrocardiogram and echocardiogram. *Anesth Analg*. 1992;75:511-514.

Saito S. Anesthesia management for electroconvulsive therapy: hemodynamic and respiratory management. *J Anesth*. 2005;19:142-149.

Tørring N, Sanghani SN, Petrided G, et al. The mortality rate of electroconvulsive therapy: a systematic review and pooled analysis. *Acta Psychiatr Scand*. 2017;135:388-397.

C.3. By what means would you attempt to maximize hemodynamic stability?

First, one should continue antihypertensive medication on the evening before and the morning of the procedure. Second, a small dose of atropine (0.4 mg) or glycopyrrolate (0.2 mg) can be given several minutes before the electrical stimulation in order to prevent bradycardia. Glycopyrrolate, which is a quaternary ammonium compound, has the advantage of not crossing the intact blood-brain barrier. In addition, the tachycardic response from the seizure is not as pronounced when glycopyrrolate is used compared with atropine. Anticholinergic pretreatment is most important during the first treatment when the electrical stimulation is being titrated, and it is likely not to progress into a generalized seizure on the first or second stimulus. If the pretreatment with an anticholinergic leaves a fragile patient with an undesirable tachycardia, it can be omitted during subsequent treatments as long as the bradycardia is not too severe or prolonged.

Similarly, medications to attenuate the sympathetic response are typically not administered until it is certain that the seizure will generalize. This results in a requirement for very fast-acting drugs to control heart rate and blood pressure. Either esmolol (0.5-1.0 mg/kg) or labetalol (5-20 mg) are usually effective. If there is a contraindication to β-blockers, diltiazem, or nicardipine can be substituted. Nitroglycerin can be particularly useful in patients with ischemic cardiac disease. Remifentanil is also effective in attenuating the sympathetic response.

A study of American Society of Anesthesiologists physical status 1 and 2 patients assessed echocardiographic and hemodynamic parameters when the sympathetic response was pretreated with intravenous β-blocker, calcium channel blocker, or nitroglycerin prior to the electrical stimulus. No new regional wall motion abnormalities were found, but β-blocker therapy seemed to be the most effective medication at attenuating fractional shortening and the entire sympathetic response.

Joung KW, Park DH, Jeong CY, Yang HS. Anesthetic care for electroconvulsive therapy. *Anesth Pain Med (Seoul)*. 2022;17:145-156.

Kadoi Y, Takahashi K, Saito S, et al. Effects of antihypertensive medication on left ventricular function during electroconvulsive therapy: study with transthoracic echocardiography. *J Clin Anesth*. 2006;18:441-445.

Saito S. Anesthesia management for electroconvulsive therapy: hemodynamic and respiratory management. *J Anesth.* 2005;19:142-149.

van Zijl DH, Gordon PC, James MF. The comparative effects of remifentanil or magnesium sulfate versus placebo on attenuating the hemodynamic responses after electroconvulsive therapy. *Anesth Analg.* 2005;101:1651-1655.

C.4. Describe the cerebral hemodynamic effects of ECT.

Electrically induced seizures lead to cerebral hyperemia (increase in cerebral blood flow) as documented by transcranial Doppler ultrasound and near-infrared spectroscopy. This response occurs even if the seizure does not generalize, suggesting that they are a result of the electric stimulation itself. The increase in cerebral blood flow is related to the degree of systemic hypertension and occurs whether bilateral or unilateral stimulus is applied. Although there is a correlation with systemic hypertension, systemically administered antihypertensives do not fully ameliorate the increase in cerebral blood flow, perhaps since these drugs have differing effects on the cerebral and systemic circulations.

Saito S. Anesthesia management for electroconvulsive therapy: hemodynamic and respiratory management. *J Anesth.* 2005;19:142-149.

C.5. How would you proceed with an induction of anesthesia for this procedure?

Anesthetic induction may be accomplished with a number of medications. Historically, methohexital (0.5-1.0 mg/kg) was the induction agent of choice because it has very little effect on seizure duration and has a rapid onset and recovery profile. Regional medication shortages have necessitated use of alternative medications. Propofol (0.5-1.0 mg/kg) or etomidate (0.2-0.3 mg/kg) are common substitutes. In research studies, etomidate provides for longer seizure duration when compared to methohexital and propofol; however, postictal hypertension is more severe and myoclonic contractions can be undesirable. In addition, there is a greater incidence of nausea, increased confusion, and prolonged recovery time. Although adrenal suppression has been reported in patients on continuous infusions of etomidate, there are no reports of adrenal suppression in patients receiving multiple bolus doses of etomidate as part of a course of ECT. While propofol reduces seizure duration, there is controversy as to how this reduction in seizure duration impacts the efficacy of therapy.

Ketamine has antidepressant effects and potentiates the early reduction of depressive symptoms when given in conjunction with ECT. Ketamine might be useful in some patients in whom a rapid decrease in depressive symptoms is essential, such as those with extreme suicidal ideation or catatonia. A randomized controlled trial of "ketofol," a combination of ketamine and propofol, determined that ketofol was associated with a longer seizure time than propofol, faster recovery than ketamine, and demonstrated good hemodynamic stability. Ketamine as a sole anesthetic agent for ECT has also been used, taking advantage of its ability to prolong seizure duration and induce a more intense seizure. Ketamine has not had widespread use for ECT due to concerns surrounding extended posttreatment disorientation and blood pressure elevations. In a study at the Sheppard Pratt Health System, ketamine was used as the anesthetic for ECT and there were no incidences of blood pressure aberrations, increase in recovery room time, or complications requiring emergency room transfer. Current investigations are focused on the optimal dosing of the optimal anesthetic agent to improve ECT efficacy.

Muscle paralysis is usually achieved with succinylcholine (0.5-1.0 mg/kg) unless there is a contraindication. In that case, a short-acting nondepolarizing neuromuscular blocking agent can be substituted.

Recent studies have demonstrated that rocuronium (0.3 mg/kg) reversed with sugammadex (1.5 mg/kg) is an acceptable alternative to succinylcholine and has an even shorter time to return to full muscle strength then succinylcholine alone.

Joung KW, Park DH, Jeong CY, Yang HS. Anesthetic care for electroconvulsive therapy. *Anesth Pain Med (Seoul).* 2022;17:145-156.

Oflezer C, Atay Ö, Kaşdoğan ZE, Özakay G, İpekçioğlu D, Bahadır H. Does the use of rocuronium-sugammadex instead of succinylcholine in electroconvulsive therapy affect seizure duration? *Psychiatry Investig.* 2022;19:824-831.

Okamoto N, Nakai T, Sakamoto K, et al. Rapid antidepressant effect of ketamine anesthesia during electroconvulsive therapy of treatment-resistant depression: comparing ketamine and propofol anesthesia. *J ECT.* 2010;26:223-227.

Wojdacz R, Święcicki Ł, Antosik-Wójcińska A. Comparison of the effect of intravenous anesthetics used for anesthesia during electroconvulsive therapy on the hemodynamic safety and the course of ECT. Porównanie wpływu anestetyków dożylnych stosowanych do znieczulenia w trakcie leczenia elektrowstrząsowego na bezpieczeństwo hemodynamiczne i przebieg zabiegów elektrowstrząsowych. *Psychiatr Pol.* 2017;51:1039-1058.

Zisselman M, Zitzmann W. A role for ketamine in electroconvulsive therapy. *J ECT.* 2019:35:e57.

C.6. How do you intend to manage his airway during each treatment?

The diagnosis of sleep apnea and the patient's body habitus raise concerns regarding the ease and effectiveness of mask ventilation. In spite of these concerns, a plan to proceed with mask ventilation as well as a backup plan of supraglottic airway or tracheal intubation is reasonable. As ECT is usually administered 3 times a week, repeated intubation can lead to airway trauma and edema. GERD can also be of concern; however, patients for ECT are not intubated solely because of GERD. Continuation of medication to reduce stomach acid and promote gastric emptying as well as a dose of preinduction sodium citrate/citric acid can be used to reduce gastric acidity.

Effective mask ventilation is important for several reasons. First, hypocapnia can lower seizure threshold and promote more effective therapy. Second, avoidance of postseizure hypercapnia is necessary as hypercapnia can exacerbate hypertension and tachycardia.

In anticipation of potential difficult ventilation during ECT, the patient is preoxygenated for 3 to 5 minutes prior to induction of anesthesia. As soon as induction is accomplished, an oral or well-lubricated nasal airway can be placed. A second person should be available in case two-person ventilation is required. A Jackson-Rees circuit can be advantageous for ventilation during ECT. It allows adjustment of the amount of positive pressure administered, and the weight of a bag-valve–mask ventilator can make maintenance of ideal mask placement difficult. Also, as the patient regains spontaneous ventilation, they can breathe comfortably and effectively through the Jackson-Rees circuit. If mask ventilation is not effective, an appropriately sized supraglottic airway can be placed. If necessary for adequate ventilation, tracheal intubation can be considered.

Saito S. Anesthesia management for electroconvulsive therapy: hemodynamic and respiratory management. *J Anesth.* 2005;19:142-149.

C.7. How might the management of a patient with recent COVID-19 or another viral respiratory virus be adjusted for patient and staff safety?

If emergency ECT is warranted despite the patient having a viral respiratory infection, the procedure should be performed as the last of the day, and staff should wear appropriate personal protective equipment (PPE) as required for the pathogen.

Since manipulation of the airway can result in aerosolization of viral particles, preoxygenation can be maximized by placing oxygen via a filtered circuit as early as possible and avoiding mask ventilation after induction of anesthesia unless hemoglobin saturation falls below to less than 92%. If positive pressure ventilation is required, it is recommended that two members of the team perform this task together: one to provide an optimal facemask seal and the other to deliver the lowest possible tidal volume to obtain minimal chest excursion (estimated at 2-3 mL/kg).

Limoncelli J, Marino T, Smetana R, et al. General anesthesia recommendations for electroconvulsive therapy during the coronavirus disease 2019 pandemic. *J ECT.* 2020;36:152-155.

Zucco L, Levy N, Ketchandji D, et al. An update on the perioperative considerations for COVID-19 severe acute respiratory syndrome coronavirus-2 (SARS-CoV-2). *Anesth Patient Saf Foundation Newslett.* 2020;35:33-68.

D. Postoperative Management

D.1. The patient is extremely agitated upon emergence. Discuss the risk factors for postictal agitation (PIA) as well as the therapeutic options.

PIA manifests as disorientation, inability to consistently follow commands, and motor agitation. Risk factors for PIA include prolonged seizure duration, bilateral *versus* unilateral ECT, and concomitant lithium therapy. Low doses of induction agent as well as very low doses of succinylcholine are considered risk factors. Use of low-dose succinylcholine can lead to excess lactate production in those patients who have greater manifestation of clinical seizure activity. Increased lactate levels were noted in patients who experienced PIA compared to those who did not.

It is of critical importance to rule out nonconvulsive status epilepticus as an etiology for PIA. Nonconvulsive status can present as agitation or conversely as mutism.

Treatment of PIA usually consists of a benzodiazepine such as midazolam 1 to 2 mg. If this is not effective, haloperidol can be added. In some circumstances, propofol as a bolus or an infusion can be effective. Current management of PIA includes use of dexmedetomidine, either as a pretreatment or postseizure therapy.

Other potential adverse effects of ECT include aspiration, headache, nausea, and dental or tongue injuries.

Aksay SS, Bumb JM, Remennick D, et al. Dexmedetomidine for the management of postictal agitation after electroconvulsive therapy after S-ketamine anesthesia. *Neuropsychiatr Dis Treat.* 2017;13:1389-1394.

Cohen MB, Stewart JT. Treatment of post-electroconvulsive therapy agitation with dexmedetomidine. *J ECT.* 2013;29:e23-e24.

Tzabazis A, Schmitt HJ, Ihmsen H, et al. Postictal agitation after electroconvulsive therapy: incidence, severity, and propofol as a treatment option. *J ECT.* 2013;29:189-195.

D.2. After three consecutive uneventful inpatient treatments, the psychiatrist asks if the patient can undergo ECT as an outpatient. Would you agree to this plan?

Outpatient ECT has become an acceptable therapeutic option for many patients. Primarily, it is used for maintenance therapy. It can also be used to complete an initial course of ECT provided that the first several treatments are uneventful medically (ie, no respiratory or cardiovascular problems) and that the patient is showing improvement in psychiatric status. Because psychiatric patients can be unreliable in following preoperative instructions, such as NPO status, they must have another adult assume responsibility for ensuring that those instructions are followed. Of course, they must also have an escort bring them home.

Finally, there needs to be close communication between the treating psychiatrist and the ECT psychiatrist to keep abreast of any change in psychiatric status or medical condition.

D.3. Are there any specific risk factors or cause for concern for postoperative mortality (within 30 days) after ECT?

In general, ECT is associated with a reduced risk of suicide and mortality from all causes in patients with severe depression. In a study from Sweden, 20,225 patients treated with ECT were reviewed to assess mortality 30 days after ECT. All-cause mortality rate was 1.07%. Medical causes of death, with cardiovascular disease being the primary cause in patients over 70 years of age, accounted for 0.61% and suicide accounted for 0.46%. It is generally agreed upon that ECT appears to be a low-risk medical procedure, with the highest risk assigned to older individuals with severe somatic diseases. Cardiac arrest, myocardial infarction, and pulmonary embolism are the most common causes of death.

Lindblad L, Nordenskjold A, Otterbeck, et al. Risk factors for mortality of medical causes within 30 days of electroconvulsive therapy. *J Affect Disord.* 2023;320:527-533.

D4. What alternative therapies are available for patients in whom ECT is relatively contraindicated?

Various alternative therapies have been investigated including transcranial direct current stimulation, repetitive transcranial magnetic stimulation, intravenous and intranasal ketamine (the latter of which is approved for use in patients with treatment-resistant depression [TRD] or major depressive disorder with suicidal ideation as esketamine [Spravato]), psilocybin (and other related ethnobotanicals), and nitrous oxide. Many of these medications are utilized in "subanesthetic" doses for treatment of TRD.

Anand A, Mathew SJ, Sanacora G, et al. Ketamine versus ECT for nonpsychotic treatment-resistant major depression. *N Engl J Med.* 2023;388:2315-2325.

Marwaha S, Palmer E, Suppes T, Cons E, Young AH, Upthegrove R. Novel and emerging treatments for major depression. *Lancet.* 2023;401:141-153.

Shao X, Yan D, Kong W, et al. Brain function changes reveal rapid antidepressant effects of nitrous oxide for treatment-resistant depression: evidence from task-state EEG. *Psychiatry Res.* 2023;322:115072.

61

Ambulatory Surgery

Justin S. Chung, Melinda Randall, and
Hugh C. Hemmings Jr.

A 71-year-old female with recently diagnosed breast cancer is scheduled for a mastectomy without reconstruction in the ambulatory surgery center. The patient has a significant family history of breast cancer in both her mother and grandmother. Her preoperative outpatient questionnaire indicates that she has hypertension that is well controlled by medication. Her surgical history includes T4-T8 laminectomy and fusion 5 years ago. She walks and exercises at greater than 4 metabolic equivalent of task (METs) 4 to 5 times per week without symptoms of chest pain or shortness of breath. She is 165 cm in height with a weight of 82 kg. The only medication she takes is lisinopril for hypertension. There is a history of postoperative nausea and vomiting (PONV) with prior anesthetics, even with monitored anesthesia care (MAC) for a bunionectomy. This patient is concerned about memory loss after anesthesia; she had some issues after colonoscopy with midazolam, fentanyl, and propofol. She also reports poor pain tolerance and is anxious about how her pain will be managed before she is discharged home.

A. Medical Disease and Differential Diagnosis

1. Is this patient morbidly obese?
2. What medical conditions can be associated with obesity and morbid obesity?
3. Is there a link to a decline in memory and thinking with anesthesia and surgery?

B. Preoperative Evaluation and Preparation

1. What advantages does outpatient surgery offer?
2. What are the goals of the preoperative evaluation of the surgical outpatient?
3. In order to thoroughly screen for disease, should one put all outpatients through a full battery of laboratory testing?
4. What preoperative laboratory testing is necessary for surgical outpatients?
5. Which outpatients should receive preoperative chest radiography?
6. In which patients is an electrocardiogram (ECG) necessary before outpatient anesthesia and surgery?
7. Would age or physical status influence the decision to perform outpatient surgery?
8. What patients are considered inappropriate for ambulatory surgery?
9. What questions are critically important to ask this patient when obtaining her history?
10. What instructions should the patient be given with regard to continuing or discontinuing lisinopril in the perioperative period?
11. What is an enhanced recovery after surgery (ERAS) protocol, and how would you apply it in the outpatient setting?
12. How would you premedicate this patient?
13. Should every outpatient receive prophylaxis against aspiration pneumonitis?
14. Is an overnight fast justified for all outpatients?

C. Intraoperative Management

1. What are the important considerations in choosing an anesthetic technique for outpatient surgery?
2. How would you monitor this patient?
3. What is the bispectral index (BIS) and what information does it convey?
4. What benefits might be derived from using a BIS monitor?
5. Is BIS monitoring applicable to children?
6. What are the major limitations of BIS monitoring?

7. What does a BIS reading of 56 mean?
8. What anesthetic agents would you use to induce and maintain general anesthesia in this patient?
9. Under what circumstances might spinal anesthesia be appropriate for outpatient surgery?
10. What nerve blocks might be beneficial in this patient?

D. Postoperative Management

1. What are the common causes of nausea and vomiting in outpatients?
2. How would you pharmacologically prevent PONV in the susceptible ambulatory patient?
3. What are the implications of using regional anesthesia on PONV in ambulatory surgery patients?
4. How is postoperative pain treated?
5. What criteria would you use to establish that a patient can be safely discharged after ambulatory surgery?
6. How would you decide when to discharge a patient after regional anesthesia?
7. What instructions should be given to an ambulatory surgical patients upon discharge?

A. Medical Disease and Differential Diagnosis

A.1. Is this patient morbidly obese?

Morbid obesity is defined by a body mass index greater than 40 kg/m^2. This patient has a body mass index of 30.2 and would, therefore, be considered obese (>30 kg/m^2) but not morbidly obese.

Fernandez-Bustamante A, Bucklin BA. Anesthesia and obesity. In: Cullen BF, Stock MC, Ortega R, et al, eds. *Barash, Cullen, and Stoelting's Clinical Anesthesia*. 9th ed. Wolters Kluwer; 2024:1229-1248.

A.2. What medical conditions can be associated with obesity and morbid obesity?

An abundance of medical conditions can be associated with obesity and morbid obesity. Obstructive sleep apnea (OSA) is the most prevalent sleep-related breathing disorder in *severely obese patients*. Screening tools such as the *STOP-BANG questionnaire* (also see Chapter 63: Morbid Obesity, Obstructive Sleep Apnea, and Bariatric Anesthesia, Section B.1) help to identify patients at high risk for OSA, and it is prudent to observe these patients for a minimum of 3 hours postoperatively in an ambulatory setting.

Obesity hypoventilation syndrome is defined as hypoventilation in an obese individual that cannot be attributed to other conditions associated with alveolar hypoventilation. These patients can exhibit hypoxemia and serum electrolyte abnormalities. Transesophageal echocardiography to assess global cardiac function, pulmonary hypertension, and specifically right heart function is recommended in these patients.

Other conditions that associate with obesity include:

- Hypertension
- Cardiovascular disease
- Diabetes mellitus type 2 is strongly associated with obesity.
- Metabolic syndrome or the co-occurrence of metabolic risk factors in both type 2 diabetes mellitus and cardiovascular disease (abdominal obesity, insulin resistance, dyslipidemia, and hypertension)
- Kidney disease

Fernandez-Bustamante A, Bucklin BA. Anesthesia and obesity. In: Cullen BF, Stock MC, Ortega R, et al, eds. *Barash, Cullen, and Stoelting's Clinical Anesthesia*. 9th ed. Wolters Kluwer; 2024:1229-1248.

A.3. Is there a link to a decline in memory and thinking with anesthesia and surgery?

Postoperative neurocognitive disorders (PNDs) including postoperative neurocognitive dysfunction (POCD) or neurocognitive decline are objectively measured declines in cognition postoperatively compared with preoperative function. Cognitive change after anesthesia was described over 100 years ago, initially as delirium and dementia. The term POCD was applied in the 1980s to refer to cognitive decline assessed purely on the basis of a change in neuropsychological test results. Increasing age, baseline cognitive impairment, and fewer years of education are consistently associated with POCD. According to the Mayo Clinic Study of Aging, 2,000 participants showed that anesthetic exposure after the age of 70 years was positively associated with long-term changes in brain physiology. The decline in cognitive function was small but significant for those who were already suffering from low cognitive function or preexisting mild impairment when exposed to general anesthesia for surgery. Older people whose clinical symptoms of cognitive dysfunction are not yet clinically symptomatic can manifest neurocognitive dysfunction if exposed to anesthesia. It is not possible to determine whether anesthesia, surgery, or the underlying conditions necessitating surgery cause the decline.

There are two anesthesia-related risks that are more common in older people: **Postoperative delirium** is a temporary condition that causes the patient to be confused, disoriented, unaware of her surroundings, and to have problems with memory and attention. It may not start until a few days after surgery, can come and go, and usually disappears after about a week. Both hyperactive and hypoactive forms exist, the latter being particularly difficult to diagnose. Many older elective orthopedic surgical patients have probable cognitive impairment preoperatively. Such impairment is associated with development of delirium postoperatively, longer hospital stay, and lower likelihood of going home upon hospital discharge. *POCD* is a more serious condition that can lead to long-term memory loss with difficulties in learning, concentration, and thinking. Because some of these problems are already common in older people, the only way to determine if a patient actually has POCD (more recently termed postoperative neurocognitive dysfunction) is to conduct cognitive testing before and after surgery/anesthesia. Certain conditions including heart disease (especially congestive heart failure), lung disease, Alzheimer disease, Parkinson disease, and previous stroke increase the risk for POCD. Also see Chapter 24: Diabetes Mellitus, Sections D.4 and D.5.

The American College of Surgeons and the American Geriatric Society have suggested that preoperative cognitive screening should be performed in older surgical patients. Recently, the clock drawing task has been promoted as a cognitive screening tool, either by asking a patient to draw a clock free hand with a specific time or handing a patient a piece of paper with a circle on it and asking them to fill it in with the numbers and time on a clock.

Culley DJ, Flaherty D, Fahey MC, et al. Poor performance on a preoperative cognitive screening test predicts postoperative complications in older orthopedic surgical patients. *Anesthesiology*. 2017;127:765-774.

Safavynia SA, Goldstein PA, Evered LA. Mitigation of perioperative neurocognitive disorders: a holistic approach. *Front Aging Neurosci*. 2022;14:949148.

Schulte PJ, Roberts RO, Knopman DS, et al. Association between exposure to anesthesia and surgery and long-term cognitive trajectories in older adults: report from the mayo clinic study of aging. *Br J Anaesth*. 2018;121:398-405.

B. Preoperative Evaluation and Preparation

B.1. What advantages does outpatient surgery offer?

Outpatient surgery typically offers greater convenience to the patient (less time away from home, family, and work), a more pleasant environment with less stress and emotional disturbance, and a reduced risk of infection, particularly for immunocompromised or pediatric patients. In addition to increasing patient satisfaction, outpatient surgery is more economical and enables more efficient use of operating rooms with greater flexibility in scheduling surgery, and does not depend on hospital bed availability. Patients also benefit from reduced health care costs, with one study estimating that patients save $684 on an average per outpatient procedure when compared to the same procedure done in a hospital setting. During the COVID-19 pandemic, hospitals shifted certain procedures to outpatient centers as they adapted to limited resources and attempted to reduce the rise of coronavirus infections.

Mancini P. Ambulatory anesthesia. In: Cullen BF, Stock MC, Ortega R, et al, eds. *Barash, Cullen, and Stoelting's Clinical Anesthesia*. 9th ed. Wolters Kluwer; 2024:818-828.

Shariq OA, Bews KA, Etzioni DA, Kendrick ML, Habermann EB, Thiels CA. Performance of general surgical procedures in outpatient settings before and after onset of the COVID-19 pandemic. *JAMA Netw Open*. 2023;6:e231198.

Young S, Osman B, Shapiro FE. Safety considerations with the current ambulatory trends: more complicated procedures and more complicated patients. *Korean J Anesthesiol*. 2023;76:400-412.

B.2. What are the goals of the preoperative evaluation of the surgical outpatient?

The objectives of the preoperative evaluation are:

- To perform necessary medical assessments, obtain data, arrange for laboratory tests and consultations as indicated, and prescreen for relevant conditions in order to optimize perioperative outcome.
- To obtain informed consent.
- To provide information and instructions to reduce patient anxiety and improve perioperative management.

Organization of preoperative screening varies among ambulatory surgical facilities. The screening process can be organized with an office or facility visit before the day of surgery, by a telephone interview or review of health questionnaire without a visit, or by preoperative screening and visit on the morning of surgery. Each of these systems has its advantages and disadvantages. Nevertheless, the system for preoperative evaluation of ambulatory surgical patients should ensure that screening is performed far enough in advance so that preexisting diseases can be evaluated, treatment optimized, and laboratory data recorded before the patient presents for anesthesia. Written instructions should be supplied to the patient in advance describing the preoperative workup, medications to be taken or held preoperatively, admission, and recovery periods.

Hata TM, Licina LK, Wyler DJ. Preoperative patient assessment and management. In: Cullen BF, Stock MC, Ortega R, et al, eds. *Barash, Cullen, and Stoelting's Clinical Anesthesia*. 9th ed. Wolters Kluwer; 2024:551-576.

Mancini P. Ambulatory anesthesia. In: Cullen BF, Stock MC, Ortega R, et al, eds. *Barash, Cullen, and Stoelting's Clinical Anesthesia*. 9th ed. Wolters Kluwer; 2024:818-828.

B.3. In order to thoroughly screen for disease, should one put all outpatients through a full battery of laboratory testing?

Extensive preoperative laboratory testing is rarely required for ambulatory surgery. The practice of routine preoperative laboratory screening for outpatient surgery has received much criticism. In addition to unnecessarily adding billions of dollars annually to the cost of health care, laboratory screening tests in asymptomatic patients are of dubious value and can actually increase complications from unnecessary follow-up procedures. History and physical examination are a better means of screening for disease and bleeding risks and should serve to reduce expensive, potentially harmful, and inappropriate tests.

Chung F, Yuan H, Yin L, et al. Elimination of preoperative testing in ambulatory surgery. *Anesth Analg*. 2009;108:467-475.

Hata TM, Licina LK, Wyler DJ. Preoperative patient assessment and management. In: Cullen BF, Stock MC, Ortega R, et al, eds. *Barash, Cullen, and Stoelting's Clinical Anesthesia*. 9th ed. Wolters Kluwer; 2024:551-576.

Hepner DL. Update on Preprocedure testing. In: Fleisher LA, ed. *Evidence-Based Practice of Anesthesiology*. 4th ed. Elsevier Saunders; 2023:55-61.

B.4. What preoperative laboratory testing is necessary for surgical outpatients?

Most outpatient surgical facilities consider the operative procedure and patient age, medical condition, medication history, and state and local regulations in determining which preoperative tests are "required." For the healthy ambulatory patient between the ages of 1 and 40 years having a minor surgical procedure, no laboratory testing might be required. Pregnancy testing is a controversial issue. Many believe that pregnancy testing should be offered to all consenting females of childbearing potential. This approach, however, does not substitute for an appropriate pregnancy history and physical examination. Hemoglobin or hematocrit determination is appropriate for surgical procedures associated with potential blood loss (unlikely in the ambulatory venue) and for patients at risk for anemia or polycythemia, such as children younger than 1 year or with suspected sickle cell disease, patients with a history of anemia, blood dyscrasia or malignancy, congenital heart disease or chronic disease, or females with heavy menstrual flow, or patients older than 60 years old.

Additional testing depends on preexisting conditions. For example, serum electrolyte testing is indicated for a patient with a history of hypertension, diabetes mellitus, renal disease, or taking diuretics, digoxin, steroids, or angiotensin-converting enzyme inhibitors (ACEIs). Likewise, measurement of the partial thromboplastin time (PTT) and the prothrombin time (PT) would be indicated in the presence of a bleeding disorder, anticoagulant use, liver disease, or poor nutritional status. Preoperative urinalysis has been shown to be not useful as a screening test and is no longer required in a routine anesthetic evaluation.

All patients with diabetes mellitus should have a point-of-care blood glucose measurement on the day of surgery when they arrive to the preoperative area. Although hemoglobin A1c (HbA1c) should be monitored in all diabetic patients, a 2024 consensus statement by the Society of Ambulatory Anesthesia did not find sufficient evidence to support postponing surgery for a HbA1c greater than 8.5, which differs from the 2022 ESC Guidelines on cardiovascular assessment and management of patients undergoing elective noncardiac surgery in hospital-based procedures.

Finegan BA, Rashiq S, McAlister FA, et al. Selective ordering of preoperative investigations by anesthesiologists reduces the number and cost of tests. *Can J Anaesth*. 2005;52:575-580.

Hepner DL. Update on Preprocedure testing. In: Fleisher LA, ed. *Evidence-Based Practice of Anesthesiology*. 4th ed. Elsevier Saunders; 2023:55-61.

Joshi GP, Chung F, Vann MA. Society for ambulatory anesthesia updated consensus statement on perioperative blood glucose management in adult patients with diabetes mellitus undergoing ambulatory surgery. *Anesth Analg*. 2024;139:459-477.

B.5. Which outpatients should receive preoperative chest radiography?

Abnormalities in the chest radiogram in asymptomatic patients are rare, and the risks to the patient probably exceed the benefits. Preoperative chest radiography is indicated only for patients with a history or clinical findings of active pulmonary disease. Extremes of age, smoking, stable chronic obstructive pulmonary disease, stable cardiac disease, or resolved recent upper respiratory infection should not be considered absolute indications.

Committee on Standards and Practice Parameters, Apfelbaum JL, Connis RT, et al. Practice advisory for preanesthesia evaluation: an updated report by the American Society of Anesthesiologists Task Force on Preanesthesia Evaluation. *Anesthesiology*. 2012;116:522-538.

Hata TM, Licina LK, Wyler DJ. Preoperative patient assessment and management. In: Cullen BF, Stock MC, Ortega R, et al, eds. *Barash, Cullen, and Stoelting's Clinical Anesthesia*. 9th ed. Wolters Kluwer; 2024:551-576.

Joo HS, Wong J, Naik VN, et al. The value of screening preoperative chest x-rays: a systematic review. *Can J Anaesth*. 2005;52:568-574.

B.6. In which patients is an electrocardiogram (ECG) necessary before outpatient anesthesia and surgery?

It has not been established that information obtained from the preoperative ECG affects clinical care. The American College of Cardiology/American Heart Association (ACC/AHA) guidelines published in 2007 were silent on the need for a preoperative ECG based on age alone. According to the 2014 ACC/AHA guideline, a preoperative ECG is "reasonable for patients with known coronary artery disease, significant arrhythmia, peripheral arterial disease, cerebrovascular disease, or other significant structural heart disease, except for those undergoing low-risk surgery." The 2014 guideline specifically states that a preoperative ECG is "not useful for asymptomatic patients undergoing low-risk surgical procedures." The 2007 ACC/AHA guidelines considered ambulatory surgery as one entity, classifying *all* ambulatory procedures as low risk, with reported cardiac mortality less than 1%. The 2014 version, however, defines a *low-risk* procedure as one in which the combined surgical and patient characteristics predict a risk of a major adverse cardiac event (MACE) of death or myocardial infarction to be less than 1%, such as cataract or plastic surgery. A further refinement in the 2014 guideline was to eliminate the separate categories of *intermediate risk* and *high risk*, substituting the category of *elevated risk*, reflecting procedures with a risk of MACE of greater than or equal to 1%. These guidelines have again been updated in 2024, and reflect the belief that in the absence of active cardiac conditions (defined as unstable coronary syndromes, decompensated heart failure, and significant arrhythmias [eg, high-degree atrioventricular block, symptomatic ventricular arrhythmias, and supraventricular tachycardia with uncontrolled ventricular rate]), cardiovascular testing in stable patients would rarely result in a change in management and it would be appropriate to proceed with surgery without further testing.

Nonetheless, Correll and colleagues found that being older than 65 years is an independent predictor of preoperative ECG abnormalities. In general, a preoperative ECG should be considered in ambulatory patients in whom there is a reasonably high likelihood of cardiac dysfunction and the results of the ECG would have the potential to influence perioperative management. The patient's history, including a thorough exploration of activity level and exercise tolerance, the physical examination, and the proposed surgical procedure are vital elements in the assessment of whether an ECG is indicated.

Correll DJ, Hepner DL, Chang C, et al. Preoperative electrocardiograms: patient factors predictive of abnormalities. *Anesthesiology*. 2009;110:1217-1222.

Fleisher LA, Beckman JA, Brown KA, et al. ACC/AHA 2007 guidelines on perioperative cardiovascular evaluation and care for noncardiac surgery: executive summary: a report of the American College of Cardiology/American Heart Association Task Force on Practice Guidelines (Writing Committee to revise the 2002 guidelines on perioperative cardiovascular evaluation for noncardiac surgery): developed in collaboration with the American Society of Echocardiography, American Society of Nuclear Cardiology, Heart Rhythm Society, Society of Cardiovascular Anesthesiologists, Society for Cardiovascular Angiography and Interventions, Society for Vascular Medicine and Biology, and Society for Vascular Surgery. *Circulation*. 2007;116:1971-1996.

Fleisher LA, Fleischmann KE, Auerbach AD, et al. 2014 ACC/AHA guideline on perioperative cardiovascular evaluation and management of patients undergoing noncardiac surgery: executive summary. *J Am Coll Cardiol*. 2014;64:2373-3405.

Halvorsen S, Mehilli J, Casses S, et al. 2022 ESC guidelines on cardiovascular assessment and management of patients undergoing non-cardiac surgery. *Eur Heart J*. 2022;43:3826.

Hepner DL. Preprocedure testing. In: Fleisher LA, ed. *Evidence-Based Practice of Anesthesiology*. 4th ed. Elsevier Saunders; 2023:55-61.

Thompson A, Fleischmann KE, Smilowitz NR, et al. 2024 AHA/ACC/ACS/ASNC/HRS/SCA/SCCT/SCMR/SVM guideline for perioperative cardiovascular management for noncardiac surgery: a report of the American College of Cardiology/American Heart Association Joint Committee on Clinical Practice Guidelines. *Circulation*. 2024;150:e351-e442.

B.7. Would age or physical status influence the decision to perform outpatient surgery?

Patients at the extremes of age (eg, younger than 6 months and older than 80 years) can be managed successfully at ambulatory centers. With the exception of the former preterm infant and newborns in the first few weeks of life, age alone should not be considered a deterrent in the selection of patients for outpatient surgery. Premature infants (gestational age at birth less than 37 weeks) who undergo general anesthesia during the first months of life are at increased risk for postoperative apnea for up to 12 hours. This risk is greatest for infants younger than 46 weeks postconceptional age, but some investigators have reported apnea in infants as old as 60 weeks postconceptional age. Unfortunately, the postconceptional age at which the former premature infant no longer has an increased risk for postoperative apnea, and therefore would be considered an acceptable candidate for an ambulatory surgical procedure, is not known. It is safest to admit to a hospital or to a 24-hour recovery unit all former premature infants less than 46 weeks postconceptional age so that they can be monitored for apnea. Many anesthesiologists are more conservative and adhere to cut-offs ranging from 52 to 60 weeks postconceptional age. If anemia, bronchopulmonary dysplasia, or other neonatal problems are present, this period may need to be extended. Postoperative apneic episodes have been described in otherwise healthy full-term infants who are anesthetized in the first few weeks of life. For this reason, many anesthesiologists are reluctant to proceed with outpatient anesthesia and surgery on a healthy full-term infant of younger than 2 to 4 weeks of age.

For geriatric patients, clinical experience has not shown an age-related effect on the duration of recovery or the incidence of postoperative complications after outpatient surgery. However, in determining the acceptability of a geriatric patient for an ambulatory surgical procedure, one must consider physiologic age and physical status, the surgical procedure, the anesthetic technique, and the quality of care that will be provided at home. Chronologic age is not a determinant of suitability for ambulatory surgery. It is becoming increasingly recognized that frailty is a better predictor of perioperative morbidity and readmissions rather than advanced age alone. Frailty encompasses multiple factors which include functional capacity, nutritional status, mental health, and cognition.

No longer is outpatient surgery restricted to patients of American Society of Anesthesiologists (ASA) physical status 1 and 2. It is increasingly common and acceptable to encounter patients that are ASA physical status 3. Although most patients who are ASA 4 or higher are generally not suitable candidates for surgery at standalone ambulatory surgical centers, those with stable comorbidities may undergo low-risk procedures requiring local or topical anesthesia such as cataract surgery.

Bentov I, Kaplan SJ, Pham TN, Reed MJ. Frailty assessment: from clinical to radiological tools. *Br J Anaesth*. 2019;123:37-50.

Everett LL. How young is the youngest infant for outpatient surgery? In: Fleisher LA, ed. *Evidence-Based Practice of Anesthesiology*. 4th ed. Elsevier Saunders; 2023:478-483.

Rajan N, Rosero EB, Joshi GP. Patient selection for adult ambulatory surgery: a narrative review. *Anesth Analg*. 2021;133:1415-1430.

Rampersad SE, Ojo B, Hansen EE, Holland EL, Feldman RM, Gentry KR. Pediatric anesthesia. In: Cullen BF, Stock MC, Ortega R, et al, eds. *Barash, Cullen, and Stoelting's Clinical Anesthesia*. 9th ed. Wolters Kluwer; 2024:1183-1214.

B.8. What patients are considered inappropriate for ambulatory surgery?

An individual can be considered inappropriate for ambulatory surgery for the following reasons:

- Existence of a condition that places an infant at risk
- History of prematurity in an infant less than 46 to 60 weeks postconceptional age
- Apneic episodes, feeding difficulty, or failure to thrive
- Respiratory distress syndrome that has required intubation and ventilatory support (may take up to a year for symptoms to resolve)
- Bronchopulmonary dysplasia with any significant decrease in pulmonary function or requirement for supplemental oxygen
- Acute concurrent illness
- ASA physical status 3 or 4 with poorly controlled disease

- Active cardiac conditions, as defined by ACC/AHA guidelines
- Acute substance misuse
- Morbid obesity with other serious systemic diseases, such as severe OSA and ventricular dysfunction
- Placement of a bare metal stent within 4 to 6 weeks of the proposed surgery
- Placement of a drug-eluting stent less than at least 1 year before the date of proposed surgery
- No available adult at home
- Refusal to have surgical procedure done as an outpatient
- Unwilling to follow instructions

The appropriateness of each patient must be evaluated on an individual basis, taking into account a combination of several factors, such as the patient's circumstances, the nature of the surgical procedure, anesthetic technique, anticipated severity of postoperative pain, and comfort level of the anesthesiologist.

American Society of Anesthesiologists Committee on Standards and Practice Parameters. Practice alert for the perioperative management of patients with coronary artery stents: a report by the American Society of Anesthesiologists Committee on Standards and Practice Parameters. *Anesthesiology*. 2009;110:22-23.

Fleisher LA, Fleischmann KE, Auerbach AD, et al. 2014 ACC/AHA guideline on perioperative cardiovascular evaluation and management of patients undergoing noncardiac surgery: executive summary. *J Am Coll Cardiol*. 2014;64:2373-3405.

Levine GN, Bates ER, Blankenship JC, et al. 2011 ACCF/AHA/SCAI guidelines for percutaneous coronary intervention: executive summary: a report of the American College of Cardiology Foundation/American Heart Association Task Force on Practice Guidelines and the Society for Cardiovascular Angiography and Interventions. *Circulation*. 2011;124:2574-2609.

Mancini P. Ambulatory anesthesia. In: Cullen BF, Stock MC, Ortega R, et al, eds. *Barash, Cullen, and Stoelting's Clinical Anesthesia*. 9th ed. Wolters Kluwer; 2024:818-828.

Motovska Z. Management of antiplatelet therapy inpatients at risk for coronary stent thrombosis undergoing non-cardiac surgery. *Drugs*. 2011;71:1797-1806.

B.9. What questions are critically important to ask this patient when obtaining her history?

It is important to rule out OSA in view of the patient's obesity, hypertension, and complaints of fatigue. Does she snore, have frequent awakenings during the night, or daytime somnolence? Not all patients with OSA are appropriate candidates for ambulatory surgery. An assessment instrument such as the STOP-BANG questionnaire is also a useful tool to evaluate the likelihood of OSA. A recent review by Ceban et al looked specifically at patients with OSA undergoing ambulatory surgery and found that these patients had 2-fold higher odds of same-day admission compared to non-OSA patients. In patients undergoing orthopedic ambulatory surgery, this risk was 2.7 fold higher than non-OSA patients. Moreover, patients who are obese with severe sleep apnea and certain associated conditions (pulmonary hypertension, ventricular dysfunction, etc.) having painful surgery under general anesthesia that might require significant amounts of opioids postoperatively for pain control are typically considered poor candidates for planned outpatient surgery.

American Society of Anesthesiologists Task Force on Perioperative Management of Patients with Obstructive Sleep Apnea. Practice guidelines for the perioperative management of patients with obstructive sleep apnea: an updated report by the American Society of Anesthesiologists Task Force on the Management of Patients with Obstructive Sleep Apnea. *Anesthesiology*. 2014;120:268-286.

Ceban F, Yan E, Pivetta B, et al. Perioperative adverse events in adult patients with obstructive sleep apnea undergoing ambulatory surgery: an updated systematic review and meta-analysis. *J Clin Anesth*. 2024;96:111464.

Chung F, Subramanyam R, Liao P, et al. High STOP-Bang score indicates a high probability of obstructive sleep apnoea. *Br J Anaesth*. 2012;108:768-775.

Joshi GP, Ankichetty SP, Gan TJ, et al. Society for ambulatory anesthesia consensus statement on preoperative selection of adult patients with obstructive sleep apnea scheduled for ambulatory surgery. *Anesth Analg*. 2012;115:1060-1068.

B.10. What instructions should the patient be given with regard to continuing or discontinuing lisinopril in the perioperative period?

This is a controversial issue, especially for ambulatory surgery patients. Significant hypotension has been reported after induction of general anesthesia in patients continuing to take ACEIs and angiotensin II subtype 1 receptor antagonists (angiotensin II receptor blockers [ARBs]) on the morning of surgery. A recent study, however, compared two groups of ambulatory and same-day admission patients who were taking either ACEIs or ARBs; one group took the ACEI or ARB on the day before surgery but not on the day of surgery, whereas the other group took the drug on the day of surgery at least 2 hours preoperatively along with other prescribed medications. Discontinuing ACEIs and ARBs on the morning of surgery did not place patients at risk for preoperative hypertension, cancellation, unplanned admission, or notable hypertension in the postanesthesia care unit. Moreover, patients who continued treatment on the day of surgery did not have more stable hemodynamics perioperatively than did those who discontinued these drugs. Although current opinion generally favors continuation of antihypertensive medications, especially β-blockers, up to the time of surgery, it appears that discontinuing ACEIs and ARBs on the day of surgery is safe and does not increase the incidence of adverse hemodynamic outcomes. Specifically, the 2014 and 2024 ACC/AHA guidelines state that continuation of ACEIs or ARBs perioperatively is "reasonable" and that if these drugs are held before surgery, it is reasonable to restart as soon as clinically feasible postoperatively.

Feinman J. Should all antihypertensive agents be continued before surgery? In: Fleisher LA, ed. *Evidence-Based Practice of Anesthesiology*. 4th ed. Elsevier Saunders; 2023:95-100.

Fleisher LA, Fleischmann KE, Auerbach AD, et al. 2014 ACC/AHA guideline on perioperative cardiovascular and management of patients undergoing noncardiac surgery: executive summary. *J Am Coll Cardiol*. 2014;64:2373-3405.

Twersky RS, Goel V, Narayan P, et al. The risk of hypertension after preoperative discontinuation of angiotensin-converting enzyme inhibitors or angiotensin receptor antagonists in ambulatory and same-day admission patients. *Anesth Analg*. 2014;118:938-944.

Wolf A, McGoldrick KE. Cardiovascular pharmacotherapeutic considerations in patients undergoing anesthesia. *Cardiol Rev*. 2011;19:12-16.

B.11. What is an enhanced recovery after surgery (ERAS) protocol, and how would you apply it in the outpatient setting?

ERAS programs are perioperative protocols of evidence-based interventions that have been grouped together with the goals of speeding functional recovery and improving postoperative outcomes. Also known as "enhanced recovery protocols" (ERPs) or "fast-track surgery," ERAS programs typically include standardized multidisciplinary and multimodal analgesic and anesthetic regimens aimed at minimizing the physiologic changes associated with surgery. Patient benefits associated with ERAS include reduction in speed to functional recovery, postoperative nausea and vomiting (PONV), postoperative opioid use, and length of stay. An enhanced recovery program includes education and engagement through the preoperative, intraoperative, and postoperative period.

Preoperative

- Preoperative medical optimization, patient education, preoperative nutrition and hydration (clear liquids up to 2 hours before scheduled arrival), and PONV prophylaxis with medications including ondansetron or aprepitant
- Multimodal analgesia given preoperative, which can be divided into pharmacologic and nonpharmacologic techniques. Systemic pharmacologic modalities involve opioids and nonopioids, such as acetaminophen, nonsteroidal anti-inflammatory drugs, *N*-methyl-D-aspartate receptor antagonist, anticonvulsants (eg, γ-aminobutyric acid analogues), β-blockers, α_2-agonists, transient receptor potential vanilloid receptor agonists (capsaicin), and glucocorticoids.

Intraoperative

- Consider total intravenous anesthesia in high PONV risk populations.
- Central neuraxial techniques, surgical site infiltration with local anesthetic and regional anesthesia
- Adjunctive techniques include acupuncture, music therapy, transcutaneous electrical nerve stimulation, and hypnosis.

Postoperative

- Early ambulation as soon as patient feel able
- Resume full diet as quickly as possible.

Afonso AM, McCormick PJ, Assel MJ, et al. Enhanced recovery programs in an ambulatory surgical oncology center. *Anesth Analg*. 2021;133:1391-1401.

Tan M, Law LS, Gan TJ. Optimizing pain management to facilitate enhanced recovery after surgery pathways. *Can J Anaesth*. 2015;62:203-218.

B.12. How would you premedicate this patient?

The use of premedication for ambulatory surgical patient has been the subject of much interest and debate. Keeping in mind that a prompt recovery is an important consideration in outpatient anesthesia, many recommend that little or no premedication (especially centrally active depressant premedicants) be given to surgical outpatients so that recovery is not prolonged. Interestingly, most prospective clinical studies have failed to demonstrate prolonged recovery following premedication with sedative-anxiolytic and analgesic drugs. However, opioid premedications have been shown to increase the incidence of postoperative nausea, which could prolong recovery time, and are not recommended unless the patient is in pain preoperatively.

Given the goals of outpatient preoperative medication, such as anxiety relief, sedation, amnesia, analgesia, vagolysis, prophylaxis against aspiration pneumonia, and prevention of PONV, premedication drugs can be safely used if needed, provided the drug and dosage are carefully chosen. Drugs commonly used for outpatients include sedative-hypnotics, opioids, anticholinergics, antacids, gastroprokinetic, H_2-receptor antagonists, and antiemetics.

Midazolam remains the most common anxiolytic used for premedication in the ambulatory setting. Most prospective studies have not found recovery to be prolonged after the use of appropriate doses of sedative premedication (eg, midazolam 1-2 mg IV). Appropriate use of premedication can actually expedite discharge by reducing postoperative side effects. Grant et al found that administration of preoperative or intraoperative midazolam is associated with a significant decrease in overall PONV, nausea, vomiting, and rescue antiemetic use. Providers might consider administration of midazolam IV as part of a multimodal approach in preventing PONV. Lorazepam's very long duration of action makes it unsuitable for use in the ambulatory surgical patient.

Gonzalez SN, Nin OC, Mehta SD. Anesthesia for ambulatory surgical procedures. In: Kaye AD, Urman RD, eds. *Cambridge Handbook of Anesthesiology*. Cambridge University Press; 2023:423-438.

Grant MC, Kim J, Page AJ, et al. The effect of intravenous midazolam on postoperative nausea and vomiting: a meta-analysis. *Anesth Analg*. 2016;122:656-663.

Hata TM, Licina LK, Wyler DJ. Preoperative patient assessment and management. In: Cullen BF, Stock MC, Ortega R, et al, eds. *Barash, Cullen, and Stoelting's Clinical Anesthesia*. 9th ed. Wolters Kluwer; 2024:551-576.

B.13. Should every outpatient receive prophylaxis against aspiration pneumonitis?

Despite early studies demonstrating that a large percentage of outpatients are potentially at risk for gastric aspiration, the actual incidence of pulmonary aspiration is very low (<1/35,000) in surgical patients with no specific risk factors. The possibility that outpatients have a greater potential for acid aspiration than inpatients prompted recommendations of some form of aspiration prophylaxis for all patients scheduled for outpatient surgery. This is costly and can result in undesired side effects. Although individual ambulatory surgery centers must determine their own policies, pharmacologic prevention of acid aspiration should not be routine but rather reserved for outpatients with predisposing factors (eg, pregnancy, symptomatic hiatal hernia, diabetes mellitus with autonomic neuropathy). When antacids are used, they should be restricted to nonparticulate antacids.

Hata TM, Licina LK, Wyler DJ. Preoperative patient assessment and management. In: Cullen BF, Stock MC, Ortega R, et al, eds. *Barash, Cullen, and Stoelting's Clinical Anesthesia*. 9th ed. Wolters Kluwer; 2024:551-576.

Practice guidelines for preoperative fasting and the use of pharmacologic agents to reduce the risk of pulmonary aspiration: application to healthy patients undergoing elective procedures: an updated report by the American Society of Anesthesiologists Task Force on preoperative fasting and the use of pharmacologic agents to reduce the risk of pulmonary aspiration. *Anesthesiology*. 2017;126:376-393.

B.14. Is an overnight fast justified for all outpatients?

Several investigators have questioned the value of the traditional overnight fast for surgical outpatients, particularly pediatric outpatients. Prolonged fasting does not guarantee an empty stomach at the time of induction of anesthesia. It does, however, cause patient discomfort and can produce significant physiologic disturbances in infants and young children. Studies in children and adults found no increase in volume or decrease in pH of gastric fluid when clear liquids were administered as late as 2 hours before induction of anesthesia. Therefore, arbitrary restrictions on the preoperative fast for surgical outpatients without risk factors for pulmonary aspiration, such as "nothing by mouth (nil per os; NPO) after midnight," appear unwarranted. Clear fluids in reasonable amounts (3 mL/kg) can be safely ingested until

2 hours before surgery. Although coffee is not transparent, it is devoid of particulate matter and is accepted as a clear liquid. There is some evidence that briefer periods of preoperative fasting (2 hours) are accompanied by less PONV as well as reduced incidence of dizziness, drowsiness, and thirst. Breast milk should be withheld for at least 4 hours in neonates and infants who are being breastfed. Intake of nonclear liquids, nonhuman milk, and solid food should be discontinued at least 6 hours before induction of anesthesia.

Mancini P. Ambulatory anesthesia. In: Cullen BF, Stock MC, Ortega R, et al, eds. *Barash, Cullen, and Stoelting's Clinical Anesthesia*. 9th ed. Wolters Kluwer; 2024:818-828.

Practice guidelines for preoperative fasting and the use of pharmacologic agents to reduce the risk of pulmonary aspiration: application to healthy patients undergoing elective procedures: an updated report by the American Society of Anesthesiologists Task Force on preoperative fasting and the use of pharmacologic agents to reduce the risk of pulmonary aspiration. *Anesthesiology*. 2017;126:376-393.

C. Intraoperative Management

C.1. What are the important considerations in choosing an anesthetic technique for outpatient surgery?

Important goals in ambulatory anesthesia include the following:

- Smooth and rapid onset of action
- Intraoperative amnesia and analgesia
- Hemodynamic stability
- Good operating conditions
- Rapid recovery period without side effects
- Cost-effectiveness

No ideal anesthetic drug or technique has been identified for outpatient anesthesia. No single agent or combination of agents, either inhaled or IV, has been clearly shown to reduce recovery time and allow faster discharge of the ambulatory surgical patient. However, with its smooth induction profile and short elimination half-life, propofol is currently the induction, if not the maintenance, agent of choice for most outpatient anesthesia. The newer halogenated ether compounds, sevoflurane and desflurane, have become increasingly popular in ambulatory anesthesia owing to their rapid onset and elimination of clinical effect. Currently, desirable anesthetic conditions with an acceptable recovery profile can be produced by a large array of pharmacologically active drugs administered in conjunction with either general, regional, or local anesthesia techniques. It is essential, however, to combine these agents in a rational manner with carefully titration to optimal effect.

Mancini P. Ambulatory anesthesia. In: Cullen BF, Stock MC, Ortega R, et al, eds. *Barash, Cullen, and Stoelting's Clinical Anesthesia*. 9th ed. Wolters Kluwer; 2024:818-828.

C.2. How would you monitor this patient?

The effects of anesthesia during ambulatory procedures should be monitored using the same standards applicable to inpatient procedures. Standard monitoring in this patient would include a blood pressure cuff, ECG, pulse oximeter, precordial or esophageal stethoscope, temperature probe, and measurement of inspired oxygen and end-tidal carbon dioxide.

Standards for basic anesthetic monitoring. Committee of origin: standards and practice parameters (approved by the ASA House of Delegates on October 21, 1986, last amended on October 20, 2010, and last affirmed on December 13, 2020). https://www.asahq.org/standards-and-practice-parameters/standards-for-basic-anesthetic-monitoring

C.3. What is the bispectral index (BIS) and what information does it convey?

The BIS monitor is a noninvasive monitoring system that is derived from a two-electrode processed electroencephalogram (EEG). Using proprietary bispectral analysis of the EEG waveform and other features within the EEG, the BIS monitor is used to detect changes in purported depth of anesthesia or hypnosis. The proprietary algorithm translates complex data generated from the analysis of the EEG over a 30-second period into a single dimensionless number between 0 (ie, no brain activity) and 100 (ie, the patient is fully awake) that is displayed on the BIS. The BIS is one of many brain function monitors that record or process brain electrical activity and convert these signals mathematically into a continuous measure, typically scaled from 0 to 100. It is important to appreciate that intraoperative awareness cannot be measured during the intraoperative phase of general anesthesia because the recall component of awareness can only be determined postoperatively by obtaining information directly from the patient. Although clinically important, intraoperative awareness under general anesthesia is a rare occurrence, with a reported incidence of 0.1% to 0.2% in adults.

American Society of Anesthesiologists Task Force on Intraoperative Awareness. Practice advisory for intraoperative awareness and brain function monitoring: a report by the American Society of Anesthesiologists Task Force on Intraoperative Awareness. *Anesthesiology*. 2006;104:847-864.

Avidan MS, Mashour GA. Prevention of intraoperative awareness with explicit recall: making sense of the evidence. *Anesthesiology*. 2013;118:449-456.

Avidan MS, Zhang L, Burnside BA, et al. Anesthesia awareness and the bispectral index. *N Engl J Med*. 2008;358:1097-1108.

Kent CD, Domino KB. Depth of anesthesia. *Curr Opin Anaesthesiol*. 2009;22:782-787.

Sebel PS, Bowdle TA, Ghoneim MM, et al. The incidence of awareness during anaesthesia: a multicenter United States study. *Anesth Analg*. 2004;99:833-839.

C.4. What benefits might be derived from using a BIS monitor?

Information about the patient's hypnotic state, or depth of anesthesia, obtained from the BIS, in combination with other monitored parameters and clinical signs, can allow balancing of hypnotic and analgesic administration. Titration of hypnotic agents based on individual requirements arguably is improved, potentially reducing the incidence of relative under- and overdosing. Furthermore, selection of anesthetic interventions (eg, administration of hypnotics, analgesics, and vasoactive drugs) can be more rational. Reduced drug usage, earlier awakening, and faster recovery have all been associated with using the BIS monitor to help guide anesthesia maintenance. This translates into a higher potential for bypassing the stage 1 postanesthesia care unit (PACU) and earlier discharge eligibility from the PACU. It is not known whether these benefits ultimately reduce medical costs significantly. A recent meta-analysis based on 1,380 subjects from 11 trials found that BIS monitoring reduced anesthetic consumption by 19%, reduced the incidence of nausea/vomiting, and reduced time in the PACU by 4 minutes. However, these benefits did not lead to a significant reduction in time until patient discharge from the ambulatory surgery unit. Additionally, BIS monitoring actually increased the cost per patient by $5.55 owing to the cost of the BIS electrodes.

There has been considerable recent interest in depth of anesthesia and 1-year mortality. The investigators in the B-Aware trial reported a secondary analysis of long-term mortality and found that the absence of low BIS values (BIS <40 for >5 minutes) was associated with improved long-term survival and reduced morbidity (myocardial infarction, stroke). However, this association does not imply causation. Preoperative comorbidity is an important independent risk factor for postoperative mortality.

Patients with a history of intraoperative awareness are at increased risk to develop the complication again. These patients, and others at high risk of intraoperative awareness (eg, use of total intravenous anesthesia [TIVA], patients having trauma surgery or cesarean delivery, patients with refractory hypotension), might benefit from BIS monitoring.

Other modalities can also be used to monitor purported anesthetic depth. These include end-tidal anesthetic concentration monitoring, auditory evoked potentials, as well as derivatives of processed EEG including EEG entropy, Narcotrend monitor, Neurosense monitor, and Patient State index. Major trials are currently underway to further elucidate the impact of these technologies on postoperative cognitive dysfunction.

Aranake A, Gradwohl S, Ben-Abdallah A, et al. Increased risk of intraoperative awareness in patients with a history of awareness. *Anesthesiology*. 2013;119:1275-1283.

Laferrière-Langlois P, Morisson L, Jeffries S, Duclos C, Espitalier F, Richebé P. Depth of anesthesia and nociception monitoring: current state and vision for 2050. *Anesth Analg*. 2024;138:295-307.

Leslie K, Myles PS, Forbes A, et al. The effect of bispectral index monitoring on long-term survival in the B-aware trial. *Anesth Analg*. 2010;110:816-822.

Liu S. Effects of bispectral index monitoring on ambulatory anesthesia: a meta-analysis of randomized controlled trials and a cost analysis. *Anesthesiology*. 2004;101:311-315.

Mashour GA, Kent C, Picton P, et al. Assessment of intraoperative awareness with explicit recall: a comparison of 2 methods. *Anesth Analg*. 2013;116:889-891.

Pavlin JD, Souter KJ, Hong JY. Effects of bispectral index monitoring on recovery from surgical anesthesia in 1,580 inpatients from an academic medical center. *Anesthesiology*. 2005;102:566-573.

C.5. Is BIS monitoring applicable to children?

The BIS was developed and tested on adults. Because the EEG in infants and young children is different from that of an adult and changes as the brain matures, BIS values might not apply directly to children. Validating the BIS monitor in infants and young children poses significant problems. Endpoints used to confirm BIS in adults, such as assessment of sedation, sleep, or purposeful movement in response to voice commands, cannot be reliably obtained in young children. Furthermore, there are serious ethical problems in recruiting healthy children as volunteers in studies of general anesthesia. Nevertheless, recent data comparing BIS values between adults and children at various clinical end points during general anesthesia, such as before anesthesia, during maintenance, at emergence, and with increasing concentrations of volatile anesthetic, suggest that BIS generally performs similarly in adults and children with respect to dose response to anesthetic agents. However, in children aged 6 months to 12 years, the BIS increased paradoxically as end-tidal sevoflurane concentration increased from 3% to 4%. BIS values showed a wide variation at the same end-tidal sevoflurane concentration, and age was considered to be a factor affecting BIS values. A consensus seems to be forming that BIS monitoring should be used with caution in infants younger than 1 year of age, and further work in this area is needed.

Definitive studies correlating level of sedation, awareness, and anesthetic outcome with BIS in children have not been published. Nonetheless, consensus is emerging that the incidence of intraoperative awareness is greater in children than adults. Children, however, seem to be less disturbed by the experience than adults who appear to be more vulnerable to the development of posttraumatic stress.

Bannister CF, Brosius KF, Sigl JC, et al. The effect of bispectral index monitoring on anesthetic use and recovery in children anesthetized with sevoflurane in nitrous oxide. *Anesth Analg*. 2001;92:877-881.

Blussé van Oud-Alblas HJ, van Dijk M, Liu C, et al. Intraoperative awareness during paediatric anaesthesia. *Br J Anaesth*. 2009;102:104-110.

Davidson AJ, Huang GH, Rebmann CS, et al. Performance of entropy and bispectral index as measures of anaesthesia effect in children of different ages. *Br J Anaesth*. 2005;95:674-679.

Davidson AJ, Smith KR, Blussé van Oud-Alblas HJ, et al. Awareness in children: a secondary analysis of five cohort studies. *Anaesthesia*. 2011;66:446-454.

Kim HS, Oh AY, Kim CS, et al. Correlation of bispectral index with end-tidal sevoflurane concentration and age in infants and children. *Br J Anaesth*. 2005;95:362-366.

C.6. What are the major limitations of BIS monitoring?

BIS is not a measure of global anesthetic depth but a measure of level of sedation and hypnotic state. As such, it helps assess the potential for patient awareness, but it cannot prevent it. In fact, use of BIS has not been proven to reduce or eliminate the risk of intraoperative awareness. BIS does not predict patient movement or hemodynamic response to noxious stimulation nor does it predict the exact moment when consciousness will return. Sedation produced by ketamine or nitrous oxide does not produce the expected decrease in BIS. The utility of BIS in patients with neurologic disease has not been adequately studied to validate its use in these patients. Finally, more work is necessary to establish whether BIS is an accurate measure of hypnosis in pediatric patients.

It is important to appreciate that a specific numerical value might not correlate with a specific depth of anesthesia. Moreover, the measured values do not have uniform sensitivity across different anesthetic drugs or types of patients. Artifacts can be introduced by electrocautery, lasers, warming devices, and other devices and circumstances. BIS cannot be relied on in all situations, including hypothermia, circulatory arrest, and brain death. Moreover, a small study recently reported that patient position can affect BIS readings, with the head-down position producing an increase in BIS value, and the head-up position being associated with a reduction in BIS values. Intraoperative monitoring of depth of anesthesia to minimize the risk of awareness should rely on multiple modalities, including clinical observations of purposeful or reflex movement, blood pressure, heart rate, end-tidal anesthetic concentration, and capnography.

The consensus of the ASA Task Force on Intraoperative Awareness is that the brain function monitoring is not routinely indicated for patients undergoing general anesthesia, and that the decision to use a brain function monitor should be made on a case-by-case basis by the individual practitioner for selected patients at increased risk.

American Society of Anesthesiologists Task Force on Intraoperative Awareness. Practice advisory for intraoperative awareness and brain function monitoring: a report by the American Society of Anesthesiologists Task Force on Intraoperative Awareness. *Anesthesiology*. 2006;104:847-864.

Avidan MS, Zhang L, Burnside BA, et al. Anesthesia awareness and the bispectral index. *N Engl J Med.* 2008;358:1097-1108.

Barr G, Jakobsson JG, Owall A, et al. Nitrous oxide does not alter bispectral index: study with nitrous oxide as sole agent and as adjunct to I.V. anaesthesia. *Br J Anaesth.* 1999;82:827-830.

Bowdle A. Can we prevent recall during anesthesia? In: Fleisher LA, ed. *Evidence-Based Practice of Anesthesiology.* 4th ed. Elsevier Saunders; 2023:309-315.

Chan MT, Gin T. What does the bispectral EEG index monitor? *Eur J Anaesthesiol.* 2000;17:146-148.

Kaki AM, Almarakbi WA. Does patient position influence the reading of the bispectral index monitor? *Anesth Analg.* 2009;109:1843-1846.

Wennervirta J, Salmi T, Hynynen M, et al. Entropy is more resistant to artifacts than bispectral index in brain-dead organ donors. *Intensive Care Med.* 2007;33:133-136.

C.7. What does a BIS reading of 56 mean?

The BIS scale is a dimensionless scale from 0 to 100. Typically, BIS values between 40 and 60 correspond with a moderate hypnotic state of general anesthesia and are associated with a low probability of patient consciousness. Deep sedation with a low probability of explicit recall occurs in the 60 to 70 BIS range, with higher values up to 85 associated with light to moderate sedation. A BIS number below 40 indicates a deep hypnotic state, with probability of EEG isoelectricity increasing as BIS approaches 0. However, there are multiple exceptions to these generalities, and the BIS is perhaps best thought of as a trend monitor rather than an absolute monitor of hypnotic depth.

Hemmerling TM, Migneault B. Falsely increased bispectral index during endoscopic shoulder surgery attributed to interferences with the endoscopic shaver device. *Anesth Analg.* 2002;95:1678-1679.

Johansen JW, Sebel PS. Development and clinical application of electroencephalographic bispectrum monitoring. *Anesthesiology.* 2000;93:1336-1344.

C.8. What anesthetic agents would you use to induce and maintain general anesthesia in this patient?

A number of anesthetic agents in a variety of combinations can be used successfully to provide general anesthesia in this ambulatory patient. A reasonable approach would be to induce anesthesia with propofol after a preinduction dose of a short-acting benzodiazepine. After tracheal intubation, anesthesia is maintained with a volatile anesthetic, such as sevoflurane or desflurane in an air-oxygen mixture, supplemented with a short-acting opioid as needed and a neuromuscular blocking agent. Alternatively, a TIVA technique with propofol as the primary agent could be used. Recent meta-analyses suggest that TIVA results in decreased PONV and pain scores when compared with volatile anesthesia. TIVA also consistently scores higher than volatile techniques in patient satisfaction surveys. Despite these benefits, surveys of anesthesiologists seem to suggest that TIVA is still not widespread in its use.

Although nitrous oxide has been thought to contribute to PONV, conclusive evidence is lacking to demonstrate an important effect of nitrous oxide on the incidence of postoperative emesis after laparoscopic cholecystectomy or pelvic laparoscopy. A recent review and meta-regression analysis reported that the increase in PONV sometimes seen with administration of nitrous oxide depends on the duration of exposure and is clinically unimportant up to at least 1 hour of exposure. Therefore, any potential benefit from its elimination for surgical cases of limited duration must be balanced against the potential increased risk of intraoperative awareness.

The Beers Criteria for Potentially Inappropriate Medication Use in Older Adults, commonly called the Beers List, are guidelines for health care professionals to help improve the safety of prescribing medications for older adults.

- *Dementia or cognitive impairment in the geriatric population: drugs to avoid*
  - Anticholinergics, benzodiazepines, H_2-receptor antagonists, nonbenzodiazepine benzodiazepine receptor agonist hypnotics (eszopiclone, zolpidem, zaleplon), antipsychotics
- *Delirium: drugs to avoid*
  - Anticholinergics, antipsychotics, benzodiazepines, chlorpromazine, corticosteroids, H_2-receptor antagonists (cimetidine, famotidine, nizatidine, ranitidine), meperidine, sedative-hypnotics

American Geriatrics Society Beers Criteria® Update Expert Panel. American Geriatrics Society 2019 Updated AGS Beers Criteria® for potentially inappropriate medication use in older adults. *J Am Geriatr Soc.* 2019;67:674-694.

Clegg A, Young JB. Which medications to avoid in people at risk of delirium: a systemic review. *Age Ageing.* 2011;40:23-29.

Diemunsch PA, Torp KD, Van Dorsselaer T, et al. Nitrous oxide fraction in the carbon dioxide pneumoperitoneum during laparoscopy under general inhaled anesthesia in pigs. *Anesth Analg*. 2000;90:951-953.

McIlroy EI, Leslie K. Total intravenous anaesthesia in ambulatory care. *Curr Opin Anaesthesiol*. 2019;32:703-707.

Peyton PJ, Wu CY. Nitrous oxide-related postoperative nausea and vomiting depends on the duration of exposure. *Anesthesiology*. 2014;120:1137-1145.

Rodriguez G, Joseph SE. Anesthesia for laparoscopic and robotic surgeries. In: Cullen BF, Stock MC, Ortega R, et al, eds. *Barash, Cullen, and Stoelting's Clinical Anesthesia*. 9th ed. Wolters Kluwer; 2024:1215-1228.

C.9. Under what circumstances might spinal anesthesia be appropriate for outpatient surgery?

Spinal anesthesia is a quick and reliable technique. Its advantages include decreased rates of PONV, lower cost, and potential reduction in perioperative morbidity in patients with comorbidities such as obesity, OSA, and chronic obstructive pulmonary disease (COPD). However, limitations to spinal anesthesia exist, including provider comfort, possible delayed ambulation, risk of urinary retention, patient unfamiliarity, postdural puncture headache, and pain after block regression. Reducing the dose of the commonly used long-acting local anesthetics can reduce recovery time, but discharge times are still prolonged compared with general anesthesia. 2-Chloroprocaine is an amino-ester local anesthetic with a very short half-life that can be used as a local anesthetic for ultra-short outpatient procedures; it is associated with a very low risk of urinary retention and transient neurologic symptoms when compared with bupivacaine or lidocaine.

Ben-David B, Maryanovsky M, Gurevitch A, et al. A comparison of minidose lidocaine-fentanyl and conventional-dose lidocaine spinal anesthesia. *Anesth Analg*. 2000;91:865-870.

Fanelli A, Ghisi D, Allegri M. Is spinal anaesthesia a suitable technique for ultra-short outpatient procedures? *Acta Biomed*. 2013;84:76-80.

Ledesma I, Stieger A, Luedi MM, Romero CS. Spinal anesthesia in ambulatory patients. *Curr Opin Anaesthesiol*. 2024;37:661-665.

C.10. What nerve blocks might be beneficial in this patient?

There are several nerve blocks that can be utilized for patients undergoing breast surgery. The paravertebral block is well established as an effective technique for analgesia but its use can be limited by its technical difficulty and potential for complication given its proximity to the pleura and spinal canal.

Pectoralis blocks (PECS) have gained in popularity as a safer and more accessible option compared to paravertebral blocks. In the originally described PECS-1 block, local anesthetic is deposited between the pectoralis major and minor to anesthetize the medial and lateral pectoral nerves. A modification of this block, called the PECS-2 block, aims to anesthetize the upper intercostal nerves as they course between the pectoralis minor and serratus anterior muscles. PECS blocks seem to provide comparable analgesia and opioid sparing to paravertebral blocks in meta-analyses.

The serratus anterior block as another option for analgesia for breast surgery. To perform a serratus anterior block (SAP), local anesthetic is deposited between the serratus anterior and latissimus dorsi under ultrasound to block the intercostobrachial nerve, long thoracic nerve, thoracodorsal nerve, and cutaneous branches of the T3-T9 intercostal nerves. While there is evidence of clear analgesic benefit when SAP is utilized compared to placebo, there is a lack of high-quality evidence that SAP is comparable to PECS blocks in breast surgery.

Innervation of the breast is complex. While nerve blocks are an extremely useful tool for analgesia, further studies are still needed to determine what block or combination of blocks is ideal for ambulatory breast surgery.

Ardon AE, George JE, Gupta K, et al. The use of pectoralis blocks in breast surgery: a practice advisory and narrative review from the Society for Ambulatory Anesthesia (SAMBA). *Ann Surg Oncol*. 2022;29:4777-4786.

Blanco R. The 'pecs block': a novel technique for providing analgesia after breast surgery. *Anaesthesia*. 2011;66:847-848.

Blanco R, Fajardo M, Parras Maldonado T. Ultrasound description of Pecs II (modified Pecs I): a novel approach to breast surgery. *Rev Esp Anestesiol Reanim*. 2012;59:470-475.

Blanco R, Parras T, McDonnell JG, Prats-Galino A. Serratus plane block: a novel ultrasound-guided thoracic wall nerve block. *Anaesthesia*. 2013;68:1107-1113.

Jacobs A, Lemoine A, Joshi GP, Van de Velde M, Bonnet F; PROSPECT Working Group Collaborators. PROSPECT guideline for oncological breast surgery: a systematic review and procedure-specific postoperative pain management recommendations. *Anaesthesia*. 2020;75:664-673.

D. Postoperative Management

D.1. What are the common causes of nausea and vomiting in outpatients?

Nausea and vomiting are significant problems after ambulatory surgery, causing patient discomfort and delayed recovery and discharge from the ambulatory center. Prolonged vomiting is one of the most frequent causes of unexpected hospital admission from the ambulatory surgical facility and is a major cause of patient dissatisfaction with their anesthesia care. Patients who have a history of motion sickness or PONV are more likely to develop postoperative symptoms of emesis, as are patients who are obese, pregnant, or have diabetes mellitus. PONV are common in children; the incidence decreases with age. Males and females are equally affected until puberty, when the incidence becomes considerably higher in females. Excessive anxiety and nonadherence to fasting can increase gastric volume and predispose patients to PONV. Interestingly, smoking has been shown to decrease the incidence of PONV.

The use of opioid analgesics, particularly morphine and meperidine, as premedication, as part of the anesthetic technique, or postoperatively to control pain, increases the incidence of PONV after outpatient anesthesia. Methohexital is less likely than either thiopental or etomidate to cause postoperative nausea. Propofol has a low incidence of emetic symptoms postoperatively and has been proposed to be antiemetic, but this is largely due to avoidance of volatile anesthetics.

Although the Apfel scoring system to predict the likelihood of PONV emphasizes female sex, nonsmoking status, history of PONV or motion sickness, and opioid administration as the major risk factors, there is no or insufficient evidence for a number of commonly held factors, such as preoperative fasting, menstrual cycle, and surgery type; using these factors might be counterproductive in assessing risk for PONV. In addition, pain, hypotension, and early ambulation are postoperative factors shown to increase PONV.

Apfel CC, Heidrich FM, Jukar-Rao S, et al. Evidence-based analysis of risk factors for postoperative nausea and vomiting. *Br J Anaesth*. 2012;109:742-753.

Apfel C, Kranke P, Eberhart LH, et al. Comparison of predictive models for postoperative nausea and vomiting. *Br J Anaesth*. 2002;88:234-240.

D.2. How would you pharmacologically prevent PONV in the susceptible ambulatory patient?

Because of concerns about medication cost and potential side effects, routine prophylactic administration of antiemetics is not considered appropriate for all ambulatory surgical patients. Instead, antiemetic prophylaxis should be reserved for patients who are considered to be susceptible to developing PONV. Many medications have been used as prophylaxis for PONV in the outpatient, some with only limited success. Unfortunately, the ideal medication for each patient is not known. Serotonin antagonists, such as ondansetron 4 to 8 mg IV in adults and 0.1 mg/kg IV in children, are highly effective, but their use as single agents in high-risk patients may not suffice. Droperidol is effective, inexpensive, and without an increase in postoperative sedation when used in low doses, such as 0.625 to 1.25 mg in adults (or as low as 10-20 μg/kg). However, the US Food and Drug Administration (FDA) issued a black box warning on the use of droperidol for antiemetic prophylaxis based on concerns about prolongation of the QTc interval and subsequent potentially dangerous ventricular arrhythmias. Charbit et al reported that droperidol and ondansetron induce similar clinically relevant QTc prolongation and concluded that the safety of 5-hydroxytryptamine type 3 (5-HT_3) antagonists might not be superior to that of low-dose droperidol. Although the serotonin antagonists are believed to lack efficacy with regard to preventing or treating nausea, the newest 5-HT_3 blocker, palonosetron, appears to reduce its severity, and the extended benefits of palonosetron can last up to 3 days given its long half-life. In addition, palonosetron purportedly has no QT-interval prolongation issues.

Prophylactic administration of dexamethasone, 1 to 10 mg IV in adults and 0.5 to 1 mg/kg IV in children, is effective in the prevention of PONV and appears to offer no evidence of clinically relevant toxicity. Combining dexamethasone with a serotonin antagonist further decreases the incidence of PONV and could prove to be the best prophylactic regimen, although optimal doses of this combination are not currently known. Transdermal scopolamine effectively reduces PONV if given well in advance of the surgery, but the high incidence of anticholinergic side effects and prolonged residual effects on cognitive performance, especially in the older adults, detract from its usefulness in the ambulatory patient.

Aprepitant is a highly selective, brain-penetrating neurokinin-1 receptor antagonist that is effective against centrally induced emesis. A recent study showed that aprepitant was superior to ondansetron for prevention of vomiting in the first 24 to 48 hours, but no notable differences were detected between aprepitant and ondansetron for nausea control, use of rescue drugs, or complete response.

Because the etiology of PONV is multifactorial, there is increasing evidence that a multimodal approach may lead to improved outcomes. Double and triple antiemetic combinations, using drugs with different mechanisms of action, are recommended for patients at high risk of PONV. Moreover, liberal hydration and effective analgesia play an important role in reducing the incidence of PONV. General anesthesia with volatile agents should be avoided, if possible, in high-risk patients. If general anesthesia is necessary, a TIVA approach with propofol can be advantageous. Moreover, if rescue therapy for PONV is needed within 6 hours of surgery, patients should not receive a repeat dose of the drug that was administered prophylactically. Rather, a rescue drug with a different mechanism of action should be selected.

Amisulpride should be used as a rescue medication for established PONV that occurs in the postanesthesia care unit. Intravenous doses of 5 and 10 mg are superior to placebo for the treatment of established PONV in patients who have received no other PONV prophylaxis or treatment. The data show a complete response rate (defined as no emesis in the period 30 minutes to 24 hours after study drug treatment and no use of rescue medication in the entire 24-hour period) of 31.4% for both 5 and 10 mg IV amisulpride groups, which was significantly different compared to the 21.5% complete response rate in the placebo group. There was no difference in adverse event profiles between the amisulpride groups and the placebo group, implying a favorable safety profile for the medication.

Apfel CC, Kranke P, Katz MH, et al. Volatile anaesthetics may be the main cause of early but not delayed postoperative vomiting: a randomized controlled trial of factorial design. *Br J Anaesth.* 2002;88:659-668.

Apfel CC, Läärä E, Koivuranta M, et al. A simplified risk score for predicting postoperative nausea and vomiting: conclusions from cross-validations between two centers. *Anesthesiology.* 1999;91:693-700.

Ashraf HA. What is the best strategy for prevention of postoperative nausea and vomiting? In: Fleisher LA, ed. *Evidence-Based Practice of Anesthesiology.* 4th ed. Elsevier Saunders; 2023:241-247.

Charbit B, Albaladejo P, Funck-Brentano C, et al. Prolongation of QTc interval after postoperative nausea and vomiting treatment by droperidol or ondansetron. *Anesthesiology.* 2005;102:1094-1100.

Gan TJ, Apfel CC, Kovac AL, et al. A randomized, double-blind comparison of the NK_1 antagonist, aprepitant, versus ondansetron for the prevention of postoperative nausea and vomiting. *Anesth Analg.* 2007;104:1082-1089.

Gan TJ, Belani KG, Bergese S, et al. Fourth consensus guidelines for the management of postoperative nausea and vomiting. *Anesth Analg.* 2020;131:411-448.

Gan TJ, Diemunsch P, Habib AS, et al. Consensus guidelines for the management of postoperative nausea and vomiting. *Anesth Analg.* 2014;118:85-113.

Gan TJ, Mouch CM. Amisulpride: a new dopamine antagonist for treatment of postoperative nausea and vomiting. *Anesth Analg.* 2019;128:1074-1076.

Kovac AL, Eberhart L, Kotarski J, et al. A randomized, double-blind study to evaluate the efficacy and safety of three different doses of palonosetron versus placebo in preventing postoperative nausea and vomiting over a 72-hour period. *Anesth Analg.* 2008;107:439-444.

Kranke P, Eberhart LH. Possibilities and limitations in the pharmacological management of postoperative nausea and vomiting. *Eur J Anaesthesiol.* 2011;28:758-765.

Ruiz JR, Kee SS, Frenzel JC, et al. The effect of an anatomically classified procedure on antiemetic administration in the postanesthesia care unit. *Anesth Analg.* 2010;110:403-409.

Sinclair DR, Chung F, Mezei G. Can postoperative nausea and vomiting be predicted? *Anesthesiology.* 1999;91:109-118.

D.3. What are the implications of using regional anesthesia on PONV in ambulatory surgery patients?

Regional anesthesia (RA) can be a useful tool in decreasing risk of PONV. The Society for Ambulatory Anesthesiology (SAMBA) recommends the use of RA as a strategy to reduce baseline risk of PONV, and suggests the use of RA in high-risk patients when possible. There is evidence that patients receiving general anesthesia are 9 times more likely to experience PONV compared to patients who receive RA, especially when patients are spared exposure to inhaled volatile anesthetics.

Many randomized controlled trials indicate that use of RA can provide excellent postoperative analgesia, reduce the use of perioperative opioids, decrease the incidence of PONV, and improve patient satisfaction in the ambulatory surgical setting. The dose-dependent relationship between perioperative opioid use and incidence of PONV is well documented. Whether this association leads to decreased times to discharge from an ambulatory surgical center remains controversial in meta-analyses.

Liu SS, Strodtbeck WM, Richman JM, Wu CL. A comparison of regional versus general anesthesia for ambulatory anesthesia: a meta-analysis of randomized controlled trials. *Anesth Analg*. 2005;101:1634-1642.

Roberts GW, Bekker TB, Carlsen HH, et al. Postoperative nausea and vomiting are strongly influenced by postoperative opioid use in a dose-related manner. *Anesth Analg*. 2005;101:1343-1348.

D.4. How is postoperative pain treated?

Pain control is one of the most important factors in determining when a surgical outpatient can be discharged. Pain should be treated preemptively, rapidly, and effectively to minimize postoperative symptoms so that ambulation and discharge are not delayed. The optimal strategy is to use a preemptive, multimodal approach. Begin controlling postoperative pain intraoperatively by supplementing the anesthetic technique with a short-acting opioid analgesic or a regional block. IV fentanyl is usually the opioid of choice for postoperative pain relief. It can be given in small doses of 25 μg at 5-minute intervals and titrated to relief of pain. Ketorolac, a nonsteroidal anti-inflammatory drug, has become increasingly popular in the management of postoperative pain in the ambulatory patient because of its lack of opioid-related side effects (eg, sedation, nausea, vomiting, respiratory depression). It is available for oral and parental administration, and its use can decrease requirements for opioid analgesics. Controversy still surrounds the perioperative use of ketorolac because of the potential for bleeding complications and renal dysfunction. Local and regional anesthetic techniques can be used to provide effective postoperative analgesia and, when used to supplement general anesthesia, facilitate a pleasant emergence and minimize the need for opioids.

When the patient has resumed intake of oral fluids, oral analgesics (eg, acetaminophen, nonsteroidal anti-inflammatory drugs, oxycodone, hydrocodone, and other opioid analgesics) can be administered for control of pain after discharge.

In 2025, Suzetrigine, a nonopioid selective voltage-gated sodium channel blocker was approved by the FDA for use in the treatment of acute pain. While the prospect of a new class of medication with low addictive potential is exciting, it has not yet been widely studied in the ambulatory surgical setting.

Golf M, Daniels SE, Onel E. A phase 3, placebo-controlled trial of DepoFoam® bupivacaine (extended-release bupivacaine local analgesic) in bunionectomy. *Adv Ther*. 2011;28:776-788.

Joshi GP. Anesthetic management for enhanced recovery after major surgery (ERAS) in adults. Accessed March 18, 2025. https://www.uptodate.com/contents/overview-of-enhanced-recovery-after-major-noncardiac-surgery-eras?search=joshi%20enhanced%20recovey%20after%20surgery&source=search_result&selectedTitle=4%7E150&usage_type=default&display_rank=4

Mancini P. Ambulatory anesthesia. In: Cullen BF, Stock MC, Ortega R, et al, eds. *Barash, Cullen, and Stoelting's Clinical Anesthesia*. 9th ed. Wolters Kluwer; 2024:818-828.

Osteen JD, Immani S, Tapley TL, et al. Pharmacology and mechanism of action of suzetrigine, a potent and selective $Na_V1.8$ pain signal inhibitor for the treatment of moderate to severe pain. *Pain Ther*. 2025;14:655-674.

D.5. What criteria would you use to establish that a patient can be safely discharged after ambulatory surgery?

For patients to be discharged from an ambulatory facility, they must satisfy specific criteria that are usually summarized on simplified checklists. Although each ambulatory surgical facility must determine its own set of criteria, generally accepted guidelines for safe discharge home after ambulatory surgery include:

- Stable vital signs
- No evidence of respiratory depression
- Oriented to person, place, and time
- Able to walk unassisted
- Able to dress unassisted
- Minimal nausea or vomiting
- No active bleeding or oozing
- Pain controllable with oral analgesics
- Responsible adult to escort patient home and to remain with the patient overnight

- Discharge by both the person who administered anesthesia and the person who performed surgery, or their designees
- Written instructions for the postoperative period at home must be supplied to the patient before discharge as well as a phone number to call in the case of emergency.

The requirement for patients to drink and void before discharge is no longer considered mandatory, except in the case of certain patients who had central neuraxial blockade.

Fridman J. Optimal discharge strategy. In: Fleisher LA, ed. *Evidence-Based Practice of Anesthesiology*. 4th ed. Elsevier Saunders; 2023:496-505.

Mancini P. Ambulatory anesthesia. In: Cullen BF, Stock MC, Ortega R, et al, eds. *Barash, Cullen, and Stoelting's Clinical Anesthesia*. 9th ed. Wolters Kluwer; 2024:818-828.

Rohi A, Olofsson MET, Jakobsson JG. Ambulatory anesthesia and discharge: an update around guidelines and trends. *Curr Opin Anaesthesiol.* 2022;35:691-697.

D.6. How would you decide when to discharge a patient after regional anesthesia?

Patients recovering from regional anesthesia must satisfy the discharge criteria listed earlier. In addition, if spinal or epidural anesthesia is used for outpatients, it is important to ensure recovery from the sympathetic and motor blocks. Hypotension and syncope on standing can be signs that the sympathetic nervous system is still blocked. An indication that the motor block is no longer functioning is the ability to move the legs and feet freely. A simple test is to have the patient run each heel up and down the opposite leg from the big toe to the knee. Ability to walk to the bathroom and void are excellent recovery tests after epidural or spinal anesthesia because these abilities reflect recovery of both the motor and the sympathetic functions.

Mulroy et al have suggested that delaying discharge for voiding after spinal or epidural anesthesia with *short-acting local anesthetics* is unnecessary in *low-risk* patients (eg, age less than 70 years; no hernia, rectal, or urologic surgery; no history of voiding problems). Nonetheless, appropriate measures must be in place for bladder catheterization if the inability to void persists after discharge home. The use of ultrasonographic monitoring of bladder volume before discharge can reduce the incidence of urinary retention after discharge.

Darrah DM, Griebling TL, Silverstein JH. Postoperative urinary retention. *Anesthesiol Clin.* 2009;27:465-484.

Fridman J. Optimal discharge strategy. In: Fleisher LA, ed. *Evidence-Based Practice of Anesthesiology*. 4th ed. Elsevier Saunders; 2023:496-505.

Mulroy MF, Salinas FV, Larkin KL, et al. Ambulatory surgery patients may be discharged before voiding after short-acting spinal and epidural anesthesia. *Anesthesiology*. 2002;97:315-319.

Pavlin DJ, Pavlin EG, Gunn HC, et al. Voiding in patients managed with or without ultrasound monitoring of bladder volume after outpatient surgery. *Anesth Analg*. 1999;89:90-97.

D.7. What instructions should be given to an ambulatory surgical patients upon discharge?

Patients should be discharged to the care of a responsible adult. Additionally, they should be instructed that after surgery, they should not ingest alcoholic beverages or depressant medications unknown to their surgeon or anesthesiologist, drive a car, or operate complex machinery for at least 24 hours. In addition, the discharge instructions should provide a list of problems that require immediate notification of the surgeon (eg, bleeding that does not stop, inability to void, and persistent PONV).

Mancini P. Ambulatory anesthesia. In: Cullen BF, Stock MC, Ortega R, et al, eds. *Barash, Cullen, and Stoelting's Clinical Anesthesia*. 9th ed. Wolters Kluwer; 2024:818-828.

Marshall SI, Chung F. Discharge criteria and complications after ambulatory surgery. *Anesth Analg*. 1999;88:508-517.

62

Magnetic Resonance Imaging

Jyun-you Liou, Dana L. Gurvitch, and
Hugh C. Hemmings Jr.

You are consulted by the pediatric intensive care unit (PICU) team for urgent magnetic resonance imaging (MRI) on an 11-year-old, 35-kg boy. Two days after undergoing a partial temporal lobectomy for seizure management, he now has altered mental status and is thrashing about in the PICU. The child has intractable seizures but no other medical history. He was able to cooperate enough to perform a computed tomography (CT) scan that showed no acute bleeding, but the team wants an MRI and does not believe he will stay still for the 1.5-hour scan. He is currently extubated, but on your review of his previous anesthetic record, you see that he required an oral airway to achieve adequate mask ventilation. On conventional direct laryngoscopy, only the epiglottis was visualized (Cormack-Lehane grade III view), but when a videolaryngoscope was used, the epiglottis, arytenoid cartilages, and posterior vocal cords were visualized (Cormack-Lehane grade IIa view) and a tracheal tube was passed atraumatically. Your patient has a left-hand 20-gauge peripheral intravenous catheter and a right radial arterial catheter for close blood pressure monitoring. He is current with all his antiepileptic medications and is appropriately taking nothing orally (NPO).

A. Medical Disease and Differential Diagnosis

1. What is MRI, and how does it work?
2. What are the major advantages of MRI in comparison to CT?
3. What are some disadvantages associated with MRI? What are some safety concerns?
4. How do you manage patients with implanted devices?
5. What are the biologic effects of clinical MRI and its contrast agents?
6. What are the anesthetic considerations for this procedure?
7. What is intraoperative MRI (iMRI)? What is real-time MRI, and in what setting can this be used?

B. Preoperative Evaluation and Preparation

1. What types of patients require sedation or general anesthesia for MRI?
2. Do all children require sedation for MRI?
3. What preoperative laboratory testing would you require for this patient?
4. How would you premedicate this patient? What are some options that can be used to premedicate other patients for MRI?

C. Intraoperative Management

1. What are some of the anesthetic options for this patient?
2. How is an MRI conducted?
3. How would you monitor this patient?
4. What special considerations apply to monitoring equipment used during MRI?
5. How would you induce and maintain general anesthesia in this patient?
6. What are ways to maintain the airway during an MRI scan?
7. What is the risk to the patient of gadolinium administration in the presence of renal insufficiency?
8. After the patient receives the contrast agent, you notice the loss of end-tidal carbon dioxide. What do you do next?
9. While you are examining the patient, he starts to desaturate and develops significant bradycardia. What do you do next?

D. Postoperative Management

1. How will you recover the patient from anesthesia?

A. Medical Disease and Differential Diagnosis

A.1. What is MRI, and how does it work?

MRI is a noninvasive diagnostic technique that uses the magnetic properties of atomic nuclei to produce high-resolution, multiplanar images of the body. It is utilized both as an aid in diagnosis and in disease therapy in lieu of conventional approaches.

The proton in hydrogen atoms, because of its "spin," behaves like a small magnet. When placed in a powerful static magnetic field (SMF) created by the MRI scanner, the protons in hydrogen atoms align themselves with the field. When a radiofrequency (RF) pulse is applied, the protons absorb energy and change their alignment according to the direction of the RF pulse. Once the RF pulse is over, the protons gradually return to their original alignment. This process is called "relaxation," during which the protons emit signals that can be detected by the MRI scanner. There are two components of relaxation, T1 and T2, which represent separate components of the process.

Most hydrogen atoms in biologic tissues exist in water and fat molecules. Because biologic tissues vary in composition and environment, their T1 and T2 signal intensities can be different. Combination of RF pulse direction, sequence, and associated magnetic field settings generates various images that help visualize and differentiate normal versus pathologic tissues.

The resolution of the image depends on the strength of the magnetic field, which is measured in tesla (T) units. Most MRI scanners have a magnetic field of 0.5 to 3.0 T, which is significantly stronger than the earth's magnetic field (5×10^{-5} T); the smaller the opening in the scanner, the stronger the magnet, and the better the resolution. Therefore, although patients prefer an "open" magnet, which induces less claustrophobia, this can compromise image resolution.

Azhar S, Chong LR. Clinician's guide to the basic principles of MRI. *Postgrad Med J.* 2023;99:894-903.

A.2. What are the major advantages of MRI in comparison to CT?

The advantages of MRI over CT are:

1. Lack of ionizing radiation
2. Use of noniodinated intravenous contrast agent, thereby reducing the risk of anaphylactic or nephrotoxic reactions
3. Excellent resolution of normal and pathologic tissues without image artifact from bone
4. Advanced image series such as brain tractography, blood and cerebrospinal fluid flow imaging, and dynamic imaging

Several real-time MR-guided interventions have also been developed.

1. MRI is superior to CT in capturing temperature-related changes. As a result, it has been used to guide cryoablation and thermoablation procedures for treating various conditions, including liver, kidney, breast, and prostate tumors, as well as uterine fibroids.
2. MRI better defines the presence and extent of cardiac scar tissue. Thus, it has become an important tool in interventional cardiac electrophysiology studies and catheter ablation procedures employed to treat atrial fibrillation or ventricular arrhythmia.
3. MRI provides a higher resolution of brain structure than CT and can assess local tissue health and metabolic status. iMRI systems are increasingly used by neurosurgeons to enhance the visualization of intracranial lesions, including gliomas, for safe and effective surgical planning. MRI systems also offer additional capabilities, such as MR spectroscopy and brain mapping (functional MRI [fMRI]), which can improve diagnostic accuracy and surgical outcomes.

Callahan MJ, MacDougall RD, Bixby SD, et al. Ionizing radiation from computed tomography versus anesthesia for magnetic resonance imaging in infants and children: patient safety considerations. *Pediatr Radiol.* 2018;48:21-30.

Claessens AJ, Hall ML. Nonoperating room anesthesia. In: Cullen BF, Stock MC, Ortega R, et al. eds. *Barash, Cullen, and Stoelting's Clinical Anesthesia.* 9th ed. Wolters Kluwer; 2023:849–865.

Cravero JP, Kaplan RF, Landrigan-Ozuna M, Coté CJ. Sedation for diagnostic and therapeutic procedures outside the operating room. In: Coté CJ, Lerman J, Anderson BJ, et al, eds. *Coté and Lerman's A Practice of Anesthesia for Infants and Children.* 6th ed. Elsevier/Saunders; 2019:1077–1094.

Eitel C, Hindricks G, Grothoff M, et al. Catheter ablation guided by real-time MRI. *Curr Cardiol Rep*. 2014;16:511.

Hall WA, Truwit CL. Intraoperative MR-guided neurosurgery. *J Magn Reson Imaging*. 2008;27:368-375.

Note: Cullen et al.'s *Barash, Cullen, and Stoelting's Clinical Anesthesia* and Coté et al.'s *A Practice of Anesthesia for Infants and Children* can be universally applied to all questions in this chapter. These references are not repeated in the list to keep the text concise.

A.3. What are some disadvantages associated with MRI? What are some safety concerns?

The major disadvantages and safety concerns of MRI include:

1. Magnetic fields
2. Limited patient access
3. Long scan time
4. Noise
5. Potential quenching event

The strong magnetic field attracts ferromagnetic objects, causing them to dislodge or behave as dangerous projectiles. Time-varying fast-switching gradient magnetic fields and RF pulses can cause electronic device malfunction or induce electric currents in metal objects, leading to thermal injury. Thermal injuries have been reported from electrocardiogram (ECG) electrodes and pulse oximeter probes. All cables and monitoring equipment should be placed in a straight manner without coiling to avoid induced currents and thermogenesis.

The magnetic field strength diminishes depending on the distance from the magnet core. Distances less than the 5-gauss line can make pacemakers malfunction, and less than the 50-gauss line can make ferromagnetic gas cylinders lethal projectile missiles (1 tesla = 10,000 gauss).

Owing to the potential for catastrophic events, recommendations for MRI safety have been proposed by the American College of Radiology. Briefly, the MRI suite should be separated into four zones:

1. Zone I is the public zone immediately outside the MRI suite.
2. Zone II is the reception area monitored by MRI personnel.
3. Zone III encompasses the control room with access restricted from the public.
4. Zone IV is the physical MRI scanner room.

To ensure safety, entry into zones III and IV must be screened by MRI personnel (**Figure 62.1**). Ferromagnetic objects should not be brought into zone III; if necessary, they should be brought in with extreme caution. Items such as credit cards, pens, keys, laryngoscopes, scissors, stethoscopes, paper clips, and ferromagnetic gas cylinders are excluded from zone IV. One important way to ensure safety is to use aluminum oxygen E-gas cylinders instead of magnetic ones. Adherence to these zones must be maintained, especially during emergent situations.

The American Society for Testing and Materials (ASTM) International developed safety terminology for devices and implants. *MR safe* refers to items with no known hazards in any MR environment. *MR conditional* refers to items that pose no known hazards in a specified MR environment (ie, the conditions present at your scanner). *MR unsafe* refers to items that pose definite hazards in all MR environments (ie, ferromagnetic scissors). MR-safe or MR-conditional monitors and machines should be used in the scanner. MR-safe or MR-conditional infusion pumps can be used in zone IV, but otherwise, pumps can be left in zone III, and the tubing is passed through a waveguide.

The relatively long scan time necessary to obtain images (as much as 15 minutes per image series, with a total scanning period of 1-3 hours) and image degradation from any motion, including cardiac contractions, respirations, cerebrospinal fluid flow, and bowel peristalsis, are additional disadvantages. MRI-safe anesthesia machines and monitoring equipment are available; however, the cost can prove prohibitive for institutions that do not regularly do MRI under anesthesia.

Another potential hazard to both patients and operators is the high-decibel sound emanating from the scanner due to RF pulses (>90 dB). Hearing protection for both is mandatory even if the patient is receiving a general anesthetic.

Quenching of the MRI machine is a rare hazard that refers to a sudden loss of superconductivity of the magnet due to loss of coolant, which can occur either spontaneously or be triggered by a significant safety event. During a quench, the temperature of the magnet coil suddenly rises, resulting in an explosive boil-off of surrounding liquid helium and deactivation of the magnet. In the event of a quench, the patient should be quickly removed from the room, as it now contains a potentially hypoxic atmosphere. The magnet should almost never be quenched on purpose because it creates a dangerous room for the patient

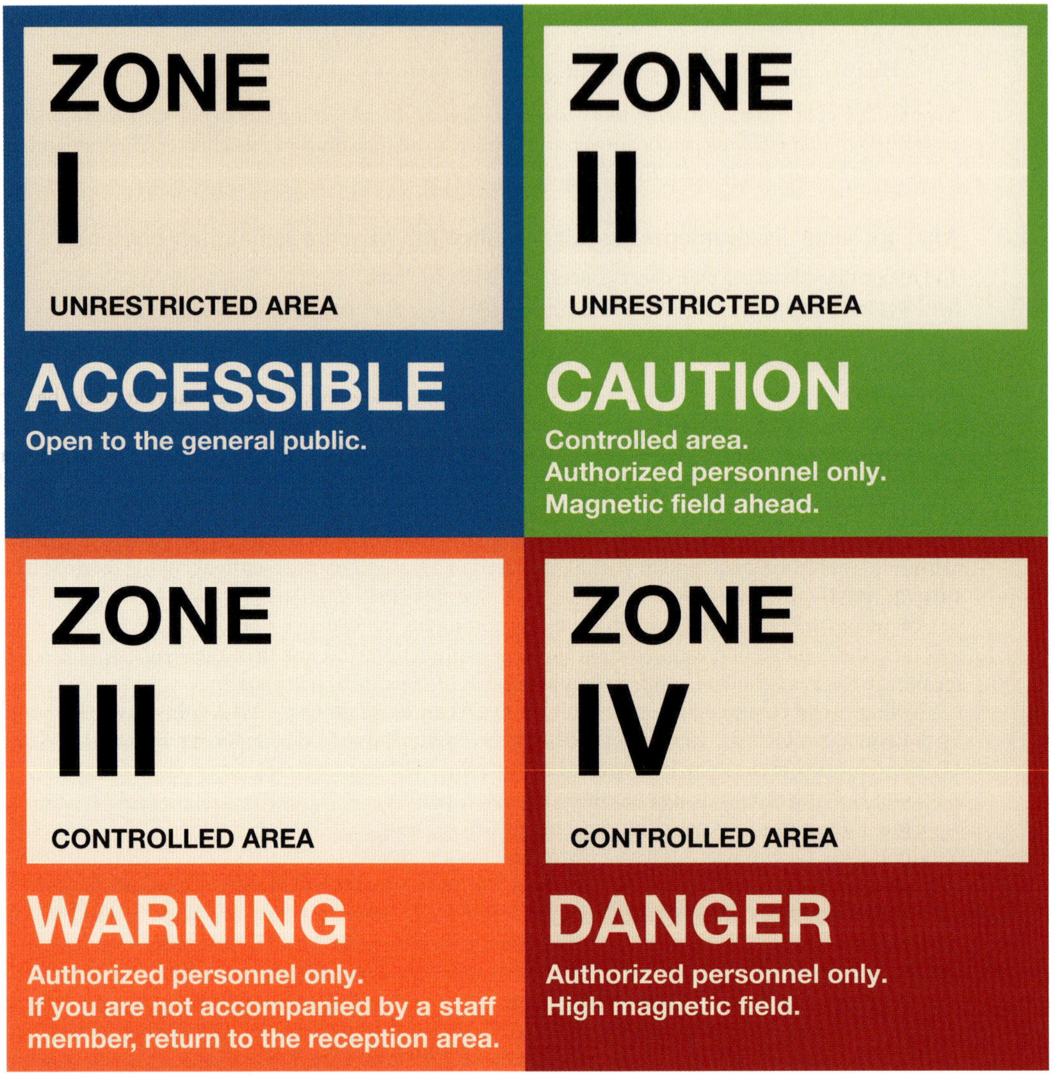

FIGURE 62.1. The MRI suite is separated into four safety zones based on the magnetic field. MRI, magnetic resonance imaging.

as well as other providers. In the case of a medical emergency for a patient, the best practice would be to remove the patient from zone II or zone III and initiate resuscitation. Once the magnet is quenched, it cannot be reactivated for days.

International Society of Magnetic Resonance in Medicine. Safety guidelines for magnetic resonance imaging equipment in clinical use. Medicines and Healthcare Products Regulatory Agency. 2014;16-17. Accessed December 21, 2019. http://www.ismrm.org/smrt/files/con2033065.pdf

Kanal E, Barkovich AJ, Bell C, et al. ACR guidance document on MR safe practices: 2013. *J Magn Reson Imaging*. 2013;37:501-530.

Ocazionez D, Dicks DL, Favinger JL, et al. Magnetic resonance imaging safety in cardiothoracic imaging. *J Thorac Imaging*. 2014;29:262-269.

Practice advisory on anesthetic care for magnetic resonance imaging: a report by the Society of Anesthesiologists Task Force on Anesthetic Care for Magnetic Resonance Imaging. *Anesthesiology*. 2009;110:459-479.

A.4. How do you manage patients with implanted devices?

The following devices need to be carefully reviewed and can be contraindicated:

1. Cardiac implantable electronic devices (CIEDs) such as pacemakers, implantable cardioverter defibrillators (ICDs), and cardiac resynchronization therapy (CRT) devices
2. Artificial heart or ventricular assist device

3. Intravascular stents, valves, and filters
4. Vascular aneurysm clips
5. Cochlear implants, ear implants, hearing aids
6. Implanted neurostimulators
7. Drug infusion pumps
8. Catheters with metallic components, such as the Swan-Ganz catheter
9. Foreign bodies, such as retained bullet fragments, tissue expanders, and artificial limbs

Patients with a CIED might be excluded from MRI studies because of the possibility of device malfunction, inactivation, or damage in the magnetic field. Currently, the American Heart Association (AHA) and the American Society of Anesthesiologists (ASA) Practice Advisory Task Force on Anesthetic Care for Magnetic Resonance Imaging regard the presence of a pacemaker or an ICD as a strong relative contraindication to routine MRI examination. In 2011, MR-conditional ICDs, pacemakers, and leads became available in the United States; they are approved in specific settings and up to 1.5 T MRI examinations. Intact pacemaker leads are unlikely to move; however, an electric current could be generated if fractured leads are exposed to the magnet, causing lethal arrhythmia.

If the benefits far outweigh the risks of the exam, MRI should be performed in an experienced center with collaboration between the cardiologist, radiologist, device manufacturer, and MRI technician. Written consent must detail all risks to the patient, including death. Full resuscitation equipment, including external defibrillators, must be readily accessible in the MRI suite in case of an arrhythmia or equipment malfunction. If the device is not MR conditional and the patient is pacemaker dependent, the device should be programmed to asynchronous pacing and ICD features deactivated. The device should be interrogated before and after the scan.

MRI is currently contraindicated in patients with an artificial heart or ventricular assist device (see Chapter 8: Cardiac Implantable Electronic Devices, Therapy Devices)

Coronary artery stents, especially after 2007, are safe for patients having an MRI procedure at less than or equal to 3 T. Most aortic stent grafts are MR safe. However, the Zenith AAA and TAA endovascular grafts (Cook Medical) are MR conditional, and their timing for scanning needs to be individualized. Coil embolization materials, such as platinum, iridium, and nitinol, are safe for MRI examinations. Most heart valves and annuloplasty rings can be safe under certain conditions (ie, ≤3 T), but, if possible, delay the scan for up to 6 weeks after implantation. Regardless, it is crucial to review the MR compatibility of coronary stents, peripheral stents, sternal wires, inferior vena cava filters, prosthetic heart valves, and annuloplasty rings in the patient's body.

Clips used in vascular surgery and neurosurgery must be verified, and the model and type of clip need to be documented. All intracranial aneurysm clips manufactured after 1995 that the company identifies as MR conditional need no further testing. Clips manufactured before 1995 require some pretesting and need the approval of an MRI-attending radiologist. Despite a prior history of MRI, variations can occur in different magnetic fields under the influence of different pulsed frequencies, so verification is still needed.

Certain cochlear implants are MR conditional and can be safe if the patient is over 8 years of age and less than or equal to 1.5 T is used.

Patients with implanted neurostimulators, such as deep brain stimulators, need to be investigated because some can be MR unsafe. Newer generations of implanted neurostimulation systems tend to be MR conditional; however, a careful review of the device manual is mandatory. MRI might be performed on a limited basis.

Swan-Ganz catheters contain temperature sensors and electrodes that are MR unsafe.

If possible, drug infusion pumps (insulin delivery, analgesic drugs, or chemotherapy pumps) should be removed.

Care must be taken for patients with retained foreign bodies, such as shrapnel and bullets; there can be potential risks if it is ferromagnetic due to movement and heating near vital organs. Although safe, orthodontic braces, dentures, tattoos, or cosmetics that contain metallic dyes can degrade the image quality significantly.

For a more thorough evaluation of these devices, please refer to the website http://www.mrisafety.com, which has a thorough list of MR-safe, conditional, and unsafe devices.

Baikoussis NG, Apostolakis E, Papakonstantinou NA, et al. Safety of magnetic resonance imaging in patients with implanted cardiac prostheses and metallic cardiovascular electronic devices. *Ann Thorac Surg*. 2011; 91:2006-2011.

Ghadimi M, Sapra A. Magnetic resonance imaging contraindications. [Updated 2023 May 1]. In: *StatPearls* [Internet]. StatPearls Publishing; 2025. https://www.ncbi.nlm.nih.gov/books/NBK551669/

SECTION 12

Indik JH, Gimbel JR, Abe H, et al. 2017 HRS expert consensus statement on magnetic resonance imaging and radiation exposure in patients with cardiovascular implantable electronic devices. *Heart Rhythm*. 2017;14:e97-e153.

Kanal E, Barkovich AJ, Bell C, et al. ACR guidance document on MR safe practices: 2013. *J Magn Reson Imaging*. 2013;37:501-530.

Ocazionez D, Dicks DL, Favinger JL, et al. Magnetic resonance imaging safety in cardiothoracic imaging. *J Thorac Imaging*. 2014;29:262-269.

Practice advisory on anesthetic care for magnetic resonance imaging: a report by the Society of Anesthesiologists Task Force on Anesthetic Care for Magnetic Resonance Imaging. *Anesthesiology*. 2009;110:459-479.

A.5. What are the biologic effects of clinical MRI and its contrast agents?

Although an area of controversy and ongoing investigation, most human data to date suggest that there are no significant deleterious effects on patients or health care professionals from short-term exposure to the SMF of an MRI machine. Among MRI personnel, however, working at greater than or equal to 3 T doubled the odds of experiencing SMF symptoms (vertigo/dizziness, nausea, metallic taste, and/or illusion of movement) as compared to working exclusively at less than or equal to 1.5 T.

Also controversial is the use of MRI during pregnancy because the effects of magnetic fields on the human fetus cannot be easily determined. Current evidence does not support the suggestion that routine clinical exposure of the pregnant patient to MRI causes fetal developmental abnormalities. Pregnant patients have undergone MRI safely during all stages of pregnancy. Nevertheless, caution is advised. Studies have shown that gadolinium-based contrast agents enter the fetal circulation and are filtered in the fetal kidneys into the amniotic fluid, which can potentially form free gadolinium ions that can theoretically pose risks to the developing fetus. The appropriateness of the MRI examination and the acuteness of the diagnostic need must be considered. Ultrasonography is preferred if it can provide equivalent diagnostic information, and consideration should be given to postponing the MRI until late in the pregnancy or until after delivery.

Chernoff D, Stark P. Principles of magnetic resonance imaging. Accessed December 16, 2021. http://www.uptodate.com/contents/principles-of-magnetic-resonance-imaging

Glans A, Wilen J, Lindgren L, Bjorkman-Burtscher IM, Hansson B. Health effects related to exposure of static magnetic fields and acoustic noise-comparison between MR and CT radiographers. *Eur Radiol* 2022;32:7896-909.

Kanal E, Barkovich AJ, Bell C, et al. ACR guidance document on MR safe practices: 2013. *J Magn Reson Imaging*. 2013;37:501-530.

A.6. What are the anesthetic considerations for this procedure?

The problems that complicate anesthetic management of any patient outside the operating room environment exist for patients requiring sedation or general anesthesia for MRI. The MRI suite is often located some distance from the operating room and the anesthesia department, thus limiting the availability of backup assistance and supplies. As with any remote anesthetizing location, the personnel might not be familiar with the requirements of anesthetized patients, thereby decreasing their ability to provide assistance. Frequently, MRI suites have been designed without consideration for anesthetic needs, such as pipeline gases, suction, or an anesthetic exhaust system. Access to a recovery suite for postanesthesia care might not be readily available, thereby necessitating transfer to the main recovery room.

In addition, there are anesthetic challenges unique to the MRI suite. Because of the bulkiness of the unit, the patient is often far removed from the anesthesiologist, and access to the airway is limited. Intravenous lines, anesthesia circuits, oxygen tubing, and monitoring cables must be of sufficient length to reach the patient deep within the scanner. The strong magnetic field necessitates the exclusion of all ferromagnetic objects and equipment. The displays of standard monitoring devices can be distorted or displaced by the magnetic field, and the monitors themselves can degrade the MR image by disturbing the signal/noise ratio. The ASA task force understands that the interpretation of the ECG can be limited due to the superimposed voltages from blood flow in a high magnetic field (ie, ST-segment interpretation is unreliable even with filters). Safe monitoring conditions must be maintained with MR-safe or MR-conditional equipment and comply with ASA standards. **Figure 62.2** shows that the anesthesiologist is watching the patient (in zone IV) and anesthesia monitors in the zone III control room during the MRI scan.

Finally, for a machine to be MR conditional, its components must be less than 2% ferromagnetic. Vaporizers themselves are not ferromagnetic; thus, conventional ones can be used.

Practice advisory on anesthetic care for magnetic resonance imaging: a report by the Society of Anesthesiologists Task Force on Anesthetic Care for Magnetic Resonance Imaging. *Anesthesiology*. 2009;110:459-479.

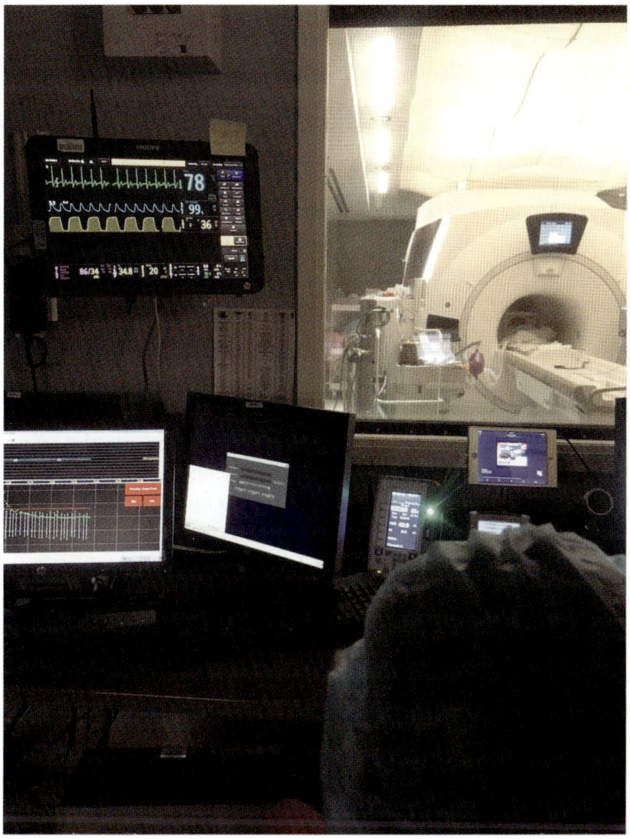

FIGURE 62.2. The anesthesiologist, in zone II, is watching the patient, who is in zone IV, and the anesthesia monitors, which are in zone III control room during an MRI scan. MRI, magnetic resonance imaging.

A.7. What is intraoperative MRI (iMRI)? What is real-time MRI, and in what setting can this be used?

Since 1993, image-guided surgery systems have been introduced that combine the resources of an operating room with MRI technology and high-performance computing. Several low-, mid-, and high-field strength interventional MRI systems have been developed that permit access to the patient by surgeons and provide near real-time imaging during surgical procedures. iMRI furnishes the surgeon with a simultaneous combination of direct vision and beyond-the-surface MRI, allowing for more accurate localization and targeting during surgery. In addition, iMRI allows the surgeon to detect the full extent of lesions, devise a safe surgical approach with less potential operative morbidity, and monitor for unseen hemorrhage. In some cases, iMRI obviates the need for postoperative imaging that necessitates additional sedation for pediatric patients. In addition to tumor resections, iMRI can be utilized in the surgical revascularization of moyamoya arteriopathy and during the management of arteriovenous malformations (AVMs), placement of deep brain stimulator for Parkinson disease and other movement disorders, evaluation of hematoma, and resection of epileptogenic foci.

Other fields of medicine that incorporate iMRI include liver, pancreas, and kidney surgeries and radiation therapy guidance when tumors shift. Not surprisingly, iMRI systems are expensive and require MRI-compatible surgical instruments and monitoring equipment. One of the most significant challenges anesthesiologists face in this setting is the high-energy iMRI-generated electric noise that can interfere with the ECG. Unlike in an MRI suite, there are multiple people and objects to account for when the iMRI unit is brought out and engaged around the patient. All personnel working in an iMRI environment must take MRI safety courses to ensure patient and personal safety. For the duration of the scan, the anesthesiologist has limited or no access to the patient. Visualization of the patient may be limited when enclosed in an electric noise shield. All ferromagnetic objects, such as laryngoscopes, stylets, and beepers, must be left outside the operating room or in a secure area. Lastly, anesthetic considerations for iMRI must also include the needs of the ongoing complex surgical procedure.

As opposed to iMRI, real-time MRI integrates exceptional soft tissue visualization in a 3D anatomic and functional manner with delineation of suspected lesions without radiation exposure. In the electrophysiology suite, real-time MRI allows catheter ablation procedures to treat various arrhythmias, reducing fluoroscopy usage. In addition, delayed enhancement (DE) MRI is the gold standard for scar and fibrosis mapping, which serves as an arrhythmogenic source for ventricular tachycardia. This preprocedural MRI may be difficult to obtain because these patients often have ICDs that are contraindicated for MRI. DE MRI can also predict potential atrial fibrillation ablation failure based on the amount of left atrial fibrosis present. After an intervention, MRI can help identify complications, such as pulmonary vein stenosis and esophageal injury. MRI thermography is another useful tool for showing tissue heating during RF ablation.

There are many hazards associated with real-time MRI and iMRI. Special MRI-conditional and MRI-safe monitors, devices, and catheters need to be utilized to avoid catastrophic complications.

Dzwonczyk R, Fujii JT, Simonetti O, et al. Electrical noise in the intraoperative magnetic resonance imaging setting. *Anesth Analg*. 2009;108:181-186.

Eitel C, Hindricks G, Grothoff M, et al. Catheter ablation guided by real-time MRI. *Curr Cardiol Rep*. 2014;16:511.

Henrichs B, Walsh RP. Intraoperative MRI for neurosurgical and general surgical interventions. *Curr Opin Anaesthesiol*. 2014;27:448-452.

B. Preoperative Evaluation and Preparation

B.1. What types of patients require sedation or general anesthesia for MRI?

Although MRI is painless, patients must remain still for the time required for each scan (as much as 15 minutes) to obtain images free of movement artifacts. Patients who cannot cooperate (eg, infants, young children, and adults who are confused, mentally ill, or intellectually compromised) usually require sedation or anesthesia to assist with the examination. Most children younger than 5 years of age and as old as 11 years of age require some form of sedation or general anesthesia, and 30% of adult patients experience some form of anxiety during MR scanning. Anesthesiologists frequently manage claustrophobic or anxious adults as well as those requiring airway protection (unconscious or critically ill patients) or mechanical ventilation (patients with head injuries or elevated intracranial pressure) to ensure that adequate examinations are obtained safely and efficiently.

B.2. Do all children require sedation for MRI?

Performing general anesthesia in neonates and children with a potentially challenging airway in a remote location is challenging and potentially dangerous. In addition, potential risks associated with neurotoxicity in the developing brain are driving methods to perform MRI scans without sedation. For instance, small infants and neonates can use the "feed and swaddle" method. Although this strategy is associated with an increased likelihood of inadequate images, it can be used as a first-line method with general anesthesia reserved as a backup. In older children, one can use multimedia, trained child life experts, and handheld device application-based technologies to calm children and help them stay still. This method can be sufficient in developmentally appropriate and cooperative children. Discussing cases with the attending radiologist is important to determine whether MRI is appropriate for the clinical question. The harms of ionizing radiation on the developing child are well known; however, the amount of radiation required to obtain quality CT images has decreased with modern CT scanners. Because CT exams are far shorter (minutes instead of hours for MRI), children likely do not need general anesthesia or sedation.

Callahan MJ, MacDougall RD, Bixby SD, et al. Ionizing radiation from computed tomography versus anesthesia for magnetic resonance imaging in infants and children: patient safety considerations. *Pediatr Radiol*. 2018;48:21-30.

Heller BJ, Yudkowitz FS, Lipson S. Can we reduce anesthesia exposure? Neonatal brain MRI: swaddling vs. sedation, a national survey. *J Clin Anesth*. 2017;38:119-122.

Runge SB, Christensen NL, Jensen JE, et al. Children centered care: minimizing the need for anesthesia with a multi-faceted concept for MRI in children aged 4-6. *Eur J Radiol*. 2018;107:183-187.

B.3. What preoperative laboratory testing would you require for this patient?

For this patient, a complete blood count (CBC) to evaluate for postoperative bleeding and a basic metabolic panel (BMP) to evaluate electrolyte derangements (particularly sodium) are appropriate to evaluate contributors to the patient's altered mental status. However, no further laboratory studies would be warranted if the patient were otherwise healthy.

B.4. How would you premedicate this patient? What are some options that can be used to premedicate other patients for MRI?

The goal of premedication is to provide anxiolysis yet not precipitate hypoxemia or hypercarbia. In this patient who already has altered mental status, long-acting sedatives should be avoided. However, other children are good candidates for premedication for anxiolysis.

At some centers, ambulatory pediatric patients are not routinely given pharmacologic premedication; rather, parents are allowed to be present at the time of induction in order to help allay anxiety and ease the induction. The most commonly used premedication in pediatrics is oral midazolam. Although the standard dose is 0.5 mg/kg, some advocate an increased dose in younger children of up to 1 mg/kg in children 1 to 3 years old. A relatively high dose is likely needed due to the poor bioavailability of the drug orally (15%). Midazolam should be administered at least 20 to 25 minutes prior to the intended onset for maximal effect. Side effects include respiratory depression, bad taste, and in some patients, paradoxical agitation.

There are other medications that can be used for anxiolysis in children, including dexmedetomidine and ketamine. Dexmedetomidine can be given either intranasally (2.5-3 μg/kg) or orally (4 μg/kg). Dexmedetomidine is a centrally acting α_2-adrenergic receptor agonist that produces sedation without respiratory depression. It is odorless and tasteless, and so can be much more palatable for children. Dexmedetomidine can also reduce the incidence of postoperative emergence delirium, an added benefit.

Ketamine can be given orally (6 mg/kg) or intramuscularly (1-2 mg/kg). The oral route is preferred because many children have a fear of needles. The side effects of ketamine include increased oral secretions, which can cause upper airway obstruction, bronchospasm, laryngospasm, and micro-aspiration (even in the presence of intact upper airway reflexes). Ketamine can also increase delirium, especially if the child is not pretreated with a benzodiazepine.

Melatonin (0.5 mg/kg) can provide comparable anxiolysis as oral midazolam (both administered 40 minutes prior to induction of general anesthesia). Melatonin is an endogenous indolamine produced and secreted by the pineal gland that regulates circadian rhythm and promotes sleep. Melatonin can reduce the dose of propofol needed for induction of anesthesia in pediatric patients.

Impellizzeri P, Vinci E, Gugliandolo MC, et al. Premedication with melatonin vs midazolam: efficacy on anxiety and compliance in paediatric surgical patients. *Eur J Pediatr*. 2017;30:947-953.

Jannu V, Mane RS, Dhorigol MG, et al. A comparison of oral midazolam and oral dexmedetomidine as premedication in pediatric anesthesia. *Saudi J Anaesth*. 2016;10:390-394.

Lerman J. Preoperative assessment and premedication in paediatrics. *Eur J Anaesthesiol*. 2013;30:645-650.

Qiao H, Xie Z, Jia J. Pediatric premedication: a double-blind randomized trial of dexmedetomidine or ketamine alone versus a combination of dexmedetomidine and ketamine. *BMC Anesthesiol*. 2017;17:158.

C. Intraoperative Management

C.1. What are some of the anesthetic options for this patient?

There are many techniques used to anesthetize children undergoing MRI or other painless radiologic procedures. This can range from moderate sedation with midazolam or fentanyl to deep sedation, with various combinations of intravenous ketamine, propofol and dexmedetomidine, or general anesthesia with inhaled anesthetics or total intravenous anesthesia (TIVA). Because conscious sedation of children is frequently insufficient to prevent patient movement, deeper levels of sedation or general anesthesia are often required to anesthetize the pediatric patient for MRI successfully. The ideal anesthetic should allow titration and maintenance of stable drug concentrations to prevent undesired patient movement during the scan and to provide rapid rates of induction and recovery with a minimal requirement for special MRI-compatible equipment.

Intravenous anesthesia with propofol can be an excellent technique for MRI. Continuous intravenous infusion of propofol allows precise, rapid titration to the desired effect and a rapid recovery. Propofol use eliminates the need for a nonferromagnetic, MRI-compatible anesthesia machine and for scavenging waste anesthetic gases, both of which are major drawbacks of an inhalational technique (but propofol still may require the use of an MRI-conditional infusion pump). However, propofol compromises muscle tone and can cause airway obstruction, a significant concern in the MRI suite due to the physical barrier between the patient and the anesthesiologist. Ketamine is another valuable drug for deep sedation while maintaining airway reflexes. However, in addition to the issue with increased secretions, ketamine can elicit undesirable myoclonic movements and emergence delirium, especially at higher doses and in ages younger than 2 years and older than 13 years. Recently, a combination regimen of ketamine and propofol has been shown to allow speedy recovery while minimizing propofol side effects.

Dexmedetomidine can be used as a maintenance agent as well as a premedication. No significant respiratory effects are known with this agent, although hemodynamic side effects can occur, especially at higher doses; however, patients receiving dexmedetomidine have a longer induction course and overall hospital times than patients receiving propofol. Due to potential hemodynamic side effects, such as hypotension and bradycardia, and life-threatening complications when used with digoxin, dexmedetomidine should be used cautiously in patients with cardiac compromise. MRI scans performed under propofol sedation lead to better image quality than those performed with dexmedetomidine alone. Dexmedetomidine is a good adjunct agent, especially in a patient where spontaneous ventilation is paramount, however, it might not be suitable as a sole agent.

Outside of the United States, oral chloral hydrate is still used for sedating children for radiology studies due to its low cost. However, because of its risk of adverse events, slow pharmacokinetics, and potential for compounding errors, it has fallen out of favor of use.

Another viable alternative to deep sedation with intravenous agents would be general anesthesia with inhalational anesthetics. General anesthesia with a secured airway might be the preferred choice for patients with comorbidities requiring or necessitating airway management.

Artunduaga M, Liu CA, Morin CE, et al. Safety challenges related to the use of sedation and general anesthesia in pediatric patients undergoing magnetic resonance imaging examinations. *Pediatr Radiol.* 2021;51:724-735.

Grissinger M. Chloral hydrate: is it still being used? Are there safer alternatives? *P T.* 2019;44:444-459.

Loh P-S, Ariffin MA, Rai V, et al. Comparing the efficacy and safety between propofol and dexmedetomidine for sedation in claustrophobic adults undergoing magnetic resonance imaging (PADAM trial). *J Clin Anesth.* 2016;34:216-222.

Schmitz A, Weiss M, Kellenberger C, et al. Sedation for magnetic resonance imaging using propofol with or without ketamine at induction in pediatrics—a prospective randomized double-blinded study. *Paediatr Anaesth.* 2018;28:264-274.

Wu J, Mahmoud M, Schmitt M, et al. Comparison of propofol and dexmedetomedine techniques in children undergoing magnetic resonance imaging. *Paediatr Anaesth.* 2014;24:813-818.

C.2. How is an MRI conducted?

The patient is placed on a long, thin table outside the scanner. After obtaining an adequate level of sedation (or anesthesia), the patient is positioned. If the head is to be examined, it is often enclosed within a small coil or tube. Next, the table with the patient is moved into the long tube of the MRI magnet. The portion of the body to be examined is usually centered in the magnet about 1 m from the end of the tube. During the examination, delivery of RF pulses produces a loud thumping noise, which can average 95 dB in a 1.5 T scanner. To obtain a high-quality scan, the patient must refrain from moving during the acquisition of an individual cut or from changing position at any time during the entire examination. An individual scan can take several minutes, and the total scanning time may range from 1 to 3 hours. Body surfaces can absorb some of the RF energy during the sequence, although this is unlikely to increase core temperature by more than 1 °C. Nevertheless, the specific absorption rate (SAR) of energy is monitored as measured in watts per kilogram. Depending on the patient, if the SAR is too high, the sequence might need to be aborted and adjusted.

C.3. How would you monitor this patient?

Reliable and accurate monitoring of an unconscious individual during MRI is essential because the patient cannot be seen adequately or easily accessed by the anesthesiologist. During sedation, ASA standard monitors including blood pressure, pulse oximetry, and ECG must be used. ECG electrodes should be placed together and toward the middle of the magnetic field, and the leads should be insulated from the patient's skin to avoid any potential thermal injuries. During general anesthesia, capnography and temperature should also be monitored. Assessment of ventilation in a spontaneously breathing patient can be difficult, especially when the patient is within the magnet and far from view. Monitoring end-tidal carbon dioxide from one limb of the nasal oxygen prongs or through a nasal catheter is frequently successful. Pulse oximetry is a marker for oxygenation and should not be used as the only marker for ventilation.

Hypothermia can be problematic, especially in pediatric patients. Because of the high airflow through the scanner cavity, the patient should be covered in blankets. Hyperthermia can also occur, and if suspected based on SAR, the sequence might need to be temporarily stopped. When feasible, temperature monitoring can be accomplished using nonferromagnetic temperature strips or probes with RF filters. It is currently not mandatory for the anesthesiologist to remain in the scanner room during the examination as long as remote monitoring with direct vision of the patient is possible.

The patient outlined in this case requires invasive blood pressure monitoring. However, one might need extension tubing, as the transducer should be placed at least 50 gausses away from the scanner, potentially leading to a dampened signal.

Practice advisory on anesthetic care for magnetic resonance imaging: a report by the Society of Anesthesiologists Task Force on Anesthetic Care for Magnetic Resonance Imaging. *Anesthesiology*. 2009;110:459-479.

C.4. What special considerations apply to monitoring equipment used during MRI?

Unshielded ferromagnetic materials, such as those within monitors and cables, or metallic pieces on patient clothing, can interfere with imaging signals, distorting MRI results and causing burns. Similarly, the RF signals can induce currents in ferromagnetic elements of monitors, causing a distortion of the monitoring signal and making the monitor unusable. MR-safe or MR-conditional monitors and equipment (eg, ECG electrodes) are preferable because they contain shielding nonferromagnetic components and filters to produce satisfactory results without major signal distortion. To avoid magnetic pull, monitors should be placed at least 5 to 8 ft from the magnet bore or permanently mounted.

The ECG can show significant changes within an SMF. In particular, T waves and late ST segments can mimic ECG changes associated with conditions such as hyperkalemia and pericarditis. This is due to induced voltage in the blood (a conducting fluid) flowing through the magnetic field. These changes are directly related to field strength but do not appear to represent any significant physiologic alteration.

Pulse oximeter cables must be nonconducting, fiberoptic, and MRI compatible. Traditional pulse oximeter probes may contain metal and can cause burns.

The high RF power used in MRI poses the risk of excessive heat at monitoring sites. This can lead to thermal injury. To minimize the risk of burns, one should:

- Inspect the insulation on all monitoring wires to ensure that it is intact.
- Place cables and lead wires in a straight alignment. Do not allow monitoring wires to form loops.
- Remove all leads or wires not in use.
- Separate cables from the patient's skin.
- Keep the cable and sensor out of the scanning area (eg, place a pulse oximeter probe on the toe of a patient whose chest is being examined).
- Avoid excessive power.
- Remove the patient's gown or any clothing that might have metal.

The anesthesiologist must confirm that all monitors used in zone IV are MR compatible. In addition, a monitor should be available to view vital signs from zone III when the anesthesia provider is not in zone IV.

C.5. How would you induce and maintain general anesthesia in this patient?

This patient will likely require general anesthesia to complete the MRI scan due to his altered mental status and the necessity to avoid hypoxemia and hypercarbia following neurosurgery. General endotracheal anesthesia can be the best option. However, the child was difficult to intubate in the operating room and required videolaryngoscopy. Therefore, it is important to ensure that help from experienced and trained anesthesiologists is available and to induce general anesthesia away from the scanner such that difficult airway equipment would be readily available. Induction can also be accomplished in the intensive care unit, and the patient can be subsequently transported to the MRI suite. Importantly, not all endotracheal tube stylets are nonferromagnetic. MR-safe stylets are required if they are used in zone IV.

Intravenous induction of anesthesia should be performed to control ventilation as quickly as possible. MRI-compatible monitors should be placed prior to induction to allow a smooth transition to the scanner. The pilot balloon on the cuff of the endotracheal tube (or supraglottic airway device, if used) must be taped away from the patient to minimize artifact from the cuff's spring. Once under general anesthesia, the child is moved into the scanner room and placed on the MRI table. The patient and monitors are carefully positioned before advancing the table into the magnet bore. Anesthesia can be maintained with either a continuous intravenous infusion of propofol or an inhalational agent combined with oxygen.

Schulte-Uentrop L, Goepfert MS. Anaesthesia or sedation for MRI in children. *Curr Opin Anaesthesiol*. 2010;23:513-517.

C.6. What are ways to maintain the airway during an MRI scan?

Securing the airway with an endotracheal tube is not required to successfully sedate a patient during an MRI scan, which can be performed with patients breathing spontaneously with a native airway. This should be considered in patients with a good natural airway whose ventilation is being monitored adequately. Infusions of propofol or dexmedetomidine can be considered in this situation. Placing a shoulder roll under the patient with the chin taped up can help prevent airway obstruction. This should only be performed when there are no contraindications, such as potential spine injuries with head and neck manipulations.

Limited access to the patient's airway is one of the most significant challenges for the anesthesiologist during MRI. In patients whose airway might be difficult, placing either an endotracheal tube or supraglottic airway device might be appropriate. Respiration can be spontaneous or controlled depending on personal preference and patient needs. However, supraglottic airway devices can alter the appearance of cervical soft tissue masses causing problems in diagnosis and should be used only after consulting with a radiologist if the neck is being imaged. It is unclear whether the use of a tracheal tube decreases the incidence of airway complications during MRI scans. As long as a plan is in place should emergencies occur, various types of anesthetics can be used to accomplish the scan.

Practice advisory on anesthetic care for magnetic resonance imaging: an updated report by the American Society of Anesthesiologists Task Force on Anesthetic Care for Magnetic Resonance Imaging. *Anesthesiology*. 2015;122:495-520.

Simpao AF, Obsekov V, Galvez JA, et al. A retrospective study of the impact of supraglottic airway devices on the appearance of neck masses in children undergoing serial magnetic resonance imaging. *Paediatr Anaesth*. 2018;28:1123-1128.

C.7. What is the risk to the patient of gadolinium administration in the presence of renal insufficiency?

Gadolinium-based contrast agents carry a risk of nephrogenic systemic fibrosis in patients undergoing renal replacement therapy, with acute kidney injury, or with stage 4 or 5 chronic kidney disease. Nephrogenic systemic fibrosis primarily involves the skin, but other organs such as the liver, heart, lungs, diaphragm, and skeletal muscle can be affected, and it can be fatal. Gadolinium-based contrast agents can be classified according to their chemical structures. Most nephrogenic systemic fibrosis cases are associated with the use of group I gadolinium-based contrast agents, which are no longer advertised in the United States and have been withdrawn from the market in many countries. Recent studies have shown that the risk of nephrogenic systemic fibrosis is low for group II gadolinium-based contrast agents. Based on these updated data, in 2021, the American College of Radiology, the European Society of Urogenital Radiology, and the Canadian Association of Radiology issued recommendations liberalizing administration of group II gadolinium-based contrast agents in high-risk patients. However, the US Food and Drug Administration (FDA) issued a "black box" warning for all gadolinium-based contrast agents in 2010, and the warning has not been rescinded. If a pediatric patient with advanced renal disease requires gadolinium, the US FDA suggests prompt hemodialysis be considered. Gadolinium-based contrast agents should also be avoided in patients with previous allergic or anaphylactoid reactions. The safety of gadolinium-based contrast agents' exposure during pregnancy has not been established, and their use during pregnancy is not recommended unless it is essential for the woman's or fetus' health, particularly during the first trimester.

Bird ST, Gelperin K, Sahin L, et al. First-trimester exposure to gadolinium-based contrast agents: a utilization study of 4.6 million US pregnancies. *Radiology*. 2019;293:193-200.

Practice advisory on anesthetic care for magnetic resonance imaging: an updated report by the American Society of Anesthesiologists Task Force on Anesthetic Care for Magnetic Resonance Imaging. *Anesthesiology*. 2015;122:495-520.

Weinreb JC, Rodby RA, Yee J, et al. Use of intravenous gadolinium-based contrast media in patients with kidney disease: consensus statements from the American College of Radiology and the National Kidney Foundation. *Radiology*. 2021;298:28-35.

C.8. After the patient receives the contrast agent, you notice the loss of end-tidal carbon dioxide. What do you do next?

The anesthesiologist must immediately request the radiology team to pause the current scanning sequence and move the patient out of the MRI scanner tunnel to gain prompt access. Even in emergencies, strictly prohibiting introduction of ferromagnetic objects into zone IV is imperative.

The time course of end-tidal CO_2 ($ETco_2$) loss can provide valuable insight into the underlying etiology. A sudden loss of $ETco_2$ can result from equipment malfunction, such as obstruction or disconnection of the endotracheal tube or the gas sampling line. However, sudden loss of pulmonary perfusion, such as cardiac arrest or massive pulmonary embolism, can present just as dramatically. A more gradual loss of $ETco_2$, ranging from several seconds to minutes, can be due to cardiac or pulmonary etiologies. Given that the patient has recently received a contrast agent, bronchospasm due to contrast allergy is a likely diagnosis. The waveform of $ETco_2$ carries significant diagnostic value in this situation.

The anesthesiologist should empirically increase the fraction of inspired oxygen (Fio_2) to 100% and provide additional ventilator support while assessing the patient. Given the remoteness of the MRI suite, the threshold for calling for help should be low.

Practice advisory on anesthetic care for magnetic resonance imaging: an updated report by the American Society of Anesthesiologists Task Force on Anesthetic Care for Magnetic Resonance Imaging. *Anesthesiology*. 2015;122:495-520.

C.9. While you are examining the patient, he starts to desaturate and develops significant bradycardia. What do you do next?

The patient should be immediately removed from zone IV. The anesthesiologist should request additional assistance. This action not only ensures complete access to the patient but also reduces the risk of bringing in ferromagnetic devices such as oxygen tanks and defibrillators into zone IV.

Given this scenario presents a high likelihood of severe bronchospasm, it is crucial to provide prompt and aggressive treatment. In addition to administering 100% oxygen with proper ventilator settings, it is reasonable to give low-dose epinephrine boluses empirically. If hemodynamics permits, also consider using propofol. Management of bradycardia (atropine or pacing) should follow the guidelines outlined in the Pediatric Advanced Life Support (PALS) protocol.

D. Postoperative Management

D.1. How will you recover the patient from anesthesia?

Postanesthesia recovery care after MRI is the same as that required after any anesthetic. This can be accomplished in a designated MRI suite area, provided adequate facilities and trained personnel are available. For most, such a facility will not be available, and the patient will require transport to the main recovery room. To transport the patient quickly and safely, one must ensure that adequate personnel and the proper equipment are organized in advance. It is useful to have the location of recovery and logistics of transport (if necessary) planned before the procedure begins.

63 Morbid Obesity, Obstructive Sleep Apnea, and Bariatric Anesthesia

Jon D. Samuels and Fun-Sun F. Yao

A 27-year-old male was scheduled for elective robotic sleeve gastrectomy. He had a past medical history significant for morbid obesity (MO) (height, 182.9 cm; weight, 272.2 kg; body mass index [BMI], 81.4 kg/m^2), pickwickian habitus, osteoarthritis, mild asthma, hypertension, adult-onset diabetes mellitus, peptic ulcer disease with symptomatic gastroesophageal reflux, and obstructive sleep apnea (OSA). He experienced daytime somnolence, heavy nighttime snoring, and had slept in a seated position for the previous 2 years. He was able to walk around the house with a cane but was unable to climb any stairs. A preoperative diagnostic polysomnography (PSG) was performed, and an apnea-hypopnea index (AHI) of 64 was calculated. Home oxygen therapy with bilevel positive airway pressure (BiPAP) settings had been started at the following settings, with symptomatic improvement: fraction of inspired oxygen (FIO_2) of 0.40, respiratory rate 10 breaths per minute, inspired positive airway pressure (IPAP) of +12 cm H_2O, and expired positive airway pressure (EPAP) of +5 cm H_2O, spontaneous mode. Cardiology clearance indicated high risk, after an echocardiogram revealed mild right-sided cardiomegaly and mild pulmonary hypertension. The patient's blood pressure was 155/82 mm Hg, pulse 60 beats per minute, and respirations 20 breaths per minute. The patient was determined to have a difficult airway. Prior to scheduling surgery, the patient was scheduled for an upper endoscopy and a Bravo procedure.

A. Medical Disease and Differential Diagnosis

1. What medical problems exist with this patient? The patient asks you if he is "high risk." What is the evidence? Is surgical therapy a safe and viable alternative for this patient?
2. Define the terms overweight, obesity, morbid obesity (MO), super obesity, super-super obesity, normal weight, ideal body weight (IBW), and lean body weight (LBW). What is the impact of obesity on society?
3. What is OSA? What are the risk factors for OSA?
4. How is OSA diagnosed? What is a sleep study or polysomnography? How are the results obtained from polysomnography used to grade the severity of OSA? What are the subtypes of OSA? Are there genetic disorders with a predisposition to OSA? What is the role of OSA screening tests in the preoperative setting?
5. How does OSA differ in the pediatric population in clinical presentation and pathogenesis?
6. What is Pickwickian syndrome? What is obesity hypoventilation syndrome (OHS)? Describe the pathogenesis of severe OSA.
7. What is the association between obesity and OSA? What is the etiology of OSA in severe obesity?
8. What metabolic problems do patients with MO typically have? What are the roles of leptin and ghrelin in obesity?
9. Describe the changes that occur in the following respiratory parameters in patients with MO.
    - Pulmonary function tests (PFTs): tidal volume (V_T), functional residual capacity (FRC), residual volume (RV), vital capacity (VC), inspiratory reserve volume (IRV), expiratory reserve volume (ERV), and total lung capacity (TLC)
    - Flow-volume loops
    - Pressure-volume loops
    - Diffusing capacity for carbon monoxide (DLCO)

- Compliances: lung (C_L), chest wall (C_{CW}), and total (C_{RS})
- Resistance: airway and total respiratory system
- Closing capacity (CC)
- Work of breathing (WOB)

10. What changes occur in $Pa{O_2}$ and $Pa{CO_2}$ in patients with MO?
11. What changes occur in intrapulmonary shunt (Q_S/Q_T) and dead space (V_D/V_T) in MO? Describe the shunt equation and the physiologic dead space, or Bohr equation.
12. What changes occur in the cardiovascular system of the patient with obesity? Discuss cardiac output, blood volume, blood pressure, and pulmonary arterial pressure.
13. Are there any other diseases commonly associated with obesity?
14. What anatomic changes that affect the airway are associated with MO and OSA?
15. What derangements of the gastrointestinal system are associated with MO?

B. Preoperative Evaluation and Preparation

1. How would this patient be optimized for surgery preoperatively? Would you use preoperative screening questionnaires to diagnose OSA? Summarize the workup for this patient.
2. Bariatric surgery patients often receive preoperative screening procedures performed in the endoscopy suite. Describe the anesthetic considerations.
3. Summarize the evidence-based workup, risk, chance of various adverse outcomes, and expected length of stay for this patient.
4. What is the role of enhanced recovery after surgery (ERAS) in bariatric surgery? How does the public find a quality bariatric surgery team and surgical facility? What is the role of robotics in bariatric surgery?
5. Would you premedicate this patient?
6. Describe the mechanism of action of each premedication in the ENERGY protocol.
7. How would you adjust doses of anesthetics in the morbidly obese?

C. Intraoperative Management

1. How would you monitor this patient?
2. The American Society of Anesthesiologists (ASA) Difficult Airway Algorithm provides a guideline for management of the difficult airway. How do the comorbidities in patients with MO and OSA modify implementation of the algorithm?
3. Why is it important to preoxygenate the patient with obesity? How would you do it? Compare the effectiveness of the four-maximum-breath and 3-minute techniques. What is the importance of continuous positive airway pressure (CPAP) during the induction of general anesthesia? Describe the use of the nasal CPAP mask and transnasal humidified oxygenation rapid-insufflation ventilatory exchange in the induction of general anesthesia.
4. There are many new airway devices in the marketplace. Which of these devices have been particularly successful in the patient with MO or OSA?
5. How would you induce anesthesia? Describe the tracheal intubation technique.
6. How would you maintain general anesthesia? What agents would you choose? How would you prepare for emergence?
7. Which neuromuscular blocking agent would you use?
8. What is the pathophysiology of pneumoperitoneum (PNP)? What is the effect on the cardiopulmonary system? How does it change perioperative care? What are the optimal ventilator strategies for patients with MO undergoing bariatric surgery?
9. What are the devices that anesthesiologists place in the upper gastrointestinal canal during laparoscopic bariatric surgery? Are there risks associated with placement and management of these devices?
10. When will you extubate the patient's trachea? Describe weight-based extubation criteria.

D. Postoperative Management

1. What are the early postoperative complications of bariatric surgical procedures?
2. What are the late complications of bariatric surgical procedures?
3. What is the effect of position on respiratory function in the patient with obesity?
4. How would you prevent postoperative atelectasis?
5. How long would you prescribe supplementary oxygen postoperatively?
6. How would you control postoperative pain? What are the sources of surgical pain? What is the role of regional anesthesia in the bariatric surgery?

A. Medical Disease and Differential Diagnosis

A.1. What medical problems exist with this patient? The patient asks you if he is "high risk." What is the evidence? Is surgical therapy a safe and viable alternative for this patient?

Preoperative significant past medical history in this patient includes of MO, OSA, possible Pickwickian syndrome, right ventricular hypertrophy, early-onset coronary artery disease, mild pulmonary hypertension, systemic hypertension, adult-onset diabetes mellitus, osteoarthritis, and severe gastroesophageal reflux disease (GERD). This patient is at increased risk of coronary artery disease, cardiac arrhythmias, left- and right-sided congestive heart failure, peripheral vascular disease, venous thrombosis and pulmonary emboli, cerebrovascular disease, hepatobiliary disease, hepatic steatosis, hepatic cirrhosis, degenerative joint disease, metabolic syndrome, socioeconomic and psychosocial impairment.

This is a patient with high risk, with increased risk of both perioperative morbidity and mortality (described in detail in Section B.3). Major anesthetic concerns include risk of difficult airway, difficult mask ventilation, decreased apneic threshold to anesthetics, sedatives and opioids, prolonged anesthesia emergence, postemergence re-sedation, positional ventilatory collapse, restrictive and obstructive lung disease, ventilation/perfusion mismatch, worsening of reactive pulmonary hypertension, and cor pulmonale. This patient must receive continuation of his preoperative oxygen therapy with CPAP in the immediate recovery period, at the values determined by his sleep study (PSG), or greater. Additional anesthetic concerns include potentially difficult monitoring, difficult vascular access, and positioning issues. Additionally, there is a risk of postoperative respiratory arrest, rhabdomyolysis with renal failure, increased risk of infection including pneumonia, and positional injuries. Meticulous attention to acute pain management is essential.

Safe perioperative care for this patient requires triage to a specialized facility with additional personnel, surgeons with advanced laparoscopic training, and anesthesiologists with advanced airway skills and optimal equipment. Overall, the evidence for the long-term effectiveness of bariatric surgical therapy is quite compelling. The most widely quoted studies are on the gastric bypass, which has the longest track record; the Swedish Obese Subjects (SOS) study, and the National Institute of Diabetes and Digestive and Kidney Diseases (NIDDK)-National Institute of Health Longitudinal Assessment of Bariatric Surgery (LABS) study. These studies showed that compared with conventional treatment, the surgery group was associated with favorable short-term (low 30-day mortality of 0.3%, low rates of adverse outcomes comparable to a laparoscopic cholecystectomy) and long-term (reduction in overall mortality, decreased incidence of diabetes mellitus, myocardial infarction, stroke, cancer) outcomes. Bariatric surgery is the most effective long-term therapy for patients with severe obesity and has been recommended in all current guidelines.

Alvarez R, Telem DA. Comparative surgical outcomes in bariatric surgery. In: Reavis K, Barrett AM, Kroh MD, eds. *The SAGES Manual of Bariatric Surgery*. Springer International Publishing AG, part of Springer Nature; 2018:339.

Bussetto L, Dicker D, Azran C, et al. Practical recommendations of the Obesity Management Task Force of the European Association for the study of obesity for the post-bariatric surgery medical management. *Obes Facts*. 2017;10:597-632.

Flum DR, Belle SH, King WC, et al. Perioperative safety in the longitudinal assessment of bariatric surgery. *N Engl J Med*. 2009;361:445-454.

Longitudinal Assessment of Bariatric Surgery (LABS) Consortium, Flum DR, Belle SH, et al. Perioperative safety in the longitudinal assessment of bariatric surgery. *N Engl J Med*. 2009;361:445-454.

Sjöström L, Narbro K, Sjöström CD, et al. Effects of bariatric surgery on mortality in Swedish obese subjects. *N Engl J Med*. 2007;357:741-752.

A.2. Define the terms overweight, obesity, morbid obesity (MO), super obesity, super-super obesity, normal weight, ideal body weight (IBW), and lean body weight (LBW). What is the impact of obesity on society?

Obesity is a multifactorial chronic disease involving social, cultural, physiologic, psychological, metabolic, endocrine, genetic, and behavioral components, resulting in excess adipose and tissue mass. The modern basis for the determination of demographics is the BMI or the Quetelet Index, after the Belgian statistician, and is measured in body weight in kilograms divided by the height in meters squared (kg/m^2). The standard for *IBW*, the sex-specific desirable weight for persons with small, middle, and large frames, is published in the Metropolitan Life Insurance Tables. *LBW* accounts for the added muscle mass supporting the added weight and corresponds to the well-perfused portion of 120% to 140% of the IBW, or 1.3 times the IBW.

- *Anorexia* is defined as a BMI of less than 17.5 in males or females.
- *Underweight* is defined as a BMI of 17.6 to 19.0 in females or 17.6 to 20.6 in males.
- *Ideal (normal) weight* is defined as a BMI of 19.1 to 25.8 in females and 20.7 to 26.4 in males.
- *Marginally overweight* is defined as a BMI of 25.9 to 27.2 in females and 26.5 to 27.8 in males.
- *Overweight* is defined as a BMI of 27.3 to 32.3 in females and 27.9 to 31.1 in males.
- *Obesity* is defined as a BMI of greater than 20% of IBW, 32.4 to 34.9 in females and 31.2 to 34.9 in males.
- *Severe obesity* is defined as a BMI of 35.0 to 39.9 in both sexes.
- Morbid obesity is defined as a BMI of greater than 40 or greater than 35 with associated comorbidities such as hypertension and diabetes mellitus. MO is the accepted medical term for all cases of severe obesity.
- *Super obesity*, a relatively new term, is defined as a BMI of 50 to 59.9. *Super-super obesity* is defined as a BMI of greater than 60.

There exist both imperial and metric system BMI tables and web-based calculators.

Occasionally, an approximate, non–sex-specific system is used. In this system, a *healthy (normal) weight* is a BMI of 18.6 to 24.9, *overweight* is a BMI of 25 to 29.9, *obesity* is a BMI of 30 to 34.9, *severe obesity* is a BMI of 35 to 39.9, and *morbid obesity* is a BMI of greater than 40.0.

Alternative systems for the determination of obesity exist. In the triceps skinfold thickness test, for example, obesity is defined as a value of greater than 23 mm in males or greater than 30 mm in females. In the Broca Index (height in cm minus 100 for males and minus 105 for females), the IBW is calculated in kg.

- Males: IBW (kg) = height (cm) − 100
- Females: IBW (kg) = height (cm) − 105

There are different patterns of distribution of obesity. In *peripheral obesity* (eg, gynoid or gluteal pattern), the individual has a pear shape, and adipose tissue deposition is predominantly in the lower body. In *central obesity* (eg, android or cushingoid), and especially upper body obesity, the individual has an apple shape, and adipose tissue deposition occurs predominantly in the upper body. Central obesity has greater associations with perioperative risk and OSA.

Much has been written on the obesity epidemic; according to the World Health Organization (WHO), obesity remains one of the most critical health challenges of the modern era. Obesity has reached epidemic proportions in the industrialized world and currently poses a greater worldwide health risk than malnourishment. In the United States alone, 65% of the US population, or 127 million adults, are obese and is annually responsible for 300,000 premature deaths.

The financial impact on society of obesity is due to direct medical costs, increased incidence disease associated with obesity, associated medical costs, cost associated with lost productivity, absenteeism, presenteeism, disability, increased health insurance issues, and increased indirect costs and have been discussed elsewhere. Together, the total cost of obesity has been estimated in 2010 at annual costs of $215 billion for the US economy and $2 trillion a year for the world economy.

Assessment Psychology Online. Metropolitan Life height-weight tables 1943, Revised 1983. Accessed May 19, 2025. http://www.assessmentpsychology.com/metlife.htm.com

James WP, Gill T. Obesity—introduction: history and the scale of the problem worldwide. In: Kopelman PG, Caterson ID, Dietz WH, eds. *Clinical Obesity in Adults and Children*. 4th ed. Wiley; 2022:3-16. Accessed May 19, 2025. https://www.wiley.com/enae/Clinical+Obesity+in+Adults+and+Children%2C+4th+Edition-p-9781119695271

The Calculator Site. Imperial and metric BMI calculator. Accessed May 19, 2025. https://thecalculatorsite.com

World Health Organization. Obesity: overview. Accessed May 19, 2025. https://www.who.int/health-topics/obesity#tab=tab_1

A.3. What is OSA? What are the risk factors for OSA?

OSA is a sleep disorder. Sleep disorders are grouped into the following types: conditions with excessive daytime somnolence (eg, OSA), conditions with disorders initiating and maintaining sleep (eg, insomnia), and circadian rhythm disorders (eg, jet lag). In the older terminology, OSA is referred to both OSA proper and to obstructive sleep hypopnea (OSH) syndrome, a milder variant. Today, it is more precise to refer to OSA and hypopnea syndrome (OSAHS) when naming the general condition.

OSA is defined as cessation of airflow for more than 10 seconds despite continuing ventilatory effort, five or more times per hour of sleep, associated with a decrease in arterial oxygen saturation (Spo_2) of greater than 4%. OSH is defined as a decrease in airflow of greater than 50% for more than 10 seconds,

15 or more times per hour of sleep, associated with a decrease in Spo_2 of greater than 4%. Both forms of OSAHS are usually associated with snoring, sleep disruption from increased ventilatory effort–induced arousal, hypersomnolence (daytime sleepiness), altered cardiovascular function, and pathophysiologic alterations, of which hypoxemia and hypercarbia are primary events, and polycythemia, systemic and pulmonary hypertension, various cardiac arrhythmias, myocardial ischemia, right and left ventricular (LV) hypertrophy, and eventually failure are secondary events.

Severe obesity is a strong independent risk factor for OSAHS. Other risk factors include male gender, middle age, evening ingestion of alcohol, and drug-induced sleep. In individuals without obesity, risk factors are craniofacial dysostosis, particularly micrognathia (absolute or relative), cartilaginous abnormalities (eg, lingual tonsillar hyperplasia), chronic nasal obstruction, and tonsillar hypertrophy.

Charchaflieh JG. Sleep-related breathing disorders. In: Hines RL, Marschall KE, eds. *Stoelting's Anesthesia and Co-existing Disease*. 7th ed. Elsevier; 2017:1-14.

Yayan J, Rasche K. A systematic review of risk factors for sleep apnea. *Prev Med Rep*. 2024;42:102750.

Yeghiazarians Y, Jneid H, Tietjens JR, et al. Obstructive sleep apnea and cardiovascular disease: a scientific statement from the American Heart Association. *Circulation*. 2021;144:e56-e67.

A.4. How is OSA diagnosed? What is a sleep study or polysomnography? How are the results obtained from polysomnography used to grade the severity of OSA? What are the subtypes of OSA? Are there genetic disorders with a predisposition to OSA? What is the role of OSA screening tests in the preoperative setting?

OSA can be suspected based on history, physical examination, or comorbidities, but definitive diagnosis requires a sleep study. The hallmark of OSA is a history of heavy snoring. Most adults with OSA have upper body obesity, increased neck circumference, micrognathia, and poor Mallampati scores on physical examination. In 90% of cases, OSA is associated with obesity. OSA, however, may result from any condition that predisposes to upper airway obstruction. Some examples are pregnancy, upper airway abnormalities (eg, deviated nasal septum, hypertrophic tonsils, and adenoids), cartilaginous abnormalities (eg, lingual tonsillar hyperplasia), craniofacial dysostoses, certain congenital and genetic conditions (eg, Prader-Willi syndrome, Down syndrome, Marfan syndrome, Pierre Robin sequence, acromegaly, muscular dystrophy, cerebral palsy), as well as certain medical conditions (hypothyroidism). The absence of a typical or compelling presentation, however, does not rule out the possibility of OSAHS.

Adult OSA consists of a continuum from asymptomatic, to paroxysmal snoring, to severe nocturnal airway closure, requiring the patient to sleep in a sitting position, and daytime somnolence. The pathophysiology of OSA is central, peripheral, or mixed. Peripheral disease is caused by redundant adipose tissue in the upper airway, in the setting of severe obesity, sometimes with a superimposed craniofacial dysostosis. The symptomatology of OSA consists of intermittent snoring, apneic episodes, with daytime somnolence. *OSH*, a milder form of OSA, can be clinically indistinguishable. *OHS* is severe OSA with chronic daytime hypoventilation, super obesity, and hypercapnia not related to pulmonary disease. *Pickwickian syndrome* is OHS with cor pulmonale.

Definitive diagnosis of OSA is made by sleep specialists with a formal sleep study. A polysomnogram (PSG), performed at a sleep study center, examines nocturnal sleeping patterns by monitoring physiologic parameters. In its most comprehensive form, the following parameters are studied: two to six electroencephalographic (EEG) channels to measure electrical activity of the brain and to document sleep cycles, two electrooculogram (EOG) channels to distinguish rapid eye movement (REM) from non-REM sleep, chin electromyogram (EMG) to monitor arousal and activity of the upper airway (genioglossus and digastric muscles), an airway microphone to monitor airflow from the nose and mouth, elastic belts placed on the chest and abdomen to monitor respiratory effort, an infrared video camera to monitor body position, one channel of electrocardiogram (ECG) to monitor cardiac activity, a pulse oximeter to monitor oxygen saturation, and two-leg EMG channels to monitor leg movements. A PSG can be ordered to definitively diagnose a sleep disorder, as part of medical management, or in the surgical workup of a high-risk population (eg, preoperative screening of bariatric surgical candidates).

A PSG will diagnose the presence of OSA, type (central, peripheral, or mixed), and grade severity. Results are reported in as the total number of apneas and hypopneas per hour of sleep or the AHI. AHI values correspond to OSA severity: 6 to 20 (mild), 21 to 40 (moderate), and greater than 40 (severe). The total number of arousals hourly is the arousal index (AI). The respiratory disturbance index (RDI) is the most accurate measure of OSA severity—calculated as the number of (respiratory-effort related arousals (RERAs) plus the number of hypopneas plus the number of apneas) times 60 divided by the total sleep time (TST). RDI includes RERAs that impact breathing during sleep. The American Academy of Sleep Medicine uses RDI to determine the severity of OSA according to the following range: 5 to 14.9 for mild, 15 to 29.9 for moderate, and greater than 30 for severe. This patient had a RDI of 36. Because the PSG is an expensive and time-consuming study that is not covered by all insurance plans, simpler tests have been proposed, such as a partial (level 2) portable polysomnography and nocturnal oximetry. OSA is primarily a clinical diagnosis. Because only a very small percentage of patients presenting for surgery have been tested, have available results, and are compliant with recommendations, great importance is placed on preoperative sleep apnea screening tools and questionnaires. Of these, the STOP-BANG questionnaire is the most widely used, the utility of which has been confirmed in a meta-analysis across different populations.

The ASA has developed official policy for the perioperative management of patients with OSA. In its most recent iteration of the practice guidelines for the Perioperative Management of Patients with Obstructive Sleep Apnea, all aspects of anesthetic care are described, including a scoring system for perioperative risk for patients with OSA, based on OSA severity, invasiveness of surgery and anesthesia, and requirement for postoperative opioids.

American Society of Anesthesiologists Task Force on Perioperative Management of Patients with Obstructive Sleep Apnea. Practice guidelines for the perioperative management of patients with obstructive sleep apnea: an updated report by the American Society of Anesthesiologists Task Force on Perioperative Management of Patients with Obstructive Sleep Apnea. *Anesthesiology*. 2014;120:268-286.

Chung F, Abdullah HR, Liao P. STOP-Bang questionnaire: a practical approach to screen for obstructive sleep apnea. *Chest*. 2016;149:631-638.

Kapur VK, Auckley DH, Chowdhuri S, et al. Clinical practice guideline for diagnostic testing for adult obstructive sleep apnea: an American Academy of Sleep Medicine clinical practice guideline. *J Clin Sleep Med*. 2017;13:479-504. https://aasm.org/resources/clinicalguidelines/diagnostic-testing-osa.pdf

Nagappa M, Liao P, Wong J, et al. Validation of the STOP-Bang questionnaire as a screening tool for obstructive sleep apnea among different populations: a systematic review and meta-analysis. *PLoS One*. 2015;10:e0143697.

A.5. How does OSA differ in the pediatric population in clinical presentation and pathogenesis?

Childhood OSA (COSA) consists of a continuum from snoring to upper airway resistance syndrome to the fully expressed syndrome. The pathophysiology of COSA is most commonly peripheral in origin due to nocturnal airway blockage from nasal pathophysiology, hypertrophic tonsils and adenoids, or craniofacial dysostoses. The symptomatology in COSA consists of snoring (usually continuous), rare daytime sleepiness, and frequent behavioral disturbances (eg, attention-deficit hyperactivity disorder [ADHD]). It is distinguished from adult OSA by the following: snoring is more continuous, there is no sex predilection, and surgery (commonly adenotonsillectomy, rarely uvulopalatopharyngoplasty [UPPP]) is curative.

COSA occurs in 2% of children. COSA can be also related to severe chronic disease, such as chronic asthma, cystic fibrosis, pulmonary fibrosis, bronchopulmonary dysplasia, or chest wall abnormality. Rarely is the basis of childhood OSA a genetic disease that has been identified. While some cases of childhood obstructive sleep apnea have a genetic component, most do not adhere to traditional patterns of inheritance. Instead, multiple genes and environmental factors likely contribute to the development of the condition. The American Academy of Pediatrics (AAP) recommends that all children be screened for snoring. Polysomnography has been recommended as the most reliable diagnostic test and has been described elsewhere in detail. The American Academy of Otolaryngology—Head and Neck Surgery has published clinical practice guidelines for polysomnography to screen children with sleep-disordered breathing prior to tonsillectomy.

Roland PS, Rosenfeld RM, Brooks LJ, et al; American Academy of Otolaryngology—Head and Neck Surgery Foundation. Clinical practice guideline: polysomnography for sleep-disordered breathing prior to tonsillectomy in children. *Otolaryngol Head Neck Surg*. 2011;145:S1-S15.

Wise MS, Nichols CD, Grigg-Damberger MM, et al. Executive summary of respiratory indications for polysomnography in children: an evidence-based review. *Sleep*. 2011;34:389-398AW.

A.6. What is Pickwickian syndrome? What is obesity hypoventilation syndrome (OHS)? Describe the pathogenesis of severe OSA.

Pickwickian syndrome was named by Burwell in 1956, as a reference to Joe, an obese, somnolent boy in *The Posthumous Papers of the Pickwick Club*, by Charles Dickens. In Joe, Dickens provided the first accurate description of the most severe type of OSA, consisting of a BMI greater than 50 kg/m^2 or super obesity, alveolar hypoventilation (hypoxemia and hypercarbia), heavy nighttime snoring with periodic respiration, hypersomnolence (daytime somnolence), secondary polycythemia, right and left ventricular hypertrophy, and right-sided heart failure.

In individuals with Pickwickian syndrome, there are repeated cycles of sleep, arousal, and sleep, accompanied by obstructed breathing, with snoring and restlessness. Hypoxemia and hypercarbia result from disruption of a normal sleep pattern, with loss of REM sleep and cardiovascular changes. Loss of REM sleep induces hypersomnolence, personality, behavior, and cognitive changes and predisposes these individuals to be accident prone. Eventually, severe OSA leads to OHS, with nocturnal, and later diurnal alterations in the control of breathing, manifested as central apneic events, or apnea without ventilatory efforts. Patients also develop an alveolar-arterial oxygen gradient by ventilation/perfusion mismatch and can develop pulmonary hypertension. The major factor in the pathogenesis of this syndrome is unknown but might be due to decreased hypoxic and hypercarbic ventilatory drive. Late in the disease process, there is progressive daytime hypoxia and hypercarbia. When cor pulmonale supervenes, Pickwickian syndrome is complete. Recently, the term Pickwickian syndrome has been abandoned in favor of OHS.

There are several cardiovascular changes in severe OSA, all related to the episodic airway closure, with hypoxemia and hypercarbia. Hypoxemia and alterations in autonomic tone can induce bradycardia during apneic episodes; in half of these patients, long sinus pauses, second-degree heart block, and ventricular ectopy result. These arrhythmias can lead to nocturnal angina and myocardial infarction in susceptible individuals. Pulmonary hypertension can be caused directly by hypoxic pulmonary vasoconstriction, or indirectly by either increased transmural pulmonary artery pressures from negative thoracic pressure created by a sustained ventilatory effort against the upper airway obstruction, or by increases in pulmonary artery tone from increased sympathetic tone created by episodic hypoxemia. Pulmonary hypertension initially causes right ventricular hypertrophy, resulting in a higher right ventricular end-diastolic pressure (RVEDP), and later culminates in right ventricular failure, or cor pulmonale. The systemic circulation is also affected by episodic increases in sympathetic tone, with systemic hypertension presenting early, and LV hypertrophy, followed by LV failure, presenting much later. Systemic hypertension may also lead to increased stroke volume.

Castro-Añón O, Pérez de Llano LA, De la Fuente Sánchez S, et al. Obesity-hypoventilation syndrome: increased risk of death over sleep apnea syndrome. *PLoS One*. 2015;10:e0117808.

De Athayde RAB, de Oliviera JRB, Filho GL, et al. Obesity hypoventilation syndrome: a current review. *J Bras Pneumol*. 2018;44:510-518.

A.7. What is the association between obesity and OSA? What is the etiology of OSA in severe obesity?

Obesity and OSAHS are both common, coexisting diseases. The prevalence of severe obesity, a strong risk factor for OSA, is 3.2% in males and 6.7% in females, according to the US population data. Incidence and severity of OSA correlates loosely with BMI, better with neck circumference, and most closely with waist circumference. OSAHS is 2.6 times more likely when the waist-to-hip ratio exceeds 1.0 in obese males and 0.85 in obese females.

Sixty to 90% of patients with OSA are obese, and it has been estimated that 9% of females and 24% of males in the United States suffer from the syndrome (a total of 18 million individuals), of which 2% of females and 4% of males are symptomatic. These figures are increasing as the demographics shift toward an older and more obese population. Many of these patients do not have a diagnosis of OSA on their medical record at the time of surgery, representing potential perioperative complications. The prevalence of OSA in morbidly obese patients presenting for weight loss surgery is 78%.

There are three reasons why severe obesity can cause or exacerbate OSAHS. First, there is an inverse relationship between obesity and pharyngeal volume. The pharyngeal area decreases in obesity from deposition of adipose tissue into pharyngeal structures. The volume of adipose in the lateral pharyngeal walls correlates with the clinical severity of airway obstruction. Increased deposition of pharyngeal adipose increases the likelihood that relaxation of the upper airway muscles will result in collapse of the soft-walled retroglossal space, between the uvula and the epiglottis. The shape of the pharynx remodels from an ellipse with the long axis transverse to an ellipse with the long axis anterior-posterior. The muscles that open the collapsible pharynx on expiration during sleep (eg, tensor palatini, genioglossus, hyoid muscles) in response to stretch receptors in the pharynx are located in the anterior pharynx and do not function well with a remodeled pharynx.

Second, patency of the collapsible pharynx is determined by the transmural pressure (the difference between the extraluminal and intraluminal pressure) and compliance of its wall. If the compliance of the pharyngeal wall and intraluminal pressure (inspiratory pressure) is constant, then the remaining important determinant of upper airway patency is extraluminal pressure. In patients with obesity, extraluminal pressure is increased by superficially located fat masses; that is, the upper airway is compressed externally. Therefore, neck circumference is greater in patients with obesity with OSAHS compared to patients with obesity without OSAHS.

Third, pharyngeal patency is partially determined by lung volume. The collapsible (particularly in a supine position) soft-walled pharynx is kept patent during sleep by lung volumes above the FRC, which displaces the carina caudally, thereby tenting open the pharynx. This is known as *the lung volume hypothesis*. Smaller lung volumes allow a cephalad displacement of the carina (by 0.5 to 1.5 cm), resulting in collapse or even telescoping of the pharynx (which results in a smaller circumferential area).

Ainge-Allen HW, Yrr BJ, Grunstein RR. Obstructive sleep apnea. In: Kopelman PG, Caterson ID, Dietz WH, eds. *Clinical Obesity in Adults and Children*. 4th ed. Wiley; 2022:192-210.

Greer MK, Venkateshiah SB. Obesity hypoventilation syndrome—a concise clinical review. Touch Respiratory. Accessed May 1, 2023. https://doi.org/10.17925/USPRD.2020.5.1.43

A.8. What metabolic problems do patients with MO typically have? What are the roles of leptin and ghrelin in obesity?

In MO, there is an increase in both low metabolically active tissue (eg, adipose) and normally active tissue (eg, muscle). In general, LBW is equal to IBW plus 20% to 40% IBW.

Morbidly obese individuals have an increase in total oxygen consumption and carbon dioxide (CO_2) production due to an increased tissue mass. Increased metabolism demonstrates a linear relation with body weight and body surface area. Basal metabolic rate, however, remains normal in obese individuals.

Patients with severely obesity often have nonalcoholic fatty liver disease (NAFLD) and nonalcoholic steatohepatitis (NASH) increasing long-term risk of hepatic cirrhosis, dyslipidemia, inflammation, insulin resistance, and atherosclerosis. Metabolic syndrome, defined as a collection of central obesity, hypertension, dyslipidemia, and impaired glucose tolerance, is present in severe cases and increases perioperative risk of morbidity and death. Metabolic syndrome is mediated through adipocytokines and prothrombotic factors (increases in plasminogen activator inhibitor-1 [PAI-1], fibrinogen, and factor VII).

Leptin is a satiety hormone secreted by adipocytes. Most obese adults have high inappropriate leptin levels or hyperleptinemia. Congenital leptin deficiency is a rare cause of obesity, caused by mutations in the *LEP* gene in an autosomal recessive pattern. Ghrelin is the hormonal stimulant of short-term hunger. In MO, there is a resistance to both leptin and ghrelin. The cellular and molecular basis for the interplay between leptin and ghrelin is an area of intense research.

Cui H, López M, Rahmouni K. The cellular and molecular bases of leptin and ghrelin resistance in obesity. *Nat Rev Endocrinol*. 2017;13:338-351.

Genetics Home Reference. Congenital leptin deficiency. Accessed May 1, 2023. http://ghr.nlm.nih.gov/condition/congenital-leptin-deficiency.

A.9. Describe the changes that occur in the following respiratory parameters in patients with MO.

- Pulmonary function tests (PFTs): tidal volume (V_T), functional residual capacity (FRC), residual volume (RV), vital capacity (VC), inspiratory reserve volume (IRV), expiratory reserve volume (ERV), and total lung capacity (TLC)
- Flow-volume loops
- Pressure-volume loops
- Diffusing capacity for carbon monoxide (DLCO)
- Compliances: lung (C_L), chest wall (C_{CW}), and total (C_{RS})
- Resistance: airway and total respiratory system
- Closing capacity (CC)
- Work of breathing (WOB)

Patients with MO have reduced lung volumes, increased WOB, and alterations in control of breathing and gas exchange. Body fat distribution, as well as BMI, determine the effects of obesity on pulmonary function.

Pulmonary mechanics. V_T is normal or increased in the obese and is decreased in OHS. Inspiratory reserve volume (IRV) is decreased. Expiratory reserve volume (ERV) is markedly decreased because the increased weight of the torso decreases the normal expansion of the rib cage and pulmonary parenchyma. Residual volume (RV) is normal. Functional residual capacity (FRC) or expiratory reserve volume (ERV) plus RV is markedly decreased because of the decrease in ERV. Vital capacity (VC) or ERV + V_T + IRV is decreased because of decreased ERV. Total lung capacity (TLC) or RV + ERV + V_T + IRV is decreased for the same reason as VC. Individuals with central, as opposed to peripheral, fat distribution have greater decreases in forced vital capacity (FVC), forced expiratory volume (FEV), and TLC. The maximum voluntary ventilation (MVV) can also be reduced.

Diffusing capacity for carbon monoxide (DLCO). DLCO is normal in individuals with obesity and mildly reduced in patients with OHS because the lung parenchyma is normal, and changes in p are due to abnormal chest wall mechanics and lower lung volumes. DLCO is a useful test to separate intrinsic lung pathology from obesity.

Compliance. There is a decrease in the total respiratory system compliance ($1/C_{RS} = 1/C_L + 1/C_{CW}$), where C_{RS} is the total compliance, C_L is the compliance of the lung, and C_{CW} is the compliance of the chest wall. Total compliance is always decreased because of the weight of the torso and abdominal contents pressing against the diaphragm creating a restrictive component, markedly decreasing the C_{CW}. Lung compliance is often normal but is decreased when pulmonary and circulatory comorbidities are present (eg, pulmonary hypertension).

Resistance. There are increases both in airway resistance (reduced elastic tension of the lung) and in total respiratory system resistance (increased elastic tension of chest wall) at lower lung volumes, which lead to reduction in the caliber of the smaller airways. The increase in total resistance is ~30% in simple obesity and 100% in OHS. Resistance increases further in the supine position, possibly due to extrinsic adipose pressure of the supralaryngeal airway and decreased FRC.

Closing capacity. FRC is reduced in patients with MO and can be below the closing capacity (CC) resulting in small airway closure, ventilation/perfusion mismatch, right-to-left shunting, and possibly hypoxemia, so-called positional ventilatory collapse. This can be worsened in the supine position, Trendelenburg position, by general anesthesia and neuromuscular block, and can be improved using lung recruitment strategies (eg, positive end-expiratory pressure [PEEP]) and reverse Trendelenburg position.

Increased work of breathing. MO is associated with a 70% increase in the WOB and a 4-fold increase in the oxygen cost of breathing (oxygen consumed by the respiratory muscles per liter of ventilation, used as a surrogate for the energy cost of breathing). This is due to decreased lung compliance, increased respiratory resistance, and threshold inspiratory load from adipose tissue mass. Morbidly obese individuals with obstructive sleep apnea syndrome (MO-OSAHS) have elevated pharyngeal and nasopharyngeal resistance, raising the WOB to 60% above that of obese and 250% that of patients without obesity.

Brinkman JE, Toro F, Sharma S. Physiology, respiratory drive. In: *StatPearls* [Internet]. StatPearls Publishing; 2025. Accessed May 19, 2025. https://www.ncbi.nlm.nih.gov/books/NBK482414/

Piper A, Yee B. Clinical manifestations and diagnosis of obesity hypoventilation syndrome. *UpToDate.* Accessed May 1, 2023. http://www.uptodate.com/contents/clinical-manifestations-and-diagnosis-of-obesity-hypoventilation-syndrome

A.10. What changes occur in $Pa{O_2}$ and $Pa{CO_2}$ in patients with MO?

In the awake patient, positional reductions in lung volume and respiratory system compliance occur when moving from an upright position to a supine position, particularly in ERV and FRC. FRC declines both with obesity and with induction of general anesthesia.

Hypoxemia is the most common blood gas abnormality in the patient with severe obesity. This is most commonly due to a low ventilation/perfusion (V_E/Q) ratio. Pulmonary perfusion is increased in the obese as a result of increased cardiac output and increased circulating blood volume. Alveolar ventilation is decreased in the obese as a result of upper airway closure. Closing volume is often greater than the ERV, particularly in the supine position, causing airway closure, resulting in right-to-left shunt and hypoxemia. These patients frequently develop atelectasis, both from cephalad position of the diaphragm and increased weight of thoracic adipose tissue. Many patients with obesity develop a restrictive respiratory pattern, with mild small-volume tachypnea, and increased use of accessory muscles of respiration.

The second most common blood gas abnormality in patients with severe obesity is a variable change in CO_2 tension ($Pa{CO_2}$), not related to lung disease, and dependent on alveolar ventilation. There are three patterns of ventilatory derangement:

- *Alveolar hyperventilation* in response to hypoxic drive. This occurs in young, active subjects. $Pa{CO_2}$ is approximately 35 mm Hg.
- *Periodic, nocturnal, alveolar hypoventilation* with normal daytime values with OSA
- *Daytime, or constant, alveolar hypoventilation* with IOHS

Lung disease, such as asthma and chronic obstructive pulmonary disease (COPD), is more common in patient population with obesity.

Onofri A, Patout M, Kaltsakas G, et al. Neural respiratory drive and cardiac function in patients with obesity hypoventilation syndrome following initiation of non-invasive ventilation. *J Thorac Dis.* 2018;10:S135-S143.

Shetty S, Parthasarathy S. Obesity hypoventilation syndrome. *Curr Pulmonol Rep.* 2015;4:42-55.

A.11. What changes occur in intrapulmonary shunt (Q_S/Q_T) and dead space (V_D/V_T) in MO? Describe the shunt equation and the physiologic dead space, or Bohr equation.

Q_S/Q_T is normally less than 5%. In MO, this is increased because of the following:

- Lower ratio
- Upper airway closure (eg, OSAHS)
- Decreased FRC from abdominal compression
- Hypoventilation (eg, OSAHS)
- Increased pulmonary circulation, from increased cardiac output, increased blood volume, and occasionally pulmonary hypertension

$$\text{Shunt equation: } Q_S/Q_T = (Cco_2 - Cao_2)/(Cco_2 - C_VO_2)$$

where Q_S is pulmonary physiology shunt (mL/min), Q_T is cardiac output (mL/min), Cco_2 is end pulmonary capillary oxygen content, Cao_2 is arterial oxygen content, and C_VO_2 is mixed venous oxygen content.

Dead space is anatomic, alveolar, or physiologic. *Anatomic dead space* is the volume of the lung and upper airway that is not involved in gas exchange. Ventilation of this area does not result in gas exchange. The volume of the anatomic dead space in milliliters is approximately the IBW in pounds. Fowler's method of measuring anatomic dead space is by analyzing nitrogen concentration after single breath 100% oxygen. *Alveolar dead space* is the volume of alveoli with ventilation and no perfusion, with a high ventilation/perfusion ($\dot{V}/\dot{Q}$) ratio, also defined as West Zone 1.. *Physiologic dead space*, the sum of anatomic and alveolar dead space, is the total area of lung plus airways not involved in gas exchange. Physiologic dead space is approximately 30% of the V_T. It is decreased in the supine position, and increased with disease states that alter, and in OHS, because the latter individuals adopt a shallow ventilatory pattern. Physiologic dead space is decreased in super obesity due to increased V_T ventilation and unchanged anatomic dead space. Physiologic dead space, or V_D/V_T, is measured by the Bohr equation, with Enghoff modification.

$$\text{Bohr equation: } V_D/V_T = (Paco_2 - P\text{ECO}_2)/P\text{ECO}_2$$

where V_D is the physiologic dead space volume (mL), V_T is the tidal volume (mL), $Paco_2$ is the partial pressure of carbon dioxide in arterial blood, and $P\text{ECO}_2$ is the partial pressure of carbon dioxide in the average mixed expired air (in mm Hg).

There are no changes in the physiologic dead space-to-V_T ratio or the alveolar-arterial oxygen gradient in patients with obesity undergoing laparoscopic gastric bypass surgery during general anesthesia compared with baseline.

Powers KA, Dhamoon AS. Physiology, pulmonary ventilation and perfusion. In: *StatPearls* [Internet]. StatPearls Publishing; 2025. Accessed May 19, 2025. https://www.ncbi.nlm.nih.gov/books/NBK539907/

A.12. What changes occur in the cardiovascular system of the patient with obesity? Discuss cardiac output, blood volume, blood pressure, and pulmonary arterial pressure.

As BMI increases, blood volume increases. Although absolute blood volume is expanded, relative blood volume is decreased. Increase in circulating blood volume and decrease in systemic vascular resistance results in increased cardiac output. Cardiac output increases by increased stroke volume, and the heart rate remains unchanged. Cardiac output and stroke volume increase in proportion to oxygen consumption and the degree of obesity but more closely to the LBW. LV wall stress increases according to the law of Laplace ($P_2 - P_1 = 2T/R$), where P is the change in arterial pressure produced by the increased volume, T is the LV wall stress, and R is the LV radius. Increased afterload from hypertension produces eccentric LV hypertrophy and eventually LV dysfunction. They are thus sensitive to acute changes in preload and afterload. Seventy percent of echocardiograms in patients with MO show abnormalities.

Hypertension is more prevalent because of increased cardiac output and increased blood volume. Hypertension is more commonly systolic in the obese. Patients with obesity and without comorbidities have normal pulmonary artery filling pressures. Those individuals with OHS and Pickwickian syndrome, however, commonly have pulmonary hypertension as a result of hypoxic pulmonary vasoconstriction and increased cardiac output. There are two major mechanisms in the pathogenesis of heart failure in these patients. Pulmonary and systemic vascular congestion develops as a consequence of chronic volume overload superimposed on diminished diastolic compliance caused by long-standing LV hypertrophy. Chronic volume overload and high cardiac output result in LV hypertrophy. The ventricular wall/cavity ratio decreases, and LV systolic dysfunction results. Obesity leads to fatty infiltration of the cardiac conduction system, predisposing to sudden death. Incidence of congestive heart failure and stroke is elevated.

Centrally, patients with obesity and normal blood pressure develop eccentric ventricular remodeling from chronic volume overload, increased diastolic pressure, increased diastolic wall stress, and chamber enlargement, in contrast to lean patients with hypertension, who develop concentric hypertrophy. The patient with obesity and hypertension can have both systolic and diastolic pressure overload and potentially earlier heart failure.

Metabolic syndrome, including central obesity, type 2 diabetes mellitus with insulin resistance, hypertension, dyslipidemia, increased sympathetic nerve activity, and OSA.

Bhupathiraju SN, Hu FB. Epidemiology of obesity and diabetes and their cardiovascular complications. *Circ Res.* 2016;118:1723-1735.

Csige I, Ujvárosy D, Szabó Z, et al. The impact of obesity on the cardiovascular system. *J Diabetes Res.* 2018;2018:3407306.

Poirier P, Giles TD, Bray GA, et al. Obesity: association with cardiovascular disease. Accessed May 1, 2023. https://www.uptodate.com/contents/obesity-weight-reduction-with-cardiovascular-disease

A.13. Are there any other diseases commonly associated with obesity?

Secondary obesity can be associated with hypothyroidism, Cushing disease, insulinoma, hypogonadism, and hypothalamic disorders. Although most patients with obesity are not diabetic, 80% to 90% of nonketotic diabetics are obese. Increased insulin secretion and insulin resistance resulting from peripheral tissue insensitivity are well characterized features of obesity. Obesity exacerbates the diabetic state. Furthermore, malignancies of breast, prostate, cervix, uterus, colon, and rectum are more common in the obese.

There is a disproportionate increase in health-related risks from obesity. Above a BMI of 25, the risk of coronary artery disease more than doubles. Above a BMI of 29, there is an increased perioperative risk of pulmonary embolus. Above a BMI of 35, there is more than a 40-fold increase in adult-onset diabetes mellitus, respiratory disease, osteoarthritis, and OSAHS. Perioperative mortality during weight reduction surgery correlates with BMI, preoperative hypertension, anastomotic leak, and pulmonary embolus.

González-Muniesa P, Mártinez-González MA, Hu FB, et al. Obesity. *Nat Rev Dis Primers.* 2017;3:17034.

Karam JG, McFarlane SI. Secondary causes of obesity. *Therapy.* 2007;4:641-650.

Lauby-Secretan B, Scoccianti C, Loomis D, et al. Body fatness and cancer—viewpoint of the IARC Working Group. *N Engl J Med.* 2016;375:794-798.

A.14. What anatomic changes that affect the airway are associated with MO and OSA?

Patient-specific anatomic changes in the MO are related to the BMI, type of obesity (peripheral *vs* central), and presence or absence of OSA. Not all patients with MO have airway involvement. The anatomic changes affecting the airway are not always easily diagnosed with routine physical examination. At a given BMI, there is more airway involvement in central obesity compared to peripheral obesity, and the most severe airway involvement occurs in patients with OSAHS.

Anatomic alterations in MO and OSA include:

- Increased adipose tissue in the airway lateral pharyngeal walls causes a decrease in the pharyngeal area.
- Increased adipose tissue external to the upper airway (lateral parapharyngeal fat pads or jowls), extrinsically compressing the airway
- Presence of hypopharyngeal adipose tissue not evident on external examination that acts as a ball valve, obstructing the upper airway and interfering with the line of sight at direct laryngoscopy
- Presence of pretracheal adipose tissue, which pushes the hyoid bone posteriorly into a less favorable position, causing the epiglottis to partially override the glottic entrance, worsening laryngoscopic view
- Change in the pharynx shape from an ellipse with the long axis lateral transverse to an ellipse with the long axis anterior-posterior
- Decreased efficiency of the anterior pharyngeal dilator muscles promotes snoring.
- The "lung volume hypothesis." Decreased FRC in the asleep or anesthetized patient displaces the tracheal carina cephalad 0.5 to 2 cm, relaxing the soft-walled hypopharynx and decreasing the internal volume. In severe cases, it can passively seal or telescope. Noninvasive positive pressure ventilation (NIPPV) tents open the hypopharynx, promoting gas exchange.

In these patients, the airway can obstruct with light-to-moderate sedation (peripheral OSA). They can be difficult to ventilate by mask. They have a higher incidence of difficult intubation and failed intubation. Head and neck adipose tissue can obscure craniofacial dysostoses (eg, micrognathia).

Barrera JE, Pau CY, Forest VI, et al. Anatomic measures of upper airway structures in obstructive sleep apnea. *World J Otorhinolaryngol Head Neck Surg.* 2017;3:85-91.

Feng Y, Keenan BT, Wang S, et al. Dynamic upper airway imaging during wakefulness in obese subjects with and without sleep apnea. *Am J Respir Crit Care Med.* 2018;198:1435-1443.

Isono S. Obstructive sleep apnea of obese adults: pathophysiology and perioperative airway management. *Anesthesiology.* 2009;110:908-921.

Kheterpal S, Martin L, Shanks AM, et al. Prediction and outcomes of impossible mask ventilation: a review of 50,000 anesthetics. *Anesthesiology.* 2009;110:891-897.

A.15. What derangements of the gastrointestinal system are associated with MO?

There are several changes in the upper gastrointestinal tract that place severely obese individuals at risk of acid aspiration pneumonitis upon induction of and emergence from general anesthesia: increase in intra-abdominal pressure with increasing body weight, increased incidence of gastroesophageal reflux disease (GERD), decreased gastric pH, increased incidence of hiatal hernia, and impaired gastroesophageal antireflux mechanism. Ninety percent of fasting patients with MO exceed Mendelson criteria, a gastric volume of greater than 0.35 mL/kg total body weight (TBW), with a pH less than 2.5. Patients with severe obesity have a normal gastric emptying rate with a larger pouch, so that after a controlled fasting (eg, 2-day liquid diet for bariatric surgery), patients should have an empty stomach.

There is a substantially higher incidence of hepatobiliary disease in the patients with MO, such as cholelithiasis, hepatitis, intrahepatic and extrahepatic cholestasis, hepatic steatosis, and cirrhosis. Seventy-five percent of the morbidly obese have hepatic steatosis. Although there is a 25% incidence of severe hepatic dysfunction in the morbidly obese, there is no clear correlation between liver function tests (LFTs) and hepatic dysfunction, complicating medical and anesthetic management. There are increased incidences of nonalcoholic fatty liver disease (NAFLD), nonalcoholic steatohepatitis (NASH), and hepatocellular carcinoma in the morbidly obese population, as well as of gallstone pancreatitis, adult-onset diabetes mellitus, and insulinoma, and a higher incidence of colorectal malignancies. Long-standing central obesity in the presence of metabolic syndrome is associated with erosive esophagitis, Barrett's esophagus, and esophageal adenocarcinoma.

Chang P, Friedenberg F. Obesity and GERD. *Gastroenterol Clin North Am.* 2014;43:161-173.

Fabbrini E, Sullivan S, Klein S. Obesity and nonalcoholic fatty liver disease: biochemical, metabolic, and clinical implications. *Hepatology.* 2010;51:679-689.

Macdonald K, Porter GA, Guernsey DL, et al. A polymorphic variant of the insulin-like growth factor type 1 receptor gene modifies risk of obesity for esophageal adenocarcinoma. *Cancer Epidemiol.* 2009;33:37-40.

National Cancer Institute. Obesity and cancer. Accessed May 1, 2023. https://www.cancer.gov/about-cancer/causes-prevention/risk/obesity/obesity-fact-sheet

Singh M, Lee J, Gupta N, et al. Weight loss can lead to resolution of gastroesophageal reflux disease symptoms: a prospective intervention trial. *Obesity.* 2013;21:284-290.

B. Preoperative Evaluation and Preparation

B.1. How would this patient be optimized for surgery preoperatively? Would you use preoperative screening questionnaires to diagnose OSA? Summarize the workup for this patient.

After the initial surgical visit, the patient was assigned an internal medicine physician, specializing in obesity medicine, with a period of medical optimization. Complete, comprehensive care, consisting of rehabilitation medicine, pharmacologic and nonpharmacologic interventions, behavior modification, and medically supervised diet, was accompanied by psychological evaluation to determine motivation and long-term perception of patient goals. This resulted in a functional improvement to 2 metabolic equivalents (METs) and weight loss to 204.1 kg, with a BMI of 61.0 kg/m^2, an approximately 25% decrease. Once the patient had been deemed optimized for surgery, and after at least 6 months, the preoperative workup was scheduled.

Preoperative evaluation includes a detailed history, review of systems, physical examination, and laboratory tests. Special attention is paid to circulatory, pulmonary, and hepatic function. Circulatory evaluation includes signs and symptoms of left or right ventricular failure, history of hypertension, and electrocardiographic abnormalities. Respiratory evaluation includes smoking history, exercise tolerance, history of hypoventilation and somnolence. Hepatic function tests include serum albumin and globulin, serum aspartate aminotransferase, serum alanine aminotransferase, direct and total bilirubin, alkaline phosphatase, prothrombin time, and cholesterol levels.

A cardiology consultation was conducted with a noninvasive assessment of cardiac function by echocardiography. Patients without an adequate echocardiographic window require radionucleotide ventriculography to assess ventricular function and morphology, as in this case. This patient was found to have mild RV hypertrophy and mild pulmonary artery hypertension. Pertinent negatives were the absence of demonstrated coronary artery disease, LV failure or RV failure. In this case, it was determined that the patient was optimized.

Physical examination focuses on the cardiovascular, pulmonary, and the upper airway. A thorough airway assessment consisting of the routine parameters documenting pretracheal adipose thickness, neck circumference, and absence or presence of hypertrophic tonsils and adenoids. Concerning findings in our patient were a large neck, increased anterior neck soft tissue, and obligate mouth breathing. Neck circumference is an independent predictor of difficult tracheal intubation; the odds ratio is 1.13 (the odds of a problematic intubation in a particular patient with a neck circumference 1 cm larger than that of another patient are 1.13 times the odds of the patient with a 1 cm smaller neck circumference). At 40 cm (15.8 in), there is a 5% chance of difficult intubation; at 60 cm (23.6 in), this increases to 35%. Pretracheal adipose tissue greater than 2.5 cm at the level of the vocal cords (determined by ultrasonography) is an independent predictor of difficult intubation. Obligate mouth breathing can be a clue that the patient has adenotonsillar hypertrophy, nasal septal blockage, or a craniofacial dysostosis. Factors that render mask ventilation problematic, such as a heavy beard, were noted.

Prior anesthetic records should be obtained. Patients with a history of heavy snoring should have a formal sleep study or polysomnogram. Severity of OSAHS, AHI, home oxygen therapy with CPAP or BiPAP, response, and compliance with NIPPV are areas to be investigated.

The STOP-BANG questionnaire is a widely used tool to screen patients for OSA; our patient had a high-risk score of 7. The ASA has devised a patient- and procedure-specific OSA perioperative risk scoring system:

A. OSA severity based on clinical indicators (0 to 3)
B. Invasiveness of surgery and anesthesia (0 to 3)
C. Need for postoperative opioids (0 to 3)

Score is based on A + B or A + C, whichever is greater. Expert consensus is that patients are at increased perioperative risk of OSA complications if the score is less than 3. In this case, A. *3 – 1 = 2 (due to patient compliance)*, B. *2*, C. *0*. OSA risk: *4 (mild increase)*. Recommendation: *Continue CPAP/BiPAP*, no need for monitored bed.

American Society of Anesthesiologists Task Force on Perioperative Management of Patients with Obstructive Sleep Apnea. Practice guidelines for the perioperative management of patients with obstructive sleep apnea: an updated report by the American Society of Anesthesiologists Task Force on Perioperative Management of Patients with Obstructive Sleep Apnea. *Anesthesiology*. 2014;120:268-286.

Nagappa M, Liao P, Wong J, et al. Validation of the STOP-BANG Questionnaire as a screening tool for obstructive sleep apnea among different populations: a systematic review and meta-analysis. *PLoS One*. 2015;10:e0143697.

Nastalek P, Polok K, Celejewska-Wojcik N, et al. Impact of bariatric surgery on obstructive sleep apnea severity and continuous positive airway pressure therapy-prospective observational study. *Sci Rep*. 2021;11:5003

Wolkove N, Baltzan M, Kamel H, et al. Long-term compliance with continuous positive airway pressure in patients with obstructive sleep apnea. *Can Respir J*. 2008;15:365-369.

B.2. Bariatric surgery patients often receive preoperative screening procedures performed in the endoscopy suite. Describe the anesthetic considerations.

Sleeve gastrectomy has emerged over the last few years to be an optimal bariatric procedure because it is simpler than the Roux-en-Y gastric bypass (RYGB), yet still highly effective. More than half of the annual bariatric surgical procedures performed in the United States in 2017 (228,000) were sleeve gastrectomies (59.39%). Patients with severe chronic GERD, however, can have worsening of symptoms after a sleeve gastrectomy. The RYGB is an alternate procedure that can improve symptoms of GERD.

Endoscopic prescreening for bariatric surgery is becoming more widely used, and is used in roughly 50% of cases. Upper endoscopy (esophagogastroduodenoscopy [EGD]), Bravo (Bravo Reflux Testing System and Endoflip impedance planimetry system, Medtronic) can help determine the appropriate surgical procedure, documenting lower esophageal pH and demonstrating signs of chronic severe GERD, and gastroesophageal dynamic contracture rings. The Bravo pH testing system is usually placed via upper endoscopy. A capsule is imbedded into the mucosa of the lower esophagus, where it remains for 48 hours and then either passes enterically or is retrieved endoscopically. Continuous pH readings can be obtained via an external device using Bluetooth wireless technology. Anesthesia for bariatric prescreening procedures is typically deep sedation via propofol bolus or infusion. In all patients for upper endoscopy, the mortality rate is 0.03% and a serious morbidity rate is 0.54%. Both high-flow nasal oxygenation (Optiflow-THRIVE) and modified nasal CPAP devices (SuperNO$_2$VA, Vyaire Medical) devices facilitate spontaneous, assisted, or controlled ventilation and provide an adequate safety margin.

American Society for Metabolic and Bariatric Surgery. Estimate of bariatric surgery numbers, 2011-2023. Accessed May 1, 2023. https://asmbs.org/resources/estimate-of-bariatric-surgery-numbers

De Palma GD, Forestieri P. Role of endoscopy in the bariatric surgery of patients. *World J Gastroenterol.* 2014;20:7777-7784.

Hendricks L, Alvarenga E, Dhanabalsamy N, et al. Impact of sleeve gastrectomy on gastroesophageal reflux disease in a morbidly obese population undergoing bariatric surgery. *Surg Obes Relat Dis.* 2016;12:511-517.

Thereaux J, Barsamian C, Bretault M, et al. pH monitoring of gastro-oesophageal reflux before and after laparoscopic sleeve gastrectomy. *Br J Surg.* 2016;103:399-406.

B.3. Summarize the evidence-based workup, risk, chance of various adverse outcomes, and expected length of stay for this patient.

The American College of Surgeons National Surgery Quality Improvement Project (NSQIP) Surgical Risk Calculator provides the latest, nationally risk-adjusted database for tracking surgical outcomes and has an online risk calculator. This calculator estimates adverse outcomes for a given surgical procedure based on their database. This patient has a laparoscopic sleeve gastrectomy (CPT code 43775, 2018/2019 ICD-10-CM Z.98.84) and has multiple risk factors (severe systemic disease, diabetes mellitus [oral medications], hypertension, class 3 obesity). A panel of expected outcomes is generated, which compares case-specific risk to average risk and chance of outcome, as follows: serious complication 3.1% (2.6%), above average; any complication 3.8% (3.3%), above average; pneumonia 0.2% (0.2%); cardiac complication 0.1% (0.1%); surgical site infection 1.4% (1.2%), above average; urinary tract infection 0.4% (0.5%), below average; venous thromboembolism 0.5% (0.4%); renal failure 0.4% (0.2%); readmission 3.8% (3.2%), above average; return to OR 1.1% (0.9%), above average; death 0.1% (0.1%); discharge to nursing or rehabilitation facility 0.4% (0.4%); and predicted length of hospital stay 2 days.

American College of Surgeons. National Surgery Quality Improvement Project (NSQIP) surgical risk calculator. Accessed May 19, 2025. https://riskcalculator.facs.org/RiskCalculator/PatientInfo.jsp

Greenstein AJ, Wahed AS, Adeniji A, et al. Prevalence of adverse intraoperative events during obesity surgery and their sequelae. *J Am Coll Surg.* 2012;215:271.e3-277.e3.

B.4. What is the role of enhanced recovery after surgery (ERAS) in bariatric surgery? How does the public find a quality bariatric surgery team and surgical facility? What is the role of robotics in bariatric surgery?

ERAS is a multimodal approach to the care of surgical patients first outlined by Danish surgeon Henrik Kehlet in 1995 for colorectal surgery. ERAS quickly evolved from several perioperative elements into a cohesive multidisciplinary team approach, and has been adopted into many surgical subspecialties including urology, obstetrics and gynecology, vascular surgery, orthopedic surgery, spine surgery, cardiac surgery, and bariatric surgery. Although originally used for laparoscopic procedures, ERAS has been applied to open and robotic surgeries. ERAS implementation has radically changed the surgical experience and results in net health care cost savings. ERAS has evolved into a multidisciplinary instrument integrating several perioperative elements. An ERAS protocol for bariatric surgery has also been termed ENERGY, for *EN* hanc*E*d *R*ecovery *G*oals in Bariatric Surger*Y*.

In 2017, The American College of Surgeons (ACS) launched a major surgical quality improvement initiative in collaboration with the Johns Hopkins Medicine Armstrong Institute for Patient Safety and Quality and the Agency for Healthcare Research and Quality (AHRQ). Separate programs of the ACS and the American Society for Metabolic and Bariatric Surgery (ASMBS) have since been combined into a single unified program to achieve one national accreditation standard for bariatric surgery centers, the Metabolic and Bariatric Surgery Accreditation and Quality Improvement Program (MBSAQIP). Participating medical centers are subjected to rigorous ongoing criteria, data registry, and reaccreditation surveys, and are high-quality. The ACS website provides timely information to the public.

American College of Surgeons. Metabolic and Bariatric Surgery Accreditation and Quality Improvement Program. Accessed May 1, 2023. https://www.facs.org/quality-programs/mbsaqip

ERAS Society. Accessed May 1, 2023. https://erassociety.org

Senturk JC, Kristo G, Gold J, et al. The development of enhanced recovery after surgery across surgical specialties. *J Laparoendosc Adv Surg Tech A*. 2017;27:863-870.

Stenberg E, Dos Reis FLF, O'Kane M, et al. Guidelines for perioperative care in bariatric surgery: Enhanced Recovery After Surgery (ERAS) Society recommendations: a 2021 update. *World J Surg*. 2022;46:729-751.

B.5. Would you premedicate this patient?

Patients at increased risk of respiratory compromise from OSA should not receive respiratory depressant medications in an unmonitored setting. A well-conducted preoperative visit will allay anxiety of both the patient and family in most cases, so this patient was not sedated before surgery.

Premedications without respiratory depressant effects can be used as part of multimodal analgesia in patients with MO; this has the potential to decrease preinduction anxiety, lower anesthetic requirements, and decrease immediate postoperative depressant effects of opioids in a high-risk population. A single loading dose of intravenous dexmedetomidine intraoperatively blunts the hemodynamic responses during laryngoscopy and reduces opioid and anesthetic requirements; it also decreases blood pressure and heart rate as well as the recovery time after the procedure. Other preoperative and perioperative medications that have been considered include acetaminophen, nonsteroidal anti-inflammatory drugs (NSAIDs), pregabalin, tramadol, ketamine, magnesium, and others. More research needs to be conducted in this area before a standard of care emerges; however, preemptive analgesia has not been adopted as a standard in the bariatric surgical population. Aprepitant, a selective human substance P/neurokinin 1 receptor antagonist, has recently been advocated as prophylaxis of postoperative nausea and vomiting (PONV).

The Society of American Gastrointestinal and Endoscopic Surgeons (SAGES) recommends the following, unless contraindicated. Two hours prior to surgery, in the holding area, subcutaneous heparin 5,000 mg, and the ENERGY protocol medications: celecoxib 400 mg PO, acetaminophen 975 mg PO, and aprepitant 40 mg PO. Despite the efficacy for reduction of PONV, use of both gabapentin and pregabalin have recently been called into question, because of minimal contribution to analgesia and adverse effects, including dizziness and visual disturbances. Despite best practice, the incidence of PONV, the most common postoperative complication in bariatric surgery, remains high.

Jones SB. Multimodal analgesia in patients with morbid obesity. Published November 26, 2013. Accessed May 1, 2023. http://bariatrictimes.com/multimodal-analgesia-in-patients-with-morbid-obesity

Kharasch ED, Clark JD, Kheterpal S. Perioperative gabapentinoids: deflating the bubble. *Anesthesiology*. 2020;133:251-254.

King AB, Spann MD, Jablonski P, et al. An enhanced recovery program for bariatric surgical patients significantly reduces perioperative opioid consumption and postoperative nausea. *Surg Obes Relat Dis*. 2018;14:849-856.

Małczak P, Pisarska M, Piotr M, et al. Enhanced recovery after bariatric surgery: systematic review and meta-analysis. *Obes Surg*. 2017;27:226-235.

Thorell A, MacCormick AD, Awad S, et al. Guidelines for perioperative care in bariatric surgery: Enhanced Recovery After Surgery (ERAS) Society recommendations. *World J Surg*. 2016;40:2065-2083.

Verret M, Lauzier F, Zarychanski R, et al. Perioperative use of gabapentinoids for the management of postoperative acute pain: a systematic review and meta-analysis. *Anesthesiology*. 2020;133:265-279.

B.6. Describe the mechanism of action of each premedication in the ENERGY protocol.

- *Celecoxib* is a highly selective reversible inhibitor of the COX-2 isoform of cyclooxygenase, which inhibits the transformation of arachidonic acid to prostaglandins, produces antipyretic, analgesic, and anti-inflammatory effects.
- *Acetaminophen*, a centrally acting cyclooxygenase inhibitor (COX-3), is a nonopioid analgesic with a rapid onset. Preincisional intravenous administration results in lower postoperative VAS scores.
- *Aprepitant* works as a selective human substance P/neurokinin 1 receptor antagonist and has been used as powerful antiemetic therapy to treat chemotherapy-induced nausea and vomiting.

Cooke FE, Samuels JD, Pomp A, et al. A randomized, double-blind, placebo-controlled trial of intravenous acetaminophen on hospital length of stay in obese individuals undergoing sleeve gastrectomy. *Obes Surg*. 2018;28:2998-3006.

DrugBank. Aprepitant. Accessed May 1, 2023. https://www.drugbank.ca/drugs/DB00673

Gong L, Thorn CF, Bartagnolli MM, et al. Celecoxib pathways: pharmacokinetics and pharmacodynamics. *Pharmacogenet Genomics*. 2012;22:310-318.

Semyonov M, Bartulovic A, Cohen N, et al. The effect of timing of intravenous paracetamol on perioperative pain and cytokine levels following laparoscopic bariatric surgery, a randomized controlled trial. *Obesity.* 2022;30:2185-2193.

U.S. Food and Drug Administration. Neurontin. Accessed May 1, 2023. https://www.accessdata.fda.gov/drugsatfda_docs/label/2009/020235s041,020882s028,021129s027lbl.pdf

B.7. How would you adjust doses of anesthetics in the morbidly obese?

Anesthetizing patients with MO requires careful consideration of changes in the pharmacokinetic and pharmacodynamic properties of numerous drugs used in anesthesia. Physiologic and anthropometric changes, such as increases in cardiac output, changes in regional blood flow, and increases in the body composition affect pharmacokinetic properties. In addition, respiratory pathophysiology such as the increased incidence of OSA and fat deposition in the oropharynx and chest wall alters pharmacodynamic properties of anesthetics.

Weight-based dosing scalars other than TBW must be considered when administering drugs to patients with MO. Administration of drugs based on TBW can result in an overdose, whereas administration based on IBW can result in a subtherapeutic dose.

With the exceptions of succinylcholine (where TBW is appropriate) and the nondepolarizing neuromuscular blocking agents (where IBW is appropriate), LBW is the optimal dosing scalar for most anesthetic agents including opioids and anesthetic induction agents, especially as cardiac output is significantly correlated to LBW, except in individuals with obesity cardiomyopathy (**Table 63.1**).

Sevoflurane is the most commonly used potent inhaled anesthetic agent. Sevoflurane is especially useful for short-duration titration of anesthetic depth and in selected patients (eg, smokers, asthma). Desflurane had been touted as having faster washout and recovery than sevoflurane, however, clinical data demonstrate that in both patients with MO and patients without obesity, the faster emergence of desflurane is only on the order of a few minutes. Desflurane use has also decreased because of greenhouse gas and global warming considerations.

Barras M, Legg A. Drug dosing in obese adults. *Aust Prescr.* 2017;40:189-193.

Hendrickx JFA, Nielsen OJ, De Hert S, De Wolf AM. The science behind banning desflurane: a narrative review. *Eur J Anaesthesiol.* 2022;39:818-824.

TABLE 63.1 Weight-Based Dosing Recommendations for Commonly Used Intravenous Anesthetics

Drug	Dosing Scalar	Comments
Propofol	Induction: LBW Maintenance: TBW	Subjects with MO given an induction dose based on LBW require similar amounts of propofol and similar times to loss of consciousness compared with lean subjects given propofol based on TBW. Volume of distribution and clearance at steady-state increases with increasing TBW.
Thiopental	Induction: LBW Maintenance: TBW	Simulations showed a 60% decrease in peak plasma concentration in subjects with MO compared with lean subjects after a 250 mg dose. Induction dose adjusted to LBW results in same peak plasma concentration as dose adjusted to CO. Volumes and clearances increase proportionally with TBW.
Fentanyl	LBW	Clearance increases linearly with “PK mass,” an arbitrary scalar highly correlated to LBW.
Remifentanil	LBW	An infusion based on LBW results in similar plasma concentrations as normal weight subjects were given an infusion based on TBW.
Succinylcholine	TBW	Administration of 1 mg/kg based on TBW resulted in a more profound block and better intubating conditions compared with doses based on IBW or LBW.
Vecuronium	IBW	Doses based on TBW result in a prolonged duration of action in obese *vs* nonobese subjects.
Rocuronium	IBW	There is an increased duration of action when the drug is given based on TBW *vs* IBW.
Atracurium, Cisatracurium	IBW	The duration of action is prolonged in obese subjects when given on the basis of TBW *vs* IBW.

CO, cardiac output; IBW, ideal body weight; LBW, lean body weight; MO, morbid obesity; PK, pharmacokinetic; TBW, total body weight.
Reprinted from Ingrande J, Lemmens HJM. Dose adjustment of anaesthetics in the morbidly obese. *Br J Anaesth.* 2010;105:i16-i23.

Ingrande J, Lemmens HJM. Dose adjustment of anaesthetics in the morbidly obese. *Br J Anaesth.* 2010;105:i16-i23.

Nightingale CE, Margarson MP, Shearer E, et al. Peri-operative management of the obese surgical patient 2015. *Anaesthesia.* 2015;70:859-876.

Seyni-Boureima R, Zhang Z, Antoine MMLK, Antoine-Frank CD. A review on the anesthetic management of obese patients undergoing surgery. *BMC Anesthesiol.* 2022;22:98.

C. Intraoperative Management

C.1. How would you monitor this patient?

In addition to the routine use of noninvasive ASA standard monitoring of heart rate, blood pressure, pulse oximetry, end-tidal CO_2, and temperature, an arterial catheter can be inserted for assessment of blood gases as well as continuous blood pressure measurement in patients with cardiac disease (as in our patient). Wrist cuffs for noninvasive blood pressure monitoring have been utilized in patients with severe obesity due to the conical shape of the upper extremity. Temperature can be monitored via tympanic probe sensors, which track core temperatures; alternatively, an esophageal stethoscope with a temperature sensor can be placed in the axilla to monitor cutaneous temperature. Esophageal stethoscopes are not used because any device placed in the esophagus can be inadvertently included in the surgical anastomosis. Urinary drainage catheters are not typically placed. A peripheral nerve stimulator is used to monitor the depth of neuromuscular blockade. A processed EEG device, such as the bispectral index or BIS (Medtronic) can be used to monitor depth of anesthesia since patients with obesity are at higher risk of perioperative awareness under general anesthesia. Intraoperative spirometry and flow-volume loops (GE Datex S/5 [System 5] series monitor [GE Datex Ohmeda]) are useful in monitoring changes in ventilation, surgical conditions and patient status. An automatic peripheral nerve stimulator (eg, IntelliVue NMT; Phillips) simplifies data acquisition and charting in the electronic medical record.

The advantages of invasive monitoring are weighed against possible complications. Laparoscopic bariatric surgeries have minimal blood loss (typically <100 mL) and fluid shifts. These are elective cases, and patients are optimized preoperatively. Invasive arterial monitoring is used rarely for the super obese with severe cardiopulmonary disease or poor fit of the noninvasive blood pressure cuff. Accurate blood pressure readings can alternatively be obtained from the wrist. Central venous access is typically used when there are difficulties obtaining peripheral access. A pulmonary artery catheter is reserved for the rare patient with severe pulmonary hypertension, cor pulmonale, or LV failure.

Fogagnolo A, Montanaro F, Al-Husinat L, Turrini C, et al. Management of intraoperative mechanical ventilation to prevent postoperative complications after general anesthesia: a narrative review. *J Clin Med.* 2021;10:2656.

Haren AP, Nair S, Pace MC, Sansone P. Intraoperative monitoring of the obese patient undergoing surgery: a narrative review. *Adv Ther.* 2021;38:3622-3651.

Mechanick JI, Apovian C, Brethauer S, et al. Clinical practice guidelines for the perioperative nutrition, metabolic, and nonsurgical support of patients undergoing bariatric procedures—2019 update: cosponsored by American Association of Clinical Endocrinologists/American College of Endocrinology, The Obesity Society, American Society for Metabolic and Bariatric Surgery, Obesity Medicine Association, and American Society of Anesthesiologists. *Obesity.* 2020;28:O1-O58.

Siddiqui M, Calhoun DA. Blood pressure measurement challenges in severely obese patients. *Am J Hypertens.* 2019; 32:139-140.

Stenberg E, Dos Reis Falcão LF, et al. Guidelines for perioperative care in bariatric surgery: Enhanced Recovery After Surgery (ERAS) Society recommendations: a 2021 update [published correction in *World J Surg.* 2022;46:752]. *World J Surg.* 2022;46:729-751.

C.2. The American Society of Anesthesiologists (ASA) Difficult Airway Algorithm provides a guideline for management of the difficult airway. How do the comorbidities in patients with MO and OSA modify implementation of the algorithm?

The ASA difficult airway algorithm provides a guideline for management of the difficult airway. It was created by a panel of experts under the direction of the ASA in 1993 and modified in 2003 (to include the laryngeal mask airway [LMA]), in 2013 (to include the supraglottic airway [SGA] and videolaryngoscopes), and in 2022 (to reflect current practice). The major changes in the most recent iteration include: factors supporting awake intubation; optimizing oxygenation throughout by factors including positioning, noninvasive ventilation, preoxygenation, and maximizing functional residual capacity (FRC);

limiting intubation attempts; considerations in awakening the patient; calling for help; and performing invasive airway access. Implementation of the algorithm can be altered in specific patient populations, according to factors such as location, patient characteristics and comorbidities, surgical requirements, equipment availability, presence of additional personnel, and importantly the skills of the anesthesiologist.

In the bariatric surgical patients with demonstrated or suspected OSA, considerations include: status as having an "empty stomach" in most cases; vulnerability to precipitous apneic deoxygenation; higher incidence of difficult mask ventilation and difficult intubation with redundant adipose tissue can obstruct the line of sight on laryngoscopy. Each of these points deserves clarification.

First, bariatric surgical candidates typically undergo upper endoscopy prior to the planned bariatric surgery procedure. We therefore know whether they have conditions associated with the need for aspiration prophylaxis, such as GERD, hiatal hernia, a gastric hypersecretory state, or achalasia. Obesity produces a moderate increase in gastric accommodation and an increase in emptying rate. Foregut surgical patients are placed on a liquid diet for 2 days and should, in most cases, have an empty stomach. Notable exceptions such as bile reflux, achalasia, gastrointestinal stromal tumors (GIST), and Zollinger-Ellison syndrome should be noted prior to the time of surgery. As part of the ENERGY ERAS protocol for bariatrics, patients receive an energy drink prior to midnight on the day prior to surgery and upon awakening. Studies have shown that gastric fluid volume and pH are unchanged after drinking a nonparticulate drink 2 hours prior to surgery.

Second, patients with severe obesity are at higher risk of early arterial apneic desaturation during induction of anesthesia. This is due to several factors, including derangement of pulmonary mechanics (decreased ERV and FRC) by cephalad displacement of the diaphragm, increased incidence of atelectasis, airway modifications, and increased frequency of hypotensive events.

Third, the standard airway assessment might not be sufficient. Physical findings suggestive of peripheral OSA (such as paratracheal adipose thickness, neck circumference, and hypertrophic tonsils and adenoids) should be sought out. Craniofacial dysostoses (eg, relative micrognathia) might be hidden by facial adipose tissue or hair. As a consequence, there is a higher incidence of both difficult mask ventilation and unanticipated difficult airway. The latest guidance is from the Difficult Airway Society 2015 guidelines for management of the unanticipated difficult intubation in the adult patient. Videolaryngoscopy and alternative airway devices, including flexible intubating scopes, can improve laryngeal view during intubation. It is important to have other options when the primary airway management technique fails.

Fourth, the importance of additional personnel needs to be stressed. The attending surgeon needs to be present at induction of anesthesia, and unopened emergency front-of-neck access (eFONA) and tracheostomy equipment should be available. When indicated, an additional anesthesiologist might be helpful. With the evolution of videolaryngoscopy and accumulating experience, use of awake techniques for securing the airway have become less common. The flexible scope remains an important part of our arsenal, however, and should be available as part of any backup plan.

Apfelbaum JL, Hagberg CA, Connis RT, Abdelmalak BB, et al. 2022 American Society of Anesthesiologists practice guidelines for management of the difficult airway. *Anesthesiology*. 2022;136:31-81.

Atterhem V, Hultin M, Myrberg T. The incidence of hemodynamic and respiratory adverse events in morbidly obese presenting for bariatric surgery. *Int J Clin Anesth Res*. 2018;2:9-17.

Cook TM, Woodall N, Frerk C. Major complications of airway management in the UK: results of the Fourth National Audit project of the Royal College of Anaesthetists and the Difficult Airway Society. Part 1: anaesthesia. *Br J Anaesth*. 2011;106:617-631.

Frerk C, Mitchell VS, McNarry AF, et al. Difficult Airway Society 2015 guidelines for management of unanticipated difficult intubation in adults. *Br J Anaesth*. 2015;115:827-848.

Kruisselbrink R, Arzola C, Jackson T, et al. Ultrasound assessment of gastric volume in severely obese individuals: a validation study. *Br J Anaesth*. 2017;118:77-82.

C.3. Why is it important to preoxygenate the patient with obesity? How would you do it? Compare the effectiveness of the four-maximum-breath and 3-minute techniques. What is the importance of continuous positive airway pressure (CPAP) during the induction of general anesthesia? Describe the use of the nasal CPAP mask and transnasal humidified oxygenation rapid-insufflation ventilatory exchange in the induction of general anesthesia.

In patients with obesity, preoxygenation is essential due to precipitous apneic deoxygenation on induction of anesthesia. Preoxygenation is optimized by semi-recumbent position and a tight-fitting face mask. In the past, two techniques of preoxygenation have been used: full, or "slow" (V_T breathing for 3 minutes), and "fast" (four-maximum-breath over 30 seconds). "Slow" preoxygenation produces higher oxygen tension. When time is of the essence, however, a modified "fast" technique (eight-maximum-breath over 60 seconds) compares favorably with the "slow" preoxygenation, both in terms of fraction of expired oxygen (FEO_2) and duration of apnea without desaturation in seconds (DAWD). Most oxygen reserve is in the FRC. The amount of time for onset of hypoxemia (SpO_2 of 90%) has been calculated for a healthy nonobese adult when breathing room air *versus* 100% oxygen starting at onset of apnea as a period of apnea of 0.9 minutes *versus* 9 minutes. The first 8.1 minutes are spent consuming FRC reserve. For the patient with MO, time to hypoxemia will be significantly shorter.

Continuous positive pressure ventilation (CPAP) increases FRC and further raises the oxygen reserve compared with nasal oxygen. This occurs both during sedation and induction of general anesthesia. CPAP works by tenting open the hypopharynx and increasing the FRC, both particularly important in the patient population with MO. Recent meta-analysis of perioperative noninvasive ventilation in patients with obesity suggests that CPAP is well tolerated and effective before induction of general anesthesia and after extubation in improving CO_2 clearance and decreasing the risk of respiratory complications.

The SuperNO$_2$VA (Vyaire Medical) is a modified nasal CPAP mask that has been favorably used during the induction of general anesthesia. Nasal positive pressure ventilation is conducted via the anesthesia ventilator during the induction sequence without steric hindrance due to the low-profile mask, and patients can be effectively ventilated while being intubated, as was our patient. This can be helpful in the event of an unexpected difficult airway. Transnasal humidified rapid-insufflation ventilatory exchange (OptiFlow-THRIVE, Fisher Paykel, NZ) extends apnea time and provides PEEP due to continuous delivery of high-flow warmed humidified oxygen from preoxygenation during the process of securing a definitive airway, and can be used during the extubation process. THRIVE has been used for known difficult airways, as well as the unexpected difficult airway.

Carron M, Zarantonello F, Tellaroli P, et al. Perioperative noninvasive ventilation in obese patients: a qualitative review and meta-analysis. *Surg Obes Relat Dis*. 2016;12:681-691.

Ghebremichael S, Gumbert SD, Vanga N, et al. Evaluation of SuperNO$_2$VA® mask technology in a clinical setting: a pilot study. *Trends Anesth Crit Care*. 2017;16:54-61.

Patel A, Nouraei SA. Transnasal humidified rapid-insufflation ventilatory exchange (THRIVE): a physiologic method of increasing apnoea time in patients with difficult airways. *Anaesthesia*. 2015;70:323-329.

Tanoubi I, Drolet P, Donati F. Optimizing preoxygenation in adults. *Can J Anaesth*. 2009;56:449-466.

C.4. There are many new airway devices in the marketplace. Which of these devices have been particularly successful in patient with MO or OSA?

Although the skill set of the clinician still appears to be the most relevant factor until the literature provides more guidance, several noteworthy advances in airway management have occurred. The first is the advent of affordable, high-quality video laryngoscopes (VL) now included in the 2022 Difficult Airway Algorithm. Particularly promising is the McGrath MAC VL (Medtronic) and the C-MAC (Karl Storz Endoskope). The McGrath is totally portable, low profile (eg, TMJ dysfunction), Macintosh-like device. Originally intended as a routine replacement of direct laryngoscopy, it could be the first airway device capable of replacing direct laryngoscopy. The C-MAC VL (Karl Storz Endoskope) is a complete difficult airway platform. Attached to a semiportable electronic module, and possessing high-quality optical resolution, it is a true difficult airway device and can also be connected to a fiberoptic scope. Single-use or reusable blades come in different sizes; most patients with MO and OSA can be intubated with either the no. 3 Macintosh-like or the hyperangulated D (Doerges) blade. The D-blade (which we used) is particularly suited to patients with increased neck circumference who are prone to lateral pharyngeal collapse. The C-MAC electronic module can be used for flexible, fiberoptic, and rigid (Storz Bonfils; Karl Storz SE & Co. KG) or articulating (Videostylet; Karl Storz SE & Co. KG) laryngoscopes. Both the McGrath and the C-MAC combine the benefits of direct laryngoscopy (DL) and videolaryngoscopy (VL). Other videolaryngoscopy devices that have been used for the morbidly obese with OSA population include the GlideScope VL (Verathon) suite of products.

The second advance in airway management is development of a new class of airway devices: the hyperangulated optical laryngoscope. The Airtraq SP (AT) (Mercury Medical) and the King Vision (KV) (Ambu) are in this category. Advantages include portability, being able to intubate in unusual positions (such as semi-Fowler position or "face-to-face"), or with limited access as an excellent conduit for fiberoptic bronchoscopy. Intubation is accomplished in a neutral neck position with little mouth opening, so temporomandibular joint limitation and cervical spine pathology are indications.

The third advance in airway management is development of better airway "bridges" and short-term ventilatory support devices. The LMA Fastrach (LMA-FT) or intubating LMA (Teleflex Medical; LMA, North America), provides a method of oxygenating and ventilating while obtaining a definitive airway. The I-Gel (Intersurgical Complete Respiratory Systems), which we had available for airway rescue, provides an uncuffed perilaryngeal airway with a gastric decompression lumen. The LMA Supreme (Teleflex Medical; LMA, North America) is an supraglottic airway salvage device with a gastric decompression port that incorporates features of the LMA Unique, ProSeal, and LMA-FT. An airway salvage device that has had success out-of-hospital by first responders and military medics, particularly in the event of gastrointestinal bleeding or for the difficult to manage airway (eg, OSA), is the King Laryngo-Tracheal-Suction-Disposable (King LTS-D) (Ambu).

The final advance in airway management is the development of high-quality, single-use metal laryngoscope blades, which appear to have superior success rates compared with their reusable counterparts (both in terms of blade and handles and plastic) when used during the induction of anesthesia, due to a predictable degree of brightness.

For the patient with MO/OSA with a challenging airway, fiberoptic bronchoscopy remains the gold standard. Fiberoptic bronchoscopy has substantial limitations, however, such as limited availability, a long learning curve, a low retention rate, equipment fragility, longer setup time, longer intubation time, and few absolute indications (mostly lower airway pathology). As the advanced airway management devices improve and the clinician experience grows, the need for fiberoptic bronchoscopy should continue to decline.

Buléon C, Parienti JJ, Lesage A, et al. Comparison of plastic and metallic single-use and metallic reusable laryngoscope blades: a randomised controlled trial. *Eur J Anaesthesiol.* 2013;30:163-169.

Hansel J, Rogers AM, Lewis AF, et al. Videolaryngoscopy versus direct laryngoscopy for adults undergoing tracheal intubation. *Cochrane Database Syst Rev.* 2022;4:CD011136.

Hoshijima H, Denawa Y, Tominaga A, et al. Videolaryngoscope versus Macintosh laryngoscope for tracheal intubation in adults with obesity: a systematic review and meta-analysis. *J Clin Anesth.* 2018;44:69-75.

Reutzler K, Rivas E, Cohen B, et al. McGrath video laryngoscope versus Macintosh direct laryngoscopy for intubation of morbidly obese patients: a randomized trial. *Anesth Analg.* 2020;131:586-593.

C.5. How would you induce anesthesia? Describe the tracheal intubation technique.

The OR should be set up with appropriate alternative noninvasive and invasive airway devices. On arrival in the OR, the patient is positioned on the OR table in a ramp position (Troop Elevation Pillow; Sharn Anesthesia Inc), placed on monitors, and administered an F_{IO_2} of 100% for 5 minutes via a tight-fitting mask. General anesthesia is gradually induced with midazolam 2 mg, fentanyl 100 μg, lidocaine 100 mg, and propofol in divided doses (300 mg). An oral airway is placed, the face mask is secured by head straps, and the patient is placed on the anesthesia ventilator with a jaw thrust. Once it has been ascertained that mask ventilation is feasible, nondepolarizing neuromuscular blockade (rocuronium 100 mg) was administered.

We elected to intubate with a Doerges, or D-blade C-MAC (Karl Storz Endoskope), with fiberoptic bronchoscopy backup. This patient was considered a difficult mask ventilation and a difficult airway, but not an aspiration risk, having a prolonged fast and no history of GERD or bile reflux.

Isono S. Obstructive sleep apnea of obese adults: pathophysiology and perioperative airway management. *Anesthesiology.* 2009;110:908-921.

Kaw R, Dupuy-McCauley K, Wong J. Screening and perioperative management of obesity hypoventilation syndrome. *J Clin Med.* 2024;13:5000.

Niu L, Wang Y, Yao C, et al. Efficacy and safety of neuromuscular blockade in overweight patients undergoing nasopharyngeal surgery. *Med Sci Monit.* 2020;26:e926452.

Seyni-Boureima R, Zhang Z, Antoine MM, et al. A review of the anesthetic management of obese patients undergoing surgery. *BMC Anesthesiol.* 2022;22:98.

C.6. How would you maintain general anesthesia? What agents would you choose? How would you prepare for emergence?

We elected to use total intravenous anesthesia (TIVA) consisting of propofol starting at 125 μg/kg/min IBW and dexmedetomidine 0.5 μg/kg/h TBW without a bolus. Depth of anesthesia was guided by a processed EEG (BIS, Medtronic). Our main criterion in choosing propofol over volatile anesthesia was anti-emesis. Sevoflurane would have been chosen in the presence of a reactive airway. Preparation for emergence included stopping propofol, acetaminophen 1,000 mg IV, and pressure-support ventilation. Dexmedetomidine was continued through tracheal extubation, only marginally increasing the CO_2 apneic threshold.

ENERGY, or ERAS for bariatric surgery (see Section B.4), has changed both the surgical and anesthetic management of these patients. More than half of the cases are sleeve gastrectomies (57% of 233,000 in 2017), a simpler surgical procedure with no anastomoses lasting about 2 to 3 hours. In consequence, anesthetic requirements are decreased, particularly for opioids. This patient received fentanyl 100 μg, with a pain score of 0/10 on arrival in the PACU. Transverse abdominus plane (TAP) blocks decrease postoperative analgesic requirements, reducing the need for postoperative opioid infusions (eg, IV-PCA), which means less PONV and less opioid-induced nausea and vomiting (OINV) as well as a more awake patient who is less likely to require NIPPV support.

Ahmed MM, Tian C, Lu J, Lee Y. Total intravenous anesthesia versus inhalation anesthesia on postoperative analgesia and nausea and vomiting after bariatric surgery: a systematic review and meta-analysis. *Asian J Anesthesiol.* 2021;59:135-151.

Awad S, Carter S, Purkayastha S, et al. Enhanced recovery after bariatric surgery (ERABS): clinical outcomes from a tertiary referral bariatric centre. *Obes Surg.* 2014;24:753-758.

Thorell A, MacCormick AD, Awad S, et al. Guidelines for perioperative care in bariatric surgery: Enhanced Recovery After Surgery (ERAS) Society recommendations. *World J Surg.* 2016;40:2065-2083.

Xu B, Zhou D, Ren L, et al. Pharmacokinetic and pharmacodynamics of intravenous of intravenous dexmedetomidine in morbidly obese patients undergoing laparoscopic surgery. *J Anesth.* 2017;31:813-820.

C.7. Which neuromuscular blocking agent would you use?

We used rocuronium, based on IBW, for tracheal intubation. Patients presenting for bariatric surgery are generally on a liquid diet for a couple of days. The rate of gastric emptying is identical to that of the nonobese subjects, although patients with MO have a larger gastric capacity. For the occasional subject requiring rapid sequence induction, succinylcholine or high-dose rocuronium are acceptable. Succinylcholine is dosed by TBW because the plasma cholinesterase activity increases in proportion to BMI. When an awake technique is chosen for securing the airway, a nondepolarizing neuromuscular blocking agent can be administered once tracheal intubation has been confirmed. Dense neuromuscular block is required for laparoscopic bariatric surgical procedures to facilitate ventilation, to maintain adequate intraperitoneal space for visualization and manipulation of the surgical instruments, and to permit the introduction of surgical instruments and the removal of excised tissues. Intraoperative contracture of the abdominal musculature due to inadequate neuromuscular block can increase intra-abdominal pressure. A peripheral nerve stimulator should be used to monitor the extent of relaxation and to avoid underdosing or overdosing. Tracheal extubation should only occur after documentation of full baseline train-of-four (T_4/T_1 >0.9) to meet extubation criteria. Reversal agents should be given in appropriate doses. Sugammadex, a modified γ-cyclodextrin developed to reverse aminosteroid nondepolarizing neuromuscular blocking agents, has had a huge impact on bariatric surgery, allowing dense anterior abdominal wall muscle relaxation until the end of surgery. It is dosed by TBW.

Erstad BL, Barletta JF. Dosing of neuromuscular blocking agents in patients with obesity: a narrative review. *Anaesth Intensive Care.* 2021;49:98-104.

Li D, Wang Y, Zhou Y, Yin C. Efficacy and safety of sugammadex doses calculated on the basis of corrected body weight and total body weight for the reversal of deep neuromuscular blockade in morbidly obese patients. *J Int Med Res.* 2021;49:300060520985679.

Radkowski P, Derkaczew MA, Jacewicz MA, Onichimowski D. The dosage of muscle relaxants in morbidly obese patients in daily practice—a narrative review. *Int J Gen Med.* 2024;17:4055-4060.

Sasakawa T, Miyasaka K, Sawa T, et al. Postoperative recurarization after sugammadex administration due to the lack of appropriate neuromuscular monitoring: the Japanese experience. *APSF Newslett.* 2020;35:33-68.

Pathmanathan A, Stewart P. Neuromuscular blocking agents in obesity. In: Sinha AC, ed. *Oxford Textbook of Anaesthesia for the Obese Patient.* Oxford University Press; 2021:63.

C.8. What is the pathophysiology of pneumoperitoneum (PNP)? What is the effect on the cardiopulmonary system? How does it change perioperative care? What are the optimal ventilator strategies for patients with MO undergoing bariatric surgery?

The majority of bariatric surgical procedures are performed laparoscopically or robotically. Benefits of laparoscopy include much smaller surgical incisions, decreased postoperative pain requirements, shorter hospital stay, and faster recovery time to baseline level of activity. CO_2 is the universally accepted gas chosen for abdominal insufflation during laparoscopy. CO_2 has documented advantages, including short half-life due to high tissue diffusion across all tissue beds, and less flammability and morbidity compared with other agents trialed (oxygen, N_2O).

Pneumoperitoneum with CO_2, however, alters physiology and complicates intraoperative anesthetic management. Altered physiology is both primary (due to CO_2 absorption) and secondary (due to increased intra-abdominal pressure). Primary physiologic changes arise from acidification of tissues from CO_2 absorption (~30-42 mL/min), which increases ventilator requirements (~30%). *Cerebral effects* arise from changes in cerebral vasoregulation due to hypercarbia: increased intracranial pressure from increased intrathoracic pressure and cerebral vasodilation, decreased cerebral oxygen saturation, and initiation of a hormonal cascade, with catecholamine and vasopressin release. *Cardiovascular effects* arise from CO_2, which mildly depresses myocardial contractility and sensitizes myocardium to the arrhythmogenic effects of catecholamines. Most of the pathophysiologic changes occur as a result of increased intra-abdominal pressure, which decreases venous return, decreasing cardiac output and blood pressure. Other *cardiac effects* are those typical of increased sympathetic output from hypercarbia, although bradycardia can result from initial peritoneal insufflation. *Pulmonary effects* are due to cephalad shift of the diaphragm, decreased FRC, increased physiologic dead space, greater ventilation/perfusion mismatch, decreased pulmonary compliance, and increased airway pressures especially peak airway pressure. Airway closure in patients with obesity causes lack of communication between proximal airways and alveoli, so tidal inflation starts only after a critical airway opening pressure is overcome. *Renal effects* are due to decreased renal perfusion; decreased urine output; and increased release of antidiuretic hormone, plasma renin, and aldosterone levels. *Hepatic effects* are due to decreased portal venous flow, which can lead to hepatic hypoperfusion, acute hepatocellular injury, and increased transaminase levels. Increased intra-abdominal pressure causes decreased venous drainage of the abdominal viscera and the lower extremities, which can result in deep venous thrombosis.

Most of the intraoperative changes caused by penumoperitoneum are well tolerated, provided that the insufflation pressure is maintained at the lowest acceptable level, approximately less than 20 mm Hg, with intraoperative recruitment maneuvers when indicated, and the following precautions: loading of intravenous fluids (500-1,000 mL), use of sequential compression devices, optimal ventilator settings, and monitoring of plateau airway pressure and intraoperative spirometry (flow-volume and pressure-volume loops). In comparison with volume control ventilation, pressure control ventilation appears to improve oxygenation, produce lower airway pressures and greater dynamic compliance, and better preserve ventilation/perfusion matching.

- *Management of ventilation in patients with MO*
    - CPAP during induction
    - FIO_2 less than 0.8
    - Recruitment maneuver after induction, then periodically
    - Pressure control-volume guaranteed (PC-VG)
    - V_T = 6 to 10 mL/kg IBW
    - PEEP 10 to 12 cm H_2O
    - Inspiration: expiration (I:E) = 1:1 longer inspiratory time to minimize atelectasis and improve gas exchange
    - Inspiratory pressure less than 30 cm H_2O
    - CPAP or iIPAP after extubation, if used preoperative, or deemed high risk (as our patient)

Grieco DL, Anzellotti GM, Russo A, et al. Airway closure during surgical pneumoperitoneum in obese patients. *Anesthesiology*. 2019;131:58-73.

Jaju R, Jaju PB, Dubey M, et al. Comparison of volume-controlled ventilation and pressure-controlled ventilation in patients undergoing robot-assisted pelvic surgeries: an open-label trial. *Indian J Anaesth*. 2017;61:17-23.

Sen O, Umutoglu T, Aydın N, Toptas M, Tutuncu AC, Bakan M. Effects of pressure-controlled and volume-controlled ventilation on respiratory mechanics and systemic stress response during laparoscopic cholecystectomy. *Springerplus*. 2016;5:298.

Wang JP, Wang HB, Liu YL, et al. Comparison of pressure- and volume-controlled ventilation in laparoscopic surgery: a meta-analysis of randomized controlled trial. *Clin Invest Med*. 2015;38:E119-E141.

C.9. What are the devices that anesthesiologists place in the upper gastrointestinal canal during laparoscopic bariatric surgery? Are there risks associated with placement and management of these devices?

Various devices have been placed in the upper gastrointestinal canal during laparoscopic bariatric surgery. The surgeon laparoscopically visualizes transit of the device through the gastrointestinal tract by gut distension on the video monitor and can help guide passage. *Orogastric tubes* are used both to decompress the stomach at the beginning of surgery and for "a leak test" after completion of the anastomosis, in which a vital dye, such as methylene blue, is injected, the stomach is inflated, and lack of "leak" documented. The amount of vital dye is documented and serves as a rough estimate of neogastric pouch size. Both *bougies* or *calibration tubes* serve as templates to delineate the feeding channel, identify landmarks for the anastomosis, and choose the staple line. Bougies come as either *graduated-tip*, which are easier to insert, or *blunt-tip*. Gastroesophageal *anvils*, *OrVil* EEA Stapler (Medtronic), are used to create the gastrojejunostomy anastomosis in RYGB. The *ViSiGi* 3D (Boehringer) can perform these functions and is used for sleeve gastrectomy; functioning as a bite block, a suction device, an insufflation device, and a calibration tube, around which the surgeon fashions the neo-stomach and gastroesophageal junction. Both the anesthetist who place these devices and the surgeon are responsible for monitoring proper function and lack of trauma at removal. When unable to place the indicated device, there are three options: placement by the surgeon, gastroscopy, or conversion to an open procedure.

Placement of these devices in the proximal gastrointestinal canal is a crucial portion of the anesthetic and surgical risk. Regardless of which device is chosen, the attending anesthesiologist should be present at the time of placement and document their findings. Orogastric tubes and esophageal temperature probes are strictly prohibited for patient monitoring during bariatric surgery since they can be stapled and left as foreign bodies resulting in major morbidity.

Abu-Gazala S, Donchin Y, Keidar A. Nasogastric tube, temperature probe, and bougie stapling during bariatric surgery: a multicenter survey. *Surg Obes Relat Dis*. 2012;8:595-600.

Boehringer. ViSiGi 3D. Accessed June 9, 2025. https://visigi.com

Ece I, Yilmaz H, Alptekin H, et al. Comparison of two different circular-stapler techniques for creation of gastrojejunostomy anastomosis in bariatric Roux-en Y gastric bypass. *Int J Clin Exp Med*. 2015;8:11032-11037.

Rosenthal RJ, Diaz AA, Arvidsson D, et al. International Sleeve Gastrectomy Expert Panel Consensus Statement: best practice guidelines based on experience of >12,000 cases. *Surg Obes Relat Dis*. 2012;8:8-19.

C.10. When will you extubate the patient's trachea? Describe weight-based extubation criteria.

Bariatric surgical patients are generally extubated in the operating room. Patients on CPAP or BiPAP should return to their therapy in the PACU and the surgical ward. Patients with an unfavorable OSA questionnaire response, a STOP-BANG score of 4 or more (see Section B.1), might require NIPPV therapy. Our patient received BiPAP +12/5 cm H_2O at 40% oxygen via a full-face mask.

Extubation criteria for patients with obesity include:

- Intact neurologic status, fully awake and alert, with head lift more than 5 seconds
- Hemodynamic stability
- Normothermia, greater than 36 °C
- Full reversal of neuromuscular blocking agents confirmed with train-of-four ratio (T_4/T_1 >0.9)
- Respiratory rate (breaths per minute) greater than 10 and less than 30
- Baseline peripheral oxygenation (Spo_2) greater than 95% on Fio_2 of 0.4
- Acceptable blood-gas results, if available (Fio_2 of 0.4; pH, 7.35 to 7.45; Pao_2, >80 mm Hg; $Paco_2$, <50 mm Hg)
- Acceptable respiratory mechanics: negative inspiratory force (NIF) greater than 25 to 30 cm H_2O; VC greater than 10 mL/kg IBW; V_T greater than 5 mL/kg IBW
- Acceptable pain control
- No demonstrated or suspected laboratory abnormalities
- No surgical complications noted

Note that patients with OSA and OHS have higher incidence of postoperative respiratory dysfunction. They require close attention during tracheal extubation, and occasionally, warrant respiratory monitoring for observation.

Extubation criteria should be used systematically in patients with obesity; in all cases, an attending anesthesiologist with advanced airway skills must be in attendance in case tracheal reintubation becomes necessary, and the surgeon should be immediately available. Patients with documented difficult airway should be extubated based on the protocol of the individual institution. A significant percentage of settled malpractice cases in the ASA Closed Claims Database (67% upon induction, 15% during surgery, 12% at extubation, and 5% during recovery) occurred at the end of surgery. Death and brain damage decreased in the periods of 1985-1992 and 1993-1999 during induction but not during extubation and recovery. The majority of bariatric surgical patients, and certainly our patient, belong in the Difficult Airway Society Extubation Guidelines "At Risk" algorithm, in which awake extubation, advanced techniques (laryngeal mask exchange, remifentanil, airway exchange catheter) are featured. We opted for an awake extubation, with preparation for possible reintubation and presence of attending surgeon.

Apfelbaum JL, Hagberg CA, Connis RT, et al. American Society of Anesthesiologists practice guidelines for management of the difficult airway. *Anesthesiology*. 2022;163:31-81.

DeJong A, Huguet H, Molinari N, et al. Non-invasive ventilation versus oxygen therapy after extubation in patients with obesity in intensive care units: the multicentre randomised EXTUB-OBESE study protocol. *BMJ Open*. 2022;12:e052712.

Difficult Airway Society. DAS extubation guidelines. Accessed May 1, 2023. https://das.uk.com

Eipe N. Anesthesia for the patient with obesity. *UpToDate*. Assessed May 19, 2025. https://www.uptodate.com/contents/anesthesia-for-the-patient-with-obesity

Thiele AW, Coudroy R, Nay M-A, et al. Beneficial effects of noninvasive ventilation after extubation in obese or overweight patients. *Am J Respir Crit Care Med*. 2022;205:440-449.

D. Postoperative Management

D.1. What are the early postoperative complications of bariatric surgical procedures?

The most quoted source of early postoperative morbidity and mortality after bariatric surgery is the Longitudinal Assessment of Bariatric Surgery (LABS) Study, a 10-center observational cohort study of bariatric surgical outcomes, consisting of 6,118 bariatric surgical patients initially from March 2005 to April 2009 and ongoing, at academic centers of excellence. The incidence of 30-day all-cause mortality was 0.3%, and the incidence of at least one major adverse outcome was 4.3%; very few of these were related to anesthesia. The most common cause of death was sepsis (33%), followed by all cardiac causes (28%) and pulmonary embolism (17%). Early surgical complications included anastomotic closure with bowel obstruction, anastomotic or staple line leak, gastrointestinal bleeding, and wound infection. LABS revealed the relationship between surgical volume and adverse outcome, at least for the RYGB.

Early postoperative complications are mostly related to the pulmonary and cardiovascular systems. Postanesthetic hypoxemia is more common in the patient with MO, with or without the presence of OSA, despite supplemental oxygen therapy. This can be due to atelectasis, or reversion to a restrictive breathing pattern with increased use of accessory muscles, as well as decreased FRC from pain ("splinting"), residual pneumoperitoneum, parietal peritoneal irritation from carbonic acid, air in the stomach, inadequate reversal of neuromuscular blockade, or pain. Other potential early postoperative complications include respiratory depression from residual anesthetic neuromuscular blockade, early ventilatory failure with need for reintubation, positional ventilatory collapse, hemodynamic instability, PONV, positional injury, and venous thromboembolism. PONV, the single most common postoperative patient complaint after bariatric surgery, is distinguished from OINV, which is more severe and more difficult to treat. Bariatric surgical procedures are highly emetogenic and frequently require prophylaxis with multiple agents. They are foregut surgical operations and interrupt peristalsis and the gastroesophageal antireflux mechanism. Severe, resistant, or recurrent PONV can be due to anastomotic kink, leak, or iatrogenic esophageal injury; when present, the surgical team should be called to examine the patient. In-hospital postoperative ventilatory insufficiency is always a risk; patients should be triaged by the perioperative team for postsurgical care. Very high-risk patients include those with severe cardiopulmonary disease or severe OSA, by either preoperative questionnaire, or who are noncompliant with NIPPV. The high-risk patient should be triaged from the PACU to a step-down unit postoperatively or rarely to an intensive care unit. All patients should be transported fully emerged from anesthesia whenever possible, and with oxygen (nasal cannula or face mask), as well as a NIPPV device if needed. The SuperNO$_2$VA nasal CPAP device (Vyaire Medical) was used to transport this patient to the PACU, and the patient was placed on NIPPV and later transferred to the surgical ward.

Belle S. Longitudinal assessment of bariatric surgery (LABS) (Version 5)[Dataset]. NIDDK Central Repository. NIDDK-CR resources for research (R4R). Accessed May 1, 2023. https://repository.niddk.nih.gov/

Husain F, Jeong H, Spight S, et al. Risk factors for early postoperative complications after bariatric surgery. *Ann Surg Treat Res*. 2018;95:100-110.

Iranmanesh P, Shah SK, Chevallay M, et al. Assessment of predictors of early postoperative complications after primary robotically assisted Roux-en-Y gastric bypass: a multicenter, retrospective cohort study. *Surg Endosc*. 2023;37:2851-2857.

Lim R, Beekley A, Johnson DC, et al. Early and late complications of bariatric operation. *Trauma Surg Acute Care Open*. 2018;3:e000219.

D.2. What are the late complications of bariatric surgical procedures?

Late (after 30 days) complications of bariatric surgical procedures are mostly surgical. They occur in up to 20% of sleeve gastrectomies, the most common procedure, and up to 40% in more complex procedures in which one or more anastomosis are created, such as the RYGB or the biliopancreatic diversion duodenal switch. For all bariatric surgical procedures, hernias occur in 10% to 20%, requiring up to 1/6 patients to have follow-up herniorrhaphies, including incisional hernias, ventral hernias, and internal hernias. Cholelithiasis is the second most common late complication.

Other late complications of bariatric surgery include persistent nausea and vomiting, marginal ulcers, small bowel obstruction, and metabolic and nutritional derangements. Some of the procedure-specific complications are gastric remnant distension, stomal stenosis, marginal ulcers, nephrolithiasis and renal failure, short bowel syndrome, dumping syndrome, postoperative hypoglycemia, failure to lose weight, weight regain, internal (usually gastro-gastric) fistulas, loss of fascial planes requiring panniculectomy, recurrent calcium oxalate urolithiasis, osteoporosis, and others. Failure to lose weight, weight regain, malnutrition, gastroesophageal reflux disease (GERD), and Barrett's esophagus are also common. Rare late complications include abscesses, delayed leak, addiction, severe nutritional deficiencies, and psychological disorders, including an increase in the suicide rate. The actual rate of late complications is hard to determine because many patients are lost to follow-up.

Auge M, Menahem B, Savey V, et al. Long-term complications after gastric bypass and sleeve gastrectomy: what information to give to patients and practitioners, and why? *J Visceral Surg*. 2022;159:298-308.

Bevilacqua LA, Obeid NR, Yang J, et al. Incidence of GERD, esophagitis, Barrett's esophagus, and esophageal adenocarcinoma after bariatric surgery. *Surg Obes Relat Dis*. 2020;16:1828-1836.

Koball AM, Ames GA, Goetze RE. Addiction transfer and other behavioral changes following bariatric surgery. *Surg Clin North Am*. 2021;101:323-333.

Lim R, Beekley A, Johnson DC, Davis KA. Early and late complications of bariatric operation. *Trauma Surg Acute Care Open*. 2018;3:e000219.

Weiss D. Long-term complications of bariatric surgery. *JAMA*. 2021;325:186-187.

D.3. What is the effect of position on respiratory function in the patient with obesity?

In the supine position, intra-abdominal contents shift the diaphragm cephalad, resulting in diaphragmatic dysfunction, decreased FRC, airway closure, increased venous admixture (Q_S/Q_T), decreased $Pa{O_2}$, and possibly, positional ventilatory collapse. The FRC, which supplies the oxygen reserve, decreases 30% in the supine position. Preoxygenation is more effective in the semi-Fowler position (head up 30°-45°) than in the supine position for preoxygenation and induction of general anesthesia in patients with severe obesity. Recovery should take place in this position as soon as patients are hemodynamically stable. Other benefits of a semi-sitting position are decreased superior vena cava pressure and decreased incidence of positional injuries, which are more common in the morbidly obese, especially ulnar neuropathy. Patients recovered in the semi-Fowler position in need of eventual emergent mask ventilation or tracheal reintubation present better conditions for the laryngoscopist. There is a higher incidence of tracheal tube misplacement in the morbidly obese; care should be taken when positioning intubated patients with MO in a semi-Fowler position.

Hasanin A, Tarek H, Amin S. Modified-ramped position: a new position for intubation of obese females: a randomized controlled study. *BMC Anesthesiology*. 2020;20:151.

Seyni-Boureima R, Zhang Z, Antoine MMLK, Antoine-Frank CD. A review of the anesthetic management of obese patients undergoing surgery. *BMC Anesthesiol*. 2022;22:98.

Troop CA. The importance of proper positioning for airway management for obese patients [Internet]. In: Hakan Erbay R. *Tracheal Intubation*. InTech; 2018. Accessed May 1, 2023. http://dx.doi.org/10.5772/intechopen.75514

D.4. How would you prevent postoperative atelectasis?

In the past, bariatric surgical procedures were often performed open, with an incidence of postoperative atelectasis of 45%. Now, approximately 90% are performed laparoscopically (with or without the use of a surgical robot), so the incidence of atelectasis might be less.

Early ambulation, chest physical ambulation with incentive spirometry, and effective coughing are encouraged to improve respiratory function in selected patients, such as the COPD or former smoker. ERAS protocols encourage smoking cessation. Prolonged recumbency is avoided whenever possible because of its adverse effects on the ventilation/perfusion (V/Q) ratio, to minimize circulatory congestion of the recumbent lung, and a cephalad position of the diaphragm which decreases the FRC, which promotes diaphragmatic inefficiency and increased use of the accessory muscles of respiration, increasing the work on the pharyngeal dilator muscles. Careful titration of postoperative analgesics is needed to prevent splinting from pain with subsequent atelectasis and hypoventilation from excessive sedation.

A recruitment maneuver followed by PEEP shortly after intubation, as indicated during the surgical procedure, and before extubation can be tried to reduce atelectasis and improve oxygenation with variable results. Among patients with obesity undergoing general anesthesia, an intraoperative mechanical ventilation strategy with a higher level of PEEP and alveolar recruitment maneuvers, compared with a strategy with a lower level of PEEP, does not reduce postoperative pulmonary complications. Incentive spirometry does not improve postoperative hypoxemia, oxygen saturation levels, or rate of pulmonary complications, and is not routinely recommended. The most important therapy for postoperative atelectasis is to get the patients out of bed as soon as possible, typically to a chair on postoperative day 1.

Bluth T, Serpa Neto A, et al. Effect of intraoperative high positive end-expiratory pressure (PEEP) with recruitment maneuvers vs low PEEP on postoperative pulmonary complications in obese patients: a randomized clinical trial. *JAMA*. 2019;321:2292-2305.

Eltorai AEM, Szabo AL, Antoci V, et al. Clinical effectiveness of incentive spirometry for the prevention of pulmonary complications. *Respir Care*. 2018;63:347-352.

Hodgson LE, Murphy PB, Hart N. Respiratory management of the obese patient undergoing surgery. *J Thorac Dis*. 2015;7:943-952.

Martin JB, Garbee D, Bonanno L. Effectiveness of positive end-expiratory pressure, decreased fraction of inspired oxygen and vital capacity recruitment maneuver in the prevention of pulmonary atelectasis in patients undergoing general anesthesia: a systematic review. *JBI Database System Rev Implement Rep*. 2015;13:211-249.

Pantel H, Hwang J, Brams D, et al. Effect of incentive spirometry on postoperative hypoxemia and pulmonary complications after bariatric surgery: a randomized clinical trial. *JAMA Surg*. 2017;152:422-428.

D.5. How long would you prescribe supplementary oxygen postoperatively?

Following bariatric surgery, patients without OSA or with uncomplicated OSA require prophylactic oxygen supplementation in a semi-sitting position. After the initial PACU stay, they can be monitored safely in a surgical ward. A low threshold for NIPPV should be maintained in the presence of respiratory distress. Patients with OSA on home CPAP or BiPAP should use their equipment in the immediate postoperative period. Patients with OHS are at high risk of respiratory adverse events. Postoperative noninvasive ventilation should be strongly considered in the presence of hypoxemia or respiratory decompensation. These patients are often recovered in a specialized unit, with respiratory monitoring and continuous pulse oximetry (as was our patient).

With the advent of ERAS, opioid administration is substantially lower, decreasing hypoxemia and respiratory depression. Most bariatric patients are discharged to home on the second or third postsurgical day.

Rosen J, Frykholm P, Fors D. Effect of high-flow nasal oxygen on postoperative oxygenation in obese patients: a randomized controlled trial. *Health Sci Rep*. 2022;5:e616.

Stenberg E, dos Reis Falcão L, Thorell A. Guidelines for perioperative care in bariatric surgery: Enhanced Recovery After Surgery (ERAS) Society recommendations: a 2021 update. *World J Surg*. 2022;46:729-751.

D.6. How would you control postoperative pain? What are the sources of surgical pain? What is the role of regional anesthesia in the bariatric surgery?

With ERAS, bariatric surgery has become less painful, at least for the surgery-naïve patient. The majority of patients are opting for laparoscopic or robotic sleeve gastrectomy (61.4% in 2020). There are three pain sources: somatic pain from the surgical portholes, pain from the mobilized proximal stomach and distal esophagus, and carbonic acid peritoneal irritation from the pneumoperitoneum. The first of these is treated by the surgeons with either porthole injections or TAP blocks. Pain from the mobilized stomach and esophagus is of short duration and generally not severe. Peritoneal irritation resembles colitis pain and is effectively treated with anti-inflammatory drugs such as dexamethasone and acetaminophen. Under ERAS, multimodal analgesia regimens reduce postoperative opioid requirements. This patient having a robotic sleeve received fentanyl 100 μg IV on induction of anesthesia, acetaminophen 1 g IV prior to surgical incision, and as needed hydromorphone 0.5 mg IV during the PACU stay. Lower opioid doses translate not only into an awake, cooperative patients without respiratory depression, but also into reduced OINV.

Patients with prior abdominal surgeries usually require higher doses of analgesics, including methadone and ketamine, both NMDA receptor antagonists, and can benefit from postoperative intravenous patient-controlled analgesia (PCA). Ketamine, whether used intraoperatively or postoperatively, decreases opioid consumption and reduces postoperative VAS scores at 4 and 8 hours and hospital length of stay. Intraoperative methadone improves quality of recovery compared with morphine, and reduces postoperative pain, opioid consumption, and the incidence of opioid-related adverse events. Methadone as the sole analgesic agent in bariatric surgery has been shown to be safe and effective, reducing postoperative opioid consumption, lowering pain scores both at rest and with movement, decreasing opioid-related nausea and vomiting, and improving patient satisfaction. PCA with hydromorphone has been shown to be safe and effective in patients with MO. Dose regimens need to be individualized according to pain control and side effect profile. The regimens for the morbidly obese are generally started for the opioid-naive, based on IBW, and dosed upwards.

- Morphine sulfate 20 μg/kg IBW
- Hydromorphone 4 to 5 μg/kg IBW
- Fentanyl 1 μg/kg IBW
- Methadone 20 μg/kg IBW

All settings are every 10 minutes, without continuous rate, at 80% of the calculated maximum doses. Although these opioids have different lipid solubilities, all have been dosed by IBW to minimize respiratory depression.

In the rare patient with a complex surgical history having an involved bariatric surgical procedure, a patient-controlled epidural analgesia (PCEA) can be helpful in order to provide adequate analgesia with minimal ventilatory depression. PCEA dosages in the morbidly obese should be decreased 75% to 80% due to decreased volume of the epidural space secondary to increased intra-abdominal pressure. Patients should be positioned in a sitting position for epidural catheter insertion, and ultrasound guidance is recommended. There is a higher rate of inadequate function, catheter migration and replacement, and variable block level. The mainstay of postoperative analgesics today is nonopioid analgesics and anti-inflammatory drugs. Intravenous opioid analgesics are reserved for breakthrough pain. Minimizing opioid exposure is associated with substantial societal benefits.

Chaouch M, Daghmouri MA, Boutron MC, et al. Ketamine as a component of multimodal analgesia for pain management in bariatric surgery: a systematic review and meta-analysis of randomized controlled trials. *Ann Med Surg (Lond)*. 2022;78:103783.

Clapp B, Ponce J, Corbett J, et al. American Society for Metabolic and Bariatric Surgery 2022 estimate of metabolic and bariatric procedures performed in the United States. *Surg Obes Relat Dis*. 2024;20:425-431.

DeUgarte DA, Fleischman R, Mccollough M. Assessment of an opioid stewardship program on perioperative opioid prescribing in a safety-net health system. *JAMA Surg*. 2023;158:318-319.

Lam KKY, Mui WLM. Multimodal analgesia model to achieve low postoperative opioid requirement following bariatric surgery. *Hong Kong Med J*. 2016;22:429-434.

Machado FC, Palmeira CCA, Torres JNL, Vieira JE, Ashmawi HA. Intraoperative use of methadone improves control of postoperative pain in morbidly obese patients: a randomized controlled study. *J Pain Res*. 2018;11:2123-2129.

Phillips JK. Pain management and the intersection of pain and opioid use disorder. In: Phillips JK, Ford MA, Bonnie RJ, eds. *Pain Management and the Opioid Epidemic: Balancing Societal and Individual Benefits and Risks of Prescription Opioid Use*. National Institutes of Health. Accessed May 1, 2023. https://www.ncbi.nlm.nih.gov/books/NBK458655/

Pontes JPJ, Braz FR, Modolo NSP, Mattar LA, Sousa JAG, Navarro ELLH. Intra-operative methadone effect on quality of recovery compared with morphine following laparoscopic gastroplasty: a randomised controlled trial. *Anaesthesia*. 2021;76:199-208.

Index

Note: Page numbers followed by *f* indicate figures; page numbers followed by *t* indicate tables.

C

D

J

K

L

M

O

P

Q

R

S